Allergy

Allergy

Edited by

ALLEN P. KAPLAN, MD
Pellegrino Professor of Medicine
Department of Medicine
State University of New York at Stony Brook
School of Medicine
Stony Brook, New York

SECOND EDITION

W.B. SAUNDERS COMPANY
A Division of Harcourt Brace & Company
Philadelphia London Toronto Montreal Sydney Tokyo

W.B. SAUNDERS COMPANY
A Division of Harcourt Brace & Company

The Curtis Center
Independence Square West
Philadelphia, Pennsylvania 19106

Library of Congress Cataloging-in-Publication Data

Allergy/edited by Allen P. Kaplan.—2nd ed.

p. cm.

Includes bibliographical references and index.

ISBN 0–7216–4974–2

1. Allergy. I. Kaplan, Allen P. [DNLM: 1. Hypersensitivity. WD 300 A432501 1997]

RC584.A345 1997 616.97′92—dc21

DNLM/DLC 96–29737

ALLERGY, SECOND EDITION ISBN 0–7216–4974–2

Printed in the United States of America.

Last digit is the print number: 9 8 7 6 5 4 3 2 1

Contributors

DAVID F. ANDERSON, M.B., B.S., F.R.C. Ophthal.
Research Registrar, University of Southampton; Registrar, Southampton Eye Unit, Southampton, England
Allergic Rhinitis, Nonallergic Rhinitis, and Ocular Allergy

JONATHAN P. ARM, M.D., M.R.C.P.
Assistant Professor of Medicine, Harvard Medical School; Consultant in Allergy, Brigham and Women's Hospital, Boston, Massachusetts
Sympathomimetic and Cholinergic Agents and Antagonists

JAMES N. BARANIUK, M.D., F.R.C.P.C.
Assistant Professor of Medicine, Department of Medicine, Division of Rheumatology, Immunology, and Allergy, Georgetown University School of Medicine, Washington, D.C.
The Autonomic Nervous System, Neuropeptides, and Allergy

I. LEONARD BERNSTEIN, M.D.
Clinical Professor of Medicine, University of Cincinnati College of Medicine, Cincinnati, Ohio
Occupation-Induced Asthma

JONATHAN A. BERNSTEIN, M.D.
Assistant Professor of Clinical Medicine, University of Cincinnati College of Medicine, Cincinnati, Ohio
Occupation-Induced Asthma

PETER J. BIANCHINE, M.D.
Medical Staff Fellow, Mast Cell Physiology Section, Laboratory of Clinical Investigation; Staff Physician, National Institute of Allergy and Infectious Diseases HIV Research Clinic, National Institute of Allergy and Infectious Diseases, National Institutes of Health, Bethesda, Maryland
Systemic Mastocytosis

MALCOLM N. BLUMENTHAL, M.D.
Clinical Professor and Director, Section of Allergy, University of Minnesota Medical School—Minneapolis, Minneapolis, Minnesota
Epidemiology and Genetics of Asthma and Allergy

BRUCE S. BOCHNER, M.D.
Associate Professor of Medicine, Department of Medicine, Division of Clinical Immunology, Johns Hopkins University School of Medicine; Johns Hopkins Asthma and Allergy Center, Baltimore, Maryland
Endothelial Cells and Cell Adhesion

LARRY BORISH, M.D.
Associate Professor of Medicine, University of Colorado School of Medicine; Associate Faculty Member, National Jewish Center for Immunology and Respiratory Medicine, Denver, Colorado
Cytokines, Interleukins, and Growth Factors

JOSHUA A. BOYCE, M.D.
Assistant Professor of Medicine and Pediatrics, Harvard Medical School; Assistant in Pediatrics, Massachusetts General Hospital; Associate Physician in Medicine, Brigham and Women's Hospital, Boston, Massachusetts
Idiopathic Hypereosinophilic Syndrome

REBECCA H. BUCKLEY, M.D.
Professor of Pediatrics, Duke University School of Medicine, Durham, North Carolina
Primary Immunodeficiency Diseases

WILLIAM W. BUSSE, M.D.
Professor of Medicine, University of Wisconsin Medical School, Madison, Wisconsin
Asthma: Pathogenesis and Treatment

THOMAS B. CASALE, M.D.
Professor of Internal Medicine, University of Iowa College of Medicine, Iowa City, Iowa
The Autonomic Nervous System, Neuropeptides, and Allergy

RICHARD A. F. CLARK, M.D.
Professor and Chair, Department of Dermatology, State University of New York at Stony Brook, School of Medicine; Chief of Service, Dermatology, University Medical Center, State University of New York at Stony Brook, Stony Brook, New York
Atopic Dermatitis

PETER S. CRETICOS, M.D.
Associate Professor of Medicine and Clinical Director, Division of Allergy and Clinical Immunology, Johns Hopkins University School of Medicine; Medical Director, Asthma and Allergic Diseases, Johns Hopkins Asthma and Allergy Center, Baltimore, Maryland
Immunotherapy

HOWARD M. DRUCE, M.D., F.A.C.P.
Clinical Associate Professor of Medicine, University of Medicine and Dentistry of New Jersey, New Jersey Medical School, Newark; Director, Clinical Research, Whitehall-Robins Healthcare Division, American Home Products Corporation, Madison, New Jersey
Imaging Techniques in Nasal Allergy and Sinusitis

LAWRENCE M. DuBUSKE, M.D.
Clinical Instructor of Medicine, Harvard Medical School; Consultant in Allergy, Brigham and Women's Hospital, Boston, Massachusetts
Sympathomimetic and Cholinergic Agents and Antagonists

STEPHEN R. DURHAM, M.D., F.R.C.P.
Reader, Allergy and Immunology, The Imperial College School of Medicine at the National Heart and Lung Institute; Honorary Consultant Physician, Royal Brompton Hospital, London, England
Late Allergic Responses

PHILIPPE A. EIGENMANN, M.D.
Assistant Professor, University of Geneva School of Medicine; Head, Pediatric Allergy, Children's Hospital, University Hospital of Geneva, Geneva, Switzerland
Adverse Reactions to Foods

JORDAN N. FINK, M.D.
Professor of Medicine, Chief, Allergy-Immunology, Medical College of Wisconsin, Milwaukee, Wisconsin
Hypersensitivity Pneumonitis

RENEE E. FOX, M.D.
Assistant Professor of Pediatrics and Director, Neonatal Intensive Care Unit, University of Maryland School of Medicine, Baltimore, Maryland
HIV-1 Infection, AIDS, and the Immune System

DEBORAH L. FRENCH, PH.D.
Assistant Professor of Medicine, Mount Sinai School of Medicine of the City University of New York, New York, New York
Immunoglobulin Structure and Genetics

JACK FUHRER, M.D.
Associate Professor of Medicine, State University of New York at Stony Brook, School of Medicine, Stony Brook, New York
HIV-1 Infection, AIDS, and the Immune System

RAIF S. GEHA, M.D.
Prince Turki bin Abdul Aziz Al-Saud Professor of Pediatrics, Harvard Medical School; Chief, Division of Immunology, Children's Hospital, Boston, Massachusetts
Structure, Function, and Synthesis of IgE

BERHANE GHEBREHIWET, D.V.M., D.SC.
Professor of Medicine and Pathology, Department of Medicine, State University of New York at Stony Brook, School of Medicine, Stony Brook, New York
The Complement System: Mechanisms of Activation, Regulation, and Biologic Functions

GERALD J. GLEICH, M.D.
Professor of Immunology and Medicine, Mayo Medical School; Consultant in Immunology and Medicine, Mayo Clinic, Rochester, Minnesota
The Eosinophil: Structure and Functions

PETER D. GOREVIC, M.D.
Professor of Medicine and Pathology, State University of New York at Stony Brook, School of Medicine, Stony Brook, New York
Drug Allergy

RONI GRAD, M.D.
Assistant Professor, University of New Mexico School of Medicine, Albuquerque, New Mexico
Cromolyn Sodium and Nedocromil Sodium

DAVID F. GRAFT, M.D.
Clinical Associate Professor of Pediatrics, Family Practice and Community Medicine, University of Minnesota School of Medicine—Minneapolis; Chairman, Department of Allergy, Park Nicollet Clinic, Minneapolis, Minnesota
Insect Sting Allergy

BARRY L. GRUBER, M.D.
Associate Professor, Department of Medicine and Department of Dermatology, State University of New York at Stony Brook, School of Medicine, Stony Brook, New York
Systemic Sclerosis (Scleroderma)

STEPHEN T. HOLGATE, M.D., F.R.C.P., D.Sc.
Professor of Immunopharmacology, University of Medicine, Southampton, England
Allergic Rhinitis, Nonallergic Rhinitis, and Ocular Allergy

MARY L. JELKS, M.D.
Clinical Assistant Professor, Department of Allergy and Immunology, University of South Florida College of Medicine, Tampa, Florida
Airborne Allergens

RICHARD S. KALISH, M.D., Ph.D.
Assistant Professor of Dermatology, Department of Dermatology, State University of New York at Stony Brook, School of Medicine; Attending Physician, Dermatology, University Medical Center, State University of New York at Stony Brook, Stony Brook, New York
Contact Dermatitis and Photoallergic Reactions

ALLEN P. KAPLAN, M.D.
Pellegrino Professor of Medicine, Department of Medicine, State University of New York at Stony Brook, School of Medicine, Stony Brook, New York
Bradykinin Formation: Plasma and Tissue Pathways; Vasculitis; Chemokines/Histamine-Releasing Factors; Urticaria and Angioedema

A. BARRY KAY, F.R.C.P., Ph.D.
Professor, Allergy and Immunology, Imperial College School of Medicine at the National Heart and Lung Institute; Honorary Consultant Physician, Royal Brompton Hospital, London, England
Late Allergic Responses

HIROHITO KITA, M.D.
Assistant Professor of Immunology, Mayo Medical School; Associate Consultant, Department of Immunology, Mayo Clinic, Rochester, Minnesota
The Eosinophil: Structure and Functions

LEONARD KRISTAL, M.D.
Clinical Assistant Professor of Dermatology, Department of Dermatology, State University of New York at Stony Brook, School of Medicine; Attending Physician, Dermatology, University Medical Center, State University of New York at Stony Brook, Stony Brook, New York
Atopic Dermatitis

TAK HONG LEE, M.D., F.R.C.P.
Professor of Allergy and Respiratory Medicine, United Medical and Dental Schools of Guy's and St. Thomas's Hospitals; Honorary Consultant Physician, Guy's Hospital, London, England
Lipid Mediators—Leukotrienes, Prostanoids, Platelet-Activating Factor, and Lipoxins

ROBERT F. LEMANSKE, Jr., M.D.
Professor of Medicine and Pediatrics, Departments of Medicine and Pediatrics, University of Wisconsin Medical School, Madison, Wisconsin
Asthma in Infants and Children

MANUEL LOPEZ, M.D.
Professor of Medicine and Chief, Section of Allergy and Clinical Immunology, Department of Medicine, Tulane University School of Medicine, New Orleans, Louisiana
Allergic Bronchopulmonary Aspergillosis

DAVID LOWRY, M.D.
Resident in Radiology, Saint Louis University School of Medicine, St. Louis, Missouri
Imaging Techniques in Nasal Allergy and Sinusitis

NICHOLAS W. LUKACS, Ph.D.
Research Investigator, Department of Pathology; Lecturer, Department of Epidemiology, University of Michigan Medical School, Ann Arbor, Michigan
Chemotactic Molecules and Cellular Activation

DAVID S. MARTIN, M.D., F.A.C.R.
Associate Professor of Radiology and Head and Neck Surgery, Saint Louis University School of Medicine; Attending Neuroradiologist, Saint Louis University Hospital and Cardinal Glennon Children's Hospital, St. Louis, Missouri
Imaging Techniques in Nasal Allergy and Sinusitis

RICHARD J. MARTIN, M.D.
Professor of Medicine, University of Colorado School of Medicine; Head, Pulmonary Division, National Jewish Center for Immunology and Respiratory Medicine, Denver, Colorado
Theophylline: Role of Importance in the Treatment of Asthma

E. R. McFADDEN, Jr., M.D.
Argyl J. Beams Professor of Medicine, Case Western Reserve University School of Medicine; Director, Division of Pulmonary and Critical Care Medicine; Program Director, General Clinical Research Center, University Hospitals of Cleveland, Cleveland, Ohio
Exercise and Asthma

DEAN D. METCALFE, M.D.
Director, Allergy and Immunology Training Program, Office of the Clinical Director; Chief, Laboratory of Allergic Diseases, National Institute of Allergy and Infectious Diseases, National Institutes of Health, Bethesda, Maryland
Systemic Mastocytosis

HENRY METZGER, M.D.
Director, Intramural Research Program, National Institute of Arthritis and Musculoskeletal and Skin Diseases, National Institutes of Health, Bethesda, Maryland
Receptor for IgE and Initiation of Allergic Reactions

FREDERICK MILLER, M.D.
Marvin Kuschner Professor and Chairman, Department of Pathology, State University of New York at Stony Brook, School of Medicine; Pathologist-in-Chief and Director of Laboratories, University Hospital, Stony Brook, New York
Autoimmunity; Vasculitis

SHIRLEY MURPHY, M.D.
Professor and Chairman, Department of Pediatrics, University of New Mexico School of Medicine, Albuquerque, New Mexico
Cromolyn Sodium and Nedocromil Sodium

ROBERT M. NACLERIO, M.D.
Professor of Surgery and Professor and Chief of Otolaryngology and Head and Neck Surgery, University of Chicago, Division of the Biological Sciences, Pritzker School of Medicine, Chicago, Illinois
Structure and Function of the Upper Airway; Rhinoscopy

S. M. SHUAIB NASSER, M.B., B.S., M.R.C.P.
Clinical Lecturer and Senior Registrar, Department of Allergy, Clinical Immunology, and Respiratory Medicine, University of Cambridge, Addenbrooke's Hospital, Cambridge, England
Lipid Mediators—Leukotrienes, Prostanoids, Platelet-Activating Factor, and Lipoxins

DEBORAH ORTEGA-CARR, M.D.
Postdoctoral Fellow, Allergy and Immunology, University of Wisconsin Medical School, Madison, Wisconsin
Asthma: Pathogenesis and Treatment

WILLIAM F. OWEN, JR., M.D.
Assistant Professor of Medicine, Harvard Medical School; Director of Dialysis Services, Brigham and Women's Hospital, Boston, Massachusetts
Idiopathic Hypereosinophilic Syndrome

NIGEL A. M. PATERSON, M.B., B.S., F.R.C.P.C.
Professor of Medicine, Professor of Pharmacology and Toxicology, and Chair, Respirology Division, University of Western Ontario Faculty of Medicine; Chief, Respirology, London Health Sciences Centre, London, Ontario, Canada
Corticosteroids and Anti-Metabolites

ECKHARD R. PODACK, M.D., PH.D.
Professor and Chairman, Department of Microbiology and Immunology, University of Miami School of Medicine; Associate Director of Basic Research, Sylvester Comprehensive Cancer Center, Miami, Florida
Natural Killer Cells

KARALASINGAM RAJAKULASINGAM, M.B., B.S., M.R.C.P. (UK)
Honorary Lecturer, The Imperial College School of Medicine at The National Heart and Lung Institute; Senior Registrar, Royal Brompton Hospital, London, England
Allergic Rhinitis, Nonallergic Rhinitis, and Ocular Allergy

SESHA R. REDDIGARI, PH.D.
Scientist, Dade International Inc., Miami, Florida
Bradykinin Formation: Plasma and Tissue Pathways

MICHAEL REDMAN, M.D.
University of Chicago, Division of the Biological Sciences, Pritzker School of Medicine, Chicago, Illinois
Structure and Function of the Upper Airway; Rhinoscopy

ROBERT R. RICH, M.D.
Distinguished Service Professor, Department of Microbiology and Immunology and Department of Medicine; Vice President and Dean of Research, Baylor College of Medicine, Houston, Texas
Antigen Presentation and the Major Histocompatibility Complex

JOHN R. RODGERS, PH.D.
Professor, Department of Microbiology and Immunology, Baylor College of Medicine, Houston, Texas
Antigen Presentation and the Major Histocompatibility Complex

LANNY J. ROSENWASSER, M.D.
Professor of Medicine, University of Colorado School of Medicine; Senior Faculty Member and Head, Division of Allergy and Clinical Immunology, National Jewish Center for Immunology and Respiratory Medicine, Denver, Colorado
Cytokines, Interleukins, and Growth Factors

JOHN E. SALVAGGIO, M.D.
Henderson Professor of Medicine and Vice Chancellor for Research, Tulane University School of Medicine, New Orleans, Louisiana
Allergic Bronchopulmonary Aspergillosis

HUGH A. SAMPSON, M.D.
Professor of Pediatrics, Division of Allergy and Immunology, Johns Hopkins University School of Medicine; Director, Pediatric Clinical Research Center, Johns Hopkins Hospital, Baltimore, Maryland
Adverse Reactions to Foods

ROBERT P. SCHLEIMER, PH.D.
Professor of Medicine, Department of Medicine, Division of Clinical Immunology, Johns Hopkins University School of Medicine; Johns Hopkins Asthma and Allergy Center, Baltimore, Maryland
Endothelial Cells and Cell Adhesion

MARY K. SCHROTH, M.D.
Assistant Professor of Pediatrics, Department of Pediatrics, University of Wisconsin Medical School, Madison, Wisconsin
Asthma in Infants and Children

LAWRENCE B. SCHWARTZ, M.D., PH.D.
Charles and Evelyn Thomas Professor of Medicine, Virginia Commonwealth University, Medical College of Virginia, Richmond, Virginia
Basophils and Mast Cells

ALBERT L. SHEFFER, M.D.
Clinical Professor of Medicine, Harvard Medical School; Director, Allergy Section, Brigham and Women's Hospital, Boston, Massachusetts
Sympathomimetic and Cholinergic Agents and Antagonists

ETHAN M. SHEVACH, M.D.
Chief, Cellular Immunology Section, Laboratory of Immunology, National Institute of Allergy and Infectious Diseases, National Institutes of Health, Bethesda, Maryland
T and B Lymphocytes

MICHAEL SILVERBERG, PH.D.
Associate Professor of Medicine, Department of Medicine, State University of New York at Stony Brook, School of Medicine, Stony Brook, New York
Bradykinin Formation: Plasma and Tissue Pathways

F. ESTELLE R. SIMONS, M.D., F.R.C.P.C.
Bruce Chown Professor and Head, Section of Allergy and Clinical Immunology, Department of Pediatrics and Child Health, University of Manitoba Faculty of Medicine, Winnipeg, Manitoba, Canada
Antihistamines

REUBEN P. SIRAGANIAN, M.D., PH.D.
Chief, Receptors and Signal Transduction Section, Laboratory of Immunology, National Institute of Dental Research, National Institutes of Health, Bethesda, Maryland
Biochemical Events in Basophil/Mast Cell Activation and Mediator Release

RAYMOND G. SLAVIN, M.D.
Professor, Internal Medicine and Microbiology, and Director, Division of Allergy and Immunology, Saint Louis University School of Medicine, St. Louis, Missouri
Nasal Polyps and Sinusitis

GERALD C. SMALDONE, M.D., PH.D.
Associate Professor of Medicine, Physiology, and Biophysics, Pulmonary/Critical Care Division, Department of Medicine; State University of New York at Stony Brook; Attending Physician, Pulmonary/Critical Care, and Director of Respiratory Therapy, University Hospital at Stony Brook, Stony Brook, New York
Respiratory Physiology in Asthma: Pulmonary Function Testing, Bronchoprovocation, and Mucociliary Clearance

WILLIAM R. SOLOMON, M.D., M.S.
Professor of Internal Medicine, University of Michigan Medical School, Ann Arbor, Michigan
Airborne Allergens

NICHOLAS A. SOTER, M.D.
Professor of Dermatology, The Ronald O. Perelman Department of Dermatology, New York University School of Medicine; Attending Physician, Tisch Hospital—The University Hospital of New York University; Medical Director, Charles C. Harris Skin and Cancer Pavilion, New York, New York
Erythema Multiforme and Stevens-Johnson Syndrome

ALFRED D. STEINBERG, M.D.
Senior Physician-Scientist, Mitretek, McLean, Virginia
Systemic Lupus Erythematosus

JEFFREY R. STOKES, M.D.
Clinical Instructor of Pediatrics, Department of Pediatrics, University of Wisconsin Medical School; Fellow in Pediatric Pulmonology, University of Wisconsin Hospitals and Clinics, Madison, Wisconsin
Asthma in Infants and Children

JOHN H. TOOGOOD, M.D., F.R.C.P.C.
Professor of Medicine, University of Western Ontario Faculty of Medicine; Allergy Clinic Associate, London Health Sciences Centre, London, Ontario, Canada
Corticosteroids and Anti-Metabolites

MARTIN D. VALENTINE, M.D.
Professor of Medicine, Johns Hopkins University School of Medicine; Clinical Professor of Medicine, University of Maryland School of Medicine, Baltimore, Maryland
Insect Sting Allergy

DONATA VERCELLI, M.D.
Chief, Molecular Immunoregulation Unit, San Raffaele Scientific Institute, Milan, Italy
Structure, Function, and Synthesis of IgE

DAVID J. VOLKMAN, PH.D., M.D.
Associate Professor of Medicine and Pediatrics, State University of New York at Stony Brook, School of Medicine, Stony Brook, New York
HIV-1 Infection, AIDS, and the Immune System

PETER A. WARD, M.D.
Professor and Chairman, Department of Pathology, University of Michigan Medical School, Ann Arbor, Michigan
Chemotactic Molecules and Cellular Activation

STEPHEN I. WASSERMAN, M.D.
The Helen M. Ranney Professor of Medicine and Chairman, Department of Medicine, University of California, San Diego, School of Medicine, La Jolla, California
Anaphylaxis

FREDERICK A. WHITE, M.D., F.R.C.P.C.
Associate Staff, Department of Medicine, Grand River Hospital, Kitchener, Ontario, Canada
Corticosteroids and Anti-Metabolites

JOHN W. YUNGINGER, M.D.
Professor of Pediatrics, Mayo Medical School; Consultant in Pediatric and Adolescent Medicine, Mayo Clinic and Foundation, Rochester, Minnesota
Diagnostic Testing: Skin Tests, IgE Quantitation

NATHAN J. ZVAIFLER, M.D.
Professor of Medicine, Division of Rheumatology, University of California, San Diego, School of Medicine, La Jolla, California
Rheumatoid Arthritis

Preface

Allergic diseases affect approximately 20% of the population and are, therefore, among the most frequent disorders treated by family practitioners, pediatricians, and general internists. Because of such an unusual prevalence of cases, our subspecialty, allergy and clinical immunology, is expected to provide a cadre of trainees and practicing physicians with expertise in the diagnosis and treatment of these disorders. The first edition of *Allergy,* published 10 years ago, was an attempt to present the latest available information regarding etiology, pathogenesis, diagnostic methods, and therapeutic modalities, and when possible prevention of disease in a focused yet thorough fashion. The emphasis was on the diseases that an allergist/clinical immunologist treats most frequently and those in which particular expertise is expected.

Now that 10 years have passed, the state of the art has evolved dramatically and the second edition has required extensive revision of all chapters. Additional chapters are also needed to explore certain areas more comprehensively. Further, because of the broadening of the specialty to include clinical immunology, I have added a new section in which selected immunologic diseases are discussed; these may overlap with other disciplines, but are nevertheless likely to be part of one's own practice.

Some of the highlights of the past decade that are emphasized in the text can be summarized as follows. Important new data regarding the genetics of allergy have been included. For example, bronchial hyperreactivity has been linked to chromosome 5q, suggesting a relationship to those factors regulating IgE synthesis and those cytokines associated with allergic inflammation. The receptor for IgE has been cloned, its structure discerned, and progress made in understanding the early steps of signal transduction and their relationship to receptor cross-linking.

Much progress has been made in associating the Th2 type of inflammatory response with the late phase reaction. The cell-to-cell communication that occurs during the late phase has in addition led to a new understanding of the role of adhesion molecules and chemotactic cytokines (chemokines) in mediating that inflammatory response.

Histamine-releasing factors and stimuli for eosinophil migration have been associated with the β chemokines. An IgE-dependent, histamine-releasing factor has been characterized that presents a further link to IgE synthesis and the evolution of the late phase reaction. This factor also defines a functional heterogeneity for IgE. Alternative forms of IgE have indeed been described, some of which are cell bound, whereas others remain in the fluid phase. These differ from the classic structure of IgE, and their function is as yet a mystery.

Available diagnostic methods have also changed over the past decade. With the advent of rhinoscopy, we can assess the nasal cavity in an improved manner. The utilization of limited MR imaging is important to the assessment of chronic sinusitis. This method represents a new approach that is also cost effective. A host of new allergens have been defined. A new era of cloned allergens and allergenic fragments, containing major epitopes, is upon us. All these materials have the potential to be used in new ways (inhalation, oral desensitization, injection protocols) to alleviate allergic reactivity. They have the potential to induce a state of true hyporesponsiveness, or anergy, and to redirect the immune response to a less inflammatory mode through direct suppression or rerouting to alternative pathways (Th1).

Because of the explosion of new inflammation and agents for treatment, the original chapters on upper respiratory diseases are now expanded to include chapters dealing with allergic rhinitis and conjunctivitis, nasal polyposis and sinusitis, asthma in infants and children, asthma in adults, exercise-induced asthma, and occupational asthma. Further, new and separate chapters review all of the therapeutic modalities we employ, including β-adrenergic agents, cholinergic antagonists, methyl xanthines, corticosteroids, immunosuppressive agents, and immunotherapy.

The new section on immunologic diseases emphasizes immunodeficiency diseases (congenital, acquired, AIDS) and autoimmunity, including separate chapters on systemic lupus erythematosus, rheumatoid arteritis, scleroderma, and vasculitis. Two proliferative disorders of cells that are typically associated with the allergic response, namely, systemic mastocytosis and hypereosinophilic syndrome, are considered.

In spite of the increased size and coverage of the subject matter, this work remains as a single volume meant to be utilized as a textbook or reference work, depending on the reader's need. Thus the clinical immunology portion is quite selective rather than comprehensive as required of a textbook of clinical immunology. We hope that the book will serve the needs of Fellows who are in training and preparing for board examinations, as well as the needs of practicing allergists and physicians in related specialties who are reviewing and updating specific subjects or concepts.

The quality of any book is based on the quality of the manuscript and, of course, the efforts of the contributors. An exceptional group of authors has contributed chapters to this volume, and I am indebted to each of them. I am also grateful for their cooperation in keeping to the timetable and for valuable suggestions and assistance in making revisions and reviewing proofs.

Finally, the staff at W.B. Saunders Company are always available for guidance and assistance. I am particularly grateful to Raymond Kersey, Senior Medical Editor, and David Kilmer, Developmental Editor, for their support during this effort.

ALLEN P. KAPLAN, M.D.

Contents

I The Immune System and Inflammation

II Assessment of Allergic Diseases

III Allergic Diseases

IV Therapeutic Modalities

V Immunologic Diseases

NOTICE

I The Immune System and Inflammation

1 Antigen Presentation and the Major Histocompatibility Complex

JOHN R. RODGERS   ROBERT R. RICH

A "good" antigen, like good art, is hard to define but easy to recognize. What constitutes an antigen is not primarily a theory of properties intrinsic to antigens but a theory of how structures are perceived by the immune system. Antigenicity is not a property of the substance per se but is *emergent* during its interaction with a responding organism.[2] This chapter summarizes the means by which the body processes biochemical structures to present them to the principal perceptive molecules of the immune system, namely, antibodies and T-cell receptors.[22, 43]

Whether a particular biochemical structure will be recognized as antigenic by an individual depends on the prior immunologic history of that individual and on the constitutive apparatus of antigen processing and presentation. The secondary antibody response to an immunogen provides a classic example of the historical effect in which the kinetics, magnitude, isotypes, and fine specificities of induced antibodies depend on the nature of the primary immunization. Historical factors determine largely what antibodies and T-cell receptors are available to the organism at the time of subsequent antigen exposure. Similarly, the route of antigen acquisition can be critical: with some exceptions, such as food allergies and effective oral vaccines, ingestion of antigens results in oral tolerance more frequently than in immunity.

Constitutive factors include the polymorphic major histocompatibility complex (MHC) class I and class II molecules that control which peptides can be presented to T-cell receptors. Other constitutive mechanisms of antigen processing and presentation also exhibit genetic polymorphism and/or can be conditioned by the immune history. These include mechanisms by which different cell types acquire antigens, modify native macromolecules into antigenic forms, and transport them into different parts of the cell.

This chapter is organized in four parts to address the chemistry of antigens, mechanisms of antigen acquisition, biochemistry of antigen processing, and the presentation process itself. The recognition of antigens also requires the active participation of T cells, discussed in Chapter 3.

SOME DEFINITIONS

An antigen is anything capable of inducing antibodies specific to the antigen.[56] This circular definition requires the substance to elicit the immune response and to serve as a ligand for the induced receptor. Antigen also refers to a substance that can elicit specific T-cell responses, although the T-cell receptor itself cannot usually bind directly to the immunizing substance but only to a derived fragment. Most antigens are proteins, but carbohydrates, nucleic acids, and occasionally lipids can also function as antigens.

Antigens as inducers of antibodies.[2, 7] Substances that bind antigen receptors and can induce those receptors are called *immunogens* or *complete antigens*. Complete antigens include the specific epitope to which elicited antibodies will bind and a *carrier* containing epitopes for helper T cells. Antibody responses to most protein antigens require cooperative interactions between T cells and antibody-producing B cells. Such antigens are termed *T dependent*. In principle, if not always in practice, multiple antigenic peptides (MAPs) can be synthesized, combining both epitopes. *T-independent (TI) antigens* induce B-cell proliferation and differentiation in the complete absence of T cells.[41] Two general types of TI antigens have been identified, based on differences in the nature of the antibody responses to them. At low doses, TI-1 antigens, such as lipopolysaccharide (LPS, endotoxin), stimulate B cells specific for the TI antigen itself. However, high doses induce polyclonal proliferation of B cells. TI-1 antigens probably cross-link surface immunoglobulins and other receptors on B cells and other cells. For example, LPS induces monocytes to secrete tumor necrosis factor α. However, TI-1 antigens cannot induce the cytokine environment required for the accelerated kinetics and isotype switching observed in typical secondary immune responses.

Responses to TI-2 antigens, such as pneumococcal capsular polysaccharides, more closely resemble those to T-dependent antigens. Although they can stimulate antigen-specific responses in athymic mice, TI-2 antigens do not stimulate polyclonal proliferation at high doses and typically produce an IgM response. They can, under the influence of interferon-γ (IFN-γ) provided by T cells or by natural killer cells, lead to Ig isotype switching.

Antigens as ligands for antibodies. The molecular assemblage of atoms bonding to the antibody is the *epitope* or determinant.[28] A surface area of 400 $Å^2$ to 600 $Å^2$ is presented to the combining site (paratope) of an antibody. This size corresponds to peptides of approximately six to eight amino acids or to carbohydrates of approximately seven sugar monomers. The interaction of epitope with paratope typically involves a few salt-bridges, up to a dozen hydrogen bonds, and 60 to 90 van der Waals bonds. Minimal chemical moieties, such as dinitrophenyl, can also react with specific antibodies and are called *haptens*.

The structure of many epitopes for antibodies is a *linear* or *continuous* array of amino acids or sugars. Immunization with synthetic peptides, MAPs, or denatured proteins typically elicits antibodies reactive with continuous epitopes. Western blots typically detect such epitopes, because they do not depend on retention of the native folding pattern of the protein. However, most epitopes detected by antibodies elicited following immunization with native protein are *discontinuous* and/or *conformational*.[6, 7] Such epitopes are found on the surface of native proteins and are lost following denaturation. Most neutralizing antibodies detect discontinuous or conformational epitopes. Sometimes, linear synthetic peptides (*mimotopes*) can be constructed that mimic the three-dimensional pattern of conformational epitopes.

Predicting epitopes for antibodies. Antigenicity depends on the ability of the organism to process, present, and perceive the antigen. A number of strategies have been proposed to predict surface epitopes in native proteins.[2] X-ray crystal structures are useful in identifying regions of relative *accessibility* or *exteriority* or *flexibility*. Analyses of crystal structures of proteins carrying known epitopes show that accessibility and flexibility account for about half of known antigenic sites. Primary sequence information can also be useful. For example, charged and polar amino acids are more likely than hydrophobic residues to be found at the surface of native proteins. Hydrophilicity, estimates of the probability of forming turns, and measures of evolutionary mutability intercorrelate and are predictive of epitopes. In practice, however, the identification of immunodominant epitopes for antibodies is empirical.

Antigens for T-cell receptors.[4, 21] T-cell receptors recognize class I or class II MHC molecules, usually with a tightly bound oligopeptide derived from self-proteins or foreign proteins. The details of these two molecules and how they bind peptides are summarized in Table 1–1.

Roughly 85% of the molecular surface area detected by a

TABLE 1–1
CLASS I AND II MHC MOLECULES COMPARED

Feature	Class I	Class II
Peptide source	Endogenous (cytoplasmic), exogenous	Endogenous (autophagy), exogenous (endocytosis)
Antigen acquisition	TAP transporter, secretory pathway, endocytosis	Autophagy, endocytosis
Peptide size	8–11	8–22
Peptide ends	Buried in cleft	Free
Expressing tissues	Most forms in virtually all tissues; low in neural tissue	Professional APC (macrophages, dendritic cells), B cells (very low in plasma cells), various cell types exposed to IFN-γ
T-cell coreceptor	CD8	CD4
T-cell type	Mostly cytolytic	T_{H1} and T_{H2}
Other responding cells	Natural killer cells	None known
Chief function of responding cells	Cytolytic	Regulatory, cytolytic
Major trafficking pathway	ER → Golgi → surface	ER → Golgi → endosome; surface ←→ endosome
Trafficking chaperones	Calnexin, BiP, TAP?	Calnexin, BiP, invariant chain, PBP72/74, DMA/B?
Number of genes	Many: 3 dozen	Few: 2–6
MHC-linked antigen processing genes	TAP1 and 2, LMP 2 and 7 (proteasome)	DMA, DMB
Response to IFN-γ	Induction	Induction (repression in B cells)
Response to IFN-α/β	Induction	Repression

From Rodgers JR, Rich RR: Antigens and antigen presentation. In Rich RR, Shearer WT, Strober W, et al (eds): Clinical Immunology: Principles and Practice. Mosby–Year Book, Inc, St. Louis, 1995.

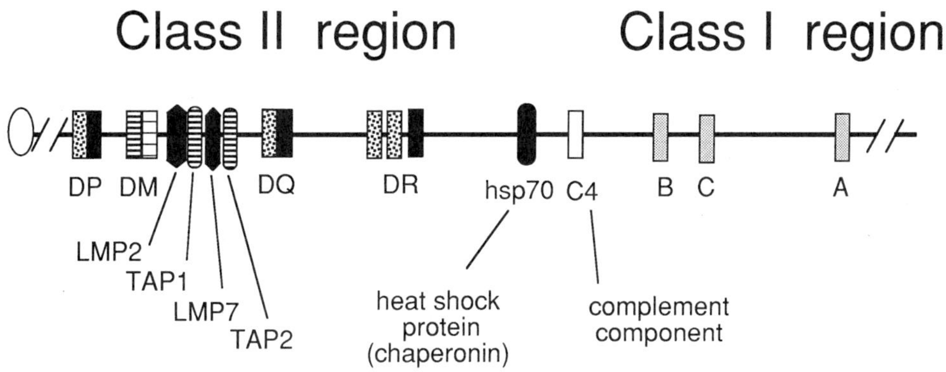

FIGURE 1–1. A simplified view of the human MHC on chromosome 6. Part of the chromosome is illustrated with some genes involved in antigen processing and presentation. The class II region contains TAP and LMP genes involved in processing for class I and DM genes involved in processing for class II. Numerous nonclassic class I-b genes and class I and II pseudogenes are not shown. Class II molecules consist of two chains (α and β), both of which are encoded within the MHC. The DR molecules consist of a single nonpolymorphic α chain complexed with either of two β chains, one of which is very polymorphic and the other oligomorphic. Class I molecules consist of a single heavy (α) chain, which is a product of the MHC, noncovalently associated with a light chain, β_2m, which is not encoded within the MHC.

T-cell receptor is provided by the MHC molecule itself; the remainder is contributed by the bound peptide. As a result, T cells are sensitive to variations in the surface of MHC molecules. The genes of the MHC are probably the most polymorphic of the genome, especially in the regions encoding peptide and T-cell receptor binding sites. There are dozens of allelic forms of each class I or class II molecule. This extreme polymorphism in the peptide/T-cell receptor interaction domains, combined with the prominent role the MHC molecule plays as a ligand for T-cell receptors, has four fundamental corollaries for antigen recognition. First, most individuals are heterozygous for genes encoding MHC molecules. Second, most individuals differ in the MHC alleles they express. Third, the pattern of self-peptides to which an individual will become tolerant varies tremendously in the population. Fourth, the pattern of foreign peptides to which an individual can respond, if that individual is not already tolerant, also varies tremendously. Proteins, and especially peptides, that are immunogenic, allergenic, or autoimmunogenic in one individual can be completely ignored in another.

MHC molecules are encoded by genes within a short chromosomal segment, the MHC (Fig. 1–1).[64] The MHC might better be called the antigen processing and presentation complex, because in addition to the better-known MHC molecules that present antigenic peptides to T cells, many other genes within the complex play critical roles in processing. Among the products of such genes are six that are especially important. Two interferon-inducible proteins, LMP2 and LMP7, are regulatory subunits of *proteasomes*.[25] Proteasomes are composed of stacks of ringlike multisubunit complexes. They render cytosolic proteins into oligopeptides preparatory to entry into the endoplasmic reticulum. Such peptides are pumped into the endoplasmic reticulum (ER), for binding by class I molecules, by an enzyme formed by two other MHC-encoded proteins; this is TAP, the peptide transporter associated with antigen processing. The *DMA* and *DMB* genes encode subunits of an MHC class II-like protein required for proper and efficient maturation of class II molecules within endosomes.[15]

Most T-cell receptors detect the composite antigen formed by a peptide imbedded within the binding groove atop a class I or class II MHC molecule (Fig. 1–2).[35] A few exceptions include reports of T cells that detect nonpeptidic antigens. For example, allergies to beta-lactam antibiotics and contact sensitivities to cosmetic metals both require antigen-specific T cells. These agents conjugate covalently or noncovalently to (haptenate) cellular proteins. Other agents, such as the lipid-containing urushiol (the agent of poison ivy), may function in the same way. Scattered reports suggest that

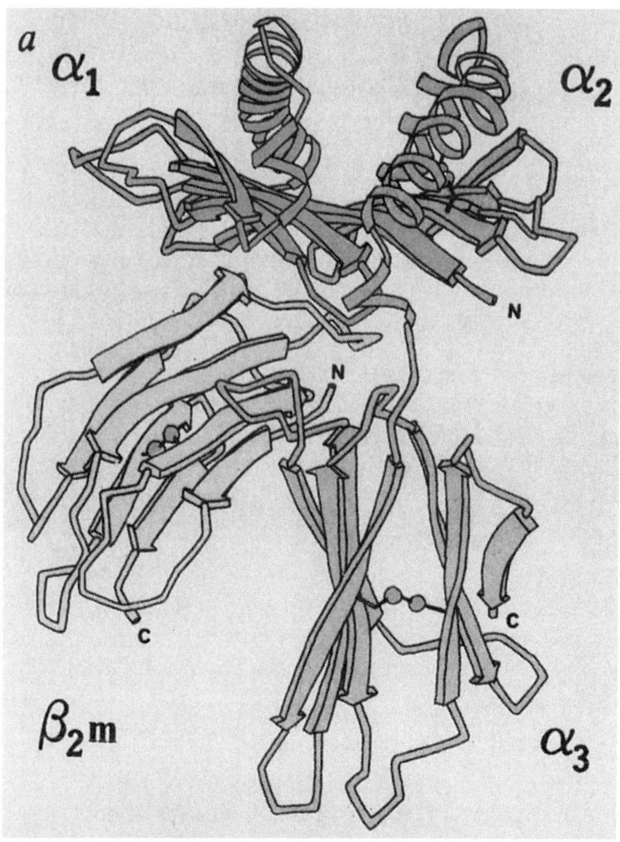

FIGURE 1–2. The class I MHC molecule, based on x-ray diffraction analysis. The peptide (not shown) binds in the cleft between the two α helixes atop the α1 and α2 domains. (From Bjorkman PJ, Saper MA, Samraoui B, et al: Structure of the human class I histocompatibility antigen, HLA-A2. Nature 329:506, 1987; Macmillan Magazines Limited: Artist, Michael Silver.)

some T cells might recognize nonpeptidic moieties bound by MHC class I molecules.[5] In contrast, some $\gamma\delta$ T cells almost certainly detect MHC molecules lacking bound peptides.[32] Superantigens are proteins that bind T-cell receptors in a family-specific but nonclonotypic fashion and consequently can activate a high proportion of T cells.[17] Although superantigens are also presented by MHC class II molecules, they bind outside the antigen-binding cleft and are perceived as native proteins rather than as processed oligopeptides. From the x-ray crystal structure of one superantigen, staphylococcal enterotoxin B (SEB), it appears that one face of the globular superantigen binds the $\alpha 1$ domain outside the binding groove and does not interfere with peptide binding.[27] Modeling studies suggest that SEB could bind to one surface of the Vβ chain of the T-cell receptor without interfering with T-cell receptor recognition of peptide presented by the class II molecule.[27]

Antigen peptides are buried deeply within the MHC binding cleft[35]; most of the molecular contacts made by the combining site or paratope of the T-cell receptor are with the MHC molecule. For most class I molecules, the bound peptide is 8 to 10 amino acids in length, whereas peptides extracted from class II molecules are longer.[18, 46] The MHC molecules contact the peptide backbone and one or two side chains, leaving the remaining side chains to contact the T-cell receptor. Adducts such as N-linked carbohydrates or haptens may also bind the T-cell receptor. The peptides themselves are derived proteolytically *(processing)* from larger proteins by pathways that are described later in this chapter.

There are few limitations on what kind of peptide can interact with a T-cell receptor, but there are severe restrictions on processing and on MHC binding. The specific binding interactions with side chains are such that each allelic form of an MHC molecule can bind only a tiny fraction of possible peptides. As a result, it has been possible to define for many class I molecules a predictive *binding motif*.[19] Nevertheless, not all predicted peptides that bind in vitro are used in vivo. This is due, at least in part, to details of proteolysis and peptide transport. Thus many peptides eluted from class II MHC molecules have a proline in the first or second position, not because they bind proline, but because proline cannot be cleaved by most aminopeptidases. Other peptides are readily cleaved by endoproteases, preventing their accumulation in quantities sufficient for immunogenicity. As an example, TAP, the polymorphic peptide transport enzyme that pumps antigenic peptides from the cytosol into the lumen of the endoplasmic reticulum to bind class I molecules, displays specificity for peptide size and amino acid composition.

ANTIGEN PRESENTATION BY CLASS I MOLECULES

The structure of class I molecules.[9, 65] The typical mature class I MHC molecule consists of a membrane-bound heavy chain that may be encoded by any of many usually polymorphic loci, a light chain, β_2-microglobulin (β_2m) encoded by a single monomorphic locus, and a short peptide (usually 8 to 10 amino acids) derived from a self-antigen or foreign antigen. The HLA-A and HLA-B loci are the most polymorphic, with dozens of alleles in most human populations. The HLA-C locus is less polymorphic, whereas HLA-G is essentially monomorphic. The heavy chain consists of three extracellular domains, $\alpha 1$, $\alpha 2$, and $\alpha 3$ (see Fig. 1–2). The last of these, and possibly all three, belong to the immunoglobulin gene superfamily. Most class I heavy chains also contain a transmembrane (TM) domain and a cytoplasmic (CYT) domain.

Antigen binding and presentation are chiefly the functions of the polymorphic $\alpha 1$ and $\alpha 2$ domains. The strands of the $\alpha 1$ and $\alpha 2$ domains interweave to form a platform of β-pleated sheets that support a peptide-binding groove, each wall of which is a long α helix donated by a single domain. The peptide nestles within this groove, its charged amino and carboxyl termini anchored within specific pockets of the cleft. The $\alpha 3$ domain, however, is much less variable between loci and alleles. The $\alpha 3$ domain of different heavy chains can, at least in some cases, be swapped with little effect on the antigen-presenting functions of the $\alpha 1$ and $\alpha 2$ domains. The $\alpha 3$ domain forms many important molecular bonds with the bottom of the $\alpha 1$ and $\alpha 2$ β-pleated sheet when the molecule is correctly folded. A short "tether" peptide, partly encoded by the $\alpha 3$ exon, connects the $\alpha 3$ domain to the TM domain. The latter is hydrophobic but otherwise unremarkable.

The cytoplasmic domain of class I MHC molecules has no known function. In some cases, it is capable of being phosphorylated upon cell activation. It may serve only to help anchor the heavy chain in the membrane. Messenger RNA (mRNA) encoding some class I molecules can be spliced in different ways, giving rise to external domains lacking a TM/CYT anchor; these are secreted in body fluids. In other cases, alternative splicing results in attachment of the three external domains to a membrane-bound phosphatidylinositol anchor. Such anchors can be cleaved in cells, such as T cells, responding to activating signals that hydrolyze phosphatidylinositol. Reciprocally, cross-linking this kind of class I molecule can deliver a mitogenic signal to T cells.

The MHC encodes a variety of class I heavy chains. The best known in humans are the HLA-A, HLA-B, and HLA-C molecules, sometimes collectively called the class I-a genes. Class I-a molecules present the majority of known epitopes and are major players in graft rejection. Their tissue distribution is often referred to as ubiquitous, but this is misleading, as the levels of constitutive expression vary greatly in different tissues. For example, lymphocytes and hepatocytes typically express relatively high and low levels, respectively. Other cell types are intermediate in expression, whereas neurons, spermatozoa, and human erythrocytes are devoid of or express very low levels of class I.

These variations in surface expression are important to antigen presentation function: even a threefold difference in surface expression can radically change the susceptibility of a cell to lysis mediated by class I–restricted cytotoxic T lymphocytes (CTL). In cells expressing intermediate or low constitutive levels of class I, higher expression may be induced by a variety of cytokines. These include type I (α and β) interferons, secreted predominantly by macrophages and fibroblasts, respectively, during virus infection, and type II interferon (IFN-γ), secreted mostly by activated T cells and by natural killer cells. Another important inducer of MHC class I expression in some tissues is tumor necrosis factor α

(TNFα), produced by macrophages and T cells. Class I expression and/or function is inhibited in a variety of clever ways by certain viruses, including some adenoviruses, herpes viruses, and retroviruses. A number of oncogenes in specific tissues, such as *N-myc* in neuroblastoma cells, can also down regulate expression of MHC class I-a genes.

Class I-a molecules dominate the landscape on most cell types but are only the tip of the iceberg of potential class I gene products.[55, 59] A large number of class I-b genes are found in mice and have also been described in humans. Many of these are also MHC linked. They tend to be oligomorphic or nonpolymorphic and are expressed at relatively low levels or on only a few cell types. In the mouse, for example, the H-2M3 locus encodes only two known alleles in wild populations, only one of which is common. As a result, most individuals are homozygous for this allele. The human class I-b molecule, HLA-G, is expressed almost exclusively on trophoblasts. Other proteins that can be included under the rubric of class I-b molecules are not encoded within the MHC. These include CD1 and FcRn, a low-affinity IgG receptor. CD1 is expressed on thymocytes, intestinal epithelial cells, and T-cell–associated dendritic cells, such as Langerhans cells. It can be recognized by specific T cells and may be involved in specialized antigen presentation functions. In contrast, FcRn, the low-affinity receptor for milk-borne maternal immunoglobulin expressed in neonatal intestinal epithelium, apparently does not interact with T cells but is required for the transcytosis of maternal Ig from the gut lumen into the blood.

With few exceptions, class I molecules cannot be expressed stably at the cell surface in the absence of bound peptide and β_2-microglobulin (β_2m), the class I light chain. β_2m is a twelve kilodalton (M_r 12 kDa) protein encoded by a single gene located outside of the MHC. It contains a single Ig-like domain and does not carry a TM or CYT region. β_2m locks the heavy chain into a stable conformation that retains a bound peptide and is resistant to cleavage by proteases. In cell lines or in mice in which the β_2m gene is disrupted, surface expression of most class I molecules is severely inhibited.[47]

The peptide binding site.[36] The entire phenomenon of MHC restriction of antigen presentation can be explained on the basis of selective peptide binding by both class I and class II MHC molecules. That is, each allelic form of an MHC molecule can bind only a small subset of the universe of possible peptides. An individual can respond only to those antigenic peptides that can be bound by his or her own MHC molecules. Similarly, a T-cell receptor can recognize an antigenic peptide only when it is presented by a particular MHC molecule. Each T cell is specific for a particular peptide presented in (restricted by) the molecular context of a particular MHC molecule.

Peptides are bound within a deep groove formed by the α1 and α2 domains. A platform composed of interwoven elements from each domain (forming a β-pleated sheet) supports two long α-helical arms, one from each domain. The α-helixes form the walls of the peptide-binding groove. X-ray crystallography reveals that peptides adopt an extended rather than helical conformation within the pocket. In general, class I MHC molecules bind peptides ranging in length from 7 to 10 amino acids, whereas class II MHC molecules bind longer peptides. The reason for the size limitation by class I molecules is that the ends of the groove are pinched off, creating binding pockets for the positively charged amino terminus and the negatively charged carboxyl terminus of the peptide (Fig. 1–3). In contrast, the groove of class II molecules is not pinched off, allowing longer peptides to bind.

Epitope prediction. Peptides that bind to class I MHC molecules engage the binding groove through the terminal anchors, the peptide backbone, and some but not all of the amino acid side chains. Because most termini and backbone residues are identical, peptide specificity is achieved by permissive and nonpermissive interactions between particular pockets of the binding groove and particular side chains of the peptide. For example, a common allele of HLA-A, HLA-A2, preferentially binds peptides of nine amino acids with a leucine in the second position and a valine in the last position. In contrast, HLA-B27 preferentially binds nonamer peptides with an arginine in the second position and either arginine or lysine in the last position. Amino acid side chains not engaged with the peptide groove itself may interact with the T-cell receptor. Detection of such binding motifs suggests that knowing the binding rules for particular MHC alleles should permit the prediction of antigenic epitopes from the

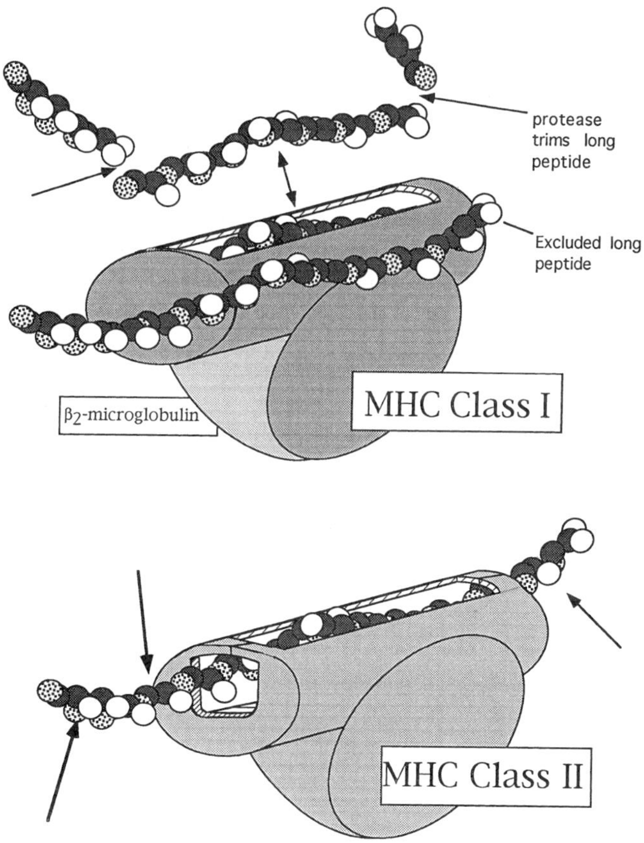

FIGURE 1–3. Size restriction on peptides binding MHC molecules. Class I molecules must engage the peptide termini, limiting the length of bound peptides. In contrast, class II molecules are free to bind long peptides, which are, however, subject to trimming by proteases. (From Rodgers JR, Rich RR: Antigens and antigen presentation. In Rich RR, Shearer WT, Strober W, et al (eds): Clinical Immunology: Principles and Practice. Mosby–Year Book, Inc, St. Louis, 1995.)

primary sequence of an antigen. Although this is true in some cases, other results suggest that epitope prediction is more difficult. Not every peptide that carries a binding motif is produced in sufficient quantities during antigen processing. Many potential epitopes closely resemble self-peptides to which the individual has become tolerant. Interactions between peptide side chains may affect the ability of the heavy chain to detect the motif.

MHC molecules can bind peptides with high affinity ($K_d \approx 1$ nM) and selectivity. They are therefore peptide antigen receptors. Only 10% to 30% of the surface area of a bound peptide is available to the T-cell receptor. Antigen presentation to T cells is mostly presentation of the MHC molecule itself, with a critical but minor component binding through the peptide. About three fourths of the interaction surface between the T-cell receptor and the peptide/MHC complex consists of the MHC molecule itself, predominantly the two α helixes. MHC restriction thus reflects the fact that the clonotypic regions of the T-cell receptor bind primarily to the allele-specific regions of the MHC molecule.

A common misapprehension is that MHC molecules and/or antigen processing somehow discriminates between self- and nonself-antigens. This is not true. Probably due to their relative abundance, the majority of peptides bound by class I and class II molecules are self-peptides. The organismic distinction between self and nonself is made by T cells, which are specifically selected during thymic education and by postthymic tolerance mechanisms.

Most, but not all, T cells whose T-cell receptors detect class I MHC molecules also carry the CD8 accessory molecule. CD8 exists as a dimer on the T-cell surface and can probably make contact simultaneously with two different class I molecules. The primary binding site for CD8 is on the highly conserved α3 domains. CD8 can bind to class I molecules independently of T-cell receptor engagement. However, coengagement is probably critical to antigen presentation, as this brings the cytoplasmic portion of CD8 into proximity with cytoplasmic domains of the T-cell receptor, permitting efficient signaling.

The biogenesis of class I molecules.[8, 45, 60] Perhaps 99% of all peptides that bind class I MHC molecules do so within the ER. Two pathways are known by which peptides enter the ER (Fig 1–4.) The major pathway is through the transporter associated with antigen processing (TAP), the genes for which are encoded within the class II region of the MHC. TAP is an ATP-dependent enzyme, composed of two subunits, that pumps peptides in the size range of 5 to 15 amino acids from the cytosol into the ER.[39] TAP-mutant cells and cells from TAP-knockout mice or from certain bare lymphocyte syndrome patients[14] that carry disrupted TAP genes are unable to acquire these peptides in the ER and display very few class I molecules at the cell surface. Although genetic variation in TAP genes does affect the pattern of peptides presented by class I molecules,[40] there is no evidence corroborating earlier reports that such polymorphisms predispose carriers to autoimmune disease.[51]

Peptides destined to be pumped by TAP enter the cytosol through several pathways. Many, of course, derive from cytosolic proteins. Others derive from surface proteins, such as the hemagglutinin protein of influenza virus. In most cases, however, only surface proteins synthesized by the cell itself

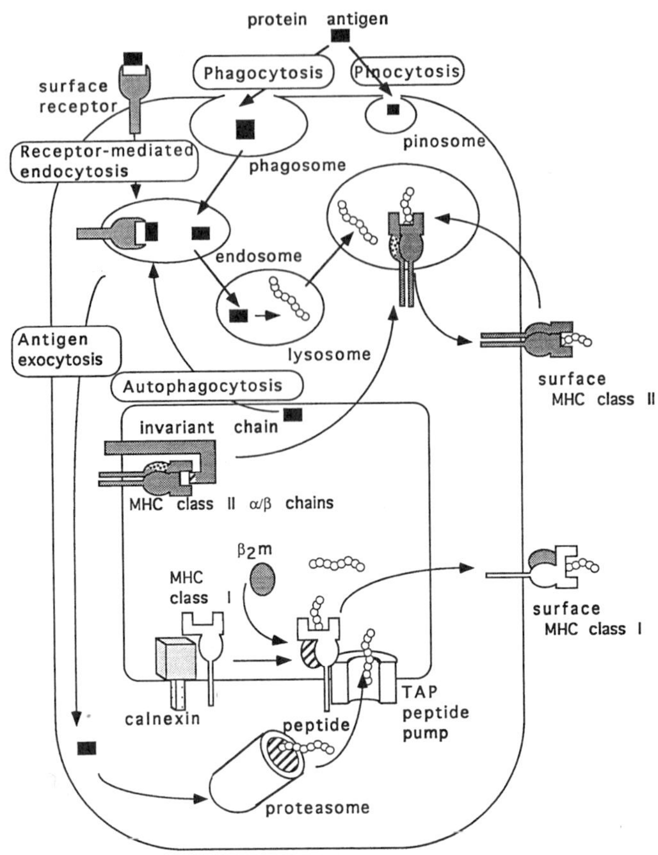

FIGURE 1–4. The major routes of antigen and MHC trafficking. Antigens (solid rectangle) enter the cell through endocytosis or are synthesized on ribosomes. The major route for loading class I molecules involves protein degradation by proteasomes and translocation into the endoplasmic reticulum via the TAP transporters. Cellular proteins enter the class II loading pathway via autophagocytosis, whereas exogenous antigens are endocytosed. Lysosomal enzymes degrade proteins to produce peptides.

are presented by class I molecules. Such proteins are made on cellular ribosomes but are diverted into the cytosol for degradation. Some truly exogenous proteins can find their way into the cytosol through an unknown pathway. Intracellular proteins are targeted for degradation by being coupled to the small protein ubiquitin before degradation within proteasomes. The latter produce peptides (8 to 14 amino acids) that are capable of translocation by TAP.

The second known pathway for antigenic peptides to enter the ER is that followed by most secretory and membrane-bound proteins: the protein secretory pathway. Most of these proteins are synthesized initially as preproteins, bearing a *signal peptide* at their *N* terminus. The signal peptide interacts with a signal recognition particle (SRP) that docks with transmembrane pore proteins. Following translocation from the cytosol into the ER, the signal peptide is cleaved by a *signal peptidase*. The remainder of the protein is translocated entirely into the lumen, although in the case of membrane-bound proteins, it may remain attached to the membrane by the hydrophobic TM domains. The signal peptides, or occasionally fragments of the translocated protein, may be bound by class I molecules. Some class I-binding peptides from the gp120 (env) protein of HIV-1 are processed through this pathway,[24] as they derive from a protein synthesized with a signal peptide, and their presentation is not TAP dependent.

MHC heavy chains enter the ER to their own assembly line through the protein secretory pathway. Signal peptidases remove the signal peptides of nascent heavy chains, and glycosyltransferases add polysaccharide side chains to certain asparagines, especially on the $\alpha 1$ and $\alpha 2$ domains. A chemically reducing environment within the ER aids an enzyme, protein disulfide isomerase, to connect the free cysteines in the $\alpha 2$ and $\alpha 3$ domains. The membrane-bound, ER-resident, calcium-dependent chaperone protein known as calnexin grabs the nascent class I molecule and retains it within the ER until it is properly folded (see Fig. 1–4). The TAP heterodimer itself binds the naked heavy chain and feeds it peptides. Peptide binding to class I molecules is favored at the neutral pH of the ER. If the heavy chain acquires an appropriate peptide, it will adopt a mature conformation, bind β_2m with high affinity, and be released by calnexin and the TAP to emigrate via the Golgi apparatus to the cell surface. Heavy chains that do not acquire peptides degrade within the ER. Peptides that do not bind to heavy chains are either degraded or returned to the cytosol. Peptides that are too long for binding may be partially degraded or trimmed within the ER to a size that can bind.

The molecular fate of the heavy chain depends on the reversible adoption of the mature conformation. Although peptide binding favors this conformation, reversible conformation means that some heavy chains will escape the ER without binding β_2m or without binding an appropriate peptide. Some of these may be caught within the *cis*-Golgi by another kind of chaperonin, in this case a 70 kilodalton heat shock protein (Hsp70) or the closely related protein BiP (see Table 1–I) that recognizes partially denatured proteins and can return them to the ER.[16] Some heavy chains may escape this checkpoint or lose their bound peptide on the way to the cell surface. These heavy chains bind peptides at the cell surface if they have retained their β_2m. The physiologic significance of acquiring peptides at the cell surface is presently uncertain but is probably important for the design of vaccines based on synthetic peptides.[66]

Most peptides that bind typical class I molecules do so within the ER and must derive from proteins synthesized within the cell. As a result, pathogen-specific CTL will lyse principally the cells that are actively infected. In some cases, however, macrophages, T-cell–associated dendritic cells, and antigen-specific B cells can present endocytosed antigens that through a currently unknown mechanism enter the cytosol for subsequent TAP-dependent movement into the ER.

ANTIGEN PRESENTATION BY CLASS II MOLECULES[13, 50, 52, 57]

Class II MHC molecules may more closely resemble the ancestral MHC molecule that gave rise by gene duplication and exon shuffling to the modern class I and class II molecules. For example, the two chains of class II molecules (α and β) each contain a single antigen-binding domain and a single membrane-proximal domain. They adopt a three-dimensional conformation resembling that of the class I heavy chain:β_2m:peptide heterotrimer. Peptide binding by class II molecules may be less specific: there are no strict requirements that peptide termini be buried within the binding cleft, and surface expression does not require the presence of the peptide.[13, 52, 57] In other respects, however, the biology of class II molecules is more specialized than that of typical class I-a molecules. For example, class II molecules are expressed on very few cell types or on others only after exposure to IFN-γ.

The structure of class II molecules.[58] Humans express three distinct subfamilies of class II genes: HLA-DR, HLA-DP, and HLA-DQ. Unlike class I molecules, whose shared light chain is encoded outside the MHC, the α and β chain genes of each class II molecule are closely linked within the MHC. The α genes are much less polymorphic than are the β chain genes. The β chain contains several regions that interact with CD4, the accessory molecule found on helper T cells. The features of interactions with the T-cell receptor are similar to those of class I molecules: most contact sites involve the two α helixes surrounding the peptide-binding cleft. In addition, class II molecules bind certain bacterial and viral proteins known as superantigens. These proteins, which are encoded by a family of related genes found in streptococci and staphylococci and by an unrelated family of genes in certain retroviruses, bind to certain families of T-cell receptor Vβ proteins and activate T cells expressing them. Although Vβ specificity differs among the superantigens, a superantigen activates a large fraction of T cells polyclonally. For example, the toxic shock syndrome toxin is a superantigen that activates T cells expressing the Vβ2 family.[17] As mentioned earlier, known superantigens bind the $\alpha 1$ domain of class II molecules but stimulate both CD4+ and CD8+ T cells.

Unlike most class I molecules, class II molecules are known to transduce activating signals. For example, exposure to superantigens in the absence of T cells can cause monocytes to release TNFα. The molecular pathways by which signal transduction occurs have not been determined.

The biogenesis of class II molecules.[13, 42, 52] Like other membrane-bound proteins, nascent class II molecules are translocated into the ER via the protein secretory pathway. Almost immediately, the α and β chains bind each other in the absence of peptide and adopt a conformation that in the absence of other events would allow them to leave the ER and migrate to the cell surface. However, a specialized chaperone protein known as an invariant chain binds the $\alpha\beta$ dimers within the ER and influences their behavior in two important ways. First, a loop of the invariant chain inserts into the peptide-binding cleft and inhibits binding by peptides within the ER. This effectively segregates the antigens presented by class I and class II molecules. Second, the invariant chain carries an intracellular trafficking signal that diverts class II migration from the Golgi into the endosomal compartment where class II molecules acquire peptides (see Fig. 1–4).

The endosomal compartment consists of a variety of vesicles constantly undergoing fusion and separation. Trapping by pinocytosis internalizes small solute molecules in all cell types. Endocytosis of surface receptors also is a constitutive process. Phagocytes internalize large particles, including opsonized viruses and bacteria, in phagosomes. Fusion of any of these endosomes with lysosomes permits exchange of vesicle contents. Autophagocytosis is the poorly understood process by which organelles such as the ER and mitochondria fuse with endosomal vesicles. Fusion of autophagosomes with lysosomes generates autophagolysosomes, which are major sites for catabolizing cellular proteins.

Whether obtained by endocytosis or autophagocytosis, proteins entering the lysosomes are exposed to denaturing acid conditions. A variety of proteases, lipases, and other catabolic enzymes degrade the proteins into peptides that can bind class II molecules.[30] Note that approximately one half of the peptides bound to class II molecules are self-peptides derived through autophagocytosis, belying the common assumption that class II molecules present only exogenous antigens. Degradation within lysosomes is sensitive to inhibition by lysosomotropic alkalinizing agents, such as chloroquine, or by cellular mutations that block acidification. Inhibition of lysosomal activity prevents class II antigens from presenting most but not all antigens.

Class II molecules bind peptides in one or more subcompartments within the endosomal network (see Fig 1–4, Table 1–1). Nascent class II molecules, newly arrived from the Golgi, must first disengage from invariant chain. This process requires entry into an acidified compartment and cleavage of the invariant chain. Dissociation of the invariant chain loop and binding most peptides require the activity of two proteins, the products of the DMA and DMB genes. These genes closely resemble class II MHC molecules and are encoded within the class II subregion of the MHC. The majority of class II molecules in cell mutants defective in lysosomal acidification or missing the DMA or DMB genes do not disgorge the invariant chain loop but instead carry it to the cell surface. These molecules cannot present antigens because they cannot bind additional peptides.

Nascent class II molecules that have lost their invariant chain loops, or mature class II molecules that have recycled from the cell surface, can bind peptides. The rules governing the binding of peptides to class II molecules have been more difficult to decipher than those related to class I molecules.[18] In particular, class II molecules do not bind peptide termini; this allows binding of peptides of disparate lengths. Peptides with long terminal extensions are subject to variable amounts of trimming, resulting in additional complexity of peptide binding.

Predicting epitopes for class II molecules from primary sequences of antigens has met with varied results. The successes of early algorithms that assumed a helical or amphipathic (charged on one face, hydrophobic on the other) helical conformation of the peptide within the binding cleft appeared perplexing after x-ray crystallography demonstrated an extended rather than helical conformation. It has proved difficult to identify binding motifs for class II molecules as is now routine for class I molecules. Discerning the rules of antigen processing may prove more fruitful. For example, many naturally processed peptides eluted from purified class II molecules have the amino acid proline in the first or second position. This finding may be explained by the fact that cellular aminopeptidases (enzymes that nibble one or two amino acids at a time from the amino terminus of a peptide) are unable to cleave beyond a proline residue. Proline is also recognized as an amino acid that disrupts regular structures, such as helixes, and is therefore often present at turns and at the beginning of loops. A reasonable speculation based on this and other observations is that immunodominant class II-binding peptides are those peptides most likely to survive rapid degradation within the endosomal compartment.

ANTIGEN ACQUISITION

A variety of cellular pathways are available for acquisition of antigens for subsequent processing and presentation. The most common means is endogenous synthesis on cellular ribosomes. The majority of peptides bound to class I molecules and approximately one half of those bound to class II molecules are self-peptides that enter the appropriate binding compartments through TAP or autophagy. Recall that a minority of self-peptides that bind class I molecules are transported into the lumen of the ER cotranslationally via the protein secretory pathway. A much larger fraction of proteins yielding class II–binding peptides also follow this route. Some of these are then transported to the endosomes from the Golgi apparatus. Others emerge at the surface before reentering the cell by endocytosis.

Endocytosis is another major pathway of entry of exogenous and some endogenous antigens into the class II pathway (Table 1–2). There are three chief mechanisms of endocytic acquisition of antigens. Soluble antigens in the fluid phase are *pinocytosed* through microinvaginations. Surface proteins, such as membrane-bound gp120 of human immunodeficiency virus, can be internalized directly by *simple endocytosis.* This results from the normal turnover of cellular membranes and involves the formation of *coated pits.* Aggregated antigens, whether denatured in antibody-antigen complexes or in the form of microorganisms, are *phagocytosed* by specialized cell types, chiefly macrophages and T-cell–associated dendritic cells (TADC). These endocytic mechanisms are all nonspecific, which means that phagocytes cannot distinguish between exogenous and endogenous antigens. This may explain why macrophages especially are active in stimulating, via the elaboration of IL-12, the cytolytic and inflammatory TH1-like cytokine pathway. Particulate antigens can sometimes be phagocytosed by monocytes and TADC for delivery to class I molecules. This pathway is insensitive to lysosomotropic inhibitors, such as chloroquine, but is dependent on the TAP peptide pumps. Because of this

TABLE 1–2
PROCESSING OF EXOGENOUS ANTIGEN

Feature	B Cells	Phagocytes
Antigen acquisition	Specific	Nonspecific
Antigen entry	Endocytosis of sIg	Pinocytosis, FcR-mediated endocytosis, phagocytosis
FcRII	Not internalized	Internalized
Antigen-presenting molecule	MHC class I and II	MHC class I and II
Cytokine produced	IL-12 in some cases	IL-12, induces IFN-γ production by T cells
T-cell response	TH2 (IL-4, IL-10)	TH1 (IL-2, IFN-γ), inflammatory CD8+CTL (IFN-γ)

From Rodgers JR, Rich RR: Antigens and antigen presentation. In Rich RR, Shearer WT, Strober W, et al (eds): Clinical Immunology: Principles and Practice. Mosby–Year Book, Inc, St. Louis, 1995.

pathway, it makes teleological sense that responding T cells treat antigen-presenting phagocytes as if they were infected, that is, by killing them.

A more discriminating pathway of acquisition of exogenous antigens occurs through *receptor-mediated endocytosis*.[33] B cells, which are nonphagocytic and poor presenters of particulate antigens, avidly acquire cognate antigens and internalize them via antigen-induced endocytosis of their own surface antibodies. As a result, antigen-specific B cells can be 10,000 times more efficient at presenting low levels of soluble antigens to T cells than are macrophages. This quality is a fundamental mechanism by which cognate helper reactions occur between immune B and T cells during secondary responses.

Receptor-mediated endocytosis of acquired antigen bound to antibodies is not limited to B cells. Different Fc receptors on different cell types can bind secreted antibodies that carry antigens (Table 1–3). The best known of these receptors is the high-affinity receptor for IgE (see Chapter 8), present in great numbers on mast cells and basophils (see Chapter 10). Mast cells and basophils respond to antigen-mediated cross-linking of their FcRε molecules by activation and degranulation. Mast cells also internalize such antigens and present them to T cells. The chief form of FcRγ present on B cells (FcRγII) cannot internalize bound antibodies. Instead of antigen presentation by the B cell, acquisition of antigen and the resulting cross-linking of the B-cell receptor (surface antibodies) with FcRγII lead to inhibition of B-cell proliferation. In contrast, an isoform of this protein found on monocytes and generated by alternative splicing of the precursor mRNA is internalized efficiently to stimulate immune responses.[1]

Among other antigen-acquiring molecules are several complement receptors that trap and internalize opsonized antigen-antibody complexes and activate phagocyte functions. Antigen acquisition through complement receptors is a major pathway. As a result, genetic deficiency in C2 expression results in severe impairment of antigen presentation. For example, opsonized particles trigger complement receptor 1 (CR1, also called CD35), which binds C3b and C4b, to induce phagocytosis in monocytes. This activation requires coligation with FcRγ receptors or cellular activation by IFN-γ. The CR2 receptor (CD21) associates tightly with the Igαβ B-cell receptor complex (the B-cell homologue of the CD3 structure found on T cells) and is required for efficient signaling through surface Ig. CR3 (CD11b) forms heterodimers with the CD18 integrin β2 subunit to produce the Mac-1 molecule present on macrophages and on some natural killer cells and CD8-positive T cells. CR3 binds the inhibitory molecule iCb3 and is the cellular receptor for the cell adhesion molecule ICAM-1 (CD54) as well as for bacterial LPS and yeast β-glucan. Signaling through CR3 activates macrophage phagocytosis and may contribute to the generation of TNFα seen following exposure to endotoxin.

Macrophages do not express a cellular Fc receptor for IgM, the major immunoglobulin present during primary and TI-antigen–induced immune responses. Indirect binding of IgM is provided instead by the C5a receptor, which binds bacteria opsonized by IgM that has interacted with C5a-containing complement factors. Signaling through the C5a receptor induces chemotaxis and phagocytosis (see Chapter 16) and up-regulates the expression of CR1 and CR3 molecules on macrophages.

Endocytosis mediated by additional receptors is important for antigen acquisition in special cases. For example, both helper T cells and macrophages acquire soluble HIV gp120 protein via CD4 molecules and internalize gp120-CD4 complexes for processing and presentation to T cells. Lysis by gp120-specific cytotoxic T cells might contribute to the loss of CD4 cells observed in AIDS.

TABLE 1–3
Fc RECEPTORS AVAILABLE FOR ANTIGEN ACQUISITION

Name	Function/Affinity	Cell Type	Subunits
αRI		Monocytes	
γRI CD64	10 nM IgG1 >G3,G4,>G2	Macrophages, neutrophils, eosinophils	α74 γ9 or 12?
γRII CD32	0.5 μM IgG1>G3,G4,G2	Macrophages, neutrophils, eosinophils, platelets, B cells	α45 β33 γ9
γRIII CD16	2 μM IgG1>G2,G3, triggers natural killer cell cytolysis	B cells, mast cells, neutrophils, eosinophils, macrophages	α in neutrophils; γ9 or ζ in natural killer cells
εRI	0.1 nM for monomeric IgE	Mast cells	α45 β33 γ9
εRII CD23	Low affinity for IgE; on follicular dendritic cells is a ligand for CD19/CR2 TAPA-1 complex of B cells	Activated B cells, eosinophils, apical FDC	α45
FcγRn	Transcytosis	Neonate gut epithelium	α $β_2m$

ANTIGEN-PRESENTING CELLS[31]

Antigen presentation occurs within a cellular context. The response of a given T cell to its antigen depends not only on its own cellular state and the concentration of the antigen on the presenting cell but also on the variety and number of accessory molecules and cytokines in the microenvironment. These different interactions are part of what has been called the two signal hypothesis governing T-cell responses.[12, 37] Signal 1 is delivered through the T-cell receptor, its strength depending on the overall avidity of antigen recognition. Signal 2 is transduced through certain nonclonotypic receptors, such as CD28, on the T cell surface. Interactions with adhesion molecules, such as ICAM-1, also add to the overall strength or avidity of the reaction. Binding of class I or class II molecules by CD8 or CD4, respectively, not only contributes to avidity but also transduces signals to the TCR.

Virgin and possibly resting T cells need to see both Signal 1 and Signal 2 to be activated. Stimulation by antigen alone (Signal 1) leads to anergy (the loss of cell responsiveness to subsequent signaling through Signals 1 and 2 together) and/or apoptosis (programmed cell death). Cells that can deliver both signals to class II-restricted (CD4) T cells are known as professional antigen-presenting cells (APC). The nature of

Signal 2 and the identity of professional APC are not understood in all cases. In many cases, it appears that Signal 2 can be delivered via the CD28 molecule on T cells. The ligand for CD28 is B7, now designated CD80, a membrane-bound molecule found on a variety of cell types, including activated B cells, monocytes, TADC, and thymic medullary epithelium.[48] Antigen presentation by resting B cells, which lack expression of CD80, to virgin T cells sometimes leads to anergy or apoptosis. Some researchers have emphasized the need for T-cell–associated interdigitated dendritic cells as true professional antigen-presenting cells for virgin and resting T cells.

Monocytes and macrophages. In terms of antigen presentation, macrophages and tissue-resident phagocytes are the first line of defense against infection. They bind opsonized bacteria and virus particles via their complement receptors (binding complement factors derived from the alternative pathway in primary infections or amplified by specific immunoglobulin in secondary infections), which are then internalized by receptor-mediated endocytosis. During the latter stages of a primary response or during a secondary response, antigens bound to secreted specific immunoglobulins are acquired and internalized via macrophage Fc receptors. Internalized antigens are degraded by an extensive lysosomal network in macrophages and presented by class II molecules to T cells. Macrophages express the CD28 ligand, B7 (CD80), and so are nominally competent to deliver Signal 2. In addition, they express membrane-bound interleukin-1 (IL1), which is required by T cells for full activation. However, Matzinger[37] has reported that under at least some conditions, macrophages deliver a "tolerizing" rather than an activating signal to virgin CD4 T cells in the mouse.

Besides their professional ability to stimulate antigen-specific T-cell proliferation, macrophages control the direction and magnitude of immune responses by secreting regulatory cytokines (see Chapter 5), principally TNFα and IL-12.[26] IL-12 induces T cells to secrete IFN-γ. This pivotal cytokine in turn affects many immune responses, including several pathways of antigen processing and presentation. IFN-γ is produced by natural killer cells, CD8 T cells, and TH1-like inflammatory T cells. IFN-γ in turn stimulates the cytolytic, inflammatory (TH1) immune pathways and suppresses the TH2 pathways.[23, 54] For example, in most cell types, IFN-γ stimulates elevated expression of antiviral genes, including oligo(A)-synthetase, and the entire MHC class I-related antigen presentation pathway, including TAP, LMP proteasome subunits, β_2m, and class I heavy chains. In many cell types, including macrophages and some endothelial cells, IFN-γ induces high levels of class II expression. IFN-γ also upregulates chemotaxis, phagocytosis, lysosomal enzyme activity, and TNFα production by macrophages. These effects obviously have a feed-forward influence on the ability of macrophages to stimulate further the same pathway. IFN-γ directly stimulates cytolytic activity carried out by macrophages, natural killer cells, and both CD8 and CD4 T cells.

Besides stimulating these inflammatory pathways, IFN-γ suppresses TH2 pathways, especially by blocking the secretion of IL4 by TH2-like T cells. In addition, IFN-γ suppresses class II expression by resting B cells. The mechanism and implications of this effect have not been fully explored. One prediction, however, is that IFN-γ should suppress secondary antibody responses by inhibiting the ability of antigen-specific memory B cells to present processed antigen to helper memory T cells. IFN-γ also inhibits allergic responses by blocking immunoglobulin gene switching to the IgE isotype.

T-cell–associated dendritic cells.[29, 38] T-cell–associated dendritic cells (TADC) are found in a variety of tissues under a variety of names: Langerhans cells in skin, veiled cells in the afferent lymph nodes, interdigitating cells in other secondary lymphoid organs, and simply dendritic cells. They are found in great numbers in airway mucosa. They should not be confused with follicular dendritic cells (FDC), occasionally called dendritic reticulum cells, of germinal center follicles. TADC are professional APC for CD4 and CD8 T cells. In contrast, FDC are a very different kind of antigen-presenting cell in that they present unprocessed antigen to B cells (discussed later).

TADC probably represent a single lineage or group of closely related, MHC class II-expressing, actively phagocytic cells. They derive almost certainly from bone marrow and differentiate from class II-negative precursors under the influence of the cytokine GM-CSF.[29] They often express the non-MHC–linked class I-b molecule, CD1, in addition to class I-a molecules. Some reports suggest that TADC belong to the myeloid lineage of cells. Others observe expression of markers in addition to CD1 that are typically associated with T cells, including CD8 and CD4. These raise the possibility that TADC may be closely related to T cells ontogenetically. However, they express other markers, such as CD40, that are otherwise found on B cells. Activation of TADC by the CD40 ligand (a membrane-bound protein normally found on T cells) increases expression of MHC class I and class II molecules and several adhesion molecules on the TADC. In most comparisons with monocytes and macrophages and even with antigen-specific B cells, TADC are much more potent APC for T cells as measured by antigen-specific T-cell proliferation, cytokine production, and help for B-cell responses. In the form of Langerhans cells, they are major if not sole stimulators of skin graft rejection. TADC are mobile and rapidly recruited to sites of inflammation.

Professional APC, including macrophages, TADC, and B cells, have traditionally been viewed as specialized for endocytosing (or phagocytosing) exogenous antigen for presentation by class II molecules. Under some conditions both macrophages and TADC can also endocytose exogenous antigens for presentation by class I molecules. It will be important to learn whether processing exogenous antigens for presentation by class I molecules is a unique function of phagocytic cells or is active in other cells, especially antigen-specific B cells, that can endocytose exogenous antigens.

B cells. B cells are good targets for T cells detecting endogenous antigens (such as those encoded by infecting viruses). However, as presenters of exogenous antigens, B cells present only those antigens for which their surface Ig molecules are specific. Although B cells express high levels of class II molecules, their surface membranes do not phagocytose or endocytose at high rates. Moreover, because of alternative splicing of mRNAs encoding the FcRγII, this receptor cannot internalize upon ligand binding. As a result, B cells are less than 1% as effective as are macrophages at presenting nonspecific antigens to T cells. In contrast, recall that B cells rapidly and efficiently internalize their own surface Ig molecules after antigen binding.[33] Thus primary responses require much higher antigen concentrations than do secondary responses in which high-affinity antibodies on memory B cells focus antigens for processing and presentation. Once internalized, antigens are processed in the endosomes of B cells just as by phagocytes. Antigen presentation by B cells may account for the experimental immunologic phenomenon known as the hapten-carrier effect. In this, antihapten antibody responses depend on cooperation between hapten-specific B cells that present antigens to MHC-restricted T cells specific for epitopes of the carrier protein. Such T cells in turn provide help to the B cells.

Mucosal epithelium.[10] The gut epithelium provides a stage for cells with interesting roles in antigen processing and presentation. The immunobiology of these cells is not well understood, but they are likely to be important in oral tolerance and oral immunity. M cells are specialized polarized epithelial cells overlying lymphoid follicles within the gut, facing the intestinal milieu. They are active in endocytosis and in a specialized form of endocytosis known as *transcytosis,* in which the contents of vesicles endocytosed on one side are actively transported and disgorged on the opposite side of polarized epithelial cells.[11]

Gut-associated epithelial cells express several special immune surface markers, suggesting a specialized role in antigen presentation that may include transcytosis. For example, for a short time soon after birth, the gut epithelium expresses a low-affinity receptor for IgG, known as FcRn.[20] Unlike other Fc receptors, which belong to a distantly related immunoglobulin-related gene superfamily, FcRn is a class I molecule. Although not encoded within the MHC, FcRn, like most other class I MHC molecules, requires β_2m for surface expression (see Table 1–3). There is no evidence that FcRn is recognized by T cells, and x-ray crystallography suggests that its "peptide-binding" groove probably cannot bind peptides. Instead, FcRn has apparently evolved a very different immune function: it binds milk-borne maternal immunoglobulin and transcytoses it across the epithelium to the blood. For example, FcRn binds IgG avidly at the low pH found in the gut and releases it under the more basic conditions of the blood. It would be fascinating to know the fate of antigens that might be bound specifically to maternal Ig and acquired by FcRn-positive epithelial cells. For example, are those antigens stripped off during transcytosis and redirected into an antigen-processing pathway, or are they co-transcytosed to the blood?

A second subfamily of unusual class I molecules expressed on gut epithelial cells are the CD1 antigens.[3, 10, 14, 44] Like FcRn, CD1 genes are not found on the same chromosome that bears the MHC. Unlike genes encoding the better-known class I molecules, such as HLA-A and HLA-B, CD1 genes also are not polymorphic but are evolutionarily conserved. Thus CD1 genes from mice and humans are more closely related to each other than are the better-known class I molecules encoded within the MHC. This finding means CD1 genes evolve more slowly than other class I molecules, suggesting a specialized function conserved over evolutionary time. Beyond the fact that CD1 can be recognized by T cells, including $\gamma\delta$ T cells,[44] the immune function of CD1 is unknown. A few additional facts support the hypothesis that any such function is highly specialized. Although CD1 binds β_2m as do other class I molecules, its surface expression depends on neither β_2m nor TAP function. CD1 molecules very likely reach the cell surface without bound peptides and may be available for binding gut peptides, other peptides derived from noncanonical pathways, or antigens such as glycopeptides.[5] It is not known whether CD1 can transcytose.

The gut is also a primary site for T cells expressing the $\gamma\delta$ T-cell receptor, a minor subset of T cells. Some $\gamma\delta$ T-cell receptor cells are called dendritic T cells due to their morphology but probably are distinct from TADC even though the latter do express several T-cell markers. It appears that the antigen ligands recognized by $\gamma\delta$ T-cell receptors include but are not limited to the short peptide ligands typically recognized by $\alpha\beta$ T-cell receptors. For example, some cloned mouse $\gamma\delta$ T cells recognize MHC molecules lacking any typical peptide,[53] and others appear to recognize carbohydrate ligands. The $\gamma\delta$ T cells may express either the CD4 or CD8 molecules. They may also express both simultaneously (double positives) or not express either one (double negatives). These observations suggest that $\gamma\delta$ T cells may be educated in a manner distinct from typical $\alpha\beta$ T cells, that their ligands may include ligands previously unrecognized, and that antigen processing and presentation of these ligands may follow unknown pathways. For example, the unusual features of the FcRn, CD1, and TL class I-b molecules suggest that these pathways could involve extracellular antigens and transcytosis.

Follicular dendritic cells.[63] Follicular dendritic cells (FDC) are a type of APC entirely distinct from TADC. Unlike the latter, which bind to T cells, FDC bind B cells. They can express MHC class II in addition to class I molecules but are nonphagocytic. They express complement and Fc receptors but lack expression of ICAM (CD54). FDC are pleiomorphic, ranging between those with filiform dendrites to those, perhaps more mature, with beaded dendrites (Fig. 1–5). The filiform dendrites acquire unprocessed antigens, presumably via their complement and Fc receptors, in a form that is partially surrounded but not endocytosed by layers of dendritic membrane. These accumulations generate beads of iccosomes that can retain antigens stably for days and perhaps much longer. FDC present these beads of concentrated and unprocessed antigens to antigen-specific B cells within the germinal center follicles, which are then able to endocytose, process, and present the antigen to T cells.

FDC are characteristic elements of germinal centers that form in lymph nodes following secondary antigenic stimulation.[34] Other key players within these centers are oligoclonal clusters of antigen-specific B cells as well as antigen-specific T helper cells. The germinal centers are the anatomic sites of somatic hypermutation of immunoglobulin genes during the secondary response. Presumably, the FDC play an important role in shaping the evolving response. Moreover, by retaining unprocessed antigen in a protected environment, FDC probably play a role in maintaining antigenic memory.

SUMMARY

The art of seeing antigens, in the vertebrate immune system, reflects multiple interacting processes that take native

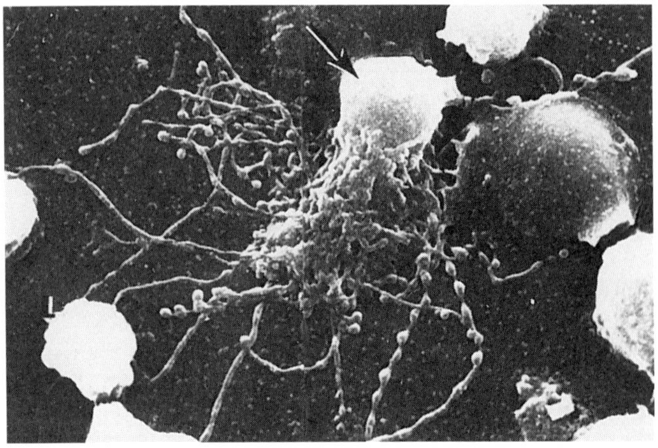

FIGURE 1–5. A scanning electron micrograph of a maturing, isolated, follicular dendritic cell (arrow). The forming beaded dendrites give rise to immune complex–coated bodies (iccosomes). Iccosomes are released in germinal centers for endocytosis by B lymphocytes (L). The iccosomal antigen is then processed and presented by the germinal center B cells to T cells. (From Szakal AK, Gieringer RL, Kosco MH, et al: Isolated follicular dendritic cells: cytochemical antigen localization, Nomarski, SEM, and TEM morphology. J Immunol 134:1349, 1985. Copyright 1985. The American Association of Immunologists.)

antigens and reduce them to small peptides for presentation to T cells via MHC class I and class II molecules. This chapter describes these pathways, emphasizing the importance of processing in determining what a good antigen is. All along these insinuating paths, manifold mechanisms of acquisition, processing, and presentation shape the biochemical quality and quantity of resulting antigenic peptides and determine in large part the character of the immune response. These pathways reflect innate as well as acquired immunity. Primary responses reflect largely nonspecific acquisition of antigens, whereas secondary responses are sensitized by the availability of specific antibodies serving as acquisition molecules. Differential sensitivity to protease attack determines the availability of specific peptides for binding to class I and class II molecules. The binding specificities of MHC molecules severely limit the number of distinct peptides that can be antigenic in each individual and result in extreme polymorphisms in antigen recognition.

REFERENCES

1. Amigorena S, Bonnerot C, Drake JR, et al: Cytoplasmic domain heterogeneity and functions of IgG Fc receptors in B lymphocytes. Science 256:1808, 1992.
2. Arnon R, Van Regenmortel MH: Structural basis of antigenic specificity and design of new vaccines. FASEB J 6:3265, 1992.
3. Balk SP, Burke S, Polischuk JE, et al: β_2-microglobulin-independent MHC class Ib molecule expressed by human intestinal epithelium. Science 265:259, 1994.
4. Barber LD, Parham P: The essence of epitopes. J Exp Med 180:1191, 1994.
5. Beckman EM, Porcelli SA, Morita CT, et al: Recognition of a lipid antigen by CD1-restricted $\alpha\beta^+$ T cells. Nature 372:691, 1994.
6. Benjamin DC, Berzofsky JA, East IJ, et al: The antigenic structure of proteins: a reappraisal. Annu Rev Immunol 2:67, 1984.
7. Berzofsky JA, Berkower IJ: Immunogenicity and antigen structure. In Paul WE (ed): Fundamental Immunology, 3rd edition. Raven Press, New York, 1993.
8. Bijlmakers MJ, Ploegh HL: Putting together an MHC class I molecule. Curr Opin Immunol 5:21, 1993.
9. Bjorkman PJ, Saper MA, Samraoui B, et al: Structure of the human class I histocompatibility antigen, HLA-A2. Nature 329:506, 1987.
10. Blumberg RS, Balk SP: Intraepithelial lymphocytes and their recognition of non-classical MHC molecules. Int Rev Immunol 11:15, 1994.
11. Bomsel M, Mostov K: Sorting of plasma membrane proteins in epithelial cells. Curr Opin Cell Biol 3:647, 1991.
12. Cohn M: The wisdom of hindsight. Annu Rev Immunol 12:1, 1994.
13. Cresswell P: Antigen presentation. Getting peptides into MHC class II molecules. Curr Biol 4:541, 1994.
14. de la Salle H, Hanau D, Fricker D, et al: Homozygous human TAP peptide transporter mutation in HLA class I deficiency. Science 265:237, 1994.
15. Denzin LK, Robbins NF, Carboy-Newcomb C, et al: Assembly and intracellular transport of HLA-DM and correction of the class II antigen-processing defect in T2 cells. Immunity 1:595, 1994.
16. Dobberstein B: On the beaten pathway. Nature 367:599, 1994.
17. Drake CG, Kotzin BL: Superantigens: biology, immunology, and potential role in disease. J Clin Immunol 12:149, 1992.
18. Engelhard VH: Structure of peptides associated with class I and class II MHC molecules. Annu Rev Immunol 12:181, 1994.
19. Englehard VH: Structure of peptides associated with MHC class I molecules. Curr Opin Immunol 6:13, 1994.
20. Gastinel LN, Simister NE, Bjorkman PJ: Expression and crystallization of a soluble and functional form of an Fc receptor related to class I histocompatibility molecules. PNAS 89:638, 1992.
21. Germain RN: MHC-dependent antigen processing and peptide presentation: providing ligands for T lymphocyte activation. Cell 76:287, 1994.
22. Germain RN, Margulies DH: The biochemistry and cell biology of antigen processing and presentation. Annu Rev Immunol 11:403, 1993.
23. Golding B, Zaitseva M, Golding H: The potential for recruiting immune responses toward type 1 or type 2 T cell help. Am J Trop Med Hyg 50(4):33, 1994.
24. Hammond SA, Bollinger RC, Tobery TW, et al: Transporter-independent processing of HIV-1 envelope protein for recognition by CD8+ T cells. Nature 364:158, 1993.
25. Howard JC, Seelig A: Antigen processing. Peptides and the proteasome. Nature 365:211, 1993.
26. Hsieh Chyi-S, Macatonia SE, Tripp CS, et al: Development of T_h1 $CD4^+$ T cells through IL-12 produced by *Listeria*-induced macrophages. Science 260:547, 1993.
27. Jardetzky TS, Brown JH, Gorga JC, et al: Three-dimensional structure of a human class II histocompatibility molecule complexed with superantigen. Nature 368:711, 1994.
28. Jerne NK: Immunological speculations. Annu Rev Microbiol 14:341, 1960.
29. Kämpgen E, Koch F, Heufler C, et al: Understanding the dendritic cell lineage through a study of cytokine receptors. J Exp Med 179:1767, 1994.
30. Katunuma N, Matsunaga Y, Saibara T: Mechanism and regulation of antigen processing by cathepsin B. Adv Enzyme Regul 34:145, 1994.
31. Knight SC, Stagg AJ: Antigen-presenting cell types. Curr Opin Immunol 5:374, 1993.
32. Kronenberg M: Antigens recognized by $\gamma\delta$ T cells. Curr Opin Immunol 6:64, 1994.
33. Lanzavecchia A: Receptor-mediated antigen uptake and its effect on antigen presentation to class II-restricted T lymphocytes. Annu Rev Immunol 8:773, 1990.
34. MacLennan IC: Germinal centers. Annu Rev Immunol 12:117, 1994.
35. Madden DR: The three-dimensional structure of peptide-MHC complexes. Annu Rev Immunol 13:587, 1995.
36. Matsumura M, Fremont DH, Peterson PA, et al: Emerging principles for the recognition of peptide antigens by MHC class I molecules. Science 257:927, 1992.
37. Matzinger P: Tolerance, danger, and the extended family. Annu Rev Immunol 12:991, 1994.
38. McWilliam AS, Nelson D, Thomas JA, et al: Rapid dendritic cell recruitment is a hallmark of the acute inflammatory response at mucosal surfaces. J Exp Med 179:1331, 1994.
39. Momburg F, Neefjes JJ, Hämmerling GJ: Peptide selection by MHC-encoded TAP transporters. Curr Opin Immunol 6:32, 1994.
40. Momburg F, Roelse J, Howard JC, et al: Selectivity of MHC-encoded

peptide transporters from human, mouse and rat. Nature 367:648, 1994.
41. Mond JJ, Lees A, Snapper CM: T cell-independent antigens Type 2. Annu Rev Immunol 13:655, 1995.
42. Morris P, Shaman J, Attaya M, et al: An essential role for HLA-DM in antigen presentation by class II major histocompatibility molecules. Nature 368:551, 1994.
43. Paul WE: Fundamental Immunology, 3rd edition. Raven Press, New York, 1993.
44. Porcelli S, Morita CT, Brenner MB: CD1b restricts the response of human $CD4^-8^-$ T lymphocytes to a microbial antigen. Nature 350:593, 1992.
45. Rajagopalan S, Xu Y, Brenner MB: Retention of unassembled components of integral membrane proteins by calnexin. Science 263:387, 1994.
46. Rammensee HG, Falk K, Rötzschke O: Peptides naturally presented by MHC class I molecules. Annu Rev Immunol 11:213, 1993.
47. Raulet DH: MHC class I-deficient mice. Adv Immunol 55:381, 1994.
48. Reiser H, Schneeberger EE: The costimulatory molecule B7 is expressed in the medullary region of the murine thymus. Immunology 81:532, 1994.
49. Rodgers JR, Rich RR: Antigens and antigen presentation. In Rich RR, Shearer WT, Strober W, et al (eds): Clinical Immunology: Principles and Practice. Mosby–Year Book, Inc, St. Louis, 1995.
50. Rötzschke O, Falk K: Origin, structure and motifs of naturally processed MHC class II ligands. Curr Opin Immunol 6:45, 1994.
51. Ronningen KS, Undlien DE, Ploski R, et al: Linkage disequilibrium between TAP2 variants and HLA class II alleles; no primary association between TAP2 variants and insulin-dependent diabetes mellitus. Eur J Immunol 23:1050, 1993.
52. Sant AJ, Miller J: MHC class II antigen processing: biology of invariant chain. Curr Opin Immunol 6:57, 1994.
53. Schild H, Mavaddat N, Litzenberger C, et al: The nature of major histocompatibility complex recognition by γδ T cells. Cell 76:29, 1994.
54. Schwarz EM, Salgame P, Bloom BR: Molecular regulation of human interleukin 2 and T-cell function by interleukin 4. PNAS 90:7734, 1993.
55. Shawar SM, Vyas JM, Rodgers JR, et al: Antigen presentation by major histocompatibility complex class I-b molecules. Annu Rev Immunol 12:839, 1994.
56. Silverstein AM: A History of Immunology. Academic Press, San Diego, CA, 1989.
57. Sinigaglia F, Hammer J: Defining rules for the peptide-MHC class II interaction. Curr Opin Immunol 6:52, 1994.
58. Stern LJ, Brown JH, Jardetsky TS, et al: Crystal structure of the human class II MHC protein HLA-DR1 complexed with an influenza virus peptide. Nature 368:215, 1994.
59. Stroynowski I, Fischer Lindahl K: Antigen presentation by non-classical class I molecules. Curr Opin Immunol 6:38, 1994.
60. Suh W-K, Cohen-Doyle MF, Fruh K, et al: Interaction of MHC class I molecules with the transporter associated with antigen processing. Science 264:1322, 1994.
61. Szakal AK, Gieringer RL, Kosco MH, et al: Isolated follicular dendritic cells: cytochemical antigen localization, Nomarski, SEM, and TEM morphology. J Immunol 134:1349, 1985.
62. Szakal AK, Kosco MH, Tew JG: Microanatomy of lymphoid tissue during humoral immune responses: structure function relationships. Annu Rev Immunol 7:91, 1989.
63. Tew JG, Kosco MH, Burton GF, et al: Follicular dendritic cells as accessory cells. Immunol Rev 117:185, 1990.
64. Trowsdale J: Genomic structure and function in the MHC. Trends Genet 9:117, 1993.
65. Wilson IA, Fremont DH: Structural analysis of MHC class I molecules with bound peptide antigens. Semin Immunol 5:75, 1993.
66. Yewdell JW, Bennink JR: Antigen processing: a critical factor in rational vaccine design. Semin Hematol 30:26, 1993.

2 Immunoglobulin Structure and Genetics

DEBORAH L. FRENCH

Immunoglobulins are expressed by B lymphocytes and defend the host against an infinite array of antigenic stimuli in the environment. These molecules bind specifically to invading pathogenic organisms or foreign substances and eliminate these invaders through the recruitment of effector mechanisms. The antigen binding and effector functions of immunoglobulins are mediated by two distinct areas of the core structure designated variable and constant regions. The variable region of the molecule carries the specific recognition site for antigenic determinants, and the constant region of the molecule carries the recognition sites for the receptors of a variety of effector systems.

Within the past 25 years, an explosion of information has been generated to elucidate the structural and molecular basis of antibody function and specificity. These studies have resulted in the identification of structural motifs and genetic mechanisms that have had a universal impact in many of the scientific disciplines, including immunology, biophysics, and molecular and evolutionary genetics. For example, the three-dimensional structure of the immunoglobulin domain (reviewed in 5, 37, 38) has been identified in a growing number of proteins, which is the basis for classification of these proteins in the immunoglobulin supergene family (reviewed in 73, 199). Another example is the elucidation of the genetic mechanisms that create the repertoire of antigen specificities of the immunoglobulin combining sites. A triumph of molecular biology was the determination of a gene rearrangement event within immunoglobulin loci (reviewed in 184), and this discovery provided evidence supporting the "two gene, one polypeptide chain" concept proposed by Dreyer and Bennett.[43] This chapter will focus on the basic features and fundamental concepts of immunoglobulin structure and genetics.

The structural aspects of immunoglobulins will include a description of the core structure of an antibody molecule, the accessory molecules that associate with membrane immunoglobulin during B lymphocyte development, the structural implications of immunoglobulin domains that have been derived from crystallography studies, and the structure and function of immunoglobulin isotypes. The molecular genetics of immunoglobulins will include a description of immunoglobulin loci, mechanisms of immunoglobulin gene rearrangement, mechanisms that generate diversity in the immunoglobulin repertoire, and mechanisms of heavy chain class switching. The transcriptional regulation of immunoglobulin genes (reviewed in 111, 171) and the signal transduction mechanisms that are mediated through the B lymphocyte antigen receptor (reviewed in 27, 28, 41, 133) will not be discussed in this chapter.

CORE ARCHITECTURE

The core structure of a prototypic immunoglobulin molecule consists of two identical covalently associated heavy chains of M_r ~50,000 or 70,000 (depending on the isotype) that are each covalently bound to identical light chains of M_r ~25,000 (Fig. 2–1). The development of this basic model evolved from early studies that subjected pooled serum globulin fractions to limited proteolysis, reduction, and denaturation. The initial studies of Heidelberger and colleagues[61] determined that the molecular weight of purified rabbit immunoglobulin was close to the principal normal globulin component of 150,000. With the development of the Tiselius electrophoretic apparatus, Elvin Kabat provided detailed information on the electrochemical properties of immune serum and purified antibodies.[182] By quantitative immunochemical analyses, Kabat demonstrated that immunoglobulin activity from a number of different species was associated with IgM and IgG classes of antibody.[77]

The basis for a structural understanding of immunoglobulin function came from the proteolytic studies of Porter[137] and Nisonoff.[124] Porter demonstrated that papain cleavage of a heterogeneous population of purified rabbit γ-globulins resulted in the production of chromatographically separable fragments. Two of the purified fragments blocked the precipitation of antigen with native purified rabbit γ-globulin and were designated Fab for fraction antigen binding (see Fig. 2–1). A fragment that did not bind antigen but crystallized in solution was designated Fc for fraction crystallizable (see Fig. 2–1).

Edelman and colleagues[48] demonstrated that the reduction of normal and abnormal immunoglobulins or myeloma proteins resulted in the dissociation of these proteins into separable subunits. They hypothesized that normal and abnormal immunoglobulins consisted of several polypeptide chains, designated heavy and light,[49] that were linked by disulfide bonds.[52] This hypothesis was strengthened with the demonstration by Nisonoff and colleagues[124] that cleavage of immunoglobulin with pepsin resulted in the formation of bivalent $F(ab)'_2$ fragments that upon reduction with sulfhydryl compounds resulted in two univalent Fab fragments. The use of heterogeneous mixtures of high molecular weight serum γ-globulins for these studies was sufficient because the overall structure and chemical nature of immunoglobulins are very similar. These heterogeneous mixtures of antibodies were not sufficient for determining the chemical basis of antigen binding and effector functions of individual immunoglobulin molecules and required a homogenous source of immunoglobulin molecules.

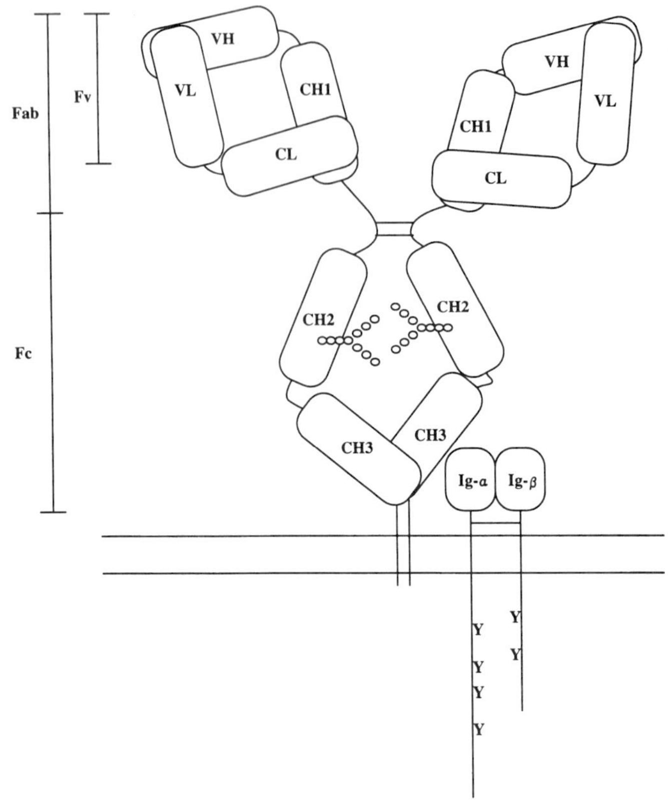

FIGURE 2–1. Prototypic multichain complex of the B-cell antigen receptor. Schematic of membrane immunoglobulin showing two identical light and heavy chains with accessory molecules Ig-α and Ig-β noncovalently associated with the heavy chain. The light and heavy chains are folded into distinct domain structures in which the variable region domains form the antigen binding site and the heavy chain constant region domains recruit various effector mechanisms. The areas of immunoglobulin heavy and light chains that comprise each of the proteolytic Fab, Fc, and Fv fragments are bracketed. The heavy chain hinge region is depicted by interchain disulfide bonds. Each C_H2 domain contains a site for N-linked glycosylation. The cytoplasmic domains of the disulfide-linked Ig-α and Ig-β chains contain tyrosine (Y) residues that are involved in signal transduction events.

A major contribution by Edelman and colleagues[51] provided the experimental evidence to demonstrate that myeloma proteins were identical to normal immunoglobulins. They demonstrated that Bence Jones proteins, originally found by Bence Jones in the urine of a patient with multiple myeloma,[9] were composed of light chains that were chemically identical to the myeloma protein of the same patient and to normal γ-globulins. Extensive antigenic cross-reactivities among myeloma proteins and normal γ-globulins had already been defined,[98, 174] and the development and characterization of plasmacytomas in mice[138] subsequently provided the animal counterpart to the human myelomas. The identification of myeloma proteins as homogeneous pools of antibodies resulted in our initial understanding of antibody structure and genetics.

This advance was followed by the advent of the hybridoma technology in 1975 by Köhler and Milstein.[94] This technology provided the means to generate an unlimited supply of monoclonal antibodies but, more importantly, provided the means to generate antigen-specific monoclonal antibodies. The antigen specificity of most myeloma proteins is not known; thus the correlation of antibody structure and genetics to antigen specificity could not be determined.

The hybridoma technology or somatic cell fusion technique resulted in major advances in our understanding of structural features between different immunoglobulin molecules and in elucidating the genetic mechanisms responsible for creating the immunoglobulin repertoire. The advances that were generated with myeloma and hybridoma cell lines and proteins included amino acid sequence analyses and identification of variable and constant regions, determination of the three-dimensional structure of an antibody molecule, the classification of immunoglobulin isotypes, the demonstration of immunoglobulin gene rearrangement events, the characterization of immunoglobulin loci, and elucidation of the genetic mechanisms of antibody diversity.

VARIABLE AND CONSTANT REGION DOMAINS

EARLY AMINO ACID SEQUENCE ANALYSES

The determination that myeloma proteins were identical to normal immunoglobulin molecules provided the initial sources of monoclonal pools of antibodies from which amino acid sequences were obtained. The amino acid sequences of three different Bence Jones proteins were determined by Hilschmann and Craig, who identified the variable and constant regions of immunoglobulin molecules.[64] They identified a striking level of sequence variation within the amino-terminal ends of the different light chains and identical sequences within the carboxy-terminal ends of the molecules. The first demonstration of the entire amino acid sequence of the heavy and light chains of an IgG_1 myeloma protein was by Edelman and colleagues.[50] From this sequence analysis, nonoverlapping regions of approximately 110 amino acid residues were identified that showed marked sequence homology. This observation led to the hypothesis that these homology regions folded into discrete three-dimensional domains and that each domain evolved to perform specific functions.[50] The exact sites of intradisulfide and interdisulfide bonds were identified. Highly conserved cysteine residues were identified within each domain and were proposed as providing intradisulfide bonds that stabilized the structural assembly of each domain.

As more amino acid sequence data of immunoglobulin fragments became available, regions of homology were apparent. In particular, the variable regions of human and mouse light chains could be divided into subgroups based on sequence identity within the amino-terminal residues.[71, 119, 123, 138] These subgroups have since been divided into families of homology-related sequences based on nucleotide cross-hybridization and sequence analyses (reviewed in 130). Current membership in a family corresponds to 80% homology at the DNA level and 75% homology at the protein level. These criteria have resulted in the division of six human heavy chain variable region gene families[12, 139] and six to seven human kappa[10, 178] and lambda[8, 190] light chain variable region gene families. The significance of these sequence homologies is that the classification of heavy and light chain variable regions into families and subfamilies extends to the individual genes. The extent of families of related genes directly reflects the germline antibody repertoire of an individual. As will be discussed later in this chapter, the families of germline genes provide the starting components from which the vast number of different antibody specificities are generated.

With all of the sequencing data that became available, attempts were made to identify the antigen binding site of antibody molecules. In an attempt to localize the precise location of the antibody combining site, Wu and Kabat performed a statistical analysis of the amino acid sequence data of 77 human and mouse myeloma proteins.[203] They hypothesized that the antibody combining sites were probably in the same location within all immunoglobulin molecules and that the enormous number of antibody combining sites were created by different amino acid residues located in defined portions of the variable region. Variability plots were determined, and three regions of hypervariability, which were widely separated in the primary sequence, were identified in the heavy and light chain variable regions.[80, 203] The authors hypothesized that the regions of hypervariability were brought into close proximity at the surface of the immunoglobulin molecule by the folding of the polypeptide chains into their native structure. The first high-resolution crystal structures of antibody fragments from myeloma proteins confirmed this hypothesis and the immunoglobulin domain theory.[135, 162, 167]

These studies showed that the hypervariable regions were located on the surface of the heavy and light chain variable region domains. These regions were brought together as contiguous loop structures on the surface of the molecule, forming the antibody combining site. Since amino acid residues within the hypervariable regions have been shown to create the antigen binding surface and form the contact sites with antigen,[6, 129] the hypervariable regions are designated complementarity determining regions (CDRs) (Fig. 2–2).[78] The amino acid residues within the variable region domains that surround the CDRs are designated as framework regions (FRs) (see Fig. 2–2).[79, 203] These residues are responsible for driving the assembly of the characteristic folding pattern of the variable region domains and positioning the CDR loop structures at the surface of the antibody molecule.

IMMUNOGLOBULIN DOMAIN STRUCTURE

The early x-ray work on myeloma Fab fragments[135, 167] and light chain dimers[162] helped to establish the structural basis of antibody function. The antibody molecule was demonstrated to be a flexible association of heavy and light chains in which each chain folded into characteristic globular

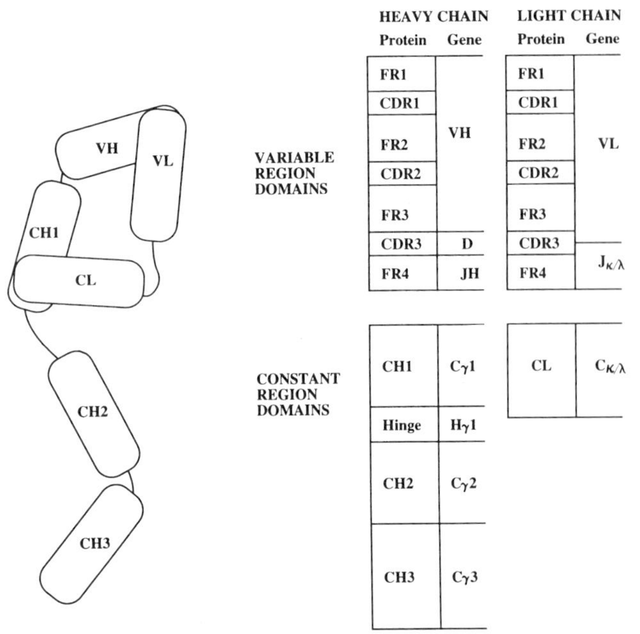

FIGURE 2–2. Variable and constant region domains of immunoglobulin heavy and light chains. The heavy and light chain variable region domains consist of complementarity-determining regions (CDR) that are surrounded by framework regions (FR). Multiple gene segments encode each of the variable region domains. The heavy chain variable region domain is encoded by three gene segments designated V_H (variable), which encodes CDR1, CDR2, FR1, FR2, and FR3; D (diversity), which encodes the middle of CDR3; and J_H (joining), which encodes FR4. The light chain variable region domain is encoded by two gene segments designated V_L, which encodes CDR1, CDR2, CDR3, FR1, FR2, and FR3; and J_L, which encodes FR4. The constant region domains, including the hinge region, are encoded by separate exons, and the protein and gene designations are given.

subunits. These globular subunits or domains are the structural building blocks of the immunoglobulin molecule and exist as independent, compact units of three-dimensional structure. X-ray diffraction studies have shown that immunoglobulin domains share a characteristic folding pattern that is known as the immunoglobulin fold (reviewed in 5, 37, 38).[135, 162, 167] This folding pattern is the basis for classification of numerous other proteins into the immunoglobulin supergene family (reviewed in 73, 199). The structural folding pattern of immunoglobulins consists of two layers of antiparallel β-sheets that are arranged in a sandwich or β-barrel. The two layers of β-pleated sheets are twisted, surround tightly packed internal hydrophobic residues, and are stabilized by the formation of an intrachain disulfide bridge.[53] The three-dimensional structure is highly conserved between immunoglobulin domains, and the conservation of invariant residues reinforces the postulate that different homology domains of immunoglobulin may have appeared during evolution through a gene duplication mechanism.[53]

In the constant region domains, the formation of the β-barrel structure consists of a total of seven antiparallel β-strands in which three β-strands form one side of the barrel and four β-strands form the other side. The variable region domains are longer than the constant region domains, and the extra residues result in the formation of two additional β-strands that form a loop structure characteristic of variable region domains (reviewed in 5, 37, 38).[53] The β-barrel structure of the variable region domain consists of nine antiparallel β-strands in which four β-strands lie on one side of the barrel and five β-strands lie on the other side. The CDRs of the variable region domains form three of the connecting segments between the β-strands. These segments are brought together in spatial proximity in the three-dimensional structure to form the antigen binding site of the immunoglobulin molecule.

DOMAIN INTERACTIONS

As previously mentioned, the highly conserved cysteine residues within each domain form stabilizing intrachain disulfide bonds (reviewed in 5, 37, 38). Other stabilizing features in the structure of immunoglobulin molecules involve noncovalent interactions between domains in different polypeptide chains and between domains within the same polypeptide chain. The noncovalent interactions between homologous domains of different polypeptide chains are extensive and result in the formation of dimeric modules such as V_L:V_H and C_L:C_H1 pairing (see Fig. 2–1). The interactions between domains within the same polypeptide chain involve a small number of contact residues that result in generally flexible interactions.[33, 136] As the complete immunoglobulin molecule is formed, the interaction of heavy and light chains results in the dimerization of homologous domains that define the smallest structural and functional units of the native antibody structure. The minimal antigen binding unit of the immunoglobulin molecule is the Fv fragment (see Fig. 2–1), which is a dimeric module of V_L and V_H domains.[60]

In homologous domain pairing, two types of associations have been identified that involve pairing of variable region domains and constant region domains (reviewed in 5, 37, 38). The pairing of variable region domains involves contact sites that are formed by key hydrophobic residues within the β-strands on one side of the variable region β-barrel structure.[53] These hydrophobic amino acids form the core of the variable region dimeric module structure that associates with a twofold axis of symmetry.[53] This geometrical arrangement is apparent whether V_L:V_L or V_L:V_H pairs are compared, and the domain associations are independent of light or heavy chain class or subclass. The loop segments that contain the CDRs generate an antigen binding surface in the three-dimensional array of V_L:V_H pairs binding globular proteins and a cavity structure of V_L:V_H or V_L:V_L pairs binding small molecules such as haptens (reviewed in 37, 39).

The constant region domain pairing also involves contact sites formed by key hydrophobic residues that are located on the opposite side of the constant region domain β-barrel structure (reviewed in 5, 37, 38). The domains associate with twofold axes of symmetry, and modular pairs include C_L:C_L, C_L:C_H1, and C_H3:C_H3 interactions. The C_H3 domains interact closely, similar to the C_H1 and C_L interactions of Fab fragments. For structural reasons, the C_H2 domains of Cγ, Cδ, and Cα and the C_H3 domains of Cμ and Cε do not interact due to the formation of four strand-four strand β-barrels instead of the characteristic three strand-four strand β-sandwich of other constant region domains.[42, 128] This structural feature of the C_H2 domain is due to sequence homology with both variable and constant region domains, and dimerization is precluded along either face.[42] In addition, conserved N-linked oligosaccharides are located in this domain and extend between the domains. With the exception of the C_H2 domain, the structural associations between homologous pairs of immunoglobulin domains are close and involve large areas of contact.

MEMBRANE AND SOLUBLE IMMUNOGLOBULINS

ISOTYPE NOMENCLATURE

The classification of antibody molecules into isotypes or classes and subtypes or subclasses was determined with antisera that were generated by immunizing mice or rabbits with purified human or murine myeloma proteins (reviewed in 55). Following absorption with other myeloma proteins, the resulting antisera were specific for antigenic determinants that are present predominantly in the constant regions of the heavy and light chains. These antisera defined the five heavy chain (γ, α, μ, ε, and δ) and two light chain (κ and λ) isotypes or classes, with some of the isotypes splitting further into subclasses such as human γ into γ1, γ2, γ3, and γ4 and α into α1 and three allelic forms of α2.[31] This nomenclature is used for the specific designation of the heavy and light chains of a particular antibody, but antibodies are commonly referred to by their heavy chain isotype or class as IgM, IgD, IgG, IgA, and IgE.

In addition to the identification of immunoglobulin isotypes, antisera were also generated by immunization of purified myeloma proteins within a given species, and two other types of antigenic determinants designated allotopes[88] and idiotopes[98] (reviewed in 16) were identified. Allotopes are determinants expressed in the constant regions of heavy and light chains and in framework portions of the variable region domains due to polymorphisms in inherited alleles. No functional significance can be attributed to these determinants, but their use in gene linkage studies provided early evidence suggesting that constant and variable region domains were encoded by separate genes.[88] Idiotopes are antigenic determinants that are present in or close to the antigen combining site of the antibody molecule (reviewed in 16).[98] The functional significance of these determinants is postulated in the network hypothesis by Niels Jerne,[75] who proposed that the interaction of anti-idiotypic antibodies with idiotopes expressed on antigen receptors of B and T cells can regulate the steady state responsiveness of these cells. A perturbation of this balance with antigen disrupts the steady state balance, resulting in the generation of an immune response.

MEMBRANE IMMUNOGLOBULINS AND ACCESSORY MOLECULES

The antigen receptor of mature B lymphocytes is membrane immunoglobulin that is generated by alternative splicing in which exons encoding a hydrophobic transmembrane domain and a short cytoplasmic domain are spliced in-frame to constant region genes of expressed immunoglobulin molecules (reviewed in 149).[3, 46] Membrane immunoglobulin is a monomer containing two identical heavy and light chains that induce vigorous signal transduction reactions when cross-linked on the cell surface (reviewed in 28).[15] Since the membrane forms of immunoglobulin have as few as three amino acid residues in their putative cytoplasmic domains (reviewed in 149), the interaction of cytoplasmic signaling components with membrane immunoglobulin was unclear. The membrane form of IgM (μ_m) is critical for B-lymphocyte development[89] and is responsible for a number of important regulatory functions of the B lymphocyte. These functions include interactions with accessory molecules Ig-α and Ig-β, which are responsible for signal transduction mechanisms during B-cell activation (reviewed in 28, 41, 133, 146, 147) and with surrogate light chain molecules during B-cell development that are important in the mechanisms regulating B-cell differentiation and allelic exclusion (reviewed in 116).

ACCESSORY MOLECULES Ig-α AND Ig-β

The chemical nature and location of polar residues within the transmembrane domains of all isotypes supported the view that this region of the molecule may, like the T-cell receptor, interact with other proteins (reviewed in 146). Accessory molecules that associate with membrane immunoglobulin on the surface of mature B lymphocytes were identified by transfection and expression studies. Reth and colleagues demonstrated that a μ_m expression vector that was transfected into a light chain secreting mouse myeloma cell line failed to yield membrane IgM on the cell surface.[68] A variant cell line was isolated that expressed membrane IgM. Immunoprecipitation of membrane IgM revealed that coprecipitating proteins were present in the variant cells but not the parental cells.[66]

The proteins, designated Ig-α and Ig-β, are expressed as a disulfide-linked heterodimer (see Fig. 2–1).[29, 69] The Ig-α protein is encoded by the *mb-1* gene,[84, 154] and the Ig-β protein is encoded by the *B29* gene.[62, 63] The Ig-α and Ig-β proteins are transmembrane polypeptides that contain extracellular immunoglobulin-like domains, transmembrane domains, and cytoplasmic domains in which Ig-α has 61 amino acids and Ig-β has 48 amino acids, including tyrosine residues in both domains (reviewed in 146). The cytoplasmic domains contain conserved sequences that are important in the signal transduction machinery of the cell. These are referred to as tyrosine-based activation motif (TAM),[159] antigen receptor homology 1 (ARH1) motif,[27, 28] or, by consensus designation, immunoglobulin tyrosine-based activation motif (ITAM).[86a] These conserved sequences are also present in accessory molecules associated with the T-cell receptor and various Fc receptors.[145]

By mutagenesis experiments, the transmembrane domain of membrane immunoglobulin (Fig. 2–3) was shown to be essential for association with Ig-α and Ig-β accessory proteins (see Fig. 2–1) and for transport of this complex from the endoplasmic reticulum to the cell surface.[200] The association of the μ_m transmembrane domain with the α-β heterodimer is thought to be mediated via the Ig-α transmembrane domain, which has polar residues on both sides of the transmembrane α-helix; the Ig-β transmembrane domain contains polar residues on only one side (reviewed in 146). This analysis suggested that the Ig-α molecule may lie between the μ_m heavy chain and the Ig-β molecule. The trans-

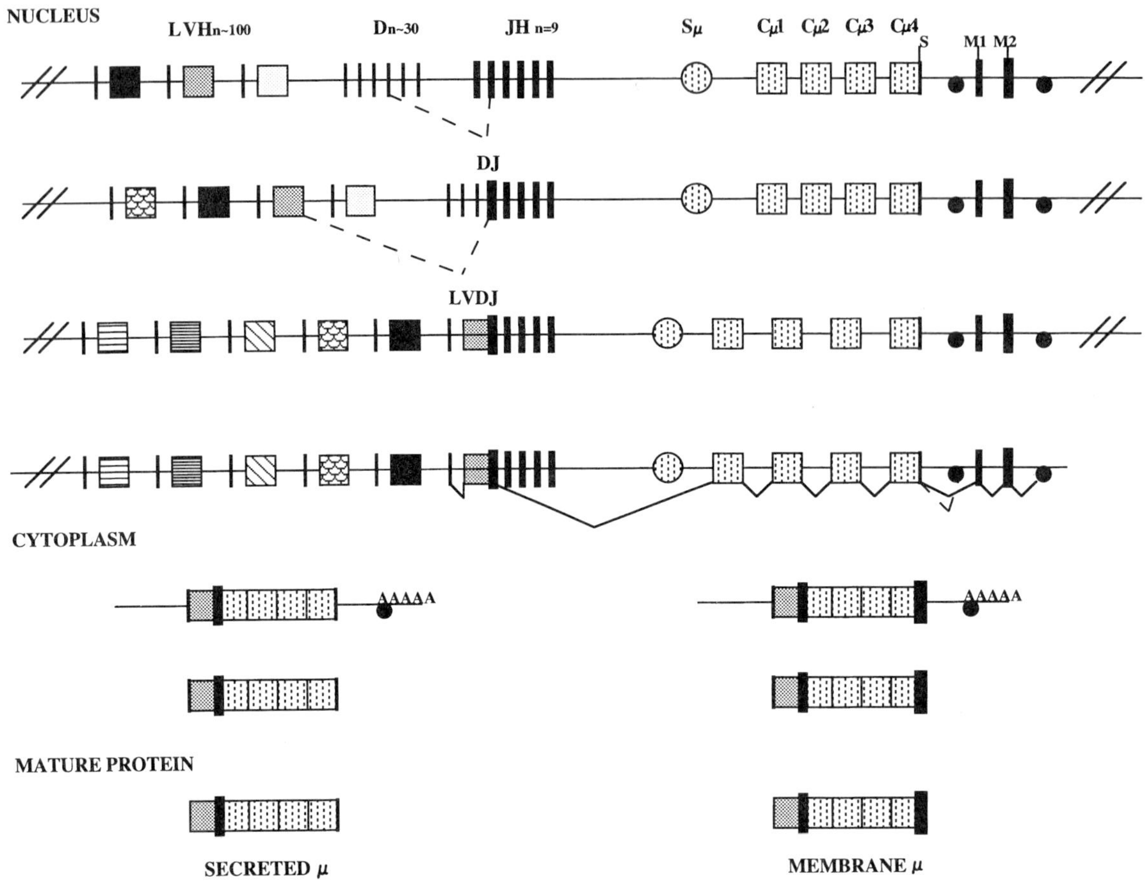

FIGURE 2–3. Immunoglobulin gene rearrangement producing membrane and secreted μ heavy chains. Schematic of the human heavy chain locus showing $V_{n\geq100}$ (including leader (L) sequence), $D_{n\geq30}$, and $J_{n=9}$ (six functional genes, three pseudogenes) gene elements upstream of constant region exons for C_μ and the C_μ switch site region (S_μ) (distances between genes and locations of gene clusters are not drawn to scale). Downstream of the constant region exons are exons M1 and M2 encoding transmembrane and cytoplasmic regions of μ_m. The $C_\mu4$ exon contains an extra piece of DNA (S) that encodes the carboxy-terminal end of the secreted heavy chain. Polyadenylation sites for secreted or membrane immunoglobulin genes are represented by dots. During B-cell development, the first gene rearrangement to occur is DJ followed by VDJ to form the complete variable region gene. Transcription of nuclear RNA is followed by splicing to form mature mRNA. The heavy chain polypeptide is translated and the leader peptide is cleaved upon expression of the mature protein (with light chain, not shown) on the cell surface or as a secreted molecule.

membrane domains of these proteins are crucial for their intracellular association and expression, but the interaction of the extracellular domains of μ_m and the accessory proteins have also been shown to be important for their expression and function.[67] Since membrane immunoglobulin is usually expressed as a complex containing two identical heavy chains, two Ig-α/Ig-β heterodimers have been proposed to associate with one immunoglobulin molecule.[67] Excellent reviews describe signal transduction pathways activated by the multichain B-lymphocyte antigen receptor complex (reviewed in 27, 28, 41, 133).

SURROGATE LIGHT CHAIN

During B-lymphocyte development, heavy chain synthesis occurs first, followed by light chain synthesis (reviewed in 34).[150] One of the defining features of a pre-B cell is the presence of cytoplasmic μ heavy chain without light chain. Once light chains are synthesized, membrane immunoglobulin can be expressed on the cell surface. A mature B lymphocyte is defined by the presence of membrane immunoglobulin, which differentiates the antigen-dependent stage from the antigen-independent stages of B-cell development (reviewed in 87). The sequential expression of immunoglobulin heavy and light chains can be explained at the level of the genes, which also undergo a sequential order of rearrangement and expression.

During the antigen-independent stage of B-lymphocyte development, the heavy chain variable region gene segments rearrange first, followed by light chain gene rearrangement (reviewed in 2). The rearranged heavy chain variable region gene is transcribed with the downstream (sequences that proceed in the direction of transcriptional expression) constant region gene, spliced, and expressed as heavy chain protein, which in a primary immune response is the membrane form of IgM. The generation of μ_m heavy chain is an important regulatory component of allelic exclusion (reviewed in 2),[91, 125, 148] which limits a single B cell to the functional assembly and expression of single heavy chain and single light chain alleles. The synthesis of μ_m is involved in signaling mechanisms that inhibit further heavy chain variable region gene rearrangement and initiate light chain gene rearrangement. The mechanism is unknown, but μ_m protein associates with other immunoglobulin-like light chains called surrogate light chains,[86, 132, 194] which may be expressed on the cell surface and interact with unknown ligands in the stroma.

The surrogate light chain proteins in the mouse are encoded by λ_5 and V_{preB} genes[96, 97, 155] and human homologs have been cloned.[161] The protein products of the λ_5 and V_{preB} genes have single immunoglobulin-like domains. The λ_5 gene encodes a protein of M_r 18,000 that is designated omega (ω).[132] This gene was designated λ_5 based on sequence homology to the J and C region genes of the λ locus. Since four functional constant region genes, which arose presumably from gene duplication events, had already been identified in the mouse λ locus, this gene became known as λ_5.[97, 155] Another gene located close to the λ_5 gene had sequence homology to V_κ and V_λ genes.[96] Both genes are expressed in pre-B cells, and the newly identified gene became known as V_{preB}.[96] The V_{preB} gene encodes a protein of M_r 14,000 that is designated iota (ι).[132]

The sequence similarity of these gene products to immunoglobulin light chains led to the hypothesis that they may bind to the μ_m polypeptide chain similar to light chains (reviewed in 116). In transfection studies using transformed cell lines, surface μ_m expression only occurs with cotransfection of λ_5 and V_{preB} genes.[188] The λ_5- and V_{preB}-encoded proteins form a noncovalent association, and this complex associates covalently with surface μ_m polypeptide chains.[81, 188] The μ_m surrogate light chain complex is capable of functioning as a receptor on the surface of transformed pre-B cell lines as shown by cross-linking experiments in which signal transduction events were induced, resulting in an increase in intracellular calcium and tyrosine phosphorylation of intracellular proteins.[120, 189]

The importance of the λ_5 gene in B-lymphocyte development was demonstrated initially by targeted disruption of this gene in transgenic mice.[90] The analysis of B-lymphocyte compartments in these mice demonstrated a significant decrease in the number and rate of production of B lymphocytes, but small numbers of mature B lymphocytes accumulated in peripheral lymphoid organs. These data suggested that λ_5-encoded protein may play a role in B-cell development, but absence of this protein did not completely eliminate B-cell development. A direct test of the requirement for membrane immunoglobulin and surrogate light chain in B-lymphocyte differentiation was performed using transgenic mice deficient in the recombinase activating gene-2 (RAG-2),[173] which is essential for immunoglobulin variable region gene rearrangement.[126] The RAG-2–deficient mouse (RAG-$2^{-/-}$) is a homozygous nonleaky mutation that inactivates the RAG-2 gene, resulting in mice that cannot initiate heavy or light chain variable region gene rearrangement.[173] The development of B and T cells is blocked at an early precursor stage. The beauty of these mice is that only B- and T-lymphocyte development is affected and other cellular components of the immune system are normal.[173]

Functional and rearranged heavy or light chain transgenes were introduced into the RAG-$2^{-/-}$ background.[83, 206] Introduction of the heavy chain transgene resulted in development of a mature monoclonal population of peripheral B lymphocytes, suggesting that T lymphocytes and a repertoire of B lymphocytes were not required for normal B-cell development.[206] Expression of light chain transgenes in these mice had no effect on B-cell development. Mice expressing heavy chain transgenes were analyzed for expression of surrogate light chain and heavy chain complexes on the cell surface of precursor B lymphocytes. The results were different from those observed using transformed pre-B cell lines.[66] Surrogate light chain and membrane immunoglobulin complexes were undetectable on the cell surface but detectable in the cytoplasm of cells, suggesting potential intracellular function.[83, 206] Interestingly, bone marrow cells of RAG-$2^{-/-}$ mice without heavy chain transgenes and normal mice expressed cell surface surrogate light chain, suggesting that expression of this protein may occur early in development prior to heavy chain expression.[83, 206] The early expression of this protein in association with proteins of molecular weights distinct from immunoglobulin heavy chain has been identified,[82] suggesting that cell surface expression of surrogate light chain may occur early in B-lymphocyte development and be down-regulated with the expression of immunoglobulin heavy chain. Transient or low-level cell surface expression of surrogate light chain and heavy chain complexes may occur, but at concentrations below current levels of detection.[206]

An intriguing finding in mice expressing heavy chain transgenes was the generation of B cells with decreased steady-state levels of λ_5 transcripts and increased levels of germline κ light chain transcripts.[206] The expression of germline light chain gene transcripts following expression of heavy chain protein correlates with the accessibility model of immunoglobulin gene rearrangement.[164] This model postulates that germline immunoglobulin genes become transcriptionally active and accessible to the recombinase enzymatic machinery, resulting in gene rearrangement forming functional variable region genes. The precise function of surrogate light chain complexes, the expression pattern of these complexes, and the nature of the possible ligand(s) that these complexes may interact with in the bone marrow stroma or within the cell are areas of ongoing research.

SOLUBLE IMMUNOGLOBULINS

Soluble immunoglobulins are secreted from plasma cells and remove pathogenic organisms by effector mechanisms such as complement lysis, antibody-dependent cell-mediated cytotoxicity (ADCC), and phagocytosis. The heavy and light chain variable region domains of all isotypes form the antibody combining site, and the heavy chain constant region domains provide the sites for activation of effector pathways. Depending on the isotype, heavy chain constant regions consist of either three or four domains.

The C_H1 domain of all isotypes interacts with the constant region domain of κ or λ light chains (C_L). No known effector functions have been associated with C_L. The Fc region of IgA, IgD, and IgG immunoglobulins consists of C_H2 and C_H3 domains, and Fc regions of IgE and IgM include C_H3 and C_H4 domains. The hinge region domain provides segmental flexibility to immunoglobulin molecules and connects the Fab arms to the Fc region in the IgA, IgD, and IgG isotypes. The hinge region in IgE and IgM isotypes is substituted by an additional heavy chain constant region domain designated $C_\epsilon 2$ and $C_\mu 2$, respectively. This substitution results in rigidity and diminished flexibility of the Fab arms. The hinge region provides the greatest sequence variation between the four subclasses of human IgG.[36, 179] IgG_1, IgG_2, and IgG_4 have hinge regions of 12–15 amino acids that are encoded by one exon, whereas IgG_3 has an extended hinge region of 62 amino acids that is encoded by four exons separated by short introns.

The hinge region can be divided into segments designated upper hinge, core, and lower hinge (reviewed in 56).[26] The upper hinge extends from the end of the C_H1 domain to the first cysteine, forming an interchain disulfide bond, and this part of the hinge correlates with segmental flexibility of the Fab arms.[36] The core contains the inter–heavy chain disulfide bridges and a high proline content. The lower hinge is the bridge to the C_H2 domain and includes the bridging residues within the C_H2 domain. Structurally, hinge regions are extended segments of peptides held together by disulfide bonds. The amino acid composition of this region provides the flexibility[36, 166] and mobility[195] of the Fab arms of the immunoglobulin molecule.

The IgG, IgD, IgA, and IgE isotypes are secreted in the blood as monomers, and IgM can be secreted in pentameric or hexameric forms.[110, 143] In glandular or mucosal secretions, IgA is present as a dimeric molecule. The polymeric molecules, except the hexameric form of IgM, are covalently linked with a single J-chain accessory molecule (reviewed in 95). A covalent bond is formed between the 20-kDa J-chain glycoprotein and a cysteine residue within the carboxy-terminal tail piece of $C\mu$ or $C\alpha$. The J chain is associated with dimeric IgA and pentameric IgM (reviewed in 95), but not with hexameric IgM.[142] The expression of J chain results in the production and secretion of predominantly pentameric IgM, whereas the absence of J chain results in the production and secretion of predominantly hexameric IgM.[142] The expression of J chain is transcriptionally regulated independent of immunoglobulin synthesis.[110, 143] Hexameric IgM is more effective in inducing complement-mediated lysis than is pentameric IgM,[143] thus the presence or absence of J chain appears to regulate the structural and functional properties of IgM.

In addition to J chain, another molecule designated secretory piece or secretory component is covalently bound to the Fc portion of secretory IgA or IgM (reviewed in 121, 183). Secretory component is the extracellular portion of the transmembrane polymeric immunoglobulin receptor (pIgR) that is located on the basolateral surface of epithelium (reviewed in 121). This receptor is part of the immunoglobulin supergene family (reviewed in 73, 199).[122] Dimeric IgA interacts with the amino-terminal domain of pIgR, and a disulfide bond forms between the hingelike domain of IgA and the receptor. This complex enters the cell via coated pits, where the carboxy-terminal domains of pIgR are proteolytically cleaved. The complex is cotransported to the apical surface of the cell and expressed as secretory IgA. In addition to secretory IgA, the J chain containing pentamer of IgM can also be presented at mucosal surfaces and in breast milk via this mechanism. The function of the secretory component probably acts as a protective shield against the proteolytic components that are present within the environment of the mucosal surfaces.

The expression of IgD in the periphery is low but expression of membrane IgD is high on the surface of mature B cells where it is coexpressed with IgM.[194a] This is a stage in B-cell development where dual isotype expression occurs and the IgD and IgM molecules express identical antigen specificities. The exact function of IgD at this stage of B-cell development is not known, but a direct role of membrane IgD in B-cell development was assessed with IgD-deficient mice generated by gene targeting.[124a, 148a] These mice developed normal antibody responses with a slight delay in affinity maturation of serum antibodies, suggesting that the antigen binding avidity of IgD may be important in the recruitment of B cells early in the immune response. The association of membrane IgD with Ig-α and Ig-β accessory molecules[198] supports a role as a B-lymphocyte receptor. The IgE isotype of immunoglobulin is a powerful mediator of allergic responses and anaphylactic reactions that can be beneficial to the host in the clearance of parasites (reviewed in 74). This molecule is described in detail in Chapter 7.

EFFECTOR MECHANISMS

The ability to activate the classic complement cascade is an important effector function of the IgM and IgG isotypes. IgG is the predominant form of serum antibody, whereas IgM is expressed in primary immune responses. The four human IgG isotypes differ markedly in their ability to activate complement. IgG_1 and IgG_3 can effectively activate the complement cascade, IgG_2 is a poor activator, and IgG_4 is completely deficient in the ability to activate complement.[23, 36] These four isotypes have very similar amino acid sequences, and the most variation occurs in the hinge region.[36, 179] The hinge region is essential for complement binding[192, 179] but does not determine the isotype-specific differences.[179]

The C_H2 domain has been suggested to be important for complement activation,[192, 205] and glycosylation of this domain has been shown to be essential.[103, 181] Three residues in this domain were shown by in vitro mutagenesis to be important for complement activation,[44] but the conservation of these residues in all four isotypes did not explain the isotype differences. By producing intradomain switch antibodies, the carboxy-terminal residues in the C_H2 domain determine the isotype-specific differences.[180] In this region, only four residues differ between IgG_1 and IgG_4, and two of the four residues are located on a β-strand in three-dimensional proximity to the three conserved residues previously identified.[180] The combination of the conserved and variant residues may form the complement binding site on IgG, and the hinge may modulate the ability of the antibody molecule to activate complement.[180] The binding site for complement on IgM has been localized to the $C\mu3$ domain, where glycosylation plays an important role.[202]

Phagocytosis and ADCC are effector functions mediated through the interaction of immunoglobulin with Fc receptors (FcR) on cells of hematopoietic origin. Isoforms of IgG binding receptors include FcγRI (CD64), which has a high binding affinity for monomeric IgG, and FcγRII (CD32) and FcγRIII (CD16), which interact with complexed IgG (reviewed in 104a, 117, 191). Three FcγRI genes designated A, B, and C encode secreted and membrane-bound forms of the receptor that are expressed on monocytes and macrophages (reviewed in 104a). At least three genes, also designated A, B, and C, encode FcγRII, which is expressed on a wide variety of cells, including monocytes, neutrophils, platelets, B cells, basophils, eosinophils, and trophoblasts (reviewed in 104a). Two genes (A and B) encode FcγRIII, and FcγRIIIA is expressed on natural killer cells and macrophages, and

FcγRIIIB is expressed on neutrophils (reviewed in 104a). The FcγRs are part of the immunoglobulin supergene family (reviewed in 72, 199). Except for FcγRIIIB, which is anchored to the neutrophil cell membrane by a glycan phosphatidylinositol moiety, the FcγRs are transmembrane proteins that transduce signaling events upon cross-linking with antigen or immune complexes (reviewed in 104a).

The hierarchy of binding of human IgG subclasses to FcγRI is IgG_1 and IgG_3 > IgG_4 >> IgG_2, which does not bind at all.[7] Sites on IgG_1 and IgG_3 that associate with human FcγRI have been mapped to noncontiguous residues that are present in the lower hinge region (amino-terminal end of the C_H2 domain) and the carboxy-terminal end of the C_H2 domain.[30] Using chimeric molecules and site-directed mutagenesis, two leucine residues in the lower hinge region and a proline residue in the C_H2 domain were shown to be critical for high-affinity binding. In the tertiary structure of the C_H2 domain, the proline residue was shown to be positioned in proximity to the lower hinge region, demonstrating that these two regions may contribute to the human high-affinity FcR binding site on IgG_1 and IgG_3. These leucine residues are not present in the C_H2 domain of IgG_2, which does not bind the receptor, and substitution of this domain with the C_H2 domain of IgG_3 resulted in a gain of binding affinity for the receptor. In IgG_3, the deletion of the hinge region abrogates FcγRI binding, suggesting that segmental flexibility of the hinge region may contribute to optimal binding affinity.

IMMUNOGLOBULIN GENE REPERTOIRE

Early investigators realized that determination of a mechanism to account for the unprecedented diversity in the immunoglobulin variable region domains and the homogeneity of the constant region domains required an analysis of immunoglobulin genes. The use of myeloma and plasmacytoma cell lines provided the source of DNA for the initial characterization of immunoglobulin gene structure and the identification of immunoglobulin gene rearrangement (reviewed in 184). A number of gene theories were proposed to explain the variability within the antibody combining site. Two of these theories were the somatic mutation[21] and germline[43] models of diversity.

The somatic mutation model proposed that a small number of genes were present in the genome and that a mutational mechanism created the diversity in the variable region sequences. The germline model proposed that all of the information to create the complete repertoire of immunoglobulin variable region genes was present in the genome. Neither of these models proved to be completely correct, but components of each model apply to the genetic mechanisms that create antibody diversity. A large number of gene segments are involved in the formation of complete variable region genes. A somatic hypermutation mechanism is active on rearranged variable region genes, resulting in amino acid substitutions that can affect the binding site of the antibody molecule (reviewed in 184).

In addition to the attention that was directed toward determining the genetic mechanisms responsible for generating the variability within the antibody combining sites, another question addressed at the time was how the constant region domains of the immunoglobulin molecule escaped the diversification process. One proposed model was that there were complete sets of variable and constant region genes in the germline genome, providing the information that was necessary for creating the entire repertoire of immunoglobulin molecules. This model was refuted by "gene counting" experiments that measured the kinetics of hybridization annealing of cDNA probes to genomic DNA.[187]

In 1965, the "two genes one polypeptide" hypothesis of Dreyer and Bennett revolutionized the dogma at the time in which all cells were thought to contain identical DNA.[43] Dreyer and Bennett proposed that a single immunoglobulin constant region gene was encoded in the germline genome separately from the variable region genes. During the development of an antibody-producing cell, these genes rearrange to encode an immunoglobulin polypeptide chain. Through the development of technical advances in molecular biology, including the Southern blot technique,[175] the unprecedented notion of separate genetic elements in the germline genome undergoing DNA rearrangement to form complete immunoglobulin genes was proven correct (reviewed in 184). These studies paved the way for the explosion of information that has elucidated the genetic mechanisms of antibody production and diversity.

VARIABLE AND CONSTANT REGION GENES

The molecular basis of antibody diversity involves a somatic assembly process of germline segments to form complete heavy and light chain variable region genes (reviewed in 2, 184). Extensive gene cloning and comparative sequence analyses of rearranged and germline immunoglobulin genes provided the database from which immunoglobulin gene structure and rearrangement were determined.[19, 20, 40, 45, 47, 113, 114, 156–158, 163, 168, 185, 186] In mammals, the heavy and two light polypeptide chains are encoded by families of genes that are located on different chromosomes. Human and mouse immunoglobulin genes are located on chromosomes 14 (human) and 12 (mouse) for the heavy chain genes, chromosomes 22 (human) and 6 (mouse) for the κ light chain genes, and chromosomes 2 (human) and 16 (mouse) for the λ light chain genes. The complete heavy chain variable region gene is generated from three distinct gene segments designated V_H (heavy chain variable region gene segment), D (diversity gene segment), and J_H (heavy chain joining gene segment) (see Figure 2–2). The complete κ or λ light chain variable region genes are generated from two distinct gene segments designated $V_{\kappa/\lambda}$ (light chain variable region gene segments) and $J_{\kappa/\lambda}$ (light chain joining gene segments) (see Figure 2–2).

Approximately 100 functional and unique V-gene segments and four to six J-gene segments are present within each of the heavy and light chain loci (reviewed in 33a, 111, 144, 170, 207). Approximately 30 D-gene segments (12, 24, 33a, 99, 109) have been identified in the heavy chain locus between the V_H- and J_H-gene segments. The V_H- and $V_{\kappa/\lambda}$-gene segments encode the CDR1, CDR2, and first three framework regions of the heavy and light chain variable region domains, respectively (see Figure 2–2). The J_H-gene segments encode FR4 of the heavy chain variable region domain, and $J_{\kappa/\lambda}$-gene segments encode CDR3 and FR4 portions of the light chain variable region domain (see Figure 2–2). The heavy chain D-gene segments encode the central portion of CDR3 (see Figure 2–2). Due to the numerous D-gene segments and the diversity generated from joining D-gene segments to V- and J-gene segments, this region of the heavy chain variable region domain confers increased sequence variability in the antigen binding site of the immunoglobulin molecule.

The heavy and light chain immunoglobulin gene segments that rearrange to form complete heavy and light chain variable region genes were identified by cloning germline genes (reviewed in 2, 184). The formation of a complete gene from multiple gene segments was unknown at the time, and the assumption was made that a germline variable region gene sequence would be the same as a rearranged variable region gene sequence from an antibody-producing cell line. This assumption was found to be incorrect because the nucleotide sequence of cloned germline variable region genes did not completely match the sequence of the rearranged variable region gene. This discrepancy led to the identification of the heavy and light chain J-gene segments[19, 156] and heavy chain D-gene segments.[45, 157, 158] Extensive cloning and sequence analyses led to an understanding of the organization of the heavy and light chain loci, which are similar with some exceptions within the λ light chain locus.

The heavy and light chain V-gene segments are located upstream (sequences in the opposite direction of transcriptional expression) of the respective J-gene segments (see Figure 2–3). The large number of V-gene segments have been divided into families that were initially derived at the protein level from amino acid homology and have since been confirmed and extended to germline V-gene segments based on nucleotide sequence homology (reviewed in 2, 184). Interestingly, the numerous gene segments that compose each of the variable region gene families in the mouse are located in clusters along the chromosome, whereas in humans the V-gene segments that compose each family are highly interspersed.[22, 93, 165, 196]

The heavy chain D-gene segments are located between the V_H- and J_H-gene segments (see Figure 2–3). The heavy chain constant region genes and the single κ light chain constant region gene are located after the heavy and light chain J-C intron (see Figure 2–3). Each of the heavy chain constant region genes are located sequentially along the chromosome. The constant region gene order in the mouse is μ, δ, γ3, γ1, γ2b, γ2a, ε,α (reviewed in 70) and in humans is μ, δ, γ3, γ1, ψε (pseudogene or nonfunctional gene), α1, ψγ, γ2, γ4, ε, α2.[57, 112] The λ light chain locus contains at least four functional constant region genes, each of which is preceded by unique J-gene segments. Analyses involving long-range mapping studies by pulsed-field electrophoresis have led to more complete determinations of gene structure and location.[17, 65, 118, 177]

A common organization of rearranged variable region gene structure was identified by comparing DNA sequences of light chain variable and constant region genes to known amino acid sequences (reviewed in 2, 184). A signal peptide is interrupted within codon -4 by a short intron of approximately 100 nucleotides. Following the intron, the remaining sequence of the signal peptide and the entire variable region gene sequence were comparable to known amino acid sequences. A large intron sequence separates variable region genes from constant region genes. The pattern of a short intron interrupting the signal peptide at codon -4 and a long intron between the variable and constant region exons, identified as the J-C intron, has been found in all rearranged heavy and light chain genes. The light chain constant region domains are encoded by single exons, whereas the heavy chain constant region domains and hinge are encoded by distinct exons (see Figure 2–3) that are separated by introns of approximately 100 to 300 base pairs. The rearranged variable region gene, including the exon encoding the leader sequence and the exons encoding the constant region domains, is transcribed, spliced, translated, and processed into mature protein (see Figure 2–3).

GENE REARRANGEMENT AND RECOMBINATION

The rearrangement of heavy chain V-gene segments occurs in a sequential and ordered manner in which D- and J_H-gene segments rearrange first, followed by V_H-gene rearrangement (reviewed in 2, 184). After transcription, intron sequences are spliced to generate mature heavy chain transcripts that are translated and processed into immunoglobulin heavy chain molecules (see Figure 2–3). The first constant region gene to be expressed in a primary immune response is the μ_m gene, resulting in the expression of the membrane form of IgM. After the μ_m heavy chain is produced, the immunoglobulin light chain variable region gene is assembled from V_L- and J_L-gene segments. This rearrangement process results in the transcription, splicing, and expression of κ or λ light chains that associate with μ_m to form the antigen receptor on the surface of mature B lymphocytes.

The expression of membrane IgM on the surface of B lymphocytes defines the antigen-dependent stage of B-cell development. Each B cell expresses a homogeneous set of receptors that are generated from the functional assembly and expression of single heavy chain and light chain alleles. The interaction of antigen with immunoglobulin receptors of the appropriate specificity and affinity is the basis of the clonal selection theory,[25] and clones of B cells activated by antigen determine the specificity of an immune response. Cross-linking of the antigen receptor results in the maturation and proliferation of B lymphocytes in which terminally differentiated plasma cells (reviewed in 34) and memory cells (reviewed in 115) are generated.

Plasma cells produce secreted immunoglobulin molecules that do not contain the carboxy-terminal sequences encoded by the membrane exons (reviewed in 4). A poly(A) addition site that is upstream of the membrane exons (see Figure 2–3) is utilized to generate the secreted molecules that also contain carboxy-terminal residues encoded by a piece of DNA contiguous to the last constant region domain (reviewed in 149).[3, 46] The mechanism that controls the balance between the membrane and secreted forms of immunoglobulin is not known, but competition between splicing of membrane exons to the carboxy-terminal constant region domain, cleavage/polyadenylation of the poly(A) addition site preceding the membrane exons, and formation of loop structures may be involved (reviewed in 111).

MECHANISM OF GENE REARRANGEMENT

Nucleotide sequence comparisons of the flanking regions between germline variable region gene segments were performed to identify clues about the mechanism of gene recombination (reviewed in 2, 184). These comparisons revealed two conserved sequence elements that are involved in the recombination event and determine the exact position where the two gene segments rearrange. These recognition sequences that mediate site-specific recombination have been found to flank all germline variable region gene segments (reviewed in 2, 4, 184). The recognition sequences consist of a highly conserved palindromic heptamer, 5′-CACAGTG-3′, a nonconserved spacer of 12 or 23 base pairs, and a conserved nanomer, 5′-ACAAAAACC-3′. The nonconserved spacer sequences were found to be very important in the recombination mechanism, and joining usually occurs only between gene segments that are flanked by heptamer and nanomer recognition sequences with unequal spacers. This requirement of unequal spacers for appropriate gene rearrangement is referred to as the 12/23 joining rule.

The recognition sequences dictate the gene elements that can join and probably prevent futile recombinations, such as between two variable region gene segments. These recognition sequences are the target of an unidentified common site-specific recombination system that has been designated the immunoglobulin recombinase (reviewed in 2, 184). At least two lymphoid-specific products encoded by genes designated RAG-1 and RAG-2[126, 160] are involved in the mechanism of gene rearrangement, but their direct or indirect involvement in the enzymatic machinery is not known (reviewed in 4). The recruitment of nonlymphoid-specific components may also be involved (reviewed in 4).

The earliest model for rearrangement of the variable region gene segments assumed that all gene segments were oriented in the same direction of transcription. When the gene segments underwent rearrangement and joining, the intervening DNA was thought to be excised and lost from the cell. This deletional mechanism of gene rearrangement was confirmed by Southern blot analysis.[169] Additional studies revealed an alternative mechanism that was identified as an inversional joining event.[1] In this mechanism, all recognition and coding gene sequences remain in the genome.[193] This type of recombination event is possible because gene segments have been identified, particularly in the κ light chain locus, that have a chromosomal orientation that is in the opposite direction of transcription (reviewed in 207). In in vitro expression systems using inversion and deletion recombination substrates (reviewed in 4), the enzymatic machinery that is responsible for immunoglobulin gene rearrangement rearranges germline gene elements by either inversion or deletion mechanisms.

A model for the mechanism of recombination by inversion or deletion proposed that the process was initiated by a precise double-strand break between the gene segments to be joined and their flanking recognition heptamers.[1] This event was followed by ligation of the two coding sequences and the two recognition sequences, resulting in either retention or deletion of recognition signal sequences in the genome. Inversional recombination results in the back-to-back ligation of heptamer recognition signal sequences, leading to inversion and retention of the intervening DNA in the chromosome (reviewed in 4).

To determine the exact sequences within the joining sites of two coding and two recognition sequences in the same piece of DNA, inversion or deletion recombination substrates were used in in vitro expression systems. In these studies, the precise ligation of noncoding heptamer signal sequences was confirmed, and heptamer fusion products were isolated as circles of DNA from the deletion recombination substrate.[59, 127] The precision observed in the joining region of two heptamer signal sequences is usually not observed in the joining region of two coding sequences, leading to the formation of amino acid residues not encoded in the germline sequence (reviewed in 2, 184). The flexibility in the joining sites of variable region gene segments contributes to increased sequence diversity within the antibody combining site of an immunoglobulin molecule.

MECHANISMS OF DIVERSITY

The creation of complete heavy and light chain variable region genes by the somatic assembly of germline gene segments contributes to the diversification of different antibody combining sites. In addition to the combining association of different heavy and light chains and the multiple distinct germline gene segments that undergo a combining assortment to form complete variable region genes, a number of other features of the somatic assembly process contribute to antibody diversity. The junctions of the coding sequences in the joining of variable region gene segments are sites of increased nucleotide sequence variability that contribute to the diversification of the antigen binding site of an immunoglobulin molecule. The junctional diversity that is created at these sites occurs by a number of different mechanisms, including the imprecise joining of the germline gene segments (reviewed in 2, 184),[100] the addition of novel bases or N regions (reviewed in 2, 184),[1] and the formation of palindrome sequences or P nucleotides that are generated following hairpin loop formation.[101]

The imprecision of joining within the coding regions of two variable region gene segments is manifested by the loss of bases from one or both coding partners that can result in an amino acid substitution or the formation of nonproductive alleles. The N regions are generated between two coding segments, and the enzyme terminal deoxynucleotide transferase (TdT) has been postulated as preferentially adding G/C nucleotides to the 3′ hydroxyl ends of the cut DNA between the heptamer and coding sequences.[102] The formation of P nucleotides occurs as a consequence of the joining reaction of coding sequences. After double-stranded DNA is cut, the coding ends ligate to form hairpin loop structures. Endonuclease activity asymmetrically opens the hairpin loop, resulting in a variable number of nucleotides added to the opposite strand of DNA. Exonuclease activity removes nucleotides, usually resulting in variability by one or two bases at the junction.[151, 152] The diversity that is generated at these sites provides the recombining flexibility required during immunoglobulin gene rearrangement to compensate for the nonproductive rearrangements that are inherent in the system yet provide the system with an immense potential repertoire.

In addition to the diversity that is generated during the somatic assembly process, a mechanism of somatic hypermutation is active on rearranged immunoglobulin genes following antigen stimulation (reviewed 2, 141, 184).[197] A general observation from analyses of antigen binding affinities of immunoglobulin molecules generated from memory cell responses is that the affinity of these molecules is higher than that of molecules generated from a primary immune response.[54] The affinity maturation of the immune response is achieved by somatic hypermutation (reviewed in 58, 184). The mechanism of somatic hypermutation is currently unknown, but the result of this mechanism is that nucleotide substitutions are generated in and around the rearranged variable region gene in an untemplated fashion (reviewed in 11, 14).

Somatic hypermutation occurs in the microenvironment of germinal centers (reviewed in 85, 108) during B-cell development when surface immunoglobulin is expressed. The mutations do not extend upstream beyond the promoter or downstream into the constant region exons, and the mutation rate has been calculated to be approximately 0.4×10^{-3} per base pair per generation. Mutations can be scattered throughout the rearranged variable region gene, but the process may not be random in that intrinsic hot spots can be found. Transgenic mice have provided important information on cis (sites on the same molecule of DNA)-acting factors influencing the somatic hypermutation mechanism. The immunoglobulin enhancer elements located within the J-C intron and 3′ of the last constant region genes are important regulators of the mechanism of somatic hypermutation.[13, 205a] The identification and regulation of this mutational mechanism within the immunoglobulin and potentially T-cell receptor loci[209] remain active areas of ongoing research.

HEAVY CHAIN CLASS SWITCHING

In a primary immune response, the first heavy chain isotype of immunoglobulin molecules expressed by B lymphocytes is IgM. In these cells, productively rearranged heavy chain variable region genes are expressed with C_μ. During the course of an immune response, the isotypes of immunoglobulin molecules produced among progeny B lymphocytes frequently switch from IgM to another heavy chain class or subclass. The expression of immunoglobulin molecules with identical heavy chain variable region genes and different constant region genes generates a population of molecules that have identical antigen binding specificities and different isotypes that exert a variety of effector functions. The association of different heavy chain constant region domains with the same variable region domain is known as heavy chain class switching (Fig. 2–4) (reviewed in 70, 153).[172] The DNA rearrangement that results in the placement of downstream constant region genes proximal to functionally rearranged variable region genes is known as switch recombination (reviewed in 70, 153).[172]

The identification of heavy chain class switching and rearrangement of constant region genes came from genetic analyses of clones of constant region genes isolated from nonlymphoid and antibody-producing cell lines. By Southern blot analyses, DNA fragments isolated from myeloma cell lines that contained variable and constant region genes expressing different immunoglobulin isotypes were compared with germline variable and constant region gene fragments (reviewed in 70, 153).[172] Additional sequences were found in the DNA isolated from the myeloma cell line that could not be identified in the corresponding germline DNA fragments (reviewed in 70, 153).[40] The sequences corresponded to upstream flanking regions of germline C_μ gene, suggesting that μ-derived DNA segments remained in the genome following gene rearrangement to downstream constant region genes. These observations led to a model suggesting that immunoglobulin heavy chain class switching involved the replacement of C_μ with a downstream constant region gene, resulting in the expression of a new isotype.[172] Another switch recombination event can then take place in which the expressed gene is replaced by another downstream constant region gene (see Fig. 2–4).

The process of somatic recombination of constant region genes is accomplished in most instances by a deletion/recombination mechanism (see Fig. 2–4) (reviewed in 70, 153).[172] Other mechanisms (reviewed in 153), however, including a trans (sites on different molecules of DNA)-RNA splicing mechanism,[131] have also been identified. The mechanism of constant region switch recombination is different than variable region gene rearrangement by several criteria (reviewed in 153). The recombination signal sequences that are utilized by variable region gene segments do not occur within the sites of heavy chain class switching. The constant region switch sites are located several kilobases 5′ of each constant region gene except C_δ and occur as clusters of tandemly repeated sequences called switch or S regions. In the mouse, the switch regions extend from 1 to 10 kilobases, and switch recombinations can occur at multiple locations within or outside of the S region. The expansive area within and outside of the S region in which switch recombination can occur is very different from the site-specific recombination of variable region gene rearrangement. Consensus sequences at sites of switch recombination have not been found, but common sequences in the area of different heavy chain switch recombination sites have been identified. An enzymatic machinery system that is involved in the mechanism of switch recombination has not been identified.

Switch recombination may occur as a targeted event as suggested in studies analyzing constant region gene structure on productive and nonproductive alleles of hybridoma cell lines expressing switched immunoglobulin isotypes. These studies demonstrated that a high frequency of switching to the same constant region gene occurred on both alleles (reviewed in 153).[72, 140, 201] The analyses of heavy chain isotypes produced during particular immune responses have suggested that heavy chain class switching may be a directed event.[35, 74] Examples include the increased levels of IgE that are induced by parasitic infections and the increased levels of murine IgG_{2a} that are produced in response to viral infections. The directed switching to specific constant region genes may be controlled by lymphokines produced by subsets of T lymphocytes.[32]

A proposed model for directed heavy chain class switching suggests that lymphokines and/or other unknown factors may target recombinase enzymes to switch regions by modulating the accessibility of particular switch sites for

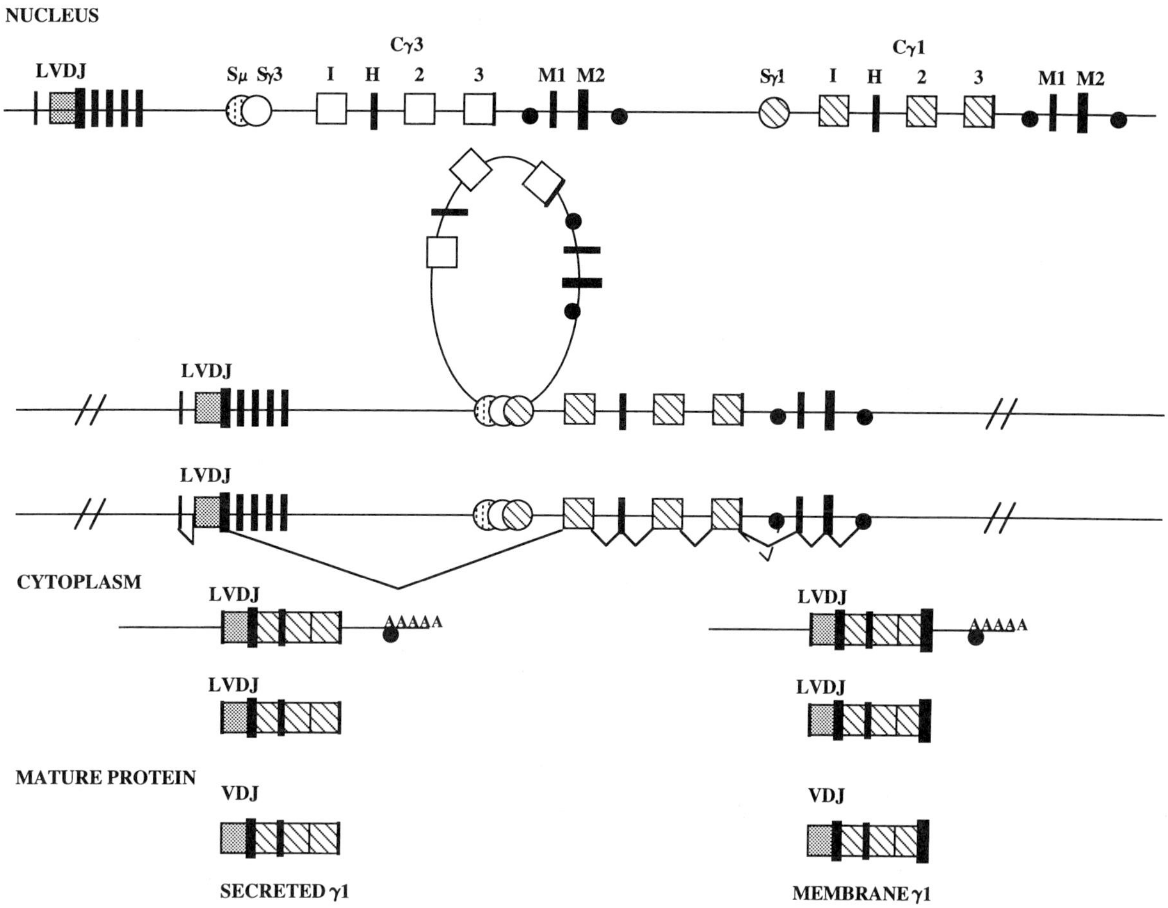

FIGURE 2–4. Heavy chain class switching by deletion recombination of immunoglobulin $C_{\gamma}3$ to $C_{\gamma}1$. Schematic showing a rearranged variable gene and the exons and switch regions for $C_{\gamma}3$ and $C_{\gamma}1$ constant region genes (distances between genes are not drawn to scale). The exons encoding each constant region domain, hinge, and membrane domain are designated I, H, 2, 3, M1, and M2. Upstream of the $C_{\gamma}3$ exons is depicted a switch site region showing partial sequence remaining from a μ switch site (S_{μ}) and a $C_{\gamma}3$ switch site ($S_{\gamma}3$). This can occur following a switch event from C_{μ} to $C_{\gamma}3$. Upstream of $C_{\gamma}1$ exons is depicted a switch site region for $C_{\gamma}1$ ($S_{\gamma}1$). Heavy chain class switching from $C_{\gamma}3$ to $C_{\gamma}1$ is shown as a deletional event in which the DNA between $S_{\gamma}3$ and $S_{\gamma}1$ switch sites is brought together, cut, and deleted, leaving partial sequences from the three switch sites. The transcription, splicing, translation, and processing of protein are the same as shown in Figure 2–3.

transcription.[176, 204] This model was proposed from observations that the isotype of immunoglobulin produced by some murine tumor cell lines switched from IgM to IgG_{2b} while the cells were grown in culture.[107] This switch event to a particular constant region gene was preceded by the appearance of germline constant region gene transcripts. A transcriptional promoter lies upstream of germline constant region genes, and analysis of cloned transcripts demonstrated common structural features.[104, 106] The constant region transcripts are processed such that an exon 5′ of the switch region, designated I exon (derived from intervening sequence) of about 100 to 500 base pairs,[106] is spliced to a constant region gene generating a switch transcript that is referred to as a germline or sterile transcript.[104, 106] This mature transcript is generated from primary transcripts that initiate at the promoter, run through the switch region, and terminate at normal sites downstream of the constant region gene (reviewed in 153). The mature transcript may be incapable of encoding protein because each I exon encodes multiple stop codons in all three reading frames.[106]

The integrity of the I exon was analyzed in transgenic mice by disruption of promoter and I exons for particular constant region genes.[76, 208] These mice were defective in switching to the targeted constant region gene, but switch events to other constant regions were normal, suggesting an important regulatory role for the production of germline transcripts. To distinguish between the potential roles of transcription alone and the formation of germline transcripts in regulating the class switch process, the promoter and I exon of the C_{ϵ} gene were replaced with an inducible enhancer and variable region gene promoter.[18] These mice expressed a low basal level of switching to IgE, but these low levels did not change upon induction of high levels of transcription through the S region. This study suggested that efficient switch recombination is not induced by transcription alone but may require other factors, including the I exon and/or promoter. Recent studies have suggested that the I exon donor splice site is necessary for the induction of normal switch recombination events.[105] These findings suggest that spliced germline transcripts or the process of splicing may play a functional role in the targeting mechanism of switch recombination to particular constant region genes. The mechanism of directed heavy chain class switching, the identification of cis- and trans-acting factors, and the enzymatic machinery responsible for the class switch event remain exciting areas of ongoing research.

SUMMARY

Immunoglobulins are bifunctional molecules that defend the host against an infinite number of pathogenic organisms in the environment. The insights gained in determining the structure of immunoglobulin molecules have endowed science with a growing immunoglobulin supergene family of related proteins that function in cell communication, development, and activation. Questions regarding the structural requirements of these proteins that result in exquisite specificity and recognition will provide further insight into protein function. The determination of the genetics responsible for creating the diverse repertoire of bifunctional immunoglobulin molecules has resulted in elucidation of unprecedented mechanisms that also function in generating the repertoire of T-cell receptors. These seminal discoveries have resulted in a basic understanding of antibody diversity leading to current studies investigating mechanisms unique to these genes. Included among the numerous discoveries to be made are the identification of mechanisms and regulatory controls of allelic exclusion, somatic hypermutation, and components involved in the enzymatic machinery and control of variable region gene rearrangement and heavy chain class switching.

REFERENCES

1. Alt FW, Baltimore D: Joining of immunoglobulin heavy chain gene segments: implications from a chromosome with evidence of three D-JH fusions. Proc Natl Acad Sci USA 79:4118, 1982.
2. Alt FW, Blackwell TK, Yancopoulos GD: Development of the primary antibody repertoire. Science 238:1079, 1987.
3. Alt FW, Bothwell ALM, Knapp M, et al: Synthesis of secreted and membrane-bound immunoglobulin μ heavy chains is directed by mRNAs that differ at their 3′ ends. Cell 20:293, 1980.
4. Alt FW, Oltz EM, Young F, et al: VDJ recombination. Immunol Today 13:306, 1992.
5. Amzel LM, Poljak RJ: Three-dimensional structure of immunoglobulins. Annu Rev Biochem 48:961, 1979.
6. Amzel LM, Poljak RJ, Saul F, et al: The three-dimensional structure of a combining region-ligand complex of immunoglobulin NEW at 3.5 Å resolution. Proc Natl Acad Sci USA 71:1427, 1974.
7. Anderson CL, Abraham GN: Characterization of the Fc receptor for IgG on a human macrophage cell line, U937. J Immunol 125:2735, 1980.
8. Anderson MLM, Szajnert MF, Kaplan JC, et al: The isolation of a human Ig V lambda gene from a recombinant library of chromosome 22 and estimation of its copy number. Nucleic Acids Res 12:6647, 1984.
9. Bence-Jones H: On a new substance occurring in the urine of a patient with "mollities ossium." Phil Tr Roy Soc Lond 138:55, 1848.
10. Bentley DB, Rabbitts TH: Human Vk immunoglobulin gene number: implications for the origin of antibody diversity. Cell 24:613, 1981.
11. Berek C, Ziegner M: The maturation of the immune response. Immunol Today 14:400, 1993.
12. Berman JE, Mellis SJ, Pollock R, et al: Content and organisation of the human Ig VH locus: definition of three new families and linkage to the Ig CH locus. EMBO J 7:727, 1988.
13. Betz AG, Milstein C, González-Fernández A, et al: Elements regulating somatic hypermutation of an immunoglobulin κ gene: critical role for the intron enhancer/matrix attachment region. Cell 77:239, 1994.
14. Betz AG, Neuberger MS, Milstein C: Discriminating intrinsic and antigen-selected mutational hotspots in immunoglobulin V genes. Immunol Today 14:405, 1993.
15. Bij terbosch MK, Meade CJ, Turner GA, et al: B lymphocyte receptors and polyphosphoinositide degradation. Cell 41:999, 1985.
16. Bona CA, Victor-Kobrin C, Manheimer AJ, et al: Regulatory arms of the immune network. Immunol Rev 79:25, 1984.
17. Bottaro A, de Marchi M, Migone N, et al: Pulsed-field gel analysis of human immunoglobulin heavy-chain constant region gene deletions reveals the extent of unmapped regions within the locus. Genomics 4:505, 1989.
18. Bottaro A, Lansford R, Xu L, et al: S region transcription per se promotes basal IgE class switch recombination but additional factors regulate the efficiency of the process. EMBO J 13:665, 1994.
19. Brack C, Hirama M, Lenhard-Schuller, et al: A complete immunoglobulin gene is created by somatic recombination. Cell 15:1, 1978.
20. Brack C, Tonegawa S: Variable and constant parts of the immunoglobulin light chain gene of a mouse myeloma cell are 1250 nontranslated bases apart. Proc Natl Acad Sci USA 74:5652, 1977.
21. Brenner S, Milstein C: Origin of antibody diversity. Nature 211:242, 1966.
22. Brodeur PH, Osman GE, Mackle JJ, et al: The organization of the mouse Igh-V locus: dispersion, interspersion, and the evolution of VH gene family clusters. J Exp Med 168:2261, 1988.
23. Brüggenmann ME, Williams GT, Bindon MR, et al: Comparisons of the effector function of human immunoglobulins using a matched set of chimeric antibodies. J Exp Med 166:1351, 1987.
24. Buluwela L, Albertson D, Sherrington P, et al: The use of chromosomal translocations to study human immunoglobulin gene organisation: mapping DH segments with 35 kb of the Cμ gene and identification of a new DH locus. EMBO J 7:2003, 1988.
25. Burnet FM: The Clonal Selection Theory of Acquired Immunity. Vanderbilt University Press, Nashville, TN, 1959.
26. Burton DR: Immunoglobulin G: functional sites. Mol Immunol 22:161, 1985.
27. Cambier JC: Signal transduction by T- and B-cell antigen receptors: converging structures and concepts. Curr Opin Immunol 4:257, 1992.
28. Cambier JC, Pleiman CM, Clark MR: Signal transduction by the B cell antigen receptor and its coreceptors. Annu Rev Immunol 12:457, 1994.
29. Campbell KS, Cambier JC: B-lymphocyte antigen receptors (mIg) are non-covalently associated with a disulfide-linked, inducibly phosphorylated glycoprotein complex. EMBO J 9:441, 1990.
30. Canfield SM, Morrison SL: The binding affinity of human IgG for its high affinity Fc receptor is determined by multiple amino acids in the C_H2 domain and is modulated by the hinge region. J Exp Med 173:1483, 1991.
31. Chintalacharuvu KR, Raines M, Morrison SL: Divergence of human α-chain region gene sequences. J Immunol 152:5299, 1994.
32. Coffman R, Seymour B, Lebman D, et al: The role of helper T cell products in mouse B cell differentiation and isotype regulation. Immunol Rev 102:5, 1988.
33. Colman PM, Deisenhofer J, Huber R, et al: Structure of the human antibody molecule Kol (Immunoglobulin G1): an electron density map at 5Å resolution. J Mol Biol 100:257, 1976.

33a. Cook GP, Tomlinson IM: The human immunoglobulin V_H repertoire. Immunol Today 16:237, 1995.

34. Cooper MD, Burrows PD: B-cell differentiation. In Honjo T, Alt FW, Rabbitts TH (eds): Immunoglobulin Genes. Academic Press, New York, 1989.
35. Coutelier J-P, Van der Logt J, Heessen F, et al: IgG2a restriction of murine antibodies elicited by viral infections. J Exp Med 165:64, 1987.
36. Dangl JL, Wensel TG, Morrison SL, et al: Segmental flexibility and complement fixation of genetically engineered chimeric human, rabbit, and mouse antibodies. EMBO J 7:1989, 1988.
37. Davies DR, Metzger H: Structural basis of antibody function. Annu Rev Immunol 1:87, 1983.
38. Davies DR, Padlan EM, Segal DM: Three-dimensional structure of immunoglobulins. Annu Rev Biochem 44:639, 1975.
39. Davies DR, Sheriff S, Padlan EA: Antibody-antigen complexes. J Biol Chem 263:10541, 1988.
40. Davis MM, Calame K, Early P, et al: An immunoglobulin heavy-chain gene is formed by at least two recombinational events. Nature 283:733, 1980.
41. DeFranco AL: Structure and function of the B cell antigen receptor. Annu Rev Cell Biol 9:377, 1993.
42. Diesenhofer J, Colman PM, Epp O, et al: Crystallographic structural studies of a human Fc fragment. Hoppe-Zeylers Z Physiol Chem 357:1421, 1976.
43. Dreyer WJ, Bennett JC: The molecular basis of antibody formation. Proc Natl Acad Sci USA 54:864, 1965.
44. Duncan AR, Winter G: The binding site for C1q on IgG. Nature 332:738, 1988.

45. Early P, Huang H, Davis M, et al: An immunoglobulin heavy chain variable region gene is generated from three segments of DNA: V_H, D, J_H. Cell 19:981, 1980.
46. Early P, Rogers J, Davis M, et al: Two mRNAs can be produced from a single μ gene by alternative RNA processing pathways. Cell 20:313, 1980.
47. Early PW, Davis MM, Kaback DB, et al: Immunoglobulin heavy chain gene organization in mice: analysis of a myeloma genomic clone containing variable and α constant regions. Proc Natl Acad Sci USA 76:857, 1979.
48. Edelman GM: Dissociation of γ-globulin. J Am Chem Soc 81:3155, 1959.
49. Edelman GM, Benacerraf B: On structural and functional relationships between antibodies and proteins of the gamma-system. Proc Natl Acad Sci USA 48:1035, 1962.
50. Edelman GM, Cunningham BA, Gall EW, et al: The covalent structure of an entire γG immunoglobulin molecule. Biochemistry 63:78, 1969.
51. Edelman GM, Gally JA: The nature of Bence-Jones proteins. Chemical similarities to polypeptide chains of myeloma globulins and normal γ-globulins. J Exp Med 116:207, 1962.
52. Edelman GM, Poulik MD: Studies on structural units of the γ-globulins. J Exp Med 113:861, 1961.
53. Edmundson AB, Ely KR, Abola EE, et al: Rotational allomerism and divergent evolution of domains in immunoglobulin light chains. Biochemistry 14:3953, 1975.
54. Eisen HN, Siskind GW: Variations in affinities of antibodies during the immune response. Biochemistry 3:996, 1964.
55. Fahey JL: Heterogeneity of γ-globulins. Adv Immunol 2:41, 1962.
56. Feinstein A, Richardson N, Taussig MJ: Immunoglobulin flexibility in complement activation. Immunol Today 7:169, 1986.
57. Flanagan JG, Rabbitts TH: Arrangement of human immunoglobulin heavy chain constant region genes implies evolutionary duplication of a segment containing γ, ϵ and α genes. Nature 300:709, 1982.
58. French DL, Laskov R, Scharff MD: The role of somatic hypermutation in the generation of antibody diversity. Science 244:1152, 1989.
59. Fujimoto S, Yamagishi H: Isolation of an excision product of T-cell receptor α-chain gene rearrangements. Nature 327:242, 1987.
60. Givol D: The minimal antigen-binding fragment of antibodies-Fv fragment. Mol Immunol 28:1379, 1991.
61. Heidelberger M, Kendall FE: Quantitative studies on antibody purification. I. Dissociation of precipitates formed by pneymococcus specific polysaccharides and homologous antibodies. J Exp Med 64:161, 1936.
62. Hermanson GG, Briskin M, Sigman D, et al: Immunoglobulin enhancer and promoter motifs 5′ of the B29 B-cell-specific gene. Proc Natl Acad Sci USA 86:7341, 1989.
63. Hermanson GG, Eisenberg D, Kincade PW, et al: A member of the immunoglobulin super-family exclusively expressed on B-lineage cells. Proc Natl Acad Sci USA 85:6890, 1988.
64. Hilschmann N, Craig LC: Amino acid sequence studies with Bence-Jones proteins. Proc Natl Acad Sci USA 53:1403, 1965.
65. Hofker MH, Walter MA, Cox DW: Complete physical map of the human immunoglobulin heavy chain constant region gene complex. Proc Natl Acad Sci USA 86:5567, 1989.
66. Hombach J, Leclercq L, Radbruch A, et al: A novel 34 kD protein co-isolated with IgM molecule in surface IgM expressing cells. EMBO J 7:3451, 1988.
67. Hombach J, Lottspeich F, Reth M: Identification of the genes encoding the IgM-α and Igβ components of the IgM antigen receptor complex by amino-terminal sequencing. Eur J Immunol 20:2795, 1990.
68. Hombach J, Sablitzky F, Rajewsky K, et al: Transfected plasmacytoma cells do not transport the membrane form of IgM to the cell surface. J Exp Med 167:652, 1988.
69. Hombach J, Tsubata T, Leclercq L, et al: Molecular components of the B cell antigen receptor complex of the IgM class. Nature 343:760, 1990.
70. Honjo T, Shimizu A, Yaoita Y: Constant-region genes of the immunoglobulin heavy chain and the molecular mechanism of class switching. In Honjo T, Alt FW, Rabbitts TH (eds): Immunoglobulin Genes. Academic Press, New York, 1989.
71. Hood L, Gray WR, Sanders BG, Dreyer WJ: Light chain evolution. Cold Spring Harb Symp Quant Biol 32:133, 1967.
72. Hummel M, Berry J, Dunnick W: Switch region content of hybridomas: two spleen IgH loci tend to rearrange to the same isotype. J Immunol 138:3539, 1987.
73. Hunkapiller T, Hood L: Diversity of the immunoglobulin gene superfamily. Adv Immunol 44:1, 1989.
74. Jarrett E, Miller H: Production and activities of IgE in helminth infection. Prog Allergy 31:178, 1982.
75. Jerne NK: The generative grammar of the immune system. Scand J Immunol 38:1, 1993.
76. Jung S, Rajewsky K, Radbruch A: Shutdown of class switch recombination by deletion of a switch region control element. Science 259:984, 1993.
77. Kabat EA: The molecular weight of antibodies. J Exp Med 69:103, 1939.
78. Kabat EA: The structural basis of antibody complementarity. Adv Protein Chem 32:1, 1978.
79. Kabat EA: Antibody diversity versus antibody complementarity. Pharmacol Rev 34:23, 1982.
80. Kabat EA, Wu TT: Attempts to locate complementarity-determining residues in the variable positions of light and heavy chains of immunoglobulins. Ann NY Acad Sci 190:382, 1971.
81. Karasuyama H, Kudo A, Melchers F: The proteins encoded by the V_{preB} and $\lambda 5$ pre-B cell-specific genes can associate with each other and with heavy chains. J Exp Med 172:969, 1990.
82. Karasuyama H, Rolink A, Melchers F: A complex of glycoproteins is associated with $V_{preB}/\lambda 5$ surrogate light chain on the surface of μ heavy chain-negative early precursor B cell lines. J Exp Med 178:469, 1993.
83. Karasuyama H, Rolink A, Shinkai Y, et al: The expression of $V_{preB}/\lambda 5$ surrogate light chain in early bone marrow precursor B cells of normal and B cell-deficient mutant mice. Cell 77:133, 1994.
84. Kashiwamura S-I, Koyama T, Matsuo T, et al: Structure of the murine mb-1 gene encoding a putative sIgM-associated molecule. J Immunol 145:337, 1990.
85. Kepler TB, Perelson AS: Cyclic re-entry of germinal center B cells and the efficiency of affinity maturation. Immunol Today 14:412, 1993.
86. Kerr WG, Cooper MD, Feng L, et al: Mu heavy chains can associate with a pseudo-light complex (ψL) in human pre-B cell lines. Int Immunol 1:354, 1989.
86a. Kim K-M, Reth M: Function of B-cell antigen receptor of different classes. Immunol Letters 44:81, 1995.
87. Kincade PW: Experimental models for understanding B lymphocyte formation. Adv Immunol 41:1987.
88. Kindt T: Rabbit immunoglobulin allotypes: structure, immunology, and genetics. Adv Immunol 21:35, 1975.
89. Kitamura D, Jürgen R, Kühn R, et al: A B cell-deficient mouse by targeted disruption of the membrane exon of the immunoglobulin μ chain gene. Nature 350:423, 1991.
90. Kitamura D, Kudo A, Schaal S, et al: A critical role of $\lambda 5$ in B cell development. Cell 69:823, 1992.
91. Kitamura D, Rajewsky K: Targeted disruption of μ chain causes loss of heavy chain allelic exclusion. Nature 356:154, 1992.
92. Klein M, Haeffner-Cavaillon N, Isenman DE, et al: Expression of biological effector functions by immunoglobulin G molecules lacking the hinge region. Proc Natl Acad Sci USA 78:524, 1981.
93. Kodaira M, Kinashi T, Umemura I, et al: Organization and evolution of variable region genes of the human immunoglobulin heavy chain. J Mol Biol 190:529, 1986.
94. Köhler G, Milstein C: Continuous cultures of fused cells secreting antibody of predefined specificity. Nature 256:495, 1975.
95. Koshland ME: The coming of age of the immunoglobulin J chain. Annu Rev Immunol 3:425, 1985.
96. Kudo A, Melchers F: A second gene, V_{pre}B in the $\lambda 5$ locus of the mouse, which appears to be selectively expressed in pre-B cells. EMBO J 6:2267, 1987.
97. Kudo A, Sakaguchi N, Melchers F: Organization of the murine Ig-related $\lambda 5$ gene transcribed selectively in pre-B lymphocytes. EMBO J 6:103, 1987 [erratum EMBO J 6:4242, 1987].
98. Kunkel HG, Mannik M, Williams RC Jr: Individual antigenic specificity of isolated antibodies. Science 140:1218, 1963.
99. Kurosawa Y, Tonegawa S: Organization, structure, and assembly of immunoglobulin heavy chain diversity DNA segments. J Exp Med 155:201, 1982.
100. Kurosawa Y, von Boehmer H, Haas W, et al: Identification of D segments of immunoglobulin heavy-chain genes and their rearrangement in T lymphocytes. Nature 290:565, 1981.
101. Lafaille JJ, DeCloux A, Bonneville M, et al: Junctional sequences of T cell receptor $\gamma\delta$ genes: implications for $\gamma\delta$ T cell lineages and for a novel intermediate of V-(D)-J joining. Cell 59:859, 1989.
102. Landau NR, Schatz DG, Rosa M, et al: Increased frequency of N-

region insertion in a murine pre-B-cell line infected with a terminal deoxynucleotidyl transferase retroviral expression vector. Mol Cell Biol 7:3237, 1987.

103. Leatherbarrow RJ, Rademacher TW, Dwek RA, et al: Effector functions of a monoclonal aglycosylated mouse IgG2a: binding and activation of complement component C1q and interaction with human monocyte Fc receptor. Mol Immunol 22:407, 1985.
104. Lennon GG, Perry RP: Cμ-containing transcripts initiate heterogeneously within the IgH enhancer region and contain a novel 5′-nontranslatable exon. Nature 318:475, 1985.
104a. Lin C-T, Shen Z, Boros P, et al: Fc receptor-mediated signal transduction. J Clin Immunol 14:1, 1994.
105. Lorenz M, Jung S, Radbruch A: Switch transcripts in immunoglobulin class swtiching. Science 267:1825, 1995.
106. Lutzker SG, Alt FW: Structure and expression of germline immunoglobulin γ2b transcripts. Mol Cell Biol 8:1849, 1988.
107. Lutzker SG, Rothman P, Pollock R, et al: Mitogen and IL-4-regulated expression of germline Ig γ2b transcripts: evidence for directed heavy chain class switching. Cell 53:177, 1988.
108. MacLennan ICM: Germinal centers. Annu Rev Immunol 12:117, 1994.
109. Matsuda F, Lee KL, Nakai A, et al: Dispersed localisation of D segments in the human immunoglobulin heavy-chain locus. EMBO J 7:1047, 1988.
110. Matsui K, Nakanishi K, Cohen DJ, et al: B cell response pathways regulated by IL5 and IL2. J Immunol 142:2918, 1989.
111. Max EE: Immunoglobulins molecular genetics. In Paul WE (ed): Fundamental Immunology, 3rd edition. Raven Press, New York, 1993.
112. Max EE, Battey J, Ney R, et al: Duplication and deletion in the human immunoglobulin ϵ genes. Cell 29:691, 1982.
113. Max EE, Maizel JV Jr, Leder P: The nucleotide sequence of a 5.5-kilobase DNA segment containing the mouse κ immunoglobulin J and C region genes. J Biol Chem 256:5116, 1981.
114. Max EE, Seidman JG, Leder P: Sequences of five recombination sites encoded close to an immunoglobulin κ constant region gene. Proc Natl Acad Sci USA 76:3450, 1979.
115. Melchers F: The many roles of immunoglobulin molecules in the development and growth control of the B-lymphocyte lineage. In Honjo T, Alt FW, Rabbitts TH (eds): Immunoglobulin Genes. Academic Press, New York, 1989.
116. Melchers F, Haasner D, Grawunder U, et al: Role of I_GH and L chains and of surrogate H and L chains in the development of cells of the B lymphocyte lineage. Annu Rev Immunol 12:209, 1994.
117. Mellman I: Relationships between structure and function in the Fc receptor family. Curr Opin Immunol 1:16, 1988.
118. Miller J, Ogden S, McMullen M, et al: The order and orientation of mouse λ-genes explain λ-rearrangement patterns. J Immunol 141:2497, 1988.
119. Milstein C: Linked groups of residues in immunoglobulin chains. Nature 216:330, 1967.
120. Misener V, Downey GP, Jongstra J: The immunoglobulin light chain related protein λ5 is expressed on the surface of mouse pre-B cell lines and can function as a signal transducing molecule. Int Immunol 3:1129, 1991.
121. Mostov KE: Transepithelial transport of immunoglobulins. Annu Rev Immunol 12:63, 1994.
122. Mostov KE, Freidlander M, Blobel G: The receptor for transepithelial transport of IgA and IgM contains multiple immunoglobulin-like domains. Nature 308:37, 1984.
123. Niall HD, Edman P: Two structurally distinct classes of κ-chains in human immunoglobulins. Nature 216:262, 1967.
124. Nisonoff A, Wissler FC, Lipman LN: Properties of the major component of a peptic digest of rabbit antibody. Science 132:1770, 1960.
124a. Nitschke L, Kosco MH, Köhler G, et al: Immunoglobulin D-deficient mice can mount normal immune responses to thymus-independent and -dependent antigens. Proc Natl Acad Sci USA 90:1887, 1993.
125. Nussenzweig MC, Shaw AC, Sinn E, et al: Allelic exclusion in transgenic mice that express the membrane form of immunoglobulin μ. Science 236:816, 1987.
126. Oettinger MA, Schatz DG, Gorka C, et al: RAG-1 and RAG-2, adjacent genes that synergistically activate V(D)J recombination. Science 248:1517, 1990.
127. Okazaki K, Davis DD, Sakano H: T cell receptor β gene sequences in the circular DNA of thymocyte nuclei: direct evidence for intramolecular DNA deletion in V-D-J joining. Cell 49:477, 1987.
128. Padlan EA, Davies DR: A model of the Fc of immunoglobulin E. Mol Immunol 10:1063, 1986.
129. Padlan EA, Davies DR, Rudikoff S, et al: Structural basis for the specificity of phosphorylcholine-binding immunoglobulins. Immunochemistry 13:945, 1976.
130. Pascual V, Capra JD: Human immunoglobulin heavy-chain variable region genes: organization, polymorphism, and expression. Adv Immunol 49:1, 1991.
131. Perlmutter AP, Gilbert W: Antibodies of the secondary response can be expressed without switch recombination in normal B cells. Proc Natl Acad Sci USA 81:7189, 1984.
132. Pillai S, Baltimore D: The omega and iota surrogate immunoglobulin light chains. Curr Top Microbiol Immunol 137:136, 1988.
133. Pleiman CM, D'Ambrosio D, Cambier JC: The B-cell antigen receptor complex: structure and signal transduction. Immunol Today 15:393, 1994.
134. Poljak RJ, Amzel LM, Avey HP, et al: Structure of Fab′ NEW at 6 Å resolution. Nature New Biol 235:137, 1972.
135. Poljak RJ, Amzel LM, Avey HP, et al: Three-dimensional structure of the FAB′ fragment of a human immunoglobulin at 2.8 Å resolution. Proc Natl Acad Sci USA 70:3305, 1973.
136. Poljak RJ, Amzel LM, Chen BL, et al: The three dimensional structure of the Fab′ fragments of a myeloma immunoglobulin at 2.0-Å resolution. Proc Natl Acad Sci USA 71:3440, 1974.
137. Porter RR: The hydrolysis of rabbit γ-globulin and antibodies with crystalline papain. Biochem J 73:119, 1959.
138. Potter M: Immunoglobulin-producing tumors and myeloma proteins of mice. Physiol Rev 52:631, 1972.
139. Rabbitts TH, Matthyssens G, Hamlyn PH: Contribution of immunoglobulin heavy-chain variable-region genes to antibody diversity. Nature 284:238, 1980.
140. Radbruch A, Muller W, Rajewsky K: Class switch recombination is IgG1 specific on the active and inactive IgH loci of IgG1-secreting B cell blasts. Proc Natl Acad Sci USA 83:3954, 1986.
141. Rajewsky K, Förster I, Cumano A: Evolutionary and somatic selection of the antibody repertoire in the mouse. Science 238:1088, 1987.
142. Randall TD, King LB, Corley RB: The biological effects of IgM hexamer formation. Eur J Immunol 20:1971, 1990.
143. Randall TD, Parkhouse RME, Corley RB: J chain synthesis and secretion of hexameric IgM is differentially regulated by LPS and IL5. Proc Natl Acad Sci USA 89:962, 1992.
144. Rathbun G, Berman J, Yancopoulos G, et al: Organization and expression of the mammalian heavy-chain variable-region locus. In Honjo T, Alt FW, Rabbitts TH (eds): Immunoglobulin Genes. Academic Press, New York, 1989.
145. Reth M: Antigen receptor tail clue. Nature 338:383, 1989.
146. Reth M: Antigen receptors on B lymphocytes. Annu Rev Immunol 10:97, 1992.
147. Reth M, Hombach J, Wienands J, et al: The B-cell antigen receptor complex. Immunol Today 12:196, 1991.
148. Reth M, Petrac E, Wiese P, et al: Activation of V_κ gene rearrangement in pre-B cells follows the expression of membrane-bound immunoglobulin heavy chain. EMBO J 6:3299, 1987.
148a. Roes J, Rajewsky K: Immunoglobulin D (IgD)-deficient mice reveal an auxiliary receptor function for IgD in antigen-mediated recruitment of B cells. J Exp Med 177:45, 1993.
149. Rogers J, Wall R: Immunoglobulin RNA arrangements in B lymphocyte differentiation. Adv Immunol 35:39, 1984.
150. Rolink A, Melchers F: Molecular and cellular origins of B lymphocyte diversity. Cell 66:1080, 1991.
151. Roth DB, Menetski JP, Nakajima PB, et al: V(D)J recombination: broken DNA molecules with covalently sealed (hairpin) coding ends in scid mouse thymocytes. Cell 70:983, 1992.
152. Roth DB, Nakajima PB, Menetski JP, et al: V(D)J recombination in mouse thymocytes: double-strand breaks near T cell receptor delta rearrangement signals. Cell 69:41, 1992.
153. Rothman P, Li SC, Alt FW: The molecular events in heavy chain class-switching. Semin Immunol 1:65, 1989.
154. Sakaguchi N, Kashiwamura S-I, Kinoto M, et al: B lymphocyte lineage restricted expression of mb-1, a gene with CD3-like structural properties. EMBO J 7:3457, 1988.
155. Sakaguchi N, Melchers F: λ5, a new light-chain-related locus selectively expressed in pre-B lymphocytes. Nature 324:579, 1986.
156. Sakano H, Hüppi K, Heinrich G, et al: Sequences at the somatic recombination sites of immunoglobulin light-chain genes. Nature 280:288, 1979.
157. Sakano H, Kurosawa Y, Weigert M, et al: Identification and nucleotide

sequence of a diversity DNA segment (D) of immunoglobulin heavy-chain genes. Nature 290:562, 1981.
158. Sakano H, Maki R, Kurosawa Y, et al: Two types of somatic recombination are necessary for the generation of complete immunoglobulin heavy-chain genes. Nature 286:676, 1980.
159. Samelson LE, Klausner RD: Tyrosine kinases and tyrosine-based activation motifs. J Biol Chem 267:24913, 1992.
160. Schatz DG, Oettinger MA, Baltimore D: The V(D)J recombination activating gene, RAG-1. Cell 59:1035, 1989.
161. Schiff C, Milili M, Bossy D, et al: Organization and expression of the pseudo-light chain genes in human B-cell ontogeny. Int Rev Immunol 8:135, 1992.
162. Schiffer M, Girling RL, Ely KR, et al: Structure of a λ-type Bence-Jones protein at 3.5 Å resolution. Biochemistry 12:4620, 1973.
163. Schilling J, Clevinger B, Davie JM, et al: Amino acid sequence of homogeneous antibodies to dextran and DNA rearrangements in heavy chain V-region gene segments. Nature 283:35, 1980.
164. Schlissel MS, Baltimore D: Activation of immunoglobulin kappa gene rearrangement correlates with induction of germline kappa gene transcription. Cell 58:1001, 1989.
165. Schroeder HWJ, Hillson JL, Perlmutter RM: Structure and evolution of mammalian VH families. Int Immunol 2:41, 1990.
166. Shumaker VN, Phillips ML, Hanson DC: Dynamic aspects of antibody structure. Mol Immunol 28:1347, 1991.
167. Segal DM, Padlan EA, Cohen GH, et al: The three-dimensional structure of a phosphorylcholine-binding mouse immunoglobulin Fab and the nature of the antigen binding site. Proc Natl Acad Sci USA 71:4298, 1974.
168. Seidman JG, Leder P: The arrangement and rearrangement of antibody genes. Nature 276:790, 1978.
169. Seidman JG, Nau MM, Norman B, et al: Immunoglobulin V/J recombination is accompanied by deletion of joining site and variable region segments. Proc Natl Acad Sci USA 77:6022, 1980.
170. Selsing E, Durdik J, Moore MW, et al: Immunoglobulin λ genes. In Honjo T, Alt FW, Rabbitts TH (eds): Immunoglobulin Genes. Academic Press, New York, 1989.
171. Sen R, Baltimore D: Factors regulating immunoglobulin-gene transcription. In Honjo T, Alt FW, Rabbitts TH (eds): Immunoglobulin Genes. Academic Press, New York, 1989.
172. Shimizu A, Honjo T: Immunoglobulin class switching. Cell 36:801, 1984.
173. Shinkai Y, Rathbun G, Lam K-P, et al: RAG-2 deficient mice lack mature lymphocytes owing to inability to initiate V(D)J rearrangement. Cell 68:855, 1991.
174. Slater RJ, Ward SM, Kunkel HG: Immunological relationships among the myeloma proteins. J Exp Med 101:85, 1955.
175. Southern E: Detection of specific sequences among DNA fragments separated by gel electrophoresis. J Mol Biol 98:503, 1975.
176. Stavnezer-Nordgren J, Sirlin S: Specificity of immunoglobulin heavy chain class switch correlates with activity of germline heavy chain genes prior to switching. EMBO J 5:95, 1986.
177. Storb U, Haasch D, Arp B, et al: Physical linkage of mouse λ genes by pulsed-field electrophoresis suggests that the rearrangement process favors proximate target sequences. Mol Cell Biol 9:711, 1989.
178. Straubinger B, Huber E, Lorenz W, et al: The human Vk locus: characterisation of a duplicated region encoding 28 different immunoglobulin genes. J Mol Biol 199:23, 1988.
179. Tan LK, Shopes RJ, Oi VT, et al: Influence of the hinge region on complement activation, C1q binding, and segmental flexibility in chimeric human immunoglobulins. Proc Natl Acad Sci USA 87:162, 1990.
180. Tao M-H, Canfield SM, Morrison SL: The differential ability of human IgG1 and IgG4 to activate complement is determined by the COOH-terminal sequence of the C_H2 domain. J Exp Med 173:1025, 1991.
181. Tao MH, Morrison SL: Studies of aglycosylated chimeric mouse-human IgG. Role of carbohydrate in the structure and effector functions mediated by the human IgG constant region. J Immunol 143:2595, 1989.
182. Tiselius A, Kabat EA: An electrophoretic study of immune sera and purified antibody preparations. J Exp Med 69:119, 1939.
183. Tomasi TB Jr, Bienenstock J: Secretory immunoglobulins. Adv Immunol 9:1, 1968.
184. Tonegawa S: Somatic generation of antibody diversity. Nature 302:575, 1983.
185. Tonegawa S, Brack C, Hozumi N, et al: Cloning of an immunoglobulin variable region gene from mouse embryo. Proc Natl Acad Sci USA 74:3518, 1977.
186. Tonegawa S, Maxam AM, Tizard R, et al: Sequence of a mouse germline gene for a variable region of an immunoglobulin light chain. Proc Natl Acad Sci USA 74:3171, 1978.
187. Tonegawa S, Steinberg C, Dube S: Evidence for somatic generation of antibody diversity. Proc Natl Acad Sci USA 71:4027, 1974.
188. Tsubata T, Reth M: The products of pre-B cell-specific genes (λ5 and V_{preB}) and the immunoglobulin μ chain form a complex that is transported onto the cell. J Exp Med 172:973, 1990.
189. Tsubata T, Tsubata R, Reth M: Crosslinking of the cell surface immunoglobulin (μ-surrogate light chains complex) on pre-B cells induces activation of V gene rearrangements at the immunoglobulin κ locus. Int Immunol 4:637, 1992.
190. Tsujimoto Y, Croce CM: Molecular cloning of a human immunoglobulin lambda chain variable sequence. Nucleic Acids Res 12:8407, 1984.
191. Unkeless JC: Function and heterogeneity of human Fc receptors for immunoglobulin G. J Clin Invest 83:355, 1989.
192. Utsumi S, Okada M, Udaka K, et al: Preparation and biologic characterization of fragments containing dimeric and monomeric C gamma 2 domain of rabbit IgG. Mol Immunol 22:811, 1985.
193. Van Ness BG, Coleclough C, Perry RP, et al: DNA between variable and joining gene segments of immunoglobulin κ light chain is frequently retained in cells that rearrange the κ locus. Proc Natl Acad Sci USA 79:262, 1982.
194. Venkitaraman A: Light chain surrogacy. Curr Biol 2:559, 1992.
194a. Vitetta ES, Uhr JW: IgD and B cell differentiation. Immunol Rev 37:50, 1977.
195. Wade RH, Taveau JC, Lamy JN: Concerning the axial flexibility of the Fab regions of immunoglobulin G. J Mol Biol 206:349, 1989.
196. Walter MA, Dosch HM, Cox DW: A deletion map of the human immunoglobulin heavy chain variable region. J Exp Med 174:335, 1991.
197. Weigert MG, Cesari IM, Yondovich SJ, et al: Variability in the lambda light chain sequences of mouse antibody. Nature 228:1045, 1970.
198. Wienands J, Hombach J, Radbruch A, et al: Molecular components of the B cell antigen receptor complex of class IgD differ partly from those of IgM. EMBO J 9:449, 1990.
199. Williams AF, Barclay AN: The immunoglobulin superfamily—domains for cell recognition. Ann Rev Immunol 6:381, 1988.
200. Williams GT, Venkitaraman AR, Gilmore DJ, et al: The sequence of the μ transmembrane segment determines the tissue specificity of the transport of immunoglobulin M to the cell surface. J Exp Med 171:947, 1990.
201. Winter E, Krawinkel U, Radbruch A: Directed Ig class-switch recombination in activated B cells. EMBO J 6:1663, 1987.
202. Wright JF, Shulman MJ, Isenman DE, et al: C1 binding by mouse IgM. J Biol Chem 265:10506, 1990.
203. Wu TT, Kabat EA: An analysis of the sequences of the variable regions of Bence Jones proteins and myeloma light chains and their implications for antibody complementarity. J Exp Med 132:211, 1970.
204. Yancopoulos G, DePinho R, Zimmerman K, et al: Secondary rearrangement events in pre-B cells: V_HDJ_H replacement by a LINE-1 sequence and directed class switching. EMBO J 5:3259, 1986.
205. Yasmeen D, Ellerson JR, Dorrington KJ, et al: The structure and function of immunoglobulin domains. IV. The distribution of some effector functions among the Cγ2 and Cγ3 homology regions of human immunoglobulin G. J Immunol 116:518, 1976.
205a. Yélamos J, Klix N, Goyenechea B, et al: Targeting of non-Ig sequences in place of the V segment by somatic hypermutation. Nature 376:225, 1995.
206. Young F, Ardman B, Shinkai Y, et al: Influence of immunoglobulin heavy- and light-chain expression on B-cell differentiation. Genes Dev 8:1043, 1994.
207. Zachau HG: Immunoglobulin light-chain genes of the κ type in man and mouse. In Honjo T, Alt FW, Rabbitts TH (eds): Immunoglobulin Genes. Academic Press, New York, 1989.
208. Zhang J, Bottaro A, Li S, et al: A selective defect in IgG2b switching as a result of targeted mutation of the Iγ2b promoter and exon. EMBO J 12:3529, 1993.
209. Zheng B, Xue W, Kelsoe G: Locus-specific somatic hypermutation in germinal centre T cells. Nature 372:556, 1994.

3 T and B Lymphocytes

ETHAN M. SHEVACH

In many respects, the immune system can be visualized as a symphony orchestra composed of many different instruments all cooperating together to generate and regulate the immune response. T and B lymphocytes are the most important players in this group and might be considered to make up the violin and viola sections, respectively. Each of these sections alone would not result in the production of a complicated musical work. On the other hand, absence of either of these sections would seriously diminish the impact of a musical composition in the same manner that deficiencies in either T or B lymphocytes result in major clinical immunodeficiency syndromes in both humans and experimental animals.

This chapter will review the structure of B and T lymphocyte receptors and summarize the developmental processes needed for production of the peripheral lymphocyte pool. In much the same manner that the violin and viola resemble each other, there are great similarities in all aspects of T and B lymphocyte function, including the structure of the receptor complexes, the associated signal transduction apparatus, and the process of positive/negative selection in which autoreactive T and B lymphocytes are deleted from the repertoire during development. The last section of the chapter focuses on cell cooperation in the immune response, not only between T and B lymphocytes themselves but also with all the other critical members of the immunologic orchestra, including lymphoid dendritic cells, macrophages, and follicular dendritic cells, whose presence is also needed to produce a finely tuned immune response.

B LYMPHOCYTES

STRUCTURE OF THE B-CELL RECEPTOR

The main function of B lymphocytes is to produce immunoglobulins, of which nine different isotypes (IgM, IgD, IgG_{1-4}, IgA_1, IgA_2, and IgE) have been isolated in humans.[3] Each of these isotypes displays specific effector functions such as binding to complement components or to fraction crystallizable (Fc) receptors whose engagement results in a wide array of biologic activities. B lymphocytes represent about 5% to 10% of the circulating lymphoid pool and are classically defined by the presence of surface immunoglobulin. Immunoglobulins play a critical role in defense against a variety of infectious microorganisms. Their complete absence is lethal if not compensated for by a repeated, lifelong reconstitution therapy.

The response of B cells to all foreign antigens is mediated through the cell surface B-cell receptor (BCR) for antigen. The BCR belongs to a class of cell surface receptors that includes the T-cell receptor (TCR) and the receptors for the Fc region of IgE and IgG.[55, 57] The immunoglobulins are inserted into the surface membrane of the B cell, where they act as specific antigen receptors. These immunoglobulins constitute the ligand portion of the receptor and are made up as a tetrameric complex of Ig heavy (H) and light (L) chains. The majority of human B cells in peripheral blood express two immunoglobulin isotypes on their surface, IgM and IgD. The antigen-binding sites of IgM and IgD are identical on a given cell. Very few cells in the circulation express IgG, IgA, or IgE, although cells expressing these isotypes are present in larger numbers in specific locations in the body, for example, IgA-bearing cells in the intestinal mucosa.

Triggering of surface IgM (sIgM) with specific antibodies had been shown in the 1970s to deliver activation signals to B cells, but it was difficult to understand how sIgM could transduce a signal as its cytoplasmic domain consisted of only three amino acids. It has been shown that surface IgM is associated with other molecules, Ig-α and Ig-β, which exist as disulfide-bonded heterodimers and function as the transducer components of the BCR (Fig. 3–1).[57] Ig-α (CD79a), a 34-kD molecule and product of the *mb-1* gene, and Ig-β (CD79b), a 39-kD product encoded by the B29 gene, are required for the transport and assembly of IgM monomers in the cell membrane. Signaling function can be mediated by both chains. Ig-γ is a truncated form of Ig-β, which lacks the C-terminus and is expressed on some resting B cells. Both Ig-α and Ig-β show similarity to components of the T-cell receptor complex and are glycosylated and phosphorylated transmembrane proteins with an extracellular Ig-like domain and a cytoplasmic tail. All classes of sIg are associated with a heterodimer that appears to be identical to that of sIgM, although some differences in glycosylation may exist.

The Ig-α and Ig-β have extensive cytoplasmic domains which couple the BCR to the cytoplasmic signaling appara-

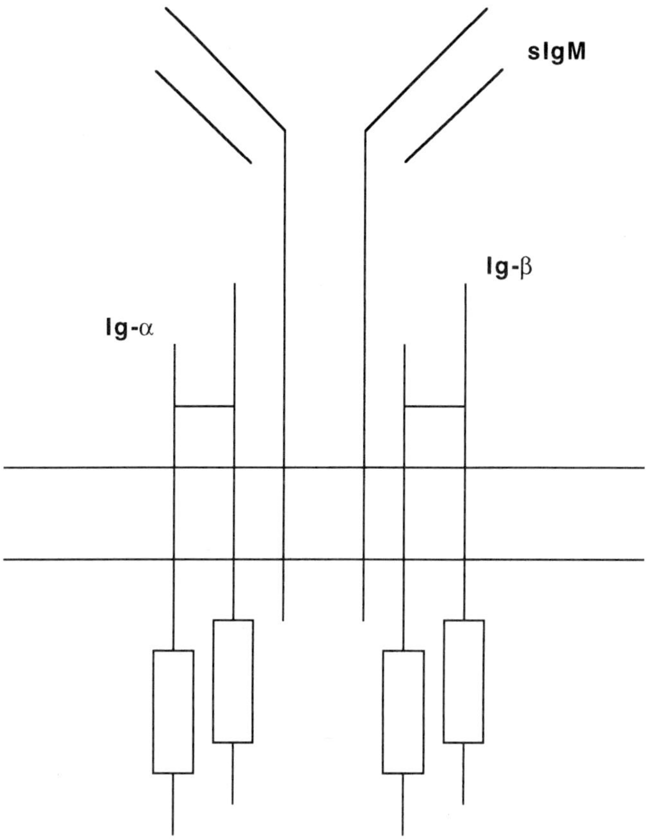

FIGURE 3–1. The BCR complex is composed of sIgM and associated invariant chains. The ITAMs present in Ig-α and Ig-β are depicted as rectangles.

tus. A 26-amino acid immunoreceptor tyrosine-based activation motif (ITAM) found in the cytoplasmic tails of many other transducer chains (TCRζ, TCRε, δ, γ, FcεR1γ, and others) is present in both Ig-α and Ig-β and contains sufficient structural information to initiate multiple signal transduction events.[5, 76] Protein tyrosine phosphorylation is important in the initiation of cellular responses by the BCR.[18] None of the BCR subunits have intrinsic protein kinase or phosphatase activity. It is therefore likely that the ITAMs interact directly with cytoplasmic protein-tyrosine kinases. Receptor engagement leads to phosphorylation of two ITAMs by an *src* family protein-tyrosine kinase. Several *src* kinase family members, including *lyn, blk, fyn,* and *lck*, have been reported to be associated with the ITAMs of the BCR.[9] ITAM phosphorylation is followed by binding of a second type of protein-tyrosine kinase, *syk*, in B cells; *syk* had previously been shown by immunoprecipitation studies to be associated with components of the BCR complex. Stimulation of the BCR induces the tyrosine phosphorylation of many cytoplasmic and membrane proteins. However, it is not known which of these proteins represent direct substrates of the protein-tyrosine kinases associated with the BCR complex. The future identification of the downstream effector molecules that regulate cellular responses in B cells should allow one to map out the pathway from the plasma membrane to the cell nucleus.

A number of other markers are expressed by both mouse and human B cells (Table 3–1).[3, 7, 63] The majority of B cells express multiple antigenic peptides (MHC) class II antigens, which are involved in cooperative interactions with T cells. In humans, these consist of DP, DQ, and DR antigens. Complement receptors for C3b (CR1, CD35) and C3d (CR2, CD21) are commonly found on B cells and are associated with cell activation. Fc receptors for exogenous IgG (FcγRII, CD32) are also present and play a role in negative signaling to the B cell. CD19, CD20, and CD22 are the main markers used to identify human B cells. Other molecules that identify human B cells are CD72 through CD78, and in the mouse B220, the high molecular weight form of CD45. CD5, which is primarily a T-cell marker, has been shown to be present on some B cells, particularly a subset (B1) that is predisposed to autoantibody production.[48] These cells are predominantly found in the peritoneal cavity of mice, and there is some evidence that they differentiate via a pathway that is distinct from conventional (B2 cells) B cells.

Some of these cell surface antigens, in addition to serving as membrane markers that facilitate identification of B cells, may also play important roles in the process of B-cell activation. CD19 is a member of the Ig gene superfamily and is expressed on B cells throughout their maturation. Although its ligand has not been identified, it interacts with various molecules on other B cells, including the receptor for the C3d component of complement, CD21/CR2.[68] When cross-linked, CD19 induces calcium mobilization in both pre–B and mature B cells. A molecular complex formed by CD19 and CD21, as well as other molecules, may play a role in the amplification of signals received by the BCR. The CD19/CD21 complex co-caps with the BCR after anti-IgM activation, and cross-linking of CD19 lowers the threshold for stimulation by anti-IgM. Anti-IgM–mediated B-cell signaling is also accompanied by tyrosine phosphorylation of CD19. Another member of the Ig gene superfamily, CD22, may also associate with surface IgM and is rapidly phosphorylated on tyrosine residues after it becomes cross-linked.[60] CD22 may

TABLE 3–1
ACCESSORY MOLECULES THAT PLAY A ROLE IN B-CELL ACTIVATION

Molecule	Molecular Weight (KD)	Ligand	Function
CD19	95	?	Regulation of B-cell proliferation
CD21	145	?	Receptor for C3d and Epstein-Barr virus; regulation of B-cell proliferation
CD40	50	CD40L (gp39)	B-cell growth and differentiation
CD22	Dimer α 130 β 140	CD45RO; CD75	Cell-cell adhesion
CD72	Homodimer 42	CD5	B-cell activation and proliferation

be required for normal signaling as intracellular calcium is not elevated after cross-linking sIg in CD22-negative B cells. CD22 also interacts with several ligands on B and T lymphocytes that contain α2,6-linked sialic acids and is likely to affect antigen-specific B-cell maturation.[66]

B-CELL DEVELOPMENT

In the chicken, primary B-cell lymphopoiesis occurs in a discrete lymphoepithelial organ, the bursa of Fabricius. The bursal rudiment develops as an outpushing of the hindgut endoderm and becomes seeded with blood-borne stem cells. There is a window for the immigration of stem cells into the bursa between days 10 and 14 of embryonic life. The putative stem cells make contact with epithelial cells; one or a few stem cells give rise to a single bursal follicle, which is composed of a cortex and medulla. Mammals do not have a specific discrete organ for B-cell lymphopoiesis. Instead, B cells develop directly from lymphoid stem cells in the hematopoietic tissue of the fetal liver by 8 to 9 weeks of gestation in humans and by about 14 days in mice. The site of B-cell production then moves from the liver to the bone marrow, where it continues into adult life.

The development of the B-cell lineage in the bone marrow is independent of T cells and antigens and occurs in a carefully programmed stepwise fashion (Fig. 3–2), which permits the commitment and maturation of a hematopoietic multipotent stem cell into mature B lymphocytes coexpressing IgM and IgD.[23] In the bone marrow, B cells mature in close association with stromal reticular cells. Stromal cells have mixed phenotypic features with similarities to fibroblasts, endothelial cells, and smooth muscle cells.[33] Stromal cells are required for the B-cell differentiation process; for example, stem cells that are removed from the bone marrow and placed into culture fail to differentiate into B cells unless stromal cells are also present.[44] At early stages, the B cells must be in direct physical contact with the stromal cells. The interaction between the CD44 antigen on the B cell with hyaluronic acid on the stromal cell[43] may facilitate the interaction of a second stromal cell surface molecule (stem cell factor) with its receptor, the c-kit molecule on the B-cell precursors[51]; the c-kit molecule has tyrosine kinase activity that stimulates the proliferation of early pre–B cells. At later stages, developing B cells respond to growth factors, particularly IL-7, that are secreted by the stromal cells.[24]

The first B-lineage committed cell is the pro–B cell, which has its immunoglobulin genes in germline configuration. Rearrangement of the heavy chain variable (V), diversity (D), and joining (J) gene segments then occurs, resulting in cytoplasmic expression of μ chains, which defines pre–B cells. The RAG-1 and RAG-2 genes encode proteins required for immunoglobulin gene rearrangement and are very active in the earliest B cells, but their activity is lost in mature B cells upon completion of gene rearrangement. The suppression of heavy chain gene rearrangement depends on the cell surface expression of the products of the rearranged genes.[41] However, the μ chain cannot be expressed on the surface in the absence of light chains. While the pre–B-cell pool expands, a special mechanism takes place that allows some of the B cells to express small amounts of a truncated surface μ chain associated with pseudo light chains V_{preB} and λ_5.[29] Both λ_5 and V_{preB} genes have sequence homology to conventional light chains, but they do not have to be rearranged before expression. It is possible that their products may play some role in the interaction of the developing B cell with stromal cells. Once the immunoglobulin-like molecule is expressed on the cell surface, it then signals the developing B cell to stop further heavy chain gene rearrangement and to begin light chain rearrangement.[17] When κ or λ light chains are synthesized, they displace the surrogate light chains from the heavy chains to form the completed cell surface IgM molecule. The immature B cell is then committed to the antigen-binding specificity of its sIgM receptor.

All progenitors, precursors, and immature B cells are short-lived, with a half-life of 1 to 4 days. The majority of B cells (75%) maturing in the bone marrow die, as they have not made productive rearrangements. Only after screening for autoreactivity do the B cells complete their maturation process and become capable of migrating to peripheral lymphoid tissues. B cells that recognize self-antigens undergo a process of programmed cell death or apoptosis and are phagocytosed by bone marrow macrophages[20]; alternatively, self-reactive B cells are rendered nonresponsive (anergic).[12] The non–self-reactive and low-affinity self-reactive cells are then induced further to express sIgD, thus defining the mature (naive or virgin) B cell. IgM and IgD are created by alternative splicing of heavy chain mRNA. It has been estimated that human bone marrow produces 10^{10} to 10^{11} B cells per day, but only 2% to 5% of the pool of immature sIgM+ B cells is selected every day to enter the peripheral, mature sIgM/sIgD compartment. Newly formed B cells in the periphery have a very short life span and are continuously replenished during life.

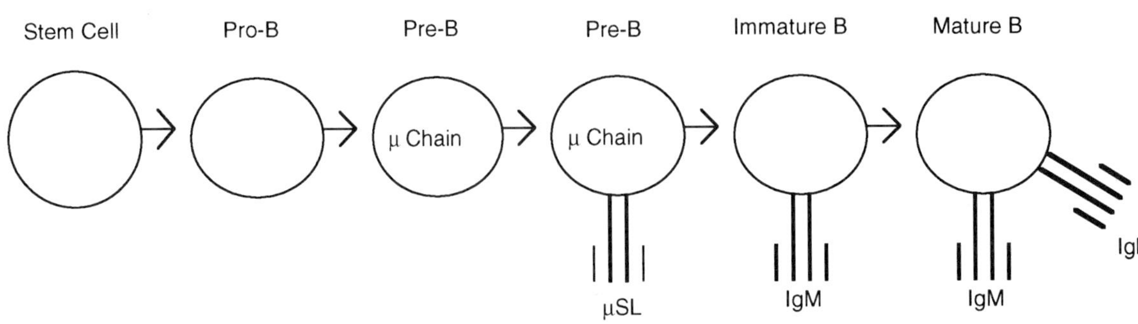

FIGURE 3–2. Development of the B-cell lineage in the bone marrow. Two stages of pre–B-cell development are shown. The earliest pre–B cell expresses only cytoplasmic μ chain, whereas the later pre–B cell also expresses surface μ chain, which is associated with the surrogate light chains (μSL).

Whereas the T-cell repertoire is shaped in the thymus and is independent of exogenous antigen, the B cell is subject to an antigen-dependent maturation process in secondary lymphoid tissue that results in an increased affinity of the immunoglobulin repertoire of memory B cells.[50] When B cells mature, they leave the bone marrow and migrate to the lymphoid follicles of lymph nodes and spleen. Mature B cells are not sessile and form part of the recirculating lymphocyte pool. Many B cells are found in gut-associated lymphoid tissues in Peyer's patches. Recirculating B cells first enter secondary lymphoid tissues via high endothelial venules or in the spleen via marginal zone sinuses. The primary encounter of B cells, T cells, and antigen-presenting cells (APC) occurs outside the follicles in the T-cell zone (Fig. 3–3). Antigen is presented by the APC to the T cells, which in turn initiate the process of B-cell activation. Following the binding of antigen to sIg, a carefully regulated and orchestrated process ultimately results in the production of highly efficient antibody-secreting plasma cells and the development of memory B cells.

In the first stage of the B-cell maturation process, some of the virgin B cells are converted to blast cells and then to short-lived plasma cells that produce genetically unmodified low-affinity IgM antibody. The production of this low-affinity antibody is critical for progression of B-cell differentiation to the second stage, which involves the generation of germinal centers. The low-affinity antibody results in the formation of antigen-antibody complexes, which are taken up by the follicular dendritic cells (FDC) in the center of the primary lymphoid follicles. The cellular origins of the FDC are not known, although they are definitely not of bone marrow origin. The FDC express both Fc receptors and complement receptors and retain antigens in the form of antigen-antibody complexes on their surface for prolonged periods of time (months or years); the retention of antigen-antibody complexes by the FDC is highly radioresistant. The accumulation of antigen on the FDC in primary follicles and the subsequent formation of germinal centers require that an early antibody response be made to the antigen; germinal centers are therefore first formed about a week after antigen stimulation. However, the development of the germinal center is a T-cell–dependent process, and the passive administration of antibody that results in the trapping of antigen by the FDC will not result in germinal center formation.

The primary function of the germinal center is to create an immunoglobulin repertoire that is of higher affinity for the eliciting antigen than is coded by germline Ig gene sequences.[22] Antigen initiates the expansion and hypermutation of the centroblasts, serves as the primary stimulus for positive selection of centrocytes, and stimulates specific T cells to provide accessory signals for all these processes. Some of the proliferating blast cells generated in the T-cell zone during their primary encounter with antigen enter primary follicles, where they proliferate in response to anti-

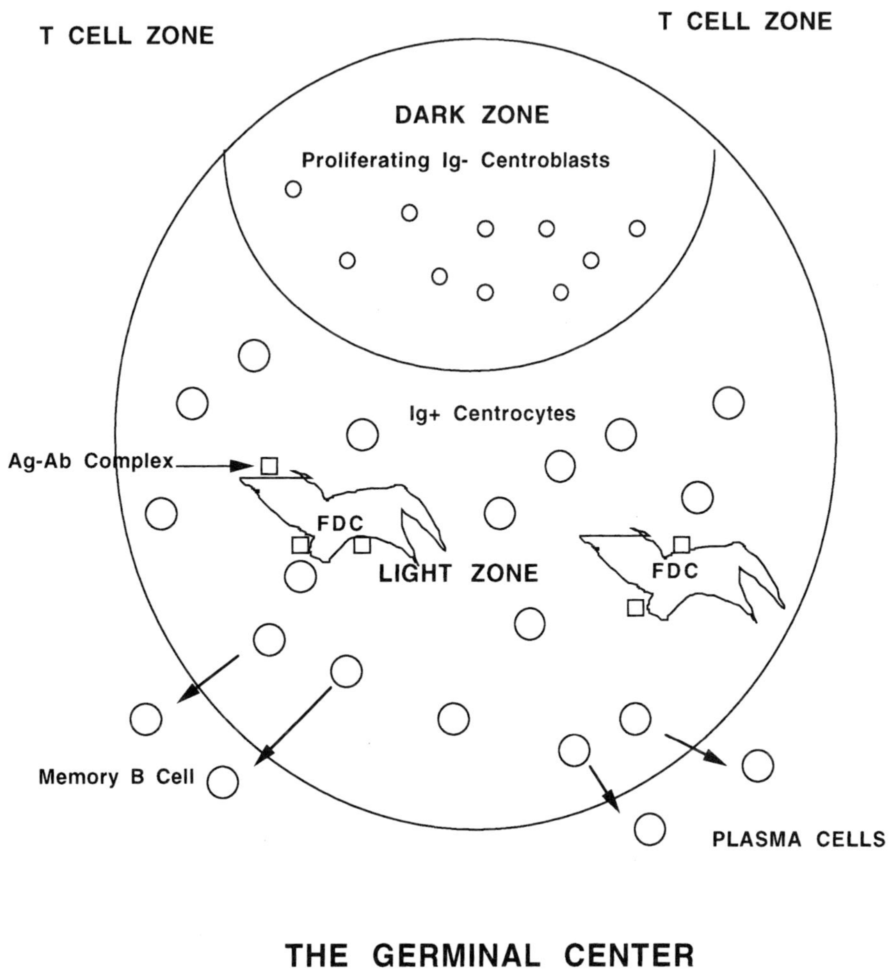

FIGURE 3–3. Organization of the germinal center. Naive B cells encounter T cells and dendritic cells primarily in the T-cell zone and then enter the lymphoid follicle to establish the germinal center. The dark zone contains rapidly dividing sIg^- centroblasts, whereas the light zone contains sIg^+ centrocytes and FDC. B cells exiting the germinal center are both sIg^- antibody-producing plasma cells and sIg^+ memory B cells.

gen that is expressed on the dense network of processes extending from the FDC.[30, 31]

The cross-linking of Ig receptors on B cells by the extensive array of antigen molecules on the FDC constitutes one of the stimuli for activated B cells to strongly replicate and undergo selection for high-affinity receptors and class switching. With further stimulation, they enter the cell cycle and begin to divide to compensate for the relatively small number of antigen-specific B cells that is normally available. B-cell blasts proliferate at a high rate and reach approximately 10^4 cells in 3 to 4 days. On the fourth day, the cells transform into centroblasts, which have no surface Ig. The visible focus of centroblasts that form in a few days within a primary lymphoid follicle is called a germinal center. These proliferating B cells form the center of a secondary follicle, and the original resting B cells of the primary follicle now form the outer mantle zone. Closely packed centroblasts form the dark zone of the germinal center (Fig. 3–3). Somatic hypermutation is induced by antigen in dividing centroblasts.

The resulting mutant receptors are expressed on the progeny of the rapidly dividing centroblasts, the centrocytes, which are all derived from the few antigen-specific progenitors that founded the germinal center. The small centrocytes then reexpress surface Ig and occupy the basal light zone of the germinal center, where they make contact with the dense network of FDC processes. The centrocytes eventually give rise to relatively long-lived antibody-secreting plasma cells. Centrocytes are programmed to die within a fixed period of time unless their surface Ig is bound to antigen. The close physical association of the centrocytes with antigen on the surface of the FDC facilitates the rescue and selection of centrocytes that bind antigen with high affinity; the interaction between these two cell types is mediated by LFA-1 (CD11a/CD18) on the lymphocytes and ICAM-1 (CD54) on the FDC. Centrocytes selected in this way for antigen binding have mutations in the complementarity-determining regions of the Ig genes. Successful interactions of centrocytes bearing high-affinity receptors for antigen presented by the FDC give rise to secondary blasts, which leave the secondary follicles either as memory cells or plasma cell precursors (plasmablasts).

The retention of antigen on the FDC membranes is strongly believed to be critical for the growth and selection of high-affinity clones of B cells, the maintenance of immunologic memory for the B cell, and the persistence of antibody formation following stimulation. Lack of centrocyte-FDC interactions leads to programmed cell death.[31] The germinal centers persist for about 3 weeks and then begin to decrease in size and lose their polarized morphology. Plasmablasts generated in these organs migrate to the medullary chords of lymph nodes, to the red pulp in the spleen, and to bone marrow, where they mature into nondividing plasma cells that secrete large amounts of antibody. The differentiation of the B cell to the plasma cell is accompanied by down-regulation of surface Ig and major histocompatibility complex (MHC) class II antigens and by morphological changes, including the presence of abundant cytoplasm with multiple layers of rough endoplasmic reticulum. Plasma cells have a limited life span after their differentiation, which results in limiting the duration of the antibody response. Once the elicting antigen has been eliminated, the B-cell blasts will stop proliferating, and rather than terminally differentiate to plasma cells, they differentiate into small memory B cells that do not secrete antibody but express novel isotypes. Memory B cells may be long-lived, and their presence ensures that those cells needed to recognize pathogens are retained to combat infection. These memory B cells rapidly proliferate and differentiate in response to a repeated specific antigenic challenge.

T LYMPHOCYTES

STRUCTURE OF THE T-CELL RECEPTOR

T-cell receptor (TCR) was first defined and purified using specific antibodies directed against clone-specific determinants on T cells. It was called the $\alpha\beta$ TCR because it was a heterodimeric molecule consisting of an α chain and a β chain linked by a disulfide bond. Independently, putative TCR α and β cDNA clones were isolated either by subtractive or differential hybridization of cDNA libraries.[1] The amino acid sequence deduced from the nucleotide sequence of cDNA clones matched the partial sequence obtained from α and β TCR proteins purified using mAbs. A second TCR, termed $\gamma\delta$, was isolated later.[56]

The $\alpha\beta$ TCR comprises a disulfide-linked heterodimer of α (40–50 kD) and β (35–47kD) subunits.[1, 47] Each polypeptide chain comprises two Ig-like domains of approximately 110 amino acids, which are anchored into the plasma membrane by a transmembrane peptide and a short cytoplasmic tail. The difference in molecular weights of the α and β chains is accounted for by the presence of extra N-linked carbohydrates on the former. The amino acid sequence variability resides in the N-terminal domain of the α and β polypeptide chains, which are homologous with the variable domain of immunoglobulins. This domain is encoded by rearranging V, D, and J gene segments of β and V and J gene segments of α. Analysis of different TCR V domain sequences has revealed areas of relatively greater variability that correspond to Ig hypervariable regions. An unusual feature of both the α and β chain transmembrane regions is the inclusion of positively charged residues. These charged residues have been implicated in the assembly and intracellular transport of the TCR complex.

The overall structure of the $\gamma\delta$ TCR is similar to that of its $\alpha\beta$ counterpart, each chain being organized into external V and C domains, a transmembrane segment containing positively charged residues, and a short cytoplasmic tail.[21] The two forms of the TCR show quite distinct anatomic locations. The $\alpha\beta$ TCR is present on more than 95% of peripheral T cells and the vast majority of TCR-expressing thymocytes. In contrast, T cells expressing the $\gamma\delta$ receptor often have defined anatomic locations. Although $\gamma\delta$ T cells are only minor proportions of the T cells in the thymus and secondary lymphoid organs, they are abundant in various epithelia, such as the epidermis (mouse but not human), intestinal epithelium, uterus, and tongue. The various distinct $\gamma\delta$ T-cell subsets differ structurally in terms of which V regions are expressed. $\gamma\delta$ T cells found in mouse skin express exclusively the Vγ3 and Vδ1 regions, whereas $\gamma\delta$ T cells in the mouse gut intraepithelial (IEL) populations express Vγ5 almost exclusively in combination with Vδ4, Vδ5, Vδ6, or Vδ7.

The αβ and γδ forms of the TCR are both associated physically with a series of at least five invariant polypeptides.[74] This association is required for expression of the TCR complex at the cell surface. These components show no amino acid variability on different T cells and thus are not associated with the diversity of the TCR. Rather, they are probably required for signal transduction following antigen recognition by the TCR heterodimer.[10] CD3 consists of at least three invariant polypeptides (Fig. 3–4). The CD3 γ, δ, and ε chains are the products of three closely linked genes and are related in their primary sequence. These polypeptides are members of the Ig superfamily, and each contains an external domain followed by a transmembrane region and a highly conserved cytoplasmic tail of 40 or more amino acids. The transmembrane regions contain a single negatively charged amino acid (glutamic acid in the CD3 γ chain and aspartic acid in the δ and ε chains) rather than being completely apolar. The ζ and η polypeptides are products of a single gene and differ at their C-terminal ends due to alternative splicing of the corresponding RNA. The ζ and η chains are encoded for by genes on a different chromosome than are γ, δ, and ε and are structurally unrelated. The ζ chain contains a small extracellular domain of only nine amino acids, a transmembrane segment including a negatively charged residue (aspartic acid), and a large cytoplasmic tail. The cytoplasmic tail of η is 42 amino acids longer than that of ζ. The ζ and η chains exist as disulfide-linked dimers. Three dimeric forms exist (ζ–ζ, η–ζ, and η–η). The precise subunit stoichiometry of the TCR-CD3 complex has not been completely established.

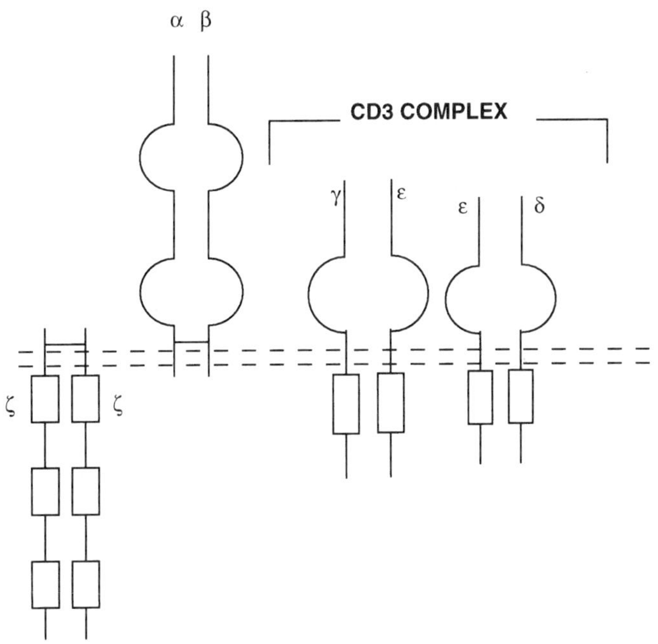

FIGURE 3–4. The TCR complex is composed of the TCR α and β chains and associated invariant chains. The CD3 complex contains the γ, δ, and ε chains; the ζ chain can be expressed as a homodimer (illustrated), as a ζ–η heterodimer, or as an η–η homodimer. The ITAMs present in the CD3 complex and in the ζ chains are depicted as rectangles. The precise stoichiometry of the TCR complex is still unknown, and the makeup of the complex may vary on different T-cell populations or even on the surface of a single T cell. It is unlikely that the δ chain can pair with the γ chain.

Because the cytoplasmic domains of the associated invariant chains are considerably larger (40–113 residues) than those of the TCR α and β chains (5 residues), it is very likely that they are responsible for coupling the TCR to the intracellular signaling machinery.[75] The γ, δ, and ε chains all contain a single ITAM (see Fig. 3–4), whereas the ζ chain has three ITAMs.[76] Following the interaction of these ITAMs with cytoplasmic protein-tyrosine kinases during the process of T-cell activation, various components of the CD3 complex become phosphorylated on their intracytoplasmic portions. The murine and human γ chains are rapidly phosphorylated upon mitogen or antigen stimulation, and minor phosphorylation of the murine δ chain also occurs. Immune activation of T cells also results in rapid and transient tyrosine phosphorylation of the ζ chain.

The major tyrosine kinases that have been implicated in the functions of the TCR are *src* family members and ZAP-70. *Lck* has the best documented role for an *src* family member in signal transduction in T cells. *Lck* interacts with cytoplasmic domains of the coreceptors CD4 and CD8 and may also interact with the TCR chains in a manner independent of CD4/CD8. The *src* family member *fyn* may also play a role in TCR signal transduction, particularly during T-cell development. ZAP-70 is a 70-kD protein-tyrosine kinase that is exclusively expressed in T cells and natural killer (NK) cells; it does not associate with the TCR in the resting state but is recruited to the ζ and CD3 chains following TCR stimulation. In order for ZAP-70 to associate with the ITAMs, they must first be phosphorylated by one of the *src* family members.[6] The interaction of ZAP-70 with phosphorylated tyrosine residues on the ITAMs is mediated by the SH2 (*src* homology 2) domain of ZAP-70. Tyrosine phosphorylation on ζ is therefore a critical step of the signal transduction pathway that communicates signals from the T-cell surface to the nucleus.

Although a minimal model of T-cell recognition of antigen would involve only the TCR and its associated complex of invariant chains interacting with a peptide bound to either MHC class I or class II molecules, the majority of T cells are equipped with a large number of cell surface molecules (Table 3–2) that assist in the process of antigen recognition by stabilizing and strengthening the binding of the T cell to the APC that bears the appropriate MHC-peptide complex. These molecules have been conveniently termed accessory molecules.[63] The two most important molecules are the coreceptors CD4 and CD8.[27] Both molecules have extracellular domains consisting of one or more Ig domains; CD4 is monomeric and CD8 is heterodimeric. The extracellular domains of CD4 and CD8 bind to MHC class I and class II molecules on APC and act as adhesion molecules to strengthen the contact between the T cell and the APC. The cytoplasmic domains of CD4 and CD8 associate with the *src* family tyrosine kinase, termed *lck*.

During the process of antigen recognition by the TCR, the CD4 and CD8 molecules cluster to the site of contact of the TCR with the MHC-antigenic peptide complex and simultaneously bind the MHC molecules and the TCR molecules. The TCR of CD4 cells binds to the outer aspect of the MHC class II molecules comprising the two helixes of the outer domains of the MHC molecule with the peptide bound in the groove between them, whereas the CD4 coreceptor binds to the lateral face of the same MHC molecule. Similarly, the

TABLE 3–2
ACCESSORY MOLECULES THAT PLAY A ROLE IN T-CELL ACTIVATION

Molecule	Molecular Weight (KD)	Ligand	Function
CD4	55	MHC II	Stabilization of TCR binding Receptor for HIV
CD8	Dimer α 32–34 β 32–34	MHC I	Stabilization of TCR binding
CD2	45	LFA-3 (CD58)	Adhesion/signal transduction
CD44	85	Hyaluronate	Adhesion to endothelium
CD45	180–270	CD22	Tyrosine protein phosphatase; may regulate *lck*
CD28	Homodimer 44	B7 (CD80/86)	Costimulation
CD11a/CD18 (LFA-1)	CD11a 180 CD18 90	ICAM-1 (CD54) ICAM-2 (CD102) ICAM-3 (CD50)	Cell-cell adhesion

CD8 molecule has been shown to facilitate the interaction of CD8⁺ T lymphocytes with class I molecules by binding to a monomorphic determinant in the α3 domain of MHC class I. This model permits CD4/CD8 and the TCR molecules to interact with MHC molecules at distinct locations. Coengagement of the TCR and coreceptor by the same MHC molecules increases the affinity of the interaction from 10- to 30-fold and results in aggregation and activation of the *lck* molecules, which play a signaling role very early in the process of signal transduction by the CD3 complex.

LFA-1 (CD11a/CD18) is a member of the Ig supergene family and plays a critical role in many intercellular interactions between T cells and other cell types.[40] LFA-1 has a wide tissue distribution and is present on most cells of lymphocytic, granulocytic, and monocytic series. mAbs to LFA-1 inhibit all T-cell functions that require cellular interactions. LFA-1 mediates its adhesive functions by binding to a number of highly related proteins, ICAM-1, ICAM-2, and ICAM-3, which are members of the Ig gene superfamily and are differentially expressed on lymphocytes, monocytes, endothelial cells, epithelial cells, and fibroblasts.[13] For example, the ICAM-3 is much better expressed than the other ICAMs on monocytes and resting lymphocytes. The interaction of LFA-1 with its ligands is also under control of signals delivered from the TCR. On resting T cells, LFA-1 exists in a low-affinity state, and its interaction with ICAM-1 is not of sufficient magnitude to stabilize cell adhesion. However, when T cells recognize antigen via their TCR, an intracellular signal is transmitted that converts LFA-1 to a high-avidity state and favors a firm LFA-1/ICAM-1 adhesion.[16]

The second most important molecule that mediates the ability of T lymphocytes to adhere to other cell types is CD2. Human T lymphocytes were first identified by their ability to form rosettes with sheep erythrocytes.[42] The CD2 molecule was later identified and shown to be the sheep erythrocyte receptor. Human CD2 is a member of the Ig gene superfamily and is a glycoprotein of 50 to 58 kD in size. CD2 mediates intercellular adhesion by binding to its ligand, LFA-3 (CD58), a 65- to 70-kD glycoprotein found on some B and T lymphocytes, all monocytes, granulocytes, and other cell types.[73] The high-affinity interactions of CD2 with LFA-3 may increase the efficiency of cell-cell interactions to a point where TCR interactions with antigen may occur efficiently. Furthermore, certain mAbs to CD2 are capable of inducing T-cell activation in the absence of other stimuli. Thus CD2 plays a dual function as both an adhesion molecule and a signal transducing molecule on T lymphocytes.

T-CELL DEVELOPMENT

In a manner similar to B cells, T cells derive from bone marrow stem cells and undergo gene rearrangements in a specialized microenvironment to produce a unique antigen receptor on each cell. However, T cells do not differentiate in the bone marrow but migrate at a very early stage to the thymus, a central lymphoid organ that provides the specialized microenvironment where receptor gene rearrangement and maturation of T cells can occur. In contrast to B cells, T cells recognize foreign antigens only in the form of peptide fragments bound to molecules encoded by the MHC. Only those T cells able to recognize the body's own MHC molecules will be capable of contributing to adaptive immune responses. Thus it is critical that T cells should be self-MHC restricted and recognize foreign peptides bound to self-MHC molecules, but the TCR should not be able to recognize self-peptides bound to MHC molecules. Self-tolerance must also exist. These dual requirements are met when T cells differentiate in the thymus.[58]

During their development as thymocytes, the cells undergo the gene rearrangements that produce the TCR and the positive and negative selection that shapes the mature receptor repertoire. The thymus contains numerous lobules, each clearly differentiated into an outer cortical region, the thymic cortex, and an inner medulla.[52] The cortex is very prominent in healthy young animals but shrinks to a thin rim in old age and in animals subjected to stress or given corticosteroids. The medulla occupies the central portion of the thymus and accounts for about 15% of thymic tissue in young animals. Cortical and medullary epithelial cells have different embryonic origins and express different cell surface markers. The developing T-cell precursors are embedded in an epithelial network known as the thymic stroma. In addition to these cell types, dendritic cells and macrophages also colonize the thymus. T-cell precursors arriving in the thymus from the bone marrow enter a phase of intense proliferation. A young adult thymus contains about 100 million cells. About 50 million cells are generated each day, but only 1 million of these will leave the thymus as mature cells. Approximately 98% of the thymocytes generated each day die within the thymus. Death occurs by a process called programmed cell death or apoptosis.

When progenitor cells enter the thymus from the bone marrow, they lack most of the surface molecules characteristic of mature T cells, and their TCR receptor genes are not rearranged. Most T-cell development takes place in the thymic cortex as only mature single positive cells are seen in the medulla. The stroma of the cortex is composed of epithelial cells with long branching processes that express MHC class II as well as MHC class I molecules. The branching processes of the thymic cortex epithelial cells make contact with most cortical thymocytes. Following interaction with the thymic stroma, the progenitors express certain T-cell surface markers such as CD2 but do not express molecules characteristic of mature T cells such as CD3, CD4/CD8. Because of the absence of CD4 and CD8, they are called double-negative (DN) thymocytes and make up about 3% to 5% of the total cells in the adult thymus (Fig. 3–5). The rapid turnover of thymocytes reflects the high rate of proliferation at the level of DN cells.[26] Very few double-positive cells or single-positive cells are in cell cycle.

The rearrangements of β and α chain genes during T-cell development closely parallel the rearrangements of Ig heavy and light chain genes during B-cell development. The β chain genes rearrange first, Dβ gene segments rearrange to Jβ gene segments, and this is followed by Vβ to DJβ gene rearrangement. The β chain protein is then expressed on the cell surface together with an invariant partner chain, which is termed the pre-TCR α chain, and the CD3 chain.[71] Although the exact role of this heterodimer has not been elucidated, like the pre–B-cell receptor complex, the heterodimer can transduce signals, trigger rapid proliferation and survival of immature T cells, and halt β chain rearrangement.

The appearance of a functional TCR β chain is accompanied by the expression of CD8 and shortly thereafter CD4. These cells are therefore called double-positive (DP) thymocytes. Early in the double-positive stage, the α chain genes

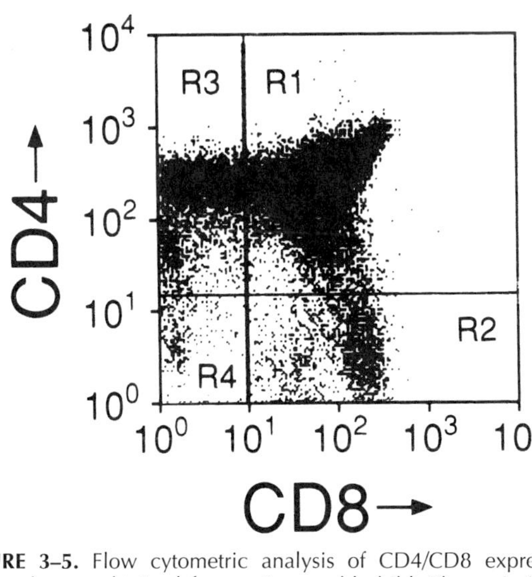

FIGURE 3–5. Flow cytometric analysis of CD4/CD8 expression of human thymus obtained from a 1-year-old child. The majority of the cells express both CD4 and CD8 (R1); there are approximately twice as many single positive CD4 cells (R3) as single positive CD8 cells (R2). Only a very small number of double negative precursors (R4) can be detected in this specimen.

rearrange, after which the complete αβ TCR complex is expressed. The TCR α chain genes are comparable to immunoglobulin κ light chain genes because they do not have D gene segments and are the second of the two chains to undergo rearrangement during normal T-cell development. Once a productive α chain rearrangement has occurred, the cells are ready to undergo selection (positive>negative) by ligands they encounter in the microenvironment of the thymus. Positive selection also determines the cell surface phenotype of the mature T cell, equipping it with the coreceptor (CD4 or CD8) that it requires for efficient antigen recognition.

The ability of thymic stromal cells to determine coreceptor specificity has suggested that the thymic stromal cell that is crucial for positive selection of thymocytes is the thymic cortical epithelial cell.[2] DP cells express only low levels of the TCR. A large percentage (about 90%) of the DP cells express receptors that cannot recognize self-MHC and therefore cannot undergo positive selection; such cells do not mature further and die. Those DP cells that do recognize self-MHC mature to express high levels of TCR and then cease to express one of the two coreceptor molecules and become either $CD4^+CD8^-$ or $CD4^-CD8^+$ single-positive thymocytes that no longer proliferate. Positive selection is also associated with termination of the TCR rearrangement process. The nature of the MHC-bound peptide that induces positive selection is still unknown. This peptide must be distinct from the peptide required for activation of mature T cells, as T cells with a TCR that recognizes a male-specific peptide can be positively selected in female mice, which lack the male antigen. Thus a process is present for positive selection of TCRs specific for peptides that do not occur in the organism.

The interaction of the TCR with self-MHC and self-peptides that leads to positive selection must differ from that for negative selection.[49] The threshold binding of MHC molecules by the TCR required to signal for positive selection is lower than the threshold required for negative selection. The TCR may send graded signals depending upon the nature and affinity of ligand binding. Weak signals are sufficient to select for survival but inadequate to delete the developing cell or to activate it once it matures. Such weak signals lead to positive selection, whereas stronger ones cause deletion. Developing T cells undergo negative selection during the transition from the double-positive stage to the single-positive stage in development. In normal mice, developing T cells in the thymus will encounter a large selection of self-peptides bound to self-MHC molecules on thymic cells, and those developing cells with receptors specific for these self-peptides will be deleted from the repertoire.

The self-peptides encountered by developing thymocytes are thought to be derived from proteins expressed in the thymus as well as from ubiquitous proteins that are brought to the thymus via the blood. Clonal deletion in the thymus, however, cannot eliminate T cells whose receptors recognize proteins found exclusively at other sites in the body that are not presented in the thymus. Immunologic tolerance to such antigens is maintained by inactivation of T cells in the periphery rather than by their deletion before they mature. The negative selection process is carried out by dendritic cells that express a high density of MHC molecules and are particularly numerous and strategically positioned at the corticomedullary junction and by macrophages that are scattered throughout the cortex but also abundant in the medulla. Both thymocytes and thymic epithelial cells also have the ability to cause deletion of self-reactive cells.

The γδ T cells arise from hematopoietic precursors like αβ T cells but differ in specificity, the pattern of expression of CD4 and CD8 coreceptors, and their anatomic distribution. The nature of the signal that initiates the decision to become an αβ T cell or a γδ T cell is unknown. It is also unknown whether this signal is delivered within the thymus or whether T-cell precursors that arrive in the thymus are committed to one pathway or another.[21] Very little is known about the function of γδ T cells, although experimental data have raised the possibility that some γδ T cells may be able to recognize antigens in the absence of MHC antigens (similar to B lymphocytes) or to recognize both classic (class I or class II) or nonclassic (TL antigens) MHC molecules in the absence of bound peptides.

Those T cells that survive both positive and negative selection are rapidly exported from the thymus to form the peripheral T-cell repertoire. Although the mechanism of cell export from the thymus is still poorly understood, most cells probably exit via veins and lymphatics at the corticomedullary junction. Peripheral T cells expressing the αβ TCR can be subdivided into two distinct nonoverlapping populations that engage in different effector functions. CD4 T lymphocytes are frequently referred to as T helper cells, as they secrete hormone-like lymphokines that support antibody production by B cells, expansion of cytotoxic T cells, and activation of macrophages as well as mast cells, basophils, and eosinophils. In contrast, CD8 lymphocytes, commonly referred to as cytotoxic T cells, function mainly as killer cells and play a major role in the destruction of virus-infected targets. Although the CD4/CD8 subsets were originally defined on the basis of these major differences in function, the critical difference in the two subsets is the nature of the antigen recognized by their TCR.[67] CD4 T cells recognize their specific ligand in the form of a peptide fragment of a non–self-protein bound to an MHC class II molecule; the peptides bound to MHC class II molecules are derived from internalized proteins as well as other proteins entering the endocytic compartment. In contrast, CD8 T cells recognize peptides mostly derived from intracellularly produced proteins, such as viral proteins, which are transported to the cell surface by peptide-binding MHC class I molecules. It is logical that cytotoxic T lymphocytes (CTL), whose primary function is to eliminate virus-infected cells, tend to recognize antigenic peptides in association with MHC class I molecules since they are expressed on all nucleated cell types.

INTERCELLULAR COMMUNICATION IN THE REGULATION OF THE IMMUNE RESPONSE

DEVELOPMENT AND DIFFERENTIATION OF EFFECTOR T CELLS

Naive CD8 T cells emerging from the thymus are already predestined to become cytotoxic cells even though they are not yet expressing any of the differentiated functions of effector cells. CD8 cells can differentiate into cytotoxic T cells by direct activation on antigen-presenting cells, which express both antigen and costimulatory molecules that directly stimulate the CD8 T cells to synthesize the IL-2 that drives their own proliferation and differentiation.[4] However, some CTL responses to viruses and tissue grafts require the presence of CD4 T cells during the priming of the CD8 cell. The CD4 T cells secrete IL-2 in response to antigen, which drives the proliferation/differentiation of the CD8 cell. The principal mechanism by which cytotoxic CD8 T cells mediate their function is by the release of secretory granules on recognition of antigen on the surface of a target cell. These secretory granules contain at least two distinct classes of protein, collectively termed cytotoxins. One of these, perforin, is a 65-kD calcium-dependent lytic protein related antigenically to the ninth component of complement.[37] Perforin can polymerize to generate transmembrane pores in cell membranes and alone can cause the rapid lysis of target cells, including red blood cells and nucleated cells. (See Chapter 4.)

The other class comprises multiple serine proteases with esterase activity, which are called granzymes.[64] CD8 cytotoxic effector cells in tissue lesions in vivo can be seen to contain granules that store perforin, and the combination of perforin and granzymes can mimic the action of CTL in vitro. Cytotoxin release from cytotoxic T cells occurs almost immediately after receptor ligation and requires no new protein or RNA synthesis. This allows cytotoxic T cells to act very rapidly on their targets, programming them for eventual lysis in a matter of minutes. However, purified granule contents cannot fully replicate killing by cytotoxic T cells. Granule-mediated killing is strictly calcium dependent, yet some cytotoxic activity of CD8 T cells survives calcium depletion.

There is a second calcium-independent mechanism of cytotoxicity that requires membrane-associated effector molecules, which like the cytokines are induced by recognition of antigen on target cells. The most important for CTL function is the Fas-ligand, which binds to a receptor called Fas on the target cell membrane.[19] Fas is a member of the TNF receptor family, and its cytoplasmic domain contains a 70 amino acid death domain that is required for transducing death signals. Most cytotoxic CD8 T cells also release IFN-γ and TNF-α, which contribute to host defense. IFN-γ has a direct effect on viral replication and induces increased expression of MHC class I antigens on infected cells, increasing the chance that infected cells will be recognized as target cells for cytotoxic attack. TNF-α and TNF-β can synergize with IFN-γ in killing some target cells by a cytokine-mediated pathway.

Most of the best understood functions of effector CD4 T cells are mediated by secreted molecules whose release is stimulated by specific recognition of antigen. In contrast to the CD8 T cells that are predestined to develop into CTL, naive CD4 T cells represent a set of relatively recent thymic emigrants that have not yet encountered antigen or responded to antigen and produce only IL-2, but no other cytokines, when initially triggered through their TCR.[53] CD4 cells can develop into Thl cells, which primarily release IFN-γ and preferentially activate macrophages, resulting in delayed hypersensitivity responses and the production of opsonizing antibodies, particularly of the IgG subclasses required for clearance of infection by intracellular organisms. Alternatively, CD4 T cells may develop into Th2 cells, which release IL-4, IL-5, IL-10, and IL-13, providing optimal help in the mouse for the production of antibodies mainly of the IgG_1 and IgE (in humans, IgG_4 and IgE) isotypes and mucosal immunity through production of growth and differentiation factors for mast cells and eosinophils and facilitation of IgA synthesis. The final decision on which of these fates the cells will follow is made rapidly during their first encounter with antigen in vivo, as immunization can yield either cell type within 7 days of priming with antigen. Some cytokines may be produced by either subset, including IL-3, GM-CSF, and TNF-α. Once established, each of these patterns of response is able to suppress the other. Thus IFN-γ from Th1 cells inhibits proliferation of Th2 cells, whereas IL-10 from Th2 cells reduces cytokine secretion from Th1 cells.

This specialization of T helper cells was first recognized in the mouse[45] but has now been clearly demonstrated in humans.[59] For example, T-cell clones from the eyelids of patients with severe pollen allergy, leading to vernal conjunctivitis, resemble Th2 cells, as do clones from the skin of patients with atopic dermatitis.[39] Clones from the CSF of patients with multiple sclerosis, a primarily IFN-γ–mediated disease, are of the Th1 type. Further support of the existence of Th1 and Th2 cells was derived from studies of T-cell clones from the same individual. Whereas the majority of clones specific for tuberculin (i.e., PPD) secreted IL-2 and IFN-γ, but not IL-4 or IL-5, most clones specific for an antigen derived from *Toxocara canis* secreted IL-4 and IL-5, but not IL-2 and IFN-γ. IL-10 and IL-13 tend to segregate less clearly among human CD4 cells than the mouse. Human Th1 and Th2 clones also differ in their responsiveness to cytokines. IL-4 potentiates the antigen-induced proliferation and cytokine production of Th2 clones, but not Th1 clones. IFN-γ selectively inhibited the response and cytokine production of Th2 clones. The majority of allergen-specific T-cell clones are of the Th2 type; however, allergen-specific clones from nonatopic individuals appear to be of the Th1 type, and PPD-specific clones from allergic individuals are of the Th2 type. This suggests that some deregulation of cytokine gene expression may be responsible for the atopic phenotype. Th2 cells from the peripheral blood are easily recruited and expanded by allergen in the airway mucosa and play a crucial role in the induction and maintenance of allergic inflammation.

The factors that determine whether a proliferating CD4 T cell will differentiate into an inflammatory Th1 cell or a helper Th2 cell are not well understood.[46] Although it was initially believed that these two cell populations with distinctive lymphokine-producing phenotypes represented distinct cell lineages that separated from one another prior to their contact with antigen, it is now clear that they are the product of a differentiation step that occurs at the time of antigen-specific activation of the cell. Thus an individual naive T cell can give rise to cells that produce both IL-4 and IFN-γ. The pre–T helper cell is multipotential, and the initial event that determines lymphokine-producing phenotype is not the selective outgrowth of already committed cells but rather the differentiation of pre–T helper cells under the influence of factors present at the time of primary stimulation (Table 3–3). The critical role of IL-4 itself in priming for IL-4 production has been best studied with T cells from TCR transgenic mice.[62] Purified naive T cells from transgenic mice proliferated and secreted IL-2 when cultured with antigen and a source of APC. The presence of IL-4 in the priming culture allowed the T cells to develop into cells that produced IL-4 upon restimulation. The type of APC used in the priming culture (B cells, macrophages, or dendritic cells) appeared to have no role in directing the development of IL-4–producing cells.

In contrast to the lack of effect of the type of APC in the priming of Th2 cells, the nature of the APC plays a major role in the priming and development of Th1 cells.[25] Activated macrophages obtained by incubation with heat-killed *Listeria monocytogenes* enhanced priming for IFN-γ production. Indeed, such macrophages enhanced priming for IFN-γ production even when they could not present antigen. A soluble factor released from the macrophages mediated this effect and was shown to be IL-12. Addition of IL-12 enhanced priming for IFN-γ production by 10-fold in the absence of any source of activated macrophages (see Table 3–3). Thus IL-4 and IL-12 play critical and opposing roles as regulators of T helper cell differentiation.[70] IL-4 blocks the priming of naive cells to develop into Th1 cells. This effect is total if IL-12 is not present in the priming culture and is significant, but incomplete, in the presence of exogenous IL-12. The in vitro differentiation of naive cells to Th2 cells under the influence of IL-4 is partially inhibitable by IFN-γ, particularly in the presence of suboptimal amounts of IL-4. IL-12 does not directly inhibit priming of IL-4 production, but since it induces IFN-γ production by both T cells and NK cells, the addition of IL-12 diminishes priming for IL-4 production indirectly.

One of the most critical questions regarding the regulation of the development of Th1/Th2 populations is the source of the IL-4 and IL-12 that controls differentiation of the precur-

TABLE 3–3
ROLE OF CYTOKINES IN THE DIFFERENTIATION OF TH1 AND TH2 SUBPOPULATIONS

First Culture			Cytokine Production in Second Culture	
T cells	*Antigen*	*Cytokine*	*IL-4*	*IFN-γ*
+	+	–	–	+ +
+	+	IL-4	+ + + +	–
+	+	IL-4 + IFN-γ	+ +	–
+	+	IL-12	–	+ + + +
+	+	IL-12 + IL-4	–	+ +

Naive T cells from TCR transgenic mice are cultured for 4 to 7 days with antigen and the indicated cytokine. They are then washed and restimulated with antigen and no added cytokines. Cytokine production in the second culture is measured after 48 hours. The presence of no added cytokine in the first culture results in a modest degree of priming for IFN-γ production. IL-4 primes for IL-4, IL-12 primes for IFN-γ, and both cytokines cross-regulate the production of the other.

sor populations. Macrophages infected with intracellular microorganisms produce IL-12. This IL-12 can act on NK cells for rapid induction of IFN-γ production by these cells and together with APC can prime naive T cells to become IFN-γ producers. Since IFN-γ is effective in inducing microbicidal activity in macrophages, it is logical that macrophages make IL-12 in response to the type of infectious microorganism that is best controlled by IFN-γ–induced macrophages.

The IFN-γ produced by both T cells and NK cells will suppress the development of IL-4–producing cells. The source of IL-4 used in the physiologic priming process is not clear. Basophils, mast cells, or both can produce IL-4 in response to cross-linkage of FcεRI or FcγRII.[54] This mechanism requires the existence of IgG or IgE antibodies specific for epitopes of the antigen for the basophil or the mast cells to be stimulated to make IL-4. IL-4 may be produced by T cells or by a specialized subpopulation of CD4 cells that bear the NK1.1 antigen.[77] It has not been determined whether the preferential ability of helminth antigens or allergens to expand Th2 cells is related to their molecular structure, to the type of APC involved in their processing, or to other microenvironmental influences at the site of immunization. Perhaps certain allergens and some parasite antigens fail to induce IL-12 production by macrophages and are poor stimulators of NK cells. Under these conditions, Th1 cells would not be induced, and if IL-4 was available, a Th2 response might be facilitated.

Although cytokines play an important role in priming of Th1 and Th2 cells, it is also possible that the immunogenic antigen can determine whether a Th1 or Th2 pattern of response will occur. Some studies have suggested that the concentration of antigen presented to the naive T cell at the time of priming may control the pattern of cytokines produced by the responding T cells.[11] Low antigen density favors differentiation to Th2 cells, high antigen density favors differentiation to Th1 cells, and very high antigen density may shut off Th1 responses to again reveal Th2 responses.

COSTIMULATION OF LYMPHOCYTE GROWTH

The activation of naive CD4 T cells by antigen may be the most important event in the initiation of adaptive immunity.[28] As antigen-specific naive lymphocytes that recognize antigen are present in the host at a very low frequency, they have to proliferate to increase their frequency before they can differentiate into effector cells that can regulate the activation of B cells, in some cases CD8 T cells and macrophages, and ultimately control the immune response that leads to the elimination of a pathogen. Naive CD4 T cells require two distinct signals to proliferate and subsequently differentiate into armed effector cells that mediate adaptive immunity.[61] One of the signals is delivered by the TCR, which recognizes peptide fragments bound to MHC class II molecules. The second signal, which is not delivered via the TCR, is not antigen specific and has been termed a costimulatory signal. Although the second signal is essential for the proliferation and differentiation of CD4 T cells into effector cells, it does not by itself induce any response in T cells.

On activation, CD4 T cells must enter the cell cycle and divide rapidly to produce large numbers of progeny that will differentiate into armed effector cells. Their proliferation and differentiation are driven by IL-2. The production of IL-2 is what determines whether a T cell will proliferate and become an armed effector cell, and the most important function of costimulation is to promote the synthesis of IL-2. The combination of antigen and costimulation induces naive T cells to express IL-2 and its receptor, and IL-2 induces clonal expansion of the naive T cell and the differentiation of its progeny into effector T cells, which are able to synthesize all the cytokines required for their specialized function as Th1, Th2, or cytotoxic cells.

More important, T cells that bind antigen, but do not receive a costimulatory signal, are thought to die or to become anergic, a state in which the cell cannot be activated even if it subsequently receives both of the signals required to activate a naive T cell (Table 3–4). The most important change in anergic T cells is their inability to produce IL-2, which prevents them from proliferating and differentiating into effector cells. Thus an encounter of T cells with antigen can lead to two distinct outcomes—proliferation and differentiation into effector cells or inactivation and death. The appropriate delivery of costimulatory signals determines the fate of antigen-specific CD4 cells.

The expression of costimulator molecules must be carefully regulated so that responses are mounted when needed but avoided when they may be harmful. It appears that CD4 T cells respond most efficiently to costimulatory molecules when they are expressed on the same cell as the ligand for the TCR.[38] Thus only cells that express costimulatory molecules can effectively activate naive CD4 T cells. In addition, when CD4 T cells encounter antigen on costimulator negative cells, they are likely to become anergic even when costimulator positive cells are also present. This process may be very important in maintaining tolerance to self-tissue cells, as it allows active costimulatory cells to coexist with costimulator negative tissue cells expressing autoantigens not found in the thymus.

Although multiple molecules may be identified that can deliver costimulatory signals to CD4 T cells, the most prominent are members of the B7 family (B7-1/CD80, B7-2/CD86) of antigens that deliver their antigen-independent costimulatory signal by binding to the T-cell surface molecule CD28.[36] CD28 is found on naive T cells, and naive T cells will also proliferate if they are stimulated by a combination of antibodies to CD3 and CD28; anti-CD28 can also provide the costimulatory signal required to block the induction of anergy. The ligation of CD28 by B7 leads to stabilization of IL-2 mRNA, which increases IL-2 synthesis 20- to 30-fold and IL-2 transcription by about 3-fold.

A second receptor for the B7 antigens, CTLA4, has also been identified.[35] CTLA4 is closely related to CD28, as both are members of the immunoglobulin superfamily and have a nucleotide sequence homology of about 75%. The genes have similar genomic organization and are chromosomally linked in both human and mouse. Although CD28 is constitutively expressed at high levels on all T cells, CTLA4 expression is not expressed on resting CD4 cells but is transiently detectable 2 to 3 days after T-cell activation. Although B7-1/B7-2 molecules exhibit only a low degree of sequence homology (15%), they have remarkably similar binding affinities for CD28 and CTLA4. Both bind approximately 100-fold better to CTLA4 than to CD28. However, CTLA4 is not

TABLE 3–4
INDUCTION OF T-CELL ANERGY BY ANTIGEN-SPECIFIC ACTIVATION IN THE ABSENCE OF COSTIMULATION

	First Culture		Second Culture
T cells	*Antigen*	*Costimulation*	*Antigen-Specific Proliferation*
+	+	+	++++
+	−	−	++
+	−	+	++
+	+	+	−

Antigen-specific T cells are cultured for 2 to 4 days in the presence or absence of antigen and the presence or absence of costimulation. They are then washed and restimulated with antigen and costimulation. T cells stimulatd with antigen and a competent source of costimulation expand and mount a strong response in the second culture. T cells cultured without antigen in the presence or absence of costimulation respond normally in the second culture. In contrast, T cells cultured with antigen in the absence of costimulation are anergic (nonresponsive) in the second culture.

found on naive T cells in normal mice or humans and is not thought to be involved in the initial stages of naive T-cell activation.

When CTLA4 is produced as a soluble fusion protein with the constant domain of immunoglobulin G (termed, CTLA4Ig), it acts as a high-affinity soluble B7 binding protein. CTLA4Ig inhibits many different CD4 T cell responses to antigens in vitro and in vivo. More important, when CD4 T cells are stimulated with specific antigen in the presence of CTLA4Ig and then challenged with the same antigen in the absence of CTLA4Ig, they no longer respond to that antigen, but the population of cells can respond to other antigens. Thus inactivation is mediated by the antigen and affects only specific T cells. This shows that stimulation of CD4 T cells with antigen in the absence of engagement of CD28 can induce a state of unresponsiveness or anergy. Moreover, CTLA4Ig can induce tolerance in vivo when given in conjunction with tissue grafts in some experimental systems.

The importance of B7 as a costimulatory molecule in vivo has been tested in several experimental systems. Nonimmunogenic transplantable tumor cells can become immunogenic if they are transfected with the B7 gene, and mice that have rejected such B7 transfected tumor cells now have active immunity against the nontransfected tumor. These responses are elicited by MHC class II negative and class II positive tumors and thus involve both CD8 and CD4 cells. It is therefore clear that CD8 T cells that recognize peptide antigens in association with MHC class I molecules can also use B7 as a costimulator and that molecules that costimulate the growth of CD4 T cells also appear to costimulate the growth of CD8 T cells. Although mice that lack CD28 are significantly compromised in their ability to mount adaptive immune responses, their defect is not absolute and they are not totally immunodeficient. Other undefined cell surface molecules may also mediate costimulatory function of T cells in these mice.

Costimulatory activity cannot be delivered by nonlymphoid cells. The expression of costimulatory molecules on the three major cell types that present antigen to CD4 T cells, B cells, macrophages, and dendritic cells is differentially regulated. Costimulatory activity appears to be expressed constitutively only by dendritic cells and perhaps by certain macrophage subpopulations. Resting B cells do not express B7 on their cell surface, but activation by a number of different stimuli, including microbial products such as lipopolysaccharide, ligation of MHC class II molecules, binding of antigen to sIg, and cross-linking of the CD40 antigen are capable of inducing the expression of B7 on B cells. In addition, there are important differences in the distribution of the two costimulatory molecules, B7-1/CD80 and B7-2/CD86. CD86 is rapidly up-regulated by activation of most cell types, whereas CD80 appears more slowly. B7 can also be induced on T cells, and activated T cells can become costimulatory for other T cells. Thus the control of the level of costimulatory activity on different types of APC may regulate which specific antigens may be presented to naive CD4 T cells.

The functional role of the second receptor for the B7 antigens on T cells, the CTLA4 antigen, has been elusive. CTLA4 cannot replace CD28 in providing costimulation in CD28 mutant mice, ruling out functional redundancy. A rampant lymphoproliferative disorder occurs in CTLA4-deficient mice, raising the possibility that this molecule is critical for the negative regulation of T-cell responses.[69] Because CTLA4 is expressed maximally on T cells only transiently for 2 days or so after activation, inhibitory signals generated by its engagement with B7 molecules on APC may be instrumental in terminating lymphokine production and the proliferation of activated T cells.[35] Thus the outcome of T-cell activation may be determined by regulation of the balance between positive signals from CD28 and negative signals from CTLA4.

All of the studies on the role of costimulatory molecules in the induction of T-cell activation have strongly supported the concept that IL-2–induced T-cell proliferation is a key determinant affecting the magnitude of the immune response. A number of immunosuppressive drugs have been shown to exert their effects by blocking steps in the IL-2 activation cascade.[65, 72] Cyclosporin and FK-506 inhibit T-cell activation by blocking TCR-initiated signals that lead to the transcription of the IL-2 gene. Following the binding of these drugs to their intracellular receptors, cyclophilin and FK-506 binding protein, respectively, the drug-receptor complex inhibits the Ca^{2+} calmodulin-dependent protein phosphatase, calcineurin. The inhibition of calcineurin results in the failure to dephosphorylate the cytoplasmic component of the T-cell–specific transcription factor, nuclear factor of activated T cells (NF-AT), with resultant inhibition of transcription of IL-2. Although the immunosuppressive drug rapamycin also binds to FK-506 binding protein, it does not block the synthesis of IL-2 but inhibits the ability of IL-2 to induce cell proliferation. Collectively, the studies on costimulation and immunosuppressive drugs confirm the dominant role of IL-2 in controlling T lymphocyte expansion and also demonstrate that suppression of the production and/or action of IL-2 is a valuable therapeutic approach to controlling graft rejection or treating autoimmune diseases.

HOW T AND B CELLS COMMUNICATE

Antibody responses to most protein antigens require T-cell help, and antigens that require T-cell help are termed thymus-dependent (TD) antigens. Thymus-independent antigens, which are microbial products, particularly bacterial polysaccharides, can directly induce B cells to make antibody in the absence of helper T cells. Surface Ig on B cells plays two roles in B-cell activation. First, like the antigen receptor on T cells, the BCR directly transmits a signal to the cell interior upon binding antigen. Second, it delivers the antigen to intracellular sites, where it is degraded and from which it is returned to the B-cell surface as peptides bound to MHC class II molecules. The peptide MHC class II molecules can then be recognized by antigen-specific helper cells that in turn secrete factors that cause the B cell to proliferate and differentiate into antibody-producing cells.[7] B cells only become effective targets for activated T cells when antigen bound by sIg is internalized and returned to the cell surface as peptides bound to MHC class II molecules. Helper T cells that recognize the peptide MHC complex can then deliver activating signals to the B cell. Thus protein antigen binding to the B cell provides both a specific signal to the B cell and a focus for T-cell help.

In TD responses, the helper T cell and the B cells recognize the same antigen, a process called linked recognition. Although the epitope recognized by the helper T cell must be linked to that recognized by the B cell, the two cells need not recognize identical epitopes. T cells can recognize internal peptides in proteins that are quite distinct from the surface epitopes recognized by B cells. Even though a B cell can bind a self-antigen and present peptides derived from it on its cell surface, if the T cells that recognize the peptides have been deleted in the thymus or rendered tolerant in the periphery, no T-cell help will be available to activate the B cell and the animal will remain tolerant.

Although all naive B cells express IgM and IgD, less than 10% of the Ig found in plasma is IgM. The effector activity of antibody is determined by the isotype of its heavy chain constant domains. A given heavy chain variable domain can become associated with the constant region of any isotype through a process called isotype switching. Most antibody is therefore produced by B cells that have undergone isotype switching. The changes in the functional properties of antibody molecules that result from isotype switching and the changes in the variable regions that allow affinity maturation depend on the interaction of antigen-stimulated B cells with helper T cells and other cells in peripheral lymphoid organs. Helper T cells control isotype switching and play a role initiating somatic hypermutation of antibody variable region genes, which is required for the affinity maturation of antibodies that occurs during a humoral response. Chickens or mice treated with anti-μ antibodies fail to develop antibodies of any immunoglobulin class, which clearly demonstrates that the cells carrying non-IgM classes are the progeny of the IgM-bearing B cells. B cells switch from IgM to the other isotypes by a process of recombination between highly repetitive switch regions 5′ to each heavy chain constant region gene.

The process of activation of helper T cells begins in the paracortical region of lymphoid tissues, where bone marrow–derived dendritic cells present MHC class II bound peptides to CD4⁺ T cells. It is likely that bone marrow–derived dendritic cells, rather than B cells themselves, are the cell type to initially present antigen to the CD4 T cell, as dendritic cells express high levels of the costimulatory molecules B7-1/B7-2 as well as the adhesion molecules ICAM-1 (CD54) and LFA-3 (CD58); resting B cells lack expression of these molecules. The CD4 and CD2 coreceptors on T cells help signaling through the TCR after binding to MHC class II and CD58, their respective ligands on the bone marrow–derived dendritic cells. Cross-linking of the TCR also activates CD11a/CD18 (LFA-1), which can then bind to its ligand ICAM-1 (CD54) on the dendritic cell.[16] Once activated, the T cells in turn promote B-cell activation both by releasing T-cell–derived cytokines and by direct intercellular contact.

The most important T-cell surface molecule induced in the process of T-cell activation that plays a critical role in the early phase of the B-cell response is the CD40 ligand (CD40L, also called gp39), a member of the TNF family of cytokines that binds to CD40 (a 45- to 50-kD protein that is a member of the TNF receptor family of cytokine receptors) on the B-cell surface.[15] Resting T cells that lack CD40L cannot help B cells. CD40 is expressed on late pre–B cells in the bone marrow, mature B cells, and a variety of accessory cells, including macrophages and both bone marrow–derived dendritic cells and FDC. Binding of CD40L to CD40 is needed for the promotion of B-cell proliferation, prevention of apoptosis of germinal center B cells, and promotion of Ig class switching. The interaction of CD40L with CD40 (Fig. 3–6) as well as the cross-linking of MHC class II on B cells by the TCR results in the up-regulation of B7-1/B7-2 expression on the responding B cells, and B7-1/B7-2 can in turn signal to the T cell via CD28.[32] Cross-linking of CD28 on activated T cells may produce a further increase in the expression of CD40L.[14]

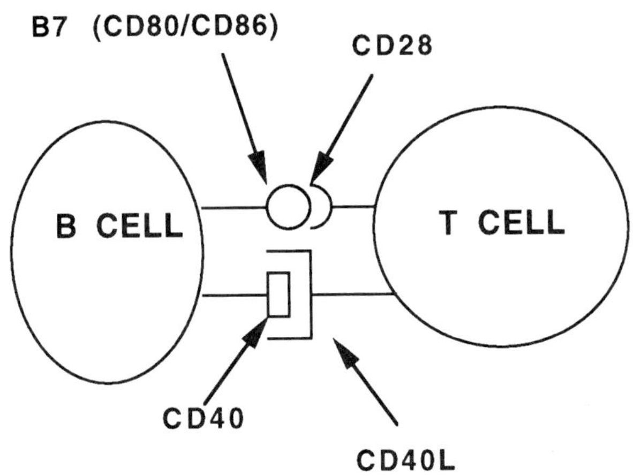

FIGURE 3–6. The interactions of CD40L/CD40 and CD28/B7 synergistically function to facilitate T-B cooperation. Activation of the T cell by antigen up-regulates the expression of the CD40L on the T-cell surface, which then binds to CD40 on the B cell. The CD40L/CD40 interaction up-regulates the expression of B7 on the B cell, which in turn binds to CD28 on the T cell, leading to enhanced expression of the CD40L.

Fully activated B cells that express high levels of B7-1/B7-2 are also highly efficient APC, which can augment T-cell activation via the TCR. This reciprocal dialogue may occur in peripheral lymphoid T-cell zones after T-cell activation or in the basal light zones of germinal centers, where CD40L$^+$ T cells have also been found. However, following the engagement of CD40L with CD40, CD40L is rapidly internalized or shed from the cell surface, ensuring that this potent interaction is short-lived. There is a great similarity in the outcome of cell signaling through CD40 on B cells or CD28 on T cells, as both signals result in cell proliferation stimulated by antigen receptor cross-linking. Both signals also prevent apoptosis or specific unresponsiveness that would occur upon engagement of the TCR or BCR. Furthermore, blockade of the interaction of B7-1/B7-2 with CD28 not only interferes with T-cell proliferation and B-cell maturation induced by T-cell cytokines but also blocks primary antibody responses.

Patients with mutations in CD40L make very weak and ineffective antibody responses and suffer from severe immunodeficiency.[34] Isotype switching does not occur in individuals with mutations of CD40L who have high levels of IgM, which is probably induced by thymus-independent antigens. Furthermore, genetic defects or reagents that block CD40L/CD40 interactions prevent formation of germinal centers and block the development of both primary and secondary antibody responses. It is not clear where the CD40L/CD40 interactions necessary for germinal center formation or class switching take place. CD40/CD40L interaction may also regulate interactions of T cells with non–B cells, as interaction of CD40L with CD40 on macrophages has been shown to promote the production of IL-12, which plays a major role in the generation of Th1 cells.

Different cytokines play roles at several steps in the interaction of the T helper cell with the B cell, and certain cytokines preferentially induce switching to different isotypes. Naive B cells must undergo a clonal expansion before they can differentiate into effector cells, and so a proliferative phase precedes the differentiation of B cells into antibody-secreting plasma cells. Activation of B cells by CD40L and IL-4 drive the clonal expansion that precedes antibody production in vivo. IL-4 also induces switching to IgG1 and IgE (in humans, IgG_4 and IgE) with suppression of the other isotypes, whereas in mouse mucosal tissues, TGF-β production by T cells preferentially induces switching to IgG2b and IgA. IL-5 induces secretion of IgA by cells that have already undergone switching. In the mouse, IFN-γ preferentially induces switching to IgG3 and IgG2a but suppresses all other isotypes. Cytokines induce isotype switching by making the switch recombination sites that lie 5′ to each CH gene accessible to switch recombinases. IL-5 and IL-6 also contribute to the later stages of B-cell activation.

The immune response to environmental allergens is mediated in a manner similar to that of all other foreign antigens.[59] Allergens are taken up by MHC class II–positive APC and presented to T helper cells. Activated T helper cells then induce B lymphocytes to produce allergen-specific antibodies mainly of the IgE class. However, the basis for the preferential IgE production in individuals genetically determined to recognize allergen epitopes is still unclear. It is widely accepted that IL-4 and IL-13 are the main regulatory cytokines responsible for IgE production. IL-4 and IL-13 induce in B cells a sterile ϵ-germline transcript, and then the interaction between CD40L on activated T cells and CD40 molecules on B cells results in a signal leading to a productive ϵ-transcript. T cells that produce high amounts of IL-4 and IL-5, but only limited amounts of IFN-γ, can be identified in the blood and/or target organs of patients with helminth infections or atopic disorders and can account for the IgE antibody formation and eosinophilia observed in these patients. Recombinant IL-4 and IL-13 can induce the synthesis of IgE in peripheral blood mononuclear cells, and this effect is inhibited by addition of IFN-γ, IFN-α, IL-12, and PGE_2. Mast cells may also secrete IL-4 and express CD40L on their surface and may play a role in the control of IgE synthesis by B cells.

REFERENCES

1. Allison JP, Lanier LL: Structure, function and serology of the T-cell antigen receptor complex. Annu Rev Immunol 5:503, 1987.
2. Anderson G, Jenkinson EJ, Moore NC, et al: MHC class II-positive epithelium and mesenchyme cells are both required for T-cell development in the thymus. Nature 362:70, 1993.
3. Banchereau J, Rousset F: Human B lymphocytes: phenotype, proliferation, and differentiation. Adv Immunol 52:125, 1992.
4. Berke G: The binding and lysis of target cells by cytotoxic lymphocytes: molecular and cellular aspects. Annu Rev Immunol 12:735, 1994.
5. Cambier JC, Pleiman CM, Clark MR: Signal transduction by the B cell antigen receptor and its coreceptors. Annu Rev Immunol 12:457, 1994.
6. Chan AC, Iwashima M, Turck CW, et al: ZAP-70: a 70 kd protein-tyrosine kinase that associates with the TCR ζ chain. Cell 71:649, 1992.
7. Clark EA, Ledbetter JA: How B and T cells talk to each other. Nature 367:425, 1994.
8. Clark EA, Lane PJL: Regulation of human B-cell activation and adhesion. Annu Rev Immunol 9:97, 1991.
9. Clark MR, Johnson SA, Cambier JC: Analysis of Ig-α–tyrosine kinase interaction reveals two levels of binding specificity and tyrosine phosphorylated Ig-α stimulation of Fyn activity. EMBO J 13:1911, 1994.
10. Clevers H, Alarcon B, Wileman T, et al: The T cell receptor/CD3 complex: a dynamic protein ensemble. Annu Rev Immunol 6:629, 1988.
11. Constant S, Pfeiffer C, Woodard A, et al: Extent of T cell receptor ligation can determine the functional differentiation of naive CD4$^+$ T cells. J Exp Med 182:1591, 1995.
12. Cyster JG, Goodnow CC: Antigen-induced exclusion from follicles and anergy are separate and complementary processes that influence peripheral B cell fate. Immunity 3:691, 1995.
13. de Fougerolles AR, Stacker SA, Schwarting R, et al: Characterization of ICAM-2 and evidence for a third counter-receptor for LFA-1. J Exp Med 174:253, 1991.
14. Ding L, Green JM, Thompson CB, et al: B7/CD28-Dependent and -independent induction of CD40 ligand expression. J Immunol 155:5124, 1995.
15. Durie FH, Foy TM, Masters SR, et al: The role of CD40 in the regulation of humoral and cell-mediated immunity. Immunol Today 15:406, 1994.
16. Dustin ML, Springer TA: T-cell receptor crosslinking transiently stimulates adhesiveness through LFA-1. Nature 341:619, 1989.
17. Ehlich A, Schaal S, Gu H, et al: Immunoglobulin heavy and light chain genes rearrange independently at early stages of B cell development. Cell 72:695, 1993.
18. Flaswinkel H, Reth M: Dual role of the tyrosine activation motif of the Ig-α protein during signal transduction via the B cell antigen receptor. EMBO J 13:83, 1994.
19. Golstein P, Marguet D, Depraetere V: Fas bridging cell death and cytotoxicity: the reaper connection. Immunol Rev 146:45, 1995.
20. Goodnow CC: Transgenic mice and analysis of B-cell tolerance. Annu Rev Immunol 10:489, 1992.
21. Haas W, Pereira P, Tonegawa S: Gamma/delta cells. Annu Rev Immunol 11:637, 1993.
22. Han S, Zheng B, Dal Porto J, et al: In situ studies of the primary immune response to (4-hydroxy-3-nitrophenyl)-acetyl IV. Affinity-de-

pendent, antigen-driven B cell apoptosis in germinal centers as a mechanism for maintaining self-tolerance. J Exp Med 182:1635, 1995.
23. Hardy RR, Carmack CE, Shinton SA, et al: Resolution and characterization of pro-B and pre–pro-B cell stages in normal mouse bone marrow. J Exp Med 173:1213, 1991.
24. Hayashi S-I, Kunisada T, Ogawa M, et al: Stepwise progression of B lineage differentiation supported by interleukin 7 and other stromal cell molecules. J Exp Med 171:1683, 1990.
25. Hsieh C-S, Heimberger AB, Gold JS, et al: Differential regulation of T helper phenotype development by interleukins 4 and 10 in an $\alpha\beta$ T-cell–receptor transgenic system. Proc Natl Acad Sci USA 89:6065, 1992.
26. Jameson SC, Hogquist KA, Bevan MJ: Positive selection of thymocytes. Annu Rev Immunol 13:93, 1995.
27. Janeway CA Jr: The T cell receptor as a multicomponent signalling machine: CD4/CD8 coreceptors and CD45 in T cell activation. Annu Rev Immunol 10:645, 1992.
28. Janeway CA Jr: Signals and signs for lymphocyte responses. Cell 76:275, 1994.
29. Karasuyama H, Rolink A, Melchers F: A complex of glycoproteins is associated with V_{pre}/λ_5 surrogate light chain on the surface of μ heavy chain-negative early precursor B cell lines. J Exp Med 178:469, 1993.
30. Kelsoe G: The germinal center reaction. Immunol Today 16:324, 1995.
31. Kelsoe G: Life and death in germinal centers (redux). Immunity 4:107, 1996.
32. Kennedy MK, Mohler KM, Shanebeck KD, et al: Induction of B cell costimulatory function by recombinant murine CD40 ligand. Eur J Immunol 24:116, 1994.
33. Kincade PW, Lee G, Pietrangeli CE, et al: Cells and molecules that regulate B lymphopoiesis in bone marrow. Annu Rev Immunol 7:111, 1989.
34. Kroczek RA, Graf D, Brugnoni D, et al: Defective expression of CD40 ligand on T cells causes "X-linked immunodeficiency with hyper-IgM (HIGM1)." Immunol Rev 138:39, 1994.
35. Krummel MF, Allison JP: CD28 and CTLA-4 have opposing effects on the response of T cells to stimulation. J Exp Med 182:459, 1995.
36. Linsley PS: Distinct roles of CD28 and cytotoxic T lymphocyte-associated molecule-4 receptors during T cell activation? J Exp Med 182:289, 1995.
37. Liu C-C, Persechini PM, Young JD-E: Perforin and lymphocyte-mediated cytolysis. Immunol Rev 146:145, 1995.
38. Liu Y, Janeway CA Jr: Cells that present both specific ligand and costimulatory activity are the most efficient inducers of clonal expansion of normal CD4 T cells. Proc Natl Acad Sci USA 89:3845, 1992.
39. Maggi E, Romagnani S: Role of T cells and T-cell–derived cytokines in the pathogenesis is allergic diseases. Ann NY Acad Sci 725:2, 1994.
40. Martz E: LFA-1 and other accessory molecules functioning in adhesions of T and B lymphocytes. Hum Immunol 18:3, 1987.
41. Melchers F, Haasner D, Grawunder U, et al: Roles of IgH and L chains and of surrogate H and L chains in the development of cells of the B lymphocyte lineage. Annu Rev Immunol 12:209, 1994.
42. Meuer SC, Hussey RE, Fabbi M, et al: An alternative pathway of T-cell activation: a functional role for the 50 kd T11 sheep erthyrocyte receptor protein. Cell 36:8997, 1984.
43. Miyake K, Medina KL, Hayashi S-I, et al: Monoclonal antibodies to Pgp-1/CD44 block lympho-hemopoiesis in long-term bone marrow cultures. J Exp Med 171:477, 1990.
44. Miyake K, Medina K, Ishihara K, et al: A VCAM-like adhesion molecule in murine bone marrow stromal cells mediates binding of lymphocyte precursors in culture. J Cell Biol 114:557, 1991.
45. Mosmann TR, Coffman RL: TH1 and TH2 cells: different patterns of lymphokine secretion lead to different functional properties. Annu Rev Immunol 7:145, 1989.
46. Mosmann TR, Sad S: The expanding universe of T-cell subsets: Th1, Th2 and more. Immunol Today 17:138, 1996.
47. Moss PAH, Rosenberg WMC, Bell JI: The human T cell receptor in health and disease. Annu Rev Immunol 10:71, 1992.
48. Murakami M, Honjo T: Involvement of B-1 cells in mucosal immunity and autoimmunity. Immunol Today 16:534, 1995.
49. Nossal GJV: Negative selection of lymphocytes. Cell 76:229, 1994.
50. Nossal GJV: Differentiation of the secondary B-lymphocyte repertoire: the germinal center reaction. Immunol Rev 137:173, 1994.
51. Ogawa M, Matsuzaki Y, Nishikawa S, et al: Expression and function of c-*kit* in hemopoietic progenitor cells. J Exp Med 174:63, 1991.
52. Owen JJT, Moore NC: Thymocyte-stromal-cell interactions and T-cell selection. Immunol Today 16:336, 1995.
53. Paul WE, Seder RA: Lymphocyte responses and cytokines. Cell 76:241, 1994.
54. Paul WE, Seder RA, Plaut M: Lymphokine and cytokine production by FcϵRI+ cells. Adv Immunol 53:1, 1992.
55. Pleiman CM, D'Ambrosio D, Cambier JC: The B-cell antigen receptor complex: structure and signal transduction. Immunol Today 15:393, 1994.
56. Raulet DH: The structure, functions, and molecular genetics of the γ/δ T cell receptor. Annu Rev Immunol 7:175, 1989.
57. Reth M: Antigen receptors on B lymphocytes. Annu Rev Immunol 10:97, 1992.
58. Robey E, Fowlkes BJ: Selective events in T cell development. Annu Rev Immunol 12:675, 1994.
59. Romagnani S: Lymphokine production by human T cells in disease states. Annu Rev Immunol 12:227, 1994.
60. Schulte RJ, Campbell M-A, Fischer WH, et al: Tyrosine phosphorylation of CD22 during B cell activation. Science 258:1001, 1992.
61. Schwartz RH: Costimulation of T lymphocytes: the role of CD28, CTLA-4, and B7/BB1 in interleukin-2 production and immunotherapy. Cell 71:1065, 1992.
62. Seder RA, Paul WE, David MM, et al: The presence of interleukin 4 during in vitro priming determines the lymphokine-producing potential of $CD4^+$ T cells from T cell receptor transgenic mice. J Exp Med 176:1091, 1992.
63. Shevach EM: Accessory molecules. In Paul WE (ed): Fundamental Immunology, 3rd edition. Raven Press, New York, 1993, p 531.
64. Shresta S, Heusel JW, Macivor DM, et al: Granzyme B plays a critical role in cytotoxic lymphocyte-induced apoptosis. Immunol Rev 146:211, 1995.
65. Sigal NH, Dumont FJ: Cyclosporin A, FK-506, and Rapamycin: pharmacologic probes of lymphocyte signal transduction. Annu Rev Immunol 10:519, 1992.
66. Stamenkovic I, Sgrol D, Aruffo A, et al: The B lymphocyte adhesion molecule CD22 interacts with leukocyte common antigen CD45RO on T cells and α2-6 sialytransferase, CD75, on B cells. Cell 66:1133, 1991.
67. Swain SL: T cell subsets and the recognition of MHC class. Immunol Rev 74:129, 1983.
68. Tedder TF, Zhou L-J, Engel P: The CD19/CD21 signal transduction complex of B lymphocytes. Immunol Today 15:437, 1994.
69. Tivol EA, Borriello F, Schweitzer AN, et al: Loss of CTLA-4 leads to massive lymphoproliferation and fatal multiorgan tissue destruction, revealing a critical negative regulatory role of CTLA-4. Immunity 3:541, 1995.
70. Trinchieri G: Interleukin-12: a proinflammatory cytokine with immunoregulatory functions that bridge innate resistance and antigen-specific adaptive immunity. Annu Rev Immunol 13:251, 1995.
71. von Boehmer H: Positive selection of lymphocytes. Cell 76:219, 1994.
72. Waldmann TA: The IL-2/IL-2 receptor system: a target for rational immune intervention. Immunol Today 14:264, 1993.
73. Wallner BP, Frey AZ, Tizard R, et al: Primary structure of lymphocyte function-associated antigen 3 (LFA-3). The ligand of the T lymphocyte CD2 glycoprotein. J Exp Med 166:923, 1987.
74. Weiss A: Molecular and genetic insights into T cell antigen receptor structure and function. Annu Rev Genet 25:487, 1991.
75. Weiss A: T cell antigen receptor signal transduction: a tale of tails and cytoplasmic protein-tyrosine kinases. Cell 73:209, 1993.
76. Weiss A, Littman DR: Signal transduction by lymphocyte antigen receptors. Cell 76:263, 1994.
77. Yoshimoto T, Paul WE: $CD4^{pos}$, $NK1.1^{pos}$ T cells promptly produce interleukin 4 in response to in vivo challenge with anti-CD3. J Exp Med 179:1285, 1994.

4 Natural Killer Cells

ECKHARD R. PODACK

Natural killer (NK) cells constitute a lymphocytic population that is part of the innate, nonadaptive immune system. As the name implies, NK cells are endowed with natural, or constitutive, cytotoxic activity. Although the original operational definition of NK cells was derived from this functional property, subsequent analysis revealed that some cell subpopulations of the T lineage were also endowed with constitutive, natural cytotoxicity. The current definition of NK cells therefore defines them as cells with natural cytotoxicity but lacking rearranged T-cell receptor gene products.

Functionally, the role of NK cells is believed to be important in the early phase of viral and other intracellular infections, prior to the onset of cytotoxic T-lymphocyte–mediated immunity, which requires 3 to 4 days for induction. NK cells may also be important physiologically for other functions, such as control of hematopoiesis or surveillance against tumor cells.

How NK cells recognize their target cells has long been an enigma and is still not fully understood. However, it is now clear that NK cells, contrary to earlier reports, are able to distinguish HLA class I molecules and that their cytolytic action is modulated, usually down-regulated, by major histocompatibility complex (MHC) expression on target cells. Thus NK cells, like T cells, use MHC molecules as guideposts for cell recognition, but with an inverse outcome regarding activation compared with T cells. Whereas T cells are turned on by MHC and costimuli, NK cells are turned off.

MHC recognition by NK cells implies education (selection) of NK cells according to the haplotype of MHC alleles expressed by individuals. Although such a mechanism must be postulated, virtually nothing is known about this process. NK cells thus continue to be one of the most enigmatic cell populations among lymphocytes, and many surprises may yet be discovered regarding their functional and molecular mechanisms.

NK-CELL ONTOGENY

A common precursor for NK cells and T cells has been identified in the thymus.[27] Culture of CD3−, CD4−, CD8−, and CD34+ thymic cells gives rise to both NK cells and T cells, depending on the culture condition. In the presence of IL-2, IL-7, and stem-cell factor, the precursor cells develop into NK cells. In fetal thymic organ culture, however, the precursor cells develop into T cells. Progenitors for the common T/NK precursor can also be detected in fetal liver. According to current analysis, the division between NK cells and T cells occurs in the thymus at a stage before T-cell receptor rearrangement (Fig. 4–1). The common progenitor expresses cytoplasmic CD3ε chains and is positive for CD34 and CD38 but negative for membrane CD3, CD4, and CD8.

CLONAL NK-CELL RECOGNITION AND NK-CELL REPERTOIRE

The notion that NK cells are a homogeneous group of cells can no longer be maintained. Increasing evidence is accumulating to point out that NK cells are endowed with MHC recognition, including the distinction between self-peptides and foreign peptides.[15] NK cells are defined as cytotoxic lymphocytes whose T-cell receptor genes are in germline configuration and hence are not expressed on the surface. Other recognition molecules on NK cells therefore must be present and may be divided into two groups: those activating the effector program of NK and those inhibiting its use.

MHC RECOGNITION BY NK CELLS RESULTS IN INHIBITORY SIGNALS

Activity-inhibiting receptors on NK cells recognize MHC class I molecules on the target cell.[13, 16, 17] Individual NK clones are able to distinguish between HLA-B and HLA-C alleles. For instance, the same target cell expressing HLA B*2705 is protected from lysis, whereas HLA*B081 or B*1402 expression is unable to prevent lysis. Although some NK clones are inhibited only by one specific group of related HLA-B or HLA-C alleles, other clones are inhibited by two or three different groups of alleles. Thus target cells expressing either one of these groups are protected from lysis. Detection and inhibition of more than one group of MHC alleles imply the possibility of more than one MHC receptor on a single NK clone. Inhibition of NK cells by HLA recognition results in the inhibition of both the lytic machinery and lymphokine secretion.

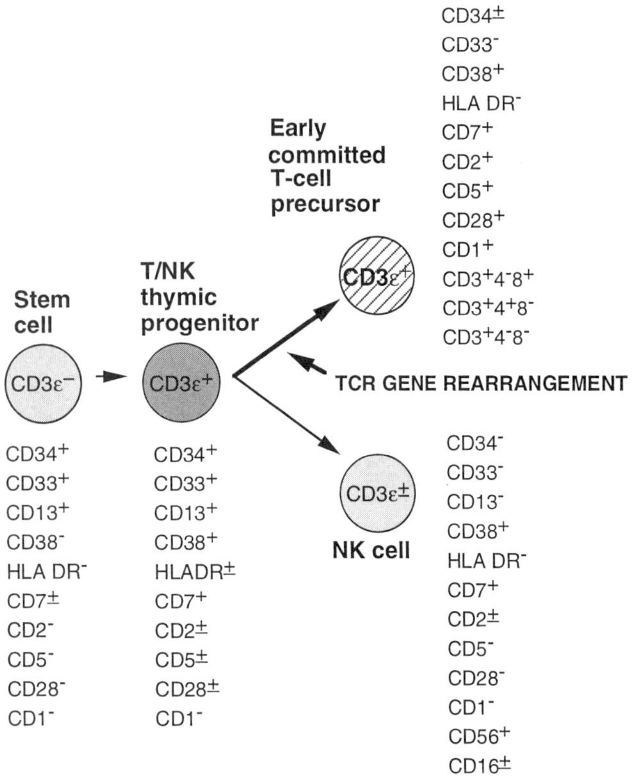

FIGURE 4–1. Schematic representation of NK- and T-cell development in the thymus from a common T/NK progenitor and distribution of phenotypic markers.

The function of MHC molecules is to present antigens to T cells. Class I molecules are specialized for the presentation of intracellularly generated peptides. Because of that property, they are crucial for the recognition by T cells of intracellular pathogens and oncogenic mutations. As is well appreciated, T cells must be selected to be able to distinguish between foreign (viral) peptides presented by MHC and self-peptides. This selection is achieved in the thymus and the periphery, where autoreactive and nonreactive T-cell receptor-bearing T cells are eliminated or anergic, respectively.

NK cells, analogous to T cells, may be capable of distinguishing different peptides presented by class I molecules. Although some self-peptides presented by class I protect these cells from lysis by NK cells, other peptides presented by the same allele do not inhibit lysis.[15] Peptide-MHC recognition by NK cells would imply NK-cell selection and elimination of those NK cells that are not inhibited by self-MHC plus self-peptide. Whether and where this selection occurs is not known. Although NK precursors are found in the thymus, NK development is not dependent on the presence of a thymus. NK cells of apparently normal function are present in athymic animals.

The molecular characterization of inhibitory NK receptors has not been completed. Several groups of apparently different protein families have only been partly characterized to date. In human NK cells, CD94, a disulfide-linked homodimer composed of 43-kD chains, is capable of interacting with HLA-B alleles. P58, a different molecule, interacts with HLA-C alleles and some HLA-B alleles. The NKB1 molecule, the third MHC receptor and a 70-kD protein, interacts with HLA-B alleles. Some monoclonal antibodies to the NK-MHC receptor molecules can abolish the protective effect of MHC class I. Other antibodies to the NK-MHC receptor, however, are able to induce protection of target cells even in the absence of the appropriate class I molecule.

A polymorphic group of about 220 amino acid–long dimeric proteins containing a C-type lectin-binding domain and termed NKG2[10] is expressed predominantly by NK cells. Although the function of this group of proteins on human NK cells has not been completely defined, it is homologous to a group of murine NK receptors, Ly49, that interacts with MHC class I molecules and mediates negative signals to murine NK cells.[3] Another group of proteins on rat NK cells is named NKR-P1.[6] NKG2 is localized on the short arm of chromosome 12, which may define an NK gene complex. The various NK molecules and their properties are summarized in Table 4–1.

NK RECEPTORS TRANSMITTING POSITIVE SIGNALS

NK cells are capable of mediating antibody-dependent cell-mediated cytotoxicity (ADCC) by virtue of their expression of the Fc receptor CD16.[20] This complex signals through CD3ζ chains and through γ chains of the Fc_{ϵ} receptor. Signals through CD16 powerfully activate the lytic program of NK cells. However, simultaneous binding of Class I MHC to p58 or monoclonal antibodies to p58 are capable of down-modulating the cytolytic activity. Apparently, positive and negative signals of cell-surface receptors on NK cells are integrated into the outcome of the final NK response.

In this context, some members of the mouse Ly49 family and the NKRP1 complex have been shown to transmit positive, activating signals. This raises the possibility that the outcome of signaling of even the inhibitory receptors is modified by the concurrent signals and previous history of the NK cells.

MHC RECOGNITION BY NK AND T CELLS ENHANCES EARLY RECOGNITION OF VIRAL INFECTIONS

It is likely that NK cells, just like T cells, continuously survey all tissues for signs of infection or oncogenic transformation. This survey relies on nonspecific adherence receptor pairs present on all cells and capable of interacting with lymphocyte receptors, such as LFA1 and ICAM1, CD2 and LFA3, and many others. NK cells are constitutively active for cytotoxicity and lymphokine secretion and, via their array of MHC receptors, survey target cell surfaces for MHC class I molecules. If the appropriate MHC molecule, recognized by the MHC receptor, is encountered, the NK cell is prevented from releasing its effector molecules and continues to scout the tissues.

Viral infection of target cells may have two different outcomes with regard to MHC class I and peptide expression by the infected cell. Many viruses down-regulate class I molecules. Alternatively, viral peptides in productively infected cells will replace the normal self-peptides presented by MHC. Either of these events is capable of activating the effector program of NK cells, usually leading to lysis of

TABLE 4–1
HUMAN NK-CELL RECEPTORS INTERACTING WITH CLASS I MHC

Human NK-cell Receptor	CD94	p58	NKB1	NKG2
Class I interaction	HLA-B HLA-C?	HLA-C	HLA-B	?
Structure	Disulfide-linked dimer 43 kD	58 kD protein	70 kD glycoprotein	Disulfide-linked dimer C-type lectin ~220A
Polymorphism	Yes?	Yes?	Yes?	Yes

the virus-infected cell and production of lymphokines γ-interferon and IL12. NK-MHC receptors thus recognize the absence of the appropriate class I molecule (down-regulation) or the absence of the appropriate peptide (replaced by viral peptides). This leads to a loss of repressive, inhibitory signals by the MHC receptor and to lysis of the target. In Figure 4–2, the putative events of NK-cell activation by deinhibition are graphically presented and compared with recognition of MHC and peptide by cytotoxic T cells.

T cells, in contrast to NK cells, recognize specific viral peptides in association with MHC via the T-cell receptor. Since only a very small number of T cells can be available for the multitude of possible peptides, activation and clonal expansion of peptide-specific T cells are required for a T-cell response to become effective. This process requires several days. During this period, NK cells may represent the only defense against viral infection or other intracellular parasites. Activation of NK cells by deinhibition is not peptide specific, because the absence of self-peptides is recognized, which may be achieved by any viral peptide that is not a self-peptide. In addition to triggering target cell lysis, deinhibition also leads to lymphokine production, mainly γ-interferon and IL12, which cooperate in the ensuing clonal activation of T cells.

NK CYTOTOXICITY

The original discovery of NK cells was based on their ability to lyse certain target cells without prior activation. The typical susceptible target for human NK-cell lysis is the erythroleukemia line K562. NK-like killing activity is also found in some T-cell populations such as γδ–cell receptor-positive T cells, CD4, CD8 double negative, and αβ–T-cell receptor-positive T cells, as well as in T cells activated in high concentrations of IL2. All of these T-cell populations lack typical MHC restriction; that is, they do not recognize MHC peptide. Whether these T cells recognize other molecules is not clear, except for γδ–T cells recognizing CD1 molecules presenting peptide and nonpeptide antigens.

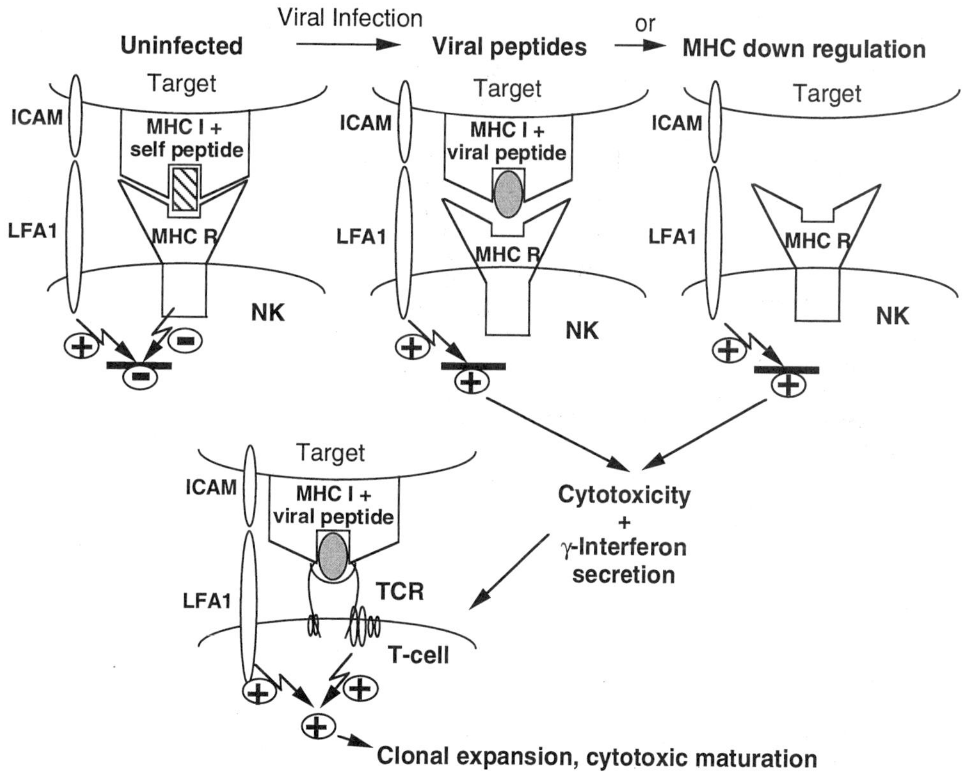

FIGURE 4–2. Recognition of the MHC and inhibition of NK cells by the MHC receptor. Binding of the MHC receptor of NK cells leads to the generation of inhibitory (negative) signals. Lack of binding of the MHC-R to viral peptides or down regulation leaves other positive signals uninhibited. MHC-R = MHC receptor (p58, CD94, NKB1).

NK cells have long been recognized as large granular lymphocytes (Fig. 4–3).[33] NK cells are constitutively endowed with granules. T cells acquire granules only during activation, a process that simultaneously leads to their acquisition of cytotoxicity. The granules contain the cytotoxic machinery of NK cells as well as cytotoxic T lymphocytes (CTL) (Table 4–2).

Membrane Damage. Cytotoxicity is mediated, upon adherence receptor–initiated killer target cell contact, through a regulated secretory process of the granules.[23] Regulated secretion of storage granules is Ca dependent and requires participation of the microtubules (see Fig. 4–3).

The primary cytotoxic molecule of granules is perforin, which is capable of perforating target membranes. Perforin binds to phospholipid head groups via calcium (perforin receptors).[35] Association with additional perforin molecules, conformational change, and insertion into the hydrocarbon core of the membrane result in the formation of a transmembrane pore of up to 16-nm diameter, which is detectable by electron microscopy (Fig. 4–4).[22] This mode of action is highly reminiscent of complement component C9, which is homologous to perforin.[21] Membrane damage mediated by perforin pores results in cell death provided that the capacity of the cell to repair transmembrane channels is overwhelmed by the number of perforin pores generated. Red cells, which are unable to repair their membrane, are highly susceptible to perforin-mediated lysis.

Through its ability to bind directly to phospholipid molecules, perforin lysis is absolutely nonspecific. Specificity of NK or CTL lysis is thus entirely conferred by the membrane receptors of the killer cell making contact with the target.

Apoptosis. Cell death mediated by NK cells or CTL of nucleated target cells usually shows signs of nuclear disintegration in addition to membrane damage.[26] DNA damage is initiated by granzymes, proteases associated with granules, and is dependent on the membrane damage perpetrated by perforin (Table 4–3).[31] In order to repair perforin pores, the target cells endocytose the perforated membrane area and inadvertently take up granzymes in the endosome, which activate the apoptotic cascade leading target cell DNA degradation. The molecular nature of the apoptotic process is unknown but in some cases may involve untimely activation of the mitotic pathway (mitotic catastrophe) or activation of interleukin-1 converting enzyme.[30]

CTL can also activate the apoptotic pathway independently of granule perforin and granzymes. This is achieved through the activation of Fas on the target cell by the Fas-ligand expressed on the CTL.[25] NK cells also express the Fas-ligand and are able to mediate target cell death via this pathway.[1] The two pathways of cytolysis are schematically represented in Figure 4–5.

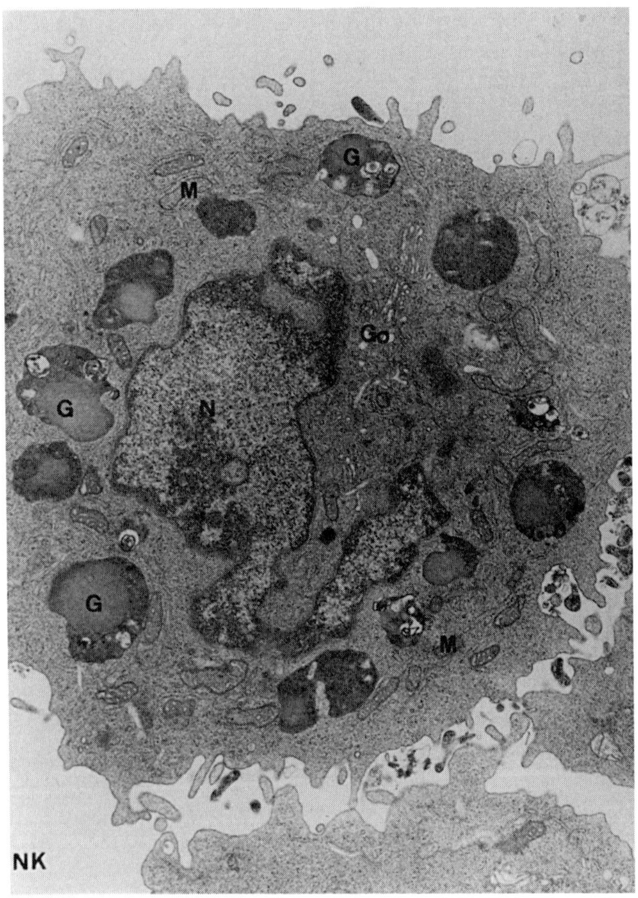

FIGURE 4–3. Electron micrograph of a cross-section through an NK cell. Note well-developed Golgi apparatus (Go), large cytoplasmic granules (G), mitochondria (M), and nucleus (N).

THE ROLE OF CYTOTOXICITY IN VIRAL CLEARANCE AND TUMOR REJECTION

NK cells and CTL mediate cytotoxic responses that are complementary in their recognition of virally infected or oncogenically transformed targets. Although the recognition molecules and mechanisms for activation differ greatly, the terminal cytotoxic events appear to be identical in their use of cytolytic granules and Fas-ligand. The importance of the granule-mediated effector pathway has recently been highlighted through the generation of perforin-deficient mice by gene knockout technology. Mice deficient in perforin do not mediate NK cytotoxicity and are restricted to Fas-ligand–induced apoptosis of target cells. An in vivo challenge of perforin-deficient mice with a small dose of lymphocytic choriomeningitis virus results in a failure of viral clearance, sustained viremia, and death by wasting within 3 weeks.[11] Normal, perforin-sufficient mice have no difficulty clearing an identical infection and establishing immunity. Similarly, perforin-deficient mice are unable to clear immunogenic tumors, which are rejected by immunocompetent mice. Table 4–4 summarizes the in vitro and in vivo defects of perforin deficiency.

Many nonimmunogenic, transplantable tumors are not recognized in mice by NK or T cells, grow rapidly, and are not rejected, thus killing the mice. Gene transfer to these cells of genes that activate the immune system often results in a dramatic increase in the tumor rejection rate. Lewis lung carcinoma (LLC), for instance, is nonimmunogenic. However, production of IL-2 by LLC, achieved through gene transfer, results in the rejection of the tumor upon transplantation into syngeneic mice.[18] Tumor rejection of LLC-IL-2 requires both NK and T cells, because nude mice and beige

TABLE 4–2
COMPOSITION OF HUMAN CYTOLYTIC GRANULES

Name	Function	Molecular Weight	Synonym	Reference
Perforin	Pore formation	70,000	C9-related protein, cytolysin	12 36 9
Granzyme 1	Protease, apoptosis	45,000	HHF,[1] BLT-esterase[2]	5, 8
Granzyme 2	Protease, apoptosis	30,000	HLP[3]	8, 28
Granzyme 3	Protease, apoptosis	25,000	—	8
TIA[4]	RNA, apoptosis	15,000–40,000	RNA binding domain	34
Proteoglycan	Packaging	200,000	Chondroitin sulfate A	32
Calreticulin	Ca-binding	60,000	—	4
Chemotactic factor	Recruitment of monocytes, PMN	?	—	24
Nucleolysis triggering factor	DNA degradation	50,000	Leukalexin	14
Lysosomal components				
β-hexosaminidase	Degradation, detoxification		—	37
β-glucuronidase	Degradation, detoxification		—	7
Aryl sulfatase	Degradation, detoxification		—	19

[1]Human Hanuka factor
[2]Benzoyl-lysyl-thioester-esterase
[3]Human leukocyte protease
[4]T-intracellular antigen

mice, lacking T cells or functional NK cells, respectively, are unable to reject the IL2-producing tumor. Similarly, perforin-deficient mice are unable to reject LLC-IL2, indicating that cytotoxicity is crucial for tumor rejection (Fig. 4–6).

The fact that both NK and T cells are required for rejection of LLC-IL2 may indicate that some tumor cells escape T-cell detection by down-regulation of MHC class I molecules but that these cells are recognized and eliminated by NK cells. Alternatively, NK cells may be required to activate the T-cell response, for instance, via γ-interferon and IL-12, a pathway well documented in virus infection.

The importance of the Fas-ligand–mediated pathway can be assessed by analyzing genetic deficiency states of Fas or the Fas-ligand. Natural deficiency of these membrane proteins leads to polyclonal lymphoproliferation associated with autoimmunity comparable to systemic lupus erythematosus. This seems to indicate that the Fas-ligand–mediated pathway of cytotoxicity is required primarily to maintain homeostasis in the lymphocytic compartment. Failure to eliminate lymphocytes by this pathway leads to a cell-mediated horror autotoxicosis. Although Fas and Fas-ligand may also participate in the removal of cells parasitized by viruses and oncogenes, their genetic deficiency does not significantly increase disease susceptibility to virus infection or tumors. It therefore appears that the two primary cytolytic pathways described serve different biological functions. The Fas-ligand eliminates self-reactive T cells and other lymphocytes in a carefully regulated process requiring cooperation of the cells to be eliminated by expressing a functional Fas signaling pathway through cell suicide.

In contrast, the granule-mediated pathway of lysis does not require participation or cooperation of the target. Targets that attempt to repair membrane damage sustained through perforin pores inevitably take up granzymes and other secreted granule proteins by repair endocytosis and consequently die by apoptosis. Cells that do not repair membrane damage will die through the inability to maintain their membrane potential and through the equilibration of the intracellular and extracellular milieu. Thus it is not a choice for the target whether to repair or not to repair; they will die in either case.

Genes protecting cells from apoptosis, such as bcl-2 or bcl-x, protect against death by the Fas pathway while not interfering with granule-mediated killing. Anti-apoptosis genes have evolved to maintain the balance, in development and in life, between cell death and survival through a genetically programmed and environmentally controlled process. The granule-mediated killing pathway, in contrast, is free of these constraints to facilitate survival of the organism by the removal of parasitized cells.

NK CELLS IN BONE MARROW REJECTION

Allogeneic bone marrow transplantation is used more and more frequently for the treatment of a variety of diseases. Complications of this procedure arise from the potential for

TABLE 4–3
ACTIONS OF GRANZYME B (MOUSE) OR GRANZYME 2 (HUMAN)

Uptake through perforin-mediated mechanism
Serine protease with Asp specificity
Activates cdc2 kinase via activation of a phosphatase or inactivation of wee 2 kinase
Results in premature mitosis and mitotic catastrophe
Apoptosis mediated by granzymes is bcl-2 resistant

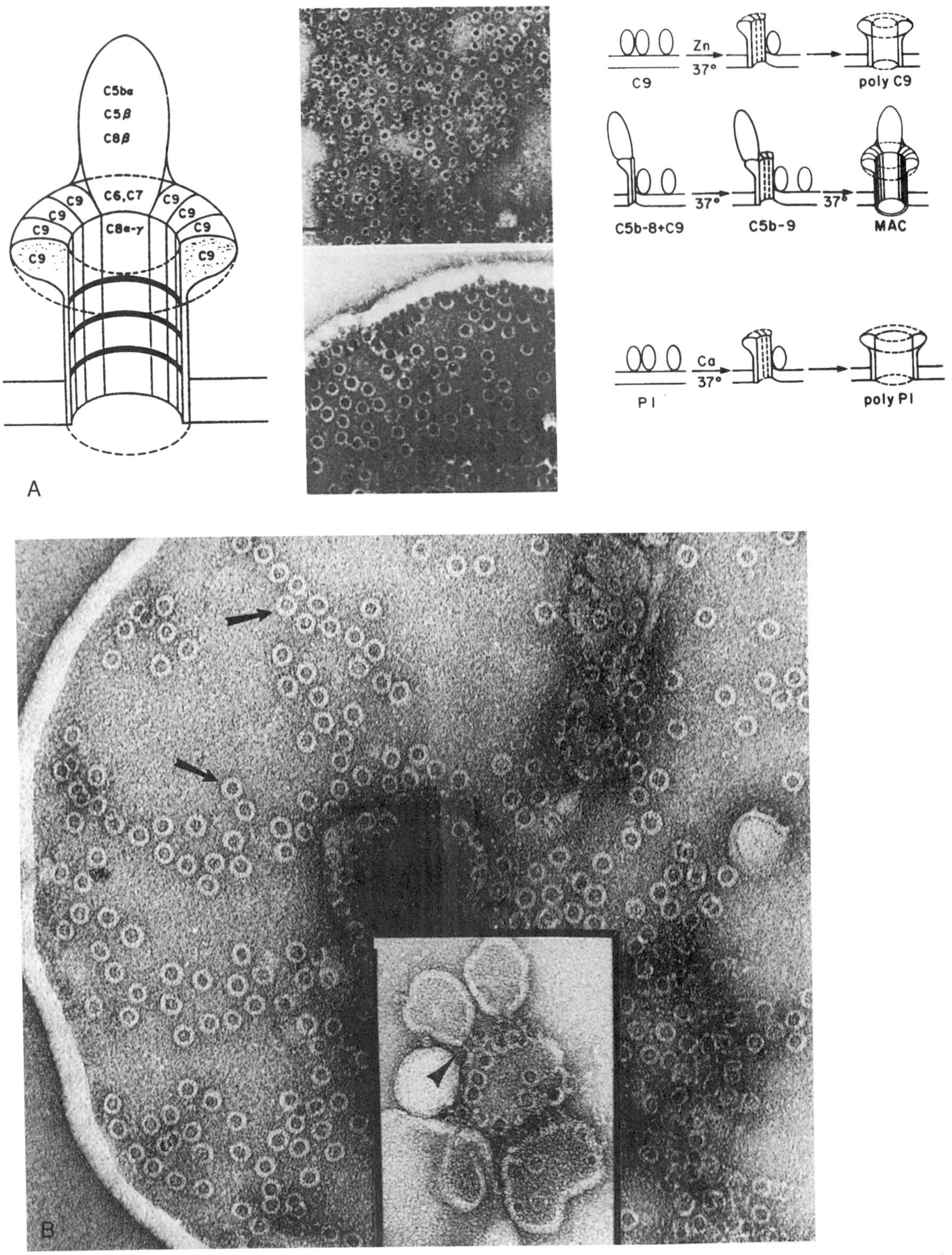

FIGURE 4–4. **(A)** Electron micrographs and schematic representation of complement membrane lesions and polyperforin membrane damage. The inner diameter of complement lesions (upper panel of electron micrographs) is 10 nm and that of polyperforin is 16 nm (lower panel). The right panels show (from top to bottom) the assembly on membranes of poly-C9, formation of the membrane attack complex from C5b-8 and C9, and polyperforin complex. C5b-8, as shown at the left, is formed by interaction of the α chain of C5b (after cleavage of C5 to liberate C5a) and the β chain of C5 (or C5b) with the β chain of C8, followed by C6, C7, and the α-γ chains of C8. Poly-C9 forms around this core (right, center). **(B)** Polyperforin lesions on a larger membrane fragment and on membrane vesicles (inset). Side views of polyperforin are indicated by the arrowhead.

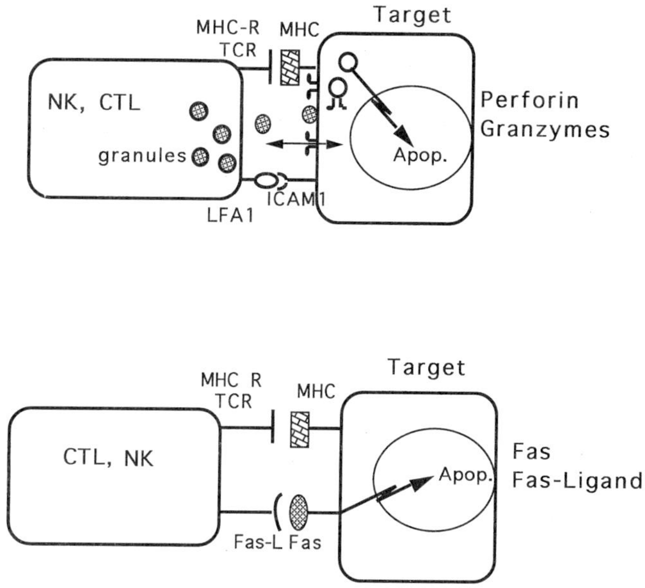

FIGURE 4–5. Schematic representation of the two major cytotoxic pathways mediated by CTL and NK cells. Although the pathways are shown separately, they are mediated by the same cell; NK cells can kill using either pathway or both combined.

graft-versus-host disease and from bone marrow rejection by the recipient. In mice, the effector cells of graft-versus-host disease may be primarily CTL, whereas bone marrow rejection is largely mediated by NK cells. In certain strain combinations of mice, a role for the Ly49 gene complex has been demonstrated, supporting the role of NK cells in bone marrow rejection. Interestingly, however, perforin deficiency does not correct allogeneic bone marrow rejection, indicating that perforin cytotoxicity is not responsible for this reaction.[2]

In graft-versus-host disease, on the other hand, perforin deficiency greatly ameliorates disease. Under appropriate conditions, bone marrow allografts are established without any sign of graft-versus-host disease. Under these conditions, specific tolerance seems to be established to the donor MHC haplotype while allowing immunity toward other antigens.[29]

SUMMARY

It has become clear that NK cells are not a homogeneous population. Clonal differences are caused by the expression of different arrays of MHC receptors, that are able to distinguish self-MHC and self-peptides from allo-MHC and foreign peptides and from missing MHC. Binding to these receptors blocks NK activation, whereas absence of MHC-receptor engagement leads to NK cytotoxicity. NK cells thus are able to detect targets that escape T-cell scrutiny by virtue of the loss of MHC expression. It is the complementarity of T and NK recognition that renders the system capable of responding to viral and oncogenic challenges even in the face of evasive strategies by the target.

The attempt by the cellular immune defense to foil evasive strategies of parasitized cells is also evident in the delineation of the mechanisms of the cytolytic process. One killing pathway of CTL and NK using Fas-ligand–mediated programmed cell death of the target is used predominantly to maintain homeostasis of the lymphocytic repertoire and possibly of other rapidly dividing hemopoietic elements. This suicide pathway, requiring target cooperation, is contrasted by the granule perforin pathway of target killing that is designed to overcome any evasive strategy of the parasitized cell.

TABLE 4–4
BIOLOGICAL EFFECTS OF PERFORIN DEFICIENCY

	In Vivo	In Vitro
Impaired	• Viral clearance absent • Tumor rejection reduced • Local inflammatory response impaired • Graft-versus-host disease upon allogeneic bone marrow transplantation ameliorated or absent	• NK-cell cytolytic activity absent • CTL MHC–restricted cytolytic activity to fibroblasts and epithelial cells absent • CTL MHC–restricted cytolytic activity to hemopoietic cells strongly reduced • LAK activity absent
Unimpaired	• Thymic selection and differentiation • Peripheral T-cell distribution • T-cell activation and proliferation • Pregnancy and fertility • Allogeneic transplant rejection	• Fas-mediated cytolytic activity

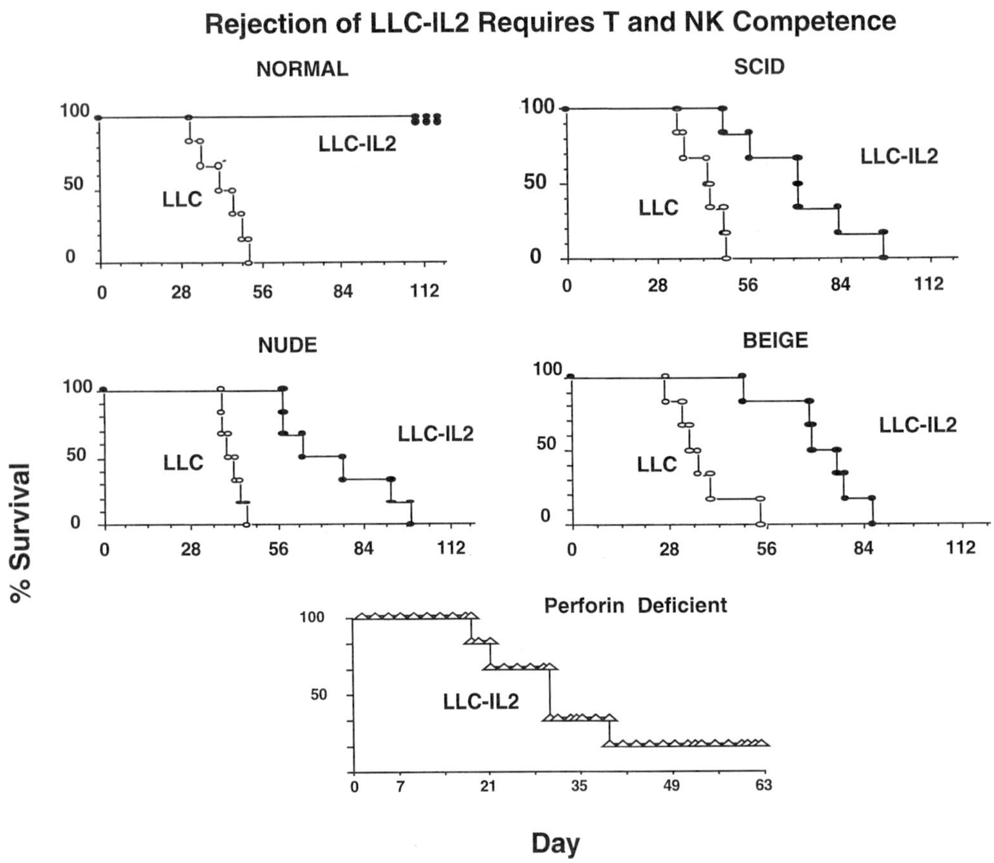

FIGURE 4–6. All mice exposed to Lewis lung carcinoma (LLC) cells die by day 56. IL2 producing LLC is rejected by normal mice (100% survival), but not by immunodeficient mice (SCID, nude) or NK deficient (beige mice) or by perforin-deficient mice.

REFERENCES

1. Arase H, Arase N, Saito T: Fas-mediated cytotoxicity by freshly isolated natural killer cells. J Exp Med 181:1235–1238, 1995.
2. Baker M, Podack ER, Levy RB: Perforin-mediated cytotoxicity is not the major effector mechanism in resistance to allogeneic bone marrow. FASEB 9:5922, 1995.
3. Brennan J, Mager D, Jefferies W, Takei F: Expression of different members of the Ly-49 gene family defines distinct natural killer cell subsets and cell adhesion properties. J Exp Med 180:2287–2295, 1994.
4. Dupuis M, Schaerer E, Krause KH, Tschopp J: The calcium-binding protein cakreticulin is a major constituent of lytic granules in cytolytic T lymphocytes. J Exp Med 177(1):1–7, 1993.
5. Gershenfeld HK, Hershberger RJ, Shows TB, Weissman IL: Cloning and chromosomal assignment of a human cDNA encoding a T-cell and natural killer cell-specific trypsin-like serine protease. Proc Natl Acad Sci USA 85:1184, 1988.
6. Giroda R, Rudert WA, Vavassori C, et al: NKR-P1, a signal transduction molecule on killer cells. Science 249:1289, 1990.
7. Grossi CE, Cadoni A, Zicca A, et al: Large granular lymphocytes in human peripheral blood: ultrastructural and cytochemical characterization of the granules. Blood 59:277, 1982.
8. Hameed A, Lowrey DM, Lichtenheld MG, Podack ER: Characterization of three serine esterases isolated from human interleukin 2 activated killer cells. J Immunol 141:3142, 1988.
9. Henkart PA: Mechanisms of lymphocyte-mediated cytotoxicity. Annu Rev Immunol 3:31–58, 1985.
10. Houchins JP, Yabe T, McSherry C, Bach FH: DNA sequences analysis of NKG2, a family of related cDNA clones encoding type II integral membrane proteins on human natural killer cells. J Exp Med 173(4):1017–1020, 1991.
11. Kägi D, Ledermann B, Bürki K, et al: Cytotoxicity mediated by T cells and natural killer cells is greatly impaired in perforin-deficient mice. Nature 369:31–37, 1994.
12. Lichtenheld MG, Olsen KJ, Lu P, et al: Structure and function of human perforin. Nature 335:448–51, 1988.
13. Litwin V, Gumperz J, Parham P, et al: NKB1: a natural killer cell receptor involved in the recognition of polymorphic HLA-B molecules. J Exp Med 180:537–543, 1994.
14. Liu CC, Steffen M, King F, Young JDE: Identification, isolation, and characterization of a novel cytotoxin in murine cytolytic lymphocytes. Cell 51:393, 1987.
15. Malnati MS, Peruzzi M, Parker KC, et al: Peptide specificity in the recognition of MHC class I by natural killer cell clones. Science 267:1016–1018, 1995.
16. Moretta A, Vitale M, Bottino C, et al: P58 molecules as putative receptors for major histocompatibility complex (MHC) class I molecules in human natural killer (NK) cells. Anti-p58 antibodies reconstitute lysis of MHC class I-protected cells in NK clones displaying different specificities. J Exp Med 178(2):597–604, 1993.
17. Moretta A, Vitale M, Sivori S, et al: Human natural killer cell receptors for HLA-class I molecules. Evidence that the Kp43 (CD94) molecule functions as receptor for HLA-B alleles. J Exp Med 180:545–555, 1994.
18. Ohe Y, Podack ER, Olsen KJ, et al: Combination effect of vaccination with IL2 and IL4 cDNA transfected cells on the induction of a therapeutic immune response against Lewis lung carcinoma cells. Int J Cancer 53:432–437, 1993.
19. Oyre E, Plum J, DeSmedt M: β-blucuronidase activity in human T and B lymphocytes and the Tμ and Tγ sub-populations. Histochemistry 81:287, 1984.
20. Perussia B, Acuto O, Terhost C, et al: Human natural killer cells analyzed by B73.1 antibody-antigen interaction on the lymphocyte membrane. J Immunol 130:2142, 1982.
21. Podack ER: Molecular composition of the tubular structure of the membrane attack complex of complement. J Biol Chem 259:8641–8647, 1984.
22. Podack ER, Dennert G: Assembly of two types of tubules with putative cytolytic function by cloned natural killer cells. Nature 302:442–445, 1983.
23. Podack ER, Kupfer A: T-cell effector functions: mechanisms for delivery of cytotoxicity and help. Annu Rev Cell Biol 7:479–504, 1991.
24. Roussel E, Greenberg AH: Identification of a macrophage-activating factor in granules of the RNK large granular lymphocyte leukemia. J Immunol 142:543, 1989.
25. Rouvier E, Luciani MF, Goldstein P: Fas involvement in Ca (2+)

independent T cell mediated cytotoxicity. J Exp Med 177(1):195–200, 1993.
26. Russell JH, Dobos CB: Mechanisms of immune lysis II. CTL-induced nuclear disintegration of the target begins within minutes of cell contact. J Immunol 125(3):1256–61, 1980.
27. Sanchez MJ, Muench MO, Roncarolo MG, et al: Identification of a common T/natural killer cell progenitor in human fetal thymus. J Exp Med 180:569–576, 1994.
28. Schmid J, Weissman C: Induction of mRNA for a serine protease and a beta-thromboglobulin-like protein in mitogen-stimulated human leukocytes. J Immunol 139:250, 1987.
29. Selvaggi G, Inverardi L, Brendel MD, et al: Tolerance without graft-versus-host disease following allotransplantation of perforin deficient bone marrow. Submitted.
30. Shi L, Nishioka WK, Th'ng J, et al: Premature p34cdc2 activation required for apoptosis. Science 263(5150):1143–1145, 1994.
31. Shiver JW, Su L, Henkart PA: Cytotoxicity with target DNA breakdown by ray basophilic leukemia cells expressing both cytolysin and granzyme A. Cell 71(2):315–322, 1992.
32. Stevens RL, Kamada MN, Serafin WE: Structure and function of the family of proteoglycans that reside in the secretory granules of natural killer cells and other effector cells of the immune response. Curr Top Membr Trans 140:93, 1989.
33. Timonen T, Saksela K: Isolation of human NK cells by density gradient centrifugation. J Immunol 36:285, 1980.
34. Tlan Q, Streuli M, Saito H, et al: A polyadennylate binding protein localized to the granules of cytolytic lymphocytes induces DNA fragmentation in target cells. Cell 67(3):629–639, 1991.
35. Tschopp J, Schafer S, Masson D, et al: Phosphorylcholine acts as a Ca2+-dependent receptor molecule for lymphocyte perforin. Nature 337(6204):272–274, 1989.
36. Zalman LS, Brothers MA, Chiu FJ, Muller-Eberhard HJ: Mechanism of cytotoxicity of human large granular lymphocytes: relationship of the cytotoxic protein to the ninth component (C9) of human complement. Proc Natl Acad Sci USA 83:5262–5266, 1986.
37. Zucker-Franklin D, Grusky G, Yang JS: Arylsulfatase in natural killer cells: its possible role in cytotoxicty. Proc Natl Acad Sci USA 80:6977, 1983.

5 *Cytokines, Interleukins, and Growth Factors*

LANNY J. ROSENWASSER LARRY BORISH

Cytokines are secreted proteins with significant growth, differentiation, and activation functions on contiguous or distant cells and tissues. Hence cytokines may influence the function of their own original cell of origin and exercise an autocrine activity. Cytokines may function locally in a concentration gradient–dependent effect from their source of origin to contiguous tissues and hence act in a paracrine function. Finally, cytokines may have distant effects on tissues and therefore act as endocrine agents.

The science of cytokine biology started in the 1960s with the identification of protein factors active in vitro in a wide range of assays and made by a variety of cells, but primarily lymphocytes. Hence the first nomenclature concerning the source of the proteins that were assessed for in vitro immunologic or inflammatory functions originally related to lymphocytes and macrophages; their products were called lymphokines and monokines. As the biology of these systems moved into the world of molecular description and molecular discovery, it became clear that cells other than immune and inflammatory cells had the capability of producing these proteins under different characteristics and with different characteristics of stimulation and activation, and the term cytokine was adopted. This designation, a broader term, refers to any protein secreted by any cell or tissue that functions in a manner previously outlined.

Cytokines are generally small proteins and are often glycoproteins. Their molecular weight is usually in the range of 5 to 40 kD. Once cytokines were identified on a molecular basis, it was easy to identify unique receptors with specific cellular distribution for the response to these cytokines in an autocrine, a paracrine, or an endocrine mode. It also became clear that there was a cascade of responses that could be seen in response to inflammation, immunity or host defense, or any of the other body functions that cytokines controlled. Often three or four cytokines were required to synergize to get an optimal function expressed. Hence the production of red cells from precursors in the bone marrow required the interaction of three or four different proteins, including erythropoietin, interleukin (IL)-3, IL-1, and IL-11. These overlapping or redundant functions clearly identify the importance of many of the cytokine activities on body economy, since elimination or lack of function of one of the particular cytokines would not then prove to be detrimental to mounting a regulatory response.

This chapter will review the major cytokine families, including the interferons (IFN), IL, chemokines, colony-stimulating factors (CSF), differentiation and growth factors, and tumor necrosis factors (TNF) (Table 5–1). Each of these families of cytokines is made up of multiple proteins and may have a number of factors that overlap function. Hence

TABLE 5–1
CYTOKINE FAMILIES

Interferons
Interleukins
Colony-stimulating factors
Growth and differentiation factors
Tumor necrosis factors
Chemokines and histamine-releasing factors

there are CSF that may behave like IL, IL that may behave like CSF, IFN that act like IL, and other possible combinations between these various protein families. Each of these families will be dealt with individually, with each of the members identified. This chapter will identify the function of these various factors in allergic responses characterized by the kinds of responses made by each particular type of cell, such as which cytokines are made by lymphocytes, macrophages, mast cells, and eosinophils. Two sections on cytokine genetics and cytokine receptors and signaling highlighting new information concerning the cell and molecular biology of these factors will also be presented.

INTERFERONS

The IFN are the first family to be described in this chapter, since they were the first family to have molecular characterization done in the late 1970s and early 1980s. There are three members for the interferon family (Table 5–2). Their initial biologic activity involved the stimulation and expression of antiviral activity measured in a wide variety of viral assays that measure viral growth or killing.

The first form of IFN that is discussed is IFN-α, also known as leukocyte IFN. IFN-α comes primarily from monocytes, macrophages, B lymphocytes, and natural killer (NK) cells. It has significant antiviral activity and a number of other important biologic actions, including up-regulation of class I major histocompatibility complex (MHC) antigens on various cell types, mediation of antitumor activity, and stimulation of immune cytotoxicity. The clinical utility of IFN-α is well established as an antiviral agent in the treatment of various viral infections, including hepatitis. It also has been used to treat a number of malignancies, including chronic myelogenous leukemia, hairy cell leukemia, and the idiopathic hypereosinophilic syndrome.

The second interferon is IFN-β. It is involved in antiviral activity and mirrors many of the biologic effects of IFN-α. It is called fibroblast IFN because the major initial cellular source is fibroblasts, although it is now clear that monocytes, macrophages, and epithelial cells also have the capability of producing IFN-β. The clinical utility of IFN-β in some autoimmune diseases, such as multiple sclerosis, is now being studied. IFN-β is secreted by T helper lymphocytes and contributes to cell-mediated immunity.

TABLE 5–2
INTERFERONS

Cytokine	Cellular Source
IFN-α	B cells NK cells Monocytes/macrophages
IFN-β	Fibroblasts Epithelial cells Macrophages
IFN-γ	T cells NK cells Macrophages

IFN-γ, otherwise known as immune IFN, is made primarily by T cells and NK cells and to a lesser degree by macrophages. In addition to increasing MHC class I antigens on various cell surfaces, it increases the surface expression of MHC class II. These MHC class II antigens are very important in mediating antigen presentation, antitumor activity, macrophage activation, and other immune functions. Those activities associated with IFN-γ and its source from T lymphocytes suggest that IFN-γ may be more of an IL than an IFN because its antiviral activity is modest compared with its immunoregulatory effects.

IFN-γ is the most important cytokine responsible for macrophage activation and therefore cell-mediated immunity.[38] It is produced primarily by T helper lymphocytes but may also be derived from cytotoxic T cells, γδ cells, and NK cells. IFN-γ mediates increased class I and II MHC and IgG receptor expression. IFN-γ stimulates antigen presentation and cytokine production by monocytes and also stimulates monocyte effector functions, including adherence, phagocytosis, secretion, the respiratory burst, nitric oxide production, and microbicidal and tumoricidal activity. The net result is the accumulation of monocytes at the site of cellular immune responses and their activation into macrophages capable of killing intracellular pathogens.

In addition to its effects on mononuclear phagocytes, IFN-γ stimulates killing by NK cells and neutrophils. It stimulates adherence of granulocytes to endothelial cells through the induction of intracellular adhesion molecule (ICAM)-1, an activity shared with IL-1 and TNF.[167] IFN-γ stimulates antigen-specific B-cell proliferation and differentiation. As with other IFN, IFN-γ inhibits viral replication. As discussed later, IFN-γ has been proposed as an inhibitor of allergic responses through its capacity to inhibit IL-4–mediated effects on B cells, thereby inhibiting IgE secretion and expression of low-affinity IgE receptors.

IFN-γ is critically important in the regulation of IgE synthesis. IFN-γ functions as an inhibitor of allergic responses through its capacity to inhibit IL-4–mediated expression of low-affinity IgE receptors and the isotype switch to IgE. The capacity of T lymphocyte clones to support IgE production is inversely proportional to their IFN-γ production. Clones producing both IL-4 and IFN-γ will support IgE production only in the additional presence of anti–IFN-γ antibodies.[23, 121, 162] Additional cytokines that have been reported to inhibit IL-4–induced IgE production are IL-12, TGF-β, and IL-8.[43, 66]

In summary, IgE production is observed when there is a combination of excessive IL-4 and IL-13 production occurring in the relative absence of IFN-γ. It is therefore thought that the immune response to allergens in atopic subjects selectively activates T helper lymphocytes to secrete IL-4 and IL-13 as opposed to IFN-γ. In support of this are experiments using a series of T lymphocyte clones directed against the dust mite allergen.[170] These clones were developed from atopic and nonatopic subjects and then assayed for their capacity to produce IFN-γ, IL-4, and IL-2. Most of the clones produced IL-2. However, allergen-specific T lymphocyte clones obtained from the atopic subjects produced IL-4, whereas similar clones generated to the same allergen but by nonatopic subjects produced IFN-γ.

INTERLEUKINS

The next family of cytokines to be described are the IL, which were the second group to be molecularly identified. IL represent a very diverse and heterogeneous group of proteins that have various effects on immune responses that spill over into other important effects on host defense and inflammation (Table 5–3).

TABLE 5–3
INTERLEUKINS

Cytokine	Cellular Source	Size
IL-1α	Macrophages	31 kD (precursor)
(EP)(LAF)	Many other tissues	17 kD
IL-β	Macrophages	31 kD (precursor)
		17 kD
IL-1ra	Macrophages	17 kD
(Irap)	Pure inhibition of IL-1α, IL-1β	
IL-2	T cells	15 kD
(TCGF)		
IL-3	T cells	22 kD
(multi-CSF)	Thymic epithelial cells	
IL-4	T cells	15 kD
(BSF-1)	Basophils	
	Mast cells	
	Eosinophils	
IL-5	T cells	14 kD
(BSGF-II)	Mast cells	
(EDF)	Eosinophils	
IL-6	T cells	26 kD
(IFN-β2)	Monocytes/macrophages	
(PGF)	Fibroblasts	
	Endothelial cells	
	Mast cells	
	Hepatocytes	
IL-7	Bone marrow stromal cells	22 kD
(LP-1)		
IL-8	T cells	8 kD
(chemokine)	Monocytes/macrophages	
	Epithelial cells	
	Fibroblasts	
IL-9	T cells	39 kD
(p40-MEA)	Mast cells	
IL-10	Monocytes/macrophages	14 kD
(CSIF)	T cells	
IL-11	Bone marrow stromal cells	22 kD
IL-12	Macrophages	α-35 kD, β-40 kD
(NKSF)	B cells	
IL-13	T cells	14 kD
(p600)	Mast cells	
	Basophils	
IL-14	T cells	39 kD
(HMW-BCGF)		
IL-15	Monocytes/macrophages	15 kD
	T cells	
IL-16	T cells	16 kD
(LCF)		

INTERLEUKIN-1

The first IL, not surprisingly, is IL-1. This is actually a family of three proteins, IL-1α, IL-1β, and IL-1 receptor antagonist (IL-1ra), which is an antagonist that has no agonist activity compared with the first two family members.[34, 35, 103] IL-1α and IL-1β are both synthesized as precursors that are then modeled and reduced from the size of the precursors, which are 31 kD, to the mature forms that have the greatest biologic impact, which are 17 kD in size. These mature forms of IL-1α and IL-1β are not only very potent enhancers of immune responses but also very potent inducers of acute phase responses and inflammation and have a wide variety of effects in both immunity, inflammation, and host defense. The identification of IL-1ra as a potential antagonist leads to some very interesting possibilities for clinical intervention with cytokine antagonists that have only begun to be explored in terms of their efficacy.

Despite the minimal sequence similarity (~25% amino acid homology), IL-1α and IL-1β have similar biologic activities, and all three proteins interact with similar affinities to the two IL-1 receptors.[34] Type I receptors have been found on T cells, fibroblasts, endothelial cells, hepatocytes, and numerous other cells. Type I receptors have an extensive cytoplasmic domain and following ligand binding transduce the biologic effects attributed to IL-1.[140] These are in contrast to type II receptors, which have been identified on B cells, neutrophils, and bone marrow cells and have a minimal intracellular domain. The capture and sequestration of IL-1 by these inactive type II receptors may subserve an anti-inflammatory function. Hence type II receptors are sometimes referred to as decoy receptors. Type II receptors are thought to function as the precursor for the soluble IL-1 binding factors, which, when shed, antagonize IL-1 activity.[119, 140] The capacity of IL-1ra to bind to the type I (proinflammatory) IL-1 receptor without transducing a biologic signal is the basis for its capacity to function as an anti-inflammatory cytokine antagonist.[8, 36, 47]

IL-1 is produced primarily by cells of the mononuclear phagocytic lineage but is also produced by endothelial cells, keratinocytes, synovial cells, astrocytes, osteoblasts, neutrophils, and glial cells. IL-1 production may be stimulated by a variety of agents, including endotoxins, other cytokines, microorganisms, and a multitude of antigens. Both IL-1α and IL-1β are synthesized without a hydrophobic leader sequence as a less active 31 kD precursor.[9] The mechanism for IL-1 secretion is unknown but is dependent on its cleavage by a specific converting enzyme into the active 17 kD form and may utilize MHC transporters with unique signal recognition particles (see Chapter 1).[18, 169]

One of the most important biologic activities of IL-1 is its function as a lymphocyte activating factor (LAF). T helper cell activation requires the interaction of the antigen MHC complex with the T-cell receptor. However, an additional noncognate signal is also required for optimal T-cell activation and proliferation, and this is generally provided by IL-1. IL-1 enhances the production of T lymphocyte–derived cytokines, such as IL-2, as well as IL-2 receptors. In the absence of IL-1, either no immune response or a state of tolerance develops. In addition to these effects on T lymphocytes, IL-1 can augment B-cell proliferation and increases immunoglobulin synthesis. IL-1 synergizes with various CSF to stimulate early bone marrow hematopoietic progenitor cell proliferation. IL-1 administration produces a bone marrow–derived neutrophilia.

The production of IL-1 during the immune response produces a spectrum of changes associated with being sick. IL-1 interacting with the central nervous system is responsible for producing fever, lethargy, slow wave sleep, anorexia, and the release of corticotrophin-releasing factor. An IL-1 hepatocyte interaction inhibits the production of housekeeping proteins, such as albumin, and stimulates in turn the synthesis of acute phase response peptides, such as amyloid peptide, C-reactive peptide, and complement. To provide the amino acids for this new protein synthesis, IL-1 stimulates the catabolism of muscle. IL-1 activity in joints stimulates synovial cell proliferation, cartilage and bone resorption, and collagen deposition. These effects of IL-1 on muscles and joints contribute to the myalgias and arthralgias associated with illness. IL-1 stimulates endothelial cell adherence of leukocytes through the up-regulation of ICAM.[167] IL-1 also acts on blood vessels to induce vasodilation, contributing to the hypotension of septic shock.

Much of the proinflammatory activities of IL-1 relates to its ability to induce arachidonate metabolism with many eicosanoids, such as prostaglandin E_2 and leukotriene B_4, functioning as second messengers. IL-1 induces the synthesis of additional cytokines, including TNF, IL-6, granulocyte-macrophage colony-stimulating factor (GM-CSF), and as a positive feedback mechanism, additional IL-1. Like TNF, IL-1 is directly cytotoxic to certain cancerous and virus-infected cells. TNF and IL-1 share numerous biologic activities, the major distinction being that TNF has no direct effect on lymphocyte proliferation.

The IL-1 receptor antagonist (IL-1ra or IL-1γ) is secreted naturally in inflammatory processes. Its production is up-regulated by many cytokines, including IL-4, IL-13, transforming growth factor (TGF)-β, and IL-1 itself. Production of IL-1ra is thought to modulate the potentially deleterious effects of IL-1 in the natural course of inflammation. IL-1ra has been utilized experimentally as an anti-inflammatory agent. In rabbits, IL-1ra prevents death from lipopolysaccharide (LP)-mediated septic shock and modulates immune complex–induced colitis.[40, 102]

INTERLEUKIN-2

IL-2 is the first IL to be molecularly cloned and identified. It is the most potent and predominant T-cell growth factor (TCGF) and stimulates the proliferation and differentiation of T lymphocytes, cytolytic activity of cytotoxic T lymphocytes (CTL), cytolytic activity of NK cells, and development of lymphokine-activated killer cells. As a result of its stimulation of other cells and other IL, IL-2 stimulates the proliferation and immunoglobulin secretion by B lymphocytes.

Stimulation of T cells by antigen in the additional presence of IL-1 induces the simultaneous secretion of IL-2 and the expression of high-affinity IL-2 receptors.[142, 152] Subsequently, the binding of secreted IL-2 to these IL-2R–positive T cells induces clonal T-cell proliferation. The requirement for both IL-2 production and IL-2R expression for T cells to proliferate assures that only T cells specific for the antigen inciting the immune response will become activated.

IL-2 receptors consist of three chains.[90] IL-2Rα (or Tac antigen or CD25) is a 55 kD transmembrane glycoprotein with only 13 of 351 amino acids located intracytoplasmically.[79] IL-2Rβ is a 75 kD glycoprotein with a large intracytoplasmic component and therefore is critical for signal transduction.[50] A third chain, IL-2Rγ, has been shown to be essential for high-affinity binding, ligand internalization, and, when approximated to the β chain, signaling.[50, 150] IL-4, IL-7, IL-9, IL-13, and IL-15 all make use of the γ chain as part of their receptor complexes. All three chains are in contact with the IL-2 ligand in the high-affinity form of the receptor. Alone, IL-2Rα has low affinity for IL-2 and is unable to transduce a signal. The αβ chains in combination produce a receptor with intermediate affinity but are still unable to activate the cell. Absence of γ chains is responsible for one form of X-linked severe combined immunodeficiency, reflecting its importance in signaling by at least six cytokines.[101]

IL-2 receptors (predominantly βγ) are also found on NK cells, through which IL-2 induces a more potent cytotoxic response, as the NK cells differentiate into one type of lymphokine-activated killer (LAK) cells.[54, 138] IL-2 also functions as a B cell, cytotoxic T cell, and macrophage activator, as well as possibly having neurotransmitter functions.[82, 164]

INTERLEUKIN-3

IL-3 is an important factor that stimulates the growth of precursors of a wide variety of mature cells, including erythrocytes, granulocytes, macrophages, mast cells, and lymphoid cells.[7] This early-acting stimulatory cofactor makes this more of a multi-CSF, another name for this particular factor, which was initially identified because of its effects on these hematopoietic cell precursors.[130] Two major sources of IL-3 are T lymphocytes and mast cells. IL-3 stimulates the early stages of hematopoietic cell differentiation. It also has synergistic activity with many other cytokines or CSF.[60, 80, 130]

INTERLEUKIN-4

IL-4 was initially described as a B-cell growth factor (BCGF-1) called B-cell stimulatory factor (BSF-1). Its primary targets were T lymphocytes, macrophages, mast cells, basophils, B lymphocytes, bone marrow precursors, and stromal cells. It is now known best as the major inducer of the differentiation of CD4 T cells into the so-called Th2 subset of T-cell development. The Th2 subset is primarily involved with the generation, proliferation, differentiation, and growth of B lymphocytes and promotes isotype antibody switching. In particular, it is involved in promoting IgE production from B lymphocytes. It also has diverse effects on many other cells and cytokines that place it in a central role not only for the regulation of IgE isotype switch and humoral immunity but also, perhaps more important, for a unique kind of allergic inflammation.[108] IL-4 is a two-edged sword, however. There is another set of activities associated with interleukin-4, namely, the suppression of some macrophage functions related to cytokine and monokine production. For example, IL-4 will significantly turn off IL-1 production by macrophages and prevent the development of other forms of activity related to the macrophage.[108]

IL-4 was originally identified as a B-cell growth factor that drives the optimal stimulation of B cells by antigen.[23, 109] In addition to production by T helper lymphocytes, IL-4 may be derived from cytotoxic T cells, mast cells, and basophils. IL-4 also stimulates MHC class II antigen, B7.1 (CD80), B7.2 (CD86), CD40, surface IgM, and low-affinity IgE receptor expression by B cells, resulting in enhanced antigen-presenting capacity of B cells.[108] However, as implied earlier, IL-4 induces the immunoglobulin isotype switch from IgM to IgE.[22, 23, 32, 121] IgE production occurs after the IL-4–mediated initiation of transcription of ϵ heavy chain transcripts. With the additional presence of signals triggered through CD40, genomic splicing occurs and mature ϵ heavy chain transcripts are synthesized. The additional presence of B-cell activating cytokines, including IL-2, IL-5, and IL-6, synergizes with IL-4 to increase the secretion of IgE.[162]

That IL-4 is absolutely essential for IgE production has been demonstrated by the ability of anti–IL-4 antibodies to abrogate the capacity of *Nippostrongylus* infection to induce IgE in mice.[158] Similarly, mice that have been genetically engineered to lack the IL-4 gene (IL-4 knock-outs) are unable to synthesize IgE.[76] In contrast to these experiments, mice that have been genetically engineered to secrete excessive IL-4 gene demonstrate elevated serum IgE levels.[154] In addition, they have a conjunctivitis that on pathology has the appearance of an allergic reaction with increased eosinophilia and infiltration with mast cells. Evidence supporting a role for IL-4 regulation of IgE synthesis in humans is derived from several observations. IL-4 induces the synthesis of IgE by B lymphocytes, and the capacity of T-cell clones to support IgE production is directly proportional to their IL-4 production.[32]

In addition to these effects on B cells, IL-4 is a growth factor for T cells, whose function in allergic inflammation will be discussed later. It enhances the production of cytotoxic T cells and activates NK and LAK cells. It has some macrophage-activating activities, enhancing expression of MHC class I and II molecules, LFA-1, and low-affinity IgE receptors.[108] In contrast to these proinflammatory effects on monocytes, IL-4 inhibits antibody-dependent cellular cytotoxicity, inhibits expression of FcγR, and down-regulates the production of NO, IL-1, IL-6, and TNF-α while stimulating the production of IL-1ra.[39] Another potentially important activity of IL-4 in allergic inflammation is its ability to induce expression of vascular cell adhesion molecule (VCAM)-1 on endothelial cells. This will produce the enhanced adhesiveness of endothelium for T cells, eosinophils, basophils, and monocytes, but not neutrophils, which is characteristic of allergic reactions.[92]

INTERLEUKIN-5

IL-5 was also identified as a T-cell reactive cytokine originally termed BCGF-2 or T-cell replacing factor. It was identified early on as an eosinophil differentiation factor and a cytotoxic cell differentiation factor. It is synthesized primarily by T cells, mast cells, and eosinophils and stimulates a growth differentiation and the activation of eosinophils from eosinophil precursors. It prolongs eosinophil survival by blocking apoptosis and is a chemotactic factor for eosinophils. It stimulates the differentiation of B cells, as well as T cells, particularly cytotoxic T cells.[125, 149]

As with IL-4, IL-5 was originally identified as a B-cell–stimulating factor that mediates the proliferation and differentiation of B lymphocytes and induces the secretion of IgM.[72, 148, 175] In addition to T helper lymphocytes, important sources for IL-5 in allergic inflammation may also be eosinophils and mast cells. IL-5 interacts with specific IL-5 receptors, which consist of a heterodimer with IL-5Rα and IL-5Rβ chains.[69] The β subunit is shared with GM-CSF and IL-3 receptors.

After cloning and generating the purified protein, human IL-5 was demonstrated to have minimal activities toward B cells. However, IL-5 has become very important to the understanding of allergic inflammation, as it is the most important eosinophilopoietin. IL-5 induces the maturation of a homogeneous population of eosinophils when exposed to bone marrow precursors, and mice transgenic for constitutive IL-5 expression develop eosinophilia.[21, 155] In addition to stimulating eosinophil production, IL-5 is chemotactic for eosinophils and activates mature eosinophils, inducing eosinophil secretion and enhanced antibody-dependent cytotoxicity. IL-5 is responsible for the generation of hypodense eosinophils and prolongs eosinophil survival while limiting apoptosis.[123] Mice injected with *Nippostrongylus* and anti–IL-5 antibodies fail to develop eosinophilia.[24] Anti–IL-5 therapy abrogates the development of eosinophilic bronchitis in animal models of asthma.[159] The importance of IL-5 in human allergic disorders is supported by the demonstration of increased serum IL-5 levels in the hypereosinophilic syndrome, the eosinophilia-myalgia syndrome, and endobronchial allergen challenges.[25, 105, 106] Additional activities of IL-5 include an interaction with T lymphocytes to mediate the maturation of CTL and a role in basophilic differentiation.[33]

In addition to IL-5, two CSF, IL-3 and GM-CSF, contribute to the activity of eosinophils in allergic inflammation through their capacities to prolong eosinophil survival and to generate activated, hypodense eosinophils.[107, 122] Additional factors that are chemotactic and activating for eosinophils are members of the chemokine family, including RANTES, monocyte inflammatory peptide (MIP)-1α, monocyte chemotactic protein (MCP)-3, and eotaxin-A.

INTERLEUKIN-6[4, 160]

IL-6, or IFN-β2, an alternative form of the IFN-β family, also has a number of other names, including plasmacytoma growth factor (PGF), hepatocyte-stimulating factor, hybridoma growth factor, and B-cell differentiation factor. It is made by monocytes, macrophages, fibroblasts, endothelial cells, and to some extent T cells. It induces the entry of primitive hematopoietic progenitor cells into the cell cycle and stimulates the production of acute phase proteins by hepatocytes. It also acts as an endogenous pyrogen. IL-6 will promote the growth of differentiation of T and B lymphocytes and stimulate the production of platelets from megakaryoyocytes. In addition, it will cause terminal differentiation of B lymphocytes into immunoglobulin-secreting plasma cells.

Mononuclear phagocytic cells are probably the most important source of IL-6. However, IL-6 is also produced by T and B lymphocytes, fibroblasts, keratinocytes, hepatocytes, glial cells, and bone marrow stromal cells. Its synthesis is induced by IL-1, IL-2, TNF, and IFN and inhibited by IL-4 and IL-13. An important biologic activity of IL-6 is its ability to stimulate the final stages of B lymphocyte maturation. Under the influence of IL-6, B lymphocytes differentiate into mature plasma cells and are stimulated to secrete immunoglobulins. IL-6 mediates T-cell activation, growth, and differentiation, including the differentiation of cytotoxic T cells. In addition to costimulating lymphocyte proliferation, IL-6 shares several activities with IL-1, including the induction of pyrexia and the acute phase response. IL-6 is considered the most important inducer of hepatocyte synthesis of acute phase proteins, such as C-reactive protein, fibrinogen, haptoglobin, and amyloid protein. IL-6 may have antiviral activity, as well as sharing IFN's capacity to induce class I MHC expression. Similar to TNF and IL-1, IL-6 may display antitumor effects. IL-6 is a neutrophil primer and synergizes with other cytokines to support bone marrow stem cell maturation.

INTERLEUKIN-7

IL-7 is a stromal factor involved in the differentiation and proliferation of B lymphocyte and T lymphocyte precursors primarily through intimate interaction with bone marrow precursors. It also stimulates the proliferation and differentiation of cytotoxic T cells and LAK cells and stimulates the tumoricidal activity of monocytes and macrophages.

INTERLEUKIN-9

IL-9 is a novel and important cytokine involved in T-cell, mast cell, megakaryocytic, and erythropoietic biology. It was originally identified as a 40 kD protein product of T-cell lines. Once the protein was cloned, it became clear that the p40 T-cell activity found in T-cell line supernatants (TCGF III) could also enhance mast cell proliferation (MEA activity) and synergize with IL-3 in megakaryocyte and erythrocyte development. The cellular source of IL-9 appears to be the Th2 subpopulation of CD4 T cells in mice, and it is presumed to be the Th2 subpopulation of CD4 T cells in humans. In mice, antigen, mitogen, and alloantigen can trigger T cells to produce IL-9.

INTERLEUKIN-10

IL-10 is a primary antagonist of a number of lymphokine-related activities and suppresses the functional activity of macrophages and T cells by inhibiting the production of proinflammatory cytokines. It enhances B-cell proliferation and immunoglobulin secretion indirectly by decreasing the synthesis of inhibitory cytokines.

IL-10, or cytokine synthesis inhibitory factor (CSIF), was initially identified in mice, in which it is a Th2 lymphocyte product that inhibits both Th1 proliferation and the production of IFN-γ and IL-2.[41] Subsequent studies have extended these activities to humans and have shown that IL-10 is also a product of various other cells, including Th1 lymphocytes, cytotoxic T cells, B lymphocytes, mast cells, and mononuclear phagocytic cells.[31, 176] In humans, monocytes may be the major source for IL-10.[165] In addition to its effects on Th1 cytokines, IL-10 acts to inhibit the production of IL-1β, IL-6, IL-8, IL-12, and TNF-α by mononuclear phagocytes, IL-4 and IL-5 by Th2 lymphocytes, and IFN-γ and TNF-α by NK cells.[26, 31, 42, 58, 118] In addition to the effects of IL-10 on monocyte-derived cytokines, IL-10 also inhibits monocyte MHC class II expression and accessory cell function. Expression of IL-10 by antigen-presenting cells may have a role in the induction and maintenance of allergen-specific tolerance in allergic disorders.[37]

Support for a modulator role for IL-10 in human atopic disease is further derived from observations that IL-10 inhibits eosinophil survival and IL-4–induced IgE synthesis.[115, 147] These inhibitory effects of IL-10 are in contrast to its effect on B lymphocytes, in which it functions as an activating factor, stimulating cell proliferation and immunoglobulin secretion.[124] IL-10 contributes to isotype switching to IgG1 and IgG3.[16] IL-10 also functions as a growth cofactor for immature T cells and is a differentiating factor for cytotoxic T cells.[20] Thus IL-10 inhibits cytokines associated with cellular immunity and allergic inflammation while stimulating humoral and cytotoxic immune responses.

The kinetics of IL-10 production differ from those of other cytokines.[176] Whereas mRNA for IL-1β, IL-2, IL-4, and IFN-γ can be identified as rapidly as 15 minutes and peaks 2 to 4 hrs after stimulation, IL-10 mRNA does not appear until 8 hours after stimulation and is maximal only at 12 to 24 hours. The appearance of IL-10 thus correlates with and may contribute to the down-regulation of the proinflammatory cytokines. Secretion of these proinflammatory cytokines may be a signal for IL-10 synthesis.[165] TNF-α, for example, is a potent stimulus for IL-10 secretion. These studies suggest a homeostatic mechanism whereby an inflammatory stimulus induces TNF-α secretion that in turn stimulates IL-10 secretion, which feeds back to turn off TNF-α synthesis. Support for an anti-inflammatory mechanism for IL-10 is suggested by knock-out mice for IL-10, which develop an inflammatory bowel disease thought to be due to uncontrolled immune responses to enteric antigens.[75]

INTERLEUKIN-11

IL-11 is another stromally derived precursor stimulatory factor. It synergizes with IL-3 and IL-4 to cause hematopoietic progenitor cells, synergizes with IL-3 and IL-6 to produce megakaryocytes, and stimulates the production of acute phase proteins. It will also cause lymphoid cells to differentiate and may be an important stimulatory factor for connective tissue cells, such as fibroblasts.

INTERLEUKIN-12

IL-12 is a very important cytokine involved in a number of activities related to monocyte and fibroblast production. It enhances cytolytic activities of cytotoxic T cells, NK cells, and lymphokine-activated killer cells. IL-12 increases the proliferation of such cells; and, most important, is a potent inducer of the IFN-γ gene by all of these different types of cells. By its ability to induce IFN-γ, it creates a milieu that causes enhanced hemopoietic stem cell differentiation and stimulates the differentiation of uncommitted CD4+ T lymphocytes into Th1 cells. Hence it is an indirect inhibitor of IgE secretion by Th2 cell interactions with B lymphocytes.[157]

IL-12 is a mononuclear phagocytic cell–derived peptide originally described as natural killer stimulatory factor.[17, 87] It is a heterodimer composed of two unrelated subunits. The larger subunit (p40) is homologous to the soluble receptor for IL-6, whereas the smaller subunit (p35) is homologous to both IL-6 and GM-CSF. IL-12 is derived from monocytes and macrophages as well as B cells and connective tissue–type mast cells. IL-12 activates and induces the proliferation of NK cells and stimulates their cytotoxicity, causes the secretion of IFN-γ and TNF-α, and increases the expression of CD56, CD2, and CD11a. Similar to IL-2, IL-12 stimulates the differentiation of NK cells into LAK cells. Other activities attributed to IL-12 include enhanced proliferation of CD4 and CD8 lymphocytes and stimulation of hematopoiesis.[12] Its counterregulatory role in allergic inflammation will be discussed later.

INTERLEUKIN-13

IL-13 is a T lymphocyte product previously known as P600, a product of the gene that stimulates B lymphocyte growth and development. It is involved in inducing the IgE isotype switch and inhibits proinflammatory cytokine production by monocytes and macrophages. IL-13 has a spectrum of activity identical to that of IL-4 except that IL-13 will not induce T-cell growth and proliferation or Th2 generation from Th0 precursors.[29, 86]

IL-13 has about 30% homology to IL-4 and shares much of the biologic activities of IL-4 on mononuclear phagocytic cells and B cells. Thus IL-13 inhibits monocyte-mediated antibody-dependent cell-mediated cytotoxicity (ADCC), proinflammatory cytokine production, and NO secretion and induces the IgE isotype switch.[86, 178] The functional IL-13 receptor is thought to represent a heterotrimer containing the IL-4R, the IL-2Rγ chain, and a unique IL-13 binding component. IL-13 is contrasted with IL-4 by different mechanisms of transcriptional regulation. IL-4 tends to be an earlier and more transient signal in comparison to IL-13. IL-13 is also distinguished from IL-4 by an absence of effects on T lymphocytes. As discussed later, IL-4 may be particularly important in allergic diseases through its ability to induce the differentiation of IL-4–producing T helper lymphocytes, an activity not shared by IL-13.

INTERLEUKIN-14

IL-14 is a name given to a high molecular weight B-cell growth factor (HMW-BCGF) made by T lymphocytes that stimulates the proliferation of activated B cells, but not resting B cells. Yet it inhibits immunoglobulin secretion from mitogen-activated B lymphocytes.[6]

INTERLEUKIN-15

IL-15 is a cytokine made primarily by monocytes and not T cells that stimulates the proliferation of T helper cells, cytotoxic T cells, and NK cells. Its biologic activity is very similar to that of IL-2. In fact, IL-15 shares most components of the IL-2 receptor for stimulation. The only differences are that IL-15 is not a T-cell product and it does not utilize IL-2Rα chain. Instead it has a unique α chain as part of the cytokine receptor signaling complex that is involved in recognition.

IL-15 is a 15 kD peptide that interacts with a heterotrimeric receptor, two components of which are also used by IL-2 (the IL-2Rβ and γ chains).[44] IL-15 competes for binding sites with IL-2, and anti–IL-2 receptor antibodies block binding of IL-15. Mononuclear phagocytic cells, epithelial cells, fibroblasts, muscle, and placenta are the best sources of IL-15.[46] Activated T lymphocytes, the most important source for IL-2, were not found to express detectable IL-15.[46] Similar to IL-2, IL-15 is a T-cell growth factor, is chemotactic for T lymphocytes, differentiates NK cells into LAK cells, and stimulates B-cell growth and differentiation. The significance of IL-15 is that this peptide represents an additional mechanism by which mononuclear phagocytic cells regulate T-cell and NK-cell proliferation and function.

After induction of T-cell activation and proliferation, depending on the repertoire of cytokines produced, either cell-mediated, humoral, or allergic immune responses will occur.

INTERLEUKIN-16

IL-16 is a T-cell–derived product made primarily by CD8+ T lymphocytes that influences the chemokinetic and chemotactic response of CD4+ lymphocytes and in fact binds to CD4. It is potentially proinflammatory and has been implicated in asthma and other pulmonary diseases.

CHEMOKINES

INTERLEUKIN-8 AND THE SMALL CYTOKINE FAMILY (CHEMOKINES)[10, 56, 104]

The chemokines are a family of structurally and functionally related proteins that include at least 14 distinct members. In addition to mononuclear phagocytic cells, chemokines are secreted by T lymphocytes, NK cells, neutrophils, keratinocytes, hepatocytes, fibroblasts, endothelium, and epithelial cells. The peptides are small (8–10 kD) secreted proinflammatory cytokines that exhibit between 20% and 50% homology in their amino acid sequences. The chemokines are characterized by the presence of four conserved cysteine residues and are subdivided into two families based on the positioning of these cysteines. The C-X-C subfamily is located on chromosome 4q, and its members are characterized by the separation of the first two cysteines by a variable amino acid. The C-C subfamily has the first two cysteine residues adjacent to each other, and its genes are located on chromosome 17q. These two families may also be distinguished by their primary target cell, with the C-X-C subfamily primarily targeting neutrophils and the C-C family targeting monocytes and T cells. A new family of chemokines has been identified that lacks the first and third C and is referred to as the C subfamily. The major chemokines and some functions are summarized in Table 5–4. They are discussed further in Chapter 6.

TABLE 5–4
CHEMOKINES AND HISTAMINE-RELEASING FACTORS

Cytokine	Cell Source	Activate
C-X-C Subfamily		
IL-8 (NAP-1)	T cells/monocytes, endothelial cells	Neutrophils Lymphocytes
GRO α, β, γ	T cells/monocytes	Neutrophils
NAP-2	Platelets	Neutrophils
CTAP-III	Platelets	Neutrophils
BTG	Platelets	Neutrophils
γIP-10	T cells/monocytes	Neutrophils
ENA-78 (MIP-2)	T cells/monocytes	Neutrophils
C-C Subfamily		
MIP-1α	T cells/monocytes	Neutrophils Eosinophils Basophils
MIP-1β	T cells/monocytes	Neutrophils
MCP-1, MCP-2, MCP-3, MCP-4	T cells/monocytes	Eosinophils Basophils
RANTES	T cells/monocytes	Eosinophils Basophils
Eotaxin	T cells/monocytes	Eosinophils

IL-8 or neutrophil activating protein 1 (NAP-1) is a chemotactic factor for neutrophils and T lymphocyte subsets. IL-8 is the most extensively studied member of the chemokine superfamily.[56, 78, 104] It is primarily derived from mononuclear phagocytes and endothelial cells but also can be synthesized by T cells, eosinophils, neutrophils, fibroblasts, keratinocytes, hepatocytes, and chondrocytes. IL-8 synthesis may be induced by lipopolysaccharide, IL-1, TNF, and viruses. IL-8 on a molar basis is one of the most potent chemoattractants for neutrophils. It also stimulates polymorphonuclear neutrophils (PMN) degranulation, the respiratory burst, and adherence to endothelial cells via CD11b/CD18. During the inflammatory response, IL-8 appears relatively late in comparison with other chemoattractants. For example, leukotriene B_4 appears within minutes of cellular activation, and its concentration peaks at 3 hours. As leukotriene B_4 concentrations decline, the newly synthesized IL-8 begins to be secreted and persists for at least 24 hours. Other members of the C-X-C chemokine family, including platelet factor 4, GRO (α, β, γ), MIP-2, and neutrophil-activating protein 2, share to a lesser extent a capacity to activate PMN. Other members of the chemokine C-C family, including RANTES, MIPIα, MIPIβ, MCP-1, and MCP-3, have unique contributions toward allergic inflammation, which will be discussed later. They all are chemotactic and activating factors for monocytes, and some act on lymphocytes. Activities on granulocytes are shown in Table 5–4.

COLONY-STIMULATING FACTORS

The most clinically efficacious cytokine is erythropoietin (EPO), made by peritubular cells of the kidney and Kupffer's cells. It is involved in the stimulation, differentiation, and growth of erythroid progenitor cells. The synergy of EPO with IL-3, IL-9, and IL-11 in producing mature erythroid cells has been appreciated. Nonetheless, in situations of anemia and chronic disease in which a defect in EPO may be related specifically to renal impairment of EPO production, EPO replacement is found to be a significant adjunct to treatment.[74]

Granulocyte colony-stimulating factor (G-CSF) made by monocytes, fibroblasts, and endothelial cells increases the production of neutrophils and accelerates their maturation and differentiation. Hence the physiologic production of mature neutrophils is enhanced. It is used in the treatment of people who have received cytotoxic agents that limit the bone marrow's ability to make neutrophils and thus has become a significant adjunct to treatment of patients with hematologic or oncologic disorders. Furthermore, in a purely hematologic disorder, namely cyclic neutropenia, G-CSF treatment has been shown to be incredibly effective in its treatment.[168]

Macrophage colony-stimulating factor (M-CSF) is another form of hematopoietic growth factor that is involved in promoting the growth and differentiation of multipotential hematopoietic progenitor cells and can stimulate the physiologic activity of neutrophils, eosinophils, monocytes, and macrophages. It is intimately involved in normal surfactant turnover and surfactant generation in the lung. M-CSF (CSF-1) is made primarily by monocytes, fibroblasts, and endothelial cells and modulates the physiologic activation and proliferation of monocytes and macrophages. It also stimulates the differentiation and proliferation of monocytes from bone marrow precursors.[168]

The final hematopoietic growth factor to be mentioned is the stem cell factor (SCF). This steel factor, or c-kit ligand, is made by bone marrow stromal cells, endothelial cells, and fibroblasts and interacts with other hematopoietic growth factors to stimulate myeloid, lymphoid, and erythroid progenitor cells and to maintain the viability of germ cells. It is a critically important factor for the generation of all forms of tissue mast cells and maintains the mast cell phenotype within tissues.[174] The major colony-stimulating factors are summarized in Table 5–5.

GROWTH AND DIFFERENTIATION FACTORS

Within this group is platelet-derived growth factor (PDGF), whose cellular source is platelets, endothelial cells, and macrophages and whose target includes smooth muscle

TABLE 5–5
COLONY-STIMULATING FACTORS—HEMATOPOIETIC GROWTH FACTORS

Cytokine	Cell Source	Size
EPO	Kidney, Kupffer's cells Liver	15 kD
GCSF	Monocytes/macrophages Fibroblasts Endothelial cells	15 kD
GM-CSF	T cells Monocytes Fibroblasts Endothelial cells	17 kD
M-CSF	Monocytes Fibroblasts Endothelial cells	14 kD
SCF (c-kit ligand) (steel factor)	Stromal cells Fibroblasts	17 kD

TABLE 5–6
GROWTH AND DIFFERENTIATION FACTORS

Cytokine	Cell Source	Size
Oncostatin M	T cell Monocytes/macrophages	12 kD
TGF-α	Macrophages/monocytes Keratinocytes Brain cells	23 kD
TGF-β	T cell Monocytes Osteoclasts Platelets, fibroblasts	25 kD
PDGF	Platelets, macrophages Endothelial cells Smooth muscle cells	22 kD
Leukemia inhibitory factor	Platelets, monocytes/macrophages Endothelial cells Smooth muscle cells	17 kD
Hepatocyte growth factor	Platelets, fibroblasts Monocytes/macrophages Endothelial cells Smooth muscle cells	18 kD
Epidermal growth factor–heparin binding	Macrophages	15 kD

and endothelial cells. This factor is important as a proliferative factor for endothelial cells and smooth muscles and therefore has an important role in vascular biology, atherosclerosis, and wound healing.[53]

Endothelial cell growth factor is also made by a variety of cells, including stromal cells. Its main function is to enhance the proliferation, growth, and differentiation of endothelial cells. Some growth and differentiation factors are given in Table 5–6. The transforming growth factors are discussed subsequently.

TGF-β is made by chondrocytes, osteoclasts, osteoblasts, fibroblasts, monocytes, and some T cells. It stimulates osteoblasts and osteoclasts, the formation of extracellular matrix, and wound-healing scar formation but inhibits NK cells and the proliferation and activation of B and T lymphocytes, as well as many other cell types. In the gut, it promotes IgA isotype switching by B lymphocytes in humans and under some circumstances can inhibit macrophage killing.

TGF-β represents a family of at least five peptides that regulate cell growth, having both stimulatory and inhibitory effects on different cell types.[144] It is produced by numerous cell types but primarily by mesenchymal cells, including platelets and osteocytes. It is synthesized as an inactive precursor that requires proteolytic cleavage to become active. Receptors for TGF-β are present on virtually all cells, and it mediates a wide range of biologic activities. In general, it is an important stimulant of fibrosis, inducing the formation of the extracellular matrix. In immunity, it is generally found to be inhibitory for B lymphocytes and T helper and cytotoxic lymphocytes. It inhibits immunoglobulin secretion by B lymphocytes and cytotoxicity of mononuclear phagocytes and NK/LAK cells.

In contrast to these anti-inflammatory effects, TGF-β is chemoattractive for macrophages and supports the α isotype switch to IgA by B cells.[30, 143] TGF-β knock-out mice do not survive secondary to diffuse inflammation of numerous organs by mononuclear cells.[137] In allergic inflammation, the expression of TGF-β may be associated with the fibrosis observed in long-standing asthma and the subendocardial fibrosis associated with the hypereosinophilic syndrome. TGF-β may lessen allergic inflammation through a capacity to inhibit ϵ germline transcription and IgE synthesis in IL-4–treated human B cells and through inhibition of mast cell proliferation.

TGF-α is made by macrophages and keratinocytes. It stimulates the proliferation of fibroblasts, induces epithelial development, and promotes angiogenesis. Hepatocyte growth factor is made by macrophages, endothelial cells, and smooth muscle cells and stimulates the growth of multiple cell types, including hepatocytes and some epithelial cells. Keratinocyte growth factor is a factor made by macrophages and stimulates the proliferation of keratinocytes and fibroblasts. Heparin-binding epidermal growth factor is made by macrophages and stimulates a proliferation of smooth muscle cells and fibroblasts. There are other factors in this category, including fibroblast growth factors and a variety of other factors, all of which are important in wound healing and the stromal ground substance development and function.[85]

TUMOR NECROSIS FACTORS

TNF-α is made primarily by macrophages. It is also known as cachectin. It has a wide variety of effects on diverse cell types due to modulation of gene expression for growth factors, cytokines, transcription factors, cell surface receptors, and acute phase proteins and plays an important role in host defense. It is an endogenous pyrogen. It can stimulate catabolism as well. The same thing can be said for lymphotoxin, or TNF-β, also made by T lymphocytes, B lymphocytes, and macrophages.

The third member of this group is a factor known as oncostatin M (OSM). OSM is a T-cell–derived factor, as well as a monocyte-derived factor, that inhibits the proliferation of solid tumors and stimulates the growth of normal fibroblasts and AIDS Kaposi sarcoma–derived cells. In addition to OSM, there is another tumor factor known as leukemia inhibitory factor (LIF), which suppresses the differentiation of lymphoid and hematopoietic stem cells but potentiates the development and differentiation of hematopoietic progenitor cells. It also enhances the production of acute phase proteins.

TNF represents two homologous 17 kD proteins, which are primarily derived from mononuclear phagocytes (TNF-α) and lymphocytes (TNF-β) (Table 5–7).[13, 163] In addition to mononuclear phagocytes, TNF-α may be produced by neutrophils, activated lymphocytes, NK cells, endothelial cells, and smooth muscle cells. The most potent inducer of TNF by monocytes is lipopolysaccharide. Numerous cytokines, including IL-1, IL-3, GM-CSF, and IFN-γ, may also induce TNF transcription. TNF-α is processed as a mem-

TABLE 5–7
TUMOR NECROSIS FACTORS

Cytokine	Cell Source	Size
TNF-α (cachectin)	Monocytes/macrophages	17 kD
TNF-β (lymphotoxin)	T cells	17 kD

brane-bound protein from which the soluble active factor is derived via cleavage of the extracellular domain.[113] TNF-β is synthesized and processed as a typical secretory protein.[100] The active form of both cytokines is as a noncovalently linked trimer. TNF-α and TNF-β have about 30% amino acid residue homology but bind to the same two distinct cell surface receptors with similar affinities and produce similar although not identical effects.[153] Virtually all cells studied demonstrate the presence of one or both of these receptors.

As its name implies, TNF was originally discovered as secreted peptides that induce antitumor immunity.[13, 113, 163] TNF is directly cytotoxic toward cancerous cells, stimulates antitumor immune responses by immune cells, and, when administered in vivo, induces hemorrhagic necrosis of tumors. A major proinflammatory activity of TNF is its ability to interact with endothelial cells to induce ICAM-1, permitting the egress of granulocytes into inflammatory loci.[167] Additional activities of TNF include stimulating bone resorption, cartilage degradation, and B-cell and monocyte activation. TNF augments the capacity of monocytes to produce inflammatory mediators, including IL-6 and IL-8. TNF is a potent activator of neutrophils and contributes to their adherence, chemotactic responsiveness, and degranulation and the respiratory burst.[70] Like IFN, TNF has antiviral activity and stimulates MHC class I and II expression.

Enthusiasm for the potential therapeutic value of TNF has been tempered by its severe side effects. TNF is responsible for the severe wasting that occurs in chronic infections and cancer, with cachexia occurring as the result of inhibition by TNF of the enzyme lipoprotein lipase.[13] Furthermore, TNF induces vascular leakage, has negative inotropic effects, and is thought to be an endogenous mediator of toxic shock and sepsis.[156]

ROLE OF CYTOKINES IN THE REGULATION OF ALLERGIC IMMUNITY AND INFLAMMATION

There are three major ways in which cytokines play a major role in allergic inflammation and immunity: regulation of IgE, eosinophil activation and biology, and mast cell development and activation (Table 5–8).

REGULATION OF IGE

The capability of B cells to undergo isotype switching to produce IgE requires plasma cell differentiation and is critically dependent on the interaction between three or four cytokines and other signals delivered to the B cell from activated T cells. These other signals include the transient expression of CD40 ligand on activated T cells that interacts with the CD40 marker on B cells. Switch recombinases are activated to utilize the antigen-specific VDJ gene segments of the immunoglobulin molecule and the constant region isotype marker structures for immunoglobulin synthesis. Induction of germline transcription of these isotype-specific response elements in the constant region of the immunoglobulin genes is dependent on the expression and activation of B cells by both IL-4 and IL-13. In fact, IL-4 and IL-13 share a gamma family receptor subunit in common with other cytokines.[29, 86]

The ability of both IL-4 and IL-13 to induce constant germline region mRNA is a necessary prerequisite to the activation of switch recombinases that utilize switch sites upstream of the isotype genes for VDJ insertion. The down-regulation of this cytokine-dependent IL-4– and IL-13–dependent IgE regulation is a negative influence on this response generally mediated by the cytokine IFN-γ or more interestingly by the IFN-γ inducer IL-12. Thus the activities of IL-12 and IFN-γ would have a net negative effect on IgE isotype switch by opposing some of the activities related to IL-4 and IL-13 function. Other nonspecific inhibitors of cytokine activity that may also interfere with IgE production are the effect of TGF-β in vitro on these systems. Some data support the idea that other T-cell–dependent cytokines, such as IL-2, IL-5, and IL-6, may synergize with IL-4 and IL-13 in the fully complete production of the IgE isotype.

EOSINOPHIL REGULATION

The major eosinophilopoietic and activating cytokines are IL-5, IL-3, and GM-CSF. All three of these cytokines have a well-known activity in terms of inducing eosinophilia from bone marrow precursors, activating eosinophils, and then

TABLE 5–8
ROLE OF CYTOKINES IN ALLERGIC RESPONSES

Allergic Response	Cytokine	Activity
IgE regulation	IL-4, IL-13	ϵ isotype switch
	IL-4	Generation of IL-4–producing T lymphocytes
	IL-2, IL-5, IL-6	Synergize with IL-4, IL-13
	IFN-γ, TGF-β	Inhibit IL-4, IL-13
	IL-12	Stimulates IFN-γ production by NK cells and T cells
		Inhibits differentiation of IL-4–producing T lymphocytes
Eosinophilia	IL-5, IL-3, GM-CSF	Eosinophilopoietins
	RANTES, MIP-1α, eotaxin, MCP-3	Eosinophil chemotaxis and activation
	IL-1, TNF	Eosinophil activation (priming)
Mast cell development	IL-3, IL-9, IL-10, nerve growth factor, hematopoietic SCF	Mast cell growth factors
	GM-CSF	Inhibits mast cell proliferation
	MIP-1α, MCP-1, MCP-3, RANTES	Basophil chemotaxis and histamine release
	IL-8	Inhibition of histamine release

prolonging eosinophil survival by interrupting apoptotic pathways triggered in the eosinophils. In addition to eosinophilopoietins and survival cytokines, a number of the chemokines are involved in eosinophil activation and chemotaxis, including RANTES, eotaxin, MIP-1α, and MCP-3.[125, 149] Finally, the proinflammatory cytokines, IL-1 and TNF, are involved in direct activation of eosinophils and may prime the cells for responsiveness to other agents. Hence through a wide variety of cytokines, including chemokines, eosinophils are recruited from bone marrow precursors and arrive at the tissues in an activated status.

MAST CELL PROLIFERATION

Increased numbers of mast cells characterize allergic responses. As is true of elevated IgE concentration or eosinophilia, this mast cell activation and increase in number is T-cell dependent. Mast cell proliferation may result from the activities of cytokines, such as IL-3, IL-4, IL-9, IL-10, SCF, and others. IL-3 supports the differentiation of multiple precursors, including those for megakaryocytes, monocytes, erythrocytes, and granulocytes. However, IL-3 is also involved in producing predominantly mast cell- and basophil-derived derivatives from progenitors of the CD34$^+$ lineage. IL-10 is included as a mast cell activator primarily because it is involved in the proliferation of mast cell lines in the mouse. It is not clear whether such a role exists for human IL-10. SCF is clearly an important proliferative and differential factor in both mice and humans. GM-CSF, however, has a negative effect on mast cell differentiation and has been shown to specifically inhibit mast cell proliferation. Furthermore, the chemokines, including MIP-1α, MCP-1, MCP-3, and RANTES, all have significant effects on basophil activation and chemotaxis and histamine release.

T HELPER LYMPHOCYTE FAMILIES

T lymphocytes do not necessarily produce all of their cytokines upon activation. Subclasses of T helper lymphocytes can therefore be identified among antigen-specific T cells on the basis of their repertoire of cytokines.[93, 170] In humans, type 1 helper cells (Th1) produce IFN-γ and TNF-β, but not IL-4 and IL-5. Type 2 helper cells (Th2) produce IL-4, IL-5, and IL-9, but not IFN-γ or TNF-β. Both classes produce GM-CSF, IL-2, IL-3, IL-10, and IL-13. These observations on human T-cell clones are in contrast to those on the mouse, insofar as production of IL-2, IL-10, and IL-13 is shared by both classes of T helper cells. Although T helper lymphocyte subclasses may be less apparent in human than in murine cells, there is an inverse relationship between the tendency of a T-cell clone to produce IFN-γ as opposed to IL-4 or IL-5. Undifferentiated Th0 cells produce primarily IL-2 but may also synthesize cytokines characteristic of both Th1 and Th2 lymphocytes.

There are, however, a number of caveats concerning this differentiation of Th1 versus Th2 lymphocytes. No firm differentiation markers exist that identify a Th1 versus a Th2 cell in either the mouse or the human. Therefore, functional characterization of enhanced cytokine production may not represent a firm state of differentiation, but rather the functional consequences of the milieu in which the cell is being stimulated.

TABLE 5–9
Th1/Th2 RESPONSES IN HUMANS AND MICE

	Th1	Th2	Th10
Murine	IL-2, IFN-γ, lymphotoxin	IL-4, IL-5, IL-6, IL-9, IL-10, IL-13	IL-3, GM-CSF
Human	IFN-γ, lymphotoxin	IL-4, IL-5, IL-9	IL-2, IL-10, IL-13, IL-3, GM-CSF

The second caveat is that there are circumstances in which the analogy of cytokine profiles between human and murine Th2- and Th1-type lymphocytes is different (Table 5–9). For example, in the human, both Th1 and Th2, as well as Th0 subsets, make IL-2, IL-10, and IL-13 in addition to GM-CSF and IL-3. Data demonstrate enhanced and significant production of IL-2 in a patient with Sézary syndrome in which there is predominant Th2-like pattern to the Sézary cell cytokine production, in Th2-like T-cell clones taken from the blood of atopic mite-sensitive individuals, and even in the bronchoalveolar lavage of patients with allergic asthma.[14, 120, 170] In addition, IL-13 in humans is not solely a product of Th2 cells but can be made by Th1 and Th0 cells as well. In humans, IL-10 is predominantly a product of macrophages but can be made by both Th1- and Th2-like cells.[31, 165, 176] Hence significant limitations concerning the clear distinction between the cytokine profiles made by Th1 and Th2 cells in humans need to be kept in mind.

Th1 lymphocytes, through their production of IL-2, TNF-β, and IFN-γ, activate T cells and monocytes and therefore promote cell-mediated immune responses. T helper lymphocytes that produce IFN-γ, IL-2, IL-6, IL-10, and IL-14 induce B-cell maturation and are important in antibody-dependent immunity. Th2 lymphocytes that produce IL-4, IL-5, and IL-13 and function in the relative absence of IFN-γ induce allergic immune responses. Support for the concept that Th2-like cells are important in mediating allergic diseases is the observation discussed previously that mite-specific T-cell clones obtained from atopic subjects were Th2-like, whereas clones derived from a nonallergic subject were Th1-like.[170]

MECHANISMS OF Th1/Th2 DIFFERENTIATION

One of the most important issues in understanding allergic disorders is to determine the basis for Th1/Th2 differentiation in response to allergen. A detailed discussion of this topic is beyond the scope of this review. Factors such as genetic predisposition, specific physiochemical nature of the offending allergen, different antigen-processing and antigen-presenting pathways, and antigen-presenting cell type, as well as usage of unique MHC restriction elements or T-cell receptor V region usage, have all been proposed as having a role. However, one of the most critical elements in determining T helper differentiation is the cytokine milieu in which the T lymphocyte is activated. The major determinant of Th2 differentiation is the cytokine IL-4.[1, 131] This has been best established in T-cell receptor transgenic mice, in which the concomitant exposure of the animal to IL-4 and the relevant antigen induces in a dose-dependent fashion increasing production of IL-4 in the responding T cells. Neutralizing antibodies to IL-4 preclude the development of IL-4–producing T lymphocytes.

A mechanism for Th1 differentiation has been shown to be dependent on IL-12. Thus IL-12 induces in a dose-dependent fashion increasing concentrations of IFN-γ and decreasing concentrations of IL-4 in the responding T-cell receptor antigen-specific T lymphocytes.[83] Similarly, concomitant infection of mice with *Leishmania* and exposure to murine IL-12 lead to the development of IFN-γ–producing T helper cells and a decrease in IL-4 production within lymph node cells.[52, 145] IL-12–mediated IFN-γ production may be required for the full expression of the Th1 phenotype.[129] In one study, IL-12 costimulated antigen-specific proliferation of established Th1 clones, but not Th0 or Th2 clones.[65] Insofar as mononuclear phagocytes are the major source for IL-12, this suggests a mechanism whereby antigens more likely to be processed by macrophages, including bacterial antigens and intracellular pathogens, produce Th1 responses. The Th1-inducing effects of IL-12 can be overcome in the additional presence of IL-4. Thus the IL-4 effects on undifferentiated Th0 cells are dominant.[19, 57] The original source for the IL-4 responsible for Th2 differentiation remains unclear. The net result, however, is that in a milieu where allergic inflammation is present, such as nasal and bronchial mucosa, more and more extensive allergenic responses (Th2-type) against bystander antigens would be expected to develop.

CYTOKINE GENETICS

A tremendous interest in the genetics of atopy and asthma has resulted in the examination of a wide variety of genetic loci for alteration related to linked inheritance of asthma and atopy in families at risk for these characteristics.[15, 84, 88] A number of the linkages have identified potential candidates for Th2-like cytokine responses on human chromosome 5 (see Chapter 24). A number of studies have shown linkages between these responses and cytokine variation. There are linkages that are worth considering. The first involves the Th2 cytokines on chromosome 5q, where the genes that code for cytokines, such as IL-4, IL-5, IL-3, IL-9, IL-12β, IL-13, GM-CSF, fibroblast growth factor α, and interferon regulatory factor 1, are all encoded. In addition to this cluster, there are a number of receptor genes in this same cluster, including the B_2-adrenergic receptor, CSF-1 receptor, PDGF receptor, and glucocorticoid receptor. This constellation of genes, all of which may be significantly dysregulated in asthma, makes chromosome location 5q an important potential hot spot in the study of the genetics of asthma and atopy.

A second area that has also been examined for potential linkage to cytokine dysregulation in asthma is the MHC itself on human chromosome 6p. Here, the genes for both TNF-α and TNF-β are expressed in conjunction with class I-class II transporter and proteasome genes, as well as complement genes, any of which might also be dysregulated in immune and inflammatory diseases, such as asthma. Finally, the two major families of chemokines, the C-X-C and the C-C, are present on human chromosome 17q and 4q, respectively.

TABLE 5–10
GENETIC LOCI FOR CYTOKINE GENES

Classes of Cytokines	Loci	Cytokine Candidate Genes
Chemokines C-X-C	4q	IL-8, NAP-2, PF-4, βTG, CTAP-III, γIP-10, MIP-2
Chemokines C-C	17q	MIP-1α, MIP-1β MCP 1–4, eotaxin, RANTES
Th2 cytokines	5q	IL-4, IL-5, IL-3, IL-9, IL-12, IL-13, GM-CSF, FGFA, β2ADR, IRF-1, CSFI-R, PDGF-R, GC-R
MHC	6p	TNF-α, TNF-β

The 4q chemokines include IL-8, NAP-2, platelet factor 4, β-thromboglobulin, CTAP-3, MIP-2, and γIP-10. The C-C subfamily on 17q includes the MIP-1α and MIP-1β genes, along with the MCP-1 and MCP-3 genes, eotaxin, and RANTES. The study in families of these two genetic loci on 17q and 4q may lead to interesting potential associations that have not yet been studied. The genetic loci for cytokine genes are summarized in Table 5–10.

CYTOKINE RECEPTORS AND RECEPTOR SIGNALING

CYTOKINE RECEPTORS

Cytokines produce their biologic activities through their linkage to signal transduction pathways mediated by high-affinity receptors present on cells throughout the body. The cellular location of these receptors and the nature of the activating cascades induced by the receptor ultimately are responsible for each cytokine's biologic activity. Cytokine receptors and signaling are unusually complex insofar as they may evoke either positive or negative signals, depending on the type and developmental state of the target cell. Alternatively, many different cytokines acting through their individual receptors may transduce identical biologic responses. The signaling cascades stimulated by receptor binding form complex networks with cross-communication. Thus a single receptor may couple to multiple transduction systems, or multiple receptors may couple to the same pathway.

Cytokine receptors are integral membrane glycoproteins, oriented with an external amino terminus and a single membrane-spanning domain. Most cytokine receptors are members of a superfamily characterized by a motif containing four conserved cysteine residues and one tryptophan residue in their extracellular portion (typical sequence of Cys-X_{9-20}-Cys-X-Tyr-X_{22-36}-Cys-X_{8-25}-Cys) and a second domain characterized by a Trp-Ser-X-Trp-Ser motif more proximal to the membrane.[11, 59, 91] These regions are critical for binding of the receptor to its respective cytokines. A second conserved domain (the box 1/box 2 motifs) is present in the membrane proximal portion of the cytoplasmic region and is essential for receptor signaling.

γ CHAIN RECEPTOR SUBFAMILY

The paradigm of this family is the high-affinity form of the IL-2 receptor.[148, 150] The IL-2R is composed of at least three distinct subunits. The α subunit is a 55 kD protein with a small cytoplasmic domain (13 amino acids) that has homology only with the IL-15Rα chain. The β and γ subunits (γc) are members of the cytokine receptor superfamily and have relatively large intracytoplasmic domains that are capable of transducing signals.[99] The β and γ chains are constitutively expressed in T cells, whereas the α chain is rapidly induced after occupation of the T-cell antigen receptor. Signal transduction is mediated by the β and γ chains, whereas the α chain acts to enhance the affinity of the IL-2R complex for the ligand. Heterodimerization of the β and γ chains of the IL-2R complex initiates signal transduction. Activated β and γ chains become associated with several activated tyrosine kinases, including *lck, lyn,* and *fyn.*[49, 151] The capacity of cytokine receptors to couple to more than one transduction pathway is exemplified by IL-2Rβ.[151]

Proliferative signals have been linked to the presence of a serine-rich intracytoplasmic region and the induction of *c-myc.* In contrast, a more distal acidic region is linked to the induction of the *c-fos* gene and to the tyrosine kinases. Studies with the IL-2Rγ chain have suggested analogous dual pathways for the induction of *c-myc* and *c-fos.* The γ chain is also a constitutive part of the high-affinity form of at least five other receptors, which may explain many of their redundant functions. With the exception of the IL-15R, which also utilizes the IL-2Rβ chain, the other four members of the γ-containing subfamily are heterodimers. The absence of γ chains is responsible for one form of X-linked severe combined immunodeficiency, reflecting its importance in signaling by these six cytokines.[62, 101]

IL-3, IL-5, AND GM-CSF RECEPTORS

The IL-3, IL-5, and GM-CSF receptors represent heterodimers that share a common 140 kD β chain and are characterized by their distinct α chains.[51, 91, 94] These α chains are homologous, and there is mutual competition for their binding to their respective cytokines. The structural similarities of these receptors help explain the overlapping functions of these cytokines, such as eosinophil activation. Both α and β chains are members of the cytokine receptor superfamily. The three ligand-binding α chains have short cytoplasmic domains that are not required for signal transduction. Signaling is mediated through ligand-induced interactions of the cytoplasmic regions of the receptors' heterodimers. As described for the β and γ chains of the IL-2R, the common β chain expresses numerous domains capable of signaling.[126] A membrane proximal region is essential for the induction of *c-myc* and *pim*-1. A second distal region is required for the activation of the ras/raf-1/MAP kinase pathway, as well as the induction of *c-fos* and *c-jun.*

IL-6 RECEPTOR SUBFAMILY SHARING GP130

IL-6, IL-11, LIF, OSM, and ciliary neutrotrophic factor (CNTF) all share structural and functional similarities.[68] A role for gp130 (β component) in IL-12 signaling is speculative but is based on the known homology of this cytokine with IL-6 and the IL-6R. The use of the shared receptor is an explanation for the functional redundancy of these ligands. The gp130 subfamily of receptors triggers signaling through the formation of homodimers and heterodimers with gp130.[96, 145] In the case of IL-6 and probably IL-11, the cytokine receptor complex serves to approximate the two gp130 moieties, resulting in the formation of enzymatically active homodimers.

The ligand-specific α components to these receptors have an insignificant cytoplasmic domain that has no role in signaling. Although gp130 is expressed on almost all tissues, it is the more limited expression of the ligand-specific α component that therefore regulates cellular responsiveness. The binding of IL-6 to the soluble form of the IL-6R (sIL-6R) (free α chain) can confer IL-6 responsiveness to gp130-expressing cells, which do not express IL-6R. This is potentially an unusual and important proinflammatory mechanism for soluble receptors, since most soluble receptors bind ligand and impede interaction with the cell surface and thus are inhibitory. This model of activity of IL-6 and IL-11 is in contrast to LIF-R and OSM-R.[146] These receptors are homologous to gp130 and have more extensive cytoplasmic domains that are necessary for signaling. These receptors form enzymatically active heterodimers with gp130 after binding their respective ligands.

INTERFERON RECEPTORS

IFN-α and IFN-β share a common receptor that has only limited sequence homology to the IFN-γ receptor.[2, 3] Both IFN receptors are heterodimers, and both proteins are essential for signaling. The IL-10R is closely related to the IFN receptors, and all three receptors are distant members of the cytokine receptor superfamily. The cascades initiated by the IFN receptors are probably the best understood of all the cytokines and will be discussed later in further detail as a model of cytokine-mediated cellular signaling.

SINGLE CHAIN RECEPTORS

Additional receptors related to the cytokine receptor superfamily are characterized by the presence of only a single signaling protein. This family includes several hematopoietic growth factors and hormones and the cytokine G-CSF.

TNF RECEPTOR SUBFAMILY

Additional cytokine receptors are not members of the cytokine receptor superfamily. TNF-α and TNF-β are structurally and functionally closely related, and each has two distinct receptors, TNFR 1 (85 kD) and TNFR II (55 kD).[45, 55] Both receptors are homologous and bind TNF with comparable affinity. Although other receptors of this family do not bind cytokines, they mediate important immune functions, including mast cell proliferation (NGF), the immunoglobulin isotype switch (CD40) and its ligand (CD39), and immune cell apoptosis (fas).[141]

IMMUNOGLOBULIN RECEPTOR SUPERFAMILY

This superfamily is unrelated to the cytokine receptor superfamily but includes the receptors for IL-1.[172] The two

IL-1 receptors bind IL-1α and IL-1β equally well and are structurally homologous. As discussed previously, the type II receptors are inactive and may subserve anti-inflammatory functions.

TYROSINE KINASE RECEPTOR FAMILY

In contrast to most of the cytokine receptors, receptors for many growth factors have large cytoplasmic domains with intrinsic tyrosine kinase activity. Physiologically, tyrosine kinase activity is initiated by receptor dimerization. Mutations that result in spontaneous tyrosine kinase activation promote oncogenesis, and these receptors are therefore proto-oncogenes. Two cytokines that bind to members of this family are M-CSF and SCF.[133, 177] The M-CSF receptor was originally identified as the proto-oncogene c-fms and is expressed primarily on mononuclear phagocytic cells. The M-CSFR is highly homologous to PDGFR, and they are closely associated on chromosome 5 in the midst of the cytokine gene cluster. SCFR was identified as the pro-oncogene c-kit in deficient mice characterized by a reduction of pluripotent hematopoietic stem cells, anemia, albinism, and absent mast cells.

SIGNAL TRANSDUCTION BY CYTOKINE RECEPTORS

In contrast to many growth factors, cytokine receptors generally do not have cytoplasmic domains with intrinsic tyrosine kinase activity. However, cytokine receptors do activate cytoplasmic tyrosine kinases and may be phosphorylated by these enzymes.[64, 89, 98, 117] The first step in the activation of cytokine receptors is ligand-induced dimerization/oligomerization. This results in approximation of the cytoplasmic regions that initiates the cascade of signaling events. In the absence of intrinsic tyrosine kinase activity, the current model is that dimerization approximates two contact surfaces, allowing their stable interaction with a cytoplasm-derived signaling molecule.[132]

The concept has emerged that a novel family of cytoplasmic protein-tyrosine kinases, termed *Janus* kinases (Jaks), uniquely function in cytokine signaling.[171] Jaks are structurally unique from other cytoplasmic protein-tyrosine kinases previously characterized. There are four Janus kinases: Jak 1, Jak 2, Jak 3, and Tyk 2. There are identifiable blocks of homology among the four family members, which include the presence of two kinase domains.[48] Interestingly, Jaks lack detectable src-homology-2 (SH2) or SH3 domains.[110] SH2 domains are binding sites that are structurally conserved and were first identified in the src oncogene. SH2 domains participate in the binding of phosphotyrosine residues, whereas SH3 domains recognize proline-rich motifs. These Jaks physically associate with membrane proximal cytoplasmic domains of the receptor (the box1/box2 domain) following ligand binding and rapidly induce tyrosine kinase activity.[97, 132]

The role for Jak family members in the pathway to gene activation was largely deduced from studies of signal transduction by the IFN receptors, IFN-α/β and IFN-γ.[28, 127, 173] A series of mutants were selected for their inability to respond to either IFN-α/β or IFN-γ. This provided the first genetic evidence that Tyk 2 was required for an IFN-α/β response and Jak 2 was required for an IFN-γ response. However, Jak 1 is essential for both IFN responses.[95, 161, 166] The current model for IFN-α/β and IFN-γ activation is as follows. Ligand-stimulated receptor dimerization increases the affinity of the cytoplasmic domain of the dimers to bind two Jaks. The two chains of the IFN-α receptor bind Jak 1 and Tyk 2, respectively, whereas the two chains of the IFN-γ receptor bind Jak 1 and Jak 2. The receptors and the Jaks themselves become phosphorylated. This phosphorylated complex becomes the catalyst for the phosphorylation of cytoplasmic substrates. The Jaks do not become phosphorylated in a kinase cascade, but rather this occurs simultaneously via cross-phosphorylation.[95, 161, 166]

Although other Jak family members may exist, it appears that receptor signaling is mediated by a limited number of highly redundant tyrosine kinases. Jak 2 is involved in GM-CSF, G-CSF, IL-6, and IL-3 signaling.[116, 139] Jak 1, Jak 3, and all of the other cytokines whose receptors are members of the γ chain family of receptors are tyrosine phosphorylated in response to IL-2 and IL-4.[63, 67] Jak 3 is physically linked to the γ chain, whereas Jak 1 is linked to the box1/box2 domains of this subfamily of receptors. This importance of Jak 3 signaling in the transduction cascades of the γ chain subfamily and other cytokines is consistent with observations that Jak 3 deficiency is responsible for one form of autosomal recessive severe combined immunodeficiency.

Once activation of a cytokine receptor has led to tyrosine phosphorylation of the receptor and of receptor-associated Jaks, the next step in signal transduction involves the phosphorylation of latent cytoplasmic transcription factors. These factors have been termed signal transducers and activators of transcription (STAT).[135] After activation, these proteins migrate to the nucleus, where they bind to specific regulatory sequences in the promoters of cytokine-responsive genes, thereby initiating gene transcription. STATs thereby transduce a signal from the cytokine receptor to a transcription regulatory element of DNA.

STAT proteins are characterized by the presence of a carboxy-terminal SH3 domain followed by an SH2 domain, which represents the phosphotyrosine-binding segment. A conserved tyrosine is found near the carboxy terminus that is phosphorylated and is essential for function.[136] As with the Jaks, the function of STATs was originally characterized with studies dealing with the biochemical events of IFN-induced gene transcription.[27, 111, 112, 161] Using mutants nonresponsive to IFN signaling, it was demonstrated that Jaks directly catalyze the tyrosine phosphorylation of STAT proteins. Ligand binding of IFN-α/β induces the formation of a cytoplasmic transcription complex termed the IFN-α–stimulated gene factor 3 complex (ISGF-3), which subsequently binds to a DNA sequence termed the IFN-stimulated response element (ISRE) present in the promoters of IFN-responsive genes. The ISGF-3 complex consists of the STAT proteins: STAT 1α (p91), STAT 1β (p84), STAT 2 (p113), and p48.[27, 111, 112, 161]

In IFN-α–stimulated cells, following phosphorylation of the ISGF-3 complex by Jak 1 and Tyk 2, the STAT 1-STAT 2 proteins dimerize and then complex with the 48 kD DNA-binding protein, all of which migrate to the nucleus and bind to the ISRE. In contrast, the stimulation of cells with

IFN-γ results in the tyrosine phosphorylation of STAT 1 by Jak 1 and Jak 2, but not STAT 2. This transcription factor, which is responsible for IFN-γ–induced gene transcription (also termed the IFN-γ activation factor or GAF), is made up of dimers of STAT 1.[134] In the nucleus, the STAT 1 homodimers form DNA-binding complexes that recognize specific DNA sequences termed γ-activated sequences (GAS) in the promoters of genes that are transcriptionally activated by IFN-γ.

The list of STAT proteins is expanding. There are currently 6 known members of the STAT family, with an estimate that ultimately there may be up to 10. STAT 3, STAT 4, and STAT 6 were identified as IL-6–, IL-12–, and IL-4–inducible peptides, respectively.[5, 61, 77, 81] Although important in cytokine signaling, STAT 5 was originally defined as a prolactin-inducible peptide. In addition to sharing homologous SH2 and SH3 regions at their carboxy terminus, STAT peptides are also characterized by the highly conserved sequences of their DNA-binding regions (consensus sequence TTCCNGGAA). These novel STAT proteins function very similarly to the way that STAT 1 and STAT 2 pathways work in IFN-mediated signal transduction. IL-4 signaling, for example, involves the phosphorylation of the substrate STAT 6 via Jak 1 and Jak 3 kinases.[114] Phosphorylation allows STAT 6 to dimerize, forming STF-IL-4 (signaling transduction factor), which then undergoes nuclear translocation. In the nucleus, STF-IL-4 binds to DNA sequences related to GAS.[71, 73, 128]

STAT 6 mediates the major biologic activities of IL-4 associated with allergic inflammation: the IgE isotype switch and Th2 differentiation. STAT 6 sites are present in the switch region of the ϵ heavy chain. STAT 6 knock-out mice, while having mature B cells capable of proliferation, are unable to synthesize IgE. Stimulation of T helper lymphocytes derived from these STAT 6 knock-outs in the presence of IL-4 fails to induce Th2 lymphocytes. These cells do not secrete IL-4 or IL-5 but develop the phenotype of Th1 cells. These studies are in contrast to those of mice deficient in functional STAT 4. Elimination of this IL-12–inducible protein prevents these mice from producing Th1 lymphocytes (J. Ihle, personal communication).

This final specificity in any gene activation is nuclear. For different protein ligands to have unique effects on cells, the activated transcription factors (both cytoplasmic and nuclear) must bind to specific promoter sites and DNA elements. Specificity of STAT activation is mediated by the presence of specific binding sites for the appropriate STAT proteins on each receptor. Compared with the number of cytokines, there are relatively few STATs. Therefore the signaling pathways of several distinct cytokines share common STAT proteins. Epidermal growth factor (EGF), PDGF, M-CSF, IL-6, IL-11, and the IFNs all activate STAT 1α. Although there are extensive redundancies in the biologic activities of cytokines that share Jak and STAT, mechanisms must also exist that specify the biologic responses to different cytokines. In part, these reflect the activities of other signaling pathways stimulated by cytokine receptors.

Although beyond the scope of this discussion, the ras-dependent pathway is also a major signaling pathway activated by members of the cytokine receptor superfamilies. In this cascade, SHC, Grb2, SOS, ras, raf-1, MEKK, and MAP kinases are sequentially phosphorylated and activated. The MAPK pathway is associated with the induction of several immediate early genes, such as *pmn-1, c-myc,* and *c-fos.* Proteins such as the transcription factor NF-IL-6 are phosphorylated by MAP kinase and are transcriptionally activated. The ras pathway is activated by several growth factors, as well as the cytokines IL-2, IL-3, IL-5, and EPO, suggesting that this pathway may play a fundamental role in a variety of cells.[131] A notable exception to the use of the ras pathway for signaling by cytokines is IL-4, which in distinction to these other cytokines activates the signaling protein insulin response substrate-1 (IRS-1). IRS-1 is required for IL-4–mediated mitogenesis, an activity not induced by STAT 6. Studies addressing the relative contribution of the Jak kinases to the ras and other signaling pathways to cytokine signaling are important areas for future research.

In summary, a generalized framework for polypeptide-dependent gene control involving Jak and STAT proteins has been developed. This signal transduction pathway is initiated by a ligand that stimulates dimerization of receptor complexes, leading to the activation of one or more Jaks in association with the membrane proximal domain of the cytokine receptor. The Jaks in turn tyrosine phosphorylate themselves and the receptor. The phosphorylated tyrosine of the receptor is the site for reversible binding of a latent cytoplasmic transcription factor, or STAT, where it is phosphorylated. The STAT proteins then dimerize, and these active transcription factors can then enter the nucleus and initiate gene transcription by binding to response elements, such as the well-described ISRE and GAS sequences.

SUMMARY

Cytokines that are important in the pathophysiology of allergic disorders are summarized in Table 5–8. The IgE isotype switch results from the activities of IL-4 and IL-13 and is inhibited by IFN-γ and TGF-β. IL-2, IL-5, and IL-6 synergize with IL-4 and IL-13 to enhance IgE secretion. IL-4 is responsible for the differentiation of IL-4–producing lymphocytes, whereas IL-12 inhibits the differentiation of IL-4–producing T cells. IL-5 is the most important eosinophilopoietin and together with GM-CSF and IL-3 prolongs the survival and activates mature eosinophils. These three cytokines are responsible for the generation of the hypodense eosinophils that characterize the asthmatic state. Eosinophilia may also result from selective recruitment by the eosinophil chemotaxins RANTES, MCP-3, MIP-1α, and eotaxin. Mast cell proliferation results from the activities of IL-3, IL-9, IL-10, nerve growth factor, and SCF. Finally, several cytokines contribute to the inflammatory state of allergic inflammatory disorders. IL-1, TNF, and IFN-γ increase expression of endothelial cell adhesion molecules and support the egress of mononuclear cells, neutrophils, and eosinophils into the lungs. Induction of VCAM-1 by IL-4 may promote the selective recruitment of eosinophils, basophils, and lymphocytes. Many cytokines may then contribute to the activation of these leukocytes once they have reached the airways.

REFERENCES

1. Abehsira-Amar O, Gibert M, Joliy M, et al: IL-4 plays a dominant role in the differential development of Th0 into Th1 and Th2 cells. J Immunol 148:3820–3829, 1992.

2. Aguet M, Dembic Z, Merlin G: Molecular cloning and expression of the human interferon-γ receptor. Cell 55:273–280, 1988.
3. Aguet M, Grobke M, Dreiding P: Various human interferon α subunits cross-react with common receptors: their binding affinities correlate with their specific biological activities. Virology 132:211–216, 1984.
4. Akina S, Taga T, Koshimoto T: Interleukin-6 in biology and medicine. Adv Immunol 54:1–78, 1993.
5. Akira S, Nishio Y, Inoue M, et al: Molecular cloning of APRF, a novel IFN-stimulated gene factor 3 p91-related transcription factor involved in the gp130-mediated signaling pathway. Cell 77(1):63–71, 1994.
6. Ambrus JL, Chesky L, Chused T: Intracellular signaling events associated with induction of proliferation of normal human B lymphocytes by two different antigenically related human B cell growth factors (high molecular weight B cell growth factor [HMW-BCGF] and the complement factor 3b). J Biol Chem 266:3702–3708, 1991.
7. Arai K, Lee F, Miyajima A, et al: Cytokines: coordinators of immune and inflammatory responses. Annu Rev Biochem 59:783–836, 1990.
8. Arend WP: Interleukin-1 receptor antagonist. Adv Immunol 54:167–227, 1993.
9. Auron PE, Warner SJ, Webb AC, et al: Studies on the molecular nature of human interleukin 1. J Immunol 138(5):1447–1456, 1987.
10. Baggiolini M, Dahinden CA: CC chemokines in allergic inflammation. Immunol Today 15(3):127–133, 1994.
11. Bazan JF: Structural design and molecular evolution of a cytokine receptor superfamily. Proc Natl Acad Sci USA 87:6934–6938, 1990.
12. Bellone G, Trinchieri G: Dual stimulatory and inhibitory effect of NK cell stimulatory factor/IL-12 on human hematopoiesis. J Immunol 153:930–937, 1994.
13. Beutler B, Cerami A: The biology of cachectin/TNF—a primary mediator of the host response. Annu Rev Immunol 7:625–655, 1989.
14. Borish L, Dishuck J, Cox L, et al: Sézary syndrome with elevated serum IgE and hypereosinophilia: role of dysregulated cytokine production. J Allergy Clin Immunol 92:123–131, 1993.
15. Borish L, Mascali JJ, Klinnert M, et al: SSC polymorphisms in interleukin genes. Hum Mol Genet 3:1710, 1994.
16. Briere F, Servet-Delprat C, Bridon JM, et al: Human interleukin 10 induces naive surface immunoglobulin D+ (sIgD+) B cells to secrete IgG1 and IgG3. J Exp Med 179:757–762, 1994.
17. Brunda MJ: Interleukin-12. Leukoc Biol 55:280–288, 1994.
18. Cerretti DP, Kozlosky CJ, Mosley B, et al: Molecular cloning of the interleukin-1β converting enzyme. Science 256(5053):97–100, 1992.
19. Chan SH, Perussia B, Gupta JW: Induction of interferon γ production by natural killer cell stimulatory factor: Characterization of the responder cells and synergy with other inducers. J Exp Med 173(4):869–879, 1991.
20. Chen WF, Zlotnik A: IL-10: a novel cytotoxic T cell differentiation factor. J Immunol 147:528–534, 1991.
21. Clutterbuck EJ, Hirst EMA, Sanderson CJ: Human interleukin 5 (IL-5) regulates the production of eosinophils in human bone marrow cultures: comparison and interaction with IL-1, IL-3, IL-6, and GM-CSF. Blood 73:1504–1512, 1989.
22. Coffman RL, Carty J: A T cell activity that enhances polyclonal IgE production and its inhibition by interferon-gamma. J Immunol 136:949–954, 1986.
23. Coffman RL, Ohara J, Bond MW, et al: B cell stimulatory factor-1 enhances the IgE response of lipopolysaccharide-activated B cells. J Immunol 136:4538–4541, 1986.
24. Coffman RL, Seymour BWP, Hudak S, et al: Antibody to interleukin-5 inhibits helminth-induced eosinophilia in mice. Science 245:308–310, 1989.
25. Corrigan CJ, Haczku A, Gemou-Engesaeth V, et al: CD4 T lymphocyte activation in asthma is accompanied by increased serum concentrations of IL-5. Effect of glucocorticoid therapy. Am Rev Respir Dis 147(3):540–547, 1993.
26. D'Andrea A, Aste-Amezaga M, Vaiante NM, et al: Interleukin 10 (IL-10) inhibits human lymphocyte interferon-γ production by suppressing natural killer cell stimulatory factor/IL-12 synthesis in accessory cells. J Exp Med 178:1041–1048, 1993.
27. Darnell JE Jr, Kerr IM, Stark GR: Jak-STAT pathways and transcriptional activation in response to IFNs and other extracellular signaling proteins. Science 264(5164):1415–1421, 1994.
28. Decker T, Lew DJ, Mirkovitch J, Darnell JE Jr: Cytoplasmic activation of GAF, an IFN-gamma-regulated DNA-binding factor. EMBO J 10(4):927–932, 1991.
29. Defrance T, Carayon P, Billian G: Interleukin 13 is a B cell stimulating factor. J Exp Med 179:135–143, 1994.
30. DeFrance T, Vanbervliet B, Briere F, et al: Interleukin 10 and transforming growth factor β cooperate to induce anti-CD40-activate naive human B cells to secrete immunoglobulin A. J Exp Med 175(3):671–682, 1992.
31. Del Prete G, De Carli M, Almerigogna F, et al: Human IL-10 is produced by both type 1 helper (Th1) and Type 2 helper (Th2) T cell clones and inhibits their antigen-specific proliferation and cytokine production. J Immunol 150:353–360, 1993.
32. Del Prete GF, Maggi E, Parronchi P, et al: IL-4 is an essential factor for IgE synthesis induced in vitro by human T cell clones and their supernatants. J Immunol 140:4193–4198, 1988.
33. Denberg JA, Silver JE, Abrams JS: Interleukin-5 is a human basophilopoietin: induction of histamine content and basophilic differentiation of HL-60 cells and of peripheral blood basophil-eosinophil progenitors. Blood 77:1462–1468, 1991.
34. Dinarello CA: Interleukin-1 and interleukin-1 antagonism. Blood 77:1627–1652, 1991.
35. Dinarello CA, Wolff SM: The role of interleukin-1 in disease. N Engl J Med 328:106–113, 1993.
36. Eisenberg SP, Evans RJ, Arend WP, et al: Primary structure and functional expression from complementary DNA of a human interleukin-1 receptor antagonist. Nature 343:341–346, 1990.
37. Enk AH, Angeloni VL, Udey MC, Katz SI: Inhibition of Langerhans cell antigen-presenting function by IL-10: a role for IL-10 in induction of tolerance. J Immunol 151:2390–2398, 1993.
38. Farrar MA, Schreiber RD: The molecular cell biology of interferon-γ and its receptor. Annu Rev Immunol 11:571–611, 1993.
39. Fenton MJ, Buras JA, Donnelly RP: IL-4 reciprocally regulates IL-1 and IL-1 receptor antagonist expression in human monocytes. J Immunol 149:1283–1288, 1992.
40. Ferretti M, Casini-Raggi V, Pizarro TT, et al: Neutralization of endogenous IL-1 receptor antagonist exacerbates and prolongs inflammation in rabbit immune colitis. J Clin Invest 94(1):449–453, 1994.
41. Fiorentino DF, Bond MW, Mosmann TR: Two types of mouse T helper cell. IV. Th2 clones secrete a factor that inhibits cytokine production by Th1 clones. J Exp Med 170:2081–2095, 1989.
42. Fiorentino DF, Zlotnik A, Mosmann TR, et al: IL-10 inhibits cytokine production by activated macrophages. J Immunol 147:3815–3822, 1991.
43. Gauchat JF, Gascan H, Malefyt RD, de Vries JE: Regulation of germ-line ϵ transcription and induction of ϵ switching in cloned EBV-transformed and malignant human B cell lines by cytokines and CD4+T cells. J Immunol 148:2291–2299, 1992.
44. Giri JG, Ahdieh M, Eisenman J, et al: Utilization of the β chain and γ chains of the IL-2 receptor by the novel cytokine IL-15. EMBO J 13(12):2822–2830, 1994.
45. Goodwin RG, Anderson D, Jerzy R: Molecular cloning and expression of the type 1 and type 2 murine receptors for tumor necrosis factor. Mol Cell Biol 11(6):3020–3026, 1991.
46. Grabstein K, Eisenman J, Shanebeck K, et al: Cloning of a T cell growth factor that interacts with the β chain of the interleukin-2 receptor. Science 264(5161):965–968, 1994.
47. Granowitz EV, Clark BD, Mancilla J, Dinarello CA: Interleukin-1 receptor antagonist competitively inhibits the binding of interleukin-1 to the type II interleukin-1 receptor. J Biol Chem 266:14147–14150, 1991.
48. Harpur AG, Andres AC, Ziemiecki A, et al: JAK2, a third member of the JAK family of protein tyrosine kinases. Oncogene 7(7):1347–1353, 1992.
49. Hatekeyama M, Kono T, Kobayashi N, et al: Interaction of the IL-2 receptor with the src-family kinase $p56^{lck}$. Identification of novel intermolecular association. Science 252:1523–1528, 1991.
50. Hatekeyama M, Minamoto S, Uchiyama T, et al: Reconstitution of functional receptor for human interleukin-2 in mouse cells. Nature 318(6045):467–470, 1985.
51. Hayashida K, Kitamura T, Gorman DM, et al: Molecular cloning of a second subunit of the receptor for human granulocyte-macrophage colony-stimulating factor (GM-CSF): reconstitution of a high-affinity GM-CSF receptor. Proc Natl Acad Sci USA 87:9655–9659, 1990.
52. Heinzel FP, Schoenhaut DS, Rerko RM, et al: Recombinant interleukin 12 cures mice infected with Leishmania major. J Exp Med 177:1505–1509, 1993.
53. Heldin CH: Structural and functional studies on platelet-derived growth factor. EMBO J 11:4251–4259, 1992.
54. Henney CS, Kuribayashi K, Kern DE, Gillis S: Interleukin-2 augments natural killer cell activity. Nature 291:335–338, 1981.

55. Hohmann H, Remy R, Brockhaus M, Van Loon APGM: Two different cell types have different major receptors for human tumor necrosis factor (TNF-α). J Biol Chem 264:14646–14652, 1989.
56. Horuk R: The interleukin-8-receptor family: from chemokines to malaria. Immunol Today 15:169–174, 1995.
57. Hseih CS, Macatonia SE, Tripp CS, et al: Development of TH1 CD4+ T cells through IL-12 produced by Listeria-induced macrophages. Science 260:547–549, 1993.
58. Hsu DH, Moore KW, Spits H: Differential effects of interleukin-4 and -10 on interleukin-2 induced interferon-γ synthesis and lymphokine-activated killer activity. Int Immunol 4:563–569, 1992.
58a. Hultner L, Druez C, Moeller J, et al: Mast cell growth–enhancing activity (MEA) is structurally related and functionally identical to the novel mouse T cell growth factor P40/TCGF III (interleukin 9). Eur J Immunol 20:1413–1416, 1990.
59. Idzerda RL, March CJ, Mosley B, et al: Human interleukin 4 receptor confers biological responsiveness and defines a novel receptor superfamily. J Exp Med 171(3):861–873, 1990.
60. Ihle JN: Interleukin-3 and hematopoiesis. Chem Immunol 51:65–106, 1992.
61. Ihle JN, Witthuhn BA, Quelle FW, et al: Signaling by the cytokine receptor superfamily: JAKs and STATs. Trends Biochem Sci 19(5):222–227, 1994.
62. Ishii N, Asao H, Kimura Y, et al: Impairment of ligand binding and growth signaling of mutant IL-2 receptor γ chains in patients with X-linked severe combined immunodeficiency. J Immunol 153(3):1310–1317, 1994.
63. Johnston JA, Kawamura M, Kirken RA, et al: Phosphorylation and activation of the Jak-3 Janus kinase in response to interleukin-2. Nature 370(6485):151–153, 1994.
64. Kanakura Y, Druker B, Cannistra SA, et al: Signal transduction of the human granulocyte-macrophage colony-stimulating factor and interleukin-3 receptors involves tyrosine phosphorylation of a common set of cytoplasmic proteins. Blood 76(4):706–715, 1990.
65. Kennedy MK, Picha KS, Shanebeck KD, et al: Interleukin-12 regulates the proliferation of Th1, but not Th2 or Th0, clones. Eur J Immunol 24:2271–2278, 1994.
66. Kiniwa M, Gately M, Gubler U, et al: Recombinant interleukin-12 suppresses the synthesis of immunoglobulin E by interleukin-4 stimulated human lymphocytes. J Clin Invest 90:262–266, 1992.
67. Kirken RA, Rui H, Malabarba MG, Farrar WL: Identification of interleukin-2 receptor-associated tyrosine kinase p116 as novel leukocyte-specific Janus kinase. J Biol Chem 269(29):19136–19141, 1994.
68. Kishimoto T, Akira S, Taga T: Interleukin-6 and its receptor: a paradigm for cytokines. Science 258:593–597, 1992.
69. Kitamura T, Sato N, Arai K, Miyajima A: Expression cloning of the human IL-3 receptor cDNA reveals a shared β subunit for the human IL-3 and GM-CSF receptors. Cell 66:1165–1174, 1991.
70. Klebanoff SJ, Vadas MA, Harlan JM, et al: Stimulation of neutrophils by tumor necrosis factor. J Immunol 136:4220–4225, 1986.
71. Kohler I, Rieber EP: Allergy-associated I epsilon and Ec epsilon receptor II (CD23b) genes activated via binding of an interleukin-4-induced transcription factor to a novel responsive element. Eur J Immunol 23(12):3066–3071, 1993.
72. Koike M, Takatsu K: IL-5 and its receptor: which role do they play in the immune response? Int Arch Allergy Immunol 104:1–9, 1994.
73. Kotanides H, Reich NC: Requirement of tyrosine phosphorylation for rapid activation of a DNA binding factor by IL-4. Science 262(5137):1265–1267, 1993.
74. Krantz SB: Erythropoietin. Blood 77:419–434, 1991.
75. Kuhn R, Lohler J, Rennick D, et al: Interleukin-10–deficient mice develop chronic enterocolitis. Cell 75(2):263–274, 1993.
76. Kuhn R, Rajewsky K, Muller W: Generation and analysis of interleukin-4 deficient mice. Science 254:707–710, 1991.
77. Larner AC, David M, Feldman GM, et al: Tyrosine phosphorylation of DNA binding proteins by multiple cytokines. Science 261(5129): 1730–1733, 1993.
78. Leonard EJ, Yoshimura T: Neutrophil attractant/activation protein-1 (NAP-1[Interleukin-8]). Am J Respir Cell Mol Biol 2:479–486, 1990.
79. Leonard WJ, Depper JM, Crabtree GR, et al: Molecular cloning and expression of cDNAs for the human interleukin-2 receptor. Nature 311(5987):626–631, 1984.
80. Lindemann A, Mertelsmann R: Interleukin-3: structure and function. Cancer Invest 11:609–623, 1993.
81. Lutticken C, Wegenka UM, Yuan J, et al: Association of transcription factor APRF and protein kinase Jak1 with the interleukin-6 signal transducer gp130. Science 263(5143):89–92, 1994.
82. Malkovsky M, Loveland B, North M, et al: Recombinant interleukin-2 directly augments the cytotoxicity of human monocytes. Nature 325:262–265, 1987.
83. Manetti R, Parronchi R, Giudizi MG, et al: Natural killer cell stimulatory factor (interleukin 12 [IL-12]) induces T helper type 1 (Th1)-specific immune responses and inhibits the development of IL-4–producing Th cells. J Exp Med 177(4):1199–1204, 1993.
84. Marsh DG, Neely JD, Breazeale DR, et al: Linkage analysis of IL-4 and other chromosome 5q31.1 markers and total serum immunoglobulin E concentrations. Science 264:1152–1156, 1994.
85. Massague J: Transforming growth factor α. J Biol Chem 265:21393–21398, 1990.
86. McKenzie AN, Culpepper JA, de Waal Malefy R, et al: Interleukin-13, a T cell-derived cytokine that regulates human monocyte and B cell function. Proc Natl Acad Sci USA 90(8):3735–3739, 1993.
87. Merberg DM, Wolf SF, Clark SC: Sequence similarity between NKSF and the IL-6/G-CSF family. Immunol Today 13:77–78, 1992.
88. Meyers DA, Postma DS, Panhuysen CIM, et al: Evidence for a locus regulating total serum IgE levels mapping to chromosome 5. Genomics 23:464–470, 1994.
89. Mills GB, May C, McGill M, et al: Interleukin 2-induced tyrosine phosphorylation. Interleukin 2 receptor beta is tyrosine phosphorylated. J Biol Chem 265(6):3561–3567, 1990.
90. Minami Y, Kono T, Miyazaki T, Taniguchi T: The IL-2 receptor complex: its structure, function, and target genes. Annu Rev Immunol 11:245–267, 1993.
91. Miyajima A, Kitamura T, Haraa N, et al: Cytokine receptors and signal transduction. Annu Rev Immunol 10:295–331, 1992.
92. Moser R, Fehr J, Bruijnzeel PLB: IL-4 controls the selective endothelium-driven transmigration of eosinophils from allergic individuals. J Immunol 149:1432–1438, 1992.
93. Mosmann TR, Coffman RL: TH1 and TH2 cells: different patterns of lymphokine secretion lead to different functional properties. Annu Rev Immunol 7:145–173, 1989.
94. Mui ALF, Miyajima A: Interleukin-3 and granulocyte-macrophage colony-stimulating factor receptor signal transduction. Proc Soc Exp Biol Med 206(3):284–288, 1994.
95. Muller M, Briscoe J, Laxton C, et al: The protein tyrosine kinase JAK1 complements defects in interferon-alpha/beta and -gamma signal transduction. Nature 366(6451):129–135, 1993.
96. Murakami M, Hibi M, Nakagawa N, et al: IL-6-induced homodimerization of gp130 and associated activation of a tyrosine kinase. Science 260(5115):1808–1810, 1993.
97. Murakami M, Narazaki M, Hibi H, et al: Critical cytoplasmic region of the interleukin 6 signal transducer gp130 is conserved in the cytokine receptor family. Proc Natl Acad Sci USA 88(24):11349–11353, 1991.
98. Murata Y, Yamaguchi N, Hitoshi Y, et al: Interleukin 5 and interleukin 3 induce serine and tyrosine phosphorylations of several cellular proteins in an interleukin 5-dependent cell line. Biochem Biophys Res Commun 173(3):1102–1108, 1990.
99. Nakamura M, Asao H, Takeshita T, Sugamura K: Interleukin-2 receptor heterotrimer complex and intracellular signaling. Semin Immunol 5:309–317, 1993.
100. Nedwid GE, Naylor SL, Sakaguchi AY, et al: Human lymphotoxin and tumor necrosis factor genes: structure, homology and chromosomal localization. Nucleic Acids Res 13:6361–6373, 1985.
101. Noguchi M, Yi H, Rosenblatt HM, et al: Interleukin-2 receptor γ chain mutation results in X-linked severe combined immunodeficiency in humans. Cell 73:147–157, 1993.
102. Ohisson K, Bjork P, Bergenfeidt M, et al: Interleukin-1 receptor antagonist reduces mortality from endotoxin shock. Nature 348:550–552, 1990.
103. Oppenheim JJ, Kovacs EJ, Matsushima K, Durum K: There is more than one interleukin 1. Immunol Today 7:45–56, 1986.
104. Oppenheim J, Zachariae COC, Mukaida N, Matsushima K: Properties of the novel proinflammatory supergene "intercrine" cytokine family. Annu Rev Immunol 9:617–647, 1991.
105. Owen WF Jr, Petersen J, Sheff DM, et al: Hypodense eosinophils and interleukin 5 activity in the blood of patients with the eosinophilia-myalgia syndrome. Proc Natl Acad Sci USA 87(21):8647–8651, 1990.
106. Owen WF Jr, Rothenberg ME, Petersen J, et al: Interleukin 5 and phenotypically altered eosinophils in the blood of patients with the idiopathic hypereosinophil syndrome. J Exp Med 170:343–348, 1989.

107. Owen WF Jr, Rothenberg ME, Silberstein DS, et al: Regulation of human eosinophil viability, density, and function by granulocyte/macrophage colony-stimulating factor in the presence of 3T3 fibroblasts. J Exp Med 166:129–141, 1987.
108. Paul WE: Interleukin-4: A prototypic immunoregulatory lymphokine. Blood 77:1859–1870, 1991.
109. Paul WE, Ohara J: B cell stimulatory factor 1/interleukin 4. Annu Rev Immunol 5:429–459, 1987.
110. Pawson T, Gish GD: SH2 and SH3 domains: from structure to function. Cell 71(3):359–362, 1992.
111. Pellegrini S, John J, Shearer M, et al: Use of a selectable marker regulated by alpha interferon to obtain mutations in the signaling pathway. Mol Cell Biol 9(11):4605–4612, 1989.
112. Pellegrini S, Schindler C: Early events in signalling by interferons. Trends Biochem Sci 18(9):338–342, 1993.
113. Perez C, Albert I, DeFay K, et al: A nonsecretable cell surface mutant of tumor necrosis factor (TNF) kills by cell-to-cell contact. Cell 63:251–258, 1990.
114. Pernis A, Witthuhn B, Keegan AD, et al: Interleukin 4 signals through two related pathways. Proc Natl Acad Sci USA 92(17):7971–7975, 1995.
115. Punnonen J, Malefyt RD, Van Vlasselaer P, et al: IL-10 and viral IL-10 prevent IL-4-induced IgE synthesis by inhibiting the accessory cell function of monocytes. J Immunol 151:1280–1289, 1993.
116. Quelle FW, Sato N, Witthuhn BA, et al: JAK2 associates with the beta c chain of the receptor for granulocyte-macrophage colony-stimulating factor, and its activation requires the membrane-proximal region. Mol Cell Biol 14(7):4335–4341, 1994.
117. Quelle FW, Wojchowski DM: Proliferative action of erythropoietin is associated with rapid protein tyrosine phosphorylation in responsive B6SUt.EP cells. J Biol Chem 266(1):609–614, 1991.
118. Ralph P, Nakoinz I, Sampson-Johannes A, et al: IL-10, T lymphocyte inhibitor of human blood cell production of IL-1 and tumor necrosis factor. J Immunol 148(3):808–814, 1992.
119. Re F, Muzio M, DeRossi M, et al: The type II "receptor" as a decoy target for interleukin 1 in polymorphonuclear leukocytes: characterization of induction by dexamethasone and ligand binding properties of the released decoy receptor. J Exp Med 179:739–743, 1994.
120. Robinson DS, Hamid Q, Ying S, et al: Predominant TH2-like bronchoalveolar T-lymphocyte population in atopic asthma. N Engl J Med 326(5):298–304, 1992.
121. Romagnani S: Regulation and deregulation of human IgE synthesis. Immunol Today 11:316–321, 1990.
122. Rothenberg ME, Owen WF, Silberstein DS, et al: Human eosinophils have prolonged survival, enhanced functional properties, and become hypodense when exposed to human interleukin 3. J Clin Invest 81:1986–1992, 1988.
123. Rothenberg ME, Petersen J, Stevens RL, et al: IL-5-dependent conversion of normodense human eosinophils to the hypodense phenotype uses 3T3 fibroblasts for enhanced viability, accelerated hypodensity, and sustained antibody-dependent cytotoxicity. J Immunol 143:2311–2316, 1989.
124. Rousset F, Garcia E, Defrance T, et al: Interleukin 10 is a potent growth and differentiation factor for activated human B lymphocytes. Proc Natl Acad Sci USA 89(5):1890–1893, 1992.
125. Sanderson CJ: Pharmacological implications of interleukin-5 in the control of eosinophilia. Adv Pharmacol 23:163–177, 1992.
126. Sato TA, Widmer MB, Finkelman FD, et al: Recombinant soluble murine IL-4 receptor can inhibit or enhance IgE responses in vivo. J Immunol 150(7):2717–2723, 1993.
127. Schindler C, Fu XY, Improta T: Proteins of transcription factor ISGF-3: one gene encodes the 91- and 84-kDa ISGF-3 proteins that are activated by interferon alpha. Proc Natl Acad Sci USA 89(16):7836–7839, 1992.
128. Schindler C, Kashleva H, Pernis A: STF-IL-4: a novel IL-4-induced signal transducing factor. EMBO J 13(6):1350–1356, 1994.
129. Schmitt E, Hoehn P, Huels C, et al: T helper type 1 development of naive CD4+ T cells requires the coordinate action of interleukin-12 and interferon-γ and is inhibited by transforming growth factor-β. Eur J Immunol 24:793–798, 1994.
130. Schrader JW: The primitive hemopoietin of activated T lymphocytes (interleukin-3). Annu Rev Immunol 4:205–230, 1986.
131. Seder RA, Paul WE, Davis MM, de St. Groth BF: The presence of interleukin 4 during in vitro priming determines the lymphokine-producing potential of CD4+ T cells from T cell receptor transgenic mice. J Exp Med 176:1091–1098, 1992.
132. Seed B: Initiation of signal transduction by receptor aggregation: role of nonreceptor tyrosine kinases. Semin Immunol 7(1):3–11, 1995.
133. Sherr SJ: Colony-stimulating factor-1 receptor. Blood 75:1–12, 1990.
134. Shuai K, Horvath CM, Huang LH, et al: Interferon activation of the transcription factor Stat91 involves dimerization through SH2-phosphotyrosyl peptide interactions. Cell 76(5):821–828, 1994.
135. Shuai K, Schindler C, Prezioso VR, Darnell JE Jr: Activation of transcription by IFN-gamma: tyrosine phosphorylation of a 91-kD DNA binding protein. Science 258(5089):1808–1812, 1992.
136. Shuai K, Stark GR, Kerr IM, Darnell JE Jr: A single phosphotyrosine residue of Stat91 required for gene activation by interferon-gamma. Science 261(5129):1744–1746, 1993.
137. Shull MM, Ormsby I, Kier A, et al: Targeted disruption of the mouse transforming growth factor-β1 gene results in multifocal inflammatory disease. Nature 359(6397):693–699, 1992.
138. Siegel JP, Sharon M, Smith PL, Leonard WJ: The IL-2 receptor β chain (p70): role in mediating signals for LAK, NK, and proliferative activities. Science 238:75–78, 1987.
139. Silvennoinen O, Witthuhn BA, Quelle FW, et al: Structure of the murine Jak2 protein-tyrosine kinase and its role in interleukin 3 signal transduction. Proc Natl Acad Sci USA 90(18):8429–8433, 1993.
140. Sims JE, Gayle MA, Slack JL, et al: Interleukin 1 signaling occurs exclusively via the type I receptor. Proc Natl Acad Sci USA 90(13):6155–6159, 1993.
141. Smith CA, Davis T, Anderson D, et al: A receptor for tumor necrosis factor defines an unusual family of cellular and viral proteins. Science 248(4958):1019–1023, 1990.
142. Smith KA: Interleukin 2. Annu Rev Immunol 2:319–333, 1984.
143. Sonoda E, Matsumoto R, Hitoshi Y, et al: Transforming growth factor beta induces IgA production and acts additively with interleukin 5 for IgA production. J Exp Med 170(4):1415–1420, 1989.
144. Sporn MB, Roberts AB: Transforming growth factor-β: recent progress and new challenges. J Cell Biol 119:1017–1021, 1993.
145. Sypek JP, Chung CL, Mayor SE, et al: Resolution of cutaneous Leishmaniasis: interleukin 12 initiates a protective T helper type 1 immune response. J Exp Med 177(6):1797–1802, 1993.
146. Taga T, Kishimoto T: Signaling mechanisms through cytokine receptors that share signal transducing receptor components. Curr Opin Immunol 7:17–23, 1995.
147. Takanaski S, Nonaka R, Xing Z, et al: Interleukin 10 inhibits lipopolysaccharide-induced survival and cytokine production by human peripheral blood eosinophils. J Exp Med 180:711–715, 1994.
148. Takatsu K: Interleukin-5. Curr Opin Immunol 4:299–306, 1992.
149. Takatsu K, Tominaga A, Harada N: T cell-replacing factor (TRF)/interleukin 5 (IL-5): molecular and functional properties. Immunol Rev 102:107–135, 1988.
150. Takeshita T, Asao H, Ohtani K, et al: Cloning of the γ chain of the human IL-2 receptor. Science 257(5068):379–382, 1992.
151. Taniguchi T, Asao H, Ohtani K: The IL-2/IL-2 receptor system: a current overview. Cell 73:5–8, 1993.
152. Taniguchi T, Fujita H, Takaoka C, et al: Structure and expression of a cloned cDNA for human interleukin-2. Nature 302:305–310, 1983.
153. Tartaglia LA, Goeddel DV: Two TNF receptors. Immunol Today 13:151–153, 1992.
154. Tepper RI, Levinson DA, Stanger BZ, et al: IL-4 induces allergic-like inflammatory disease and alters T cell development in transgenic mice. Cell 62:457–467, 1990.
155. Tominaga A, Takaki S, Koyama N, et al: Transgenic mice expressing a B cell growth and differentiation factor gene (interleukin 5) develop eosinophilia and autoantibody production. J Exp Med 173(2):429–437, 1991.
156. Tracey KJ, Fong Y, Hesse DG, et al: Anti-cachectin/TNF monoclonal antibodies prevent septic shock during lethal bacteraemia. Nature 330:662–664, 1987.
157. Trinchieri G: Interleukin-12: a cytokine produced by antigen-presenting cells with immunoregulatory functions in the generation of T-helper cells type 1 and cytotoxic lymphocytes. Blood 84:4008–4026, 1994.
158. Urban J, Katona IM, Paul WE, Finkelman FD: Interleukin 4 is important in protective immunity to a gastrointestinal nematode infection in mice. Proc Natl Acad Sci USA 88:5513–5517, 1991.
159. Van Oosterhout AJ, Ladenius AR, Savelkoul HF, et al: Effect of anti-IL-5 and IL-5 on airway hyperreactivity and eosinophils in guinea pigs. Am Rev Respir Dis 147(3):548–552, 1993.
160. Van Snick J: Interleukin 6: an overview. Annu Rev Immunol 8:253–278, 1990.

161. Velazquez L, Fellous M, Stark GR, Pellegrini S: A protein tyrosine kinase in the interferon alpha/beta signaling pathway. Cell 70(2):313–322, 1992.
162. Vercelli D, Geha RS: Regulation of IgE synthesis: from the membrane to the genes. Springer Semin Immunopathol 15:5–16, 1993.
163. Vilcek J, Lee TH: Tumor necrosis factor: new insights into the molecular mechanisms of its multiple actions. J Biol Chem 266:7313–7316, 1991.
164. Waldmann TA, Goldman CK, Robb RJ, et al: Expression of interleukin 2 receptors on activated B cells. J Exp Med 160(5):1450–1466, 1984.
165. Wanidworanun C, Strober W: Predominant role of tumor necrosis factor-α in human monocyte IL-10 synthesis. J Immunol 151:6853–6861, 1993.
166. Watling D, Guschin D, Muller M, et al: Complementation by the protein tyrosine kinase JAK2 of a mutant cell line defective in the interferon-gamma signal transduction pathway. Nature 366(6451): 166–170, 1993.
167. Wegner CD, Gundel RH, Reilly P, et al: Intercellular adhesion molecule-1 (ICAM-1) in the pathogenesis of asthma. Science 247:456–459, 1990.
168. Weisbart RH, Golde DW: Physiology of granulocyte and macrophage colony-stimulating factors in host defense. Hematol Oncol Clin North Am 3:401–409, 1989.
169. Weldmann B, Sakai H, Davis TA, Wiedmann M: A protein complex required for signal-sequence-specific sorting and translocation. Nature 370:434–440, 1994.
170. Wierenga EA, Snoek M, deGroot C, et al: Evidence for compartmentalization of functional subsets of CD4+ T lymphokines in atopic patients. J Immunol 144(12):4651–4656, 1990.
171. Wilks AF, Harpur AG, Kurban RR, et al: Two novel protein-tyrosine kinases, each with a second phosphotransferase-related catalytic domain, define a new class of protein kinase. Mol Cell Biol 11(4):2057–2065, 1991.
172. Williams AF, Barclay AN: The immunoglobulin superfamily—domains for cell surface recognition. Annu Rev Immunol 6:381–405, 1988.
173. Williams BR: Transcriptional regulation of interferon-stimulated genes. Eur J Biochem 200(1):1–11, 1991.
174. Williams DE, De Vries P, Namen AE, et al: The steel factor. Dev Biol 151:368–376, 1992.
175. Yokota T, Coffman RL, Hagiwara H, et al: Isolation and characterization of lymphokine cDNA clones encoding mouse and human IgA-enhancing factor and eosinophil colony-stimulating factor activities. Relationship to interleukin 5. Proc Natl Acad Sci USA 84(21):7388–7392, 1987.
176. Yssel H, de Waal Malefyt R, Roncarolo M-G, et al: IL-10 is produced by subsets of human CD4+ T cell clones and peripheral blood T cells. J Immunol 149(7):2378–2384, 1992.
177. Zsebo KM, Williams D, Geissler E: Stem cell factor (SCF) is encoded at the SI locus of the mouse and is the ligand for the *c-kit* tyrosine kinase receptor. Cell 63:213–224, 1990.
178. Zurawski G, de Vries JE: Interleukin 13, an interleukin 4-like cytokine that acts on monocytes and B cells, but not on T cells. Immunol Today 15:19–26, 1994.

6 Chemokines/Histamine-Releasing Factors

ALLEN P. KAPLAN

Chemokines are defined as cytokines that are also chemotactic factors whose actions are thought to be responsible, in part, for cellular recruitment during the inflammatory response. These particular cytokine-like molecules are all structurally related and belong to two subfamilies, designated α and β (Table 6–1). Although the entire group of proteins are structurally related, those within a particular subfamily (α or β) are, in general, more homologous.

Chemokines have a molecular weight between 8 and 10 kD and are all heparin-binding proteins, but the two subfamilies are encoded on different chromosomes. The α-chemokines are located at the q12–21 region of chromosome 4,[84] and the β-chemokines are found at the q11–21 region of chromosome 17.[54] All chemokines have four cysteines at the amino-terminal end that are almost identical in position. However, the first two cysteines in the α subfamily are separated by a single amino acid and designated C-X-C, whereas the first two cysteines in the β subfamily are adjacent and designated C-C. Thus the C-X-C or C-C chemokines are terms used interchangeably with α and β. It is likely that chemokines were derived from a single generic sequence that duplicated and translocated to differing chromosomes, and each one replicated several times. Each sequence then evolved separately to yield the individual member of the two subfamilies.

PROPERTIES OF SPECIFIC α-CHEMOKINES

Interleukin-8 (IL-8), or neutrophil activating peptide-1 (NAP-1), is perhaps the best characterized of the chemokines. It is one of the most potent chemotactic factors for neutrophils, a property it shares with virtually all other α-chemokines (Table 6–2).[116, 166] It is also chemotactic for a subpopulation of lymphocytes, which includes CD4+ and CD8+ cells.[69, 72] IL-8 can be found throughout the body

TABLE 6–1
THE CHEMOKINE CYTOKINES

Subfamily A	Subfamily B
Platelet factor 4	MCAF/MCP-1
CTAP III/β-thromboglobulin/NAP-2	MCP-2
IL-8	MCP-3
Melanoma growth factor (MGF)	RANTES
Macrophage inflammatory peptide-2 (MIP-2)	MIP1-α
IP-10	MIP1-β
	I-309
	Eotaxin
Chromosome 4	Chromosome 17
8–10 kD	8–10 kD
Bind heparin	Bind heparin
4 cysteines (Cys-X-Cys)	4 cysteines (Cys-Cys)
Free N-terminus	Blocked N-terminus

because it is produced by a wide variety of cells, including neutrophils,[137] endothelial cells,[117, 137] monocytes,[69, 119, 120, 137, 148, 167, 168] keratinocytes,[17, 68, 70, 118] and fibroblasts.[70] The precursor has 99 amino acids, whereas after processing, the secreted form of IL-8 generally has 71 amino acids. However, longer, intermediate forms at 79 and 77 amino acids have been described, as well as a truncated form at 69 amino acids apparently due to varying degrees of proteolysis.

The protein has no carbohydrate, and it dimerizes at high concentrations via hydrogen bonds.[30, 37] It is interesting to note that the three-dimensional structure of monocyte chemotactic and activating factor (MCAF) (a β-chemokine) can be superimposed upon that of IL-8 despite only about 21% homology, but its dimeric structures do not superimpose.[31] It has been theorized that this change with dimerization relates to its distinct interactions with receptors that bind either α- or β-chemokines, but not both. However, Baggiolini and colleagues[15] have reported that an N-methyl substitution of a leucine required for dimerization yields a monomeric analog of IL-8 that retains function; thus an alternative explanation regarding α versus β specificity must be sought. An amino terminal Glu-Leu-Arg has been identified as critical for interaction with the IL-8 receptor.[15]

Neutrophils were originally shown to have approximately 20,000 receptors/cells for IL-8 with an affinity constant (K_d) of 8×10^{-10}M.[108] This receptor is distinct from receptors for other cytokines, as well as receptors for C5a, leukotrienes, platelet activating factor (PAF), or β-chemokines. But the IL-8 receptor can respond to some of the other α-chemokines such as GRO/MGSA and MIP-2.[95] After binding to neutrophils, the IL-8 receptor complex is internalized within 10 minutes at 37°C[109] and degraded intracellularly. If the ligand is removed, receptors rapidly reappear at the cell surface. Two forms of the IL-8 receptor have been described, each coupled to GTP-binding proteins. In these studies, the average neutrophil receptor number was 64,500 ± 14,000 with a KD of 01.8 ± 0.07 × 10^{-10}M, which is comparable to that reported earlier. One high-affinity receptor binds IL-8 strongly but has low affinity for NAP-2 or GROα[14, 85, 123] and is termed IL-8 RI. The second receptor, IL-8 RII, binds all three with high affinity. Cloning studies yield two cDNAs conforming to these two receptor subtypes.

Signal transduction is clearly dependent upon a receptor-G protein interaction, which is inhibitable by pertussis toxin.[42, 142] Receptor binding leads to a rapid rise in cystolic-free calcium, which occurs within a few seconds,[119, 142] and a respiratory burst[83, 120, 142, 153] is seen that is dependent upon protein kinase C activation and is inhibitable by 17-hydroxywortmannin and staurosporine.[142] Cytosolic proteins at 48 and 65 KD are phosphorylated,[115] and cytoskeleton proteins such as F-actin polymerize.[95] The receptor sites on lymphocytes are far fewer (about 300/cell), but are of very high affinity, and respond to lower concentrations of IL-8 than do receptors on neutrophils.[31, 93]

IL-8 genomic DNA consists of four exons and three introns with single "TATA"- and "CAT"-like structures. The 5′ flanking region has a variety of potential binding sites for regulating proteins that may be involved with induction by cytokines.[70, 82, 129, 143] Addition of cycloheximide leads to enhancement of IL-8 mRNA rather than the expected inhibition; thus protein synthesis may be regulated by an inhibitory element whose inactivation therefore enhances the response.[86] Suppressive agents for the synthesis of IL-8 as well as other α-chemokines are corticosteroids, TGF-β, and cyclosporine.[95, 170] Induction of IL-8 mRNA is stimulated by IL-1 and TNF-α in cells such as neutrophils, fibroblasts, and keratinocytes,[16, 121] as well as monocytes and endothelial cells[82, 117, 137] and peaks, in vitro, at approximately 3 hours after stimulation.

IL-8 is not only chemotactic for neutrophils but also activates them to secrete lysosomal enzymes[119, 142, 153] and

TABLE 6–2
CHEMOTACTIC ACTIVITIES

	Neutrophils	Monocytes	T cells	Basophils	Eosinophils
α-Chemokines					
PF4	+	+			
IL-8	++		+		
NAP-2	+				
β-Chemokines					
MCP-1		++		++	
MCP-2		++		+	+
MCP-3		++		++	++
RANTES		+	+	+	++
MIP-1α	+	+	+ (CD8)	+	+/−
MIP-1β	+	+	+ (CD4)	+/−	
Eotaxin					++

leucotriene B_4,[115] and the respiratory burst is stimulated to produce reactive oxygen intermediates. Adherence to endothelial cells is enhanced,[27, 38] and the neutrophils express complement receptors CR1 and CR3 and the integrin CD11b/CD18.[38, 46, 97] L-Selectin, by contrast, is shed from the cell surface.[39] Increased concentrations of IL-8 are found in body fluids reflecting a variety of inflammatory conditions, including synovial fluid of rheumatoid arthritics[22]; in bronchoalveolar lavage fluid of patients with acute respiratory distress syndrome; and within keratinocytes of psoriatic scales.[119] Lung diseases with high neutrophil influx are of obvious interest. Increased IL-8 mRNA has been seen in alveolar macrophages of patients with idiopathic pulmonary fibrosis and correlates with neutrophilic influx as well as disease severity.[26] Thus IL-8 may be a major mediator of alveolitis when characterized by early neutrophil influx.[75] In cystic fibrosis, neutrophil elastase induces IL-8 production by bronchial epithelial cells.[88] Finally, injection of IL-8 into skin produces a neutrophilic infiltrate,[71, 147] although very low concentrations may yield some lymphocytes as well.

GRO was initially described as an oncogene growth-related factor[10] and was soon shown to be identical to a melanoma growth-stimulating factor, hence the alternative abbreviation MGSA (see Table 6–1).[102] It is also a potent neutrophil chemotactic factor,[156] competes with IL-8 for the same receptor (IL-8 RII),[120] and can be extracted from human psoriatic scales.[120] GRO/MGSA has also been shown to stimulate fibroblast growth.[120] There are now three separate GRO proteins, designated GRO-α, GRO-β, or GRO-γ, and these have comparable activities. Macrophage inflammatory peptide-2 (MIP-2) has activities similar to GRO/MGSA and/or IL-8, but it is a murine protein and not clearly distinguished in humans.[160]

Platelet factor four (PF4) was actually the first protein discovered that is a member of the α-chemokine family, and it is produced virtually exclusively by platelets. It is a weak chemotactic factor for neutrophils[40] and monocytes[40] but a potent chemotactic factor for fibroblasts.[171] It also stimulates fibroblasts to proliferate and stimulates chondrocytes to synthesize proteoglycans (aggrecan).[125] Platelets produce another α-chemokine known as platelet basic protein, which is inactive but can be digested to yield a variety of active products.[152]

Removal of the first nine amino acids produces connective tissue activating peptide III (CTAP III), which stimulates fibroblasts and chondrocytes to produce collagen and proteoglycans.[125] Removal of four more amino acids yields β-thromboglobulin, which is a potent chemoattractant for fibroblasts.[125] Removal of the next 15 amino acids from CTAP III or 11 amino acids from β-thromboglobulin yields neutrophil activating peptide 2 (NAP-2), which is a neutrophil chemoattractant and activator,[151, 152] although it is about 100-fold less potent than IL-8. A variable degree of competition for the IL-8 receptors or cross-deactivation between IL-8/NAP-1 and IL-8/NAP-2 is seen.[71] There is disagreement regarding the details of this point, which may relate to the two receptor subtypes.

Another α-chemokine termed IP-10 is an interferon-γ–inducible protein,[74] which can be synthesized by macrophages, endothelial cells, keratinocytes, and fibroblasts and has been shown to be a chemotactic factor for human monocytes and T lymphocytes. It also promotes T-cell adhesion to endothelial cells.[140] It seems that IP-10 is an exception; it has activities more consistent with those of the β-chemokine family.

In summary, the α-chemokines have, as a group, activity on neutrophils with the potency being IL-8 > GRO/MGSA > NAP-2 > PF4. Some α-chemokines derived primarily from platelets are active on fibroblasts or chondrocytes, and these include CTAP III, NAP-2, and β-thromboglobulin. IL-8 is the only one with significant chemotactic activity for a subpopulation of lymphocytes. None of these are known to be active on eosinophils. Activity on basophils is present but very weak compared to the β-chemokines, as described in the section on histamine-releasing factors.

β-CHEMOKINES

A major characteristic of β-chemokines is their ability to attract and activate monocytes and various subpopulations of lymphocytes (see Tables 6–1 and 6–2). Some β-chemokines are also potent chemotactic factors for eosinophils and basophils and activate them as well. The β-chemokines have little or no activity on neutrophils or fibroblasts and are thereby distinguished from the α-chemokines. They typically have a three exon/two intron structure in which the first exon contains the 5′ untranslated sequence and coding nucleotides for the leader peptide. The second exon encodes the N-terminal half of the mature protein, and the third exon encodes the carboxyl portion of the protein and the 3′ untranslated region.[127] Many receptors for these agents are being described that interact with one or more β-chemokines; thus a complex heterogeneity of response elements is anticipated. The prototype is known as monocyte chemotactic and activating factor (MCAF) or monocyte chemotactic protein-1 (MCP-1).[164, 166] It has no activity on neutrophils.

MCAF/MCP-1 was originally purified from a stimulated myelomonocytic cell line THP-1[81] and cloned from a cDNA library from the HL-60 cell line.[48] It was also isolated from culture supernatants of PHA-stimulated human mononuclear cells, fibroblasts, a T-cell hybridoma, and a glioblastoma cell line.[162, 164, 165, 168] It has a molecular weight of 8.7 KD but has anomalous behavior on SDS gels and migrates as if it were considerably larger. As is true of most of the β-chemokines and in contradistinction to the α-chemokines, it has a blocked N-terminus with pyroglutamic acid and therefore cannot be sequenced from the N-terminal end unless first treated with enzymes or digested to yield an internal fragment. The open reading frame is 99 amino acids (as is IL-8). It has a signal leader peptide of 23 amino acids and a secreted protein moiety of 76 residues. Its four half-cysteines are at position 11, 12 (C–C), 36, and 52, and the other β-chemokines have cysteines at the same positions.

MCAF/MCP-1 is a potent chemotactic factor for human monocytes[104, 164] and is active at the 10^{-9}M range. It is produced by monocytes (an autacoid)[83, 146]; endothelial cells once activated by cytokines such as IL-1, TNF-α, interferon-γ, and IL-4[103, 105, 136, 138]; fibroblasts[71, 139]; keratinocytes[50]; and human mesangial cells.[107] MCP-1 stimulates adhesion molecules (integrins CD11b/CD18 and CD11c/CD18)[55] and the synthesis of IL-1 and IL-6 by monocytes.[55] Lysosomal enzymes are secreted and the respiratory burst is stimulated. Macrophage colony-stimulating factor stimulates endothelial cells to produce MCAF/MCP-1 and augments monocyte–endothelial cell adhesion.[128] MCAF/MCP-1 is also chemotactic for basophils[73] and is the major histamine-releasing factor (HRF) based upon its ability to degranulate basophils. It is also a prominent cytokine found in the subendothelial layers of early atherosclerotic plaques, where it appears to stimulate monocyte chemotaxis and phagocytosis of lipids to generate "foam" cells.[90, 91] In addition, it is produced by cultured synoviocytes,[150] cytokine-stimulated chondrocytes,[149] and synovial tissue of patients with rheumatoid arthritis.[60] It is also upregulated in conditions producing pulmonary fibrosis.[169]

Two other proteins, MCP-2 and MCP-3, that were subsequently purified and cloned are closely homologous to MCAF/MCP-1 and have activities that overlap with it (see Table 6–1).[146] Both are chemotactic for basophils and activate them to secrete histamine, although MCP-3 is the more potent and approximately equal to MCP-1 on a molar basis.[2] MCP-1, however, is far more plentiful. MCP-3 is further distinguished by it's chemoattractant activity for eosinophils.[34] All three factors, MCP-1, MCP-2, and MCP-3, are chemotactic for T lymphocytes, and responding cells include both CD4 and CD8 subpopulations.[141]

Another major member of this β-chemokine family is RANTES, a term meaning regulated in activation, normal T cells expressed and secreted, which was originally isolated from a subtracted cDNA library.[111] It was found as a product of both helper and cytotoxic T lymphocytes.[111] RANTES has a molecular weight of 8 KD. It is not glycosylated and is a chemoattractant for blood monocytes and T lymphocytes of the CD4, CD45RO phenotype, i.e., memory helper cells.[89, 111] It can also be expressed by a wide variety of cell types, including monocytes,[112] synovial fibroblasts,[100] and platelets.[56] In fibroblasts, its synthesis can be induced by IL-1 and TNF-α.

RANTES is one of the histamine-releasing factors[67] and a potent chemoattractant for eosinophils.[8, 56, 106] RANTES also activates purified eosinophils so as to induce a respiratory burst as detected by the biphasic chemiluminescence response, as well as secretion of eosinophil cationic protein (Fig. 6–1). The cells adopt a hypodense phenotype, which is often seen with activation, and increase surface adhesion

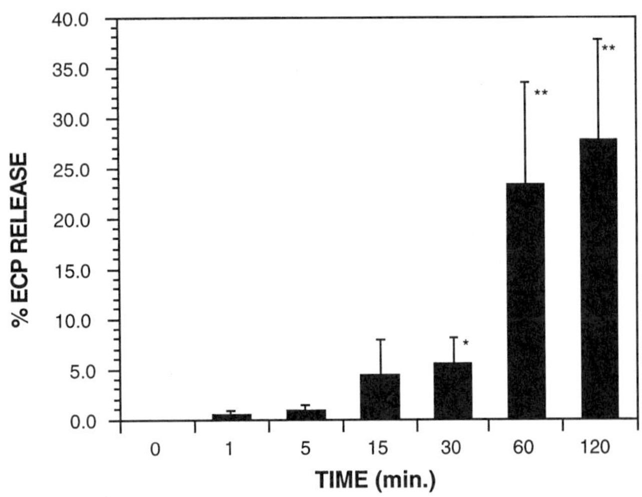

FIGURE 6–1. Time course of release of eosinophil cationic protein upon stimulation of purified human eosinophils with 10^{-7} M RANTES.

molecules.[8, 57, 106] Priming with IL-5 clearly augments the eosinophil response to RANTES, although there is some disagreement regarding the dose response (typically 10^{-8}–10^{-6}M) before versus after IL-5 treatment.[124] In assays of transendothelial migration, RANTES is strikingly positive, and the response is potentiated by IL-5.[44] Chemokines that have no effect upon eosinophil migration when tested in the same assay were IL-8, PF4, β-thromboglobulin, IP-10, MCAF/MCP-1, MIP-1α, and MIP-1β. RANTES, as well as MCP-1 and MIP-1α (but not MIP-1β), is also among the first described chemotactic factors for natural killer (NK) cells.[79]

MIP-1 proteins. These were originally described in rodents as products of endotoxin-stimulated mouse macrophages,[36, 37] which induce fever that is independent of prostaglandins. The activity was attributable to two distinct but closely homologous proteins, MIP-1α and MIP-1β, which designate two macrophage inflammatory peptides encoded by separate genes.[158] Originally, MIP-1 was found to be a neutrophil chemoattractant,[50, 159] but very high concentrations were needed, and this is unlikely to be of physiologic significance.

The human homologues to MIP-1α and MIP-1β are now designated Hu MIP-1α and Hu MIP-1β and have 70% homology to the murine proteins. However, there have been a multiplicity of clones and closely related proteins that correspond to Hu MIP-1α and Hu MIP-1β, which causes considerable confusion regarding nomenclature. For example, LD78, SIS-α or SIS-β, and GOS19 all relate to Hu MIP-1α, whereas ACT2, HC21, and MAD5 relate to Hu MIP-1β. Some are truncated forms of the same protein, but there may also be multiple nonallelic forms of these genes, which would account for considerable microvariability.

In general, MIP proteins are produced by T and B lymphocytes[170] as well as monocytes. They are chemotactic for monocytes and in a murine system activate them (particularly MIP-1α) to secrete IL-1, TNF-α, and IL-6.[45] Of particular interest is their distinct activity upon lymphocyte subpopulations. MIP-1α proteins are chemotactic for CD8+ lymphocytes, whereas MIP-1β proteins are chemotactic for CD4+ lymphocytes.[114, 139]

As is true of some of the other B-chemokines, expression of MIP-1α is enhanced in fibrosing diseases of the lung in which monocyte infiltration is prominent, such as sarcoidosis, idiopathic pulmonary fibrosis, and bleomycin-induced fibrosis.[132, 135] Recent evidence indicates that neutrophils can also be a source of MIP-1α[58] and that both MIP-1α and MIP-1β costimulate growth of mature bone marrow progenitor cells in combinations with GM-CSF or M-CSF but not G-CSF.[24] Thus the precursor of monocytes and granulocytes would differentiate to favor a monocytic lineage. MIP-1α, but not MIP-1β, inhibits growth of early progenitor stem cells.[11, 51]

HC14 is a β-chemokine with about 10% homology to MCAF/MCP-1, which is induced in monocytes by interferon-γ. It has no known function. I-309 is a cDNA clone originally isolated from a γδT-cell line; but unlike MCP-1, it is not found in endothelial cells, fibroblast, or monocytes. Its function is uncertain.

The newest human C-C chemokine is eotaxin, which is selectively chemotactic for eosinophils, is as potent as

RANTES and MCP-3, and shares an eosinophil receptor with them.[99a]

A chemokine with potent and seemingly selective activity on lymphocytes has been described in the mouse. It is of potential importance because it lacks two of the four cysteines and defines a third chemokine family, the "C" chemokines.[59a]

REGULATORY ELEMENTS AND RECEPTORS OF β-CHEMOKINES

A variety of regulatory elements may control expression of β-chemokines, but the best studied is the synthesis of MCAF/MCP-1. Among the described elements is an AP-1 binding site, an octamer transcription factor binding site, an NF-kβ enhancer element, an interferon consensus sequence, and a lymphokine decanucleotide core sequence.[113] Some data for Hu MIP-1α and I-309 suggest similar regulatory sites. However, the contribution and mechanism by which these elements can modulate MCAF/MCP-1 secretion are unknown.

A variety of β-chemokine receptors have been described, but few have been well characterized on a molecular level. The first is a "promiscuous" receptor that resides on red blood cells and binds not only β-chemokines, such as MCP-1 and RANTES, but also α-chemokines, including IL-8, GRO-α, and NAP-2. It does not bind all chemokines, however; for example, it does not interact with MIP-1α or MIP-1β. This receptor corresponds to the Duffy antigen, a protein of 34 KD known to be the receptor for invasion of erythrocytes by *Plasmodium vivax*.[93, 94] The protein has been cloned and appears to belong to the seven-transmembrane–spanning receptor suprafamily, but it does not transduce a signal.[94] It may function to maintain low plasma levels of chemokines. IL-8 bound to red blood cells does not activate neutrophils, thus the Duffy antigen (receptor) may limit available chemokine activity. Red blood cell contamination in in vitro studies has also lead to underestimates of chemokine activity on some cells, e.g., the effects of RANTES on human basophils.

Direct binding studies with radiolabeled MCAF/MCP-1, RANTES, MIP-1α, and MIP-1β have identified high-affinity binding sites on human monocytes (KD < 400 pM).[148, 154, 161] Neote and colleagues[92] described a receptor on HL-60 cells that binds MIP-1α and RANTES with high affinity and MIP-1β and MCAF/MCP-1 with lower affinity. It has seven transmembrane domains, is linked to a pertussis-sensitive G protein, and has 32% homology to the IL-8 receptor but is not stimulated by IL-8. The gene for this MIP-1α/RANTES receptor has also been isolated from leucocyte libraries by homology cloning strategies.[49]

Wang and colleagues[154] characterized a high-affinity receptor for RANTES in the human monocyte leukemia cell line THP-1, which can also react with MCAF/MCP-1 and MIP-1α. However, preincubation with MCAF/MCP-1 desensitized the cells to RANTES, but preincubation with RANTES did not desensitize to the other factors. Such results suggest the presence of a shared receptor and a specific RANTES receptor. These same cells also appear to have a specific high-affinity receptor for MCP-1 alone.[148] Charo and colleagues[29] have cloned two distinct isoforms of the MCP-1 receptor formed by alternative splicing of the carboxy-terminal tails. Other studies suggest a separate receptor shared by MIP-1α and MIP-1β that does not bind any of the other β-chemokines.[155] Five human β-chemokine receptors have been defined and their genes cloned. Binding specificities are summarized in Table 16–2.

HISTAMINE-RELEASING FACTORS

Thueson and colleagues first described the existence of a substance present in mononuclear cell supernatants that activates basophils to release histamine and could be distinguished from C5a.[144, 145] Platelets are also a source of histamine-releasing factors (HRF) and often contaminate mononuclear cell preparations.[96] Chromatographic separation of HRF revealed three major fractions with activity.[12] Purification of the first fraction revealed an 8- to 10-KD protein, which upon amino acid sequencing was identified to be a mixture of CTAP III and its proteolytic derivative NAP-2.[13] Thus it appeared that HRF was within the chemokine group of cytokines. However, when a monoclonal antibody was used to remove CTAP III/NAP-2 from purified HRF, a major portion of the activity passed through the column. It had a very similar mobility to CTAP III/NAP-2 upon SDS gel electrophoresis but was not evident upon amino acid sequencing of the purified material because its N-terminus was blocked. This protein was MCAF/MCP-1, which demonstrated that although some α-chemokines have weak activity on basophils, the major factors would be within the β-chemokine subfamily.

Kuna and colleagues[64] and Alam and colleagues[6] first demonstrated that MCAF/MCP-1 is a potent basophil activator and accounts for 50% to 60% of the histamine-releasing capability of mononuclear cell supernatants (Fig. 6–2). It is also chemotactic for basophils.[163] Histamine release is G protein dependent and is exceedingly rapid, with a half-life of approximately 30 seconds. Its potency is equal to that of antigen plus IgE antibody. Its activity is also independent of the donor's atopic status, and virtually all basophils respond. Since the late-phase reaction is characterized by basophil infiltration and protracted histamine release, MCAF/MCP-1 production must be considered to be one of the contributory factors. Separate studies by Bischoff and colleagues[21] also

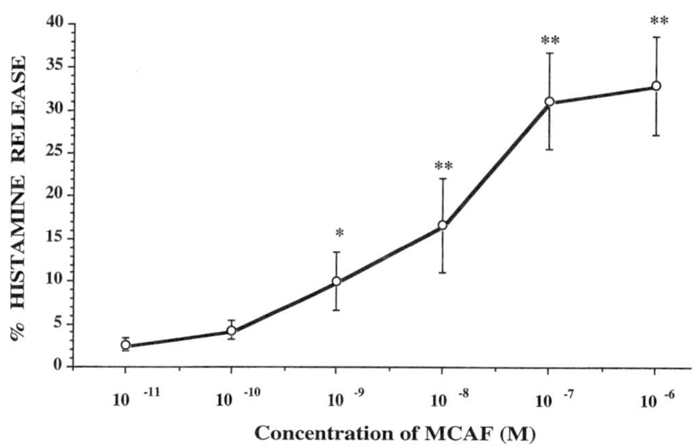

FIGURE 6–2. Dose response of basophil histamine release upon incubation with various concentrations of MCAF/MCP-1.

demonstrated the activity of MCAF/MCP-1 upon basophils. MCP-2 is a trace protein possessing about half the activity of MCP-1. MCP-3, however, is equipotent with MCAF/MCP-1[34] but also less plentiful. Their relative contribution to the total activity of mononuclear cell supernatants is uncertain.

We next tested recombinant RANTES for histamine-releasing capability. It had the same dose response range (10^{-9}–10^{-7}M) with equally rapid histamine release, but on average the percent histamine release was half that seen with MCAF/MCP-1.[67] Whereas virtually all subjects responded to MCAF/MCP-1 whether atopic or not, about 80% of subjects responded to RANTES, and the atopic subjects were clearly more responsive. MIP-1α has been reported to have HRF activity on the basophils of atopic subjects (14 of 20 responded at 10^{-9}–10^{-7}M),[4] which is similar to our activity of RANTES. Our own studies of both MIP-1α and MIP-1β found only 6 of 20 responders, the potency being 30% to 40% of RANTES.[66] Both RANTES and MIP-1α have been shown to be chemotactic for basophils.[4] IL-8 has been reported to possess histamine-releasing activity upon basophils if they are first primed with IL-3, IL-5, or GM-CSF.[18, 20, 35] Release of both histamine and LTC_4 has been reported, although the primary effect is upon LTC_4 secretion. Our own data, however, are negative for histamine secretion[66] whether basophils are primed or not. The relative potency of chemokines with HRF activity compared with a variety of other basophil-activating agents is shown in Figure 6–3.

PRIMING BASOPHILS FOR HRF-INDUCED SECRETION

The responsiveness of basophils to HRF can be modulated by preincubation with low concentrations of cytokines, which themselves are unable to induce secretion. Thus preincubation of basophils with (10^{-9}–10^{-8}M) IL-3 or IL-5 or GM-CSF can augment the release of histamine by a subsequent exposure to 10^{-7}M MCAF/MCP-1 or 10^{-7}M RANTES.[18, 20, 64] The overlapping activities (in this instance priming) by this group of cytokines may be related to the

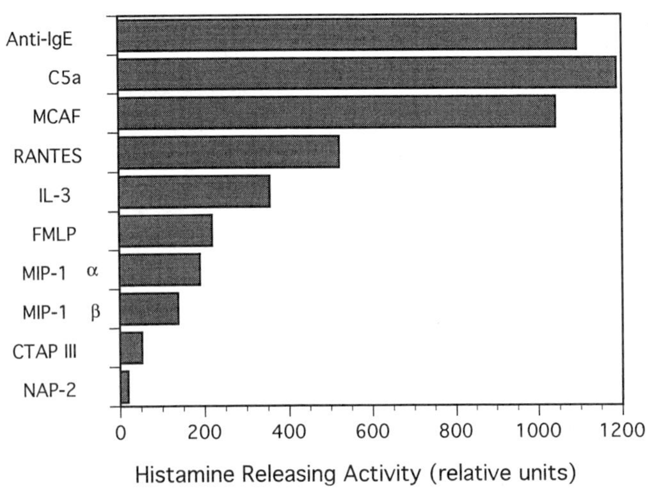

FIGURE 6–3. Relative potency of the various histamine-releasing chemokines relative to other secretagogues such as C5a, anti-IgE, and f-met-leu-phe as well as the nonchemokine IL-3. Not shown is MCP-3, which is equivalent to MCAF, and MCP-2, which is equivalent to RANTES.

TABLE 6–3
PRIMERS VERSUS CHEMOTACTIC FACTORS AND ACTIVATORS OF BASOPHILS AND EOSINOPHILS

Primers	Chemotactic Factors/Activators
Basophils	
IL-3	MCP-1
IL-5	MCP-3
GMCSF	RANTES
Interferon-γ	MIP-1α
IL-1	C5a
Eosinophils	
IL-3	MCP-3
IL-5	Eotaxin
GMCSF	RANTES
	MIP-1α
	C5a
	IL-5

fact that the receptors for these cytokines share a subunit; that is, they consist of an α chain that is specific for each and a common β chain. Higher concentrations of IL-3, and to a lesser degree GM-CSF, can directly induce histamine release from basophils.[52, 66, 77] In general, the responsive subjects are atopic individuals whose cells are likely primed in vivo. Immunoabsorption of IL-3 from cell supernatants depletes HRF activity by about 15% to 20%. This is likely due to the priming effect of IL-3 rather than its ability to induce secretion directly based on the relative concentrations required. IL-3 is therefore unusual in that it is the only cytokine that is not a chemokine that can cause basophil secretion and contributes significantly to HRF activity (see Fig. 6–3). Immunoabsorption of MCAF/MCP-1, RANTES, and IL-3 accounts for a 75% to 80% reduction in the total HRF activity of mononuclear cells/platelet-derived supernatants.

Other primers of basophils include IL-1[80] and interferon-γ,[53] which have been tested using agonists such as antigen or anti-IgE. A summary indicating primers versus chemotactic factors and activators of basophils and eosinophils (including the complement fragment C5a) is shown in Table 6–3.

CHEMOKINE-DEPENDENT INHIBITION OF BASOPHIL HISTAMINE RELEASE

Soon after the concept of HRF evolved, mononuclear cell supernatants were found to contain an inhibitor of HRF-dependent histamine release, and the activity was designated histamine release inhibitory factor (HRIF).[5] IL-8 has been thought to fulfill the function attributed to HRIF since preincubation of basophils with concentrations ranging from 10^{-11} to 10^{-8} M inhibit HRF-induced histamine release[63] as well as histamine release due to recombinant MCAF. Subsequently, preincubation with low concentrations of RANTES has been shown to inhibit HRF- or MCAF-induced histamine release,[3] suggesting that inhibition may be a more general phenomenon. However, the mechanism is unclear since there are little data available regarding chemokine receptors.

It is of interest that preincubation of basophils with concentrations of MCAF that are insufficient to cause histamine secretion prevent secretion by a subsequent challenge with 10^{-7}M MCAF. Washing the cells after the initial incubation does not reverse the process, suggesting either receptor blockade by a high-affinity ligand that cannot be removed by simple washing or induction of some active process that inhibits secretion. This phenomenon is referred to as homologous desensitization, as is seen with ligand-receptor interactions that are coupled to G proteins and well described for chemotactic factors. Preincubation with RANTES similarly desensitizes itself.

However, we have found that preincubation of basophils with a wide variety of α- or β-chemokines tested at 5×10^{-9}M inhibits subsequent secretion by optimal MCAF/MCP-1 (10^{-7}M). Washing the cells after the initial incubation reverses the inhibition. Inhibition by RANTES was 69%, by MIP-1α 49%, by MIP-1β 43%, by PF4 57%, by IL-8 41%, by CTAP III 27%, and by IP-10 15%.[65] This may reflect "receptor class desensitization," in which the agonists act on different receptors that couple to the same or very similar G proteins. The kinase that phosphorylates the occupied receptor to uncouple it from the G protein also acts on other nonoccupied receptors to uncouple them also and diminish the response to alternative ligands.

An IgE-dependent form of HRF has also been described that differs from antibody in that it is not anti-IgE, an anti-IgE receptor, or a chemokine.[157] This factor has been purified[78] and appears to activate basophils by binding to carbohydrate moieties on IgE antibody. IgE of approximately 50% of atopic subjects (IgE+) is responsive,[76] whereas IgE of nonatopics or the other 50% of atopic subjects (IgE−) is not responsive. This is thought to reflect some previously unsuspected IgE heterogeneity perhaps due to carbohydrate. Thus this form of HRF may have lectin-like properties.

HRF was defined using human basophils as responder cells; however, activation of cutaneous mast cells by cytokines, chemokines, or other factors is of particular interest. Lung mast cells appear responsive to supernatants containing HRF[122] but are less responsive than basophils. Thus far, human cutaneous mast cells are not responsive to the β-chemokines, whereas rodent skin mast cells appear to respond to MIP-1α.[4] Mast cell activating factor (c-kit ligand) is the only agonist thus far described that is active on human mast cells.[19, 33] Its function on basophils is unclear; one study is negative,[19] and a second indicates that it is a primer of basophils at low concentrations and an activator at 10- to 50-fold higher levels.[33]

Relationship to Allergic Diseases

One of the areas of particular relevance to the activities of β-chemokines is the allergic late-phase response, which is characterized by a mixture of neutrophils, eosinophils (in abundance), basophils, and mononuclear cells.[43, 133] More recent studies have examined this cellular infiltrate in detail[28] and describe basophils (particularly in nasal mucosa),[17] eosinophils,[99] monocytes, and T lymphocytes of the CD4+, Th2 subtype.[47] Studies of histamine release during late-phase reactions indicate that elevated levels persist over a 12-hour period.[98, 101, 126] In some instances, a second peak is seen between 4 and 8 hours.[87] Since most cell tryptase is elevated primarily within the first hour of such reactions, the source of the histamine is presumed to be the basophil. Chemokines are prime candidates as activators of basophils in such reactions.

Some data suggest that HRF is functionally present in cutaneous late-phase reactions[157] and that injection of chemokines in rodents can elicit a response that resembles the late phase.[4] HRF activity has been found in nasal washings of allergic subjects,[130] which decreases with topical steroid therapy[131] or immunotherapy.[25] It is also found in bronchoal-

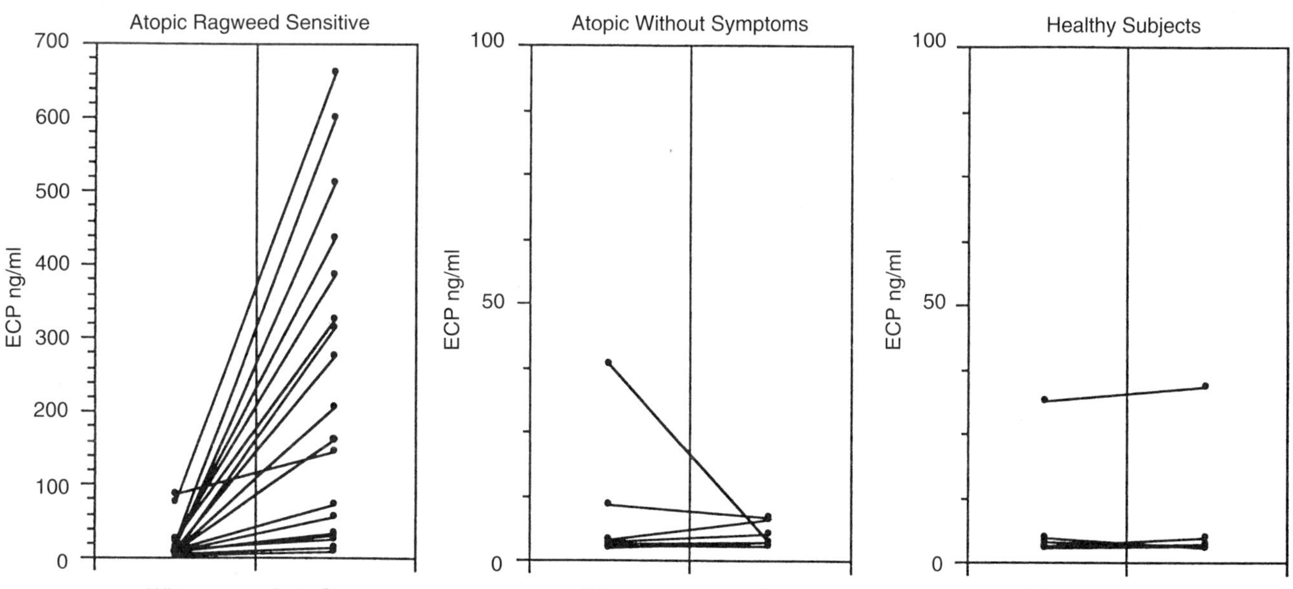

FIGURE 6–4. Individual results of MCAF/MCP-1 concentration changes in the ragweed season in subjects sensitive to ragweed (n = 18) compared with atopic subjects without symptoms (n = 9) and nonatopic controls (n = 6). MCAF/MCP-1 concentrations were determined in the winter (preseason) and late summer (season). Note lower scale in the central and right panels for asymptomatic atopics and nonatopic controls.

veolar lavage fluids.[23] Some initial studies of asthma have examined the possibility that HRF, as an inflammatory agonist, and HRIF, as a control mechanism, are important contributors to symptoms and that the relative ratio of the two might determine the clinical course. Alam and Rozniecki[7] demonstrated that stimulation of patients' lymphocytes with allergen or with a nonspecific mitogen augmented secretion of HRF-like activity into the supernatant. A later study of immunotherapy for allergic rhinitis (grass pollen) demonstrated inhibition of spontaneous HRF production and the augmented antigen-induced HRF production when patients' mononuclear cells were cultured overnight.[62]

The aforementioned studies, although suggestive of a role for HRF in allergic reactions, do not examine the presence of particular proteins and relate only to net effects upon histamine release. They also do not include studies of eosinophil recruitment. Assays are now commercially available for many factors using monoclonal antibodies or monospecific polyclonal antigen (MCAF/MCP-1, IL-8, RANTES, MIP-1α), allowing quantitation in body fluids. In one study of nasal washings of ragweed-sensitive versus normal controls during the allergy season, we demonstrated a striking increase in MCAF/MCP-1 (Fig. 6–4) with a concomitant decline in IL-8 that was strikingly correlated with the change in symptoms. During the off-season (winter), the IL-8/MCAF ratio was markedly augmented, indicating a relative abundance of IL-8 and diminished MCAF secretion, i.e., a "quiescent" chemokine distribution (Fig. 6–5). Thus the chemokine profile during the allergy season is consistent with an increase in basophil agonists and a decline in basophil inhibition.[1]

Other recent studies have attempted to obtain information regarding the synthesis of particular chemokines in allergic late-phase reactions or by specific tissues. A variety of positive results have been reported. Allergen-induced transcription of mRNA for MCP-3 and RANTES was shown in the skin of atopic subjects during the late phase,[59] increased MCP-1 protein and mRNA were found in bronchoalveolar lavage fluid of asthmatics,[134] and bronchial and nasal epithelial cells were shown to synthesize RANTES.[9, 41] Finally, nasal inhalation of RANTES caused an influx of eosinophils, basophils, and monocytes.[61] Eosinophils are also present at sites of eotaxin up-regulation.[99a] Thus data implying in vivo production of these specific factors are accumulating. There is also evidence that the IgE-dependent form of HRF can contribute to cutaneous late-phase reactions,[76] and its foundation correlates with exacerbations of atopic dermatitis in children whose symptoms can be produced by hypersensitivity to foods.[110]

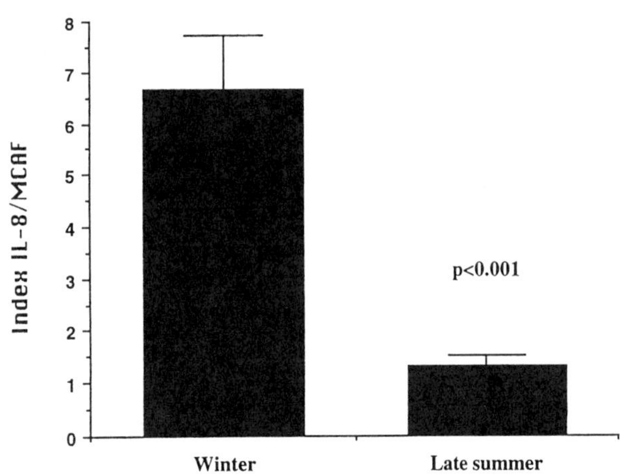

FIGURE 6–5. The ratio of the IL-8 level to the MCAF/MCP-1 level in atopic symptomatic subjects with ragweed hay fever in the winter or late summer. During the symptomatic period, the ratio declines as IL-8 decreases and MCAF/MCP-1 increases.

REFERENCES

1. Kuna P, Lazarovich M, Kaplan AP: Chemokines in seasonal allergic rhinitis. J Allergy Clin Immunol 97:104, 1996.
2. Alam R, Forsythe P, Stafford S, et al: Monocyte chemotactic protein-2, monocyte chemotactic protein-3, and fibroblast-induced cytokine. Three new chemokines induce chemotaxis and activation of basophils. J Immunol 153:3155, 1994.
3. Alam R, Forsythe PA, Lett-Brown MA, et al: Interleukin 8 and RANTES inhibit basophil histamine release induced with monocyte chemotactic and activating factor/monocyte chemotactic protein-1 and histamine releasing factor. Am J Respir Cell Mol Biol 7:427, 1992.
4. Alam R, Forsythe PA, Stafford S, et al: Macrophage inflammatory protein Iα activates basophils and mast cells. J Exp Med 176:781, 1992.
5. Alam R, Grant JA, Lett-Brown MA: Identification of a histamine releasing inhibitory factor produced by human mononuclear cells in vitro. J Clin Invest 82:2056, 1988.
6. Alam R, Lett-Brown MA, Forsythe PA, et al: Monocyte chemotactic and activating factor is a potent histamine-releasing factor for basophils. J Clin Invest 89:723, 1992.
7. Alam R, Rozniecki J: A mononuclear cell-derived histamine releasing factor in asthmatic patients. Allergy 40:124, 1985.
8. Alam RS, Stafford P, Forsythe R, et al: RANTES is a chemotactic and activating factor for human eosinophils. J Immunol 150:3442, 1993.
9. Altman LC, Baker C, Luchtel DL: RANTES synthesis by cultured human nasal epithelial cells (HNE). J Allergy Clin Immunol 95:219, 1995.
10. Anisowicz A, Bardwell L, Sager R: Constitutive expression of a growth-regulated gene in transformed Chinese hamster and human cells. Proc Natl Acad Sci USA 84:7188, 1987.
11. Avalos BR, Bartynski KJ, Elder PJ, et al: The active monomeric form of macrophage inflammatory protein Iα interacts with high and low affinity classes of receptors in human hematopoietic cells. Blood 84:1790, 1994.
12. Baeza ML, Reddigari SR, Haak-Frendscho M, et al: Purification and further characterization of human mononuclear cell histamine releasing factor. J Clin Invest 83:1204, 1989.
13. Baeza ML, Reddigari SR, Kornfeld D, et al: Relationship of one form of human histamine releasing factor to connective tissue activating peptide-III. J Clin Invest 85:1516, 1990.
14. Baggiolini M, DeWald B, Moser B: Interleukin 8 and related chemotactic cytokines—CXC and CC chemokines. Adv Immunol 55:97, 1994.
15. Baggiolini M, Loetscher P, Moser P: Interleukin 8 and the chemokine family. Int J Immunopharmacol 17:103, 1995.
16. Barker JNWN, Sarma V, Mitra RS, et al: Marked synergism between tumor necrosis factor-α and interferon gamma in regulation of keratinocyte-derived adhesion molecules and chemotactic factors. J Clin Invest 85:605, 1990.
17. Bascom R, Wachs M, Naclerio RM, et al: Basophil influx occurs after nasal antigen challenge: effects of topical corticosteroid treatment. J Allergy Clin Immunol 81:580, 1988.
18. Bischoff SC, Brunner T, deWeck AL, et al: Interleukin 5 modifies histamine release and leukotriene generation by human basophils in response to diverse agonists. J Exp Med 172:1577, 1990.
19. Bischoff SC, Dahinden CA: c-kit ligand: a unique potentiator of mediator release by human lung mast cells. J Exp Med 175:237, 1992.
20. Bischoff SC, deWeck AL, Dahinden CA: Interleukin 3 and granulocyte/macrophage-colony-stimulating factor render human basophil responsive to low concentration of complement component C3a. Proc Natl Acad Sci USA 87:6813, 1990.
21. Bischoff SC, Krieger M, Brunner T, et al: Monocyte chemotactic protein 1 is a potent activator of human basophils. J Exp Med 175(5):1271, 1992.

22. Brennan FM, Zachariae COC, Chantry D, et al: Detection of interleukin 8 (IL 8) biological activity in synovial fluids from patients with rheumatoid arthritis and production of IL 8 mRNA by isolated synovial cells. Eur J Immunol 20:2141, 1990.
23. Broide DH, Smith CM, Wasserman SI: Mast cells and pulmonary fibrosis. Identification of histamine releasing factor in bronchoalveolar lavage fluid. J Immunol 145:1838, 1990.
24. Broxmeyer HE, Sherry B, Lu L, et al: Myelopoietic enhancing effects of murine macrophage inflammatory protein 1 and 2 on colony formation in vitro by murine and human bone marrow granulocyte/macrophage progenitor cells. J Exp Med 170:1583, 1989.
25. Brunet C, Bedard P-M, Lavoie A, et al: Allergic rhinitis to ragweed pollen II. Modulation of histamine releasing factor production by specific immunotherapy. J Allergy Clin Immunol 89:87, 1992.
26. Carre PC, Mortenson RL, King TE, et al: Increased expression of the interleukin-8 gene by alveolar macrophages in idiopathic pulmonary fibrosis. A potential mechanism for the recruitment and activation of neutrophils in lung fibrosis. J Clin Invest 88:1802, 1991.
27. Carveth HJ, Bohnsack JF, McIntyre TM, et al: Neutrophil activating factor (NAF) induces polymorphonuclear leukocyte adherence to endothelial cells and to subendothelial matrix proteins. Biochem Biophys Res Comm 162:387, 1989.
28. Charlesworth CN, Hood AF, Soter NA, et al: Cutaneous late-phase response to allergen. Mediator release and inflammatory cell infiltration. J Clin Invest 83:1519, 1989.
29. Charo IF, Myers SJ, Herman A, et al: Molecular cloning and functional expression of two monocyte chemoattractant protein 1 receptors reveals alternative splicing of the carboxy-terminal tails. Proc Natl Acad Sci USA 91:2752, 1994.
30. Clore CM, Appella E, Yamada M, et al: Determination of the secondary structure of interleukin 8 by nuclear magnetic resonance spectroscopy. J Biol Chem 264:18907, 1989.
31. Clore GM, Gronenborn AM: Three dimensional structure of α and β chemokines. Fed Proc 9:57, 1995.
32. Clore MG, Appella E, Yamada M, et al: Three dimensional structure of interleukin 8 in solution. Biochemistry 29:1689, 1990.
33. Columbo M, Horowitz EM, Botana LM, et al: The human recombinant c-kit receptor ligand, rh SCF, induces mediator release from human cutaneous mast cells and enhances IgE-dependent mediator release from both skin mast cells and peripheral blood basophils. J Immunol 149:599, 1992.
34. Dahinden CA, Geiser T, Brunner T, et al: Monocyte chemotactic protein 3 is a most effective basophil and eosinophil-activating chemokine. J Exp Med 179:751, 1994.
35. Dahinden CA, Kurimoto Y, deWeck AL, et al: The neutrophil-activating peptide NAF/NAP-1 induces histamine release and leukotriene release by interleukin 3-primed basophils. J Exp Med 170:1787, 1989.
36. Davatelis G, Tekamp-Olson P, Wolpe SD, et al: Cloning and characterization of a c-DNA for murine macrophage inflammatory protein (MIP), a novel monokine with inflammatory and chemokinetic properties. J Exp Med 117:1939, 1988.
37. Davatelis G, Wolpe SD, Sherry B, et al: Macrophage inflammatory protein-1: a prostaglandin-independent endogenous pyrogen. Science 243:1066, 1989.
38. Detmers PA, Lo SK, Olsen-Egbert E, et al: Neutrophil-activating protein 1/interleukin 8 stimulates the binding of the leukocyte adhesion receptor CD11b/CD18 on human neutrophils. J Exp Med 171:1155, 1990.
39. Detmers PA, Powell DE, Waltz A, et al: Differential effects of neutrophil-activating peptide 1/IL8 and its homologues on leukocyte adhesion and phagocytosis. J Immunol 147:4211, 1991.
40. Deuel TF, Senior RM, Chang D, et al: Platelet factor 4 is chemotactic for neutrophils and monocytes. Proc Natl Acad Sci USA 78:4584, 1981.
41. Devalia JL, Wang JH, Sapsford RJ, et al: Human bronchial epithelial cells synthesize RANTES. J Allergy Clin Immunol 95:218, 1995.
42. Dewald B, Thelen B, Baggiolini M: Two transduction sequences are necessary for neutrophil activation by receptor agonists. J Biol Chem 263:16179, 1988.
43. Dolovich J, Hargreave FE, Chalmers R, et al: Late cutaneous allergic responses in isolated IgE-dependent reactions. J Allergy Clin Immunol 52:38, 1973.
44. Ebisawa M, Yamada T, Bickel C, et al: Eosinophil transendothelial migration induced by cytokines III. Effect of the chemokine RANTES. J Immunol 153:2153, 1994.
45. Fahey TJI, Tracey KJ, Tekamp-Olsen P, et al: Macrophage inflammatory protein-1 modulates macrophage function. J Immunol 148:2764, 1992.
46. Farina PR, DeLeon R, Graham A, et al: Monocyte-derived neutrophil chemotactic factor (MDNCF): a stimulator of neutrophil function. FASEB J 3:A1333, 1989.
47. Frew AJ, Kay AB: Eosinophils and T lymphocytes in late-phase allergic reactions. J Allergy Clin Immunol 85:533, 1990.
48. Furutani Y, Nomura H, Notake M, et al: Cloning and sequencing of the cDNA for human monocyte chemotactic and activating factor (MCAF). Biochem Biophys Res Comm 159:249, 1989.
49. Gao JL, Kuhns DB, Tiffany HL, et al: Structure and functional expression of the human macrophage inflammatory protein 1α/RANTES receptor. J Immunol 150:3022, 1993.
50. Gillitzer R, Wolff K, Tong D, et al: MCP-1 mRNA expression in basal keratinocytes of psoriatic lesions. J Invest Dermatol 101:127, 1993.
51. Graham GJ, Wright EG, Hewick R, et al: Identification and characterization of an inhibitor of hematopoietic stem cell proliferation. Nature 344:442, 1990.
52. Haak-Frendscho M, Arai N, Arai K-I, et al: Human recombinant granulocyte-macrophage colony-stimulating factor and interleukin 3 cause basophil histamine release. J Clin Invest 82:17, 1988.
53. Hernandez-Asensio M, Hooks JJ, Ida S, et al: Interferon-induced enhancement of IgE-mediated histamine release from human basophils requires RNA synthesis. J Immunol 122:1601, 1979.
54. Irving SG, Zipfel PF, Balke J, et al: Two inflammatory mediator cytokine genes are closely linked and variably amplified on chromosome 179. Nucleic Acids Res 18:3261, 1990.
55. Jiang Y, Beller DI, Frend LG, et al: Monocyte chemoattractant protein-1 regulates adhesion molecule expression and cytokine production in human monocytes. J Immunol 148:2423, 1992.
56. Kameyoshi Y, Dorschner A, Mallet AI, et al: Cytokine RANTES released by thrombin-stimulated platelets is a potent attractant for human eosinophils. J Exp Med 176:587, 1992.
57. Kapp A, Zeck-Kapp G, Czech W, et al: The chemokine RANTES is more than a chemoattractant: characterization of its effect in human eosinophil oxidative metabolism and morphology in comparison with IL5 and GM-CSF. J Invest Dermatol 102:906, 1994.
58. Kasama T, Strieter RM, Standiford TJ, et al: Expression and regulation of human neutrophil-derived macrophage inflammatory protein Iα. J Exp Med 178:63, 1993.
59. Kay AB, Taborada-Barata L, Meng Q, et al: Allergen-induced transcription of messenger RNA for monocyte chemotactic protein-3 (MCP-3) and RANTES in the skin of human atopic subjects. J Allergy Clin Immunol 95:217, 1995.
59a. Kelner GS, Kennedy J, Bacon KB, et al: Lymphotactin: a cytokine that represents a new class of chemokine. Science 266:1395, 1994.
60. Koch AE, Kunkel LS, Harlow LA, et al: Enhanced production of monocyte chemoattractant protein-1 in rheumatoid arthritis. J Clin Invest 90:772, 1992.
61. Kuna P, Alam R, Gorski P, et al: RANTES induces eosinophil, basophil, lymphocyte, and monocyte influx after nasal challenge in vivo. J Allergy Clin Immunol 95:218, 1995.
62. Kuna P, Alam R, Kuzminska B, et al: The effect of preseasonal immunotherapy on the production of histamine releasing factor (HRF) by mononuclear cells from patients with seasonal asthma: results of a double blind placebo-controlled, randomized study. J Allergy Clin Immunol 83:816, 1989.
63. Kuna P, Reddigari SR, Kornfeld D, et al: Interleukin 8 inhibits histamine release from human basophils induced by histamine releasing factors, connective tissue activating peptide III, and interleukin 3. J Immunol 147:1920, 1991.
64. Kuna P, Reddigari SR, Rucinski D, et al: Monocyte chemotactic and activating factor is a potent histamine-releasing factor for human basophils. J Exp Med 175:489, 1992.
65. Kuna P, Reddigari SR, Rucinski D, et al: Chemokines of the α and β subclass inhibit human basophils' responsiveness to monocyte chemotactic and activating factor/monocyte chemoattractant protein-I. J Allergy Clin Immunol 95:574, 1995.
66. Kuna P, Reddigari SR, Schall TJ, et al: Characterization of the human response to cytokines, growth factors, and histamine releasing factor of the intercrine/chemokine family. J Immunol 150:1932, 1993.
67. Kuna P, Reddigari SR, Schall TJ, et al: RANTES, A monocyte and

T lymphocyte chemotactic cytokine releases histamine from human basophils. J Immunol 149:636, 1992.
68. Kunkel SL, Strieter RM, Chensue SW, et al: Regulation of tumor necrosis factor-alpha and neutrophil activating protein-1 gene expression: potential role of cytokine directed cell communication during multiple organ injury. In Bringham K, Stahlmann M (eds): Respiratory Distress Syndrome: Molecular to Man. Vanderbilt Press, Nashville, TN, 1989.
69. Larsen CG, Anderson AO, Appella E, et al: Neutrophil activating protein (NAP-1) is also chemotactic for T lymphocytes. Science 243:1464, 1989.
70. Larsen CG, Anderson AO, Oppenheim JJ, et al: Production of interleukin 8 by human dermal fibroblasts and keratinocytes in response to interleukin 1 or tumor necrosis factor. Immunology 68:31, 1989.
71. Leonard E, Yoshimura T: Neutrophil attractant/activation protein 1 (NAP-1/IL8). Am J Respir Cell Mol Biol 2:479, 1990.
72. Leonard EJ, Skeel A, Yoshimura T, et al: Leukocyte specificity and binding of human neutrophil attractant/activating protein 1. J Immunol 144:1323, 1990.
73. Leonard EJ, Yoshimura T: Human monocyte chemoattractant protein-1 (MCP-1). Immunol Today 11:97, 1990.
74. Luster AS, Unkeless JC, Ravetch JV: Gamma-interferon transcriptionally regulates an early-response gene containing homology to platelet proteins. Nature 315:672, 1985.
75. Lynch JP III, Standiford TJ, Rolfe MW, et al: Neutrophilic alveolitis in idiopathic pulmonary fibrosis: the role of interleukin 8. Am Rev Respir Dis 145:1433, 1992.
76. MacDonald SM, Lichtenstein LM, Proud D, et al: Studies of IgE-dependent histamine releasing factors: heterogeneity of IgE. J Immunol 139:506, 1987.
77. MacDonald SM, Schleimer RP, Kagey-Sobotka A, et al: Recombinant IL-3 induces histamine release from human basophils. J Immunol 142:3527, 1989.
78. MacDonaldsin Rafnai T, Langdon MS, et al: Molecular identification of the IgE dependent histamine releasing factor. J Allergy Clin Immunol 95:175, 1995.
79. Maghazachi AA, Al-Aoukaty A, Schall JJ: C-C chemokines induce the chemotaxis of NK and IL-2–activated NK cells. J Immunol 153:4969, 1994.
80. Massey WA, Randall TC, Kagey-Sabotka A, et al: Recombinant human IL-1α and -1β potentiate IgE-mediated histamine release from human basophils. J Immunol 143:1875, 1989.
81. Matsushima K, Larsen CG, DuBois GC, et al: Purification and characterization of a novel monocyte chemotactic and activating factor produced by a human myelomonocytic cell line. J Exp Med 169:1485, 1989.
82. Matsushima K, Morishita K, Yoshimura T, et al: Molecular cloning of a human monocyte-derived neutrophil chemotactic factor (MDNCF) and the induction of MDNCF mRNA by interleukin 1 and tumor necrosis factor. J Exp Med 167:1883, 1988.
83. Matsushima K, Oppenheim JJ: Interleukin 8 and MCAF: novel inflammatory cytokines inducible by IL1 and TNF. Cytokine 1:2, 1989.
84. Modi WS, Dean M, Seuanez HN, et al: Monocyte derived neutrophil chemotactic factor (MDNCF/IL-8) resides in a gene cluster along with several other members of the platelet factor 4 gene superfamily. Hum Genet 84:185, 1990.
85. Moser B, Schumacher C, Tscharner V, et al: Neutrophil activating peptide-2 and gro/melanoma growth stimulating activity interact with neutrophil activating peptide/interleukin 8 receptors on human neutrophils. J Biol Chem 266:10666, 1991.
86. Mukaida N, Hishinuma A, Zachariae COC, et al: Regulation of IL 8 gene expression and binding of several other members of the intercrine family to receptors for IL 8. In Westwick J (ed): Second International Symposium in Chemotactic Cytokines. Humana 31, 1990.
87. Naclerio RM, Proud D, Togias AG, et al: Inflammatory mediators in late antigen-induced rhinitis. N Engl J Med 313:65, 1985.
88. Nakamura H, Yoshimura K, McElvaney NG, et al: Neutrophil elastase in respiratory epithelial lining fluid of individuals with cystic fibrosis induces interleukin 8 gene expression in a human bronchial epithelial cell line. J Clin Invest 89:1478, 1992.
89. Napalitano M, Seamon KB: Identification of cell surface receptors for Act-2 cytokines. J Exp Med 17:285, 1990.
90. Navab M, Imes SS, Hama SY, et al: Monocyte transmigration induced by modification of low density lipoprotein in cocultures of human aortic wall cells is due to induction of monocyte chemotactic protein 1 synthesis and is abolished by high density lipoprotein. J Clin Invest 88:2039, 1991.
91. Nelken NA, Coughlin SR, Gordon D, et al: Monocyte chemoattractant protein-1 in human atheromatous plaques. J Clin Invest 88:1121, 1991.
92. Neote K, DiGregorio D, Mak JY, et al: Molecular cloning, functional expression, and signaling characteristics of a C-C chemokine receptor. Cell 72:415, 1993.
93. Neote K, Darbonne W, Ogez J, et al: Identification of a promiscuous inflammatory peptide receptor on the surface of red blood cells. J Biol Chem 268:12247, 1993.
94. Neote K, May JY, Kolakowski LF Jr, et al: Functional and biochemical analysis of the cloned Duffy antigen: identity with the red blood cell chemokine receptor. Blood 84:44, 1994.
95. Oppenheim JJ, Zachariae COC, Mukaida N, et al: Properties of the novel proinflammatory supergene "intercrine" cytokine family. Annu Rev Immunol 9:617, 1991.
96. Orchard MA, Kagey-Sobotka A, Proud D, et al: Basophil histamine release induced by a substance from stimulated platelets. J Immunol 136:2240, 1986.
97. Paccaud JP, Schifferli JA, Baggiolini M: NAP-1/IL 8 induces up-regulation of CR1 receptors in human neutrophil leukocytes. Biochem Biophys Res Comm 166:187, 1990.
98. Pienkowski MM, Adkinson NF Jr, Plaut M, et al: Prostaglandin D_2 and histamine during the immediate and late phase components of allergic cutaneous responses. J Allergy Clin Immunol 82:95, 1988.
99. Pipkorn U, Karlsson G, Enerback L.: The cellular response of the human allergic mucosa to natural allergen exposure. J Allergy Clin Immunol 82:1046, 1988.
99a. Ponath PD, Qin S, Ringler DJ, et al: Cloning of the human eosinophil chemoattractant, eotaxin. J Clin Invest 97:604, 1996.
100. Rathanaswami F, Hachicha M, Sadick M, et al: Expression of cytokine RANTES in human synovial fibroblasts: differential regulation of RANTES and interleukin 8 genes by inflammatory cytokines. J Biol Chem 268:5834, 1993.
101. Reshef A, Kagey-Sobotka A, Adkinson NF Jr, et al: The pattern and kinetics in human skin of erythema and mediators during the acute and late-phase response (LPR). J Allergy Clin Immunol 84:678, 1989.
102. Richmond A, Balentien E, Thomas HG, et al: Molecular characterization and chromosomal mapping of melanoma growth stimulatory activity, a growth factor structurally related to b-thromboglobulin. EMBO J 7:2025, 1988.
103. Rollins BJ, Pober JS: Interleukin-4 induces the synthesis and secretion of MCP-1/JE by human endothelial cells. Am J Path 138:1315, 1991.
104. Rollins BJ, Walz A, Baggiolini M: Recombinant human MCP-1/JE induces chemotaxis, calcium flux, and the respiratory burst in human monocytes. Blood 136:1112, 1990.
105. Rollins BJ, Yoshimura T, Leonard EJ, et al: Cytokine-activated human endothelial cells synthesize and secrete a monocyte chemoattractant, MCP-1/JE. Am J Path 136:1229, 1990.
106. Rot A, Krieger M, Brunner T, et al: RANTES and macrophage inflammatory protein I alpha induce the migration and activation of human eosinophil granulocytes. J Exp Med 176:1489, 1992.
107. Rovin BH, Yoshimura T, Tan L: Cytokine-induced production of monocyte chemoattractant protein-1 by cultured human mesangial cells. J Immunol 148:2148, 1992.
108. Samanta AK, Oppenheim JJ, Matsushima K: Identification and characterization of specific receptors for monocyte derived neutrophil chemotactic factor (MDNCF) on human neutrophils. J Exp Med 169:1185, 1989.
109. Samanta AK, Oppenheim JJ, Matsushima K: Interleukin 8 (MDNCF) dynamically regulates its own receptor expression on human neutrophils. J Biol Chem 265:183, 1989.
110. Sampson HA, Broadbent KR, Bernhisel-Broadbent J: Spontaneous release of histamine from basophils and histamine-releasing factor in patients with atopic dermatitis and food hypersensitivity. N Engl J Med 321:228, 1989.
111. Schall T, Jongestra J, Dyer BJ, et al: A human T cell-specific molecule is a member of a new gene family. J Immunol 141:1018, 1988.
112. Schall T, Lu LH, Gillett N, et al: RANTES/SIS cytokine gene expression in rheumatoid synovium as analyzed by in situ hybridization. Arth Rheum 34(Abst):117, 1991.
113. Schall TJ: Biology of the RANTES/SIS cytokine family. Cytokine 3:156, 1991.
114. Schall TJ, Bacon K, Camp RDR, et al: Human macrophage inflamma-

tory protein α (MIP-1α) and MIPIβ chemokines attract distinct populations of lymphycytes. J Exp Med 177:1821, 1993.
115. Schroeder JM: The monocyte-derived neutrophil activating peptide (NAP-1/interleukin 8) stimulated human neutrophil arachidonate-5-lipoxygenase, but not the release of cellular arachidonate. J Exp Med 170:847, 1989.
116. Schroeder JM, Christophers E: Identification of C5a des arg and an anionic neutrophil-activating peptide (ANAP) in psoriatic scales. J Invest Dermatol 87:53, 1986.
117. Schroeder JM, Christophers E: Secretion of novel and homologous neutrophil-activating peptides by LPS-stimulated human endothelial cells. J Immunol 142:244, 1989.
118. Schroeder JM, Mrowietz, U, Christophers E: Identification of different charged species of a human monocyte derived neutrophil activating peptide (MONAP). Biochem Biophys Res Comm 152:277, 1988.
119. Schroeder JM, Mrowietz U, Morita E, et al: Purification and partial biochemical characterization of a human monocyte-derived, neutrophil-activating peptide that lacks interleukin 1 activity. J Immunol 139:3474, 1987.
120. Schroeder JM, Pearson NLM, Christophers E: Lipopolysaccharide-stimulated human monocytes secrete, apart from neutrophil-activating peptide 1/interleukin 8, a second neutrophil-activating protein. J Exp Med 171:1791, 1990.
121. Schroeder JM, Sticherling M, Hennicke JJ, et al: IL 1α or tumor necrosis factor α stimulate release of three NAP-1IL 8-related neutrophil chemotactic proteins in human dermal fibroblasts. J Immunol 144:2223, 1990.
122. Schulman ES, Liu PC, Proud D, et al: Human lung macrophages induce histamine release from basophils and mast cells. Am Rev Respir Dis 131:230, 1985.
123. Schumacher C, Clark-Lewis I, Baggiolini M, et al: High and low affinity binding of GROα and neutrophil activating peptide-2 to interleukin 8 receptors on human neutrophils. Proc Natl Acad Sci USA 89:10542, 1992.
124. Schweizer RC, Welmers BAC, Raaijmakers JAM, et al: RANTES and interleukin 8-induced responses in normal human eosinophils: effects of priming with interleukin 5. Blood 12:3697, 1994.
125. Senior RM, Griffin GL, Huang JS, et al: Chemotactic activity of a platelet alpha granule protein for fibroblasts. J Cell Biol 96:382, 1983.
126. Shalit M, Schwartz LB, vonAllmen C, et al: Release of histamine and tryptase during cutaneous and interrupted cutaneous challenge with allergen in humans. J Allergy Clin Immunol 86:117, 1990.
127. Shyy Y-J, Li Y-S, Lolattakady PE: Structures of human genes coding for cytokine LD78 and their expression. Biochem Biophys Res Commun 169:346, 1990.
128. Shyy Y-J, Wickham LL, Hagan JP, et al: Human monocyte colony-stimulating factor stimulates the gene expression of monocyte chemotactic protein-1 and increases the adhesion of monocytes to endothelial monolayers. J Clin Invest 92:1745, 1993.
129. Sica A, Matsushima K, Wang JM, et al: IL 1 transcriptionally activates the monocyte-derived neutrophil chemotactic factor/IL 8 gene in endothelial cells. Immunology 69:548, 1990.
130. Sim TC, Alam R, Forsythe PA, et al: Measurement of histamine-releasing factor activity in individual nasal washings: relationship with atopy, basophil response, and membrane-bound IgE. J Allergy Clin Immunol 89:1157, 1992.
131. Sim TC, Hilsmeier RA, Alam R, et al: Effect of topical corticosteroids on the recovery of histamine releasing factors in nasal washings of patients with allergic rhinitis. Am Rev Respir Dis 145:1316, 1992.
132. Smith RE, Strieter RM, Phan SH, et al: Production and function of murine macrophage inflammatory-1α in bleomycin-induced lung injury. J Immunol 153:4704, 1994.
133. Solley GO, Gleich GJ, Jordan RE, et al: The late phase of the immediate wheal and flare skin reaction. Its dependence upon IgE antibodies. J Clin Invest 58:408, 1976.
134. Stafford S, Sim J, Boyars M, et al: Increased levels of monocyte chemotactic peptide-1 (MCP-1) in the bronchoalveolar lavage (BAL) fluid and mRNA in the lavage cells from patients with asthma. J Allergy Clin Immunol 95:218, 1995.
135. Standiford TJ, Rolfe MW, Kunkel SL, et al: Macrophage inflammatory protein-1α expression in interstitial lung disease. J Immunol 151:2852, 1993.
136. Strieter RM, Chensue SW, Standiford TJ, et al: Disparate gene expression of chemotactic cytokines by human mononuclear phagocytes. Biochem Biophys Res Comm 166:886, 1990.
137. Strieter RM, Kunkel SL, Showell HJ, et al: Endothelial cell gene expression of a neutrophil chemotactic factor by TNFα, LPS and IL 1β Science 243:1467, 1989.
138. Strieter RM, Wiggins R, Phan SH, et al: Monocyte chemotactic protein gene expression by cytokine-treated human fibroblasts and endothelial cells. Biochem Biophys Res Comm 162:694, 1989.
139. Taub DD, Conlon K, Lloyd AR, et al: Preferential migration of activated CD4+ and CD8+ T cells in response to MIP Iα and MIP Iβ. Science 260:355, 1993.
140. Taub DD, Lloyd AR, Conlon K, et al: Recombinant human interferon–inducible protein 10 is a chemoattractant for human monocytes and T lymphocytes and promotes T cell adhesion to endothelial cells. J Exp Med 147:1809, 1993.
141. Taub DD, Proost P, Murphy WJ, et al: Monocyte chemotactic protein-1 (MCP-1) -2, and -3 are chemotactic for human T lymphocytes. J Clin Invest 95:1370, 1995.
142. Thelen M, Peveri P, Kernen P, et al: Mechanism of neutrophil activation by NAF, a novel monocyte-derived peptide agonist. FASEB J 2:2702, 1988.
143. Thornton AJ, Strieter RM, Lindley I, et al: Cytokine-induced gene expression of a neutrophil chemotactic factor/IL 8 in human hepatocytes. J Immunol 144:2609, 1990.
144. Thueson DO, Speck LS, Lett-Brown MA, et al: Histamine-releasing activity (HRA). I. Production by mitogen or antigen stimulated human mononuclear cells. J Immunol 122:623, 1979.
145. Thueson DO, Speck LS, Lett-Brown MA, et al: Histamine-releasing activity (HRA). II. Interaction with basophils and physicochemical characterization. J Immunol 123:633, 1979.
146. Van Damme J, Proost P, Lenaertz JP, et al: Structural and functional identification of two human, tumor-derived monocyte chemotactic proteins (MCP-2 and MCP-3) belonging to the chemokine family. J Exp Med 176:59, 1992.
147. Van Damme J, Van Beeumen J, Opdenakker G, et al: A novel NH_2-terminal sequence-characterized human monokine possessing neutrophil chemotactic, skin-reactive, and granulocytosis-promoting activity. J Exp Med 167:1364, 1988.
148. Van Riper G, Siciliano S, Fischer PA, et al: Characterization and species distribution of high affinity GTP-coupled receptors for human RANTES and monocyte chemoattractant 1. J Exp Med 177:851, 1993.
149. Villiger PM, Terkeltaub R, Lotz M: Monocyte chemoattractant protein-1 (MCP-1) expression in human articular cartilage. J Clin Invest 90:488, 1992.
150. Villiger PM, Terkeltaub R, Lotz M: Production of monocyte chemoattractant protein-1 by inflamed synovial tissue and cultured synoviocytes. J Immunol 149:722, 1992.
151. Walz A, Baggiolini M: Generation of the neutrophil activating peptide NAP-2 from basic platelet protein or connective tissue-activating peptide III through monocyte protease. J Exp Med 171:449, 1990.
152. Walz A, Dewald B, Tscharner V, et al: Effects of the neutrophil activating peptide NAP-2, platelet basic protein, connective tissue activating peptide III, and platelet factor 4 on human neutrophils. J Exp Med 170:1745, 1989.
153. Walz A, Peveri P, Achauer AO, et al: Purification and amino acid sequencing of NAF, a novel neutrophil activating factor produced by monocytes. Biochem Biophys Res Commun 149:755, 1987.
154. Wang JM, McVicar DW, Oppenheim JJ, et al: Identification of RANTES receptors on human monocyte cells: competition for binding and desensitization by homologous chemotactic chemokines. J Exp Med 177:699, 1993.
155. Wang JM, Sherry B, Fivash MJ, et al: Human recombinant macrophage inflammatory protein-1α and β and monocyte chemotactic and activating factor utilize common and unique receptors on human monocytes. J Immunol 150:3022, 1993.
156. Wantanabe K, Kinishi K, Fujioka M, et al: The neutrophil chemoattractant produced by the rat kidney epithelial cell line, NRK-52E is a protein related to KC/GRO protein. J Biol Chem 264:19559, 1989.
157. Warner JA, Pienkowski MM, Plaut M, et al: Identification of histamine releasing factor(s) in the late phase of cutaneous IgE-mediated reactions. J Immunol 136:2583, 1986.
158. Wolpe SD, Cerami A: Macrophage inflammatory proteins 1 and 2: members of a novel superfamily of cytokines. FASEB J 3:2565, 1989.
159. Wolpe SD, Davatelis G, Sherry B, et al: Macrophages secrete a novel heparin-binding protein with inflammatory and neutrophil chemokinetic properties. J Exp Med 167:570, 1988.
160. Wolpe SD, Sherry B, Juers D, et al: Identification and characterization

of macrophage inflammatory protein 2. Proc Natl Acad Sci USA 86:612, 1988.

161. Yoshimura T, Leonard EJ: Identification of high affinity receptors for human MCP-1 on human monocytes. J Immunol 145:292, 1990.
162. Yoshimura T, Leonard EJ: Secretion by human fibroblasts of monocyte chemoattractant protein-1, the product of gene JE. J Immunol 144:2377, 1990.
163. Yoshimura T, Matsushima Y, Tanaka S, et al: Purification of a human monocyte-derived neutrophil chemotactic factor that has peptide sequence similarity to other host defense cytokines. Proc Natl Acad Sci USA 84:9233, 1987.
164. Yoshimura T, Robinson EA, Tanaka S, et al: Purification and amino acid analysis of two human monocyte chemoattractants produced by phyohemagglutinin-stimulated human blood mononuclear leukocytes. J Immunol 142:1956, 1989.
165. Yoshimura T, Yuhki N, Moore SK, et al: Human monocyte chemoattractant protein-1 (MCP-1): full length cDNA cloning, expression in mitogen stimulated blood mononuclear leukocytes and similarity to mouse competence gene, JE. FEBS Lett 244:487, 1989.
166. Yoshimura TK, Matsushima K, Oppenheim JJ, et al: Neutrophil chemotactic factor produced by lipopolysaccharide (LPS)-stimulated human blood mononuclear leukocytes: partial characterization and separation from interleukin 1 (IL1). J Immunol 139:788, 1987.
167. Yoshimura TK, Matsushima K, Tanaka S, et al: Purification of human monocyte-derived neutrophil chemotactic factor that shares sequence homology with other host defense cytokines. Proc Natl Acad Sci USA 84:9233, 1987.
168. Yoshizuka N, Yoshimura M, Tsuchiya S, et al: Macrophage chemotactic factor (MCF) produced by a human T cell hybridoma clone. Cell Immunol 123:212, 1989.
169. Zhang K, Gharaee-Kermani M, Jones ML, et al: Lung monocyte chemoattractant protein-1 gene expression in bleomycin-induced pulmonary fibrosis. J Immunol 153:4733, 1994.
170. Zipfel PF, Balke J, Irving SG, et al: Mitogenic activation of human T cells induces two closely related genes which share structural similarities with a new family of secreted factors. J Immunol 142:1582, 1989.
171. Zucker MB, Katz IR, Thorbecke GJ, et al: Immunoregulatory activity of peptides related to platelet factor 4. Proc Natl Acad Sci USA 86:7571, 1989.

7 Structure, Function, and Synthesis of IgE

DONATA VERCELLI RAIF S. GEHA

Immunoglobulin E (IgE) plays a key role in the pathogenesis of allergic disease (reviewed in 105, 106). Studies on the cellular basis of IgE regulation have provided important insights into a disease that affects a considerable proportion of the population worldwide. More recently, the molecular events underlying IgE synthesis have been actively investigated, inasmuch as they represent an ideal model to characterize the signals involved in isotype-specific regulation of Ig synthesis. This chapter will discuss the cells, cytokines, and molecular mechanisms involved in human IgE synthesis.

ROLE OF CELLS AND CYTOKINES IN THE INDUCTION OF IgE SYNTHESIS

TWO-SIGNAL MODEL FOR THE INDUCTION OF IgE SYNTHESIS

During an immune response, a B lymphocyte can express different Ig heavy chain isotypes sharing the same VDJ region. This phenomenon (isotype switching) allows a single B-cell clone to produce antibodies with the same fine specificity but different effector functions. In order to switch to a particular isotype, a B cell needs to receive two signals. Signal 1 is cytokine dependent, results in the activation of transcription at a specific region of the Ig locus, and thus determines isotype specificity. Signal 2 activates the recombination machinery, resulting in DNA switch recombination.

The two signals required for switching to IgE are delivered to B cells by T cells through a complex series of interactions. Allergen-specific B cells capture the antigen via their surface Ig molecules, internalize it, and process it into peptides, which are then presented on the B-cell surface in association with MHC class II molecules. Recognition of the antigen/MHC class II complex by the T-cell receptor leads to two crucial events: the secretion of lymphokines, in particular IL-4, which provides the first signal for IgE induction, and the expression of CD40 ligand (CD40L) (Fig. 7–1). Notably, CD40L is absent on resting T cells, and it is the expression of this molecule following activation that renders T cells fully competent to induce IgE. Engagement of CD40 on B cells by its ligand on T cells delivers the signal that triggers switch recombination to IgE. Amplification circuits involving accessory molecules then lead to high-rate IgE synthesis.

Signal 1: IL-4 and IL-13. The interaction between IL-4 and IL-4 receptors (R) delivers the first signal for switching to IgE. Evidence from different lines of inquiry consistently

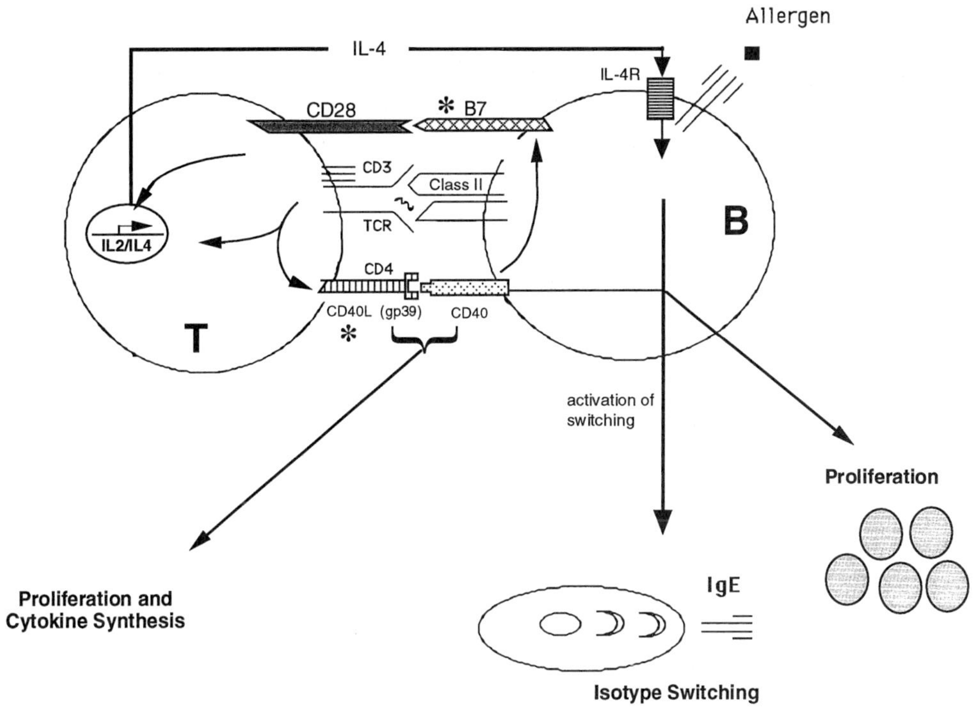

FIGURE 7–1. T-B cell interactions in IgE synthesis.

shows that IL-4 is essential for IgE production. IL-4 was the only cytokine able to induce IgE synthesis in vitro, when added in recombinant form; injection of an anti–IL-4 antibody abolished IgE production in parasite-infected mice.[28] IL-4R exist in vivo not only as cell-bound molecules but also in a soluble, circulating form. A recombinant extracellular IL-4R domain blocked switching to IgE by blocking IL-4/IL-4R interactions.[32] The same result was obtained using an IL-4 mutant in which a tyrosine at position 124 was replaced by aspartic acid.[6] The mutation preserves the ability to bind IL-4R but destroys the capacity to transmit a signal upon receptor binding.[117] Both experiments show that it is sufficient to block the IL-4 signal in order to block isotype switching to IgE and IgE production.

The most compelling evidence for the central role of IL-4 in IgE induction comes from gene-targeting experiments. Mice in which the IL-4 gene had been knocked out by homologous recombination (IL-4 KO mice) were unable to mount an anti-parasite IgE response. The IgG1 response was also suppressed, although to a lesser extent, whereas the production of other isotypes was unaffected.[61] Furthermore, genetic linkage analysis has shown that IL-4, or a nearby gene in the 5q31.1 region (IL-13, IL-5, IL-9), is responsible for the regulation of overall IgE production.[74] Polymorphism in the regulatory region of the gene may result in a predisposition to secrete abnormally high levels of IgE-inducing cytokines in response to antigen.

More recently, it has become clear that another cytokine, IL-13, shares many of the functional properties of IL-4, including the ability to induce IgE synthesis.[77] Although the sequence homology between IL-13 and IL-4 is only about 30%, all residues that contribute to the hydrophobic core of IL-4 are conserved or have conservative hydrophobic replacements in IL-13.[117] Indeed, an IL-4 mutant protein, which binds IL-4R with high affinity, competitively inhibits receptor binding of both IL-4 and IL-13 and blocks induction of IgE synthesis by both cytokines.[6] However, IL-4 and IL-13, as well as their receptors, are by no means identical. IL-13 does not bind to the 130 KD IL-4–binding protein and, unlike IL-4, has no effects on human T cells.[117] Furthermore, the IL-13 receptor does not share the γ chain subunit common to IL-2, IL-4, IL-7, IL-9, and IL-15 receptors.[56] The elucidation of the respective roles of IL-4 and IL-13 in physiologic conditions will require information about the structure and distribution of IL-13R, as well as a detailed analysis of the mechanisms that control the expression of these cytokines. The molecular events dependent on the delivery of signal 1 will be discussed.

Signal 2: CD40/CD40L interactions. The engagement of CD40 on B cells by CD40L expressed on T cells provides the second signal required for switching to IgE. CD40L can be replaced in vitro by anti-CD40 monoclonal antibodies (mAbs). Indeed, this was the first experimental system in which the B-cell activating signal for human IgE synthesis was delivered by antibody-induced engagement of a discrete B-cell surface antigen.

CD40 is a 50 KD surface glycoprotein expressed on human B lymphocytes,[110] cytokine-activated monocytes,[3] follicular dendritic cells,[12] and epithelial cells (including thymic epithelium)[31] and by certain carcinomas and melanomas, but not by T cells.[62, 82] CD40 plays a key role in the survival, growth, and differentiation of B cells. Signaling through CD40 rescues B cells from apoptosis induced by Fas (CD95) or by cross-linking of the IgM complex.[65, 101] Selected anti-CD40 mAbs trigger significant proliferation of highly purified resting B cells in the absence of other costimuli.[39]

CD40 belongs to the tumor necrosis factor receptor (TNFR) superfamily, which includes TNFRI and TNFRII, nerve growth factor receptor (NGFR), CD30, CD27, and Fas (CD95) (reviewed in 7). Members within this family share sequence similarity through their extracellular regions that contain multiple cysteine-rich repeats. The common structural framework of the extracellular domain is reflected by the ability of the TNFR superfamily members to interact with a parallel family of TNF-related molecules, which includes the ligands for CD40, CD27, and CD30, TNF-α, and lymphotoxin (TNF-β). CD40L is a 261 aa type 2 membrane glycoprotein, which is transiently expressed on activated, but not resting, Th1 and Th2 cells.[5] Cells transfected with CD40L induced IgE synthesis by both murine[5] and human B cells[99] in the presence of IL-4, whereas a soluble CD40-Ig fusion protein inhibited IL-4–dependent IgE synthesis in human peripheral blood mononuclear cells (PBMC).[26] These results clearly indicated that CD40/CD40L interactions are critical in delivering the second signal required for IgE production.

The central role of the CD40/CD40L pathway in IgE synthesis, and more generally in isotype switching, was confirmed by the finding that defective switching in patients with X-linked hyper-IgM (HIM) syndrome is due to mutations in CD40L, which result in impaired CD40/CD40L interactions.[4, 30] Furthermore, no IgG, IgA, and IgE response to thymus-dependent antigens was detectable in CD40[11, 51] and CD40L[113] KO mice, and no germinal centers were recognizable in lymphoid organs. In contrast, responses to thymus-independent antigens were preserved. Finally, the inability of human newborn B cells to switch has been ascribed to the decrease observed in both CD40L expression[29] and responses to CD40 agonists.[24] Thus data from a number of in vitro and in vivo models consistently point to the crucial role of CD40/CD40L interactions in germinal center formation, B-cell activation, isotype switching, and antibody production. The molecular events that lead to isotype switching following CD40 engagement will be discussed.

The interactions between CD40 and CD40L are tightly regulated. T cells only become competent to activate B cells via CD40 after they express CD40L, and this in turn requires TCR-dependent T-cell activation. The latter process seems to be anatomically constrained, in that CD40L is only expressed in secondary lymphoid tissues at the site of cognate T/B-cell interactions. Interestingly, a subset of CD4+ memory T cells in germinal centers contains preformed CD40L that is rapidly, but transiently, expressed on the cell surface after TCR-mediated activation.[10] The speed at which T cells can express CD40L on their surface may be crucial in germinal centers because centrocytes either leave the light zone within a few hours of activation or die by apoptosis in situ. On the other hand, the availability of CD40L is drastically limited because the interaction with CD40 induces rapid endocytosis of surface CD40L[114] and release of soluble CD40 by B cells down-regulates CD40L mRNA.[104]

CD40L, γ/δ T cells, and IgE regulation. CD40L has been shown to be expressed by both α/β- and γ/δ-activated T cells.[33, 40] Because CD40L expression is lower on γ/δ than α/β T cells, γ/δ T cells are less efficient in inducing IgE synthesis, but they are competent to induce isotype switching to IgE in vitro in the presence of exogenous IL-4. The recent finding that mice congenitally deficient in α/β T cells produce Ig of all isotypes, with high levels of IgE and IgG1,[111] suggests that γ/δ T cells play a role in directing isotype switching in vivo as well. The potential role of γ/δ T cells in the induction of IgE responses is further stressed by the observation that γ/δ T cells are able to discriminate early in infection between Th1- and Th2-inducing pathogens and produce cytokines associated with the appropriate pattern of response. Cytokines produced by γ/δ T cells may not only aid in the direct elimination of certain pathogens but also contribute to the cytokine milieu that influences the differentiation of CD4+ T cells into either Th1 or Th2.[27]

Interestingly, adoptive transfer of small numbers of γ/δ T cells from OVA-tolerant mice selectively suppressed Th2-dependent IgE synthesis without affecting IgG responses. These γ/δ cells were CD8+ and produced large amounts of interferon γ (IFN-γ). These findings confirm the potential role of γ/δ T cells in the regulation of IgE responses, pointing to potentially different roles in different models.

Accessory molecules and amplification circuits. Several pairs of accessory molecules (CD28/B7, LFA-1/ICAM-1, CD2/CD58) have been shown to participate in T/B-cell interactions conducive to IgE synthesis. Interactions within these ligand/receptor pairs complement and/or up-regulate the T-cell–dependent activation of B cells that follows the engagement of CD40 by CD40L. A major accessory role is likely to be played by the CD28/B7 ligand receptor pair. CD28 KO mice have reduced basal Ig levels and decreased class switching after infection with viruses.[96] Both CD28 on T cells and its B-cell counterreceptor, B7, are part of a reciprocal amplification mechanism that amplifies T/B-cell interactions mediated via CD40/CD40L. Engagement of CD40 is known to result in B7 expression on B cells.[86] On the other hand, engagement of CD28 results in increased expression of CD40L on T cells[57] and, most importantly, in increased IL-4 secretion[57] and Th2 differentiation.[54] IL-4 in turn up-regulates B7 expression.[102] Thus CD28/B7 interactions may enhance both IL-4 secretion and CD40-mediated B-cell activation and would ultimately potentiate both signal 1 and signal 2. Consistent with this view, IgE synthesis has been shown to be inhibited by anti-CD28 blocking mAbs.[64]

A marked increase in B7 expression is also induced by cross-linking MHC class II molecules on B cells, particularly when ICAM-1 is simultaneously engaged. Thus interactions through MHC class II and ICAM-1 complement T-cell help provided via CD40/CD40L interactions.[84] In contrast, the weak IgE-inducing signal provided by engagement of CD58 (LFA-3) seems to be independent of the CD40 pathway.[22]

Amplification of IgE synthesis. Human basophils and mast cells have been reported to secrete IL-4[9, 94] and to express CD40L.[37] Thus basophils and mast cells may, in principle, provide both signal 1 and signal 2 for IgE synthesis. However, these non–T cells conceivably play a role in IgE amplification rather than IgE induction. The optimal physiologic stimulus for secretion of IL-4 and IL-13 seems to be allergen-dependent cross-linking of receptor-bound, allergen-specific IgE.[9, 94] Thus cytokine secretion would be predicated on the production of allergen-specific IgE, and this in turn requires the signals and cells (including allergen-specific T cells) discussed previously. Once IgE has been produced, it can recruit basophils and mast cells by binding to their IgE receptors, thus inducing IL-4/IL-13 secretion and CD40L expression. Only at this point may non–T cells trigger an IgE response, which would not necessarily be allergen specific but may be polyclonal as well. This scenario is consistent with the observation that a significant proportion of the IgE response in hyper-IgE states is frequently polyclonal rather than allergen specific.

CD40L was found to be constitutively expressed on eosinophils from one patient with the hypereosinophilic syndrome; however, these cells were not able to induce IgE synthesis in the presence of exogenous IL-4.[36] The significance of this isolated observation therefore remains to be understood.

Addendum: B-cell-centered terminology. The complexity in the interplay between T cells, B cells, and cytokines involved in IgE induction makes it difficult to unambiguously establish a chronology of the events leading to IgE synthesis. On the other hand, molecular studies clearly point to a hierarchy in the steps to IgE induction and in the signals that trigger such steps. The initial event in switching to IgE is the determination of isotype specificity through cytokine (IL-4)-dependent induction of ϵ germline transcription, which is followed by CD40-mediated DNA switch recombination. Our terminology of signal 1 and signal 2 therefore reflects a B-cell–centered perspective, although high-rate IL-4 secretion (signal 1) and full B-cell activation via CD40/CD40L (signal 2) may well enhance each other and require CD28/B7 interactions.

Th1/Th2 DICHOTOMY AND POTENTIAL Th2 MARKERS

Studies with T-cell clones obtained from patients with atopic disease and parasitic infections clearly indicate that the lymphokine profile of T-cell clones specific for an antigen is determined by both the nature of the antigen and the genetic background of the individual (reviewed in 89). The majority of helper T-cell clones specific for parasitic antigens, isolated from patients with no history of atopic disease, had a Th2 lymphokine profile; that is, they produced high levels of IL-4, low IL-2 and IFN-γ, and induced vigorous IgE synthesis. On the other hand, allergen-specific CD4+ T-cell clones established from atopic patients had a Th2 lymphokine profile and provided help for IgE synthesis; whereas helper T-cell clones from the same patients, specific for nonallergenic antigens, or CD4+ clones from nonatopic individuals had a Th1 profile.[20, 50, 81] Thus antigens such as those expressed on parasites seem to be able to evoke a Th2/IgE response regardless of the genetic background. In contrast, the genetic background seems to be critical for the generation of a Th2/IgE response against allergens.

The factors ultimately responsible for skewing the T-helper repertoire toward Th1 or Th2 will be discussed elsewhere in this book. Here, it is important to underline the existence of complex cytokine amplification loops, which significantly influence both T-helper differentiation and IgE regulation. Th2-derived IL-4 markedly inhibits IFN-γ production by human T cells[83, 109] and furthermore directs the differentiation of precursor T cells into Th2 cells, which will secrete more IL-4.[70, 93] By contrast, IFN-γ promotes the differentiation of CD4+ T cells into Th1 cells.[70] Thus once an antigen has initially triggered a response—which will be Th1 or Th2 depending on the nature of the antigen and the genetic background of the individual—the antigen-specific T cell repertoire will be progressively skewed and more T cells with the same lymphokine profile will be recruited. IL-13, an IgE-inducing Th2 lymphokine, may represent an exception, in that it is not active on T cells[117] and therefore does not contribute to Th2 skewing. The inability of IL-13 to promote Th2 differentiation may explain why Th2 responses were severely impaired in mice in which the IL-4 gene had been disrupted but the IL-13 gene was intact.[59, 61]

IL-12 has been shown to skew the profile of the Th response toward Th1.[73] IL-12 may provide a link between natural and specific immune responses because some viruses and intracellular bacteria have the ability to stimulate macrophages to produce IL-12, which in turn induces IFN-γ production by both T cells and NK cells. Thus Th cells may be simultaneously presented with processed antigen plus cytokines that induce them to differentiate toward a Th1 phenotype.[88]

Further understanding of the mechanisms underlying the Th1/Th2 dichotomy may be provided by ongoing studies aimed at identifying potential markers for Th1 and Th2 cells. It has been proposed that the ability of Th clones to produce Th2-type lymphokines may correlate positively or negatively with the expression of two molecules, CD30 and CD27, which belong to the TNFR superfamily. The majority of human Th2 clones stimulated with the relevant allergen express CD30 and concomitantly secrete IL-4 and IL-5,[19] suggesting that CD30 may be associated with the differentiation/activation pathway of human T cells producing Th2-type cytokines. Furthermore, CD30 was expressed on Th2-like T-cell clones isolated from HIV patients with hyper-IgE syndrome.[72] These clones produced IL-4 and provided help for IgE synthesis, in spite of their CD8 phenotype.[69, 80] These findings suggest that CD30 may be a marker for CD8+ T cells that have switched to the production of type-2 helper cytokines.

In patients with atopy or filariasis, the proliferative response to allergens[18] and the secretion of IL-4 and IL-5[25] have been reported to be confined to a memory T-cell population that expresses CD4 and CD45R0, but not CD27. This seems to be true for both peripheral blood T cells and T-cell clones. Because little is known about Th2 physiology, it is not yet clear how the expression of CD30 and/or the lack of expression of CD27 may result in a Th2 phenotype.

T-CELL–INDEPENDENT IgE INDUCTION BY EPSTEIN-BARR VIRUS (EBV) AND GLUCOCORTICOIDS

It has been shown that stimulation with IL-4 and EBV induces T-cell–independent IgE synthesis in human B cells.[47, 100] IgE production results from de novo induction of isotype switching rather than from expansion of a precommitted $sIgE^+$ B-cell population that has switched to IgE in vivo.[47]

The role played by EBV in IgE induction is not entirely clear. However, a clue was provided by the characterization of CD40 receptor-associated factor 1 (CRAF-1), a novel component of the CD40 signaling pathway.[14, 42] The C-terminus of CRAF-1 interacts directly and specifically with the cytoplasmic tail of CD40. Interestingly, the C-terminus of CRAF-1 is homologous to the TNF-α receptor-associated factors 1 and 2 (TRAF-1 and TRAF-2), which can complex with the cytoplasmic tail of the related TNF-α receptor II.[90] The

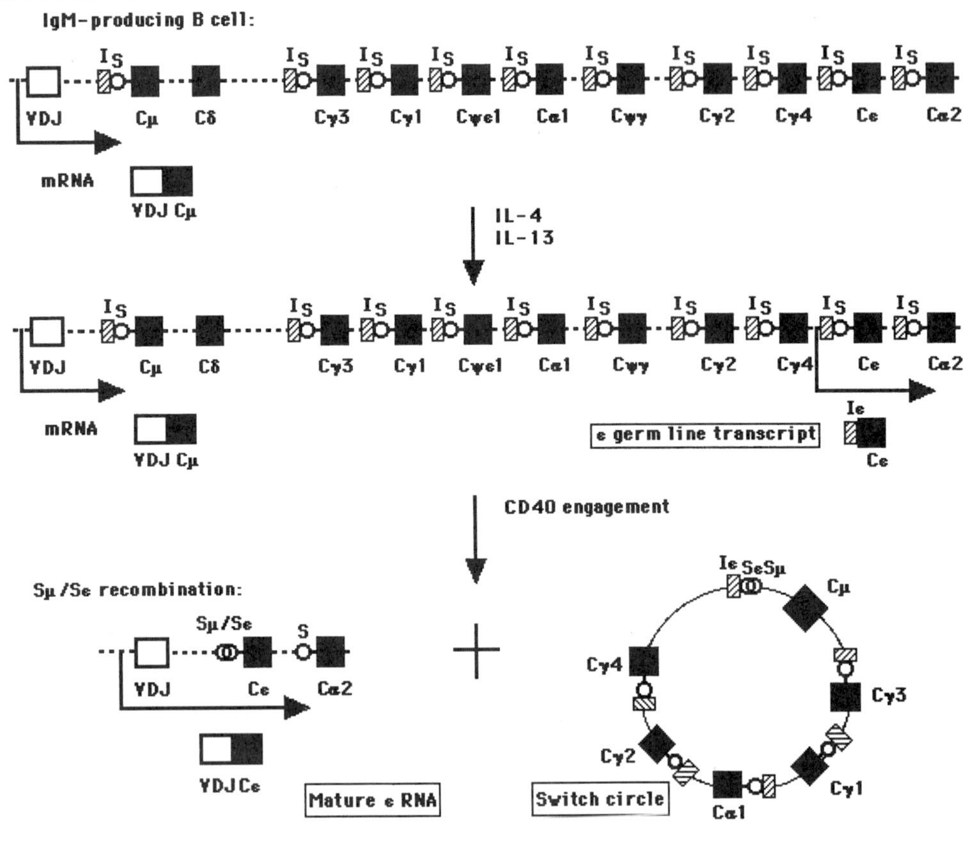

FIGURE 7–2. Isotype switching from an IgM-producing B cell to an IgE-producing cell. IL-4 plus IL-13 induces the IεCε germline transcript. CD4D engagement switches Cε for Cμ by Sμ/Sε recombination. Mature εRNA and the switch circle remains.

TRAF-C (for COOH-terminal) domain shared by CRAF-1, TRAF-1, and TRAF-2 is necessary and sufficient for CD40 binding and for homodimerization. It is likely that other members of the TNFR superfamily use CRAF-related proteins in their signal transduction process. Interestingly, CRAF-1 also interacts with the cytoplasmic domain of EBV latent infection membrane protein 1 (LMP1),[78] an EBV-encoded integral membrane protein that is critical for B lymphocyte transformation and, most importantly, is the only EBV gene that has transforming effects in nonlymphoid cells. The IgE-inducing properties of EBV may indeed result from the ability of EBV-encoded protein(s) to activate the CD40 signaling pathway, thus providing B cells with signal 2.

IgE synthesis can be induced in highly purified, sIgE-negative normal[45] and leukemic[91] B cells by a combination of IL-4 and glucocorticoids (hydrocortisone). The effects of hydrocortisone are specific, inasmuch as steroid sex hormones have no influence on IL-4–dependent IgE synthesis.[112] The mechanisms by which hydrocortisone synergizes with IL-4 remain unknown. Paradoxically, prolonged topical steroid treatment in vivo inhibits IL-4 production.[75] The observation that hormone-receptor interactions can provide a second signal for IgE synthesis warrants further investigation.

MOLECULAR EVENTS IN THE INDUCTION OF IgE SYNTHESIS

ROLE OF GERMLINE TRANSCRIPTS IN ISOTYPE SWITCHING

Isotype switching results from a DNA recombination event that juxtaposes different downstream CH genes to the expressed V(D)J gene. Considerable evidence indicates that isotype switching is not a random event but is directed by cytokines in conjunction with the regulation of B-cell proliferation and differentiation. Molecular analysis has shown that induction of isotype switching to a particular CH gene almost invariably correlates with the transcriptional activation of the same gene in its germline configuration (reviewed in 16, 107). The germline transcripts (GLT) that result from this process initiate a few kilobases (kb) upstream of the switch (S) region and proceed through one or more short exons (I exons) that are spliced to the first exon of the CH gene (Fig. 7–2). GLT are unable to code for any mature protein of significant length because the I exon contains multiple stop codons in all three reading frames. Therefore, GLT are also referred to as sterile transcripts. Alternatively, GLT are referred to as truncated transcripts because the I exon is usually 200 to 300 base pairs (bp) shorter than the VDJ exon present in mature transcripts. Although there is no significant conservation of the sequences of GLT of different isotypes, their overall structure is conserved.[16]

Expression of GLT is thought to play a key role in modulating the accessibility of a particular S region to a putative common switch recombinase, thus directing switching to the corresponding isotype. The role of GLT in the regulation of isotype switching has been tested by gene knockout experiments. Deletion of the mouse Iγ1[48] or Iγ2b[115] exons and their promoter resulted in inhibition of class switching to the corresponding genes, indicating that transcription in the S region is necessary to direct switch recombination. However, it is apparently not sufficient: replacement of Iε with a B-cell–specific promoter cassette containing the murine Eμ intronic enhancer and a VH promoter, without the Iε splice donor site, resulted in only marginal switch recombination to IgE at about 1% of the frequency induced by IL-4.[8] In contrast, replacement of all known IL-4–inducible control elements in the Sγ1 region with the heterologous human metallothioneine IIA promoter did not impair switch recombination to mouse IgG1, provided that the Iγ1 splice donor site was included in the construct, thus allowing for the induction of artificial but processed GLT.[66] These data indicate that artificial induction of structurally conserved, spliced GLT can target switch recombination, whereas transcription in the S region as such cannot; and that spliced switch transcripts (or the process of splicing) have a functional role in switch recombination.[66] The most intriguing speculation is that GLT are part of the switch recombinase, providing the specificity to target distinct S regions.

TRANSCRIPTION FACTORS INVOLVED IN THE REGULATION OF ε GLT EXPRESSION

Expression of ε GLT is regulated at the transcriptional level by nuclear factors that bind to the Iε promoter and adjacent regions (Fig. 7–3). Nuclear factors specifically bind to relatively short (10–20 bp) DNA sequences, functionally defined as responsive elements (RE). Among the proteins that bind the ε GLT promoter, some are constitutively expressed, and others are induced by specific cytokines. The specificity in the induction of nuclear factors provides a molecular basis for the specificity of cytokine-induced GLT expression and isotype switching.

BSAP, a transcription factor expressed in B but not T cells,[1] binds to a highly conserved region upstream of the Iε transcription initiation site and has been shown to contribute to the regulation of GLT expression (see Fig. 7–3).[63] An IL-4 RE more upstream has been found to bind the IL-4–inducible factor NF-IL-4, a member of the C/EBP family, and NF-κB p50.[21] It has been proposed that these factors may have to interact physically in order to induce ε GLT expression.[21] The role of NF-κB in the induction of murine GLT has been confirmed by the finding that expression of GLT for several isotypes, including IgE, and switching to the same isotypes, is severely impaired in NF-κB p50 KO mice (Snapper, personal communication).[95]

STAT6 (NF-IL-4) binds close to the Iε transcription initiation site and exhibits a unique pattern of rapid activation.[60, 92] STAT6 belongs to the newly identified family of signal transducers and activators of transcription (STAT).[41, 44] Binding of IL-4 to its receptor leads to activation by tyrosine phosphorylation of two receptor-associated cytoplasmic tyrosine kinases, Janus kinase (JAK)-3 and, to a lesser extent, JAK-1.[71] These kinases are believed to rapidly (within minutes) phosphorylate STAT6, a latent cytoplasmic factor. The phosphorylated STAT6 would homodimerize, translocate to the nucleus, and bind to one or possibly two regions in the murine ε GLT promoter, contributing to the activation of transcription.[41] The discovery of JAKs and STATs has finally provided an explanation for the apparent paradox that the IL-4R, as well as the receptors for a number of other cytokines, lacks kinase domains and yet couples ligand binding to tyrosine phosphorylation.[44] STAT6 is not B-cell specific and is induced by IL-4 in monocytes, where it participates

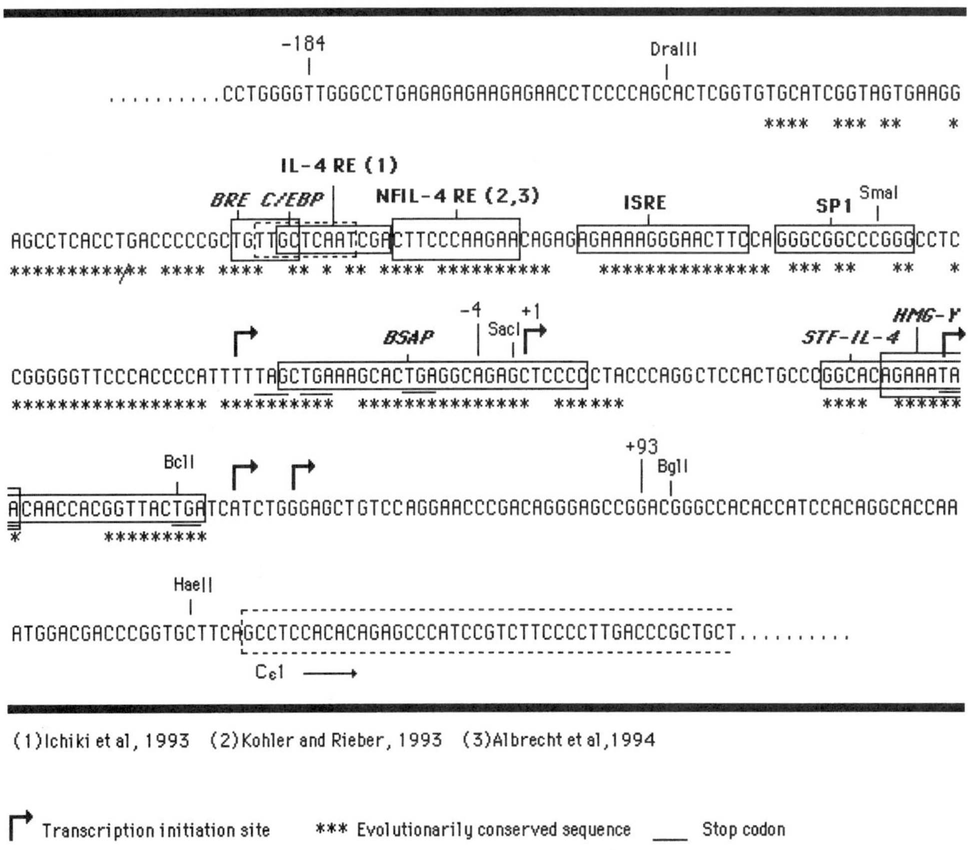

FIGURE 7–3. Regulatory elements in the ε GLT promoter indicated by boxed nucleotides. BSAP binds just "upstream" of the Ie transcription start site (+1). The beginning of Ce is shown by the dotted box at the bottom (+142). STAT6 (NF-IL4) and NF-κB bind to the IL-4 response elements shown. ISRE is a response element for γ interferon. Sites of cleavage by restriction enzymes are indicated by fine lettering.

in the transcriptional regulation of the IL-4–inducible CD23b promoter. STAT6 binding sites have been identified in the promoters of a number of IL-4–responsive genes, such as CD23, Cγ1, and MHC class II.[58, 60] The presence of homologous RE in the promoter of different genes underlies the concerted regulation of these genes by a single cytokine. Thus the concerted increase in the expression of ϵ GLT, CD23, and MHC class II in B cells stimulated with IL-4 is mediated by IL-4 RE located 5′ of each of these genes.

The requirements for the induction of ϵ GLT seem to be somewhat different in mice and humans. Two signals, IL-4 and LPS, are required for murine ϵ GLT expression in most murine B-cell lines, whereas IL-4 alone is sufficient in humans. The interactions between the human ϵ GLT promoter and transcription factors are only incompletely defined. Two contiguous IL-4 RE have been identified upstream of Iϵ in a region of high human/mouse homology.[43, 58] The most 3′ site binds STAT6, which also interacts with a 9-bp binding motif in the promoter of CD23.[58] The role of both IL-4 responsive elements has been validated in reporter assays.[2, 43] However, the minimal set of elements in the human ϵ GLT promoter required to confer full IL-4 inducibility to a heterologous promoter has not been unambiguously determined. Interestingly, the STAT6 binding site in the human ϵ GLT promoter[2] resembles the murine HMG-I(Y) site,[52] in that deletion or mutation results in a marked increase in basal promoter activity and in loss of IL-4 inducibility. Thus these elements seem to have a bifunctional activity: they repress the activity of the promoter in the absence of IL-4, but they are required for IL-4–induced promoter activation.

DNA SWITCH RECOMBINATION

Although IL-4 (signal 1) is by itself sufficient for the initiation of transcription through the ϵ locus, switching and expression of mature Cϵ transcripts (containing VDJ spliced to Cϵ1–4) require signal 2 (engagement of CD40 by CD40 ligand). The molecular events that follow the delivery of the second signal for switching to IgE have been characterized (see Fig. 7–2). The classic model, according to which switching occurs via loop-out and deletional recombination between highly repetitive S regions (reviewed in 76), was challenged in the late 1980s, at least for the IgE isotype. Indeed, it was reported that IgE could be produced by B cells in which the immunoglobulin locus was retained in germline configuration.[13, 68] Thus it became important to characterize the molecular mechanisms that underlie the expression of mature VDJ-Cϵ mRNA in normal human B cells.

This issue was investigated using polymerase chain reaction (PCR)-based approaches that allow for amplification, cloning, and sequencing of Sμ/Sϵ switch fragments or of switch circles, their reciprocal products. DNA sequencing of Sμ/Sϵ switch fragments amplified from IgE-producing B-cell cultures formally proved that deletional switch recombination had occurred. Most of the switch fragments represented direct joining of Sμ to Sϵ. The recombination sites within Sμ were clustered within 900 bp at the 5′ end of the S region, suggesting that there are hot spots for recombination within Sμ. In contrast, the Sϵ recombination sites were scattered throughout the Sϵ region.[46, 97, 98]

Interestingly, some fragments amplified from B cells stimulated with IL-4 and hydrocortisone contained insertions at the Sμ/ϵ junction that were derived from Sγ4.[46] The presence of an Sγ4-derived insertion suggested that some B cells had undergone sequential isotype switching from IgM to IgG4 to IgE. Indeed, IL-4 has been shown to induce isotype switching to IgG4,[67] as well as to IgE, and single B cells can give rise to clones that secrete IgG4 and IgE.[34]

Because a B cell that first switches to IgG4 and then to IgE may lose Sγ4-derived sequences during the second switch recombination, it became important to assess whether sequential and direct switching coexist. Switch circles generated in B cells triggered to switch to IgE by IL-4 and anti-CD40 mAb were PCR amplified. Sequencing of the circles showed the presence of μ–γ–ϵ switching, and of sequential events even more complex (μ–α1–γ–ϵ), but μ–ϵ circles representing direct switching events were also found at high frequency.[116] Likewise, sequence analysis of Sμ/Sϵ switch fragments from patients with atopic dermatitis showed a predominance of direct Sμ/Sϵ joining.[103]

The importance of sequential switching in vivo was investigated by examining switching to IgE in mutant mice that lacked the Sγ1 region,[48] and were therefore unable to support sequential switching via IgG1 (note that mouse IgG1 is most similar to human IgG4). In these mice, the frequency of switching to IgE was not affected.[49] These results indicated that sequential switching merely reflects the simultaneous accessibility of two acceptor S regions for switch recombination induced by one cytokine. The apparent dominance of sequential switching observed in the generation of murine IgE-expressing cells following IL-4 stimulation is due to the parallel activation of Sγ1 and Sϵ by IL-4, Sγ1 being intrinsically more accessible to recombination with Sμ.[48, 49] Thus the overall low frequency of IgE switching is an autonomously determined intrinsic feature of Sϵ and its control elements. This may explain why, in the presence of saturating concentrations of IL-4 in vitro, the frequency of IgE switching reaches at most 10% of the frequency of switching to IgG1, which is also induced by IL-4.

CYTOKINE-DEPENDENT MODULATION OF IL-4–INDUCED IgE SYNTHESIS

Although IL-4 and IL-13 are the only cytokines capable of inducing IgE synthesis, cellular studies have shown that IL-4/IL-13–induced IgE production can be further enhanced, or inhibited, by a number of cytokines (Table 7–1). However, the mechanisms responsible for the effects of these cytokines, and the events that are targeted, are still mostly unclear.

TNF-α, IL-6, and IL-9 enhance IL-4–dependent IgE synthesis.[23, 35, 108] IgE potentiation by TNF-α and IL-6 is detectable in both T-cell–dependent and T-cell–independent systems. The increase in IgE synthesis induced by TNF-α is mediated by enhanced ϵ GLT expression, whereas this step is not affected by IL-6 and IL-9.[35] IL-6 is not isotype specific[79] and induces IgG secretion by selective accumulation of mRNA for the secreted form of the molecule, and possibly through differential mRNA stabilization.[87] IgE secretion might be amplified by similar mechanisms, but no direct evidence is available. Notably, engagement of CD40 triggers IL-6 and TNF-α secretion by B cells[15] and monocytes.[3]

TABLE 7–1
CYTOKINES MODULATE MOLECULAR EVENTS IN IgE INDUCTION

	T-cell Dependent			T-cell Independent		
	GLT	***mature RNA***	***IgE***	***GLT***	***mature RNA***	***IgE***
TNF-α	↑	↑	↑	↑	↑	↑
IL-6	↔	↑	↑	↔	↑	↑
IL-9	↔	ND	ND	ND	ND	↑
TGF-β	↓	↓	↓	↓	↓	↓
IFN-γ	↔	↔	↔	↓	↓	↓
IFN-α	↔	↔	↔	↓	↓	↓
IL-8	ND	ND	↓	ND	ND	↓
IL-12	ND	ND	↔	↔	↓	↓
PAF-acether	ND	ND	ND	↓	↓	↓
IL-10*	↔	↔	↔	↓	↓	↓

*Monocyte dependent

All the other cytokines listed in Table 7–1 inhibit IgE synthesis. Interestingly, only TGF-β has been shown to act on B cells by targeting ϵ GLT expression.[35] IL-8 also inhibits IgE production by purified B cells,[53] but the molecular targets remain unknown. The other cytokines are either inactive on germline transcription or uncharacterized so far. Interestingly, IFN-α, IFN-γ, and IL-12 inhibit IgE secretion only when tested in T-cell–dependent systems,[35, 38, 55] and IL-10 only suppresses IgE synthesis in the presence of monocytes.[85] Thus none of these cytokines act directly on B cells.

REFERENCES

1. Adams B, Dörfler P, Aguzzi A, et al: Pax-5 encodes the transcription factor BSAP and is expressed in B lymphocytes, the developing CNS, and adult testis. Genes Dev 6:1589–1607, 1992.
2. Albrecht B, Peiritsch S, Woisetschläger M: A bifunctional control element in the human IgE germline promoter involved in repression and IL-4 activation. Int Immunol 6:1143–1151, 1994.
3. Alderson M R, Armitage R J, Tough T W, et al: CD40 expression by human monocytes: regulation by cytokines and activation of monocytes by the ligand for CD40. J Exp Med 178:669–674, 1993.
4. Allen R C, Armitage R J, Conley M E, et al: CD40 ligand gene defects responsible for X-linked Hyper-IgM syndrome. Science 259:990–993, 1993.
5. Armitage R J, Fanslow W C, Strockbine L, et al: Molecular and biological characterization of a murine ligand for CD40. Nature 357:80–82, 1992.
6. Aversa G, Punnonen J, Cocks B G, et al: An IL-4 mutant protein inhibits IL-4 or IL-13 induced human IgG4 and IgE synthesis and B cell proliferation: support for a common component shared by IL-4 and IL-13 receptors. J Exp Med 178:2213–2216, 1993.
7. Banchereau J, Bazan F, Blanchard D, et al: The CD40 antigen and its ligand. Annu Rev Immunol 12:881–922, 1994.
8. Bottaro A, Lansford R, Xu L, et al: S region transcription *per se* promotes basal IgE class switch recombination but additional factors regulate the efficiency of the process. EMBO J 13:665–674, 1994.
9. Burd P R, Thompson W C, Max E E, et al: Activated mast cells produce interleukin 13. J Exp Med 1373–1380, 1995.
10. Casamayor-Palleja M, Khan M, MacLennan I C M: A subset of CD4+ memory T cells contains preformed CD40 ligand that is rapidly but transiently expressed on their surface after activation through the T cell receptor complex. J Exp Med 181:1293–1301, 1995.
11. Castigli E, Alt F W, Davidson L, et al: CD40 deficient mice generated by RAG-2 deficient blastocyst complementation. Proc Natl Acad Sci USA 91:12135–12139, 1994.
12. Caux C, Massacrier C, Vanbervliet B, et al: Activation of human dendritic cells through CD40 cross-linking. J Exp Med 180:1263–1272, 1994.
13. Chan M A, Benedict S H, Dosch H-M, et al: Expression of IgE from a nonrearranged ϵ locus in cloned B-lymphoblastoid cells that also express IgM. J Immunol 144:3563–3568, 1990.
14. Cheng G, Cleary A M, Ye Z-s, et al: Involvement of CRAF1, a relative of TRAF, in CD40 signaling. Science 267:1494–1498, 1995.
15. Clark E A, Shu G: Association between IL-6 and CD40 signaling. IL-6 induces phosphorylation of CD40 receptors. J Immunol 145:1400–1406, 1990.
16. Coffman R L, Lebman D A, Rothman P: The mechanism and regulation of immunoglobulin isotype switching. Adv Immunol 54:229–269, 1993.
17. Cogné M, Lansford R, Bottaro A, et al: A class switch control region at the 3′ end of the immunoglobulin heavy chain locus. Cell 77:737–747, 1994.
18. de Jong R, Brouwer M, Hooibrink B, et al: The CD27-subset of peripheral blood memory CD4+ lymphocytes contains functionally differentiated T lymphocytes that develop by persistent antigenic stimulation in vivo. Eur J Immunol 22:993–999, 1992.
19. Del Prete G, De Carli M, Almerigogna F, et al: Preferential expression of CD30 by human CD4+ T cells producing Th2-type cytokines. FASEB J 9:81–86, 1995.
20. Del Prete G F, De Carli M, Mastromauro C, et al: Purified protein derivative of Mycobacterium tubercolosis and excretory-secretory antigen(s) of Toxocara canis expand in vitro human T cells with stable and opposite (type 1 T helper or type 2 T helper) profile of cytokine production. J Clin Invest 88:346–350, 1991.
21. Delphin S, Stavnezer J: Characterization of an IL-4 responsive region in the immunoglobulin heavy chain germline ϵ promoter: regulation by NF-IL-4, a C/EBP family member, and NF-kB/p50. J Exp Med 181:181–192, 1995.
22. Diaz-Sanchez D, Chegini S, Zhang K, et al: CD58 (LFA-3) stimulation provides a signal for human isotype switching and IgE production distinct from CD40. J Immunol 153:10–20, 1994.
23. Dugas B, Renauld J C, Péne J, et al: Interleukin-9 potentiates the interleukin-4–induced immunoglobulin (IgG, IgM, and IgE) production by normal human B lymphocytes. Eur J Immunol 1687–1692, 1993.
24. Durandy A, de Saint Basile G, Lisowska-Grospierre B, et al: Undetectable CD40 ligand expression on T cells and low B cell responses to CD40 binding agonists in human newborns. J Immunol 154:1560–1568, 1995.
25. Elson L H, Shaw S, Van Lier R A W, et al: T cell subpopulation phenotypes in filarial infections: CD27 negativity defines a population greatly enriched for Th2 cells. Int Immunol 6:1003–1009, 1994.
26. Fanslow W C, Anderson D M, Grabstein K H, et al: Soluble forms of CD40 inhibit biologic responses of human B cells. J Immunol 149:655–660, 1992.
27. Ferrick D A, Schrenzel M D, Mulvania T, et al: Differential production of interferon-γ and interleukin-4 in response to Th1- and Th2-stimulating pathogens by γδ T cells in vivo. Nature 373:255–257, 1995.
28. Finkelman F D, Katona I M, Urban J F, et al: Suppression of in vivo polyclonal IgE responses by monoclonal antibody to the lymphokine B-cell stimulatory factor 1. Proc Natl Acad Sci USA 83:9675–9678, 1986.
29. Fuleihan R, Ahern D, Geha R S: Decreased expression of the ligand for CD40 in newborn lymphocytes. Eur J Immunol 24:1925, 1994.

30. Fuleihan R, Ramesh N, Loh R, et al: Defective expression of the CD40 ligand in X-chromosome-linked immunoglobulin deficiency with normal or elevated IgM. Proc Natl Acad Sci USA 90:2170–2173, 1993.
31. Galy A H, Spits H: CD40 is functionally expressed on human thymic cells. J Immunol 149:775–782, 1992.
32. Garrone P, Djossou O, Galizzi J-P, et al: A recombinant extracellular domain of the human interleukin 4 receptor inhibits the biological effects of interleukin 4 on T and B lymphocytes. Eur J Immunol 21:1365–1369, 1991.
33. Gascan H, Aversa G C, Gauchat J-F, et al: Membranes of activated CD4+ T cells expressing T cell receptor (TcR) αβ or TcR γδ induce IgE synthesis by human B cells in the presence of interleukin-4. Eur J Immunol 22:1133–1141, 1992.
34. Gascan H, Gauchat J-F, Aversa G, et al: Anti-CD40 monoclonal antibodies or CD4+ T cell clones and IL-4 induce IgG4 and IgE switching in purified human B cells via different signaling pathways. J Immunol 147:8–13, 1991.
35. Gauchat J-F, Aversa G, Gascan H, et al: Modulation of IL-4 induced germline ϵ RNA synthesis in human B cells by tumor necrosis factor-α, anti-CD40 monoclonal antibodies or transforming growth factor-β correlates with levels of IgE production. Int Immunol 4:397–406, 1992.
36. Gauchat J-F, Henchoz S, Fattah D, et al: CD40 ligand is functionally expressed on human eosinophils. Eur J Immunol 25:863–865, 1995.
37. Gauchat J-F, Henchoz S, Mazzei G, et al: Induction of human IgE synthesis in B cells by mast cells and basophils. Nature 365:340–343, 1993.
38. Gauchat J-F, Lebman D A, Coffman R L, et al: Structure and expression of germline ϵ transcripts in human B cells induced by interleukin 4 to switch to IgE production. J Exp Med 172:463–473, 1990.
39. Gruber M F, Bjorndahl J M, Nakamura S, et al: Anti-CD45 inhibition of human B cell proliferation depends on the nature of activation signals and the state of B cell activation. J Immunol 142:4144–4152, 1989.
40. Horner A A, Jabara H, Ramesh N, et al: γ/δ T lymphocytes express CD40 ligand and induce isotype switching in B lymphocytes. J Exp Med 181:1239–1244, 1995.
41. Hou J, Schindler U, Henzel W J, et al: An interleukin-4-induced transcription factor: IL-4 Stat. Science 265:1701–1706, 1994.
42. Hu H M, O'Rourke K, Boguski M S, et al: A novel RING finger protein interacts with the cytoplasmic domain of CD40. J Biol Chem 269:30069–30072, 1994.
43. Ichiki T, Takahashi W, Watanabe T: Regulation of the expression of human Cϵ germline transcript—identification of a novel IL-4 responsive element. J Immunol 150:5408–5417, 1993.
44. Ihle J N, Kerr I M: Jaks and Stats in signaling by the cytokine receptor superfamily. Trends Genet 11:69–74, 1995.
45. Jabara H H, Ahern D J, Vercelli D, et al: Hydrocortisone and IL-4 induce IgE isotype switching in human B cells. J Immunol 147:1557–1560, 1991.
46. Jabara H H, Loh R, Ramesh N, et al: Sequential switching from μ to ϵ via γ4 in human B cells stimulated with IL-4 and hydrocortisone. J Immunol 151:4528–4533, 1993.
47. Jabara H H, Schneider L C, Shapira S K, et al: Induction of germ-line and mature Cϵ transcripts in human B cells stimulated with rIL-4 and EBV. J Immunol 145:3468–3473, 1990.
48. Jung S, Rajewsky K, Radbruch A: Shutdown of class switch recombination by deletion of a switch region control element. Science 259:984–987, 1993.
49. Jung S, Siebenkotten G, Radbruch A: Frequency of immunoglobulin E class switching is autonomously determined and independent of prior switching to other classes. J Exp Med 179:2023–2026, 1994.
50. Kapsenberg M L, Wierenga E A, Bos J D, et al: Functional subsets of allergen-reactive human CD4+ T cells. Immunol Today 12:392–395, 1991.
51. Kawabe T, Naka T, Yoshida K, et al: The immune responses in CD40-deficient mice: impaired immunoglobulin class switching and germinal center formation. Immunity 1:167–178, 1994.
52. Kim J, Reeves R, Rothman P, et al: The non-histone chromosomal protein HMG-I(Y) contributes to repression of the immunoglobulin heavy chain germ-line ϵ RNA promoter. Eur J Immunol 25:798–807, 1995.
53. Kimata H, Yoshida A, Ishioka C, et al: Interleukin-8 selectively inhibits immunoglobulin E production induced by IL-4 in human B cells. J Exp Med 176:1227–1231, 1992.
54. King C L, Stupi R J, Craighead N, et al: CD28 activation promotes Th2 subset differentiation by human CD4+ cells. Eur J Immunol 25:587–595, 1995.
55. Kiniwa M, Gately M, Gubler U, et al: Recombinant interleukin-12 suppresses the synthesis of immunoglobulin E by interleukin-4 stimulated human lymphocytes. J Clin Invest 90:262–266, 1992.
56. Kishimoto T, Taga T, Akira S: Cytokine signal transduction. Cell 76:253–262, 1994.
57. Klaus S J, Pinchuk L M, Ochs H D, et al: Costimulation through CD28 enhances T cell-dependent B cell activation via CD40-CD40L interaction. J Immunol 152:5643–5652, 1994.
58. Köhler I, Rieber E P: Allergy-associated Iϵ and Fcϵ receptor II (CD23b) genes activated via binding of an interleukin-4-induced transcription factor to a novel responsive element. Eur J Immunol 23:3066–3071, 1993.
59. Kopf M, Le Gros G, Bachmann M, et al: Disruption of the murine IL-4 gene blocks Th2 cytokine responses. Nature 362:245–248, 1993.
60. Kotanides H, Reich N C: Requirement of tyrosine phosphorylation for rapid activation of a DNA binding factor by IL-4. Science 262:1265–1267, 1993.
61. Kühn R, Rajewsky K R, Müller W: Generation and analysis of interleukin-4 deficient mice. Science 254:707–710, 1991.
62. Ledbetter J A, Clark E A, Norris N A, et al: Expression of a Functional B-Cell Receptor CDw40 (Bp50) on Carcinomas. Oxford University Press, Oxford, 1987, p 432.
63. Liao F, Birshtein B K, Busslinger M, et al: The transcription factor BSAP (NF-HB) is essential for immunoglobulin germ-line ϵ transcription. J Immunol 152:2904–2911, 1994.
64. Life P, Aubry J-P, Estoppey S, et al: CD28 functions as an adhesion molecule and is involved in the regulation of human IgE synthesis. Eur J Immunol 25:333–339, 1995.
65. Liu Y-J, Joshua D E, Williams G T, et al: Mechanism of antigen-driven selection in germinal centres. Nature 342:929–931, 1989.
66. Lorenz M, Jung S, Radbruch A: Switch transcripts in immunoglobulin class switching. Science 267:1825–1828, 1995.
67. Lundgren M, Persson U, Larsson P, et al: Interleukin 4 induces synthesis of IgE and IgG4 in human B cells. Eur J Immunol 19:1311–1315, 1989.
68. MacKenzie T, Dosch H M: Clonal and molecular characteristics of the human IgE-committed B cell subset. J Exp Med 169:407–430, 1989.
69. Maggi E, Giudizi M G, Biagiotti R, et al: Th2-like CD8+ T cells showing B cell helper function and reduced cytolytic activity in human immunodeficiency virus type 1 infection. J Exp Med 180:489–495, 1994.
70. Maggi E, Parronchi P, Manetti R, et al: Reciprocal regulatory effects of IFN-γ and IL-4 on the in vitro development of human Th1 and Th2 clones. J Immunol 148:2142–2147, 1992.
71. Malabarba M G, Kirken R A, Rui H, et al: Activation of JAK3, but not JAK1, is critical to interleukin-4 stimulated proliferation and requires a membrane proximal region of IL-4 receptor α. J Biol Chem 270:9630–9637, 1995.
72. Manetti R, Annunziato F, Biagiotti R, et al: CD30 expression by CD8+ T cells producing type 2 helper cytokines. Evidence for large numbers of CD8+CD30+ T cell clones in human immunodeficiency virus infection. J Exp Med 180:2407–2411, 1994.
73. Manetti R, Parronchi P, Giudizi M G, et al: Natural killer cell stimulatory factor (interleukin 12) induces T helper type 1-specific immune responses and inhibits the development of IL-4-producing Th cells. J Exp Med 177:1199–1204, 1993.
74. Marsh DG, Neely JD, Breazeale DR, et al: Linkage analysis of IL4 and other chromosome 5q31.1 markers and total serum immunoglobulin E concentrations. Science 264:1152–1156, 1994.
75. Masuyama K, Jacobson MR, Rak S, et al: Topical glucocorticosteroid (fluticasone propionate) inhibits cells expressing cytokine mRNA for interleukin-4 in the nasal mucosa in allergen-induced rhinitis. Immunology 82:192–199, 1994.
76. Max EE: Immunoglobulins: Molecular Genetics. Raven Press, New York, 1989, pp 235–290.
77. McKenzie ANJ, Culpepper JA, de Waal Malefyt R, et al: Interleukin 13, a T-cell-derived cytokine that regulates human monocyte and B-cell function. Proc Natl Acad Sci USA 90:3735–3739, 1993.
78. Mosialos G, Birkenbach M, Yalamanchili R, et al: The Epstein-Barr virus transforming protein LMP1 engages signaling proteins for the tumor necrosis factor receptor family. Cell 80:389–399, 1995.
79. Muraguchi A, Hirano T, Tang B, et al: The essential role of B cell

stimulatory factor 2 (BSF-2/IL-6) for the terminal differentiation of B cells. J Exp Med 167:332–344, 1988.

80. Paganelli R, Scala E, Ansotegui I J, et al: CD8+ T lymphocytes provide helper activity for IgE synthesis in human immunodeficiency virus-infected patients with hyper-IgE. J Exp Med 181:423–428, 1995.
81. Parronchi P, Macchia D, Piccinni M-P, et al: Allergen- and bacterial antigen-specific T-cell clones established from atopic donors show a different profile of cytokine production. Proc Natl Acad Sci USA 88:4538–4542, 1991.
82. Paulie S, Ehlin-Henriksson B, Mellstedt H, et al: A p50 surface antigen restricted to human urinary bladder carcinomas and B-lymphocytes. Cancer Immunol Immunother 20:23–30, 1985.
83. Peleman R, Wu J, Fargeas C, et al: Recombinant interleukin 4 suppresses the production of interferon γ by human mononuclear cells. J Exp Med 170:1751–1756, 1989.
84. Poudrier J, Owens T: CD54/intercellular adhesion molecule 1 and major histocompatibility complex II signaling induces B cells to express interleukin 2 receptors and complements help provided through CD40 ligation. J Exp Med 179:1417–1427, 1994.
85. Punnonen J, de Waal Malefyt R, van Vlasselaer P, et al: IL-10 and viral IL-10 prevent IL-4-induced IgE synthesis by inhibiting the accessory cell function of monocytes. J Immunol 151:1280–1289, 1993.
86. Ranheim E A, Kipps T J: Activated T cells induce expression of B7/BB1 on normal or leukemic B cells through a CD40-dependent signal. J Exp Med 177:925–935, 1993.
87. Raynal M-C, Liu Z, Hirano T, et al: Interleukin 6 induces secretion of IgG1 by coordinated transcriptional activation and differential mRNA accumulation. Proc Natl Acad Sci USA 86:8024–8028, 1989.
88. Romagnani S: Induction of TH1 and TH2 responses: a key role for the "natural" immune response? Immunol Today 13:379–381, 1992.
89. Romagnani S: Lymphokine production by human T cells in disease states. Annu Rev Immunol 12:227–257, 1994.
90. Rothe M, Wong S C, Henzel W J, et al: A novel family of putative signal transducers associated with the cytoplasmic domain of the 75 KDa tumor necrosis factor receptor. Cell 78:681–692, 1994.
91. Sarfati M, Luo H, Delespesse G: IgE synthesis by chronic lymphocytic leukemia cells. J Exp Med 170:1775–1780, 1989.
92. Schindler C, Kashleva H, Pernis A, et al: STF-IL-4: a novel signal transducing factor. EMBO J 13:1350–1356, 1994.
93. Schmitz J, Thiel A, Kühn R, et al: Induction of interleukin-4 (IL-4) expression in T helper (Th) cells is not dependent on IL-4 from non Th-cells. J Exp Med 179:1349–1353, 1994.
94. Schroeder JT, MacGlashan DW, Kagey-Sobotka A, et al: IgE-dependent IL-4-secretion by human basophils—the relationship between cytokine production and histamine release in mixed leukocyte cultures. J Immunol 153:1808–1817, 1994.
95. Sha WC, Liou H-C, Tuomanen EI, et al: Targeted disruption of the p50 subunit of NF-κB leads to multifocal defects in immune responses. Cell 80:321–330, 1995.
96. Shahinian A, Pfeffer K, Lee KP, et al: Differential T cell costimulatory requirements in CD28-deficient mice. Science 261:609–612, 1993.
97. Shapira SK, Jabara HH, Thienes CP, et al: Deletional switch recombination occurs in IL-4 induced isotype switching to IgE expression by human B cells. Proc Natl Acad Sci USA 88:7528–7532, 1991.
98. Shapira SK, Vercelli D, Jabara HH, et al: Molecular analysis of the induction of IgE synthesis in human B cells by IL-4 and engagement of CD40 antigen. J Exp Med 175:289–292, 1992.
99. Spriggs MK, Armitage RJ, Strockbine L, et al: Recombinant human CD40 ligand stimulates B cell proliferation and immunoglobulin E secretion. J Exp Med 176:1543–1550, 1992.
100. Thyphronitis G, Tsokos GC, June CH, et al: IgE secretion by Epstein-Barr virus-infected purified human B lymphocytes is stimulated by interleukin 4 and suppressed by interferon γ. Proc Natl Acad Sci USA 86:5580–5584, 1989.
101. Tsubata T, Wu J, Honjo T: B-cell apoptosis induced by antigen receptor crosslinking is blocked by a T-cell signal through CD40. Nature 364:645–648, 1993.
102. Vallé A, Aubry J-P, Durand I, et al: IL-4 and IL-2 upregulate the expression of antigen B7, the B cell counterstructure to T cell CD28: an amplification mechanism for T-B cell interactions. Int Immunol 3:229–235, 1991.
103. van der Stoep N, Korver W, Logtenberg T: In vivo and in vitro IgE isotype switching in human B lymphocytes: evidence for a predominantly direct IgM to IgE class switch program. Eur J Immunol 24:1307–1311, 1994.
104. van Kooten C, Gaillard C, Galizzi J-P, et al: B cells regulate expression of CD40 ligand on activated T cells by lowering the mRNA level and through the release of soluble CD40. Eur J Immunol 24:787–792, 1994.
105. Vercelli D, Geha RS: Regulation of IgE synthesis in humans: a tale of two signals. J Allergy Clin Immunol 88:285–295, 1991.
106. Vercelli D, Geha RS: Regulation of IgE synthesis in man. J Clin Immunol 9:75–83, 1989.
107. Vercelli D, Geha RS: Regulation of isotype switching. Curr Opin Immunol 4:794–797, 1992.
108. Vercelli D, Jabara HH, Arai K, et al: Endogenous IL-6 plays an obligatory role in IL-4 induced human IgE synthesis. Eur J Immunol 19:1419–1424, 1989.
109. Vercelli D, Jabara HH, Lauener RP, et al: Interleukin-4 inhibits the synthesis of interferon-γ and induces the synthesis of IgE in mixed lymphocyte cultures. J Immunol 144:570–573, 1990.
110. Wang CY, Fu SM, Kunkel HG: Isolation and immunological characterization of a major surface glycoprotein (gp54) preferentially expressed on certain human B cells. J Exp Med 149:1424–1437, 1979.
111. Wen L, Roberts SJ, Viney JL, et al: Immunoglobulin synthesis and generalized autoimmunity in mice congenitally deficient in αB(+) cells. Nature 369:654–658, 1994.
112. Wu CY, Sarfati M, Heusser C, et al: Glucocorticoids increase the synthesis of immunoglobulin E by interleukin-4-stimulated human lymphocytes. J Clin Invest 87:870–877, 1991.
113. Xu J, Foy TM, Laman JD, et al: Mice deficient for the CD40 ligand. Immunity 1:423–431, 1994.
114. Yellin MJ, Sippel K, Inghirami G, et al: CD40 molecules induce down-modulation and endocytosis of T cell surface T cell-B cell activating molecule/CD40 ligand. Potential role in regulating helper effector function. J Immunol 152:598–608, 1994.
115. Zhang J, Bottaro A, Li S, et al: Targeted mutation in the Ig2b exon results in a selective Iγ2b deficiency in mice. EMBO J 12:3529–3537, 1993.
116. Zhang K, Mills FC, Saxon A: Switch circles from IL-4-directed ε class switching from human B lymphocytes—evidence for direct, sequential and multiple step sequential switch from μ to ε Ig heavy chain gene. J Immunol 152:3427–3435, 1994.
117. Zurawski SM, Vega F, Huyghe B, et al: Receptors for interleukin-13 and interleukin-4 are complex and share a novel component that functions in signal transduction. EMBO J 12:2663–2670, 1993.

8 Receptor for IgE and Initiation of Allergic Reactions

HENRY METZGER

A variety of cells synthesize membrane glycoproteins that can bind the Fc portion of immunoglobulins with more or less specificity and with variable affinity. Such Fc receptors mediate a variety of cellular functions.[31, 56, 66]

This chapter principally describes the Fc receptor found on mast cells and basophils, which has a high affinity for monomeric IgE. According to the accepted nomenclature for Fc receptors, it is dubbed FcεRI. This receptor appears to be the most important one for initiating IgE-mediated allergic reactions.[18, 76] In the concluding section, the properties of another Fc receptor for IgE are compared.

Extensive studies have been performed on the high-affinity receptor found on a neoplastic line of rat mucosal mast cells, called RBL because it was initially thought to represent a line of basophilic leukemia cells. I do not distinguish between the receptors from such cells and those on normal mast cells and basophils except where there is evidence for a difference. For convenience, I refer to this receptor as the IgE receptor.

HIGH-AFFINITY RECEPTOR

BINDING PROPERTIES

It is important to understand the binding properties of IgE for the receptor both because they can explain certain clinical features and because the binding reaction is a potential target for new therapeutic measures. Most binding studies have been performed using IgE labeled with radioisotopes and analyzing its interaction with the receptor on intact (rodent) cells. However, solubilized receptors or genetic constructs of the IgE-binding portion of the receptor are also available for study. So far, no significant differences have been observed from such alternative analyses. Similarly, the results comparing rodent and human receptors are quantitatively similar.

Mechanism of Binding and Binding Affinity

The binding of monomeric IgE to the receptor obeys the kinetics expected for a simple, reversible bimolecular reaction[46]:

$$\text{IgE} + \text{R} \rightleftharpoons \text{IgE:R}$$

where IgE, R, and IgE:R refer to the molar concentrations of IgE, receptors, and IgE-receptor complexes, respectively. The second-order (bimolecular) forward rate constant, k_{+1}, is not unusual compared with other protein-cell interactions, being about $10^5\ M^{-1}\ sec^{-1}$. However, the first-order (unimolecular) reverse rate constant, k_{-1}, is unusually small, $10^{-5}\ sec^{-1}$. The affinity (K_A) of the receptor for the IgE is defined by the ratio k_{+1}/k_{-1} and is therefore $10^{10}\ M^{-1}$.

For such reactions, the time required for one half of the complexes to dissociate, $t_{1/2}$, is given by the relation

$$t_{1/2} = 0.69/k_{-1}$$

so that for $k_{-1} = 10^{-5}\ sec^{-1}$, $t_{1/2}$ calculates out to be approximately 20 hours. Even this rate of dissociation is likely to be an underestimate. Other studies on cells or with solubilized receptors suggest that dissociation can be more prolonged, with half-times of the order of 100 to 200 hours (4–8 days). This slow dissociation and the fact that molecules that have dissociated from a cell are unaltered and can rebind to neighboring cells account adequately for the prolonged reactivity of cells observed experimentally and clinically. It also makes it unlikely that inhibitors of the binding reaction will be therapeutically useful for interfering with an ongoing reaction since they can only block rebinding of the slowly dissociating IgE. Thus the binding properties suggest that inhibitors of binding will have their chief application in preventing rather than reversing sensitization.

Except for IgE-derived fragments and other immunoglobulins, there are no known inhibitors of the binding reaction, nor have any requirements for cofactors been identified. Experimentally, the IgE can be stripped off the cells using mildly acidic buffers. This confirms that the IgE is noncovalently bound to the receptors and is a useful procedure for a variety of investigations.

Binding Sites on IgE

There is continuing research to define the sites on IgE that interact with the receptor because that information may assist the development of inhibitors that could block sensitization of mast cells and basophils. There is increasing evidence that the so-called Cϵ3 domain (the penultimate constant region domain of the ϵ heavy chain of IgE) contains the critical sites of interaction (reviewed in 31), but more distal parts of the molecule also appear to be required to maintain the sites in Cϵ3 in an active configuration. Despite the bilateral symmetry of the IgE (that each IgE contains two such Cϵ3 domains), the experimental evidence indicates that only a single receptor binds to an IgE at a time.[37, 40]

For human IgE, the smallest fragment that shows reproducible activity is composed of the entire Fc region; reports of activity by smaller peptides[13, 28, 29] either have been refuted[10] or have not yet been replicated by others.[6] Even if no IgE-derived small peptide retaining potent inhibitory activity can be isolated, this does not preclude the possibility that nonpeptidic small compounds can be effective in this respect.

Binding Sites on the High-Affinity Receptor

This subject will be discussed in the context of the description of the IgE-binding alpha subunit of the receptor.

Specificity

In general, monomeric IgE from one species binds with high affinity only to IgE receptors of the same (or closely related) species. An exception is that rodent IgE binds well to the human receptor.[16] Because monoclonal mouse IgE antibodies against a specific antigen can be readily induced, this cross-reactivity is useful for investigating activation of human cells. Likewise, it is now possible to "transfect" the human IgE-binding subunit into rodent cells,[58] so that the absence of useful human lines no longer obviates easy study of the binding of human IgE.

The question of whether other immunoglobulin isotypes, such as IgG, can inhibit the binding of IgE to the high-affinity receptor is not completely resolved. Nevertheless, it can be safely concluded that only high concentrations of aggregated IgG can interfere substantially with the binding of IgE. There are additional receptors on mast cells as well as on other cells that have a much lower affinity for monomeric IgE and to which the binding of IgE and IgG is much more competitive. Nevertheless, mice genetically engineered to lack the ability to produce IgE (IgE knockout mice) can exhibit anaphylactic reactions presumably mediated by the high-affinity IgE receptors.[60] This suggests that alternate immunoglobulins can bind to FcϵRI with sufficient avidity to produce pathophysiologic effects.

DISTRIBUTION, NUMBER, LOCATION, MOBILITY, AND VALENCE

FcϵRI are found on a wider variety of cells than originally thought. In addition to mast cells and basophils, they have been observed on monocytic cells,[53] Langerhans cells in the skin,[11, 77] eosinophils,[24] and so-called non-B/non-T cells.[9] Binding studies can be used to determine the number of receptors per cell. These investigations have given estimates of 10^3 to 10^6 receptors per cell using different cell preparations. Indirect studies have suggested that human basophils from individuals with high levels of IgE in their serum have an increased number of receptors.[51] These findings need confirmation by direct studies; no evidence for such regulation of the number of receptors on RBL cells grown in the absence or presence of IgE has been found.

Electron microscopic and other studies indicate that the receptors are distributed diffusely over the surface of the cell[61] and that there is no substantial pool of receptors in the cytoplasm.[68] The receptors are mobile in the plane of the membrane,[54, 69] and most studies suggest that the receptors move independently.[55] Those data also indicated that the receptors are univalent[55]—one receptor binds one IgE. The latter finding has been corroborated by studies on solubilized receptors.[40, 59]

STRUCTURE OF THE RECEPTOR

The structure of FcϵRI and the genes that code for its subunits have been extensively studied in three species, rat, mouse, and human. Because rat FcϵRI have been investigated most completely, they will be the principal focus of this discussion.

Genes and Proteins

ALPHA CHAINS

The alpha chain, FcϵRIα, historically was the first to be characterized. There is one per receptor, and it contains the binding site for IgE. Its principal characteristics are listed in Table 8–1. The sequence of amino acid residues deduced from its genetic sequence suggests three distinctive regions or domains. By a variety of criteria, these regions can be reliably assigned to a particular topological arrangement with respect to the lipid bilayer of the plasma membrane,[44, 71] and I refer to the domains accordingly.

Ectodomain. The ectodomain refers to that portion of a plasma membrane protein that is exposed to the exterior of the cell. The single ectodomain of the alpha chain is at its amino-terminal end and contains approximately 180 amino acids. It consists of two similar regions, ED1 and ED2, each

TABLE 8–1
PROPERTIES OF THE SUBUNITS OF FcϵRI*

Characteristic	Subunit α	β	γ
Number per receptor	1	1	2
Peptide mol. wt. (kD)	25–26	26–27	8
Carbohydrate	+	—	—
Ig-like domains	2	0	0
Binding site for IgE	1	0	0
ITAMs per subunit	0	1	1
Chromosomal site of gene	1q(h), 1(m)	11q(h), 19(m)	1q(h), 1(m)

*Data are for human (h), rat, and mouse (m) FcϵRI.
Abbreviations: kD-kilodalton; Ig-like-immunoglobulin-like; ITAM-immune tyrosine activation motif.

bearing a considerable homology to members of the so-called immunoglobulin superfamily. By genetic engineering, the ectodomain can be synthesized separately from the remainder of FcεRI[12] or as chimeric proteins in which the ectodomain is fused to an irrelevant, easily expressed protein.[27, 32] Binding studies of such isolated ectodomains have revealed that their binding properties are qualitatively and quantitatively essentially indistinguishable from those of the whole FcεRI. These studies also showed that the carbohydrate residues, which make up roughly 30% of the molecular weight of the intact alpha chains, do not contribute to the binding characteristics.

Because of the intense interest in developing inhibitors of IgE binding, there has been extensive exploration of which regions of the ectodomains are most critical. Multiple regions in both ED1 and ED2 have been implicated.[31] Only the kind of detailed study of the IgE: alpha chain interaction made possible by x-ray diffraction (or conceivably nuclear magnetic resonance) is likely to yield the information required to synthesize optimum inhibitors. No such data on either of the components or on the complex have been reported. However, such data are available for the ectodomains of several lymphocyte glycoproteins that have domains structurally related to ED1 and ED2. Using the known conformation of these and the sequence of the corresponding portions of FcεRIα, plausible models of the latter have been proposed.[7, 30]

Transmembrane Domain. The transmembrane domain is that portion of certain membrane proteins that traverses the lipid bilayer. A single such domain, as is present in alpha chains, generally consists of a relatively hydrophobic peptide, 20 to 22 amino acids in length and in an alpha helical conformation. This region of the alpha chain contains a particular sequence motif of seven amino acids that has been implicated in the interaction of the alpha chain with the gamma subunits. A corresponding region has been found in other Fc receptors that contain gamma chains. Within this motif is a critical aspartic acid residue.

Cytoplasmic Domain. The short cytoplasmic domain of the alpha chain shows the greatest variability among different species. It is characterized by a concentration of positive charges the significance of which is unknown. Truncation of this cytoplasmic tail by genetic engineering has failed so far to reveal any functional or structural role for this region.[3]

BETA CHAINS

The beta chain, of which there is one per FcεRI, was the second subunit to be discovered. Its sequence resembles that of several other membrane proteins that share its topological arrangement.[1] It contains three cytoplasmic domains and two ectodomains separated from each other by four trans-

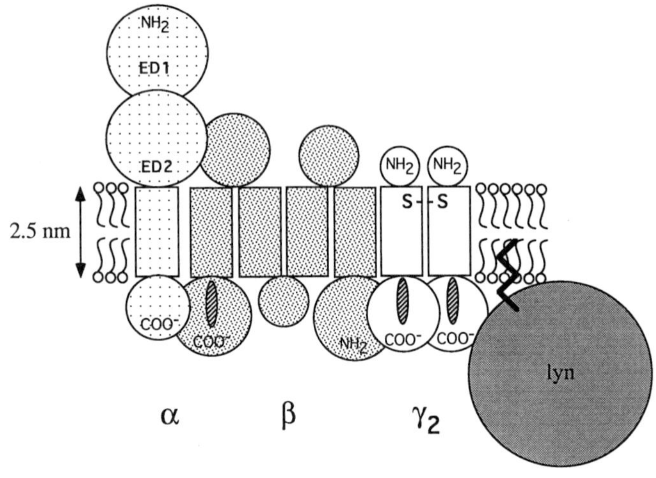

FIGURE 8–1. Schematic model of the high-affinity receptor for IgE. The receptor is shown embedded in the plasma membrane in association with the src-like kinase, lyn (speckled circle). The orientation is such that the outside of the cell is toward the top. The circles and rectangles represent spheres and cylinders whose volumes are proportional to the relative masses of the various domains of the individual polypeptide chains (see text). The domains containing the amino-terminal (NH_2) and carboxy-terminal (COO^-) ends of the polypeptide chains are indicated. The relative position of the disulfide bond that links the two gamma chains together is also indicated. The shaded ovals represent the ITAM motifs. The jagged line attached to the kinase represents one or more lipid tails by which the amino-terminal end of the enzyme is tethered to the inner lipid layer of the membrane.

membrane domains (Fig. 8–1).[43] The amino-terminal domain is the largest and is rich in proline and serine residues. Truncation of this domain produced no apparent functional alterations.[3]

The carboxy-terminal cytoplasmic domain contains a so-called immune receptor tyrosine activation motif (ITAM), a sequence of 26 amino acids discovered by Michael Reth.[67] The consensus (ITAM) sequence can be represented as shown at the bottom of the page.

The letters D, E, Y, L, and I refer to aspartic, glutamic, tyrosine, leucine, and isoleucine residues, respectively, and X is a variable residue. In the β subunit, the central portion of this motif (residues 9–16) is particularly well conserved across species. The tyrosine residues in these motifs are subject to phosphorylation by protein tyrosine kinases generating the sites to which proteins bearing src homology region 2 (SH2) domains[45] can bind. There is good evidence that these are the boards on which FcεRI and related receptors play their signaling games. The precise role of this motif in the beta chain is being investigated.[20, 36, 73] Receptors engineered to contain a beta chain missing virtually the entire carboxyl-terminal cytoplasmic domain show a variety of functional deficiencies.[3, 52] It is likely that the beta chain plays a supportive rather than mandatory role in at least certain aspects of signal transduction since related receptors

1	2	3	4	5	6	7	8	9	10	11	12	13	14	15	16	17	18	19	20	21	22	23	24	25	26
D	X	X	X	X	X	X	X	D	X	X	Y	X	X	X	L	X	X	X	X	X	X	Y	D	X	L
E								E															E		I

that contain no beta chain are active. Likewise, FcεRI containing a human FcεRIα chain, and which can be expressed in the absence of beta, are partially active.

One group of investigators has correlated susceptibility to atopy with a variant sequence at the amino-terminal end of the fourth transmembrane domain of human beta.[72] In the variant, the isoleucine at position 181 is substituted with a leucine. The latter is the residue found in the rat sequence. There is as yet no direct evidence that such a change affects either the function of the receptor or the allergic status of the individual harboring such a change.

GAMMA CHAINS

A single FcεRI contains two disulfide-linked gamma chains.[64] Each gamma chain resembles the alpha chain topologically, but the ectodomain is very small and variable between species, whereas the cytoplasmic domain is highly conserved and extensive. The cytoplasmic domain contains one ITAM, and experiments utilizing truncation[3] or chimeric constructs[20, 36, 41, 73] indicate that the cytoplasmic domains of FcεRIγ are essential for activity of the receptor. The gamma chains are highly homologous to the zeta and eta chains of the multisubunit, antigen-specific receptor of thymus-derived lymphocytes.[62] The latter chains each contain three ITAMs in their cytoplasmic domains and appear to play an analogous role in the activity of the receptors of which they are subunits.[42]

RECEPTOR-MEDIATED ACTIVATION OF CELLS

When monomeric IgE binds to the receptor on mast cells or basophils, no perturbation of the cells occurs. However, if an antigen that can react with the cell-bound IgE is added, a cascade of biochemical changes can be detected immediately, which lead to a variety of cellular changes that are described elsewhere in this text. Here, the role of the receptor in the initiation of this cascade is described exclusively.

Role of IgE

Like other immunoglobulins, IgE has separate regions that are specialized to react with antigens (Fab) and with a variety of biologic effector systems (Fc). Although virtually no studies have been performed on IgE itself, by analogy with other immunoglobulins, it is unlikely that reaction of an antigen with the Fab region initiates any allosteric signal that is transmitted to the Fc region and hence to the receptor to which the IgE is bound.[56] Instead, the antigen-induced activation of the cell appears to be initiated solely by the aggregation of the cell-bound IgE that occurs as a consequence of the latter's interaction with a multivalent antigen. Indeed, any maneuver that leads to aggregation of the Fc regions of the IgE is effective in initiating degranulation.

Aggregation of the Fc regions pari passu leads to aggregation of the receptors to which they are bound. It is this aggregation of the receptors that constitutes the critical event. Thus antibodies to the receptor, even in the total absence of IgE, can stimulate release because they can cluster the receptor.[34, 35] From experiments employing defined, preformed oligomers of IgE, it is known that the association of receptors into dimers is sufficient to initiate both inactivating and activating signals.[70] There is also evidence that the system can distinguish between clusters of varying multiplicity—larger clusters generating more numerous (or effective) positive and negative stimuli.[22] With such larger clusters, only a small fraction (likely less than 0.01) of the total receptors are required to yield substantial release.[22]

As with other immunoglobulins, the Fc regions of IgE are attached to Fab regions that can express the full repertoire of diversity that the immune system is capable of generating. It is apparent, therefore, that a single cell can bind to its surface IgE molecules with diverse antigen-combining sites. The mobility of the receptors to which the IgE is bound ensures that multiple receptors can be clustered when the IgE on some of them reacts with a given antigen.

Consequences of Receptor Aggregation

Considerable progress has been made in clarifying how FcεRI and other multichain immune response receptors[38] as well as numerous other receptors[57] convert a topological perturbation (aggregation) into chemical signals that initiate biochemical cascades. A common feature of all of these is that phosphorylation of tyrosines is the first detectable event. Receptors such as those for various growth factors have a tyrosine kinase encoded in their cytoplasmic domains. There is mounting evidence that upon ligand-induced aggregation, these domains phosphorylate each other by a process of transphosphorylation.[48] Although FcεRI has no intrinsic tyrosine kinase (nor any other enzyme) encoded in any of its cytoplasmic domains, there is now evidence that it utilizes a similar mechanism. It appears that the FcεRI is constitutively associated with an src-like tyrosine kinase.[19, 33] In RBL cells, which have been studied most intensively, this appears to be lyn kinase.[19, 78] At any point in time, only a small fraction of the receptors appear to be constitutively associated with the kinase.[78] The lack of a one:one stoichiometry is not because there is a shortage of total cellular lyn kinase; at least in the RBL cells where this has been studied, there are many more molecules of lyn than of receptor. This kinase phosphorylates tyrosines exclusively on an exogenously added peptide but exhibits little activity toward the unaggregated receptor itself or toward any other proteins associated with the receptor.

Tyrosines of both the beta and gamma chains of the receptors become rapidly phosphorylated when FcεRI are aggregated on the cell.[49, 63] When isolated, such aggregated receptors exhibit increases in lyn kinase and kinase activity not only toward an exogenous substrate but also toward the receptor and several associated proteins.[19, 49, 65] When disaggregated in vitro, such receptors retain a substantial fraction of their increased lyn kinase and their enhanced ability to phosphorylate an exogenous peptide substrate but lose almost completely their ability to promote phosphorylation of the subunits of the receptor and of the associated proteins. From these results, it appears that the physical approximation of the receptors in the aggregates is essential for the phosphorylation of the receptors and their associated proteins and initiates the subsequent events.

These and other results are incorporated in the model

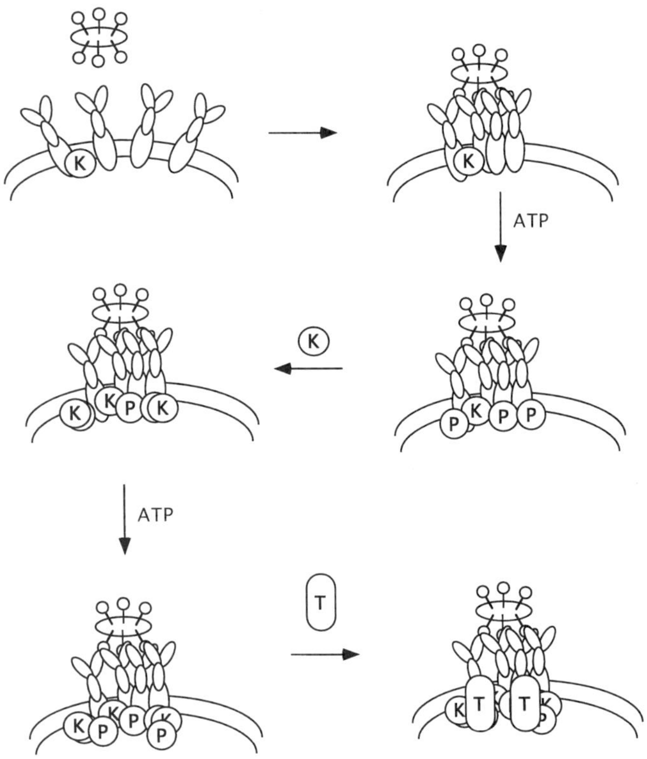

FIGURE 8–2. Initiation of signal transduction by aggregation of FcϵRI. The flow diagram shows the receptor-bound IgE interacting with a multivalent antigen, which leads to an association of multiple receptors. The constitutively associated kinase (K) phosphorylates the receptor, (P) leading to recruitment of additional kinase, further phosphorylation, and association with newly recruited targets (T).

shown in Figure 8–2. It proposes that the constitutively associated kinase initiates the phosphorylation of the receptor when aggregation promotes the formation of enzyme: substrate complexes. This leads to recruitment of further molecules of kinase, additional phosphorylation, and recruitment of further molecular targets, such as syk kinase (see Chapter 9).[33]

As already noted, several laboratories are using genetic manipulation of the receptor and other methods to try to determine the role of the individual cytoplasmic domains, the critical sequence motifs, and the downstream targets. There is not yet a complete consensus, but the conflicting findings are likely to be resolved soon. In addition, parallel studies are being pursued on the structurally related antigen receptors of B and T lymphocytes. Although the details show considerable variation, overall, a very similar picture is emerging from those studies.[25]

The initial events stimulated by the receptor are attractive targets for therapeutic agents. To the extent that such agents would interfere with the early events in which the receptor itself is involved, their sites of action may be fairly circumscribed and side effects would be minimized. Importantly, such agents could in principle be effective even after sensitization of the mast cells and basophils with IgE antibody.

Some additional experiments give insight into an important aspect of the control of the IgE receptor system. So far, I have focused on the initiation of signal transduction but have said nothing about its persistence. Studies with chemically cross-linked size-fractionated oligomers of IgE (e.g., dimers or trimers) have allowed one to examine the functional lifetime and other characteristics of the aggregates of FcϵRI they induce upon binding to the cell. The results show unambiguously that small receptor aggregates continue to initiate signals for prolonged periods.[39] Notably, the aggregates appear to be dynamically phosphorylated and dephosphorylated. It is apparent then that in this system, the extent and persistence of aggregation determine the signal strength. In turn, it can be shown that in principle, the persistence of aggregates is directly related to the affinity of the ligand whose binding to the IgE-receptor complex initiates the aggregation of the latter.

The system is likely to be more complex than suggested by the relatively simple model illustrated in Figure 8–2. For example, it is known that if it is too extensive, aggregation can actually reduce or even abrogate cellular activation.[8, 21, 50, 74] This finding may be related to a topological redistribution of aggregates and their interaction with cytoskeletal structures.

LOW-AFFINITY RECEPTOR FOR IgE

A glycoprotein that binds IgE with much lower affinity than FcϵRI and is expressed by a variety of cells has been studied extensively in mice and humans. Named FcϵRII, it is also known as CD23 (where CD refers to cluster of differentiation, a systematic nomenclature based on the common reactivity of groups of monoclonal antibodies with particular cell surface proteins on lymphocytes).[14, 15, 17] In humans, this protein has been observed on granulocytes (eosinophils, but not mast cells), monocytic-type cells (monocytes, follicular dendritic cells, Langerhans cells), platelets, and lymphocytes (T and B).

BINDING PROPERTIES

FcϵRII binds IgE 1,000-fold less firmly than does FcϵRI due largely to the much higher dissociation rate constant, $k_{-1} \approx 10^{-3}$. The binding site is located on its extensive ectodomain, and soluble fragments, some as small as 16 kD, show equivalent binding activity. There is evidence that FcϵRII can form oligomers with a 50- to 100-fold enhanced avidity, presumably because of multivalent interactions.[5, 14] Some studies have revealed that the receptor also binds N-linked oliosaccharides on CD21.[4] This large cell surface protein consists of 16 so-called complement control protein domains, and the gene is a member of a cluster of genes whose products form a family of complement factor 3/complement factor 4–binding proteins. CD21 is implicated in the regulation of B-cell function.[2]

STRUCTURE AND GENE

The structure of FcϵRII is entirely different from that of FcϵRI (reviewed in 14, 17). It consists of a single transmembrane polypeptide chain whose carboxy-terminus rather than amino-terminus forms the ectodomain. The latter contains carbohydrate and is 277 amino acid residues in length. The sequence is homologous to a family of carbohydrate-binding proteins that includes the adherence molecules selectins and the asialoglycoprotein-binding receptor prominently found on hepatic cells. The ectodomain is joined to a 20-residue-long transmembrane domain followed by a 23-reside-long cytoplasmic domain. A stalk region between the lectin homology domain and the transmembrane segment contains a heptad motif characteristic of an α-helical coiled coil.

Through the utilization of two different promoters that govern two distinctive first exons, the single gene (on chromosome 19) that codes for human FcεRII can generate two distinctive transcripts. These distinctive transcripts lead to discrete isoforms, FcεRIIa and FcεRIIb, that differ in their cytoplasmic domains and are expressed in a tissue-specific manner.

BIOLOGIC ROLE

Early on in the exploration of FcεRII, its presence on lymphocytes suggested it might play a role in regulating the IgE responses. There is now extensive literature on this subject both with respect to the membrane-bound and the soluble, IgE-binding, forms of the receptor.[23, 26, 75, 79] In some cases, an implied role was suggested by the up-regulation of FcεRII associated with stimulated IgE responses. However, at least in part, this is simply due to the receptor-bound IgE protecting FcεRII from proteolytic cleavage.[47]

It is possible that antigen interaction with IgE bound to FcεRII can activate those cells possessing this receptor. This finding is addressed briefly in subsequent chapters, but the data are preliminary and FcεRI may also be present, which complicates the interpretation of any functional changes observed.

REFERENCES

1. Adra CN, Lelias JM, Kobayashi H, et al: Cloning of the cDNA for a hematopoietic cell-specific protein related to CD20 and the beta subunit of the high-affinity IgE receptor: evidence for a family of proteins with four membrane-spanning regions. Proc Natl Acad Sci USA 91:10178, 1994.
2. Ahearn JM, Fearon DT: Structure and function of the complement receptors, CR1 (CD35) and CR2 (CD21). Adv Immunol 46:183, 1989.
3. Alber G, Miller L, Jelsema C, et al: Structure/function relationships in the mast cell high-affinity receptor for IgE (FcεRI): role of cytoplasmic domains. J Biol Chem 266:22613, 1991.
4. Aubry J-P, Pochon S, Graber P, et al: CD21 is a ligand for CD23 and regulates IgE production. Nature 358:505, 1992.
5. Bartlett WC, Kelly AE, Johnson CM, et al: Analysis of murine soluble FcεRII sites of cleavage and requirements for dual-affinity interaction with IgE. J Immunol 154:4240, 1995.
6. Basu M, Hakimi J, Dharm E, et al: Purification and characterization of human recombinant IgE-Fc fragments that bind to the human high affinity IgE receptor. J Biol Chem 268:13118, 1993.
7. Beavil AJ, Beavil RL, Chan CMW, et al: Structural basis of the IgE-FcεRI interaction. Biochem Soc Trans 21:968, 1993.
8. Becker KE, Ishizaka T, Metzger H, et al: Surface IgE on human basophils during histamine release. J Exp Med 138:394, 1973.
9. Ben-Sasson SZ, Le Gros G, Conrad DH, et al: Cross-linking Fc receptors stimulate splenic non-B, non-T cells to secrete interleukin 4 and other lymphokines. Proc Natl Acad Sci USA 87:1421, 1990.
10. Bennich H, Ragnarsson U, Johansson SG, et al: Failure of the putative IgE pentapeptide to compete with IgE for receptors on basophils and masts cells. Intl Arch Allergy Appl Immunol 53:459, 1977.
11. Bieber T, De la Salle H, De la Salle C, et al: Expression of the high-affinity receptor for IgE (FcεRI) on human Langerhans cells: the end of a dogma. J Invest Dermatol 99:10S, 1992.
12. Blank U, Ra C, Kinet J-P: Characterization of truncated α chain products from human, rat, and mouse high affinity receptor for immunoglobulin E. J Biol Chem 266:2639, 1991.
13. Burt DS, Stanworth DR: Inhibition of binding of rat IgE to rat mast cells by synthetic IgE peptides. Eur J Immunol 17:437, 1987.
14. Conrad DH: FcεRII/CD23: the low affinity receptor for IgE. Annu Rev Immunol 8:623, 1990.
15. Conrad DH, Campbell KA, Bartlett WC, et al: Structure and function of the low affinity IgE receptor. Adv Exp Med Biol 347:17, 1994.
16. Conrad DH, Wingard JR, Ishizaka T: The interaction of human and rodent IgE with the human basophil IgE receptor. J Immunol 130:327, 1983.
17. Delespesse G, Suter U, Mossalayi D, et al: Expression, structure, and function of the CD23 antigen. Adv Immunol 49:149, 1991.
18. Dombrowicz D, Flamand V, Brigman KK, et al: Abolition of anaphylaxis by targeted disruption of the high affinity immunoglobulin E receptor α chain gene. Cell 75:969, 1994.
19. Eiseman E, Bolen JB: Engagement of the high-affinity IgE receptor activates *src* protein-related tyrosine kinases. Nature 355:78, 1992.
20. Eiseman E, Bolen JB: Signal transduction by the cytoplasmic domains of FcεRI-gamma and TCR-zeta in rat basophilic leukemia cells. J Biol Chem 267:21027, 1992.
21. Fewtrell C: Activation and desensitization of receptors for IgE on tumor basophils. In Rubin RP, Weiss GP, Putney JW Jr (eds): Calcium in Biological Systems. Plenum Publishing Corporation, New York, 1985, pp 129–135.
22. Fewtrell C, Metzger H: Larger oligomers of IgE are more effective than dimers in stimulating rat basophilic leukemia cells. J Immunol 125:701, 1980.
23. Fujiwara H, Kikutani H, Suematsu S, et al: The absence of IgE antibody-mediated augmentation of immune responses in CD23-deficient mice. Proc Natl Acad Sci USA 91:6835, 1994.
24. Gounni AS, Lamkhioued B, Ochiai K, et al: High-affinity IgE receptor on eosinophils is involved in defence against parasites. Nature 367:183, 1994.
25. Gupta S, Paul WE, DeFranco A, Perlmutter R (eds): Mechanisms of Lymphocyte Activation and Immune Regulation V. Plenum, New York, 1994, pp 1–264.
26. Gustavsson S, Hjulstrom S, Liu T, et al: CD23/IgE-mediated regulation of the specific antibody response in vivo. J Immunol 152:4793, 1994.
27. Hakimi J, Seals C, Kondas JA, et al: The α subunit of the human IgE receptor (FcεRI) is sufficient for high affinity IgE binding. J Biol Chem 265:22079, 1990.
28. Hamburger RN: Peptide inhibition of the Prausnitz-Kustner reaction. Science 189:389, 1975.
29. Helm B, Marsh P, Vercelli D, et al: The mast cell binding site on human immunoglobulin E. Nature 331:180, 1988.
30. Hogarth PM, Hulett MD, Ierino FL, et al: Identification of the immunoglobulin binding regions (IBR) of Fc gamma RII and Fc epsilon RI. Immunol Rev 125:21, 1992.
31. Hulett MD, Hogarth PM: Molecular basis of Fc receptor function. Adv Immunol 57:1, 1994.
32. Hulett MD, McKenzie IFC, Hogarth PM: Chimeric Fc receptors identify immunoglobulin-binding regions in human FcgammaRII and FcεRI. Eur J Immunol 23:640, 1993.
33. Hutchcroft JE, Geahlen RL, Deanin GG, et al: FcεRI-mediated tyrosine phosphorylation and activation of the 72-kDa protein-tyrosine kinase, PTK72, in RBL-2H3 rat tumor mast cells. Proc Natl Acad Sci USA 89:9107, 1992.
34. Isersky C, Taurog JD, Poy G, et al: Triggering of cultured neoplastic mast cells by antibodies to the receptor for IgE. J Immunol 121:549, 1978.
35. Ishizaka T, Chang TH, Taggart M, et al: Histamine release from rat mast cells by antibodies against rat basophilic leukemia cell membrane. J Immunol 119:1589, 1977.
36. Jouvin M-HE, Adamczewski M, Numerof R, et al: Differential control of the tyrosine kinases lyn and syk by the two signaling chains of the high affinity immunoglobulin E receptor. J Biol Chem 269:5918, 1994.
37. Kanellopoulos J, Rossi G, Metzger H: Preparative isolation of the cell receptor for immunoglobulin E. J Biol Chem 254:7691, 1979.
38. Keegan AD, Paul WE: Multichain immune recognition receptors: similarities in structure and signaling pathways. Immunol Today 13:63, 1992.
39. Kent UM, Mao S-Y, Wofsy C, et al: Dynamics of signal transduction after aggregation of cell-surface receptors: studies on the type I receptor for IgE. Proc Natl Acad Sci USA 91:3087, 1994.

40. Keown MB, Ghirlando R, Young RJ, et al: Hydrodynamic studies of a complex between the Fc fragment of human IgE and a soluble fragment of the FcεRI α chain. Proc Natl Acad Sci USA 92:1841, 1995.
41. Kihara H, Siraganian RP: Src homology 2 domains of Syk and Lyn bind to tyrosine-phosphorylated subunits of the high affinity IgE receptor. J Biol Chem 269:22427, 1994.
42. Kinet J-P: The gamma-zeta dimers of Fc receptors as connectors to signal transduction. Curr Opin Immunol 4:43, 1992.
43. Kinet J-P, Blank U, Ra C, et al: Isolation and characterization of cDNAs coding for the beta subunit of the high-affinity receptor for immunoglobulin E. Proc Natl Acad Sci USA 85:6483, 1988.
44. Kinet J-P, Metzger H, Hakimi J, et al: A cDNA presumptively coding for the alpha subunit of the receptor with high affinity for immunoglobulin E. Biochemistry 26:4605, 1987.
45. Koch CA, Anderson D, Moran MF, et al: SH2 and SH3 domains: elements that control interactions of cytoplasmic signaling proteins. Science 252:668, 1991.
46. Kulczycki A Jr, Metzger H: The interaction of IgE with rat basophilic leukemia cells. II. Quantitative aspects of the binding reaction. J Exp Med 140:1676, 1974.
47. Lee WT, Rao M, Conrad DH: The murine lymphocyte receptor for IgE. IV. The mechanism of ligand-specific receptor upregulation on B cells. J Immunol 139:1191, 1987.
48. Lemmon MA, Schlessinger J: Regulation of signal transduction and signal diversity by receptor oligomerization. Trends Biochem Sci 19:459, 1994.
49. Li W, Deanin GG, Margolis B, et al: FcεR1-mediated tyrosine phosphorylation of multiple proteins, including phospholipase Cgamma1 and the receptor βgamma$_2$ complex, in RBL-2H3 rat basophilic leukemia cells. Mol Cell Biol 12:3176, 1992.
50. Maeyama K, Hohman RJ, Ali H, et al: Assessment of IgE-receptor function through measurement of hydrolysis of membrane inositol phospholipids. New insights on the phenomena of biphasic antigen concentration-response curves and desensitization. J Immunol 140: 3919, 1988.
51. Malveaux FJ, Conroy MC, Adkinson NF Jr, et al: IgE receptors on human basophils. Relationship to serum IgE concentration. J Clin Invest 62:176, 1978.
52. Mao S-Y, Alber G, Rivera J, et al: Interaction of aggregated native and mutant IgE receptors with the cellular skeleton. Proc Natl Acad Sci USA 89:222, 1992.
53. Maurer D, Fiebiger E, Reininger B, et al: Expression of functional high affinity immunoglobulin E receptors (FcεRI) on monocytes of atopic individuals. J Exp Med 179:745, 1994.
54. McCloskey MA, Liu Z-Y, Poo M-M: Lateral electromigration and diffusion of Fc(epsilon) receptors on rat basophilic leukemia cells: effects of IgE binding. J Cell Biol 99:778, 1984.
55. Mendoza GR, Metzger H: Distribution and valency of receptor for IgE on rodent mast cells and related tumour cells. Nature 264:548, 1976.
56. Metzger H: General aspects of antibody action. In Metzger H (ed): Fc Receptors and the Action of Antibodies. American Society of Microbiology, Washington, DC, 1990, pp 7–11.
57. Metzger H: Transmembrane signaling: the joy of aggregation. J Immunol 149:1477, 1992.
58. Miller L, Blank U, Metzger H, et al: Expression of high-affinity binding of human immunoglobulin E by transfected cells. Science 244:334, 1989.
59. Newman SA, Rossi G, Metzger H: Molecular weight and valence of the cell-surface receptor for immunoglobulin E. Proc Natl Acad Sci USA 74:869, 1977.
60. Oettgen HC, Martin TR, Wynshaw-Boris A, et al: Active anaphylaxis in IgE-deficient mice. Nature 370:367, 1994.
61. Oliver JM, Seagrave J, Stump RF, et al: Signal transduction and cellular response in RBL-2H3 mast cells. Prog Allergy 42:185, 1988.
62. Orloff DG, Ra C, Frank SJ, et al: Family of disulfide-linked dimers containing the zeta and eta chains of the T-cell receptor and the gamma chain of Fc receptors. Nature 347:189, 1990.
63. Paolini R, Jouvin M-H, Kinet J-P: Phosphorylation and dephosphorylation of the high-affinity receptor for immunoglobulin E immediately after receptor engagement and disengagement. Nature 353:855, 1991.
64. Perez-Montfort R, Kinet J-P, Metzger H: A previously unrecognized subunit of the receptor for immunoglobulin E. Biochemistry 22:5722, 1983.
65. Pribluda VS, Pribluda C, Metzger H: Transphosphorylation as the mechanism by which the high-affinity receptor for IgE is phosphorylated upon aggregation. Proc Natl Acad Sci USA 91:11246, 1994.
66. Ravetch JV, Kinet J-P: Fc receptors. Annu Rev Immunol 9:457, 1991.
67. Reth M: Antigen receptor tail clue [letter]. Nature 338:383, 1989.
68. Rossi G, Newman SA, Metzger H: Assay and partial characterization of the solubilized cell surface receptor for immunoglobulin E. J Biol Chem 252:704, 1977.
69. Schlessinger J, Webb WW, Elson EL, et al: Lateral motion and valence of Fc receptors on rat peritoneal mast cells. Nature 264:550, 1976.
70. Segal DM, Taurog JD, Metzger H: Dimeric immunoglobulin E serves as a unit signal for mast cell degranulation. Proc Natl Acad Sci USA 74:2993, 1977.
71. Shimizu A, Tepler I, Benfey PN, et al: Human and rat mast cell high-affinity immunoglobulin E receptors: characterization of putative alpha-chain gene products. Proc Natl Acad Sci USA 85:1907, 1988.
72. Shirakawa T, Li A, Dubowitz M, et al: Association between atopy and variants of the β subunit of the high-affinity immunoglobulin E receptor. Nature Genet 7:125, 1994.
73. Shiue L, Green J, Green OM, et al: Interaction of p72^{syk} with the gamma and β subunits of the high-affinity receptor for immunoglobulin E, FcεRI. Mol Cell Biol 15:272, 1995.
74. Sobotka AK, Dembo M, Goldstein B, et al: Antigen-specific desensitization of human basophils. J Immunol 122:511, 1979.
75. Stief A, Texido G, Sansig G, et al: Mice deficient in CD23 reveal its modulatory role in IgE production but no role in T and B cell development. J Immunol 152:3378, 1994.
76. Takai T, Li M, Sylvestre D, et al: FcR gamma chain deletion results in pleiotrophic effector cell defects. Cell 76:519, 1994.
77. Wang B, Rieger A, Kilgus O, et al: Epidermal Langerhans cells from normal human skin bind monomeric IgE via FcεRI. J Exp Med 175:1353, 1992.
78. Yamashita T, Mao S-Y, Metzger H: Aggregation of the high-affinity IgE receptor and enhanced activity of p53/56^{lyn} protein-tyrosine kinase. Proc Natl Acad Sci USA 91:11251, 1994.
79. Yu P, Kosco-Vilbois M, Richards M, et al: Negative feedback regulation of IgE synthesis by murine CD23. Nature 369:753, 1994.

9 Biochemical Events in Basophil/Mast Cell Activation and Mediator Release

REUBEN P. SIRAGANIAN

Mast cells and basophils were first described by Paul Ehrlich more than 100 years ago as cells with prominent cytoplasmic granules and staining with basic dyes. Still, it was many years before it was recognized that mast cells and basophils play a critical role in immediate hypersensitivity reactions and that they contain histamine and other inflammatory mediators.

CHARACTERISTICS OF MAST CELLS AND BASOPHILS

Mast cells and basophils have several features in common. Both have prominent cytoplasmic granules containing histamine and other inflammatory mediators. Both cell types have surface receptors (FcεRI) that bind the Fc portion of IgE with high affinity. These cells are stimulated to secrete mediators when the IgE on their surface reacts with multivalent antigen.

There are several differences between basophils and mast cells. Basophils differentiate and mature in the bone marrow, then enter the circulation and rarely migrate into tissues. They are short lived (<2 weeks) and are probably end cells. In contrast, mast cells are distributed in connective tissue often located next to blood vessels and beneath epithelial surfaces such as in the gastrointestinal and respiratory tracts and the skin. Mast cells normally do not circulate, are long lived, and appear to retain the capacity to proliferate. Studies in mammalian species suggest an inverse quantitative relationship between basophils and mast cells; namely, species that have abundant mast cells have few basophils. Humans, however, have a large number of both mast cells and basophils.

The stimulation of basophils or mast cells is initiated by the interaction of secretagogues with cell surface receptors. This results in a series of biochemical events that culminate in the release of biologically active mediators. This chapter reviews our current knowledge of the mechanisms involved in the activation of these cells to release mediators. Some older literature and other aspects of mast cell biology are summarized in several reviews.[118, 181, 214, 265, 416, 431]

MEDIATORS FROM BASOPHILS AND MAST CELLS

Basophils and mast cells secrete substances that mediate allergic reactions. The mediators released from basophils and mast cells are either preformed and stored in secretory granules or newly generated (see Chapter 10). Preformed mediators include the biogenic amines such as histamine and serotonin that on a molar basis are the major components of the secretory granules. Human basophils and mast cells contain only histamine; however, serotonin is present in the mast cells of some species (e.g., rodents). The amount of histamine in mast cells is greater than that in basophils; human basophils contain approximately 1 to 3 μg of histamine per 10^6 cells, whereas human mast cells appear to have 5- to 10-fold higher concentrations. In the granule, histamine is associated with the carboxyl groups of proteoglycans and/or other proteins by ionic binding. During secretion, the interior of the granule is exposed to the extracellular ions and histamine is released by a cation exchange mechanism from these binding sites. Other granular contents include the neutral proteases, proteoglycans, several acid hydrolases (such as β-hexosaminidase and β-glucuronidase), and chemotactic molecules.

Several mediators are newly generated when mast cells or basophils are activated by an appropriate stimulus. During the release process, arachidonic acid is released from cellular phospholipids due to the activation of phospholipase enzymes. The metabolism of this arachidonic acid can then proceed along different pathways depending on the enzymes present. If it is metabolized along the cyclooxygenase pathway, it results in the formation of prostaglandins, whereas the lipoxygenase pathway leads to the formation of leukotrienes. Platelet-activating factor (1-O-alkyl-2-acetyl-sn-glyceryl-3-phosphorylcholine) is generated from alkyl phospholipids following cell activation. It has many potent biologic activities. These pathways and the resulting mediators are discussed in detail in Chapter 12.

Activation of mast cells and, to a lesser degree, basophils also results in an increased RNA expression and/or the release of several cytokines.[131, 359, 487] Some of these factors are IL-1, IL-3, IL-4, IL-5, IL-6, IFN-γ, GM-CSF, macrophage inflammatory peptides α and β, T-cell activation gene 3, and tumor necrosis factor α. Thus besides inflammatory

TABLE 9–1
MODEL SYSTEMS FOR STUDY OF MEDIATOR RELEASE

- Heterogeneous cell population
  - Organ fragments, e.g., lung
  - Peripheral leukocytes containing basophils
- Purified cells
  - Mast cells
  - Basophils
- Cell lines
  - Transformed cells, e.g., rat basophilic leukemia cell line (RBL-2H3)
  - Primary growth factor–dependent lines, e.g., bone marrow–derived mast cells
  - Transfected cells, e.g., RBL-2H3 with human FcεRI

mediators, mast cells and basophils are also a source of growth and regulatory factors. Interestingly, FcεRI aggregation also results in the stimulation of mast cell proliferation that could be due to the autocrine activity of factors released from these cells.[446] Thus antigen stimulation of mast cells may play a role in their proliferation. There may be differences in the regulation of the release of these different groups of mediators. Most of the current information is about secretion of the preformed and newly generated mediators.

MODEL SYSTEMS

Progress in the understanding of the biology of basophils and mast cells has been due largely to the development of techniques to obtain large numbers of these cells. Basophils and mast cells are sparsely distributed in the blood or tissues. Therefore, the earliest experiments with human materials used peripheral blood leukocytes or organ fragments in which only a small fraction of the cells were basophils or mast cells. Methods have been described to obtain purified basophils or mast cells from either peripheral blood or lung fragments (Table 9–1). Still, even with these techniques, the number of cells obtained are small and few biochemical studies can be performed.[258, 403] In contrast, rat peritoneal mast cells can be purified easily and usually yield about 1×10^6 cells per rat. This low number limits the biochemical studies that can be undertaken; a further complication is that conclusions drawn from experiments with rat mast cells might not be applicable to human basophils or mast cells.

The development of cultured cell lines has had an important influence on mast cell and basophil studies.[21, 22] A cloned rat basophilic leukemia cell line has been established that can be activated for histamine release.[21] Variants of these cells have also been isolated that are incapable of release and can be used in the characterization of the biochemical events in the release process.[422] Unlike these cell lines that were established from tumors, the use of growth factors has allowed the isolation of untransformed cell lines.[322] The culture of mouse bone marrow or spleen cells with IL-3, a growth factor from T lymphocytes, stimulates pluripotential stem cells to grow and differentiate into mast cells.[401] The cells require the continued presence of growth factors. Using growth factors, cells similar to human mast cells or basophils have been grown from cord blood or bone marrow.[111, 178, 212, 338] However, unlike the murine system, the human model has not been well standardized. In cultured cell lines, phenotypic differences are not as distinct because the characteristics of the cell depend on the culture conditions. The gene for the human α chain of FcεRI has been introduced into RBL-2H3 cells and could induce secretion.[126] These cells will be useful for further studies of the structure-function relationship of the receptor and other related surface molecules that are critical for cell activation.[133, 215, 341, 430]

The study of the FcεRI has been facilitated by several factors. First was the isolation and characterization of IgE and the availability of large amounts of IgE myeloma proteins and hybridomas from several species (e.g., human, rat, and mouse). Second was the availability of cell lines that have IgE receptors. The most extensive biochemical and molecular biologic studies have been with the rat basophilic leukemia RBL-2H3 cells; however, more recent work has also used human and mouse cultured lines that have IgE receptors. Some studies have used short-term cultured cell lines or mast cells and basophils purified from blood or tissue, but their use has been more problematic due to the difficulty of recovering adequate numbers of cells.

STIMULI FOR MAST CELL OR BASOPHIL SECRETION

Many different stimuli can activate basophils and mast cells (Table 9–2). Both of these cells respond to physiologically relevant stimulation through the IgE receptor. Still, there appear to be differences in their response to other secretagogues; for example, compound 48/80 causes histamine release from rat mast cells and human cutaneous mast cells but not from human lung mast cells or basophils.[262] There are also differences in the response of mast cells or basophils from different species to the same stimulus. Different secretagogues can activate distinct biochemical pathways in the release process. Parts of these pathways are probably different, whereas other parts are presumably common events in degranulation.

IgE Receptor-Mediated. A characteristic of mast cells and basophils is the presence of FcεRI on their cell surface, which bind IgE with high affinity ($K_A > 10^{10}\ M^{-1}$). The IgE binds through the Fc portion of the molecule, whereas the Fab are available for interacting with antigen. Activation of the cell is due to bridging of the IgE molecules by antigen.[421]

TABLE 9–2
PATHWAYS FOR MAST CELL/BASOPHIL ACTIVATION

- IgE receptor
  - Cell-bound IgE
    - Antigen
    - Anti-IgE
    - Concanavalin A
    - Protein A
  - Anti-IgE receptor antibody
- IgG receptor
- C5a receptor
- C3a receptor?
- Lymphokines/cytokines/chemokines
- Formyl methionine tripeptide receptor
- Eosinophil granule major basic protein
- Other compounds, e.g., 48/80

Antibodies to the IgE receptor can activate cells in the absence of IgE.[23] Therefore, IgE functions to confer antigenic specificity to the FcεRI. The sera of some patients with chronic urticaria have anti-FcεRIα antibodies that may play a role in their disease.

In experimental systems, basophils and mast cells also can be activated to release with heterologous antisera that react with the IgE on the cell surface (e.g., antibody that recognizes the immunoglobulin light or heavy chain). Such reactions could occur in vivo with autoimmune antibodies that react with IgE on cells. Mitogens such as concanavalin A or phytohemagglutinin (PHA) can cross-link cell surface IgE by binding to the carbohydrates on the IgE molecules.[423] Protein A from *Staphylococcus aureus* also can react with IgE to release histamine. Some mononuclear cell-derived factors react with IgE on the basophil surface and release histamine.[253] Only the IgE from some donors is effective as a substrate for these factors, and this could be due to differences in glycosylation.

IgG Receptor-Mediated. Basophils and mast cells besides FcεRI have FcγRII and FcγRIII that bind human IgG.[183, 408, 449] The binding of IgG to these FcγR is of much lower affinity than the binding of IgE to the FcεRI. The IgG bound to the receptor easily dissociates from the cell surface unless it is in the form of antigen-IgG complexes.[76, 106, 408] Basophils or mast cells, especially from rodents, can be activated through the FcγRIII to release histamine.[3, 199] However, this is a less efficient system and requires much more antibody than does the IgE receptor. Some subclasses of rodent IgG antibodies can also stimulate mast cells by binding to FcεRI.[30]

Alloantisera directed toward the major histocompatibility complex can trigger mast cells. In mouse cells, these IgG alloantisera bind to the mast cell surface by their Fab and trigger the cell through the Fc portion of the molecule binding to Fcγ receptors. The digestion of the alloantibodies to remove the Fc portion abolished the reaction.

Complement Receptors. The two major complement-derived anaphylatoxins, C5a and C3a, can release mediators from mast cells and basophils.[159, 165] Whereas there is a distinct receptor for C5a, the release by C3a could be similar to other basic molecules and not be receptor mediated.[318] On a molar basis, C5a is much more potent than C3a in stimulating cells for histamine release. Both mast cells and basophils have C3b receptors, but these do not cause the activation of cells to release. With human basophils, the activation of the C3b receptor results in enhancement of IgE-mediated histamine release.[455, 456]

Cytokines. Several histamine-releasing factors have been identified in the supernatants of T and B lymphocytes, mononuclear cells, platelets, and human lung macrophages.[196] Some of these molecules might release histamine by reacting with IgE on the cell surface.[254, 475] Purification and testing of recombinant proteins have shown that a number of different chemokines that are related to interleukin 8 (IL-8) release histamine from human basophils. These include the following, in order of decreasing potency: monocyte chemotactic protein-1 (MCP-1), MCP-3, RANTES, macrophage inflammatory protein-1α (MIP-1α), and IL-8.[16, 196, 221] These probably act through several different receptors that are members of the seven transmembrane family that activate GTP-binding proteins.

A few lymphokines, for example the interferons, enhance the IgE-mediated histamine release from human basophils.[169, 170, 394] These effects of interferons are due to the induction of new RNA synthesis in the cells.[149] Such modulation of mediator release could be important at sites of inflammation and during viral infections. Other cytokines can bind to cell surface receptors and modulate the extent of histamine release; for example, human basophils have IL-3 receptors,[466] and the addition of IL-3 results in enhancement of histamine secretion by both IgE- and nonreceptor-mediated mechanisms.[152, 255, 394, 466] IL-5 and GM-CSF act similarly and share a common receptor subunit.[171] Similarly, the addition of granulocyte or macrophage CSF, IL-1α, and IL-1β enhances release.[152, 279] In contrast, IL-4 has no effect on secretion. Some of these lymphokines can release histamine directly at high concentrations.[2] The lymphokines also can change the response spectrum of the mediators released on stimulation; for example, basophils stimulated with C5a do not release leukotrienes unless the cells have been pretreated with IL-3.[224] Similarly, platelet-activating factor induces histamine release only after such priming.

Formyl Methionine Peptides. Formyl methionine–containing tripeptides are chemotactic for some cells and have similarities to chemotactic factors produced by bacteria. They bind to specific receptors and induce histamine release from human basophils but not from rat mast cells.[157, 419] The morphology of this release has some of the characteristics of piecemeal degranulation.[98]

Eosinophilic Granule-Derived Proteins. Approximately half the eosinophil granule protein consists of the arginine-rich major basic protein. This protein has been shown to damage cells and activates basophils and mast cells for noncytotoxic histamine release.[495]

Other Compounds. Many compounds activate mast cells or basophils for histamine release. Ionophores are lipophilic compounds that insert themselves into cell membranes and transport ions across the membrane. The Ca^{2+} ionophore A23187 triggers mediator release from basophils and mast cells in the presence of Ca^{2+} in the medium. Other compounds that are of experimental interest are tumor promoters, such as phorbol myristic acid, which releases histamine from human basophils without a requirement for extracellular calcium.[395, 396] This compound binds and activates PKC (see discussion on the role of phosphatidylinositol in the release pathway). Other secretagogues include polycationic compounds like polymyxin B, compound 48/80, polylysine, and polyarginine. Other compounds that cause mediator release are neuropeptides such as substance P, luteinizing hormone-releasing hormone, morphine, codeine, tubocurarine, adenosine triphosphate, dextran, mellitin, chymotrypsin, and proteins released from neutrophils.[128] Human basophils and subtypes of mast cells (see Chapter 10) differ considerably in responsiveness to these various agents.

BIOCHEMICAL MECHANISMS OF THE RELEASE REACTION

The initial event in the stimulation of the basophil and mast cell is the interaction of antigen with IgE on the cell surface. The antigen then bridges two IgE molecules to initiate a series of biochemical events that eventually result in the secretion of mediators from the cells (Table 9–3). Therefore, the optimal conditions for the release of histamine depend on the concentration of antigen-specific IgE antibody on the membrane, the concentration of the antigen, and the affinity of the IgE for the antigen.[53, 81–83] In vitro, as little as 1 ng of ragweed antigen E (2.5×10^{-11} M) can activate basophils from ragweed-allergic individuals. The release of histamine and other mediators is a rapid process that is complete in less than 30 minutes. Mediator release is a secretory (exocytotic) event that is noncytotoxic and does not require serum. However, there is an absolute requirement for the presence of Ca^{2+} in the medium for the IgE-receptor–mediated release reactions. The release reaction is temperature dependent with optimal release at 37°C.

Aggregation of FcεRI results in many biochemical events in the basophil and mast cell. As FcεRI does not have any intrinsic enzymatic activity, the activation of cellular biochemical events is due to the interaction of the aggregated receptors with other cytoplasmic or membrane proteins.

The FcεRI is a tetramer composed of an IgE-binding α chain, a β chain, and a homodimer formed of disulfide-linked γ chains (see Chapter 8). The receptor subunits lack any known enzymatic activity, and thus FcεRI must rely on associated molecules for transducing intracellular signals (Table 9–4). The extracellular domain of the α chain of FcεRI binds IgE, whereas its relatively short cytoplasmic domain probably does not play a role in cell signaling. In contrast, the COOH-terminal cytoplasmic domains of both the β and γ subunits are important in FcεRI-mediated signal transduction. For example, truncation of the COOH-terminal of either the β or γ cytoplasmic domain abolishes FcεRI-mediated signaling in transfected P815 mast cells (a murine cell line derived from a mastocytoma). The cytoplasmic domains of the β and γ subunits of FcεRI contain a motif (a sequence of amino acids) that is important for signal transduction. Although previously called TAM (tyrosine activation motif) or ARAM (antigen recognition activation motif), the preferred terminology is ITAM (immunoreceptor tyrosine-based activation motif) (Fig. 9–1). This motif is present in the β and γ chains of FcεRI, in the ζ subunit of the T-cell receptor complex, and in Igβ and Igα of the B-cell receptor.[52, 54] The ligand-binding domains of the receptors on these cells lack intrinsic enzymatic activity but associate with transducing subunits that contain this cytoplasmic motif that is critical for cell activation.[371, 389, 479] Chimeric proteins with the cytoplasmic domain of ζ of the T-cell receptor or β or γ of FcεRI linked to the extracellular and transmembrane domains of other proteins have been used for signal transduction studies.[100, 173, 188, 232, 379] Aggregation of these chimeric molecules by antibodies to their extracellular domains results in cell activation. The γ component appears to be the essential receptor subunit for signaling cells for secretion. Aggregation of chimeric molecules prepared with FcεRIγ or TCRζ, but not with FcεRIβ, induces secretion in RBL-2H3 cells.[188] By analogy to studies in T cells, the critical signaling is probably due to the ITAM motif contained in the cytoplasmic domain of the γ subunit.[172, 378]

By gene transfer, FcεRI has been expressed in cells that do not normally have the receptor.[42] The receptor expressed in monkey kidney Cos 7 cells results in normal IgE binding; yet it is incapable of activating any of the biochemical events that accompany receptor aggregation (e.g., increase in $[Ca^{2+}]_i$ or phosphatidyl inositol (PtdIns) hydrolysis). However, if expressed in mast cells that do not have IgE receptors (mouse mastocytoma P815 cells), they can activate some early receptor-mediated signaling events.[302] These experiments demonstrate that molecules besides FcεRI are present in mast cells and play a critical role for propagating intracellular signals.

The following sections will describe the biochemical events that have been discussed under basophil and mast cell activation (see Table 9–3). The recognition of biochemical events has been either by direct measurement or by studying the action of inhibitors on the release process. Examples of direct measurement of changes induced by stimulation would be the rise in intracellular Ca^{2+} or the

TABLE 9–4
COMPONENTS OF FcεRI

Molecule	Characteristics
α	IgE binding component.
β	ITAM motif. Lyn associates with it before FcεRI aggregation. Increased interaction after β is tyrosine phosphorylated. PKC-δ also associates with it. Phosphorylated on Tyr and Ser after activation.
γ	ITAM motif. Phosphorylated on Tyr and Thr after receptor aggregation. Syk associates with it after it is Tyr phosphorylated. Phosphorylated by PKC on Thr.

TABLE 9–3
BIOCHEMICAL EVENTS DURING BASOPHIL/MAST CELL SECRETION

In Absence of Ca^{2+} in Medium
- IgE reacting with receptors on the cell surface
- IgE aggregation
- Immobilization of receptors
- Internalization of receptors
- Morphological changes
- Protein tyrosine phosphorylations
- Hydrolysis of phosphatidyl inositides
- Changes in membrane potential
- Role for GTP-binding proteins
- Activation of protease enzymes
- Release of Ca^{2+} from intracellular stores
- Rise in cAMP

Later Events (Ca^{2+} Dependent)
- Activation of methyl transferase
- Hydrolysis of phosphatidyl inositides
- Influx of Ca^{2+}
- Phosphorylation of proteins on Tyr, Ser, and Thr
- Release of arachidonic acid—activation of phospholipase A2, C, and D
- Changes in the cytoskeleton
- Fusion of the granular membrane to the plasma membrane
- Opening of the granule to the extracellular space—release of granular contents

$$(\text{Asp/Glu})\text{-}X_2\text{-}\underset{*}{\textbf{Tyr}}\text{-}X_2\text{-Leu-}X_{6\text{-}8}\text{-}\underset{*}{\textbf{Tyr}}\text{-}X_2\text{-Leu/Iso}$$

FIGURE 9–1. The *i*mmunoreceptor *t*yrosine-based *a*ctivation *m*otif (ITAM). The Tyr residues are phosphorylated in activated cells (asterisk). X refers to any amino acid.

phosphorylation of proteins. In contrast, evidence for the activation of protease enzymes is deduced from the inhibition of secretion by inhibitors of proteolytic enzymes. The measurement of a biochemical change is the most unequivocal result because of the notorious nonspecific activity of most inhibitors. Thus several inhibitors block release only in some cell types. Some of these biochemical events are bypassed when cells are activated by different secretagogues or by nonphysiologic means; for example, the Ca^{2+} ionophores by directly transporting Ca^{2+} into the cell bypass early receptor-mediated steps in cell activation.

The studies of the different biochemical changes do not unequivocally lead to a hypothesis of the sequence of events that occur in the cell. However, many of these biochemical events occur without added Ca^{2+} in the medium. Some of these Ca^{2+}-independent events transmit the early signals that then activate other downstream molecules that eventually result in degranulation. These steps in the release process are described in more detail in the following sections.

FcεRI RECEPTOR BRIDGING, AGGREGATION, AND INTERNALIZATION

The FcεRI are distributed diffusely over the surface of the cell without any significant pool of receptors in the cytoplasm. The monomeric IgE-receptor complex is freely mobile in the plane of the membrane.[291, 399, 496] By photobleaching recovery techniques, the diffusion coefficient of the IgE receptor was similar to other membrane proteins.[399] By this method, the IgE receptors were univalent (one IgE bound per receptor) and independently mobile,[295] although cointernalization studies suggest that there is some interaction between different IgE receptors.[116] Several different proteins are in close proximity to the receptor and may interact with the receptor components.[215, 273, 332, 426] Furthermore, specialized gangliosides on the mast cells may play a role in the association of the receptor with protein tyrosine kinases.[133, 305] Such molecules may be critical for receptor-mediated signaling.

The presence of monomeric IgE bound to the FcεRI decreases the rate of receptor turnover.[115] The half-life of receptors on the RBL-2H3 cells is 8 to 13 hours.[115, 363] If occupied with IgE, the half-life is much longer, with estimates of greater than 32 hours.[115] However, these results do not distinguish between the possibility that there are changes in the lability of the receptor or that IgE protects FcεRI from digestion when the complex is exposed to lysosomal enzymes following internalization.[299]

The estimate of the number of FcεRI has varied between 10^3 and 10^6 per cell on different cell preparations.[66, 262, 433] Basophils from individuals with high levels of serum IgE have increased numbers of FcεRI.[67, 272] Similarly in culture, the presence of IgE in the medium increased the number of IgE receptors on the RBL-2H3 cells.[115, 363] This up-regulation of the FcεRI number by the presence of IgE is different from the observation with many other receptor systems where an increased concentration of the ligand causes a down-regulation in the receptor number.

The addition of antigen or anti-IgE to basophils or mast cells results in the bridging of the IgE molecules with the initial formation of aggregates, with progression into patching and capping at one pole of the cell. There is eventual internalization and degradation of these complexes.[29, 231] Such internalization of aggregated surface receptors is a common phenomenon of many aggregated cell surface receptors.

Binding of multivalent antigen with IgE on the cell surface results in the immobilization of the receptor.[297, 298] This immobilization does not require the presence of Ca^{2+} in the medium. Immobilization is due to the interaction of the receptors with cytoskeletal elements in the cell.[298]

The internalization and recycling of the IgE receptors on RBL-2H3 cells have been studied in detail.[112–114, 116, 174, 175, 373] The aggregation of IgE with multivalent antigen results in rapid internalization of the complexes; the $t_{1/2}$ for this reaction is 3 to 5 minutes. Internalization is through coated pits and results in degradation of the aggregates. Unlike histamine release, internalization does not require external Ca^{2+}. Even when the internalization reaction has gone to completion, a significant portion of the IgE is left on the cell surface. IgE dimers can initiate the internalization process, although they are less efficient than larger oligomers. During endocytosis of IgE-antigen aggregates, there is cointernalization of receptors that have bound monomeric IgE. However, this is not due to random cointernalization of membrane proteins. Internalization of FcεRI can also be induced by activation of protein kinase C, although this enzyme does not appear to be directly involved in aggregated receptor internalization.[365] Because internalization of cross-linked receptors occurs in the absence of Ca^{2+} in the medium, it must be an event that precedes and/or is independent of other biochemical changes that accompany secretion, such as the influx of Ca^{2+} into the cell and the hydrolysis of phospholipids. However, internalization probably does not play a role in signaling the cell for secretion. The cytoplasmic domains of the three subunits of FcεRI are not required for aggregation-induced internalization of FcεRI.[274, 469]

Studies with defined-length bivalent haptens have shown that bridging of two IgE molecules initiates the cell-triggering signal.[421] Small bivalent haptens with a different antigenic site at each end will activate cells, suggesting that the bridging is between adjacent IgE molecules on the cell surface.[421] Different length rigid bivalent haptens can activate RBL-2H3 cells most effectively when the molecules are separated by 80 to 240 Å, whereas there is a poor response when they are less than 50 Å apart.[191, 192] Monoclonal anti-FcεRI antibodies activate cells to release, again demonstrating that receptor bridging is the critical event.[17, 23] However, there appear to be orientational constraints, and not all aggregates are equally effective in signaling for secretion.[342] Preformed, chemically cross-linked IgE dimers are active in triggering both rodent mast cells and human basophils.[190, 409] In contrast, with RBL-2H3 cells, IgE-dimers are much less effective than trimers in releasing histamine.[104] With human basophils, the dimeric triggering signal is qualitatively different from stimulation by trimers or oligomers.[261] Basophils from some donors respond to dimers as well as to larger oligomers, whereas basophils from other donors require at least trimers to release mediators.[260] This difference in response correlates with the capacity of the cells to release histamine, a parameter that has been called releasability (see discussion on releasability). Therefore, dimers are the unit signal for activating cells of only some donors. The variation in response of basophils from different donors could be due to intracellular changes that modify the sensitivity of a cell to an external stimulus.

Dimers once bound to the cell surface can coalesce to form larger aggregates due to intrinsic changes in the receptor or due to the interaction of the IgE-receptor complex with the cytoskeleton.[296]

NUMBER OF AGGREGATES FOR CELL ACTIVATION

Activation of basophils or mast cells requires the bridging of a very few IgE molecules on the cell surface. Studies suggest that bridging of 100 or fewer IgE molecules will completely activate the cell for histamine release. As mast cells and basophils have approximately 10^5 receptors per cell, it is obvious that bridging of less than 1% of the total IgE molecules on the cell surface results in degranulation.[81, 82, 104, 270] In rat mast cells, the addition of secretagogues immobilized on beads induced localized degranulation; therefore full secretion from the cell requires the bridging of IgE molecules on different sectors of the cell surface.[230]

CHANGES IN RECEPTOR MOBILITY

The IgE receptors are diffusely distributed on the cell surface.[29] The interaction of IgE with multivalent antigen results in the interaction of the receptors with the cytoskeleton.[375] There is the formation of clusters, aggregates, and patches and finally capping of these into one pole of the cell. The addition of wheat germ agglutinin to cells results in binding to FcϵRIα, the association of the receptor with the insoluble cytoskeleton, and a decrease in receptor-mediated signaling.[290] Thus the ability of receptors to be freely mobile in the membrane is important for signal transduction.

MORPHOLOGICAL STUDY OF DEGRANULATION

Microscopic studies have detected changes that occur in mast cells and basophils during mediator release.[119, 226] Under phase contrast microscopy, when antigen is added to basophils in vitro, the cells lose their oriented motility and spread, extending pseudopodia in several directions.[144] Some cells that exhibit this change do not go on to degranulate. Degranulating basophils develop small vesicles in their cytoplasm that rapidly increase in size and coalesce. Accompanying the increase in the vesicles is a decrease in the number of specific granules. The basophils remain sticky but regain their motility. By electron microscopy, the surface of the RBL-2H3 cells shows many microvilli.[357] Within seconds of the addition of antigen, the microvillus surface transforms to a plicated appearance; the cells spread with increased adhesion to the substrate. There is also increased fluid pinocytosis. These changes occur in the absence of degranulation.[150, 340]

Transmission microscopic studies have described the changes that occur in basophils or mast cells of different species during secretion. The stimulation of human basophils with antigen to release histamine results in a series of characteristic morphological changes. The granular membranes fuse with the plasma membrane around the circumference of the cell, resulting in the extrusion of the granular material to the outside. The diameters of the openings to the exterior are variable. There are occasional interconnected chains of granules within the cell that open to the exterior at a single point on the cell surface. The granule matrix is released as a whole to the outside, but the granule membrane is left behind. Frequently, membrane-free granular contents are seen attached to the cell exterior. In a fully degranulated basophil, there is a complete loss of recognizable cytoplasmic granules. In contrast, a different morphological picture of degranulation is seen in basophils infiltrating sites of delayed hypersensitivity reactions. The process has been termed piecemeal degranulation; the granules never fuse with the cell membrane and lose their matrix in piecemeal manner over a period of days. This type of degranulation probably does not occur in immediate hypersensitivity reactions.

The degranulation of human mast cells following IgE-receptor activation has similar morphological characteristics.[96, 97] After stimulation, a dimple forms in the plasma membrane in areas that contact the secretory granule membrane. This area becomes clear of proteins, and electrophysiologic measurements demonstrate the formation of a small fusion pore, which is stable for variable lengths of time.[74] The earliest event in degranulation is this formation of narrow-necked pores joining the membranes of the granules with the plasma membrane.[57] There is swelling of the individual granules accompanied by a change in the electron-dense granular contents. However, the swelling of the secretory granule is not the driving force for membrane fusion.[497] In contrast to basophils, the individual granular contents fuse with each other to form an interconnected chain filled with altered granule matrix. These channels then open to the exterior by fusion with the plasma membrane. The granule fusion does not have to be an all-or-nothing event but can be due to partial release.[10] During the release process, there are prominent cytoplasmic filaments observed close to the granules. The granule membrane is under tension, and this results in a net transfer of membrane from the plasma membrane to the secretory granules when they are connected by fusion pores.[310] This tension also is the force that causes the expansion of the fusion pore.[311] There are differences in the degranulation-induced morphological changes observed in human skin as compared with lung mast cells.[96] Interestingly, the full reconstitution of granules in rat mast cells after a secretory event can take up to 4 weeks.[141]

REQUIREMENT FOR METABOLIC ENERGY

Energy is required for maintaining general cell functions and for the secretion of mediators. Several inhibitors block energy utilization in mast cells and basophils; these include anoxia in the absence of glucose, as well as cyanide, 2-deoxy-D-glucose, or antimycin A. Such experiments suggest that energy for histamine release may be from either aerobic or anaerobic glycolysis. Direct experiments have also demonstrated energy use during mediator release with isolated cell systems in which oxidative phosphorylation (aerobic glycolysis) plays the dominant role.[186, 187] The depletion of intracellular ATP by mitochondrial inhibitors blocks the increase in $[Ca^{2+}]_i$, the influx of Ca^{2+}, and secretion.[309] Interestingly, during secretion, there is the release of ATP that then reacts with specific ATP receptors on cell surfaces and propagates the cell activation signal to other cells.[343]

CHANGES IN TRANSMEMBRANE POTENTIAL AND INTRACELLULAR pH

In many cells, there are changes in the transmembrane potential as an early step in stimulus-response coupling. Cell membrane potential depends on the ionic gradient of K^+ maintained across the plasma membrane. For human basophils, changing the K^+ in the medium has no effect on the release of histamine, although it results in membrane depolarization in other cells. Similarly, there is no other monovalent cation or anion requirement for histamine release from human basophils as long as Ca^{2+} is available in the medium.[158] However, incubation of RBL-2H3 cells in a high K^+ medium results in depolarization and inhibition of the increase in $[Ca^{2+}]_i$ and of secretion.[307] Membrane potential changes have been observed in rat mast cells and RBL-2H3 cells following cell stimulation for histamine release.[194, 383] The plasma membrane potential of RBL-2H3 cells is set in part by the activity of the Na^+ pump and in part by the K^+ conductance, whereas for rat mast cells, it is set predominantly by the Na^+ pump.[49] In rat mast cells, there is increased Na^+/K^+ pump activity following secretion that may be related to the recovery of the cells from the secretory event.[216] There is depolarization when cells are stimulated with the calcium ionophore A23187, whereas there is hyperpolarization with compound 48/80.[51] There is also activation of a chloride channel that may not be essential for exocytosis but may enhance secretion after suboptimal stimulation.[86, 107, 377] In RBL-2H3 cells, both FcϵRI and Ca^{2+} ionophore stimulation results in hyperpolarization followed by depolarization that is dependent on Ca^{2+} influx.[19, 306] The membrane potential changes in the RBL-2H3 cells have been interpreted either as due to true membrane potential change or as secondary to Ca^{2+} uptake by the mitochondria and may be dependent on extracellular Ca^{2+}. Still, the repolarization is dependent on a K^+ channel and is critical for secretion.[225] There is a rise in intracellular pH that is a synergistic signal to the increase in $[Ca^{2+}]_i$ and PtdIns hydrolysis for exocytosis.[4] There is an outwardly rectifying K^+ current that is activated after FcϵRI aggregation, which may be closed by the rise in $[Ca^{2+}]_i$. The changes in membrane potential may be important for regulating Ca^{2+} entry after cell activation.[216, 292] Thus there are changes in transmembrane potential and in the intracellular pH during secretion.

ACTIVATION OF PROTEASE ENZYMES

Both protease inhibitors and substrates of proteolytic enzyme block secretion from mast cells and basophils.[181] These inhibitors include serine protease inhibitors such as diisopropyl flurophosphate and some trypsin and chymotrypsin substrates. These chemicals block the rise in $[Ca^{2+}]_i$, the cAMP increase, and cell secretion.[181] In some experimental systems, the inhibitors are only effective if present during cell stimulation; that is, if cells are incubated with the inhibitor and washed before the addition of the secretagogue, there is normal release. This suggests that the proteolytic enzyme is activated only after the start of the secretory process. The activation of this protease is Ca^{2+} independent. There may also be a different protease that is involved in cell desensitization (see discussion on desensitization). The activation of this second protease occurs in the absence of Ca^{2+} and is sensitive to lower concentrations of the inhibitors.[182, 203] Studies with rat mast cell membrane fragments suggest that a membrane-associated proteolytic enzyme might be a very early step.[180]

ACTIVATION OF METHYLTRANSFERASES

Methylation reactions require methyltransferase enzymes that transfer methyl groups from S-adenosylmethionine (a high-energy methyl donor) to lipids, proteins, or nucleic acids. These reactions regulate reactions such as chemotaxis and gene expression. Inhibitors of methylation reactions block FcϵRI-mediated secretion from a variety of mast cells and basophils.[70, 71, 177, 179] There is also inhibition of the increase in $[Ca^{2+}]_i$ and abrogation of the early rise in cAMP levels and of the release of arachidonic acid.[70, 71, 180, 294] This inhibition is limited to the FcϵRI-mediated cell activation but not to stimulation with either compound 40/80, the Ca^{2+} ionophore A23187, formyl methionine peptides, or C5a.[155, 314, 315]

It was suggested that phospholipid methyl transferase enzymes may play a critical role in signal transduction.[154] In this model, two different phospholipid methyltransferase enzymes present in the plasma membrane would generate phosphatidylcholine in a stepwise fashion from phosphatidylethanolamine. Although most of the cellular phosphatidylcholine is synthesized through the UDP-choline pathway, the small fraction generated by this methylation pathway was postulated to play a role in signal transduction.

Several studies observed an early transient increase in phospholipid but not protein methylation following IgE-receptor activation of mast cells or basophils.[70, 71, 179, 181, 284] This transient increase temporally preceded the $[Ca^{2+}]_i$ increase and histamine secretion.[71] Variants of the RBL-2H3 cells were identified that were defective in either one of the two phospholipid methyltransferase enzyme activities and did not demonstrate increased phospholipid methylation, Ca^{2+} influx, or histamine release after FcϵRI-mediated cell stimulation. Fusion of these lines restored the IgE-receptor activation and resulted in Ca^{2+} influx and histamine release.[293] However, questions have been raised about the role of phospholipid methylation in secretion. First, the two different phospholipid methyltransferase enzymes have never been purified from mammalian tissues, although two such enzymes have been identified by genetic analysis and the cDNA isolated in yeast. Second, the early experiments measured the total incorporation of radioactive counts into a lipid-soluble fraction. The number of counts found in this fraction is a very small percentage of the total added and incorporated into the cell. In experiments where the different phospholipids were fractionated, the predicted changes in the phospholipids were not observed.[36, 37, 312] Third, the effect of the methyltransferase inhibitors could be at multiple sites in the cell.[316] Therefore, although inhibitors of the methylation reaction block histamine release, the mechanism of their action is not clear.

PHOSPHORYLATION OF CELLULAR PROTEINS

In many biologic systems, extracellular ligands bind to cell surface receptors and activate protein kinase enzymes, which then phosphorylate cellular proteins. Many protein kinases have been described, including cAMP-dependent protein kinase, cGMP-dependent protein kinase, Ca^{2+}-dependent protein kinase that requires either calmodulin or phospholipids, and protein tyrosine kinases. The phosphorylated proteins are dephosphorylated by phosphatases that limit the effect of the phosphorylated proteins. This phosphorylation-dephosphorylation of proteins regulates many intracellular processes. This section will discuss some of the early studies on phosphorylation of proteins. Sections that follow will discuss the protein tyrosine phosphorylation and protein kinase C, the Ca^{2+} phospholipid-dependent enzyme that is activated by DAG generated by the breakdown of PtdIns.

Early studies in the 1970s and 1980s observed that stimulation of rat mast cells for secretion results in the phosphorylation of several proteins (78, 68, 59, and 42 kD).[413] The phosphorylation of the three lower molecular weight proteins is rapid and parallels the rate of histamine release. In contrast, the phosphorylation of the 78-kD protein is slower than histamine secretion. Several inhibitors of mast cell secretion, including cromolyn, transiently increase the phosphorylation of a 78-kD protein that might be identical with that phosphorylated during cell stimulation.[414, 454] Interestingly, the inhibitory effect of cromolyn on mast cell secretion is also transient. Therefore, the phosphorylation of this 78-kD protein may be the turnoff signal for secretion. In RBL-2H3 cells, IgE- or ionophore-mediated histamine release is accompanied by the rapid phosphorylation of a 92-kD protein.[145] This phosphorylation requires the presence of extracellular Ca^{2+} in the medium, although it is not due to the rise in the $[Ca^{2+}]_i$. The phosphorylation of several other proteins, some in the absence of extracellular Ca^{2+}, was also observed in these early studies.[101, 382, 452] As the identity of the phosphorylated amino acid was not determined in these early studies, we cannot know the class of the involved kinase.

Several cell surface receptors, such as the insulin and epidermal factor receptors, have kinase activity. However, none of the components of the FcεRI have kinase activity or structural similarity to kinases. There is a tyrosine kinase, however, that associates with the receptor during purification.[364] This results in the tyrosine phosphorylation of the β and γ components in partially purified receptor preparations. The α chain of the FcεRI on rat mast cells is normally phosphorylated (probably on Ser), and there is a further increase during mast cell activation.[148] However, these changes in the α component have not been observed with the RBL-2H3 cells.[103, 354] There is also phosphorylation of this subunit in mast cells following ionophore A23187 stimulation, suggesting that it could be secondary to intracellular changes in Ca^{2+}. The β and γ components of the FcεRI are normally phosphorylated on Ser and Thr residues, respectively.[103, 354] Following receptor activation, there is approximately a 45% increase in the Ser phosphorylation of the β subunit, whereas there is a 35% decrease in the Thr phosphorylation of the γ component.[354] However, only a small fraction of the receptors incorporate labeled phosphate. In later studies, FcεRI cross-linking was found to result in Tyr and Ser phosphorylation of the β subunit and on Tyr and Thr residues of the γ component.[346] This suggests that there is activation of both serine and tyrosine kinases that phosphorylate the IgE receptor. The next section discusses the tyrosine phosphorylation events that have become the focus of studies on signal transduction in mast cells.

PROTEIN TYROSINE PHOSPHORYLATION

Protein tyrosine phosphorylation is an early event in signal transduction not only by growth factor receptors that are protein tyrosine kinases but also by other immune receptors, such as FcεRI, that themselves have no intrinsic enzymatic activity. These receptors associate and/or activate several non-receptor protein tyrosine kinases that are critical for cell activation. The tyrosine phosphorylation of a protein is important because it results in conformational changes in the protein, changes in enzymatic activity, and changes in interaction of the protein with other proteins.

The study of protein tyrosine phosphorylation has provided major insights into signaling pathways in cells. An important theme is that there are defined domains in proteins that are critical for protein-protein interactions (Table 9–5). These protein domains form compact units that maintain their structure in isolation[217, 282, 348] and occur in many enzymes, including protein kinases, lipid kinases, protein phosphatases, and phospholipases. They are also present on

TABLE 9–5
PROTEIN DOMAINS PRESENT IN MOLECULES THAT ARE IMPORTANT IN SIGNAL TRANSDUCTION

Domains	Characteristics
SH2 (Src homology 2)	
Structure:	~100 amino acid residues
Distribution:	Many protein tyrosine kinases; protein tyrosine phosphatases; phospholipase C-γ; activators of Ras-like GTPases; molecules that regulate cytoskeletal function.
Specificity:	Phosphorylated Tyr residues; specificity of binding determined by amino acid residues immediately C-terminal of pTyr.
PTB (Phosphotyrosine Binding)	
Structure:	~ 200 amino acid residues
Distribution:	Shc adaptor protein; IRS-1.
Specificity:	Phosphorylated Tyr residues; specificity of binding determined by the residues immediately N-terminal of pTyr; Asn-Pro-X-pTyr.
SH3 (Src homology 3)	
Structure:	~50 amino acid residues
Distribution:	Many proteins in tyrosine phosphorylation pathway also cytoskeletal proteins.
Specificity:	Proline-rich peptides approximately 10 amino acids in length.
PH (Pleckstrin domain)	
Structure:	~ 100 amino acid residues
Distribution:	Many proteins, including Ser/Thr and Tyr kinases, their substrates, and cytoskeletal proteins.
Specificity:	Unclear; may localize signaling molecules to the membrane.

adaptor proteins, which have no enzymatic function but act to aggregate other proteins. Some of these domains (SH3 and PH) are present on cytoskeletal proteins where they may play a role in regulating cell shape. The approximately 100 amino acid residue Src homology 2 (SH2) domain is present on many protein tyrosine kinases and other molecules. The SH2 domains mediate the interaction with specific phosphorylated tyrosine residues in other proteins. The three-dimensional structure of SH2 domains in different proteins are very similar, and each binds to a distinct sequence of amino acids surrounding a phosphotyrosine residue. The three amino acids immediately C-terminal to the phosphotyrosine are critical for the specificity of binding. The SH3 domain, in contrast, is slightly smaller (approximately 55 to 70 residues) but is also present in a large number of proteins. It selectively binds to proline-rich sequences in other proteins, with different SH3 domains binding to different proline-rich sequences. The described *p*hosphorylated *t*yrosine *b*inding (PTB) domain is present in adaptor molecules (e.g., Shc and IRS-1) and interacts with proteins that are tyrosine phosphorylated. Its binding specificity is determined by residues N-terminal to the phosphorylated tyrosine.[348] The PH (pleckstrin) domain is found on many proteins, including protein Tyr and Ser and Thr kinases and was originally described in pleckstrin, a substrate of protein kinase C. This domain may be involved in binding of proteins to phospholipids, although its crystal structure would suggest that is not likely. It may function in holding molecules close to the membrane.

The first observation in mast cells was that aggregation of the FcεRI results in rapid protein tyrosine phosphorylations, the most prominent being a 72-kD protein.[31] The phosphorylation of this 72-kD protein (pp72) correlated by both time course and antigen dose with histamine release. PKC activation by phorbol ester or an increase of $[Ca^{2+}]_i$ by ionophore A23187 did not induce tyrosine phosphorylation of pp72. Furthermore, in the absence of extracellular Ca^{2+}, there was FcεRI-mediated phosphorylation of pp72 but no degranulation. Activation of G proteins resulted in PtdIns hydrolysis and secretion of histamine without pp72 tyrosine phosphorylation. The tyrosine kinase inhibitor genistein efficiently blocked both tyrosine phosphorylation of pp72 and secretion without inhibiting PtdIns hydrolysis. This suggested that phosphorylation of pp72 was a distinct, independent signaling pathway induced specifically by aggregation of the FcεRI.[429] The very rapid time course of tyrosine phosphorylation of proteins after FcεRI aggregation, the coupling to FcεRI aggregation, and the fact that tyrosine kinase inhibitors block secretion emphasize the importance of protein tyrosine phosphorylation in FcεRI-mediated secretion.[201, 227, 429]

The following sections will discuss the protein tyrosine kinases involved, the substrates that are tyrosine phosphorylated, and the protein tyrosine phosphatases that limit or reverse these reactions. Some of these classifications are arbitrary; for example, a tyrosine kinase could also be a substrate for another kinase, or a protein tyrosine phosphatase can itself get tyrosine phosphorylated.

Protein Tyrosine Kinases (Table 9–6)

Src Family Kinases. The Src family kinases are associated with the inner surface of the plasma membrane and appear to function in signal transduction, especially of transmembrane receptors that lack intrinsic enzymatic activity.[45] They contain a region that is unique for each member of the family, followed by SH3, SH2, kinase, and COOH-terminal regulatory domains. The regulatory domain has tyrosine phosphorylation sites that can be phosphorylated by a specific tyrosine kinase, Csk. The tyrosine phosphorylation of these regulatory sites by Csk results in the intramolecular interaction of the regulatory region with the SH2 domain, resulting in an inactive kinase. Conversely, the dephosphorylation of this site by a specific tyrosine phosphatase results in activation of the kinase.

TABLE 9–6
PROTEIN TYROSINE KINASE IN BASOPHILS AND MAST CELLS

Molecule	Characteristics
Lyn	Src family PTK; SH2 and SH3 domains. Associated with the plasma membrane and FcεRI. Regulatory domain at COOH-terminal region is tyrosine phosphorylated. Activated after FcεRI aggregation.
Src	Similar to Lyn. Activated after FcεRI aggregation. Not FcεRI associated.
Syk	Two SH2 domains; cytosolic. Activated by FcεRI aggregation. Binds to the tyrosine phosphorylated ITAM γ subunit of FcεRI.
Btk	PH, SH3, and SH2 domains; cytosolic. PH domain at its amino terminus. Interacts with PKC. Phosphorylated and activated by FcεRI aggregation and translocates to the membrane.
FAK	Activated by both integrin and FcεRI aggregation; normally localizes to focal adhesion sites. Associates with β integrins, paxillin, Src, Csk, Grb2, and PI3-K. Binds cytoskeletal protein vinculin.
Csk and Ctk	Tyrosine kinase with SH2 and SH3 domains. Phosphorylates Lyn in regulatory site and down-regulates its activity.

Lyn. The Src family protein tyrosine kinase $p53/56^{lyn}$ is coprecipitated with FcεRI from RBL-2H3 cells, whereas in mouse PT18 mast cells, another Src kinase, $p62^{c\text{-}yes}$, associates with the receptor.[100] The association of Lyn with the receptor is in both nonstimulated and activated cells.[361, 490] Unique α-galactosyl derivatives of the GD1b ganglioside present on mast cells may play a role in the association of Lyn with FcεRI.[305] Only a small fraction of FcεRI is associated with Lyn, and there is a threefold to fourfold increase in associated Lyn kinase after receptor aggregation. The phosphorylation of the receptor by Lyn is due to transphosphorylation similar to the reaction that has been described for receptors that are protein tyrosine kinases. The association of Lyn appears to be between the kinase and the COOH-terminal cytoplasmic domain of β but not with the γ subunit of FcεRI.[188] Replacement of the tyrosine residues in the ITAM motif of FcεRIβ with Phe produces only a modest decrease in the amount of associated $p53/56^{lyn}$. This suggests that the interaction between $p53/56^{lyn}$ and the β subunit is only partially, if at all, mediated by the tyrosine residues of the ITAM motif in FcεRIβ. The SH2 domain of $p53/56^{lyn}$ binds to tyrosine phosphorylated β but not the γ subunit of FcεRI. Thus SH2 domains of $p53/56^{lyn}$ may enhance the binding of $p53/56^{lyn}$ to the β subunit after receptor activation. Although FcεRI aggregation induces rapid tyrosine phosphorylation of $p53/56^{lyn}$ and an increase in its kinase activity, there is no direct evidence that this kinase is responsible for tyrosine phosphorylation of the β or γ subunits.

Src. The aggregation of FcεRI also results in the rapid tyrosine phosphorylation of $pp60^{c\text{-}src}$, which like $p53/56^{lyn}$ is a tyrosine kinase that has SH2 and SH3 domains and is associated with the plasma membrane due to myristoylation. Tyrosine phosphorylation of $pp60^{c\text{-}src}$ is apparent within 30 seconds after FcεRI aggregation and correlates with the increase in its tyrosine kinase activity. However, unlike $p53/56^{lyn}$, this kinase does not associate with FcεRI.

Syk Family. The Syk/ZAP-70 family protein tyrosine kinases have two tandem SH2 domains in the N-terminal half of the molecule.[56, 211, 450] Aggregation of FcεRI results in tyrosine phosphorylation of the protein tyrosine kinase $p72^{syk}$ and its association with the γ subunit of FcεRI.[32, 167, 211] Although there may be some association of Syk with the receptor in the nonstimulated state, the predominant interaction is with receptors that are aggregated and therefore tyrosine phosphorylated.[55] The in vivo tyrosine phosphorylation of Syk is rapid and parallels the in vitro increase in the kinase activity of $p72^{syk}$. With cell activation, there is association of $p72^{syk}$ with the γ subunit of FcεRI and minimal, if any, association with the β subunit. Chimeric proteins with the cytoplasmic domain of ζ or FcεRIγ fused to the extracellular and transmembrane domains of other proteins have been used for signal transduction studies. The chimeric molecules are then aggregated by antibodies to their extracellular domains. In such experiments, the cytoplasmic domains of FcεRIγ but not FcεRIβ result in in vivo tyrosine phosphorylation of $p72^{syk}$ and its activation. However, the chimeric molecules that contain γ are not themselves tyrosine phosphorylated. Thus tyrosine phosphorylation of the γ subunit by FcεRI aggregation may not be essential for the tyrosine phosphorylation of $p72^{syk}$ and degranulation.

The SH2 domains of $p72^{syk}$ bind strongly to the tyrosine-phosphorylated (but not to nonphosphorylated) γ subunit and less efficiently to the β subunit of FcεRI.[211, 412] This binding requires the two SH2 domains of Syk and suggests that the binding occurs when the two tandem SH2 domains form a bidentate association with closely spaced phosphorylated tyrosines of the same ITAM motif. In contrast, the SH2 domain of $p53/56^{lyn}$ binds only to the tyrosine-phosphorylated β subunit. The binding of $p53/56^{lyn}$ and $p72^{syk}$ to different subunits of FcεRI is probably due to the differences in the amino acid sequence of the ITAM motif on the β and γ subunits.

The Syk/ZAP-70 tyrosine kinases that are bound to the ITAMs are usually tyrosine phosphorylated and activated.[55, 56, 69] In transient transfection experiments, the activation of Syk/ZAP-70 requires the presence of the Src family kinase.[184] It is therefore postulated that the Src family kinase may tyrosine phosphorylate the Syk/ZAP-70 and induce activation.[184] Binding of Syk to a diphosphorylated ITAM peptide results in a conformational change and an increase in kinase activity. This change is likely involved in the downstream propagation of activation signals.[33] Aggregation of Syk introduced into mast cells as a chimeric transmembrane protein containing the extracellular and transmembrane domains of another molecule results in its tyrosine phosphorylation and in degranulation.[374] Therefore Syk is a critical component in signaling in mast cells.

Bruton Tyrosine Kinase (Btk). This is a 77-kD cytosolic protein that contains SH2, SH3, and PH domains. Btk is rapidly tyrosine phosphorylated and activated after FcεRI aggregation.[202] FcεRI aggregation also results in the translocation of Btk from the cytosol to the membrane, although it does not associate with FcεRI. However, Btk associates with several protein kinase C isoforms in vitro but only with PKC β1 in vivo. This association of BTK with protein kinase C is independent of FcεRI aggregation.[491] Btk is a substrate for PKC in vitro, and PKC-mediated phosphorylation on Ser results in the down-regulation of the enzymatic activity of BTK. FcεRI aggregation in PKC-depleted cells results in enhanced tyrosine phosphorylation of Btk, suggesting that PKC may modulate FcεRI-induced phosphorylation of Btk.

Focal Adhesion Kinase $pp125^{FAK}$. This is a nonreceptor protein tyrosine kinase that accumulates at focal adhesion sites.[143, 392] Focal adhesion sites, also called adhesion plaques, are areas where the plasma membrane of cells is attached to the extracellular matrix. Many other proteins, including integrins, localize to these sites. The $pp125^{FAK}$ kinase has a central catalytic domain and amino- and carboxyl-terminal noncatalytic regions. It is a cytosolic protein that lacks SH2 and SH3 domains and membrane localization signals. There is constitutive tyrosine phosphorylation of $pp125^{FAK}$ in adherent RBL-2H3 cells.[136] This phosphorylation is enhanced by treatment of the cells with PMA or Ca^{2+} ionophore. The aggregation of FcεRI in nonadherent RBL-2H3 cells induces the tyrosine phosphorylation of $pp125^{FAK}$ and enhances this phosphorylation in adherent cells. A monoclonal antibody to an FcεRI-associated ganglioside induces tyrosine phosphorylation of FcεRIβ, FcεRIγ, $p53/56^{lyn}$, PLCγ1, and $p72^{syk}$ but not of $pp125^{FAK}$.[440] This antibody, however, does not induce significant degranulation, suggesting a role for $pp125^{FAK}$ in secretion from mast cells. $pp125^{FAK}$ associates with a 77-kD protein in RBL-2H3 that is not Btk.[139] In vitro kinase reaction of Fak immunoprecipitates results in strong tyrosine phosphorylation of this protein, suggesting that it may be a substrate of $pp125^{FAK}$. As this 77-kD protein is tyrosine phosphorylated in vivo after FcεRI, it may play a role in FcεRI signaling and secretion.

Csk (Carboxy-Terminal Src Kinase). Csk is a tyrosine kinase that phosphorylates the regulatory tyrosine in Src family kinases such as Lyn. This results in down-regulation of the enzymatic activity of the kinase. This kinase has SH3 and SH2 domains and associates with Fak and paxillin. A second member of this family is Ctk. Both of these kinases are present in RBL-2H3 cells and may function to regulate the activity of Lyn.

Substrates

Substrates are proteins that are tyrosine phosphorylated after FcεRI aggregation (Tables 9–7, 9–8).

TABLE 9–7
SHE2/SH3-CONTAINING MOLECULES IN BASOPHIL/MAST CELL SIGNALING

Molecule	Characteristics
PLC-γ	Phospholipase: hydrolyzes inositol phospholipids such as PIP_2 forming DAG and IP_3. PLC-γ has two SH2, one SH3, and one PH domain; is tyrosine phosphorylated after FcεRI aggregation.
Nck	Has one SH2 and three SH3 domains; tyrosine phosphorylated after FcεRI activation.
HS1 (SPY75)	Consists of helix-turn-helix motif, nuclear localization signal, and SH3 domain. Tyrosine phosphorylated after FcεRI aggregation.
PI-3K	Lipid kinase specific for phosphatidyl inositol on the D3 position. Two subunits; 85 kD (85α) subunit has two SH2 domains and an SH3 domain that associates with a 110-kD enzymatic subunit. Is tyrosine phosphorylated after FcεRI aggregation.
RasGAP	GTPase-activating protein (GAP) for Ras contains two SH2 domains and an SH3 and PH domain. Deactivates Ras.
Crk	Has an SH2 domain and two SH3 domains. Associates with paxillin.

FcεRI. Aggregation of FcεRI in the RBL-2H3 cells results in the rapid tyrosine phosphorylation of the β and γ subunits of FcεRI.[241, 346] Interestingly, the β and γ subunits are phosphorylated on tyrosine only in aggregated FcεRI. This tyrosine phosphorylation of both subunits is rapidly reversed by the addition of hapten to disaggregate the receptors. Mutations of the β subunit in which Tyr residues in the ITAM sequence are replaced with Phe markedly decrease the in vivo and in vitro tyrosine phosphorylation of the γ subunit.[188] This suggests that tyrosine phosphorylation of the β subunit, presumably by $p53/56^{lyn}$, plays an important role in the tyrosine phosphorylation of FcεRIγ. Furthermore, these results suggest that tyrosine residues in the ITAM motif of FcεRIβ may promote the further binding of either the same or a different protein tyrosine kinase that subsequently phosphorylates the γ subunit.

The tyrosine phosphorylation of FcεRIβ and FcεRIγ subunits by the aggregation of FcεRI renders both subunits accessible for interacting with SH2-containing molecules and further propagating the receptor-mediated signals. Both p53/$p56^{lyn}$ and $p72^{syk}$ contain SH2 domains. As discussed above, the SH2 domains of $p72^{syk}$ bind strongly to the tyrosine-phosphorylated (but not to nonphosphorylated) γ subunit and less efficiently to the β subunit of FcεRI.[211] In contrast, the SH2 domains of $p53/56^{lyn}$ bind only to the β subunit, and this is enhanced when this subunit is tyrosine phosphorylated.

Several observations suggest a role for the tyrosine phosphorylation of FcεRIγ and FcεRβ in receptor-mediated signaling and secretion. First, tyrosine phosphorylation of both subunits is rapid. Second, when the Tyr residues in the ITAM motif of β are replaced with Phe, not only is the FcεRI-induced tyrosine phosphorylation of β blocked, but there is also a decrease in the tyrosine phosphorylation of FcεRIγ and other intracellular proteins. Third, SH2 domains of $p72^{syk}$ or $p53/56^{lyn}$ bind only to tyrosine-phosphorylated γ and β. Fourth, aggregating the extracellular domain of chimeric proteins containing the cytoplasmic domain of the γ subunit induces signaling and secretion in RBL-2H3 mast cells, although it is unclear whether this chimeric molecule is itself tyrosine phosphorylated. Fifth, deletion of the C-terminal cytoplasmic tail of β that contains an ITAM motif abrogates activation responses.

Phospholipase C-γ1. Another SH2-containing protein that is rapidly phosphorylated on tyrosine after FcεRI aggregation is phospholipase C-γ1 (PLCγ1).[108, 241, 347, 400] This PLCγ contains two SH2 domains and one SH3 domain and catalyzes the hydrolysis of phosphatidylinositol 4,5-bisphosphate, resulting in the generation of inositol 1,4,5-trisphosphate and 1,2,diacylglycerol (DAG). These second messengers release Ca^{2+} from internal stores and activate PKC, respectively. Both events are essential for FcεRI-mediated secretion. Incubation of RBL-2H3 cells or mouse bone marrow culture-derived mast cells with inhibitors of protein tyrosine kinase activity (e.g., genistein) blocked FcεRI-mediated tyrosine phosphorylation of PLC, the generation of inositol phosphates, and secretion. These results suggest that FcεRI cross-linking activates PLCγ1 and stimulates PtdIns hydrolysis by increasing the tyrosine phosphorylation of PLCγ1 and its association with the plasma membrane. However, in other experiments, genistein markedly decreased the total cellular protein tyrosine phosphorylations without inhibiting PtdIns hydrolysis. The protein tyrosine kinase responsible for phosphorylating PLCγ1 is not known, although by analogy to lymphocytes, it is probably the Syk kinase. A 44-kD protein tyrosine kinase has been found to be associated with PLCγ1

TABLE 9–8
OTHER MOLECULES PROBABLY INVOLVED IN BASOPHIL/MAST CELL SIGNALING

Molecule	Characteristics
PKC	Family of Ser/Thr kinases; β and δ critical for secretion; α and ε inhibit secretion; β associates with FcεRI-β and phosphorylated FcεRI-γ on Thr. Activated by DAG and calcium.
IP_3R	Receptor for IP_3 in the ER; a Ca^{2+} channel protein; composed of four subunits. Binding of IP_3 opens channel and releases Ca^{2+} to the cytosol.
Paxillin	Cytoskeletal protein, accumulates at focal adhesion sites. Associates with Lyn, Src, Csk, Fak, and Crk. Binds to vinculin, another cytoskeletal protein, which itself interacts with other cytoskeletal proteins, including talin, tensin, and actin filaments.
Vav	Two SH3, one SH2, PH, acidic CDC24 homology region and a region homologous to the DAG-binding site of PKC. Binds to activated receptors and is itself tyrosine phosphorylated after FcεRI aggregation. May activate Ras.
Vimentin	Intermediate cytoskeletal proteins; phosphorylated on Ser probably by PKC after stimulation.
cPLA2	Cytoplasmic phospholipase A2; phosphorylated on Ser by MAPK. Translocates to the membrane in activated cells; releases arachidonic acid.
Myosin	Light chain and heavy chain of myosin phosphorylated by PKC on Ser by cell activation.

in mouse bone marrow culture-derived mast cells.[108] This 44-kD kinase phosphorylates PLCγ1 on tyrosine in vitro. Aggregation of FcεRI activates the kinase as determined by the increase in its in vitro autophosphorylation and the increased in vitro phosphorylation of PLCγ1. The activation parallels the increase in the in vivo phosphorylation of PLCγ1 by FcεRI aggregation. It is possible that this 44 kD is a proteolytic fragment of Syk that is frequently observed in experiments.

Paxillin. Paxillin is a cytoskeletal protein that accumulates at focal adhesion sites. It has several sequence motifs, including binding sites for SH2 domains, SH3 domains, vinculin, and $pp125^{FAK}$. Tyrosine phosphorylation of paxillin by FcεRI is slower than that of other proteins such as subunits of FcεRI and of Syk. The optimal tyrosine phosphorylation of paxillin by FcεRI aggregation requires PKC and extracellular Ca^{2+}. In vitro, paxillin is phosphorylated on tyrosine by $pp125^{FAK}$. This suggests that the activation of $pp125^{FAK}$ by FcεRI aggregation may be responsible for the in vivo tyrosine phosphorylation of paxillin. In vitro, paxillin interacts with other proteins that have SH2 and SH3 domains. $p53/56^{lyn}$ proteins produced by molecular biologic techniques bind in vitro to several tyrosine-phosphorylated proteins from RBL-2H3 cells, one of which is paxillin. This binding is mediated by the SH2 domain of $p53/56^{lyn}$, and there is binding only with tyrosine-phosphorylated paxillin.[304] Thus paxillin binds to several tyrosine kinases and to cytoskeletal proteins and could play an important role in signal transduction from FcεRI to the cytoskeleton.

Other Substrates. The aggregation of FcεRI also induces the tyrosine phosphorylation of many other proteins. Among those that have been identified are HS1 (also called SPY75), $p95^{vav}$, and Nck. All these proteins are phosphorylated on tyrosine residues after FcεRI cross-linking in RBL-2H3 cells or in bone marrow–derived mast cells. As several of these proteins have SH2 and/or SH3 domains and because they become phosphorylated on tyrosine, they can associate with other molecules during signal transduction and therefore may play a role in protein-protein interactions during FcεRI signaling.

Nck consists almost exclusively of three SH3 domains and one SH2 domain.[242] HS1 has one SH3 domain close to its C-terminal and putative nuclear localization signal and repetitive helix-turn-helix motifs found in many DNA-binding proteins.[110, 303]

$p95^{vav}$ is expressed only in cells of the hematopoietic lineage.[275] It has several sequence motifs similar to signaling molecules, including one SH2 domain, two SH3 domains, and a PH domain, as well as acidic regions and a putative diacylglycerol/phorbol ester-binding domain. Vav can bind to tyrosine-phosphorylated proteins through its SH2 domain and itself is tyrosine phosphorylated after cell activation. Although some reports have suggested that tyrosine-phosphorylated Vav may activate Ras due to its guanine nucleotide dissociation stimulator function (i.e., it exchanges GDP for GTP), these observations were not confirmed by other investigators. Vav also contains a Cys-rich region that may be involved in binding to DAG. It is also tyrosine phosphorylated after c-Kit receptor stimulation on mast cells.[1] SH2 of Vav associates with ZAP70 in T cells[200] and also interacts with the adaptor protein Grb2.[492] Thus Vav may link tyrosine phosphorylation with subsequent signal transduction events.

Hematopoietic protein tyrosine phosphatase (HePTP) is a protein tyrosine phosphatase that is present in RBL-2H3 cells and is tyrosine phosphorylated after cell activation.[442] This phosphatase is also tyrosine phosphorylated after stimulation of cells with calcium ionophore, suggesting that its phosphorylation is a later event in degranulation.

Phosphatidylinositol 3-kinase (PI 3-kinase) is a heterodimer consisting of an 85-kD regulatory subunit (p85) and a 110-kD catalytic subunit. The p85 subunit has an SH3 and two SH2 domains and is tyrosine phosphorylated after FcεRI aggregation. The interaction of p85 with tyrosine-phosphorylated proteins stimulates the PI 3-kinase activity of the p110 catalytic subunit. PI 3-kinase interacts with several proteins and is required for membrane ruffling.

Other proteins, also, are tyrosine phosphorylated during secretion. For example, the tyrosine phosphorylation of a 110-kD protein is induced by different cell activation signals, including FcεRI, Ca^{2+} ionophore, G protein, and PKC.[34] The phosphorylation of this protein is a later event in exocytosis.

Protein tyrosine kinase activation can regulate downstream signaling by several mechanisms. First, tyrosine phosphorylation of proteins, including enzymes, can regulate their activity. For example, the serine/threonine kinase activity of Raf-1 is activated by tyrosine phosphorylation.[317] Similarly, the tyrosine phosphorylation of phospholipase C-γ1 results in increased catalytic activity,[331] although in some cells there can be increased tyrosine phosphorylation of phospholipase-Cγ1 without the concomitant hydrolysis of PtdIns.[233] Second, there is recruitment of the SH2 domain containing proteins to the phosphorylated residues on the receptor. Third, recruitment of these molecules then results in activation of signaling by a variety of mechanisms, including tyrosine phosphorylation (e.g., phospholipase C-γ1), conformational changes (e.g., Syk, p85α, and SH-PTP2 tyrosine phosphatase), and translocation to the membrane (e.g, PLC-γ).

Protein Tyrosine Phosphatases

The induction of protein tyrosine phosphorylation after stimulation does not necessarily indicate activation of protein tyrosine kinases. Rather, tyrosine phosphorylation depends on the dynamic balance between competing reactions: increased phosphorylation by the protein tyrosine kinase versus dephosphorylation by protein tyrosine phosphatase.[105, 166] The protein tyrosine phosphatases are a growing family of molecules, some of which are receptor-like, as best characterized by CD45 (leukocyte common antigen),[63, 457] whereas others have no extracellular domains. The CD45 molecule plays an important role in T-cell signaling,[9, 380] probably by dephosphorylating the Src-related tyrosine kinase $p56^{lck}$ that associates with the CD4 and CD8 molecules.[463]

There are many different protein tyrosine phosphatases in mast cells, including CD45, a transmembrane protein that may play a role in mast cell activation (Table 9–9).[39, 156] In the earliest experiments, addition of monoclonal antibodies to CD45 to human basophils blocked IgE-mediated histamine release but not that induced by fMet peptide, Ca^{2+} ionophore A23187, or phorbol myristic acetate. It is likely

TABLE 9–9
PROTEIN TYROSINE PHOSPHATASES IDENTIFIED IN BASOPHILS AND MAST CELLS

Molecule	Characteristics
CD45	Protein tyrosine phosphatase with an extracellular domain and two intracellular phosphatase domains. Dephosphorylates Lyn at its regulatory site, resulting in activation.
HePTP	Hematopoietic protein tyrosine phosphatase; cytosolic. Tyr phosphorylated after mast cell activation.
PTP1C (SH-PTP1)	Cytosolic phosphatase, has two SH2 domains; binds to activated c-KIT receptor. Is tyrosine phosphorylated in growth factor–stimulated cells.
Syp (SH-PTP2)	Cytosolic phosphatase, has two SH2 domains; binds to activated c-KIT receptor. Binds to Grb2 and to activated protein tyrosine kinase receptors.

that binding of the anti-CD45 antibodies results in changes in the intracellular protein tyrosine phosphatase activity. If protein tyrosine phosphorylation is a critical signal for secretion, then an increase in tyrosine phosphatase activity could result in a decrease in the intracellular protein tyrosine phosphorylation and thus block secretion. Mast cells have been derived from mice in which CD45 was genetically inactivated.[39] These cells secrete when activated with calcium ionophores but not when stimulated through FcεRI. However, the exact nature of the defect in these cells and whether there is inhibition of the early tyrosine phosphorylation steps have not been determined.

There are several other protein tyrosine phosphatases in basophils and mast cells.[442] These include the two SH2 containing protein tyrosine phosphatases, PTP1C (also called SH-PTP1), and Syp (also called SH-PTP2, PTP1D, and PTP2C). Both PTP1C and Syp have two SH2 domains and bind several growth factor receptors that are protein tyrosine kinases, including the c-Kit receptor. Both are tyrosine phosphorylated after growth factor stimulation of cells and associate with several proteins, including Grb2. There is also a protein tyrosine phosphatase associated with the high-affinity receptor that is not CD45 or the SH2 containing protein tyrosine phosphatases.[441] This phosphatase dephosphorylated both the tyrosine phosphorylated β and γ subunits but not Lyn or Syk. Therefore, this phosphatase may be involved in regulating the steady-state tyrosine phosphorylation level of the FcεRI subunits. There is also protein tyrosine phosphatase activity that is increased after cell stimulation either by FcεRI aggregation or with Ca^{2+} ionophores and is dependent on the increase in $[Ca^{2+}]_i$, suggesting that it may play a role in degranulation.[142] Altogether, these data suggest that protein tyrosine kinases and phosphatases play critical roles in the FcεRI-mediated signaling in basophils and mast cells.

The following model of the early tyrosine phosphorylation events in mast cells has emerged (Fig. 9–2). Aggregation of the receptor results in activation of protein tyrosine kinase(s). This is most likely the Src family protein tyrosine kinase Lyn that is associated with the receptor. The mechanism of this

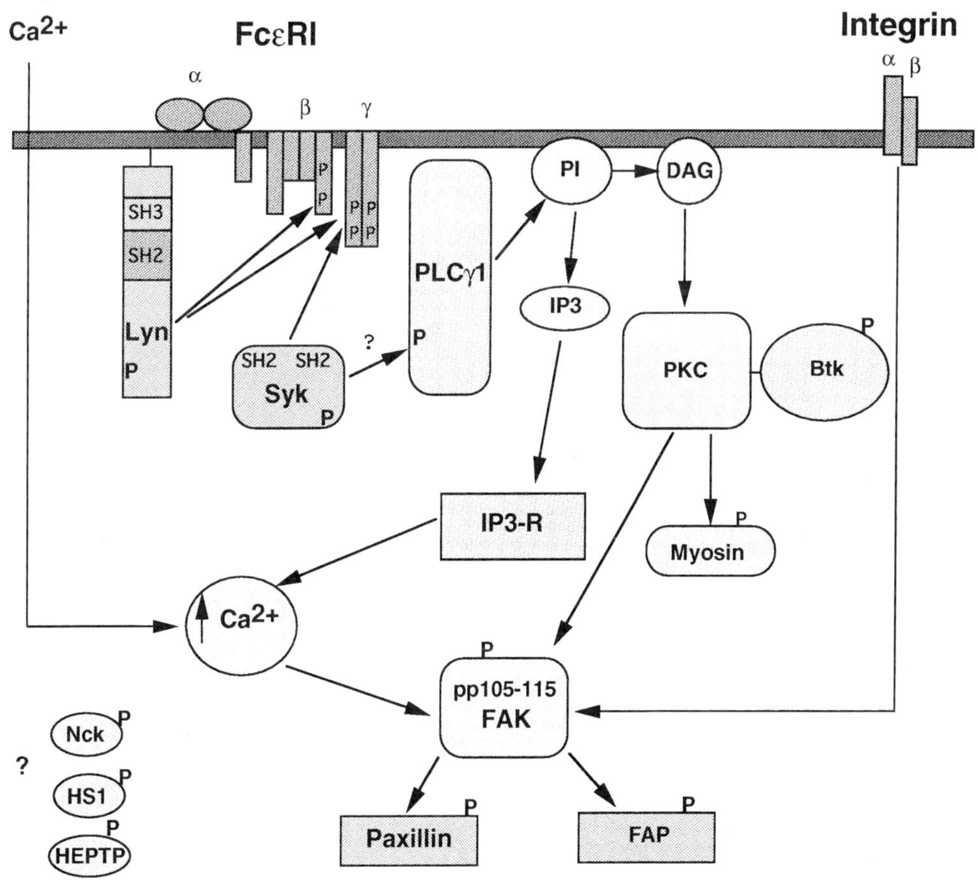

FIGURE 9–2. Early FcεRI-mediated signaling pathways. Arrows indicate both the interaction of molecules and the enzymatic products. Proteins that are phosphorylated are marked with P. Arrows do not always indicate a direct interaction but may include intervening steps. Other proteins that are phosphorylated are listed in the lower left corner; the exact interaction of these with the other molecules is still unclear.

activation is unclear but may involve the dephosphorylation of Lyn at its regulatory site by a protein tyrosine phosphatase. The activation of Lyn results in intermolecular phosphorylation at the autophosphorylation sites. Alternatively, aggregation of the receptor may exclude a protein tyrosine phosphatase that normally maintains the ITAMs of FcεRI in the dephosphorylated state. Activation of Lyn would result in phosphorylation of the Tyr residues in the ITAMs of both the β and γ subunits of the receptor. Phosphorylation of the two tyrosines in the ITAM recruits Syk to the receptor. The binding and activation of the Syk kinase result in the tyrosine phosphorylation of downstream substrates. A number of other protein tyrosine kinases, such as Btk and Fak, are also activated during cell stimulation.

ROLE OF GTP-BINDING PROTEINS

The GTP-binding proteins are a family of molecules that are the transducers of signals from many membrane hormone receptors to intracellular effectors.[434] These GTP-binding proteins (or GTPases) are classified into two groups: the high molecular weight or heterotrimeric GTP-binding proteins (G proteins) and the low molecular weight monomeric GTP-binding proteins (e.g., ras). Both types of proteins are widely distributed in different tissues. Several high molecular weight heterotrimeric G proteins are well characterized and include G_s, G_i, G_o, and transducin. Whereas G_s and G_i appear to be present in most cells, G_o is described in the brain and transducin in the retina. These heterotrimers consist of three proteins: the α chain of 39 to 52 kD that has guanine, nucleotide binding activity, the β chain of 35 to 36 kD, and the γ chain of 7 to 10 kD. The three components associate when GDP is bound to the α chain (forming the GDPαβγ complex). This complex is inactive and membrane bound. Ligand binding to a receptor results in a conformational change and triggers G protein activation by exchanging GTP for the bound GDP. This results in the dissociation of the α chain from the other two components, leaving the βγ complex. Both the Gα and dissociated Gβγ subunits can transduce cellular signals. There are four subfamilies of the G protein α subunit and multiple G protein β and γ subunits. The α chain of the G proteins can be specifically ADP ribosylated by bacterial toxins: the G_s with cholera toxin and the G_i with pertussis toxin. G proteins are coupled to different second messengers and ion channels within the cell. The activation of this pathway can result in either the stimulation (by G_s) or inhibition (by G_i) of adenylate cyclase or in the hydrolysis of PtdIns.

Many receptors (including those for muscarinic, adrenergic, or C5a) are coupled to G proteins.[415] These receptors have a characteristic topological structure with seven membrane-spanning domains and amino acid sequence similarity. Although the three components of the FcεRI together have seven transmembrane-spanning domains, they do not have any amino acid similarity to the G protein–coupled receptor family.

There is evidence for a role for G proteins in exocytosis from mast cells.[129] In permeabilized rat mast cells, nonhydrolyzable GTP analogs stimulate secretion of histamine. Similarly, there is exocytosis if these compounds are introduced into mast cells through patch pipettes.[102] There appear to be two different sites for the action of these molecules within the cell; one site is postulated to be in the plasma membrane and activates PtdIns hydrolysis, whereas a second site is distal to the action of Ca^{2+} and PKC.[64, 80, 352] This second GTP-binding protein, G_E, may be an integral part of the membrane fusion mechanism and may activate exocytosis.[14, 130] The G protein coupled to PtdIns hydrolysis results in Ca^{2+} signals in the cell.[470] In RBL-2H3 cells, the Ca^{2+} influx appears to be more dependent on G proteins than does PtdIns hydrolysis.[485] Microinjection of stable GTP analogues into rat mast cells results in degranulation if there is Ca^{2+} in the medium.[61] Therefore, the signals generated by GTP together with Ca^{2+}-mediated signals induce exocytosis.

There is also evidence for a role of G proteins in the FcεRI-mediated degranulation. In RBL-2H3 cells, stimulation of G proteins by either AlF_4^+ complexes or GTPγS (a nonhydrolyzable GTP analogue) induces both PtdIns hydrolysis and histamine release.[5, 73] Furthermore, GDPβS (an inhibitor of G protein activation) decreases both PtdIns hydrolysis and histamine secretion induced by either FcεRI cross-linking or GTPγS.[4] Similarly, the depletion of GTP by mycophenolic acid inhibits the FcεRI-mediated cell activation.[485] Still, the G protein responsible for coupling the FcεRI to PtdIns-PLC has not been identified. Studies with bacterial toxins in RBL-2H3 cells suggest that FcεRI activation is pertussis toxin–insensitive, although there is ADP ribosylation of a cellular protein.[6] Therefore, the coupling of FcεRI to PtdIns-PLC must require a pertussis toxin–resistant Gα subunit. By contrast, in bone marrow–derived cultured mouse mast cells, PtdIns-PLC activation is independent of G proteins.[387]

Toxins that ADP-ribosylate some G proteins have been used to inhibit histamine release. In most experimental systems, pertussis toxin does not inhibit the FcεRI-mediated release.[323, 388] Still, it does inhibit the release induced by other secretagogues. For example, in rat mast cells, pertussis toxin inhibits 48/80-induced Ca^{2+} uptake, arachidonic acid, and histamine release.[222, 324] This suggests that a pertussis toxin–sensitive G protein is involved in activating the Ca^{2+} channel with this secretagogue. Similarly, in bone marrow–derived mast cells, it inhibited the thrombin-mediated but not the IgE-mediated degranulation.[388] With human basophils, pertussis toxin inhibits the fMet peptide- and C5a-mediated but not the IgE-mediated release.[47, 476] Therefore, the receptors for some of these other secretagogues are coupled to pertussis toxin–sensitive G proteins.

The small G proteins are associated with signal transduction from the cell surface[204] and may also play a role in mast cell or basophil secretion. The microinjection into rat mast cells of the Ras oncogene, which is a member of this family of GTP-binding proteins, results in exocytosis.[18] The Rab small GTP-binding protein is present in mast cells, and intracellular injection of peptides based on the Rab3a structure results in degranulation.[335, 336] However, even the extracellular addition of these peptides induced intracellular Ca^{2+} changes and secretion.[228] Two other small G proteins, Rac and Rho (Table 9–10), may also play a role in secretion[362] through their action on regulating cytoskeletal rearrangements.

In rat mast cells, compound 48/80 and peptides such as mastoparan or LHRH induce exocytosis by directly activating

TABLE 9–10
SMALL GTP-BINDING PROTEINS THAT MAY BE INVOLVED IN BASOPHIL AND MAST CELL SECRETION

Molecule	Characteristics
Rab3a	Microinjection of peptides based on structure induces secretion.
Ras	Activated in basophils and mast cells (see Table 9–11).
Rho, Rac	Participate in changes in the cytoskeleton. Rho essential for stress fiber formation, RAC for membrane ruffles.

G proteins.[13] In permeabilized cells, the introduction of a synthetic peptide corresponding to the COOH-terminal end of the sequence of $G\alpha_{i3}$ blocked this secretion.

TABLE 9–11
COMPONENTS OF RAS ACTIVATION PATHWAY

Molecule	Characteristics
Shc	Has PTB and SH2 domains. Is tyrosine phosphorylated in RBL-2H3 cells; but no change in phosphorylation after FcεRI aggregation.
Grb2	SH3-SH2-SH3 adaptor protein that links receptors to Ras activation. Associates with tyrosine phosphorylated proteins (including receptor subunits and Fak) by SH2 domain and with SOS by the SH3 domain.
mSOS	Converts inactive Ras-GDP to active Ras-GTP. Binds to SH3 domain of Grb2.
Vav	Two SH3, one SH2, PH, acidic CDC24 homology region and a region homologous to the DAG binding site of PKC. Binds to activated receptors and is itself tyrosine phosphorylated after FcεRI aggregation. May activate Ras.

RAS PATHWAY

In this pathway, a small guanine nucleotide–binding protein links signals from the early tyrosine phosphorylation events at the membrane to a cytosolic protein kinase cascade (Fig. 9–3). Activation of Ras is an important intermediary in this pathway. It is activated to the GTP form by guanine nucleotide exchange. This results from signals generated from tyrosine phosphorylation after cell activation. By analogy to T cells, activation of Ras by FcεRI would be downstream of the activation of the nonreceptor protein tyrosine kinases of the Src and Syk families such as Lyn and Syk. The next section will describe the members of this pathway (Tables 9–11, 9–12; also see Fig. 9–3).

Shc. Shc is a 46- and 52-kD adaptor protein with a carboxy-terminal SH2 domain that binds to activated growth factor receptors that are tyrosine kinases and an N-terminal PTB domain. The Shc gene encodes two overlapping, widely expressed proteins of 46 and 52 kD. A minor and variably expressed 66 kD protein is encoded by a distinct Shc transcript. Stimulation of T and B cells results in tyrosine phosphorylation of Shc and the formation of a complex that

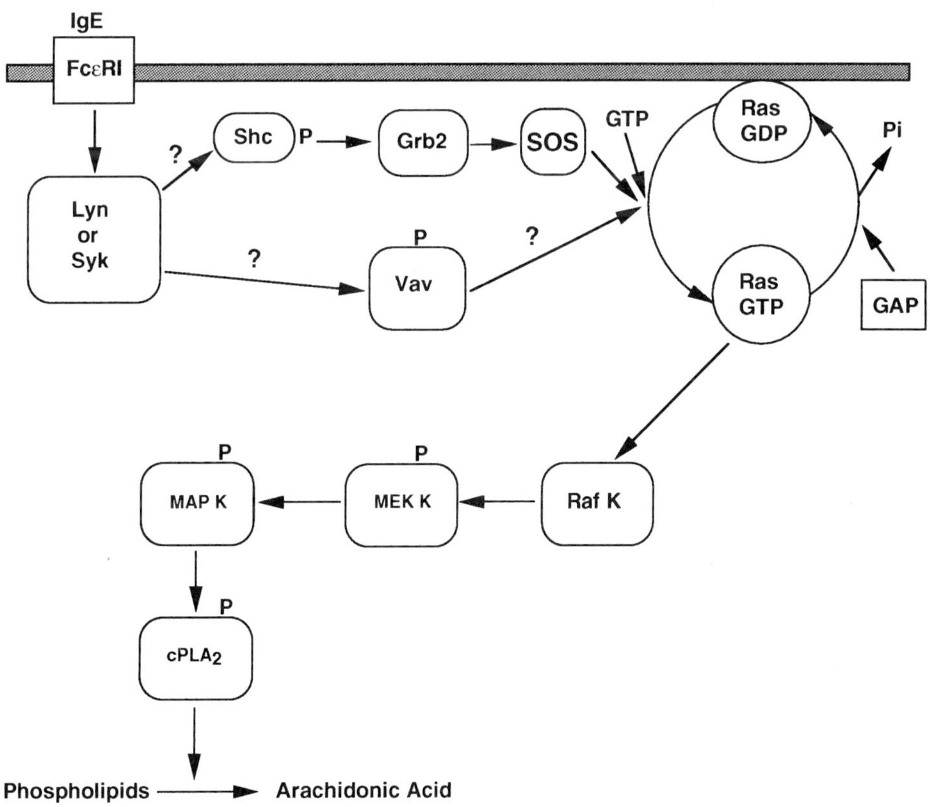

FIGURE 9–3. Pathways of activation of Ras and MAP kinase. Characteristics of these molecules are described in the tables, especially Tables 9–11 and 9–12.

TABLE 9–12
RAS PATHWAY FOR ACTIVATION OF MAP KINASE

Molecule	Characteristics
Ras	21 kD protein, member of small GTPase superfamily. Activated by guanine nucleotide exchange factor (e.g., SOS); inactivated by Ras-GAP. Binds Raf.
Raf	70–75 kD proteins. Ser/Thr protein kinase; kinase domain in the COOH-terminal half and a regulatory domain in the rest. Binds to activated Ras. Activated by recruitment to the membrane and by tyrosine phosphorylation?
MEK	41–45 kD proteins. A dual specificity kinase that phosphorylates both Tyr and Thr residues. It is activated by Ser phosphorylation by Raf. There are several isoforms (MEK-1a, MEK-1b, and MEK-2).
MAP (ERK-1, ERK-2)	40–44 kD proteins. Ser/Thr kinase. Activated by dual phosphorylation on Tyr and Ser by MEK. Are activated by FcεRI aggregation. Substrates include cPLA2, transcription factors, RSK kinase.
RSK	90 kD (by cDNA 70) Ser/Thr kinase. Activated by Thr phosphorylation by MAPK. Has two kinase domains in COOH-terminal region. Substrates include S6 ribosomal protein, and transcription factors c-Fos and GSK-3 kinase.

contains Shc, Grb2, and Sos.[366, 391, 424] However, in RBL-2H3 cells, Shc is constitutively tyrosine phosphorylated and associated with Grb2.[462] Furthermore, FcεRI aggregation does not result in an increase in its phosphorylation.[462]

Grb2. Grb2 is a 23-kD adaptor protein that does not get tyrosine phosphorylated. It has an SH2 and two SH3 domains. The SH2 domain of Grb2 binds to tyrosine-phosphorylated Shc. Grb2 also binds to Fak through its SH2 domain. Grb2 associates through one of its SH3 domains with Sos (the mammalian homologue of the *Drosophila* son of sevenless). Sos is constitutively associated with Grb2; this complex is usually cytosolic but gets membrane associated after cell activation and therefore can act on Ras. Sos is a guanine nucleotide exchange factor that activates Ras to the GTP form by the promotion of guanine nucleotide exchange. Thus Shc binds to tyrosine-phosphorylated receptors and recruits the adaptor protein Grb2, which then binds Sos. Vav also has guanine nucleotide exchange factor activity and may play a role in activating Ras. Thus two pathways, one mediated by Shc-Grb2-Sos and the other by Vav, could result in the activation of Ras.

Ras. Ras is a member of the small GTPase superfamily. In the inactive state, Ras has bound GDP. It is activated by the dissociation of GDP and the binding of GTP, a step that is facilitated by guanine nucleotide exchange factor such as Sos. This results in the activation of downstream kinases. Ras is then deactivated by GTPase-activating proteins (GAP), which results in the hydrolysis of GTP. Ras can activate several effector pathways, which may involve the Raf, Jun, and p38 pathways. Only the Raf pathway is known to be activated in mast cells.

Raf. Raf is a 70- to 75-kD cytosolic protein Ser/Thr kinase. The activation of Raf by tyrosine kinase pathways requires $p21^{ras}$. Activated Ras binds Raf and thus recruits Raf to the plasma membrane where another tyrosine kinase–mediated signal results in its activation. Two signals are required; one is RasGTP, and the other is unknown. There is tyrosine phosphorylation of Raf that may play a role in its activation. However, Ras also activates other effector pathways that lead to Jun kinase activation.

MEK. Mitogen-activated ERK-activating kinase (MEK), also called MAP-kinase kinase, is activated by Raf, which phosphorylates two Ser that are four amino acids apart.[410] MEKs are dual specificity kinases that activate the ERKs by phosphorylating them on both the Tyr and Thr residues.

ERK. Extracellular signal-regulated kinase (ERK), also called mitogen-activated protein kinase (MAPK), is activated in this pathway. There are other MAPK that are activated by stress signals to the cell. The substrates of ERK1 ($p44^{MAPK}$) and ERK2 ($p42^{MAPK}$) include transcription factors such as c-Jun, c-Fos, and the RSK ($p90^{rsk}$) kinase. Activated ERK1/ERK2 can phosphorylate SOS and Raf and may regulate their functions. As discussed later, these also phosphorylate cPLA2. In mast cells, FcεRI aggregation and also stimulation of the c-Kit receptor result in the phosphorylation and activation of ERK1 and ERK2.[109, 337, 390, 460] The phosphorylation of these proteins may require activation of protein kinase C. The activation of ERK/MAPK appears to be a late event in exocytosis and correlates with the extent of secretion. Not only FcεRI activation but also calcium ionophores and activation of G protein–mediated receptors all result in activation of MAPK.

RSK. RSK is a protein Ser/Thr kinase that is activated by Ser phosphorylation. It has two distinct kinase domains that are located in its COOH-terminal part. Its substrates include the ribosomal protein S6, which may not be physiologically relevant. Other substrates are the transcription factor c-Fos. It is also phosphorylated after FcεRI aggregation.[460]

Aggregation of FcεRI results in nuclear events such as the accumulation of nuclear transcription factors of the Fos and Jun families and the induction of a number of genes.[20, 88, 461] The ERK-mediated phosphorylation of the transcription factors of the c-Jun and c-Fos families allows their nuclear migration and the induction of new genes. However, protein kinase C is also important for the phosphorylation and activation of these nuclear factors.[370] The Ras pathway leading from FcεRI aggregation to nuclear transcription factors may play an important role in the induction of cytokine genes in stimulated mast cells.

ACTIVATION OF ADENYLATE CYCLASE

Adenylate cyclase is a membrane-associated enzyme that is regulated by activated G proteins. It results in the formation of cyclic 3′,5′-adenosine monophosphate (cAMP) that acts as an intracellular second messenger. In some pathways, an increased level of cAMP provides a signal for cell activation.

There are conflicting reports on whether a rise in cAMP is present and/or plays any role in signal transduction in basophils and mast cells.[8, 445] Some investigators have observed an increase in intracellular cAMP on FcεRI stimulation of human and rat mast cells or basophils.[181, 182, 262, 350, 437] When reported, the cAMP rise is an early, rapid response, can be blocked by both methylation and protease inhibitors, and occurs in the absence of extracellular Ca^{2+} and before the increase in $[Ca^{2+}]_i$.[176, 177, 181, 182, 438] A late rise in cAMP has also been observed; this is a secondary effect due to the PGD_2 released from cells,[240, 448] occurs in a different compartment, and inhibits secretion. In contrast, in RBL-2H3 cells, the FcεRI-mediated stimulation does not result in an increase in the intracellular cAMP levels.[315] Therefore, a rise in cAMP is not essential for secretion but might modulate other intracellular events.

The level of cAMP appears to modulate the secretion of mediators from mast cells and basophils.[48, 350, 439, 486] Several pharmacologic agents bind to specific cell surface receptors, activate adenylate cyclase, and increase intracellular cAMP levels. These compounds include the β-adrenergic agents, prostaglandins, and histamine acting through the H2 receptors. The intracellular levels of cAMP also can be raised by the addition of exogenous cAMP or its analogue, 8-bromocyclic AMP, and by the addition of inhibitors of the phosphodiesterase enzyme involved in the breakdown of cAMP. These agents have been reported to inhibit mediator release in a variety of in vitro systems, including human basophils and mast cells. Therefore, the increased cAMP levels could be a normal turnoff signal for secretion in these cells.

The intracellular effects of cAMP are mediated by the cAMP-dependent protein kinases. Increased intracellular cAMP levels activate cAMP-dependent protein kinases that phosphorylate their respective protein substrates on Ser/Thr residues. In the rat mast cell, both type I and type II cAMP-dependent protein kinase activity is present in the cytoplasm and is activated after IgE-mediated cell triggering.[486] The resulting phosphorylation of cellular proteins could then modulate the release process. However, the increased intracellular cAMP levels following the addition of PGD_2 or theophylline do not activate the protein kinase enzymes.

HYDROLYSIS OF PHOSPHATIDYL INOSITIDES AND PHOSPHOLIPID TURNOVER

The activation of many different types of receptors results in the hydrolysis of myoinositol-containing phospholipids due to the activation of phospholipase C, resulting in the generation of products that are intracellular second messengers.[40, 271, 333] There are three myoinositol-containing phosphatides: phosphatidylinositol (PtdIns), phosphatidylinositol 4-phosphate (PIP), and phosphoinositol 4,5-bisphosphate (PIP2). They account for less than 10% of the total phospholipid of the cell, with PtdIns accounting for over 90% of the inositides. Receptor stimulation results in the hydrolysis of phosphoinositides with the release of water-soluble inositol phosphates and 1,2-diacylglycerol (DAG). These two then are important synergistic second messengers within the cell; DAG activates PKC, whereas some inositol phosphates release Ca^{2+} from the endoplasmic reticulum. For example, the hydrolysis of phosphatidylinositol 4,5-bisphosphate results in the formation of inositol 1,4,5-trisphosphate (IP_3) that releases Ca^{2+} from ATP-dependent Ca^{2+} stores in the endoplasmic reticulum of the cell. Hydrolysis of other phosphoinositides and the interconversion of the inositol phosphates and their degradation products also occur and might be secondary to the rise in intracellular Ca^{2+}. These enzymatic pathways result in the rapid conversion of inositol 1,4,5-trisphosphate to inositol 1,3,4,5-tetrakisphosphate and subsequently to inositol 1,3,4-trisphosphate.[25] Several of these molecules appear to have the capacity to release Ca^{2+} from intracellular stores.

The FcεRI stimulation of RBL-2H3 cells results in a rapid breakdown of PtdIns.[27, 270] Although some of this PtdIns hydrolysis precedes the rise in intracellular Ca^{2+},[25, 72, 360] the major hydrolysis of PtdIns is a Ca^{2+}-dependent event. Once the hydrolysis of PtdIns has started, it is no longer dependent on external Ca^{2+} for continuation, although secretion of histamine is totally dependent on external Ca^{2+}.[269] There is some hydrolysis of PtdIns following stimulation with the Ca^{2+} ionophore A23187 that correlates with secretion.[250] There is also hydrolysis of PtdIns in permeabilized cells and cytoplasts that are devoid of organelles.[25, 91] In permeabilized cells, there is release of inositol 1,4,5-trisphosphate by either stimulation of FcεRI or activation of G proteins by GTP-γ-S.[5] In these cells, there is also formation of inositol 1,4-bisphosphate, suggesting that both phosphatidylinositol 4-monophosphate and 4,5-bisphosphate are substrates for the activated phospholipase C. An increase in inositol 1,4,5-trisphosphate alone is not sufficient or essential for histamine release.[123] Thus although inositol phosphates probably play a critical role in signal transduction, other biochemical events are also important.

The hydrolysis of membrane inositol phospholipids is due to the activation of phospholipase C (PLC). There are at least five different PLC enzymes with a diversity in structure and tissue distribution.[372] There are different mechanisms for coupling of the activation of different cell surface receptors to PLC; in one pathway, the receptor that is usually a protein tyrosine kinase directly phosphorylates PtdIns-specific PLC-γ1 and PLC-γ2 on tyrosine residues. Although after FcεRI aggregation the PLC-γ are tyrosine phosphorylated, this phosphorylation by itself is not the signal for the hydrolysis of the cellular PtdIns but may induce translocation of the phospholipase to the plasma membrane, which then may be crucial for the increased hydrolysis of membrane lipids.[15] An alternative pathway utilized by some other receptors is by using a G protein. The evidence for a role for G protein in FcεRI-mediated activation of PLC is discussed in the section on G proteins. The data suggest that this pathway utilizes G proteins distinct from the well-characterized molecules such as G_s, G_i, and transducin. The activation of phospholipase C by FcεRI aggregation occurs in plasma membrane vesicles from RBL-2H3 cells and is dependent on ATP and Mg^{2+} and enhanced by the addition of phosphoenolpyruvate and creatine phosphate.[89–91]

The activation of rat mast cells results in increased turnover of PtdIns, phosphatidylcholine, and phosphatidic acid.[208] The changes in phosphatidic acid occur before the onset of mediator release and could be generated by several pathways, such as phospholipase C or D pathways (discussed later). In these cells, there is increase in DAG following cell activation but this appears to be slower than the time course of histamine release.[209] There is parallel inhibition of mediator release and phospholipid turnover with several pharmacologic agents. The changes in phospholipids are also blocked by drugs that increase intracellular cAMP levels.[207]

ACTIVATION OF PROTEIN KINASE C (PKC)

Protein kinase C is an essential transducer of signals for secretion in mast cells.[11, 344] Besides PKC, there are a large number of Ser/Thr kinases in mast cells,[109] some of which are part of the Ras pathway described previously. The protein kinase C family is a group of proteins with multiple subspecies that phosphorylate proteins on either Ser or Thr residues.[333] Some of these isoforms are activated by the increase in $[Ca^{2+}]_i$ and phospholipids such as DAG that result from cell activation. Protein kinase C also can be directly activated by the binding of phorbol esters. This could be the mechanism by which phorbol esters stimulate secretion from basophils and mast cells.[381, 385, 396] Permeabilized rat mast cells release histamine upon the addition of Ca^{2+} or GTP-γ-S but rapidly lose their capacity to respond unless they have been pretreated with phorbol esters before permeabilization.[62, 163, 219] Furthermore, the sensitivity of the cells to these stimulatory signals is increased by PKC activation. Therefore, PKC-mediated protein phosphorylation may be essential to maintain the cells in a primed condition for release.[163]

The RBL-2H3 cells contain the Ca^{2+}-dependent α and β and the Ca^{2+}-independent δ, ϵ, and ζ isoforms of PKC.[164, 344] In nonstimulated cells, most of the PKC is in the cytoplasm; after FcϵRI activation, PKC isoforms translocate to various extent to the membrane fractions.[50, 344, 481, 483] PKC isozymes are probably necessary for optimal FcϵRI-mediated secretion, as shown by the following experiments. First, overnight incubation of cells with phorbol esters depletes some of the different PKC isoforms and decreases but does not abolish secretion. The addition of PKC inhibitors blocks secretion in these cells. Second, there is no secretion in washed permeabilized RBL-2H3 cells that lose all the PKC isozymes.[344] The secretory response is reconstituted by the addition of either the β or δ isozymes of PKC, but the response still requires the presence of Ca^{2+}. In these permeabilized cells, the addition of α and ϵ isozymes of PKC inhibits the FcϵRI-induced hydrolysis of inositol phospholipids[345] probably by reducing the tyrosine phosphorylation of phospholipase C-γ1. Therefore, there are distinct roles for both Ca^{2+} and PKC in the secretory pathway.

In RBL-2H3 cells, the activation of PKC by phorbol esters enhances the Ca^{2+} ionophore A23187–induced release but does not directly activate the cells for secretion.[381, 384, 488] The FcϵRI-mediated signals are not mimicked by the action of phorbol esters together with the Ca^{2+} ionophore A23187,[73] thus suggesting that the activation of PKC and the influx of Ca^{2+} are not the only signals generated by receptor cross-linking. The role of PKC also could be in the modulation of the secretory event; thus the treatment of RBL-2H3 cells with phorbol esters results in the inhibition of PtdIns hydrolysis but the enhancement of exocytosis.[124] There is a 45-kD protein phosphorylated by PKC after IgE or phorbol ester stimulation; both the phosphorylation of this protein and the secretion is inhibited by staurosporine, a PKC inhibitor.[482] In RBL-2H3 cells, there is a PKC-induced phosphorylation on Ser of myosin light and heavy chains.[252] In nonstimulated cells, the myosin light chain is monophosphorylated at Ser 19 by the Ca^{2+}/calmodulin-dependent myosin light chain kinase.[58] Stimulation results in further phosphorylations due to this kinase (at position Ser 18) and by protein kinase C (at Ser 1 and 2). These phosphorylations are closely associated with degranulation.

The γ chain of FcϵRI is phosphorylated by PKC on Thr residues after receptor aggregation.[125] This phosphorylation is probably due to the calcium-independent PKC δ that associates with the β subunit of the receptor. This phosphorylation may signal receptor internalization.

In human basophils, FcϵRI aggregation with anti-IgE results in a total rise in cellular PKC activity due to an increase in membrane-associated PKC. This is only partially dependent on extracellular Ca^{2+} and does not correlate with histamine release. However, there is a redistribution of cytoplasmic PKC induced by fMet peptide–mediated but not FcϵRI-mediated cell activation.[472, 473]

The phosphorylations induced by PKC are reversed by Ser/Thr phosphatases present in cells. These phosphatases are inhibited by okadaic acid.[351] The addition of this inhibitor blocks the release of both histamine and LTC_4 in mast cells.

PHOSPHOLIPASE D ACTIVATION

In cells, DAG is formed either by a direct pathway by the action of phospholipase C on phosphoinositides or indirectly by a step that requires phospholipase D. This enzyme digests phosphatidylcholine to yield phosphatidic acid and choline. Phosphatidic acid can act as a second messenger in cells and directly activate PKC. Phosphatidic acid can also be enzymatically converted to DAG, which also activates PKC. The enzymes for this indirect pathway are present in mast cells and may be important for the generation of DAG. Evidence for this is that after activation less than 25% of the DAG in mast cells is from the phospholipase C pathway of phosphoinositides hydrolysis.[205, 206] FcϵRI activation also results in a 3- to 10-fold increase in phospholipase D activity.[87, 132, 247, 248] Similarly, there is also activation of phospholipase D by Ca^{2+} ionophores. The activation of phospholipase D is probably downstream of PKC activation and the rise in $[Ca^{2+}]_i$.[246, 489] In FcϵRI-stimulated cells, there is a biphasic increase in the production of DAG; the initial phase, which is related to cell activation, is not due to the PLD pathway.[244] The second phase is generated by PLD and may play a role in most of the activation of PKC. Tyrosine kinase inhibitors block only the second wave of DAG formation.[245] Altogether, the results indicate that there is activation of the PLD pathway during cell stimulation and it could play a role in degranulation.

CHANGES IN INTRACELLULAR CALCIUM

A requirement for Ca^{2+} has long been recognized as essential for secretion from mast cells and basophils. The following is the evidence for the essential role of Ca^{2+} in the release process. First, Ca^{2+} chelators inhibit the release process. Second, different Ca^{2+} ionophores such as A23187 or ionomycin transport Ca^{2+} into cells and initiate secretion. Third, the introduction of Ca^{2+} into the cytoplasm by microinjection, by the fusion of cells with Ca^{2+}-containing vesicles, or after permeabilization of the cell membrane results usually in secretion.[35, 329, 453] Fourth, measurements with isotopic Ca^{2+} demonstrate the uptake of this cation into the cell before the release of mediators.[71] Fifth, measurement of $[Ca^{2+}]_i$ with fluorescent dyes demonstrates an increase in the $[Ca^{2+}]_i$ when the cells are stimulated.[28, 480] The low $[Ca^{2+}]_i$ concentrations of about 100 nM in the cytoplasm, compared with 2 mM in the extracellular space, are maintained by an energy-dependent pump that moves Ca^{2+} out of the cell. Following FcεRI stimulation, there is a dramatic increase in $[Ca^{2+}]_i$ in basophils and mast cells.[22, 263] In human basophils, the rise is from 85 nM to 190 nM and precedes the release of histamine.[263] In studies with individual cells, FcεRI stimulation results in rapid increases in $[Ca^{2+}]_i$ with different lag periods and heterogeneity in the extent of the increase.[301] After FcεRI aggregation, there are oscillations in $[Ca^{2+}]_i$ especially in basophils.[266] The rise in $[Ca^{2+}]_i$ depends on the presence of Ca^{2+} in the medium. A variant RBL-2H3 cell line has been isolated that can be stimulated to release mediators without a measurable increase in the $[Ca^{2+}]_i$ levels.[488] Even in this cell line, release is dependent on the presence of extracellular Ca^{2+}.

Immediately after receptor cross-linking, there is a rapid initial rise in $[Ca^{2+}]_i$ that is independent of extracellular Ca^{2+}.[308, 435] This release of Ca^{2+} from the endoplasmic reticulum is due to inositol 1,4,5-trisphosphate binding to specific receptors.[79, 478, 493, 494] The intracellular application of inositol 1,4,5-trisphosphate results in the release of Ca^{2+} from intracellular sources and in the influx of Ca^{2+}.[281] The Ca^{2+} released from intracellular sources is usually not sufficient to induce secretion.[308] The initial rise in $[Ca^{2+}]_i$ is followed by the sustained influx of Ca^{2+} from the medium by either increased permeability of the plasma membrane to Ca^{2+} or the opening of specific channels.[151, 281, 353, 447] In the absence of extracellular Ca^{2+}, there is uptake of isotopic Na^{+} from the medium after FcεRI aggregation, suggesting that the plasma membrane channels are specific for Ca^{2+} only at mM concentrations of Ca^{2+}.[195] By micropipette measurements, the Ca^{2+} influx is via both Ca^{2+}-specific and nonspecific channels.[281] These channels are activated by the intracellular application of either inositol 1,4,5-trisphosphate or GTP-γ-S. Thus the hypothesis is that G proteins couple receptor activation to the stimulation of phospholipase C with the generation of inositol phosphates that are then responsible for the stimulation of the changes in intracellular Ca^{2+}. However, the effects of G proteins also could be independent of inositol phosphates; thus cholera toxin enhances the rise in $[Ca^{2+}]_i$ and the rate of Ca^{2+} influx in the absence of PtdIns hydrolysis.[328]

The release of calcium from the endoplasmic reticulum is followed by an increase in the entry of calcium into the cell. The mechanism for this is not understood, but there are two competing hypotheses. The first suggests that there is a direct link between the receptor for InsP3 and a putative surface Ca^{2+} channel, whereas the second suggests that a diffusible second messenger is released from the endoplasmic reticulum and gates a Ca^{2+} channel at the plasma membrane. Electrophysiologic measurements have characterized a calcium-selective current (I_{CRAC}) that is activated by depletion of the intracellular Ca^{2+} stores.[161, 162, 499] This current is very selective for Ca^{2+} (Ca^{2+} versus Na^{+} or K^{+} selectivity of 1,000:1). It is not activated by cyclic AMP, cyclic GMP, GTP, InsP4, or several other molecules. The biochemical nature of this channel is unknown. However, the sustained elevation of $[Ca^{2+}]_i$ could be due to cAMP or to Ca^{2+}-activated chloride channels.[280, 353] This activation of the chloride channel could provide the force for the entry of Ca^{2+} into the cell.[280, 377]

The increase in $[Ca^{2+}]_i$ starts at the periphery of the cytoplasm and then spreads to the nucleus.[160, 197] The rise in the nucleus is secondary to the rise in the cytoplasm.[7] In human basophils, the increase in $[Ca^{2+}]_i$ due to influx from extracellular Ca^{2+} is blocked by agents that increase cAMP.[46] The IgE-receptor activation of RBL-2H3 cells also results in the stimulation of Ca^{2+} efflux from the cell.[307, 447] This would function to return $[Ca^{2+}]_i$ levels to normal.

Although an increase in $[Ca^{2+}]_i$ is a prominent signal in mast cells or basophils, it alone is not sufficient to trigger exocytosis. For example, the Ca^{2+} ionophore A23187 can induce an equivalent increase in intracellular Ca^{2+} without inducing secretion.[26] Similarly, activation of PKC together with the increase of $[Ca^{2+}]_i$ to these levels is not enough of a secretory signal. The microinjection of 1,4,5,-trisphosphate induced a rise in intracellular calcium, but there is no secretion unless a stable analogue of GTP is also present. Similarly, addition of GTP-γ-S alone induces slow secretion unless $[Ca^{2+}]_i$ is also elevated. Therefore, multiple signals are essential for optimal degranulation.

A series of investigations suggests that there is a specific Ca^{2+} channel-forming protein in RBL-2H3 cells.[283–289] These studies are based on the observation that the drug cromolyn inhibits mediator release from mast cells due to inhibition of Ca^{2+} channels. Both rat mast cells and RBL-2H3 cells bind to cromolyn immobilized on beads.[286] By using immobilized cromolyn, a protein was isolated from RBL-2H3 cells and used for producing monoclonal antibodies.[284] There were conductance changes when the monoclonal antibody was added to the purified protein reconstituted into planar bilayers.[289] A variant RBL-2H3 cell line was isolated that did not bind cromolyn and did not secrete. The addition of the purified cromolyn-binding protein in vesicles restored the secretory capacity of these cells.[283, 285] In experiments when both purified IgE receptors and this protein were reconstituted into planar membranes, there were conductance changes when the IgE receptors were aggregated.[68, 287] Still, it is unclear how these findings relate to the cytosolic enzyme nucleoside 5′-diphosphate kinase that binds immobilized cromoglycate.[146, 147] It is also difficult to reconcile these findings with other observations.[299] For example, patch-clamp techniques with whole RBL-2H3 cells have not resulted in activation of a Ca^{2+} channel.[249] Furthermore, it is difficult to envision why inhibitors block the rise in $[Ca^{2+}]_i$[465] if aggregation of the FcεRI directly interacts with and opens Ca^{2+} channels.

Many of the intracellular regulatory functions of Ca^{2+} are mediated by the ubiquitous Ca^{2+}-binding protein calmodulin. This protein has a molecular weight of 17,000 and contains four Ca^{2+} binding sites. The binding of Ca^{2+} to any one of the four binding sites results in a conformational change that brings about the association of the complex with enzymes. The Ca^{2+}-calmodulin complex regulates many enzyme systems, including phospholipase A2 and microtubule assembly. A few inhibitors (e.g., trifluoperazine) bind to calmodulin and inhibit its action in isolated systems; still, when these inhibitors are added to cells, they probably affect several other systems.

RELEASE OF ARACHIDONIC ACID

The activation of basophils or mast cells also results in the release of arachidonic acid (an unsaturated fatty acid) from cellular phospholipids.[70, 294] Arachidonic acid is commonly present in the sn-2 position on the glycerol backbone of phospholipids. The major membrane phospholipid is phosphatidylcholine, with lesser amounts of phosphatidylethanolamine, phosphatidylserine, and PtdIns. There are different pools of phospholipids in cells, and the source from which the arachidonic acid is released depends on the stimulus.

There are several possible pathways for the release of arachidonic acid during cell activation. This results in the stimulation of phospholipase C and phospholipase A2 enzymes. The phospholipase C acts on phosphatidyl inositides, resulting in the formation of DAG. This DAG can then be hydrolyzed by DAG lipase to release arachidonic acid. In the second pathway, arachidonic acid is released by phospholipase A2 acting on different phospholipids, including phosphatidylcholine, phosphatidylethanolamine, and phosphatidylinositol. There is evidence for the activation of both the phospholipase C and phospholipase A2 pathways in stimulated rat mast cells and RBL-2H3 cells.[121, 209] The activation of both pathways may include the participation of a G protein.[327]

In the RBL-2H3 cells, the time course of the release of arachidonic acid parallels the release of histamine but is slower than the increase in $[Ca^{2+}]_i$.[70, 294] The release is observed only in the presence of extracellular Ca^{2+}, suggesting the importance of the phospholipase A2 pathway. Phospholipase A2 activation is present in cell homogenates following cell activation.[122] In permeabilized cells, GTP-γ-S induces phospholipase A2 activation, indicating that G proteins can activate this enzyme.[327] Although arachidonic acid is released by both IgE and Ca^{2+} ionophore stimulation of cells, there are several differences in the release induced by these two secretagogues. With the Ca^{2+} ionophore, more of the total cellular arachidonic acid is released, and it is derived predominantly from the cellular phosphatidylethanolamine.[121] In contrast, with IgE-mediated release, the major source of the arachidonic acid is phosphatidylinositol/phosphatidylserine. Therefore, either different phospholipase enzymes are activated by the two stimulants or there are different pools of phospholipids that are accessible to the activated enzymes.

Mast cells and basophils contain at least three different phospholipase A2 (PLA2) enzymes.[320, 325] The low molecular weight secreted form called sPLA2 does not participate in the generation of the arachidonic acid–derived eicosanoids.[319] The major phospholipase in mast cells is the high molecular weight PLA2, which is referred to as cytosolic or cPLA2. The FcεRI-mediated release of arachidonic acid is regulated by this cPLA2, which has a Ca^{2+}-dependent phospholipid-binding domain, a single serine-containing consensus site for phosphorylation by mitogen-activated protein (MAP) kinase. Cell stimulation with the increase in $[Ca^{2+}]_i$ results in the translocation of this enzyme from the cytosol to membranes. Phosphorylation on Ser activates the phospholipase activity of the molecule.[75, 243, 325] This phosphorylation is by MAPK through the Ras/Raf/MEK1 pathway.[153] cPLA2 is also phosphorylated and activated by protein kinase C, an event that is critical for secretion.[498]

The arachidonic acid released by cell stimulation can be metabolized by either the cyclooxygenase or lipoxygenase pathways (see Chapter 12). In mast cells and basophils, the cyclooxygenase pathway leads predominantly to the formation of prostaglandin D2 with formation of some thromboxane A2 and prostacyclin. There are two isoforms of prostaglandin endoperoxide synthase (cyclooxygenase) that are regulated by cytokines such as c-Kit, IL-3, and IL-10.[321] The products of the lipoxygenase pathway are the leukotrienes. Some experiments suggest that a product from this lipoxygenase pathway plays a role in cell secretion.[223] Inhibitors of arachidonic acid metabolism block histamine release, whereas the selective inhibition of the cyclooxygenase pathway (with indomethacin or aspirin) by diverting the arachidonic acid to the lipoxygenase pathway enhances histamine release.[276, 278, 330, 355, 436] In contrast, lipoxygenase inhibition blocks release.[330] Furthermore, several lipoxygenase products (e.g., 5-HPETE, 5-HETE, and 12-HETE) enhance IgE-mediated release, and 5-HPETE can release histamine in the presence of cytochalasin B, an agent that disrupts microfilaments.[355, 428] However, with RBL-2H3 cells, the inhibition of the cyclooxygenase pathway with indomethacin has no effect on histamine release.[294] Therefore, the role of the lipoxygenase products in the release process is not clearly established.

Secretion is not always accompanied by arachidonic acid release. For example, with human basophils, several secretagogues (e.g., C5a and phorbol esters) release histamine but not LTC_4,[474] whereas substance P and codeine release histamine but not PGD_2 or LTC_4 from cutaneous mast cells. In permeabilized rat mast cells, there is release of arachidonic acid that is derived primarily from phosphatidylcholine and parallels the release of granular contents. Still, by manipulating the system, it is possible to release granule content without releasing arachidonic acid. Therefore, phospholipase A2 activation is not an essential requirement for secretion.[60] Similarly, in PT18 cells, slight increases in cAMP result in inhibition of arachidonic acid production but not in inhibition of the increase in $[Ca^{2+}]_i$ or of histamine release.[464] Therefore, the release of arachidonic acid is an independent pathway during secretion.

Glucocorticoids inhibit mediator release in in vitro models of allergic reactions. With human basophils, inhibition is limited to FcεRI-mediated activation but not stimulation with other secretagogues, such as Ca^{2+} ionophore A23187, fMetLeuPhe, or the phorbol ester.[77, 376, 397, 398] There is no inhibition of the IgE-mediated release of histamine or prostaglandin D_2 from human mast cells, although there are decreases in the release of some cyclooxygenase products.[393] In both mouse mast cells and RBL-2H3 cells, dexamethasone inhibits histamine and arachidonic acid release, the increased influx of Ca^{2+}, and PtdIns hydrolysis.[38, 77, 358, 376, 484] There is also evidence for inhibition of phospholipase A2. Secretion and PtdIns hydrolysis are not blocked in permeabilized cells, suggesting that inhibition by steroids is due to a cytosolic factor.[65] Inhibition requires the exposure of these cells to the steroid for several hours, probably due to a requirement for the synthesis of a phospholipase A2 inhibitory protein. Although such an inhibitor can explain the decrease in arachidonic acid release, it does not explain the inhibition of the Ca^{2+} entry into the cells nor the inhibition of the IgE-receptor–mediated PtdIns hydrolysis. Therefore, steroids must be inhibiting the coupling of the receptor aggregation to subsequent early events such as PtdIns hydrolysis and Ca^{2+} influx.

CYTOSKELETAL INVOLVEMENT

The cytoskeletal structures consisting of the microtubules, actin filaments, and intermediate filaments specify the characteristic shape of eukaryotic cells. These structures are not static but undergo rapid changes that are responsible for cell motility and for movement in the cytoplasm. The cytoskeletal components insert either directly or through other proteins into the cell membrane and also bind to granules. Receptors in the cell membrane may exist in two interconvertible states: free, where they can diffuse in the cell membrane, or bound in some way to the microtubular or microfilament structures in the cell. Therefore, the distribution of cell surface receptors is influenced by their interaction with the cytoskeleton. Conversely, the binding of ligands to cell surface receptors influences the organization of the cytoskeleton. The cytoskeletal elements are involved in the aggregation of receptors into patches and their eventual coalescence into caps at one end of the cell.

Cytoskeletal reorganizations probably play a role in granule migration and in regulation of the access of secretory vesicles to the plasma membrane. The cytoskeletal changes could be secondary to changes in $[Ca^{2+}]_i$, phosphorylation of cellular proteins, and/or activation of GTP-binding proteins. As discussed in previous sections, GTP-binding proteins can act indirectly by production of secondary messengers (e.g., Ca^{2+}, cAMP, cGMP, activation of PKC, or PI hydrolysis). GTP-binding proteins can also be acting directly. Two Ras-related small GTPases, Rho and Rac, are essential for the formation of stress fibers and membrane ruffles, respectively. The addition of GTP-γ-S, a slowly hydrolyzable GTP analogue, to permeabilized mast cells results in reorganization of actin filaments.[218, 334] The content of filamentous (F) actin is reduced in the cortical region and increased in the cell interior. This appearance of actin filaments in the interior of the cell depends on Rac and Rho. Rho is responsible for actin polymerization, and Rac for the entrapment of actin filaments in the interior of the cell.[334]

Microtubules are present in mast cells and basophils. They have a characteristic tubular structure of heterodimers formed from α- and β-tubulin polypeptides. The microtubules are filamentous protein polymers that are labile structures and are in a state of constant dynamic equilibrium with the pool of tubulin subunits. The assembly of the tubules is controlled by the level of Ca^{2+} and the oxidation state of tubulin sulfhydryl groups and cyclic nucleotides. There are several microtubule-associated proteins that may play a role in regulating the polymerization of tubulin. Microtubules are inserted into both the cell membrane and granules, thus they could be either passive direction markers for the secretion of granules or actively involved in the movement of the granule. Colchicine and vinblastine bind to tubulin dimers and prevent their polymerization into microtubules. Colchicine also binds to cell surface proteins and inhibits nucleoside transport into the cell. Colchicine and vinblastine inhibit histamine release from both basophils and mast cells. Conversely, deuterium oxide (heavy water) stabilizes microtubules and enhances IgE-mediated histamine release.[127] However, heavy water also enhances PtdIns hydrolysis, suggesting that it also could have effects at early steps of the release process.[270] Inhibitors of microtubular function block the release of arachidonic acid without affecting the increase in $[Ca^{2+}]_i$.[465] Therefore, the coupling of the IgE receptor and Ca^{2+} influx to phospholipase activation requires the microtubular system.

Microfilaments are filamentous structures observed in many cells and are usually distributed close to the cell surface. They are thought to be actin-like polymers, and there is some evidence that they interact with the cell membrane. The cytochalasins are fungal products that inhibit cellular movement. Although they were thought originally to act directly on microfilaments, more recent studies suggest that they have several effects, including inhibition of membrane transport systems. Cytochalasin B inhibits the lateral diffusion of IgE molecules in the membrane of cells. These agents also enhance FcϵRI-mediated histamine release from mast cells or basophils but inhibit leukotriene formation. The disruption of the microfilaments in RBL-2H3 cells with cytochalasin B increased histamine release but did not change the receptor-mediated PtdIns hydrolysis or Ca^{2+} influx.[326] In permeabilized cells, it also enhanced the GTP-γ-S–induced release, suggesting that microtubules regulate a late step in the release process. From these data with inhibitors, it appears that microtubules and microfilaments are probably involved in the secretory function of basophils and mast cells.

There is redistribution of cytoskeletal elements during activation of mast cells and basophils.[339, 386] In nonstimulated RBL-2H3 cells, actin is localized to the cell periphery just under the plasma membrane. After stimulation, it is in the periphery, concentrated under the membrane ruffles that appear after stimulation. There is also redistribution of the intermediate filaments and microtubules throughout the cell body. Vimentin, an intermediate cytoskeletal protein, is normally distributed around granules. After stimulation, it is phosphorylated on Ser, probably by PKC, and becomes diffusely distributed in the cytoplasm.[185] The decrease in the detergent solubility of the receptor proteins is not due to changes in the microfilaments.[12] The large-scale clustering and capping of receptors is due to their interaction with the membrane skeleton (e.g., F-actin).[407] There are increased adhesive properties of cells with the formation of actin plaques that contain phosphorylated proteins.[356] The detergent insolubility of cross-linked receptors correlates inversely with secretion; at the highest antigen concentration, there is maximal insolubility and minimal secretion.[406] Cytoskeletal-inhibiting agents do not block the generation of inositol phosphates but inhibit the release of Ca^{2+} from intracellular stores.[451] Therefore, microtubules are not involved in the early activation steps of signaling but play a role in the Ca^{2+} release process.

RELEASABILITY

There is wide variation in the extent of histamine release from the cells of both atopic and nonatopic individuals; this has been termed the releasability of the cells.[420] The extent of stimulated histamine release from the cells of any one individual can vary from as low as no different from the spontaneous release to values as high as 90% to 100% of total cellular histamine. The releasability of the cells can also be different with different secretagogues; that is, the cells of one individual may release well with an IgE-mediated stimulus but poorly with another secretagogue (e.g., fMetLeuPhe or C5a), and vice versa.[157, 418, 419] Similarly, there are differences in the extent of release from basophils compared with mast cells. The release by FcεRI-mediated activation of the cells has drawn the most interest because it may relate to clinical allergy. There is no correlation between the number of IgE molecules present on the surface of basophils and releasability.[67, 268] Variations have also been observed over time as to the releasability of the cells of the same donor. In comparing cells from monozygotic and dizygotic twins, there was good correlation in IgE-induced histamine release only when the basophils were from monozygotic twins.[277]

Evidence suggests that these differences in secretion are regulated by intracellular factors. For example, studies have shown that basophils of individuals who are high responders release histamine with chemically cross-linked IgE dimers, whereas the cells of the low responders release with chemically cross-linked trimers but very poorly with dimers.[260] The sensitivity of cells to different stimuli is set by differences in intracellular signaling mechanisms. It can be modified by factors such as adherence of the cells to other cells or extracellular matrix proteins, by lymphokines, by steroids, or by dietary lipids that are incorporated into the membranes. The effect of adhesion and lymphokines will be discussed in the next two sections.

ADHESION

Adhesion of cells to other cells and to the extracellular matrix regulates developmental, cellular, and immunologic processes.[427] Such adherence is mediated by cell surface receptors.[168, 427] Adherence also activates intracellular signals that not only evoke new cellular responses but also modulate the response of cells to other stimuli.[189] Both basophils and mast cells have surface adherence receptors that can mediate binding to other cells and to extracellular matrix glycoproteins.[43, 138, 467] This adherence has effects on cellular functions and may be important for controlling the releasability of these cells.

Adherence of basophils and mast cells is mediated by several classes of adhesion molecules such as the integrins, many of which have been identified on these cells.[138] There are changes in the expression of integrins in murine mast cells cultured with different growth factors, suggesting modulation of integrin expression during mast cell differentiation.[93, 134] There is also enhanced adherence of cells after stimulation, which may be due to the redistribution of surface adhesion receptors, their enhanced expression on the cell surface, and/or the modulation of their affinity to ligands.[44, 458]

Adherence of cells not only may control their migration and localization at sites of inflammation but also may regulate their proliferation and phenotype. Adherence of cells results in the aggregation of adhesion receptors and the transduction of intracellular signals that includes reorganization of the cytoskeleton and changes in intracellular signaling and in the degranulating capacity of the cells. These signals are mediated by intracellular changes induced by adhesion such as protein tyrosine phosphorylations, phosphatidylinositol hydrolysis, changes in intracellular pH or calcium, and the expression of new genes.[189] Adherence of mast cells can transduce signals that affect cell growth, differentiation, and cell secretion. For example, culture of mature human or rat mast cells on fibroblasts maintains their phenotype, viability, and secretory function.[234, 235, 237, 239] Mast cells that are derived by the culture of mouse bone marrow cells in IL-3 (BMMC) are immature progenitors of serosal and mucosal mast cells, although they are more similar to mucosal mast cells in morphology, histochemistry, biochemistry, and responses to secretagogues. When transferred to feeder layers of mouse 3T3 fibroblasts, these cells persist in the absence of IL-3. If IL-3 is added to these cocultures, however, they acquire a more serosal phenotype with an increase in the content of mediators and a switch from synthesizing predominantly chondroitin sulfate proteoglycans to mostly heparin proteoglycans.[78] Many of these effects are due to the interaction of the fibroblast product, stem cell factor, with its receptor (c-Kit) on mast cells.[120, 443] Coculture of mast cells with fibroblasts regulates secretory function.[117, 431, 443] When activated, BMMC produce sulfidopeptide leukotrienes, whereas after coculture with fibroblasts, there is a shift to PGD_2.[236, 238] The coculture of BMMC with fibroblasts results in an increase in surface expression of FcγRIII and enhanced degranulation by FcγR activation.[198, 199] RBL-2H3 cells lack responsiveness to compound 48/80 and substance P. However, when these cells are cultured for 2 weeks on fibroblasts, they release histamine in response to these compounds.[444] Therefore, adherence of mast cells to fibroblasts modulates secretory function.

The adherence of mast cells results in changes in the cytoskeleton, cell spreading, and the redistribution of secretory granules to the periphery of the cell.[140, 193, 459] These changes may play an important role in intracellular signaling and degranulation. Thus there is enhanced secretion from RBL-2H3 cells that are adherent to surfaces coated with fibronectin.[140] The enhancement of release requires immobilized fibronectin. Cell adherence and FcεRI aggregation synergistically regulate tyrosine phosphorylation of 105- to 115-kD proteins.[137] The nonreceptor protein tyrosine kinase, $pp125^{FAK}$, is one of these pp105-115 proteins.[136] Thus adherence may regulate the extent of mast cell and basophil degranulation by modulating intracellular protein tyrosine phosphorylations.

LYMPHOKINES

Several lymphokines such as IL-3, IL-5, interferon-γ, G-CSF, or M-CSF enhance both FcεRI- and nonreceptor-mediated histamine release from human basophils.[152, 196] Monoclonal antibodies to CD11b (anti-αMβ2 integrin) but not CD11a (anti-αLβ2 integrin) or CD18 (β2 integrin family) inhibit the IL-3–enhanced anti-IgE–induced histamine release, suggesting a role for adhesion molecules.[477] Thus the enhancement of release with these cytokines may be due to changes in cell adherence.

DESENSITIZATION FOR THE RELEASE REACTION

Cross-linking of IgE receptors on the basophil or mast cell results in the activation of biochemical reactions that not only result in degranulation but also function to regulate the extent of the release reaction. This process is called desensitization. In in vitro experiments, desensitization is initiated by the addition of a secretagogue under conditions that do not result in secretion. For example, mast cells are first exposed to the secretagogue in the absence of Ca^{2+}, and after a defined incubation period, the permissive conditions are restored by the addition of Ca^{2+}. In such experiments, desensitization has been observed when the secretagogue has been added without Ca^{2+}, when the concentration of the antigen has been supraoptimal, or when the reaction temperature is nonoptimal.[83–85, 92, 106, 417] When different secretagogues are used with human basophils, the desensitization is specific for the stimulus. For example, desensitization for IgE-mediated release does not inactivate the cells for release with C5a or with the formyl-methionine peptides.[418, 419] The FcεRI-mediated desensitization requires receptor aggregation and can be initiated by dimers, although larger oligomers are more effective. In experiments with FcεRI-mediated release, the desensitization can be either specific to the antigen that is used for the desensitization process or nonspecific, in which case the cells do not respond to challenge with any antigen.[425] There is specific desensitization at low densities of IgE on basophils but nonspecific desensitization at high IgE levels.[259] Because desensitization occurs in the absence of added Ca^{2+}, it must involve a step independent of the influx of Ca^{2+}. Further evidence for such an early step is the observation that in desensitized cells rechallenged by an IgE-mediated reaction there is no increase in Ca^{2+} influx.[182] Desensitization is an active process with similarities to the events that result in cell secretion. The desensitization reaction can be blocked by the addition of some inhibitors; with human basophils, but not with lung mast cells, the serine esterase inhibitor DFP at a narrow concentration range decreased desensitization and enhanced release.[203, 267] With mouse mast cells, both DFP and inhibitors of methylation blocked desensitization.[182] There is a decrease in the receptor-mediated Ca^{2+} response of desensitized human mast cells, again suggesting that desensitization involves early steps of the release process.[267] Still, the changes in Ca^{2+} influx cannot alone explain desensitization,[264] and basophils desensitized for an anti-IgE response have an increased response on activation with PMA.[471]

The mechanism of desensitization is uncertain. It is not due to a loss from the cell surface of antigen-specific IgE caused by endocytosis or shedding of IgE-antigen complexes.[256, 257] Although there is rapid endocytosis of IgE-antigen complexes from the cell surface, there are still enough IgE-receptor complexes remaining on the cell surface to initiate release. With human basophils, endocytosis of the antigen-receptor complexes from the cell surface does not occur in the absence of Ca^{2+}, although this is not true for the RBL-2H3 cells. In desensitized cells, there is still the continued capacity of antigen to bind to IgE on the cell surface.[257] Similarly, nonspecific desensitization is not due to the cointernalization of all cell surface IgE when the specific IgE is aggregated. Studies with human basophils suggest that specific desensitization is due to alteration in a very early biochemical event, whereas the nonspecific desensitization is due to changes in more distal events. Desensitization could be due to the decay of an unstable intermediate formed by the aggregated receptors interacting with another protein.[84, 85]

Degranulation of cells results from a balance between activation and deactivation signals.[24] Clearly, membrane and intracellular signals are generated after receptor cross-linking that results in secretion; these signals are degraded by enzymatic pathways. If the signals cannot be processed due to unfavorable experimental conditions (e.g., absence of Ca^{2+} in the medium), there is decay in the signal.

HETEROGENEITY IN MAST CELL AND BASOPHIL RELEASE REACTIONS

HETEROGENEITY IN MAST CELL POPULATIONS AND IN THE MEDIATORS RELEASED

The concept of heterogeneity in the population of mast cells is based principally on studies in rodents.[41, 117, 213, 443] Histologic studies dating back to Maximow in 1905 described some atypically staining mast cells in the rat intestinal mucosa. These staining differences can now be explained by the different proteoglycans present in the granules of these cells.

There appear to be two major populations of mast cells in rats and mice. The atypical mast cells in intestinal mucosa are frequently called mucosal mast cells in contrast with those that are predominantly in connective tissues (e.g., the peritoneal cavity). Several differences are seen in their staining characteristics. Berberine binds well to heparin and stains the connective type of mast cells. With alcian blue safranin, the mucosal mast cells stain blue, whereas the connective tissue type has a red-blue color. The mucosal mast cells, as the name implies, are found predominantly in the intestinal wall. They are about half the size of the connective tissue type and contain approximately 1.3 μg of histamine/10^6 cells. In contrast, the connective tissue type has about 10-fold more histamine. The in vitro culture of bone marrow or spleen cells with IL-3 results in the development of cells that resemble the mucosal type of mast cells. There is also histologic and histochemical evidence for the presence of different types of mast cells in human tissues.

There are differences in the granular content of these two murine mast cell populations. The proteoglycan in the connective tissue mast cells is heparin (750 kD), whereas the mucosal type of mast cells have chondroitin sulfates (200 kD).[367, 432] Similarly, there are differences in the content of the serine protease enzyme present in the different mast cells; the connective tissue type contains the rat mast cell protease I (also called chymase), whereas the mucosal cells have rat mast cell protease II. Interestingly, RBL-2H3 cells contain a chondroitin sulfate and rat mast cell protease II, suggesting that they have homology with mucosal mast cells.[210, 411] Human mast cells can also be distinguished by enzyme content, such as T versus TC subtypes, which have some analogy to the mucosal and connective tissue type of mast cells in the rodent, but the nature of their development from mast cell precursors is unsettled.

Different secretagogues may be used to demonstrate differences between the mucosal and connective tissue types of mast cells. Both cell types respond to IgE-receptor or ionophore stimulation with the release of mediators. However, compound 48/80 or a bee venom peptide causes histamine release from the connective tissue mast cell but not from the mucosal type. Similarly, some other compounds cause secretion from the connective tissue type of mast cells only; these include bradykinin, vasoactive polypeptide, somatostatin, endorphins, and opiate-type drugs. Considerable differences exist, however, in reactivity of such cells. This depends upon the particular tissue source. Skin mast cells have the broadest range of response. Phosphatidylserine enhances the release from the connective type of mast cells but has no effect on the secretion from mucosal cells.

There are also differences in mediators generated by the two cell types. Both mucosal and connective tissue mast cells release histamine, and in rodents they contain and release serotonin. The predominant arachidonic acid metabolite made by rat connective tissue mast cell is PGD_2, whereas the mucosal mast cells generate more lipoxygenase products.[368, 369] Human mast cells make PGD_2 but also produce LTC_4 and other leukotrienes. In contrast, human basophils do not generate PGD_2 and produce only small amounts of the leukotrienes.

The observations described suggest that there are differences in mast cells isolated from different tissues. These results should be interpreted in the light of two important observations. First, the two types of mast cells can change their phenotype from one to the other depending on microenvironmental factors. Second, mast cells at different stages in their cell cycle or maturation can respond differently to various secretagogues.[300, 402]

HETEROGENEITY IN THE MECHANISM OF RELEASE

An important question is whether the mechanism for mediator release is similar in the various cell systems studied, such as human mast cells compared with basophils or rat mast cells. There are differences in the response of various cells to diverse nonphysiologic stimuli. For example, rat mast cells and human skin mast cells can be stimulated with compound 48/80, whereas human basophils do not respond. Still, all systems respond to the physiologically relevant system of IgE antigen. There are differences in the rate of release with different cells; for example, the rate with human mast cells is faster than that with human basophils.

Basophils are smaller cells that enter the circulation and have a short half-life in comparison with mast cells that are located in tissues. There are morphological differences in degranulation as observed by electron microscopy; that of mast cells is of the compound type with granules fusing with each other, whereas granules in basophils fuse directly with the plasma membrane. Mast cells require higher concentrations of anti-IgE for activation than do basophils. When tested with different secretagogues, several differences have been observed between mast cells and basophils. Basophils and skin mast cells respond to C5a and fMet peptides, whereas lung mast cells do not release with these stimuli.[404] Basophils also release when activated with the phorbol ester TPA, whereas this has no effect on lung mast cells. Similarly, the lipoxygenase product 5-HPETE releases histamine from basophils but not from lung mast cells. There are also differences in mast cells isolated from different tissues. Skin mast cells respond to compound 48/80, bradykinin, substance P, and morphine (similar to rat peritoneal mast cells).[59, 229] However, lung, intestinal, and synovial mast cells do not respond to these compounds.[220, 251] Even in cells from one tissue, there is some heterogeneity; human basophils separated by density show functional differences in response to FcϵRI- and nonreceptor-mediated activation.[313] There is also density heterogeneity of human lung mast cells with some differences in the quantitative but not qualitative response to secretagogues.[405, 468] These variations could be due to differences in the maturation of the cells.

There are also differences in the capacity of pharmacologic agents to inhibit FcϵRI-mediated secretion from basophils compared with mast cells. Inhibitors of the cyclooxygenase pathway enhance release from basophils but not from mast cells. The H2 agonists inhibit release from basophils but have no effect on mast cells, whereas PGD_2 enhances the release from human basophils but is without effect on mast cells.[262] Other differences include the effect of dexamethasone, which inhibits mediator release from human basophils but not from human mast cells. Adenosine inhibits the release from basophils but slightly enhances the release from mast cells.[349] Some of these differences in the effects of pharmacologic agents could be due to the presence or absence of agonist-specific receptors on these cells.

Differences have also been observed in the mediators released by mast cells compared with basophils. In contrast with mast cells, human basophils release very little if any of the cyclooxygenase-derived products of arachidonic acid such as PGD_2. Yet both mast cells and basophils release the leukotriene LTC_4. These are secondary mediators generated by enzymes acting on released arachidonic acid. The differences between basophils and mast cells could be due to the presence or absence of the enzymes involved in the production of these metabolites. Although there are differences between the basophil and mast cell, there is little evidence to suggest that the secretory process is fundamentally different in the two cell types.

SUMMARY

A better understanding of signaling in mast cells and basophils is crucial for advancing our knowledge of immediate hypersensitivity reactions. As discussed in this chapter, there have been major advances in understanding the biochemistry of secretion in these cells. Knowledge of the mechanisms involved in the secretion of mediators from mast cells and basophils could allow a more rational development of pharmacologic agents capable of abrogating this secretory event.

REFERENCES

1. Alai M, Mui AL, Cutler RL, et al: Steel factor stimulates the tyrosine phosphorylation of the proto-oncogene product, $p95^{vav}$, in human hemopoietic cells. J Biol Chem 267:18021, 1992.

2. Alam R, Welter JB, Forsythe PA, et al: Comparative effect of recombinant IL-1, -2, -3, -4, and -6, IFN-γ, granulocyte-macrophage-colony-stimulating factor, tumor necrosis factor-α, and histamine-releasing factors on the secretion of histamine from basophils. J Immunol 142:3431, 1989.
3. Alber G, Kent UM, Metzger H: Functional comparison of FcεRI, FcγRII, and FcγRIII in mast cells. J Immunol 149:2428, 1992.
4. Ali H, Collado-Escobar DM, Beaven MA: The rise in concentration of free Ca^{2+} and of pH provides sequential, synergistic signals for secretion in antigen-stimulated rat basophilic leukemia (RBL-2H3) cells. J Immunol 143:2626, 1989.
5. Ali H, Cunha-Melo JR, Beaven MA: Receptor-mediated release of inositol 1,4,5-trisphosphate and inositol 1,4-bisphosphate in rat basophilic leukemia RBL-2H3 cells permeabilized with streptolysin O. Biochim Biophys Acta 1010:88, 1989.
6. Ali H, Cunha-Melo JR, Saul WF, Beaven MA: Activation of phospholipase C via adenosine receptors provides synergistic signals for secretion in antigen-stimulated RBL-2H3 cells. Evidence for a novel adenosine receptor. J Biol Chem 265:745, 1990.
7. Allbritton NL, Oancea E, Kuhn MA, Meyer T: Source of nuclear calcium signals. Proc Natl Acad Sci USA 91:12458, 1994.
8. Alm E, Bloom GD: Cyclic nucleotide involvement in histamine release from mast cells—a reevaluation. Life Sci 30:213, 1982.
9. Altman A, Coggeshall KM, Mustelin T: Molecular events mediating T cell activation. Adv Immunol 48:227, 1990.
10. Alvarez de Toledo G, Fernandez-Chacon R, Fernandez JM: Release of secretory products during transient vesicle fusion. Nature 363: 554,1993.
11. Amon U, Von Stebut E, Subramanian N, Wolff HH: CGP 41251, a novel protein kinase inhibitor with in vitro selectivity for protein kinase C, strongly inhibits immunological activation of human skin mast cells and human basophils. Pharmacology 47:200, 1993.
12. Apgar JR: Antigen-induced cross-linking of the IgE receptor leads to an association with the detergent-insoluble membrane skeleton of rat basophilic leukemia (RBL-2H3) cells. J Immunol 145:3814, 1990.
13. Aridor M, Rajmilevich G, Beaven MA, Sagi-Eisenberg R: Activation of exocytosis by the heterotrimeric G protein Gi3. Science 262:1569, 1993.
14. Aridor M, Sagi-Eisenberg R: Neomycin is a potent secretagogue of mast cells that directly activates a GTP-binding protein involved in exocytosis. J Cell Biol 111:2885, 1990.
15. Atkinson TP, Kaliner MA, Hohman RJ: Phospholipase C-γ1 is translocated to the membrane of rat basophilic leukemia cells in response to aggregation of IgE receptors. J Immunol 148:2194, 1992.
16. Baggiolini M, Dahinden CA: CC chemokines in allergic inflammation. Immunol Today 15:127, 1994.
17. Baniyash M, Alkalay I, Eshhar Z: Monoclonal antibodies specific to the alpha-subunit of the mast cell's FcεR block IgE binding and trigger histamine release. J Immunol 138:2999, 1987.
18. Bar-Sagi D, Gomperts BD: Stimulation of exocytotic degranulation by microinjection of the *ras* oncogene protein into rat mast cells. Oncogene 3:463, 1988.
19. Barajas-Lopez C, Huizinga JD: Immunoglobulin E mediated membrane conductance changes in rat basophilic leukemia cells. Can J Physiol Pharmacol 66:328, 1988.
20. Baranes D, Lewin I, Razin E: Serum modulates mast cell responses to IgE antigen stimulation. Eur J Immunol 23:291, 1993.
21. Barsumian EL, Isersky C, Petrino MG, Siraganian RP: IgE-induced histamine release from rat basophilic leukemia cell lines: isolation of releasing and nonreleasing clones. Eur J Immunol 11:317, 1981.
22. Barsumian EL, McGivney A, Basciano LK, Siraganian RP: Establishment of four mouse mastocytoma cell lines. Cell Immunol 90:131, 1985.
23. Basciano LK, Berenstein EH, Kmak L, Siraganian RP: Monoclonal antibodies that inhibit IgE binding. J Biol Chem 261:11823, 1986.
24. Baxter JH, Adamik R: Control of histamine release: effects of various conditions on rate of release and rate of cell desensitization. J Immunol 114:1034, 1975.
25. Beaven MA, Cunha-Melo JR: Membrane phosphoinositide-activated signals in mast cells and basophils. Prog Allergy 42:123, 1988.
26. Beaven MA, Guthrie DF, Moore JP, et al: Synergistic signals in the mechanism of antigen-induced exocytosis in 2H3 cells: evidence for an unidentified signal required for histamine release. J Cell Biol 105:1129, 1987.
27. Beaven MA, Moore JP, Smith GA, et al: The calcium signal and phosphatidylinositol breakdown in 2H3 cells. J Biol Chem 259: 7137, 1984.
28. Beaven MA, Rogers J, Moore JP, et al: The mechanism of the calcium signal and correlation with histamine release in 2H3 cells. J Biol Chem 259:7129, 1984.
29. Becker KE, Ishizaka T, Metzger H, et al: Surface IgE on human basophils during histamine release. J Exp Med 138:394, 1973.
30. Benhamou M, Berenstein EH, Jouvin M, Siraganian RP: The receptor with high affinity for IgE on rat mast cells is a functional receptor for rat IgG2a. Mol Immunol 31:1089, 1994.
31. Benhamou M, Gutkind JS, Robbins KC, Siraganian RP: Tyrosine phosphorylation coupled to IgE receptor-mediated signal transduction and histamine release. Proc Natl Acad Sci USA 87:5327, 1990.
32. Benhamou M, Ryba NJP, Kihara H, et al: Protein-tyrosine kinase $p72^{syk}$ in high affinity IgE receptor signaling. Identification as a component of pp72 and association with the receptor γ chain. J Biol Chem 268:23318, 1993.
33. Benhamou M, Siraganian RP: Protein-tyrosine phosphorylation: an essential component of FcεRI signaling. Immunol Today 13:195, 1992.
34. Benhamou M, Stephan V, Robbins KC, Siraganian RP: High-affinity IgE receptor-mediated stimulation of rat basophilic leukemia (RBL-2H3) cells induces early and late protein-tyrosine phosphorylations. J Biol Chem 267:7310, 1992.
35. Bennett JP, Cockcroft S, Gomperts BD: Rat mast cells permeabilized with ATP secrete histamine in response to calcium ions buffered in the micromolar range. J Physiol (Lond) 317:335, 1981.
36. Benyon RC, Church MK, Holgate ST: IgE-dependent activation of mast cells is not associated with enhanced phospholipid methylation. Biochem Pharmacol 35:2535, 1986.
37. Benyon RC, Church MK, Holgate ST: IgE-dependent activation of human lung mast cells is not associated with increased phospholipid methylation. J Immunol 141:954, 1988.
38. Berenstein EH, Garcia-Gil M, Siraganian RP: Dexamethasone inhibits receptor-activated phosphoinositide breakdown in rat basophilic leukemia (RBL-2H3) cells. J Immunol 138:1914, 1987.
39. Berger SA, Mak TW, Paige CJ: Leukocyte common antigen (CD45) is required for immunoglobulin E-mediated degranulation of mast cells. J Exp Med 180:471, 1994.
40. Berridge MJ: Inositol trisphosphate and calcium signalling. Nature 361:315, 1993.
41. Bienenstock J: An update on mast cell heterogeneity. J Allergy Clin Immunol 81:763, 1988.
42. Blank U, Ra C, Miller L, et al: Complete structure and expression in transfected cells of high affinity IgE receptor. Nature 337:187, 1989.
43. Bochner BS, Schleimer RP: The role of adhesion molecules in human eosinophil and basophil recruitment. J Allergy Clin Immunol 94:427, 1994.
44. Bochner BS, Sterbinsky SA: Altered surface expression of CD11 and Leu 8 during human basophil degranulation. J Immunol 146:2367, 1991.
45. Bolen JB, Rowley RB, Spana C, Tsygankov AY: The Src family of tyrosine protein kinases in hemopoietic signal transduction. FASEB J 6:3403, 1992.
46. Botana LM, MacGlashan DW: Differential effects of cAMP-elevating drugs on stimulus-induced cytosolic calcium changes in human basophils. J Leukoc Biol 55:798, 1994.
47. Bourne HR, Lehrer RI, Lichtenstein LM, et al: Effects of cholera enterotoxin on adenosine 3′,5′-monophosphate and neutrophil function. Comparison with other compounds which stimulate leukocyte adenyl cyclase. J Clin Invest 52:698, 1973.
48. Bourne HR, Lichtenstein LM, Melmon KL, et al: Modulation of inflammation and immunity by cyclic AMP. Science 184:19, 1974.
49. Bronner C, Mousli M, Eleno N, Landry Y: Resting plasma membrane potential of rat peritoneal mast cells is set predominantly by the sodium pump. FEBS Lett 255:401, 1989.
50. Buccione R, Di Tullio G, Caretta M, et al: Analysis of protein kinase C requirement for exocytosis in permeabilized rat basophilic leukaemia RBL-2H3 cells: a GTP-binding protein(s) as a potential target for protein kinase C. Biochem J 298:149, 1994.
51. Cabado AG, Vieytes MR, Botana LM: Effect of ion composition on the changes in membrane potential induced with several stimuli in rat mast cells. J Cell Physiol 158:309, 1994.
52. Cambier JC, Pleiman CM, Clark MR: Signal transduction by the B cell antigen receptor and its coreceptors. Annu Rev Immunol 12:457, 1994.

53. Chabay R, DeLisi C, Hook WA, Siraganian RP: Receptor cross-linking and histamine release in basophils. J Biol Chem 255:4628, 1980.
54. Chan AC, Desai DM, Weiss A: The role of protein tyrosine kinases and protein tyrosine phosphatases in T cell antigen receptor signal transduction. Annu Rev Immunol 12:555, 1994.
55. Chan AC, Irving BA, Fraser JD, Weiss A: The ζ chain is associated with a tyrosine kinase and upon T-cell antigen receptor stimulation associates with ZAP-70, a 70-kDa tyrosine phosphoprotein. Proc Natl Acad Sci USA 88:9166, 1991.
56. Chan AC, Iwashima M, Turck CW, Weiss A: ZAP-70: a 70 kd protein-tyrosine kinase that associates with the TCR ζ chain. Cell 71:649, 1992.
57. Chandler DE, Heuser JE: Arrest of membrane fusion events in mast cells by quick-freezing. J Cell Biol 86:666, 1980.
58. Choi OH, Adelstein RS, Beaven MA: Secretion from rat basophilic RBL-2H3 cells is associated with diphosphorylation of myosin light chains by myosin light chain kinase as well as phosphorylation by protein kinase C. J Biol Chem 269:536, 1994.
59. Church MK, Lowman MA, Robinson C, et al: Interaction of neuropeptides with human mast cells. Int Arch Allergy Appl Immunol 88:70, 1989.
60. Churcher Y, Allan D, Gomperts BD: Relationship between arachidonate generation and exocytosis in permeabilized mast cells. Biochem J 266:157, 1990.
61. Churcher Y, Gomperts BD: ATP-dependent and ATP-independent pathways of exocytosis revealed by interchanging glutamate and chloride as the major anion in permeabilized mast cells. Cell Regul 1:337, 1990.
62. Churcher Y, Kramer KM, Gomperts BD: Evidence for protein dephosphorylation as a permissive step in GTP-γ-S-induced exocytosis from permeabilized mast cells. Cell Regul 1:523, 1990.
63. Clark EA, Ledbetter JA: Leukocyte cell surface enzymology: CD45 (LCA, T200) is a protein tyrosine phosphatase. Immunol Today 10:225, 1989.
64. Cockcroft S, Gomperts BD: Role of guanine nucleotide binding protein in the activation of polyphosphoinositide phosphodiesterase. Nature 314:534, 1985.
65. Collado-Escobar D, Cunha-Melo JR, Beaven MA: Treatment with dexamethasone down-regulates IgE-receptor-mediated signals and up-regulates adenosine-receptor-mediated signals in a rat mast cell (RBL-2H3) line. J Immunol 144:244, 1990.
66. Conrad DH, Wingard JR, Ishizaka T: The interaction of human and rodent IgE with the human basophil IgE receptor. J Immunol 130:327, 1983.
67. Conroy MC, Adkinson NF Jr, Lichtenstein LM: Measurement of IgE on human basophils: relation to serum IgE and anti-IgE-induced histamine release. J Immunol 118:1317, 1977.
68. Corcia A, Schweitzer-Stenner R, Pecht I, Rivnay B: Characterization of the ion channel activity in planar bilayers containing IgE-Fc epsilon receptor and the cromolyn-binding protein. EMBO J 5:849, 1986.
69. Couture C, Baier G, Altman A, Mustelin T: $p56^{lck}$-independent activation and tyrosine phosphorylation of $p72^{syk}$ by T-cell antigen receptor/CD3 stimulation. Proc Natl Acad Sci USA 91:5301, 1994.
70. Crews FT, Morita Y, Hirata F, et al: Phospholipid methylation affects immunoglobulin E-mediated histamine and arachidonic acid release in rat leukemia basophils. Biochem Biophys Res Commun 93:42, 1980.
71. Crews FT, Morita Y, McGivney A, et al: IgE-mediated histamine release in rat basophilic leukemia cells: receptor activation, phospholipid methylation, Ca^{2+} flux, and release of arachidonic acid. Arch Biochem Biophys 212:561, 1981.
72. Cunha-Melo JR, Dean NM, Moyer JD, et al: The kinetics of phosphoinositide hydrolysis in rat basophilic leukemia (RBL-2H3) cells varies with the type of IgE receptor cross-linking agent used. J Biol Chem 262:11455, 1987.
73. Cunha-Melo JR, Gonzaga HM, Ali H, et al: Studies of protein kinase C in the rat basophilic leukemia (RBL-2H3) cell reveal that antigen-induced signals are not mimicked by the actions of phorbol myristate acetate and Ca^{2+} ionophore. J Immunol 143:2617, 1989.
74. Curran MJ, Cohen FS, Chandler DE, et al: Exocytotic fusion pores exhibit semi-stable states. J Membr Biol 133:61, 1993.
75. Currie S, Roberts EF, Spaethe SM, et al: Phosphorylation and activation of Ca^{2+}-sensitive cytosolic phospholipase A2 in MCII mast cells mediated by high-affinity Fc receptor for IgE. Biochem J 304:923, 1994.
76. Daeron M, Couderc J, Ventura M, et al: Anaphylactic properties of mouse monoclonal IgG2a antibodies. Cell Immunol 70:27, 1982.
77. Daeron M, Sterk AR, Hirata F, Ishizaka T: Biochemical analysis of glucocorticoid-induced inhibition of IgE-mediated histamine release from mouse mast cells. J Immunol 129:1212, 1982.
78. Dayton ET, Pharr P, Ogawa M, et al: 3T3 fibroblasts induce cloned interleukin 3-dependent mouse mast cells to resemble connective tissue mast cells in granular constituency. Proc Natl Acad Sci USA 85:569, 1988.
79. De Smedt H, Missiaen L, Parys JB, et al: Determination of relative amounts of inositol trisphosphate receptor mRNA isoforms by ratio polymerase chain reaction. J Biol Chem 269:21691, 1994.
80. Deckmyn H, Tu SM, Majerus PW: Guanine nucleotides stimulate soluble phosphoinositide-specific phospholipase C in the absence of membranes. J Biol Chem 261:16553, 1986.
81. DeLisi C, Siraganian RP: Receptor cross-linking and histamine release. II. Interpretation and analysis of anomalous dose response patterns. J Immunol 122:2293, 1979.
82. DeLisi C, Siraganian RP: Receptor cross-linking and histamine release. I. The quantitative dependence of basophil degranulation on the number of receptor doublets. J Immunol 122:2286, 1979.
83. Dembo M, Goldstein B: A model of cell activation and desensitization by surface immunoglobulin: the case of histamine release from human basophils. Cell 22:59, 1980.
84. Dembo M, Goldstein B, Sobotka AK, Lichtenstein LM: Degranulation of human basophils: quantitative analysis of histamine release and desensitization, due to a bivalent penicilloyl hapten. J Immunol 123:1864, 1979.
85. Dembo M, Goldstein B, Sobotka AK, Lichtenstein LM: Histamine release due to bivalent penicilloyl haptens: the relation of activation and desensitization of basophils to dynamic aspects of ligand binding to cell surface antibody. J Immunol 122:518, 1979.
86. Dietrich J, Lindau M: Chloride channels in mast cells: block by DIDS and role in exocytosis. J Gen Physiol 104:1099, 1994.
87. Dinh TT, Kennerly DA: Assessment of receptor-dependent activation of phosphatidylcholine hydrolysis by both phospholipase D and phospholipase C. Cell Regul 2:299, 1991.
88. Dogar JH, Nemeth GG, Durdik JM, Dreskin SC: FcεRI-mediated expression of mRNA for c-fos in rat basophilic leukemia cells does not require ongoing aggregation of the receptor. Cell Signal 5:605, 1993.
89. Dreskin SC, Kuhn DE, Huang Y: Phosphoenolpyruvate and creatine phosphate augment ATP and magnesium-dependent, FcεRI-mediated activation of phospholipase C in RBL cell ghosts. J Immunol 151:3199, 1993.
90. Dreskin SC, Metzger H: FcεRI-mediated hydrolysis of phosphoinositides in ghosts derived from rat basophilic leukemia cells. J Immunol 146:3102, 1991.
91. Dreskin SC, Pribluda VS, Metzger H: IgE receptor-mediated hydrolysis of phosphoinositides by cytoplasts from rat basophilic leukemia cells. J Immunol 142:4407, 1989.
92. Drobis JD, Siraganian RP: Histamine release from cultured human basophils: lack of histamine resynthesis after antigenic release. J Immunol 117:1049, 1976.
93. Ducharme LA, Weis JH: Modulation of integrin expression during mast cell differentiation. Eur J Immunol 22:2603, 1992.
94. Dvorak AM: Similarities in the ultrastructural morphology and developmental and secretory mechanisms of human basophils and eosinophils. J Allergy Clin Immunol 94 Suppl:1103, 1994.
95. Dvorak AM, Lett-Brown MA, Thueson DO, et al: Histamine-releasing activity (HRA). III. HRA induces human basophil histamine release by provoking noncytotoxic granule exocytosis. Clin Immunol Immunopathol 32:142, 1984.
96. Dvorak AM, Massey W, Warner J, et al: IgE-mediated anaphylactic degranulation of isolated human skin mast cells. Blood 77:569, 1991.
97. Dvorak AM, Schulman ES, Peters SP, et al: Immunoglobulin E-mediated degranulation of isolated human lung mast cells. Lab Invest 53:45, 1985.
98. Dvorak AM, Warner JA, Kissell S, et al: F-met peptide-induced degranulation of human basophils. Lab Invest 64:234, 1991.
99. Eiseman E, Bolen JB: Signal transduction by the cytoplasmic domains of FcεRI-γ and TCR-ζ in rat basophilic leukemia cells. J Biol Chem 267:21027, 1992.
100. Eiseman E, Bolen JB: Engagement of the high-affinity IgE receptor activates src protein-related tyrosine kinases. Nature 355:78, 1992.
101. Essani N, Essani K, Siraganian RP: Protein phosphorylation in rat basophilic leukemia cells following stimulation for histamine release. Fed Proc 45:243, 1986.

102. Fernandez JM, Neher E, Gomperts BD: Capacitance measurements reveal stepwise fusion events in degranulating mast cells. Nature 312:453, 1984.
103. Fewtrell C, Goetze A, Metzger H: Phosphorylation of the receptor of immunoglobulin E. Biochemistry 21:2004, 1982.
104. Fewtrell C, Metzger H: Larger oligomers of IgE are more effective than dimers in stimulating rat basophilic leukemia cells. J Immunol 125:701, 1980.
105. Fischer EH, Charbonneau H, Tonks NK: Protein tyrosine phosphatases: a diverse family of intracellular and transmembrane enzymes. Science 253:401, 1991.
106. Fox PC, Basciano LK, Siraganian RP: Mouse mast cell activation and desensitization for immune aggregate-induced histamine release. J Immunol 129:314, 1982.
107. Friis UG, Johansen T, Hayes NA, Foreman JC: IgE-receptor activated chloride uptake in relation to histamine secretion from rat mast cells. Br J Pharmacol 111:1179, 1994.
108. Fukamachi H, Kawakami Y, Takei M, et al: Association of protein-tyrosine kinase with phospholipase C-γ1 in bone marrow-derived mouse mast cells. Proc Natl Acad Sci USA 89:9524, 1992.
109. Fukamachi H, Takei M, Kawakami T: Activation of multiple protein kinases including a MAP kinase upon FcεRI cross-linking. Int Arch Allergy Immunol 102:15, 1993.
110. Fukamachi H, Yamada N, Miura T, et al: Identification of a protein, SPY75, with repetitive helix-turn-helix motifs and an SH3 domain as a major substrate for protein tyrosine kinase(s) activated by FcεRI cross-linking. J Immunol 152:642, 1994.
111. Furitsu T, Saito H, Dvorak AM, et al: Development of human mast cells in vitro. Proc Natl Acad Sci USA 86:10039, 1989.
112. Furuichi K, Ra C, Isersky C, Rivera J: Comparative evaluation of the effect of pharmacological agents on endocytosis and coendocytosis of IgE by rat basophilic leukaemia cells. Immunology 58:105, 1986.
113. Furuichi K, Rivera J, Buonocore LM, Isersky C: Recycling of receptor-bound IgE by rat basophilic leukemia cells. J Immunol 136:1015, 1986.
114. Furuichi K, Rivera J, Isersky C: The fate of IgE bound to rat basophilic leukemia cells. III. Relationship between antigen-induced endocytosis and serotonin release. J Immunol 133:1513, 1984.
115. Furuichi K, Rivera J, Isersky C: The receptor for immunoglobulin E on rat basophilic leukemia cells: effect of ligand binding on receptor expression. Proc Natl Acad Sci USA 82:1522, 1985.
116. Furuichi K, Rivera J, Triche T, Isersky C: The fate of IgE bound to rat basophilic leukemia cells. IV. Functional association between the receptors for IgE. J Immunol 134:1766, 1985.
117. Galli SJ: New insights into "the riddle of the mast cells": microenvironmental regulation of mast cell development and phenotypic heterogeneity. Lab Invest 62:5, 1990.
118. Galli SJ: New concepts about the mast cell. N Engl J Med 328:257, 1993.
119. Galli SJ, Dvorak AM, Dvorak HF: Basophils and mast cells: morphologic insights into their biology, secretory patterns, and function. Prog Allergy 34:1, 1984.
120. Galli SJ, Tsai M, Wershil BK: The c-kit receptor, stem cell factor, and mast cells. Am J Pathol 142:965, 1993.
121. Garcia-Gil M, Siraganian RP: Source of the arachidonic acid released on stimulation of rat basophilic leukemia cells. J Immunol 136:3825, 1986.
122. Garcia-Gil M, Siraganian RP: Phospholipase A2 stimulation during cell secretion in rat basophilic leukemia cells. J Immunol 136:259, 1986.
123. Gat-Yablonski G, Sagi-Eisenberg R: Differential down-regulation of protein kinase C selectively affects IgE-dependent exocytosis and inositol trisphosphate formation. Biochem J 270:679, 1990.
124. Gat-Yablonski G, Sagi-Eisenberg R: Evaluation of the role of inositol trisphosphate in IgE-dependent exocytosis. Biochem J 270:685, 1990.
125. Germano P, Gomez J, Kazanietz MG, et al: Phosphorylation of the γ chain of the high affinity receptor for immunoglobulin E by receptor-associated protein kinase C-δ. J Biol Chem 269:23102, 1994.
126. Gilfillan AM, Kado-Fong H, Wiggan GA, et al: Conservation of signal transduction mechanisms via the human FcεRI-α after transfection into a rat mast cell line, RBL 2H3. J Immunol 149:2445, 1992.
127. Gillespie E, Lichtenstein LM: Histamine release from human leukocytes: studies with deuterium oxide, colchicine, and cytochalasin B. J Clin Invest 51:2941, 1972.
128. Goetzl EJ, Chernov T, Renold F, Payan DG: Neuropeptide regulation of the expression of immediate hypersensitivity. J Immunol 135:802s, 1985.
129. Gomperts BD: GE: a GTP-binding protein mediating exocytosis. Annu Rev Physiol 52:591, 1990.
130. Gomperts BD, Barrowman MM, Cockcroft S: Dual role for guanine nucleotides in stimulus-secretion coupling. Fed Proc 45:2156, 1986.
131. Gordon JR, Burd PR, Galli SJ: Mast cells as a source of multifunctional cytokines. Immunol Today 11:458, 1990.
132. Gruchalla RS, Dinh TT, Kennerly DA: An indirect pathway of receptor-mediated 1,2-diacylglycerol formation in mast cells. I. IgE receptor-mediated activation of phospholipase D. J Immunol 144:2334, 1990.
133. Guo NH, Her GR, Reinhold VN, et al: Monoclonal antibody AA4, which inhibits binding of IgE to high affinity receptors on rat basophilic leukemia cells, binds to novel α-galactosyl derivatives of ganglioside GD1b. J Biol Chem 264:13267, 1989.
134. Gurish MF, Bell AF, Smith TJ, et al: Expression of murine β-7, α-4, and β-1 integrin genes by rodent mast cells. J Immunol 149:1964, 1992.
135. Haak-Frendscho M, Arai N, Arai K, et al: Human recombinant granulocyte-macrophage colony-stimulating factor and interleukin 3 cause basophil histamine release. J Clin Invest 82:17, 1988.
136. Hamawy MM, Mergenhagen S, Siraganian RP: Tyrosine phosphorylation of $pp125^{FAK}$ by the aggregation of high affinity immunoglobulin E receptors requires cell adherence. J Biol Chem 268:6851, 1993.
137. Hamawy MM, Mergenhagen SE, Siraganian RP: Cell adherence to fibronectin and the aggregation of the high affinity IgE receptor synergistically regulate tyrosine phosphorylation of 105-115 kDa proteins. J Biol Chem 268:5227, 1993.
138. Hamawy MM, Mergenhagen SE, Siraganian RP: Adhesion molecules as regulators of mast cell and basophil function. Immunol Today 15:62, 1994.
139. Hamawy MM, Minoguchi K, Swaim WD, et al: A 77-kDa protein associates with $pp125^{FAK}$ in mast cells and becomes tyrosine-phosphorylated by high affinity IgE receptor aggregation. J Biol Chem 270:12305, 1995.
140. Hamawy MM, Oliver C, Mergenhagen SE, Siraganian RP: Adherence of rat basophilic leukemia (RBL-2H3) cells to fibronectin-coated surfaces enhances secretion. J Immunol 149:615, 1992.
141. Hammel I, Lagunoff D, Kruger PG: Recovery of rat mast cells after secretion: a morphometric study. Exp Cell Res 184:518, 1989.
142. Hampe CS, Pecht I: Protein tyrosine phosphatase activity enhancement is induced upon Fcε receptor activation of mast cells. FEBS Lett 346:194, 1994.
143. Hanks SK, Calalb MB, Harper MC, Patel SK: Focal adhesion protein-tyrosine kinase phosphorylated in response to cell attachment to fibronectin. Proc Natl Acad Sci USA 89:8487, 1992.
144. Hastie R: The antigen-induced degranulation of basophil leucocytes from atopic subjects, studied by phase-contrast microscopy. Clin Exp Immunol 8:45, 1971.
145. Hattori Y, Siraganian RP: Rapid phosphorylation of a 92,000 MW protein on activation of rat basophilic leukemia cells for histamine release. Immunology 60:573, 1987.
146. Hemmerich S, Sijpkens D, Pecht I: A novel cell-permeable cromoglycate derivative inhibits type I Fcε receptor mediated Ca^{2+} influx and mediator secretion in rat mucosal mast cells. Biochemistry 30:1523, 1991.
147. Hemmerich S, Yarden Y, Pecht I: A cromoglycate binding protein from rat mast cells of a leukemia line is a nucleoside diphosphate kinase. Biochemistry 31:4574, 1992.
148. Hempstead BL, Parker CW, Kulczycki A Jr: Selective phosphorylation of the IgE receptor in antigen-stimulated rat mast cells. Proc Natl Acad Sci USA 80:3050, 1983.
149. Hernandez-Asensio M, Hooks JJ, Ida S, et al: Interferon-induced enhancement of IgE-mediated histamine release from human basophils requires RNA synthesis. J Immunol 122:1601, 1979.
150. Hesketh TR, Beaven MA, Rogers J, et al: Stimulated release of histamine by a rat mast cell line is inhibited during mitosis. J Cell Biol 98:2250, 1984.
151. Hide M, Beaven MA: Calcium influx in a rat mast cell (RBL-2H3) line. Use of multivalent metal ions to define its characteristics and role in exocytosis. J Biol Chem 266:15221, 1991.
152. Hirai K, Morita Y, Misaki Y, et al: Modulation of human basophil histamine release by hemopoietic growth factors. J Immunol 141:3958, 1988.
153. Hirasawa N, Santini F, Beaven MA: Activation of the mitogen-activated protein kinase/cytosolic phospholipase A2 pathway in a rat mast cell line. Indications of different pathways for release of arachidonic acid and secretory granules. J Immunol 154:5391, 1995.

154. Hirata F, Axelrod J: Phospholipid methylation and biological signal transmission. Science 209:1082, 1980.
155. Hirata F, Axelrod J, Crews FT: Concanavalin A stimulates phospholipid methylation and phosphatidylserine decarboxylation in rat mast cells. Proc Natl Acad Sci USA 76:4813, 1979.
156. Hook WA, Berenstein EH, Zinsser FU, et al: Monoclonal antibodies to the leukocyte common antigen (CD45) inhibit IgE-mediated histamine release from human basophils. J Immunol 147:2670, 1991.
157. Hook WA, Schiffmann E, Aswanikumar S, Siraganian RP: Histamine release by chemotactic, formyl methionine-containing peptides. J Immunol 117:594, 1976.
158. Hook WA, Siraganian RP: Influence of anions, cations and osmolarity on IgE-mediated histamine release from human basophils. Immunology 43:723, 1981.
159. Hook WA, Siraganian RP, Wahl SM: Complement-induced histamine release from human basophils. I. Generation of activity in human serum. J Immunol 114:1185, 1975.
160. Horikoshi Y, Furuno T, Teshima R, et al: Thapsigargin-induced nuclear calcium signals in rat basophilic leukaemia cells. Biochem J 304:57, 1994.
161. Hoth M, Penner R: Depletion of intracellular calcium stores activates a calcium current in mast cells. Nature 355:353, 1992.
162. Hoth M, Penner R: Calcium release-activated calcium current in rat mast cells. J Physiol (Lond) 465:359, 1993.
163. Howell TW, Kramer IM, Gomperts BD: Protein phosphorylation and the dependence on Ca^{2+} and GTP-γ-S for exocytosis from permeabilized mast cells. Cell Signal 1:157, 1989.
164. Huang FL, Yoshida Y, Cunha-Melo JR, et al: Differential down-regulation of protein kinase C isozymes. J Biol Chem 264:4238, 1989.
165. Hugli TE, Muller-Eberhard HJ: Anaphylatoxins: C3a and C5a. Adv Immunol 26:1, 1978.
166. Hunter T: Protein-tyrosine phosphatases: the other side of the coin. Cell 58:1013, 1989.
167. Hutchcroft JE, Geahlen RL, Deanin GG, Oliver JM: FcεRI-mediated tyrosine phosphorylation and activation of the 72-kDa protein-tyrosine kinase, PTK72, in RBL-2H3 rat tumor mast cells. Proc Natl Acad Sci USA 89:9107, 1992.
168. Hynes RO: Integrins: versatility, modulation, and signaling in cell adhesion. Cell 69:11, 1992.
169. Ida S, Hooks JJ, Siraganian RP, Notkins AL: Enhancement of IgE-mediated histamine release from human basophils by viruses: role of interferon. J Exp Med 145:892, 1977.
170. Ida S, Hooks JJ, Siraganian RP, Notkins AL: Enhancement of IgE-mediated histamine release from human basophils by immune-specific lymphokines. Clin Exp Immunol 41:380, 1980.
171. Ihle JN, Witthuhn BA, Quelle FW, et al: Signaling through the hematopoietic cytokine receptors. Annu Rev Immunol 13:369, 1995.
172. Irving BA, Chan AC, Weiss A: Functional characterization of a signal transducing motif present in the T cell antigen receptor zeta chain. J Exp Med 177:1093, 1993.
173. Irving BA, Weiss A: The cytoplasmic domain of the T cell receptor ζ chain is sufficient to couple to receptor-associated signal transduction pathways. Cell 64:891, 1991.
174. Isersky C, Rivera J, Mims S, Triche TJ: The fate of IgE bound to rat basophilic leukemia cells. J Immunol 122:1926, 1979.
175. Isersky C, Rivera J, Segal DM, Triche T: The fate of IgE bound to rat basophilic leukemia cells. II. Endocytosis of IgE oligomers and effect on receptor turnover. J Immunol 131:388, 1983.
176. Ishizaka T: Biochemical analysis of triggering signals induced by bridging of IgE receptors. Fed Proc 41:17, 1982.
177. Ishizaka T, Conrad DH, Schulman ES, et al: Biochemical analysis of initial triggering events of IgE-mediated histamine release from human lung mast cells. J Immunol 130:2357, 1983.
178. Ishizaka T, Dvorak AM, Conrad DH, et al: Morphologic and immunologic characterization of human basophils developed in cultures of cord blood mononuclear cells. J Immunol 134:532, 1985.
179. Ishizaka T, Hirata F, Ishizaka K, Axelrod J: Stimulation of phospholipid methylation, Ca^{2+} influx, and histamine release by bridging of IgE receptors on rat mast cells. Proc Natl Acad Sci USA 77:1903, 1980.
180. Ishizaka T, Hirata F, Sterk AR, et al: Bridging of IgE receptors activates phospholipid methylation and adenylate cyclase in mast cell plasma membranes. Proc Natl Acad Sci USA 78:6812, 1981.
181. Ishizaka T, Ishizaka K: Activation of mast cells for mediator release through IgE receptors. Prog Allergy 34:188, 1984.
182. Ishizaka T, Sterk AR, Daeron M, et al: Biochemical analysis of desensitization of mouse mast cells. J Immunol 135:492, 1985.
183. Ishizaka T, Sterk AR, Ishizaka K: Demonstration of Fcγ receptors on human basophil granulocytes. J Immunol 123:578, 1979.
184. Iwashima M, Irving BA, Van Oers NSC, et al: Sequential interactions of the TCR with two distinct cytoplasmic tyrosine kinases. Science 263:1136, 1994.
185. Izushi K, Fujiwara Y, Tasaka K: Identification of vimentin in rat peritoneal mast cells and its phosphorylation in association with histamine release. Immunopharmacology 23:153, 1992.
186. Johansen T: Further observations on the utilization of adenosine triphosphate in rat mast cells during histamine release induced by the ionophore A23187. Br J Pharmacol 69:657, 1980.
187. Johansen T: Dependence of anaphylactic histamine release from rat mast cells on cellular energy metabolism. Eur J Pharmacol 72:281, 1981.
188. Jouvin MHE, Adamczewski M, Numerof R, et al: Differential control of the tyrosine kinases Lyn and Syk by the two signaling chains of the high affinity immunoglobulin E receptor. J Biol Chem 269:5918, 1994.
189. Juliano RL, Haskill S: Signal transduction from the extracellular matrix. J Cell Biol 120:577, 1993.
190. Kagey-Sobotka A, Dembo M, Goldstein B, et al: Qualitative characteristics of histamine release from human basophils by covalently cross-linked IgE. J Immunol 127:2285, 1981.
191. Kane P, Erickson J, Fewtrell C, et al: Cross-linking of IgE-receptor complexes at the cell surface: synthesis and characterization of a long bivalent hapten that is capable of triggering mast cells and rat basophilic leukemia cells. Mol Immunol 23:783, 1986.
192. Kane PM, Holowka D, Baird B: Cross-linking of IgE-receptor complexes by rigid bivalent antigens greater than 200 Å in length triggers cellular degranulation. J Cell Biol 107:969, 1988.
193. Kaneko Y, Takenawa J, Yoshida O, et al: Adhesion of mouse mast cells to fibroblasts: adverse effects of steel (S1) mutation. J Cell Physiol 147:224, 1991.
194. Kanner BI, Metzger H: Crosslinking of the receptors for immunoglobulin E depolarizes the plasma membrane of rat basophilic leukemia cells. Proc Natl Acad Sci USA 80:5744, 1983.
195. Kanner BI, Metzger H: Initial characterization of the calcium channel activated by the cross-linking of the receptors for immunoglobulin E. J Biol Chem 259:10188, 1984.
196. Kaplan AP, Reddigari S, Baeza M, Kuna P: Histamine releasing factors and cytokine-dependent activation of basophils and mast cells. Adv Immunol 50:237, 1991.
197. Katagiri S, Takamatsu T, Minamikawa T, Fujita S: Secretagogue-induced calcium wave shows higher and prolonged transients of nuclear calcium concentration in mast cells. FEBS Lett 334:343, 1993.
198. Katz HR, Arm JP, Benson AC, Austen KF: Maturation-related changes in the expression of FcγRII and FcγRIII on mouse mast cells derived in vitro and in vivo. J Immunol 145:3412, 1990.
199. Katz HR, Raizman MB, Gartner CS, et al: Secretory granule mediator release and generation of oxidative metabolites of arachidonic acid via Fc-IgG receptor bridging in mouse mast cells. J Immunol 148: 868,1992.
200. Katzav S, Sutherland M, Packham G, et al: The protein tyrosine kinase ZAP-70 can associate with the SH2 domain of proto-Vav. J Biol Chem 269:32579, 1994.
201. Kawakami T, Inagaki N, Takei M, et al: Tyrosine phosphorylation is required for mast cell activation by FcεRI cross-linking. J Immunol 148:3513, 1992.
202. Kawakami Y, Yao L, Miura T, et al: Tyrosine phosphorylation and activation of bruton tyrosine kinase upon FcεRI cross-linking. Mol Cell Biol 14:5108, 1994.
203. Kazimierczak W, Meier HL, MacGlashan DW Jr, Lichtenstein LM: An antigen-activated DFP-inhibitable enzyme controls basophil desensitization. J Immunol 132:399, 1984.
204. Kaziro Y, Itoh H, Kozasa T, et al: Structure and function of signal-transducing GTP-binding proteins. Annu Rev Biochem 60:349, 1991.
205. Kennerly DA: Diacylglycerol metabolism in mast cells. Analysis of lipid metabolic pathways using molecular species analysis of intermediates. J Biol Chem 262:16305, 1987.
206. Kennerly DA: Phosphatidylcholine is a quantitatively more important source of increased 1,2-diacylglycerol than is phosphatidylinositol in mast cells. J Immunol 144:3912, 1990.
207. Kennerly DA, Secosan CJ, Parker CW, Sullivan TJ: Modulation of stimulated phospholipid metabolism in mast cells by pharmacologic agents that increase cyclic 3′,5′ adenosine monophosphate levels. J Immunol 123:1519, 1979.

208. Kennerly DA, Sullivan TJ, Parker CW: Activation of phospholipid metabolism during mediator release from stimulated rat mast cells. J Immunol 122:152, 1979.
209. Kennerly DA, Sullivan TJ, Sylwester P, Parker CW: Diacylglycerol metabolism in mast cells: a potential role in membrane fusion and arachidonic acid release. J Exp Med 150:1039, 1979.
210. Kido H, Izumi K, Otsuka H, et al: A chymotrypsin-type serine protease in rat basophilic leukemia cells: evidence for its immunologic identity with atypical mast cell protease. J Immunol 136:1061, 1986.
211. Kihara H, Siraganian RP: Src homology 2 domains of Syk and Lyn bind to tyrosine-phosphorylated subunits of the high affinity IgE receptor. J Biol Chem 269:22427, 1994.
212. Kirshenbaum AS, Goff JP, Dreskin SC, et al: IL-3-dependent growth of basophil-like cells and mastlike cells from human bone marrow. J Immunol 142:2424, 1989.
213. Kitamura Y: Heterogeneity of mast cells and phenotypic change between subpopulations. Annu Rev Immunol 7:59, 1989.
214. Kitamura Y, Kasugai T, Arizono N, Matsuda H: Development of mast cells and basophils: processes and regulation mechanisms. Am J Med Sci 306:185, 1993.
215. Kitani S, Berenstein E, Mergenhagen S, et al: A cell surface glycoprotein of rat basophilic leukemia cells close to the high affinity IgE Receptor (FcεRI). Similarity to human melanoma differentiation antigen ME491. J Biol Chem 266:1903, 1991.
216. Knudsen T, Ferjan I, Johansen T: Activation of the Na^+/K^+-pump in rat peritoneal mast cells following histamine release: a possible role in cell recovery. Br J Pharmacol 108;120, 1993.
217. Koch CA, Anderson D, Moran MF, et al: SH2 and SH3 domains: elements that control interactions of cytoplasmic signaling proteins. Science 252:668, 1991.
218. Koffer A, Tatham PE, Gomperts BD: Changes in the state of actin during the exocytotic reaction of permeabilized rat mast cells. J Cell Biol 111:919, 1990.
219. Koopmann WR Jr, Jackson RC: Calcium- and guanine-nucleotide-dependent exocytosis in permeabilized rat mast cells. Modulation by protein kinase C. Biochem J 265:365, 1990.
220. Kopicky-Burd JA, Kagey-Sobotka A, Peters SP, et al: Characterization of human synovial mast cells. J Rheumatol 15:1326, 1988.
221. Kuna P, Reddigari SR, Schall TJ, et al: Characterization of the human basophil response to cytokines, growth factors, and histamine releasing factors of the intercrine/chemokine family. J Immunol 150:1932, 1993.
222. Kuno M, Kawaguchi J, Mukai M, Nakamura F: PT pretreatment inhibits 48/80-induced activation of Ca^{2+}-permeable channels in rat peritoneal mast cells. Am J Physiol 259:C715, 1990.
223. Kuno M, Kawawaki J, Shibata T, Gotani H: Inhibitors of the arachidonic acid cascade dissociate 48/80-induced Ca^{2+} influx and Ca^{2+} release in mast cells. Am J Physiol Cell Physiol 264:C912, 1993.
224. Kurimoto Y, De Weck AL, Dahinden CA: Interleukin 3-dependent mediator release in basophils triggered by C5a. J Exp Med 170:467, 1989.
225. Labrecque GF, Holowka D, Baird B: Antigen-triggered membrane potential changes in IgE-sensitized rat basophilic leukemia cells: evidence for a repolarizing response that is important in the stimulation of cellular degranulation. J Immunol 142:236, 1989.
226. Lagunoff D, Chi EY: Cell biology of mast cells and basophils. Glynn LE, Houck JC, Weissman G (eds): The Cell Biology of Inflammation. Handbook of Inflammation. Elsevier/North Holland, New York, 1980, p 217.
227. Lavens SE, Peachell PT, Warner JA: Role of tyrosine kinases in IgE-mediated signal transduction in human lung mast cells and basophils. Am J Respir Cell Mol Biol 7:637, 1992.
228. Law GJ, Northrop AJ, Mason WT: Rab3-peptide stimulates exocytosis from mast cells via a pertussis toxin-sensitive mechanism. FEBS Lett 333:56, 1993.
229. Lawrence ID, Warner JA, Cohan VL, et al: Induction of histamine release from human skin mast cells by bradykinin analogs. Biochem Pharmacol 38:227, 1989.
230. Lawson D, Fewtrell C, Raff MC: Localized mast cell degranulation induced by concanavalin A-sepharose beads. Implications for the Ca^{2+} hypothesis of stimulus-secretion coupling. J Cell Biol 79:394, 1978.
231. Lawson D, Raff MC, Gomperts B, et al: Molecular events during membrane fusion. A study of exocytosis in rat peritoneal mast cells. J Cell Biol 72:242, 1977.
232. Letourneur F, Klausner RD: T-cell and basophil activation through the cytoplasmic tail of T-cell-receptor ζ family proteins. Proc Natl Acad Sci USA 88:8905, 1991.
233. Lev S, Givol D, Yarden Y: A specific combination of substrates is involved in signal transduction by the kit-encoded receptor. EMBO J 10:647, 1991.
234. Levi-Schaffer F, Austen KF, Caulfield JP, et al: Fibroblasts maintain the phenotype and viability of the rat heparin-containing mast cell in vitro. J Immunol 135:3454, 1985.
235. Levi-Schaffer F, Austen KF, Caulfield JP, et al: Co-culture of human lung-derived mast cells with mouse 3T3 fibroblasts: morphology and IgE-mediated release of histamine, prostaglandin D2, and leukotrienes. J Immunol 139:494, 1987.
236. Levi-Schaffer F, Austen KF, Gravallese PM, Stevens RL: Coculture of interleukin 3-dependent mouse mast cells with fibroblasts results in a phenotypic change of the mast cells. Proc Natl Acad Sci USA 83:6485, 1986.
237. Levi-Schaffer F, Bar-Shavit Z: Osteoblast-like cell line maintains in vitro rat peritoneal mast cell viability and functional activity. Immunology 69:145, 1990.
238. Levi-Schaffer F, Dayton ET, Austen KF, et al: Mouse bone marrow-derived mast cells cocultured with fibroblasts. Morphology and stimulation-induced release of histamine, leukotriene B4, leukotriene C4, and prostaglandin D2. J Immunol 139:3431, 1987.
239. Levi-Schaffer F, Shalit M: Long-term cultures of mast cells: a new model for studying the allergic response. Pharmacol Res 24:307, 1991.
240. Lewis RA, Holgate ST, Roberts LJ 2d, et al: Effects of indomethacin on cyclic nucleotide levels and histamine release from rat serosal mast cells. J Immunol 123:1663, 1979.
241. Li W, Deanin GG, Margolis B, et al: FcεR1-mediated tyrosine phosphorylation of multiple proteins, including phospholipase C, γ1 and the receptor β,γ2 complex, in RBL-2H3 rat basophilic leukemia cells. Mol Cell Biol 12:3176, 1992.
242. Li W, Hu P, Skolnik EY, et al: The SH2 and SH3 domain-containing Nck protein is oncogenic and a common target for phosphorylation by different surface receptors. Mol Cell Biol 12:5824, 1992.
243. Lin LL, Wartmann M, Lin AY, et al: cPLA2 is phosphorylated and activated by MAP kinase. Cell 72:269, 1993.
244. Lin P, Fung WJ, Gilfillan AM: Phosphatidylcholine-specific phospholipase D-derived 1,2-diacylglycerol does not initiate protein kinase C activation in the RBL 2H3 mast-cell line. Biochem J 287:325, 1992.
245. Lin P, Fung WJC, Li S, et al: Temporal regulation of the IgE-dependent 1,2-diacylglycerol production by tyrosine kinase activation in a rat (RBL 2H3) mast-cell line. Biochem J 299:109, 1994.
246. Lin P, Gilfillan AM: The role of calcium and protein kinase C in the IgE-dependent activation of phosphatidylcholine-specific phospholipase D in a rat mast (RBL 2H3) cell line. Eur J Biochem 207:163, 1992.
247. Lin PY, Wiggan GA, Gilfillan AM: Activation of phospholipase D in a rat mast (RBL 2H3) cell line. A possible unifying mechanism for IgE-dependent degranulation and arachidonic acid metabolite release. J Immunol 146:1609, 1991.
248. Lin PY, Wiggan GA, Welton AF, Gilfillan AM: Differential effects of propranolol on the IgE-dependent, or calcium ionophore-stimulated, phosphoinositide hydrolysis and calcium mobilization in a mast (RBL 2H3) cell line. Biochem Pharmacol 41:1941, 1991.
249. Lindau M, Fernandez JM: IgE-mediated degranulation of mast cells does not require opening of ion channels. Nature 319:150, 1986.
250. Lo TN, Saul W, Beaven MA: The actions of Ca^{2+} ionophores on rat basophilic (2H3) cells are dependent on cellular ATP and hydrolysis of inositol phospholipids. A comparison with antigen stimulation. J Biol Chem 262:4141, 1987.
251. Lowman MA, Rees PH, Benyon RC, Church MK: Human mast cell heterogeneity: histamine release from mast cells dispersed from skin, lung, adenoids, tonsils, and colon in response to IgE-dependent and nonimmunologic stimuli. J Allergy Clin Immunol 81:590, 1988.
252. Ludowyke RI, Peleg I, Beaven MA, Adelstein RS: Antigen-induced secretion of histamine and the phosphorylation of myosin by protein kinase C in rat basophilic leukemia cells. J Biol Chem 264:12492, 1989.
253. MacDonald SM, Lichtenstein LM, Proud D, et al: Studies of IgE-dependent histamine releasing factors: heterogeneity of IgE. J Immunol 139:506, 1987.
254. MacDonald SM, Rafnar T, Langdon J, Lichtenstein LM: Molecular identification of an IgE-dependent histamine-releasing factor. Science 269:688, 1995.
255. MacDonald SM, Schleimer RP, Kagey-Sobotka A, et al: Recombinant IL-3 induces histamine release from human basophils. J Immunol 142:3527, 1989.

256. MacGlashan D Jr, Lichtenstein LM: Studies of antigen binding on human basophils. I. Antigen binding and functional consequences. J Immunol 130:2330, 1983.
257. MacGlashan D Jr, Mogowski M, Lichtenstein LM: Studies of antigen binding on human basophils. II. Continued expression of antigen-specific IgE during antigen-induced desensitization. J Immunol 130:2337, 1983.
258. MacGlashan DW Jr, Lichtenstein LM: The purification of human basophils. J Immunol 124:2519, 1980.
259. MacGlashan DW Jr, Lichtenstein LM: The transition from specific to nonspecific desensitization in human basophils. J Immunol 127: 2410, 1981.
260. MacGlashan DW Jr, Peters SP, Warner J, Lichtenstein LM: Characteristics of human basophil sulfidopeptide leukotriene release: releasability defined as the ability of the basophil to respond to dimeric cross-links. J Immunol 136:2231, 1986.
261. MacGlashan DW Jr, Schleimer RP, Lichtenstein LM: Qualitative differences between dimeric and trimeric stimulation of human basophils. J Immunol 130:4, 1983.
262. MacGlashan DW Jr, Schleimer RP, Peters SP, et al: Comparative studies of human basophils and mast cells. Fed Proc 42:2504, 1983.
263. MacGlashan D Jr: Single-cell analysis of Ca^{2+} changes in human lung mast cells: graded vs. all-or-nothing elevations after IgE-mediated stimulation. J Cell Biol 109:123, 1989.
264. MacGlashan D Jr: Single cell analysis of free cytosolic calcium changes in human lung mast cells—II. The relationship between desensitization and the cellular regulation of calcium changes. Mol Immunol 28:585, 1991.
265. MacGlashan D Jr: Signal transduction: mechanisms in basophils. J Allergy Clin Immunol 94 Suppl:1146, 1994.
266. MacGlashan D Jr, Guo CB: Oscillations in free cytosolic calcium during IgE-mediated stimulation distinguish human basophils from human mast cells. J Immunol 147:2259, 1991.
267. MacGlashan D Jr, Lichtenstein LM: Basic characteristics of human lung mast cell desensitization. J Immunol 139:501, 1987.
268. MacGlashan DW Jr: Releasability of human basophils: cellular sensitivity and maximal histamine release are independent variables. J Allergy Clin Immunol 91:605, 1993.
269. Maeyama K, Hohman RJ, Ali H, et al: Assessment of IgE-receptor function through measurement of hydrolysis of membrane inositol phospholipids. New insights on the phenomena of biphasic antigen concentration-response curves and desensitization. J Immunol 140;3919, 1988.
270. Maeyama K, Hohman RJ, Metzger H, Beaven MA: Quantitative relationships between aggregation of IgE receptors, generation of intracellular signals, and histamine secretion in rat basophilic leukemia (2H3) cells. Enhanced responses with heavy water. J Biol Chem 261:2583, 1986.
271. Majerus PW, Ross TS, Cunningham TW, et al: Recent insights in phosphatidylinositol signaling. Cell 63:459, 1990.
272. Malveaux FJ, Conroy MC, Adkinson NF Jr, Lichtenstein LM: IgE receptors on human basophils. Relationship to serum IgE concentration. J Clin Invest 62:176, 1978.
273. Mao S, Yamashita T, Metzger H: Chemical cross-linking of IgE-receptor complexes in RBL-2H3 cells. Biochemistry 34:1968, 1995.
274. Mao SY, Varin-Blank N, Edidin M, Metzger H: Immobilization and internalization of mutated IgE receptors in transfected cells. J Immunol 146:958, 1991.
275. Margolis B, Hu P, Katzav S, et al: Tyrosine phosphorylation of vav proto-oncogene product containing SH2 domain and transcription factor motifs. Nature 356:71, 1992.
276. Marone G, Kagey-Sobotka A, Lichtenstein LM: Effects of arachidonic acid and its metabolites on antigen-induced histamine release from human basophils in vitro. J Immunol 123:1669, 1979.
277. Marone G, Poto S, Celestino D, Bonini S: Human basophil releasability. III. Genetic control of human basophil releasability. J Immunol 137:3588, 1986.
278. Marquardt DL, Nicolotti RA, Kennerly DA, Sullivan TJ: Lipid metabolism during mediator release from mast cells: studies of the role of arachidonic acid metabolism in the control of phospholipid metabolism. J Immunol 127:845, 1981.
279. Massey WA, Randall TC, Kagey-Sobotka A, et al: Recombinant human IL-1α and -1β potentiate IgE-mediated histamine release from human basophils. J Immunol 143:1875, 1989.
280. Matthews G, Neher E, Penner R: Chloride conductance activated by external agonists and internal messengers in rat peritoneal mast cells. J Physiol (Lond) 418:131, 1989.
281. Matthews G, Neher E, Penner R: Second messenger-activated calcium influx in rat peritoneal mast cells. J Physiol (Lond) 418:105, 1989.
282. Mayer BJ, Baltimore D: Signalling through SH2 and SH3 domains. Trends Cell Biol 3:8, 1993.
283. Mazurek N, Bashkin P, Loyter A, Pecht I: Restoration of Ca^{2+} influx and degranulation capacity of variant RBL-2H3 cells upon implantation of isolated cromolyn binding protein. Proc Natl Acad Sci USA 80:6014, 1983.
284. Mazurek N, Bashkin P, Pecht I: Isolation of a basophilic membrane protein binding the anti-allergic drug cromolyn. EMBO J 1:585, 1982.
285. Mazurek N, Bashkin P, Petrank A, Pecht I: Basophil variants with impaired cromoglycate binding do not respond to an immunological degranulation stimulus. Nature 303:528, 1983.
286. Mazurek N, Berger G, Pecht I: A binding site on mast cells and basophils for the anti-allergic drug cromolyn. Nature 286:722, 1980.
287. Mazurek N, Dulic V, Pecht I, et al: The role of the Fcϵ receptor in calcium channel opening in rat basophilic leukemia cells. Immunol Lett 12:31, 1986.
288. Mazurek N, Geller-Bernstein C, Pecht I: Affinity of calcium ions to the anti-allergic drug, dicromoglycate. FEBS Lett 111:194, 1980.
289. Mazurek N, Schindler H, Schurholz T, Pecht I: The cromolyn binding protein constitutes the Ca^{2+} channel of basophils opening upon immunological stimulus. Proc Natl Acad Sci USA 81:6841, 1984.
290. McCloskey MA: Immobilization of Fcϵ receptors by wheat germ agglutinin: receptor dynamics in IgE-mediated signal transduction. J Immunol 151:3237, 1993.
291. McCloskey MA, Liu ZY, Poo MM: Lateral electromigration and diffusion of Fcϵ receptors on rat basophilic leukemia cells: effects of IgE binding. J Cell Biol 99:778, 1984.
292. McCloskey MA, Qian Y: Selective expression of potassium channels during mast cell differentiation. J Biol Chem 269:14813, 1994
293. McGivney A, Crews FT, Hirata F, et al: Rat basophilic leukemia cell lines defective in phospholipid methyltransferase enzymes, Ca^{2+} influx, and histamine release: reconstitution by hybridization. Proc Natl Acad Sci USA 78:6176, 1981.
294. McGivney A, Morita Y, Crews FT, et al: Phospholipase activation in the IgE-mediated and Ca^{2+} ionophore A23187-induced release of histamine from rat basophilic leukemia cells. Arch Biochem Biophys 212:572, 1981.
295. Mendoza G, Metzger H: Distribution and valency of receptor for IgE on rodent mast cells and related tumour cells. Nature 264:548, 1976.
296. Menon AK, Holowka D, Baird B: Small oligomers of immunoglobulin E (IgE) cause large-scale clustering of IgE receptors on the surface of rat basophilic leukemia cells. J Cell Biol 98:577, 1984.
297. Menon AK, Holowka D, Webb WW, Baird B: Clustering, mobility, and triggering activity of small oligomers of immunoglobulin E on rat basophilic leukemia cells. J Cell Biol 102:534, 1986.
298. Menon AK, Holowka D, Webb WW, Baird B: Cross-linking of receptor-bound IgE to aggregates larger than dimers leads to rapid immobilization. J Cell Biol 102:541, 1986.
299. Metzger H, Alcaraz G, Hohman R, et al: The receptor with high affinity for immunoglobulin E. Annu Rev Immunol 4:419, 1986.
300. Meyer C, Wahl LM, Stadler BM, Siraganian RP: Cell cycle associated changes in histamine release from rat basophilic leukemia cells separated by counterflow centrifugal elutriation. J Immunol 131:911, 1983.
301. Millard PJ, Gross D, Webb WW, Fewtrell C: Imaging asynchronous changes in intracellular Ca^{2+} in individual stimulated tumor mast cells. Proc Natl Acad Sci USA 85:1854, 1988.
302. Miller L, Alber G, Varin-Blank N, et al: Transmembrane signaling in P815 mastocytoma cells by transfected IgE receptors. J Biol Chem 265:12444, 1990.
303. Minoguchi K, Benhamou M, Swaim WD, et al: Activation of protein tyrosine kinase $p72^{syk}$ by FcϵRI aggregation in rat basophilic leukemia cells: $p72^{syk}$ is a minor component but the major protein tyrosine kinase of pp72. J Biol Chem 269:16902, 1994.
304. Minoguchi K, Kihara H, Nishikata H, et al: Src family tyrosine kinase Lyn binds several proteins including paxillin in rat basophilic leukemia cells. Mol Immunol 31:519, 1994.
305. Minoguchi K, Swaim WD, Berenstein EH, Siraganian RP: Src family tyrosine kinase $p53/p56^{lyn}$, a serine kinase and FcϵRI associate with alpha-galactosyl derivatives of ganglioside GD1b in rat basophilic leukemia RBL-2H3 cells. J Biol Chem 269:5249, 1994.

306. Mohr FC, Fewtrell C: IgE receptor-mediated depolarization of rat basophilic leukemia cells measured with the fluorescent probe bis-oxonol. J Immunol 138:1564, 1987.
307. Mohr FC, Fewtrell C: Depolarization of rat basophilic leukemia cells inhibits calcium uptake and exocytosis. J Cell Biol 104:783, 1987.
308. Mohr FC, Fewtrell C: The relative contributions of extracellular and intracellular calcium to secretion from tumor mast cells. Multiple effects of the proton ionophore carbonyl cyanide m-chlorophenylhydrazone. J Biol Chem 262:10638, 1987.
309. Mohr FC, Fewtrell C: The effect of mitochondrial inhibitors on calcium homeostasis in tumor mast cells. Am J Physiol 258:C217, 1990.
310. Monck JR, Alvarez de Toledo G, Fernandez JM: Tension in secretory granule membranes causes extensive membrane transfer through the exocytotic fusion pore. Proc Natl Acad Sci USA 87:7804, 1990.
311. Monck JR, Oberhauser AF, Alvarez de Toledo G, Fernandez JM: Is swelling of the secretory granule matrix the force that dilates the exocytotic fusion pore? Biophys J 59:39, 1991.
312. Moore JP, Johannsson A, Hesketh TR, et al: Calcium signals and phospholipid methylation in eukaryotic cells. Biochem J 221:675, 1984.
313. Morita Y, Asakawa M, Hirai K, et al: Functional differences of human basophils with different densities. Int Arch Allergy Appl Immunol 88:332, 1989.
314. Morita Y, Chiang PK, Siraganian RP: Effect of inhibitors of transmethylation on histamine release from human basophils. Biochem Pharmacol 30:785, 1981.
315. Morita Y, Siraganian RP: Inhibition of IgE-mediated histamine release from rat basophilic leukemia cells and rat mast cells by inhibitors of transmethylation. J Immunol 127:1339, 1981.
316. Morita Y, Siraganian RP, Tang CK, Chiang PK: Inhibition of histamine release and phosphatidylcholine metabolism by 5′-deoxy-5′-isobutylthio-3-deazaadenosine. Biochem Pharmacol 31:2111, 1982.
317. Morrison DK, Kaplan DR, Escobedo JA, et al: Direct activation of the serine/threonine kinase activity of Raf-1 through tyrosine phosphorylation by the PDGF beta-receptor. Cell 58:649, 1989.
318. Mousli M, Hugli TE, Landry Y, Bronner C: A mechanism of action for anaphylatoxin C3a stimulation of mast cells. J Immunol 148:2456, 1992.
319. Murakami M, Kudo I, Suwa Y, Inoue K: Release of 14-kDa group-II phospholipase A2 from activated mast cells and its possible involvement in the regulation of the degranulation process. Eur J Biochem 209:257, 1992.
320. Murakami M, Kudo I, Umeda M, et al: Detection of three distinct phospholipases A2 in cultured mast cells. J Biochem (Tokyo) 111:175, 1992.
321. Murakami M, Matsumoto R, Austen KF, Arm JP: Prostaglandin endoperoxide synthase-1 and -2 couple to different transmembrane stimuli to generate prostaglandin D2 in mouse bone marrow-derived mast cells. J Biol Chem 269:22269, 1994.
322. Nagao K, Yokoro K, Aaronson SA: Continuous lines of basophil/mast cells derived from normal mouse bone marrow. Science 212:333, 1981.
323. Nakamura T, Ui M: Suppression of passive cutaneous anaphylaxis by pertussis toxin, an islet-activating protein, as a result of inhibition of histamine release from mast cells. Biochem Pharmacol 32:3435, 1983.
324. Nakamura T, Ui M: Simultaneous inhibitions of inositol phospholipid breakdown, arachidonic acid release, and histamine secretion in mast cells by islet-activating protein, pertussis toxin. A possible involvement of the toxin-specific substrate in the Ca2+-mobilizing receptor-mediated biosignaling system. J Biol Chem 260:3584, 1985.
325. Nakatani Y, Murakami M, Kudo I, Inoue K: Dual regulation of cytosolic phospholipase A2 in mast cells after cross-linking of Fcε-receptor. J Immunol 153:796, 1994.
326. Narasimhan V, Holowka D, Baird B: Microfilaments regulate the rate of exocytosis in rat basophilic leukemia cells. Biochem Biophys Res Commun 171:222, 1990.
327. Narasimhan V, Holowka D, Baird B: A guanine nucleotide-binding protein participates in IgE receptor-mediated activation of endogenous and reconstituted phospholipase A2 in a permeabilized cell system. J Biol Chem 265:1459, 1990.
328. Narasimhan V, Holowka D, Fewtrell C, Baird B: Cholera toxin increases the rate of antigen-stimulated calcium influx in rat basophilic leukemia cells. J Biol Chem 263:19626, 1988.
329. Neher E: The influence of intracellular calcium concentration on degranulation of dialysed mast cells from rat peritoneum. J Physiol (Lond) 395:193, 1988.
330. Nemeth EF, Douglas WW: Lipoxygenase inhibitors exert secretagogue-specific effects on mast cell exocytosis. Eur J Pharmacol 79:315, 1982.
331. Nishibe S, Wahl MI, Hernandez-Sotomayor SM, et al: Increase of the catalytic activity of phospholipase C-γ1 by tyrosine phosphorylation. Science 250:1253, 1990.
332. Nishikata H, Oliver C, Mergenhagen SE, Siraganian RP: The rat mast cell antigen AD1 (homologue to human CD63 or melanoma antigen ME491) is expressed in other cells in culture. J Immunol 149:862, 1992.
333. Nishizuka Y: The molecular heterogeneity of protein kinase C and its implications for cellular regulation. Nature 334:661, 1988.
334. Norman JC, Price LS, Ridley AJ, et al: Actin filament organization in activated mast cells is regulated by heterotrimeric and small GTP-binding proteins. J Cell Biol 126:1005, 1994.
335. Oberhauser AF, Balan V, Fernandez-Badilla CL, Fernandez JM: RT-PCR cloning of Rab3 isoforms expressed in peritoneal mast cells. FEBS Lett 339:171, 1994.
336. Oberhauser AF, Monck JR, Balch WE, Fernandez JM: Exocytotic fusion is activated by Rab3a peptides. Nature 360:270, 1992.
337. Offermanns S, Jones SVP, Bombien E, Schultz G: Stimulation of mitogen-activated protein kinase activity by different secretory stimuli in rat basophilic leukemia cells. J Immunol 152:250, 1994.
338. Ogawa M, Nakahata T, Leary AG, et al: Suspension culture of human mast cells/basophils from umbilical cord blood mononuclear cells. Proc Natl Acad Sci USA 80:4494, 1983.
339. Oliver JM, Seagrave J, Stump RF, et al: Signal transduction and cellular response artifact in RBL-2H3 mast cells. Prog Allergy 42:185, 1988.
340. Oliver JM, Seagrave JC, Pfeiffer JR, et al: Surface functions during mitosis in rat basophilic leukemia cells. J Cell Biol 101:2156, 1985.
341. Ortega Soto E, Pecht I: A monoclonal antibody that inhibits secretion from rat basophilic leukemia cells and binds to a novel membrane component. J Immunol 141:4324, 1988.
342. Ortega E, Schweitzer-Stenner R, Pecht I: Possible orientational constraints determine secretory signals induced by aggregation of IgE receptors on mast cells. EMBO J 7:4101, 1988.
343. Osipchuk Y, Cahalan M: Cell-to-cell spread of calcium signals mediated by ATP receptors in mast cells. Nature 359:241, 1992.
344. Ozawa K, Szallasi Z, Kazanietz MG, et al: Ca^{2+}-dependent and Ca^{2+}-independent isozymes of protein kinase C mediate exocytosis in antigen-stimulated rat basophilic RBL-2H3 cells. Reconstitution of secretory responses with Ca^{2+} and purified isozymes in washed permeabilized cells. J Biol Chem 268:1749, 1993.
345. Ozawa K, Yamada K, Kazanietz MG, et al: Different isozymes of protein kinase C mediate feedback inhibition of phospholipase C and stimulatory signals for exocytosis in rat RBL-2H3 cells. J Biol Chem 268:2280, 1993.
346. Paolini R, Jouvin MH, Kinet JP: Phosphorylation and dephosphorylation of the high-affinity receptor for immunoglobulin E immediately after receptor engagement and disengagement. Nature 353:855, 1991.
347. Park DJ, Min HK, Rhee SG: IgE-induced tyrosine phosphorylation of phospholipase C-γ1 in rat basophilic leukemia cells. J Biol Chem 266:24237, 1991.
348. Pawson T: Protein modules and signalling networks. Nature 373: 573, 1995.
349. Peachell PT, Lichtenstein LM, Schleimer RP: Differential regulation of human basophil and lung mast cell function by adenosine. J Pharmacol Exp Ther 256:717, 1991.
350. Peachell PT, MacGlashan DW Jr, Lichtenstein LM, Schleimer RP: Regulation of human basophil and lung mast cell function by cyclic adenosine monophosphate. J Immunol 140:571, 1988.
351. Peachell PT, Munday MR: Regulation of human lung mast cell function by phosphatase inhibitors. J Immunol 151:3808, 1993.
352. Penner R: Multiple signaling pathways control stimulus-secretion coupling in rat peritoneal mast cells. Proc Natl Acad Sci USA 85:9856, 1988.
353. Penner R, Matthews G, Neher E: Regulation of calcium influx by second messengers in rat mast cells. Nature 334:499, 1988.
354. Perez-Montfort R, Fewtrell C, Metzger H: Changes in the receptor for immunoglobulin E coincident with receptor-mediated stimulation of basophilic leukemia cells. Biochemistry 22:5733, 1983.
355. Peters SP, Kagey-Sobotka A, MacGlashan DW Jr, et al: The modulation of human basophil histamine release by products of the 5-lipoxygenase pathway. J Immunol 129:797, 1982.
356. Pfeiffer JR, Oliver JM: Tyrosine kinase-dependent assembly of actin plaques linking FcεR1 cross-linking to increased cell substrate adhesion in RBL-2H3 tumor mast cells. J Immunol 152:270, 1994.

357. Pfeiffer JR, Seagrave JC, Davis BH, et al: Membrane and cytoskeletal changes associated with IgE-mediated serotonin release from rat basophilic leukemia cells. J Cell Biol 101:2145, 1985.
358. Pitton C, Michel L, Salem P, et al: Biochemical and morphological modifications in dexamethasone-treated mouse bone marrow-derived mast cells. J Immunol 141:2437, 1988.
359. Plaut M, Pierce JH, Watson CJ, et al: Mast cell lines produce lymphokines in response to cross-linkage of FcεRI or to calcium ionophores. Nature 339:64, 1989.
360. Pribluda VS, Metzger H: Calcium-independent phosphoinositide breakdown in rat leukemia cells. Evidence for an early rise in inositol 1,4,5-trisphosphate which precedes the rise in other inositol phosphates and in cytoplasmic calcium. J Biol Chem 262:11449, 1987.
361. Pribluda VS, Pribluda C, Metzger H: Transphosphorylation as the mechanism by which the high-affinity receptor for IgE is phosphorylated upon aggregation. Proc Natl Acad Sci USA 91:11246, 1994.
362. Price LS, Norman JC, Ridley AJ, Koffer A: The small GTPases Rac and Rho as regulators of secretion in mast cells. Curr Biol 5:68, 1995.
363. Quarto R, Kinet JP, Metzger H: Coordinate synthesis and degradation of the α-, β- and γ-subunits of the receptor for immunoglobulin E. Mol Immunol 22:1045, 1985.
364. Quarto R, Metzger H: The receptor for immunoglobulin E: examination for kinase activity and as a substrate for kinases. Mol Immunol 23:1215, 1986.
365. Ra C, Furuichi K, Rivera J, et al: Internalization of IgE receptors on rat basophilic leukemic cells by phorbol ester. Comparison with endocytosis induced by receptor aggregation. Eur J Immunol 19:1771, 1989.
366. Ravichandran KS, Lee KK, Songyang Z, et al: Interaction of Shc with the ζ chain of the T cell receptor upon T cell activation. Science 262:902, 1993.
367. Razin E, Ihle JN, Seldin D, et al: Interleukin 3: a differentiation and growth factor for the mouse mast cell that contains chondroitin sulfate E proteoglycan. J Immunol 132:1479, 1984.
368. Razin E, Mencia-Huerta JM, Stevens RL, et al: IgE-mediated release of leukotriene C4, chondroitin sulfate E proteoglycan, β-hexosaminidase, and histamine from cultured bone marrow-derived mouse mast cells. J Exp Med 157:189, 1983.
369. Razin E, Romeo LC, Krilis S, et al: An analysis of the relationship between 5-lipoxygenase product generation and the secretion of preformed mediators from mouse bone marrow-derived mast cells. J Immunol 133:938, 1984.
370. Razin E, Szallasi Z, Kazanietz MG, et al: Protein kinases C-β and C-ε link the mast cell high-affinity receptor for IgE to the expression of c-fos and c-jun. Proc Natl Acad Sci USA 91:7722, 1994.
371. Reth M: Antigen receptor tail clue. Nature 338:383, 1989.
372. Rhee SG, Suh PG, Ryu SH, Lee SY: Studies of inositol phospholipid-specific phospholipase C. Science 244:546, 1989.
373. Rivera J, Mullins JM, Furuichi K, Isersky C: Endocytosis of aggregated immunoglobulin G by rat basophilic leukemia cells; rate, extent, and effects on the endocytosis of immunoglobulin E. J Immunol 136:623, 1986.
374. Rivera VM, Brugge JS: Clustering of Syk is sufficient to induce tyrosine phosphorylation and release of allergic mediators from rat basophilic leukemia cells. Mol Cell Biol 15:1582, 1995.
375. Robertson D, Holowka D, Baird B: Cross-linking of immunoglobulin E-receptor complexes induces their interaction with the cytoskeleton of rat basophilic leukemia cells. J Immunol 136:4565, 1986.
376. Robin JL, Seldin DC, Austen KF, Lewis RA: Regulation of mediator release from mouse bone marrow-derived mast cells by glucocorticoids. J Immunol 135:2719, 1985.
377. Romanin C, Reinsprecht M, Pecht I, Schindler H: Immunologically activated chloride channels involved in degranulation of rat mucosal mast cells. EMBO J 10:3603, 1991.
378. Romeo C, Amiot M, Seed B: Sequence requirements for induction of cytolysis by the T cell antigen/Fc receptor ζ chain. Cell 68:889, 1992.
379. Romeo C, Seed B: Cellular immunity to HIV activated by CD4 fused to T cell or Fc receptor polypeptides. Cell 64:1037, 1991.
380. Rudd CE, Anderson P, Morimoto C, et al: Molecular interactions, T-cell subsets and a role of the CD4/CD8: p56^{lck} complex in human T-cell activation. Immunol Rev 111:225, 1989.
381. Sagi-Eisenberg R, Lieman H, Pecht I: Protein kinase C regulation of the receptor-coupled calcium signal in histamine-secreting rat basophilic leukaemia cells. Nature 313:59, 1985.
382. Sagi-Eisenberg R, Mazurek N, Pecht I: Ca^{2+} fluxes and protein phosphorylation in stimulus-secretion coupling of basophils. Mol Immunol 21:1175, 1984.
383. Sagi-Eisenberg R, Pecht I: Membrane potential changes during IgE-mediated histamine release from rat basophilic leukemia cells. J Membr Biol 75:97, 1983.
384. Sagi-Eisenberg R, Pecht I: Protein kinase C, a coupling element between stimulus and secretion of basophils. Immunol Lett 8:237, 1984.
385. Sagi-Eisenberg R, Pecht I: Resolution of cellular compartments involved in membrane potential changes accompanying IgE-mediated degranulation of rat basophilic leukemia cells. EMBO J 3:497, 1984.
386. Sahara N, Siraganian RP, Oliver C: Morphological changes induced by the calcium ionophore A23187 in rat basophilic leukemia (2H3) cells. J Histochem Cytochem 38:975, 1990.
387. Saito H, Ishizaka K, Ishizaka T: Effect of nonhydrolyzable guanosine phosphate on IgE-mediated activation of phospholipase C and histamine release from rodent mast cells. J Immunol 143:250, 1989.
388. Saito H, Okajima F, Molski TF, et al: Effect of cholera toxin on histamine release from bone marrow-derived mouse mast cells. Proc Natl Acad Sci USA 85:2504, 1988.
389. Samelson LE, Klausner RD: Tyrosine kinases and tyrosine-based activation motifs. Current research on activation via the T cell antigen receptor. J Biol Chem 267:24913, 1992.
390. Santini F, Beaven MA: Tyrosine phosphorylation of a mitogen-activated protein kinase-like protein occurs at a late step in exocytosis. Studies with tyrosine phosphatase inhibitors and various secretagogues in rat RBL-2H3 cells. J Biol Chem 268:22716, 1993.
391. Saxton TM, Van Oostveen I, Bowtell D, et al: B cell antigen receptor cross-linking induces phosphorylation of the p21ras oncoprotein activators SHC and mSOS1 as well as assembly of complexes containing SHC, GRB-2, mSOS1, and a 145-kDa tyrosine-phosphorylated protein. J Immunol 153:623, 1994.
392. Schaller MD, Borgman CA, Cobb BS, et al: pp125^{FAK}, a structurally distinctive protein-tyrosine kinase associated with focal adhesions. Proc Natl Acad Sci USA 89:5192, 1992.
393. Schleimer RP, Davidson DA, Lichtenstein LM, Adkinson NF Jr: Selective inhibition of arachidonic acid metabolite release from human lung tissue by antiinflammatory steroids. J Immunol 136:3006, 1986.
394. Schleimer RP, Derse CP, Friedman B, et al: Regulation of human basophil mediator release by cytokines. I. Interaction with antiinflammatory steroids. J Immunol 143:1310, 1989.
395. Schleimer RP, Gillespie E, Daiuta R, Lichtenstein LM: Release of histamine from human leukocytes stimulated with the tumor-promoting phorbol diesters. II. Interaction with other stimuli. J Immunol 128:136, 1982.
396. Schleimer RP, Gillespie E, Lichtenstein LM: Release of histamine from human leukocytes stimulated with the tumor-promoting phorbol diesters. I. Characterization of the response. J Immunol 126:570, 1981.
397. Schleimer RP, Lichtenstein LM, Gillespie E: Inhibition of basophil histamine release by anti-inflammatory steroids. Nature 292:454, 1981.
398. Schleimer RP, MacGlashan DW Jr, Gillespie E, Lichtenstein LM: Inhibition of basophil histamine release by anti-inflammatory steroids. II. Studies on the mechanism of action. J Immunol 129:1632, 1982.
399. Schlessinger J, Webb WW, Elson EL, Metzger H: Lateral motion and valence of Fc receptors on rat peritoneal mast cells. Nature 264:550, 1976.
400. Schneider H, Cohen-Dayag A, Pecht I: Tyrosine phosphorylation of phospholipase C-γ1 couples the Fcε receptor mediated signal to mast cells secretion. Int Immunol 4:447, 1992.
401. Schrader JW: The panspecific hemopoietin of activated T lymphocytes (interleukin-3). Annu Rev Immunol 4:205, 1986.
402. Schulman ES, Kagey-Sobotka A, MacGlashan DW Jr, et al: Heterogeneity of human mast cells. J Immunol 131:1936, 1983.
403. Schulman ES, MacGlashan DW Jr, Peters SP, et al: Human lung mast cells: purification and characterization. J Immunol 129:2662, 1982.
404. Schulman ES, Post TJ, Henson PM, Giclas PC: Differential effects of the complement peptides, C5a and C5a des Arg on human basophil and lung mast cell histamine release. J Clin Invest 81:918, 1988.
405. Schulman ES, Post TJ, Vigderman RJ: Density heterogeneity of human lung mast cells. J Allergy Clin Immunol 82:78, 1988.
406. Seagrave J, Oliver JM: Antigen-dependent transition of IgE to a detergent-insoluble form is associated with reduced IgE receptor-dependent secretion from RBL-2H3 mast cells. J Cell Physiol 144:128, 1990.
407. Seagrave J, Pfeiffer JR, Wofsy C, Oliver JM: Relationship of IgE receptor topography to secretion in RBL-2H3 mast cells. J Cell Physiol 148:139, 1991.

408. Segal DM, Sharrow SO, Jones JF, Siraganian RP: Fc (IgG) receptors on rat basophilic leukemia cells. J Immunol 126:138, 1981.
409. Segal DM, Taurog JD, Metzger H: Dimeric immunoglobulin E serves as a unit signal for mast cell degranulation. Proc Natl Acad Sci USA 74:2993, 1977.
410. Seger R, Krebs EG: The MAPK signaling cascade. FASEB J 9:726, 1995.
411. Seldin DC, Adelman S, Austen KF, et al: Homology of the rat basophilic leukemia cell and the rat mucosal mast cell. Proc Natl Acad Sci USA 82:3871, 1985.
412. Shiue L, Green J, Green OM, et al: Interaction of $p72^{syk}$ with the γ and β subunits of the high-affinity receptor for immunoglobulin E, FcϵRI. Mol Cell Biol 15:272, 1995.
413. Sieghart W, Theoharides TC, Alper SL, et al: Calcium-dependent protein phosphorylation during secretion by exocytosis in the mast cell. Nature 275:329, 1978.
414. Sieghart W, Theoharides TC, Douglas WW, Greengard P: Phosphorylation of a single mast cell protein in response to drugs that inhibit secretion. Biochem Pharmacol 30:2737, 1981.
415. Simon MI, Strathmann MP, Gautam N: Diversity of G proteins in signal transduction. Science 252:802, 1991.
416. Siraganian RP: Mast cells and basophils. In Gallin JI, Goldstein IM, Snyderman R (eds): Inflammation: Basic Principles and Clinical Correlates. Raven Press, Ltd, New York, 1988, p 513.
417. Siraganian RP, Hazard KA: Mechanisms of mouse mast cell activation and inactivation for IgE-mediated histamine release. J Immunol 122:1719, 1979.
418. Siraganian RP, Hook WA: Complement-induced histamine release from human basophils. II. Mechanism of the histamine release reaction. J Immunol 116:639, 1976.
419. Siraganian RP, Hook WA: Mechanism of histamine release by formyl methionine-containing peptides. J Immunol 119:2078, 1977.
420. Siraganian RP, Hook WA: Histamine release and assay methods for the study of human allergy. In Rose NR, Friedman M, Fahey JL (eds): Manual of Clinical Laboratory Immunology, 3rd edition. American Society for Microbiology, Washington, DC, 1986.
421. Siraganian RP, Hook WA, Levine BB: Specific in vitro histamine release from basophils by bivalent haptens: evidence of activation by simple bridging of membrane bound antibody. Immunochemistry 12:149, 1975.
422. Siraganian RP, McGivney A, Barsumian EL, et al: Variants of the rat basophilic leukemia cell line for the study of histamine release. Fed Proc 41:30, 1982.
423. Siraganian RP, Siraganian PA: Mechanism of action of concanavalin A on human basophils. J Immunol 114:886, 1975.
424. Smit L, De Vries-Smits AMM, Bos JL, Borst J: B cell antigen receptor stimulation induces formation of a Shc-Grb2 complex containing multiple tyrosine-phosphorylated proteins. J Biol Chem 269:20209, 1994.
425. Sobotka AK, Dembo M, Goldstein B, Lichtenstein LM: Antigen-specific desensitization of human basophils. J Immunol 122:511, 1979.
426. Soto EO, Pecht I: A monoclonal antibody that inhibits secretion from rat basophilic leukemia cells and binds to a novel membrane component. J Immunol 141:4324, 1988.
427. Springer TA: Adhesion receptors of the immune system. Nature 346:425, 1990.
428. Stenson WF, Parker CW, Sullivan TJ: Augmentation of IgE-mediated release of histamine by 5-hydroxyeicosatetraenoic acid and 12-hydroxyeicosatetraenoic acid. Biochem Biophys Res Commun 96:1045, 1980.
429. Stephan V, Benhamou M, Gutkind JS, et al: FcϵRI-induced protein tyrosine phosphorylation of pp72 in rat basophilic leukemia cells (RBL-2H3). Evidence for a novel signal transduction pathway unrelated to G protein activation and phosphatidylinositol hydrolysis. J Biol Chem 267:5434, 1992.
430. Stephan V, Guo N, Ginsburg V, Siraganian RP: Immunoprecipitation of membrane proteins from rat basophilic leukemia cells by the anti-ganglioside monoclonal antibody AA4. J Immunol 146:4271, 1991.
431. Stevens RL, Austen KF: Recent advances in the cellular and molecular biology of mast cells. Immunol Today 10:381, 1989.
432. Stevens RL, Otsu K, Austen KF: Purification and analysis of the core protein of the protease-resistant intracellular chondroitin sulfate E proteoglycan from the interleukin 3-dependent mouse mast cell. J Biol Chem 260:14194, 1985.
433. Stracke ML, Basciano LK, Siraganian RP: Binding properties and histamine release in variants of rat basophilic leukemia cells with changes in the IgE receptor. Immunol Lett 14:287, 1987.
434. Stryer L, Bourne HR: G proteins: a family of signal transducers. Ann Rev Cell Biol 2:391, 1986.
435. Stump RF, Oliver JM, Cragoe EJ Jr, Deanin GG: The control of mediator release from RBL-2H3 cells: roles for Ca^{2+}, Na^{+}, and protein kinase C1. J Immunol 139:881, 1987.
436. Sullivan TJ, Parker CW: Possible role of arachidonic acid and its metabolites in mediator release from rat mast cells. J Immunol 122:431, 1979.
437. Sullivan TJ, Parker KL, Eisen SA, Parker CW: Modulation of cyclic AMP in purified rat mast cells. II. Studies on the relationship between intracellular cyclic AMP concentrations and histamine release. J Immunol 114:1480, 1975.
438. Sullivan TJ, Parker KL, Kulczycki A Jr, Parker CW: Modulation of cyclic AMP in purified rat mast cells. III. Studies on the effects of concanavalin A and anti-IgE on cyclic AMP concentrations during histamine release. J Immunol 117:713, 1976.
439. Sullivan TJ, Parker KL, Stenson W, Parker CW: Modulation of cyclic AMP in purified rat mast cells. I. Responses to pharmacologic, metabolic, and physical stimuli. J Immunol 114:1473, 1975.
440. Swaim WD, Minoguchi K, Oliver C, et al: The anti-ganglioside monoclonal antibody AA4 induces protein tyrosine phosphorylations, but not degranulation, in rat basophilic leukemia cell. J Biol Chem 269:19466, 1994.
441. Swieter M, Berenstein EH, Siraganian RP: Protein tyrosine phosphatase coprecipitates with the high affinity IgE receptor and dephosphorylates the receptor subunits but not Lyn or Syk. J Immunol 155:5330, 1995.
442. Swieter M, Berenstein EH, Swaim WD, Siraganian RP: Aggregation of IgE receptors in rat basophilic leukemia 2H3 cells induces tyrosine phosphorylation of the cytosolic protein-tyrosine phosphatase HePTP. J Biol Chem 270:21902, 1995.
443. Swieter M, Mergenhagen SE, Siraganian RP: Microenvironmental factors that influence mast cell phenotype and function. Proc Soc Exp Biol Med 199:22, 1992.
444. Swieter M, Midura RJ, Nishikata H, et al: Mouse 3T3 fibroblasts induce rat basophilic leukemia (RBL-2H3) cells to acquire responsiveness to compound 48/80. J Immunol 150:617, 1993.
445. Sydbom A, Fredholm B, Uvnas B: Evidence against a role of cyclic nucleotides in the regulation of anaphylactic histamine release in isolated rat mast cells. Acta Physiol Scand 112:47, 1981.
446. Takagi M, Nakahata T, Koike K, et al: Stimulation of connective tissue-type mast cell proliferation by crosslinking of cell-bound IgE. J Exp Med 170:233, 1989.
447. Takaishi T, Siraganian RP: Changes in $^{45}Ca^{2+}$ flux following the activation of rat basophilic leukemia cells for histamine release. Annals Allergy 55:353, 1985.
448. Takei M, Endo K: Histamine release and calcium concentrations in rat mast cells are dependent on intracellular ATP: effects of prostaglandin D2. Prostaglandins Leukot Essent Fatty Acids 50:357, 1994.
449. Takizawa F, Adamczewski M, Kinet JP: Identification of the low affinity receptor for immunoglobulin E on mouse mast cells and macrophages as FcγRII and FcγRIII. J Exp Med 176:469, 1992.
450. Taniguchi T, Kobayashi T, Kondo J, et al: Molecular cloning of a porcine gene syk that encodes a 72-kDa protein-tyrosine kinase showing high susceptibility to proteolysis. J Biol Chem 266:15790, 1991.
451. Tasaka K, Mio M, Fujisawa K, Aoki I: Role of microtubules on Ca^{2+} release from the endoplasmic reticulum and associated histamine release from rat peritoneal mast cells. Biochem Pharmacol 41:1031, 1991.
452. Teshima R, Ikebuchi H, Terao T: Ca^{2+}-dependent and phorbol ester activating phosphorylation of a 36K-dalton protein of rat basophilic leukemia cell membranes and immunoprecipitation of the phosphorylated protein with IgE anti-IgE system. Biochem Biophys Res Commun 125:867, 1984.
453. Theoharides TC, Douglas WW: Secretion in mast cells induced by calcium entrapped within phospholipid vesicles. Science 201:1143, 1978.
454. Theoharides TC, Sieghart W, Greengard P, Douglas WW: Antiallergic drug cromolyn may inhibit histamine secretion by regulating phosphorylation of a mast cell protein. Science 207:80, 1980.
455. Thomas LL, Findlay SR, Lichtenstein LM: Augmentation of antigen-stimulated histamine release from human basophils by serum-treated zymosan particles. II. Dependence on IgE-mediated release. J Immunol 123:1468, 1979.
456. Thomas LL, Lichtenstein LM: Augmentation of antigen-stimulated histamine release from human basophils by serum-treated zymosan

particles. I. Characteristics of enhancement. J Immunol 123:1462, 1979.
457. Thomas ML: The leukocyte common antigen family. Annu Rev Immunol 7:339, 1989.
458. Thompson HL, Burbelo PD, Metcalfe DD: Regulation of adhesion of mouse bone marrow-derived mast cells to laminin. J Immunol 145:3425, 1990.
459. Thompson HL, Burbelo PD, Segui-Real B, et al: Laminin promotes mast cell attachment. J Immunol 143:2323, 1989.
460. Tsai M, Chen RH, Tam SY, et al: Activation of MAP kinases, $pp90^{rsk}$ and pp70-S6 kinases in mouse mast cells by signaling through the c-kit receptor tyrosine kinase or FcεRI: rapamycin inhibits activation of pp70-S6 kinase and proliferation in mouse mast cells. Eur J Immunol 23:3286, 1993.
461. Tsai M, Tam SY, Galli SJ: Distinct patterns of early response gene expression and proliferation in mouse mast cells stimulated by stem cell factor, interleukin-3, or IgE and antigen. Eur J Immunol 23:867, 1993.
462. Turner H, Reif K, Rivera J, Cantrell DA: Regulation of the adapter molecule Grb2 by the FcεR1 in the mast cell line RBL2H3. J Biol Chem 270:9500, 1995.
463. Turner JM, Brodsky MH, Irving BA, et al: Interaction of the unique N-terminal region of tyrosine kinase $p56^{lck}$ with cytoplasmic domains of CD4 and CD8 is mediated by cysteine motifs. Cell 60:755, 1990.
464. Undem BJ, Torphy TJ, Goldman D, Chilton FH: Inhibition by adenosine 3′:5′-monophosphate of eicosanoid and platelet-activating factor biosynthesis in the mouse PT-18 mast cell. J Biol Chem 265:6750, 1990.
465. Urata C, Siraganian RP: Pharmacologic modulation of the IgE or Ca^{2+} ionophore A23187 mediated Ca^{2+} influx, phospholipase activation, and histamine release in rat basophilic leukemia cells. Int Arch Allergy Appl Immunol 78:92, 1985.
466. Valent P, Besemer J, Muhm M, et al: Interleukin 3 activates human blood basophils via high-affinity binding sites. Proc Natl Acad Sci USA 86:5542, 1989.
467. Valent P, Bettelheim P: Cell surface structures on human basophils and mast cells: biochemical and functional characterization. Adv Immunol 52:333, 1992.
468. Van Overveld FJ, Houben LA, Schmitz du Mo, et al: Mast cell heterogeneity in human lung tissue. Clin Sci 77:297, 1989.
469. Varin-Blank N, Metzger H: Surface expression of mutated subunits of the high affinity mast cell receptor for IgE. J Biol Chem 265:15685, 1990.
470. von Zur M, Eckstein F, Penner R: Guanosine 5′-[beta-thio]triphosphate selectively activates calcium signaling in mast cells. Proc Natl Acad Sci USA 88:926, 1991.
471. Warner J, MacGlashan D Jr: Persistence of early crosslink-dependent signal transduction events in human basophils after desensitization. Immunol Lett 18:129, 1988.
472. Warner JA, MacGlashan DW Jr: Protein kinase C (PKC) changes in human basophils. IgE-mediated activation is accompanied by an increase in total PKC activity. J Immunol 142:1669, 1989.
473. Warner JA, MacGlashan DW Jr: Signal transduction events in human basophils. A comparative study of the role of protein kinase C in basophils activated by anti-IgE antibody and formyl-methionyl-leucyl-phenylalanine. J Immunol 145:1897, 1990.
474. Warner JA, Peters SP, Lichtenstein LM, et al: Differential release of mediators from human basophils: differences in arachidonic acid metabolism following activation by unrelated stimuli. J Leukoc Biol 45:558, 1989.
475. Warner JA, Pienkowski MM, Plaut M, et al: Identification of histamine releasing factor(s) in the late phase of cutaneous IgE-mediated reactions. J Immunol 136:2583, 1986.
476. Warner JA, Yancey KB, MacGlashan DW Jr: The effect of pertussis toxin on mediator release from human basophils. J Immunol 139:161, 1987.
477. Watanabe A, Tominaga T, Tsuji J, et al: Effects of anti-CD11a, anti-CD11b and anti-CD18 on histamine release from human basophils primed with IL-3. Int Arch Allergy Immunol 98:308, 1992.
478. Watras J, Moraru I, Costa DJ, Kindman LA: Two inositol 1,4,5-trisphosphate binding sites in rat basophilic leukemia cells: relationship between receptor occupancy and calcium release. Biochemistry 33:14359, 1994.
479. Weiss A: T cell antigen receptor signal transduction: a tale of tails and cytoplasmic protein-tyrosine kinases. Cell 73:209, 1993.
480. White JR, Ishizaka T, Ishizaka K, Sha'afi R: Direct demonstration of increased intracellular concentration of free calcium as measured by quin-2 in stimulated rat peritoneal mast cell. Proc Natl Acad Sci USA 81:3978, 1984.
481. White JR, Pluznik DH, Ishizaka K, Ishizaka T: Antigen-induced increase in protein kinase C activity in plasma membrane of mast cells. Proc Natl Acad Sci USA 82:8193, 1985.
482. White JR, Zembryki D, Hanna N, Mong S: Differential inhibition of histamine release from mast cells by protein kinase C inhibitors: staurosporine and K-252a. Biochem Pharmacol 40:447, 1990.
483. White KN, Metzger H: Translocation of protein kinase C in rat basophilic leukemic cells induced by phorbol ester or by aggregation of IgE receptors. J Immunol 141:942, 1988.
484. White MV, Igarashi Y, Lundgren JD, et al: Hydrocortisone inhibits rat basophilic leukemia cell mediator release induced by neutrophil-derived histamine releasing activity as well as by anti-IgE. J Immunol 147:667, 1991.
485. Wilson BS, Deanin GG, Standefer JC, et al: Depletion of guanine nucleotides with mycophenolic acid suppresses IgE receptor-mediated degranulation in rat basophilic leukemia cells. J Immunol 143:259, 1989.
486. Winslow CM, Austen KF: Role of cyclic nucleotides in the activation-secretion response. Prog Allergy 34:236, 1984.
487. Wodnar-Filipowicz A, Heusser CH, Moroni C: Production of the haemopoietic growth factors GM-CSF and interleukin-3 by mast cells in response to IgE receptor-mediated activation. Nature 339:150, 1989.
488. WoldeMussie E, Ali H, Takaishi T, et al: Identification of variants of the basophilic leukemia (RBL-2H3) cells that have defective phosphoinositide responses to antigen and stimulants of guanosine 5′-triphosphate-regulatory proteins. J Immunol 139:2431, 1987.
489. Yamada K, Kanaho Y, Miura K, Nozawa Y: Antigen-induced phospholipase D activation in rat mast cells is independent of protein kinase C. Biochem Biophys Res Commun 175:159, 1991.
490. Yamashita T, Mao S, Metzger H: Aggregation of the high-affinity IgE receptor and enhanced activity of $p53/p56^{lyn}$ protein-tyrosine kinase. Proc Natl Acad Sci USA 91:11251, 1994.
491. Yao L, Kawakami Y, Kawakami T: The pleckstrin homology domain of Bruton tyrosine kinase interacts with protein kinase C. Proc Natl Acad Sci USA 91:9175, 1994.
492. Ye ZS, Baltimore D: Binding of Vav to Grb2 through dimerization of Src homology 3 domains. Proc Natl Acad Sci USA 91:12629, 1994.
493. Yoshii N, Mio M, Akagi M, Tasaka K: Role of endoplasmic reticulum, an intracellular Ca^{2+} store, in histamine release from rat peritoneal mast cell. Immunopharmacology 21:13, 1991.
494. Yoshii N, Mio M, Tasaka K: Ca^{2+} uptake and Ca^{2+} releasing properties of the endoplasmic reticulum in rat peritoneal mast cells. Immunopharmacology 16:107, 1988.
495. Zheutlin LM, Ackerman SJ, Gleich GJ, Thomas LL: Stimulation of basophil and rat mast cell histamine release by eosinophil granule-derived cationic proteins. J Immunol 133:2180, 1984.
496. Zidovetzki R, Bartholdi M, Arndt-Jovin D, Jovin TM: Rotational dynamics of the Fc receptor for immunoglobulin E on histamine-releasing rat basophilic leukemia cells. Biochemistry 25:4397, 1986.
497. Zimmerberg J, Curran M, Cohen FS, Brodwick M: Simultaneous electrical and optical measurements show that membrane fusion precedes secretory granule swelling during exocytosis of beige mouse mast cells. Proc Natl Acad Sci USA 84:1585, 1987.
498. Zor U, Her E, Harell T, et al: Arachidonic acid release by basophilic leukemia cells and macrophages stimulated by Ca^{2+} ionophores, antigen and diacylglycerol: essential role for protein kinase C and prevention by glucocorticosteroids. Biochim Biophys Acta 1091:385, 1991.
499. Zweifach A, Lewis RS: Mitogen-regulated Ca^{2+} current of T lymphocytes is activated by depletion of intracellular Ca^{2+} stores. Proc Natl Acad Sci USA 90:6295, 1993.

10 Basophils and Mast Cells

LAWRENCE B. SCHWARTZ

Mast cells and possibly basophils are the principal cell types that initiate the humoral and cellular inflammatory responses seen in immediate hypersensitivity reactions (Type I). The early phase of these reactions (5 to 30 minutes), depending on the target tissue, elicits local edema, smooth muscle contraction, vasodilation, and increased permeability of post-capillary venules. The late phase of immediate hypersensitivity recruits and activates basophils, eosinophils, and other cell types. Mediators of mast cells and basophils that are stored preformed inside secretory granules (Table 10–1) are released by degranulation with cell activation, a process also termed regulated secretion. Other mediators that are not present preformed are synthesized (see Table 10–1) and secreted without a significant intracellular storage phase.

In humans, the principal preformed mediators of mast cells include histamine, proteoglycans (heparin, chondroitin sulfates), and neutral proteases (tryptase, chymase, cathepsin G-like protease, carboxypeptidase). Basic fibroblast growth factor (bFGF) also may reside preformed in at least some mast cells. In contrast, basophils contain histamine, chondroitin sulfate, and a newly described protein called the 2D7 ligand, named after the mAb that recognizes it. The major newly generated mediators include the arachidonic acid metabolites, prostaglandin D_2 (PGD_2) and leukotriene C_4 (LTC_4) for mast cells but only LTC_4 for basophils. Also, Th2-like cytokines such as interleukin (IL)-4, IL-5, IL-6, and IL-13 and tumor necrosis factor-α (TNF-α) are produced by activated mast cells and basophils (see Table 10–1). Together, these products of mast cells account for much of the phlogistic response observed with immediate hypersensitivity reactions.

Mast cells occupy a sentinel position in tissues where noxious substances might attempt entry and immediate hypersensitivity reactions typically begin. Basophils normally reside in the circulation but enter tissues at sites of inflammation, particularly during the late phase of allergic reactions and the early phase of delayed hypersensitivity reactions. These are the two cell types that constitutively express substantial quantities of the high-affinity receptor for IgE (FcεRI) in an active form and store histamine in their secretory granules. Adding to the complexity of mast cells, two phenotypes have been observed in human tissues based on the protease composition of their secretory granules. The selected participation of basophils and different types of mast cells in various clinical conditions as well as the duration, intensity, and tissue distribution of a particular response will depend on various characteristics of the agonist, the immunologic sensitivity of the host, the target tissue involved, and any underlying pathology. This chapter will focus on the different types of human mast cells and the human basophils because of their obvious relevance to human disease.

TABLE 10–1
MEDIATORS OF HUMAN MAST CELLS AND BASOPHILS

Mediator	MC_{TC} Cell	MC_T Cell	Basophil
Preformed (granules)			
Histamine	++	++	++
Tryptase	++	++	±
Chymase	++	–	–
Carboxypeptidase	++	–	–
Cathepsin G	++	–	–
Heparin	+	+	–
Chondroitin sulfate E	+	+	–
Chondroitin sulfate A			+
Newly generated			
Arachidonic acid metabolites			
Lipoxygenase metabolite			
LTC4	++	++	++
LTB4	+	+	+
Cyclooxygenase metabolite			
PGD2	++	++	–
Cytokines			
TNF-α	++	++	++
IL-5, IL-6, IL-9	+	++	++
IL-4	+	+	++
IL-13	++	++	+

DIFFERENT TYPES OF MAST CELLS

HISTOCHEMISTRY, COMPOSITION, DISTRIBUTION, AND MORPHOLOGY

Two distinct types of human mast cells have been described based on different protease compositions of the secretory granules. Mast cells of the MC_{TC} type contain chymase, mast cell carboxypeptidase, cathepsin G, and tryptase; those of the MC_T type contain only tryptase (see Table 10–1).[75] These proteases appear to reflect qualitative differences because those of the MC_T type, although morphologically mature, appear to lack chymase mRNA as well as the enzyme.[189] In histologically normal tissues (Table 10–2), mast cell concentrations are particularly high in the human alveolar wall, bowel mucosa, dermis, and nasal and conjunctival mucosa and around blood vessels, reflecting the target tissue distribution of allergic diseases. MC_T cells are the predominant, but not exclusive, type of mast cell found in the lung, particularly alveoli, and in the small intestinal mucosa, whereas MC_{TC} cells are the predominant type found in the skin and the gastrointestinal submucosa.[79] The relative abundance of MC_{TC} and MC_T cells may change with tissue inflammation or fibrosis, making it impossible to base a subtype designation on location alone.

As shown in Figure 10–1, mature mast cells of all types have a nucleus without deeply divided lobes, numerous cytoplasmic granules, and thin elongated folds of their plasma membrane.[47] Human basophils are polymorphonuclear, contain larger and less numerous granules, and exhibit a comparatively smooth plasma membrane contour. Among mature, unstimulated MC_{TC} and MC_T cells, differences in granule morphology correspond to differences in protease composition[39, 41]; MC_T granules often are scroll rich, whereas MC_{TC} granules have gratings and lattices and are scroll poor. Basophil secretory granules typically exhibit a particulate appearance. All granules in both mast cell types contain tryptase and heparin; all granules in MC_{TC} cells also contain chymase.

TABLE 10–2
CHARACTERISTICS OF HUMAN MC_{TC} AND MC_T TYPES OF MAST CELLS

Characteristic	MC_{TC} Cell	MC_T Cell
Normal tissue distribution		
Skin	++	–
Intestinal submucosa	++	+
Intestinal mucosa	+	++
Alveolar wall	–	++
Bronchi/bronchioles	+	++
Nasal mucosa	++	++
Conjunctiva	++	+
Combined immunodeficiency or AIDS (small intestine)	Amounts unchanged	Amounts decreased
Granule morphology	Grating/lattice, scroll poor	Scroll rich

FUNCTIONAL AND PHARMACOLOGIC DIFFERENCES

Although immunologic stimulation (IgE and allergen) as well as calcium ionophores activate all tissue-derived mast cells and peripheral blood basophils, nonimmunologic agonists of biologic importance show selectivity for mast cells from different tissue sites, independent of the protease phenotype of the mast cell or of basophils. Mast cells derived from human skin release histamine in response to morphine sulfate, substance P, vasoactive intestinal peptide (VIP), somatostatin, calcitonin gene-related protein (CGRP), and the anaphylatoxins C5a and C3a; whereas mast cells from lung, tonsils and adenoids, and colon, even when of the MC_{TC} type, do not.[14, 34, 50, 55, 144] Mast cells from heart uniquely respond to C5a but not to substance P.[117, 164] In contrast, basophils respond to C5a and C3a but not to substance P. Unlike all mast cells, basophils respond to f-Met-Leu-Phe. Basophils do not respond to morphine or codeine. The desArg derivatives of C3a and C5a are inactive on skin mast cells but still show limited agonist activity against basophils.[24, 50]

Although in some cases these peptides may activate mast cells and basophils through stereospecific receptor interactions, a common feature of many of these peptides is their basic nature and their capacity to perturb the cell membranes through ionic interactions.[107] For example, complement anaphylatoxin activation of rodent mast cells is abolished if sialic acid residues are removed from the membrane surface and may act as a direct stimulator of pertussis-sensitive G proteins,[106] whereas substance P activity is blocked by a receptor antagonist. Differences in the secretory response between mast cells isolated from different tissues may relate to microenvironmental influences rather than to lineage. For example, the RBL cell line, reflecting rat mucosal mast cells, acquires responsiveness to substance P when cocultured with 3T3 fibroblasts without otherwise changing its phenotype.[171] Such microenvironmental influences may result from intrinsic changes in the mast cells stimulated by neighboring cells or through the passive acquisition by mast cells of new membrane components from neighboring cells.

Histamine-releasing factors provide an alternative mechanism to FcεRI-mediated activation of basophils and possibly mast cells.[8] Mononuclear-derived proteins of the chemokine family, initially discovered because of their abilities to attract predominantly monocytes or neutrophils, include potent basophil histamine-releasing agents. Active chemokines include monocyte chemotactic protein (MCP)-1, MCP-2, and MCP-3; RANTES; monocyte inflammatory peptide (MIP)-1α and MIP-1β; human inflammatory protein-1α and -1β; connective tissue–activating peptide (CTAP)-III; neutrophil-activating peptide (NAP)-2; and fibroblast-induced cytokine (FIC).[2, 3, 42, 88] Nonactivating chemokines may inhibit those that activate by competing for the same binding sites on the basophil cell surface.[87] Although the abilities of these cytokines to activate human mast cells are less well known, some basophil-activating chemokines possess chemotactic activity for mast cells without causing degranulation in both human[111] and rodent[65] studies. Whether MC_T and MC_{TC} or mast cells from different tissue sites exhibit different response patterns remains to be determined.

Pharmacologic responsiveness of mast cells also varies

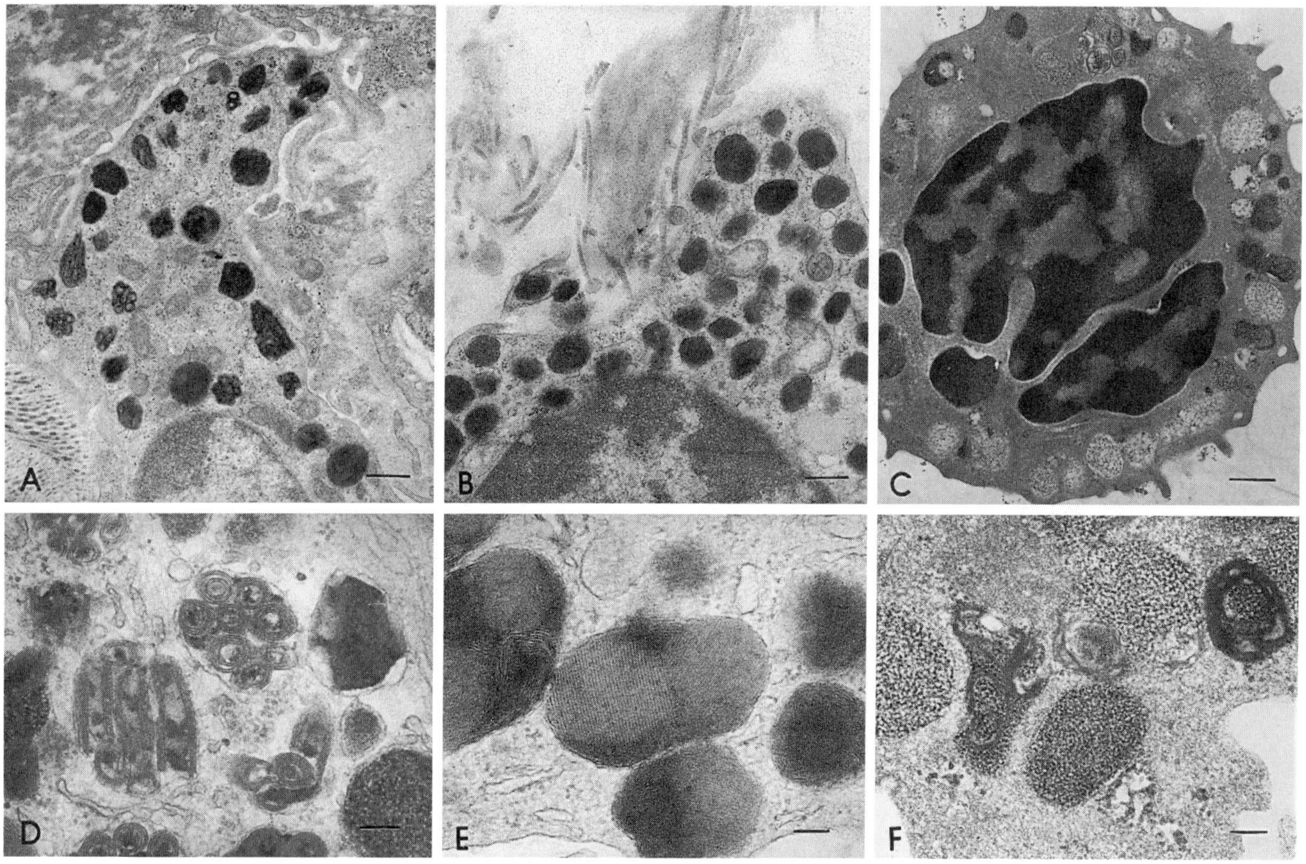

FIGURE 10–1. Ultrastructural features of human mast cells and basophils. Electron micrographs show **(A)** an MC_T cell from lung, **(B)** an MC_{TC} cell from skin, **(C)** a basophil from peripheral blood, and **(D–F)** their corresponding secretory granules at a higher magnification. Bars are 0.5 μm in **A–C** and 0.1 μm in **D–F**. (Courtesy of Dr. Shirley S. Craig, Virginia Commonwealth University, Richmond, VA.)

depending on the tissue source. Disodium cromoglycate and nedocromil, each used for the treatment of allergic asthma, rhinitis, and conjunctivitis, at high concentrations are weak inhibitors of lung-derived mast cells but do not inhibit those from skin and intestine.[113] β-Adrenoceptor agonists, at concentrations theoretically achievable on the airway surface with inhaled medication, produce 10% to 50% inhibition of IgE-dependent histamine release in vitro from dispersed human lung mast cells,[32, 121] whereas generation of LTC_4 and PGD_2 is inhibited to a greater extent.[175] Whether mast cell activation is inhibited in vivo, particularly on the airway surface, is uncertain.

Cyclosporin A and FK-506, which form complexes with cyclophyllin and FK-binding protein, respectively, that inhibit the phosphatase activity of calcineurin, produce rapid and long-lasting inhibition of IgE-dependent histamine release from human basophils and skin- and lung-derived mast cells.[25, 35, 45, 95, 167] Rapamycin interferes with the inhibitory activity of FK-506 by competing for the same FK-binding protein but by itself does not inhibit calcineurin or mast cell or basophil activation. In rodents, cyclosporin A and FK-506 prevent induction of cytokine mRNA and TNF-α protein production,[56, 85, 186] presumably because calcineurin phosphatase is inhibited from dephosphorylating transcription factors stored in the cytoplasm, thereby preventing their translocation to response elements on DNA in the nucleus.

Adenosine added to antigen or calcium ionophore–stimulated human mast cells at low concentrations augments ongoing release of both histamine and LTC_4 but has little to no effect on mediator release from unstimulated mast cells.[118] In contrast, release of these mediators from human basophils is inhibited by adenosine. Dexamethasone in vitro inhibits activation-secretion by human basophils[142] but not by human lung-derived mast cells.[143] In vivo, local instillation of nasal glucocorticosteroids diminished mediator release during the immediate response to nasal allergen challenge,[122] perhaps due to the capacity for local steroids to diminish mast cell concentrations as demonstrated in the synovium,[94] skin,[89] and rectal mucosa[58] or to prevent the superficial migration of mast cells that apparently occurs in atopic subjects during the allergy season.[10, 52] In each case, the duration of steroid exposure as well as steroid potency may be important factors.

MAST CELLS, MAST CELL TYPES, AND HUMAN DISEASE

Alterations in the numbers or distribution of mast cells may occur in human disease, although hyperplasia is not necessarily associated with diseases in which mast cell activation is evident. For example, pulmonary tissue from asthmatic subjects shows little evidence for mast cell hyperplasia overall,[17, 46] although increased numbers of mast cells in the involved epithelial lining of the airway and in the lumen, due at least in part to increased epithelial shedding, have been reported.[115] Mast cell numbers in lesions of chronic urticaria, when examined in one study by sensitive immunohistochemical techniques, are no different than in nonlesional sites or in normal controls.[161] However, this point remains controversial, because other studies have shown increased mast cell concentrations in urticarial lesions.[109] In contrast, involvement of mast cells in disorders of inflammation and fibrosis has been suggested based on observing mast cell hyperplasia and activation in fibrotic lung diseases,[62, 71, 84, 119] rheumatoid arthritis, often near sites of cartilage erosion,[76, 184] and keloids.[162]

In scleroderma lung, mast cell numbers or activation may correlate to the level of pulmonary impairment as judged by the chest x-ray.[28] Although mast cell numbers in scleroderma skin are not elevated, the cells often appear fragmented, perhaps reflecting a cytotoxic factor.[74] Studies of the tight skin mouse (Tsk) model of human scleroderma suggest that mast cell hyperplasia may correlate to the severity of the fibrosis but not to its initiation.[53]

Experimentally, bidirectional effects have been noted between mast cells and fibroblasts. Mouse skin-derived 3T3 fibroblasts prolong the survival of human lung mast cells[90] and rodent mast cells. The maturational effect is consistent with previous findings in mice,[43] suggesting that mast cell differentiation from noncommitted cells depends on factors secreted by T lymphocytes, whereas maturation of granules depends on fibroblast factors. The production of stem cell factor by fibroblasts accounts for a substantial portion of the fibroblast effect on mast cell growth and differentiation. Cultured rat embryonic skin fibroblasts also phagocytose granules released from cocultured rat mast cells.[170] Degranulation of lymph node–derived murine mast cells cocultured with murine embryonic skin fibroblasts resulted in structural alterations in the fibroblast monolayer.[57] Mouse 3T3 fibroblasts cocultured with mouse bone marrow–derived mast cells lose their contact inhibition.[44]

Tryptase also enhances proliferation of fibroblasts, although contact inhibition is maintained.[66] The ability of purified tryptase to activate latent collagenase derived from rheumatoid synovium[64] and of tryptase[66, 133] and bFGF[126] to stimulate fibroblasts may be relevant to these observations. In mice, production of transforming growth factor-β (TGF-β) and TNF-α by mast cells is associated with increased collagen production by neighboring fibroblasts.[61] Understanding the biologic relevance of these in vitro findings is problematic. For example, fibrosis is not associated with chronic urticaria, in spite of repeated episodes of mast cell activation; and lesions of urticaria pigmentosa, containing excessive numbers of mast cells, do not exhibit fibrosis. Thus mast cell activation and hyperplasia alone may not be sufficient to cause fibrosis in vivo but may influence the fibrotic process once it begins.

GROWTH AND DIFFERENTIATION OF MAST CELLS

Both mast cells and basophils originate from hematopoietic stem cells. Basophils, like most myeloid cells, complete their differentiation in the bone marrow, whereas mast cells complete their differentiation in peripheral tissues (Fig. 10–2). Basophils develop largely under the influence of IL-3,[49, 178] a process that is augmented by TGF-β.[158] Mast cells differentiate under the influence of stem cell factor (SCF),[78, 105, 179] the ligand for Kit, a product of the c-*kit* proto-oncogene. IL-3 has little direct influence on the differentiation of human mast cells but does expand the pool of hematopoietic progenitor cells capable of becoming mast cells. In contrast, rodent mast cells use IL-3 as an important growth and differentiation factor. Mast cell progenitors identified in peripheral blood have been clearly distinguished from baso-

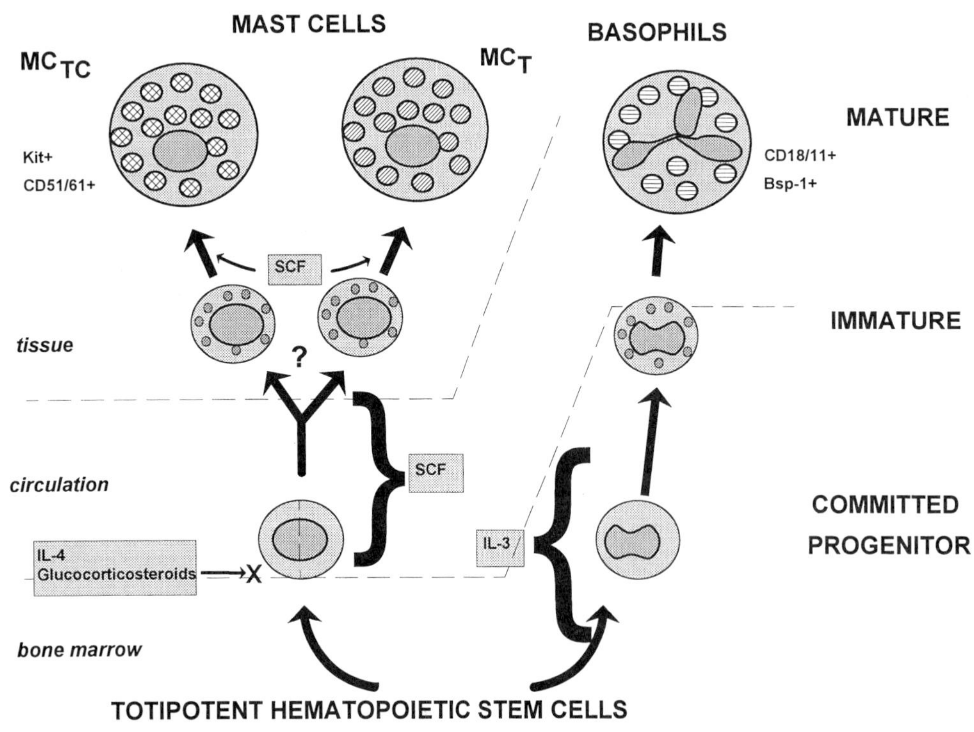

FIGURE 10–2. Developmental pathways for human mast cells and basophils.

phils, monocytes, or other leukocytes[1, 177] and thus represent a distinct myeloid lineage.

Conditions that influence the selective development or recruitment of MC_{TC} and MC_T cells at their respective tissue sites are not yet understood. However, commitment to a particular mast cell phenotype apparently occurs by the time granules begin to form.[40] Unlike other myelocytes that stop expressing Kit as they mature, mast cells express increasing amounts of Kit as they develop. Thus SCF affects properties of mast cells throughout their development, including differentiation, survival,[72, 112, 191] chemotaxis,[96, 111] activation,[37, 165] and priming.[12, 37] The effects on differentiation and survival are particularly evident in certain strains of mice with defects either in Kit or in SCF in which a profound mast cell deficiency results. Removal of SCF from mast cells in mice,[72, 191] and presumably humans,[112] results in apoptosis. Of potential interest is the observation that TGF-β inhibits the ability of SCF to rescue murine mast cells from apoptosis.[97]

Why mast cells fail to develop in the bone marrow where SCF clearly exerts an effect on other lineages is an enigma. Either the bone marrow microenvironment lacks an accessory factor present in peripheral sites, or the microenvironment contains additional factors that are not permissive for mast cell development to occur. The latter seems in part to be the case, because IL-4 appears to prevent the SCF-dependent development of mast cells from progenitors in vitro[112, 159] but has little effect on more mature mast cells. The capacity for IL-4 to down-regulate expression of Kit may explain this observation.[160] Glucocorticosteroids have a similar inhibitory effect on mast cell development, whereas mature mast cells are relatively resistant.[77]

Two experiments suggest that MC_{TC} and MC_T cells develop among distinct pathways. First, in humans with inherited combined immunodeficiency disease and in those with acquired immunodeficiency syndrome, marked and selective decreases in MC_T cell concentrations occur in the bowel, whereas the concentration and distribution of MC_{TC} cells are unaffected.[80] This suggests that the appearance in tissues of MC_T cells is dependent on functional T lymphocytes and that MC_{TC} cell development proceeds independently. Second, immature MC_T cells contain granules with complete scrolls and tryptase alone, whereas MC_{TC} cells have granules with electron dense cores surrounded by a less electron dense matrix and tryptase together with chymase.[40] Thus commitment to a particular mast cell type occurs by the time granules begin to form.

MEDIATORS OF MAST CELLS AND BASOPHILS

PREFORMED GRANULE-ASSOCIATED MEDIATORS (see Table 10–1)

Biogenic Amines

Histamine is the sole biogenic amine in human mast cells and basophils. Histamine (β-imidazolylethylamine) is formed from histidine[9] by histidine decarboxylase in the cytoplasm (Fig. 10–3).[137, 190] Histamine then diffuses into granules

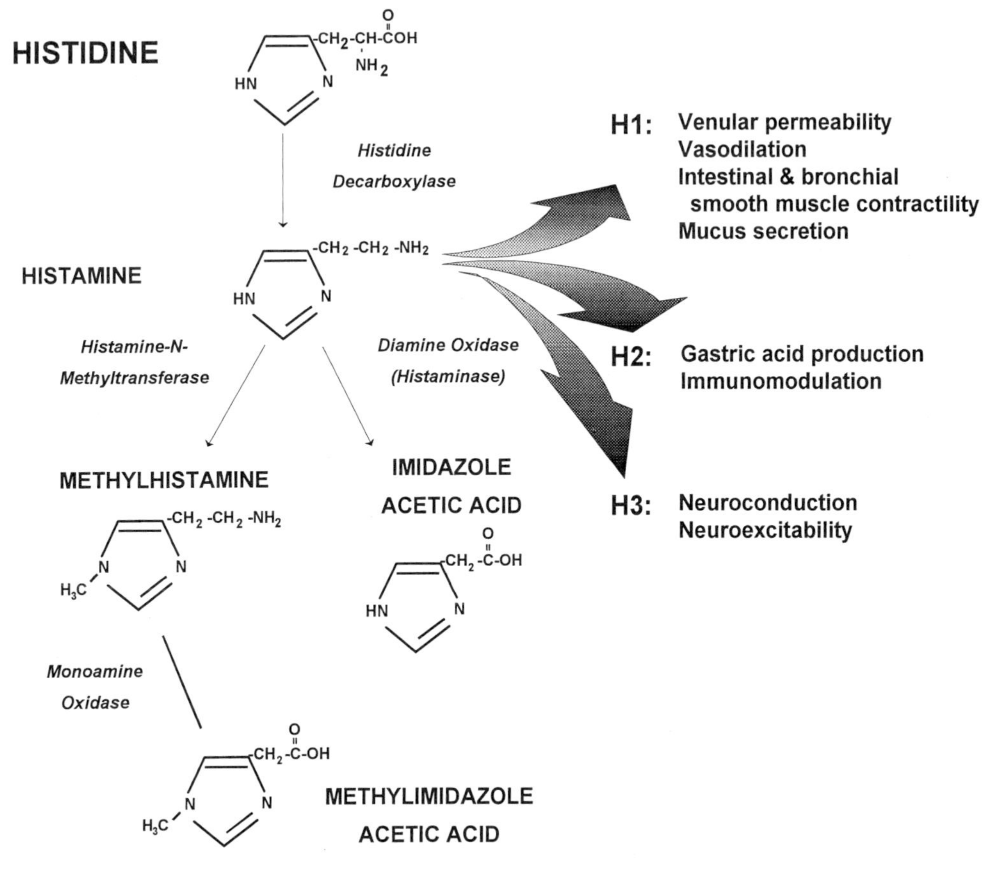

FIGURE 10–3. The synthesis, degradation, and biology of histamine.

where the acid pH confers a positive charge to the molecules. The charged moiety is not free to diffuse out of the granule but instead causes histamine to bind to carboxyl and sulfate groups on proteins and proteoglycans. Histamine is thereby stored in secretory granules but is completely solubilized during degranulation when histamine is exposed to a neutral pH. Histamine is the only preformed mediator of human mast cells with direct potent vasoactive and smooth muscle spasmogenic effects. Extracellular histamine is metabolized within minutes of release, suggesting that it is destined to act quickly and locally.

Human mast cells and basophils contain 1 to 3 pg of histamine per cell, implying histamine concentrations of about 0.1 M inside secretory granules. In contrast, histamine concentrations of about 2 nM exist in plasma. Intermediate concentrations in samples obtained from other sites, such as nasal lavage fluid, reflect local rates of production and removal. Elevated levels of histamine in plasma or urine are detected after anaphylactic reactions to allergens or radiocontrast dyes and in a portion of subjects with mastocytosis, consistent with mast cell involvement in each case. However, subjects in septic shock and those with hereditary angioneurotic edema during attacks do not exhibit elevated histamine levels, consistent with a lack of mast cell involvement.

Histamine exerts its biologic and pathobiologic effects through its interactions with cell-specific receptors designated H1, H2, and H3,[6, 13, 124] which initially were defined with the recognition of specific agonists and antagonists. H1 receptors are blocked by chlorpheniramine, H2 receptors by cimetidine, and H3 receptors by thioperamide. Previously described H2 effects based on using burimimide or impromidine, which show H3 cross-antagonism, need to be reconsidered. Examples of receptor-specific agonists include 2-methylhistamine at H1 receptors, dimaprit at H2 receptors, and α-methylhistamine at H3 receptors.

Effects of histamine (see Figure 10–3) mediated by H1 receptors include enhanced permeability of postcapillary venules, vasodilation, contraction of bronchial and gastrointestinal smooth muscle, and increased mucus secretion at mucosal sites. Increased vasopermeability will facilitate the tissue deposition of factors from plasma that may be important for tissue growth and repair and of foreign material or immune complexes that result in tissue inflammation.

H2 receptor agonists stimulate gastric acid secretion by parietal cells, explaining why peptic ulcers are a common problem in patients with systemic mastocytosis. H2 agonists also inhibit mediator secretion by cytotoxic lymphocytes and granulocytes; augment suppression by T lymphocytes[98]; enhance epithelial permeability across human airways[18]; stimulate chemokinesis of neutrophils and eosinophils and expression of eosinophil C3b receptors; suppress eosinophil chemotaxis[36]; and activate endothelial cells to release a potent inhibitor of platelet aggregation, PGI_2 (prostacyclin). Stimulation of H3 receptors affects neurotransmitter release and histamine formation in the central and peripheral nervous system.[5] They are postulated, but not proven, to be involved in cross-talk between mast cells and peripheral nerves. Bronchial hyperreactivity in atopics with asthma to irritant stimuli, such as exercise or cold air, may in part be mediated by histamine-mediated neurogenic hyperexcitability.

The combined effects of H1 and H2 receptor–mediated activities of histamine are required for the full expression of vasoactivity. For example, the triple response caused by an intradermal injection of histamine—namely, a central erythema within seconds (histamine arteriolar vasodilation) followed by circumferential erythema (axon reflex vasodilation mediated by neuropeptides) and a central weal (histamine vasopermeability, edema) peaking at about 15 minutes—is mostly blocked by H1 receptor antagonists but is completely blocked only with a combination of H1 and H2 receptor antagonists.[131] Analogous results have been observed for the tachycardia, widened pulse pressure, diastolic hypotension, flushing, and headaches observed during intravenous administration of histamine.[83]

Neutral Proteases

Neutral proteases cleave peptide bonds near neutral pH. Such enzymes are the dominant protein components of secretory granules in human and rodent mast cells.[145] In addition, such enzymes serve as selective markers that distinguish mast cells from other cell types, including basophils, and different mast cell subpopulations from one another.

Tryptase, a serine-class protease, accounts for most of the trypsin-like activity first detected in human mast cells by histochemical techniques.[69, 150] Substantial amounts of tryptase are present in MC_{TC} cells derived from foreskin (35 pg/cell) and in MC_T cells derived from lung (10 pg/cell). Tryptase resides in secretory granules and is released in parallel with histamine during degranulation.[151] Negligible amounts have been measured in human basophils (0.04 pg/cell), where tryptase mRNA levels approximately 10^5-fold lower than tissue mast cells have been measured.[189] Other cell types have no detectable tryptase protein or mRNA. Thus the enzyme is a discriminating marker of human mast cells.

Tryptase is a tetramer of 134,000 daltons with N-glycosylated subunits of 31,000 to 34,000 daltons, each with an active enzymatic site.[150] Although at least two homologous tryptase cDNA molecules (α and β) and corresponding genes have been identified on human chromosome 16,[103, 104, 182] β-tryptase homotetramers appear to account for all of the enzymatically active tryptase. A mutation in the leader sequence of α-tryptase prevents processing to a mature form. Thus tryptase enzymatic activity is accounted for by β-tryptase, whereas immunoreactive tryptase is composed of both α- and β-tryptase. β-Tryptase is the principal form stored in secretory granules and thus is the best indicator of mast cell degranulation. α-Tryptase is the principal form detected in serum or plasma under nonacute clinical conditions and thus is thought to be constitutively secreted. α-Tryptase levels are elevated in blood collected from patients with systemic mastocytosis, presumably reflecting the increased burden of mast cells.

Tryptase activity is measured by hydrolysis of synthetic trypsin-like substrates. The absence of inhibition by the biologic inhibitors of serine proteases present in plasma, lung, and urine clearly distinguishes tryptase from pancreatic trypsin and from most other serine proteases. Tryptase is stored fully active in secretory granules, uniquely stabilized in its active tetrameric through its strong ionic association with heparin.[147] However, the acid pH (~5.5) of secretory granules suppresses the activity of the mature enzyme against

TABLE 10–3
POTENTIAL BIOLOGIC PROPERTIES OF HUMAN TRYPTASE AND CHYMASE

Protease	Property
Tryptase	Fibrinogenolysis High molecular weight kininogen destruction Neuropeptide degradation Prostromelysin activation Cellular activation: fibroblast proliferation and pulmonary smooth muscle hyperreactivity to histamine
Chymase	Generation of angiotensin II Procollagenase activation Basement membrane degradation Glandular mucus secretion Neuropeptide degradation

most protein substrates but facilitates the heparin-dependent processing of preprotryptase to protryptase and protryptase to the mature tetramer. When free in a physiologic salt solution, tryptase subunits rapidly dissociate from one another into inactive monomers, irreversible under physiologic conditions, but without any evidence for autodegradation.[4]

Potential biologic activities of tryptase have been examined in vitro (Table 10–3). Tryptase rapidly inactivates fibrinogen as a coagulable substrate for thrombin[148]; the lack of fibrin deposition and rapid resolution of urticaria/angioedema reactions may in part reflect this same activity in vivo. Tryptase sensitizes airway smooth muscle to the contractile effects of histamine[156] and degrades the intrinsic bronchodilating neuropeptide called vasoactive intestinal peptide (VIP). These effects are of potential importance in asthma. Tryptase activates latent collagenase derived from rheumatoid synovial cells, apparently by first activating prostromelysin (metalloproteinase III),[64] which in turn activates latent collagenase. The increased numbers of mast cells found in rheumatoid synovium[94] and in inflammatory cutaneous lesions of scleroderma[67] together with the increased tissue turnover that occurs in each condition suggest a related role for tryptase. Also of interest are the abilities of tryptase to stimulate smooth muscle cells[21] and fibroblasts.[66] The recent availability of tryptase inhibitors as potential therapeutics should provide better information on the biologic and pathobiologic roles of this enzyme in humans.

Chymase is the principal enzyme accounting for the chymotrypsin-like activity present in human cutaneous mast cells. The enzyme was purified from human skin,[138] and the corresponding gene was cloned and localized to human chromosome 14.[27] Chymase was selectively localized to a subpopulation of mast cells by enzymatic and immunohistochemical techniques.[79] Dispersed MC_{TC} cells obtained from skin contain 4.5 pg of chymase per mast cell.

Human chymase is a monomeric serine esterase of 30,000 daltons with chymotryptic activity on synthetic substrates. Like tryptase, chymase is bound to heparin and/or chondroitin sulfate E, stored fully active in mast cell secretory granules, and processed from preprochymase by a heparin-dependent mechanism.[108, 176] Unlike tryptase, chymase stability is not substantially affected by heparin,[136] and its activity is inhibited by classic biologic inhibitors of serine proteinases, such as α_1-antichymotrypsin, α_1-proteinase inhibitor, and α_2-macroglobulin.[141] Neither chymotrypsin-like enzymatic activity nor chymase mRNA is detected in MC_T cells.[189]

Potential biologic activities of chymase, like those of tryptase, are based on in vitro observations (see Table 10–3). Chymase is a potent activator of angiotensin I[188] and procollagenase,[134] inactivates bradykinin,[127] releases latent TGF-β from connective tissue matrixes,[172] and attacks the lamina lucida of the basement membrane at the dermal-epidermal junction of human skin.[19] Chymase degrades substance P as well as VIP and probably other neuropeptides.[26, 33] The physiologic importance of angiotensin II generation by mast cell chymase is supported by a study in marmosets showing that administration of an angiotensin derivative capable of being activated by chymase, but not by angiotensin-converting enzyme, raises arterial blood pressure. Dog chymase has been shown to stimulate mucus production from glandular cells in vitro,[163] suggesting a similar role in asthma and allergic rhinitis, where release of chymase in proximity to glandular tissue might promote the state of hypersecretion.

Human mast cell cathepsin G is a serine-class neutral protease found in mast cells as well as neutrophils and monocytes. The enzyme resides with chymase in MC_{TC} cells[139, 140] and exhibits a molecular weight of 30,000.

Human mast cell carboxypeptidase resides with chymase and cathepsin G in secretory granules of MC_{TC} cells.[73] Stored fully active, when released it cleaves the carboxy-terminal His[9]/Leu[10] bond of angiotensin I. It behaves like a zinc metalloexopeptidase and is inhibited by *o*-phenanthroline.[60] Human mast cells dispersed from skin contain 5 to 16 pg of carboxypeptidase per cell.[59] Human mast cell carboxypeptidase is a monomer with a molecular weight of 34,500.[59] Based on analysis of the cDNA-derived amino acid sequence and gene structure,[128] the human enzyme is more homologous to human pancreatic carboxypeptidase B than A, but the catalytic site is more homologous to human pancreatic carboxypeptidase A, as are its substrate specificities for carboxyterminal Phe and Leu residues.

Proteoglycans

Highly sulfated proteoglycans in secretory granules of mast cells and basophils result in metachromasia when these cells are stained with basic dyes. Proteoglycans are composed of glycosaminoglycan side chains (repeating unbranched disaccharide units of a uronic acid and hexosamine moieties that are variably sulfated) covalently linked to a single-chain protein core via a specific trisaccharide-protein linkage region consisting of -gal-gal-xyl-ser. Their synthesis begins in the endoplasmic reticulum and continues during transport through the Golgi apparatus, where association with certain proteases may occur prior to trafficking to secretory granules in pregranules that bud off of the Golgi. Heparin and chondroitin sulfate E are the major intracellular proteoglycans of human mast cells,[169, 173] heparin being found in all mature mast cells.[38] Chondroitin sulfate A is the predominant type in human basophils[99] but is also found in many other cell types.

The characteristic disaccharide units of heparin, chondroitin sulfate E, and chondroitin sulfate A are shown in Figure 10–4. The average number of sulfate residues per respective disaccharide is 2.5, 1.5, and 1.0. Susceptibility of heparin to nitrous acid is due to attack at the N-sulfate residue; chon-

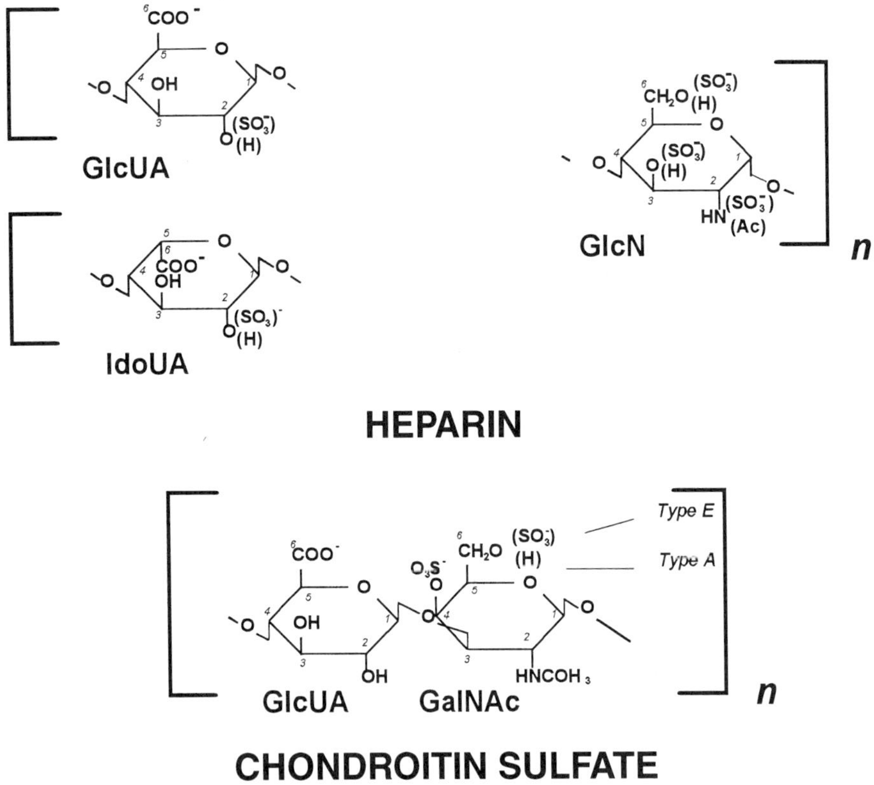

FIGURE 10–4. Structural characteristics of mast cell and basophil proteoglycans.

droitin sulfates lack this residue and are resistant to nitrous acid.

The same peptide core is associated with heparin and chondroitin sulfate proteoglycans, and both proteoglycan types may reside in the same cell and even on the same peptide core. In humans, the core protein is 17,600 daltons in size and contains a glycosaminoglycan attachment region of 18 amino acids,[168] composed largely of Ser-Gly dipeptide repeats, where two to three glycosaminoglycans of about 20,000 daltons are attached to Ser residues.[100, 101] The core peptide gene is located on chromosome 10.

The biologic functions of endogenous mast cell proteoglycans are somewhat speculative. These proteoglycans bind to histamine, neutral proteases, and acid hydrolases at the acidic pH inside mast cell secretory granules. Heparin facilitates processing of chymase and tryptase precursors to their active forms, chondroitin sulfate glycosaminoglycans being inactive. Uptake and packaging of these proteases and histamine into secretory granules may be proteoglycan dependent. The stabilizing effect of heparin, and to a lesser degree chondroitin sulfate E, on human tryptase activity[4, 147] may be crucial for the full expression of mast cell–mediated events. Heparin, and chondroitin sulfate E to a lesser extent, expresses anticoagulant, anticomplement, and antikallikrein activities but can catalyze autoactivation of Hageman factor.

Heparin neutralizes the ability of eosinophil-derived major basic protein to kill schistosomula and enhances the binding of fibronectin to collagen. Heparin protects and facilitates fibroblast growth factor activity,[166] which appears to reside in cutaneous mast cells,[126] and modulates the cell adhesion properties of matrix proteins such as vitronectin, fibronectin, and laminin. Binding of heparin to L- and P-selectins inhibits inflammation,[110] perhaps by blocking leukocyte rolling. The anticoagulant activities of human and commercial porcine heparin are similar and depend on a specific pentasaccharide sequence.[116] However, when heparin is saturated with tryptase and other mast cell proteases, these activities may be attenuated.

NEWLY GENERATED LIPID MEDIATORS

Liberation of the 20-carbon polyunsaturated fatty acid called arachidonic acid from cellular lipid stores by phospholipase A occurs with mast cell activation, whereupon it is either reincorporated into lipids, released, or oxidatively metabolized. Unstimulated human mast cells derived from lung incorporate exogenous arachidonic acid into neutral lipids and phospholipids in a ratio of about 7:2[120] and store these lipids in membranes and cytoplasmic lipid bodies.[48] Arachidonate released by hydrolysis of these lipids is then metabolized along either the cyclooxygenase pathway to prostaglandins (PGs) and thromboxanes (TXs) or the 5-, 12-, or 15-lipoxygenase pathway to monohydroxyl fatty acids, leukotrienes (LTs) that include both LTB_4 and the sulfidopeptides LTC_4, LTD_4, and LTE_4 (slow-reacting substances of anaphylaxis, SRS-A), and lipoxins. Platelet-activating factor, made by acetylating the lysophospholipid remaining after arachidonic acid departs, has not been shown to be a major secretory product of human mast cells but may be a secretory product of human basophils. The major eicosanoid products of mast cells and selected properties are shown in Figure 10–5.

Dispersed and purified preparations of human mast cells obtained from lung, skin, and intestine, upon activation, produce PGD_2 in excess over LTC_4.[132] Smaller amounts of

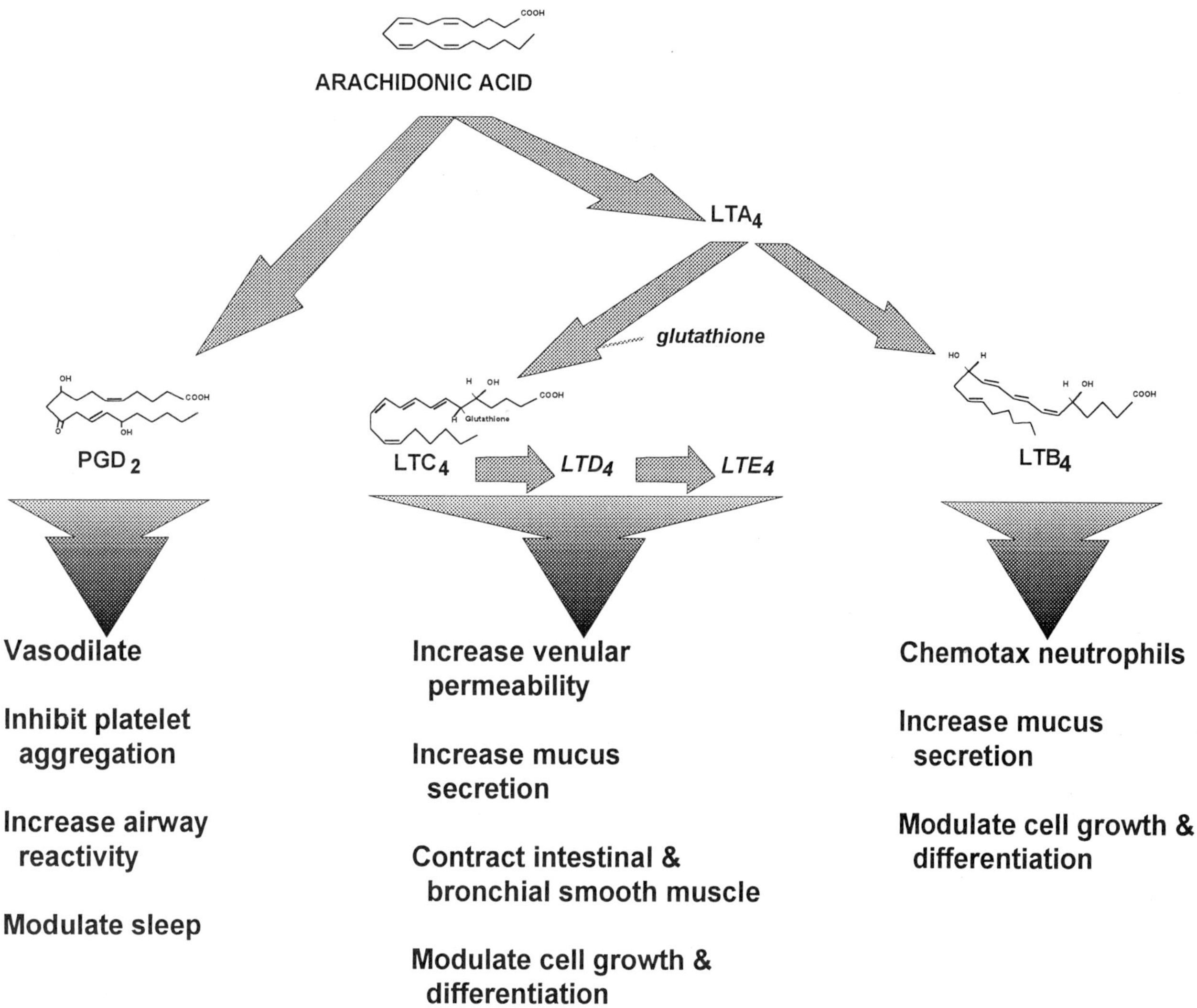

FIGURE 10–5. Major leukotriene and prostaglandin products of mast cells and basophils.

LTB_4 are also produced. Ratios of these metabolites cannot be used to distinguish MC_T from MC_{TC} cell activation. In contrast, peripheral blood basophils obtained from normal human subjects, when activated, synthesize LTC_4 but no PGD_2.[93] However, cells other than mast cells and basophils produce PGD_2 and LTC_4. Thus when these products are detected in a complex biologic milieu, there may be ambiguity as to their cell source.

The biologic importance of mast cell–derived products of arachidonic acid has gained support with the advent of 5-lipoxygenase inhibitors and LTD_4 inhibitors, both of which are helpful in atopic and aspirin-induced asthma, each condition also involving activation of mast cells.[81] A metabolite of PGD_2 has been detected in the urine of patients with active systemic mastocytosis but not in normal subjects.[130] The importance of PGD_2 production in the subgroup of these patients with recurrent hypotensive episodes was suggested when administration of aspirin inhibited generation of the PGD_2 metabolite and led to clinical improvement.

CYTOKINES (see Table 10–1)

Human mast cells and basophils, when activated, produce a diverse array of cytokines. This includes up-regulation of the IL-4 gene cluster on human chromosome 5 (IL-4, IL-5, IL-6, IL-9, and IL-13 and GM-CSF) and of TNF-α on human chromosome 6.[16, 23, 183] Comparison of IL-4 and IL-13 production reveals that mast cells preferentially produce the latter and basophils the former. Cytokine production occurs minutes to hours after mast cells or basophils are activated, in marked variance to anaphylactic degranulation that occurs within minutes and the generation of arachidonic acid metabolites beginning within minutes and lasting up to about 30 minutes. These cytokines serve to activate endothelial cells to recruit eosinophils and other cell types during the late-phase response of immediate hypersensitivity reactions. They provide a mechanism for mast cell involvement in sustaining allergic inflammation hours after release of granule mediators may have finished and also may modulate the local distribution of Th1 and Th2 types of T lymphocytes.

ACTIVATION AND REGULATED SECRETION

Immunologic activation of mast cells and basophils begins when IgE bound to the high-affinity Fcε receptor (FcεR1,

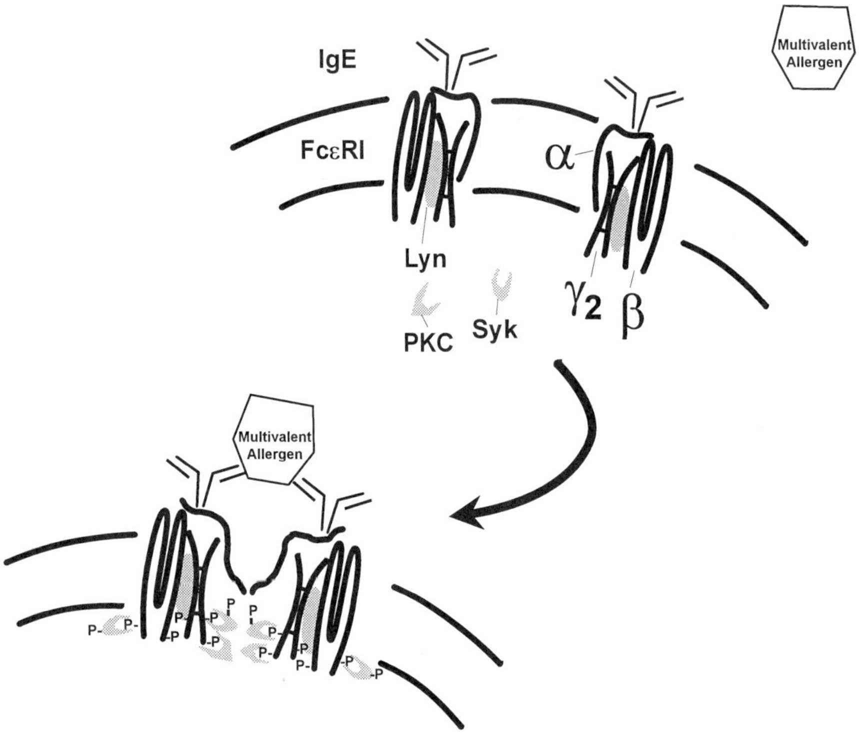

FIGURE 10–6. Early biochemical steps involved in the activation of mast cells.

Ka = 10^9 M^{-1}) is cross-linked by multivalent allergen (Fig. 10–6). The FcεR1 receptor is composed of four subunits,[102] $\alpha\beta\gamma_2$, shown schematically in Figure 10–6. The α chain contains the IgE-binding domain. The β and two disulfide-linked γ chains are not accessible on the surface. The γ chains of FcεR1 (different from the γ chain of IL-2R) are involved in signal transduction and also are present in the CD16, FcγRIII receptors of natural killer cells and may substitute for the TCR ζ chain. In vivo, autoantibodies against FcεRIα[68] and against IgE[63] in subjects with idiopathic urticaria have been detected, suggesting an autoimmune etiology in some patients with this disorder.

Regulated secretion by mast cells and basophils also may be induced by nonimmunologic agonists. Multivalent lectins, like bivalent concanavalin A, bind carbohydrate residues to cross-link membrane FcεRI or IgE. Calcium ionophores activate by translocating calcium into the cells. Basic biomolecules such as compound 48/80, C3a, C5a, morphine, mellitin, eosinophil-derived major basic protein, and various neuropeptides such as substance P directly perturb the plasma membrane of human mast cells derived from skin but are inactive against mast cells derived from most other tissues or against basophils. The peptide f-Met-Leu-Phe activates human basophils but not mast cells. Various histamine-releasing factors, particularly chemokines, derived from monocytes, lymphocytes, platelets, and neutrophils also have been described that are of potential clinical significance. An IgE-dependent histamine-releasing factor termed p23 has recently been identified that stimulates basophils carrying a particular type of IgE, termed IgE^+,[92] and appears to be linked to the severity of atopic dermatitis in children[135] and to the intensity of the late-phase immediate hypersensitivity response.

The earliest biochemical events involved in signal transduction after FcεR1 aggregation involve phosphorylation of the β and γ chains of the high-affinity receptor (see Fig. 10–6). Phosphorylation of tyrosines in membrane proteins often occurs on a special motif consisting of six conserved amino acids (two Tyr residues) distributed over a 26–amino acid stretch called ITAM (immunoreceptor tyrosine activation motif), previously called ARH1 for antigen receptor homology 1, ARAM for antigen receptor activation motif, and TAM for tyrosine activation motif. These ITAMs associate with and activate Src-family protein tyrosine kinases (PTKs). Activated PTKs phosphorylate Tyr residues in the ITAMs and phosphorylate and activate downstream effector molecules such as phospholipase Cγ (PLC-γ), Ras, and phosphatidyl inositol-3 kinase (PI3-k).

ITAMs reside on both γ and β, and these two subunits are phosphorylated within seconds after receptor cross-linking and dephosphorylated almost immediately upon disruption of the receptor aggregates. The PTK Lyn associates with the β and γ chains when the cells are at rest and initiates phosphorylation of these chains after receptor aggregation.[187] A calcium-independent isoform of protein kinase C appears to associate with and phosphorylate Ser in the γ chain. Phosphorylation of these sites increases the affinity of cytoplasmic PTK Syk for these chains. Syk is then phosphorylated by Lyn and possibly by itself and is required for mast cell activation.[114, 129, 180] These early events also are regulated by CD45, a protein tyrosine phosphatase, because mast cells from CD45 knock-out mice do not exhibit IgE-dependent activation.[11] The cytoplasmic hemopoietic cytoplasmic phosphatase (HCP) also is thought to down-regulate Lyn-dependent events. Phosphorylated Syk then carries the activation signal to pathways involving PLCγ, MAP kinase,[174] and PI-3 kinase.

Degranulation is associated with activation of small G proteins that cause actin polymerization and actin relocalization. Metabolism of phospholipids, which mostly reside in secretory granules,[31] occurs early during the secretory response, is necessary for the later secretion of lipid mediators, and may be important for regulated secretion to ensue. Generation of IP_3 and diacylglycerol after FcεRI receptor aggregation occurs and results in release of calcium from the endoplasmic reticulum. This in turn stimulates calcium-dependent isoforms of protein kinase C[22] and may directly facilitate fusion of lipid bilayers as exocytosis proceeds.

BIOLOGY AND PATHOBIOLOGY OF HUMAN MAST CELLS

A precise assessment of mast cell involvement in various diseases has been facilitated by use of monoclonal antibodies that selectively recognize the proteases specific to this cell type. The finding of a secretory granule marker for human basophils,[86] called 2D7 ligand, holds promise that similar tests for basophil involvement will become available.

SYSTEMIC ANAPHYLAXIS AND MASTOCYTOSIS

Specific sandwich immunoassays for tryptase have been developed to quantify total amounts of the enzyme in complex biologic fluids as a reflection of mast cell activation and mast cell number (Table 10–4). One immunoassay[51] uses the G5 mAb for capture. This antibody detects primarily β-tryptase,[153] the primary species of tryptase stored in secretory granules. Thus elevated levels of tryptase in serum or other biologic fluids with the G5 capture assay reflect mast cell activation. Baseline levels of tryptase with the G5 capture assay are less than 1 ng/ml but rise during systemic anaphylaxis if clinical severity is sufficient to cause hypotension.[152, 154] Peak levels of tryptase correlate closely to the drop in mean arterial pressure seen with systemic anaphylaxis to insect stings,[181] suggesting that the extent of mast cell degranulation is a major determinant of clinical severity in bee sting–induced systemic anaphylaxis. Elevated levels of tryptase by the G5 assay in postmortem serum have been used to suggest premortem anaphylaxis as a cause of death[192] and have implicated anaphylaxis as a cause of death in a substantial number of victims of sudden infant death syndrome.[123] In patients with severe or even fatal food-induced anaphylaxis diagnosed clinically, many will show no elevation in serum tryptase levels, suggesting that a mast cell–independent form of anaphylaxis should be considered.

TABLE 10–4
CLINICAL CONSIDERATIONS OF IMMUNOASSAYS FOR TRYPTASE

Condition	G5 Assay	B12 Assay
Tryptase type recognized	β	α + β
Tissue mast cells	+ +	+ +
Normal serum or plasma	<1 ng/ml	5 ng/ml
Acute systemic anaphylaxis	>5 ng/ml	>10 ng/ml (B12/G5 ratio <5)
Systemic mastocytosis (nonacute)	≥1 ng/ml (~50% of patients)	≥20 ng/ml (B12/G5 ratio >10)

The other immunoassay[149] uses the B12 mAb for capture. B12 detects both α- and β-tryptase.[153] Baseline levels of tryptase with the B12 assay are about 5 ng/ml, indicating that the predominant form of tryptase in baseline serum is α-tryptase. The presence of α-tryptase mRNA but little if any α-tryptase protein in skin- and lung-derived mast cells raised the hypothesis that this form of tryptase is constitutively secreted. α-Tryptase is markedly elevated in subjects with systemic mastocytosis[153] but only modestly elevated in those with cutaneous disease alone. In contrast, patients with active allergic rhinitis or active urticaria show B12 and G5 assay levels that are no different from normal controls.

ASTHMA

Tryptase levels in bronchoalveolar lavage fluid have been used to provide a measure of mast cell activation in various forms of asthma. Trypase levels,[185] like those of PGD_2,[91] are elevated in the asthmatic airway, indicating ongoing mast cell activation. Other supporting evidence for constitutive mast cell activation is the ultrastructural appearance of airway mast cells observed in biopsy material[70] and adenosine hyperresponsiveness of the airway.[125] Adenosine augments ongoing mast cell degranulation but does not initiate degranulation from a mast cell at rest. After bronchial challenge of sensitive subjects with allergen, tryptase levels rise during the early phase of the response but return to baseline during the late phase of the response when eosinophil activation is evident.[155] Histamine also rises during the early phase but does not return to baseline during the late phase, suggesting that basophils may be the source of histamine during this portion of the response.

In aspirin-sensitive asthmatics, it has not yet been possible to collect bronchial lavage fluid during the bronchospastic response; however, tryptase levels in serum rise when the response to aspirin extends beyond the airway to include the skin and intestine,[15] and tryptase levels rise in nasal lavage fluids in airway responders.[54] Thus mast cell activation appears to occur during aspirin-induced bronchospasm as well as aspirin-induced anaphylaxis. Of greater surprise is the observation that mast cell mediator levels, including those of histamine, tryptase, PGD_2, and LTC_4, do not rise in airway fluid after exercise-induced bronchospasm in atopic asthmatics.[20, 82] These data contrast with pharmacologic studies indicating that inhibitors of mast cell mediators suppress the exercise-induced response of the airway. A unifying hypothesis is that attenuation of bronchospasm with inhibitors of leukotrienes, prostaglandins, or histamine occur by raising the threshhold at which irritant-responsive nerve fibers are activated by exercise. This threshhold should have been lowered prior to exercise challenge by the elevated levels of these mediators known to be present at baseline in the airways of atopic asthmatics.

CUTANEOUS ALLERGY

The skin chamber model has been used to study mast cell involvement in response to allergen challenge. As in the airway, mast cell degranulation occurs during the immediate phase but not during the late phase of the response as measured by the tryptase concentration in skin chamber fluid.[146, 157] The persistent elevation of histamine during the late phase of the response to continuous allergen challenge is consistent with basophil recruitment and activation. Further, when allergen is removed after 1 hour, referred to as interrupted challenge, rechallenge at 4 to 6 hours with the same allergen results in histamine release but not tryptase release, again consistent with recruitment of sensitive basophils; whereas mast cells were desensitized to the second challenge by the first challenge. Supportive of this interpretation are the findings that basophils are observed during the late phase of the cutaneous response to allergen,[29] that pretreatment with glucocorticosteroids blocks the late-phase release of histamine and basophils,[7, 30] and that codeine challenge (codeine stimulates skin mast cells but not basophils) during the late phase causes a marked release of tryptase.[157]

REFERENCES

1. Agis H, Willheim M, Sperr WR, et al: Monocytes do not make mast cells when cultured in the presence of SCF: characterization of the circulating mast cell progenitor as a c-*kit*⁺, CD34⁺, Ly⁻, CD14⁻, CD17⁻, colony-forming cell. J Immunol 151:4221, 1993.
2. Alam R, Forsythe P, Stafford S, et al: Monocyte chemotactic protein-2, monocyte chemotactic protein-3, and fibroblast-induced cytokine: three new chemokines induce chemotaxis and activation of basophils. J Immunol 153:3155, 1994.
3. Alam R, Kumar D, Anderson-Walters D, et al: Macrophage inflammatory protein-1α and monocyte chemoattractant peptide-1 elicit immediate and late cutaneous reactions and activate murine mast cells in vivo. J Immunol 152:1298, 1994.
4. Alter SC, Metcalfe DD, Bradford TR, et al: Regulation of human mast cell tryptase. Effects of enzyme concentration, ionic strength and the structure and negative charge density of polysaccharides. Biochem J 248:821, 1987.
5. Arrang JM, Devaux B, Chodkiewicz JP, et al: H3-receptors control histamine release in human brain. J Neurochem 51:105, 1988.
6. Arrang JM, Garbarg M, Lancelot JC, et al: Highly potent and selective ligands for histamine H3-receptors. Nature 327:117, 1987.
7. Atkins PC, Schwartz LB, Adkinson NF, et al: In vivo antigen-induced cutaneous mediator release: simultaneous comparisons of histamine, tryptase, and prostaglandin D_2 release and the effect of oral corticosteroid administration. J Allergy Clin Immunol 86:360, 1990.
8. Baggiolini M, Dahinden CA: CC chemokines in allergic inflammation. Immunol Today 15:127, 1994.
9. Bauza MT, Lagunoff D: Histidine transport by isolated rat peritoneal mast cells. Biochem Pharmacol 30:1271, 1981.
10. Bentley AM, Jacobson MR, Cumberworth V, et al: Immunohistology of the nasal mucosa in seasonal allergic rhinitis: increases in activated eosinophils and epithelial mast cells. J Allergy Clin Immunol 89:877, 1992.
11. Berger SA, Mak TW, Paige CJ: Leukocyte common antigen (CD45) is required for immunoglobulin E-mediated degranulation of mast cells. J Exp Med 180:471, 1994.
12. Bischoff SC, Dahinden CA: c-*kit* Ligand: a unique potentiator of mediator release by human lung mast cells. J Exp Med 175:237, 1992.
13. Black JW, Duncan WAM, Durant CJ, et al: Definition and antagonism of histamine H2-receptors. Nature 236:385, 1972.
14. Bloch JG, Asch L, Landry Y, et al: Effects of different secretagogues on synovial fluid mast cells from patients with rheumatoid arthritis. Agents Actions Suppl 36:C290, 1992.
15. Bosso JV, Schwartz LB, Stevenson DD: Tryptase and histamine release during aspirin-induced respiratory reactions. J Allergy Clin Immunol 88:830, 1991.
16. Bradding P, Feather IH, Wilson S, et al: Immunolocalization of cytokines in the nasal mucosa of normal and perennial rhinitic subjects. The mast cell as a source of IL-4, IL-5, and IL-6 in human allergic mucosal inflammation. J Immunol 151:3853, 1993.
17. Bradley BL, Azzawi M, Jacobson M, et al: Eosinophils, T-lymphocytes, mast cells, neutrophils, and macrophages in bronchial biopsy specimens from atopic subjects with asthma: comparison with biopsy specimens from atopic subjects without asthma and normal control subjects and relationship to bronchial hyperresponsiveness. J Allergy Clin Immunol 88:661, 1991.
18. Braude S, Coe C, Royston D, et al: Histamine increases lung permeability by an H2-receptor mechanism. Lancet 2:372, 1984.
19. Briggaman RA, Schechter NM, Fraki J, et al: Degradation of the epidermal-dermal junction by a proteolytic enzyme from human skin and human polymorphonuclear leukocytes. J Exp Med 160:1027, 1984.
20. Broide DH, Eisman S, Ramsdell JW, et al: Airway levels of mast cell-derived mediators in exercise-induced asthma. Am Rev Respir Dis 141:563, 1990.
21. Brown JK, Jones CA, Tyler CL, et al: Tryptase-induced mitogenesis in airway smooth muscle cells: potency, mechanisms, and interactions with other mast cell mediators. Chest 107(suppl):95S, 1995.
22. Buccione R, Di Tullio G, Caretta M, et al: Analysis of protein kinase C requirement for exocytosis in permeabilized rat basophilic leukaemia RBL-2H3 cells: a GTP-binding protein(s) as a potential target for protein kinase C. Biochem J 298:149, 1994.
23. Burd PR, Thompson WC, Max EE, et al: Activated mast cells produce interleukin 13. J Exp Med 181:1373, 1995.
24. Bürgi B, Brunner T, Dahinden CA: The degradation product of the C5a anaphylatoxin $C5a_{desarg}$ retains basophil-activating properties. Eur J Immunol 24:1583, 1994.
25. Casolaro V, Spadaro G, Patella V, et al: In vivo characterization of the anti-inflammatory effect of cyclosporin A on human basophils. J Immunol 151:5563, 1993.
26. Caughey GH: Roles of mast cell tryptase and chymase in airway function. Am J Physiol 257:L39, 1989.
27. Caughey GH, Zerweck EH, Vanderslice P: Structure, chromosomal assignment, and deduced amino acid sequence of a human gene for mast cell chymase. J Biol Chem 266:12956, 1991.
28. Chanez P, Lacoste J-Y, Guillot B, et al: Mast cells' contribution to the fibrosing alveolitis of the scleroderma lung. Am Rev Respir Dis 147:1497, 1993.
29. Charlesworth EN, Hood AF, Soter NA, et al: Cutaneous late-phase response to allergen. Mediator release and inflammatory cell infiltration. J Clin Invest 83:1519, 1989.
30. Charlesworth EN, Kagey-Sobotka A, Schleimer RP, et al: Prednisone inhibits the appearance of inflammatory mediators and the influx of eosinophils and basophils associated with the cutaneous late-phase response to allergen. J Immunol 146:671, 1991.
31. Chock SP, Schmauder-Chock EA: Phospholipid storage in the secretory granule of the mast cell. J Biol Chem 264:2862, 1989.
32. Church MK, Hiroi J: Inhibition of IgE-dependent histamine release from human dispersed lung mast cells by anti-allergic drugs and salbutamol. Br J Pharmacol 90:421, 1987.
33. Church MK, Lowman MA, Robinson C, et al: Interaction of neuropeptides with human mast cells. Int Arch Allergy Appl Immunol 88:70, 1989.
34. Church MK, Pao GJK, Holgate ST: Characterization of histamine secretion from mechanically dispersed human lung mast cells: effects of anti-IgE, calcium ionophore A 23187, compound 48/80, and basic polypeptides. J Immunol 129:2116, 1982.
35. Cirillo R, Triggiani M, Siri L, et al: Cyclosporin A rapidly inhibits mediator release from human basophils presumably by interacting with cyclophilin. J Immunol 144:3891, 1990.
36. Clark RA, Gallin JI, Kaplan AP: The selective eosinophil chemotactic activity of histamine. J Exp Med 142:1462, 1975.
37. Columbo M, Horowitz EM, Botana LM, et al: The human recombinant c-*kit* receptor ligand, rhSCF, induces mediator release from human cutaneous mast cells and enhances IgE-dependent mediator release from both skin mast cells and peripheral blood basophils. J Immunol 149:599, 1992.
38. Craig SS, Irani A-MA, Metcalfe DD, et al: Ultrastructural localization of heparin to human mast cells of the MC_{TC} and MC_T types by labeling with antithrombin III-gold. Lab Invest 69:552, 1993.
39. Craig SS, Schechter NM, Schwartz LB: Ultrastructural analysis of human T and TC mast cells identified by immunoelectron microscopy. Lab Invest 58:682, 1988.
40. Craig SS, Schechter NM, Schwartz LB: Ultrastructural analysis of maturing human T and TC mast cells in situ. Lab Invest 60:147, 1989.

41. Craig SS, Schwartz LB: Human MC_{TC} type of mast cell granule: the uncommon occurrence of discrete scrolls associated with focal absence of chymase. Lab Invest 63:581, 1990.
42. Dahinden CA, Geiser T, Brunner T, et al: Monocyte chemotactic protein 3 is a most effective basophil- and eosinophil-activating chemokine. J Exp Med 179:751, 1994.
43. Davidson SMA, Mansour A, Gallily R, et al: Mast cell differentiation depends on T cells and granule synthesis on fibroblasts. Immunology 48:439, 1983.
44. Dayton ET, Caulfield JP, Hein A, et al: Regulation of the growth rate of mouse fibroblasts by IL-3-activated mouse bone marrow-derived mast cells. J Immunol 142:4307, 1989.
45. De Paulis A, Stellato C, Cirillo R, et al: Anti-inflammatory effect of FK-506 on human skin mast cells. J Invest Dermatol 99:723, 1992.
46. Djukanovic R, Wilson JW, Britten KM, et al: Quantitation of mast cells and eosinophils in the bronchial mucosa of symptomatic atopic asthmatics and healthy control subjects using immunohistochemistry. Am Rev Respir Dis 142:863, 1990.
47. Dvorak AM: The fine structure of human basophils and mast cells. In Holgate ST (ed): Mast Cells, Mediators and Disease. Kluwer Academic Publishers, London, 1988, p 29.
48. Dvorak AM, Dvorak HF, Peters SP, et al: Lipid bodies: cytoplasmic organelles important to arachidonate metabolism in macrophages and basophils. J Immunol 131:2965, 1983.
49. Dvorak AM, Saito H, Estrella P, et al: Ultrastructure of eosinophils and basophils stimulated to develop in human cord blood mononuclear cell cultures containing recombinant human interleukin-5 or interleukin-3. Lab Invest 61:116, 1989.
50. El-Lati SG, Dahinden CA, Church MK: Complement peptides C3a- and C5a-induced mediator release from dissociated human skin mast cells. J Invest Dermatol 102:803, 1994.
51. Enander I, Matsson P, Nystrand J, et al: A new radioimmunoassay for human mast cell tryptase using monoclonal antibodies. J Immunol Methods 138:39, 1991.
52. Enerbäck L, Paipkorn U, Granerus G: Intraepithelial migration of nasal mucosal mast cells in hay fever. Int Archs Allergy Appl Immunol 80:44, 1986.
53. Everett ET, Pablos JL, Harley RA, et al: The role of mast cells in the development of skin fibrosis in tight-skin mutant mice. Comp Biochem Physiol (A) 110A:159, 1995.
54. Fischer AR, Rosenberg MA, Lilly CM, et al: Direct evidence for a role of the mast cell in the nasal response to aspirin in aspirin-sensitive asthma. J Allergy Clin Immunol 94:1046, 1994.
55. Fox CC, Dvorak AM, Peters SP, et al: Isolation and characterization of human intestinal mucosal mast cells. J Immunol 135:483, 1985.
56. Fruman DA, Bierer BE, Benes JE, et al: The complex of FK506-binding protein 12 and FK506 inhibits calcineurin phosphatase activity and IgE activation-induced cytokine transcripts, but not exocytosis, in mouse mast cells. J Immunol 154:1846, 1995.
57. Ginsburg H, Amira M, Padawer J, et al: Structural alterations in fibroblast monolayers caused by mast cell degranulation. J Leukocyte Biol 45:491, 1989.
58. Goldsmith P, McGarity B, Walls AF, et al: Corticosteroid treatment reduces mast cell numbers in inflammatory bowel disease. Dig Dis Sci 35:1409, 1990.
59. Goldstein SM, Kaempfer CE, Kealey JT, et al: Human mast cell carboxypeptidase: purification and characterization. J Clin Invest 83:1630, 1989.
60. Goldstein SM, Kaempfer CE, Proud D, et al: Detection and partial characterization of a human mast cell carboxypeptidase. J Immunol 139:2724, 1987.
61. Gordon JR, Galli SJ: Promotion of mouse fibroblast collagen gene expression by mast cells stimulated via the $Fc_\epsilon RI$. Role for mast cell-derived transforming growth factor β and tumor necrosis factor α. J Exp Med 180:2027, 1994.
62. Goto T, Befus D, Low R, et al: Mast cell heterogeneity and hyperplasia in bleomycin-induced pulmonary fibrosis in rats. Am Rev Resp Dis 130:797, 1984.
63. Gruber BL, Baeza ML, Marchese MJ, et al: Prevalence and functional role of anti-IgE autoantibodies in urticarial syndromes. J Invest Dermatol 90:213, 1988.
64. Gruber BL, Marchese MJ, Suzuki K, et al: Synovial procollagenase activation by human mast cell tryptase dependence upon matrix metalloproteinase 3 activation. J Clin Invest 84:1657, 1989.
65. Harris RB, You JL, Milton CF, et al: The role of propeptide hormone protein conformation in limited endoproteolysis. Processing mammalian hypothalamic progonadotropin-releasing hormone (GnRH) precursor protein. In Hedin PA, Menn JJ, Hollingworth RM (eds): Natural and Engineered Pest Management Agents. American Chemical Society, Washington, DC, 1994, p 230.
66. Hartmann T, Ruoss SJ, Raymond WW, et al: Human tryptase as a potent, cell-specific mitogen: role of signaling pathways in synergistic responses. Am J Physiol Lung Cell Mol Physiol 262:L528, 1992.
67. Hawkins RA, Claman HN, Clark RA, et al: Increased dermal mast cell populations in progressive systemic sclerosis: a link in chronic fibrosis. Ann Intern Med 102:182, 1985.
68. Hide M, Francis DM, Grattan CE, et al: Autoantibodies against the high-affinity IgE receptor as a cause of histamine release in chronic urticaria. N Engl J Med 328:1599, 1993.
69. Hopsu VK, Glenner GG: A histochemical enzyme kinetic system applied to the trypsin-like amidase and esterase activity in human mast cells. J Cell Biol 17:503, 1963.
70. Howarth PH, Wilson J, Djukanovic R, et al: Airway inflammation and atopic asthma: a comparative bronchoscopic investigation. Int Arch Allergy Appl Immunol 94:266, 1991.
71. Hunt LW, Colby TV, Weiler DA, et al: Immunofluorescent staining for mast cells in idiopathic pulmonary fibrosis: quantification and evidence for extracellular release of mast cell tryptase. Mayo Clin Proc 67:941, 1992.
72. Iemura A, Tsai M, Ando A, et al: The c-*kit* ligand, stem cell factor, promotes mast cell survival by suppressing apoptosis. Am J Pathol 144:321, 1994.
73. Irani A-MA, Goldstein SM, Wintroub BU, et al: Human mast cell carboxypeptidase: selective localization to MC_{TC} cells. J Immunol 147:247, 1991.
74. Irani A-MA, Gruber BL, Kaufman LD, et al: Mast cell changes in scleroderma: presence of MC_T cells in the skin and evidence of mast cell activation. Arthritis Rheum 35:933, 1992.
75. Irani AA: Tissue and developmental variation of protease expression in human mast cells. In Caughey GH (ed): Mast Cell Proteases in Immunology and Biology. Marcel Dekker, New York, 1995, p 127.
76. Irani AA, Golzar N, DeBlois G, et al: Distribution of mast cell subsets in rheumatoid arthritis and osteoarthritis synovia. Arthritis Rheum 30:66, 1987. Abstract.
77. Irani AA, Nilsson G, Ashman LK, et al: Dexamethasone inhibits the development of mast cells from dispersed human fetal liver cells cultured in the presence of recombinant human stem cell factor. Immunology 84:72, 1995.
78. Irani AA, Nilsson G, Miettinen U, et al: Recombinant human stem cell factor stimulates differentiation of mast cells from dispersed human fetal liver cells. Blood 80:3009, 1992.
79. Irani AA, Schechter NM, Craig SS, et al: Two types of human mast cells that have distinct neutral protease compositions. Proc Natl Acad Sci USA 83:4464, 1986.
80. Irani AM, Craig SS, DeBlois G, et al: Deficiency of the tryptase-positive, chymase-negative mast cell type in gastrointestinal mucosa of patients with defective T lymphocyte function. J Immunol 138:4381, 1987.
81. Israel E, Rubin P, Kemp JP, et al: The effect of inhibition of 5-lipoxygenase by Zileuton in mild-to-moderate asthma. Ann Intern Med 119:1059, 1993.
82. Jarjour NN, Calhoun WJ, Stevens CA, et al: Exercise-induced asthma is not associated with mast cell activation or airway inflammation. J Allergy Clin Immunol 89:60, 1992.
83. Kaliner M, Shelhamer JH, Ottesen EA: Effects of infused histamine: correlation of plasma histamine levels and symptoms. J Allergy Clin Immunol 69:283, 1982.
84. Kawanami O, Ferrans V, Fulmer JD, et al: Ultrastructure of pulmonary mast cells in patients with fibrotic lung disorders. Lab Invest 40:717, 1979.
85. Kaye RE, Fruman DA, Bierer BE, et al: Effects of cyclosporin A and FK506 on Fc_ϵ receptor type I-initiated increases in cytokine mRNA in mouse bone marrow-derived progenitor mast cells: resistance to FK506 is associated with a deficiency in FK506-binding protein FKBP12. Proc Natl Acad Sci USA 89:8542, 1992.
86. Kepley CL, Craig SS, Schwartz LB: Identification and partial characterization of a unique marker for human basophils. J Immunol 154:6548, 1995.
87. Kuna P, Reddigari SR, Rucinski D, et al: Chemokines of the α, β-subclass inhibit human basophils' responsiveness to monocyte chemo-

tactic and activating factor/monocyte chemoattractant protein-1. J Allergy Clin Immunol 95:574, 1995.
88. Kuna P, Reddigari SR, Schall TJ, et al: Characterization of the human basophil response to cytokines, growth factors, and histamine releasing factors of the intercrine/chemokine family. J Immunol 150:1932, 1993.
89. Lavker RM, Schechter NM: Cutaneous mast cell depletion results from topical corticosteroid usage. J Immunol 135:2368, 1985.
90. Levi-Schaffer F, Austen KF, Caulfield JP, et al: Co-culture of human lung-derived mast cells with mouse 3T3 fibroblasts: morphology and IgE-mediated release of histamine, prostaglandin D2, and leukotrienes. J Immunol 139:494, 1987.
91. Liu MC, Bleecker ER, Lichtenstein LM, et al: Evidence for elevated levels of histamine, prostaglandin D_2, and other bronchoconstricting prostaglandins in the airways of subjects with mild asthma. Am Rev Respir Dis 142:126, 1990.
92. MacDonald SM, Rafnar T, Langdon J, et al: Molecular identification of an IgE-dependent histamine-releasing factor. Science 269:688, 1995.
93. MacGlashan DW Jr, Peters SP, Warner J, et al: Characteristics of human basophil sulfidopeptide leukotreine release: releasability defined as the ability of basophils to respond to dimeric cross-links. J Immunol 136:2231, 1986.
94. Malone DG, Wilder RL, Saavedra-Delgado AM, et al: Mast cell numbers in rheumatoid synovial tissues. Correlations with quantitative measures of lymphotic infiltration and modulation by anti-inflammatory therapy. Arthritis Rheum 30:130, 1987.
95. Marone G, Triggiani M, Cirillo R, et al: Cyclosporin A inhibits the release of histamine and peptide leukotriene C4 from human lung mast cells. Ric Clin Lab 18:53, 1988.
96. Meininger CJ, Yano H, Rottapel R, et al: The *c-kit* receptor ligand functions as a mast cell chemoattractant. Blood 79:958, 1992.
97. Mekori YA, Metcalfe DD: Transforming growth factor-β prevents stem cell factor-mediated rescue of mast cells from apoptosis after IL-3 deprivation. J Immunol 153:2194, 1994.
98. Melmon KL, Rocklin RE, Rosenkranz RP: Autacoids as modulators of the inflammatory and immune response. Am J Med 71:100, 1981.
99. Metcalfe DD, Bland CE, Wasserman SI: Biochemical and functional characterization of proteoglycans isolated from basophils of patients with chronic myelogenous leukemia. J Immunol 132:1943, 1984.
100. Metcalfe DD, Lewis RA, Silbert JE, et al: Isolation and characterization of heparin from human lung. J Clin Invest 64:1537, 1979.
101. Metcalfe DD, Soter NA, Wasserman SI, et al: Identification of sulfated mucopolysaccharides including heparin in the lesional skin of a patient with mastocytosis. J Invest Dermatol 74:210, 1980.
102. Metzger H, Alcarez G, Hohman R, et al: The receptor with high affinity for immunoglobulin E. Ann Rev Immunol 4:419, 1986.
103. Miller JS, Moxley G, Schwartz LB: Cloning and characterization of a second complementary DNA for human tryptase. J Clin Invest 86:864, 1990.
104. Miller JS, Westin EH, Schwartz LB: Cloning and characterization of complementary DNA for human tryptase. J Clin Invest 84:1188, 1989.
105. Mitsui H, Furitsu T, Dvorak AM, et al: Development of human mast cells from umbilical cord blood cells by recombinant human and murine C-kit ligand. Proc Natl Acad Sci USA 90:735, 1993.
106. Mousli M, Hugli TE, Landry Y, et al: A mechanism of action for anaphylatoxin C3a stimulation of mast cells. J Immunol 148:2456, 1992.
107. Mousli M, Hugli TE, Landry Y, et al: Peptidergic pathway in human skin and rat peritoneal mast cell activation. Immunopharmacology 27:1, 1994.
108. Murakami M, Karnik SS, Husain A: Human prochymase activation. A novel role for heparin in zymogen processing. J Biol Chem 270:2218, 1995.
109. Natbony SF, Phillips ME, Elias JM, et al: Histologic studies of chronic idiopathic urticaria. J Allergy Clin Immunol 71:177, 1983.
110. Nelson RM, Cecconi O, Roberts WG, et al: Heparin oligosaccharides bind L- and P-selectin and inhibit acute inflammation. Blood 82:3253, 1993.
111. Nilsson G, Butterfield JH, Nilsson K, et al: Stem cell factor is a chemotactic factor for human mast cells. J Immunol 153:3717, 1994.
112. Nilsson G, Miettinen U, Ishizaka T, et al: Interleukin-4 inhibits the expression of Kit and tryptase during stem cell factor-dependent development of human mast cells from fetal liver cells. Blood 84:1519, 1994.
113. Okayama Y, Benyon RC, Rees PH, et al: Inhibition profiles of sodium cromoglycate and nedocromil sodium on mediator release from mast cells of human skin, lung, tonsil, adenoid and intestine. Clin Exp Allergy 22:401, 1992.
114. Oliver JM, Burg DL, Wilson BS, et al: Inhibition of mast cell FcεR1-mediated signaling and effector function by the Syk-selective inhibitor, piceatannol. J Biol Chem 269:29697, 1994.
115. Ollerenshaw SL, Woolcock AJ: Characteristics of the inflammation in biopsies from large airways of subjects with asthma and subjects with chronic airflow limitation. Am Rev Respir Dis 145(4 Pt 1):922, 1992.
116. Oscarsson LG, Pejler G, Lindahl U: Location of the antithrombin-binding sequence in the heparin chain. J Biol Chem 264:296, 1989.
117. Patella V, Marinò I, Lampärter B, et al: Human heart mast cells: isolation, purification, ultrastructure, and immunologic characterization. J Immunol 154:2855, 1995.
118. Peachell PT, Lichtenstein LM, Schleimer RP: Differential regulation of human basophil and lung mast cell function by adenosine. J Pharmacol Exp Ther 256:717, 1991.
119. Pesci A, Bertorelli G, Gabrielli M, et al: Mast cells in fibrotic lung disorders. Chest 103:989, 1993.
120. Peters SP, MacGlashan DW, Schulman ES, et al: Arachidonic acid metabolism in purified human lung mast cells. J Immunol 132:1972, 1984.
121. Peters SP, Schulman ES, Schleimer RP, et al: Dispersed human lung mast cells. Pharmacologic aspects and comparison with human lung tissue fragments. Am Rev Respir Dis 126:1034, 1982.
122. Pipkorn U, Proud D, Lichtenstein LM, et al: Inhibition of mediator release in allergic rhinitis by pretreatment with topical glucocorticosteroids. N Engl J Med 316:1506, 1987.
123. Platt MS, Yunginger JW, Sekula-Perlman A, et al: Involvement of mast cells in sudden infant death syndrome. J Allergy Clin Immunol 94:250, 1994.
124. Polk RE, Healy DP, Schwartz LB, et al: Vancomycin and the red-man syndrome: pharmacodynamics of histamine release. J Infect Dis 157:502, 1988.
125. Polosa R, Ng WH, Crimi N, et al: Release of mast-cell-derived mediators after endobronchial adenosine challenge in asthma. Am J Respir Crit Care Med 151:624, 1995.
126. Reed JA, Albino AP, McNutt NS: Human cutaneous mast cells express basic fibroblast growth factor. Lab Invest 72:215, 1995.
127. Reilly CF, Tewksbury DA, Schechter NM, et al: Rapid conversion of angiotensin I to angiotensin II by neutrophil and mast cell proteinases. J Biol Chem 257:8619, 1982.
128. Reynolds DS, Gurley DS, Stevens RL, et al: Cloning of cDNAs that encode human mast cell carboxypeptidase A, and comparison of the protein with mouse mast cell carboxypeptidase A and rat pancreatic carboxypeptidases. Proc Natl Acad Sci USA 86:9480, 1989.
129. Rivera VM, Brugge JS: Clustering of Syk is sufficient to induce tyrosine phosphorylation and release of allergic mediators from rat basophilic leukemia cells. Mol Cell Biol 15:1582, 1995.
130. Roberts LJ, II, Sweetman BJ, Lewis RA, et al: Increased production of prostaglandin D2 in patients with systemic mastocytosis. N Engl J Med 303:1400, 1980.
131. Robertson I, Greaves MW: Responses of human skin blood vessels to synthetic histamine analogues. Brit J Clin Pharmacol 5:319, 1978.
132. Robinson C: Mast cells and newly-generated lipid mediators. In Holgate ST (ed): Immunology and Medicine: Mast Cells, Mediators and Disease. Kluwer Academic Publishers, London, 1988, p 149.
133. Ruoss SJ, Hartmann T, Caughey GH: Mast cell tryptase is a mitogen for cultured fibroblasts. J Clin Invest 88:493, 1991.
134. Saarinen J, Kalkkinen N, Welgus HG, et al: Activation of human interstitial procollagenase through direct cleavage of the Leu^{83}-Thr^{84} bond by mast cell chymase. J Biol Chem 269:18134, 1994.
135. Sampson HA, Broadbent KR, Bernhisel-Broadbent J: Spontaneous release of histamine from basophils and histamine-releasing factor in patients with atopic dermatitis and food hypersensitivity [see comments]. N Engl J Med 321:228, 1989.
136. Sayama S, Iozzo RV, Lazarus GS, et al: Human skin chymotrypsin-like proteinase chymase. Subcellular localization to mast cell granules and interaction with heparin and other glycosaminoglycans. J Biol Chem 262:6808, 1987.
137. Schayer RW: Histidine decarboxylase in mast cells. Ann NY Acad Sci 103:164, 1963.
138. Schechter NM, Fraki JE, Geesin JC, et al: Human skin chymotryptic protease. Isolation and relation to cathepsin G and rat mast cell proteinase. J Biol Chem 258:2973, 1983.
139. Schechter NM, Irani A-MA, Sprows JL, et al: Identification of a

cathepsin G-like proteinase in the MC_{TC} type of human mast cell. J Immunol 145:2652, 1990.
140. Schechter NM, Mei Wang Z, Blacher RW, et al: Determination of the primary structures of human skin chymase and cathepsin G from cutaneous mast cells of urticaria pigmentosa lesions. J Immunol 152:4062, 1994.
141. Schechter NM, Sprows JL, Schoenberger OL, et al: Reaction of human skin chymotrypsin-like proteinase chymase with plasma proteinase inhibitors. J Biol Chem 264:21308, 1989.
142. Schleimer RP, Lichtenstein LM, Gillespie E: Inhibition of basophil histamine release by anti-inflammatory steroids. Nature 292:454, 1981.
143. Schleimer RP, Schulman ES, MacGlash DW, et al: Effects of dexamethasone on mediator release from human lung fragments and purified human lung mast cells. J Clin Invest 71:1830, 1983.
144. Schmutzler W, Delmich K, Eichelberg D, et al: The human adenoidal mast cell. Susceptibility to different secretagogues and secretion inhibitors. Int Archs Allergy Appl Immunol 77:177, 1985.
145. Schwartz LB: In Schwartz LB (ed): Monographs in Allergy: Neutral Proteases of Mast Cells. Karger, Basel, 1990.
146. Schwartz LB, Atkins PC, Bradford TR, et al: Release of tryptase together with histamine during the immediate cutaneous response to allergen. J Allergy Clin Immunol 80:850, 1987.
147. Schwartz LB, Bradford TR: Regulation of tryptase from human lung mast cells by heparin. Stabilization of the active tetramer. J Biol Chem 261:7372, 1986.
148. Schwartz LB, Bradford TR, Littman BH, et al: The fibrinogenolytic activity of purified tryptase from human lung mast cells. J Immunol 135:2762, 1985.
149. Schwartz LB, Bradford TR, Rouse C, et al: Development of a new, more sensitive immunoassay for human tryptase: use in systemic anaphylaxis. J Clin Immunol 14:190, 1994.
150. Schwartz LB, Lewis RA, Austen KF: Tryptase from human pulmonary mast cells. Purification and characterization. J Biol Chem 256:11939, 1981.
151. Schwartz LB, Lewis RA, Seldin D, et al: Acid hydrolases and tryptase from secretory granules of dispersed human lung mast cells. J Immunol 126:1290, 1981.
152. Schwartz LB, Metcalfe DD, Miller JS, et al: Tryptase levels as an indicator of mast-cell activation in systemic anaphylaxis and mastocytosis. N Engl J Med 316:1622, 1987.
153. Schwartz LB, Sakai K, Bradford TR, et al: The α form of human tryptase is the predominant type present in blood at baseline in normal subjects, and is elevated in those with systemic mastocytosis. J Clin Invest 96:2702, 1995.
154. Schwartz LB, Yunginger JW, Miller JS, et al: The time course of appearance and disappearance of human mast cell tryptase in the circulation after anaphylaxis. J Clin Invest 83:1551, 1989.
155. Sedgwick JB, Calhoun WJ, Gleich GJ, et al: Immediate and late airway response of allergic rhinitis patients to segmental antigen challenge: characterization of eosinophil and mast cell mediators. Am Rev Respir Dis 144:1274, 1991.
156. Sekizawa K, Caughey GH, Lazarus SC, et al: Mast cell tryptase causes airway smooth muscle hyperresponsiveness in dogs. J Clin Invest 83:175, 1989.
157. Shalit M, Schwartz LB, von Allmen C, et al: Release of histamine and tryptase during continuous and interrupted cutaneous challenge with allergen in humans. J Allergy Clin Immunol 86:117, 1990.
158. Sillaber C, Geissler K, Scherrer R, et al: Type β transforming growth factors promote interleukin-3 (IL-3)-dependent differentiation of human basophils but inhibit IL-3-dependent differentiation of human eosinophils. Blood 80:634, 1992.
159. Sillaber C, Sperr WR, Agis H, et al: Inhibition of stem cell factor dependent formation of human mast cells by interleukin-3 and interleukin-4. Int Arch Allergy Immunol 105:264, 1994.
160. Sillaber C, Strobl H, Bevec D, et al: IL-4 regulates c-*kit* proto-oncogene product expression in human mast and myeloid progenitor cells. J Immunol 147:4224, 1991.
161. Smith CH, Kepley C, Schwartz LB, Lee TH: Mast cell number and phenotype in chronic idiopathic urticaria. J Allergy Clin Immunol 96:360, 1995.
162. Smith CJ, Smith JC, Finn MC: The possible role of mast cells (allergy) in the production of keloid and hypertrophic scarring. J Burn Care Rehabil 8:126, 1987.
163. Sommerhoff CP, Caughey GH, Finkbeiner WE, et al: Mast cell chymase. A potent secretagogue for airway gland serous cells. J Immunol 142:2450, 1989.
164. Sperr WR, Bankl HC, Mundigler G, et al: The human cardiac mast cell: localization, isolation, phenotype, and functional characterization. Blood 84:3876, 1994.
165. Sperr WR, Czerwenka K, Mundigler G, et al: Specific activation of human mast cells by the ligand for c-kit: comparison between lung, uterus and heart mast cells. Int Arch Allergy Immunol 102:170, 1993.
166. Spivak-Kroizman T, Lemmon MA, Dikic I, et al: Heparin-induced oligomerization of FGF molecules is responsible for FGF receptor dimerization, activation, and cell proliferation. Cell 79:1015, 1994.
167. Stellato C, De Paulis A, Ciccarelli A, et al: Anti-inflammatory effect of cyclosporin A on human skin mast cells. J Invest Dermatol 98:800, 1992.
168. Stevens RL, Avraham S, Gartner MC, et al: Isolation and characterization of a cDNA that encodes the peptide core of the secretory granule proteoglycan of human promyelocytic leukemia HL-60 cells. J Biol Chem 263:7287, 1988.
169. Stevens RL, Fox CC, Lichtenstein LM, et al: Identification of chondroitin sulfate E proteoglycans and heparin proteoglycans in the secretory granules of human lung mast cells. Proc Natl Acad Sci USA 85:2284, 1988.
170. Subba Rao PV, Friedman MM, Atkins FM, et al: Phagocytosis of mast cell granules by cultured fibroblasts. J Immunol 130:341, 1983.
171. Swieter M, Midura RJ, Nishikata H, et al: Mouse 3T3 fibroblasts induce rate basophilic leukemia (RBL-2H3) cells to acquire responsiveness to compound 48/80. J Immunol 150:617, 1993.
172. Taipale J, Lohi J, Saarinen J, et al: Human mast cell chymase and leukocyte elastase release latent transforming growth factor-β1 from the extracellular matrix of cultured human epithelial and endothelial cells. J Biol Chem 270:4689, 1995.
173. Thompson HL, Schulman ES, Metcalfe DD: Identification of chondroitin sulfate E in human lung mast cells. J Immunol 140:2708, 1988.
174. Tsai M, Chen R-H, Tam S-Y, et al: Activation of MAP kinases, $pp90^{rsk}$ and pp70-S6 kinases in mouse mast cells by signaling through the c-*kit* receptor tyrosine kinase or $Fc_{\epsilon}RI$: rapamycin inhibits activation of pp70-S6 kinase and proliferation in mouse mast cells. Eur J Immunol 23:3286, 1993.
175. Undem BJ, Peachell PT, Lichtenstein LM: Isoproterenol-induced inhibition of immunoglobulin E-mediated release of histamine and arachidonic acid metabolites from the human lung mast cell. J Pharmacol Exp Ther 247:209, 1988.
176. Urata H, Karnik SS, Graham RM, et al: Dipeptide processing activates recombinant human prochymase. J Biol Chem 268:24318, 1993.
177. Valent P: The phenotype of human eosinophils, basophils, and mast cells. J Allergy Clin Immunol 94(suppl):1177, 1994.
178. Valent P, Schmidt G, Besemer J, et al: Interleukin-3 is a differentiation factor for human basophils. Blood 73:1763, 1989.
179. Valent P, Spanblöauchl E, Sperr WR, et al: Induction of differentiation of human mast cells from bone marrow and peripheral blood mononuclear cells by recombinant human stem cell factor/*kit*-ligand in long-term culture. Blood 80:2237, 1992.
180. Vallé A, Kinet J-P: *N*-acetyl-L-cysteine inhibits antigen-mediated Syk, but not Lyn tyrosine kinase activation in mast cells. FEBS Lett 357:41, 1995.
181. Van der Linden PG, Hack CE, Poortman J, et al: Insect-sting challenge in 138 patients: relation between clinical severity of anaphylaxis and mast cell activation. J Allergy Clin Immunol 90:110, 1992.
182. Vanderslice P, Ballinger SM, Tam EK, et al: Human mast cell tryptase: multiple cDNAs and genes reveal a multigene serine protease family. Proc Natl Acad Sci USA 87:3811, 1990.
183. Walsh LJ, Trinchieri G, Waldorf HA, et al: Human dermal mast cells contain and release tumor necrosis factor α, which induces endothelial leukocyte adhesion molecule 1. Proc Natl Acad Sci USA 88:4220, 1991.
184. Wasserman SI: The mast cell and synovial inflammation. Or, what's a nice cell like you doing in a joint like this. Arthritis Rheum 27:841, 1984.
185. Wenzel SE, Fowler AA 3d, Schwartz LB: Activation of pulmonary mast cells by bronchoalveolar allergen challenge. In vivo release of histamine and tryptase in atopic subjects with and without asthma. Am Rev Respir Dis 137:1002, 1988.
186. Wershil BK, Furuta GT, Lavigne JA, et al: Dexamethasone or cyclosporin A suppress mast cell-leukocyte cytokine cascades: multiple mechanisms of inhibition of IgE- and mast cell-dependent cutaneous inflammation in the mouse. J Immunol 154:1391, 1995.

187. Wilson BS, Kapp N, Lee RJ, et al: Distinct functions of the FcεRI gamma and β subunits in the control of FcεR1-mediated tyrosine kinase activation and signaling responses in RBL-2H3 mast cells. J Biol Chem 270:4013, 1995.
188. Wintroub BU, Schechter NB, Lazarus GS, et al: Angiotensin I conversion by human and rat chymotryptic proteinases. J Invest Dermatol 83:336, 1984.
189. Xia H-Z, Kepley CL, Sakai K, et al: Quantitation of tryptase, chymase, FcεRIα, and FcεRIgamma mRNAs in human mast cells and basophils by competitive reverse transcription-polymerase chain reaction. J Immunol 154:5472, 1995.
190. Yamauchi K, Sato R, Tanno Y, et al: Nucleotide sequence of the cDNA encoding L-histidine decarboxylase derived from human basophilic leukemia cell line, KU-812-F. Nucleic Acids Res 18:5891, 1990.
191. Yee NS, Paek I, Besmer P: Role of *kit*-ligand in proliferation and suppression of apoptosis in mast cells: basis for radiosensitivity of *white spotting* and *Steel* mutant mice. J Exp Med 179:1777, 1994.
192. Yunginger JW, Nelson DR, Squillace DL, et al: Laboratory investigation of deaths due to anaphylaxis. J Forensic Sci 36:857, 1991.

11 *The Eosinophil: Structure and Functions*

HIROHITO KITA GERALD J. GLEICH

The existence of a distinctive granulated peripheral blood leukocyte was first recognized by Wharton-Jones in 1846. Ehrlich's use of dyes to stain blood leukocytes gave the eosinophil its name in 1879 and provided a tool to readily identify the cell.[177] By the 1890s, increased numbers of eosinophils were associated with bronchial asthma, cutaneous diseases, and parasitic diseases. In 1912, eosinophil infiltration into the lungs of guinea pigs was demonstrated following anaphylaxis, and the notion that the eosinophil was concerned with anaphylaxis appeared. During the following decades, the dominant concept for eosinophil function involved counteracting the effects of anaphylaxis by neutralization of mast cell–associated mediators, such as histamine. However, proinflammatory functions of eosinophils have since been observed. Information suggests that eosinophils are not bystanders but play important roles in allergic reactions, such as bronchial asthma and atopic dermatitis. Here, we summarize the basic immunology and cell biology of eosinophils and their correlates to the pathophysiology of bronchial asthma.

Portions of this chapter have been taken, in part, and used with permission from Gleich GJ, et al: The eosinophil. In Gallin JI, Goldstein IM, Snyderman R (eds): Inflammation: Basic Principles and Clinical Correlates, 2nd edition. Raven Press, New York, 1992; Sur S, et al: Eosinophils: Biochemical and Cellular Aspects. In Middleton E Jr, et al (eds): Allergy: Principles and Practice, 4th edition. Mosby, St Louis, 1993; and Gleich GJ, et al: Eosinophils. In Frank MM, et al (eds): Samter's Immunology Diseases, 5th edition. Little, Brown and Company, Boston, 1995.

EOSINOPHIL GROWTH AND DIFFERENTIATION

EOSINOPHILOPOIESIS

It is generally accepted that in humans eosinophils are produced in the bone marrow.[20, 27, 151, 183, 463] The mature bone marrow eosinophil is considered a nondividing cell, forming a reserve for release into the peripheral circulation, and is morphologically indistinguishable from the peripheral blood eosinophil.[183, 262, 302, 464]

Eosinophil differentiation is based on the existence of totipotent hematopoietic stem cells[127, 298, 467] that give rise to pluripotent stem cells that in turn give rise to committed progenitors of progressively more restricted potential.[242, 262, 301] Eosinophils are derived from a progenitor that is different from that of the neutrophil/monocyte cell lineage.[105, 485] A single progenitor is capable of giving rise to mixed colonies of basophils and eosinophils, pure basophil colonies, or pure eosinophil colonies,[92] suggesting that a common progenitor exists for these cells but that the degree of differentiation toward one or the other lineage is stochastic. A common eosinophil-basophil progenitor is further supported by several observations. Charcot-Leyden crystal (CLC) protein and major basic protein (MBP), two proteins previously considered unique to eosinophils, are also found in mature basophils.[5, 8, 19] Normal cord blood precursors cultured with interleukin (IL)-3 and IL-5 in a plastic vessel coated with Matrigel developed into hybrid cells with both eosinophil and basophil characteristics.[49]

Production of eosinophils in human bone marrow involves a cascade of interdependent regulatory events that are cytokine driven or assisted. Among various hematopoietic factors, those important for eosinophil proliferation and differentiation are IL-3,[186] granulocyte-macrophage colony-stimulating factor (GM-CSF),[268, 269] and IL-5. IL-3 has the broadest specificity and can act directly on the CD34+ stem cell. IL-3 leads to the expansion of megakaryocytes, erythrocytes, monocytes, and neutrophils, with eosinophils representing 10% of total colonies.[49, 120] When infused in the cynomolgus monkey, IL-3 alone led to a modest leukocytosis, with more than a 10-fold increase in levels of circulating eosinophils.[103] It is thought that GM-CSF acts on an overlapping but more mature precursor population. In vitro stimulation of human bone marrow precursors with GM-CSF induces the formation of eosinophil, neutrophil, and macrophage colonies, with eosinophils representing up to 25% of all colonies.[268, 410] In AIDS patients, GM-CSF administration induced a major increase in circulating and bone marrow eosinophils and neutrophils, with a modest increase in circulating monocytes.[150] Thus IL-3 and GM-CSF are relatively nonspecific with regard to cell lineage stimulation and stimulate proliferation of neutrophils and basophils, as well as eosinophils.

Lymphocytes and their secreted products are implicated in the regulation of eosinophilopoiesis in vivo.[36, 431] Construction of a T-cell hybrid and analyses of its products showed the existence of a cytokine specific for eosinophil differentiation.[345, 439] Subsequently, this activity was purified to homogeneity and its cDNA cloned, resulting in the recognition of IL-5.[344, 395] IL-5 potently stimulates eosinophil production by the bone marrow. For example, IL-5 forces differentiation of human basophil/eosinophil progenitors into the eosinophil lineage in vitro.[343, 345] Transgenic mice constitutively expressing the IL-5 gene have a striking increase in eosinophils, up to 265-fold higher than normal mice,[97, 178, 408] suggesting that IL-5 expression in vivo is able to control the production of eosinophil progenitors and is sufficient to induce striking eosinophilia. In agreement with these findings, systemic neutralization of IL-5 by treatment with monoclonal antibody nearly abolished eosinophil production.[77, 360] In humans with eosinophilia, it has been possible to document high plasma levels of IL-5, including patients with episodic angioedema with eosinophilia,[57] recombinant IL-2 therapy,[424] and *Onchocerca volvulus* infection.[384]

Some evidence exists that certain cytokines can inhibit eosinophil progenitor growth and differentiation. Transforming growth factor-β suppresses the eosinophil pathway and aids in the switch from eosinophil to basophil commitment.[367] Interferon (IFN)-α inhibits colony formation by human bone marrow multipotential, erythroid, granulocyte-macrophage, and eosinophil progenitor cells in vitro[52] and has been utilized for the treatment of certain patients with eosinophilia.[58]

LIFE CYCLE OF EOSINOPHILS

The life cycle of the eosinophil may be divided into bone marrow, blood, and tissue phases. Although the eosinophil is a formed element of the peripheral circulation, it is primarily a tissue-dwelling cell. For example, the tissue eosinophil to blood eosinophil ratio in rats is about 200:1 to 300:1[341] and in humans is about 100:1.[305] Thus eosinophils in the peripheral circulation represent only a small fraction of the total number of these cells; eosinophils are regarded as passing through the circulation en route to the tissues.

In bone marrow, studies of eosinophil kinetics suggested the existence of two populations of cells with differing proliferative activity, one with a rapid bone marrow emergence time of about 10 hours and the second with a slow emergence time of about 80 hours.[312] Another study found a mean bone marrow maturation and storage time of 4.3 days.[385] There is a large reserve of bone marrow eosinophils, suggesting that rapid mobilization of eosinophils is possible.[379] Once in the blood, the eosinophil has a short half-life, estimated in normal rats at 6 to 12 hours.[128, 379] In humans, mean half-lives ranging from about 8 hours[312] to 18 hours[385] have been reported. After circulating in the blood, eosinophils migrate into the tissues at endothelial junctions[334] by a mechanism involving cytokines and adhesion molecules (vide infra). Eosinophils tend to reside in those tissues whose epithelial surfaces are exposed to the external environment. For example, in the adult rat, the organs with the greatest density of eosinophils (eosinophils/mm^3) include the lamina propria of the stomach and ileum, the perivascular and peribronchial tissue of the lungs, and the uterine cavity during estrus.[341] It will be interesting in the future to examine whether these preferential localizations of eosinophils bear any physiologic significance for host defense and inflammation.

Once in the tissues, it is thought that the majority of eosinophils do not recirculate.[183] The tissue life span of eosinophils ranges from 2 to 5 days, depending partly on the tissue studied.[14, 128] Several possibilities for clearing of eosinophils from the tissues include shedding of cells across mucosal surfaces into the lumina of the gut, as described in the rat,[402] or into the respiratory tract; engulfment of apoptotic eosinophils by macrophages[334]; and lysis and/or degranulation with accompanying cell degeneration. That eosinophil degranulation occurs in tissues is shown by the striking extracellular deposition of granule proteins, often in the virtual absence of intact eosinophils.[208, 245]

MORPHOLOGY AND RECEPTOR EXPRESSION

MORPHOLOGY

The normal peripheral blood eosinophil is characterized by its distinctive acidophilic granules, is slightly larger than the neutrophil, and usually has a bilobed nucleus. They contain crystalloid granules and small granules. In bone marrow, electron microscopy of eosinophilic promyelocytes shows characteristic primary granules that are round and uniformly electron dense.[486] During differentiation, these granules develop cores and are then called secondary or specific granules.[114] When eosinophils become mature, the secondary or specific granules consist of an electron dense core and an electron lucent matrix (Fig. 11–1).[273] The granule core shows a periodicity in both longitudinal and cross-

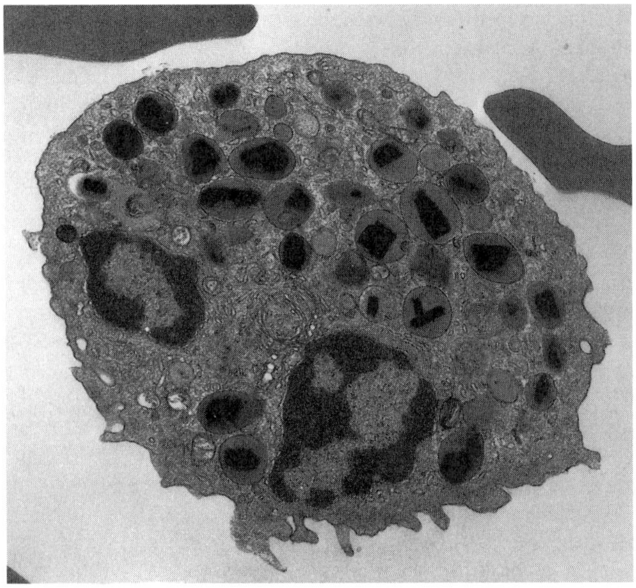

FIGURE 11–1. Electron photomicrograph of a human eosinophil (X11,500). (From Gleich GJ, Adolphson CR, Leiferman KM: The eosinophil. In Gallin JI, Goldstein IM, Snyderman R (eds): Inflammation: Basic Principles and Clinical Correlates, 2nd edition. Raven Press, New York, 1992, pp 663–700.)

sectional dimensions and therefore has been termed a crystalloid. Peroxidase activity is localized to the granule matrix of this crystalloid granule. Small granules have a round or elongated profile and stain homogeneously in standard electron micrographs. Small granules are reported to contain acid phosphatase and arylsulfatase B, although peroxidase activity is equivocal.[311]

EOSINOPHIL RECEPTORS

Like other leukocytes, eosinophils express various membrane receptors through which they communicate with the extracellular environment. These molecules involve adhesion receptors, receptors for the Fc portion of immunoglobulins (Fc receptors), and receptors for soluble mediators, such as cytokines and lipid mediators. Table 11–1 summarizes various surface structures on human eosinophils and compares their expression on human neutrophils. In this section, we describe Fc receptors and receptors for soluble mediators. Eosinophil adhesion receptors are described later in this chapter.

IMMUNOGLOBULIN RECEPTORS

Published reports suggest that eosinophils possess receptors for IgG, IgE, and IgA.[15, 156, 158, 167, 378] These receptors are associated with effector functions of eosinophils. A 1994 study, performed as part of The 5th International Workshop and Conference on Human Leukocyte Differentiation Antigens, found that all peripheral blood eosinophils (isolated from mildly allergic donors) express $Fc_\gamma RII$ (CD32). In contrast, the number of eosinophils expressing receptors for IgA (CD89) and IgE (CD23) was 5% or less of the entire eosinophil population.[116]

IgG Receptors

Receptors recognizing the Fc portion of IgG ($Fc_\gamma R$) on eosinophils have been extensively studied by their abilities to mediate eosinophil functions, including phagocytosis,[252] antigen-dependent cytotoxicity,[419] oxygen metabolism,[25] LTC_4 production,[359] and degranulation.[2] Although most of these studies have been performed using IgG-coated targets, Graziano and colleagues showed that $Fc_\gamma R$ directly mediated the eosinophil cytotoxicity.[149] In their system, eosinophils, preincubated with GM-CSF, killed both an anti-$Fc_\gamma RII$–bearing hybridoma cell line and chicken erythrocytes coated with antichicken erythrocyte antibody covalently coupled to Fab fragments of anti-$Fc_\gamma RII$. However, eosinophils could not kill hybridoma expressing anti-$Fc_\gamma RI$ or anti-$Fc_\gamma RIII$. The interaction between IgG and $Fc_\gamma RII$ may also be important in the eosinophil degranulation in allergic diseases. The sera from patients with hay fever contained elevated levels of allergen-specific IgG1 and IgG3, and these antibodies caused eosinophil degranulation in vitro in an allergen-dependent manner. This reaction was abolished when eosinophil $Fc_\gamma RII$ was blocked by a monoclonal antibody.[202]

Studies using flow cytometry analyses of human cells revealed that freshly isolated eosinophils possess only $Fc_\gamma RII$ (CD32),[167] monocytes possess $Fc_\gamma RI$ (CD64) and $Fc_\gamma RII$, and neutrophils possess $Fc_\gamma RII$ and $Fc_\gamma RIII$ (CD16).[423] The expression of $Fc_\gamma R$ is regulated by cytokines. For example, treatment of eosinophils with IFN γ for more than 24 hours enhances their expression of $Fc_\gamma RII$ and thus augments $Fc_\gamma RII$-mediated tumor cell killing by eosinophils.[419] IFN-γ also induces the expression of $Fc_\gamma RIII$ (a phosphatidylinositol-linked form), as well as $Fc_\gamma RI$, on eosinophils.[168] Moreover, the effects of IFN-γ are augmented by a membrane-permeable cyclic AMP (cAMP) analogue, dibutyryl cAMP.[292] In contrast, culture with IL-3 causes an up-regulation of $Fc_\gamma RII$ but does not induce expression of $Fc_\gamma RI$ or $Fc_\gamma RIII$.[168] Thus characterized by its effects on the expression of $Fc_\gamma R$, IFN-γ appears to be a unique activator of eosinophils.

IgE Receptors

Several reports suggest that eosinophils have IgE receptors that stimulate the eosinophil's cytotoxic function and degranulation. Eosinophil killing of schistosomula is dependent on IgE antibody or a factor that resembles IgE.[65, 226] Human eosinophils, isolated from patients with eosinophilia, form rosettes with IgE-coated erythrocytes, and rosette formation is inhibited by aggregated IgE.[63, 65] IgE bound to the eosinophil's surface has been demonstrated on human peripheral blood eosinophils and tissue eosinophils.[61, 62, 101] Anti-IgE, as well as specific antigen, induces eosinophil peroxidase release from hypodense eosinophils isolated from parasite-infected patients.[210, 407]

Eosinophils can express three types of IgE receptors. First, a monoclonal antibody has been produced by immunization with eosinophils from patients with eosinophilia, and this antibody completely inhibits IgE-dependent cytotoxicity and the binding of IgE to eosinophils.[64] This antibody, called BB10, has identified 10^5 binding sites per eosinophil and recognized different determinants than those recognized by antibodies to CD23, the low-affinity IgE receptor on B cells

TABLE 11–1
EOSINOPHIL SURFACE MOLECULES AND THEIR EXPRESSION ON NEUTROPHILS

Eosinophil Structures	Surface Molecules (CD designation)	Ligand	Expressed on Neutrophils
Immunoglobulin Receptors	$Fc_{\alpha}R$ (CD89)[277]	IgA	Yes
	$Fc_{\gamma}RI$ (CD64)*[168]	IgG	No
	$Fc_{\gamma}RII$ (CD32)[167]	IgG	Yes
	$Fc_{\gamma}RIII$ (CD16)*[168]	IgG	Yes
	$Fc_{\epsilon}RI$†[147]	IgE	No
	$Fc_{\epsilon}RII$†[199]	IgE	No
	ϵBP (Mac-2)[413]	IgE	Yes
Complement Receptors	C3a receptor[83]	C3a	No
	C5a receptor (CD88)[138]	C5a	Yes
	CR1 (CD35)[70]	C3b	Yes
	CR3 (Mac-1, CD11b/CD18)[15]	C3bi, ICAM-1	Yes
	p150, 95 (CD11c/CD18)[167]	C3bi	Yes
	MCP (CD46)[116, 418]	Measles virus	Yes
	DAF (CD55)[116, 418]		Yes
	MACIF (CD59)[116, 418]		Yes
Integrins	LFA-1 (CD11a/CD18)[167]	ICAM-1, ICAM-2	Yes
	Mac-1, CR3 (CD11b/CD18)[167]	C3bi, ICAM-1	Yes
	p150, 95 (CD11c/CD18)[167]	C3bi	Yes
	VLA-4 (CD49d/CD29)[45, 433]	VCAM-1, fibronectin	No
	VLA-6 (CD49f/CD29)[137]	Laminin	Yes
	Act-1, $\alpha 4\beta 7$[116]	MAdCAM-1, VCAM-1, fibronectin	Yes
Selectins	L-selectin[267]	GlyCAM-1, CD34	Yes
Carbohydrates	$Lewis^{x}$ (CD15)[448]	P-selectin	Yes
	Sialyl-$Lewis^{x}$ (CD15s)‡[46]	E-selectin, P-selectin	Yes
	Sialyl-dimeric $Lewis^{x}$[46]	E-selectin	Yes
	Leukosialin (CD43)[116, 418]	ICAM-1	Yes
	Pgp-1 (CD44)[163]	Hyaluronic acid	Yes
Immunoglobulin-like	PECAM-1 (CD31)[116]	PECAM, heparan sulfate	Yes
	ICAM-1 (CD54)*[166]	LFA-1	Yes
	ICAM-3 (CD50)[116]	LFA-1	Yes
	LFA-3 (CD58)[116, 418]	CD2	Yes
	CD4[254]	LCF (IL-16), gp120	No
Enzymes	p24 kinase (CD9)[116, 418]		No
	Tyrosine phosphatase (CD45)[234]		Yes
	Aminopeptidase N (CD13)[116, 418]		Yes
Cytokine Receptors§	IL-1 receptor (CDw121)[319]		Yes
	IL-2 receptor α(CD25)*[330]		No
	IL-3 receptor[250]		No
	IL-4 receptor (CD124)[418]		nt
	IL-5 receptor (CD125)[71]		No
	IL-8 receptor (CD128)[418]		Yes
	GM-CSF receptor (CDw116)[250]		Yes
	IFN-γ receptor (CDw119)[419]		Yes
	TNF-receptor (CD120)[419]		Yes
	RANTES receptor[201]		No
	MCP-2 receptor[444a]		nt
	MCP-3 receptor[84]		nt
	MIP-1α receptor[335]		No
Miscellaneous	FAS (CD95)[116]		Yes
	CAMPATH-1 (CD52)[116]		Yes
	gp53 (CD63)[267]		Yes
	CD69*[170, 297]		Yes
	HLA Class I[116]		Yes
	HLA-DR*[166, 255]		Yes
	Prostaglandin E receptor[213]		Yes
	PAF receptor[417a]		Yes
	Leukotriene B receptor[258, 296]		Yes
	Leukotriene D receptor[376]		No?
	fMLP receptor[24]		Yes
	β-adrenergic receptor[480]		Yes
	Histamine receptor[72]		Yes

*Expressed only on activated eosinophils.
†Controversial findings.
‡Levels of expression are very low compared with neutrophils.
§Expression of cytokine receptors is partially based on biologic activities of the cytokines.
Abbreviations: ICAM-1 = intercellular cell adhesion molecule-1; VCAM-1 = vascular cell adhesion molecule-1; MadCAM-1 = mucosal adressin cell adhesion molecule-1; GlyCAM-1 = glycosylated cell adhesion molecule-1; PECAM-1 = platelet-endothelial cell adhesion molecule-1; MCP = membrane cofactor protein; DAF = decay accelerating factor; MACIF = membrane attack complex inhibitory factor; LCF = lymphocyte chemoattractant factor; nt = not tested.

and monocytes.[148, 199] Second, eosinophils from patients with eosinophilia express another lectin-type low-affinity IgE-binding molecule, Mac-2/ϵBP, and the cytotoxic function of eosinophils against parasites was abolished by the antibody against this molecule.[413] Third, it has been claimed that the high-affinity IgE receptor, $Fc_{\epsilon}RI$, is present on eosinophils from patients with eosinophilia, and various functions of eosinophils, including degranulation and parasite cytotoxicity, are mediated through this receptor.[147] Interestingly, another group showed that preincubation of normal eosinophils with platelet-activating factor (PAF) for 30 minutes resulted in increases in IgE binding and in IgE-mediated cytotoxicity against parasites without demonstrable IgE receptors.[280] Taken together, these results suggest that IgE binding sites and/or IgE receptors are important molecules in the interaction of eosinophils with parasites. However, at least in our hands, peripheral blood eosinophils from normal subjects and patients with allergy do not stain with a panel of monoclonal antibodies directed against IgE receptors. The nature of eosinophil IgE binding therefore remains to be clarified. In addition, the possible heterogeneity of eosinophils among different classes of diseases (e.g., eosinophilia and allergic diseases) and from different source organs (e.g., tissue, bronchoalveolar lavage [BAL], or peripheral blood) needs to be considered.

IgA Receptors

Evidence from flow cytometric analyses and degranulation studies suggests that eosinophils have IgA receptors.[2, 67] Comparison of neutrophils with eosinophils suggests that neutrophils express much higher levels of $Fc_{\alpha}R$ (CD89), detected by the binding of IgA and by anti-$Fc_{\alpha}R$ antibody.[277] The $Fc_{\alpha}R$ on eosinophils has a higher molecular mass (70–100 kD) than that on neutrophils (55–75 kD). The $Fc_{\alpha}R$ on eosinophils and neutrophils is likely highly glycosylated because removal of N-linked carbohydrates reveals a major protein core of 32 kD for both cell types. Interestingly, eosinophils from allergic individuals displayed enhanced $Fc_{\alpha}R$ expression whereas neutrophils did not.[277] Eosinophils can be activated in vitro in an IgA-dependent manner. Sepharose 4B beads coated with IgA or secretory IgA (sIgA) induce degranulation of eosinophils.[2] When compared with IgE, IgG, and IgA, sIgA is the most potent immunoglobulin stimulant for eosinophil degranulation.[2] Why sIgA is a more potent stimulus than IgA is unknown; secretory components may play a key role. To support this hypothesis, purified secretory component has been shown to bind to a 15-kD protein on eosinophils, suggesting the presence of a receptor for secretory component on eosinophils.[241] This finding, along with the localization of eosinophils at epithelial surfaces, suggests an important role for sIgA in mediating the eosinophil effector function in vivo.[305, 341] Indeed, in a patient with asthma, IgA deposition was observed on alveolar membranes in association with eosinophils and viral particles.[321]

COMPLEMENT RECEPTORS

Eosinophils express the CR1 and CR3 (Mac-1, CD11b/18) complement receptors (see Table 11–1); these levels of expression can be increased by incubating eosinophils with leukotriene (LT)B_4,[125] *N*-formyl-methionyl-leucyl-phenylalanine (FMLP), PAF, or GM-CSF.[409] Furthermore, compared with neutrophils, eosinophils have a larger total pool of CR3 (Mac-1) within the cells, which is mobilized to the cell surface in response to IL-5.[256] CR3 (Mac-1) plays a critical role in the eosinophil effector functions, especially as a versatile adhesion molecule.

The complement anaphylatoxins, C3a and C5a, are well known for their abilities to activate human neutrophils through a receptor-mediated process. C3a and C5a also activate eosinophils. Both C3a and C5a induce the increase in $[Ca^{2+}]_i$ and cause degranulation and production of oxygen radicals from eosinophils.[83, 119, 209, 393] C3a and C5a also induce chemotaxis of eosinophils.[83, 123] Two C5a receptor populations are present on human eosinophils: a high-affinity receptor with 15,000 to 20,000 sites per cell and a K_d of 30 pM and a low-affinity receptor with approximately 375,000 sites per cell and a K_d of 100 nM. Parallel experiments with neutrophils indicate the presence of a single receptor population with approximately 90,000 sites per cell and a K_d of 480 pM.[138] Autoradiography of ^{125}I-C5a–labeled eosinophil receptor protein indicates the presence of a dominant C5a-eosinophil receptor with an apparent mass of 60 to 65 kD; the C5a-neutrophil receptor complex has a mass of 50 to 52 kD. Thus human eosinophils have a receptor for C5a that appears to be distinct from the C5a receptor present on human neutrophils.

PLATELET-ACTIVATING FACTOR RECEPTOR

Platelet-activating factor (PAF) receptors on human leukocytes have been cloned and expressed, and the resulting transfectants were stimulated by PAF and bound radiolabeled PAF.[291] Because [^{3}H]PAF caused cell activation and receptor down-regulation, the radioligand-binding study of PAF receptors on eosinophils has used metabolically stable, hydrophilic PAF antagonists, such as [^{3}H]apafant (WEB2086) and [^{3}H]L-659,989.[185] On guinea pig and human eosinophils, [^{3}H]apafant labeled homogeneous binding sites with a density of approximately 35,000 sites per cell.[417a] The observations that [^{3}H]apafant binding is concentration dependent, saturable, reversible, of high affinity (K_d = 17 nM), and antagonized by the natural ligand C_{16}-PAF indicate that these binding sites are PAF receptors. The action of PAF on eosinophils has been investigated in a number of in vitro studies. For example, PAF is one of the most potent chemoattractants for eosinophils and selectively induces the migration of eosinophils over neutrophils.[50, 364] PAF increases the binding of IgE to human eosinophils and enhances cytotoxicity toward schistosomula of *Schistosoma mansoni*.[280] Furthermore, PAF evokes the release of granule proteins,[227, 228, 232] reactive oxygen species,[227, 362] and LTC_4 from eosinophils.[397] In spite of these in vitro activities, the physiologic roles of PAF still need to be elucidated.

LEUKOTRIENE RECEPTORS

Studies of the LTB_4 receptors of eosinophils were performed using guinea pig alveolar and peritoneal eosinophils.[258, 296] [^{3}H]LTB_4 labeled a heterogeneous population of binding sites on guinea pig alveolar eosinophils. Approximately 1,000 sites per cell bound LTB_4 with high affinity (K_d = 1 nM), whereas 5,500 sites per cell bound with low affinity (K_d = 63 nM). The binding was inhibited by various metabolites of LTB_4 with a rank order of potency corresponding to their ability to induce eosinophil chemotaxis.[258] In contrast to these data, [^{3}H]LTB_4 interacted with a homogeneous population of binding sites on guinea pig peritoneal eosinophils with a K_d of 2.8 nM and 40,000 sites per cell.[296] The reason for this apparent discrepancy between these observations is unknown but may be due to differences in the concentrations of the radiolabeled ligand used in the experiments. LTB_4 induces several functional responses of eosinophils. LTB_4 potently stimulates chemotaxis and chemokinesis in guinea pig eosinophils and elicits arachidonic acid metabolism.[258, 296, 326] Although LTB_4 stimulates a respiratory burst in human and guinea pig eosinophils,[310, 387] LTB_4 does not seem to induce degranulation of eosinophils as assessed by the release of β-glucuronidase.[296]

N-FORMYL-METHIONYL-LEUCYL-PHENYLALANINE RECEPTOR

Normal human eosinophils respond to a chemotactic tetrapeptide, *N*-formyl-methionyl-leucyl-phenlyalanine (FMLP), at concentrations greater than 10^{-7} M with increases in intracellular free calcium ($[Ca^{2+}]_i$) and oxygen metabolism.[473] Eosinophils isolated from patients with atopy show a stronger response to FMLP compared with eosinophils from normal individuals.[54, 223] FMLP also stimulates PAF synthesis in human eosinophils, although 100-fold less PAF is produced compared with the eosinophil's response to A23187.[411] Thus eosinophils respond to FMLP, but the response is relatively small and varies with the source of the cells (disease status of patients). Compared with neutrophils, the maximum response of eosinophils to FMLP is smaller. To have a response equivalent to neutrophils, eosinophils require 10-fold more FMLP, suggesting that FMLP receptors on eosinophils are lower affinity and/or less abundant compared with neutrophils.

The actions of FMLP on guinea pig eosinophils are receptor mediated because they are blocked by the FMLP receptor antagonist BOC-FMLP.[233] A low number of binding sites for [^{3}H]FMLP have been identified on guinea pig eosinophils.[24] However, if guinea pig eosinophils are cultured overnight with mononuclear cells or in mononuclear cell–conditioned medium, FMLP is rendered a potent and an effective activator of eosinophils.[24] Although the mechanism of enhanced FMLP response is obscure, it likely involves the receptor itself because the binding of [^{3}H]FMLP is increased approximately sixfold during culture of eosinophils in the conditioned medium.[24] Interestingly, when human eosinophils were cultured for 3 days with GM-CSF, the FMLP-induced elevation of $[Ca^{2+}]_i$ was increased threefold, whereas the response induced by PAF was not changed.[473] Similarly, eosinophils, activated in vivo and isolated from BAL fluid 48 hours after the segmental antigen challenge, showed enhanced superoxide production and elevated $[Ca^{2+}]_i$ when stimulated by FMLP but not when stimulated by PAF,[354] suggesting a differential modulation of FMLP and PAF reactivity by cytokines.

EOSINOPHIL MEDIATORS

Eosinophils generate an array of inflammatory mediators, including granule proteins, proteolytic enzymes, lipid mediators, oxygen metabolites, and cytokines. These are summarized in Table 11–2.

GRANULE PROTEINS

Eosinophils contain two main types of secretory granules: the specific and the small granules. The specific granules consist of major basic protein (MBP), which is localized in the crystalloid core of granules. Eosinophil cationic protein (ECP), eosinophil peroxidase (EPO), eosinophil-derived neurotoxin (EDN), and β-glucuronidase are found in the matrix of specific granules. In contrast, the small granules contain enzymes, including acid phosphatase and arylsulfatase B.

Major Basic Protein

MBP consists of a single polypeptide chain of 117 amino acids; it is rich in arginine and has a molecular mass of 14 kD and a calculated isoelectric point of 10.9.[30] The initial MBP translation product (proMBP) is synthesized in eosinophil precursors with a cleavable 90 amino acid acidic region that is thought to complex with the basic residues and

TABLE 11–2
SECRETORY PRODUCTS OF EOSINOPHILS

Granule Proteins	Lipid Mediators
Major basic protein	Leukotriene B_4 (small amount)
Eosinophil peroxidase	Leukotriene C_4
Eosinophil cationic protein	5-HETE
Eosinophil-derived neurotoxin	5, 15- and 8, 15-diHETE
β-glucuronidase	5-oxo-15-hydroxy 6,8,11,13 ETE
Acid phosphatase	Prostaglandin E1 and E2
Arylsulfatase B	6-keto-Prostaglandin F1
Cytokines	Thromboxane B2
IL-1	PAF
IL-3	**Enzymes**
IL-5	Elastase (questionable)
IL-6	Charcot-Leyden crystal protein
IL-8	Collagenase
GM-CSF	92 kD Gelatinase
RANTES	
TNF-α	
TGF-α	
TGF-β1	
MIP-1α	
Reactive Oxygen Intermediates	
Superoxide radical anion	
H_2O_2	
Hydroxy radicals	

Abbreviations: HETE = hydroxy eicosatetraenoic acid; ETE = eicosatetraenoic acid; diHETE = dihydroxy eicosatetraenoic acid; TNF = tumor necrosis factor; TGF = transforming growth factor; MIP = macrophage inflammatory protein; PAF = platelet-activating factor.

protect the eosinophils from the toxic effects of MBP during synthesis and storage.[30] No synthesis of MBP occurs after eosinophils become mature.[153] MBP is highly toxic to various cells by a mechanism that disrupts the integrity of lipid bilayers.[3] For example, purified MBP damages parasites, such as schistosomula of *S. mansoni*,[59] *Trichinella spiralis*, and *Brugia pahangi*.[160, 161] MBP also can kill bacteria, such as *Staphylococcus aureus* and *Escherichia coli*.[244] MBP is toxic to human epithelial cells[143] and causes ciliostasis and exfoliation of respiratory epithelial cells[131]; this latter effect mimics the pathology of asthma.[129]

In addition to its toxicity, MBP has a number of pharmacologic properties. Incubation of human peripheral blood leukocytes with MBP causes a dose-dependent release of histamine that is calcium-, temperature-, and energy-dependent,[300] suggesting noncytotoxic activation of basophils by MBP. Similarly, MBP activates mediator release from rat mast cells,[300] neutrophils,[285] alveolar macrophages,[331] platelets,[333] and eosinophils by themselves.[217] MBP affects ion transport in tracheal epithelium and thus may change the volume and composition of respiratory tract fluid.[193] MBP reduces the activity of ciliary cells possibly by inhibition of ATPase activity.[171]

In vivo, MBP is known to be an allosteric antagonist of the inhibitory muscarinic M2 receptor, a finding that has implications for the pathogenesis of asthma.[194] BAL performed after intratracheal instillation of MBP showed increased levels of kallikrein-like activity and immunoreactive kinins.[79] Topical application of MBP to the hamster cheek pouch caused increased vascular permeability at nanomolar concentrations.[275] Application of MBP to respiratory epithelium causes increased reactivity of respiratory smooth muscle to cholinergic agonists, likely through an action on the epithelium.[50, 126, 459] Furthermore, instillation of MBP causes bronchial hyperresponsiveness in primates in vivo.[155] This MBP-induced airway hyperresponsiveness was inhibited by acidic polyamino acids.[29] With these cytotoxic and pharmacologic properties, MBP is likely playing an important role in the pathophysiologic mechanisms of bronchial asthma.[144, 368] In fact, MBP is present in high concentrations in sputum specimens from patients with asthma.[130] MBP is deposited at sites of tissue damage in patients dying from bronchial asthma.[124] Blood and bronchial eosinophilia are correlated with bronchial hyperreactivity both in patients with asthma[110, 187, 401, 436] and in an experimental model of asthma in primates.[126]

Eosinophil Cationic Protein

ECP consists of a single polypeptide chain of 133 amino acids (derived from the 160 amino acid initial translation product) with a calculated molecular mass of 15 kD. ECP has a molecular mass of 18 to 21 kD after glycosylation and an isoelectric point of approximately 10.8.[30] It shares some of the properties of MBP but also has some discrete functions. ECP is a potent toxin for schistosomula of *S. mansoni*[263] and is approximately 10 times more active than MBP.[4] ECP produces complete fragmentation and disruption of the schistosomula, whereas MBP produces distinctive ballooning and detachment of the tegumental membrane (these resemble the effects of eosinophils themselves). ECP possesses a marked bactericidal activity.[244] In contrast, it seems likely that ECP has much less activity on mammalian cells, such as epithelial cells, basophils, and platelets, when compared with MBP. Unlike MBP, both ECP and EDN produce a neurotoxic reaction when injected into the cerebrospinal fluid of rabbits.[109] An interesting feature of ECP is its structural and functional similarities to RNase from many species.[141, 369] During secretion, ECP has been thought to undergo a conformational change. This difference has been used to distinguish between resting eosinophils and activated eosinophils, in which monoclonal antibody EG1 recognizes the stored form from resting eosinophils and the monoclonal antibody EG2 recognizes the activated state.[391] However, one study suggests that this is not likely the case and is an unreliable distinction.[195]

Eosinophil-Derived Neurotoxin

The cDNA for EDN has been cloned; the amino acid sequence specifies a 134 amino acid polypeptide with a calculated molecular mass of 15 kD that is increased to 18 to 19 kD by glycosylation,[162] and it is identical to human urinary RNase and human liver RNase.[40, 373] The amino acid sequence of EDN revealed marked homology to ECP with identity at 37 of 54 *N*-terminal residues, although its net basic charge is not as great (isoelectric point of EDN is 8.9).[141] EDN possesses greater RNase activity than does ECP[369] but lesser toxicity to parasite targets.[4] The most striking activity of EDN is its neurotoxicity. When EDN is injected intrathecally into rabbits or guinea pigs, it causes the Gordon phenomenon, a syndrome that begins with stiffness and mild ataxia, followed by incoordination and marked ataxia.[109] Although the mechanism of neurotoxicity of EDN is not completely understood, it is most likely that both the RNase activity and the basic charge are required.[372] Other pharmacologic properties of EDN have not been studied extensively. EDN does not induce histamine release from basophils or mast cells.[481] Purified EDN also reacts with the EG2 but not the EG1 monoclonal antibody, suggesting that the recognition site of the EG2 monoclonal antibody is common to both ECP and EDN.[391]

Eosinophil Peroxidase

EPO consists of two subunits in 1:1 stoichiometry; the molecular masses of the heavy and light subunits are 53 and 12 kD, respectively, and their calculated isoelectric points are 10.8 and 10.7, respectively.[343] The promoter for EPO has been localized in −122 to −45 bp region of the EPO gene.[471] Although EPO is structurally related to neutrophil myeloperoxidase (MPO) (69% homology), EPO differs from MPO in its absorption spectrum and its heme prosthetic groups.[47] In the presence of H_2O_2, EPO is able to oxidize halides to form reactive hypohalous acids.[48] Analyses of EPO's halide preference showed that eosinophils preferentially utilize bromide over chloride.[261] This EPO/H_2O_2/halide system kills a variety of microorganisms, such as schistosomula of *S. mansoni* and *E. coli*.[197, 259] Studies of cultured human pneumocytes,[21] nasal epithelial cells,[22] and tumor cells[196] indicate that the EPO/H_2O_2/halide system causes toxicity to mammalian cells. Because eosinophils by themselves can generate H_2O_2,[26, 320] this EPO/H_2O_2/halide system is an effective system to mediate toxicity toward numerous targets. Interestingly, thiocyanate is preferred as a substrate for oxidation over bromide, and addition of physiologic levels of thiocyanate abolishes the bromide-dependent toxicity of EPO to endothelial cells in vitro.[370]

In the absence of H_2O_2 and halide, EPO is also toxic to some targets, although greater concentrations are required. EPO and MBP are stimuli for human platelets[333] and eosinophils.[217] They cause airway constriction and hyperresponsiveness[155] and are antagonists of the inhibitory muscarinic M2 receptor.[194]

CHARCOT-LEYDEN CRYSTAL PROTEIN

The hexagonal, bipyramidal crystals, Charcot-Leyden crystals (CLC), have been observed for over a century in biologic fluids or tissues associated with eosinophilia, including asthma and parasitic diseases. This unique crystal-forming protein was shown to possess lysophospholipase activity.[450, 456] CLC protein is a polypeptide of 117 to 119 amino acids[142] with a molecular mass of 17 kD.[451] The cloning of the cDNA-coding CLC protein revealed that CLC protein is related to the superfamily of S-type β-galactoside–binding animal lectins, including certain IgE- and laminin-binding proteins.[6] However, the significance of these sequence similarities needs to be determined.

CLC protein is a major product of basophils as well as eosinophils.[8] In eosinophils, CLC protein has been localized to a set of granules discrete from the crystalloid granules.[113] It was also possible to detect CLC protein in the nuclear matrix and the cytoplasm of eosinophils derived from IL-5–induced umbilical cord blood cultures.[111] Furthermore, in transfected COS cells expressing the recombinant form of the molecule, CLC protein was detectable in the nucleus, cytoplasm, and plasma membrane.[482] The role of CLC protein in eosinophil function is unknown; however, the lysophospholipase activity may protect the cells from the lytic effects of lysophospholipids generated at the site of inflammation by inflammatory cells.[482] Alternately, this lysophospholipase activity may degrade pulmonary surfactant lysophospholipid and alter the surface tensile properties of surfactant and, in turn, contribute to the development of focal atelectasis.[9]

PROTEASE AND OTHER ENZYMES

In addition to CLC protein (lysophospholipase), EPO, and the RNase activity associated with EDN and ECP, a variety of other enzymes have been associated with the eosinophil.[18, 34, 139, 398, 443, 449, 457, 461, 483] Arylsulfatase B[398, 443, 449] is located predominantly in the small granules of the eosinophil[311] and is present in eosinophils in greater amounts than in neutrophils. β-glucuronidase activity in eosinophils is about twice that in neutrophils,[259] and exposure of eosinophils to opsonized zymosan particles releases up to 24% of the total cellular β-glucuronidase. Although the eosinophil was thought to be deficient in lysozyme and phagocytin,[18, 457] lysozyme can be localized to both normal and abnormal eosinophil granules and is present within the eosinophil crystalloids of normal eosinophils.[283] Neutrophil elastase has been identified in human eosinophils and can be localized to eosinophil granules.[257] This is a controversial issue, however, and we could not detect elastase in eosinophils by immunohistochemistry.[132a]

Because the eosinophil has been recognized as a proinflammatory cell in various human diseases, a number of studies have analyzed eosinophil proteases. Eosinophil collagenase degrades type I and type III collagen, the two major connective tissue components of human lung parenchyma.[87, 176] Eosinophils are present during wound healing, and its collagenase could be important in tissue remodeling.[28] Using in situ hybridization and immunohistochemistry, it was demonstrated that eosinophils are a major source of a 92-kD metalloproteinase, a gelatinase, in basal cell carcinoma lesions.[381, 382] This gelatinase was localized to eosinophils infiltrating into the lesions of patients with bullous pemphigoid,[383] and it cleaved type XVII collagen, a transmembrane molecule of the epidermal hemidesmosome, suggesting that production and release of gelatinase by eosinophils contribute to tissue damage of bullous pemphigoid. However, the role of these proteinases for the pathophysiology of asthma is unknown.

LIPID MEDIATORS

Phospholipase A_2 (PLA_2) hydrolyses membrane phospholipids, phosphatidylcholine (PC), and/or phosphatidylethanolamine (PE) to produce arachidonic acid (AA) and lyso PC and/or PE. AA may be metabolized by cyclooxygenase or 5-lipoxygenase/5-lipoxygenase–activating protein (FLAP) into prostaglandins or leukotrienes, as well as lipoxins and 5-hydroxy eicosatetraenoic acid (5-HETE). Lyso PC is acetylated to form PAF.[93] Furthermore, 5-lipoxygenase has been localized by immunocytochemical staining to eosinophils.[287, 417] Evidence shows that lipid bodies in eosinophils serve as sites for AA storage in the form of esterified arachidonate, which would be available for eicosanoid synthesis.[453]

In eosinophils, the predominant metabolite via the 5-lipoxygenase pathway is LTC_4, which, in turn, is metabolized to LTD_4 and the inactive LTE_4.[454] Eosinophils can generate relatively large amounts of LTC_4 but only negligible amounts of LTB_4.[454] This finding is in contrast to neutrophils, which can produce large amounts of LTB_4 but little, if any, LTC_4. The other major 5-lipoxygenase metabolite of eosinophils is 5-HETE, which can be metabolized to LTC_4.[100] These mediators contract airway smooth muscle, promote secretion of mucus, alter vascular permeability, and elicit eosinophil and neutrophil infiltration. In eosinophils stimulated by the addition of exogenous AA, 15-lipoxygenase metabolites are detectable, including 5,15- and 8,15-diHETEs and a novel chemotactic lipid, 5-oxo-15-hydroxy 6,8,11,13 eicosatetraenoic acid.[278, 350, 414, 415] Stimulation with eicosapentanoic acid enhances leukotriene synthesis and induces synthesis of LTC_5.[404] The activation of the PLA_2 and 5-lipoxygenase pathway is tightly regulated by the intracellular calcium concentration and is described in detail later.

There have been few studies of eosinophil cyclooxygenase metabolism. It appears that eosinophils from patients with hypereosinophilic syndrome synthesize prostaglandin E1, E2, 6-keto-PGF1, and thromboxane B2.[122, 184, 190]

Analysis shows that eosinophils contain high levels of ether phospholipids (the stored precursor to PAF), about fourfold more than do neutrophils, suggesting that the eosinophil is a good PAF producer.[388] Much of this material is in the form of 1-alkyl-2-lyso-*sn*-glycero-3-phosphocholine. Eosinophils produce PAF by an acetylation reaction using the enzyme 1-alkyl-2-lyso-*sn*-glycero-3-phosphocholine:acetyl-CoA acetyl transferase.[15] Eosinophils produce at least three molecular species of PAF, the predominant species being 1-hexadecyl-2-acetyl-glycero-3-phosphocholine (16:0). Much of the PAF produced by eosinophils remains cell associated.[80] PAF has a number of important pharmacologic activities, including the activation of platelets and neutrophils and the induction of bronchoconstriction. However, the roles of PAF produced by eosinophils in asthma need further investigation.

OXIDATIVE PRODUCTS

The oxidative products of eosinophils include superoxide anion, hydroxyl radicals, H_2O_2, and singlet oxygen.[204, 317] When challenged with an appropriate stimulus, eosinophils, like neutrophils and monocytes, produce oxygen-derived free radicals. This is the result when membrane-associated oxidase is activated, which then catalyzes the single electron reduction of oxygen using NADPH as an electron donor. The product of the NADPH:O_2 oxidoreductase-catalyzed reaction is the superoxide radical anion, O_2^-, a powerful oxidizing and reducing agent with bactericidal properties.[23] Superoxide anions can undergo spontaneous oxidation to O_2 or reduction to H_2O_2 in the presence of superoxide dismutase. H_2O_2 produced by eosinophils shows potent biologic activity in conjunction with EPO, as described earlier. Furthermore, in the presence of ferrous ions, the superoxide radical anion and H_2O_2 interact to form the membrane-perturbating hydroxy radical, a reactive and unstable oxidizing species. The activity of the NADPH:O_2 oxidoreductase is significantly higher in eosinophils than it is in neutrophils,[352, 472] which may be relevant to the pathophysiology of eosinophil-mediated diseases such as bronchial asthma.[322] Eosinophil oxidative metabolism is stimulated by a variety of stimuli, including FMLP,[473] PAF,[352] LTB_4,[310] C3a,[119] zymosan,[224] IgG-coated surfaces,[25] calcium ionophore A23187,[352] and phorbol myristate acetate (PMA).[352]

CYTOKINES

Until fairly recently, the role of the eosinophil in immunoregulatory networks has been viewed as a target of cytokines. However, observations indicate that eosinophils elaborate cytokines; these results are summarized in Table 11–2. An early report showed that murine peritoneal eosinophils stimulated with lipopolysaccharide (LPS) were positive for IL-1 mRNA by in situ hybridization and released IL-1 bioactivity.[91] Subsequently, human eosinophils infiltrating intestinal tissues and eosinophils from patients with eosinophilia were found to express TGF-α[466] and TGF-β1.[465] Eosinophils from nasal polyps also expressed TGF-β1, suggesting that TGF-β1 synthesis by eosinophils may contribute to the structural abnormalities of nasal polyps, such as stromal fibrosis and basement thickening.[303]

Evidence exists that eosinophils also produce cytokines with the ability to act on eosinophils themselves, the so-called autocrine cytokines, including IL-3, IL-5, and GM-CSF. For example, human eosinophils stimulated in vitro with IFN-γ or the calcium ionophore, A23187, or ionomycin, produce GM-CSF and IL-3 protein.[212, 281] Eosinophils produced approximately one half as much IL-3 and one fifth as much GM-CSF as did ionomycin-stimulated mononuclear cells, suggesting that eosinophils are able to produce quantities of cytokines roughly comparable to T cells.[212] Production of GM-CSF was also observed with eosinophils stimulated by lipopolysaccharide, and this production was inhibited by IL-10.[394] Interestingly, fibronectin-coated surfaces enhanced eosinophil survival by a mechanism that depends on the interaction between fibronectin and VLA-4 on eosinophils. This phenomenon was inhibited by antibodies to GM-CSF and IL-3, suggesting an autocrine production of these cytokines by eosinophils.[16]

GM-CSF may be stored in eosinophils from asthmatic subjects in association with crystalloid granules.[247] That eosinophils might actually produce these cytokines in vivo is shown by studies of nasal polyp tissues where GM-CSF mRNA and protein were present.[304] Furthermore, some of the BAL eosinophils derived from asthma patients after allergen challenge were positive for IL-5 and GM-CSF mRNA.[51] By in situ hybridization, IL-5 mRNA was also detected in the intestinal tissues of patients with coeliac disease, eosinophilic cystitis, and hypereosinophilic syndrome.[99, 107] Furthermore, it was claimed that IL-5 was released after stimulation with IgA-, IgE-, or IgG-immune complexes.[107] In contrast, in nasal biopsy tissues from atopic rhinitis subjects after allergen exposure, most cells expressing IL-5 mRNA were T cells, with much smaller contributions from mast cells and eosinophils.[474] Together, these findings indicate that eosinophils have the capacity to synthesize IL-3, GM-CSF, and IL-5; however, the physiologic significance of these observations needs to be clarified.

By reverse transcription polymerase chain reaction (RT-PCR), constitutive expression of IL-6 mRNA was detected in peripheral blood eosinophils.[265] Transcription and synthesis of IL-6 by eosinophils were enhanced by IFN-γ.[164] Reports suggest that C5a and FMLP in the presence of cytochalasin B,[276] eosinophil MBP,[217] and GM-CSF plus RANTES or PAF[477] can stimulate eosinophils to produce IL-8. Increased levels of intracellular IL-8 were observed with eosinophils from patients with asthma or atopic dermatitis.[477] Furthermore, eosinophils from the peripheral blood of normal individuals or patients with the hypereosinophilic syndrome expressed proinflammatory cytokine, TNF-α, and the chemokine, macrophage inflammatory protein-1α (MIP-1α).[78] Eosinophils thereby have the potential to generate a number of cytokines. In the future, whether these cytokines elaborated by eosinophils participate in the cytokine network and actually control the inflammatory process of various diseases needs to be studied.

EOSINOPHIL RECRUITMENT

ADHESION RECEPTORS AND LIGANDS

Leukocyte migration through the endothelium is a process involving sequential steps. Initially, the cells are lightly tethered to the endothelium and roll along its surface. This is followed by leukocyte activation, which allows a firmer bond to develop between the leukocyte and the endothelial cell, resulting in successful adhesion and transmigration. The receptors and mediators involved in eosinophil migration have been characterized. A family of adhesion receptors termed selectins and their carbohydrate ligands are thought to mediate the initial attachment and rolling steps. Integrins expressed on eosinophils bind to adhesion receptors belonging to the immunoglobulin superfamily on endothelial cells and are implicated in the subsequent firmer adhesion.[43]

The selectin adhesion family comprises three receptors: E-selectin (ELAM-1) is expressed on endothelium, P-selectin (GMP-140) is expressed on endothelium and platelets, and L-selectin (LECAM-1) is expressed on leukocytes. As shown in Table 11–1, eosinophils constitutively express L-selectin; furthermore, they shed it on cell activation.[267] The selectins have a common structure characterized by an *N*-terminal calcium-dependent (C type) lectin domain, which binds sugars consisting of a family of sialylated, fucosylated glycosaminoglycans typified by the carbohydrate moiety sialyl-Lewis^X.[377] Ligands for L-selectin consist of heavily O-glycosylated, mucin-like glycoprotein receptors, in which large amounts of O-linked sugars are presented on a rigid protein backbone.[360] The inhibition assay using a panel of monoclonal antibodies suggests that eosinophils utilize a different functional epitope of L-selectin for this ligand binding than do neutrophils.[222]

The counterligands for endothelial selectins are also different for eosinophils and neutrophils. Neutrophils bind more avidly than do eosinophils to purified E-selectin.[46] Neutrophils express large amounts of sialyl-Lewis^X, whereas the expression of this epitope on eosinophils is extremely low or undetectable. A major proportion of the E-selectin ligand on the surface of eosinophils appears to be sialyl-dimeric Lewis^X.[46] The counterligands for P-selectin on eosinophils and neutrophils are similarly sialylated, protease-sensitive, endo-beta-galactosidase–resistant structures.[448] Eosinophil binding to E- and P-selectin does not appear to be affected by the state of cell activation. Furthermore, the levels of expression of L-selectin were decreased in eosinophils activated in vivo or in vitro by lipid mediators or cytokines.[293]

Integrins are composed of α and β transmembrane subunits selected from among 16 α and 8 β subunits that heterodimerize to produce more than 20 different receptors.[73] Unlike selectins, ligand recognition by integrins requires cellular activation. Cells are able to regulate the function of integrins by signaling in the opposite direction (inside-out signaling), and the receptors are converted from a form with low affinity for their ligands to one with high affinity. This so-called activation of the integrin is required for firm interaction between integrins and their ligands,[102] and this is also the case with eosinophils. The levels of expression of integrins are also dependent on the activation state of the cells. Eosinophils express several integrins that can bind to immunoglobulin family receptors expressed on the endothelium and to components of extracellular matrix proteins (see Table 11–1). The resultant bond is much firmer than the selectin carbohydrate bond and results in the eosinophils' flattening and transmigration between endothelial cells.[434] Eosinophils express β1 (CD29),[45, 433] β2 (CD18),[167] and β7 integrins. Among the β1 integrins, VLA-4 (CD49d/CD29), which binds the vascular cell adhesion molecule-1 (VCAM-1), plays an important role for eosinophil migration from the bloodstream into the tissues. Among the β2 integrins, LFA-1 (CD11a/CD18) and Mac-1 (CD11b/CD18) integrins both bind the intercellular adhesion molecule-1 (ICAM-1) expressed on various types of cells and play important roles for eosinophil migration as well as effector functions of the cells. Integrins also function as receptors for extracellular matrix proteins and plasma proteins, such as laminin, fibronectin, and fibrinogen, and many integrins recognize a common sequence in these proteins.

MECHANISMS OF EOSINOPHIL ROLLING, ADHESION, AND TRANSMIGRATION IN VITRO

Eosinophil adhesion to cytokine-stimulated human umbilical vein endothelial cells (HUVEC) was inhibited by blocking monoclonal antibodies against E-selectin and L-selectin.[221, 222, 455] When viewing microvascular endothelial cells in the rabbit mesentery with intravital video microscopy, eosinophils were found to roll in venules. This rolling was stimulated by activating endothelial cells with IL-1. Eosinophil rolling was mediated by L-selectin and VLA-4, whereas neutrophil rolling was predominantly mediated by L-selectin.[380] Eosinophil adhesion to nasal polyp tissues placed on a rotating platform (Stamper-Woodruff assay) was almost totally inhibited by an antibody against P-selectin.[390] Antibodies against ICAM-1, VCAM-1, E-selectin, L-selectin, VLA-4, and LFA-1 had no effect, whereas an antibody against Mac-1 had a modest effect. These findings suggest that E-selectin, L-selectin, P-selectin, and VLA-4 are involved in eosinophil interactions with activated endothelial cells in a flow condition. However, in allergic inflammation, P-selectin may be the principal receptor involved in the rolling stage of eosinophil adhesion to vascular endothelium.

In a static condition, Mac-1 appears to be the major receptor involved in eosinophil adhesion to unstimulated HUVEC. Eosinophil adhesion to unstimulated HUVEC was enhanced by PAF and other eosinophil-active inflammatory mediators, including IL-3, IL-5, and TNF, and their enhancement was totally inhibited by monoclonal antibody to the leukocyte integrin, Mac-1.[211, 240] Hypodense eosinophils exhibited significantly greater ability to adhere spontaneously to endothelial cells than did normodense eosinophils.[446] PAF stimulation increased adhesiveness of hypodense eosinophils; this could virtually be completely blocked by monoclonal antibody to CD18, thus implicating β2 integrin in the adhesion process.[211] In contrast, eosinophil adhesion to IL-1– or TNF-α–stimulated HUVEC was inhibited by monoclonal antibodies against ICAM-1 and VCAM-1 on the endothelial cells and LFA-1, Mac-1, and VLA-4 on the eosinophils, suggesting that both β1 integrin and β2 integrins are involved in adhesion of eosinophils to the activated endothelial cells.[45, 104, 433, 455]

Eosinophil transmigration through endothelial cells has been investigated with artificial models of the blood vessel wall. In these studies, eosinophils from allergic donors showed an increased migration capacity, and this was mimicked by in vitro culture of eosinophils from normal donors with GM-CSF, IL-3, or IL-5.[279] The receptors that mediate transmigration of eosinophils through IL-1– or TNF-α–stimulated HUVEC appear to be the LFA-1 and Mac-1 on eosinophils binding to ICAM-1 on the endothelium.[115] In contrast, eosinophil migration through IL-4–stimulated HUVEC was inhibited by anti–VLA-4 antibody, as well as by antibodies against β2 integrins.[284] Further, the combinations of IL-1 and IL-4 or TNF and IL-4, which are synergistic for VCAM-1 expression, were also synergistic in their abilities to enhance endothelial transmigration.[347] Conversely, an antibody to the β1 integrin chain, which activates β1 integrins into a high-avidity binding state by freezing β1 integrins in an activated state, inhibited eosinophil migration across extracellular matrix or endothelial cells.[235] Thus both the β2 and β1 integrins appear to be involved in the eosinophil transmigration through IL-4–activated endothelial cells.[284]

Because neutrophils do not express VLA-4 (see Table 11–1), and because IL-4 is presumably produced during the inflammatory reaction associated with asthma, the ability of IL-4 to up-regulate VCAM-1[405] is an attractive mechanism by which eosinophils could be selectively recruited into the airways. This hypothesis has been strengthened by the observation that eosinophil, but not neutrophil, adhesion and transmigration through HUVEC were enhanced by IL-4.[346] In contrast, however, the expression of VCAM-1 in allergic inflammation is relatively weak compared with the other adhesion molecules, such as selectins and ICAM-1.[237] Therefore, the evidence that selective expression of adhesion molecules is responsible for eosinophil localization in tissues of allergic diseases is still contradictory.

EOSINOPHIL CHEMOTAXIS

It has been thought that an essential component of eosinophil migration into the tissues in allergic reactions is an effective and selective chemoattractant.[117] Because of the association of immediate hypersensitivity reactions with tissue eosinophilia, considerable attention has been focused on mast cell–derived chemotactic factors, such as histamine and LTB_4.[145, 206, 207, 444] Histamine has been claimed to show chemotactic and chemokinetic activities for eosinophils in vitro.[72, 416] However, in vivo experiments do not appear to support histamine as a significant eosinophilotactic agent.[121] A lipoxygenase-derived product, LTB_4 is chemotactic for eosinophils and neutrophils.[44, 76, 288] Several groups have reported the existence of LTB_4 receptors on guinea pig eosinophils.[258, 296, 356] Moreover, in sensitized guinea pigs after respiratory challenge, structural analogues of LTB_4 inhibited lung eosinophilia, and LTB_4 could be detected in BAL fluids.[332, 400]

Although LTB_4 is chemotactic for both eosinophils and neutrophils, late evidence suggests that LTD_4 is chemotactic for eosinophils but not neutrophils in the under-agarose leukocyte assay.[376] In this assay, LTD_4 was chemotactic at as low as 10^{-10} M, suggesting that LTD_4 may be a potent and selective chemoattractant for eosinophils at physiologically relevant concentrations. Two other lipoxygenase-derived products, the diHETEs,[355] also have chemotactic activity for eosinophils. Interestingly, inhaled LTE_4 generated airway eosinophilia, although it is not clear whether this was a direct or an indirect effect.[238]

PAF, which is produced by various types of cells, including mast cells, neutrophils, macrophages, eosinophils, and endothelial cells, is more potent as an eosinophil chemotactic factor than are histamine and LTB_4 over a dose range of 10^{-8} to 10^{-6} M.[396, 437] PAF is one of the most potent chemoattractants for eosinophils and selectively induces the migration of eosinophils over neutrophils.[364, 437] In vivo, PAF injected into the skin caused the accumulation of eosinophils in atopic individuals, but neutrophils were prominent in nonatopic individuals.[174] Increased numbers of neutrophils, but not eosinophils, appeared in BAL fluid 4 to 6 hours after the inhalation of PAF in a group of normal subjects.[438] Interestingly, IL-5–induced chemotaxis of guinea pig eosinophils was inhibited by a PAF receptor antagonist, WEB2086.[75] In addition, eosinophils desensitized to PAF-acether failed to migrate to IL-5, but those desensitized to LTB_4 did respond to IL-5. Taken together, these findings suggest that eosinophil migration induced by IL-5 involves PAF, presumably produced by eosinophils by themselves. Thus PAF, which is released to the local milieu by the activated eosinophils, may costimulate the chemotaxis of eosinophils.

T-cell products also play a role in eosinophil chemotaxis. Studies have shown that IL-5, GM-CSF, and IL-3 possess eosinophil chemotactic activity, albeit at nanomolar concentrations.[435, 442, 470] In the Boyden chamber, these cytokines were chemotactic for eosinophils from normal individuals, but not for eosinophils from allergic subjects, possibly as a result of in vivo desensitization.[357] Although the chemotactic activities of these cytokines are relatively weak compared with well-established eosinophil chemoattractants, such as PAF, they can effectively prime eosinophils for enhanced chemotactic responsiveness to suboptimal concentrations of PAF and LTB_4 and enhance the generally negligible activity that FMLP and IL-8 have for unactivated eosinophils.[357] For example, preincubation of eosinophils with GM-CSF caused an increased response to LTB_4 and induced a response toward IL-8 and FMLP. Similarly, preincubation of eosinophils with IL-3, IL-5, or GM-CSF enhanced PAF-induced chemotaxis.[75, 441] These stimulatory effects of cytokines appear to be relevant in vivo because eosinophils from allergic subjects are more responsive to some chemotactic stimuli than are eosinophils from normal subjects.[441]

Despite the relative lack of activity of IL-5 in the in vitro system, inhalation of IL-5 in animals and humans leads to eosinophil recruitment.[192, 403, 427] Antibodies against IL-5 have been effective in inhibiting eosinophil migration into the lungs of allergen-challenged guinea pigs.[260, 425] Interestingly, the airway eosinophilia caused by IL-5 inhalation in mice was followed by airway hyperreactivity and mucosal exudation, suggesting that IL-5 is sufficient to provoke pathologic changes in the airway.[427] It is possible that a selective priming by IL-5 combined with a nonselective but highly effective chemoattractant results in selective eosinophil migration in allergic inflammation.

An exciting development in the area of eosinophil migration has been made by the identification of relatively cell-specific chemotactic proteins termed chemokines. Chemokines are 6- to 10-kD proteins that have 20% to 55% similarities in their amino acid sequences. The family is divided into two subfamilies, C-X-C and C-C, by the position of the first two of the conserved cysteines. The C-X-C subfamily, typified by IL-8, is particularly active on neutrophils, although IL-8 has chemotactic activity for primed eosinophils.[363] The C-C subfamily, typified by regulated upon activation in normal T cells expressed and secreted (RANTES), is potently chemotactic for eosinophils, as well as lymphocytes, but not for neutrophils.[201]

An in vitro study compared the chemotactic activity of four members of the C-C subfamily: monocyte chemotactic peptide (MCP)-1, RANTES, macrophage inflammatory protein-1α (MIP-1α), and MIP-1β.[335] In this study, RANTES strongly attracted human eosinophils with a potency similar to C5a. MIP-1α also induced eosinophil migration in vitro but with lower efficiency than RANTES.[335] In contrast, MCP-1 and MIP-1β did not induce eosinophil migration.[335] These findings suggest that RANTES is the most potent chemokine for eosinophils. In fact, intradermal injections of RANTES in dogs resulted in eosinophil-rich infiltrations within several hours; injection of IL-8 caused neutrophil infiltration.[271] Studies of MCP-2 and MCP-3 also show that they have effects on eosinophils similar to RANTES, although MCP-2 was less potent than MCP-3 and RANTES.[84, 444a] Interestingly, the expression of MCP-3 mRNA, but not RANTES mRNA, correlated with eosinophil infiltration in allergic skin reactions.[475]

Another C-C subfamily chemokine, eotaxin, is interesting because it was originally identified in BAL fluids from allergen-challenged guinea pigs and therefore is of direct relevance to allergic diseases.[198, 339] The chemokine receptors are members of the G protein–linked, seven-transmembrane receptor family,[295] and there appears to be sharing of receptors among the chemokines.[85] Thus these studies indicate the existence of eosinophil-specific chemoattractants (because they had no chemotactic activity for neutrophils), providing a possible explanation for eosinophil-enriched inflammatory infiltrates.

Activation of the complement system generates proteolytic fragments, such as C5a and C3a, which are chemotactic for eosinophils.[123] Although C5a is chemotactic for both eosinophils and neutrophils, C3a is chemotactic only for eosinophils.[83] C3a acts on eosinophils via a receptor that is distinct from the C5a receptor.

Activated eosinophils can express CD4[254] and thus can interact with the lymphocyte chemoattractant factor (LCF, IL-16),[82] a tetrameric glycoprotein of M_r 56,000 produced by activated T lymphocytes. Migration of eosinophils was elicited by LCF at low concentrations, ED_{50} 10^{-12} to 10^{-11} M, concentrations 100- to 1,000-fold lower than the ED_{50} for C5a and PAF.[329] Although IL-2 does not affect viability or other functions of eosinophils, it was found that IL-2 is a potent attractant for eosinophils, with an ED_{50} of 10^{-12} M. It was also possible to detect p55/CD25 low-affinity IL-2 receptors on the eosinophil's surface.[330] These findings collectively suggest that a mechanism involving lymphocyte-derived chemotactic cytokines may contribute to eosinophil accumulation in tissues. Other workers report these interleukins to be chemokinetic, but not strictly chemotactic (see Chapter 16).

MECHANISMS OF EOSINOPHIL RECRUITMENT IN ALLERGIC DISEASES

Animal models of allergic inflammation have provided information on the relative importance of selectins, integrins, and their ligands in eosinophil migration. There are few, if any, published studies on the roles of P- and L-selectin on eosinophil migration into sites of allergic inflammation. However, some research with E-selectin used wild but caught cynomolgus monkeys with a natural sensitivity to ascaris antigen. The airway eosinophilia and increased bronchial hyperresponsiveness (BHR) after multiple allergen challenge to these monkeys were inhibited by an antibody against ICAM-1 but not by antibody against E-selectin.[446] In contrast, the airway neutrophilia generated by a single challenge was inhibited by anti–E-selectin but not by anti–ICAM-1.[154] These findings suggest that, in this model at least, BHR is associated with an airway eosinophilia that is mediated by ICAM-1, whereas the late airway neutrophilia is mediated by E-selectin.

Interaction between VLA-4 on eosinophils and VCAM-1 on endothelial cells may also play an important role for eosinophil migration in vivo. In guinea pigs, anti–VLA-4 antibody inhibited the migration of eosinophils into the skin after injection of chemotactic factors and after passive cutaneous anaphylaxis.[445] Anti–VLA-4 antibody also inhibited allergen-induced eosinophil infiltration into the airways and bronchial hyperreactivity.[323] In sensitized mice, anti–VLA-4 antibody inhibited eosinophil infiltration into the trachea after ovalbumin challenge[290]; anti–VCAM-1 antibody was also effective.[290] Unlike the monkey model, anti–ICAM-1 and anti–LFA-1 monoclonal antibodies were ineffective at inhibiting eosinophil migration. Lastly, aerosolized anti–VLA-4 antibody inhibited allergen-induced BAL eosinophilia and BHR in rabbits sensitized to house dust mites.[270]

CD4+ T cells, presumably T-helper type II cells, and the cytokines released by such T cells play a crucial role for allergen-induced recruitment of eosinophils into lung tissues. When guinea pig lungs were injected with Sephadex particles, airway eosinophilia was totally blocked by anti–IL-5 monoclonal antibody and a combination of anti-CD18 and anti–VLA-4 antibodies, suggesting important roles for IL-5 and these integrins in the development of airway eosinophilia in this model.[86] Allergen-induced airway eosinophilia and BHR were largely mediated by IL-5 and were abrogated by anti–IL-5 administration.[425] In mice, CD4+ T cells and IL-5 mediated allergen-induced eosinophil infiltration into the mouse trachea.[289] IFN-γ inhibited this allergen-induced eosinophil infiltration by inhibiting CD4+ T-cell infiltration.[191] In humans, IL-5 and to a lesser extent GM-CSF were the predominant eosinophil-active cytokines in the allergen-induced pulmonary late-phase reaction.[302] The accumulation of eosinophils in tissues, as in chronic asthma or acute allergen challenge in the lungs, correlated with measures of local T-cell activation. For instance, increases in numbers of activated T lymphocytes and eosinophils and increased expression of cytokine mRNA for IL-5 and GM-CSF have been documented in bronchial biopsy samples after allergen inhalation challenge of atopic asthmatics.[41] Thus these findings point to important roles for VLA-4 and Mac-1 on eosinophils and ICAM-1, and possibly VCAM-1, on endothelial cells in eosinophil recruitment in allergic inflammation. Cytokines, especially IL-5, are also likely playing critical roles in eosinophil infiltration.

EOSINOPHIL INTERACTION WITH EXTRACELLULAR MATRIX PROTEINS

After migration through the endothelium, eosinophils come into contact with the extracellular matrix proteins. As shown in Table 11–1, fibronectin binds to eosinophils through VLA-4 ($\alpha_4\beta_1$) and Act-1 ($\alpha_4\beta_7$),[16] laminin through VLA-6,[137] and hyaluronate through CD44.[163] This adhesion of eosinophils to matrix proteins modifies the functions of the cells. For example, as a result of autocrine stimulation of IL-3 and GM-CSF production, eosinophils survived for prolonged periods when cultured on fibronectin.[16] Hyaluronic acid stimulates the growth of CD34+ umbilical cord blood cells into specifically differentiated mature eosinophils.[163] However, the effects of extracellular matrix proteins on eosinophil effector functions are contradictory.

Dri and colleagues[106] demonstrated that eosinophil superoxide production induced by FMLP or substance P is decreased when tissue culture wells are coated with fibronectin or laminin. We also found that fibronectin and laminin inhibited eosinophil degranulation stimulated by PAF, C5a, and IL-5 but not by PMA.[216] In contrast, Anwar and colleagues[17] demonstrated enhancement of calcium ionophore–stimulated LTC_4 generation by eosinophils adherent to fibronectin. Neeley and colleagues[294] have reported that VLA-4–mediated interaction with fibronectin results in increased degranulation of eosinophils stimulated by FMLP in the presence of cytochalasin B. Obviously, the secretagogues and detection methods are important in determining the effects of matrix proteins on eosinophil functions. More studies are needed, but extracellular matrix proteins are likely playing important roles in the regulation of eosinophil activation in the tissues and bloodstream.

EOSINOPHIL ACTIVATION

Eosinophils are tissue resident cells, and it is presumed that they are most active within the tissues. While they are infiltrating into the tissue lesions, eosinophils adhere to the endothelium, migrate through the blood vessels, and move toward the targets. During these processes, eosinophils are primed (partially activated), and they exert their full function at the site of the inflammation. In this section, the mechanism and regulation of these steps are described.

EFFECTS OF CYTOKINES ON MATURE EOSINOPHILS

Several cytokines have a marked effect on eosinophil function. IL-3, IL-5, and GM-CSF, besides being growth and maturation factors for eosinophils, also stimulate a number of mature human eosinophil functions. Eosinophils possess receptors for IL-3, IL-5, and GM-CSF (approximately 1,000 receptors per cell).[71, 250] The receptors for these cytokines consist of two noncovalently associated chains, namely, a ligand-specific alpha chain that binds the cognate ligand with low affinity (K_d = 10 nM)[136, 218, 286, 399] and a common beta chain that confers high-affinity binding to the ligand and signal transduction.[172] The affinity of the complete GM-CSF receptor (K_d = 44 pM)[250] on human eosinophils is approximately 10 times higher than that for IL-3 (K_d = 470 pM)[250] and IL-5 (K_d = 518 pM).[71] The sharing of a common beta chain among the receptors for GM-CSF, IL-3, and IL-5 may explain, in part, the cross-competition between these cytokines; this competition may be viewed as the sequestering of the common beta chain by excess heterologous competitor.[251] The beta chain is likely present in numbers similar to each of the alpha chains but fewer than the three alpha chains combined.

Interestingly, the association constant for the binding of ^{125}I-labeled IL-5 to human hypodense eosinophils was higher than that for the binding of IL-5 to normodense cells; the number of receptor sites per cell was similar.[71] Human eosinophils also bind murine IL-5, and this binding is rapid and saturable in keeping with the ability of murine IL-5 to act on human eosinophils.[178] Among human peripheral blood leukocytes, eosinophils are the only cells having detectable levels of IL-5 receptors in agreement with the specific action of IL-5 on human eosinophils, whereas IL-3 and GM-CSF have less selective activities.[188, 272] The promoter regulating the genes for the IL-5 receptor alpha chain was localized in a promyelocytic leukemia cell line committed to eosinophil lineage.[389]

IL-5, IL-3, and GM-CSF antagonize the programmed cell death of eosinophils in culture, thus prolonging survival in vitro.[39, 175, 252, 337, 338, 386] The effects of these cytokines on eosinophils are inhibited by glucocorticoids, including dexamethasone and methylprednisolone.[239, 430] IL-5 has been reported as chemotactic for eosinophils,[435] and preincubation of eosinophils with low concentrations of IL-5 induces a significant chemotactic response of eosinophils toward IL-8 or RANTES.[349, 440] IL-5 also enhances the integrin-dependent adhesion of eosinophils to plasma-coated glass and human microvascular endothelial cells.[434] IL-5 activates various effector functions of eosinophils, such as LTC_4 and superoxide generation, phagocytosis, and helminthotoxic activity,[253, 338] as well as Ig-induced degranulation.[132] Eosinophils cultured for 7 days with IL-5 released up to 50% of all granule proteins into culture fluids.[214] IL-5 provokes biochemical changes in human eosinophils, including activation of various kinases, such as Jak-2, lyn, Ras, Raf-1, and mitogen-activated protein (MAP) kinase, and induction of a DNA-binding complex containing STAT-1 protein,[313, 314, 422] providing pharmacologic bases for the action of IL-5 on eosinophils. It will be interesting to know which of these molecules are playing crucial roles in the IL-5 effects on eosinophils.

IL-5 is present in various biologic fluids, including BAL fluids from patients with allergic rhinitis after endobronchial challenge[351] and sera from patients with eosinophilia of various etiologies.[57, 302, 306] Moreover, IL-5 appears to be the predominant eosinophil-active cytokine in the antigen-induced pulmonary late-phase reaction.[302] A role for IL-5 in bronchial asthma has been studied with experimental animal models and with neutralizing antibodies and soluble receptors. In these studies, administration of either anti–IL-5 antibodies or soluble IL-5 receptors has prevented airway eosinophilia and bronchial hyperreactivity in a variety of models involving antigen or virus challenges.[118, 425, 426, 469] Conversely, IL-5 inhalation in mice caused airway eosinophilia followed by airway hyperreactivity and mucosal exudation.[427] Thus IL-5 enhances various functions of eosinophils as inflammatory cells, including adhesion, chemotaxis, survival, and mediator release. IL-5 is detected in the biologic fluids associated with eosinophilia, and antagonism of IL-5 prevents pathologic changes associated with eosinophilia in vivo. Therefore, IL-5 may be the most critical cytokine in the pathophysiology of eosinophil-associated inflammation.

GM-CSF also activates and enhances eosinophil function, such as cytotoxic killing,[252] superoxide production,[253] leukotriene production,[365] phagocytosis of serum-opsonized zymosan,[252] and immunoglobulin-induced degranulation.[132] In a similar manner, IL-3 enhances eosinophil cytotoxicity, phagocytosis, superoxide production (in response to stimulation with FMLP),[337] and Ig-induced degranulation.[132] When eosinophils are maintained in culture with murine fibroblasts and GM-CSF, they synthesize and express CD4[254] and the class II MHC protein, human leukocyte antigen (HLA)-DR.[255] These eosinophils, therefore, are able to respond to the CD4 ligand, LCF,[329] and to present antigen to CD4+ lymphocytes.[90, 166, 452] CD69, which is expressed on activated T cells and natural killer cells, is also expressed on eosinophils cultured with GM-CSF or IL-3.[297]

IFN-γ activates eosinophils, but does so in a delayed manner.[419] For example, in short-term cytotoxicity assays, eosinophils were maximally activated by GM-CSF followed in order of potency by IL-3, IL-5, TNF-α, and IL-4. After a 24-hour incubation, maximal eosinophil activation was caused by IFN-γ followed by GM-CSF, IL-3, and IL-5. IFN-α and IFN-β enhanced cytotoxicity as well. Furthermore, culture of eosinophils with IFN-γ for 1 to 2 days caused expression of $Fc_\gamma RIII$ (CD16) (not expressed on freshly isolated peripheral blood eosinophils)[168] and a significant increase in $Fc_\gamma RII$ (CD32) expression.[419] In contrast, treatment of eosinophils with IFN-γ for 1 hour inhibited release of H_2O_2 induced by opsonized zymosan and decreased eosinophil binding to complement-sensitized erythrocytes.[342] The degranulation response of eosinophils to sIgA-coated Sepharose beads was also inhibited by preincubation with IFN-γ for 3 hours.[132] Thus IFN-γ appears to inhibit eosinophil activation over short incubation times and to stimulate function and receptor expression when incubation is prolonged for days.

The proinflammatory cytokines TNF-α and IL-1 also modulate eosinophil functions. TNF-α prolonged eosinophil survival in vitro,[419] enhanced eosinophil synthesis of LTC_4,[340] increased eosinophil toxicity toward *S. mansoni* larvae,[365] and increased eosinophil adhesion for endothelial cells.[371] Although it is clear that TNF-α itself has only modest activity toward eosinophils compared with the eosinophil hemopoietins (e.g., IL-5),[406] the activity of TNF-α synergizes with that of IL-5. For example, TNF-α and IL-5 synergistically induced the expression of ICAM-1 on mature eosinophils.[166] Therefore, the mechanism of action of TNF-α on eosinophils seems to be different from that of the eosinophil hemopoietin. The effects of IL-1 on eosinophils are more complex. IL-1 increased or decreased eosinophil release of superoxide or the granule arylsulfatase and β-glucuronidase depending on the choice and concentration of PMA or calcium ionophore as costimuli.[319] Although enzyme release from IgG-stimulated eosinophils is inhibited by preincubation with IL-1β, the enzyme release from IgE-stimulated eosinophils is enhanced by IL-1β.[33]

The discovery of cytokines belonging to the chemokine superfamily has led to the identification of chemotactic peptides with rather restricted target cell specificity.[246] One group, classified on the basis of cysteine residues, is referred to as C-C and includes RANTES, MIP-1α, and MCP-3; these cytokines are chemotactic for mononuclear cells.[246] RANTES and MCP-3 are strong chemoattractants for eosinophils[84, 201, 335] as is the eotoxin described since 1994.[198, 339] The chemotactic activities of these chemokines were described in detail earlier. The chemokines also modulate eosinophil effector function. RANTES, MCP-3, and MIP-1α all induced elevations of intracellular Ca^{2+} and, at relatively high cytokine concentrations, caused ECP release from eosinophils.[335] IL-8, which belongs to another group of chemokines called C-X-C, is also chemotactic for eosinophils when eosinophils are primed by the eosinophil hemopoietins in vitro or in vivo.[363]

Little information is available regarding cytokines that inhibit the functions of eosinophils. Transforming growth factor-β (TGF-β), an anti-inflammatory cytokine,[361, 412] has been shown to decrease the number of eosinophils in human bone marrow suspension cultures.[367] TGF-β activity was exerted at the level of mRNA expression. TGF-β also inhibited eosinophil survival induced by the eosinophil hemopoietins in vitro.[13] These results suggest that TGF-β may play an important regulatory role in eosinophil-associated inflammation. IL-4 reduces human eosinophil expression of IgG, but not IgE, receptors and IgG-dependent release of granule enzymes or cytotoxic functions. This effect is moderate in degree and requires at least an 8-hour incubation of eosinophils with IL-4 before the effect can be observed.[32] The functions of eosinophil-active cytokines are summarized in Table 11–3.

PRIMING AND PARTIAL ACTIVATION OF EOSINOPHILS

Hypodense Eosinophils

Initial studies of eosinophil density revealed that human blood often contained a population of eosinophils that differed in density from normal eosinophils. When blood specimens from patients with eosinophilia were compared with those from normal individuals, two density populations of eosinophils were revealed.[35, 98, 135, 324, 325, 462] Eosinophils of lower density were termed light density or hypodense cells, and those of normal density were termed normodense cells. Eosinophils from normal individuals had a peak density of approximately 1.088 g/ml with fewer than 10% having a density below 1.082 g/ml. In contrast, light density eosinophils had a peak density of 1.075 to 1.082 g/ml.[135, 462] As well shown in individuals experimentally infected with hookworm larvae, *Necator americanus,* the numbers of light density eosinophils are correlated with the degree of peripheral blood eosinophilia.[458] Similar results have been obtained in rats infected with *T. spiralis.*[159] In general, hypodense eosinophils have been detected in blood from patients with parasitic diseases, idiopathic hypereosinophilic syndrome, bronchial asthma, and other allergic diseases. Furthermore, blood from patients receiving cytokine therapy and fluids from tissues, such as BAL, show relatively elevated numbers of light density eosinophils, corresponding to their eosinophilia.

Morphologically, hypodense eosinophils of patients with blood eosinophilia differed from normodense eosinophils of normal persons; individual granules were smaller, and the total granule area of the cell was smaller.[68, 173, 316] Hypodense eosinophils contained less MBP per 10^6 cells than did normo-

TABLE 11–3
ACTIVATORS AND REGULATORS OF EOSINOPHIL FUNCTION

Activators and Regulators	Degranulation	Production of Lipid Mediators	Superoxide Production	Cytotoxicity Against Ab-Coated Targets	Priming*	Chemotaxis	Adhesion	Survival	Cytokine Production
Immunoglobulins									
IgG	↑	↑	↑	↑			↑		↑
IgE	↑	↑		↑					↑
IgA	↑							↑	
Secretory IgA	↑								↑
Complement									
C3a	↑		↑			↑			
C5a	↑					↑			↑ †
Zymosan	↑	↑	↑						
Lipid Mediators & Small Molecules									
PAF	↑	↑	↑	↑	↑	↑	↑		↑ ‡
LTB_4			↑			↑			
FMLP	↑	↑	↑		↑	↑			↑ †
Cytokines									
IL-1	↑ ↓		↑ ↓						
IL-3	↑		↑	↑	↑	↑ §	↑	↑	
IL-4	↓			↓					
IL-5	↑	↑	↑	↑	↑	↑ §	↑	↑	
GM-CSF	↑	↑	↑	↑	↑	↑ §	↑	↑	↑ ‡
TNF-α		↑		↑			↑	↑	
IFN-γ	↑ ↓			↑				↑	↑
TGF-β								↓	
Chemokines									
IL-8						↑ ‡			
RANTES	↑ §					↑			↑ ‡
MCP-3	↑ §					↑			
MIP-1α	↑ §					↑			

Induction and/or up-regulation of eosinophil function is indicated by ↑, and inhibition of function is indicated by ↓.
*Priming means enhancement of eosinophil function (e.g., superoxide production and chemotaxis) induced by other agonists.
†In the presence of cytochalasin B.
‡In the presence of priming factors.
§At high concentrations.

dense cells[214]; EPO levels also may be reduced in hypodense cells.[152] One explanation for the generation of hypodense eosinophils in patients with eosinophilia invokes a premature release of eosinophils from the marrow.[133] Hypodense eosinophils, derived by culturing normodense eosinophils in vitro, showed significantly increased numbers of lucent granules, granule fusion, slightly decreased plasma membrane surface area-to-cell volume ratio, and increased volume.[68, 214] Thus a series of changes that include cell swelling, a decrease in the volume of the cytoplasm occupied by granules, and an increase in granule lucency appear to contribute to the generation of hypodense eosinophils in vitro, whereas a reduction in eosinophil granule size appears to be the principal determinant of the reduced density in vivo.

Numerous studies have investigated the induction of hypodense eosinophils in vitro. Purified human peripheral blood eosinophils have prolonged viability and become hypodense when cultured with growth factors,[39] including GM-CSF,[252, 308] IL-3,[337] IL-5,[338] and IFN-γ,[419] or with either endothelial cells[336] or fibroblasts.[308, 309, 338] Stimuli that are known to induce eosinophil activation also generate hypodense eosinophils, including calcium ionophore A23187, serum-treated zymosan, PAF, and FMLP.[220, 478]

Considerable evidence suggests that light density eosinophils are activated cells. Light density eosinophils are metabolically more active than normodense eosinophils by showing increased oxygen consumption,[462] increased uptake of radioactive phosphorus,[236] and increased ability to generate superoxide anion.[318] Light density eosinophils also show increased production and/or releasability of LTC_4[200, 358] and potent cytotoxic activity for antibody-coated cells.[324] In contrast, hypodense eosinophils have a similar profile of leukocyte integrin and $Fc_\gamma R$ receptor expression compared with normal density cells.[167] Furthermore, normal density cells from individuals with eosinophilia are more activated than normal density eosinophils from normal individuals. Normal density eosinophils infiltrating into an inflammation site are also more activated than the eosinophils in peripheral blood of the same individuals. Normal density eosinophils, when stimulated with an eosinophil hemopoietin, acquire enhanced cytotoxic function and LTC_4 synthesis days in advance of a shift in density. Therefore, hypodense eosinophils are not necessarily activated in every category of eosinophil function, and activated eosinophils are not necessarily hypodense. Nonetheless, most evidence suggests that hypodensity generally represents a primed or partially activated phenotype.

Phenotypic Changes of Activated Eosinophils

An interesting feature of the eosinophil is its ability to express receptors de novo after prolonged culture with certain cytokines. For example, after culture with GM-CSF alone, IL-5 plus TNF-α, or IL-3 plus IFN-γ, eosinophils express HLA-DR antigen and increased amounts of ICAM-1, giving these eosinophils the capacity to process and present antigens to T cells.[166, 452] In fact, both murine and human eosinophils can function as HLA-DR–dependent, MHC-restricted antigen-presenting cells in stimulating proliferation of human T cells or T-cell clones in vitro.[90, 452] Surface expression of the IL-2 receptor α chain (p55, CD25) increased during culture of normal eosinophils with GM-CSF.[330] In vitro stimulation of peripheral blood eosinophils with various hemopoietins, such as IL-3, IL-5, and GM-CSF, induced the expression of an early activation antigen, CD69,[170] and up-regulation of the expression of the β2 integrin, CD11b.[169] Interestingly, eosinophils that had transmigrated through an endothelial cell monolayer in vitro showed further up-regulation of CD11b.[429]

Eosinophils from patients with asthma or allergy show similar phenotypic changes to those activated in vitro. For example, peripheral blood eosinophils from patients with asthma overexpress an adhesion molecule, CD11b.[167] Eosinophils in sputa or BAL fluids from patients with asthma express ICAM-1, CD69, and human histocompatibility HLA-DR, all of which are not normally expressed on blood eosinophils.[165, 170, 354] After allergen challenge, eosinophils in BAL fluids from patients with allergic asthma show even more dramatic changes. These eosinophils, compared with blood eosinophils, show up-regulation of CD11b, CD11c, CD69, and a granule-associated antigen, CD63, and down-regulation of L-selectin, suggesting a degranulation activity in vivo.[266, 267] In contrast, the levels of CD32, CD11a, and CD45 seem to show no change and remain similar between the blood and BAL eosinophils.[234] Thus eosinophils from patients with asthma, especially those derived from the lungs, show some activated phenotypes, and these phenotypic changes may be associated with functional activation.

Concept and Mechanism of Priming

The best example of priming is the eosinophil's response to the chemotactic peptide, FMLP. The eosinophil respiratory burst is induced by FMLP, using two different mechanisms. First, at high concentrations, FMLP by itself can cause a respiratory burst in eosinophils.[473] Second, with suboptimal concentrations of FMLP, the respiratory burst is markedly enhanced after pretreatment of eosinophils with PAF.[484] This latter phenomenon is called priming.[224] In addition to PAF, several cytokines appear to prime eosinophils. For example, after preincubation with eosinophil growth factors, such as IL-3 and IL-5, eosinophils produced LTC_4 on stimulation by FMLP, C5a, and PAF; the FMLP-induced LTC_4 production was strikingly enhanced.[392] In contrast, normal eosinophils produce LTC_4 after stimulation with FMLP but not with C5a or PAF. Priming of eosinophils by cytokines also enhances the chemotactic and adhesion responses to chemotactic factors and chemotactic cytokines.[349, 440]

Eosinophils can also be primed in vivo. One strategy to obtain in vivo primed eosinophils is segmental allergen challenge followed by BAL in patients with upper airway allergy. Eosinophils in the BAL after allergen challenge show a greater respiratory burst and adherence response to FMLP.[354] Stimulation of these BAL eosinophils with FMLP causes a sustained elevation in $[Ca^{2+}]_i$; stimulation of blood eosinophils with FMLP causes only transient elevations in $[Ca^{2+}]_i$. Because eosinophils are exposed to the local cellular milieu consisting of cytokines, chemotactic factors, and extracellular matrix proteins before reaching their targets, priming of eosinophils is important to understand the pathophysiology of diseases.[351]

What is the mechanism of priming? Consider the model in which PAF added to eosinophils enhances their respiratory burst triggered by opsonized particles. After pretreatment with PAF, the initial respiratory response of eosinophils is sensitive to inhibition of protein kinase (PK) C (by staurosporine) and is accompanied by accumulation of diglycerides and a sustained increase in $[Ca^{2+}]_i$.[224] In contrast, eosinophils not pretreated with PAF and stimulated by opsonized particles show an initial phase of the respiratory burst that is not sensitive to staurosporine and is not accompanied by accumulation of diglycerides and changes in $[Ca^{2+}]_i$. These results suggest that PKC is involved in the priming of eosinophils with PAF. Although the processes leading to diglyceride formation and PKC activation are unknown, one can speculate that PAF and the transient increase in $[Ca^{2+}]_i$ cause the translocation of phospholipases from the cytosol to the plasma membrane, and these are needed to start diglyceride production.[348]

Similar differences in biochemical events are observed with cytokine-primed eosinophils. For example, incubation of eosinophils with IL-5 does not induce elevated $[Ca^{2+}]_i$. In contrast, preincubation of eosinophils with IL-5 and a suboptimal concentration (10 nM) of PAF induces a marked rise in $[Ca^{2+}]_i$.[75] In addition, $[Ca^{2+}]_i$-depleted eosinophils were still primed by IL-5 for a respiratory burst induced by opsonized zymosan, and this priming was accompanied by tyrosine phosphorylation of a few intracellular proteins.[420] Thus eosinophils are primed by a transient rise in $[Ca^{2+}]_i$ or the activation of tyrosine kinases, and the priming mechanism likely involves the activation of PKC. In fact, the PKC activity of BAL low-density eosinophils, as measured by the phosphorylation of a protein substrate, histone type IIIS, tends to be greater than that of BAL high-density eosinophils.[37]

EOSINOPHIL EFFECTOR FUNCTIONS

Eosinophil Degranulation

The striking feature of the eosinophil-rich inflammatory reaction is the marked deposition of granule proteins, often in the presence of relatively small numbers of intact eosinophils. However, the mechanism of eosinophil secretion in vivo is still poorly understood. Electron microscopic studies suggest that the release of granule proteins from eosinophils involves three different mechanisms: cell injury, regulated secretion, and piecemeal degranulation. The cell injury is often seen in biopsy samples from patients with hypereosinophilic syndrome, episodic angioedema with eosinophilia, bullous pemphigoid, and IgE-mediated cutaneous late-phase reactions.[112, 143a, 245a] Eosinophils display centralization of granules, plasma and organelle membrane breakage, and chromatolysis of nuclei. The regulated secretion resembles the secretion of granulated secretory cells, especially the anaphylactic degranulation of mast cells and basophils.[114] The individual granule membranes and portions of the plasma membrane fuse around the periphery of cells, and specific granule matrix and core contents are extruded through these degranulation pores. Occasionally, granule membranes may fuse with each other within the cytoplasm to form degranulation chambers. These chambers also open to the cell exterior through degranulation pores. Piecemeal degranulation is characterized by vesicular transport of granule contents and partially empty granule chambers in the cytoplasm.[114] Small, smooth membrane-bound vesicles are seen within empty granule chambers. Thus eosinophils can employ three different mechanisms to release granule proteins; however, it is unknown whether any of these degranulation mechanisms are regulated by different stimuli and signal transduction mechanisms. Most observations suggest that the cell injury (cytotoxic degranulation) occurs frequently in vivo.

Initial studies of eosinophil degranulation in vitro were performed using parasitic infection as a model. When eosinophils were incubated with antiserum-coated schistosomula of *S. mansoni,* they degranulated, as evidenced by release of MBP.[59, 60] However, investigation of eosinophil degranulation in this system was complicated by the presence of the viable worm. Therefore, large surfaces (e.g., Sepharose 4B beads) coated with immunoglobulins have been used as an in vitro model of eosinophil degranulation. Current evidence suggests that Sepharose beads coated with IgG, IgA, and sIgA stimulate eosinophil degranulation.[2, 67, 132] Among these immunoglobulins, sIgA is the most effective inducer of degranulation. Studies of antibody-dependent eosinophil killing of *S. mansoni,* making use of chimeric mouse/human antibodies, demonstrate that IgA_2 is a highly potent stimulus for eosinophils.[108] IgE also seems important for eosinophil activation. Eosinophils isolated from patients with eosinophilia degranulated in response to anti-IgE antibody or IgE-coated parasites.[65] However, it is still uncertain whether a similar response to IgE is observed with eosinophils from normal subjects or patients with allergy.

By using sera from patients with ragweed-sensitive hay fever, we found that ragweed-specific IgG, but not IgE, is important for allergen-dependent eosinophil degranulation in vitro.[202] Among the IgG subclasses tested, IgG1 and IgG3 induced eosinophil degranulation, whereas IgG4 did not. The ability of IgG2 to induce degranulation was dependent on donors of eosinophils, consistent with the expression of Fc_γRII on eosinophils and polymorphism of the Fc_γRIIA gene.[248] Furthermore, the ability of eosinophils to secrete granule proteins is markedly enhanced by priming with relatively low concentrations of soluble mediators such as chemotactic factors and cytokines. For example, IL-5, GM-CSF, and IL-3, but not IL-1, IL-2, IL-4, IL-6, and TNF, increased sIgA- or IgG-induced eosinophil degranulation.[132]

Eosinophil degranulation can also be induced by soluble stimuli. Cytokines, especially those with eosinophilopoietic activity, cause eosinophil degranulation. For example, eosinophils incubated for 4 days with IL-5 release 30% to 60% of their granule proteins.[214] GM-CSF also potently induces eosinophil degranulation after several hours of incubation when CD11b/CD18-dependent cellular adhesion is available, suggesting costimulatory effects of cytokines and adhesion molecules on eosinophil degranulation.[180] The release of granule proteins during culture with IL-5 may be an important mechanism for deposition of these cationic toxins in various diseases in which IL-5 plays a role. Eosinophil-chemotactic cytokines, such as RANTES and MIP-1α, also induce eosinophil degranulation, although the effects are less pronounced than those of IL-5 or GM-CSF.[12, 335] Interestingly, eosinophil granule proteins themselves, including MBP and EPO, stimulate eosinophils and cause degranulation in a noncytotoxic manner, suggesting an autocrine mechanism of eosinophil degranulation.[217] The other stimuli for eosinophil degranulation include the serum-opsonized zymosan,[463] FMLP,[473] lipid mediator PAF,[232] complement fragments C5a and C3a,[83, 209, 393] the naturally occurring peptides substance P and mellitin,[233] calcium ionophore A23187,[215] and PMA.[215] Although LTB_4 stimulates a respiratory burst in human and guinea pig eosinophils,[310, 387] LTB_4 does not seem to induce degranulation of eosinophils as assessed by the release of β-glucuronidase (see Table 11–3).[296]

Adhesion molecules, particularly Mac-1 ($\alpha_M\beta_2$, CD11b/CD18), likely play critical roles for eosinophil degranulation (see Table 11–1). Historically, receptor ligands immobilized to relatively large surfaces, such as IgG-coated Sepharose beads and parasites, but not particulate ligands, such as aggregated IgG and bacteria, are effective stimuli for eosinophil degranulation.[60, 189] The interaction of Mac-1 ligands on the targets with Mac-1 on the eosinophils is important in the eosinophil-mediated damage of opsonized parasites.[66] By using IgG immobilized to tissue culture plates or Sepharose beads, we found that β2 integrins, especially Mac-1, play a crucial role in the activation of eosinophils stimulated by IgG.[203] Similarly, the eosinophil functional response to PAF is greatly influenced by the availability of cellular adhesion. We found that PAF induced eosinophils to release EDN when the eosinophils were incubated in stationary wells of tissue culture plates and the degranulation was blocked by antibody against Mac-1 on eosinophils.[180] In contrast, the ability of PAF to induce eosinophil degranulation was minimal when cells were kept in suspension by continuous mixing.[180] These findings suggest that eosinophil adhesion, especially that mediated by Mac-1, plays an important role for eosinophil degranulation.

Mac-1 (CD11b/CD18) not only serves as an adhesion molecule but also may interact together with Fc_γR to trigger effector functions of eosinophils. As expected from the low affinity of Fc_γRII for IgG, the ability of freshly isolated eosinophils to form rosettes with IgG-sensitized erythrocytes (EA-IgG) is negligible.[225] In contrast, eosinophils ingest opsonized yeast organisms (with bound IgG and C3bi) as vigorously as neutrophils after stimulation by GM-CSF.[252] Addition of GM-CSF, IL-3, or IL-5 causes an increase in EA-IgG rosettes without significant change in Fc_γRII expression.[225]

The kinetics of activation of Fc_γRII binding to EA-IgG are paralleled by the activation of the binding of Mac-1 (CD11b/18) to EA-C3bi. Furthermore, binding via Fc_γRII is inhibited by anti-CD11b monoclonal antibody.[225] In addition, zymosan particles coated with either IgG or C3bi poorly induce eosinophil PAF production, whereas those coated with both IgG and C3bi strongly activate eosinophils.[421] These observations suggest that the binding activity and function of Fc_γRII on eosinophils may be regulated by Mac-1 (CD11b/18). Indeed, endothelial and epithelial cells express a Mac-1 ligand,

ICAM-1. Extracellular matrix proteins, such as fibrinogen, can serve as another ligand for Mac-1 on eosinophils. Mac-1 may therefore play a key role in the pathophysiology of diseases associated with tissue eosinophilia.

Some in vivo experiments suggest that these molecules may be important in bronchial asthma. For example, in cynomolgus monkeys that had been allergen challenged several times, anti–Mac-1 monoclonal antibody inhibited the development of BHR and reduced the levels of ECP in the BAL fluid but did not inhibit the airway eosinophilia. These results suggest that Mac-1 is not essential to eosinophil migration but may be involved in triggering eosinophil activation and mediator release.[447] Similar findings were observed with a sheep model of allergen challenge. Anti–VLA-4 inhibited the late response to allergen challenge and the development of BHR when given either by intravenous methods or by inhalation. Little difference existed between the antibody-treated animals and control animals in the recruitment of eosinophils into BAL. One explanation for this discrepancy between airway physiology and eosinophilia may be that anti–VLA-4 treatment inhibited eosinophil activation and mediator release in a manner similar to that observed with the anti–Mac-1 treatment.

Production of Lipid Mediators

Eosinophils produce the sulfidopeptides LTC_4 and LTD_4 in response to calcium ionophore A23187,[307] FMLP,[307] PAF,[55] and IgG-dependent stimuli.[358] Furthermore, eosinophils release LTC_4 on exposure to *S. mansoni* coated with parasite-specific IgE or IgG antibodies.[282] In these experiments, hypodense eosinophils (low-density eosinophils) produced LTC_4 after stimulation by both IgE- and IgG-coated schistosomula, whereas normodense eosinophils (high-density eosinophils) were not stimulated by IgE-coated schistosomula. Eosinophils from patients with asthma produced substantially larger quantities of LTC_4 than did eosinophils from normal subjects.[179] These results suggest that eosinophils produce LTC_4 in response to various physiologic and pharmacologic stimuli and that the behavior of eosinophils varies and is dependent on their source.

Furthermore, stimulated eosinophils release substantial quantities of PAF.[80, 243, 388] Analysis shows that eosinophils contain high levels of ether phospholipids (the stored precursor of PAF)—about fourfold more than neutrophils. The secretion of PAF from eosinophils is caused by stimulation with chemotactic stimuli, such as C5a, as well as zymosan and A23187.[15] PAF biosynthesis by eosinophils is increased threefold to fourfold by preincubation of eosinophils with GM-CSF for 72 hours. PAF has a number of important pharmacologic activities, such as the activation of platelets, neutrophils, and eosinophils and the induction of bronchoconstriction, suggesting possible roles for eosinophil-derived PAF in the pathophysiology of bronchial asthma.

The synthesis of lipid mediators is tightly regulated by intracellular calcium concentration. Stimulation of $[^3H]$AA-labeled guinea pig eosinophils with calcium ionophore A23187 resulted in the release of AA in parallel to the hydrolysis of endogenous phosphatidylcholine (PC).[89] This ionophore-induced AA release was inhibited by the chelation of intracellular calcium, but not extracellular calcium, suggesting that PLA_2 activity is dependent on the mobilization of intracellular calcium.

INTRACELLULAR MECHANISM OF EOSINOPHIL ACTIVATION

The receptor ligation of eosinophils activates several second messengers, including cAMP, inositol triphosphate (IP_3), intracellular calcium ($[Ca^{2+}]_i$), diacylglycerol (DAG), phosphatidic acid (PA), and AA (Fig. 11–2). These second messengers activate target enzymes, which, in turn, lead to the effector functions of eosinophils. In addition to these second messengers, eosinophils also possess a variety of serine/threonine kinases (e.g., PKC) and tyrosine kinases.[182] Many of these kinases are targets for specific second messengers; conversely, these kinases can regulate production of second messengers. Thus the activation of kinases and production of second messengers are important events for transducing signals and functions of eosinophils.

Phospholipases

Some of the second messengers are generated, either directly or indirectly, as a consequence of the activation of phospholipases. The phospholipases that are involved in eosinophil activation include PLA_2, which hydrolyses phosphatidylcholine (PC) and/or phosphatidylethanolamine (PE) to produce AA and lyso PC and/or lyso PE; phospholipase C (PLC), which hydrolyses phosphatidylinositol-4,5-bisphosphate (PIP_2) to produce DAG and inositol triphosphate (IP_3); and phospholipase D (PLD), which hydrolyses PC to produce PA and choline.[182] In eosinophils, there are several lines of evidence to suggest that all of these enzymes are involved in the activation of eosinophils.

The activity of PLA_2 was first confirmed in guinea pig eosinophils.[89] Later, the respiratory burst of bovine eosinophils was shown to be enhanced by AA and inhibited by a PLA_2 inhibitor.[10] Similarly, PLA_2 inhibitors inhibited degranulation, LTC_4 production, and respiratory burst of human eosinophils stimulated by FMLP plus cytochalasin B.[460] The effects of the PLA_2 inhibitor were reversed by the addition of AA. Thus PLA_2 may activate the eosinophil secretory process by either directly acting on eosinophils or inducing the generation of bioactive AA and phospholipid metabolites, such as PAF.

In numerous receptor systems, ligand binding triggers a rapid increase in phosphoinositide hydrolysis induced by PLC activation.[74] PLC-mediated hydrolysis of PIP_2 generates two second messengers, IP_3 and DAG, which, in turn, trigger $[Ca^{2+}]_i$ mobilization and PKC activation, respectively (see Fig. 11–2).[1] Several agonists, including PAF, LTB_4, C5a, and cross-linking of $Fc_\gamma R$ by anti-IgG $F(ab')_2$, elicited a rapid and transient increase in IP_3 in murine eosinophils, suggesting that PLC is activated after receptor ligation of eosinophils.[88, 230, 231] In human eosinophils, secretory IgA and IgG immobilized to Sepharose 4B beads and FMLP caused hydrolysis of PIP_2. Conversely, inhibition of PLC activity by neomycin resulted in inhibition of both IP_3 and LTC_4 production in murine eosinophils.[88] Similarly, treatment of human eosinophils with pertussis toxin inhibited both degranulation and

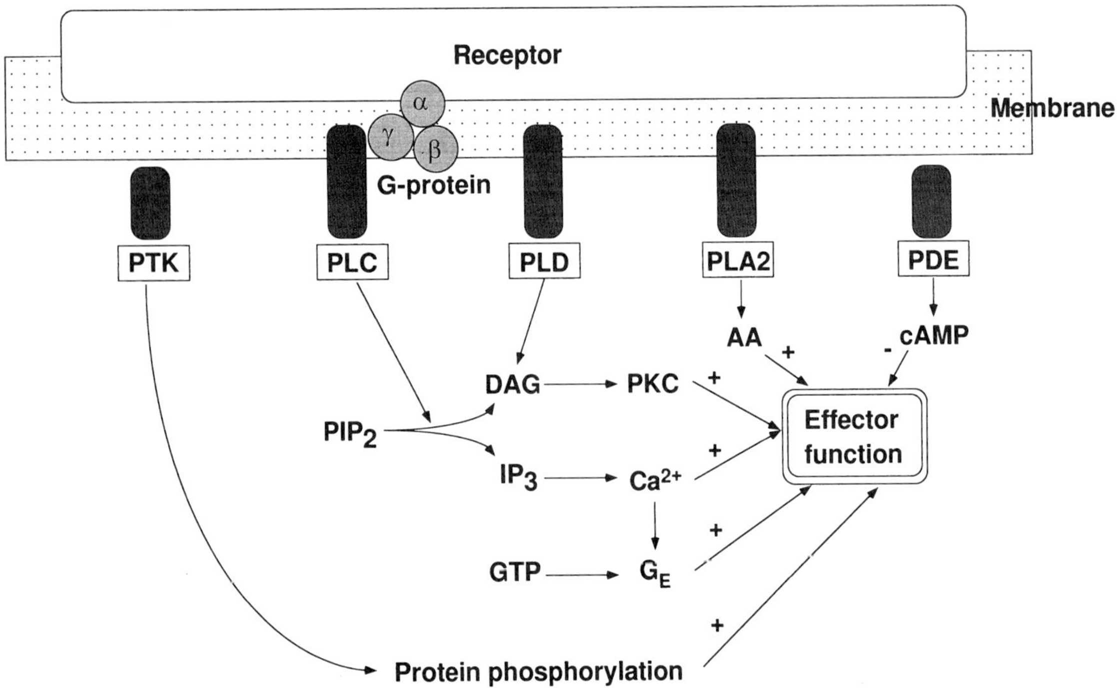

FIGURE 11–2. The intracellular mechanism of eosinophil activation. PTK = protein tyrosine kinase; PLC = phospholipase C; PLD = phospholipase D; PLA2 = phospholipase A2; PDE = phosphodiesterase; PIP_2 = phosphatidylinositol-4,5-bisphosphate; DAG = diacylglycerol; IP_3 = inositol triphosphate; PKC = protein kinase C; AA = arachidonic acid; cAMP = cyclic adenosine monophosphate; G protein = GTP-binding protein; G_E = G protein associated with exocytosis.

IP_3 production of eosinophils stimulated by sIgA- and IgG-coated Sepharose beads.[214] Thus PLC likely plays an important role for the activation of eosinophils.

The activation of PLD generates PA and choline from cellular PC, and the resultant PA is then dephosphorylated by PA phosphohydrolase to form DAG (see Fig. 11–2). There is evidence to suggest that PLD in eosinophils can also be activated following receptor ligation and involved in the zymosan-induced respiratory burst of human eosinophils.[224, 274]

Cyclic AMP (cAMP)

The activation of adenylate cyclase, generation of cAMP, and subsequent activation of protein kinase A (PKA) are known to regulate activities of various types of cells. Although PKA and its substrate are still not identified in eosinophils, pharmacologic evidence suggests that cAMP is playing an important regulatory role in eosinophil function (see Fig. 11–2). Human eosinophils possess a homogeneous population of β2-adrenoreceptors with very high affinity (K_d ~ 26 pM, 4,300 sites per cell).[480] These data are compatible with the finding that a selective β-adrenoreceptor agonist, salbutamol, induced the elevation of intracellular cAMP in human eosinophils.[213, 480] Functionally, β-adrenoreceptor agonists suppressed eosinophil function.[213, 327] The inhibitory effects of β-adrenoreceptor agonists were potentiated by a phosphodiesterase (PDE) inhibitor, supporting the evidence that these compounds are both acting on the adenylate cyclase system.[213] The inhibitory effects of the adenylate cyclase system on eosinophil function are further supported by lipophilic cAMP analogues.[213]

Cyclic nucleotide-PDE hydrolyses the 3′-ribose phosphate bond of 3′,5′-cyclic monophosphate to form the biologically inert 5′-nucleoside monophosphates. Guinea pig eosinophils express predominantly a high-affinity, membrane-bound cAMP PDE with the characteristics of a PDE IV.[374] Drugs that have been categorized as PDE IV antagonists (rolipram and denbufylline) potently increase intracellular cAMP concentration, ablate the respiratory burst, diminish PAF-induced Ca^{2+} mobilization, and decrease degranulation of guinea pig eosinophils.[95, 374, 375] Nonselective PDE inhibitors, such as theophylline, also showed inhibitory effects on eosinophil function.[213, 479] Furthermore, a potent PDE inhibitor, 3-isobutyl-1-methylxanthine (IBMX), inhibited sIgA- and IgG-induced eosinophil degranulation.[213] Thus PDE inhibitors, especially PDE IV inhibitors, down-regulate the various effector functions of eosinophils. With the advent of molecular biology, evidence now available suggests the presence of 20 to 30 different mammalian PDE isoenzymes. Although the precise significance and tissue/cell localization of these isoenzymes are still unknown, this diversity provides a unique therapeutic opportunity for the highly selective PDE inhibitors to dampen the functions of specific cells, such as eosinophils.

Protein Kinases and Protein Phosphorylation

Protein phosphorylation is one of the mechanisms that cells use to respond to extracellular signals. A number of eosinophil intracellular proteins are phosphorylated following receptor-mediated or nonreceptor-mediated stimulation of eosinophils.[328] The incorporation of ^{32}P into the protein bands of low-density eosinophils is more intense than that of the high-density eosinophils from the same individuals, suggesting that protein phosphorylation depends on the activation stage of the cells.[236]

Among the various phosphorylation events involved in the activation of cells, tyrosine phosphorylation initiated by protein-tyrosine kinase (PTK) is recognized as a critical event in a variety of cellular signaling pathways.[69, 315] Protein tyrosine phosphorylation also seems to be an early physiologic change in activated eosinophils. Stimulation of eosinophils with sIgA or IgG immobilized to Sepharose beads rapidly induces the tyrosine phosphorylation of a number of eosinophil proteins within several minutes after stimulation.[205] A number of intracellular proteins, including MAP kinase, Jak-2 (a tyrosine kinase), and STAT-1 (a nuclear factor), were tyrosine phosphorylated during activation of eosinophils by IL-3, IL-5, or GM-CSF.[38, 313, 420]

Furthermore, tyrosine phosphorylation of proteins is likely important in the effector functions of eosinophils. For example, tyrosine phosphorylation was blocked by PTK inhibitors, such as genistein and herbimycin A, and the ability of eosinophils to degranulate in response to immobilized sIgA and IgG was abolished.[205] Conversely, when the tyrosine phosphorylation of eosinophil proteins was enhanced by the tyrosine phosphatase inhibitor pervanadate, eosinophil degranulation was enhanced.[205] Tyrosine kinases also seem to be involved in the signaling of eosinophils stimulated by growth factors. Survival of eosinophils induced by IL-5 and GM-CSF was inhibited by genistein and herbimycin A.[181, 476] Conversely, increased tyrosine phosphorylation using the protein-tyrosine-phosphatase inhibitor phenylarsine oxide induced prolonged survival of eosinophils in the absence of exogenous cytokines.[476] Furthermore, the activity of PLC was inhibited by genistein and enhanced by pervanadate, suggesting that tyrosine kinases are involved in early signal transduction of eosinophils.[205] These observations suggest that PTK is activated when eosinophils are stimulated with immobilized Ig or growth factors and that protein tyrosine phosphorylation likely plays a critical role in eosinophil functions, such as degranulation and survival. More studies are needed to identify the specific PTK coupled to the specific receptor and function of eosinophils.

PKC is a serine/threonine kinase and a target for most of the known second messengers generated in leukocytes (e.g., Ca^{2+}, DAG, PA, and AA). PKC is a family of eight isoforms, and the β isoform of PKC, but not α or γ, was detected in eosinophils.[37] Whereas the PKC activity of resting eosinophils is similar to that of neutrophils, low-density eosinophils have greater PKC activity than do high-density eosinophils.[37] There are several lines of indirect evidence suggesting that PKC is important for eosinophil activation. For example, the PKC activator PMA induces a variety of eosinophil functions, such as adhesion,[104] respiratory burst,[353] and degranulation.[215] Eosinophil degranulation induced by PMA is insensitive to a G protein modulator, a pertussis toxin,[215] or a tyrosine kinase inhibitor—genistein,[205] suggesting that PKC is involved either directly in the exocytosis machinery or in the distal part of eosinophil signal transduction.

Calcium and the Calcium Mobilization System

Several agonists can induce the elevation of $[Ca^{2+}]_i$ in eosinophils from various species. In guinea pig peritoneal eosinophils, the resting $[Ca^{2+}]_i$ is 120 nM and $[Ca^{2+}]_i$ increases rapidly following stimulation of the cells by PAF.[229] This effect of PAF is transient, peaking after 10 to 15 seconds of exposure, and returns to resting levels within 60 seconds.[229] In addition to PAF, LTB_4, complement fragment C5a, FMLP, and chemokines, such as RANTES and MCP3, also induce elevations in $[Ca^{2+}]_i$ in guinea pig and human eosinophils.[209, 233] This rise of $[Ca^{2+}]_i$ is likely from both the endoplasmic reticulum and extracellular milieu; mobilization into the cells is probably mediated by IP_3.[42] The rise in $[Ca^{2+}]_i$ induced by PAF is preceded by an increase in IP_3, consistent with a causal relationship of these two parameters.[231] Other agonists, including LTB_4 and C5a, also promote the accumulation of IP_3 in guinea pig eosinophils.[231]

A rise in $[Ca^{2+}]_i$ is one of the prerequisite signals for eosinophil activation. For example, in eosinophils, a calcium ionophore, A23187, induces degranulation, respiratory burst,[134, 352] and the production of LTC_4 by eosinophils.[307] In streptolysin O-permeabilized guinea pig peritoneal eosinophils, the exocytotic process depends on both $[Ca^{2+}]_i$ and a guanine nucleotide.[81] Some research suggests the importance of a gradient in $[Ca^{2+}]_i$ for the chemotaxis of eosinophils.[53] Although Ca^{2+} is likely required for the degranulation and chemotaxis of eosinophils, calcium seems to be not as critical for some other functions of the cells. For example, the shape change of eosinophils stimulated by PAF and C5a is independent of the extracellular Ca^{2+}.[209] The respiratory burst of eosinophils also can occur without the involvement of calcium.[387, 468] In the future, it will be important to characterize and differentiate the signaling involved in the different functions of eosinophils.

G Proteins

Despite advances in knowledge about the role of eosinophils in health and disease, little is known about the mechanisms that regulate their secretory processes. The introduction of the nonhydrolyzable GTP analogue GTPγS into eosinophils was shown to elicit an exocytotic degranulation of the cell, suggesting an important role of GTP-binding proteins for granule release from eosinophils.[299] This GTP-binding protein, called G_E, is likely of small molecular weight, is distinctive from the membrane-bound G proteins coupled to PLC activity, and may directly stimulate exocytotic machinery of eosinophils.[146]

Studies have defined transmembrane receptors that regulate various second messenger–generating enzymes through intermediate G proteins.[140] In contrast to intracellular small G proteins, such as G_E, the G proteins implicated in receptor-mediated signaling are membrane-bound $\alpha\beta\gamma$-heterotrimers.[140] We found that the eosinophil degranulation response induced by sIgA and IgG immobilized to Sepharose 4B beads was inhibited by exposure of eosinophils to pertussis toxin, which specifically disrupts certain heterotrimeric G proteins.[215] A 41-kD protein representing a G protein α subunit (possibly G_{i2}-α) was found in human eosinophils.[11, 215] In addition, several other agonists utilize a pertussis toxin–sensitive G protein, including FMLP, PAF,[96] C5a,[393] RANTES,[119] and C3a[119] in eosinophils.

It seems clear that the functions of eosinophils, similar to other leukocytes, are regulated by various molecules, including phospholipases, secondary and tertiary messengers, G proteins, and protein phosphorylation (see Fig. 11–2). Further refinement of biochemical and pharmacologic techniques together with the application of molecular biology will allow better understanding of the receptors and signal transduction unique to eosinophils, and possibly the development of pharmacologic tools capable of attenuating the activation of the cells.

SUMMARY

The realization that eosinophils release proinflammatory mediators, such as PAF and eicosanoids, and the observation that eosinophil granule proteins are potent toxins and cytostimulants have led to a consensus that eosinophils are major effector cells for tissue damage in bronchial asthma and could cause many of the pathologic features of the disease. In bronchial asthma, cytokines and adhesion molecules appear to play important roles for eosinophil recruitment to and activation in the site of inflammation. In addition, along with advances in molecular biology and pharmacology, the mechanisms of activation and effector functions of eosinophils have been gradually elucidated. Future studies will likely shed additional light on the pathophysiologic roles of eosinophils in bronchial asthma, the mechanisms of the inflammatory process of the diseases associated with eosinophilia, and the means to disrupt the inflammatory process caused by eosinophils.

ACKNOWLEDGMENTS

The authors' studies have been supported, in part, by grants (AI 31155, AI 15231, AI 09728, AI 34577, and AI 34486) from the National Institutes of Health and by the Mayo Foundation. The authors wish to thank Cheryl Adolphson and Linda Arneson for excellent editorial and secretarial assistance in the preparation of this chapter.

REFERENCES

1. Abdel-Latif AA: Calcium-mobilizing receptors, polyphosphoinositides, and the generation of second messengers. Pharmacol Rev 38:227, 1986.
2. Abu-Ghazaleh RI, Fujisawa T, Mestecky J, et al: IgA-induced eosinophil degranulation. J Immunol 142:2393, 1989.
3. Abu-Ghazaleh RI, Gleich GJ, Prendergast FG: Interaction of eosinophil granule major basic protein with synthetic lipid bilayers: a mechanism for toxicity. J Membr Biol 128:153, 1992.
4. Ackerman SJ, Gleich GJ, Loegering DA, et al: Comparative toxicity of purified human eosinophil granule cationic proteins for schistosomula of *Schistosoma mansoni*. Am J Trop Med Hyg 34:735, 1985.
5. Ackerman SJ, Kephart GM, Habermann TM, et al: Localization of eosinophil granule major basic protein in human basophils. J Exp Med 158:946, 1983.
6. Ackerman SJ, Corrette SE, Rosenberg HF: Molecular cloning and characterization of human eosinophil Charcot-Leyden crystal protein (lysophospholipase). J Immunol 150:456, 1993.
7. Ackerman SJ, Loegering DA, Gleich GJ: The human eosinophil Charcot-Leyden crystal protein: biochemical characteristics and measurement by radioimmunoassay. J Immunol 125:2118, 1980.
8. Ackerman SJ, Weil GJ, Gleich GJ: Formation of Charcot-Leyden crystals by human basophils. J Exp Med 155:1597, 1982.
9. Ackerman SJ, Clark MA, Zhou Z, et al: Human eosinophil lysophospholipase (Charcot-Leyden crystal protein): molecular cloning, expression, and potential functions in asthma. In Gleich GJ, Kay AB (eds): Eosinophils in Allergy and Inflammation. Marcel Dekker, Inc, New York, 1994, pp 21–54.
10. Aebischer CP, Pasche I, Jorg A: Nanomolar arachidonic acid influences the respiratory burst in eosinophils and neutrophils induced by GTP-binding protein. A comparative study of the respiratory burst in bovine eosinophils and neutrophils. Eur J Biochem 218:669, 1993.
11. Agrawal DK, Ali N, Numao T: PAF receptors and G-proteins in human blood eosinophils. J Lipid Mediat 5:101, 1992.
12. Alam R, Stafford S, Forsythe P, et al: RANTES is a chemotactic and activating factor for human eosinophils. J Immunol 150:3442, 1993.
13. Alam R, Forsythe P, Stafford S, et al: Transforming growth factor beta abrogates the effects of hematopoietins on eosinophils and induces their apoptosis. J Exp Med 179:1041, 1994.
14. Andersen V, Bro-Rasmussen F: Autoradiographic studies of the kinetics of eosinophils. Semin Hematol 1:33, 1968.
15. Anwar ARE, Kay AB: Membrane receptors for IgG and complement (C4, C3b and C3d) on human eosinophils and neutrophils and their relation to eosinophilia. J Immunol 119:976, 1977.
16. Anwar AR, Moqbel R, Walsh GM, et al: Adhesion to fibronectin prolongs eosinophil survival. J Exp Med 177:839, 1993.
17. Anwar AR, Walsh GM, Cromwell O, et al: Adhesion to fibronectin primes eosinophils via alpha 4 beta 1 (VLA-4). Immunology 82:222, 1994.
18. Archer GR, Hirsch JG: Isolation of granules from eosinophil leucocytes and study of their enzyme content. J Exp Med 118:277, 1963.
19. Archer GT, Blackwood A: Formation of Charcot-Leyden crystals in human eosinophils and basophils and study of the composition of isolated crystals. J Exp Med 122:173, 1965.
20. Archer RK: The Eosinophil Leukocytes. FA Davis Co, Philadelphia, 1963, p 205.
21. Ayars GH, Altman LC, Gleich GJ, et al: Eosinophil- and eosinophil granule-mediated pneumocyte injury. J Allergy Clin Immunol 76:595, 1985.
22. Ayars GH, Altman LC, McManus MM, et al: Injurious effect of the eosinophil peroxide-hydrogen peroxide-halide system and major basic protein on human nasal epithelium in vitro. Am Rev Respir Dis 140:125, 1989.
23. Babior BM, Kipnes RS, Curnette JT: Biological defense mechanisms: the production by leukocytes of superoxide, a potential bactericidal agent. J Clin Invest 52:741, 1973.
24. Bach MK, Brashler JR: FMLP is a potent activator of guinea pig eosinophils but its activity is dependent on the prior overnight in vitro culture of the cells (facilitation). Immunology 75:680, 1992.
25. Bach MK, Brashler JR, Petzold EN, et al: Superoxide production by human eosinophils can be inhibited in an agonist-selective manner. Agents Actions 35:1, 1992.
26. Baehner RL, Johnston RB Jr: Metabolic and bactericidal activities of human eosinophils. Br J Haematol 20:277, 1971.
27. Bainton DF, Farquhar MG: Segregation and packaging of granule enzymes in eosinophilic leukocytes. J Cell Biol 45:54, 1970.
28. Baker JR, Bassett EG, de Souza P: Eosinophils in healing dermal wounds. J Anat 121:401a, 1976. Abstract.
29. Barker RL, Gundel RH, Gleich GJ, et al: Acidic polyamino acids inhibit human eosinophil granule major basic protein toxicity: evidence of a functional role for proMBP. J Clin Invest 88:798, 1991.
30. Barker RL, Loegering DA, Ten RM, et al: Eosinophil cationic protein cDNA. Comparison with other toxic cationic proteins and ribonucleases. J Immunol 143:952, 1989.
31. Barker RL, Gleich GJ, Pease LR: Acidic precursor revealed in human eosinophil granule major basic protein cDNA. J Exp Med 168:1493, 1988.
32. Baskar P, Silberstein DS, Pincus SH: Inhibition of IgG-triggered human eosinophil function by IL-4. J Immunol 144:2321, 1990.
33. Baskar P, Pincus SH: Selective regulation of eosinophil degranulation by interleukin 1 beta. Proc Soc Exp Biol Med 199:249, 1992.
34. Bass DA, Lewis JC, Szejda P, et al: Activation of lysosomal acid phosphatase of eosinophil leukocytes. Lab Invest 44:403, 1981.
35. Bass DA, Grover WH, Lewis JC, et al: Comparison of human eosinophils from normals and patients with eosinophilia. J Clin Invest 66:1265, 1980.
36. Basten A, Beeson PB: Mechanism of eosinophilia. II. Role of the lymphocyte. J Exp Med 131:1288, 1970.
37. Bates ME, Bertics PJ, Calhoun WJ, et al: Increased protein kinase C activity in low density eosinophils. J Immunol 150:4486, 1993.

38. Bates ME, Bertics PJ, Busse WW: IL-5 induces tyrosine (Y) phosphorylation of peripheral blood eosinophil (EOS) proteins including a 45-kDa protein immunoreactive with MAP-kinase antibodies. J Allergy Clin Immunol 93:268, 1994.
39. Begley CG, Lopez AF, Nicola NA, et al: Purified colony-stimulating factors enhance the survival of human neutrophils and eosinophils in vitro: a rapid and sensitive microassay for colony-stimulating factors. Blood 68:162, 1986.
40. Beintema JJ, Hofsteenge J, Iwama M, et al: Amino acid sequence of the nonsecretory ribonuclease of human urine. Biochemistry 27:4530, 1988.
41. Bentley AM, Meng Q, Robinson DS, et al: Increases in activated T lymphocytes, eosinophils, and cytokine mRNA expression for interleukin-5 and granulocyte/macrophage colony-stimulating factor in bronchial biopsies after allergen inhalation challenge in atopic asthmatics. Am J Respir Cell Mol Biol 8:35, 1993.
42. Berridge MJ: Inositol triphosphate and diacylglycerol: two interacting second messengers. Annu Rev Biochem 56:159, 1987.
43. Bevilacqua MP: Endothelial-leukocyte adhesion molecules (review). Annu Rev Immunol 11:767, 1993.
44. Bisgaard H, Helqvist S, Boudet L, et al: Chemotactic activity of LTB_4 in man. Allergy 41:365, 1986.
45. Bochner BS, Luscinskas FW, Gimbrone MA Jr, et al: Adhesion of human basophils, eosinophils and neutrophils to IL-1-activated human vascular endothelial cells: contribution of endothelial cell adhesion molecules. J Exp Med 173:1553, 1991.
46. Bochner BS, Sterbinsky SA, Bickel CA, et al: Differences between human eosinophils and neutrophils in the function and expression of sialic acid-containing counterligands for E-selectin. J Immunol 152:774, 1994.
47. Bolscher BGJM, Plat H, Wever R: Some properties of human eosinophil peroxidase, a comparison with other peroxidases. Biochim Biophys Acta 784:177, 1984.
48. Bos AJ, Wever R, Hamers MN, et al: Some enzymatic characteristics of eosinophil peroxidase from patients with eosinophilia and from healthy donors. Infect Immun 32:427, 1981.
49. Boyce JA, Friend D, Matsumoto R, et al: Differentiation in vitro of hybrid eosinophil basophil granulocytes—autocrine function of an eosinophil developmental intermediate. J Exp Med 182:49, 1995.
50. Brofman JD, White SR, Blake JS, et al: Epithelial augmentation of trachealis contraction caused by major basic protein of eosinophils. J Appl Physiol 66:1867, 1989.
51. Broide DH, Paine MM, Firestein GS: Eosinophils express interleukin 5 and granulocyte macrophage-colony-stimulating factor mRNA at sites of allergic inflammation in asthmatics. J Clin Invest 90:1414, 1992.
52. Broxmeyer HE, Lu L, Platzer E, et al: Comparative analysis of the influences of human γ, α, and β interferons on human multipotential (CFU-GEMM), erythroid (BFU-E) and granulocyte-macrophage (CFU-GM) progenitor cells. J Immunol 131:1300, 1983.
53. Brundage RA, Fogarty KE, Tuft RA, et al: Calcium gradients underlying polarization and chemotaxis of eosinophils. Science 254:703, 1991.
54. Bruijnzeel PLB, Kuijper PH, Rihs S, et al: Eosinophil migration in atopic dermatitis. I: increased migratory responses to N-formyl-methionyl-leucyl-phenylalanine, neutrophil-activating factor, platelet-activating factor, and platelet factor 4. J Invest Dermatol 100:137, 1993.
55. Bruijnzeel PLB, Kok PT, Hamelink ML, et al: Platelet-activating factor induces leukotriene C_4 synthesis by purified human eosinophils. Prostaglandins 34:205, 1987.
56. Burke LA, Crea AE, Wilkinson JR, et al: Comparison of the generation of platelet-activating factor and leukotriene C_4 in human eosinophils stimulated by unopsonized zymosan and by the calcium ionophore A23187: the effects of nedocromil sodium. J Allergy Clin Immunol 85:26, 1990.
57. Butterfield JH, Leiferman KM, Abrams J, et al: Elevated serum levels of interleukin-5 in patients with the syndrome of episodic angioedema and eosinophilia. Blood 79:688, 1992.
58. Butterfield JH, Gleich GJ: Interferon-α treatment of six patients with the idiopathic hypereosinophilic syndrome. Ann Intern Med 121:648, 1994.
59. Butterworth AE, Wassom DL, Gleich GJ, et al: Damage to schistosomula of *Schistosoma mansoni* induced directly by eosinophil major basic protein. J Immunol 122:221, 1979.
60. Butterworth AE, Vadas MA, Wassom DL, et al: Interactions between human eosinophils and schistosomules of *Schistosoma mansoni*. II. The mechanism of irreversible eosinophil adherence. J Exp Med 150:1456, 1979.
61. Capron M, Kusnierz JP, Prin L, et al: Cytophilic IgE on human blood and tissue eosinophils: detection by flow microfluorometry. J Immunol 134:3013, 1985.
62. Capron M, Kusnierz JP, Prin L, et al: Cytophilic IgE on human blood and tissue eosinophils. Int Arch Allergy Appl Immunol 77:246, 1985.
63. Capron M, Capron A, Dessaint JP, et al: Fc receptors for IgE on human and rat eosinophils. J Immunol 126:2087, 1981.
64. Capron M, Jouault T, Prin L, et al: Functional study of a monoclonal antibody to immunoglobulin E Fc receptor of eosinophils, platelets and macrophages. J Exp Med 164:72, 1986.
65. Capron M, Spiegelberg HL, Prin L, et al: Role of IgE receptors in effector function of human eosinophils. J Immunol 132:462, 1984.
66. Capron M, Kazatchkine MD, Fisher E, et al: Functional role of the α-chain of complement receptor type 3 in human eosinophil-dependent antibody-mediated cytotoxicity against schistosomes. J Immunol 139:2059, 1987.
67. Capron MM, Tomassini M, Van Der Vorst E, et al: Existence and function of receptor for immunoglobulin A on human eosinophils. CR Acad Sci III 307:397, 1989.
68. Caulfield JP, Hein A, Rothenberg ME, et al: A morphometric study of normodense and hypodense human eosinophils that are derived in vivo and in vitro. Am J Pathol 137:27, 1990.
69. Chan AC, Desai DM, Weiss A: The role of protein tyrosine kinases and protein tyrosine phosphatases in T cell antigen receptor signal transduction. Annu Rev Immunol 12:555, 1994.
70. Changehan PS, Fearon DT: Tissue-specific phosphorylation of complement receptors CR1 and CR2. J Exp Med 163:101, 1986.
71. Chihara J, Plumas J, Gruart V, et al: Characterization of a receptor for interleukin 5 on human eosinophils: variable expression and induction by granulocyte-macrophage colony-stimulating factor. J Exp Med 172:1347, 1990.
72. Clark RAF, Gallin JI, Kaplan AP: The selective eosinophil chemotactic activity of histamine. J Exp Med 142:1462, 1975.
73. Clark EA, Brugge JS: Integrins and signal transduction pathways: the road taken (review). Science 268:233, 1995.
74. Cockcroft S: G-protein-regulated phospholipase C, D and A_2 mediated signalling in neutrophils. Biochim Biophys Acta 1113:135, 1992.
75. Coeffier E, Joseph D, Vargaftig BB: Activation of guinea pig eosinophils by human recombinant IL-5: selective priming to platelet-activating factor-acether and interference of its antagonists. J Immunol 147: 2595, 1991.
76. Coeffier E, Joseph D, Vargaftig BB: LTB_4, a potent chemotactic factor for purified guinea-pig eosinophils: interference of PAF-acether antagonists. Int J Immunopharmacol 13:273, 1991.
77. Coffman RL, Seymour MW, Hudak S, et al: Antibody to interleukin-5 inhibits helminth-induced eosinophilia in mice. Science 245:308, 1989.
78. Costa JJ, Matossian K, Resnick MB, et al: Human eosinophils can express the cytokines tumor necrosis factor-α and macrophage inflammatory protein-1α. J Clin Invest 91:2673, 1993.
79. Coyle AJ, Ackerman SJ, Burch R, et al: Human eosinophil-granule major basic protein and synthetic polycations induce airway hyperresponsiveness in vivo dependent on bradykinin generation. J Clin Invest 95:1735, 1995.
80. Cromwell O, Wardlaw AJ, Champion A, et al: IgG dependent generation of platelet-activating factor by normal and low density human eosinophils. J Immunol 145:3862, 1990.
81. Cromwell O, Bennett JP, Hide I, et al: Mechanisms of granule enzyme secretion from permeabilized guinea-pig eosinophils. Dependence on Ca^{2+} and guanine nucleotide. J Immunol 147:1905, 1991.
82. Cruikshank WW, Berman JS, Theodore AC, et al: Lymphokine activation of $T4^+$ T lymphocytes and monocytes. J Immunol 138:3817, 1987.
83. Daffern PJ, Pfeifer PH, Ember JA, et al: C3a is a chemotaxin for human eosinophils but not for neutrophils. 1. C3a stimulation of neutrophils is secondary to eosinophil activation. J Exp Med 181:2119, 1995.
84. Dahinden CA, Geisen T, Bunner T, et al: Monocyte chemotactic protein 3 is a most effective basophil- and eosinophil-activating chemokine. J Exp Med 179:751, 1994.
85. Baggiolini M, Dahinden CA: CC chemokines in allergic inflammation. Immunol Today 15:127, 1994.
86. Das AM, Williams TJ, Lobb R, et al: Lung eosinophilia is dependent

on IL-5 and the adhesion molecules CD18 and VLA-4, in a guinea-pig model. Immunology 84:41, 1995.

87. Davis WB, Fells GA, Sun XH, et al: Eosinophil-mediated injury to lung parenchymal cells and interstitial matrix. J Clin Invest 74:269, 1984.
88. De Andres B, Del Pozo V, Cardaba B, et al: Phosphoinositide breakdown is associated with Fc-$_{\gamma}$RII mediated activation of 5′-lipoxygenase in murine eosinophils. J Immunol 146:1566, 1991.
89. Debbaghi A, Hidi R, Vargaftig BB, et al: Inhibition of phospholipase A2 activity in guinea pig eosinophils by human recombinant IL-1 beta. J Immunol 149:1374, 1992.
90. Del Pozo V, De Andres B, Martin E, et al: Eosinophil as antigen-presenting cell: activation of T cell clones and T cell hybridoma by eosinophils after antigen processing. Eur J Immunol 22:1919, 1992.
91. Del Pozo V, De Andres B, Martin E, et al: Murine eosinophils and IL-1: α IL-1 mRNA detection by in situ hybridization. Production and release of IL-1 from peritoneal eosinophils. J Immunol 144:3117, 1990.
92. Denburg JA, Telizyn S, Messner H, et al: Heterogeneity of human peripheral blood eosinophil-type colonies: evidence for a common basophil-eosinophil progenitor. Blood 66:312, 1985.
93. Dennis EA, Rhee SG, Billah MM, et al: Role of phospholipases in generating lipid second messengers in signal transduction. FASEB J 5:2068, 1991.
94. Dent G, Ukena D, Chanez P, et al: Characterization of platelet activating factor (PAF) receptors on human neutrophils and eosinophils. Am Rev Respir Dis 137:A236, 1988.
95. Dent G, Giembycz MA, Rabe KF, et al: Inhibition of eosinophil cyclic nucleotide PDE activity and opsonized zymosan-stimulated respiratory burst by 'type IV'-selective PDE inhibitor. Br J Pharmacol 103:1339, 1991.
96. Dent G, Barnes PJ: Platelet activating factor stimulates a pertussis toxin-sensitive GTPase activity in guinea-pig eosinophil membrane. Br J Pharmacol 104:86P, 1991.
97. Dent LA, Strath M, Mellor AL, et al: Eosinophilia in transgenic mice expressing interleukin 5. J Exp Med 172:1425, 1990.
98. DeSimone C, Donnelli G, Meli D, et al: Human eosinophils and parasitic diseases. II. Characterization of two cell fractions isolated at different densities. Clin Exp Immunol 48:249, 1982.
99. Desreumaux P, Janin A, Colombel JF, et al: Interleukin 5 messenger RNA expression by eosinophils in the intestinal mucosa of patients with coeliac disease. J Exp Med 175:293, 1992.
100. Dessein AJ, Lee TH, Elsas P, et al: Enhancement by monokines of leukotriene generation by human eosinophils and neutrophils stimulated with calcium ionophore A23187. J Immunol 136:3829, 1986.
101. Di Prisco MC, Perez M: Surface IgE and phagocytic activity of eosinophils from patients with American cutaneous leishmaniasis: relation to cell density. J Invest Allergol Clin Immunol 1:253, 1991.
102. Diamond MS, Springer TA: The dynamic regulation of integrin adhesiveness (review). Curr Biol 4:506, 1994.
103. Donahue RE, Seehra J, Metzger M, et al: Human IL-3 and GM-CSF act synergistically in stimulating hematopoiesis in primates. Science 241:1820, 1988.
104. Dobrina A, Menegazzi R, Carlos TM, et al: Mechanisms of eosinophil adherence to cultured vascular endothelial cells: eosinophils bind to the cytokine-induced endothelial ligand vascular cell adhesion molecule-1 via the very late antigen-4 integrin receptor. J Clin Invest 88:20, 1991.
105. Dresch C, Johnson GR, Metcalf D: Eosinophil colony formation in semisolid cultures of human bone marrow cells. Blood 49:835, 1977.
106. Dri P, Cramer R, Spessotto P, et al: Eosinophil activation on biologic surfaces: production of oxygen in response to physiologic soluble stimuli is differentially modulated by extracellular matrix components and endothelial cells. J Immunol 147:613, 1991.
107. Dubucquoi SP, Desreumaux P, Janin A, et al: Interleukin 5 synthesis by eosinophils: association with granules and immunoglobulin-dependent secretion. J Exp Med 179:703, 1994.
108. Dunne DW, Richardson BA, Jones FM, et al: The use of mouse/human chimaeric antibodies to investigate the roles of different antibody isotypes, including IgA_2, in the killing of *Schistosoma mansoni* schistosomula by eosinophils. Parasite Immunol 15:181, 1993.
109. Durack DT, Sumi SM, Klebanoff SJ: Neurotoxicity of human eosinophils. Proc Natl Acad Sci USA 76:1443, 1979.
110. Durham SR, Kay AB: Eosinophils, bronchial hyperreactivity and late-phase asthmatic reactions. Clin Allergy 40:411, 1985.
111. Dvorak AM, Furitsu T, Letourneau L, et al: Mature eosinophils stimulated to develop in human cord blood mononuclear cell cultures supplemented with recombinant human interleukin-5: Part I. Piecemeal degranulation of specific granules and distribution of Charcot-Leyden crystal protein. Am J Pathol 138:69, 1991.
112. Dvorak AM, Weller PF, Monahan-Earley RA, et al: Ultrastructural localization of Charcot-Leyden crystal protein, lysophospholipase, and peroxidase in macrophages, eosinophils, and extracellular matrix of the skin in the hypereosinophilic syndrome. Lab Invest 62:590, 1990.
113. Dvorak AM, Letourneau L, Login GR, et al: Ultrastructural localization of the Charcot-Leyden crystal protein, lysophospholipase, to a distinct crystalloid-free granule population in mature human eosinophils. Blood 72:150, 1988.
114. Dvorak AM, Furitsu T, Estrella P, et al: Ultrastructural localization of major basic protein in the human eosinophil lineage in vitro. J Histochem Cytochem 42:1443, 1994.
115. Ebisawa M, Bochner BS, Georas SN, et al: Eosinophil transendothelial migration induced by cytokines. I. Role of endothelial and eosinophil adhesion molecules in IL-1β-induced transendothelial migration. J Immunol 149:4021, 1992.
116. Ebisawa M, Schleimer RP, Bickel C, et al: Phenotyping of purified peripheral blood eosinophils using the blind panel of monoclonal antibodies. In Schlossman S, Boumsell L, Gilks W, et al (eds): Leukocyte Typing V: White Cell Differentiation Antigens. Oxford University Press, Oxford, 1995, p 1036.
117. Eidinger D, Wilkinson R, Rose B: A study of cellular responses in immune reactions utilizing the skin window technique. I. Immediate hypersensitivity reaction. J Allergy 35:77, 1964.
118. Elbon CL, Jacoby DB, Fryer AD: Pretreatment with an antibody to interleukin-5 prevents loss of pulmonary M_2 muscarinic receptor function in antigen-challenged guinea pigs. Am J Respir Cell Mol Biol 12:320, 1995.
119. Elsner J, Oppermann M, Czech W, et al: C3a activates reactive oxygen radical species production and intracellular calcium transients in human eosinophils. Eur J Immunol 24:518, 1994.
120. Emerson SG, Yang YC, Clark SC, et al: Human recombinant granulocyte-macrophage colony stimulating factor and interleukin 3 have overlapping but distinct hematopoietic activities. J Clin Invest 82:1282, 1988.
121. Fadel R, Herpin-Richard N, Rihoux JP, et al: Inhibitory effect of cetirizine dihydrochloride on eosinophil migration in vivo. Clin Allergy 17:373, 1987.
122. Foegh ML, Maddox YT, Ramwell PW: Human peritoneal eosinophils and formation of arachidonate cyclooxygenase products. Scand J Immunol 23:599, 1986.
123. Fernandez HN, Henson PM, Otani A, et al: Chemotactic response to human C3a and C5a anaphylatoxins. I. Evaluation of C3a and C5a leukotaxis in vitro and under simulated in vivo conditions. J Immunol 120:109, 1978.
124. Filley WV, Holley KE, Kephart GM, et al: Identification by immunofluorescence of eosinophil granule major basic protein in lung tissues of patients with bronchial asthma. Lancet 2:11, 1982.
125. Fischer E, Capron M, Prin L, et al: Human eosinophils express CR1 and CR3 complement receptors for cleavage fragments of complement C3. Cell Immunol 97:297, 1986.
126. Flavahan NA, Slifman NR, Gleich GJ, et al: Human eosinophil major basic protein causes hyperreactivity of respiratory smooth muscle. Role of the epithelium. Am Rev Respir Dis 138:685, 1988.
127. Fleischman RA, Custer RP, Mintz B: Totipotent hematopoietic stem cells: normal self-renewal and differentiation after transplantation between mouse fetuses. Cell 30:351, 1982.
128. Foot EC: Eosinophil turnover in the normal rat. Br J Haematol 11:439, 1965.
129. Frigas E, Gleich GJ: The eosinophil and the pathophysiology of asthma. J Allergy Clin Immunol 77:527, 1986.
130. Frigas E, Loegering DA, Solley GO, et al: Elevated levels of the eosinophil granule major basic protein in the sputum of patients with bronchial asthma. Mayo Clin Proc 56:345, 1981.
131. Frigas E, Loegering DA, Gleich GJ: Cytotoxic effects of the guinea pig eosinophil major basic protein on tracheal epithelium. Lab Invest 42:35, 1980.
132. Fujisawa T, Abu-Ghazaleh R, Kita H, et al: Regulatory effect of cytokines on eosinophil degranulation. J Immunol 144:642, 1990.
132a. Fujisawa T, Kephart GM, Gray BH, et al: The neutrophil and chronic allergic inflammation: immunochemical localization of neutrophil elastase. Am Rev Respir Dis 141:689, 1990.

133. Fukuda T, Gleich GJ: Heterogeneity of human eosinophils. J Allergy Clin Immunol 83:369, 1989.
134. Fukuda T, Ackerman SJ, Reed CE, et al: Calcium ionophore A23187 calcium-dependent cytolytic degranulation in human eosinophils. J Immunol 135:1349, 1985.
135. Fukuda T, Dunnette S, Reed CE, et al: Increased numbers of hypodense eosinophils in the blood of patients with bronchial asthma. Am Rev Respir Dis 132:981, 1985.
136. Gearing DP, King JA, Gough NM, et al: Expression cloning of a receptor for human granulocyte-macrophage colony-stimulating factor. EMBO J 8:3667, 1989.
137. Georas SN, McIntyre BW, Ebisawa M, et al: Expression of a functional laminin receptor (alpha 6 beta 1, very late activation on antigen-6) on human eosinophils. Blood 82:2872, 1993.
138. Gerard NP, Hodges MK, Drazen JM, et al: Characterization of a receptor for C5a anaphylatoxin on human eosinophils. J Biol Chem 264:1760, 1989.
139. Ghidoni JJ, Goldberg AF: Light and electron microscopic localization of acid phosphatase activity in human eosinophils. Am J Clin Pathol 45:402, 1967.
140. Gilman AG: G proteins: transducers of receptor-generated signals. Ann Rev Biochem 56:615, 1987.
141. Gleich GJ, Loegering DA, Bell MP, et al: Biochemical and functional similarities between human eosinophil-derived neurotoxin and eosinophil cationic protein: homology with ribonuclease. Proc Natl Acad Sci USA 83:3146, 1986.
142. Gleich GJ, Loegering DA, Mann KG, et al: Comparative properties of the Charcot-Leyden crystal protein and the major basic protein from human eosinophils. J Clin Invest 57:633, 1976.
143. Gleich GJ, Frigas E, Loegering DA, et al: Cytotoxic properties of the eosinophil major basic protein. J Immunol 123:2925, 1979.
143a. Gleich GJ, Schroeter AL, Marcoux JP, et al: Episodic angioedema associated with eosinophilia. N Engl J Med 310:1621, 1984.
144. Gleich GJ: The eosinophil and bronchial asthma: current understanding. Review article. J Allergy Clin Immunol 85:422, 1990.
145. Goetzl EJ, Austen KF: Purification and synthesis of eosinophilotactic tetrapeptides of human lung tissue: identification as eosinophil chemotactic factor of anaphylaxis. Proc Natl Acad Sci USA 2:4123, 1975.
146. Gomperts BD: G_E: a GTP-binding protein mediating exocytosis. Annu Rev Physiol 52:591, 1990.
147. Gounnl AS, Lamkhloued B, Ochiai K, et al: High-affinity IgE receptor on eosinophils is involved in defence against parasites. Nature 367:183, 1994.
148. Grangette C, Gruart V, Ouaissi MA, et al: IgE receptor on human eosinophils, $Fc_\epsilon RII$: comparison with B cell CD23 and association with an adhesion molecule. J Immunol 143:3580, 1989.
149. Graziano RF, Looney RJ, Shen L, et al: $Fc_\gamma R$-mediated killing by eosinophils. J Immunol 142, 230, 1989.
150. Groopman JE, Mitsuyasu RT, DeLeo MJ: Effect of recombinant human granulocyte-macrophage colony-stimulating factor on myelopoiesis in the acquired immunodeficiency syndrome. N Engl J Med 317:593, 1987.
151. Gross R: The eosinophils. In Braunsteiner H, Zucker-Franklin D (eds): The Physiology and Pathology of Leukocytes. Grune & Stratton, Inc, New York, 1962.
152. Gruart V, Ballol JM, Prin L, et al: Variations in protein expression related to human eosinophil heterogeneity. J Immunol 142:4416, 1989.
153. Gruart V, Truong MJ, Plumas J, et al: Decreased expression of eosinophil peroxidase and major basic protein messenger RNAs during eosinophil maturation. Blood 79:2592, 1992.
154. Gundel RH, Wegner CD, Torcellini CA, et al: Endothelial leukocyte adhesion molecule-1 mediates antigen-induced acute airway inflammation and late-phase airway obstruction in monkeys. J Clin Invest 88:1407, 1991.
155. Gundel RH, Letts LG, Gleich GJ: Human eosinophil major basic protein induces airway constriction and airway hyperresponsiveness in primates. J Clin Invest 87:1470, 1991.
156. Gupta S, Ross GD, Goad RA, et al: Surface markers of human eosinophils. Blood 48:755, 1976.
157. Gutt L, Greenberger PA, Liotta JL: Serum IgA antibodies to *Aspergillus fumigatus* in various stages of allergic bronchopulmonary aspergillosis. J Allergy Clin Immunol 78:98, 1986.
158. Hamada A, Greene GM: C1q enhancement of IgG-dependent eosinophil-mediated killing of schistosomula in vitro. J Immunol 138:1240, 1987.
159. Hamada A, Watanabe N, Kobayashi A: Occurrence and characteristics of hypodense eosinophils in rats infected with *Trichinella spiralis*. Parasite Immunol 14:503, 1992.
160. Hamann KJ, Barker RL, Loegering DA, et al: Comparative toxicity of purified human eosinophil granule proteins for newborn larvae of *Trichinella spiralis*. J Parasitol 73:523, 1987.
161. Hamann KJ, Gleich GJ, Checkel JL, et al: In vitro killing of microfilariae of *Brugia pahangi* and *Brugia malayi* by eosinophil granule proteins. J Immunol 144:3166, 1990.
162. Hamann KJ, Barker RL, Loegering DA, et al: Sequence of human eosinophil-derived neurotoxin cDNA: identity of deduced amino acid sequence with human nonsecretory ribonucleases. Gene 83:161, 1989.
163. Hamann KJ, Dowling TL, Neeley SP, et al: Hyaluronic acid enhances cell proliferation during eosinopoiesis through the CD44 surface antigen. J Immunol 154:4073, 1995.
164. Hamid Q, Barkans J, Meng Q, et al: Human eosinophils synthesize and secrete interleukin-6, in vitro. Blood 80:1496, 1992.
165. Hansel TT, Braunstein JB, Walker C, et al: Sputum eosinophils from asthmatics express ICAM-1 and HLA-DR. Clin Exp Immunol 86:271, 1991.
166. Hansel TT, De Vries IJ, Carballido JM, et al: Induction and function of eosinophil intercellular adhesion molecule-1 and HLA-DR. J Immunol 149:2130, 1992.
167. Hartnell A, Moqbel R, Walsh GM, et al: Fcγ and CD11/18 receptor expression on normal density and low density human eosinophils. Immunology 69:264, 1990.
168. Hartnell A, Kay AB, Wardlaw AJ: IFN-gamma induces expression of Fc gamma RIII (CD16) on human eosinophils. J Immunol 148:1471, 1992.
169. Hartnell A, Kay AB, Wardlaw AJ: Interleukin-3–induced up-regulation of CR3 expression on human eosinophils is inhibited by dexamethasone. Immunology 77:488, 1992.
170. Hartnell A, Robinson DS, Kay AB, et al: CD69 is expressed by human eosinophils activated in vivo in asthma and in vitro by cytokines. Immunology 80:281, 1993.
171. Hastie AT, Loegering DA, Gleich GJ, et al: The effect of purified human eosinophil major basic protein on mammalian ciliary activity. Am Rev Respir Dis 135:848, 1987.
172. Hayashida K, Kitamura T, Gorman DM, et al: Molecular cloning of a second subunit of the receptor for human granulocyte-macrophage colony-stimulating factor (GM-CSF): reconstitution of a high-affinity GM-CSF receptor. Proc Natl Acad Sci USA 87:9655, 1990.
173. Henderson WR, Harley JB, Fauci AS, et al: Hypereosinophilic syndrome human eosinophil degranulation induced by soluble and particulate stimuli. Br J Haematol 69:13, 1988.
174. Henocq E, Vargaftig BB: Accumulation of eosinophils in response to intracutaneous PAF-acether and allergens in man (letter). Lancet 1:1378, 1986.
175. Her E, Frazer J, Austen KF, et al: Eosinophil hematopoietins antagonize the programmed cell death of eosinophils. Cytokine and glucocorticoid effects on eosinophils maintained by endothelial cell-conditioned medium. J Clin Invest 88:1982, 1991.
176. Hibbs MS, Mainardi CL, Kang AH: Type-specific collagen degradation by eosinophils. Biochem J 207:621, 1982.
177. Hirsch JG, Hirsch BI: Paul Ehrlich and the discovery of the eosinophil. In Mahmoud AAF, Austen KF (eds): The Eosinophil in Health and Disease. Grune & Stratton, Inc, New York, 1980, pp 3–23.
178. Hitoshi Y, Yamaguchi N, Korenaga M, et al: In vivo administration of antibody to murine IL-5 receptor inhibits eosinophilia of IL-5 transgenic mice. Int Immunol 3:135, 1991.
179. Hodges MK, Weller PF, Gerard NP, et al: Heterogeneity of leukotriene C_4 production by eosinophils from asthmatic and from normal subjects. Am Rev Respir Dis 138:799, 1988.
180. Horie S, Kita H: CD11b/CD18 (Mac-1) is required for degranulation of human eosinophils induced by human recombinant granulocyte-macrophage colony-stimulating factor and platelet-activating factor. J Immunol 152:5457, 1994.
181. Hossain M, Okubo Y, Sekiguchi M: Effects of various drugs (staurosporine, herbimycin A, ketotifen, theophylline, FK506 and cyclosporin A) on eosinophil viability. Arerugi-Jpn J Allergol 43:711, 1994.
182. Huang C-K: Protein kinases in neutrophils: a review. Membr Biochem 8:61, 1989.
183. Hudson G: Quantitative study of the eosinophil granulocytes. Semin Hematol 5:166, 1968.
184. Hubscher T: Role of the eosinophil in the allergic reactions. II. Release

of prostaglandins from human eosinophilic leukocytes. J Immunol 114:1389, 1975.

185. Hwang SB, Lam M-Y, Hsu HM: Characterization of platelet activating factor (PAF) receptor by specific binding of [^{3}H]L-659,989, a PAF receptor antagonist, to rabbit platelet membrane: possible conformational states of a single PAF receptor. J Pharmacol Exp Ther 254:48, 1989.
186. Ihle JN, Keller J, Oroszlan S, et al: Biologic properties of homogeneous interleukin 3. I. Demonstration of WEHI-3 growth factor activity, mast cell growth factor activity, p cell-stimulating factor, colony-stimulating factor activity, and histamine-producing cell-stimulating factor activity. J Immunol 131:282, 1983.
187. Iijima M: Relationship between airway hyperreactivity and various atopic factors in bronchial asthma. Jpn J Allergol 34:226, 1985.
188. Ingley E, Young IG: Characterization of a receptor for interleukin-5 on human eosinophils and the myeloid leukemia line HL-60. Blood 78:339, 1991.
189. Ishikawa T, Wicher K, Arbesman CE: In vitro and in vivo studies on uptake of antigen-antibody complexes by eosinophils. Int Arch Allergy Appl Immunol 46:230, 1974.
190. Itoh K, Mukaiyama O, Satoh T, et al: Effects of CS-518, a thromboxane synthase inhibitor, on eosinophil function. Eur J Pharmacol, 239:150, 1993.
191. Iwamoto I, Nakajima H, Endo H, et al: Interferon regulates antigen-induced eosinophil recruitment into the mouse airways by inhibiting the infiltration of CD4+ T cells. J Exp Med 177:573, 1993.
192. Iwama T, Nagai H, Suda H, et al: Effect of murine recombinant interleukin-5 on the cell population in guinea-pig airways. Br J Pharmacol 105:19, 1992.
193. Jacoby DB, Ueki IF, Widdicombe JH, et al: Effect of human eosinophil major basic protein on ion transport in dog tracheal epithelium. Am Rev Respir Dis 137:13, 1988.
194. Jacoby DB, Gleich GJ, Fryer AD: Human eosinophil major basic protein is an endogenous allosteric antagonist at the inhibitory muscarinic M2 receptor. J Clin Invest 91:1314, 1993.
195. Jahnsen FL, Brandtzaeg P, Halstensen TS: Monoclonal antibody EG2 does not provide reliable immunohistochemical discrimination between resting and activated eosinophils. J Immunol Methods 175:23, 1994.
196. Jong EC, Klebanoff SJ: Eosinophil-mediated mammalian tumor cell cytotoxicity: role of the peroxidase system. J Immunol 124:1949, 1980.
197. Jong EC, Henderson WR, Klebanoff SJ: Bactericidal activity of eosinophil peroxidase. J Immunol 124:1378, 1980.
198. Jose PJ, Griffiths-Johnson DA, Collins PD, et al: Eotaxin: a potent eosinophil chemoattractant cytokine detected in a guinea pig model of allergic airways inflammation. J Exp Med 179:881, 1994.
199. Jouault T, Capron M, Balloul JM, et al: Quantitative and qualitative analysis of the Fc receptor for IgE, Fc$_\epsilon$RII, on human eosinophils. Eur J Immunol 18:237, 1988.
200. Kajita T, Yui Y, Mita H, et al: Release of leukotriene C_4 from human eosinophils and its relation to the cell density. Int Arch Allergy Appl Immunol 78:406, 1985.
201. Kameyoshi Y, Dorschner A, Mallet AI, et al: Cytokine RANTES released by thrombin-stimulated platelets is a potent attractant for human eosinophils. J Exp Med 176:587, 1992.
202. Kaneko M, Swanson MC, Gleich GJ, et al: Allergen-specific IgG1 and IgG3 through Fc$_\gamma$RII induce eosinophil degranulation. J Clin Invest 95:2813, 1995.
203. Kaneko M, Horie S, Kato M, et al: A crucial role for β2 integrin in the activation of eosinophils stimulated by IgG. J Immunol 155:2631, 1995.
204. Kanofsky JR, Hoogland H, Wever R, et al: Singlet oxygen production by human eosinophils. J Biol Chem 263:9692, 1988.
205. Kato M, Abraham RT, Kita H: Tyrosine phosphorylation is required for eosinophil degranulation induced by immobilized immunoglobulins. J Immunol 155:357, 1995.
206. Kay AB, Austen KF: The IgE-mediated release of an eosinophil leukocyte chemotactic factor from human lung. J Immunol 107:899, 1971.
207. Kay AB, Stechschulte DJ, Austen KF: An eosinophil leukocyte chemotactic factor of anaphylaxis. J Exp Med 133:602, 1971.
208. Kephart GM, Gleich GJ, Connor DH, et al: Deposition of eosinophil granule major basic protein onto microfilariae of *Onchocerca volvulus* in the skin of patients treated with diethylcarbamazine. Lab Invest 50:51, 1984.
209. Kernen P, Wymann MP, Von Tscharner V, et al: Shape changes, exocytosis, and cytosolic free calcium changes in stimulated human eosinophils. J Clin Invest 87:2012, 1991.
210. Khalife J, Capron M, Cesbron JY, et al: Role of specific IgE antibodies in peroxidase (EPO) release from human eosinophils. J Immunol 137:1659, 1986.
211. Kimani G, Tonnesen MG, Henson PM: Stimulation of eosinophil adherence to human vascular endothelial cells in vitro by platelet-activating factor. J Immunol 140:3161, 1988.
212. Kita H, Ohnishi T, Okubo Y, et al: Granulocyte/macrophage colony-stimulating factor and interleukin 3 release from human peripheral blood eosinophils and neutrophils. J Exp Med 174:745, 1991.
213. Kita H, Abu-Ghazaleh RI, Gleich GJ, et al: Regulation of Ig-induced eosinophil degranulation by cyclic AMP. J Immunol 146:2712, 1991.
214. Kita H, Weiler DA, Abu-Ghazaleh RI, et al: Release of granule proteins from eosinophils cultured with IL-5. J Immunol 149:629, 1992.
215. Kita H, Abu-Ghazaleh RI, Gleich GJ, et al: Role of pertussis toxin–sensitive G proteins in stimulus-dependent human eosinophil degranulation. J Immunol 147:3466, 1991.
216. Kita H, Horie S, Gleich GJ: Laminin and fibronectin inhibit adhesion and degranulation of eosinophils. J Allergy Clin Immunol 93:212, 1994.
217. Kita H, Abu-Ghazaleh RI, Sur S, et al: Eosinophil major basic protein induces degranulation and IL-8 production by human eosinophils. J Immunol 154:4749, 1995.
218. Kitamura T, Sato N, Arai K, et al: Expression cloning of the human IL-3 receptor cDNA reveals a shared β subunit for the human IL-3 and GM-CSF receptors. Cell 66:1165, 1991.
219. Kitani S, Ito K, Miyamoto T: IgG, IgA, and IgM antibodies to mite in sera and sputa from asthmatic patients. Ann Allergy 55:612, 1985.
220. Kloprogge E, de Leeuw AJ, de Monchy JG, et al: Hypodense eosinophilic granulocytes in normal individuals and patients with asthma: generation of hypodense cell populations in vitro. J Allergy Clin Immunol 83:393, 1989.
221. Knol EF, Kansas GS, Tedder TF, et al: Human eosinophils use L-selectin to bind to endothelial cells under non-static conditions. J Allergy Clin Immunol 91:334, 1993.
222. Knol EF, Tackey F, Tedder TF, et al: Comparison of human eosinophil and neutrophil adhesion to endothelial cells under nonstatic conditions. Role of L-selectin. J Immunol 153:2161, 1994.
223. Koenderman L, Bruijnzeel PLB: Increased sensitivity of the chemoattractant-induced chemiluminescence in eosinophils isolated from atopic individuals. Immunology 67:534, 1989.
224. Koenderman L, Tool ATJ, Roos D, et al: Priming of the respiratory burst in human eosinophils is accompanied by changes in signal transduction. J Immunol 145:3883, 1990.
225. Koenderman L, Hermans SW, Capel PJ, et al: Granulocyte-macrophage colony-stimulating factor induces sequential activation and deactivation of binding via a low-affinity IgG Fc receptor, Fc gamma RII, on human eosinophils. Blood 81:2413, 1993.
226. Kojima S, Yamamoto N, Kanazawa T, et al: Monoclonal IgE-dependent eosinophil cytotoxicity to haptenated schistosomula of *Schistosoma japonicum*: enhancement of the cytotoxicity and expression of Fc receptors for IgE by *Nippostrongylus brasiliensis* infection. J Immunol 134:2719, 1985.
227. Kroegel C, Yukawa T, Westwick J, et al: Evidence for two platelet activating factor receptors on eosinophils: dissociation between PAF-induced intracellular calcium mobilization degranulation and superoxides anion generation in eosinophils. Biochem Biophys Res Commun 162:511, 1989.
228. Kroegel C, Yukawa T, Dent G, et al: Platelet-activating factor induces eosinophil peroxidase release from purified human eosinophils. Immunology 64:559, 1988.
229. Kroegel C, Pleass R, Yukawa T, et al: Characterization of platelet activating factor–induced elevation of cytosolic free calcium concentration in eosinophils. FEBS Lett 243:41, 1989.
230. Kroegel C, Chilvers ER, Barnes PJ: Platelet activating factor (PAF) stimulates phosphoinositide (PI) metabolism in guinea-pig eosinophils. Clin Sci 76:54P, 1990.
231. Kroegel C, Chilvers ER, Giembycz MA, et al: Platelet-activating factor stimulates a rapid accumulation of inositol, 1,4,5 triphosphate in guinea pig eosinophils: relationship to calcium mobilization and degranulation. J Allergy Clin Immunol 88:114, 1991.
232. Kroegel C, Yukawa T, Dent G, et al: Stimulation of degranulation from human eosinophils by platelet-activating factor. J Immunol 142: 3518, 1989.

233. Kroegel C, Giembycz MA, Barnes PJ: Characterization of eosinophil cell activation by peptides: differential effects of substance P, melittin, and FMET-leu-phe. J Immunol 145:2581, 1990.
234. Kroegel C, Liu MC, Hubbard WC, et al: Blood and bronchoalveolar eosinophils in allergic subjects after segmental antigen challenge: surface phenotype, density heterogeneity, and prostanoid production. J Allergy Clin Immunol 93:725, 1994.
235. Kuijpers TW, Mul EP, Blom M, et al: Freezing adhesion molecules in a state of high-avidity binding blocks eosinophil migration. J Exp Med 178:279, 1993.
236. Kurosawa M, Shimizu Y, Tsukagoshi H: Human peripheral blood hypodense eosinophil proteins are more labeled with phosphorus-32 than the normodense eosinophil proteins. Int Arch Allergy Immunol 97:283, 1992.
237. Kyan-Aung U, Haskard DO, Poston RN, et al: Endothelial leukocyte adhesion molecule-1 and intercellular adhesion molecule-1 mediate the adhesion of eosinophils to endothelial cells in vitro and are expressed by endothelium in allergic cutaneous inflammation in vivo. J Immunol 146:521, 1991.
238. Laitinen LA, Laitinen A, Haahtela T, et al: Leukotriene E4 and granulocytic infiltration into asthmatic airways. Lancet 341:989, 1993.
239. Lamas AM, Leon OG, Schleimer RP: Glucocorticoids inhibit eosinophil responses to granulocyte-macrophage colony-stimulating factor. J Immunol 147:254, 1991.
240. Lamas AM, Mulroney CM, Schleimer RP: Studies on the adhesive interaction between purified human eosinophils and cultured vascular endothelial cells. J Immunol 140:1500, 1988.
241. Lamkhioued B, Gounni AS, Gruart V, et al: Human eosinophils express a receptor for secretory component—role in secretory IgA-dependent activation. Eur J Immunol 25:117, 1995.
242. Leary AG, Ogawa M, Strauss LC, et al: Single cell origin of multilineage colonies in culture. J Clin Invest 74:2193, 1984.
243. Lee T, Lenihan DJ, Malone B, et al: Increased biosynthesis of platelet-activating factor in activated human eosinophils. J Biol Chem 259:5526, 1984.
244. Lehrer RI, Szlarek D, Barton D, et al: Anti-bacterial properties of eosinophil major basic protein (MBP) and eosinophil cationic protein (ECP). J Immunol 142:4428, 1989.
245. Leiferman KM, Ackerman SJ, Sampson HA, et al: Dermal deposition of eosinophil-granule major basic protein in atopic dermatitis. N Engl J Med 313:282, 1985.
245a. Leiferman KM, Fujisawa T, Gray BH, et al: Extracellular deposition of eosinophil and neutrophil granule proteins in the IgE-mediated cutaneous late phase reaction. Lab Invest 62:579, 1990.
246. Leonard EJ, Yoshimura T: Human monocyte chemoattractant protein-1 (MIP-1). Immunol Today 11:97, 1990.
247. Levischaffer F, Lacy P, Severs NJ, et al: Association of granulocyte-macrophage colony-stimulating factor with the crystalloid granules of human eosinophils. Blood 85:2579, 1995.
248. Looney RJ, Ryan DH, Takahashi K: Identification of a second class of IgG Fc receptors on human neutrophils. A 40 kilodalton molecule also found on eosinophils. J Exp Med 163:826, 1986.
249. Lopez AF, To LB, Yang YC, et al: Stimulation of proliferation, differentiation and function of human cells by primate interleukin 3. Proc Natl Acad Sci USA 84:2761, 1987.
250. Lopez AF, Eglinton JM, Gillis D, et al: Reciprocal inhibition of binding between interleukin 3 and granulocyte-macrophage colony-stimulating factor to human eosinophils. Proc Natl Acad Sci USA 86:7022, 1989.
251. Lopez AF, Elliott MJ, Woodcock J, et al: GM-CSF, IL-3 and IL-5: cross-competition on human haemopoietic cells. Immunol Today 13:495, 1992.
252. Lopez AF, Williamson DJ, Gamble JR, et al: Recombinant human granulocyte-macrophage colony-stimulating factor stimulates in vitro mature human neutrophil and eosinophil function, surface receptor expression, and survival. J Clin Invest 78:1220, 1986.
253. Lopez AF, Sanderson CJ, Gamble JR, et al: Recombinant human interleukin 5 is a selective activator of human eosinophil function. J Exp Med 167:219, 1988.
254. Lucey DR, Dorsky DI, Nicholson-Weller A, et al: Human eosinophils express CD4 protein and bind human immunodeficiency virus 1 gp 120. J Exp Med 169:327, 1989.
255. Lucey DR, Nicholson-Weller A, Weller PF: Mature human eosinophils have the capacity to express HLA-DR. Proc Natl Acad Sci USA 86:1348, 1989.
256. Lundahl J, Hallden G, Hed J: Differences in intracellular pool and receptor-dependent mobilization of the adhesion-promoting glycoprotein Mac-1 between eosinophils and neutrophils. J Leukoc Biol 53:336, 1993.
257. Lungarella G, Menegazzi A, Gardi C, et al: Identification of elastase in human eosinophils: immunolocalization, isolation, and partial characterization. Arch Biochem Biophys 292:128, 1992.
258. Maghni K, de Brum-Fernandes AJ, Foldes-Filep E, et al: Leukotriene B4 receptors on guinea pig alveolar eosinophils. J Pharmacol Exp Ther 258:784, 1991.
259. Marshall T, Shult P, Busse WW: Release of lysosomal enzyme beta-glucuronidase from isolated human eosinophils. J Allergy Clin Immunol 82:550, 1988.
260. Mauser PJ, Pitman A, Witt A: Inhibitory effect of the TRFK-5 anti IL-5 antibody in a guinea pig model of asthma. Am Rev Respir Dis 148:1623, 1993.
261. Mayeno AN, Curran AJ, Roberts RL, et al: Eosinophils preferentially use bromide to generate halogenating agents. J Biol Chem 264:5660, 1989.
262. McCulloch EA: Stem cells in normal and leukemic hemopoiesis (Henry Stratton Lecture, 1982). Blood 62:1, 1983.
263. McLaren DJ, McKean JR, Olsson I, et al: Morphological studies on the killing of schistosomula of *Schistosoma mansoni* by human eosinophil and neutrophil cationic proteins in vitro. Parasite Immunol 3:359, 1981.
264. McPhil LC, Strum SL, Leone PA, et al: The neutrophil respiratory burst mechanism. In Coffey R (ed): Granulocyte Responses to Cytokines: Basic and Clinical Research. Marcel Dekker Inc, New York, 1992, p 47.
265. Melani C, Mattia GF, Silvani A, et al: Interleukin-6 expression in human neutrophil and eosinophil peripheral blood lymphocytes. Blood 81:2744, 1993.
266. Mengelers HJ, Maikoe T, Hooibrink B, et al: Down modulation of L-Selectin expression on eosinophils recovered from bronchoalveolar lavage fluid after allergen provocation. Clin Exp Allergy 23:196, 1993.
267. Mengelers HJ, Maikoe T, Brinkman L, et al: Immunophenotyping of eosinophils recovered from blood and BAL of allergic asthmatics. Am J Respir Crit Care Med 149:345, 1994.
268. Metcalf D, Begley CG, Johnson GR, et al: Biologic properties in vitro of a recombinant human granulocyte-macrophage colony-stimulating factor. Blood 67:37, 1986.
269. Metcalf D: The molecular biology and functions of granulocyte-macrophage colony-stimulating factors (review). Blood 67:257, 1986.
270. Metzger WJ, Ridger V, Tollefson V, et al: Anti-VLA4 antibody and CS-1 peptide inhibitor modifies airway inflammation and bronchial airway hyperresponsiveness (BHR) in the allergic rabbit. J Allergy Clin Immunol 93:183, 1994.
271. Meurer R, Van Riper G, Feeney W, et al: Formation of eosinophilic and monocytic intradermal inflammatory sites in the dog by injection of human RANTES but not human monocyte chemoattractant protein 1, human macrophage inflammatory protein 1 alpha, or human interleukin 8. J Exp Med 178:1913, 1993.
272. Migita M, Yamaguchi N, Mita S, et al: Characterization of the human IL-5 receptors on eosinophils. Cell Immunol 133:484, 1991.
273. Miller F, DeHarven E, Palade GE: The structure of the eosinophil leukocyte granules in rodents and in man. J Cell Biol 31:349, 1966.
274. Minnicozzi M, Anthes JC, Siegel MI, et al: Activation of phospholipase D in normodense human eosinophils. Biochem Biophys Res Commun 170:540, 1990.
275. Minnicozzi M, Duran WN, Gleich GJ, et al: Eosinophil granule proteins increase microvascular macromolecular transport in the hamster cheek pouch. J Immunol 153:2664, 1994.
276. Miyamasu M, Hirai K, Takahashi Y, et al: Chemotactic agonists induce cytokine generation in eosinophils. J Immunol 154:1339, 1995.
277. Monteiro RC, Hostoffer RW, Cooper MD, et al: Definition of immunoglobulin A receptors on eosinophils and their enhanced expression in allergic individuals. J Clin Invest 92:1681, 1993.
278. Morita E, Schroder J-M, Christophers E: Identification of a novel and highly potent eosinophil chemotactic lipid in human eosinophils treated with arachidonic acid. J Immunol 144:1893, 1990.
279. Moser R, Fehr J, Olgiati L: Migration of primed human eosinophils across cytokine-activated endothelial cell monolayers. Blood 79: 2937, 1992.
280. Moqbel R, Walsh GM, Nagakura T, et al: The effect of platelet activating factor on IgE binding to, and IgE-dependent biological properties of human eosinophils. Immunology 70:251, 1990.

281. Moqbel R, Hamid Q, Ying S, et al: Expression of mRNA and immunoreactivity for the granulocyte/macrophage colony-stimulating factor in activated human eosinophils. J Exp Med 174:749, 1991.
282. Moqbel R, MacDonald AJ, Cromwell O, et al: Release of leukotriene C_4, (LTC_4), from human eosinophils following adherence to IgE- and IgG-coated schistosomula of *Schistosoma mansoni*. Immunology 69:435, 1990.
283. Moscinski LC, Kasnic G Jr, Saker A Jr: The significance of an elevated serum lysozyme value in acute myelogenous leukemia with eosinophilia. Am J Clin Pathol 97:195, 1992.
284. Moser R, Fehr J, Bruijnzeel PLB: IL-4 controls the selective endothelium-driven transmigration of eosinophils from allergic individuals. J Immunol 149:1432, 1992.
285. Moy JN, Gleich GJ, Thomas LL: Noncytotoxic activation of neutrophils by eosinophil granule major basic protein: effect on superoxide anion generation and lysosomal enzyme release. J Immunol 145:2626, 1990.
286. Murata Y, Takaki S, Migita M, et al: Molecular cloning and expression of the human interleukin 5 receptor. J Exp Med 175:341, 1992.
287. Nadel JA, Conrad DJ, Ueki IF, et al: Immunocytochemical localization of arachidonate 15-lipoxygenase in erythrocytes, leukocytes, and airway cells. J Clin Invest 87:1139, 1991.
288. Nagy L, Lee TH, Goetzl EJ, et al: Complement receptor enhancement and chemotaxis of human neutrophils and eosinophils by leukotrienes and other lipoxygenase products. Clin Exp Immunol 47:511, 1982.
289. Nakajima H, Iwamoto I, Tomoe S, et al: CD4-positive T-lymphocytes and interleukin-5 mediate antigen-induced eosinophil infiltration into the mouse trachea. Am Rev Respir Dis 146:374, 1992.
290. Nakajima H, Sano H, Nishimura T, et al: Role of vascular cell adhesion molecule 1/very late activation antigen 4 and intercellular adhesion molecule 1/lymphocyte function-associated antigen 1 interactions in antigen-induced eosinophil and T cell recruitment into the tissue. J Exp Med 179:1145, 1994.
291. Nakamura M, Honda Z, Izumi T, et al: Molecular cloning and expression of platelet-activating factor receptor from human leukocytes. J Biol Chem 266:20400, 1991
292. Nambu M, Watanabe H, Kim KM, et al: Regulation of Fc gamma receptor subtype expression on a human eosinophilic leukemia cell line EoL-3: participation of cAMP and protein kinase C in the effects of interferon-gamma and phorbol ester. Cell Immunol 133:27, 1991.
293. Neeley SP, Hamann KJ, White SR, et al: Selective regulation of expression of surface adhesion molecules Mac-1, L-selectin, and VLA-4 on human eosinophils and neutrophils. Am J Respir Cell Mol Biol 8:633, 1993.
294. Neeley SP, Hamann KJ, Dowling TL: Augmentation of stimulated eosinophil degranulation by VLA-4 (CD49d)–mediated adhesion to fibronectin. Am J Respir Cell Mol Biol 11:206, 1994.
295. Neote K, DiGregorio D, Mak JY: Molecular/cloning, functional expression, and signaling characteristics of a C-C chemokine receptor. Cell 72:415, 1993.
296. Ng CF, Sun FF, Taylor BM, et al: Functional properties of guinea pig eosinophil leukotriene B4 receptor. J Immunol 147:3096, 1991.
297. Nishikawa K, Morii T, Ako H, et al: In vivo expression of CD69 on lung eosinophils in eosinophilic pneumonia: CD69 as a possible activation marker for eosinophils. J Allergy Clin Immunol 90:169, 1992.
298. Nowell PC, Hirsch BE, Fox DH, et al: Evidence for the existence of multipotential lympho-hematopoietic stem cells in the adult rat. J Cell Physiol 75:151, 1970.
299. Nusse O, Lindau M, Cromwell O, et al: Intracellular application of guanosine-5′-O-(3-thiotriphosphate) induces exocytotic granule fusion in guinea pig eosinophils. J Exp Med 171:775, 1990.
300. O'Donnell MC, Ackerman SJ, Gleich GJ, et al: Activation of basophil and mast cell histamine release by eosinophil granule major basic protein. J Exp Med 157:1981, 1983.
301. Ogawa M, Porter PN, Nakahata T: Renewal and commitment to differentiation of hemopoietic stem cells (an interpretive review). Blood 61:823, 1983.
302. Ohnishi T, Kita H, Weiler D, et al: IL-5 is the predominant eosinophil-active cytokine in the antigen-induced pulmonary late-phase reaction. Am Rev Respir Dis 147:901, 1993.
303. Ohno I, Lea RG, Flanders KC: Eosinophils in chronically inflamed human upper airway tissues express transforming growth factor β 1 gene (TGF β 1). J Clin Invest 89:1662, 1992.
304. Ohno I, Lea RG, Finotto S, et al: Granulocyte/macrophage colony-stimulating factor (GM-CSF) gene expression by eosinophils in nasal polyposis. Am J Respir Cell Mol Biol 5:505, 1991.
305. Osgood EE: Number and distribution of human hemic cells. Blood 9:1141, 1954.
306. Owen WF, Rothenberg ME, Petersen J, et al: Interleukin 5 and phenotypically altered eosinophils in the blood of patients with the idiopathic hypereosinophilic syndrome. J Exp Med 170:343, 1989.
307. Owen WF Jr, Soberman RJ, Yoshimoto T, et al: Synthesis and release of leukotriene C_4 by human eosinophils. J Immunol 138:532, 1987.
308. Owen WF Jr, Rothenberg ME, Silberstein DS, et al: Regulation of human eosinophil viability, density, and function by granulocyte-macrophage colony-stimulating factor in the presence of 3T3 fibroblasts. J Exp Med 166:129, 1987.
309. Owen WF Jr, Petersen J, Austen KF: Eosinophils altered phenotypically and primed by culture with granulocyte-macrophage colony-stimulating factor and 3T3 fibroblasts generate leukotriene C_4 in response to FMLP. J Clin Invest 87:1958, 1991.
310. Palmblad J, Gyllenhammar H, Lindgren JA, et al: Effects of leukotrienes and f-Met-Leu-Phe on oxidative metabolism of neutrophils and eosinophils. J Immunol 132:3041, 1984.
311. Parmley RT, Spicer SS: Cytochemical and ultrastructural identification of a small type granule in human late eosinophils. Lab Invest 30:557, 1974.
312. Parwaresch MR, Walle AJ, Arndt D: The peripheral kinetics of human radiolabelled eosinophils. Virchows Arch Cell Pathol 21:57, 1976.
313. Pazdrak K, Stafford S, Alam R: The activation of the JAK-STAT 1 signaling pathway by IL-5 in eosinophils. J Immunol 155:397, 1995.
314. Pazdrak K, Schreiber D, Forsythe P, et al: The intracellular signal transduction mechanism of interleukin 5 in eosinophils—the involvement of Lyn tyrosine kinase and the Ras-Raf-1-Mek-microtubule–associated protein kinase pathway. J Exp Med 181:1827, 1995.
315. Perlmutter RM, Levin SD, Appleby MW, et al: Regulation of lymphocyte function by protein phosphorylation. Annu Rev Immunol 11:451, 1993.
316. Peters MS, Gleich GJ, Dunnette SL, et al: Ultrastructural study of eosinophils from patients with the hypereosinophilic syndrome: a morphological basis of hypodense eosinophils. Blood 71:780, 1988.
317. Petreccia DC, Nauseef WM, Clark RA: Respiratory burst of normal human eosinophils. J Leukoc Biol 41:283, 1987.
318. Pincus SH, Schooley WR, DiNapoli AM, et al: Metabolic heterogeneity of eosinophils from normal and hypereosinophilic patients. Blood 58:1175, 1981.
319. Pincus SH, Whitcomb EA, Dinarello CA: Interaction of IL1 and TPA in modulation of eosinophil function. J Immunol 137:3509, 1986.
320. Pincus SH: Hydrogen peroxide release from eosinophils: quantitative, comparative studies of human and guinea-pig eosinophils. J Invest Dermatol 80:278, 1983.
321. Popper H, Pongratz M, Lanzer G: IgA_2-alveolitis and eosinophilic pneumonia—a possibly virus-triggered allergy. Allergol Immunopathol (Madr) 10:177, 1982.
322. Postma DS, Renkema TEJ, Noordhoek JA, et al: Association between non-specific bronchial hyperresponsiveness and superoxide anion generation by polymorphonuclear leukocytes in chronic airway obstruction. Am Rev Respir Dis 137:57, 1988.
323. Pretolani M, Ruffie C, Lapa e Silva JR, et al: Antibody to very late activation antigen 4 prevents antigen-induced bronchial hyperreactivity and cellular infiltration in the guinea pig airways. J Exp Med 180:795, 1994.
324. Prin L, Capron M, Tonnel AB, et al: Heterogeneity of human peripheral blood eosinophils: variability in cell density and cytotoxic ability in relation to the level and the origin of hypereosinophilia. Int Arch Allergy Appl Immunol 72:336, 1983.
325. Prin L, Charon J, Capron M, et al: Heterogeneity of human eosinophils. II. Variability of respiratory burst activity related to cell density. Clin Exp Immunol 57:735, 1984.
326. Rabe KF, Giembycz MA, Dent G, et al: Induction of thromboxane biosynthesis in guinea-pig eosinophils stimulated with leukotriene B_4. Br J Pharmacol 101:526P, 1990.
327. Rabe KF, Giembycz MA, Dent G, et al: β_2-adrenoceptor agonists and respiratory burst activity in guinea-pig and human eosinophils. Fundam Clin Pharmacol 5:402, 1991.
328. Ramesh KS, Rocklin RE, Pincus SH: Phosphorylation and dephosphorylation of soluble proteins in human eosinophils. J Cell Biochem 34:203, 1987.
329. Rand TH, Cruikshank WW, Center DM, et al: CD4-mediated stimulation of human eosinophils: lymphocyte chemoattractant factor and other CD4-binding ligands elicit eosinophil migration. J Exp Med 173:1521, 1991.

330. Rand TH, Silberstein DS, Kornfeld H, et al: Human eosinophils express functional interleukin 2 receptors. J Clin Invest 88:825, 1991.
331. Rankin JA, Harris P, Ackerman SJ: The effects of eosinophil-granule major basic protein on lung macrophage superoxide anion generation. J Allergy Clin Immunol 89:746, 1992.
332. Richards IM, Sun FF, Taylor BM, et al: Contribution of leukotriene B_4 to airway inflammation and the effect of agonists. Ann NY Acad Sci 629:274, 1991.
333. Rohrbach MS, Wheatley CL, Slifman NR, et al: Activation of platelets by eosinophil granule proteins. J Exp Med 172:1271, 1990.
334. Ross R, Klebanoff SJ: The eosinophilic leukocyte. Fine structure studies of changes in the uterus during the estrous cycle. J Exp Med 124:653, 1966.
335. Rot A, Krieger M, Brunner T, et al: RANTES and macrophage inflammatory protein 1α induce the migration and activation of normal human eosinophil granulocytes. J Exp Med 176:1489, 1992.
336. Rothenberg ME, Owen WF Jr, Silberstein DS, et al: Eosinophils cocultured with endothelial cells have increased survival and functional properties. Science 237:645, 1987.
337. Rothenberg ME, Owen WF Jr, Silberstein DS, et al: Human eosinophils have prolonged survival, enhanced function properties, and become hypodense when exposed to human interleukin 3. J Clin Invest 81:1986, 1988.
338. Rothenberg ME, Petersen J, Stevens RL, et al: IL-5-dependent conversion of normodense human eosinophils to the hypodense phenotype uses 3T3 fibroblasts for enhanced viability, accelerated hypodensity, and sustained antibody-dependent cytotoxicity. J Immunol 143:2311, 1989.
339. Rothenberg ME, Luster AD, Lilly CM, et al: Constitutive and allergen-induced expression of eotaxin mRNA in the guinea pig lung. J Exp Med 181:1211, 1995.
340. Roubin R, Elsas PP, Fiers W, et al: Recombinant human tumor necrosis factor (rTNF) enhances leukotriene biosynthesis in neutrophils and eosinophils stimulated with the Ca^{2+} ionophore A23187. Clin Exp Immunol 70:484, 1987.
341. Rytomaa T: Organ distribution and histochemical properties of eosinophil granulocytes in rat. Acta Pathol Microbiol Scand 50:1, 1960.
342. Saito H, Hayakawa T, Yui Y, et al: Effect of human interferon on different functions of human neutrophils and eosinophils. Int Arch Allergy Appl Immunol 82:133, 1987.
343. Saito H, Hatake K, Dvorak AM, et al: Selective differentiation and proliferation of hematopoietic cells induced by recombinant human interleukins. Proc Natl Acad Sci USA 85:2288, 1988.
344. Sanderson CJ, Campbell HD, Young IG: Molecular and cellular biology of eosinophil differentiation factor (interleukin-5) and its effects on human and mouse B cells. Immunol Rev 102:29, 1988.
345. Sanderson CJ, Warren DJ, Strath M: Identification of a lymphokine that stimulates eosinophil differentiation in vitro: its relationship to interleukin 3, and functional properties of eosinophils produced in cultures. J Exp Med 162:60, 1985.
346. Schleimer RP, Sterbinsky SA, Kaiser J, et al: IL-4 induces adherence of human eosinophils and basophils but not neutrophils to endothelium. J Immunol 148:1086, 1992.
347. Schleimer RP, Ebisawa M, Georas SN, et al: The role of adhesion molecules and cytokines in eosinophil recruitment. In Gleich GJ, Kay AB (eds): Eosinophils in Allergy and Inflammation. Marcel Dekker, Inc, New York, 1994, p 99.
348. Schonhardt T, Ferber E: Translocation of phospholipase A_2 from cytosol to membranes induced by 1-oleoyl-2-acetyl-glycerol in serum free cultured macrophages. Biochem Biophys Res Commun 149:769, 1987.
349. Schweizer RC, Welmers BA, Raaijmakers JA, et al: RANTES- and interleukin-8-induced responses in normal human eosinophils: effects of priming with interleukin-5. Blood 83:3697, 1994.
350. Schwenk U, Morita E, Engel R, et al: Identification of 5-oxo-15-hydroxy-6,8,11,13-eicosatetraenoic acid as a novel and potent human eosinophil chemotactic eicosanoid. J Biol Chem 267:12482, 1992.
351. Sedgwick JB, Calhoun WJ, Gleich GJ, et al: Immediate and late airway response of allergic rhinitis patients to segmental antigen challenge. Characterization of eosinophil and mast cell mediators. Am Rev Respir Dis 144:1274, 1991.
352. Sedgwick JB, Vrtis RF, Gourley MF, et al: Stimulant-dependent differences in superoxide anion generation by normal human eosinophils and neutrophils. J Allergy Clin Immunol 81:876, 1988.
353. Sedgwick JB, Geiger KM, Busse WW: Superoxide generation by hypodense eosinophils from patients with asthma. Am Rev Respir Dis 142:120, 1990.
354. Sedgwick JB, Calhoun WJ, Vrtis RF, et al: Comparison of airway and blood eosinophil function after in vivo antigen challenge. J Immunol 149:3710, 1992.
355. Sehmi R, Cromwell O, Taylor GW, et al: Identification of guinea pig eosinophil chemotactic factor of anaphylaxis as leukotriene B_4 and 8(S),15(S)-dihydroxy-5,9,11,13(Z,E,Z,E)-eicosatetraenoic acid. J Immunol 147:2276, 1991.
356. Sehmi R, Rossi AG, Kay AB, et al: Identification of receptors for leukotriene B4 expressed on guinea pig peritoneal eosinophils. Immunology 77:129, 1992.
357. Sehmi R, Wardlaw AJ, Cromwell O, et al: Interleukin-5 selectively enhances the chemotactic response of eosinophils obtained from normal but not eosinophilic subjects. Blood 79:2952, 1992.
358. Shaw RJ, Walsh GM, Cromwell O, et al: Activated human eosinophils generate SRS-A leukotrienes following IgG-dependent stimulation. Nature 316:150, 1985.
359. Sher A, Coffman RL, Heiny S, et al: Interleukin 5 is required for the blood and tissue eosinophilia but not granuloma formation induced by infection with *Schistosoma mansoni*. Proc Natl Acad Sci USA 87:61, 1990.
360. Shimizu Y, Shaw S: Cell adhesion. Mucins in the mainstream (news; comment). Nature 366:630, 1993.
361. Shull MM, Ormsby I, Kier AB, et al: Targeted disruption of the mouse transforming growth factor-β1 gene results in multifocal inflammatory disease. Nature 359:693, 1992.
362. Shute JK, Rimmer SJ, Ackerman CL, et al: Studies of cellular mechanisms for the generation of superoxide by guinea-pig eosinophils and its dissociation from granule peroxidase release. Biochem Pharmacol 40:2013, 1990.
363. Shute J: Interleukin-8 is a potent eosinophil chemo-attractant [editorial]. Clin Exp Allergy 24:203, 1994.
364. Sigal CE, Valone FH, Holtzman J, et al: Preferential human eosinophil chemotactic activity of the platelet activating factor (PAF): 1-*O*-hexadecyl-2-acetyl-*sn*-glyceryl-3-phosphocholine (AGEPC). J Clin Immunol 7:179, 1987.
365. Silberstein DS, David JR: Tumor necrosis factor enhances eosinophil toxicity to *Schistosoma mansoni* larvae. Proc Natl Acad Sci USA 83:1055, 1986.
366. Silberstein DS, Owen WF, Gasson JC, et al: Enhancement of human eosinophil cytotoxicity and leukotriene synthesis by biosynthetic (recombinant) granulocyte-macrophage colony-stimulating factor. J Immunol 137:3290, 1986.
367. Sillaber C, Geissler K, Scherrer R, et al: Type beta transforming growth factors promote interleukin-3 (IL-3)–dependent differentiation of human basophils but inhibit IL-3–dependent differentiation of human eosinophils. Blood 80:634, 1992.
368. Slifman NR, Adolphson CR, Gleich GJ: Eosinophils: biochemical and cellular aspects. In Middleton E Jr, Reed CE, Ellis EF, et al (eds): Allergy Principles and Practice, 3rd edition. Vol 1. CV Mosby Co, St Louis, 1988, p 179.
369. Slifman NR, Venge P, Peterson CGB, et al: Human eosinophil-derived neurotoxin and eosinophil protein X are likely the same protein. J Immunol 143:2317, 1989.
370. Slungaard A, Mahoney JR Jr: Bromide-dependent toxicity of eosinophil peroxidase for endothelium and isolated working rat hearts: a model for eosinophilic endocarditis. J Exp Med 173:117, 1991.
371. Slungaard A, Vercellotti GM, Walker G, et al: Tumor necrosis factor alpha/cachectin stimulates eosinophil oxidant production and toxicity towards human endothelium. J Exp Med 171:2025, 1990.
372. Sorrentino S, Glitz DG, Hamann KJ, et al: Eosinophil-derived neurotoxin and human liver ribonuclease: identity of structure and linkage of neurotoxicity to nuclease activity. J Biol Chem 267:14859, 1992.
373. Sorrentino S, Tucker GK, Glitz DG: Purification and characterization of a ribonuclease from human liver. J Biol Chem 263:16125, 1988.
374. Souness JE, Carter CM, Diocee BK, et al: Characterization of guinea-pig eosinophil phosphodiesterase activity. Assessment of its involvement in regulating superoxide generation. Biochem Pharmacol 42:937, 1991.
375. Souness JE, Maslen C, Webber S, et al: Suppression of eosinophil function by RP73401, a potent and selective inhibitor of cyclic AMP-specific phosphodiesterase: comparison with rolipram. Br J Pharmacol 115:39, 1995.
376. Spada CS, Nieves AL, Krauss AH-P, et al: Comparison of leukotriene

B_4 and D_4 effects on human eosinophil and neutrophil motility in vitro. J Leukoc Biol 55:183, 1994.
377. Springer TA, Lasky LA: Sticky sugars for selectins. Nature 349:196, 1991.
378. Spry CJF, Tai P-C: Studies on blood eosinophils. II. Patients with Loffler's cardiomyopathy. Clin Exp Immunol 24:423, 1976.
379. Spry CJF: Mechanism of eosinophilia. VI. Eosinophil mobilization. Cell Tissue Kinet 4:265, 1971.
380. Sriramarao P, von Andrian UH, Butcher EC, et al: L-selectin and very late antigen-4 integrin promote eosinophil rolling at physiological shear rates in vivo. J Immunol 153:4238, 1994.
381. Stahle-Backdahl M, Sudbeck BD, Eisen AZ, et al: Expression of 92-kDa type IV collagenase mRNA by eosinophils associated with basal cell carcinoma. J Invest Dermatol 99:497, 1992.
382. Stahle-Backdahl M, Parks WC: 92-kd gelatinase is actively expressed by eosinophils and stored by neutrophils in squamous cell carcinoma. Am J Pathol 142:995, 1993.
383. Stahle-Backdahl M, Inoue M, Guidice GJ, et al: 92-kD gelatinase is produced by eosinophils at the site of blister formation in bullous pemphigoid and cleaves the extracellular domain of recombinant 180-kD bullous pemphigoid autoantigen. J Clin Invest 93:2022, 1994.
384. Steel C, Nutman TB: Regulation of IL-5 in onchocerciasis. A critical role for IL-2. J Immunol 150:5511, 1993.
385. Steinbach KH, Schick P, Trepel F, et al: Estimation of kinetic parameters of neutrophilic, eosinophilic, and basophilic granulocytes in human blood. Blutalkohol 39:27, 1979.
386. Stern M, Meagher L, Savill J, et al: Apoptosis in human eosinophils. Programmed cell death in the eosinophil leads to phocytosis by macrophages and is modulated by IL-5. J Immunol 148:3543, 1992.
387. Subramanian N: Leukotriene B_4 induced steady state calcium rise and superoxide anion generation in guinea pig eosinophils are not related events. Biochem Biophys Res Commun 187:670, 1992.
388. Sugiura T, Mabuchi K, Ojima-Uchiyama A, et al: Synthesis and action of PAF in human eosinophils. J Lipid Mediat 5:151, 1992.
389. Sun Z, Yergeau DA, Tuypens T, et al: Identification and characterization of a functional promoter region in the human eosinophil IL-5 receptor alpha subunit gene. J Biol Chem 270:1462, 1995.
390. Symon FA, Walsh GM, Watson SR, et al: Eosinophil adhesion to nasal polyp endothelium is P-selectin-dependent. J Exp Med 180:371, 1994.
391. Tai P-C, Spry CJ, Peterson C, et al: Monoclonal antibodies distinguish between storage and secreted forms of eosinophil cationic protein. Nature 309:182, 1984.
392. Takafuji S, Bischoff SC, De Weck AL, et al: IL-3 and IL-5 prime normal human eosinophils to produce leukotriene C4 in response to soluble agonists. J Immunol 147:3855, 1991.
393. Takafuji S, Tadokoro K, Ito K, et al: Degranulation of eosinophils stimulated with C3a and C5a. Int Arch Allergy Appl Immunol 104:27, 1994.
394. Takanaski S, Nonaka R, Xing Z, et al: Interleukin 10 inhibits lipopolysaccharide-induced survival and cytokine production by human peripheral blood eosinophils. J Exp Med 180:711, 1994.
395. Takatsu K, Tominaga A, Harada N, et al: T cell-replacing factor (TRF)/interleukin 5 (IL-5): molecular and functional properties. Immunol Rev 102:107, 1988.
396. Tamura N, Agrawal DK, Suliaman FA, et al: Effects of platelet activating factor on the chemotaxis of normodense eosinophils from normal subjects. Biochem Biophys Res Commun 142:638, 1987.
397. Tamura N, Agrawal DK, Townley RG: Leukotriene C4 production from human eosinophils in vitro. Role of eosinophil chemotactic factors on eosinophil activation. J Immunol 141:4291, 1988.
398. Tanaka KR, Valentine WN, Fredricks RE: Human leucocyte arylsulphatase activity. Br J Haematol 8:86, 1962.
399. Tavernier J, Devos R, Cornelis S, et al: A human high affinity interleukin-5 receptor, IL5R, is composed of an IL5-specific alpha chain and a beta chain shared with the receptor for GM-CSF. Cell 66:1175, 1991.
400. Taylor BM, Crittenden NJ, Bruden MN, et al: Biological activity of leukotriene B4 analogs: inhibition of guinea pig eosinophil migration in vitro by the 2,6-disubstituted pyridine analogs U-75302 and U-75485. Prostaglandins 42:211, 1991.
401. Taylor KJ, Luksza AR: Peripheral blood eosinophil counts and bronchial responsiveness. Thorax 42:452, 1987.
402. Teir H, Rytomaa T, Cederberg A, et al: Studies on the elimination of granulocytes in the intestinal tract in rat. Acta Pathol Microbiol Scand 59:311, 1963.
403. Terada N, Konno A, Tada H, et al: The effect of recombinant human interleukin-5 on eosinophil accumulation and degranulation in human nasal mucosa. J Allergy Clin Immunol 90:160, 1992.
404. Thien FC, Hallsworth MP, Soh C, et al: Effects of exogenous eicosapentaenoic acid on generation of leukotriene C4 and leukotriene C5 by calcium ionophore-activated human eosinophils in vitro. J Immunol 150:3546, 1993.
405. Thornhill MH, Wellicome SM, Mahiouz DL, et al: Tumor necrosis factor combines with IL-4 or IFN-gamma to selectively enhance endothelial cell adhesiveness for T cells. The contribution of vascular cell adhesion molecule-1–dependent and –independent binding mechanisms. J Immunol 146:592, 1991.
406. Thorne KJ, Richardson BA, Taverne J, et al: A comparison of eosinophil-activating factor (EAF) with other monokines and lymphokines. Eur J Immunol 16:1143, 1986.
407. Tomassini M, Tsicopoulos A, Tai PC, et al: Release of granule proteins by eosinophils from allergic and nonallergic patients with eosinophilia on immunoglobulin-dependent activation. J Allergy Clin Immunol 88:365, 1991.
408. Tominaga T, Takaki S, Koyama N, et al: Transgenic mice expressing a B cell growth and differentiation gene (interleukin 5) develop eosinophilia and autoantibody production. J Exp Med 173:429, 1991.
409. Tomioka K, MacGlashan DW Jr, Lichtenstein LM, et al: GM-CSF regulates human eosinophil responses to F-met peptide and platelet activating factor. J Immunol 151:4989, 1993.
410. Tomonaga M, Golde DW, Gasson JC: Biosynthetic (recombinant) human granulocyte-macrophage colony-stimulating factor: effect on normal bone marrow and leukemia cell lines. Blood 67:31, 1986.
411. Triggiani M, Schleimer RP, Tomioka K, et al: Characterization of platelet-activating factor synthesized by normal and granulocyte-macrophage colony-stimulating factor-primed human eosinophils. Immunology 77:500, 1992.
412. Tsunawaki S, Sporn M, Ding A, et al: Deactivation of macrophages by transforming growth factor-β. Nature 334:260, 1991.
413. Tuong MJ, Gruart V, Liu FT, et al: IgE-binding molecules (Mac-2/e-BP) expressed by human eosinophils—implication in IgE-dependent eosinophil cytotoxicity. Eur J Immunol 23:3230, 1993.
414. Turk J, Rand TH, Maas RL, et al: Identification of lipoxygenase products from arachidonic acid metabolism in stimulated murine eosinophils. Biochim Biophys Acta 750:78, 1983.
415. Turk J, Maas RL, Brash AR, et al: Arachidonic acid 15-lipoxygenase products from human eosinophils. J Biol Chem 257:7068, 1982.
416. Turnbull LW, Kay AB: Eosinophils and mediators of anaphylaxis. Histamine and imidazole acetic acid as chemotactic agents for human eosinophil leucocytes. Immunology 31:797, 1976.
417. Ueda N: Biochemical studies on arachidonate 5-lipoxygenase. Vitam Horm 64:699, 1990.
417a. Ukena D, Krogel C, Dent G, et al: PAF-receptors on eosinophils: identification with a novel ligand, [^{3}H] WEB 2086. Biochem Pharmacol 38:1702, 1989.
418. Valent P: The phenotype of human eosinophils, basophils and mast cells. J Allergy Clin Immunol 94:1177, 1994.
419. Valerius T, Repp R, Kalden JR, et al: Effects of IFN on human eosinophils in comparison with other cytokines. A novel class of eosinophil activators with delayed onset of action. J Immunol 145:2950, 1990.
420. van der Bruggen TP, Kok PT, Raaijmakers JAM, et al: Cytokine priming of the respiratory burst in human eosinophils is Ca^{2+} independent and accompanied by induction of tyrosine kinase activity. J Leukoc Biol 53:347, 1993.
421. van der Bruggen T, Kok PT, Raaijmakers JA, et al: Cooperation between Fc gamma receptor II and complement receptor type 3 during activation of platelet-activating factor release by cytokine-primed human eosinophils. J Immunol 153:2729, 1994.
422. Vanderbruggen T, Caldenhoven E, Kanters D, et al: Interleukin-5 signaling in human eosinophils involves JAK2 tyrosine kinase and STAT1-alpha. Blood 85:1442, 1995.
423. van de Winkel JGJ, Capel PJA: Human IgG Fc receptor heterogeneity: molecular aspects and clinical implications. Immunol Today 14:215, 1993.
424. van Haelst-Pisani C, Kovach JS, Kita H, et al: Administration of IL-2 results in increased plasma concentrations of IL-5 and eosinophilia in patients with cancer. Blood 78:1538, 1991.
425. van Oosterhout AJM, Ladenius ARC, Savelkoul HFJ, et al: Effect of anti–IL-5 and IL-5 on airway hyperreactivity and eosinophils in guinea-pig. Am Rev Respir Dis 147:548, 1993.

426. van Oosterhout AJM, van Ark I, Folkerts G, et al: Antibody to IL-5 inhibits virus-induced airway hyperresponsiveness to histamine in guinea pigs. Am J Resp Crit Care Med 131:177, 1994.
427. van Oosterhout AJM, Fattah D, Van Ark I: Eosinophil infiltration precedes development of airway hyperreactivity and mucosal exudation after intranasal instillation of interleukin-5 to mice. J Allergy Clin Immunol 96:104, 1995.
428. Vanto T, Viander M, Koivikko A: Humoral and cell mediated immune response to dog dander and hair in asthmatic children. Allergy 38:103, 1983.
429. Walker C, Riha A, Braun RK, et al: Increased expression of CD11b and functional changes in eosinophils after migration across endothelial cell monolayers. J Immunol 150:4061, 1993.
430. Wallen N, Kita H, Weiler D, et al: Glucocorticoids inhibit cytokine-mediated eosinophil survival. J Immunol 147:3490, 1991.
431. Walls RS, Basten A, Leuchars E, et al: Mechanisms for eosinophilic and neutrophilic leucocytoses. Br Med J 3:157, 1971.
432. Walsh GM, Kay AB: Binding of immunoglobulin classes and subclasses to human neutrophils and eosinophils. Clin Exp Immunol 63:466, 1986.
433. Walsh GM, Mermod JJ, Hartnell A, et al: Human eosinophil, but not neutrophil adherence to IL-1 stimulated HUVEC is $\alpha_4\beta_1$ (VLA-4) dependent. J Immunol 146:3419, 1991.
434. Walsh GM, Hartnell A, Wardlaw AJ, et al: IL-5 enhances the in vitro adhesion of human eosinophils, but not neutrophils, in a leucocyte integrin (CD11/18)-dependent manner. Immunology 71:258, 1990.
435. Wang JM, Rambaldi A, Biondi A, et al: Recombinant human interleukin 5 is a selective eosinophil chemoattractant. Eur J Immunol 19:701, 1989.
436. Wardlaw AJ, Dunnette S, Gleich GJ, et al: Eosinophils and mast cells in bronchoalveolar lavage in subjects with mild asthma: relationship to bronchial hyperreactivity. Am Rev Respir Dis 137:62, 1988.
437. Wardlaw AJ, Moqbel R, Cromwell O, et al: Platelet-activating factor. A potent chemotactic and chemokinetic factor for human eosinophils. J Clin Invest 78:1701, 1986.
438. Wardlaw AJ, Chung KF, Moqbel R, et al: Effects of inhaled PAF in humans on circulating and bronchoalveolar lavage fluid neutrophils. Relationship to bronchoconstriction and changes in airway responsiveness. Am Rev Respir Dis 141:386, 1990.
439. Warren DJ, Sanderson CJ: Production of a T-cell hybrid producing a lymphokine stimulating eosinophil differentiation. Immunology 54:615, 1985.
440. Warringa RAJ, Schweizer RC, Maikoe T, et al: Modulation of eosinophil chemotaxis by interleukin-5. Am J Respir Cell Mol Biol 7:631, 1992.
441. Warringa RAJ, Mengelers HJ, Kuijper PH, et al: In vivo priming of platelet-activating factor-induced eosinophil chemotaxis in allergic asthmatic individuals. Blood 79:1836, 1992.
442. Warringa RAJ, Koenderman L, Kok PT, et al: Modulation and induction of eosinophil chemotaxis by granulocyte-macrophage colony-stimulating factor and interleukin-3. Blood 77:2694, 1991.
443. Wasserman SI, Goetzl EJ, Austen KF: Inactivation of slow reacting substance of anaphylaxis by human eosinophil arylsulfatase. J Immunol 114:645, 1975.
444. Wasserman SI, Goetzl EJ, Austen KF: Preformed eosinophil chemotactic factor of anaphylaxis (ECF-A). J Immunol 112:351, 1974.
444a. Weber M, Uguccioni M, Ochensberger B, et al: Monocyte chemotactic protein MCP-2 activates human basophil and eosinophil leukocyte similar to MCP-3. J Immunol 154:4166, 1995.
445. Weg VB, Williams TJ, Lobb RR, et al: A monoclonal antibody recognizing very late activation antigen-4 inhibits eosinophil accumulation in vivo. J Exp Med 177:561, 1993.
446. Wegner CD, Gundel RH, Reilly P, et al: Intercellular adhesion molecule-1, ICAM-1, in the pathogenesis of asthma. Science 247:456, 1990.
447. Wegner CD, Gundel R, Churchill L, et al: Adhesion glycoproteins as regulators of airway inflammation: emphasis on the role of ICAM-1. In Holgate ST, Austen KF, Lichtenstein LM, Kay AB (eds): Asthma: Physiology, Pharmacology and Treatment. Academic Press, London, 1993, p 227.
448. Wein M, Sterbinsky SA, Bickel CA, et al: Comparison of human eosinophil and neutrophil ligands for P-selectin: ligands for P-selectin differ from those for E-selectin. Am J Respir Cell Mol Biol 12:315, 1995.
449. Weller PF, Austen KF: Human eosinophil arylsulfatase B. Structure and activity of the purified tetrameric lysosomal hydrolase. J Clin Invest 71:114, 1983.
450. Weller PF, Bach D, Austen KF: Human eosinophil lysophospholipase: the sole protein component of Charcot-Leyden crystals. J Immunol 128:1346, 1982.
451. Weller PF, Bach DS, Austen KF: Biochemical characterization of human eosinophil Charcot-Leyden crystal protein (lysophospholipase). J Biol Chem 259:15100, 1984.
452. Weller PF, Rand TH, Barrett T, et al: Accessory cell function of human eosinophils. HLA-DR-dependent, MHC-restricted antigen-presentation and IL-1α expression. J Immunol 150:2554, 1993.
453. Weller PF, Monahan-Earley RA, Dvorak HF, et al: Cytoplasmic lipid bodies of human eosinophils: subcellular isolation and analysis of arachidonate incorporation. Am J Pathol 138:141, 1991.
454. Weller PF, Lee CW, Foster DW, et al: Generation and metabolism of 5-lipoxygenase pathway leukotriene by human eosinophils: predominant production of leukotriene C_4. Proc Natl Acad Sci USA 80:7626, 1983.
455. Weller PF, Rand TH, Goelz SE, et al: Human eosinophil adherence to vascular endothelium mediated by binding to vascular cell adhesion molecule 1 and endothelial leukocyte adhesion molecule 1. Proc Natl Acad Sci USA 88:7430, 1991.
456. Weller PF, Goetzl EJ, Austen KF: Identification of human eosinophil lysophospholipase as the constituent of Charcot-Leyden crystals. Proc Natl Acad Sci USA 77:7440, 1980.
457. West BV, Gleb NA, Rosenthal AS: Isolation and partial characterization of human eosinophil granules. Am J Pathol 81:575, 1975.
458. White CJ, Maxwell CJ, Gallin JI: Changes in the structural and functional properties of human eosinophils during experimental hookworm (*Necator americanus*) infection. J Infect Dis 154:778, 1986.
459. White SR, Ohno S, Munoz NM, et al: Epithelium-dependent contraction of airway smooth muscle caused by eosinophil MBP. Am J Physiol (Lung Mol Cell Physiol) 259(3):L294, 1990.
460. White SR, Strek ME, Kulp GV, et al: Regulation of human eosinophil degranulation and activation by endogeneous phospholipase A2. J Clin Invest 91:2118, 1993.
461. Williams DM, Linder JE, Hill MW, et al: Ultrastructural localization of alkaline phosphatase in rat eosinophil leucocytes. J Histochem Cytochem 26:862, 1978.
462. Winqvist I, Olofsson T, Olsson I, et al: Altered density, metabolism and surface receptors of eosinophils in eosinophilia. Immunology 47:531, 1982.
463. Winqvist I, Olofsson T, Olsson I: Mechanisms for eosinophil degranulation: release of the eosinophil cationic protein. Immunology 51:1, 1984.
464. Lee GR, Bithell TC, Foerster J, et al (eds): Wintrobe's Clinical Hematology, 9th edition. Lea & Febiger, Philadelphia, 1993.
465. Wong DT, Elovic A, Matossian K, et al: Eosinophils from patients with blood eosinophilia express transforming growth factor beta 1. Blood 78:2702, 1991.
466. Wong DT, Weller PF, Galli SJ, et al: Human eosinophils express transforming growth factor alpha. J Exp Med 172:673, 1990.
467. Wu AM, Till JE, Siminovitch L, et al: Cytological evidence for a relationship between normal hematopoietic colony-forming cells and cells of the lymphoid system. J Exp Med 127:455, 1968.
468. Wymann MP, Kernen P, Vontscharner V, et al: Activation of the respiratory burst in eosinophil leucocytes—a transduction sequence decoupled from cytosolic Ca^{2+} rise. Eur J Clin Invest 25:25, 1995.
469. Yamaguchi S, Nagai H, Tanaka H, et al: Time course study for antigen-induced airway hyperreactivity and the effect of soluble IL-5 receptor. Life Sci 54:471, 1994.
470. Yamaguchi Y, Hayashi Y, Sugama Y, et al: Highly purified murine interleukin 5, IL-5, stimulates eosinophil function and prolongs in vitro survival: IL-5 as an eosinophil chemotactic factor. J Exp Med 167:1737, 1988.
471. Yamaguchi Y, Zhang DE, Sun Z, et al: Functional characterization of the promoter for the gene encoding human eosinophil peroxidase. J Biol Chem 269:19410, 1995.
472. Yamashita T, Someya A, Hara E: Response of superoxide anion production by guinea-pig eosinophils to various soluble stimuli: comparison to neutrophils. Arch Biochem Biophys 241:447, 1985.
473. Yazdanbakhsh M, Eckman CM, Koenderman L, et al: Eosinophils do respond to FMLP. Blood 70:379, 1987.
474. Ying S, Durham SR, Barkans J, et al: T cells are the principal source of interleukin-5 mRNA in allergen-induced rhinitis. Am J Respir Cell Mol Biol 9:356, 1993.

475. Ying S, Tabordabarata L, Meng Q, et al: The kinetics of allergen-induced transcription of messenger RNA for monocyte chemotactic protein-3 and RANTES in the skin of human atopic subjects—relationship to eosinophil, T cell, and macrophage recruitment. J Exp Med 181:2153, 1995.
476. Yousefi S, Green DR, Blaser K, et al: Protein-tyrosine phosphorylation regulates apoptosis in human eosinophils and neutrophils. Proc Natl Acad Aci USA 91:10868, 1994.
477. Yousefi S, Hemmann S, Weber M, et al: IL-8 is expressed by human peripheral blood eosinophils. Evidence for increased secretion in asthma. J Immunol 154:5481, 1995.
478. Yukawa T, Kroegel C, Evans P, et al: Density heterogeneity of eosinophil leukocytes: induction of hypodense eosinophils by platelet-activating factor. Immunology 68:140, 1989.
479. Yukawa T, Kroegel C, Dent G, et al: Effect of theophylline and adenosine on eosinophil function. Am Rev Respir Dis 140:327, 1989.
480. Yukawa T, Ukena D, Kroegel C, et al: Beta$_2$-adrenergic receptors on eosinophils. Binding and functional studies. Am Rev Respir Dis 141:1446, 1990.
481. Zheutlin LM, Ackerman SJ, Gleich GJ, et al: Stimulation of basophil and rat mast cell histamine release by eosinophil granule-derived cationic proteins. J Immunol 133:2180, 1984.
482. Zhou Z-Q, Tenen DG, Dvorak AM, et al: The gene for human eosinophil Charcot-Leyden crystal protein directs the expression of lysophospholipase activity and crystallization in transfected COS cells. J Leukoc Biol 52:588, 1992.
483. Ziegler RS, Yurdin DL, Colten HR: Histamine metabolism. II. Cellular and subcellular localization of the catabolic enzymes, histaminase and histamine methyl transferase, in human leukocytes. J Allergy Clin Immunol 58:172, 1976.
484. Zoratti EM, Sedgwick JB, Bates ME, et al: Platelet-activating factor primes human eosinophil generation of superoxide. Am J Respir Cell Mol Biol 6:100, 1992.
485. Zucker-Franklin D, Grusky G: Ultrastructural analysis of hematopoietic colonies derived from human peripheral blood. J Cell Biol 63:855, 1974.
486. Zucker-Franklin D: Eosinophil structure and maturation. In Mahmoud AAF, Austen KF (eds): The Eosinophil in Health and Disease. Grune & Stratton, Inc, New York, 1980, pp 43–59.

12 Lipid Mediators—Leukotrienes, Prostanoids, Platelet-Activating Factor, and Lipoxins

S. M. SHUAIB NASSER TAK HONG LEE

Enormous scientific interest and research has centered on the products of oxygenated fatty acid metabolism known collectively as lipid mediators. Among this family are the prostaglandins and thromboxanes, which are expressed in virtually every mammalian cell, the leukotrienes, which are found almost exclusively in cells of myeloid lineage, and the dual lipoxygenase products known as lipoxins. Physiologically, these products of arachidonic acid metabolism participate in many normal processes, which include body temperature regulation, the coagulation cascade, control of parturition, blood pressure maintenance, and mediation of the immune system. Pathologically, these lipid mediators have been incriminated in a wide range of disease processes, including asthma, rhinosinusitis, psoriasis, ischemic heart disease, rheumatoid arthritis, inflammatory bowel disease, and malignancy.

The original work on these compounds began in 1930 when Raphael Kurzrok and Charles Lieb studied the ability of human semen either to relax or to contract isolated strips of uterine tissue.[234] Three years later, Goldblatt and von Euler independently observed a similar phenomenon using human seminal plasma and extracts from sheep seminal vesical glands.[161, 425] Von Euler therefore coined the term prostaglandin believing that he had isolated a product of the prostate gland. Further work on prostaglandins was carried out by three groups led by Sune Bergstrom, Bengt Samuelsson, and John Vane. Bergstrom determined the structure and biologic role of the prostaglandins and discovered that they are synthesized in vivo from dietary polyunsaturated fatty acids; Samuelsson determined the metabolic fate and disposition of the prostaglandins; and Vane demonstrated the ability of anti-inflammatory substances, such as aspirin, to inhibit prostaglandin synthesis.

Leukotrienes were discovered during the elucidation of a mixture of compounds referred to as the slow-reacting substance of anaphylaxis (SRS-A). In 1940, Kellawey and Trethewie found that as a product of immediate hypersensitivity, this isolate had the ability to constrict smooth muscle tissue more slowly than did histamine and therefore called it SRS-A.[214] In 1980, the composition of SRS-A was finally elucidated by Samuelsson and colleagues, Morris and colleagues, and Lewis, Austen, and colleagues to be a mixture of leukotriene C_4 (LTC_4) and its biologically active metabolites, LTD_4 and LTE_4.[253, 297, 367] The term leukotriene was finally conceived by Samuelsson to describe a family of compounds, each containing three conjugated double bonds and derived from the metabolism of arachidonic acid by 5-lipoxygenase (5-LO) in leukocytes. He subjected arachidonic acid to the actions of various lipoxygenases and found that rabbit PMNs metabolized arachidonate to a family of dihydroxy acids with triple spectrophotometric absorption peaks at 259, 269, and 279 nm. These characteristic triple peaks suggested the existence of triple-conjugated double bonds in these compounds.

Unlike many bioactive mediators such as histamine, the lipid mediators are not preformed but are generated de novo upon cell activation. The primary substrate fatty acid that acts as a precursor for leukotrienes, prostanoids, and lipoxins is 5,8,11,14-eicosatetraenoic acid (arachidonic acid). Arachidonic acid is released from nuclear membrane phospholipids. Subsequent oxidative metabolism of this polyunsaturated fatty acid by the 5-LO pathway yields the leukotrienes and lipoxins and by the cyclooxygenase pathway leads to prostanoid biosynthesis.

THE LEUKOTRIENES

BIOSYNTHESIS

Arachidonic acid is a 20-carbon polyunsaturated fatty acid released from membrane phospholipids by the action of phospholipase A_2. The enzyme 5-LO catalyzes the first dedicated step in arachidonic acid metabolism (Fig. 12–1) by oxygenation at the carbon 5 (C5) position to generate the unstable intermediate 5S-hydroperoxyeicosatetraenoic acid (5-HPETE). This is either reduced to the alcohol 5S-hydroxyeicosatetraenoic acid (5-HETE) or converted by a second 5-LO step via a dehydrase to a C5,6-transepoxide with three conjugated (7,9-trans,11-cis) olefinic bonds and a fourth unconjugated double bond at C14. This compound was the first leukotriene described and therefore designated LTA_4.

Further metabolism of LTA_4 takes place via two alternative enzymatic pathways. The first is by an epoxide hydrolase to 5S,12R-dihydroxyeicosatetraenoic acid (LTB_4), and the second is by a glutathione s-transferase termed LTC_4 synthase to LTC_4. LTA_4 may also degrade spontaneously in the absence of either activated enzyme system to 6-trans-LTB_4, which has significantly less bioactivity. LTC_4 is subsequently cleaved by removal of glutamic acid from the peptide by γ-glutamyltranspeptidase to form the 6R-S-cysteinylglycine analogue, LTD_4. Further cleavage of LTD_4 occurs by a dipeptidase, which removes glycine to form its 6R-S-cysteinyl analogue, LTE_4. These latter three compounds are known collectively as the sulfidopeptide or cysteinyl leukotrienes because of the presence of a peptide linked to the eicosanoid backbone through a thioether link at C6. The sulfidopeptide leukotrienes constitute the activity previously recognized as the slow-reacting substance of anaphylaxis.

ENZYMES INVOLVED IN LEUKOTRIENE BIOSYNTHESIS

5-Lipoxygenase

Borgeat, Hamberg, and Samuelsson[35] provided the first evidence of 5-LO by describing the transformation of arachidonic acid to 5-HPETE by rabbit peritoneal neutrophils. The enzyme contains dual 5-lipoxygenase/LTA_4 synthase activity and acts first by stereospecifically inserting molecular oxygen at C5 leading to the formation of 5-HPETE followed by the stereospecific removal of the pro-R C10 hydrogen followed by epoxide formation (LTA_4). This was first shown using 5-LO purified from potato tubers[378] and subsequently confirmed in human leukocytes.[359] Calcium and ATP were shown to be required for maximal activity.[361, 377] There is some support for the concept of 5-LO residing in the cytosol in the resting cell and upon activation translocating to the nuclear membrane.[358, 368, 444, 447] However, the membrane-bound 5-LO was found to be enzymatically inactive,[358, 444] suggesting that translocation to a membrane site may lead to suicide inactivation of the enzyme or that a further step such as the presentation of arachidonic acid by 5-LO activating protein (FLAP) is required for 5-LO activation. Furthermore, it has been demonstrated that in a cell-free system using homogenized leukocytes and in the presence of calcium that there is membrane association of the enzyme, which reverses upon calcium withdrawal.[362]

The cDNA encoding human 5-LO has been cloned from a dimethyl sulfoxide differentiated HL-60 cell cDNA library[106] and a human placenta cDNA library.[278] The nucleotide sequence predicts an enzyme of 673 amino acid residues with a calculated molecular weight of 78 kD. The overall predicted structure of 5-LO is hydrophilic, but one central portion encoded by exon 7 (amino acids 278–326) corresponds to the most hydrophobic region and could represent an important structural domain or region associated with the catalytic site.[151, 278] A short amino acid sequence shares some homology with the interfacial binding domain of human lipoprotein lipase and rat hepatic lipase,[106] and this may be responsible for membrane binding in the absence of predictions for transmembrane domains. 15-Lipoxygenase displays 61% sequence similarity with human 5-LO with greatest identity at the middle and carboxyl-terminal regions.[379] It is unknown at present how these similarities and differences affect the specificity of the different lipoxygenases.

The human 5-LO gene was isolated from one cosmid and three different bacteriophage genomic libraries.[151] The gene is single copy and spans greater than 82 kb of DNA organized into 14 exons and 13 introns. The size range of the exons was found to be 82 to 613 base pairs and 200 to 26,000 base pairs for the introns. The putative promoter region of the 5-LO gene seems to share a number of characteristics commonly found in housekeeping genes. For example, it lacks typical TATA and CCAAT boxes in the expected positions upstream of the major transcription initiation sites of which there are one major and several potential minor sites. Instead, this region is GC rich and contains eight potential sites for binding of the Sp 1 transcription factor. This is rather surprising as 5-LO is not constitutively expressed but is assumed to be primarily present in cells of myeloid lineage.

Five-Lipoxygenase Activating Protein (FLAP)

Although the enzyme 5-LO provides the first dedicated step for leukotriene formation, it requires the association of an additional factor. Mammalian osteosarcoma cells transfected with 5-LO express active enzyme in broken cell preparations but no leukotriene metabolites on stimulation with the calcium ionophore A23187.[360] In addition, a new class of indole leukotriene biosynthesis inhibitor, MK-886,

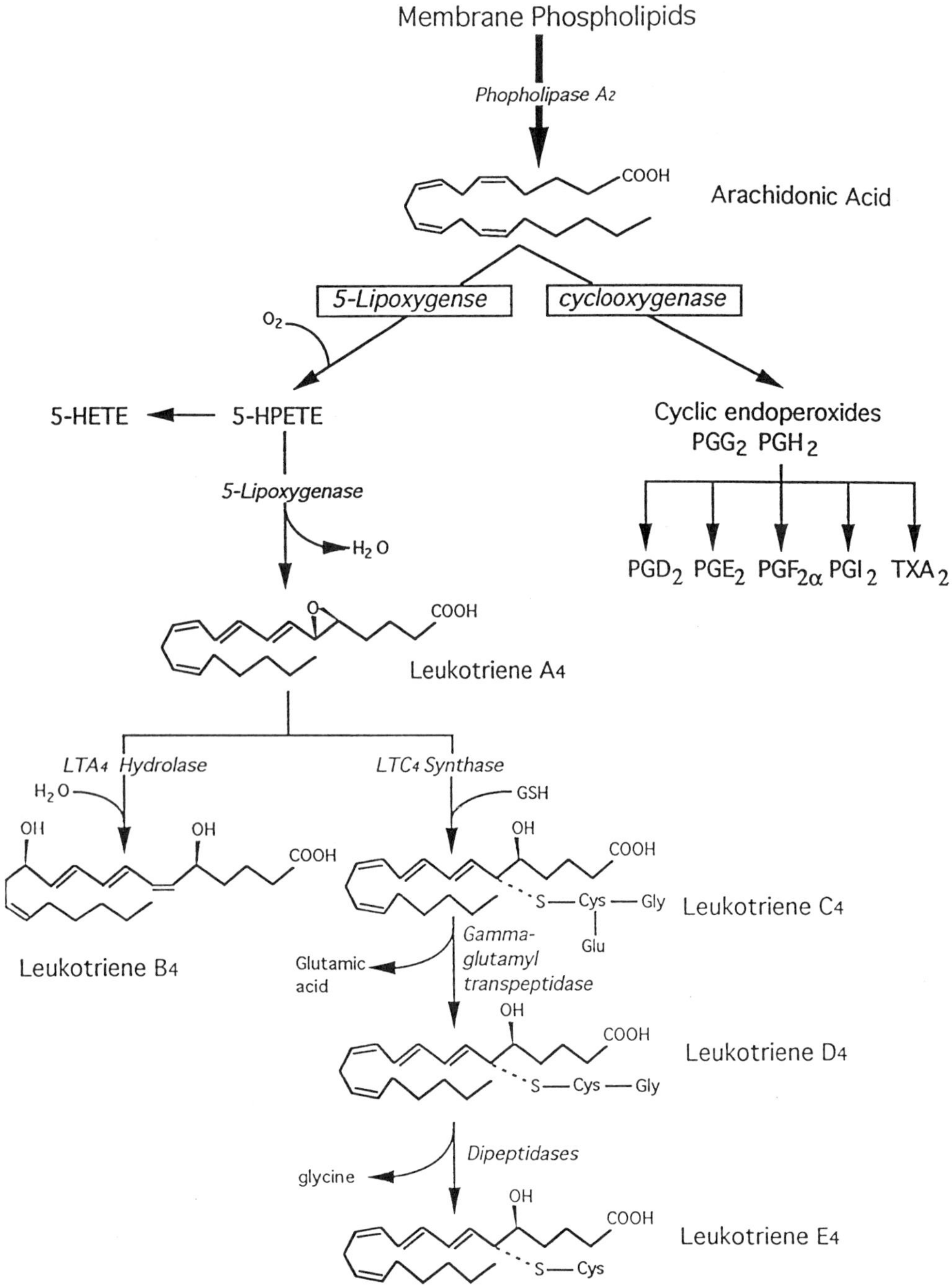

FIGURE 12–1. Leukotriene biosynthesis from nuclear membrane phospholipids and arachidonic acid via the 5-lipoxygenase (5-LO) pathway. LTA_4 = leukotriene A_4; LTC_4 = leukotriene C_4; 5-HPETE = 5-hydroperoxyeicosatetraenoic acid; 5-HETE = 5-hydroxyeicosatetraenoic acid.

was found to act only on intact PMNs but had no direct inhibitory effect on 5-LO activity in cell-free systems.[160] A membrane protein with high affinity for MK-886 of relative molecular mass 18 kD was identified from rat and human leukocytes[293] and subsequently the cDNA encoding FLAP.[105] Because the expression of both 5-LO and 5-LO activating protein (FLAP) was required for leukotriene synthesis in intact cells, it was termed FLAP.

Using hydrophobic moment analysis, three hydrophobic regions of 20 to 30 residues were proposed, which predicted three membrane-spanning domains connected by two hydrophilic loops. The human gene for FLAP was isolated from two different genomic libraries and found to span greater than 31 kb consisting of five small exons and four large introns. The putative promoter region contains a possible TATA box (TGTAAT) and possible AP-2 and glucocorticoid receptor binding sites.[215] In osteosarcoma cells transfected with 5-LO or FLAP alone and stimulated with the calcium ionophore A23187, no arachidonic acid metabolites were detected. By contrast, A23187 stimulation of cell lines expressing both 5-LO and FLAP resulted in significant production of 5-LO products.[107] The human promyelocytic cell line U937 expresses FLAP but not 5-LO and is unable to synthesize leukotrienes after A23187 stimulation but does so after transfection by a retroviral vector encoding 5-LO mRNA.[211] Five T-cell lines were found to express FLAP but not 5-LO and therefore were unable to generate leukotrienes upon cell activation.[198]

Leukotriene C_4 Synthase

Leukotriene C_4 synthase is responsible for conjugation of LTA_4 to reduced glutathione (GSH) to form the parent LTC_4 for the cysteinyl leukotriene family. The cDNA of LTC_4 synthase was cloned in 1994[237] from a KG-1 cDNA expression library, which was screened using a sensitive fluorescence-linked immunoassay for LTC_4 after transfection of COS cells and the addition of substrate LTA_4. This identified individual clones with maximal LTC_4 synthase activity that contained a 694-bp cDNA insert. The open reading frame of 450 bp encoded a 16.5-kD protein, and hybridization with a cDNA probe demonstrated an mRNA transcript of 700 bp in RNAs from human eosinophils and myelocytic KG-1 cells that contain LTC_4 synthase. The deduced amino acid sequences of the LTC_4 synthase cDNA showed no significant homology to GSH *S*-transferases but share 31% overall and 44% N-terminal two-thirds amino acid identity with FLAP. This was in agreement with a previous study that distinguished LTC_4 synthase activity from that of the cytosolic and other microsomal GSH *S*-transferases.[450] Subsequently, LTC_4 synthase activity was found to exist as an 18-kD integral membrane protein from the myeloid KG-1 cell line[326] and from the THP-1 monocytic leukemia cell line.[306]

The amino acid sequence of LTC_4 synthase cDNA contains two cysteine residues (positions 56 and 82) and two consensus protein kinase phosphorylation sites (residues 28–30 and 111–113). Hydrophobicity analysis of the deduced amino acid sequence predicts three transmembrane domains. When the LTC_4 synthase protein was aligned with FLAP, the predicted transmembrane domains of the consensus LTC_4 synthase overlapped with the membrane-spanning domains of FLAP, supporting the structural homology between these two proteins. In addition, the hydrophilic loops between the transmembrane domains were found to be of identical length. Furthermore, an inhibitor of FLAP, MK-886, was found to inhibit LTC_4 synthase activity from transfected COS cells in a dose-related fashion.[237] An explanation to account for the homologous regions in these two enzymes is that this may be the site of arachidonic acid binding to FLAP for presentation to 5-LO[267] and LTA_4 binding to LTC_4 synthase for conjugation with GSH.

LTA_4 Hydrolase

Leukotriene A_4 is an unstable epoxide intermediate that is enzymatically hydrolyzed by LTA_4 hydrolase to generate the dihydroxy acid LTB_4. LTA_4 hydrolase, a cytosolic monomeric protein of molecular weight 68–70 kD, was first purified from human peripheral leukocytes.[342] Subsequently, the presence of LTA_4 hydrolase was reported in human erythrocytes,[282] human lung,[318] and rat neutrophils.[120] The substrate requirements of LTA_4 hydrolase are quite specific and include a free carboxylic acid moiety, 5,6-epoxide, and the tetraene structure with the 7,9-trans-11,14 cis configuration.[317] In addition, it is likely that different isoforms of the enzyme exist with erythrocyte LTA_4 hydrolase of lower molecular weight (54 kD) compared with the leukocyte isoenzyme (68–71 kD).[282] Covalent binding of LTA_4 to LTA_4 hydrolase has been observed during catalysis,[122] and this probably accounts for the characteristic suicide inactivation of the enzyme.[282]

Funk and colleagues[152] immunoscreened a human lung λgt11 expression library using a polyclonal antiserum to isolate a 1910 nucleotide cDNA clone containing the complete protein-coding region of LTA_4 hydrolase. Minami and colleagues[294] used a 48-base probe based on the known partial amino acid sequence from the human leukocyte enzyme and isolated a cDNA clone encoding LTA_4 hydrolase from a human spleen library with an open reading frame of 1.8 kb. From the deduced primary structure, LTA_4 hydrolase is a compound of 610 amino acids and molecular weight 69 kD and shares no apparent homology with other epoxide hydrolases or with any other known proteins. Unlike 5-LO, LTA_4 hydrolase is found in virtually all human tissues. For example, the human diploid fibroblast and Burkitt's lymphoma Raji B-cell line contain LTA_4 hydrolase mRNA, which is actively translated into immunodetectable protein, but lacks both 5-LO mRNA and protein.[289] This suggests that transcellular metabolism of LTA_4 to LTC_4 as demonstrated in neutrophils acting in conjunction with endothelial cells[124] or platelets,[261] or to LTB_4 with erythrocytes[283] may be physiologically important.

CELLULAR ACTIVATION

The mechanism of cellular activation and subsequent leukotriene biosynthesis is believed to arise as a result of translocation of 5-LO from cytosolic to membrane compartments and to bring the enzyme into close proximity with FLAP, which acts as an anchor for 5-LO and provides access to substrate and other components of leukotriene synthesis. In osteosarcoma cells expressing 5-LO but not FLAP, 5-LO is able to associate with cell membranes following A23187 stimulation, and this is not inhibited by MK-886. This led the authors to conclude that 5-LO membrane association and activation can be divided into a two-stage process: (1) calcium-dependent movement of 5-LO to membrane without product formation, which can occur in the absence of FLAP, and (2) activation of 5-LO with product formation, which is FLAP dependent and inhibited by MK-886.[212] High levels of FLAP were expressed in SF9 insect cells transfected with recombinant baclovirus, and this system was used to demonstrate that FLAP specifically binds [^{125}I] L-739,059, a photoaffinity analogue of arachidonic acid. This binding is inhibited by both arachidonic acid and MK-886 and suggests that FLAP may activate 5-LO by bringing enzyme and substrate together.[267] Ultracentrifugation[331] and immunoelectron microscopy studies have demonstrated that on cellular activation 5-LO translocates to the nuclear envelope, which is also the site of FLAP.[447] The situation in resting cells is still uncertain, and 5-LO may be located in the cytosol[358] or nuclear euchromatin.[446]

CELLULAR ORIGIN

The cellular synthesis of leukotrienes is limited by the requirement to express both 5-LO and FLAP. Cells of myeloid lineage provide the major source of leukotriene production, although B lymphocytes also have been shown to be capable of generating small amounts of leukotrienes.[197] Cells can be divided by their ability to preferentially synthesize LTB_4 or the cysteinyl leukotrienes, LTC_4, LTD_4, and LTE_4, depending on the intracellular predominance of either LTA_4 hydrolase or LTC_4 synthase.

Monocytes, alveolar macrophages, and peripheral blood neutrophils preferentially generate LTB_4, whereas eosinophils, mast cells, and basophils preferentially generate cysteinyl leukotriene products. Monocytes and macrophages have the capacity to generate both LTB_4 and LTC_4. On stimulation with the ionophore A23187, peripheral blood monocytes in adherent monolayers produce 68 ng LTB_4 and 30 ng LTC_4 per 10^6 cells.[443] The major lipoxygenase product of alveolar macrophages is LTB_4, which generates 17 to 30 ng/10^6 cells in response to calcium ionophore A23187 stimulation.[126] Peripheral blood neutrophils from normal donors produce about 48 ng LTB_4/10^6 cells with only one seventh as much LTC_4/10^6 cells after A23187 stimulation.

Eosinophils from normal subjects preferentially synthesize LTC_4 and in response to A23187 stimulation produce 38 ng LTC_4/10^6 cells and about 6 ng LTB_4/10^6 cells.[437] Human lung mast cells release 22 ng LTC_4/10^6 cells with similar amounts released in response to either IgE– or calcium ionophore A23187–mediated degranulation.[330] Basophils obtained from the peripheral blood of patients with chronic myelogenous leukemia are found to release LTB_4.[356] Basophils also release LTC_4 but unlike mast cells do not produce PGD_2.

Local instillation of specific allergen into the nasal mucosa of sensitive subjects leads to recovery of histamine, PGD_2, and LTC_4 from nasal secretions during the early phase but only histamine and LTC_4 during the late phase reaction. These findings suggest that mast-cell degranulation is important in the early phase response to allergen and that basophils mediate the late reaction.[80, 299] Human B-lymphocyte lines and normal human tonsillar B lymphocytes produce small amounts of LTB_4 and 5-HETE upon stimulation with A23187[197] in comparison with the amounts produced by the sonicates of these cells. However, pre-incubation with a glutathione-depleting agent prior to stimulation leads to similar amounts of LTB_4 generated by the intact cells as are formed by the sonicated cells. T lymphocytes only express the FLAP gene but not the 5-LO gene and are therefore unable to generate leukotrienes.[198]

Guinea pig lung parenchyma has been shown to convert LTA_4 to LTB_4 and the cysteinyl leukotrienes,[380] suggesting the presence of LTA_4 hydrolase and LTC_4 synthase. Human lung parenchyma converts LTC_4 to LTD_4 and LTE_4.[6, 77] Unlike 5-LO, LTC_4 synthase and LTA_4 hydrolase, which convert LTA_4 to LTC_4 and LTB_4, respectively, are widely distributed in mammalian cells. Thus LTA_4 released by a cell capable of generating 5-LO products may be utilized for further metabolism by other cells without the enzyme 5-LO (Fig. 12–2).

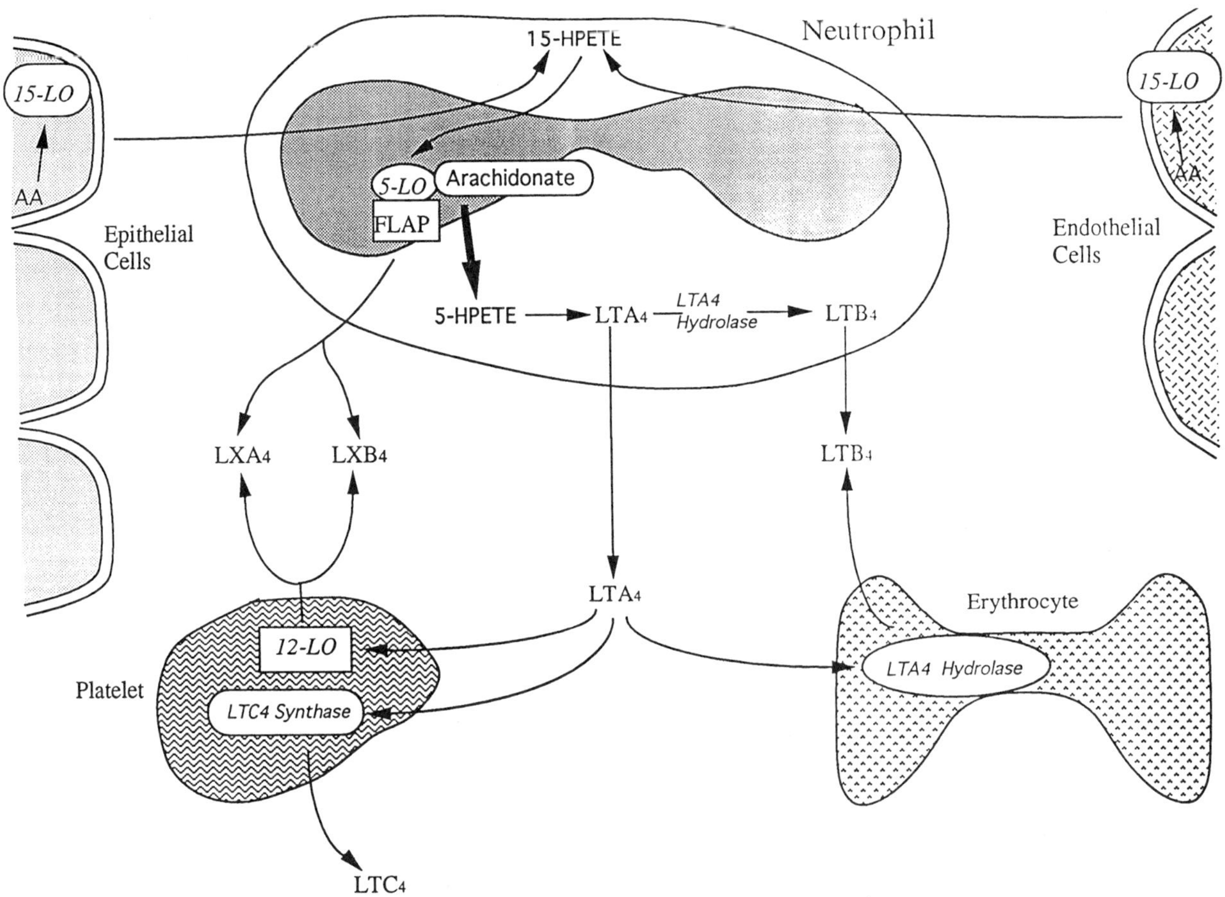

FIGURE 12–2. Transcellular biosynthesis of leukotrienes and lipoxins by cell-cell interaction between PMN leukocytes and platelets for cysteinyl leukotriene production or PMN leukocytes and either platelets or epithelial or endothelial cells for lipoxin generation. Human 5-lipoxygenase (5-LO) is located in the cytosol or nuclear euchromatin of the resting cell and upon activation is translocated to form a complex with 5-lipoxygenase activating protein (FLAP) to express enzymatic activity. Endothelial and epithelial cells contain 15-lipoxygenase (15-LO), and platelets contain both 12-lipoxygenase (12-LO) and LTC_4 synthase activity.

Such transcellular metabolism involves the supply of LTA_4 by neutrophils and to the generation of LTC_4 by platelets,[116, 262] mast cells,[85] airway epithelium, and vascular endothelial cells[125] or to the generation of LTB_4 by erythrocytes.[284]

METABOLISM AND ELIMINATION

Rapid inactivation and removal of the leukotrienes from sites of inflammation requires metabolism by specific and appropriately located enzymes. LTB_4-20-hydroxylase (P-450_{LTB}) is located exclusively in neutrophil microsomes and converts LTB_4 by ω-oxygenation to 20-OH-LTB_4, which is substantially less chemotactic for neutrophils than LTB_4. This is further metabolized by oxidation to 5S,12R-dihydroxy,20-aldehyde-6,14-cis-8,10-trans-eicosatetraenoic acid (20-CHO LTB_4), which has no biologic activity. This is followed by irreversible conversion to 20-carboxy-6,14-cis-8,10-trans-eicosatetraenoic acid (20-COOH-LTB_4). 20-CHO LTB_4 can also be metabolized via an alternative pathway by an aldehyde reductase in the microsomes back to 20-OH-LTB_4, thereby allowing tightly regulated LTB_4 degradation.

Three major metabolic pathways are involved in LTC_4 metabolism. The first comprises conversion of LTC_4 by peptide cleavage to LTD_4 and then to LTE_4 by the action of γ-glutamyl transpeptidase and one of a variety of dipeptidases, respectively. This does not require activation of the cells involved and may only result in some loss of biologic activity.

The second pathway involves the oxidative metabolism of the cysteinyl leukotrienes and depends on the production of hydrogen peroxide (H_2O_2) and superoxide anion (O_{2-}) by the respiratory burst and secretion of eosinophil peroxidase (EPO) from eosinophils and myeloperoxidase (MPO) from neutrophils or monocytes. This leads to oxidative degradation of the cysteinyl leukotrienes and acts as a control over their biologic effects. EPO or MPO catalyze the oxidation of halides by H_2O_2 to form hypohalous acids such as HOCl, HOBr, or HOI, which readily degrade LTC_4, LTD_4, and LTE_4 to their respective inactive sulfoxide derivatives and to the 6-trans-diastereoisomers of LTB_4.[174, 175] Each of the S-diastereomeric sulfoxides (SO) is then converted to its respective sulfone (SO_2), which results in considerable loss of bioactivity. The 6-trans-LTB_4-diastereoisomers are nonspasmogenic, but the sulfoxides retain approximately 5% of the spasmogenic activity of the parent compounds.

The third pathway involves β-oxidation and elimination leading to carboxylation, hydroxylation, and the gradual shortening of the ω-segment of the molecule. A fraction of infused LTE_4 is eliminated unchanged in urine, and because this fraction remains constant, urinary concentrations of LTE_4 have been used to reflect systemic synthesis of LTC_4.[266, 364] It is likely that cellular activation leads not only to enhanced leukotriene release but also to the increased capacity to degrade them.

BIOLOGIC ACTIONS

LTB_4

The actions of LTB_4 are summarized in Table 12–1. LTB_4 is a proinflammatory compound and acts on the microvasculature by increasing leukocyte adherence to endothelium[184] and enhancing cutaneous microvascular permeability by the secondary action of an unidentified neutrophil-derived factor.[38, 194] Other actions include potent chemotaxis for neutrophils, mediated by a subset of high-affinity receptors and chemokinetic and weak chemotactic activity for eosinophils.[300, 322] LTB_4 is also chemokinetic for monocytes[322]; aggregates neutrophils[139]; enhances expression of CR1 and CR3 receptors on neutrophils and eosinophils[247, 300]; and releases lysosomal enzymes and generates superoxide via a subset of low-affinity receptors.[163] LTB_4 has bronchoconstrictor activity, especially when administered intravenously, and this action is mediated indirectly through the action of thromboxane (TX) A_2 synthesized locally in lung tissues.[381] LTB_4 also has immunoregulatory functions. It induces increased numbers of suppressor T lymphocytes from precursors.[14] At concentrations of 10^{-12}M to 10^{-8}M, LTB_4 significantly enhances natural killer cytotoxicity for virus-infected cells and the tumor cell line K-562.[354] It directly increases IgG production by highly purified human tonsillar B lymphocytes and augments IL-2 and IFN-γ production in human T lymphocytes.[355]

TABLE 12–1
BIOLOGIC ACTIVITY OF LEUKOTRIENE B_4

Increase leukocyte adherence to endothelium[184]
Increase microvascular permeability (secondary action)[38, 194]
Neutrophil chemotaxis and weak eosinophil chemotaxis[300, 322]
Monocyte chemokinesis[322]
Enhanced expression of CR1 and CR3 receptors on neutrophils and eosinophils[247, 300]
Neutrophil aggregation[139]
Lysosomal release and superoxide generation[163]
Bronchoconstriction via 2° release of TXA_2[381]
Enhanced NK-cell cytotoxicity for virus-infected and tumor cells[354]
Induction of suppressor T lymphocytes[14]
Enhances IgG production by human B lymphocytes and augments IL-2 and IFN-γ production by T lymphocytes[355]

Cysteinyl Leukotrienes

The biologic actions of the cysteinyl leukotrienes are summarized in Table 12–2. The cysteinyl leukotrienes are potent

TABLE 12–2
BIOLOGIC ACTIVITY OF CYSTEINYL LEUKOTRIENES

Augment postcapillary dermal vascular permeability in guinea pigs[111, 253]
Increased microvascular permeability[111, 210]
Increased leukocyte adhesion to endothelial cells[285]
Increased mucus secretion[272]
Potent contractile agonist for bronchial smooth muscle[91]
Enhances smooth muscle contractile responsiveness to other agonists[13, 244, 312]
Vasoconstriction[46, 399]
Coronary vasoconstriction in sheep[292]
Systemic vasoconstriction in rats[332]
Renal vasoconstriction in rats[16]
Recruit granulocytes into the lamina propria of asthmatic airways (LTE_4)[236]

contractile agonists for bronchial smooth muscle in isolated human lobar and segmental bronchi, with LTC_4 and LTD_4 reported to be approximately 1,000 times more potent than histamine in contracting human bronchi in vitro.[94] Local administration to guinea pigs of LTD_4 and with lesser potency LTC_4 and LTE_4 has been shown to enhance postcapillary dermal venular permeability, as shown by the leakage of intravenously administered dye.[111, 254] The cysteinyl leukotrienes increase microvascular permeability, producing contraction of adjacent endothelial cells,[111, 210] and augment leukocyte adhesion to endothelial cells.[285] From studies of bronchial mucosal explants, as little as 10^{-9}M LTC_4 and LTD_4 has been proposed to stimulate mucus secretion, and this may contribute to the excess mucus secretion found in bronchial asthma.[273]

In studies of both normal and asthmatic subjects, the use of inhaled cysteinyl leukotrienes has demonstrated the potency of these mediators in causing bronchoconstriction, with LTC_4 the most and LTE_4 the least potent.[4, 11, 109] Subcutaneous injection of the cysteinyl leukotrienes in humans produces dermal edema sustained for 2 to 4 hours.[399] LTC_4 and to a lesser extent LTD_4 constrict arterioles, although they increase permeability of postcapillary venules. They have vasoconstrictor properties, as demonstrated in guinea pig skin after intradermal injection[111, 254] and in normal human skin by blanching of an elicited wheal at the injection site.[46, 399] Coronary vasoconstriction has been demonstrated in sheep after direct infusion of LTD_4 into a coronary vessel in vivo.[292] In the rat, intravenous infusion of LTC_4 led to systemic[332] and renal vasoconstriction.[16] In a study of four asthmatic subjects, LTE_4 has been shown to recruit granulocytes, particularly eosinophils, 4 hours after inhalation into the lamina propria of bronchial biopsy specimens (Fig. 12–3).[236]

RECEPTORS

The development of novel pharmacologic antagonists has indicated that leukotrienes mediate their actions through stereospecific receptor interactions.

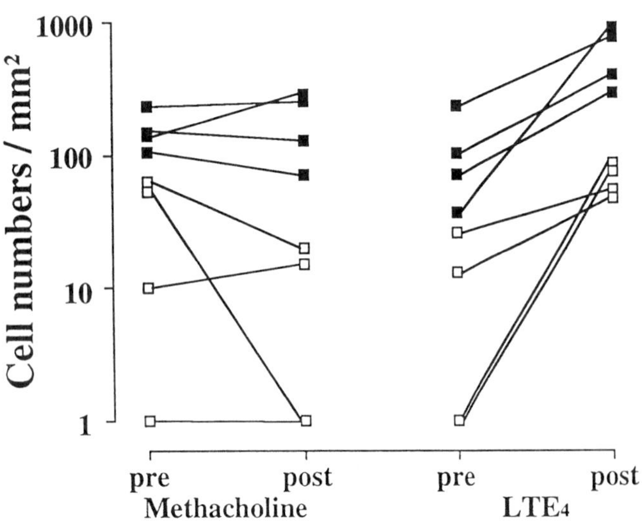

FIGURE 12–3. Change in the number of eosinophils (closed squares) and neutrophils (open squares) in the lamina propria of airways mucosa before and after provocation with inhaled LTE_4 or methacholine. (From Laitinen LA, Laitinen A, Haahtela T, et al: Leukotriene E_4 and granulocytic infiltration into asthmatic airways. Lancet 341:989–990, 1983. © by The Lancet Ltd. 1983.)

Peptide Leukotriene Receptors

Much of the evidence for the existence of distinct receptors for LTC_4, LTD_4, and LTE_4 comes from work carried out in the guinea pig lung and is supported by differences in biologic activity of the individual leukotrienes, the effects of leukotriene receptor antagonists, and radioligand-binding studies. The evidence for separate cysteinyl leukotriene receptors in human tissue is more limited and remains a matter of debate. Certainly in human lung, a ligand-specific and stereospecific LTD_4 receptor is recognized, and this is known to be regulated by GTP, implying association with a GTP-binding protein. In guinea pig lung, the use of physiologic and radioligand-binding studies has demonstrated the existence of separate receptors for LTC_4, LTD_4, and LTE_4. The rank order of potency of the sulfidopeptide leukotrienes for contracting tracheal spirals ($LTE_4 > LTD_4 = LTC_4$) is different from that for contracting parenchymal strips ($LTD_4 > LTE_4 > LTC_4$), thereby suggesting three separate receptors.[113, 244] Furthermore, in peripheral airway strips, whereas LTC_4 and LTE_4 elicit monophasic contraction, LTD_4 evokes a biphasic response.[112]

Evidence for a separate LTE_4 receptor in guinea pig lung is provided by the reported enhanced histamine responsiveness by LTE_4 in a time- and dose-dependent manner, an effect that could not be reproduced by LTC_4 and LTD_4 despite eliciting the same magnitude of contraction of tracheal smooth muscle as LTE_4.[244] Studies in guinea pig lung tissue in the presence of L-serine borate, which blocks the conversion of LTC_4 to LTD_4, showed that the LTD_4/LTE_4 antagonist FPL 55712 was unable to antagonize the contractile activity of LTC_4.[397] Other selective LTD_4 antagonists have been shown to inhibit LTD_4-induced contraction of guinea pig tracheal strips but had little or no effect on the contractile effects mediated by LTC_4.[138, 396] In guinea pig uterus, specific binding of $[^3H]LTD_4$ could not be detected, but specific and saturable binding of $[^3H]LTC_4$ was observed and reversed with unlabeled LTC_4.[251] The binding of $[^3H]LTD_4$ and $[^3H]LTE_4$ but not $[^3H]LTC_4$ in guinea pig lung was enhanced by divalent ions, and the rate of dissociation was accelerated by either NaCl or GTP, again strengthening the case for a multireceptor theory.[339]

Despite the evidence for distinct receptor subtypes, it is likely that cross-reactivity exists between the different cysteinyl leukotrienes and their receptor types. Several studies have now provided evidence for heterogeneity of LTD_4 receptors in the guinea pig lung as well as across other tissues and species.[137, 185, 228] Radioligand receptor–binding assays with guinea pig trachea[228] and lung membranes,[5] using specific LTD_4 receptor antagonists, support the existence of at least two distinct receptors for LTD_4, with LTE_4 preferentially interacting with only a subset of LTD_4 receptors. This contrasts with the evidence in studies of human airways. Responses elicited by LTC_4 and LTD_4 are inhibited to a similar degree by agents that are selective LTD_4 receptor antagonists, with the inference that all the biologic effects attributed to LTC_4 can be explained by the bioconversion of LTC_4 to LTD_4.[110] Using radiolabeled binding displacement assays, a good correlation was demonstrated between the ability of LTC_4, LTD_4, LTE_4, FPL 55712, and arachidonic acid to inhibit radiolabeled LTD_4 and LTE_4 binding in selected tissue and guinea pig crude lung membrane, suggesting that LTE_4 binds to the identical receptor as LTD_4.[56]

LTB_4 receptors

The LTB_4 receptor was first demonstrated in PMN leukocytes and later in eosinophils, monocytes, and lymphocytes. Scatchard analysis of the binding of [^{3}H]LTB_4 to freshly isolated PMN leukocytes has demonstrated the expression of two distinct subsets of receptors. A high-affinity (kD of 0.5–5 nM), low-density (20 × 10^3 sites per neutrophil) receptor has been identified, and a low-affinity (kD of 15–500 nM), high-density (40–400 × 10^3 sites per neutrophil) class has been identified.[162] These two receptor subtypes for LTB_4 also differ in their stereospecificity for stereoisomers of 5,12-diHETE. Preincubation of neutrophils with 1 × 10^{-8} LTB_4 followed by washing leads to a selective loss of high-affinity receptors and a decreased chemotactic response to subsequent LTB_4 termed deactivation, indicating that this high-affinity receptor mediates chemotactic migration and aggregation.

Degranulation and superoxide generation are elicited in the presence of cytochalasin B in chemotactically deactivated PMN leukocytes that do not express high-affinity receptors. The requirement of significantly higher concentrations of LTB_4 than for chemotaxis implies that degranulation is mediated by the low-affinity receptor for LTB_4.[163] Using differentiated HL-60 cells that respond by chemotaxis to LTB_4, it was found that LTB_4 stimulated a dose-dependent increase in GTP hydrolysis and guanosine 5′[γ-thio]triphosphate binding. This indicates that LTB_4 receptors on HL-60 cells are coupled to a G protein. Both pertussis and cholera toxin were able to inhibit this effect, indicating that the G protein contains an α subunit.[287]

BRONCHIAL ASTHMA

BRONCHOCONSTRICTOR ACTIVITY

The ability of SRS-A to produce lasting contraction of smooth muscle at very low concentrations generated the initial interest in these lipid compounds as putative mediators in bronchial asthma. Isolated tracheal, bronchial, or parenchymal tissues from guinea pigs,[337] dogs,[201] and rats[416] have been found to contract in response to LTC_4 at nanomolar concentrations. LTC_4 and LTD_4 are approximately equipotent as contractile agonists of guinea pig tissue, with EC_{50} values of 0.1 to 1 nM. In the same model, LTE_4 is less potent, with EC_{50} values of 30 to 100 nM.[88, 110]

In Vitro Studies

Similar effects of the cysteinyl leukotrienes have been demonstrated during in vitro studies of human bronchus[91] and tracheal smooth muscle.[207] The contractile actions of LTC_4 and LTD_4 are approximately equipotent and at least 1,000 times more potent than those of histamine in causing muscle contraction. An early study using smooth muscle strips of human bronchus, pulmonary artery, and vein found a lower contractile activity of LTC_4 and LTD_4 than of histamine.[167] This contrasts with the findings of Chagnon and coworkers,[51] who showed that LTA_4, LTC_4, and LTD_4 are at least 200 times more potent than histamine in human lung parenchyma in vitro. The release of the cysteinyl leukotrienes was demonstrated in vitro in isolated bronchi from two birch pollen–sensitive asthmatic subjects after antigen challenge, and the amount of leukotriene release was found to correlate with the contraction evoked by allergen.[90] In the guinea pig, pretreatment with a cyclooxygenase inhibitor lead to diminished LTC_4- and LTD_4-induced contraction in isolated perfused lung, suggesting that bronchoconstrictor prostanoids are released by leukotriene action and contribute significantly to their contractile activity.[337] By contrast, in isolated human lung tissue, indomethacin pretreatment has no effect on the contractile response to antigen induced by leukotriene release, which could be abolished by a leukotriene biosynthesis inhibitor.[90]

Normal Subjects

The use of inhaled leukotrienes in human subjects has demonstrated potent contraction of the airways in both normal and asthmatic subjects. Inhalation of nebulized solutions of leukotrienes leads to airway obstruction measured by falls in specific airway conductance (SGaw) or flow ($\dot{V}$), as measured from full or partial expiratory flow-volume curves. In five normal subjects, the potency of LTC_4 was 600 to 9,500 times greater than that of histamine, with approximately 20 μg/ml LTC_4 and 2 to 10 mg/ml histamine concentrations required to produce a 30% fall in expiratory flow rate at 30% of baseline vital capacity above residual volume ($\dot{V}_{30}$).[434] In the same study, LTD_4 was 6,000-fold more potent than histamine.[435] When data from different sources are combined,[4, 20, 30, 181, 216, 391, 434, 435] inhaled LTC_4 and LTD_4 in normal subjects are 2,000 times more potent than histamine or methacholine in producing airway obstruction. LTE_4, on the other hand, is only 40- to 60-fold more potent than histamine but produces a longer lasting bronchoconstriction.[96, 311]

Although the potencies of LTC_4 and LTD_4 are similar, they have different time courses of action. LTC_4 has a slower onset of action (10–15 minutes) than do LTD_4 and LTE_4 (4–6 minutes), but the response for LTC_4 is more prolonged (20–40 minutes).[109, 435] The reason for this difference in time course response is unclear but may be either related to the action of the cysteinyl leukotrienes at different receptor sites or because LTC_4 requires metabolism to LTD_4 prior to stimulation of the peptide leukotriene receptor. The discrepancy in the literature of the potency of the cysteinyl leukotrienes using a variety of measures of bronchoconstriction is likely due to the different parameters used as measures of constriction at distinct sites within the lung. Changes in FEV_1 and SGaw are mediated by bronchoconstricting agonists considered to act at a central site of action, whereas $\dot{V}_{30}$ is a measure of a more peripheral site of action. Inhalation of LTC_4 and LTD_4 in normal subjects produced a fall in $\dot{V}_{30}$ with little effect of FEV_1.[181] Similarly, Weiss[436] demonstrated that a 50-fold greater concentration of LTC_4 was required to achieve a 20% fall in FEV_1 compared with the concentration required to cause a 30% fall in $\dot{V}_{30}$. These studies on normal subjects have suggested a predominantly peripheral site of action for LTC_4 and LTD_4. By contrast in asthmatic subjects, inhalation of LTC_4 and LTD_4 showed similar effects on SGaw and $\dot{V}_{30}$,[22, 216, 391] indicating that the site of LTC_4 and LTD_4 bronchoconstrictor activity in asthma is likely to be in both central and peripheral airways.[295, 336]

Asthmatic Subjects

Asthmatics' airways also respond by bronchoconstriction to inhaled leukotrienes but in contrast to normal airways exhibit smaller responses when compared with a reference agonist such as histamine or methacholine. LTC_4 and LTD_4 have been reported to be 40-fold[4] to 140-fold[164] more potent than histamine or methacholine in bronchoconstrictor effect on asthmatic airways, which compares with 600- to 9,500-fold for LTC_4[434] and 6,000-fold for LTD_4[435] in normal airways compared with histamine. A correlation between the airway responsiveness to methacholine[4] and histamine[21] with the airway responsiveness to LTC_4 and LTD_4 has been established, but these studies also confirmed the relative lack of airway responsiveness to LTC_4 and LTD_4 in asthmatic compared with normal subjects.[21] Less data for LTE_4 are available. Using $\dot{V}_{30}$ as a measure of airway obstruction, LTE_4 was 39-fold more potent than histamine in normal subjects and 14-fold more potent than histamine in asthmatic subjects.[96] However, using a 35% fall in SGaw as a measure of bronchoconstriction, the relative potency of LTE_4 was found to be two to three times greater in asthmatic than in normal individuals.[311]

In view of the discordance in the literature, a more extensive study was performed to compare the relative potencies of LTC_4, LTD_4, LTE_4, histamine, and methacholine in the same normal and asthmatic subjects.[11] The airways of the subjects with asthma were approximately 14-, 15-, 6-, 9-, and 219-fold more responsive to histamine, methacholine, LTC_4, LTD_4, and LTE_4, respectively, than were those of normal subjects. Furthermore, as the airway hyperresponsiveness to histamine and methacholine increased, so did the potency of LTE_4 in contrast with LTC_4 and LTD_4, which decreased. Therefore, the results of these studies taken together suggest that compared with normals, asthmatic airways are relatively less responsive to LTC_4 and LTD_4 but have a disproportionate hyperresponsiveness to the bronchoconstricting effects of LTE_4.[10, 11] This indicates an important role for LTE_4 in bronchial asthma, which may be due to its relative stability among the cysteinyl leukotrienes and because it persists for the longest time at the site of release.[238]

Aspirin-Sensitive Asthma (ASA)

Approximately 10% to 20% of asthmatics develop bronchospasm on ingestion of aspirin and other inhibitors of cyclooxygenase such as the nonsteroidal anti-inflammatory drugs (NSAIDs). These subjects are singularly sensitive to the bronchoconstrictor effects of inhaled LTE_4, which was found to be 1,870 times more potent than histamine in aspirin-sensitive subjects and only 145 times more potent than histamine in asthmatics who are aspirin tolerant.[12] The individuals with aspirin sensitivity were desensitized to aspirin by the ingestion of incremental doses of aspirin, following which there was a mean 20-fold decrease in airway responsiveness to LTE_4 but no change in histamine responsiveness. In aspirin-sensitive subjects, this selective hyperresponsiveness is exclusive to LTE_4 and not found with LTC_4,[58] suggesting an important role in this form of asthma.

AIRWAY RESPONSIVENESS

In Vitro Studies

Bronchial hyperresponsiveness to contractile agonists such as histamine and methacholine and to nonspecific irritants is a key pathophysiologic feature of asthma. SRS-A was found to enhance the contractile response to histamine during in vitro studies on guinea pig ileum.[42] Pretreatment of guinea pig tracheal spirals with a contracting dose of LTE_4 accentuated the subsequent contractile response to histamine in a time- and dose-dependent fashion.[244] LTC_4 and LTD_4 did not enhance histamine responsiveness in parenchymal strips. Pretreatment with the cyclooxygenase inhibitor indomethacin abolished the hyperresponsiveness to histamine despite a lack of effect on the contractile activity of LTE_4.

In a further study of guinea pig tracheal spirals, enhanced contractile activity to histamine was demonstrated following LTC_4 only in the presence of 0.1 mM calcium ions, and this effect was blocked by the leukotriene antagonist FPL 55712.[79] A similar airway hyperresponsiveness was not found with carbachol or substance P. This airway hyperresponsiveness to histamine is blocked not only by indomethacin but also by a thromboxane A_2/prostaglandin H_2 (TP) receptor antagonist (GR32191). Pretreatment of isolated human bronchus with LTE_4 induces a similar effect, with a fourfold left-ward displacement of the histamine dose-response curve. This effect is blocked by GR32191, suggesting that the observed LTC_4/LTE_4-induced hyperresponsiveness to histamine found in human and guinea pig trachea is mediated by the secondary generation of cyclooxygenase products.[196]

Normal Subjects

Inhalation of either a subthreshold dose of LTD_4[21] or bronchoconstricting doses of LTC_4, LTD_4, or LTE_4 in normal subjects[13, 312] did not significantly enhance airway responsiveness to subsequent histamine inhalation. Inhalation of a bronchoconstricting dose of LTD_4 led to significantly increased airway methacholine responsiveness which was maximal at 7 days in six of eight subjects and persisted for 2 to 3 weeks in five subjects.[213] Interestingly, in the same study, the degree and duration of changes in methacholine airway responses were similar to those found after platelet-activating factor (PAF) inhalation.

Asthmatic Subjects

In asthmatic subjects, preinhalation of LTE_4, which caused a 41% fall in specific airway conductance, led to both a dose- and time-dependent increase in histamine respon-

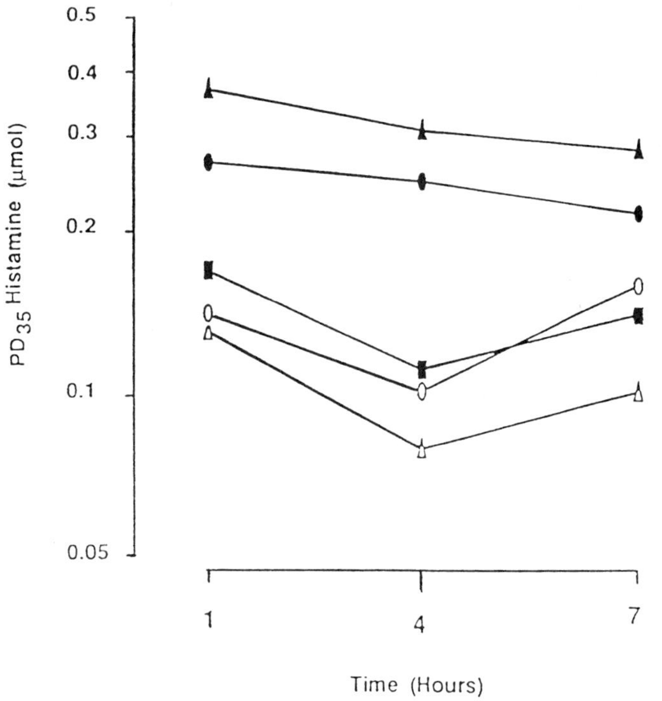

FIGURE 12–4. Time course of changes in airway histamine responsiveness after inhalation of phosphate-buffered saline (closed triangles), methacholine (closed circles), LTC_4 (open triangles), LTD_4 (closed squares), and LTE_4 (open circles). Each point represents the geometric mean for seven subjects with asthma. (From O'Hickey SP, Hawksworth RJ, Fong CY, et al: Leukotrienes C_4, D_4, and E_4 enhance histamine responsiveness in asthmatic airways. Am Rev Respir Dis 144:1053–1057, 1991.)

siveness, which reached a peak of 3.5-fold at 7 hours after LTE_4 inhalation.[13] In a subsequent study of seven asthmatic subjects, inhalation of the cysteinyl leukotrienes, LTC_4, LTD_4, and LTE_4, produced approximately a threefold to fourfold increase in histamine responsiveness at 4 hours (Fig. 12–4).[312] The magnitude of this enhanced histamine responsiveness is similar to that observed after inhaled allergen challenge.[50, 71] In nine asthmatic subjects, preinhalation of LTC_4 was shown to have no effect on airway responsiveness to subsequent inhalation of distilled water.[32] Indomethacin given before inhaled LTE_4 significantly inhibited the expected hyperresponsiveness to histamine in eight asthmatic subjects.[57] Indomethacin was also found to inhibit the increase in airway responsiveness following inhaled allergen provocation in seven atopic subjects but had no effect on either the early or late asthmatic reactions.[221] This suggests that the cysteinyl leukotrienes are important mediators of the enhanced airway responsiveness that is an attribute of clinical asthma and that they may exert part of this effect through the secondary generation of prostanoids from the cyclooxygenase pathway.

BRONCHIAL MUCOSAL SECRETIONS

Abnormal airway mucociliary function in bronchial asthma is suggested by the clinical observation of excessive tracheobronchial secretions, which are difficult to clear and may contribute to bronchial obstruction. The cysteinyl leukotrienes can influence mucus composition and secretion as well as mucociliary transport within the airways. Cultured human airway explants increased the rate of secretion of radiolabeled glucosamine as part of a high molecular weight glycoprotein in response to LTC_4 and LTD_4 by 15% and 26%, respectively.[75, 272] There was diminished radiolabeled product secretion with repeated stimulation of the explants, and the ratio of bound radiolabel to protein remained unchanged, suggesting that LTC_4 and LTD_4 stimulate secretion rather than de novo mucus synthesis.[272]

LTC_4 was found to have 1,000-fold more potent secretagogue effects on mucus secretion than was LTD_4 when injected into the artery supplying the cervical canine trachea.[200] Physiologic concentrations of LTC_4 and LTD_4 on cultured airway goblet cells demonstrated enhanced mucin release.[219] LTC_4 and LTD_4 also mediate an increase in chloride flux of isolated canine tracheal epithelium, which induces an increase in the short-circuit ionic current[249] and is accompanied by enhanced fluid secretion.[201] A reduction in tracheal mucus velocity is seen in sheep allergic to *Ascaris suum* with concentrations of LTD_4 as low as 25 μg/ml, with the maximum effect observed at 3 hours after leukotriene challenge.[363] The overall effect of the cysteinyl leukotrienes therefore leads to an increased mucus gel layer with decreased mucus clearance.

Cysteinyl leukotrienes were detected in the sputum of 16 of 25 patients with cystic fibrosis and in 1 of 5 patients with chronic bronchitis.[81] A more recent study of 30 children with cystic fibrosis demonstrated a correlation between urinary and sputum levels of LTE_4. One third of these children had urinary LTE_4 greater than 200 pmol/mol creatinine compared with only 3% of normal children.[365] A further study by the same group reported that in 13 children with cystic fibrosis the logarithm of sputum LTE_4 and total cysteinyl leukotriene levels correlated with the overall severity of pulmonary disease as assessed by Chrispin-Norman chest radiograph scores.[405] These findings suggest that cysteinyl leukotrienes may play a role in the sputum abnormalities characteristic of cystic fibrosis and chronic bronchitis.

RELEASE OF LEUKOTRIENES

Sensitive assay systems such as high-performance liquid chromatography, radioimmunoassay, and fast-atom bombardment mass spectrometry have been employed to detect picograms amounts of leukotrienes in a variety of biologic fluids (Table 12–3). Bronchoalveolar lavage (BAL) has been utilized to obtain fluid in pulmonary disease states. The ratio of the volume of lavage fluid instilled to that recovered is not always constant, and therefore BAL suffers from the drawback that it is not always easy to interpret the values given. The results from BAL are usually expressed in terms of amounts per volume recovered. Urine is a more reliable biologic fluid, and amounts of mediator are easily standardized by expressing quantities per milligram of creatinine, which is excreted in relatively constant fashion throughout a 24-hour period.[390]

An infusion of three doses of radiolabeled LTC_4 in three subjects demonstrated a constant recovery of 4.1% to 6.3%, regardless of the amount infused, in the form of LTE_4, the most stable of the cysteinyl leukotrienes.[266] Radiolabeled

TABLE 12–3
RELEASE OF LEUKOTRIENES INTO BIOLOGIC FLUIDS

Disease	Biologic Fluid	Leukotriene Release
Asthma		
Clinical	BAL	LTE_4 detected in mild/severe disease
Symptomatic	BAL	LTB_4/LTC_4
Acute	Urine	LTE_4, highest levels in patients responding to β_2-agonist treatment
Allergen challenge (EAR)	BAL	LTC_4 increases ninefold
	Urine	LTE_4 increases 2–4 hours after allergen challenge
Aspirin in sensitive patients	Urine	LTE_4 sixfold higher at baseline and increases a further fourfold after aspirin challenge
	Nasal lavage	LTC_4 levels increase after lysine-aspirin challenge
Exercise induced	BAL	LTB_4 rises 12-fold and LTC_4 rises fivefold after isocapnic hyperventilation
	Urine	LTE_4 found to increase 1.7-fold in only one study of children with severe asthma
Cryptogenic fibrosing alveolitis	BAL	LTB_4 detected
Persistent pulmonary hypertension	BAL	LTC_4 and LTD_4 detected in newborn infants
Adult respiratory distress syndrome	Pulmonary edema fluid	LTD_4 increased fourfold
Rheumatoid arthritis	Synovial fluid	LTB_4 detected in active disease
Gouty arthritis	Joint fluid	LTB_4 levels significantly increased
Psoriasis	Skin chamber fluid	LTB_4, LTC_4, and LTD_4 levels detected in increased quantities
Inflammatory bowel disease	Intestinal mucosal fluid	LTB_4 detected in both ulcerative colitis and Crohn's disease
Acute myocardial infarction	Urine	LTE_4 levels raised and return to normal by day 3
Hepatorenal syndrome	Urine	LTE_4 levels elevated threefold

LTC_4 instilled into the airways of asthmatics, nonasthmatics, and asthmatics challenged with allergen was found to be excreted in a constant fashion in all three groups, with LTE_4 as the major metabolite.[442] A further study found a significant correlation between the dose of inhaled LTC_4 and the amounts excreted as urinary LTE_4.[63] These studies provide strong evidence for the utility of urinary LTE_4 as an easily accessible marker of pulmonary cysteinyl leukotriene release.

CLINICAL ASTHMA

Fifteen out of 17 asthmatic subjects with mild to severe disease were found to have detectable LTE_4 in bronchoalveolar lavage fluid, but there was no correlation between LTE_4 levels and pulmonary function. This compared with undetectable LTE_4 levels in the control group of nine normal subjects.[239] Another study found that 8 symptomatic asthmatic subjects had significantly higher levels of BAL, LTB_4, and LTC_4 than did a control group of 14 healthy individuals.[431] A comparison of 11 healthy and 11 atopic asthmatic subjects found no difference in cysteinyl leukotriene, histamine, or PAF levels between the two groups, but there was a higher level of PGD_2 and a lower level of LTB_4 in the asthmatic group.[78] These findings are in contrast with the two previous studies and may be due to selection of very mild asthmatic subjects. Smith and colleagues found no difference in baseline urinary levels of LTE_4 between 17 normal and 31 asthmatic subjects. In addition, no correlation was found between urinary LTE_4 levels measured in picograms per milligram of creatinine and baseline airway responsiveness to histamine or FEV_1 as a percent of predicted values.[390]

Drazen and coworkers[114] examined 72 subjects presenting to the emergency room and classified 22 patients with a doubling of peak expiratory flow rate (PEFR) following nebulized albuterol as responders and 19 patients with less than a 25% increase in PEFR as nonresponders. Urinary LTE_4 levels were compared in these two groups with 13 normal controls. Levels of urinary LTE_4 were found to be significantly higher in responders compared with nonresponders or normal subjects. The authors concluded that the highest levels of LTE_4 found in those subjects with acute reversible airflow obstruction were consistent with a bronchospastic role for cysteinyl leukotrienes in spontaneous acute asthma.

ALLERGEN-INDUCED ASTHMA

Leukotriene release has been measured in studies employing various bronchial challenge procedures. The predominant leukotriene assayed by HPLC in BAL fluid of atopic asthmatic subjects after endobronchial allergen challenge was shown to be LTC_4, with approximately a ninefold rise in levels compared with baseline. Measurable levels of LTC_4 at baseline were found in 9 of 11 atopic asthmatic subjects but only in 1 of 7 atopic nonasthmatic subjects and 1 of 6 nonatopic subjects. There was only a slight rise in BAL LTC_4 levels after allergen in the atopic nonasthmatic group and no change in the nonatopic samples.[438]

In a followup study, PGD_2, TXB_2, LTC_4, and histamine levels were measured in BAL fluid before and 5 minutes after endobronchial allergen challenge in three groups of atopic subjects: seven nonasthmatic subjects, six asthmatic subjects without a late asthmatic response, and six asthmatic subjects with a late asthmatic response. At baseline, LTC_4 was detected in 9 of the 12 asthmatic subjects but only in 1 of 7 subjects without asthma. There were significant increases in all mediator levels in both groups with asthma postallergen challenge compared with the nonasthmatic group. The asthmatic group without a late asthmatic response recorded significantly higher levels of all four mediators postallergen challenge than the other two groups.[439]

In a study of 17 allergic asthmatic subjects undergoing allergen provocation, there was a fall in FEV_1 of 25% to 59% within the first 2 hours, accompanied by a rise in urinary LTE_4 levels from 46 to 92 ng during the 12-hour collection period. Methacholine challenge alone, which led to similar falls in FEV_1, did not significantly alter urinary LTE_4 excretion. A significant correlation was detected between the decrease in FEV_1 during the early asthmatic response (EAR), the excretion of urinary LTE_4, and the airway reactivity. However, no correlation was found between urinary LTE_4 excretion and the severity of the late response to allergen, although in those patients with the most severe late asthmatic responses, urinary LTE_4 excretion remained elevated for a longer period.[441]

In a separate study, 18 asthmatic subjects were divided into three groups: those with an isolated EAR, those with an isolated late asthmatic response (LAR), and those with a dual asthmatic response (DAR). Urinary LTE_4 rose significantly from baseline values only in the two groups with an EAR, with a rise from 150 to 1,816 pg/mg creatinine in the group with an isolated EAR and a rise from 66 to 174 pg/mg creatinine in the group with an EAR preceding a LAR. There was no increase in urinary LTE_4 in the group with an isolated LAR. Furthermore, the degree of maximum bronchoconstriction during the EAR correlated with urinary LTE_4 release, suggesting that the cysteinyl leukotrienes are only released during the EAR and that they contribute significantly to the bronchoconstriction found during this phase of the asthmatic response.[269] A number of subsequent studies have also documented urinary LTE_4 release 2 to 4 hours following specific inhaled allergen challenge.[187, 232, 305, 419]

ASPIRIN-SENSITIVE ASTHMA

A considerable body of evidence supports the role of the cysteinyl leukotrienes in the pathogenesis of aspirin-sensitive asthma (ASA). Resting mean urinary LTE_4 levels in ASA subjects are significantly higher than in normals or nonaspirin sensitive asthmatics. Smith and colleagues reported that baseline urinary LTE_4 levels in 10 ASA subjects were 101 pg/mg creatinine compared with 43 pg/mg creatinine in 31 nonaspirin-sensitive asthmatic subjects and 34 pg/mg creatinine in 17 normals. There was substantial overlap between the groups, and no correlation was found between urinary LTE_4 and histamine PD_{20} or baseline FEV_1. Thus measurement of LTE_4 in a single sample of urine does not predict the degree of resting airflow obstruction or of bronchial hyperresponsiveness or diagnosed aspirin sensitivity.[390]

Christie and colleagues reported sixfold higher urinary LTE_4 levels in aspirin-sensitive subjects compared with nonaspirin-sensitive asthmatic controls. Furthermore, oral aspirin challenge, which led to a mean 21% fall in FEV_1 in six ASA subjects, resulted in a fourfold increase in urinary LTE_4 above baseline values. There was no fall in FEV_1 and no increase in urinary LTE_4 levels in the control subjects following aspirin ingestion.[64] Subsequent studies have confirmed that ASA subjects have higher baseline urinary LTE_4 excretion, which rises further after aspirin challenge.[224, 232, 387] It has also been reported that urinary LTE_4 levels increase in ASA subjects following lysine-aspirin bronchial challenge.[62, 386]

Nasal lavage mediator levels have been studied in aspirin-sensitive rhinosinusitis. Following nasal instillation of lysine-aspirin, increased levels of both histamine and LTC_4 were detected in nasal lavage samples in three of four ASA subjects who experienced both naso-ocular symptoms and a bronchospastic reaction. There was no increase in these mediator levels in normals or nonaspirin-sensitive asthmatics or aspirin-sensitive subjects in whom lysine-aspirin did not provoke naso-ocular symptoms.[127, 335]

EXERCISE-INDUCED ASTHMA

Using isocapnic hyperventilation as a model for exercise-induced asthma, Pliss and coworkers reported increases in BAL fluid levels of LTB_4 from 10 to 121 pg/ml and immunoreactive cysteinyl leukotrienes from 46 to 251 pg/ml. There were also increases in eosinophil and epithelial cell numbers, but no changes in prostaglandin or histamine levels were detected.[338] A further study of seven atopic asthmatic subjects undergoing treadmill exercise was unable to find evidence for mast cell–derived mediator release or an increase in BAL fluid histamine, tryptase, PGD_2, or LTC_4. However, the LTC_4 assay in this study may have lacked sufficient sensitivity to detect BAL fluid LTC_4.[43] In a study of six asthmatic subjects after treadmill exercise leading to a mean 22% fall in FEV_1, no increase in urinary levels of LTE_4 was detected.[389] However, Kikawa and colleagues[218] reported small increases in urinary LTE_4 (14.3 before and 24.3 ng/mg creatinine after exercise) in 8 of 10 children with severe asthma following exercise, which produced a mean 60% fall in FEV_1 but no increase in urinary LTE_4 in 7 children with moderate asthma who experienced only a 24% fall in FEV_1.

Despite the conflicting evidence, pharmacologic studies have indicated an important role for cysteinyl leukotrienes in exercise-induced bronchospasm. It is likely that our inability to detect these mediators consistently in biologic fluids after exercise may be because whole body cysteinyl leukotriene release only rises modestly and currently employed detection systems are not sensitive enough. Further confounding variables that hinder detection of leukotriene release also come into play after exercise, which are not present in other forms of asthma, such as changes in bronchial or pulmonary blood flow in response to airway cooling and local changes in pH and osmolarity, which may lead to alterations in leukotriene metabolism and elimination.

OTHER DISEASES

The release of leukotrienes has also been detected in a number of other nonallergic diseases.

Lung Disease

In patients with cryptogenic fibrosing alveolitis, increased quantities of LTB_4 in BAL fluid correlated with the recovery of neutrophils, suggesting that leukotriene release may be responsible for granulocyte recruitment in this disease.[431] Lung lavage fluids of newborn infants with persistent pulmonary hypertension requiring assisted ventilation have increased concentrations of LTC_4 and LTD_4.[408] In the adult respiratory distress syndrome (ARDS), LTD_4 was detected in fourfold higher concentrations in pulmonary edema fluid compared with patients with cardiogenic pulmonary edema. Furthermore, the LTD_4 levels correlated with the ratio of edema fluid to plasma concentrations of albumin, suggesting that cysteinyl leukotrienes contribute to the permeability defect that allows accumulation of protein-rich fluid in ARDS.[279]

Joint Disorders

In active rheumatoid arthritis, small quantities of LTB_4 have been detected in synovial joint fluid.[97] In gouty joint effusions, significantly higher quantities of LTB_4 are detected than those found in either normal or rheumatoid joints. This may be due in part to monosodium urate crystals, which have been shown to inhibit the metabolic deactivation of LTB_4 by polymorphonuclear granulocytes.[343]

Inflammatory Bowel Disease

When supplied with exogenous arachidonate, intestinal mucosa obtained from patients with ulcerative colitis and Crohn's disease generate and release greater quantities of both LTB_4 and the cysteinyl leukotrienes.[241, 329, 376] Using HPLC, it was found that intestinal mucosa from patients with inflammatory bowel disease contained 50-fold higher quantities of LTB_4 per gram of tissue than did normal mucosa.[376] The use of rectal pouches has allowed the measurement of mediator levels in vivo in inflammatory bowel disease and has demonstrated significantly higher LTB_4 levels in active ulcerative colitis.[211] Prednisone or aminosalicylic acid treatment in patients with ulcerative colitis reduced the generation of LTB_4 in vivo, and this was associated with clinical improvement. Pretreatment rectal pouch fluid levels of both PGE_2 and LTB_4 were significantly higher in patients not responding to prednisolone or 5-aminosalicylic acid treatment. The authors of the study suggested that intraluminal levels of these mediators are more useful predictors of relapsing ulcerative colitis than they are clinical indexes of disease severity.[240]

Psoriasis

Skin chamber fluid from abraded psoriatic skin lesions contains significantly higher quantities of LTB_4[36] and immunoreactive LTC_4 and LTD_4[37] than that from normal skin. This may partly explain the characteristic intraepidermal neutrophil infiltration and local vasodilation found in psoriasis. Picomolar to nanomolar concentrations of LTB_4 were found to increase DNA synthesis in cultured epidermal keratinocytes using incorporation of radiolabeled thymidine as a measure. The peptide leukotrienes LTC_4 and LTD_4 were also found to stimulate keratinocyte DNA synthesis, although they were less potent than LTB_4. This finding may relate to the excessive epidermal hyperplasia seen in psoriasis.[225]

Ischemic Heart Disease

Elevated levels of urinary LTE_4 were found in a study of 16 patients presenting with acute myocardial infarction, and these levels returned to normal by day 3. Similar raised levels of urinary LTE_4 were found in unstable angina, with a reduction to normal levels once the chest pain had resolved. There was a faster decline in urinary LTE_4 levels in patients treated with thrombolytic agents leading to early coronary reperfusion compared with those who did not receive such treatment. This suggests that cardiac ischemia and necrosis may be responsible for cysteinyl leukotriene release.[49]

Hepatic Disease

In hepatorenal syndrome and decompensated liver disease, the rate of urinary LTE_4 excretion per hour is threefold higher than that found in compensated liver disease. The additional finding of reduced excretion of a radiolabeled LTC_4 infusion in one such patient suggested that the increased excretion of urinary LTE_4 is due to excessive production or reduced metabolism of LTE_4 and not due to increased renal clearance of LTE_4.[296]

Renal Disorders

Leukotriene C_4 and LTD_4 are potent renal vasoconstrictors, which implicates these mediators as modulators of glomerular function and suggests their possible involvement in the pathogenesis of renal disease.

DEVELOPMENTS IN ANTILEUKOTRIENE THERAPY

With the realization of the proinflammatory properties of leukotrienes, the pharmaceutical industry has worked toward the development of antileukotriene therapies. This has provided scientists with novel tools for further investigation of the role of leukotrienes in the test tube and in clinical disease by allowing the modulation of both leukotriene action and biosynthesis.

Most of the work with leukotriene antagonists and 5-LO inhibitors has focused on asthma, employing allergen provocation, aspirin challenge in aspirin-sensitive subjects, and various forms of exercise challenge. However, because these models may only mirror the acute inflammatory effects of asthma and bear little relationship to the chronic structural changes characteristic of the disease, the developmental process of these drugs has placed greater emphasis on the investigation of day-to-day asthmatic symptoms and the steroid-sparing and bronchodilator effects of these agents. Increasingly, other diseases are being studied using these therapeutic agents as their wider import is recognized.

Leukotriene action may be pharmacologically modulated by antagonism at the receptor site or by biosynthesis inhibition (Fig. 12–5). Leukotriene B_4 receptor antagonists have so far not been evaluated in humans, but LTD_4 receptor antagonists have been developed for use in human trials (Table 12–4). Inhibition of 5-LO biosynthesis is effected either by direct interference with its enzymatic properties or by secondary inhibition of its interaction with FLAP.

RECEPTOR ANTAGONISTS

A potent LTD_4 receptor antagonist must display a rightward shift of the dose-response curve to inhaled LTD_4 of at

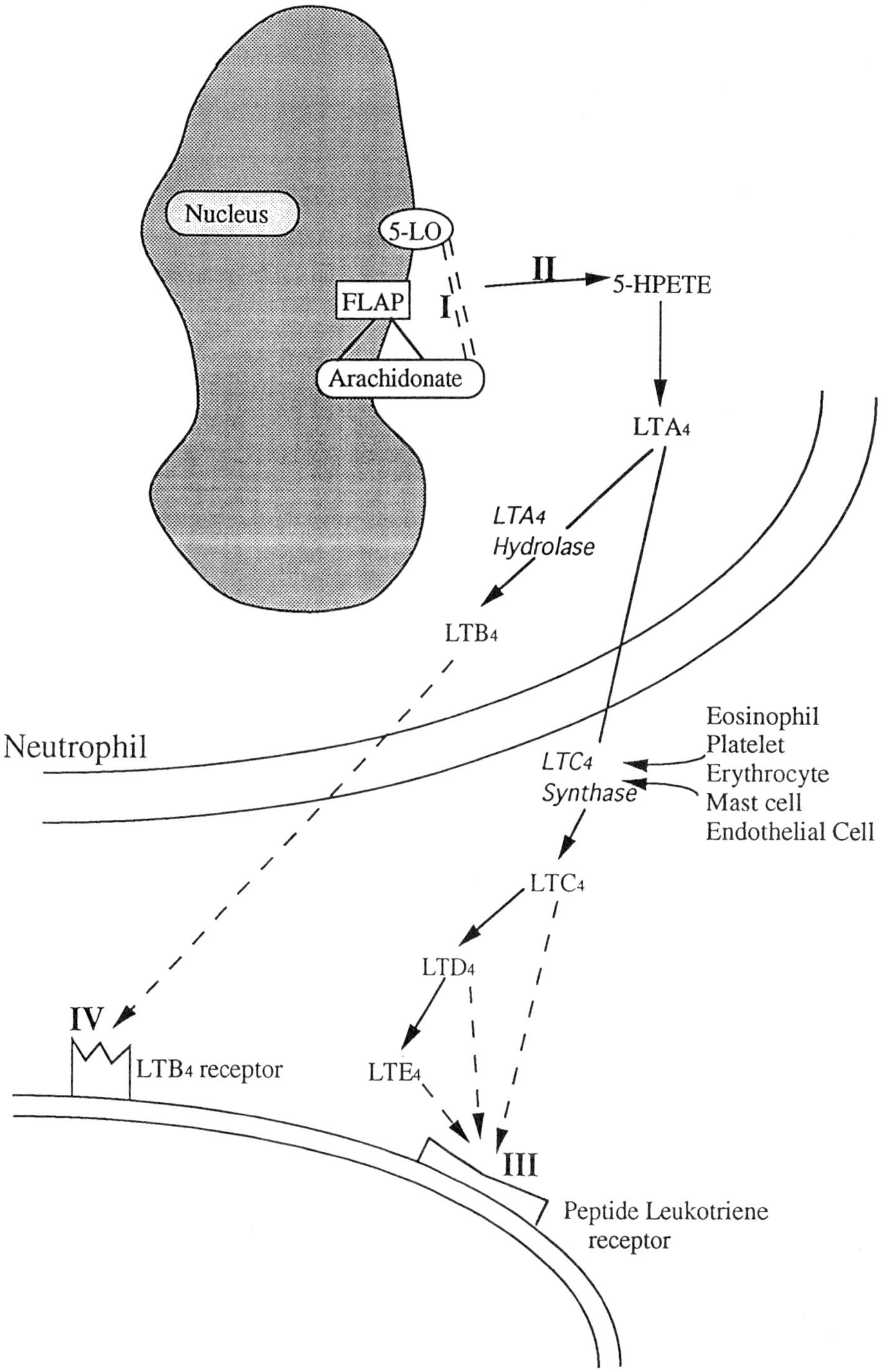

FIGURE 12–5. The sites at which novel therapeutic agents inhibit leukotriene action. Inhibition of the interaction of 5-lipoxygenase with FLAP (I); direct inhibition of the action of 5-lipoxygenase (II); peptide leukotriene receptor antagonism (III); and LTB_4 receptor antagonism (IV).

least 20-fold for adequate inhibition of cysteinyl leukotriene effects in humans. The first antagonist to be evaluated was the hydroxyacetophenone FPL 55712, which had selective activity as an inhibitor of SRS-A even before the chemical structure of SRS-A was elucidated.[15] However, it proved disappointing in clinical trials of asthma because of low potency, a short half-life, and bioavailability only by inhalation.[248] Other first-generation LTD_4 antagonists evaluated in humans include L-648,051,[208] L-649,923,[19] LY-171,883,[334] LY-170,680,[445] and SK&F 104,353.[209] These compounds were of modest potency, with a right-ward shift in the LTD_4 dose-response curve of 3- to 10-fold and poor to moderate clinical efficacy in early trials.

Second-generation, highly selective LTD_4 antagonists have been developed with up to 100-fold greater potency than FPL 55712. The most potent of these compounds include ICI 204,219, which has up to 1,000-fold greater potency than FPL 55712 in inhibiting contraction of guinea pig tracheal and parenchymal strips[227]; ONO 1078, which inhibits both LTC_4 and LTD_4 in guinea pigs and demonstrates 100-fold greater potency than FPL 55712 in isolated human bronchus[448]; and MK-571, MK-679, and MK-476, which

TABLE 12–4
CLINICAL DATA ON LEUKOTRIENE RECEPTOR ANTAGONISTS

Antagonist	Clinical Data
Allergen-Induced Asthma	
LY 171,883	Reduction of early asthmatic response (EAR)[147]
ICI 204,219 (oral)	Reduction in EAR by 80% and in late asthmatic response (LAR) by 50%; inhibition of the rise in bronchial hyperreactivity[420]
ICI 204,219 (inhaled)	10-fold rightward shift in dose-response curve (DRC) to cat-allergen[129] Inhibition of EAR; no effect on LAR[313]
MK-571	Reduction of EAR by 88% and LAR by 63%[345]
Exercise/Isocapnic Hyperventilation	
LY-171,883	20% increase in respiratory heat loss for a given fall in FEV[192]
MK-571	70% reduction of exercise-induced bronchoconstriction; reduction in recovery time from 33 to 8 minutes[271]
SK&F 104,353	Exercise-induced bronchoconstriction reduced from 29% to 20%[353]
ICI 204,219 (oral)	Exercise-induced bronchoconstriction reduced from 36% to 22%[132]
ICI 204,219 (inhaled)	50% reduction of exercise-induced bronchoconstriction[264]
Aspirin-Induced Asthma	
SK&F 104,353	Bronchoconstriction inhibited by 47% in five out of six subjects[59]
MK-0679	Improvement in baseline lung function; 4.4-fold rightward shift of DRC to lysine-aspirin[233]
Baseline Lung Function	
ICI 204,219	Significant bronchodilation; additive effect with inhaled albuterol[186]
MK-571	22% bronchodilation; additive effect with inhaled albuterol[154]
MK-0679	16% improvement in baseline FEV_1 after intravenous infusion[188]
Chronic Asthma	
LY-171,883	10% increase in FEV_1; reduction in wheeze and β_2 agonist use[70]
MK-571	14% increase in FEV_1; reduction in symptoms and albuterol use[153]
RG 12525	Improvement in FEV_1 additive to inhaled corticosteroids[426]
ONO-1078	Improvement in methacholine-PC_{20} FEV_1[143]
ICI 204,219	Improvement in FEV_1; reduction in symptoms and albuterol use[401]

are members of a whole family of quinolone-derived LTD_4 antagonists that demonstrate a 44- to 84-fold right-ward shift in the LTD_4 dose-response curve in asthmatic subjects.[220]

ALLERGEN-INDUCED ASTHMA

In early studies, LY-171,883, which has a structure similar to that of FPL 55712 and L-649,923, demonstrated a slight reduction of the EAR but had no effect on baseline lung function or the late asthmatic response.[41, 147] In a study of 10 asthmatics, a single oral dose of 40 mg ICI 204,219, a highly selective and potent LTD_4 antagonist, attenuated the EAR by 80% and the LAR by 50% and suppressed the allergen-induced rise in nonspecific bronchial reactivity at 6 hours postchallenge (Fig. 12–6).[420] An inhaled formulation of ICI 204,219 was less effective but still significantly inhibited the EAR though not the LAR.[313] A further study using a single inhaled dose of 40 mg ICI 204,219 displaced the allergen dose-response curve to inhaled cat allergen 10-fold compared with placebo.[129] The same inhaled formulation has been shown to shorten the recovery time of the EAR from 60 to 40 minutes.[87] In a study of asthmatic subjects, the quinolone derivative MK-571 substantially inhibited the EAR by 88% and the LAR by 63%.[345]

ASPIRIN-SENSITIVE ASTHMA

Current evidence suggests that aspirin-induced asthma is the most leukotriene-dependent model presently available for the evaluation of antileukotriene therapy in asthma. The weak LTD_4 antagonist SK&F 104,353, administered by the inhaled route, demonstrated inhibition of the bronchoconstrictor response to ingested aspirin by a mean 47% in five of six subjects.[59] In a study of eight subjects with aspirin-sensitive asthma, MK-0679 improved baseline pulmonary function and significantly attenuated the airway obstruction produced by inhaled lysine-aspirin, with a median 4.4-fold right-ward shift in the dose-response curve.[233]

EXERCISE CHALLENGE AND ISOCAPNIC HYPERVENTILATION

Provided that the respiratory heat exchange is matched in a time-dependent manner, the degree of bronchospasm achieved by exercise can be mimicked by controlled isocapnic hyperventilation. Exercise and isocapnic hyperventilation are considered to stimulate similar if not identical pathologic

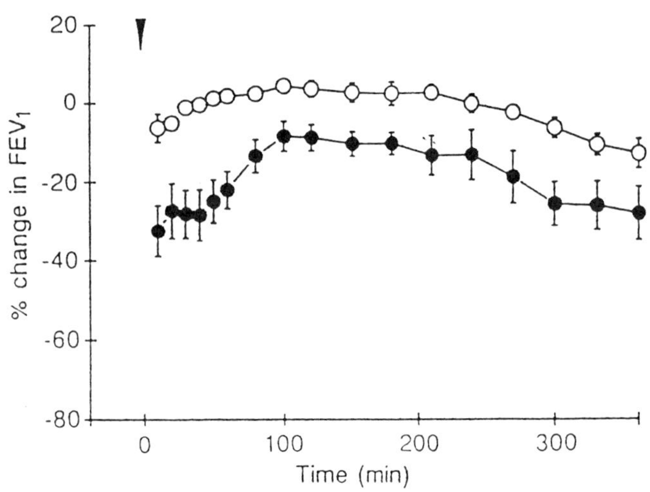

FIGURE 12–6. Effect of ICI 204,219 (open circles) compared with placebo (closed circles) on allergen-induced early and late responses. (From Taylor IK, O'Shaughnessy KM, Fuller RW, et al: Effect of cysteinyl-leukotriene receptor agonist ICI 204,219 on allergen-induced bronchoconstriction and airway hyperreactivity in atopic subjects. Lancet 337:690–694, 1991. © by The Lancet Ltd. 1991.)

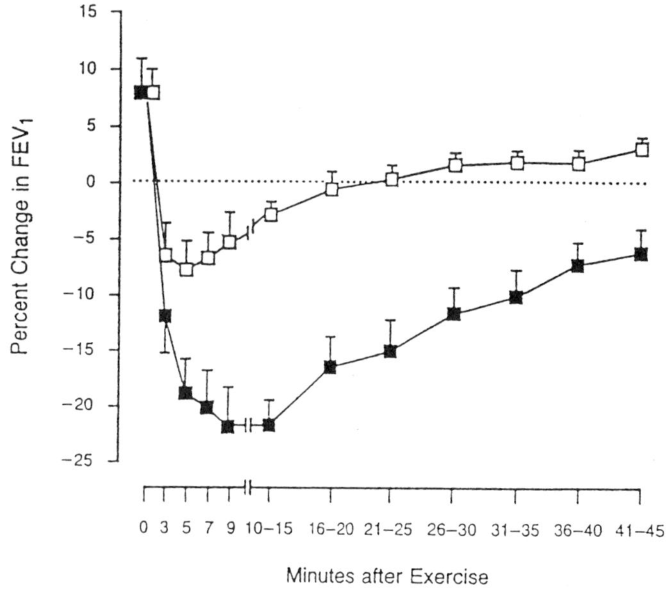

FIGURE 12–7. Mean percent change in FEV_1 over time after exercise following treatment with MK-571 (open squares) or placebo (closed squares). (From Manning PJ, Watson RM, Margolskee DJ, et al: Inhibition of exercise-induced bronchoconstriction by MK-571, a potent leukotriene D_4-receptor antagonist. N Engl J Med 323:1736–1739, 1990. Reprinted by permission of *The New England Journal of Medicine*. 1990, Massachusetts Medical Society.)

effector mechanisms for the initiation of bronchoconstriction. In a study of 20 asthmatic subjects treated for 2 weeks with LY-171,883, there was an increase in the geometric mean respiratory heat loss required to reduce FEV_1 by 20% and a marginal reduction of bronchoconstriction induced by isocapnic hyperventilation of cold air. In this study, the most reactive subjects demonstrated greatest protection.[192] Inhaled SK&F 104,353, a weak LTD_4 antagonist, reduced the exercise-induced bronchoconstrictor response from 29% to 20%, with similar efficacy to disodium cromoglycate.[353]

In eight asthmatic subjects respiring cold dry air, an oral dose of 20 mg of ICI 204,219 reduced the fall in FEV_1 induced by treadmill exercise challenge from 36% to 21.6%.[132] In a study of nine subjects undergoing exercise challenge, inhaled ICI 204,219 reduced the exercise-induced fall in FEV_1.[264] MK-571 produced similar results, with a 70% attenuation of the exercise-induced decrease in FEV_1 in 12 asthmatic subjects and a marked reduction in recovery time from 33 to 8 minutes (Fig. 12–7).[271] Despite their potency, these LTD_4 antagonists were unable to completely inhibit the bronchoconstrictor response to exercise. This suggests that other mediators, such as mast cell–derived histamine or prostaglandins, are involved in the pathogenesis of exercise-induced asthma.

BRONCHODILATION

Ellis and Undem found that isolated human bronchi of 3 to 12 mm in diameter had a high degree of intrinsic bronchomotor tone, which was on average more than 50% of the available maximal constrictor response to 30 mM of $BaCl_2$. In the presence of the LTD_4 antagonists ICI 204,219 or SKF 104,353, there was relaxation of the bronchi that was additive with a histamine H_1 antagonist, leading to the conclusion that intrinsic bronchomotor tone is due to the continual production of cysteinyl leukotrienes and histamine.[118] Further clinical studies have been carried out to support a role for cysteinyl leukotrienes in the maintenance of intrinsic bronchial muscle tone.

An intravenous infusion of the LTD_4 antagonist MK-0679 in nine asthmatic patients with baseline FEV_1 ranging from 40% to 80% of predicted values produced an increase in FEV_1 of 15.8% and 7.8% with 500 mg and 125 mg, respectively, and a fall of 2.6% 15 minutes after placebo infusion.[188] In a separate study, an oral dose of 40 mg of ICI 204,219 produced a significant resting increase in FEV_1 compared with placebo that persisted after inhaled albuterol.[186]

In a study of 12 male asthmatic patients, there was further confirmation of the additive effect of inhaled β_2-agonist administration (Fig. 12–8). The maximum bronchodilation achieved from the start of a 6-hour intravenous infusion of MK-571 was 22% compared with 1.3% after placebo. Administration of albuterol at 5 to 6 hours from the start of the infusion produced additional bronchodilatation. The overall degree of bronchodilation was inversely correlated with baseline FEV_1, suggesting a major contribution from

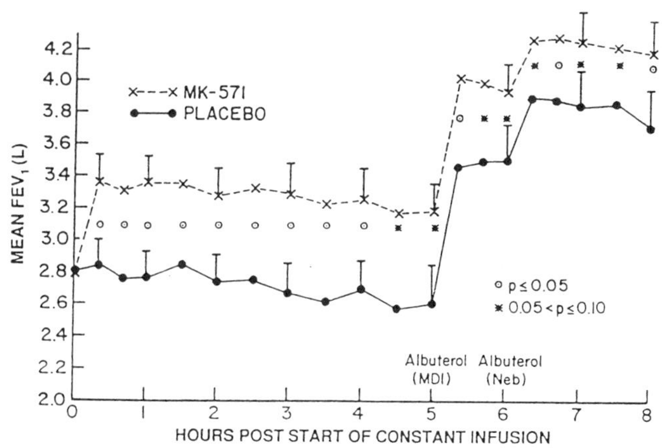

FIGURE 12–8. Mean change in FEV_1 over time in asthmatic patients with existing airway obstruction after treatment with intravenous MK-571 (x) or placebo (closed circles) and subsequent response to inhaled albuterol. (From Gaddy JN, Margolskee DJ, Bush RK, et al: Bronchodilation with a potent and selective leukotriene D_4 (LTD_4) receptor antagonist (MK-571) in patients with asthma. Am Rev Respir Dis 146:358–363, 1992.)

cysteinyl leukotrienes in resting airway tone.[154] In aspirin-sensitive asthma, the magnitude of cysteinyl leukotriene effect on intrinsic airway tone has been reported in one study using a single dose of 825 mg of MK-0679 in eight subjects. This produced a mean peak increase in FEV_1 of 18%, with a range of 5% to 34%, and strongly correlated with the severity of asthma.[86]

CHRONIC ASTHMA

The leukotriene antagonists have shown considerable efficacy in models of experimental asthma. Prior to product registration, however, much greater emphasis is placed on the demonstration of efficacy in large numbers of patients in their normal environment. There are still relatively few leukotriene antagonists that have reached this stage in the development process, and few studies have been reported. In a multicenter placebo-controlled study, 138 patients with asthma received 1,200 mg per day of LY-171,883 for 6 weeks. In the treatment group, mean FEV_1 rose significantly compared with placebo from 73.8% to 83.3% of predicted values. There were also significant improvements in the severity of daytime and nocturnal wheeze and breathlessness, with a reduction in β_2-agonist use, although there was no change in symptoms of cough or chest tightness.[70]

In a separate study, treatment with 225 mg of MK-571 three times a day for 2 weeks followed by 4 weeks of treatment with 150 mg three times a day produced a mean 8% to 14% improvement in FEV_1 and a 30% reduction in morning and evening symptom scores accompanied by a 30% reduction in albuterol usage.[153] One week of treatment with ONO-1078 in a crossover study of 11 asthmatic subjects produced a significant improvement in methacholine PC_{20}-FEV_1 compared with placebo, but there was no change in either resting FEV_1 or FVC during that period.[143]

In a placebo-controlled dose-ranging study of 266 subjects with moderate asthma treated twice daily with ICI 204,219, administration with 40 mg was linearly more effective than 20 mg or 10 mg without any increase in adverse effects. Compared with placebo, there was a significant reduction in nocturnal awakenings (by 46%), first morning asthma symptoms, daytime asthma scores (by 26%), and albuterol use (by 30%) and an increase in FEV_1 (11%) and evening peak expiratory flow rates.[401] The only reported study that has added an LTD_4 receptor antagonist to existing therapy with inhaled steroids was one using 10 days of treatment with RG 12525, which significantly improved FEV_1 in stable asthmatic subjects.[426]

Further and larger scale studies are required to accurately predict the future role of leukotriene antagonists in asthma therapy and to determine whether their major role is as bronchodilators or anti-inflammatory agents or whether they can replace existing treatments such as inhaled corticosteroids or theophyllines.

LEUKOTRIENE BIOSYNTHESIS INHIBITORS

Inhibitors of leukotriene biosynthesis were postulated to be more effective than LTD_4 receptor antagonists in preventing the pathophysiologic consequences of leukotriene release within the airways because of the dual inhibition of both LTB_4 and cysteinyl leukotriene generation. Current evidence suggests that 5-LO contains a nonheme iron that is normally in the dormant ferrous state (Fe^{2+}) and is converted to the active ferric form (Fe^{3+}) upon activation by hydroperoxides, adenosine triphosphate (ATP), and calcium. The activated 5-LO translocates (possibly due to a change from a hydrophilic to a hydrophobic conformation) to the nuclear membrane, where it comes into contact with the membrane-spanning cofactor FLAP, thus allowing access to the substrate. The enzyme complex then acts on arachidonic acid, which is oxidized stereoselectively by a free radical process involving removal of the 7H(S) hydrogen followed by peroxidation and then oxidation of Fe^{2+} in 5-LO with simultaneous reduction of the hydroperoxide radical to give 5-HPETE. There are therefore a number of possible mechanisms by which 5-LO may be inhibited.

Direct inhibition of the enzyme can be accomplished by redox inhibitors, which can act by either chelation or reduction of the nonheme iron (e.g., acetohydroxamic acids such as BW A4C and hydroxyurea derivatives such as zileuton and BW70C), or by a nonredox mechanism through antioxidant/free radical scavenger activity on radical intermediates of 5-LO (e.g., flavonoids, nafazatrom [BAY-G576], naphthalene derivatives such as RS-43,179 and Wy-47,288, and the enantioselective, competitive, and reversible inhibitor ZD2138, a methoxytetrahydropyran). A further mechanism is to use substrate analogues such as eicosatetraynoic acid (ETYA) and prostacyclin analogues.

Indirect 5-LO inhibition is achieved by using compounds that bind with high affinity to FLAP and probably act by preventing arachidonic acid presentation to 5-LO, such as the indole derivative MK-886 and the quinolone/indole hybrid MK-0591. Some 5-LO inhibitors have more than one mode of action. At low concentrations of racemic Wy-50,295, inhibition of 5-LO binding to FLAP predominates; but at higher concentrations, its activity as an arachidonic acid analogue becomes more significant.[121] Hydroxamic acids and hydroxyureas act primarily by chelating the essential iron at the active site of the enzyme, but it is likely that they also have additional antioxidant activity.[157] Clinical trials involving 5-LO inhibitors have followed the pattern set by the cysteinyl leukotriene antagonists, with earlier studies using compounds with weak inhibitory activity such as piriprost, which demonstrated little clinical utility,[268] and later more potent compounds reported to have useful activity.

ALLERGEN-INDUCED ASTHMA

In a single-dose placebo-controlled crossover study, nine asthmatic subjects received the iron chelator zileuton (A64077). Despite almost complete inhibition of ex vivo whole blood LTB_4 generation and 50% reduction of the rise of urinary LTE_4, there was no significant attenuation of the early or late asthmatic response and no decrease of the airway responsiveness to methacholine.[187] The potent and selective nonredox 5-LO inhibitor ZD2138 was evaluated in a study of eight asthmatic subjects. Although there was an 82% reduction of ex vivo LTB_4 generation in whole blood and an overall 72% inhibition of the rise in urinary LTE_4

excretion, again there was no inhibition of the allergen-induced early or late asthmatic response.[305]

In a separate placebo-controlled study of eight atopic men, 500 mg of the FLAP inhibitor MK-886 was given 1 hour before and 250 mg 2 hours after allergen inhalation. MK-886 inhibited the early asthmatic response by 58% and the late asthmatic response by 44%. This was accompanied by a 54.2% inhibition of A23187-stimulated whole blood LTB_4 generation and a 51.5% inhibition of the rise in urinary LTE_4 during the early and 80% during the late asthmatic response. However, compared with placebo, no significant change in airway responsiveness to histamine was observed 30 hours after allergen challenge.[141] The FLAP inhibitor MK-0591 (250 mg) was administered 24, 12, and 1.5 hours before allergen inhalation. Over the 24-hour period following allergen inhalation, LTB_4 generation was inhibited by 96% and urinary LTE_4 excretion by 84%. The early asthmatic response to allergen was inhibited by 79% and the late asthmatic response delayed by 3 hours, but no effect was observed on airway responsiveness to histamine 24 hours postallergen challenge.[104]

ASPIRIN-INDUCED ASTHMA

Eight subjects with aspirin-sensitive asthma and hyperexcretion of urinary LTE_4 were premedicated with zileuton or placebo, and the effect of aspirin ingestion was examined. Zileuton reduced baseline urinary LTE_4 excretion by 70% and prevented the fall in FEV_1 in response to aspirin challenge. In addition, there was protection against the development of nasal, gastrointestinal, and dermal symptoms in response to aspirin ingestion.[191] In a separate study, seven subjects with aspirin-induced asthma and hyperexcretion of urinary LTE_4 were premedicated with a single dose of 350 mg of ZD2138, which provided substantial inhibition of both LTB_4 generation and urinary LTE_4 excretion (Fig. 12–9).

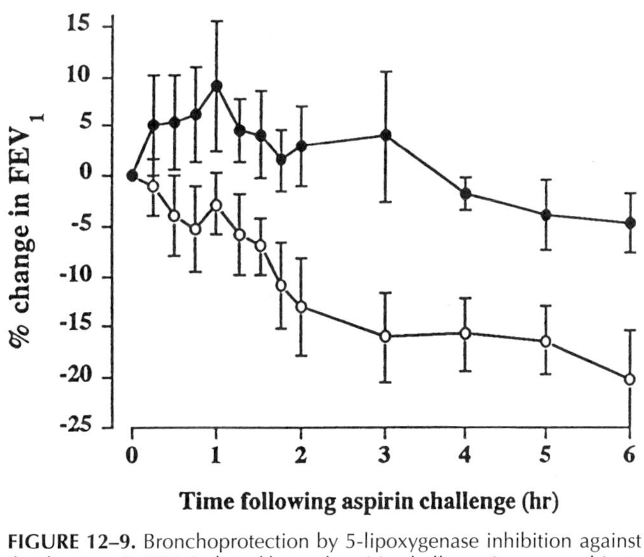

FIGURE 12–9. Bronchoprotection by 5-lipoxygenase inhibition against the decrease in FEV_1 induced by oral aspirin challenge in seven subjects with aspirin-sensitive asthma. The subjects were premedicated with either the 5LO inhibitor ZD2138 (closed circles) or placebo (open circles). (From Nasser SM, Bell GS, Foster S, et al: Effect of the 5-lipoxygenase inhibitor ZD2138 on aspirin-induced asthma. Thorax 49:749–756, 1994.)

In response to oral aspirin challenge, the mean maximum fall in FEV_1 was 20.3% after placebo and 4.9% following ZD2138 premedication, and this was associated with a reduction in systemic symptoms.[304]

EXERCISE-INDUCED ASTHMA

A single dose of 800 mg of zileuton administered to 13 asthmatic subjects inhibited ex vivo whole blood LTB_4 generation by 74% without affecting TXB_2 levels. This produced a 47% increase in the amount of cold, dry air required to reduce FEV_1 by 10%, with an increase in minute ventilation from 27.5 l/min to 39.8 l/min.[190] A further study of 24 subjects with mild asthma premedicated for 2 days with 2.4 g/day of zileuton demonstrated a 40% inhibition of exercise-induced bronchospasm. This study also demonstrated a significant protection against the fall in FVC compared with placebo.[291]

BRONCHODILATION

In a study of chronic asthma in patients treated with albuterol only, baseline FEV_1 increased by 15% within 1 hour of zileuton administration.[193] In aspirin-sensitive asthmatic subjects, administration of ZD2138 produced approximately a 10% increase in FEV_1 compared with placebo within 3 hours. However, baseline FEV_1 was significantly lower than that on the placebo day, and bronchodilation may have represented a regression to normal values.[304] It is likely that 5-LO inhibitors demonstrate their greatest effect in subjects in whom leukotriene-dependent bronchospasm plays a major role, such as those with acute severe asthma and aspirin-sensitive asthma.

CHRONIC ASTHMA

As part of a multicenter study, 139 asthmatic patients who were not taking oral or inhaled corticosteroids and had baseline FEV_1 values of 40% to 75% of normal were placed on 2.4 or 1.6 g/day of zileuton or placebo for 4 weeks. Patients treated with zileuton had a statistically significant 13.6% improvement in FEV_1 after 4 weeks of therapy. There was also a significant improvement in asthmatic symptom scores and a reduction in β_2-agonist use in subjects on the higher dose of zileuton.[193] In an extension of this study, 398 asthmatic patients with moderately severe asthma (baseline FEV_1 61%) who had been previously stabilized on albuterol were treated for 13 weeks with either 2.4 or 1.6 g/day of zileuton or placebo. In the subjects taking 2.4 g/day, there was a sustained increase in FEV_1 of 0.25 l compared with 0.08 l in the patients receiving placebo.

In a separate study, 109 asthmatic subjects taking 400 to 1600 μg of either beclomethasone or budesonide who had baseline FEV_1 values of 50% to 75% were placed on placebo or 125 mg of MK-0591 twice daily. After 4 weeks of treatment, FEV_1 increased 6.8% in the MK-0591 treated group compared with 0.6% in the placebo treated group. In addition, there was an increase in morning and evening PEFR of 19% and 13%, respectively, in the MK-0591 treated group compared with a fall in morning and evening PEFR of 5% and 6%, respectively, in the placebo group. Furthermore, subjects on active treatment reported a reduction in β_2-agonist use.[53]

OTHER DISEASES

Allergic Rhinitis

Oral administration of a single dose of 800 mg of zileuton in a double-blind placebo-controlled study of eight patients suffering from allergic rhinitis produced a significant attenuation of allergen-induced nasal congestion, and this was associated with inhibition of leukotriene release into nasal lavage fluid.[223]

Rheumatoid Arthritis

Placebo or 800 mg of zileuton twice daily was administered to 24 patients with active rheumatoid arthritis for 4 weeks. There was an improvement in clinical variables in both groups, with a nonstatistically significant trend toward greater improvement in the joint swelling index and patient assessment of the number of painful joints in the zileuton group.[433]

Inflammatory Bowel Disease

Treatment with 800 mg of zileuton for 28 days in an open study of 11 subjects with active ulcerative colitis resulted in a reduction of symptom scores in all patients and an improvement in gross mucosal appearance, although no histologic improvement was demonstrated.[76]

Psoriasis

Psoriatic plaques were treated for 28 days with a 2% topical ointment of lonapalene (6-chloro-2,3-dimethoxynaphthalene-dio-diacetate), a selective inhibitor of 5-LO. Compared with vehicle treated sites, there was a significant reduction in skin chamber fluid LTB_4 levels by 4 days, with an improvement in clinical scores in seven of nine subjects at both 14 and 28 days.[203] A 2% ointment of R 68,151, a selective 5-LO inhibitor, was applied twice daily for 4 weeks on psoriatic plaques in 44 patients and the results compared with placebo ointment in another 44 patients. The active group experienced an improvement in mean symptom scores for scaling of 46% against 6% for the placebo group and 34% for erythema compared with a deterioration of 3% for the placebo treated group. In the active group, 27% of subjects experienced either disappearance or marked improvement of lesions compared with 8% for the vehicle treated plaques.[98]

In conclusion, there are many theoretic reasons to suggest that leukotriene biosynthesis inhibitors would be more effective than cysteinyl leukotriene receptor antagonists. Biosynthesis inhibitors block generation of the full spectrum of 5-LO products, which include not only cysteinyl leukotrienes but also other inflammatory mediators such as LTB_4 and 5-HETE,[206] as well as some of the effects of platelet-activating factor.[8, 258] Conversely, leukotriene antagonists can only effectively prevent the action of one leukotriene. In addition, it is possible that cysteinyl leukotriene receptor antagonists may prolong the half-lives of leukotrienes by interfering with their elimination.[101]

However, in clinical studies, leukotriene receptor antagonists have proven to be more effective in inhibiting cysteinyl leukotriene–mediated disease processes. Several mechanisms may account for this. First, although there is good inhibition of ex vivo whole blood LTB_4 and urinary LTE_4 release, current 5-LO inhibitors may not provide sufficiently effective inhibition of leukotriene biosynthesis at the site of disease. Second, even small quantities of locally generated leukotrienes may be sufficient to exert pathologic effects. Third, inhibition of 5-LO could interfere with the synthesis of dual lipoxygenase products such as lipoxin A_4, which may have a moderating influence on cysteinyl leukotriene action.[61] Fourth, 5-LO inhibition may theoretically lead to shunting of arachidonic acid toward generation of proinflammatory cyclooxygenase products. It has been speculated that the ideal compound to modulate the effects of leukotrienes in asthma would possess both leukotriene receptor antagonism and 5-LO synthesis inhibitory activity[395] because these activities may be functionally additive.[347]

Over the next few years, the place of antileukotriene therapy in the treatment of asthma is likely to be established. However, more clinical studies are required to define whether they possess corticosteroid-sparing activity, lead to long-term symptomatic improvement, or affect the underlying disease process. The promise shown by these compounds must be tempered with a note of caution. Leukotrienes are just one of many proinflammatory mediators in asthma, and monotherapy with these agents may not prove sufficient.

PROSTAGLANDINS AND THROMBOXANES

BIOSYNTHESIS AND CELLULAR SOURCE

The enzyme prostaglandin H synthase (PGHS) is also known as cyclooxygenase and, in contrast to 5-LO, is found almost universally in mammalian cells. Prostanoid synthesis (Fig. 12–10) is initiated by hormone-activated mobilization of esterified arachidonic acid from one or more of a number of precursor phospholipids by phospholipase activity. Arachidonic acid is converted by the cyclooxygenase action of PGHS to the prostaglandin endoperoxides PGG_2 and PGH_2. This is then followed by rapid isomerization or reduction of PGH_2 by cell-specific synthases (isomerases) or reductases to the major biologically active prostanoids prostaglandin (PG) D_2, $PGF_{2\alpha}$, and thromboxane (TX) A_2, which have bronchoconstrictor properties, and PGE_2 and prostacyclin (PGI_2), which have inhibitory or bronchoprotective properties.[366, 423]

Despite the ubiquitous distribution of PGHS, there is great variation in the specific products generated by different cell sources. Mast cells preferentially synthesize PGD_2; platelets predominantly generate thromboxane TXA_2; vascular endothelial cells and both vascular and nonvascular smooth muscle synthesize prostacyclin (PGI_2); macrophages generate

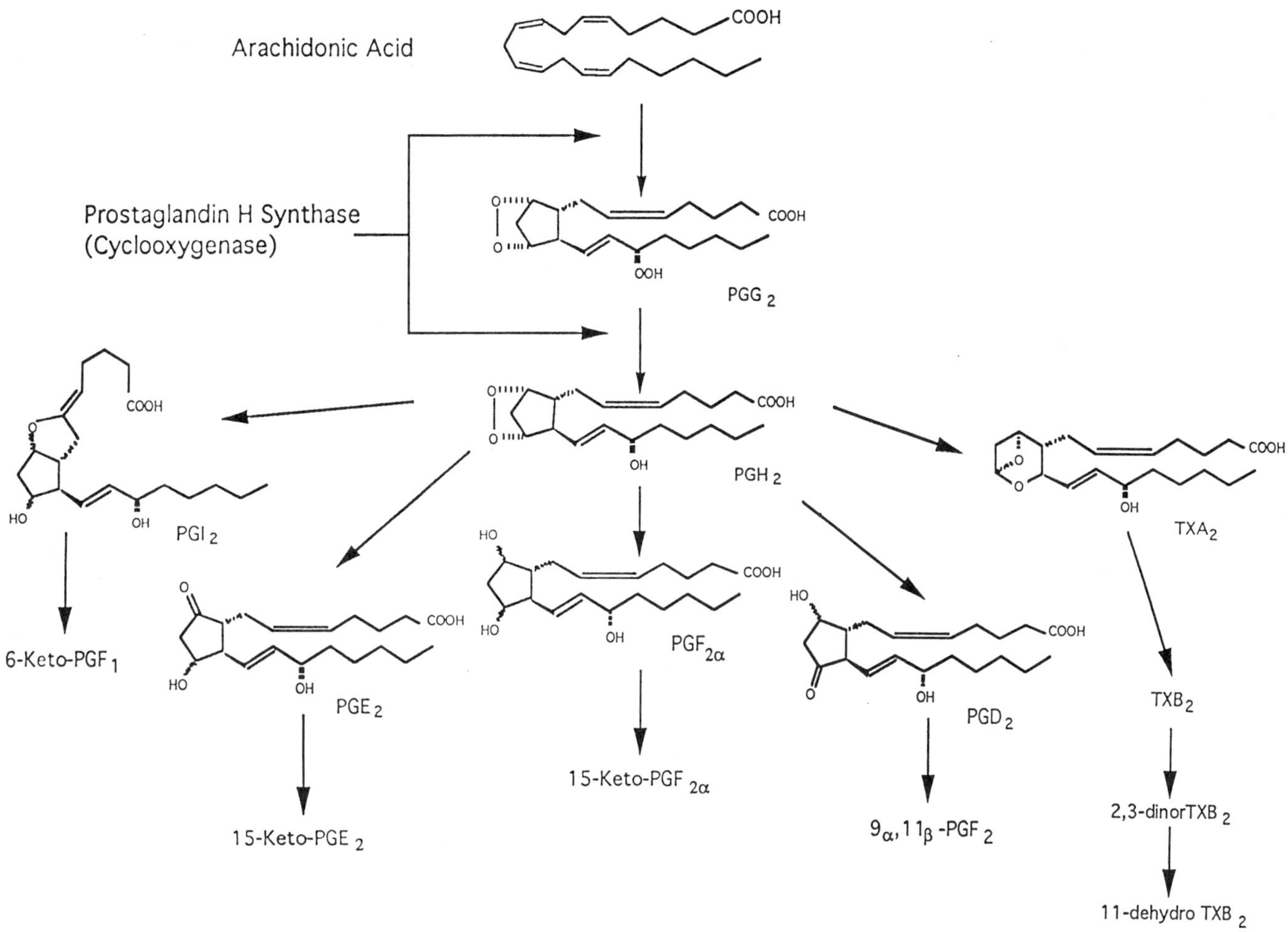

FIGURE 12–10. Prostanoid biosynthetic pathway. Cyclooxygenase catalyses the first two steps and converts arachidonic acid to the endoperoxides PGG_2 and PGH_2, which are then enzymatically transformed to prostaglandins, prostacyclin, and thromboxanes by the action of the respective synthases.

$PGF_{2\alpha}$, PGE_2, and TXA_2; and epithelial cells generate PGE_2. Mast cells are the source of PGD_2 released from human lung fragments[180, 255] in response to IgE-dependent and calcium ionophore A23187 stimulation, and this is then metabolized by an NADPH-dependent 11-ketoreductase to the active metabolite $9_\alpha,11_\beta$-PGF_2, which has bronchoconstrictor activity.[26] Neutrophils, eosinophils, and basophils do not generate prostanoid products in significant quantities.

PROSTAGLANDIN H SYNTHASE

Mammalian cells contain two isoforms of PGHS referred to as PGHS-1 and PGHS-2, with 61% homology between their amino acid sequences.[178] The amino acid sequences required for both cyclooxygenase and peroxidase functions are conserved between the two isoforms, and both have similar affinity for and capacity to convert arachidonic acid to PGH_2.[288] The differences between the two isoforms of PGHS involve their regulation and cell expression. PGHS-1 is constitutively expressed at varying levels in virtually all mammalian tissues. For example, vascular endothelial cells[103] and platelets[149] express high baseline levels of enzyme, with only minor increases of twofold to fourfold induced by hormonal or growth factor stimulation.[102, 320] PGHS-2, by contrast, is relatively undetectable in the majority of tissues, but its expression increases substantially in situations associated with differentiation and cell replication and in response to inflammation and mitogenic stimuli with typical up-regulation of 10- to 80-fold.[230, 231] For example, endotoxin can stimulate PGHS-2 expression in monocytes and macrophages,[242, 314] and growth factors such as phorbol esters and interleukin-1 induce PGHS-2 in fibroblasts.[230, 308]

Although only a limited number of tissues have been examined and shown to express PGHS-2 activity, it is likely to be present under appropriate stimulatory conditions in as many cell types as PGHS-1. A further regulatory property of PGHS-2 is that its induced expression can be completely inhibited by anti-inflammatory glucocorticoids such as dexamethasone.[275] It has therefore been hypothesized that the constitutively expressed PGHS-1 is a housekeeping gene involved in the production of prostanoids that regulate normal cellular function and that inducible PGHS-2 is involved in the production of prostanoids that mediate inflammatory and mitogenic responses.

PROSTANOID RECEPTORS

The mode of cellular egress of the prostanoids following intracellular biosynthesis probably involves facilitated diffusion.[392] Once outside the cell, the prostanoids can act on either the parent or neighboring cells through specific G protein–linked prostanoid receptors to effect changes in second messenger levels.[393] Initially, five different receptor classes were described and designated DP, EP, FP, IP, and TP on the basis of preferential sensitivity to PGD_2, PGE_2, $PGF_{2\alpha}$, PGI_2, and TXA_2.[72] With the availability of more selective agonists and antagonists, this classification has now been extended using radioligand-binding studies at these sites. The biologic actions mediated at the different prostanoid receptors are shown in Table 12–5.

EP Receptors

Further subclassification of EP receptors was required to explain the disparate actions of PGE_2, which include contraction or relaxation of vascular and nonvascular smooth muscle and stimulation and suppression of neurotransmitter and hormonal release. Three pharmacologically distinct receptor subtypes are now recognized and known as EP_1, EP_2, and EP_3. All display high affinity for PGE_2 but show differences in their affinities to various synthetic agonists and antagonists. Their heterogeneous actions are mediated by coupling to a variety of signal transduction pathways. The stimulatory/contractile actions occur at EP_1, the relaxant/inhibitory actions occur at EP_2, and the EP_3 receptor is proposed to have stimulatory actions in some tissues and inhibitory effects in others.[73, 108] Activation of the EP_1 receptor results in an increase in inositol trisphosphate and intracellular calcium, activation of the EP_2 receptor subtype leads to an increase in intracellular cAMP, and activation of the EP_3 receptor results in a decrease in intracellular cAMP. The mouse and human EP_1,[432] mouse and human EP_2,[182] and mouse and rat EP_3[413, 418] receptor subtypes have now been cloned.

TABLE 12–5
PROSTANOID ACTIONS MEDIATED AT DIFFERENT RECEPTOR SITES

Receptor	Actions
EP_1	Contraction of smooth muscle in GI and respiratory tracts, uterus, vas deferens, and iris sphincter Stimulates neurotransmitter release Inhibits absorption from small intestine
EP_2	Relaxation of smooth muscle in GI tract, uterus, renal blood vessels, iris sphincter Stimulates stomach and small bowel secretion Control of intraocular pressure Regulation of bone reabsorption Proinflammatory actions: edema and hyperanalgesia
EP_3	Contraction of smooth muscle in uterus Inhibition of gastric secretion Neurotransmitter release Lipolysis in adipose tissue Na^+ and H_2O reabsorption in the renal tubule
TP	Contraction of smooth muscle in respiratory tract and blood vessels
FP	Contraction of smooth muscle in GI and respiratory tracts, uterus, and blood vessels Luteolytic properties Reduces intraocular pressure
IP	Relaxation of smooth muscle in blood vessels Inhibits platelet activation Regulates renal blood flow, renin release, and glomerular filtration rate Stimulates stomach and small bowel secretion Modulates myocardial neurotransmitter release Proinflammatory actions: edema, hyperanalgesia, hyperemia, and pyrexia

EP_1

EP_1 receptors are postulated to mediate contraction of smooth muscle in a variety of tissues such as the gastrointestinal and respiratory tracts, myometrium, vas deferens, and iris sphincter. Other possible functions include stimulation of neurotransmitter release and inhibition of absorption from the small intestine. The functional EP_1 receptor was isolated from a human erythroleukemia cell cDNA library probed with a polymerase chain reaction fragment of the human TP receptor using low stringency.[150] The EP_1 receptor, comprising 402 amino acids with a predicted molecular mass of 42 kD and like all other G protein–coupled receptors, has 7 membrane-spanning segments. Activation of EP_1 by PGE_2 results in elevation of intracellular Ca^{2+}.

EP_2

The EP_2 receptor is reported to be present in the vasculature, the kidney, and the gastrointestinal, tracheobronchial, and reproductive tracts as well as the sphincter dilator and ciliary muscles of the eye. The actions mediated through the EP_2 receptor subtype include maintenance of homeostatic smooth muscle relaxation. Further putative roles include stimulation of secretion in the stomach and small intestine, control of intraocular pressure, and regulation of bone reabsorption. The EP_2 receptor may also mediate a variety of proinflammatory actions, including vasodilation, hyperanalgesia, edema formation, modulation of the immune system, and breakdown of bone and cartilage associated with disorders such as rheumatoid arthritis.

The cDNA clone encoding the human EP_2 receptor was isolated from a human lung library.[25] The 1.9 Kbp cDNA was found to encode for a 488–amino acid sequence with a predicted molecular weight of 53 kD and had 7 putative transmembrane domains characteristic of G protein–linked receptors. This receptor subtype is functionally coupled to adenylate cyclase mediating increased intracellular cAMP. Northern blot analysis showed that EP_2 is expressed as a 3.8 Kb mRNA in a number of human tissues, with the highest expression present in the small intestine.

EP_3

It has been proposed that actions mediated by the EP_3 receptor include contraction of the uterus,[226] inhibition of gastric acid secretion,[55] neurotransmitter release,[316] lipolysis in adipose tissue,[348] and sodium and water reabsorption in the kidney tubule.[303, 398] In the mouse, functional cDNA clones for three further isoforms of the EP_3 receptor have been reported. The three isoforms $EP_{3\alpha}$, $EP_{3\beta}$, and $EP_{3\gamma}$ are

G protein–linked rhodopsin-type receptors that are coupled to adenylate cyclase[414] and differ only in their carboxy-terminal tails. The difference in amino acid sequence results in different efficiencies for activation of the coupled inhibitory G protein (G_i) and inhibition of adenylate cyclase.[413]

The three receptor isoforms have identical ligand-binding properties, but the EP_3-selective agonist M&B 28767 increased basal cAMP levels and inhibited the forskolin-induced increase in cAMP levels in $EP_{3\gamma}$, whereas it decreased both the basal and forskolin-elevated cAMP levels in $EP_{3\alpha}$ and $EP_{3\beta}$. The M&B 28767-stimulated GTPase activity consisted of pertussis toxin–sensitive and cholera toxin–sensitive portions in the $EP_{3\gamma}$-expressing cell membrane, suggesting that $EP_{3\gamma}$ is coupled to both inhibitory and stimulatory G proteins. This indicates that $EP_{3\alpha}$ and $EP_{3\beta}$ are exclusively coupled to inhibition of adenylate cyclase, whereas $EP_{3\gamma}$ is coupled to both stimulation and inhibition of adenylate cyclase.[189] Cloning of the human EP_3 receptor has not yet been reported.

TP Receptor

The PG endoperoxides and TXA_2 share common molecular recognition sites in the airways. From studies of a large range of selective receptor agonists with differing activity profiles, it is likely that at least two subclasses of TXA/PGH (TP) receptor exist. There is likely to be cross-reactivity between the various prostanoid receptors. For example, in guinea pig trachea, the contractile responses evoked by PGD_2, $PGF_{2\alpha}$,[205] and $9_\alpha,11_\beta$-PGF_2[74] can be partially blocked by TP receptor antagonists, suggesting that a significant proportion of the contractile activity of PGD_2 and its active metabolite $9_\alpha,11_\beta$-PGF_2 is mediated through this receptor. The human platelet TP receptor was purified to apparent homogeneity by using a stable analogue of TXA_2. With the use of an oligonucleotide probe corresponding to the partial amino acid sequence of the TP receptor, a cDNA clone was isolated from a human placental cDNA library. This was found to encode a protein of 343 amino acids with 7 putative transmembrane domains, and when expressed in *Xenopus* oocytes and stimulated with an agonist, it mobilized intracellular Ca^{2+}.[177]

FP Receptor

$PGF_{2\alpha}$ is a potent luteolytic compound in a number of animal species. Analogues of $PGF_{2\alpha}$ are implicated as having a regulatory role in the flow of aqueous humor in the eye and thereby reducing intraocular pressure. Other actions include contraction of smooth muscle in the myometrium, gastrointestinal and respiratory tracts, and possibly the vasculature. The human functional cDNA clone encoding the FP receptor was isolated from a uterus cDNA library.[2] The FP receptor was found to consist of 359 amino acid residues with a predicted molecular mass of 40 kD and was shown to possess 7 putative transmembrane segments. Challenge of *Xenopus* oocytes expressing the FP receptor with either $PGF_{2\alpha}$ or a synthetic agonist resulted in an increase in intracellular Ca^{2+}, confirming that the isolated cDNA encodes a functional prostanoid receptor coupled to the Ca^{2+} signaling pathway.

IP Receptor

Prostacyclin plays a major homeostatic role as an inhibitor of platelet aggregation, degranulation, and shape change and as a potent mediator of vasodilation. Other postulated roles for PGI_2 include regulation of renal blood flow, renin release, and glomerular filtration rate in the renal cortex; stimulation of stomach and small intestinal secretion; and modulation of neurotransmitter release in the myocardium. The distribution of IP receptors has been well characterized using radioligand-binding studies. IP receptors have been shown to be present in the myocardium, myometrium, penile erectile tissue, and iris sphincter muscle, as well as arterial preparations from coronary, renal, and pulmonary vessels.

The cDNA clone encoding the functional IP receptor was isolated from a lung cDNA library using a synthesized oligonucleotide probe based on nine highly conserved amino acid residues from the transmembrane domain of other cloned prostanoid receptors.[34] The receptor was found to consist of 386 amino acid residues with a predicted molecular mass of 41 kD and had 7 putative transmembrane domains characteristic of G protein–linked receptors.

Challenge of *Xenopus* oocytes expressing the IP receptor with a synthetic analogue resulted in an increase in intracellular cAMP, confirming that the isolated cDNA encoded a functional IP receptor coupled to adenylate cyclase. Northern blot analysis showed that the IP receptor mRNA was most abundantly expressed in kidney, with lesser amounts present in lung and liver.

DETECTION OF PROSTANOIDS IN BIOLOGIC FLUIDS

Bronchoalveolar Lavage Fluid

The release of prostanoids has been measured in biologic fluids in asthma both in disease and in response to allergen challenge. Levels of the bronchoconstrictor prostanoids PGD_2, $9_\alpha,11_\beta$-PGF_2, and $PGF_{2\alpha}$ were simultaneously profiled in BAL fluid using gas chromatography–mass spectrometry in 12 normal, 11 allergic rhinitis subjects, and 15 mild asthmatic individuals.[257] The levels of these prostanoids were found to be 12 to 22 times higher in asthmatic airways compared with normal individuals. Levels of PGD_2 and $9_\alpha,11_\beta$-PGF_2 were 10-fold higher in asthmatic subjects compared with patients with allergic rhinitis, distinguishing subjects with lower airways disease from other atopic conditions. When all three groups were considered together, there was an inverse correlation between the dose of methacholine required to decrease FEV_1 by 20% and the levels of BAL bronchoconstrictor mediators.

Endobronchial allergen challenge was performed in a study involving patients with chronic stable asthma. This resulted in a 150-fold increase in BAL fluid levels of PGD_2 within 9 minutes of the challenge.[298] Bronchoalveolar fluid levels of the bronchoconstrictor prostanoids PGD_2 and thromboxane and the bronchoprotective prostanoid PGE_2 and the stable metabolite of PGI_2, 6-keto-$PGF_{1\alpha}$, were measured before and 5 minutes after endobronchial allergen challenge. Although there were no differences in prechallenge prostanoid levels between asthmatic and nonasthmatic subjects following allergen challenge, the asthmatic subjects showed a 10-fold rise in PGD_2 levels and a 3-fold rise in thromboxane levels, with a 20-fold increase in histamine levels. There was no increase in PGI_2 and 6-keto-$PGF_{1\alpha}$ levels in these individuals. Furthermore, no change was detected in levels of either bronchoconstrictor or bronchoprotective prostanoids in the nonasthmatic subjects.[440] In a study of 10 aspirin-sensitive and 6 nonaspirin-sensitive asthmatic subjects, there were significantly greater baseline BAL fluid levels of PGE_2 and TXB_2 in the aspirin-sensitive group.[386]

Urine

In a study of acute severe asthma, the urinary excretion of the TXA_2 metabolites TXB_2, 2,3 dinor TXB_2, and 11-dihydro TXB_2 and of the prostacyclin metabolites 6-oxo-$PGF_{1\alpha}$ and 2,5 dinor-6-oxo-$PGF_{1\alpha}$ was measured using gas chromatography–mass spectrometry. The levels of both the TXB_2 and prostacyclin metabolites were significantly higher in patients with acute severe asthma compared with a nonsmoking control population.[421]

Urinary metabolites of the major prostanoid released by platelets, TXA_2, were measured using the technique of gas chromatography–negative ion, chemical ionization–mass spectrometry in a study of seven atopic asthmatic subjects predosed with either low-dose aspirin or placebo followed by allergen challenge. After placebo predosing followed by allergen challenge, there was a threefold rise in urinary excretion of 2,3-dinor-TXB_2 and a twofold rise in 11-dehydro-TXB_2. Predosing with low-dose aspirin reduced baseline excretion of thromboxane metabolites and prevented the rise in the urinary excretion of TXA_2 metabolites without altering the level of bronchoconstriction after allergen inhalation. This suggests that although platelets are activated by allergen challenge, the platelet-derived product TXA_2 is not important in the early bronchoconstrictor response.[259] In a similar study of 10 atopic asthmatics, there was a threefold increase in urinary levels of 11-dehydro TXB_2 2 hours following allergen provocation but no increase during the late phase response.[385]

Plasma

Plasma concentrations of the stable metabolite of $PGF_{2\alpha}$ were measured using radioimmunoassay in 15 children during acute asthma. The mean level of 13,14-dihydro-15-keto$_2$ $PGF_{2\alpha}$ was 1470 ng/l compared with 25.5 ng/l after resolution of airway obstruction, with the highest levels obtained from those infants positive for respiratory syncytial virus.[383] A further study reported similar results using 13,14-dihydro-15-keto$_2$ $PGF_{2\alpha}$ but also found that baseline levels of this metabolite of $PGF_{2\alpha}$ were similar in normal and asthmatic children.[384]

PHARMACOLOGIC PROPERTIES OF PROSTANOIDS IN ASTHMA

Prostaglandin D_2

The endoperoxide PGH_2 undergoes nonoxidative isomerization to PGD_2 by the action of glutathione-dependent and glutathione-independent PGD synthases.[394] Prostaglandin D_2 was shown to be released from activated rat peritoneal mast cells[349] and during pulmonary anaphylaxis in the guinea pig.[352] PGD_2 is the most abundant eicosanoid generated from anti-IgE–stimulated[255] and ionophore-stimulated[179] human pulmonary mast cells. The possible bronchoactive role of PGD_2 was initially demonstrated in dogs in which it caused bronchoconstriction.

PGD_2 is a potent contractile agent when administered by aerosol to both normal and asthmatic subjects and elicits rapidly developing bronchoconstriction.[26, 27, 171] In a study of asthmatic subjects, PGD_2 was found to have a potency approximately 3.5- and 10-fold greater than $PGF_{2\alpha}$ and histamine, respectively, with the maximal effect evident 3 minutes following inhalation. Moreover, there was a significant correlation between airway responsiveness to PGD_2 and methacholine.[171]

Inhaled PGD_2 was administered to six mild asthmatic subjects in a dose that caused no measurable bronchoconstriction, immediately before each dose of histamine or methacholine. The results demonstrated approximately a twofold enhancement of bronchial responsiveness to subsequent histamine and methacholine inhalation.[148] A further study conducted in asthmatic subjects suggested that sequential doses of PGD_2 followed by histamine are additive, and therefore enhanced airway responsiveness was a physiologic rather than a pharmacologic effect.[169] There is also some evidence to suggest that PGD_2 may enhance the bronchoconstrictor activity of LTC_4 in asthmatic airways.[333] Metabolism of PGD_2 yields $9_\alpha,11_\beta$-PGF_2, which has similar bronchoconstrictor potency to PGD_2 and may play a significant role in the biologic activity of PGD_2.[26]

Prostaglandin $F_{2\alpha}$

Under resting conditions, human lung parenchyma and to a lesser extent bronchial tissue fragments spontaneously release $PGF_{2\alpha}$, leading to the suggestion that this prostanoid together with PGE_2 may be important in maintaining bronchial tone.[84, 369] $PGF_{2\alpha}$ has contractile activity on isolated human airway tissue[319, 415] and causes bronchoconstriction in vivo, with asthmatic subjects demonstrating greater sensitivity to the effects of inhaled $PGF_{2\alpha}$ than do nonasthmatics. In a study of 10 asthmatic and 10 normal controls, it was reported that the asthmatics were 10 times more sensitive to histamine but 8,000 times more sensitive to the bronchoconstrictor action of inhaled $PGF_{2\alpha}$.[277] Other studies have reported similar responses to $PGF_{2\alpha}$ inhalation in asthmatic subjects but with wide interstudy variation of the degree of hyperreactivity ranging from 150-[388] to 8,000-fold[277] greater sensitivity compared with nonasthmatic subjects. Furthermore, whereas the healthy controls demonstrated reproducible decreases in SGaw in response to repeated $PGF_{2\alpha}$ challenge, the asthmatic subjects displayed tachyphylaxis.[276]

Thromboxane A_2

The conversion of PGH_2 to TXA_2 is catalyzed by TXA synthases that have been cloned from human platelets[449] and lung[315] and confirmed as members of the cytochrome P-450 family. The in vivo half-life of TXA_2 is only about 30 seconds, and therefore much of the information about its biologic activity comes from studies of stable synthetic analogues such as the long-acting thromboxane mimetic U46619. TXA_2 is readily degraded to its more stable and relatively inactive metabolite TXB_2, which can be measured in biologic fluids such as BAL and urine.

In a study of isolated human bronchus, the rank order of contractile potency for prostanoids was U46619 >> $9_{\alpha},11_{\beta}$-PGF_2 = $PGF_{2\alpha}$ > PGD_2 > PGE_2 > PGI_2.[74] Interestingly, this is almost exactly the reverse of the rank order for the magnitude of spontaneous prostanoid release from lung parenchymal fragments, which is 6-keto-$PGF_{1\alpha}$ (stable metabolite of prostacyclin) > PGE_2 = $PGF_{2\alpha}$ > PGD_2 > TXB_2.[369] In a study of nine asthmatic subjects, a single oral dose of the specific and potent TP receptor antagonist GR 32191 had no effect on basal airway caliber and produced no effect on the position or slope of the dose-response curve to methacholine.[28] Taken together, these studies suggest that under resting conditions the most potent bronchoconstricting prostanoids are released in the smallest quantities and are therefore unlikely to play a role in resting airway tone.

The TP receptor antagonist AH 23848 was shown to antagonize the contractile activity of the prostanoids in bronchial smooth muscle but demonstrated no activity against carbachol-induced contractions,[74] suggesting that the major bronchoconstrictor action of the prostanoids is mediated through the TP receptor. In a study of 13 asthmatic and 6 normal subjects, the bronchoconstricting potency of U46619 was found to be 178-fold greater than that of methacholine. Inhalation of a subthreshold dose of U46619 increased the subsequent bronchoconstrictor response to methacholine by twofold. This effect was transient and only apparent if methacholine challenge took place within 1 hour before U46619 inhalation.[204]

Prostaglandin E_2

Human bronchial smooth muscle and lung parenchymal tissue spontaneously release PGE_2.[369] Cellular sources of PGE_2 include macrophages,[260] epithelial cells,[69] and endothelial cells. Prostanoids of the E series are usually described as having relaxant properties on airway smooth muscle. Inhalation of 55 μg PGE_1 and PGE_2 in normal subjects increased SGaw by 10% and 18%, respectively, and in asthmatic subjects by 41% and 39%, respectively.[388] However, the effect of PGE_2 on human smooth muscle is much more complex.

Inhalation in normal subjects produces an initial bronchoconstriction within 5 minutes followed by bronchodilation peaking at 15 minutes and persisting at 60 minutes. The degree of initial bronchoconstriction to inhaled PGE_2 was inversely related to resting airway tone, with the bronchoconstrictor effect enhanced when the airways were predilated by removing vagal tone with a large dose of the anticholinergic agent ipratropium bromide.[429] PGE_2 also has paradoxical effects against the bronchoconstrictor activity of histamine and methacholine, protecting against bronchoconstriction during the bronchodilator phase and enhancing bronchial responsiveness to these reference agents if they are administered after the end of this phase.[428]

Further evidence of the possible modulatory role played by PGE_2 in bronchial asthma and other inflammatory diseases comes from its in vitro effect in reducing mucus secretion.[274] The effect of PGE_2 has been examined in various models of asthma. Inhaled PGE_2 reduced the maximal decrease in exercise-induced FEV_1 by 63% and reduced the duration of exercise-induced bronchoconstriction.[290] This effect is comparable to that found with leukotriene receptor antagonists,[271] sodium cromoglycate,[353] and β_2-agonists.[9] Inhaled PGE_2 has also been shown to protect against the early and late phase bronchoconstriction induced by allergen,[325] inhalation of ultrasonically nebulized distilled water, and sodium metabisulfite[324] and against the allergen-induced rise in bronchial responsiveness.[323] Despite the apparent clinical utility of PGE_2, which appears to play a bronchoprotective role in asthma, its therapeutic use is unfortunately limited by its short half-life, the initial cough and bronchoconstrictor effect, and retrosternal soreness following inhalation.

Prostaglandin I_2 (Prostacyclin)

Macrophages and endothelial cells generate prostacyclin, which has potent cyclic AMP-dependent smooth muscle relaxant activity important for the maintenance of homeostatic vascular patency. The hydrolysis product of PGI_2, 6-keto-$PGF_{1\alpha}$, is released into biologic fluids such as BAL and provides a reliable index of PGI_2 generation and release. This metabolite is the major cyclooxygenase product released from both resting and allergen-stimulated fragments of human bronchi, although their cellular source remains unidentified.[369]

In studies of airway smooth muscle, PGI_2 produced relaxation of guinea pig tracheal strips and of isolated precontracted human bronchus, although smooth muscle contraction was also sometimes seen.[155] In a study of 8 asthmatic and 10 normal controls, the effects of inhaled PGI_2 and its hydrolysis product 6-oxo-$PGF_{1\alpha}$ on airway caliber were examined. No consistent effect was found in either group, except for reproducible bronchodilation in two asthmatic subjects, but inhalation of both cyclooxygenase products caused cough and retrosternal discomfort.[168]

The same authors went on to examine the effect of doubling doses of both prostanoids using different parameters of airway caliber in mild asthmatic subjects. In doses of up to 500 μg/ml PGI_2, there was no effect on SGaw in any of the subjects, but a concentration-dependent fall in FEV_1 and reduction in the maximum flow rate at 30% of vital capacity ($\dot{V}_{max30}$) were observed. In two of the four subjects, there was a reduction in vital capacity and an increase in residual volume without a change in total lung capacity. Furthermore, PGI_2 but not 6-oxo-$PGF_{1\alpha}$ protected against PGD_2- and methacholine-provoked bronchoconstriction as measured using any parameter of airway caliber.[170] An explanation of these seemingly paradoxical results may be that the principal action of PGI_2 in the airways is to cause vasodilatory mucosal engorgement and hence a reduction in small airway caliber as measured by FEV_1 and $\dot{V}_{max30}$. At the same time, PGI_2 may protect against the spasmogenic effects of other mediators because the increased blood flow caused by PGI_2 may increase the clearance of other agonists from receptor sites.

DEVELOPMENTS IN ANTIPROSTANOID THERAPY

Until recently, the only means to affect either the biosynthesis or the action of specific prostanoids has been with the use of the extensive range of cyclooxygenase inhibitors known as the nonsteroidal anti-inflammatory drugs (NSAIDs). Given the distinct biologic profile of individual prostanoid compounds, this deficiency of the pharmacologic repertoire has hindered investigation into the role of the prostanoids in allergic disease.

More recently, thromboxane synthesis inhibitors and receptor antagonists have been developed to inhibit the action of bronchoconstricting prostanoids while sparing the bronchoprotective compounds such as PGE_2 and PGI_2. The cloning of individual receptor subtypes will allow us to develop further compounds to selectively modulate prostanoid action at specific sites. Furthermore, the elucidation of the differential amino acid sequences of PGHS-1 and PGHS-2 will speed the development of more selective inhibitors of each isoform and provide the opportunity to test new hypotheses.

RESTING AIRWAY CALIBER

In mechanically ventilated guinea pigs, pretreatment with indomethacin demonstrated augmentation of the dose-dependent decrement in dynamic compliance and pulmonary conductance in response to LTC_4.[250] A similar effect has not been found in studies using human bronchial tissue.[40, 84] In addition, there was no effect on the resting airway caliber of asthmatic subjects treated with either cyclooxygenase inhibitors,[82] thromboxane synthetase inhibitors,[142, 146] or thromboxane receptor antagonists.[145]

ALLERGEN CHALLENGE

Predosing with 50 mg of indomethacin for 4 days in asthmatic subjects significantly increased the airway response to allergen when measures of PD_{20} FEV_1 and PD_{35} SGaw were used as measures of airway caliber.[135] In a separate study of seven asthmatic subjects exhibiting dual asthmatic responses, 2 days of pretreatment with 50 mg of indomethacin twice daily had no effect on the allergen-induced early or late asthmatic responses.[222]

By way of contrast to these results, Curzen and coworkers reported the effects of pretreatment with the more potent cyclooxygenase inhibitor, flurbiprofen, on the allergen-induced bronchoconstrictor response. At a dose of 150 mg daily for 3 days, flurbiprofen and terfenadine reduced the mean maximal fall in FEV_1 by 21% and 43%, respectively. However, pretreatment with the combination of the two drugs did not produce an additive effect on allergen-induced bronchoconstriction.[82] The thromboxane receptor antagonist GR 32191 administered at a dose of 80 mg to asthmatic subjects produced a variable degree of inhibition of the EAR to inhaled allergen.[28] In a study of 12 asthmatic subjects, the specific thromboxane synthetase inhibitor CGS 13080 was administered at a dose of 200 mg 4 times daily for 2 days before and 1 day after allergen challenge. Despite significant attenuation of the rise in serum TXB_2 levels after allergen, there was only a small though significant attenuation of the EAR, but no effect on the late response to allergen was found.[270]

BRONCHIAL HYPERRESPONSIVENESS

The involvement of prostanoids in bronchial hyperresponsiveness is supported by considerable scientific data. Indomethacin administered at 50 mg four times daily for 3 days to asthmatic subjects significantly reduced the airway sensitivity to inhaled histamine.[427] This was supported by a further clinical study in which flurbiprofen was administered to asthmatic subjects at a dose of 150 mg daily for 3 days and produced a mean 3.3-fold reduction in airway response to histamine.[82] However, the specific thromboxane synthetase inhibitor CGS 13080 did not alter baseline or postallergen airway responsiveness to histamine.[270] The thromboxane synthetase inhibitor OKY-046 in both oral[146] and inhaled[142] forms reduced the bronchial hyperresponsiveness to acetylcholine in open clinical studies of asthmatic subjects.

Early studies using cyclooxygenase inhibitors failed to demonstrate any effect on the airway hyperresponsiveness to methacholine.[82] Similarly, treatment for 3 weeks with 160 mg daily of the TP receptor antagonist GR32191[411] and in a separate study 1 week of treatment with the thromboxane synthetase inhibitor UK-38,485[156] demonstrated no reduction in the airway sensitivity to inhaled methacholine. In contrast to these findings, the TP receptor antagonist AA-2414 was found to reduce methacholine-induced airway responsiveness in asthmatic subjects[145] but not in patients with chronic bronchitis or bronchiectasis.[144]

EXERCISE-INDUCED ASTHMA

The potent cyclooxygenase inhibitor flurbiprofen, given as a single dose of 150 mg 2 hours before exercise, inhibited the mean maximal fall in FEV_1 by 31%.[130] However, the less potent cyclooxygenase inhibitor indomethacin administered at a dose of 50 mg for 3 days provided no protection against the exercise-induced fall in FEV_1.[309] Similarly, the TP receptor antagonist GR32191 administered to 12 asthmatic subjects as a single dose of 120 mg 1 hour prior to treadmill exercise did not protect against the bronchoconstrictor response compared with placebo.[131] In a separate study, BAY U3405, also a TP receptor antagonist, produced no effect on exercise-induced bronchoconstriction despite demonstrating effective inhibition of PGD_2-induced bronchoconstriction.[263] Part of the mechanism of exercise-induced asthma is therefore likely to involve vascular dilatation, which may involve prostacyclin. This is supported by the limited available data indicating the possible benefit of cyclooxygenase inhibitors and the ineffectiveness of TP receptor blockade.

REFRACTORY PERIOD

Following repeated challenges to a variety of stimuli such as exercise, inhaled hypertonic saline, and distilled water, a refractory period occurs during which there is a reduced bronchoconstrictor response to a subsequent challenge. The release of prostanoids may be involved in this process. Pretreatment with indomethacin in asthmatic subjects abolishes the refractoriness to exercise,[309] hypertonic saline challenge,[172] and distilled water challenge.[280]

LIPOXINS

Lipoxins are trihydroxytetraene lipids that comprise a more recently described addition to the eicosanoid family and possess both vascular and immunomodulatory actions.

BIOSYNTHESIS AND CELLULAR SOURCE

Human leukocytes isolated from the buffy coat were incubated with the calcium ionophore A23187, leading to the generation of novel tetraene compounds with maximum absorption at 301 nm on UV spectroscopy.[371] Using reverse-phase HPLC, it was possible to resolve these compounds into several individual peaks with retention times different from the previously characterized leukotrienes. Using purified neutrophils,[372, 374] the yield of these compounds was considerably reduced, probably reflecting the subsequently defined importance of cell-cell interaction and transcellular formation of key intermediates in the generation of lipoxins. Lipoxins or lipoxygenase interaction products received their name because of the requirement of two or more lipoxygenase enzymes for biosynthesis. It is now recognized that 5-, 12-, and 15-lipoxygenase can all participate in the generation of lipoxins. An important feature of these trihydroxy lipid mediators is the myriad of alternative biosynthetic routes that can potentially lead to their formation. The two major routes in human cells are shown in Figure 12–11.

Arachidonic acid is converted in leukocytes by the action of 15-lipoxygenase to 15(S)-HPETE. Both this product and its peroxidase metabolite 15(S)-HETE can be rapidly transformed by the action of 5-LO to yield a 5(6)-epoxytetraene. This is then hydrolysed by the action of putative epoxide hydrolases to either 5S,6R,15S-trihydroxyeicosatetraenoic acid (LXA_4),[374] 5S,14R,15S-trihydroxyeicosatetraenoic acid (LXB_4),[372] or 7-cis-11-LXA_4.[307]

Eosinophils contain large quantities of 15-LO and generate peptido-lipoxins by the action of glutathione-S-transferase from 15S-HETE.[406] Because the peptide configuration of these compounds is similar to the cysteinyl leukotrienes, they have been termed LXC_4, LXD_4, and LXE_4 in a fashion analogous to LTC_4, LTD_4, and LTE_4. Human nasal polyps and bronchial tissue express 15-LO and can convert the 5-LO product of arachidonic acid, LTA_4, into the intermediate 5(6)-epoxytetraene for further transformation into lipoxins.[117, 256] Human alveolar macrophages transform 15S-HETE to lipoxins, with levels generated by macrophages from asthmatic subjects being twofold greater than those released from normal subjects.[54] Airway tracheal epithelial cells are known to generate 15S-HETE, which may be the source of the substrate utilized by alveolar macrophages.[92]

Transcellular mechanisms of lipoxin production are likely to be the major route of lipoxin biosynthesis in mammalian cells, which takes place in a similar way to the transcellular formation of leukotrienes (see Fig. 12–2). Platelets are an abundant source of 12-lipoxygenase, which is also able to oxygenate both at C-12 of arachidonic acid to give rise to 12S-HPETE and at C-15 to form 15S-HPETE. LTA_4 added to platelets is rapidly converted to lipoxins by the action of platelet 12-lipoxygenase,[375] suggesting that transcellular provision of LTA_4 released from 5-LO bearing cells may be an important source of lipoxin biosynthesis. Further evidence for this comes from experiments in which platelets coincubated with neutrophils and stimulated with calcium ionophore are able to synthesize lipoxins.[115] Similarly, coincubation of pulmonary tissue with PMNs and stimulated with A23187 leads to lipoxin formation.[117, 256] Exogenous LTA_4 added to rat renal mesangial cells[158] and isolated platelets[115] is converted to both LXA_4 and LXB_4.[159]

LIPOXIN RECEPTOR

Perez and colleagues[327] screened a single donor human bone marrow cDNA library containing 4.5×10^5 plaques using the open reading frame from the formyl peptide receptor (FPR) cDNA as a probe. Of 22 clones isolated, the size of 1 clone was 1.8 Kb. Northern blot analysis using mRNA derived from differentiated HL-60 cells[328] demonstrated that the cDNA coding for the receptor related to the FPR hybridized strongly to a 1.8 Kb band, indicating that the cDNA was of full length. This orphan receptor cDNA coded for a 351-aa seven transmembrane domain receptor. With the knowledge that functional LXA_4 receptors are inducible in promyelocytic lineages (HL-60 cell),[134] the group led by Serhan investigated whether this orphan receptor cDNA, which displayed general sequence homology to the FMLP receptor, could encode an LXA_4 receptor. Chinese hamster ovary (CHO) cells transfected with this cDNA displayed specific binding with LXA_4, with a kd of 5.6 nM. There was no similar high-affinity binding with several other related seven transmembrane orphan receptors.

Permeabilization of these transfected cells produced no significant change in kd values but led to a significant increase in the number of receptor sites present per cell with an approximate one log increase in B_{max} values, suggesting that a significant proportion of the orphan cDNA-encoded protein is expressed intracellularly. Only LTD_4 proved effective in displacing tritiated LXA_4 binding with the orphan cDNA-transfected CHO cells, with a K_i of approximately 80 nM. Furthermore, LXA_4 was shown to specifically induce GTPase activity and release esterified ^{3}H-arachidonic acid in the transfected CHO cells, suggesting that this putative receptor is able to transduce LXA_4 signals and strengthen its candidacy for a functional LXA_4 receptor.

BIOLOGIC ACTIVITY

The lipoxins have distinct biologic properties that produce effects at concentrations of 10^{-8} to 10^{-10} M.[29, 407] Several studies have reported vasoactive effects for the lipoxins (Table 12–6). Lipoxin A_4 has shown vasodilatory activity in the hamster cheek pouch that was not mediated by prostanoid action[93] and in the rat renal microcirculation that was partially reversed by aspirin or indomethacin,[18] indicating that lipoxin action was mediated by prostanoid formation. Conversely, LXA_4 and LXB_4 administered intravenously caused

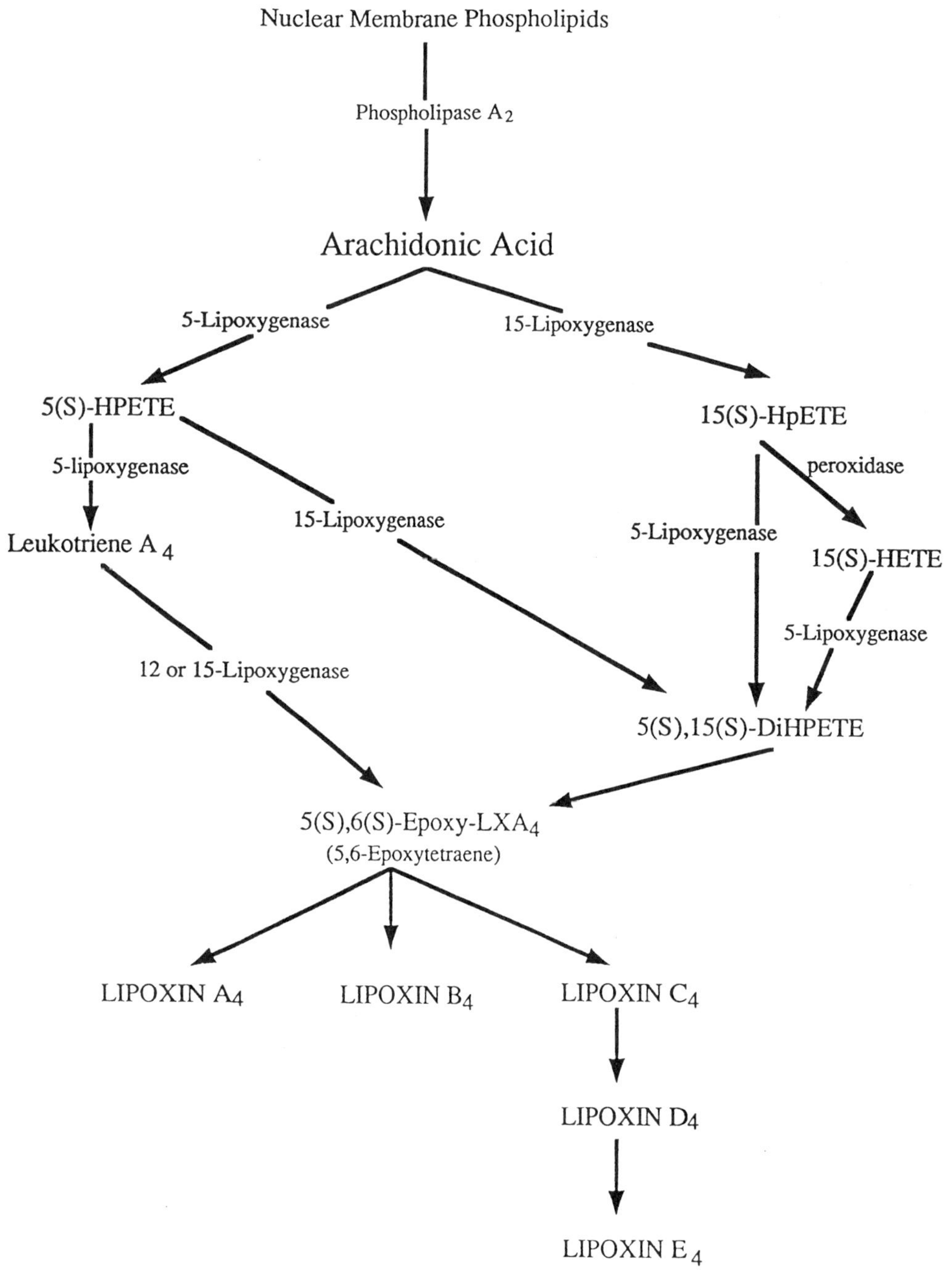

FIGURE 12–11. Lipoxin biosynthesis from membrane phospholipids demonstrating the two major pathways for lipoxin generation. This requires double oxygenation both at carbon-5 by 5-lipoxygenase and carbon-15 by the action of either 12-lipoxygenase or 15-lipoxygenase. LXA_4 = lipoxin A_4; LTC_4 = leukotriene C_4; 5(S)-HPETE = 5(S)-hydroperoxyeicosatetraenoic acid; 5(S)-HETE = 5(S)-hydroxyeicosatetraenoic acid; 15(S)-HETE = 15(S)-hydroxyeicosatetraenoic acid.

mesenteric vasoconstriction in conscious rats.[128] In human tissue, lipoxins provoke endothelium-dependent vasorelaxation of the pulmonary artery.[95]

Lipoxins demonstrate contractile activity in studies using guinea pig parenchymal lung strips.[93, 195] LXA_4 prepared by total chemical synthesis has been shown to constrict parenchymal strips over a concentration range of 1×10^{-8} to 1×10^{-5} M.[195] The contractile activity of LXA_4 was slow in onset, did not plateau for 20 minutes, and was approximately 10,000 times less potent than that of LTD_4. The contraction was not mediated through secondary generation of cyclooxygenase products or the secondary release of cysteinyl leukotrienes. It has been postulated that the activity of LXA_4 may be elicited via an interaction with an LTD_4 receptor. This is supported by a number of studies. LXA_4 (1×10^{-7} M) prevented mesangial cell inositol trisphosphate (IP_3) generation induced by LTD_4.[17] At concentrations between 1×10^{-8} and 1×10^{-5} M, LXA_4 induced the generation of mesangial IP_3, which was abolished by a leukotriene receptor antagonist SK&F 104,353. LXA_4 competed with [^{3}H] LTD_4 for specific binding to cultured rat glomerular mesangial cells. In vivo, it antagonized the LTD_4-induced decrease in glomerular filtration rate.

Dahlén and coworkers have reported that LXA_4 at a concentration of 1×10^{-6} M was able to shift the log dose-response curve of LTC_4 on guinea pig lung strip to the right.[89] Bjorck and colleagues showed that LXA_4 at concentrations between 1 and 30×10^{-6} M produced a dose-dependent contraction of human bronchi and antagonized LTC_4-induced contractions.[33] In a study of eight subjects,

TABLE 12–6
ACTIONS OF LIPOXIN A_4

Tissue	Action
Hamster cheek pouch	Vasodilation[93]
Rat renal microcirculation	Vasodilation (inhibited by aspirin)[18]
Rat mesenteric circulation	Vasoconstriction[128]
Human pulmonary artery	Vasodilation, endothelium dependent[95]
Guinea pig lung	Bronchoconstriction[195]
Mesangial cell	Antagonizes LTD_4-induced IP_3 generation[17]
Guinea pig lung	Inhibits LTC_4-induced contraction[89]
Human bronchi	Inhibits LTC_4-induced contraction[33]
Human lung in vivo	Rightward shift of the dose response curve to inhaled LTC_4[60]
Human bone marrow	Synergy with GM-CSF on myeloid colony formation[407]
Human NK cells	Inhibits cytotoxic activity[344]
Hamster cheek pouch	Inhibits LTB_4-induced neutrophil migration[173]
Human neutrophil-eosinophil	Inhibits chemotactic response to LTB_4, FMLP, and PAF[246, 400]

inhalation of 1×10^{-4} M LXA_4 was found to have no effect on resting SGaw, rate of airflow at 25% vital capacity ($\dot{V}_{25}$), blood pressure, pulse rate, or asthmatic symptoms. However, LXA_4 preinhalation was found to shift the SGaw and $\dot{V}_{25}$ dose-response curve to inhaled LTC_4 significantly to the right.[60] The combined evidence therefore suggests that LXA_4 may modulate LTC_4-induced airway obstruction in vivo and may act both as a partial agonist at the same or similar site as the cysteinyl leukotrienes and as an endogenous receptor antagonist to the cysteinyl leukotrienes.

Lipoxins have a variety of immunomodulatory actions. Both LXA_4 and LXB_4 synergize with GM-CSF to stimulate myeloid colony formation with human bone marrow,[407] and LXB_4 stimulates colony formation of mononuclear cells.[340] Lipoxin A_4 inhibits the cytotoxic activity of human NK cells[344] and displays moderate leukocyte chemoattractant effects.[321] Lipoxin A_4 has demonstrated inhibition of LTB_4-induced neutrophil migration and plasma extravasation in the hamster cheek pouch.[173, 346] Prior exposure of neutrophils or eosinophils to 10^{-9} to 10^{-6} M LXA_4 inhibited the chemotactic responsiveness to LTB_4, formyl-methionyl-leucyl-phenylalanine (FMLP), and PAF in a dose-dependent manner.[246, 400]

DETECTION IN BIOLOGIC FLUIDS

Bronchoalveolar fluid (BALF) was analyzed for LXA_4 using gas chromatography–mass spectrometry with selective ion monitoring and for sulfidopeptide leukotrienes using HPLC and radioimmunoassay in a study of 12 subjects with a variety of pulmonary diseases and 6 normal subjects. Lipoxin A_4 was detected in 9 of 12 subjects with a variety of pulmonary diseases, including infective bronchopneumonia, asthma, carcinoma of the lung, and sarcoidosis, with the higest levels in patients with sarcoidosis, but was not detected in any of the normal subjects. In addition, it was noted that in patients with detectable LXA_4 in BALF, the ratio of LXA_4: sulfidopeptide leukotriene levels ranged from 1.9 to 62 with a mean of 19.[245]

The findings of this study were important for two reasons. First, it established that lipoxins are released into biologic fluids in vivo. Second, the codetection of lipoxins and sulfidopeptide leukotrienes in the airways strengthens the case for an immunomodulatory role for these mediators. Lipoxin A_4 has also been detected in response to aspirin challenge in aspirin-sensitive subjects.[252] Granulocytes from hypereosinophilic syndrome[373] and human bone marrow subjects[407] also generate LXA_4. In patients undergoing percutaneous transluminal coronary angioplasty for atherosclerotic plaques of greater than 70% stenosis, the procedure was found to stimulate release of LXA_4 and sulfidopeptide leukotrienes within 10 seconds of the procedure.[39]

PLATELET-ACTIVATING FACTOR (PAF)

One of the most potent lipid autacoids so far described is platelet-activating factor (PAF), which is a member of a family of ether-linked cholineglycerophosphatides. The term PAF is misleading as this lipid mediator has a broad range of biologic activities and acts on a variety of cells. In 1972, Benveniste, Henson, and Cochrane[31] reported the potent aggregation of platelets when leukocytes obtained from IgE-sensitized rabbits were exposed to the specific antigen. They postulated that upon stimulation, IgE-sensitized basophils degranulated and then released a soluble factor that was responsible for platelet aggregation and therefore conceived the term platelet-activating factor for this factor.

Muirhead and colleagues also isolated a substance with similar properties as PAF from renal medulla, which had a hypotensive effect in the Goldblatt rat model of hypertension. They therefore called it antihypertensive polar renal lipid (APRL). In 1979, Demopoulos, Pinckard, and Hanahan[99] described a semisynthetic phosphoacylglycerol, 1-*O*-alkyl-2-acetyl-*sn*-glycero-3-phosphocholine (AGEPC), which was able to aggregate platelets and release serotonin and had the same physicochemical properties as PAF. In 1980, Hanahan and colleagues purified and characterized PAF from activated basophils and concluded that AGEPC and PAF comprised the same compound.[166]

BIOSYNTHESIS

Although the structure of PAF (Fig. 12–12) is described as a single molecule, it should perhaps be more appropriately considered to form a family of structurally related autacoid phospholipids synthesized by inflammatory cells that have platelet-stimulating and neutrophil-priming activity and whose main members include 1-*O*-hexadecyl-2-acetyl-*sn*-glycero-3-phosphorylcholine and 1-*O*-octadecyl-2-acetyl-*sn*-glycero-3-phosphorylcholine. At present, there is no generally accepted nomenclature to classify the extensive molecular heterogeneity of PAF.

Cell stimulation leads to the release of alkylacylglycerophosphocholine from cell membranes that can be converted

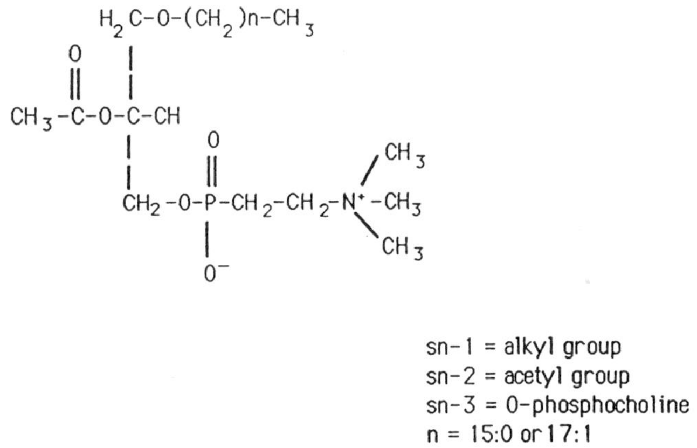

FIGURE 12–12. Chemical structure of PAF.

to PAF by one of two metabolic pathways (Fig. 12–13). The remodeling pathway involves a structural modification of a preexisting ether-linked phospholipid that forms part of the structure of cellular membranes. The initial step involves catalysis by phospholipase A_2 on the membrane phospholipid 1-alkyl-2-acyl-glycerophosphocholine.[165, 412] This deacylation step leads to the generation of lyso-PAF and the release of arachidonic acid, which has phospholipase A_2 inhibitory activity, thereby reducing further PAF synthesis. The released arachidonic acid may also act as the substrate in subsequent eicosanoid biosynthesis reactions. Lyso-PAF can then be acetylated by a specific lyso-PAF acetyltransferase to form 1-*O*-alkyl-2-acetyl-*sn*-glycero-3-phosphocholine (PAF) or subsequently remetabolized back to its precursor lyso-PAF by the action of a specific PAF-acetylhydrolase.

The de novo pathway comprises the other route for PAF biosynthesis and involves a highly specific sequence of reactions commencing with an intermediate in the synthesis of ether-linked membrane phospholipids. This is acetylated by a specific acetyltransferase, and the phosphate is removed by a phosphohydrolase from the sn-3 carbon to form alkylacetylglycerol, which is subsequently converted by cholinephosphotransferase to PAF. Degradation and inactivation of PAF are largely catalyzed by PAF acetylhydrolase in plasma to yield lyso-PAF and by the action of an arachidonyl-specific transferase in target cells to form alkylacylglycerophosphocholine. It is therefore likely that both the synthesis and inactivation of PAF are closely coupled with arachidonate metabolism.

CELLULAR RELEASE

Specific agonist-receptor interactions on the surface of a variety of cell types can lead to PAF generation. Many phagocytic stimuli such as bacteria and parasites opsonized by IgG or complement, immune complexes, complement chemotactic factors C5a and C3a, and eosinophil chemotactic factors can stimulate inflammatory cells to initiate PAF synthesis. Antigen- or IgE-stimulated mast cells and basophils generate PAF,[370] supporting a role for PAF in the pathogenesis of acute anaphylaxis. PAF is synthesized by peripheral blood monocytes in response to 4β-phorbol 12 myristate 13 acetate (PMA), opsonized zymosan, or the calcium ionophore A23187, an effect regulated by protein kinase C.[119] Macrophages activated by opsonized zymosan and by immune complex in hypersensitivity reactions are capable of PAF synthesis. Neutrophils stimulated with opsonized zymosan, A23187, and FMLP generate PAF.[382] Both unopsonized zymosan and A23187 induce a dose- and time-dependent increase in PAF synthesis by eosinophils.[44] Endothelial cells also produce PAF in response to specific stimuli such as vasopressin, angiotensin II, thrombin, bradykinin, and histamine.[47, 286, 341] Lymphocytes are unable to synthesize PAF. However, natural killer cells may produce PAF in response to IgG binding to Fc receptors.[265] Cytokines such as interleukin-1 and tumor necrosis factor stimulate macrophages, neutrophils, and endothelial cells to generate PAF.[45, 48]

PAF RECEPTOR

The first lipid mediator receptor to be cloned was the PAF receptor. A guinea pig lung cDNA library was screened using a phage clone shown to induce PAF-dependent responses in *Xenopus laevis* oocytes.[183] The identity of the receptor was confirmed based on its pharmacologic properties when expressed in COS-7 cells or oocytes and using known PAF receptor agonists and antagonists. A 3,020 nucleotide sequence was reported, and the 342 amino acid sequence was deduced from the longest open reading frame of the cloned cDNA. The existence of seven hydrophobic transmembrane domains was predicted based on a hydropathy profile plot. This suggested that, like previously described receptors such as adrenergic and acetylcholine muscarinic receptors, the PAF receptor belongs to the G protein–coupled receptor superfamily.

The human PAF receptor cDNA was first isolated from a human leucocyte cDNA library probed with a 0.8 Kb fragment of the guinea pig PAF receptor cDNA. Both the guinea pig and human PAF receptors were predicted to possess seven transmembrane domains, and both contained 342 amino acid residues with an 83% homology in amino acid sequence.[301] Activation of the receptor yielded inositol 1,4,5-trisphosphate (IP_3) in the transfected oocytes and COS-7 cells. Guanosine 5′-O-(2-thio)biphosphate injection into these cells inhibited PAF-induced Cl^- current, providing evidence that PAF stimulates phosphoinositide turnover via G proteins. When expressed in Chinese hamster ovary (CHO) cells, the PAF receptor couples with a number of second messenger systems, leading to phospholipase C activation, inhibition of adenylate cyclase, and activation of the MAP kinase cascade and arachidonate release. A subsequent study identified the PAF receptor cytoplasmic tail as not being required for forward signal transduction. The several phosphorylation sites on the cytoplasmic tail were postulated to play a critical role in the rapid agonist-induced desensitization so characteristic of PAF activity.[417]

BIOLOGIC ACTIVITY

Soon after the identification of this proinflammatory phospholipid mediator, PAF was demonstrated to possess a unique profile of biologic effects beyond the originally described platelet aggregation (Table 12–7). Furthermore, it

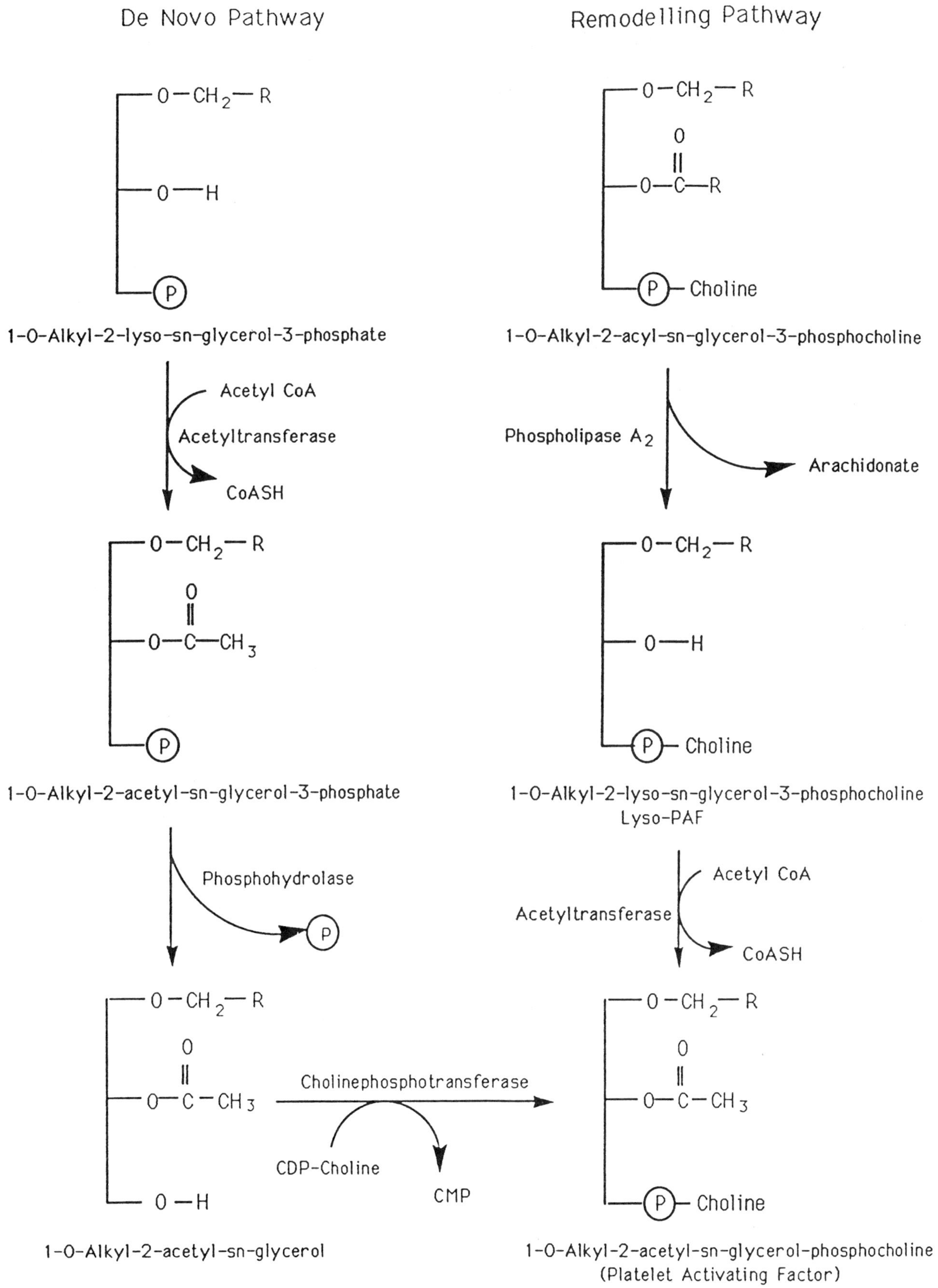

FIGURE 12–13. Biosynthetic pathways of PAF denoting the de novo and remodeling routes.

TABLE 12–7
PAF-ELICITED CELLULAR RESPONSES

	Platelets	Neutrophils	Eosinophils	Macrophages	Lymphocytes	Hepatocytes	Endothelial Cells
Degranulation	+	+					
Aggregation	+	+	+				
Chemotaxis/ chemokinesis		+	+				
Superoxide generation		+		+			
Ca^{2+} uptake	+	+					+
Arachidonic acid turnover	+	+					+
Protein kinase C activation	+	+		+			
IL-2 down-regulation					+		
TNF synthesis				+			
Glycogenolysis						+	

was found to be the most potent lipid mediator known, with biologic responses detectable at concentrations as low as 10^{-14} M and an ED_{50} value for guinea pig platelet activation of about 3×10^{-10} M. The actions of PAF include the recruitment and activation of inflammatory cells, particularly eosinophils and neutrophils.[23] PAF has potent in vivo bronchoconstrictor activity, but in vitro effects on smooth muscle preparations are negligible, suggesting that airway narrowing may be the result of secondary release of spasmogens or induction of airway edema secondary to microvascular leakage.[65, 83, 100] Inhalation of PAF induces bronchoconstriction within 2 to 3 minutes, which is followed by the rapid development of tachyphylaxis.[83]

Initial studies involving pretreatment with PAF in the guinea pig[281] and the dog[65] demonstrated increased airway responsiveness to reference agonists such as histamine and methacholine. Later studies observed that inhaled PAF induced a long-lasting increase in airway responsiveness in normal subjects, and other investigators subsequently reported similar findings.[67, 213] However, the majority of clinical studies on normal subjects have found that the increase in bronchial responsiveness was either absent or only transient.[199, 404] In asthmatic subjects, however, inhalation of PAF does not increase airway responsiveness[66] or lead to late asthmatic responses.[235]

PAF has a 1,000-fold greater potency than histamine to produce receptor-mediated increases in airway microvascular leakage.[123] The precise role of PAF in asthma has not yet been defined, but PAF has been detected in bronchoalveolar lavage fluid from asthmatic airways.[409] Inhalation of PAF aerosol leads to a twofold increase in neutrophil recovery from bronchoalveolar lavage fluid but no change in eosinophil numbers in normal volunteers.[430] Intracutaneous injection of PAF induces a dual skin response in human subjects similar to that observed after allergen[24] and an eosinophil-rich infiltrate into the skin of allergic subjects but not of normal subjects.[176] This raises the possibility of a selective recruitment of eosinophils in allergic subjects. Furthermore, eosinophils from atopic subjects release more PAF than do those from normal subjects, thus providing a possible positive feedback loop for continuing inflammation.[243]

The activation of inflammatory cells also leads to the release of other inflammatory mediators, such as the products of both the cyclooxygenase[65] and the lipoxygenase,[424] pathways and the release of oxygen free radicals.[357] This may alter the effects of PAF, which can act either synergistically with or through the secondary action of other released mediators, and may modulate the activity of PAF by stimulation of degradation. A number of studies have identified the link between PAF and leukotriene synthesis. PAF inhalation stimulates increased biosynthesis of the bronchoconstrictor eicosanoid TXA_2 and the cysteinyl leukotrienes.[422] LTD_4 receptor antagonists reduce the bronchoconstrictor response to inhaled PAF in normal volunteers,[217, 403] whereas GR 32191B, a thromboxane receptor antagonist, demonstrates little effect.[410] This suggests that the cysteinyl leukotrienes may be important in mediating the bronchoconstrictor effects to PAF.

RECEPTOR ANTAGONISTS

PAF is an inflammatory mediator that mimics many of the characteristic features of asthma, but its role in this disease remains unproven. PAF and its metabolite lyso-PAF have been demonstrated in BAL fluid from stable atopic asthmatic subjects[409] and in plasma from asthmatic subjects during both early[52] and late responses to inhaled allergen.[302] Using potent and specific PAF receptor antagonists, it should be possible to further elucidate the role of PAF in the pathophysiology of asthma. A number of PAF receptor antagonists have now been evaluated.

The ginkgolide mixture BN 52063 inhibits PAF-induced wheal and flare and platelet aggregatory responses ex vivo.[68] In a subsequent study, this compound demonstrated inhibitory activity against the late phase cutaneous response to allergen in atopic subjects but with only a 50% reduction of the early wheal response. This effect may have resulted from the inhibition of cutaneous eosinophil infiltration.[351] However, in a study of eight normal subjects,[350] inhaled PAF induced an immediate bronchoconstrictor response with a maximum fall in flow at 30% of vital capacity from a partial flow-volume maneuver ($\dot{V}p_{30}$) of 47% after placebo, with the maximum bronchoconstrictor response significantly attenuated to 35% 2 hours after ingestion of BN 52063. The characteristic neutropenia that occurs within a few minutes of PAF inhalation and the rebound neutrophilia were not affected by the PAF receptor antagonist.

WEB 2086 is a hetrazepine compound that inhibits the allergen-induced late response in allergic sheep.[1] In normal human subjects, WEB 2086 prevents PAF-induced bronchoconstriction.[3] In isolated human airway preparations, it prevents both the contractile response and the histamine hyperresponsiveness induced by PAF.[202] In a study of eight mild atopic asthmatic subjects, 1 week of treatment with 300 mg daily of WEB 2086 did not attenuate the allergen-induced early or late responses or the subsequent histamine bronchial hyperresponsiveness.[140] In a larger study involving 65 asthmatic subjects, 6 weeks of treatment with 120 mg daily of WEB 2086 did not significantly reduce the requirement for inhaled corticosteroids compared with placebo treatment.[402]

The dihydropyridine compound UK,74505 is a specific and potent PAF receptor antagonist that demonstrates 10-fold greater inhibition of PAF-induced aggregation of washed rabbit platelets than does WEB 2086.[7] In 12 normal subjects, inhalation of PAF induced bronchoconstriction for 60 minutes, neutropenia at 5 minutes, and rebound neutrophilia at 2 hours and stimulated the production of urinary eicosanoids. Premedication with the PAF antagonist UK,74505 completely abolished the bronchoconstrictor response, neutropenia, and rebound neutrophilia and significantly reduced urinary levels of LTE_4 and 2,3-dinor-TXB_2.[310] However, in a separate study of eight atopic asthmatic subjects, there was no inhibition of the early and late response to allergen and no difference in histamine airway responsiveness following the late response.[229] In conclusion, therefore, PAF receptor antagonists have so far demonstrated no clinically useful activity in asthma despite proving their potency by effectively inhibiting the response to inhaled PAF.

REFERENCES

1. Abraham WM, Stevenson JS, Garrido R: A possible role for PAF in allergen-induced late responses: modification by a selective antagonist. J Appl Physiol 66:2351–2357, 1989.
2. Abramovitz M, Boie Y, Nguyen T, et al: Cloning and expression of a cDNA for the human prostanoid FP receptor. J Biol Chem 269:2632–2636, 1994.
3. Adamus WS, Heuer HO, Meade CJ, et al: Inhibitory effects of the new PAF acether antagonist WEB-2086 on pharmacologic changes induced by PAF inhalation in human beings. Clin Pharmacol Ther 47:456–462, 1990.
4. Adelroth E, Morris MM, Hargreave FE, et al: Airway responsiveness to leukotrienes C_4 and D_4 and to methacholine in patients with asthma and normal controls. N Engl J Med 315:480–484, 1986.
5. Aharony D, Catanese CA, Falcone RC: Kinetic and pharmacologic analysis of [^{3}H]leukotriene E_4 binding to receptors on guinea pig lung membranes: evidence for selective binding to a subset of leukotriene D_4 receptors. J Pharmacol Exp Ther 248:581–588, 1989.
6. Aharony D, Dobson PT, Krell RD: In vitro metabolism of [^{3}H]-peptide leukotrienes in human and ferret lung: a comparison with the guinea pig. Biochem Biophys Res Commun 131:892–898, 1985.
7. Alabaster VA, Keir RF, Parry MJ, et al: UK-74,505, a novel and selective PAF antagonist, exhibits potent and long lasting activity in vivo. Agents Actions Suppl 34:221–227, 1991.
8. Anderson GP, Fennessy MR: Lipoxygenase metabolites as mediators of platelet activating factor-induced increased airways responsiveness to histamine in the guinea-pig. Agents Actions Suppl 23:195–200, 1988.
9. Anderson S, Seale JP, Ferris L, et al: An evaluation of pharmacotherapy for exercise-induced asthma. J Allergy Clin Immunol 64:612–624, 1979.
10. Arm JP, O'Hickey SP, Spur BW, Lee TH: Airway responsiveness to histamine and leukotriene E_4 in subjects with aspirin induced asthma. Am Rev Respir Dis 140:148–153, 1989.
11. Arm JP, O'Hickey SP, Hawksworth RJ, et al: Asthmatic airways have a disproportionate hyperresponsiveness to LTE_4, as compared with normal airways, but not to LTC_4, LTD_4, methacholine, and histamine. Am Rev Respir Dis 142:1112–1118, 1990.
12. Arm JP, O'Hickey SP, Spur BW, et al: Airway responsiveness to histamine and leukotriene E_4 in subjects with aspirin-induced asthma. Am Rev Respir Dis 140:148–153, 1989.
13. Arm JP, Spur BW, Lee TH: The effects of inhaled leukotriene E_4 on the airway responsiveness to histamine in subjects with asthma and normal subjects. J Allergy Clin Immunol 82:654–660, 1988.
14. Atluru D, Goodwin JS: Leukotriene B_4 causes proliferation of interleukin 2-dependent T cells in the presence of suboptimal levels of interleukin 2. Cell Immunol 99:444–452, 1986.
15. Augstein J, Farmer JB, Lee TB, et al: Selective inhibitor of slow reacting substance of anaphylaxis. Nature New Biol 245:215–217, 1973.
16. Badr KF, Baylis C, Pfeffer JM, et al: Renal and systemic hemodynamic responses to intravenous infusion of leukotriene C_4 in the rat. Circ Res 54:492–499, 1984.
17. Badr KF, DeBoer DK, Schwartzberg M, et al: Lipoxin A_4 antagonizes cellular and in vivo actions of leukotriene D_4 in rat glomerular mesangial cells: evidence for competition at a common receptor. Proc Natl Acad Sci USA 86:3438–3442, 1989.
18. Badr KF, Serhan CN, Nicolaou KC, et al: The action of lipoxin-A on glomerular microcirculatory dynamics in the rat. Biochem Biophys Res Commun 145:408–414, 1987.
19. Barnes N, Piper PJ, Costello J: The effect of an oral leukotriene antagonist L-649,923 on histamine and leukotriene D_4-induced bronchoconstriction in normal man. J Allergy Clin Immunol 79:816–821, 1987.
20. Barnes NC, Piper PJ, Costello JF: Comparative effects of inhaled leukotriene C_4, leukotriene D_4, and histamine in normal human subjects. Thorax 39:500–504, 1984.
21. Barnes NC, Piper PJ, Costello JF: Actions of inhaled leukotrienes and their interactions with other allergic mediators. Prostaglandins 28:629–630, 1984.
22. Barnes NC, Watson A, Piper PJ, et al: Action of inhaled leukotriene C and D on large and small airways. Effect of pre-inhalation of leukotriene D on histamine dose-response curve. Am Rev Respir Dis 129:A1, 1984.
23. Barnes PJ, Chung KF, Page CP: Platelet-activating factor as a mediator of allergic disease. J Allergy Clin Immunol 81:919–934, 1988.
24. Basran GS, Page CP, Paul W, et al: Platelet-activating factor: a possible mediator of the dual response to allergen? Clin Allergy 14:75–79, 1984.
25. Bastien L, Sawyer N, Grygorczyk R, et al: Cloning, functional expression, and characterization of the human prostaglandin E_2 receptor EP_2 subtype. J Biol Chem 269:11873–11877, 1994.
26. Beasley CR, Robinson C, Featherstone RL, et al: 9 alpha,11 beta-prostaglandin F_2, a novel metabolite of prostaglandin D_2 is a potent contractile agonist of human and guinea pig airways. J Clin Invest 79:978–983, 1987.
27. Beasley CR, Varley J, Robinson C, et al: Cholinergic-mediated bronchoconstriction induced by prostaglandin D_2 and its initial metabolite 9α, 11β-PGF_2 and $PGF_{2\alpha}$ in asthma. Am Rev Respir Dis 136:1140–1144, 1987.
28. Beasley RC, Featherstone RL, Church MK, et al: Effect of a thromboxane receptor antagonist on PGD_2- and allergen-induced bronchoconstriction. J Appl Physiol 66:1685–1693, 1989.
29. Beckman BS, Despinasse BP, Spriggs L: Actions of lipoxins A_4 and B_4 on signal transduction events in Friend erythroleukemia cells. Proc Soc Exp Biol Med 201:169–173, 1992.
30. Bel EH, van der Veen H, Kramps JA, et al: Maximal airway narrowing to inhaled leukotriene D_4 in normal subjects. Comparison and interaction with methacholine. Am Rev Respir Dis 136:979–984, 1987.

31. Benveniste J, Henson PM, Cochrane CG: Leukocyte-dependent histamine release from rabbit platelets. The role of IgE, basophils, and a platelet-activating factor. J Exp Med 136:1356–1377, 1972.
32. Bianco S, Robuschi M, Vaghi A, et al: Effects of leukotriene C_4 on the bronchial response to an ultrasonic mist of water. In Herzog H, Perruchoud AP (eds): Progress in Respiratory Research. Volume 19: Asthma and Bronchial Hyperreactivity. Karger, Basel, 1985, p 82.
33. Björck T, Nicolaou KC, Dahlén S-E: Lipoxin A_4 interacts with leukotriene C_4 in human bronchi. Am Rev Respir Dis 139:A78, 1989.
34. Boie Y, Rushmore TH, Darmon-Goodwin A, et al: Cloning and expression of a cDNA for the human prostanoid IP receptor. J Biol Chem 269:12173–12178, 1994.
35. Borgeat P, Hamberg M, Samuelsson B: Transformation of arachidonic acid and homo-gamma-linolenic acid by rabbit polymorphonuclear leukocytes. Monohydroxy acids from novel lipoxygenases. J Biol Chem 251:7816–7820, 1976.
36. Brain S, Camp R, Dowd P, et al: The release of leukotriene B_4-like material in biologically active amounts from the lesional skin of patients with psoriasis. J Invest Dermatol 83:70–73, 1984.
37. Brain SD, Camp RD, Black AK, et al: Leukotrienes C_4 and D_4 in psoriatic skin lesions. Prostaglandins 29:611–619, 1985.
38. Bray MA, Cunningham FM, Ford-Hutchinson AW, et al: Leukotriene B_4: a mediator of vascular permeability. Br J Pharmacol 72:483–486, 1981.
39. Brezinski DA, Nesto RW, Serhan CN: Angioplasty triggers intracoronary leukotrienes and lipoxin A_4. Impact of aspirin therapy. Circulation 86:56–63, 1992.
40. Brink C, Grimaud C, Guillot C, et al: The interaction between indomethacin and contractile agents on human isolated airway muscle. Br J Pharmacol 69:383–388, 1980.
41. Britton JR, Hanley SP, Tattersfield AE: The effect of an oral leukotriene D_4 antagonist L-649,923 on the response to inhaled antigen in asthma. J Allergy Clin Immunol 79:811–816, 1987.
42. Brocklehurst WE: Slow reacting substance and related compounds. Prog Allergy 6:539–558, 1962.
43. Broide DH, Eisman S, Ramsdell JW, et al: Airway levels of mast cell-derived mediators in exercise-induced asthma. Am Rev Respir Dis 141:563–568, 1990.
44. Burke LA, Crea AE, Wilkinson JR, et al: Comparison of the generation of platelet-activating factor and leukotriene C_4 in human eosinophils stimulated by unopsonized zymosan and by the calcium ionophore A23187: the effects of nedocromil sodium. J Allergy Clin Immunol 85:26–35, 1990.
45. Bussolino F, Camussi G, Baglioni C: Synthesis and release of platelet-activating factor by human vascular endothelial cells treated with tumor necrosis factor or interleukin 1 alpha. J Biol Chem 263:11856–11861, 1988.
46. Camp RDR, Coutts AA, Greaves MW, et al: Response of human skin to intradermal injection of leukotrienes C_4, D_4 and B_4. Br J Pharmacol 80:497–502, 1983.
47. Camussi G, Aglietta M, Malavasi F, et al: The release of platelet-activating factor from human endothelial cells in culture. J Immunol 131:2397–2403, 1983.
48. Camussi G, Bussolino F, Salvidio G, et al: Tumor necrosis factor/cachectin stimulates peritoneal macrophages, polymorphonuclear neutrophils, and vascular endothelial cells to synthesize and release platelet-activating factor. J Exp Med 166:1390–1404, 1987.
49. Carry M, Korley V, Willerson JT, et al: Increased urinary leukotriene excretion in patients with cardiac ischemia. In vivo evidence for 5-lipoxygenase activation. Circulation 85:230–236, 1992.
50. Cartier A, Thomson NC, Frith PA, et al: Allergen-induced increase in bronchial responsiveness to histamine: relationship to the late asthmatic response and change in airway caliber. J Allergy Clin Immunol 70:170–177, 1982.
51. Chagnon M, Gentile J, Gladu M, et al: The mechanism of action of leukotrienes A_4, C_4 and D_4 on human lung parenchyma in vitro. Lung 163:55–62, 1985.
52. Chan-Yeung M, Lam S, Chan H, et al: The release of platelet-activating factor into plasma during allergen-induced bronchoconstriction. J Allergy Clin Immunol 87:667–673, 1991.
53. Chapman KR, Friedman BS, Shingo S, et al: The efficacy of an oral inhibitor of leukotriene synthesis (MK-0591) in asthmatics treated with inhaled steroids. Am J Respir Crit Care Med 149:A215, 1994.
54. Chavis C, Godard P, Crastes de Paulet A, et al: Formation of lipoxins and leukotrienes by human alveolar macrophages incubated with 15(S)-HETE: a model for cellular cooperation between macrophages and airway epithelial cells. Eicosanoids 5:203–211, 1992.
55. Chen MC, Amirian DA, Toomey M, et al: Prostanoid inhibition of canine parietal cells: mediation by the inhibitory guanosine triphosphate-binding protein of adenylate cyclase. Gastroenterology 94:1121–1129, 1988.
56. Cheng JB, Townley RG: Evidence for a similar receptor site for binding of [^{3}H] leukotriene E_4 and [3H] leukotriene D_4 to the guinea-pig crude lung membrane. Biochem Biophys Res Commun 122:949–954, 1984.
57. Christie PE, Hawksworth R, Spur BW, et al: Effect of indomethacin on leukotriene E_4-induced histamine hyperresponsiveness in asthmatic subjects. Am Rev Respir Dis 146:1506–1510, 1992.
58. Christie PE, Schmitz-Schumann M, Spur BW, et al: Airway responsiveness to leukotriene C_4 (LTC_4), leukotriene E_4 (LTE_4) and histamine in aspirin-sensitive asthmatic subjects. Eur Respir J 6:1468–1473, 1993.
59. Christie PE, Smith CM, Lee TH: The potent and selective sulfidopeptide leukotriene antagonist, SK&F 104353, inhibits aspirin-induced asthma. Am Rev Respir Dis 144:957–958, 1991.
60. Christie PE, Spur BW, Lee TH: The effects of lipoxin A_4 on airway responses in asthmatic subjects. Am Rev Respir Dis 145:1281–1284, 1992.
61. Ibid.
62. Christie PE, Tagari P, Ford-Hutchinson AW, et al: Urinary leukotriene E_4 after lysine-aspirin inhalation in asthmatic subjects. Am Rev Respir Dis 146:1531–1534, 1992.
63. Christie PE, Tagari P, Ford-Hutchinson AW, et al: Increased urinary LTE_4 excretion following inhalation of LTC_4 and LTE_4 in asthmatic subjects. Eur Respir J 7:907–913, 1994.
64. Christie PE, Tagari P, Ford-Hutchinson AW, et al: Urinary leukotriene E_4 concentrations increase after aspirin challenge in aspirin-sensitive asthmatic subjects. Am Rev Respir Dis 143:1025–1029, 1991.
65. Chung KF, Aizawa H, Leikauf GD, et al: Airway hyperresponsiveness induced by platelet-activating factor: role of thromboxane generation. J Pharmacol Exp Ther 236:580–584, 1986.
66. Chung KF, Barnes PJ: Effects of platelet activating factor on airway caliber, airway responsiveness, and circulating cells in asthmatic subjects. Thorax 44:108–115, 1989.
67. Chung KF, Cuss FM, Barnes PJ: Platelet activating factor: effects on bronchomotor tone and bronchial responsiveness in human beings. Allergy Proc 10:333–337, 1989.
68. Chung KF, Dent G, McCusker M, et al: Effect of a ginkgolide mixture (BN 52063) in antagonising skin and platelet responses to platelet activating factor in man. Lancet 1:248–251, 1987.
69. Churchill L, Chilton FH, Resau JH, et al: Cyclooxygenase metabolism of endogenous arachidonic acid by cultured human tracheal epithelial cells. Am Rev Respir Dis 140:449–459, 1989.
70. Cloud ML, Enas GG, Kemp J, et al: A specific LTD_4/LTE_4-receptor antagonist improves pulmonary function in patients with mild, chronic asthma. Am Rev Respir Dis 140:1336–1339, 1989.
71. Cockcroft DW, Ruffin RE, Dolovich J, et al: Allergen-induced increase in non-allergic bronchial reactivity. Clin Allergy 7:503–513, 1977.
72. Coleman RA, Humphrey PPA, Kennedy I, et al: Prostanoid receptors—the development of a working classification. Trends Pharmacol Sci 5:303–306, 1984.
73. Coleman RA, Kennedy I, Sheldrick RLG: New evidence with selective agonists and antagonists for the subclassification of PGE_2-sensitive (EP) receptors. In Samuelsson B, Paoletti R, Ramwell PW (eds): Advances in Prostaglandin, Thromboxane and Leukotriene Research. Vol 17, Prostanoids and Related Compounds. Raven Press, New York, 1987, p 467.
74. Coleman RA, Sheldrick RLG: Prostanoid-induced contraction of human bronchial smooth muscle is mediated by TP-receptors. Br J Pharmacol 96:688–692, 1989.
75. Coles SJ, Neill KH, Reid LM, et al: Effects of leukotrienes C_4 and D on glycoprotein and lysozyme secretion by human bronchial mucosa. Prostaglandins 25:155–170, 1983.
76. Collawn C, Rubin P, Perez N, et al: Phase II study of the safety and efficacy of a 5-lipoxygenase inhibitor in patients with ulcerative colitis. Am J Gastroenterol 87:342–346, 1992.
77. Conroy DM, Piper PJ, Samhoun MN, et al: Metabolism and generation of cysteinyl containing leukotrienes by human airways in vitro. Br J Pharmacol 96:72P, 1989.
78. Crea AE, Nakhosteen JA, Lee TH: Mediator concentrations in bronchoalveolar lavage fluid of patients with mild asymptomatic bronchial asthma. Eur Respir J 5:190–195, 1992.

79. Creese BR, Bach MK: Hyperreactivity of airways smooth muscle produced in vitro by leukotrienes. Prostaglandin Leukotriene Med 11:161–169, 1983.
80. Creticos PS, Peters SP, Adkinson NF Jr, et al: Peptide leukotriene release after antigen challenge in patients sensitive to ragweed. New Engl J Med 310:1626–1630, 1984.
81. Cromwell O, Walport MJ, Taylor GW, et al: Identification of leukotrienes in the sputum of patients with cystic fibrosis. Adv Prostaglandin Thromboxane Leukot Res 9:251–257, 1982.
82. Curzen N, Rafferty P, Holgate ST: Effects of a cyclo-oxygenase inhibitor, flurbiprofen, and an H_1 histamine receptor antagonist, terfenadine, alone and in combination on allergen induced immediate bronchoconstriction in man. Thorax 42:946–952, 1987.
83. Cuss FM, Dixon CM, Barnes PJ: Effects of inhaled platelet activating factor on pulmonary function and bronchial responsiveness in man. Lancet 2:189–192, 1986.
84. Cuthbert NJ, Gardiner PJ: Endogenous generation of cyclooxygenase products by human isolated lung tissue. Br J Pharmacol 80:496P, 1983.
85. Dahinden CA, Clancy RM, Gross M, et al: Leukotriene C_4 production by murine mast cells: evidence for a role for extracellular leukotriene A_4. Proc Natl Acad Sci USA 82:6632–6636, 1985.
86. Dahlén B, Margolskee DJ, Zetterstrom O, et al: Effect of the leukotriene receptor antagonist MK-0679 on baseline pulmonary function in aspirin sensitive asthmatic subjects. Thorax 48:1205–1210, 1993.
87. Dahlén B, Zetterstrom O, Bjorck T, et al: The leukotriene-antagonist ICI-204,219 inhibits the early airway reaction to cumulative bronchial challenge with allergen in atopic asthmatics. Eur Respir J 7:324–331, 1994.
88. Dahlén S-E: Pulmonary effects of leukotrienes. Acta Physiol Scand Suppl 512:1–51, 1983.
89. Dahlén S-E, Franzen L, Raud J, et al: Actions of lipoxin A_4 and related compounds in smooth muscle preparations and on the microcirculation in vivo. Adv Exp Med Biol 229:107–130, 1988.
90. Dahlén S-E, Hansson G, Hedqvist P, et al: Allergen challenge of lung tissue from asthmatics elicits bronchial contraction that correlates with the release of leukotrienes C_4, D_4, and E_4. Proc Natl Acad Sci USA 80:1712–1716, 1983.
91. Dahlén S-E, Hedqvist P, Hammarström S, et al: Leukotrienes are potent constrictors of human bronchi. Nature 288:484–486, 1980.
92. Dahlén S-E, Kumlin M, Bjorck T, et al: Lipoxins and other lipoxygenase products with relevance to inflammatory reactions in the lung. Ann NY Acad Sci 629:262–273, 1991.
93. Dahlén S-E, Raud J, Serhan CN, et al: Biological activities of lipoxin A include lung strip contraction and dilation of arterioles in vivo. Acta Physiol Scand 130:643–647, 1987.
94. Ibid (1980).
95. Dahlén S-E, Serhan CN: Lipoxins. In Wong A, Crooke ST (eds): Lipoxygenases and Their Products. Academic Press, San Diego, 1991, p 235.
96. Davidson AB, Lee TH, Scanlon PD, et al: Bronchoconstrictor effects of leukotriene E_4 in normal and asthmatic subjects. Am Rev Respir Dis 135:333–337, 1987.
97. Davidson EM, Rae SA, Smith MJ: Leukotriene B_4, a mediator of inflammation present in synovial fluid in rheumatoid arthritis. Ann Rheum Dis 42:677–679, 1983.
98. Degreef H, Dockx P, De Doncker P, et al: A double-blind vehicle-controlled study of R 68 151 in psoriasis: a topical 5-lipoxygenase inhibitor. J Am Acad Dermatol 22:751–755, 1990.
99. Demopoulos CA, Pinckard RN, Hanahan DJ: Platelet-activating factor. Evidence for 1-O-alkyl-2-acetyl-sn-glyceryl-3-phosphorylcholine as the active component (a new class of lipid chemical mediators). J Biol Chem 254:9355–9358, 1979.
100. Denjean A, Arnoux B, Masse R, et al: Acute effects of intratracheal administration of platelet-activating factor in baboons. J Appl Physiol Respir Environ Exercise Physiol 55:799–804, 1983.
101. Denzlinger C, Grimberg M, Kapp A, et al: Effect of the leukotriene receptor antagonists FPL 55712, LY 163443, and MK-571 on the elimination of cysteinyl leukotrienes in the rat. Br J Pharmacol 102:865–870, 1991.
102. DeWitt DL: Prostaglandin endoperoxide synthase: regulation of enzyme expression. Biochim Biophys Acta 1083:121–134, 1991.
103. DeWitt DL, Day JS, Sonnenburg WK, et al: Concentrations of prostaglandin endoperoxide synthase and prostaglandin I_2 synthase in the endothelium and smooth muscle of bovine aorta. J Clin Invest 72:1882–1888, 1983.
104. Diamant Z, Timmers MC, van der Veen H, et al: The effect of MK-0591, a potent oral leukotriene biosynthesis inhibitor, on allergen-induced airway responses in asthmatic subjects. Am Rev Respir Dis 147:A446, 1993.
105. Dixon RA, Diehl RE, Opas E, et al: Requirement of a 5-lipoxygenase-activating protein for leukotriene synthesis. Nature 343:282–284, 1990.
106. Dixon RA, Jones RE, Diehl RE, et al: Cloning of the cDNA for human 5-lipoxygenase. Proc Natl Acad Sci USA 85:416–420, 1988.
107. Dixon RAF, Diehl RE, Opas E, et al: Requirement of a 5-lipoxygenase-activating protein for leukotriene synthesis. Nature 343:282–284, 1990.
108. Dong YJ, Jones RL, Wilson NH: Prostaglandin E receptor subtypes in smooth muscle: agonist activities of stable prostacyclin analogues. Br J Pharmacol 87:97–107, 1986.
109. Drazen JM: Comparative contractile responses to sulfidopeptide leukotrienes in normal and asthmatic human subjects. Ann NY Acad Sci USA 524:289–297, 1988.
110. Drazen JM, Austen KF: Leukotrienes and airway responses. Am Rev Respir Dis 136:985–998, 1987.
111. Drazen JM, Austen KF, Lewis RA, et al: Comparative airway and vascular activities of leukotrienes C-1 and D in vivo and in vitro. Proc Natl Acad Sci USA 77:4354–4358, 1980.
112. *Ibid.*
113. Drazen JM, Lewis RA, Austen KF, et al: Pulmonary pharmacology of the SRS-A leukotrienes. In Berti F, Folco G, Velo GP (eds): Leukotrienes and Prostacyclin. Plenum Press, New York, 1983, p 125.
114. Drazen JM, O'Brien J, Sparrow D, et al: Recovery of leukotriene E_4 from the urine of patients with airway obstruction. Am Rev Respir Dis 146:104–108, 1992.
115. Edenius C, Haeggstrom J, Lindgren JA: Transcellular conversion of endogenous arachidonic acid to lipoxins in mixed human platelet-granulocyte suspensions. Biochem Biophys Res Commun 157:801–807, 1988.
116. Edenius C, Heidvall K, Lindgren JA: Novel transcellular interaction: conversion of granulocyte-derived leukotriene A_4 to cysteinyl-containing leukotrienes by human platelets. Eur J Biochem 178:81–86, 1988.
117. Edenius C, Kumlin M, Bjork T, et al: Lipoxin formation in human nasal polyps and bronchial tissue. FEBS Lett 272:25–28, 1990.
118. Ellis JL, Undem BJ: Role of cysteinyl-leukotrienes and histamine in mediating intrinsic tone in isolated human bronchi. Am J Respir Crit Care Med 149:118–122, 1994.
119. Elstad MR, McIntyre TM, Prescott SM, et al: Protein kinase C regulates the synthesis of platelet-activating factor by human monocytes. Am J Respir Cell Mol Biol 4:148–155, 1991.
120. Evans JF, Dupuis P, Ford-Hutchinson AW: Purification and characterisation of leukotriene A_4 hydrolase from rat neutrophils. Biochim Biophys Acta 840:43–50, 1985.
121. Evans JF, Leville C, Mancini JA, et al: 5-lipoxygenase-activating protein is the target of a quinolone class of leukotriene biosynthesis inhibitors. Mol Pharmacol 40:22–27, 1991.
122. Evans JF, Nathaniel DJ, Zamboni RJ, et al: Leukotriene A3. A poor substrate but a potent inhibitor of rat and human neutrophil leukotriene A_4 hydrolase. J Biol Chem 260:10966–10970, 1985.
123. Evans TW, Chung KF, Rogers DF, et al: Effect of platelet-activating factor on airway vascular permeability: possible mechanisms. J Appl Physiol 63:479–484, 1987.
124. Feinmark SJ, Cannon PJ: Endothelial cell leukotriene C_4 synthesis results from intercellular transfer of leukotriene A_4 synthesized by polymorphonuclear leukocytes. J Biol Chem 261:16466–16472, 1986.
125. Feinmark SJ, Cannon PJ: Endothelial cell leukotriene C_4 synthesis results from intercellular transfer of leukotriene A_4 synthesized by polymorphonuclear leukocytes. J Biol Chem 261:16466–16472, 1986.
126. Fels AO, Pawlowski NA, Cramer EB, et al: Human alveolar macrophages produce leukotriene B_4. Proc Natl Acad Sci USA 79:7866–7870, 1982.
127. Ferreri NR, Howland WC, Stevenson DD, et al: Release of leukotrienes, prostaglandins, and histamine into nasal secretions of aspirin-sensitive asthmatics during reaction to aspirin. Am Rev Respir Dis 137:847–854, 1988.
128. Feuerstein G, Siren AL: Mesenteric vascular responses to i.v. administration of lipoxin A_4 and lipoxin B_4 in the conscious rat. FEBS Lett 232:51–55, 1988.

129. Findlay SR, Barden JM, Easley CB, et al: Effect of the oral leukotriene antagonist, ICI 204,219, on antigen-induced bronchoconstriction in subjects with asthma. J Allergy Clin Immunol 89:1040–1045, 1992.
130. Finnerty JP, Holgate ST: Evidence for the roles of histamine and prostaglandins as mediators in exercise-induced asthma: the inhibitory effect of terfenadine and flurbiprofen alone and in combination. Eur Respir J 3:540–547, 1990.
131. Finnerty JP, Twentyman OP, Harris A, et al: Effect of GR32191, a potent thromboxane receptor antagonist, on exercise induced bronchoconstriction in asthma. Thorax 46:190–192, 1991.
132. Finnerty JP, Wood-Baker R, Thomson H, et al: Role of leukotrienes in exercise-induced asthma. Inhibitory effect of ICI 204219, a potent leukotriene D_4 receptor antagonist. Am Rev Respir Dis 145:746–749, 1992.
133. Fiore S, Maddox JF, Perez HD, et al: Identification of a human cDNA encoding a functional high affinity lipoxin A_4 receptor. J Exp Med 180:253–260, 1994.
134. Fiore S, Romano M, Reardon EM, et al: Induction of functional lipoxin A_4 receptors in HL-60 cells. Blood 81:3395–3403, 1993.
135. Fish JE, Ankin MG, Adkinson F Jr, et al: Indomethacin modification of immediate-type immunologic airway responses in allergic asthmatic and non-asthmatic subjects. Am Rev Respir Dis 123:609–614, 1981.
136. Fitzgerald GA, Maas RL, Lawson JA, et al: Aspirin inhibits endogenous prostacyclin and thromboxane biosynthesis in man. Adv Prostaglandin Thromboxane Leukot Res 11:265–266, 1983.
137. Fleisch JH, Rinkema LE, Baker SR: Evidence for multiple leukotriene D_4 receptors in smooth muscle. Life Sci 31:577–581, 1982.
138. Fleisch JH, Rinkema LE, Haisch KD, et al: LY171883, 1-<2-hydroxy-3-propyl-4<4-(tetrazol-5-yl) butoxy>phenyl>ethanone, an orally active leukotriene D_4 antagonist. J Pharm Exp Ther 233:148–157, 1985.
139. Ford-Hutchinson AW, Bray MA, Doig MV, et al: Leukotriene B, a potent chemokinetic and aggregating substance released from polymorphonuclear leukocytes. Nature 286:264–265, 1980.
140. Freitag A, Watson RM, Matsos G, et al: Effect of a platelet activating factor antagonist, WEB 2086, on allergen induced asthmatic responses. Thorax 48:594–598, 1993.
141. Friedman BS, Bel EH, Buntinx A, et al: Oral leukotriene inhibitor (MK-886) blocks allergen-induced airway responses. Am Rev Respir Dis 147:839–844, 1993.
142. Fujimura M, Nishioka S, Kumabashiri I, et al: Effects of aerosol administration of a thromboxane synthetase inhibitor (OKY-046) on bronchial responsiveness to acetylcholine in asthmatic subjects. Chest 98:276–279, 1990.
143. Fujimura M, Sakamoto S, Kamio Y, et al: Effect of a leukotriene antagonist, ONO-1078, on bronchial hyperresponsiveness in patients with asthma. Respir Med 87:133–138, 1993.
144. Fujimura M, Sakamoto S, Matsuda T: Attenuating effect of a thromboxane synthetase inhibitor (OKY-046) on bronchial responsiveness to methacholine is specific to bronchial asthma. Chest 98:656–660, 1990.
145. Fujimura M, Sakamoto S, Saito M, et al: Effect of a thromboxane A_2 receptor antagonist (AA-2414) on bronchial hyperresponsiveness to methacholine in subjects with asthma. J Allergy Clin Immunol 87:23–27, 1991.
146. Fujimura M, Sasaki F, Nakatsumi Y, et al: Effects of a thromboxane synthetase inhibitor (OKY-046) and a lipoxygenase inhibitor (AA-861) on bronchial responsiveness to acetylcholine in asthmatic subjects. Thorax 41:955–959, 1986.
147. Fuller RW, Black PN, Dollery CT: Effect of the oral leukotriene D_4 antagonist LY171883 on inhaled and intradermal challenge with antigen and leukotriene D_4 in atopic subjects. J Allergy Clin Immunol 83:939–944, 1989.
148. Fuller RW, Dixon CM, Dollery CT, et al: Prostaglandin D_2 potentiates airway responsiveness to histamine and methacholine. Am Rev Respir Dis 133:252–254, 1986.
149. Funk CD, Funk LB, Kennedy ME, et al: Human platelet/erythroleukemia cell prostaglandin G/H synthase: cDNA cloning, expression, and gene chromosomal assignment. FASEB J 5:2304–2312, 1991.
150. Funk CD, Furci L, Fitzgerald GA, et al: Cloning and expression of a cDNA for the human prostaglandin E receptor EP_1 subtype. J Biol Chem 268:26767–26772, 1993.
151. Funk CD, Hoshiko S, Matsumoto T, et al: Characterization of the human 5-lipoxygenase gene. Proc Natl Acad Sci USA 86:2587–2591, 1989.
152. Funk CD, Radmark O, Fu JY, et al: Molecular cloning and amino acid sequence of leukotriene A_4 hydrolase. Proc Natl Acad Sci USA 84:6677–6681, 1987.
153. Gaddy J, McCreedy W, Margolskee D, et al: A potent leukotriene D_4 antagonist (MK-571) significantly reduces airway obstruction in mild to moderate asthma. J Allergy Clin Immunol 87:306, 1991. Abstract.
154. Gaddy JN, Margolskee DJ, Bush RK, et al: Bronchodilation with a potent and selective leukotriene D_4 (LTD_4) receptor antagonist (MK-571) in patients with asthma. Am Rev Respir Dis 146:358–363, 1992.
155. Gardiner PJ, Collier HOJ: Specific receptors for prostaglandins in airways. Prostaglandins 19:819–841, 1980.
156. Gardiner PV, Young CL, Holmes K, et al: Lack of short-term effect of the thromboxane synthetase inhibitor UK-38,485 on airway reactivity to methacholine in asthmatic subjects. Eur Respir J 6:1027–1030, 1993.
157. Garland LG, Salmon JA: Hydroxamic acids and hydroxureas as inhibitors of arachidonate 5-lipoxygenase. Drugs Future 16:547–558, 1991.
158. Garrick R, Shen SY, Ogunc S, et al: Transformation of leukotriene A_4 to lipoxins by rat kidney mesangial cell. Biochem Biophys Res Commun 162:626–633, 1989.
159. Garrick R, Wong PY: Enzymatic formation and regulatory function of lipoxins and leukotriene B_4 in rat kidney mesangial cells. Adv Exp Med Biol 314:361–369, 1991.
160. Gillard J, Ford-Hutchinson AW, Chan C, et al: L-663,536 (MK-886) (3-[1-(4-chlorobenzyl)-3-t-butyl-thio-5-isopropylindol-2-yl]-2,2-dimethylpropanoic acid), a novel, orally active leukotriene biosynthesis inhibitor. Can J Physiol Pharmacol 67:456–464, 1989.
161. Goldblatt MW: A depressor substance in seminal fluid. J Soc Chem Ind 52:1056–1061, 1933.
162. Goldman DW, Goetzl EJ: Specific binding of leukotriene B_4 to receptors on human polymorphonuclear leukocytes. J Immunol 129:1600–1604, 1982.
163. Goldman DW, Goetzl EJ: Selective transduction of human polymorphonuclear leukocyte functions by subsets of receptors for leukotriene B_4. J Allergy Clin Immunol 74:373–377, 1984.
164. Griffin M, Weiss JW, Leitch AG, et al: Effects of leukotriene D on the airways in asthma. N Engl J Med 308:436–439, 1983.
165. Hanahan DJ: Platelet activating factor: a biologically active phosphoglyceride. Ann Rev Biochem 55:483–509, 1986.
166. Hanahan DJ, Demopoulos CA, Liehr J, et al: Identification of platelet activating factor isolated from rabbit basophils as acetyl glyceryl ether phosphorylcholine. J Biol Chem 255:5514–5516, 1980.
167. Hanna CJ, Bach MK, Pare PD, et al: Slow-reacting substances (leukotrienes) contract human airway and pulmonary vascular smooth muscle in vitro. Nature 290:343–344, 1981.
168. Hardy C, Robinson C, Lewis RA, et al: Airway and cardiovascular responses to inhaled prostacyclin in normal and asthmatic subjects. Am Rev Respir Dis 131:18–21, 1985.
169. Hardy CC, Bradding P, Robinson C, et al: The combined effects of two pairs of mediators, adenosine with methacholine and prostaglandin D_2 with histamine, on airway caliber in asthma. Clin Science 71:385–392, 1986.
170. Hardy CC, Bradding P, Robinson C, et al: Bronchoconstrictor and antibronchoconstrictor properties of inhaled prostacyclin in asthma. J Appl Physiol 64:1567–1574, 1988.
171. Hardy CC, Robinson C, Tattersfield AE, et al: The bronchoconstrictor effect of inhaled prostaglandin D_2 in normal and asthmatic men. New Eng J Med 311:209–213, 1984.
172. Hawksworth RJ, O'Hickey SP, Lee TH: The effects of indomethacin on the refractory period to hypertonic saline-induced bronchoconstriction. Eur Respir J 5:963–966, 1992.
173. Hedqvist P, Raud J, Palmertz U, et al: Lipoxin A_4 inhibits leukotriene B_4-induced inflammation in the hamster cheek pouch. Acta Physiol Scand 137:571–572, 1989.
174. Henderson WR, Jorg A, Klebanoff SJ: Eosinophil peroxidase-mediated inactivation of leukotrienes B_4, C_4, and D_4. J Immunol 128:2609–2613, 1982.
175. Henderson WR, Klebanoff SJ: Leukotriene production and inactivation by normal, chronic granulomatous disease and myeloperoxidase-deficient neutrophils. J Biol Chem 258:13522–13527, 1983.
176. Henocq E, Vargaftig BB: Skin eosinophilia in atopic patients. J Allergy Clin Immunol 81:691–695, 1988.
177. Hirata M, Hayashi Y, Ushikubi F, et al: Cloning and expression of cDNA for a human thromboxane A2 receptor. Nature 349:617–620, 1991.
178. Hla T, Neilson K: Human cyclooxygenase-2 cDNA. Proc Natl Acad Sci USA 89:7384–7388, 1992.

179. Holgate ST, Burns GB, Robinson C, et al: Anaphylactic- and calcium-dependent generation of prostaglandin D_2 (PGD_2), thromboxane B_2 and other cyclooxygenase products of arachidonic acid by dispersed human lung mast cells and relationship to histamine release. J Immunol 133:2138–2144, 1984.
180. Ibid.
181. Holroyde MC, Altounyan REC, Cole M, et al: Bronchoconstriction produced in man by leukotrienes C and D. Lancet 2:17–18, 1981.
182. Honda A, Sugimoto Y, Namba T, et al: Cloning and expression of a cDNA for mouse prostaglandin E subtype. J Biol Chem 268:7759–7762, 1993.
183. Honda Z, Nakamura M, Miki I, et al: Cloning by functional expression of platelet-activating factor receptor from guinea-pig lung. Nature 349:342–346, 1991.
184. Hoover RL, Karnovsky MJ, Austen KF, et al: Leukotriene B_4 action of endothelium mediates augmented neutrophil/endothelial adhesion. Proc Natl Acad Sci USA 81:2191–2193, 1984.
185. Hua XY, Dahlén SE, Lundberg JM, et al: Leukotrienes C_4, D_4 and E_4 cause widespread and extensive plasma extravasation in the guinea pig. Naunyn Schmiedebergs Arch Pharmacol 330:136–141, 1985.
186. Hui KP, Barnes NC: Lung function improvement in asthma with a cysteinyl-leukotriene receptor antagonist. Lancet 337:1062–1063, 1991.
187. Hui KP, Taylor IK, Taylor GW, et al: Effect of a 5-lipoxygenase inhibitor on leukotriene generation and airway responses after allergen challenge in asthmatic patients. Thorax 46:184–189, 1991.
188. Impens N, Reiss TF, Teahan JA, et al: Acute bronchodilation with an intravenously administered leukotriene D_4 antagonist, MK-679. Am Rev Respir Dis 147:1442–1446, 1993.
189. Irie A, Sugimoto Y, Namba T, et al: Third isoform of the prostaglandin-E-receptor EP_3 subtype with C-terminal tail coupling to both stimulation and inhibition of cyclase. Eur J Biochem 217:313–318, 1993.
190. Israel E, Dermarkarian R, Rosenberg M, et al: The effects of a 5-lipoxygenase inhibitor on asthma induced by cold, dry air. New Engl J Med 323:1740–1744, 1990.
191. Israel E, Fischer AR, Rosenberg MA, et al: The pivotal role of 5-lipoxygenase products in the reaction of aspirin-sensitive asthmatics to aspirin. Am Rev Respir Dis 148:1447–1451, 1993.
192. Israel E, Juniper EF, Callaghan JT, et al: Effect of a leukotriene antagonist, LY171883, on cold air-induced bronchoconstriction in asthmatics. Am Rev Respir Dis 140:1348–1353, 1989.
193. Israel E, Rubin P, Kemp JP, et al: The effect of inhibition of 5-lipoxygenase by zileuton in mild-to-moderate asthma. Ann Intern Med 119:1059–1066, 1993.
194. Issekutz AC: Vascular responses during acute neutrophilic inflammation. Their relationship to in vivo neutrophil emigration. Lab Invest 45:435–441, 1981.
195. Jacques CA, Spur BW, Crea AE, et al: The contractile activities of lipoxin A_4 and lipoxin B_4 for guinea-pig airway tissues. Br J Pharmacol 95:562–568, 1988.
196. Jacques CA, Spur BW, Johnson M, et al: Mechanism of LTE_4-induced histamine hyperresponsiveness in guinea-pig tracheal and human bronchial smooth muscle, in vitro. Br J Pharmacol 104:859–866, 1991.
197. Jakobsson PJ, Odlander B, Steinhilber D, et al: Human B lymphocytes possess 5-lipoxygenase activity and convert arachidonic acid to leukotriene B_4. Biochem Biophys Res Commun 178:302–308, 1991.
198. Jakobsson PJ, Steinhilber D, Odlander B, et al: On the expression and regulation of 5-lipoxygenase in human lymphocytes. Proc Natl Acad Sci USA 89:3521–3525, 1992.
199. Jenkins JR, Lai CKW, Holgate ST: Effect of increasing doses of platelet-activating factor (PAF) on normal human airways. J Allergy Clin Immunol 83:282, 1989.
200. Johnson HG, McNee ML: Secretogogue responses of leukotriene C_4, D_4: comparison of potency in canine trachea in vivo. Prostaglandins 25:237–243, 1983.
201. Johnson HG, McNee ML, Johnson MA, et al: Leukotriene C_4 and dimethylphenyl-piperazinium-induced responses in canine airway tracheal muscle contraction and fluid secretion. Int Arch Allergy Appl Immunol 71:214–218, 1983.
202. Johnson PR, Armour CL, Black JL: The action of platelet activating factor and its antagonism by WEB 2086 on human isolated airways. Eur Respir J 3:55–60, 1990.
203. Jones GH, Venuti MC, Young JM, et al: Topical nonsteroidal antipsoriatic agents. 1. 1,2,3,4-Tetraoxygenated naphthalene derivatives. J Med Chem 29:1504–1511, 1986.
204. Jones GL, Saroea HG, Watson RM, et al: Effect of an inhaled thromboxane mimetic (U46619) on airway function in human subjects. Am Rev Respir Dis 145:1270–1274, 1992.
205. Jones RL, Peesapati V, Wilson NH: Antagonism of the thromboxane-sensitive contractile systems of the rabbit aorta, dog saphenous vein and guinea-pig trachea. Br J Pharmacol 76:423–438, 1982.
206. Jones TR, Charette L, Denis D: Antigen-induced contraction of guinea-pig isolated trachea: studies with novel inhibitors and antagonists of arachidonic acid metabolites. [Published erratum appears in Br J Pharmacol 96(1), 1989.] Br J Pharmacol 95:309–321, 1988.
207. Jones TR, Davis C, Daniel EE: Pharmacological study of the contractile activity of leukotriene C_4 and D_4 on isolated human airway smooth muscle. Can J Physiol Pharmacol 60:638–643, 1982.
208. Jones TR, Guindon Y, Young R, et al: L-648,051,sodium 4-[3-(4-acetyl-3-hydroxy-2-propylphenoxy)-propylsulfonyl]-gamma-oxo-benzenebutanoate: a leukotriene D_4 receptor antagonist. Can J Physiol Pharmacol 64:1535–1542, 1986.
209. Joos GF, Kips JC, Pauwels RA, et al: The effect of aerosolized SK&F 104353-Z2 on the bronchoconstrictor effect of leukotriene D_4 in asthmatics. Pulm Pharmacol 4:37–42, 1991.
210. Joris I, Majno G, Corey EJ, et al: The mechanism of vascular leakage induced by leukotriene E_4. Endothelial contraction. Am J Pathol 126:19–24, 1987.
211. Kargman S, Rousseau P, Reid GK, et al: Leukotriene synthesis in U937 cells expressing recombinant 5-lipoxygenase. J Lipid Mediat 7:31–45, 1993.
212. Kargman S, Vickers PJ, Evans JF: A23187-induced translocation of 5-lipoxygenase in osteosarcoma cells. J Cell Biol 119:1701–1709, 1992.
213. Kaye MG, Smith LJ: Effects of inhaled leukotriene D_4 and platelet-activating factor on airway reactivity in normal subjects. Am Rev Respir Dis 141:993–997, 1990.
214. Kellawey CH, Trethewie WR: The liberation of a slow reacting smooth muscle stimulating substance of anaphylaxis. Q J Exp Physiol 30:124–145, 1940.
215. Kennedy BP, Diehl RE, Boie Y, et al: Gene characterization and promoter analysis of the human 5-lipoxygenase-activating protein (FLAP). J Biol Chem 266:8511–8516, 1991.
216. Kern R, Smith LJ, Patterson R, et al: Characterization of the airway response to inhaled leukotriene D_4 in normal subjects. Am Rev Respir Dis 133:1127–1132, 1986.
217. Kidney JC, Ridge SM, Chung KF, et al: Inhibition of platelet-activating factor-induced bronchoconstriction by the leukotriene D_4 receptor antagonist ICI 204,219. Am Rev Respir Dis 147:215–217, 1993.
218. Kikawa Y, Hosoi S, Inoue Y, et al: Exercise-induced urinary excretion of leukotriene E_4 in children with atopic asthma. Pediatr Res 29:455–459, 1991.
219. Kim KC, Nassiri J, Brody JS: Mechanisms of airway goblet cell mucin release: studies with cultured tracheal surface epithelial cells. Am J Respir Cell Mol Biol 1:137–143, 1989.
220. Kips JC, Joos GF, De Lepeleire I, et al: MK-571, a potent antagonist of leukotriene D_4-induced bronchoconstriction in the human. Am Rev Respir Dis 144:617–621, 1991.
221. Kirby JG, Hargreave FE, Cockcroft DW, et al: Effect of indomethacin on allergen-induced asthmatic responses. J Appl Physiol 66:578–583, 1989.
222. Ibid.
223. Knapp HR: Reduced allergen-induced nasal congestion and leukotriene synthesis with an orally active 5-lipoxygenase inhibitor. New Engl J Med 323:1745–1748, 1990.
224. Knapp HR, Sladek K, Fitzgerald GA: Increased excretion of leukotriene E_4 during aspirin-induced asthma. J Lab Clin Med 119:48–51, 1992.
225. Kragballe K, Desjarlais L, Voorhees JJ: Leukotrienes B_4, C_4 and D_4 stimulate DNA synthesis in cultured human epidermal keratinocytes. Br J Dermatol 113:43–52, 1985.
226. Krall JF, Barrett JD, Jamgotchian N, et al: Interaction of prostaglandin E_2 and beta-adrenergic catecholamines in the regulation of uterine smooth muscle motility and adenylate cyclase in the rat. J Endocrinol 102:329–336, 1984.
227. Krell RD, Aharony D, Buckner CK, et al: The preclinical pharmacology of ICI 204,219. A peptide leukotriene antagonist. Am Rev Respir Dis 141:978–987, 1990.
228. Krell RD, Tsai BS, Berdoulay A, et al: Heterogeneity of leukotriene receptors in guinea-pig trachea. Prostaglandins 25:171–178, 1983.

229. Kuitert LM, Hui KP, Uthayarkumar S, et al: Effect of the platelet-activating factor antagonist UK-74,505 on the early and late response to allergen. Am Rev Respir Dis 147:82–86, 1993.
230. Kujubu DA, Fletcher BS, Varnum BC, et al: TIS10, a phorbol ester tumor promoter-inducible mRNA from Swiss 3T3 cells, encodes a novel prostaglandin synthase/cyclooxygenase homologue. J Biol Chem 266:12866–12872, 1991.
231. Kujubu DA, Reddy ST, Fletcher BS, et al: Expression of the protein product of the prostaglandin synthase-2/TIS10 gene in mitogen-stimulated Swiss 3T3 cells. J Biol Chem 268:5425–5430, 1993.
232. Kumlin M, Dahlén B, Bjorck T, et al: Urinary excretion of leukotriene E_4 and 11-dehydro-thromboxane B_2 in response to bronchial provocations with allergen, aspirin, leukotriene D_4, and histamine in asthmatics. Am Rev Respir Dis 146:96–103, 1992.
233. Kumlin M, Johansson H, Larsson C, et al: The leukotriene antagonist MK-0679 improves baseline pulmonary function and blocks aspirin-induced airways obstruction in aspirin-sensitive asthmatics. Am Rev Respir Dis 145:A15, 1992.
234. Kurzrok R, Lieb CC: Biochemical studies of human semen: II. The action of semen on the human uterus. Proc Soc Exp Biol Med 28:268–272, 1930.
235. Lai CK, Jenkins JR, Polosa R, et al: Inhaled PAF fails to induce airway hyperresponsiveness to methacholine in normal human subjects. J Appl Physiol 68:919–926, 1990.
236. Laitinen LA, Laitinen A, Haahtela T, et al: Leukotriene E_4 and granulocytic infiltration into asthmatic airways. Lancet 341:989–990, 1993.
237. Lam BK, Penrose JF, Freeman GJ, et al: Expression cloning of a cDNA for human leukotriene C_4 synthase, an integral membrane protein conjugating reduced glutathione to leukotriene A_4. Proc Natl Acad Sci USA 91:7663–7667, 1994.
238. Lam S, Chan H, LeRiche JC, et al: Release of leukotrienes in patients with bronchial asthma. J Allergy Clin Immunol 81:711–717, 1988.
239. Ibid.
240. Lauritsen K, Laursen LS, Bukhave K, et al: Effects of topical 5-aminosalicylic acid and prednisolone on prostaglandin E_2 and leukotriene B_4 levels determined by equilibrium in vivo dialysis of rectum in relapsing ulcerative colitis. Gastroenterology 91:837–844, 1986.
241. Lauritsen K, Laursen LS, Bukhave K, et al: In vivo effects of orally administered prednisolone on prostaglandin and leukotriene production in ulcerative colitis. Gut 28:1095–1099, 1987.
242. Lee SH, Soyoola E, Chanmugam P, et al: Selective expression of mitogen-inducible cyclooxygenase in macrophages stimulated with lipopolysaccharide. J Biol Chem 267:25934–25938, 1992.
243. Lee TC, Lenihan DJ, Malone B, et al: Increased biosynthesis of platelet activating factor in activated human eosinophils. J Biol Chem 259:5526–5530, 1984.
244. Lee TH, Austen KF, Corey EJ, et al: Leukotriene E_4-induced airway hyperresponsiveness of guinea pig tracheal smooth muscle to histamine and evidence for three separate sulfidopeptide leukotriene receptors. Proc Natl Acad Sci USA 81:4922–4925, 1984.
245. Lee TH, Crea AE, Gant V, et al: Identification of lipoxin A_4 and its relationship to the sulfidopeptide leukotrienes C_4, D_4, and E_4 in the bronchoalveolar lavage fluids obtained from patients with selected pulmonary diseases. Am Rev Respir Dis 141:1453–1458, 1990.
246. Lee TH, Horton CE, Kyan-Aung U, et al: Lipoxin A_4 and lipoxin B_4 inhibit chemotactic responses of human neutrophils stimulated by leukotriene B_4 and N-formyl-L-methionyl-L-leucyl-L-phenylalanine. Clin Sci 77:195–203, 1989.
247. Lee TH, Sethi T, Crea AE, et al: Characterization of leukotriene B_3: comparison of its biological activities with leukotriene B_4 and leukotriene B_5 in complement receptor enhancement, lysozyme release and chemotaxis of human neutrophils. Clin Sci 74:467–475, 1988.
248. Lee TH, Walport MJ, Wilkinson AH, et al: Slow reacting substance of anaphylaxis antagonist FPL 55712 in chronic asthma. Lancet 2:304–305, 1981.
249. Leikauf GD, Ueki IF, Widdicombe JH, et al: Alteration of chloride secretion across canine tracheal epithelium by lipoxygenase products of arachidonic acid. Am J Physiol 250:F47-F53, 1986.
250. Leitch AG, Corey EJ, Austen KF, et al: Indomethacin potentiates the pulmonary response to aerosol leukotriene C_4 in the guinea pig. Am Rev Respir Dis 128:639–643, 1983.
251. Levinson SL: Peptidoleukotriene binding in guinea pig uterine membrane preparations. Prostaglandins 28:229–240, 1984.
252. Levy BD, Bertram S, Tai HH, et al: Agonist-induced lipoxin A_4 generation: detection by a novel lipoxin A_4-ELISA. Lipids 28:1047–1053, 1993.
253. Lewis RA, Austen KF, Drazen JM, et al: Slow reacting substance of anaphylaxis: identification of leukotriene C-1 and D from human and rat sources. Proc Natl Acad Sci USA 77:3710–3714, 1980.
254. Lewis RA, Drazen JM, Austen KF, et al: Identification of the C(6)-S-conjugate of leukotriene A with cysteine as a naturally occuring slow reacting substance of anaphylaxis (SRS-A). Importance of the 11-cis-geometry for biological activity. Biochem Biophys Res Commun 96:271–277, 1980.
255. Lewis RA, Soter NA, Diamond PT, et al: Prostaglandin D_2 generation after activation of rat and human mast cells with anti-IgE. J Immunol 129:1627–1631, 1982.
256. Lindgren JA, Edenius C, Kumlin M, et al: Conversion of leukotriene A_4 to lipoxins by human nasal polyps and bronchial tissue. Adv Prostaglandin Thromboxane Leukot Res 21A:89–92, 1991.
257. Liu MC, Bleecker ER, Lichtenstein LM, et al: Evidence for elevated levels of histamine, prostaglandin D_2, and other bronchoconstricting prostaglandins in the airways of subjects with mild asthma. Am Rev Respir Dis 142:126–132, 1990.
258. Lundgren JD, Kaliner M, Logun C, et al: Platelet activating factor and tracheobronchial respiratory glycoconjugate release in feline and human explants: involvement of the lipoxygenase pathway. Agents Actions 30:329–337, 1990.
259. Lupinetti MD, Sheller JR, Catella F, et al: Thromboxane biosynthesis in allergen-induced bronchospasm. Evidence for platelet activation. Am Rev Respir Dis 140:932–935, 1989.
260. Macdermot J, Kelsey CR, Waddell KA, et al: Synthesis of leukotriene B_4, and prostanoids by human alveolar macrophages: analysis by gas chromatography/mass spectrometry. Prostaglandins 27:163–179, 1984.
261. Maclouf JA, Murphy RC: Transcellular metabolism of neutrophil-derived leukotriene A_4 by human platelets. A potential cellular source of leukotriene C_4. J Biol Chem 263:174–181, 1988.
262. Ibid.
263. Magnussen H, Boerger S, Templin K, et al: Effects of a thromboxane-receptor antagonist, BAY u 3405, on prostaglandin D_2- and exercise-induced bronchoconstriction. J Allergy Clin Immunol 89:1119–1126, 1992.
264. Makker HK, Lau LC, Thomson HW, et al: The protective effect of inhaled leukotriene D_4 receptor antagonist ICI 204,219 against exercise-induced asthma. Am Rev Respir Dis 147:1413–1418, 1993.
265. Malavasi F, Tetta C, Funaro A, et al: Fc receptor triggering induces expression of surface activation antigens and release of platelet-activating factor in large granular lymphocytes. Proc Natl Acad Sci USA 83:2443–2447, 1986.
266. Maltby NH, Taylor GW, Ritter JM, et al: Leukotriene C_4 elimination and metabolism in man. J Allergy Clin Immunol 85:3–9, 1990.
267. Mancini JA, Abramovitz M, Cox ME, et al: 5-lipoxygenase-activating protein is an arachidonate binding protein. FEBS Lett 318:277–281, 1993.
268. Mann JS, Robinson C, Sheridan AQ, et al: Effect of inhaled piriprost (U-60, 257) a novel leukotriene inhibitor, on allergen and exercise induced bronchoconstriction in asthma. Thorax 41:746–752, 1986.
269. Manning PJ, Rokach J, Malo JL, et al: Urinary leukotriene E_4 levels during early and late asthmatic responses. J Allergy Clin Immunol 86:211–220, 1990.
270. Manning PJ, Stevens WH, Cockcroft DW, et al: The role of thromboxane in allergen-induced asthmatic responses. Eur Respir J 4:667–672, 1991.
271. Manning PJ, Watson RM, Margolskee DJ, et al: Inhibition of exercise-induced bronchoconstriction by MK-571, a potent leukotriene D_4-receptor antagonist. N Engl J Med 323:1736–1739, 1990.
272. Marom Z, Shelhamer JH, Bach MK, et al: Slow-reacting substances, leukotrienes C_4 and D_4, increase the release of mucus from human airways in vitro. Am Rev Respir Dis 126:449–451, 1982.
273. Ibid.
274. Marom Z, Shelhamer JH, Kaliner M: Effects of arachidonic acid, monohydroxy-eicosatetraenoic acid and prostaglandins on the release of mucous glycoproteins from human airways in vitro. J Clin Invest 67:1695–1702, 1981.
275. Masferrer JL, Seibert K, Zweifel B, et al: Endogenous glucocorticoids regulate an inducible cyclooxygenase enzyme. Proc Natl Acad Sci USA 89:3917–3921, 1992.

276. Mathe AA, Hedqvist P: Effect of prostaglandins F_2 alpha and E_2 on airway conductance in healthy subjects and asthmatic patients. Am Rev Respir Dis 111:313–320, 1975.
277. Mathe AA, Hedqvist P, Holmgren A, et al: Bronchial hyperreactivity to prostaglandin F_2 and histamine in patients with asthma. Br Med J 1:193–196, 1973.
278. Matsumoto T, Funk CD, Radmark O, et al: Molecular cloning and amino acid sequence of human 5-lipoxygenase. [Published erratum appears in Proc Natl Acad Sci USA 85:3406, 1988.] Proc Natl Acad Sci USA 85:26–30, 1988.
279. Matthay MA, Eschenbacher WL, Goetzl EJ: Elevated concentrations of leukotriene D_4 in pulmonary edema fluid of patients with the adult respiratory distress syndrome. J Clin Immunol 4:479–483, 1984.
280. Mattoli S, Foresi A, Corbo GM, et al: The effect of indomethacin on the refractory period occurring after the inhalation of ultrasonically nebulized distilled water. J Allergy Clin Immunol 79:678–683, 1987.
281. Mazzoni L, Morley J, Page CP, et al: Induction of airway hyperreactivity by platelet activating factor in the guinea pig. J Physiol 365:107P, 1985.
282. McGee J, Fitzpatrick F: Enzymatic hydration of leukotriene A_4. Purification and characterization of a novel epoxide hydrolase from human erythrocytes. J Biol Chem 260:12832–12837, 1985.
283. McGee JE, Fitzpatrick FA: Erythrocyte-neutrophil interactions: formation of leukotriene B_4 by transcellular biosynthesis. Proc Natl Acad Sci USA 83:1349–1353, 1986.
284. Ibid.
285. McIntyre TM, Zimmerman GA, Prescott SM: Leukotrienes C_4 and D_4 stimulate human endothelial cells to synthesize platelet-activating factor and bind neutrophils. Proc Natl Acad Sci USA 83:2204–2208, 1986.
286. McIntyre TM, Zimmerman GA, Satoh K, et al: Cultured endothelial cells synthesize both platelet-activating factor and prostacyclin in response to histamine, bradykinin, and adenosine triphosphate. J Clin Invest 76:271–280, 1985.
287. McLeish KR, Gierschik P, Schepers T, et al: Evidence that activation of a common G-protein by receptors for leukotriene B_4 and N-formylmethionyl-leucyl-phenylalanine in HL-60 cells occurs by different mechanisms. Biochem J 260:427–434, 1989.
288. Meade EA, Smith WL, DeWitt DL: Expression of the murine prostaglandin (PGH) synthase-1 and PGH synthase-2 isozymes in cos-1 cells. J Lipid Mediat 6:119–129, 1993.
289. Medina JF, Odlander B, Funk CD, et al: B-lymphocytic cell line Raji expresses the leukotriene A_4 hydrolase gene but not the 5-lipoxygenase gene. [Published erratum appears in Biochem Biophys Res Commun 167:1413, 1990.] Biochem Biophys Res Commun 161:740–745, 1989.
290. Melillo E, Woolley KL, Manning PJ, et al: Effect of inhaled PGE_2 on exercise-induced bronchoconstriction in asthmatic subjects. Am J Respir Crit Care Med 149:1138–1141, 1994.
291. Meltzer SS, Rechsteiner EA, Johns MA, et al: Inhibition of exercise-induced asthma by zileuton, a 5-lipoxygenase inhibitor. Am J Respir Crit Care Med 149:$A_2$15, 1994.
292. Michelassi F, Landa L, Hill RD, et al: Leukotriene D_4: a potent coronary artery vasoconstrictor associated with impaired ventricular contraction. Science 217:841–843, 1982.
293. Miller DK, Gillard JW, Vickers PJ, et al: Identification and isolation of a membrane protein necessary for leukotriene production. Nature 343:278–281, 1990.
294. Minami M, Ohno S, Kawasaki H, et al: Molecular cloning of a cDNA coding for human leukotriene A_4 hydrolase. Complete primary structure of an enzyme involved in eicosanoid synthesis. J Biol Chem 262:13873–13876, 1987.
295. Molfino NA, Slutsky AS, Hoffstein V, et al: Changes in cross-sectional airway areas induced by methacholine, histamine, and LTC_4 in asthmatic subjects. Am Rev Respir Dis 146:577–580, 1992.
296. Moore KP, Taylor GW, Maltby NH, et al: Increased production of cysteinyl leukotrienes in hepatorenal syndrome. J Hepatol 11:263–271, 1990.
297. Morris HR, Taylor GW, Piper PJ, et al: Structure of slow reacting substance of anaphylaxis from guinea-pig lung. Nature 285:104–106, 1980.
298. Murray JJ, Tonnel AB, Brash AR, et al: Release of prostaglandin D_2 into human airways during acute antigen challenge. N Engl J Med 315:800–804, 1986.
299. Naclerio RM, Meier HL, Kagey-Sobotka A, et al: Mediator release after nasal airway challenge with allergen. Am Rev Respir Dis 128:597–602, 1983.
300. Nagy L, Lee TH, Goetzl EJ, et al: Complement receptor enhancement and chemotaxis of human neutrophils and eosinophils by leukotrienes and other lipoxygenase products. Clinical Exp Immunol 47:541–547, 1982.
301. Nakamura M, Honda Z, Izumi T, et al: Molecular cloning and expression of platelet-activating factor receptor from human leukocytes. J Biol Chem 266:20400–20405, 1991.
302. Nakamura T, Morita Y, Kuriyama M, et al: Platelet-activating factor in late asthmatic response. Int Arch Allergy Appl Immunol 82:57–61, 1987.
303. Nakao A, Allen ML, Sonnenburg WK, et al: Regulation of cAMP metabolism by PGE_2 in cortical and medullary ascending limb of Henle's loop. Am J Physiol 256:C652–C657, 1989.
304. Nasser SM, Bell GS, Foster S, et al: Effect of the 5-lipoxygenase inhibitor $ZD_2$138 on aspirin-induced asthma. Thorax 49:749–756, 1994.
305. Nasser SM, Bell GS, Hawksworth RJ, et al: Effect of the 5-lipoxygenase inhibitor $ZD_2$138 on allergen-induced early and late asthmatic responses. Thorax 49:743–748, 1994.
306. Nicholson DW, Ali A, Vaillancourt JP, et al: Purification to homogeneity and the N-terminal sequence of human leukotriene C_4 synthase: a homodimeric glutathione S-transferase composed of 18-kDa subunits. Proc Natl Acad Sci USA 90:2015–2019, 1993.
307. Nicolaou KC, Marron BE, Veale CA, et al: Identification of a novel 7-cis-11-trans-lipoxin A_4 generated by human neutrophils: total synthesis, spasmogenic activities and comparison with other geometric isomers of lipoxins A_4 and B_4. Biochim Biophys Acta 1003:44–53, 1989.
308. O'Banion MK, Winn VD, Young DA: cDNA cloning and functional activity of a glucocorticoid-regulated inflammatory cyclooxygenase. Proc Natl Acad Sci USA 89:4888–4892, 1992.
309. O'Byrne PM, Jones GL: The effect of indomethacin on exercise-induced bronchoconstriction and refractoriness after exercise. Am Rev Respir Dis 134:69–72, 1986.
310. O'Connor BJ, Uden S, Carty TJ, et al: Inhibitory effect of UK,74505, a potent and specific oral platelet activating factor (PAF) receptor antagonist, on airway and systemic responses to inhaled PAF in humans. Am J Respir Crit Care Med 150:35–40, 1994.
311. O'Hickey SP, Arm JP, Rees PJ, et al: The relative responsiveness to inhaled leukotriene E_4, methacholine and histamine in normal and asthmatic subjects. Eur Respir J 1:913–917, 1988.
312. O'Hickey SP, Hawksworth RJ, Fong CY, et al: Leukotrienes C_4, D_4, and E_4 enhance histamine responsiveness in asthmatic airways. Am Rev Respir Dis 144:1053–1057, 1991.
313. O'Shaughnessy KM, Taylor IK, O'Connor B, et al: Potent leukotriene D_4 receptor antagonist ICI 204,219 given by the inhaled route inhibits the early but not the late phase of allergen-induced bronchoconstriction. Am Rev Respir Dis 147:1431–1435, 1993.
314. O'Sullivan MG, Chilton FH, Huggins EM Jr, et al: Lipopolysaccharide priming of alveolar macrophages for enhanced synthesis of prostanoids involves induction of a novel prostaglandin H synthase. J Biol Chem 267:14547–14550, 1992.
315. Ohashi K, Ruan KH, Kulmacz RJ, et al: Primary structure of human thromboxane synthase determined from the cDNA sequence. J Biol Chem 267:789–793, 1992.
316. Ohia SE, Jumblatt JE: Prejunctional inhibitory effects of prostanoids on sympathetic neurotransmission in the rabbit iris-ciliary body. J Pharmacol Exp Therap 255:11–16, 1990.
317. Ohishi N, Izumi T, Minami M, et al: Leukotriene A_4 hydrolase in the human lung. Inactivation of the enzyme with leukotriene A_4 isomers. J Biol Chem 262:10200–10205, 1987.
318. Ibid.
319. Orehek J, Douglas JS, Lewis AJ, et al: Prostaglandin regulation of airway smooth muscle tone. Nature New Biol 245:84–85, 1973.
320. Oshima T, Yoshimoto T, Yamamoto S, et al: cAMP-dependent induction of fatty acid cyclooxygenase mRNA in mouse osteoblastic cells (MC3T3-E_1). J Biol Chem 266:13621–13626, 1991.
321. Palmblad J, Gyllenhammar H, Ringertz B, et al: The effects of lipoxin A and lipoxin B on functional responses of human granulocytes. Biochem Biophys Res Commun 145:168–175, 1987.
322. Palmer RMJ, Stepney RJ, Higgs GA, et al: Chemokinetic activity of arachidonic acid lipoxygenase products on leukocytes of different species. Prostaglandins 20:411–418, 1980.

323. Pasargiklian M, Bianco S, Allegra L: Clinical, functional and pathogenetic aspects of bronchial reactivity to prostaglandins F_2alpha, E_1, and E_2. Adv Prostaglandin Thromboxane Res 1:461–475, 1976.
324. Pavord ID, Wisniewski A, Mathur R, et al: Effect of inhaled prostaglandin E_2 on bronchial reactivity to sodium metabisulphite and methacholine in patients with asthma. Thorax 46:633–637, 1991.
325. Pavord ID, Wong CS, Williams J, et al: Effect of inhaled prostaglandin E_2 on allergen-induced asthma. Am Rev Respir Dis 148:87–90, 1993.
326. Penrose JF, Gagnon L, Goppelt-Struebe M, et al: Purification of human leukotriene C_4 synthase. Proc Natl Acad Sci USA 89:11603–11606, 1992.
327. Perez HD, Holmes R, Kelly E, et al: Cloning of a cDNA encoding a receptor related to the formyl peptide receptor of human neutrophils. Gene 118:303–304, 1992.
328. Perez HD, Kelly E, Holmes R: Regulation of formyl peptide receptor expression and its mRNA levels during differentiation of HL-60 cells. J Biol Chem 267:358–363, 1992.
329. Peskar BM, Dreyling KW, Peskar BA, et al: Enhanced formation of sulfidopeptide-leukotrienes in ulcerative colitis and Crohn's disease: inhibition by sulfasalazine and 5-aminosalicylic acid. Agents Actions 18:381–383, 1986.
330. Peters SP, MacGlashan DW Jr, Schulman ES, et al: Arachidonic acid metabolism in purified human lung mast cells. J Immunol 132:1972–1979, 1984.
331. Peters-Golden M, McNish RW: Redistribution of 5-lipoxygenase and cytosolic phospholipase A_2 to the nuclear fraction upon macrophage activation. Biochem Biophys Res Commun 196:147–153, 1993.
332. Pfeffer MA, Pfeffer JM, Lewis RA, et al: Systemic hemodynamic effects of leukotrienes C_4 and D_4 in the rat. Am J Physiol 244:H628–H633, 1983.
333. Phillips GD, Holgate ST: Interaction of inhaled LTC_4 with histamine and PGD_2 on airway caliber in asthma. J Appl Physiol 66:304–312, 1989.
334. Phillips GD, Rafferty P, Robinson C, et al: Dose-related antagonism of leukotriene D_4-induced bronchoconstriction by p.o. administration of LY-171883 in nonasthmatic subjects. J Pharmacol Exp Ther 246:732–738, 1988.
335. Picado C, Ramis I, Rosellò J, et al: Release of peptide leukotriene into nasal secretions after local instillation of aspirin in aspirin-sensitive asthmatic patients. Am Rev Respir Dis 145:65–69, 1992.
336. Pichurko BM, Ingram RH Jr, Sperling R, et al: Localization of the site of the bronchoconstrictor effects of leukotriene C_4 compared with that of histamine in asthmatic subjects. Am Rev Respir Dis 140:334–339, 1989.
337. Piper PJ, Samhoun MN: The mechanism of action of leukotrienes C_4 and D_4 in guinea-pig isolated perfused lung and parenchymal strips of guinea pig, rabbit and rat. Prostaglandins 21:793–803, 1981.
338. Pliss LB, Ingenito EP, Ingram RH Jr, et al: Assessment of bronchoalveolar cell and mediator response to isocapnic hyperpnea in asthma. Am Rev Respir Dis 142:73–78, 1990.
339. Pong SS, DeHaven RN: Characterization of a leukotriene D_4 receptor in guinea pig lung. Proc Natl Acad Sci USA 80:7415–7419, 1983.
340. Popov GK, Nekrasov AS, Khshivo AL, et al: Effects of lipoxin B on colony-forming capacity of human peripheral blood mononuclear cells in diffusion chambers. Byulleten Eksperimentalnoi Biologii i Meditsiny 107:80–83, 1989.
341. Prescott SM, Zimmerman GA, McIntyre TM: Human endothelial cells in culture produce platelet-activating factor (1-alkyl-2-acetyl-sn-glycero-3-phosphocholine) when stimulated with thrombin. Proc Natl Acad Sci USA 81:3534–3538, 1984.
342. Radmark O, Shimizu T, Jornvall H, et al: Leukotriene A_4 hydrolase in human leukocytes. Purification and properties. J Biol Chem 259:12339–12345, 1984.
343. Rae SA, Davidson EM, Smith MJ: Leukotriene B_4, an inflammatory mediator in gout. Lancet 2:1122–1124, 1982.
344. Ramstedt U, Ng J, Wigzell H, et al: Action of novel eicosanoids lipoxin A and B on human natural killer cell cytotoxicity: effects on intracellular cAMP and target cell binding. J Immunol 135:3434–3438, 1985.
345. Rasmussen JB, Eriksson LO, Margolskee DJ, et al: Leukotriene D_4 receptor blockade inhibits the immediate and late bronchoconstrictor responses to inhaled antigen in patients with asthma. J Allergy Clin Immunol 90:193–201, 1992.
346. Raud J, Palmertz U, Dahlén SE, et al: Lipoxins inhibit microvascular inflammatory actions of leukotriene B_4. Adv Exp Med Biol 314:185–192, 1991.
347. Redkar-Brown DG, Aharony D: Inhibition of antigen-induced contraction of guinea pig trachea by ICI 198,615. Eur J Pharmacol 165:113–121, 1989.
348. Richelsen B, Beck-Nielsen H: Decrease of prostaglandin E_2 receptor binding is accompanied by reduced antilipolytic effects of prostaglandin E_2 in isolated rat adipocytes. J Lipid Res 26:127–134, 1985.
349. Roberts LJ, Lewis RA, Oates JA, et al: Prostaglandin thromboxane, and 12-hydroxy-5,8,10,14-eicosatetraenoic acid production by ionophore-stimulated rat serosal mast cells. Biochim Biophys Acta 575:185–192, 1979.
350. Roberts NM, McCusker M, Chung KF, et al: Effect of a PAF antagonist, BN52063, on PAF-induced bronchoconstriction in normal subjects. Br J Clin Pharmacol 26:65–72, 1988.
351. Roberts NM, Page CP, Chung KF, et al: Effect of a PAF antagonist, BN52063, on antigen-induced, acute, and late-onset cutaneous responses in atopic subjects. J Allergy Clin Immunol 82:236–241, 1988.
352. Robinson C, Hoult JR, Waddell KA, et al: Total profiling by GC/NICIMS of the major cyclo-oxygenase products from antigen and leukotriene-challenged guinea-pig lung. Biochem Pharmacol 33:395–400, 1984.
353. Robuschi M, Riva E, Fuccella LM, et al: Prevention of exercise-induced bronchoconstriction by a new leukotriene antagonist (SK&F 104353). A double-blind study versus disodium cromoglycate and placebo. Am Rev Respir Dis 145:1285–1288, 1992.
354. Rola-Pleszczynski M: Differential effects of leukotriene B_4 on T4+ and T8+ lymphocyte phenotype and immunoregulatory functions. J Immunol 135:1357–1360, 1985.
355. Rola-Pleszczynski M, Chavaillaz PA, Lemaire I: Stimulation of interleukin 2 and interferon gamma production by leukotriene B_4 in human lymphocyte cultures. Prostaglandins Leukotrienes Med 23:207–210, 1986.
356. Rothenberg ME, Caulfield JP, Austen KF, et al: Biochemical and morphological characterization of basophilic leukocytes from two patients with myelogenous leukemia. J Immunol 138:2616–2625, 1987.
357. Rouis M, Nigon F, Chapman MJ: Platelet activating factor is a potent stimulant of the production of active oxygen species by human monocyte-derived macrophages. Biochem Biophys Res Commun 156:1293–1301, 1988.
358. Rouzer CA, Kargman S: Translocation of 5-lipoxygenase to the membrane in human leukocytes challenged with ionophore A_23187. J Biol Chem 263:10980–10988, 1988.
359. Rouzer CA, Matsumoto T, Shimizu T, et al: The human leukocyte 5-lipoxygenase: enzyme purification, multi-component regulatory system, and LTA_4 synthase activity. Adv Prostaglandin Thromboxane Leukot Res 16:3–16, 1986.
360. Rouzer CA, Rands E, Kargman S, et al: Characterization of cloned human leukocyte 5-lipoxygenase expressed in mammalian cells. J Biol Chem 263:10135–10140, 1988.
361. Rouzer CA, Samuelsson B: On the nature of the 5-lipoxygenase reaction in human leukocytes: enzyme purification and requirement for multiple stimulatory factors. Proc Natl Acad Sci USA 82:6040–6044, 1985.
362. Rouzer CA, Samuelsson B: 5-Lipoxygenase from human leukocytes associates with membrane in the presence of calcium. Adv Prostaglandin Thromboxane Leukot Res 17A:60–63, 1987.
363. Russi EW, Abraham WM, Chapman GA, et al: Effects of leukotriene D_4 on mucociliary and respiratory function in allergic and nonallergic sheep. J Appl Physiol 59:1416–1422, 1985.
364. Sala A, Voelkel N, Maclouf J, et al: Leukotriene E_4 elimination and metabolism in normal human subjects. J Biol Chem 265:21771–21778, 1990.
365. Sampson AP, Spencer DA, Green CP, et al: Leukotrienes in the sputum and urine of cystic fibrosis children. Br J Clin Pharmacol 30:861–869, 1990.
366. Samuelsson B, Goldyne M, Granström E, et al: Prostaglandins and thromboxanes. Ann Rev Biochem 47:997–1029, 1978.
367. Samuelsson B, Hammarstrom S, Murphy RC, et al: Leukotrienes and slow reacting substance of anaphylaxis (SRS-A). Allergy 35:375–381, 1980.
368. Samuelsson B, Rouzer CA, Matsumoto T: Human leukocyte 5-lipoxygenase: an enzyme possessing dual enzymatic activities and a multi-component regulatory system. Adv Prostaglandin Thromboxane Leukot Res 17A:1–11, 1987.
369. Schulman ES, Adkinson NF Jr, Newball HH: Cyclooxygenase metabolites in human lung anaphylaxis: airway vs. parenchyma. J Appl Physiol Respir Environ Exercise Physiol 53:589–595, 1982.

370. Schulman ES, MacGlashan DW Jr, Schleimer RP, et al: Purified human basophils and mast cells: current concepts of mediator release. Eur J Respir Dis Suppl 128:53–61, 1983.
371. Serhan CN, Hamberg M, Samuelsson B: Trihydroxytetraenes: a novel series of compounds formed from arachidonic acid in human leukocytes. Biochem Biophys Res Commun 118:943–949, 1984.
372. Serhan CN, Hamberg M, Samuelsson B, et al: On the stereochemistry and biosynthesis of lipoxin B. Proc Natl Acad Sci USA 83:1983–1987, 1986.
373. Serhan CN, Hirsch U, Palmblad J, et al: Formation of lipoxin A by granulocytes from eosinophilic donors. FEBS Lett 217:242–246, 1987.
374. Serhan CN, Nicolaou KC, Webber SE, et al: Lipoxin A. Stereochemistry and biosynthesis. J Biol Chem 261:16340–16345, 1986.
375. Serhan CN, Sheppard KA: Lipoxin formation during human neutrophil-platelet interactions. Evidence for the transformation of leukotriene A_4 by platelet 12-lipoxygenase in vitro. J Clin Invest 85:772–780, 1990.
376. Sharon P, Stenson WF: Enhanced synthesis of leukotriene B_4 by colonic mucosa in inflammatory bowel disease. Gastroenterology 86:453–460, 1984.
377. Shimizu T, Izumi T, Seyama Y, et al: Characterization of leukotriene A_4 synthase from murine mast cells: evidence for its identity to arachidonate 5-lipoxygenase. Proc Natl Acad Sci USA 83:4175–4179, 1986.
378. Shimizu T, Radmark O, Samuelsson B: Enzyme with dual lipoxygenase activities catalyzes leukotriene A_4 synthesis from arachidonic acid. Proc Natl Acad Sci USA 81:689–693, 1984.
379. Sigal E, Craik CS, Highland E, et al: Molecular cloning and primary structure of human 15-lipoxygenase. Biochem Biophys Res Commun 157:457–464, 1988.
380. Sirois P, Brousseau Y, Salari H, et al: Correlation between the myotropic activity of leukotriene A_4 on guinea-pig lung, trachea and ileum and its biotransformation in situ. Prostaglandins 30:21–36, 1985.
381. Sirois P, Roy S, Borgeat P, et al: Evidence for a mediator role of thromboxane A_2 in the myotropic action of leukotriene B_4 (LTB_4) on the guinea-pig lung. Prostaglandins Leukot Med 8:157–170, 1982.
382. Sisson JH, Prescott SM, McIntyre TM, et al: Production of platelet-activating factor by stimulated human polymorphonuclear leukocytes. Correlation of synthesis with release, functional events, and leukotriene B_4 metabolism. J Immunol 138:3918–3926, 1987.
383. Skoner DP, Fireman P, Davis HW, et al: Increases in plasma concentrations of a prostaglandin metabolite in acute airway obstruction. Arch Dis Child 64:1112–1117, 1989.
384. Skoner DP, Page R, Asman B, et al: Plasma elevations of histamine and a prostaglandin metabolite in acute asthma. Am Rev Respir Dis 137:1009–1014, 1988.
385. Sladek K, Dworski R, Fitzgerald GA, et al: Allergen-stimulated release of thromboxane A_2 and leukotriene E_4 in humans. Effect of indomethacin. Am Rev Respir Dis 141:1441–1445, 1990.
386. Sladek K, Dworski R, Soja J, et al: Eicosanoids in bronchoalveolar lavage fluid of aspirin-intolerant patients with asthma after aspirin challenge. Am J Respir Crit Care Med 149:940–946, 1994.
387. Sladek K, Szczeklik A: Cysteinyl leukotrienes overproduction and mast cell activation in aspirin-provoked bronchospasm in asthma. Eur Respir J 6:391–399, 1993.
388. Smith AP, Cuthbert MF, Dunlop LS: Effects of inhaled prostaglandins E_1, E_2, and F_2alpha on the airway resistance of healthy and asthmatic man. Clin Sci Mol Med 48:421–430, 1975.
389. Smith CM, Christie PE, Hawksworth RJ, et al: Urinary leukotriene E_4 levels after allergen and exercise challenge in bronchial asthma. Am Rev Respir Dis 144:1411–1413.
390. Smith CM, Hawksworth RJ, Thien FC, et al: Urinary leukotriene E_4 in bronchial asthma. Eur Respir J 5:693–699, 1992.
391. Smith LJ, Greenberger PA, Patterson R, et al: The effect of inhaled leukotriene D_4 in humans. Am Rev Respir Dis 131:368–372, 1985.
392. Smith WL: Prostaglandin biosynthesis and its compartmentation in vascular smooth muscle and endothelial cells. Annu Rev Physiol 48:251–262, 1986.
393. Smith WL: The eicosanoids and their biochemical mechanisms of action. Biochem J 259:315–324, 1989.
394. Smith WL, Marnett LJ, DeWitt DL: Prostaglandin and thromboxane biosynthesis. Pharmacol Ther 49:153–179, 1991.
395. Snyder DW, Fleisch JH: Leukotriene receptor antagonists as potential therapeutic agents. Annu Rev Pharmacol Toxicol 29:123–143, 1989.
396. Snyder DW, Giles RE, Keith RA, et al: In vitro pharmacology of ICI 198,615: a novel, potent selective peptide leukotriene antagonist. J Pharmacol Exp Ther 243:548–556, 1987.
397. Snyder DW, Krell RD: Pharmacological evidence for a distinct leukotriene C_4 receptor in guinea-pig trachea. J Pharmacol Exp Ther 231:616–622, 1984.
398. Sonnenburg WK, Smith WL: Regulation of cyclic AMP metabolism in rabbit cortical cells by prostaglandins. J Biol Chem 263:6155–6160, 1988.
399. Soter NA, Lewis RA, Corey EJ, et al: Local effects of synthetic leukotrienes (LTC_4, LTD_4, LTE_4, and LTB_4) in human skin. J Invest Dermatol 80:115–119, 1983.
400. Soyombo O, Spur BW, Lee TH: Effects of lipoxin A_4 on chemotaxis and degranulation of human eosinophils stimulated by platelet-activating factor and N-formyl-L-methionyl-L-leucyl-L-phenylalanine. Allergy 49:230–234, 1994.
401. Spector SL, Smith LJ, Glass M, et al: Effects of 6 weeks therapy with oral doses of ICI 204,219, a leukotriene D_4 receptor antagonist in subjects with bronchial asthma. Am J Respir Crit Care Med 150:618–623, 1994.
402. Spence DP, Johnston SL, Calverley PM, et al: The effect of the orally active platelet-activating factor antagonist WEB 2086 in the treatment of asthma. Am J Respir Crit Care Med 149:1142–1148, 1994.
403. Spencer DA, Evans JM, Green SE, et al: Participation of the cysteinyl leukotrienes in the acute bronchoconstrictor response to inhaled platelet activating factor in man. Thorax 46:441–445, 1991.
404. Spencer DA, Green SE, Evans JM, et al: Platelet activating factor does not cause a reproducible increase in bronchial responsiveness in normal man. Clin Exp Allergy 20:525–532, 1990.
405. Spencer DA, Sampson AP, Green CP, et al: Sputum cysteinyl-leukotriene levels correlate with the severity of pulmonary disease in children with cystic fibrosis. Pediatr Pulmonol 12:90–94, 1992.
406. Steinhilber D, Roth HJ: New series of lipoxins isolated from human eosinophils. FEBS Lett 255:143–148, 1989.
407. Stenke L, Mansour M, Edenius C, et al: Formation and proliferative effects of lipoxins in human bone marrow. Biochem Biophys Res Commun 180:255–261, 1991.
408. Stenmark KR, James SL, Voelkel NF, et al: Leukotriene C_4 and D_4 in neonates with hypoxemia and pulmonary hypertension. N Engl J Med 309:77–80, 1983.
409. Stenton SC, Court EN, Kingston WP, et al: Platelet-activating factor in bronchoalveolar lavage fluid from asthmatic subjects. Eur Respir J 3:408–413, 1990.
410. Stenton SC, Ward C, Duddridge M, et al: The actions of GR32191B, a thromboxane receptor antagonist, on the effects of inhaled PAF on human airways. Clin Exp Allergy 20:311–317, 1990.
411. Stenton SC, Young CA, Harris A, et al: The effect of GR32191 (a thromboxane receptor antagonist) on airway responsiveness in asthma. Pulm Pharmacol 5:199–202, 1992.
412. Sturk A, ten Cate JW, Hosford D, et al: The synthesis, catabolism, and pathophysiological role of platelet-activating factor. Adv Lipid Res 23:219–276, 1989.
413. Sugimoto Y, Namba T, Honda A, et al: Cloning and expression of a cDNA for mouse prostaglandin E receptor EP_3 subtype. J Biol Chem 267:6463–6466, 1992.
414. Sugimoto Y, Negishi M, Hayashi Y, et al: Two isoforms of the EP_3 receptor with different identical ligand binding properties and different coupling Gi proteins. J Biol Chem 268:2712–2718, 1993.
415. Sweatman WJ, Collier HO: Effects of prostaglandins on human bronchial muscle. Nature 217:69, 1968.
416. Szarek JL, Evans JN: Pharmacologic responsiveness of rat parenchymal strips, bronchi, and bronchioles. Exp Lung Res 14:575–585, 1988.
417. Takano T, Honda Z, Sakanaka C, et al: Role of cytoplasmic tail phosphorylation sites of platelet-activating factor receptor in agonist-induced desensitization. J Biol Chem 269:22453–22458, 1994.
418. Takeuchi K, Abe T, Takahashi N, et al: Molecular cloning and intrarenal localization of rat prostaglandin E_2 receptor EP_3 subtype. Biochem Biophys Res Commun 194:885–891, 1993.
419. Taylor GW, Taylor I, Black P, et al: Urinary leukotriene E_4 after antigen challenge and in acute asthma and allergic rhinitis. Lancet 1:584–588, 1989.
420. Taylor IK, O'Shaughnessy KM, Fuller RW, et al: Effect of cysteinyl-leukotriene receptor antagonist ICI 204.219 on allergen-induced bronchoconstriction and airway hyperreactivity in atopic subjects. Lancet 337:690–694, 1991.
421. Taylor IK, Ward PS, O'Shaughnessy KM, et al: Thromboxane A_2

biosynthesis in acute asthma and after antigen challenge. Am Rev Respir Dis 143:119–125, 1991.
422. Taylor IK, Ward PS, Taylor GW, et al: Inhaled PAF stimulates leukotriene and thromboxane A_2 production in humans. J Appl Physiol 71:1396–1402, 1991.
423. Uotila P, Vapaatalo H: Synthesis, pathways and biological implications of eicosanoids. Ann Clin Res 16:226–233, 1984.
424. Voelkel NF, Worthen S, Reeves JT, et al: Nonimmunological production of leukotrienes induced by platelet-activating factor. Science 218:286–289, 1982.
425. von Euler US: History and development of prostaglandins. Gen Pharmacol 14:3–6, 1933.
426. Wahedna I, Wisniewski AFZ, Wong CS, et al: Effect of multiple doses of RG 12525, an oral leukotriene D_4 antagonist, in chronic asthma. Am Rev Respir Dis 145:A16, 1992.
427. Walters EH: Prostaglandins and the control of airways responses to histamine in normal and asthmatic subjects. Thorax 38:188–194, 1983.
428. Walters EH, Bevan C, Parrish RW, et al: Time-dependent effect of prostaglandin E_2 inhalation on airway responses to bronchoconstrictor agents in normal subjects. Thorax 37:438–442, 1982.
429. Walters EH, Davies BH: Dual effect of prostaglandin E_2 on normal airways smooth muscle in vivo. Thorax 37:918–922, 1982.
430. Wardlaw AJ, Chung KF, Moqbel R, et al: Effects of inhaled PAF in humans on circulating and bronchoalveolar lavage fluid neutrophils. Relationship to bronchoconstriction and changes in airway responsiveness. Am Rev Respir Dis 141:386–392, 1990.
431. Wardlaw AJ, Hay H, Cromwell O, et al: Leukotrienes, LTC_4 and LTB_4, in bronchoalveolar lavage in bronchial asthma and other respiratory diseases. J Allergy Clin Immunol 84:19–26, 1989.
432. Watabe A, Sugimoto Y, Honda A, et al: Cloning and expression of cDNA for a mouse EP1 subtype of prostaglandin E receptor. J Biol Chem 268:20175–20178, 1993.
433. Weinblatt ME, Kremer JM, Coblyn JS, et al: Zileuton, a 5-lipoxygenase inhibitor in rheumatoid arthritis. J Rheumatol 19:1537–1541, 1992.
434. Weiss JW, Drazen JM, Coles N, et al: Bronchoconstrictor effects of leukotriene C in humans. Science 216:196–198, 1982.
435. Weiss JW, Drazen JM, McFadden ER Jr, et al: Airway constriction in normal humans produced by inhalation of leukotriene D. Potency, time course, and effect of aspirin therapy. JAMA 249:2814–2817, 1983.
436. Weiss JW, Drazen JM, McFadden ER Jr, et al: Comparative bronchoconstrictor effects of histamine, leukotriene C, and leukotriene D in normal human volunteers. Trans Assoc Am Physicians 95:30–35, 1982.
437. Weller PF, Lee CW, Foster DW, et al: Generation and metabolism of 5-lipoxygenase pathway leukotrienes by human eosinophils: predominant production of leukotriene C_4. Proc Natl Acad Sci USA 80:7626–7630, 1983.
438. Wenzel SE, Larsen GL, Johnston K, et al: Elevated levels of leukotriene C_4 in bronchoalveolar lavage fluid from atopic asthmatics after endobronchial allergen challenge. Am Rev Respir Dis 142:112–119, 1990.
439. Wenzel SE, Westcott JY, Larsen GL: Bronchoalveolar lavage fluid mediator levels 5 minutes after allergen challenge in atopic subjects with asthma: relationship to the development of late asthmatic responses. J Allergy Clin Immunol 87:540–548, 1991.
440. Wenzel SE, Westcott JY, Smith HR, et al: Spectrum of prostanoid release after bronchoalveolar allergen challenge in atopic asthmatics and in control groups. An alteration in the ratio of bronchoconstrictive to bronchoprotective mediators. Am Rev Respir Dis 139:450–457, 1989.
441. Westcott JY, Smith HR, Wenzel SE, et al: Urinary leukotriene E_4 in patients with asthma. Effect of airways reactivity and sodium cromoglycate. Am Rev Respir Dis 143:1322–1328, 1991.
442. Westcott JY, Voelkel NF, Jones K, et al: Inactivation of leukotriene C_4 in the airways and subsequent urinary leukotriene E_4 excretion in normal and asthmatic subjects. Am Rev Respir Dis 148:1244–1251, 1993.
443. Williams JD, Czop JK, Austen KF: Release of leukotrienes by human monocytes on stimulation of their phagocytic receptor for particulate activators. J Immunol 132:3034–3040, 1984.
444. Wong A, Hwang SM, Cook MN, et al: Interactions of 5-lipoxygenase with membranes: studies on the association of soluble enzyme with membranes and alterations in enzyme activity. Biochemistry 27:6763–6769, 1988.
445. Wood-Baker R, Phillips GD, Lucas RA, et al: The effect of inhaled LY-170,680 on leukotriene D_4-induced bronchoconstriction in healthy volunteers. Drug Invest 3:239–247, 1991.
446. Woods JW, Coffey MJ, Singer II, et al: 5-lipoxygenase is located in the euchromatin of the nucleus in resting human alveolar macrophages and translocates to the nuclear envelope with cell activation. Am J Respir Crit Care Med 149:$A_2$33, 1994.
447. Woods JW, Evans JF, Ethier D, et al: 5-lipoxygenase and 5-lipoxygenase-activating protein are localized in the nuclear envelope of activated human leukocytes. J Exp Med 178:1935–1946, 1993.
448. Yamaguchi T, Kohrogi H, Honda I, et al: A novel leukotriene antagonist, ONO-1078, inhibits and reverses human bronchial contraction induced by leukotrienes C_4 and D_4 and antigen in vitro. Am Rev Respir Dis 146:923–929, 1992.
449. Yokoyama C, Miyata A, Ihara H, et al: Molecular cloning of human platelet thromboxane A synthase. Biochem Biophys Res Commun 178:1479–1484, 1991.
450. Yoshimoto T, Soberman RJ, Lewis RA, et al: Isolation and characterization of leukotriene C_4 synthetase of rat basophilic leukemia cells. Proc Natl Acad Sci USA 82:8399–8403, 1985.

13 The Complement System: Mechanisms of Activation, Regulation, and Biologic Functions

BERHANE GHEBREHIWET

The complement system (reviewed in 99, 128, 132, 163) is a complex biologic entity that constitutes a major part of the immune system through which an animal can recognize foreign substances and defend itself against infection by pathogenic organisms. Complement is activated primarily when antigen-antibody complexes are formed in either plasma or tissues. As a consequence, secondary activation peptides are generated that play an important role in many types of immunologic reactions and inflammatory processes. It consists of a group of serum proteins that, together with an intricate array of modulators and regulators, constitutes one of the proteolytic cascade systems of blood plasma. Activation of complement requires an initial contact with and recognition of an activator. This in turn triggers a series of protein-protein interactions involving, in part, the conversion of proteolytic zymogens to active proteinases and the assembly of protein complexes on the surface of the activator particle. If the activating agent is a virus, a bacterium, or a tumor cell, activation of complement may lead to the destruction of that particle by causing irreversible structural and functional impairment of its membrane.

There are two well-characterized independent pathways of complement activation and a more recently identified third pathway, plus a self-assembling, nonenzymatic cascade referred to as the membrane attack complex (MAC). The MAC is common to the first two pathways, and most likely to the third, and is responsible for the well-known complement-mediated lesions on biologic membranes. The classical pathway is initiated by immune complexes of the IgG and IgM types and results in the sequential interactions of nine distinct complement components, designated numerically and in their order of participation in the sequence as C1, C4, C2, C3, C5, C6, C7, C8, and C9 (Table 13–1). Three of these components—C1r, C1s, and C2—constitute the classical pathway serine proteases.

Terminology used to describe the complement proteins is that agreed on by the World Health Organization (1968). Thus components are named by uppercase letters followed by a number (e.g., C1). Fragments derived from a component are denoted by a lowercase letter after the component from which it was derived (e.g., C3a). A bar over a component or complexes indicates an enzyme (e.g., $C\overline{1}$). Some alternative pathway components are designated by uppercase letters only: Factors B, D, I (C3b-INA), and H (β1H) and P (properdin).

The alternative pathway is activated by IgA antibodies or certain complex polysaccharides of bacterial and microbial cell walls such as bacterial endotoxins, inulin (a polyfructose from plant cell walls), zymosan (an insoluble residue of yeast cell walls), or cobra venom factor (a glycoprotein from cobra venom), which is the cobra equivalent of C3b. Six proteins can be considered components proper of the alternative pathway: C3, Factor B, Factor $\overline{D}$, Factor H (β1H), Factor I (C3b-INA), and properdin (P). Factors B and $\overline{D}$ belong to the class of serine proteases and represent the alternative pathway enzymes. Factor I is an unusual enzyme that is resistant to the classical serine protease inhibitor diisopropylphosphofluoridate, although sequence evidence suggests that it too is a serine protease.[104, 163] Factor B and perhaps Factor C2 of the classical pathway are examples of a new type of serine protease with catalytic peptide chains of about 60,000 molecular weight (MW).[163] Factor $\overline{D}$ is believed to be the only complement enzyme that circulates in plasma in its active form ($\overline{D}$).

Although its physiologic relevance has yet to be determined, a third pathway, tentatively designated MBL (mannan-binding lectin or mannan-binding protein) pathway, has been described.[111, 173, 193] MBL belongs to the group III of a family of Ca^{2+}-dependent carbohydrate-binding lectins, which include the plasma proteins, conglutinin, collectin-43, and two lung surfactant proteins, SP-A and SP-D.[114, 191, 193] These proteins, collectively known as collectins (collagen-containing lectins), are structurally similar to C1q and consist of 12 to 18 polypeptide chains with N-terminal collagen-like regions and C-terminal globular heads containing the carbohydrate recognition domain (CRD). Through its globular heads, MBL can recognize and bind to surface structures containing mannose and *N*-acetylglucosamine, thereby triggering a carbohydrate-mediated, antibody-independent activation of complement in a manner that involves a C1r/C1s-like serine enzyme(s) designated MASP (MBL-associated serine protease). MASP, C1r, and C1s have functional and structural similarity. Therefore, the C1q-$C1r_2C1s_2$, and MBL-MASP pathways may function similarly and may have similar overall regulatory mechanisms.

For a meaningful activation to occur, all three pathways more or less must obey the same sequential steps of molecular organization:

TABLE 13–1
PLASMA PROTEINS OF THE COMPLEMENT SYSTEM

Components	MW (kD)	Electrophoretic Mobility	Polypeptide Chains	Chromosome Location	Mean Serum Concentration (μg/ml)
Classic pathway					
C1q	462	γ_2	18	1p34.1	80
C1r	83	β	2	12p13	50
C1s	83	α	1	12p13	50
C2	102	β_2	1	6p21.3	25
C3	185	β_2	2	19	1600
C4	205	β_1	3	6p21.3	550
MBP pathway					
MBP	540	—	18	10	1–5
MASP	100	—	1	3q27–q28	—
Alternative pathway					
C3	185	β_2	2	19	1600
Factor B	93	β_2	1	6p21.3	200
Factor D	25	β–γ	1	—	—
Factor H	150	β	1	1q	500
Factor I	88	β	2	4q24	35
Properdin	225	γ	4	Xp11.23	25
Membrane attack					
C5	190	β_1	2	9q32–34	75
C6	120	β_2	1	5q	60
C7	110	β_2	1	5q	55
C8*	150	γ_1	3 (α,β,γ)	(1p34,1p34,9q)	80
C9	71	γ	1	5p13	60
Control proteins					
C1–INH	110	α_2	1	11p11.2	200
C4–bp	500	β_1	?	1q32	250
AI	310	α	multiple	—	50
S-protein	83	α	1	17q11	600
Sp40,40	80	—	1	8p21	50

Chromosome location is given for each chain in the order shown.
Abbreviations: MBP = mannan-binding protein; MASP = MBP-associated serine protease; AI = anaphylatoxin inactivator.

1. An initial contact with and recognition of an activator
2. Conversion of proteolytic zymogens to active proteinases
3. Enzymatic cleavage and exposure of new, labile binding sites in target or substrate proteins
4. Assembly of newly formed protein-protein complexes
5. Formation of a lytic molecular complex (MAC)

ACTIVATION AND REGULATION OF THE CLASSICAL PATHWAY

Activation of the classical pathway of complement is entirely dependent on the ability of the first component, C1, to bind to polymeric structures of activating substances such as circulating immune complexes, bacteria, viruses, and other activating substances of diverse origin (Fig. 13–1).[15] Although in vivo it is generally agreed that immune complexes of the IgG (IgG_1, IgG_2, and IgG_3 subclasses) and IgM isotypes are particularly effective initiators of the classical pathway, activation can proceed without mediation by immunoglobulins. For example, direct activation of C1 can occur by certain biologic particles such as RNA tumor viruses,[17] vesicular stomatitis virus,[124] complexes of C reactive protein and pneumococcal polysaccharide,[198] the lipid A region of certain lipopolysaccharides,[19] *Toxoplasma*,[176] and plasma enzymes such as kallikrein,[18] Hageman factor fragment (HFf, Factor XIIf),[55, 56] and plasmin.[165]

The first component of complement (C1, MW 740,000–775,000)[118, 189, 205] is a 15S to 16S glycoprotein and actually consists of three distinct glycoprotein subunits—C1q, C1r, and C1s[108]—which are held together by calcium ions. The molecular composition of C1 consists of one molecule of C1q, two noncovalently linked polypeptide chains of C1r (dimer), and two Ca^{++} ion-linked polypeptide chains of C1s to give a structural formula of $C1q\text{-}C1r_2C1s_2$.[162, 163] However, because C1 in serum is readily dissociable into C1q and the Ca^{++}-dependent tetrameric structure $C1r_2C1s_2$, it may be regarded as a macromolecular assembly of these two weakly interacting proteins.[203]

During activation of the classical pathway, the C1q subunit of the C1 macromolecule functions as the recognition unit.[128] C1q is a collagen-like molecule[11] with six flower-like globular heads that constitute the binding sites[181] for the C_H2 domain of IgG[93] and C_H3 or C_H4 domains of IgM,[87, 151] respectively. Each globular head contains the carboxyl-terminal ends of three similar but distinct polypeptide chains, A, B, and C, of 28,000, 25,000, and 24,000 MW, respectively, that occur six times in the molecule, forming six structural and functional subunits.[128, 162, 168] The three chains of C1q are the product of three distinct genes that are aligned 5′→3′ in the same orientation in the order A-C-B on a 24-kb stretch of DNA on human chromosome 1p.[180] The amino-terminal regions of each chain are collagen-like and associate to form a triple helical configuration that represents the binding site for $C1r_2C1s_2$.[167, 168] Thus C1q has a valence of six; that is, one

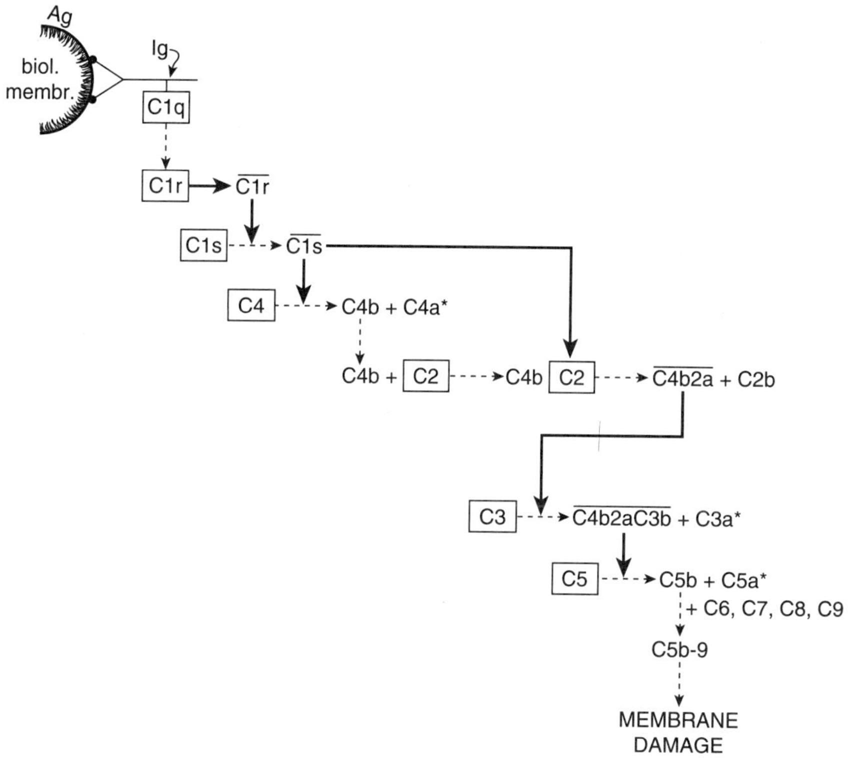

FIGURE 13–1. Activation sequence of the classical pathway of complement. Activation is initiated when C1q within the C1 macromolecule binds to the Fc portion of Ig bound to an antigen. This interaction initiates an intramolecular change within the C1 that leads to the conversion of proenzyme C1r first to an intermediate form C1r* and then to the fully activated proteolytic form $\overline{\text{C1r}}$. Activated C1r enzymatically converts C1s to $\overline{\text{C1s}}$ to complete activation of C1 and thus trigger the activation of the complement cascade. Although the model depicts C1q binding to a single Ig, activation actually occurs only when C1q binds to polymeric Ig via at least two of its globular heads (i.e., multiple Ig molecules binding to one molecule of C1q) while remaining in complex with C1r and C1s. The asterisk indicates an anaphylatoxin, and the overbar shows an enzyme.

molecule of C1q can bind a maximum of six molecules of IgG.[181] This interaction with Ig initiates a series of intramolecular changes within the C1 macromolecule that lead to the conversion of the proenzyme C1r to its proteolytic form ($\overline{\text{C1r}}$).

The conversion of C1r to an active protease is the first step in the initiation of the classical pathway. The mechanism by which this occurs is unclear. However, it has been proposed that complex formation induces a conformational change in the C1q within the C1 macromolecule[65] and that this change somehow exposes a proteolytic site in C1r prior to peptide bond cleavage, converting it to an intermediate active zymogen form designated C1r*.[163] This form of C1r, in turn, would catalyze the conversion of C1r or C1r* to the active form, $\overline{\text{C1r}}$.[163] When activation of C1r occurs, each of its polypeptide chains is cleaved from a single chain of MW 90,000 to a two-chain structure in which a heavy chain of MW 60,000 is disulfide linked to an MW 30,000, carboxy-terminal end light chain, which bears the catalytic site (Fig. 13–2). This site was found to contain three active residues (His, Asp, Ser) that are common to all serine proteases.[3] Such activated C1r ($\overline{\text{C1r}}$) enzymatically converts C1s to $\overline{\text{C1s}}$, which is accomplished by cleavage within a disulfide bridge in a fashion similar to that described for C1r (see Fig. 13–2).[163]

In spite of their structural and functional similarities, $\overline{\text{C1r}}$ and $\overline{\text{C1s}}$ are two distinct and specific enzymes with entirely different proteins as their substrates. The only natural substrate known for $\overline{\text{C1r}}$ is C1s, whereas both C4 and C2 represent the natural substrates for $\overline{\text{C1s}}$. Thus $\overline{\text{C1}}$ ($\overline{\text{C1s}}$) cleaves the fourth (C4) and second (C2) components of complement, each of which is sequentially cleaved into two fragments. For continuity of the cascade, however, cleavage of C4 must precede cleavage of C2. Furthermore, whereas $\overline{\text{C1s}}$ in free solution can cleave free or C4b-bound C2, the cell-bound enzyme does not cleave C2 unless it is bound to C4b.[197]

C4 consists of three disulfide-linked chains (each of which is a distinct gene product) of differing MWs (α = 93,000, β = 75,000, γ = 33,000) in which a single cleavage of the largest chain (termed α) by $\overline{\text{C1s}}$ activates the molecule so that a labile binding site for cells (on the α chain) is revealed and firm binding to C2 via the 33,000-dalton γ chain can proceed.[129, 177] The active site in the α chain of C4b is a reactive acyl group that has the capacity to bind covalently to hydroxyl or amino groups on any biologic membrane. C4 is digested to liberate a fragment of 8,650 daltons termed C4a,[10, 67] which has been shown to have anaphylatoxic activity.[66, 67] Anaphylatoxins are important mediators of inflammation because they have the capacity to react with basophils and mast cells, causing them to degranulate (reviewed in 83, 84). In this fashion, histamine and other mediators typical of allergic reactions can be released into tissues, resulting in vascular permeability and contraction of smooth muscle.

The larger fragment, C4b (MW 198,000), that results from this digestion (whether cell bound or in solution) can bind C2 in the presence of Mg^{++}. If the binding of C2 to C4b occurs in the vicinity of activated C1, then C4b acts as a cofactor for the next enzymatic step of the cascade in which C2 becomes cleaved by $\overline{\text{C1}}$ to yield two fragments: the C-terminal catalytic fragment C2a (MW 74,000) and the noncatalytic N-terminal piece C2b (MW 34,000).[61] The larger fragments, C4b and C2a, form a bimolecular complex ($\overline{\text{C4b2a}}$) to form the next enzyme in the cascade, the C3 convertase.[131] The active site resides on the C2a portion of the molecule,[16] and C4b functions to facilitate C2 cleavage by $\overline{\text{C1s}}$[63] and stabilize the C2a enzymatic site.[64] C4b also

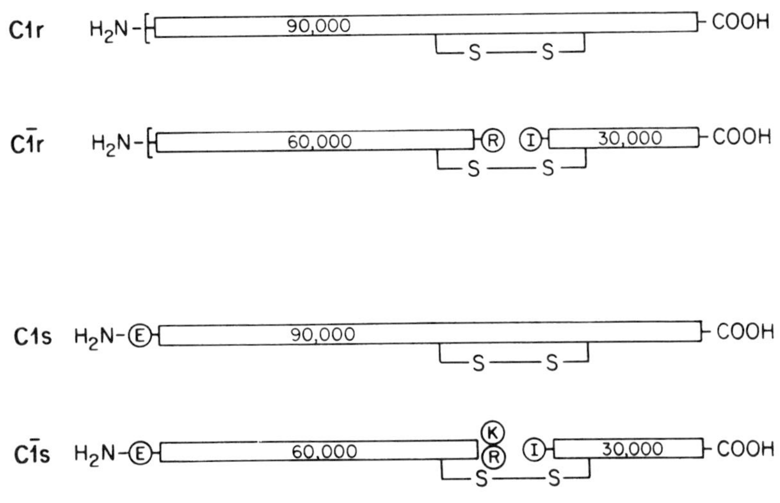

FIGURE 13–2. Proteolytic cleavage and activation of C1r and C1s. The activation patterns of C1r and C1s are almost identical. Cleavage of C1r occurs at a single site between arginine (R) and isoleucine (I) to give two chains of MW 60,000 and MW 30,000, which remain disulfide bonded. The smaller fragment contains the catalytic site of the molecule, which converts C1s to $C\overline{1s}$ by a single peptide bond cleavage between Arg-Ile or Lys-Ile. Again, the active site of the $C\overline{1s}$ molecule resides in the smaller chain at the carboxy-terminal end.

possesses a metastable binding site by which the $\overline{C4b2a}$ enzyme can attach to target cells. C2 has not been shown to possess any biologic activity of its own. It has been proposed, however, that a kinin-like peptide is released as a consequence of C2 cleavage.[27, 95] This would represent another way in which a potent vasodilator is released as a consequence of complement activation. However, these results could not be confirmed by the findings of three independent laboratories.[20, 43, 183]

Of the more than 20 distinct plasma proteins recognized to date as constituents of the complement system, the third component of complement, C3, is the most versatile and fulfills a pivotal role in the functions of both the classical and the alternative pathways. All the pathways leading to the sequential activation of complement and generation of MAC merge at the C3 step. Therefore, complete deficiency of C3 would have a devastating, but not necessarily fatal, consequence on the individual since the complement-dependent lytic machinery would be impaired and opsonic fragments, which play such a significant role in phagocytosis and immune clearance, would not be generated.[182] It circulates in plasma in its inactive but activatable form at a concentration of about 1.6 mg/ml.[128] It also functions as a subunit of the initial C3 convertase of the alternative pathway. It is no surprise, therefore, that the structure, molecular biology, and functions of C3 have been the subject of much study.[182] The chain structure and cleavage pattern during complement activation have been substantially worked out (Fig. 13–3). C3 is a 9.5S β-globulin consisting of two nonidentical polypeptide chains, α and β, with MWs of 110,000 to 120,000 and 75,000 daltons, respectively, that are held together by disulfide bonds and noncovalent forces.[5, 190] Serine has been found to be the N-terminal amino acid residue of both chains, as well as the C-terminal residue of the α chain, whereas alanine constitutes the C-terminal residue of the β chain.[190] C3 is synthesized in the liver[2, 9, 14] by monocytes and macrophages[30, 116] as a single polypeptide chain that, after translation, is processed in the cytoplasm to the two-chain molecule that occurs in serum.[9, 30, 116]

Several individuals have been described with a homozygous C3 deficiency. These individuals have been reported to have had numerous episodes of infection caused by pathogenic bacteria, including septicemia and meningococcal meningitis.[101, 182] In addition, deficiency in C3 results in suppression of complement-mediated functions, such as hemolytic and bactericidal activity, opsonization of bacteria, and mobilization of leukocytes in response to chemotactic stimuli.[22]

Native C3 is cleaved by the classical or alternative pathway C3 convertase into two fragments, C3a and C3b,[22] by hydrolysis of peptide bond 77 (Arg-Ser) of the α chain.[84, 190] The activation peptide C3a is a 9,000 MW basic peptide that constitutes one of the three complement-derived anaphylatoxins. C4a and C5a are the others and are derived by a

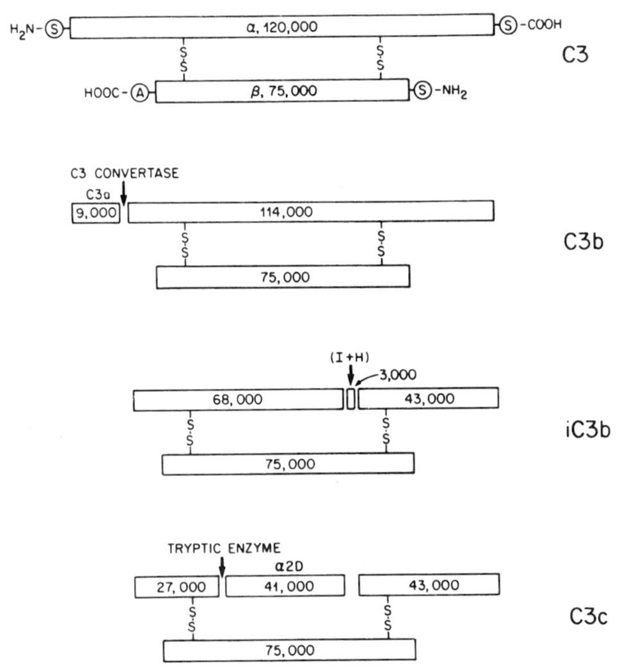

FIGURE 13–3. Structure and activation pattern of human C3. The C3 convertase of either pathway removes a 9,000-dalton fragment, C3a, by a single peptide bond cleavage (Arg-Ser) of the α chain. The α chain of C3b is further cleaved by the regulatory protein, Factor I, which in the presence of Factor H removes a 3,000-dalton fragment, C3f, leaving 68,000- and 43,000-dalton fragments disulfide bonded to the β chain to give an inactivated C3b (iC3b). iC3b is, at this stage, susceptible to proteolytic cleavage by trypticlike enzymes to generate C3c and C3dg (α2D). S = serine; A = alanine.

TABLE 13–2
PHYSIOLOGIC CLEAVAGE PRODUCTS OF C3 AND THEIR KNOWN BIOLOGIC ACTIVITIES

Cleavage Product	Number of Polypeptide Chains	MW	Biologic Activities
C3a	1	9,000	Anaphylatoxin Release of histamine from mast cells Release of enzymes from PMNs Smooth muscle contraction Suppression of immune responses (T cells) Secretion of IL-1 from macrophages Stimulation of prostaglandin and thromboxane production (macrophages)
C3b	2	170,000–186,000	Opsonization of biologic particles Recognition unit of the alternative pathway Subunit of C3/C5 convertase of the alternative pathway Subunit of the C5 convertase of the classical pathway Receptor for P and Factor H Ligand for cellular receptors (CR1 receptor) (PMNs, erythrocytes, monocytes, B lymphocytes) Potentiation of antibody-dependent cellular cytotoxicity (ADCC)
iC3b	3	170,000–186,000	Ligand for PMN, monocyte, and B lymphocyte receptors (CR3 receptor) Potentiation of ADCC Enhancement of phagocytosis
C3c	3	140,000	Precursor of C3e
C3d	1	25,000–35,000	Ligand for cellular receptors (CR2 receptor) Potentiation of ADCC
C3g	1	8,000	None
C3d–k*	1	40,000	Suppression of T-cell functions Leukocytosis
C3e*	1	10,000–12,000	Induction of leukocytosis Enhanced vascular permeability Release of lysosomal enzymes Ligand for PMNs and monocytes (?)

*These are two of the late degradation fragments that are derived from iC3b by trypsin-like enzymes.

single cleavage of an Arg-X bond in the α chain of their respective proteins. As such, C3a is an important mediator of acute inflammatory responses (Tables 13–2, 13–3). Doses as low as 1×10^{-12} mol are active, and when compared on a molar basis, C3a is less potent than C5a but more potent than C4a (C5a>C3a>C4a). It causes release of histamine from mast cells, induces smooth muscle contraction of guinea pigs, causes release of lysosomal enzymes from neu-

TABLE 13–3
PROPERTIES OF HUMAN ANAPHYLATOXINS

Properties	C3a	C4a	C5a
Electrophoretic mobility	+2.1	+2.1	−1.7
Molecular weight			
Total	9,000	8,650	11,200
Protein	9,000	8,650	8,200
Carbohydrate	0	0	3,000
Amino acid residues	77	77	74
NH-terminus	Serine	Asparagine	Threonine
COOH-terminus	Arginine	Arginine	Arginine
α-Helical structure	50%	54%	45%
Biologic activity			
Ileum contraction	1×10^{-8} M	1×10^{-8} M	5×10^{-10} M
*Chemotaxis	1×10^{-9} M	None	3×10^{-9} M
Histamine release	1×10^{-6} M	—	1×10^{-6} M
Lethal shock (guinea pig)	1×10^{-8} mol	—	1×10^{-9} mol
Edema and erythema	1×10^{-12} mol	1×10^{-9} mol	1×10^{-15} mol
Immunopotentiation	None	—	10–100 ng/ml
Immunosuppression	100–500 ng/ml	—	None

*C5a—neutrophils, eosinophils, and monocytes; C3a—eosinophils.

trophils, and upon intracutaneous injection into humans or guinea pigs enhances vascular permeability (reviewed in 83, 84, 109). It has been found that C3a suppresses both specific and polyclonal antibody responses by induction of a suppressor T-cell population, indicating that C3a may be involved in a nonspecific immunoregulatory network capable of suppressing ongoing immune responses.[200]

In vivo, the functions of C3a are controlled by serum carboxypeptidase N (anaphylatoxin inactivator), which removes the essential C-terminal arginyl residue.[6] Its structure has been found to be homologous to that of C4a[66, 67] and C5a,[41] with a 45% α-helical conformation.[82] The large fragment, C3b, like C4b, has a metastable binding site,[138, 141, 172] and the reactive group appears to be an intramolecular thiolester bond

$$(\text{—}\overset{\overset{\text{O}}{\|}}{\text{C}}\text{—S—})$$

capable of covalently binding with any nucleophile, including H_2O, and the hydroxyl or amino groups of any biologic surface. Such interaction converts the thiolester to

$$(\text{—}\overset{\overset{\text{O}}{\|}}{\text{C}}\text{—OH}\quad\text{HS—})$$

C3b performs several biologically significant in vivo functions (see Table 13–2). First, there are receptors for C3b on numerous cells, including neutrophils, eosinophils, macrophages, monocytes, and B lymphocytes (reviewed in 35, 104, 175). Because neutrophils and macrophages (and to a lesser degree eosinophils) are phagocytic cells, interaction of these cells with immune complexes to which C3b is attached appears to be sufficient to trigger phagocytosis. In this fashion, immune complexes are ingested. As a consequence of this reaction, secretion of enzymes that can destroy tissue is initiated. Second, C3b is capable of distinguishing between an activator and a nonactivator of the alternative pathway, as reflected by the differential accessibility of bound C3b to the regulator (Factor H) and the C3b inactivator (Factor I). Factor I cleaves the α′ chain at two arginyl-serine peptide bonds, removing a 3,000-dalton fragment designated C3f[77], and leaving 68,000- and 43,000-dalton α′ fragments that remain disulfide bonded to the β chain (see Fig. 13–3).[143] Such inactivated C3b is termed iC3b and at this stage is extremely susceptible to further enzymatic degradation by tryptic-like enzymes; these cleave the α′ chain in the N-terminal region, removing a 41,000-dalton α2D piece (C3dg) that contains the C3d and C3g fragments (Fig. 13–4).[100]

C3d contains a particle-binding site and remains bound, whereas C3c is in the fluid phase. Although the physiologic fragments of C3b (iC3b, C3dg, and C3d) do not participate further in the activation process, they nevertheless fulfill a diversity of immunoregulatory functions, including clearance and solubilization of immune complexes and stimulation of immune responses, by interacting with specific cell surface receptors such as CR2 (for C3dg and C3d) and CR3 (for iC3b). The larger fragment, C3c (140,000 MW), is the precursor of a 10,000 MW fragment, C3e, which appears to be derived, late in the degradation process, from the α chain by a yet unidentified plasma, leukocyte, or bacterial-derived enzyme.[52, 53] Although its exact chemical structure has not been elucidated, C3e is of particular interest, as it has been shown to induce leukocytosis in rabbits upon intravenous injection and when injected intradermally[52] causes increased vascular permeability (Fig. 13–5) with cellular infiltration. It has also been shown that polymorphonuclear neutrophils (PMNs) possess specific receptors for C3e, and upon interaction with the peptide they are induced to release lysosomal enzymes, one of which is an enzyme capable of generating a chemotactic activity when incubated with highly purified C5 (Table 13–4).[49] Another fragment expressing similar biologic properties as C3e has also been generated from iC3b by limited proteolytic digestion with kallikrein.[123] This fragment, designated C3dK, also induces leukocytosis, and it is postulated that both C3e and C3dK may share overlapping sequence homology. Figure 13–4 summarizes the chain structure of C3 and its physiologic split products, and Table 13–2 outlines their biologic activities.

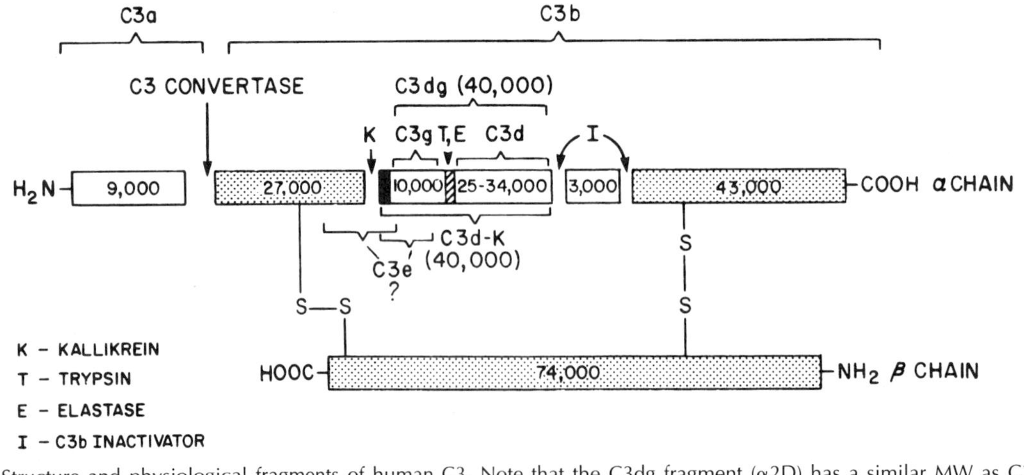

FIGURE 13–4. Structure and physiological fragments of human C3. Note that the C3dg fragment (α2D) has a similar MW as C3d-K, which is a fragment generated by kallikrein from iC3b. However, whereas C3d-K is capable of inducing leukocytosis, C3dg is devoid of such activity. The position of C3e, which contains the leukocytosis-inducing activity, is located to the left of C3d-K as part of C3c, with its active site probably shared by both C3d-K and C3e. (From Hugli TE: Biological activities of fragments derived from human complement components. In Yamamura Y, Tada T (eds): Progress in Immunology. Academic Press, New York, 1983.)

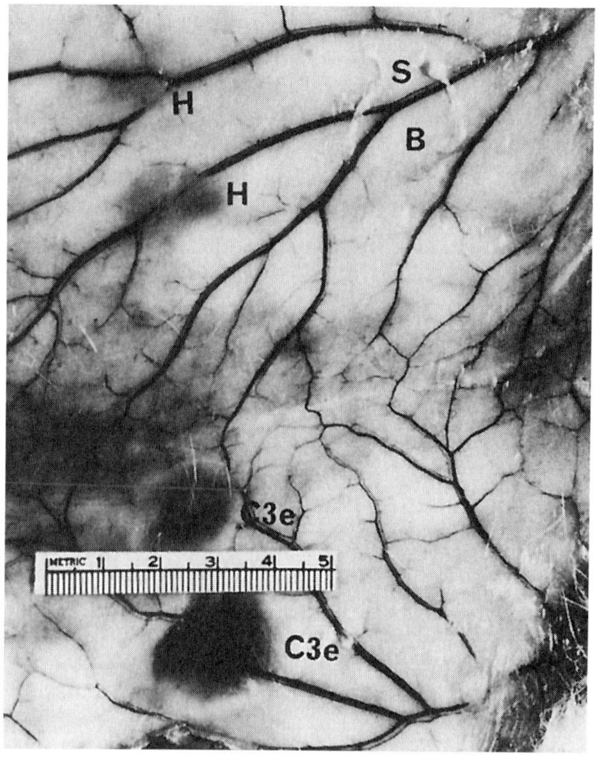

FIGURE 13–5. C3e-dependent vascular permeability. Rabbits were first given 1 ml of 2.5% Evans blue, followed by intradermal injection of 5 and 10 μg in 100 μl pyrogen-free PO_4 buffer, pH 7.1, immediately thereafter. Histamine phosphate (H) (12 μg/ml in pyrogen-free saline) was used as a positive control and saline (S) or phosphate buffer (B) as a negative control. (From Ghebrehiwet B, Müller-Eberhard HJ: C3e: an acidic fragment of human C3 with leukocytosis inducing activity. J Immunol 123:616, 1979. Copyright 1979. *The American Association of Immunologists.)*

Another important physiologic function of C3b is that it forms a subunit of the C5 converting enzymes of both the classical and alternative pathways.[128] Formation of C3b in the vicinity of a $\overline{\text{C4b2a}}$ complex confers upon this enzyme the ability to activate and cleave C5, thereby changing its specificity.[132] This $\overline{\text{C4b2a3b}}$ enzyme is the classical pathway C5 convertase and releases a 12,000-dalton peptide from C5, called C5a, and generates C5b, the first protein of the membrane attack portion of the cascade (Fig. 13–1). C5a possesses two important activities: it shares with C3a[13] and C4a the property of being an anaphylatoxin,[41] and it is a potent chemotactic factor that can attract neutrophils, eosinophils, and monocytes into the vicinity of an inflammatory reaction. Because the predominant cell in the circulation is the neutrophil, it is the most prominent cell seen in C5a-dependent inflammatory reactions. Furthermore, other findings indicate that, in contrast to C3a, which suppresses immune responses, addition of C5a to cultures results in the enhancement of specific and nonspecific humoral responses.[200] C5a has been shown to augment antigen- and alloantigen-induced T-cell proliferative responses but not mitogen-induced proliferative responses.[126] In addition, the adjuvant effects exerted by C5a were found to occur within the first 24 hours of culture, with T cells being involved in the C5a-mediated enhancement of humoral immune responses (reviewed in 201).

Homeostatic regulation of the classical pathway occurs through a number of regulatory mechanisms, including the intrinsic lability of the activated or assembled proteins. For example, activated C1 is unstable and the $\overline{\text{C4b2a}}$ enzyme decays in serum with a half-life of only 5 minutes. Regulation can occur by serum inhibitors. For example, $\text{C}\overline{1}$-INH (or α_2-neuraminoglycoprotein) provides the main control mechanism for activated C1 by binding irreversibly to $\text{C}\overline{\text{1r}}$ and $\text{C}\overline{\text{1s}}$ and dissociating them from the C1 macromolecule.[103, 204] Furthermore, C1-INH plays a crucial role in the homeostatic regulation of C1 by preventing its dissociation, which otherwise results in the autocatalytic activation of C1r.[203] Genetic deficiency in C1-INH, which is inherited as an autosomal dominant trait, results in a potentially fatal disease called hereditary angioneurotic edema (HANE or HAE), and it is postulated that a kinin-like activity derived from C2 as well as bradykinin may play a crucial role in perpetuating the symptoms of this disease. There is also regulation by proteolytic digestion of certain components such as cleavage of C4b by C4-binding protein (C4-bp) and Factor I and digestion of C3 by Factor I in the presence of Factor H. The C4-bp, like DAF (decay accelerating factor), has the property of accelerating the dissociation of $\overline{\text{C4b2a}}$ complex and is an essential cofactor for the cleavage of C4b by Factor I.[45, 62] In this respect, its action is analogous to that of Factor H in the alternative pathway. In addition, membrane proteins such as CR1 (receptor for C3b) and MCP (membrane cofactor protein) can serve as cofactors for Factor I in the cleavage of C3b and C4b.[104, 105]

ALTERNATIVE PATHWAY OF COMPLEMENT ACTIVATION

The alternative pathway of complement serves as one of the first lines of host defense because, unlike the classical pathway, it is capable of neutralizing a variety of potential pathogens in the total absence of antibody.[138, 179] Six proteins are necessary for activation of the alternative pathway: C3, properdin (P), and Factors B, $\overline{\text{D}}$, I, and H (see Table 13–1).[132] The most critical and essential component of the alternative pathway, however, is surface-bound C3b, as by virtue of its discriminatory interaction with biologic surface structures, it

TABLE 13–4
PROPERTIES OF HUMAN C3e

Molecular weight	
Gel electrophoresis	12,000 daltons
Amino acid analysis	10,014 daltons
Electrophoretic mobility, pH 8.6	-7.5×10^{-5} cm² volts^{-1} sec^{-1}
Isoelectric point	4.3
Number of amino acid residues	101
Biologic activity	
Induction of leukocytosis (rabbits)	10 μg/kg intravenously
Increased vascular permeability with leukocyte infiltration	5 μg intradermally
Release of lysosomal enzmes (PMNs)	4–25 μg/ml
Ligand for PMNs	62,000 sites/cell*
Ligand for monocytes	43,400 sites/cell*

*Unpublished data.

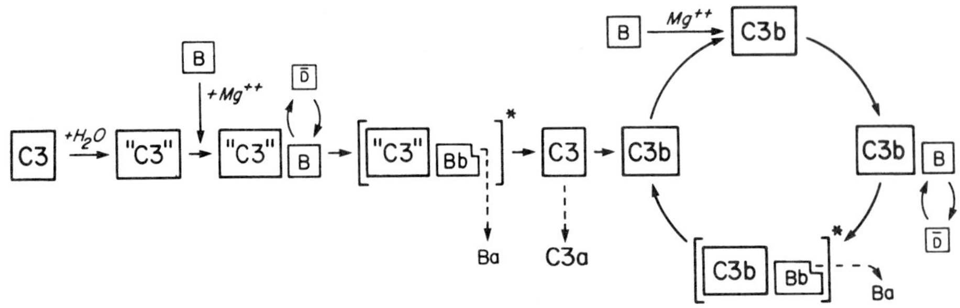

FIGURE 13–6. Alternative pathway of complement: initiation, activation, and amplification of the C3b-dependent positive feedback mechanism. Native C3 interacts with H_2O to form a C3b-like C3, "C3," which is capable of interacting with Factor B in the presence of Mg^{++} to form a loose complex "C3"B. This complex becomes cleaved by Factor $\overline{D}$ to give $[\text{"C3"}\overline{Bb}]^*$, which constitutes the initial, fluid-phase C3 convertase. The first few molecules of C3b generated by this enzyme can bind to biologic surfaces; and dependent on the ability of that surface to provide a sheltered microenvironment, the C3b molecules can initiate the amplification loop by forming a particle-bound C3 convertase $[\text{C3b}\overline{Bb}]^*$. This in turn initiates activation of the alternative pathway. Properdin (not shown) stabilizes C3bBb as the complex PC3bBb. Failure of a surface to provide a suitable microenvironment results in displacement of Bb by Factor H and inactivation of C3b by Factors I and H. Initiation is thus aborted.

serves as a recognition unit and dictates whether the pathway is triggered or aborted.[132] Initiation and activation of this pathway therefore require the initial deposition of C3b molecules on a biologic surface and recognition of this surface by the C3b molecules as an activator or a nonactivator. However, generation of C3b molecules cannot occur unless C3 is acted on by a C3 converting enzyme.

For many years, a difficult and controversial question has been where the initial C3 converting enzyme comes from. According to a currently recognized theory, a C3b-like C3 [C3(H_2O) or "C3"] arises by nonenzymatic, spontaneous thiolester bond hydrolysis of C3 so that a low steady-state concentration of the initial C3 convertase (C3 Bb) of the alternative pathway[140, 141, 171] is always present (Fig. 13–6). This C3b-like C3 ("C3"), which has undergone thiolester hydrolysis without the loss of its C3a fragment, behaves functionally like C3b with respect to Factors B and H binding, its susceptibility to cleavage by Factor I, and most importantly, its ability to form a fluid-phase C3 convertase in the presence of Factors B and $\overline{D}$ and Mg^{++}. Thus hydrated C3 and Factor B bind in the presence of Mg^{++}, and Factor B is cleaved by Factor $\overline{D}$ to generate the initial fluid-phase C3 converting enzyme—the $\overline{\text{"C3" Bb}}$ complex.[132] The first molecule of C3b produced by this enzyme thus sets in motion the C3b-dependent positive-feedback mechanism in which a molecule of C3b and Factor B[68] form a loose complex in the presence of Mg^{++}. This complex, in which C3b serves as a cofactor,[130] interacts with Factor $\overline{D}$,[86] which cleaves Factor B into two fragments: Ba (MW 30,000) is released into the medium and has been shown to have chemotactic activity,[74] whereas Bb remains bound to C3b to form the $\overline{\text{C3bBb}}$ complex. This is the C3 convertase of the alternative pathway, and the larger fragment Bb (MW 93,000) bears the active site for C3 cleavage. In addition, Bb has been reported to cause monocytes or macrophages to spread on surfaces.[4]

Because factor $\overline{D}$ is not incorporated into the $\overline{\text{C3bBb}}$ complex, it can thus generate multiple C3 convertases in a short time. However, $\overline{\text{C3bBb}}$ is labile and in the presence of Factor H dissociates to form an inactive Bb (iBb) plus C3bH. This enzyme can be stabilized upon addition of the cofactor properdin (P), which binds reversibly to C3b and forms a more stable $\overline{\text{PC3bBb}}$ enzyme.[40, 119] This stabilized enzyme then digests C3 to yield C3a and C3b. By analogy with the classical pathway, addition of a second C3b molecule to this complex forms $\overline{\text{P (C3b)}_2\text{Bb}}$, which then acts as a C5 convertase.[119] The C5 convertases (like the C3 convertases) of both pathways share the same specificity.[40, 119] There is therefore considerable structural and functional similarity between the enzymes of the alternative and classical pathways.[163] Factor B is the equivalent of C2, and C3b acts like C4b.[163] However, C2 is cleaved by $\overline{\text{C1s}}$ even in the absence of C4b, but Factor B is cleaved by Factor $\overline{D}$ only when it is complexed with C3b. The remainder of the cascade (formation and assembly of the MAC) proceeds essentially as that seen with the classical pathway and is described below.

Initiation of the alternative pathway differs, however, from that of the classical pathway in that the initiating enzyme, Factor $\overline{D}$, appears to circulate as an active enzyme and has no precursor or proenzyme form.[110] However, unless the substrate of $\overline{D}$ is assembled properly on a surface, activation does not proceed. Although the alternative pathway can be activated immunologically, it can also be triggered by a variety of other nonimmunologic agents, such as endotoxin (lipopolysaccharide),[48] inulin (polyfructose), zymosan,[128] rabbit erythrocytes,[150] or certain lymphoblastoid cells. In addition, activation can be triggered by immune complexes involving IgA antibody or by IgG antiviral antibody complexed to cells infected with virus.[90] This last reaction has been demonstrated using measles, mumps, influenza, and herpes simplex viruses and suggests that IgG-containing immune complexes (including IgG_4) can activate it as well.

Of particular interest is the special function played by two plasma regulators in controlling initiation and amplification of the alternative pathway. One protein, Factor H, is a 150,000 MW, single-chain molecule that binds to C3b[171] and can therefore dissociate Bb from $\overline{\text{C3bBb}}$. Once dissociated, Bb is inactive (iBb) and cannot bind ($\overline{\text{C3bBb}}$ + Factor H →C3bH + iBb), thus dissassembling the C3 convertase. Another regulator is Factor I, which can cleave C3b to form iC3b, which can no longer interact with Bb to form a viable enzyme.[143] However, cleavage of fluid-phase C3b by Factor I is dependent on the presence of Factor H,[202] and inactivation of surface-bound C3b is greatly enhanced by Factor H.[202] It has been shown that surfaces that initiate the alternative pathway have the property of excluding or preventing the reactions involving Factors I and H so that initiation by $\overline{D}$ proceeds, whereas nonactivating surfaces allow these inhibitors to function and activation is prevented.[39, 138, 139]

In one model system, it has been shown that rabbit erythrocytes can initiate the human alternative pathway and sheep erythrocytes cannot. Treatment of sheep erythrocytes with neuraminidase to remove sialic acid converts the sheep erythrocytes into an initiator.[36, 139, 141] As predicted, rabbit cells were relatively deficient in sialic acid. It therefore appears that the presence of sialic acid, as well as polyanions such as heparan sulfate favors binding of Factor H to the surface so that initiation of the alternative complement pathway is inhibited. Thus although a large number of cells are capable of binding C3b, only those that are capable of providing the C3b molecule with a microenvironment protected from the actions of Factors H and I can succeed in promoting a self-destructive event, that is, activation of complement on their surface.

One of the mechanisms by which bystander cells are protected against accidental lysis by complement may be due to the presence of two types of regulatory proteins with Factor H-like activities that have been isolated from human erythrocytes. The first of these proteins is a 205,000 MW glycoprotein that constitutes the C3b receptor or CR1[37] and is present in B cells, PMNs, monocytes,[38] and a certain subpopulation of T cells (reviewed in 35). It is characterized by its ability to dissociate the $\overline{C3bBb}$ and $\overline{C4b2b}$ enzymes, bind C3b, block binding of Factor B to C3b, and modulate C3b and C3bi cleavage by Factor I[21, 38, 79, 88, 117, 120, 121, 170] to form C3c plus α_2D (C3dg). The second is a 70,000 MW glycoprotein that has been named the decay-accelerating factor (DAF)[135] as it can efficiently cause the decay dissociation of both the classical and alternative pathway C3 converting enzymes.[37] Another cell surface protein with complement regulatory properties has been identified.[122] This molecule, designated membrane cofactor protein (MCP), can also serve as a cofactor for Factor I in the cleavage of C3b and C4b and, like DAF, has a wide tissue distribution.

The biologic significance of these regulators was recognized when it was shown that 44% of the red blood cells from a patient with paroxysmal nocturnal hemoglobinuria (PNH) that were susceptible to lysis by acidified complement were found to be devoid of DAF even though CR1 antigen was present.[142, 143] The molecular defect underlying the clinical manifestations of PNH may thus be due, in part, to the absence of membrane-associated DAF.[143] DAF is therefore the critical factor for dissociation of cell-bound C4b2a or C3bBb, although CR1 or fluid-phase C4b-bp and Factor H are capable of doing the same thing. CR1 binding seems critical as a Factor I cofactor, a property it shares with C4b-bp and Factor H. DAF dissociates the convertases by binding C3b or C4b and displacing Bb or 2a, respectively, but does not serve as a cofactor for Factor I cleavage of C3b or C4b. Systemic lupus erythematosus (SLE) patients have been shown to have an inherited partial deficiency in erythrocyte C3b receptors. In addition, some SLE patients with proliferative glomerulonephritis had an absence of glomerular C3b receptors. These deficiencies were postulated to contribute to systemic and organ-specific abnormalities in the clearance of immune complexes and thereby contribute to the pathogenesis of this disease.[35]

MEMBRANE ATTACK COMPLEX

Complement-induced membrane damage and cytolysis is the final step of both the classical and alternative pathways (and probably of the MBP pathway) and is entirely dependent on the activation and assembly of five structurally and functionally related precursor proteins, C5, C6, C7, C8, and C9, which have the capacity of undergoing a hydrophilic-amphiphilic transition. The C8 molecule is a heterotrimer composed of α, β, and γ chains, which are the products of three distinct genes and organized in the molecule such that the α and γ subunits are disulfide linked with each other whereas the β subunit is noncovalently associated with the α, γ dimer. A remarkably striking feature of all the members of the membrane attack complex (MAC), with the exception of C8γ, is that they contain several structural and functional modules, including a thrombospondin (TSR) module, an LDLr module, an EGF module, a MAC-specific domain, and a lytic domain that is approximately 200 residues in length. Whereas C8α and C8β have an extra TSR module at the C-terminal end, C8γ, which is not required for hemolytic function, is structurally different from the other members of MAC and therefore does not contain these modules.[24, 25, 71, 72, 80, 164]

Enzymatic cleavage of a single peptide bond in C5 initiates self-assembly of these proteins into a supramolecular organization designated the MAC of complement.[98] Assembly proceeds from formation of the stable bimolecular complex C5b-6 to the reaction of C5b-6 with C7. This results in formation of the intermediate complex C5b-7, which possesses a strong binding site for biologic membranes.[152] After the three-chain C8 molecule is bound to the C5b-7 via its C5b recognition site on the β-chain, the C5b-8 complex reacts with multiple C9 molecules leading to the formation of MAC.[194, 195]

No enzymatic function has been attributed to C8; however, C6 has been reported to contain a catalytic site that can hydrolyze acetyl glycyl-lysine-methyl ester and is inactivated by DFP[97]; it is assumed that C7 might have similar properties.[96] In the fluid phase, C8 has a single binding site for C9, and the interaction is reversible (Ka $\simeq 10^7$ M^{-1}).[161] However, several C9 molecules are bound to a target cell–bound C5b-8, and this association is virtually irreversible (Ka $\simeq 10^{11}$ M^{-1}).[161] Binding of a molecule of C9 to C5b-8 further facilitates C9-C9 interaction. The energy derived from this interaction effects the unfolding of monomeric C9 (long axis changes from 80 to 160 Å)[161] as it polymerizes to form poly-C9. Poly-C9 is amphiphilic and capable of inserting itself into hydrophobic environments such as lipid bilayers.[161] Individually spaced C5b-8 molecules can bind 12 to 16 molecules of C9, and clusters of C5b-8 molecules can bind 6 to 8 molecules. It appears that a larger poly-C9 is generated by an individually spaced C5b-8, and as few as two C5b-8 form a poly-C9[158] with fewer molecules.

Assembly of MAC results in the expression of hydrophobicity by the otherwise hydrophilic proteins. This property seems to be responsible for the insertion of C5b-7 into target membranes[156] and for membrane damage caused by the binding of C8 and C9 to C5b-7 complexes.[81, 159] Membrane damage and cytolysis caused by MAC has been attributed to lipid bilayer perturbation[34, 153] and transmembrane channel[115, 157] formation,[115, 158, 194] followed by osmotic lysis due to ion exchange with the external environment, with uptake of water accompanying sodium influx. Each lesion on the target cell membrane actually consists of (C5b-8) poly-C9 and is visualized by electron microscopy as a circular hollow structure $\simeq$ 12 nm above the membrane surface with inner and outer diameters of 10 to 11 nm and 21 nm, respectively.[85] Although it is not an essential component of immune hemolysis, C9 markedly increases the rate of lysis of cells bearing C5b-8 (erythrocytes, *Escherichia coli*,[177] Raji cells,[157, 179] and other nucleated cells). C9 is also a critical component of the MAC-induced ultrastructural membrane lesions.[28, 155]

Without C9, the C5b-8 complex possesses a certain degree of membranolytic activity as it can destroy *Neisseria gonorrhoeae*,[76] and individuals with homozygous C9 deficiency do not suffer from infections.[73, 106, 107, 144, 185] Apparently, the phospholipid binding capacity and the ability of the complex to organize and thereby weaken membrane structures are sufficient to impair the normal function of some structures.[153, 156]

It has also been shown that isolated C9 could undergo spontaneous polymerization at 37° C to form circular polymers resembling the ultrastructure of MAC.[195] Such poly-C9 can become an integral membrane protein having membranolytic activity and the ultrastructural appearance characteristic of complement-induced membrane lesions.[160] Circular poly-C9 forms spontaneously upon prolonged incubation of C9 at 37°C but requires greater activation energy than that mediated by C5b-8.[160] Ultrastructurally, poly-C9 is described as a 160 Å long tubule with an internal diameter of 100 to 110 Å rimmed on one end by a torus with a 210 Å outer diameter terminated on the opposite end by a membrane-binding hydrophobic domain.[160] Polymerization is accompanied by a change in secondary structure, with doubling of its axis from 80 Å (C9 monomer) to 160 Å, and by a hydrophilic-amphiphilic transition, enabling C9 to insert itself into phospholipid bilayers.[160] One unique characteristic of poly-C9 is that it becomes extremely resistant to SDS as well as protease digestion. It is suggested that this resistance may be a prerequisite for its function as the cytotoxic unit of the MAC complex.[161]

MAC is under control of several plasma (S-protein, SP40,40) or membrane-associated (HRF, CD59) proteins that closely regulate the undesired assembly of MAC on homologous surfaces. The S-protein (vitronectin, MW 80,000) binds to C5b-7 complex and prevents C8 from binding. Similarly, the apolipoprotein SP40,40, also known as clusterin (MW 80,000), inhibits C5b-7 activity and is found at high concentrations in seminal fluid, where it is thought to play an important role in protecting spermatozoa from complement attack.[105] The cell surface molecules HRF (homologous restriction factor, MW 65,000) and CD59 (also known as HRF20, MW 19,000) both bind to C8 and interfere with the formation of MAC assembly by preventing C9 polymerization.[105] CD59 has a GPI anchor and is present on the membrane of many cell types and tissues. Its absence in PNH is a second critical abnormality (in addition to DAF) leading to hemolysis.

Complement-mediated and cytotoxic cell–mediated membrane lesions have striking similarities, which were further confirmed when two types (T1 and T2, 16 and 5 nm diameter, respectively) of complement-like membrane lesions were observed using cloned mouse natural killer (NK) cells as effectors and rabbit erythrocytes as target cells.[154] The lesions apparently arise by membrane insertion of tubular complexes, called perforins, that are assembled from subunits during the cytolytic action. Perforin, like MAC, has a lytic domain of approximately 200 amino acid residues and is about 25% identical to that of MAC. Unlike MAC, however, perforin does not appear to require other proteins for its assembly and lytic function but does require Ca^{2+} for its function (see Chapter 4).

COMPLEMENT-DERIVED BIOLOGICALLY ACTIVE FRAGMENTS AND THEIR RECEPTORS

One of the many striking features of the complement system is that its activation results not only in the destruction of a marked target cell but also in the concomitant generation of several biologically active cleavage products. That such fragments play an important role in various types of immune reactions, such as phagocytosis, chemotaxis, anaphylaxis, acute shock, and acute allergic reactions, as well as several other inflammatory responses, is well documented.[83] It was also shown that certain active peptides can interact with the immune system and modulate the immune response.[200]

Activation of the classical pathway leads to the generation of most of the presently well characterized fragments. Enzymatic digestion of C4 by $C\overline{1}$ produces two fragments: C4a (MW 8,650) and C4b (MW 198,000). Isolated C4a was found to be spasmogenic (guinea pig ileum at 1 μM), to cause muscle desensitization with respect to C3a but not C5a (tachyphylaxis at 0.33 μM), and to enhance vascular permeability (human skin, 1 nmol), with immediate erythema and edema formation.[66, 67] Because the spasmogenic, tachyphylactic, and vascular activities of C4a were abrogated by removal of the COOH-terminal arginine, a property that is characteristic of C3a and C5a, it was concluded that C4a represents yet another complement-derived anaphylatoxin.

All three anaphylatoxins, C3a, C4a, and C5a, are generated by proteolytic cleavage in the course of complement activation and as such share several structural and functional properties. First, except for chemotactic activity, which is a property of C5a and C5a des Arg (C5a minus carboxy-terminal arginine), or C3a[20a] expression of most other biologic activities depends on the presence of the COOH-terminal arginine residue (see Table 13–3). The activity of C5a des Arg requires the presence of a cochemotaxin that has been identified as the vitamin D–binding protein.[149] Second, partial sequence analysis suggests that there is structural homology between these polypeptides with a helical conformation of 50, 54, and 45% for C3a, C4a, and C5a, respectively.[41, 66, 67] In addition, C3a, C4a, and C5a are capable of inducing histamine release from mast cells and release of hydrolytic enzymes from neutrophils, causing contraction of smooth muscle, and enhancing vascular permeability.[83]

It has also become apparent that these activation peptides can play a role in immune regulation. For example, when cultures of human peripheral blood lymphocytes were incubated with human C3a, the ability of these cells to produce polyclonal antibody was suppressed. Addition of C3a des Arg failed to cause any significant suppression,[127] suggesting that the COOH-terminal arginine was required for this activity. In contrast to C3a, however, highly purified preparations of C5a or C5a des Arg were found to enhance the primary in vitro anti-SRBC responses of both human and mouse lymphocytes.[126] Concentrations of C5a as low as 10 ng/ml significantly increased the response of mouse spleen cells.[126]

Another complement-derived fragment capable of exhibiting certain types of immunoregulatory functions is C3d-K, which is a cleavage product derived from iC3b by kallikrein (see Fig. 13–4) and as such represents a novel peptide with biologic functions.[123] C3d-K was found to inhibit mitogen-antigen and alloantigen-induced T lymphocyte proliferation. Furthermore, this fragment induced leukocytosis when injected intravenously into mice or rabbits. Because leukocytosis-mobilizing activity is a property ascribed to C3e,[52] a 10,000 MW fragment derived late in the degradation process from C3c, it is postulated that C3d-K possesses some of the functional domains of C3e.[123]

In addition to its ability to induce leukocytosis, the C3e fragment causes vascular permeability (see Fig. 13–5) with cellular infiltration when injected intradermally,[52] and causes the release of lysosomal enzymes from PMNs.[49] These enzymes can generate chemotactic activity when incubated with highly purified human C5.[49] PMNs and monocytes are also known to express receptors for C3e.[49] Because the fragment can be generated from serum by certain types of gram-negative bacteria, such as *Pseudomonas aeruginosa,*[52] the current theory is that it represents a late degradative polypeptide that is released during bacterial infections and septicemia (see Table 13–4) (B. Ghebrehiwet, unpublished data).

The larger cleavage products also participate in several immunologic reactions. The well-known complement-dependent immune adherence reactions, for instance, are mediated largely by the covalent bound complement cleavage products (C3b and C4b), which react with receptors of various types of cell. Such cell-bound C3b and C4b are capable of mediating the opsonization of target cells and thus facilitating phagocytosis, release of lysosomal enzymes from a variety of cells (including PMNs, macrophages, and platelets), and potentiation of cell-mediated cellular cytotoxicity.[51, 145]

From studies of the mechanism of phagocytosis,[29] it became clear that macrophages possess membrane receptors for Fc and C3b. Ingestion of sensitized erythrocytes depends on the interaction between these receptors and the red blood cell–associated ligands C3b and IgG.[137] Furthermore, it was observed that these receptors have synergistic roles in phagocytosis: C3b receptors mainly promote adherence of the sensitized particles to phagocytes, and the Fc receptors promote ingestion of the particles (reviewed in 137). It appears that C4b reacts with the same receptor and has similar biologic effects, although the amount of C4b bound to the complement fixation site is smaller than that of C3b and thus of less in vivo significance. In addition, C3b and C4b have a role in the solubilization of immune complexes. This solubilization apparently results from the intercalation of these proteins into the immune complex lattice.[137] Deposition of immune complexes is known to be a major mechanism of tissue injury and inflammation. Thus the interaction of complement-derived peptides with cellular receptors and its contribution to the clearance of immune complexes is of great potential significance.[137]

A variety of cell types from different animal species are known to possess distinct cell surface receptors for various complement components (reviewed in 175). These interactions elicit a variety of biologic responses that have a major role in the mechanisms involved in host defense and certain types of inflammatory reactions. The most studied of these are the receptors for the C3 fragments, such as C3b (CR1; erythrocytes, PMNs, monocytes, and B lymphocytes), C3d (CR2; B lymphocytes, K cells with T-cell markers, and lymphoblastoid cells), and C3bi (CR3; PMNs, monocytes, and B lymphocytes). C3b in serum or on the surface of activating particles is rapidly cleaved to iC3b by Factor I and its serum or cell surface cogactors.[105, 122, 183] The subsequent conversion of iC3b to the two physiologic fragments, C3c and C3dg, is relatively slow, however. Therefore, the most important receptor in terms of opsonization and phagocytosis may be CR3, the receptor for iC3b (see Table 13–3). CR3 (CD11a/CD11b) belongs to a β_2 subgroup of $\alpha\beta$ heterodimeric adhesion molecules known as integrins, in which their β_2 subunit interacts with one of the three α chains to give CR3 or Mac-1 ($\alpha M\beta_2$), LFA-1 antigen ($\alpha L\beta_2$), and p150,95 ($\alpha X\beta_2$). The significance of complement receptors in immune complex clearance is well documented, especially in immune complex–mediated diseases, where complement deficiency is known to perpetuate the inflammatory process. The most abundant cell type in the blood of primates expressing CR1, the receptor for C3b and C4b, is the red cell (platelets on nonprimates), which upon encountering complement-bearing immune complexes, shuttles them to the liver and spleen. Here, they are dislodged from the erythrocytes and digested by macrophage enzymes while the erythrocyte recirculates into the blood.

Other complement receptors that have been well characterized include the receptors for C5a and C1q. The C5a receptor (C5a-R) is a member of the rhodopsin superfamily of proteins that are characterized by having seven transmembrane helixes. The C5a receptor acts via a GTP-binding protein complex and has approximately 35% sequence identity with the f-Met-Leu-Phe receptor, and both mediate similar but not identical responses in monocytes and neutrophils. Contrary to the previously held theory that there are two types of anaphylatoxin receptors, one for C5a and the other common to both C3a and C4a, studies have suggested that there are indeed two distinct receptors for C3a and C4a, at least on monocytes and macrophages. Furthermore, although neither the structure of C3a-R nor that of C4a-R has been elucidated, the structure of C3a-R, at least, is likely to be similar to that of C5a-R since C3a activates the respiratory burst[31, 32, 46, 47] and stimulates Ca^{2+} influx in neutrophils[31, 32, 135] via a pertussis toxin–sensitive G protein (reviewed in 31, 47, 201).

The C1q receptor (C1q-R), on the other hand, is ubiquitously expressed.[57, 58] The cellular responses elicited as a result of C1q interaction with cells are also as diverse as the type of cells that express C1q receptors,[8, 53, 70, 146, 147] each cell type utilizing the receptor for a specific function within a defined microenvironment.[50, 192] These functions include promotion of cell adhesion of fibroblasts, induction of antiproliferative response on B and T cells, stimulation of Ca^{2+}-activated $K+$ channels and initiation of chemotaxis on mouse fibroblasts and mast cells, and enhancement of phagocytosis by neutrophils.[50, 54] There are at least three single-chain, highly acidic, noncross-reacting cell surface molecules that bind to human C1q: a 60-kD calreticulin-like glycoprotein that binds to the collagen-like tail of C1q,[50, 54, 70, 112, 113] a 126-kD monocyte/neutrophil-expressed protein that also binds to the collagen-like tail of C1q,[69, 192] and a 33-kD glycoprotein with affinity for the globular heads of the C1q molecule.[58] The 60-kD and 33-kD molecules are referred to as cC1q-R and gC1q-R, respectively, and are coexpressed on a wide range of cell types.[54, 58] The gC1q-R molecule, which was first isolated from Raji cells, has been cloned and expressed in *Escherichia coli*, and the unglycosylated, recombinant protein was found to retain its C1q-binding properties.[58] The 60-kD, cClq-R has not been molecularly cloned but is believed to be a surface-expressed homologue of the high affinity Ca^{2+}-binding protein, calreticulin.[113, 186]

INTERACTION BETWEEN THE COMPLEMENT SYSTEM AND THE INTRINSIC COAGULATION PATHWAYS

A remarkable similarity exists between the mechanisms involved in the activation of the complement system and those of the Hageman factor–dependent pathways that lead to blood coagulation, fibrinolysis, and kinin formation. Both systems require initial contact with an activator, which in turn initiates a cascade of reactions involving the sequential activation and conversion of zymogens to their proteolytic form. The inhibitor of $C\overline{1}$ ($C\overline{1}$-INH), which inactivates $C\overline{1}$ by binding to the $C\overline{1r}$ and $C\overline{1s}$ subcomponents of the molecule, is also a major plasma inhibitor[44, 75, 166, 167] of activated Hageman factor (HFa or XIIa),[44, 75, 166, 167] Hageman factor fragment (HFf),[174] Factor XIa,[44, 78] and kallikrein[63, 166] by the formation of stoichiometric complexes. It is a minor inhibitor of plasmin.[75, 166] This inhibitor is known to be functionally absent in patients with hereditary angioedema,[26] a disease inherited as an autosomal-dominant mendelian character that manifests by swelling and recurrent attacks of mucosal edema of the gastrointestinal and upper respiratory tracts.

Uninhibited activation of HF may trigger the kinin system by conversion of prekallikrein to kallikrein, which in turn cleaves bradykinin from high molecular weight (HMW) kininogen. In the absence of $C\overline{1}$-INH, therefore, any tissue injury that might trigger activation of the intrinsic coagulation cascade would generate large amounts of bradykinin, a potent mediator that causes increased vascular permeability.[92] Because the autoactivation of HF, the conversion of prekallikrein to kallikrein, and the effects of kallikrein on HF and HMW kininogen would be augmented[91] in the absence of $C\overline{1}$-INH, it is of particular interest to know that HFf,[55, 56] plasmin,[165] and to a very small degree HFa (B. Ghebrehiwet, M. Silverberg, and A. P. Kaplan, unpublished data) can activate complement via the classical pathway, whereas kallikrein[11, 23] activates both the classical and alternative pathways.

In terms of potency, the major complement activator appears to be HFf, which enzymatically cleaves C1r to form $C\overline{1r}$.[55] Activation of complement leads to the production and release of vasoactive peptides such as C4a, and perhaps a C2-derived[27] or a C2-dependent peptide with kinin-like activity. Data suggest the presence of a peptide sequence within C2b with kinin-like activity. Cleavage of C2b to release this peptide has not been demonstrated, although it is postulated that this peptide may be a product of cleavage of C2b by plasmin.[188] The inactivation of bradykinin in plasma is dependent on carboxypeptidase N (kininase I), which cleaves the C-terminal arginine from bradykinin and inactivates it.[33] This is the same protein known as the anaphylatoxin inactivator,[6] which inactivates C3a, C4a, and C5a. Because the anaphylatoxins lead to histamine release from basophils and mast cells, this plasma carboxypeptidase acts to control two types of vasodilators that have similar phlogistic properties. In contrast, kininase II, which inactivates bradykinin, is also capable of generating the vasoconstrictor angiotensin II from angiotensin I.[92]

Interaction of these pathways is also seen in acute gout. In this case, monosodium urate crystals are believed to initiate the inflammatory reaction.[59, 126] In addition to activation of the classic[59, 133] and alternative[42] pathways of complement, urate crystals have been shown to activate HF in human plasma and synovial fluid.[64] That complement participates in the pathogenesis of gout has been reported previously.[94, 199] In view of these findings, it is possible to postulate that activated HF plays a role in the pathogenesis of this disease through either the generation of bradykinin or activation of complement to produce vasoactive peptides. In general, the absence of an inhibitor such as $C\overline{1}$-INH may upset homeostatic mechanisms that involve more than one pathway and are more likely to lead to severe disease than does the absence of a proenzyme, particularly if the function of the latter can be bypassed by some other pathway.

ACKNOWLEDGMENTS

This revised chapter was supported by grant 94405 from the American Heart Association (New York Affiliate) and IM 771 from the American Cancer Society and was written while the author was on a Wellcome Research Fellowship (0001) at the MRC Immunochemistry Unit, Department of Biochemistry, University of Oxford, United Kingdom.

REFERENCES

1. Alper CA, Colten HR, Rosen FS, et al: Homozygous deficiency of C3 in a patient with repeated infections. Lancet 2:1179, 1972.
2. Alper CA, Johnson AM, Cirtch AG, Moore FD: Human C3: evidence for the liver as the primary site of synthesis. Science 16:286, 1969.
3. Arlaud GJ, Gagnon J, Porter RR: The catalytic chain of human complement subcomponent $C\overline{1r}$. Biochem J 201:49, 1982.
4. Bianco C, Gotze O, Cohn ZA: Regulation of macrophages migration by products of the complement system. Proc Natl Acad Sci USA 76:888, 1979.
5. Bokisch VA, Dierich MP, Müller-Eberhard HJ: Third component of complement (C3): structural properties in relation to function. Proc Natl Acad Sci USA 72:1989, 1975.
6. Bokisch VA, Müller-Eberhard HJ: Anaphylatoxin inactivator of human plasma: its isolation and characterization as a carboxypeptidase. J Clin Invest 49:2427, 1970.
7. Bokisch VA, Müller-Eberhard HJ, Cochrane CG: Isolation of a fragment (C3a) of the third component of human complement containing anaphylatoxin and chemotactic activity and description of an anaphylatoxin inactivator of human serum. J Exp Med 129:1109, 1969.
8. Bordin S, Smith M, Ghebrehiwet B, et al: Smooth muscle and epithelial cells express specific binding sites for the C1q component of complement. Clin Immunol Immunopathol 63:51, 1992.
9. Brade V, Fries W, Bently C: Identification of properdin, B, D, and C3 as biosynthetic products of guinea pig peritoneal macrophages and influence of culture conditions on their secretion. J Immunol 120:1766, 1978.
10. Budzko DB, Müller-Eberhard HJ: Cleavage of the fourth component of human complement (C4) by C1 esterase: isolation and characterization of the low molecular weight product. Immunochemistry 7:227, 1970.

11. Calcott MA, Müller-Eberhard HJ: C1q protein of human complement. Biochemistry 11:3443, 1972.
12. Chenoweth DE, Hugli TE: Demonstration of specific C5a receptor on intact human polymorphonuclear leukocytes. Proc Natl Acad Sci USA 75:3943, 1978.
13. Cochrane CG, Müller-Eberhard HJ: The derivation of two distinct anaphylatoxin activities from the third and fourth components of human complement. J Exp Med 127:371, 1968.
14. Colten HR: Ontogeny of the human complement system: in vitro biosynthesis of individual complement components by fetal tissue. J Clin Invest 51:725, 1972.
15. Cooper NR: Activation and regulation of the first complement component. Fed Proc 42:134, 1983.
16. Cooper NR: Enzymatic activity of the second component of complement. Biochemistry 14:4245, 1975.
17. Cooper NR, Jensen RC, Welsh RM, Oldstone M: Lysis of RNA tumor viruses by human serum: direct antibody independent triggering of the classical complement pathway. J Exp Med 144:970, 1976.
18. Cooper NR, Miles LA, Griffin JH: Effects of plasma kallikrein and plasmin on the first component of complement. J Immunol 124:1517, 1980.
19. Cooper NR, Morrison DC: Binding and activation of the first component of human complement by the lipid A region of lipopolysaccharides. J Immunol 120:1862, 1978.
20. Curd JG, Yelvington M, Burridge N, et al: Generation of bradykinin during incubation of hereditary angioedema plasma. Mol Immunol 19:1365, 1982.
20a. Daffern PJ, Pfeifer PH, Ember JA, et al: C3a is a chemotaxin for human eosinophils but not for neutrophils. C3a stimulation of neutrophils is secondary to eosinophil activation. J Exp Med 181:2119, 1995.
21. Daha MR, Kok DJ, Van Es LA: Regulation of the C3 nephritic factor stabilized C3/C5 convertase of complement by purified human erythrocyte C3b receptor. Clin Exp Immunol 50:209, 1982.
22. Dias Da Silva W, Eisele JW, Lepow LH: Complement as a mediator of inflammation. III. Purification of the activity with anaphylatoxin properties generated by interaction of the first four components of complement and its identification as a cleavage product of C3. J Exp Med 126:1027, 1967.
23. DiScipio RG: The activation of the alternative pathway C3 convertase by human plasma kallikrein. Immunology 45:587, 1982.
24. DiScipio RG, Chakravarti DN, Müller-Eberhard HJ, Fey GH: The structure of human complement component C7 and the C5b-7 complex. J Biol Chem 263:549, 1988.
25. DiScipio RG, Hugli TE: The molecular architecture of human complement C6. J Biol Chem 264:16197, 1989.
26. Donaldson VH, Evans LR: A biochemical abnormality in hereditary angioneurotic edema. Am J Med 35:37, 1963.
27. Donaldson VH, Ratnoff OD, DaSilva WD, Rosen FS: Permeability increasing activity in hereditary angioneurotic edema plasma. II. Mechanism of formation and partial characterization. J Clin Invest 48:642, 1969.
28. Dourmashkin RR: The structural events associated with the attachment of complement components to cell membranes in reactive lysis. Immunology 35:205, 1978.
29. Ehlenberger AG, Nussenzweig V: The role of membrane receptors for C3b and C3d in phagocytosis. J Exp Med 145:345, 1977.
30. Eisenstein LP, Hansen PJ, Ballow M, et al: Biosynthesis of the third component of complement (C3) in vitro by monocytes from both normal and homozygous C3 deficient humans. J Clin Invest 60:963, 1977.
31. Elsner J, Oppermann M, Czech W, Kapp A: C3a activates the respiratory burst in human polymorphonuclear neutrophilic leukocytes via pertussis toxin-sensitive G-proteins. Blood 83:3324, 1994.
32. Elsner J, Oppermann M, Czech W, et al: C3a activates reactive oxygen radical species production and intracellular calcium transients in human eosinophils. Eur J Immunol 24:518, 1994.
33. Erdos EG, Sloane EM: An enzyme in human blood plasma that inactivates bradykinin and kallidins. Biochem Pharmacol 11:585, 1962.
34. Esser AF, Kolb WP, Podak ER, Müller-Eberhard HJ: Molecular reorganization of lipid bilayers by complement: a possible mechanism for membranolysis. Proc Natl Acad Sci USA 76:1410, 1979.
35. Fearon DT: Identification of the membrane glycoprotein that is the C3b receptor of the human erythrocyte, polymorphonuclear leukocyte, B lymphocyte, and monocyte. J Exp Med 152:20, 1980.
36. Fearon DT: Regulation by membrane sialic acid of β1H-dependent decay-dissociation of amplification C3 convertase of the alternative complement pathway. Proc Natl Acad Sci USA 75:1971, 1978.
37. Fearon DT: Regulation of the amplification C3 convertase of human complement by an inhibiting protein isolated from human erythrocyte membrane. Proc Natl Acad Sci USA 76:5867, 1979.
38. Fearon DT: The human C3b receptor. Springer Semin Immunopathol 6:159, 1983.
39. Fearon DT, Austen KF: Activation of the alternative complement pathway due to resistance of zymosan-bound amplification convertase to endogenous regulatory mechanisms. Proc Natl Acad Sci USA 74:1683, 1977.
40. Fearon DT, Austen KF: Properdin: binding to C3b and stabilization of the C3b-dependent convertase. J Exp Med 142:856, 1975.
41. Fernandez HM, Hugli TE: Primary structural analysis of the polypeptide portion of human C5a anaphylatoxin. J Biol Chem 253:6955, 1978.
42. Fields TR, Abramson SB, Weissmann G, et al: Activation of the alternative pathway of complement by monosodium urate crystals. Clin Immunol Immunopathol 26:249, 1983.
43. Fields TR, Ghebrehiwet B, Kaplan AP: Kinin formation in hereditary angioedema plasma: evidence against kinin derivation from C2 and in support of "spontaneous" formation of bradykinin. J Allergy Clin Immunol 72:54, 1983.
44. Forbes CO, Pensky J, Ratnoff OD: Inhibition of activated Hageman factor and activated plasma thromboplastin antecedent by purified C1 inactivator. J Lab Clin Med 76:809, 1970.
45. Fujita T, Nussenzweig V: The role of C4-binding protein β1H in proteolysis of C4b and C3b. J Exp Med 150:267, 1979.
46. Gerard C, Gerard NP: C5a anaphylatoxin and its seven transmembrane-segment receptor. Annu Rev Immunol 12:775, 1994.
47. Gerard C, Gerard NP: The pro-inflammatory seven transmembrane segment receptors of the leukocyte. Curr Opin Immunol 6:140, 1994.
48. Gewurz H, Pickering RJ, Synderman R, et al: Interactions of the complement system with endotoxic lipopolysaccharides in immunoglobulins deficient sera. J Exp Med 128:817, 1968.
49. Ghebrehiwet B: The release of lysosomal enzymes from human polymorphonuclear leukocytes by human C3e. Clin Immunol Immunopathol 30:321, 1984.
50. Ghebrehiwet B: Functions associated with the C1q receptor. Behring Inst Mitt 84:204, 1989.
51. Ghebrehiwet B, Medicus RB, Müller-Eberhard HJ: Potentiation of antibody-dependent cell-mediated cytotoxicity by target-cell-bound C3b. J Immunol 123:1285, 1979.
52. Ghebrehiwet B, Müller-Eberhard HJ: C3e: an acidic fragment of human C3 with leukocytosis inducing activity. J Immunol 123:616, 1979.
53. Ghebrehiwet B, Müller-Eberhard HJ: Lysis of C1q-coated chicken erythrocytes by human lymphoblastoid cell lines. J Immunol 120:27, 1978.
54. Ghebrehiwet B, Peerschke EIB: The C1q-R participates in immunoregulation and signal transduction. Behring Inst Mitt 93:236, 1993.
55. Ghebrehiwet B, Randazzo BP, Dunn JT, et al: Mechanisms of activation of the classical pathway of complement by Hageman factor fragment. J Clin Invest 71:1450, 1983.
56. Ghebrehiwet B, Silverberg M, Kaplan AP: Activation of the classical pathway of complement by Hageman factor fragment. J Exp Med 153:665, 1981.
57. Ghebrehiwet B, Silvestri L, McDevitt C: Identification of the Raji cell membrane-derived C1q inhibitor as a receptor for human C1q. Purification and immunochemical characterization. J Exp Med 160:1375, 1984.
58. Ghebrehiwet B, Lim B-L, Peerschke EIB, et al: Isolation, cDNA cloning, and overexpression of a 33-kD cell surface glycoprotein that binds to the globular "heads" of C1q. J Exp Med 179:1809, 1994.
59. Giclas PC, Ginsberg MH, Cooper NR: Immunoglobulin G independent activation of the classical complement pathway by monosodium urate crystals. J Clin Invest 63:759, 1979.
60. Gigli I, Austen KF: Fluid phase destruction of $C2^{hu}$ by $C1^{hu}$. I. Its enhancement and inhibition by homologous and heterologous C4. J Exp Med 128:679, 1969.
61. Gigli I, Austen KF: Fluid phase destruction of $C2^{hu}$ by $C1^{hu}$. II. Unmasking by $C4i^{hu}$ of $C1^{hu}$ specificity for $C2^{hu}$. J Exp Med 130:833, 1969.
62. Gigli I, Fujita T, Nussenzweig V: Modulation of the classical pathway

C3 convertase by plasma proteins C4 binding protein and C3b inactivator. Proc Natl Acad Sci USA 76:6596, 1979.

63. Gigli I, Kaplan A, Austen KF: Alteration in complement component utilization following the interaction of $C1^{hu}$ with kallikrein fragment. J Immunol 107:311, 1971.
64. Ginsberg MH, Jaques B, Cochrane CG, Griffin JH: Urate crystal-dependent cleavage of Hageman factor in human plasma and synovial fluid. J Lab Clin Med 95:497, 1980.
65. Golan M, Burger R, Loos M: Detection of conformational changes within the C1q molecule with monoclonal anti-C1q antibodies. Mol Immunol 19:1371, 1982.
66. Gorski JP, Hugli TE, Müller-Eberhard HJ: C4a; the third anaphylatoxin of the human complement system. Proc Natl Acad Sci USA 76:5299, 1979.
67. Gorski JP, Hugli TE, Müller-Eberhard HJ: Structural and biological properties of human C4a. Fed Proc 38:1010, 1979.
68. Götze O, Müller-Eberhard HJ: The C3 activator system in an alternative pathway of complement activation. J Exp Med 134S:90, 1971.
69. Guan E, Burgess WH, Robinson SL, et al: Phagocytic cell molecules that bind the collagen-like region of C1q. Involvement in the C1q-mediated enhancement of phagocytosis. J Biol Chem 266:20345, 1991.
70. Habicht GS, Beck G, Ghebrehiwet B: Characterization of C1q-induced inhibitors of interleukin 1. Complement 4:163, 1987.
71. Haefliger JA, Tscopp J, Vial N, Jenne DE: Complete primary structure and functional characterization of the sixth component of the human complement system. J Biol Chem 264:18041, 1989.
72. Haefliger JA, Tscopp J, Naedlli D, et al: Complementary DNA cloning of complement C8β and its sequence homology to C9. Biochemistry 26:3551, 1987.
73. Haeney MR, Thompson RA, Faulkner J, et al: Recurrent bacterial meningitis in patients with genetic defects of terminal complement components. Clin Exp Immunol 40:16, 1980.
74. Hamuro J, Hadding V, Bitter-Suermann D: Fragments Ba and Bb derived guinea pig factor B of the properdin system: purification, characterization and biological activities. J Immunol 120:438, 1978.
75. Harpel PD, Cooper NR: Studies on human plasma C1 inactivator—enzyme interactions. I. Mechanisms of interaction with $\overline{C1s}$, plasmin and trypsin. J Clin Invest 55:593, 1975.
76. Harriman GR, Esser AF, Podack ER, et al: The role of C9 in complement-mediated killing of Neisseria. J Immunol 127:2386, 1981.
77. Harrison RA, Lachmann PJ: The physiological breakdown of the third component of human complement. Mol Immunol 17:9, 1980.
78. Heck WH, Kaplan AP: Substrates of Hageman factor. I. Isolation and characterization of human factor XI (PTA) and inhibition of the activated enzyme by α1-antitrypsin. J Exp Med 140:1615, 1974.
79. Hoffmann EM: Inhibition of complement by a substance isolated from human erythrocytes. II. Studies on the site and mechanism of action. Immunochemistry 6:405, 1969.
80. Howard OMZ, Rao AG, Sodetz JM: Complementary DNA and derived amino acid sequence of the β subunit of the human complement protein C8: identification of a close structural and ancestral relationship to the α subunit and C9. Biochemistry 26:3565, 1987.
81. Hu VW, Esser AF, Podack ER, Wisnieski BJ: The membrane attack of complement: photolabeling reveals insertion of terminal proteins into target membranes. J Immunol 127:380, 1981.
82. Hugli TE: Human anaphylatoxin (C3a) from the third component of complement: primary structure. J Biol Chem 250:8293, 1975.
83. Hugli TE: The structural basis for anaphylatoxin and chemotactic functions of C3a, C4a, C5a. CRC Crit Rev Immunol 2:321, 1981.
84. Hugli TE, Müller-Eberhard HJ: Anaphylatoxins: C3a and C5a. Adv Immunol 26:1, 1978.
85. Humphrey JH, Dourmashkin RR: The lesions in cell membranes caused by complement. Adv Immunol 11:75, 1969.
86. Hunsicker LG, Ruddy S, Austen KF: Alternative complement pathway factors involved in cobra venom factor (CoVF) activation of the third component (C3). J Immunol 110:128, 1973.
87. Hurst MM, Volanakis JE, Hester RB, et al: The structural basis for binding of complement by immunoglobulin M. J Exp Med 140:1117, 1974.
88. Ida K, Nussenzweig V: Complement receptor is an inhibitor of the complement cascade. J Exp Med 153:1138, 1981.
89. Ji Y, Fujita T, Hatsuse H, et al: Activation of the C4 and C2 components of complement by a proteinase in serum bactericidal factor, Ra-reactive factor. J Immunol 150:171, 1993.
90. Joseph BS, Cooper NR, Oldstone MBA: Immunologic injury of cultured cells infected with measles virus. I. Role of IgG antibody and the alternative complement pathway. J Exp Med 141:761, 1975.
91. Kaplan AP: Initiation of the intrinsic coagulation and fibrinolytic pathways of man: the role of surfaces, Hageman factor, prekallikrein, high molecular weight kininogen and factor XI. Prog Hemost Thromb 4:127, 1978.
92. Kaplan AP, Ghebrehiwet B, Silverberg M, Sealy JE: The intrinsic coagulation-kinin pathway, complement cascades, plasma renin-angiotension system and their interrelationships. CRC Crit Rev Immunol 3:75, 1981.
93. Kehoe JM, Faugerau M: Immunoglobulin peptide with complement fixing activity. Nature 224:1212, 1969.
94. Kellerman RW, Naff GB: Chemical mediators of inflammation in acute gouty arthritis. Arthritis Rheum 18:765, 1975.
95. Klemperer MR, Donaldson VH, Rosen FS: The vasopermeability response in man to purified C1 esterase. J Clin Invest 46:1079, 1967.
96. Kolb LM, Kolb WP: Expression of antithrombin III (AT111) antigenic determinants by the fluid phase SC5b-9 attack complex of human complement. Fed Proc 41:486, 1982.
97. Kolb WP, Kolb LM, Savary JR: Biochemical characterization of the sixth component (C6) of human complement. Biochemistry 21:294, 1982.
98. Kolb WP, Müller-Eberhard HJ: The membrane attack mechanism of complement: verification of a stable C5b-9 complex in free solution. J Exp Med 138:438, 1973.
99. Lachmann PJ: Complement. In Sela M (ed): The Antigens. Vol. 5. Academic Press, London, 1979, p 283.
100. Lachmann PJ, Pangburn MK, Oldroyd RG: Breakdown of C3 after complement activation: identification of a new fragment, C3g, using monoclonal antibodies. J Exp Med 156:205, 1982.
101. Lachmann PJ, Rosen FS: Genetic defects of complement in man. Springer Semin Immunopathol 1:339, 1978.
102. Lambris JD, Ross GD: Characterization of the lymphocyte membrane receptor for factor H (β1H-globulin) with an antibody to anti-factor H idiotype. J Exp Med 155:1400, 1982.
103. Laurell AB, Johnson U, Martenson U, Sjoholm AG: Formation of complexes composed of $\overline{C1r}$, $\overline{C1s}$ and $\overline{C1}$-inactivator in human serum on activation of C1. Acta Pathol Microbiol Immunol Scand [C] 6:299, 1978.
104. Law SKA, Reid KBM: Complement. In Male D (ed): Focus, 2nd edition. IRL Press at Oxford University Press, Oxford, 1995.
105. Law SK, Lichsenberg NA, Levin RP: Evidence for an ester linkage between the labile binding site of C3b and receptive surfaces. J Immunol 123:1388, 1979.
106. Lee TJ, Schmoyer A, Snyderman R, et al: Familial deficiencies of the sixth and seventh components of complement associated with bacteremic Neisserial infections. In Brooks GF, Gotschlich EC, Holmes KK, et al (eds): Immunology of Neisseria Gonorrhoeae. American Society for Microbiology, Washington, DC, 1978, pp 204–206.
107. Lee TJ, Utsinger PD, Snyderman R, et al: Familial deficiency of the seventh component of complement associated with recurrent bacteremic infections due to Neisseria. J Infect Dis 138:355, 1978.
108. Lepow IH, Naff GB, Todd EW, et al: Chromatographic resolution of the first component of human complement into three activities. J Exp Med 11:483, 1963.
109. Lepow IH, Williams-Kretschmer K, Patrick RA, Rosen FS: Cross and ultrastructural observations on lesions produced by intradermal injection of human C3a in man. Am J Pathol 61:13, 1970.
110. Lesavre PH, Müller-Eberhard HJ: Mechanisms of action of factor D of the alternative complement pathway. J Exp Med 148:1498, 1978.
111. Lu J, Wiedeman H, Timpl R, Reid KBM: Similarity in structure between C1q and the collectins as judged by electron microscopy. Behring Inst Mitt 93:6, 1993.
112. Malhotra R, Thiel S, Reid KBM, Sim RB: Human leukocyte C1q receptor binds other soluble proteins with collagen domains. J Exp Med 172:955, 1990.
113. Malhotra R, Willis AC, Jensenius J-C, et al: Structure and homology of human C1q receptor (collectin receptor). Immunology 78:341, 1993.
114. Matsushita M, Fujita T: Activation of the classical pathway by mannose-binding protein in association with a novel C1s-like serine protease. J Exp Med 176:1497, 1992.
115. Mayer MM: Mechanisms of cytolysis by complement. Proc Natl Acad Sci USA 69:2954, 1972.
116. McClelland DBL, Van Furth R: In vitro synthesis of β_1C/β_1A globulin

(the C3 component of complement) by tissues and leukocytes in mice. Immunology 31:855, 1976.
117. Medicus RG, Arnaout MA: Release of C3c from bound C3bi by C3b inactivator. Mol Immunol 19:1386, 1982.
118. Medicus RG, Chapuis RM: The first component of complement. I. Purification and properties of native C1. J Immunol 125:390, 1980.
119. Medicus RG, Gotze O, Müller-Eberhard HJ: Alternative pathway of complement: recruitment and precursor properdin by the labile C3/C5 convertase and the potentiation of the pathway. J Exp Med 144:1076, 1976.
120. Medof ME, Prince GM, Mold C: Release of soluble immune complexes from immune adherence receptors on human erythrocytes is mediated by C3b inactivator independently of β1H and is accompanied by generation of C3c. Proc Natl Acad Sci USA 79:5047, 1982.
121. Medof ME, Prince GM, Oger JJ: Kinetics of interaction of immune complexes with complement receptors on human blood cells: modification of complexes during interaction with red cells. Clin Exp Immunol 48:715, 1982.
122. Medof ME, Lublin DM, Holers VM, et al: Cloning and characterization of cDNAs encoding the complete sequence of decay-accelerating factor of human complement. Proc Nat Acad Sci USA 84:2007, 1987.
123. Meuth JL, Morgan EL, DiScipio RG, Hugli TE: Suppression of T-lymphocyte functions by human C3 fragments: inhibition of human T cell proliferative responses by a kallikrein cleavage fragment of human iC3b. J Immunol 130:2605, 1983.
124. Mills BJ, Cooper NR: Antibody-independent neutralization of vesicular stomatitis virus by human complement. I. Complement requirements. J Immunol 121:1549, 1978.
125. Minta JO, Ward PA: The complement system of man. In Movat HZ (ed): Inflammation Immunity and Hypersensitivity: Cellular and Molecular Mechanisms, 2nd edition. Harper & Row, New York, 1979.
126. Morgan EL, Thoman ML, Weigle WO, Hugli TE: Anaphylatoxin-mediated immune response. II. C5a-mediated enhancement of human humoral and T cell-mediated immune responses. J Immunol 130:1257, 1983.
127. Morgan EL, Weigle WO, Hugli TE: Anaphylatoxin-mediated regulation of the immune response. I. C3a-mediated suppression of human and murine humoral immune responses. J Exp Med 155:1412, 1982.
128. Müller-Eberhard HJ: Complement: molecular mechanisms, regulation and biologic function. In Berlin R, Hermann H, Lepow I, Tanzer J (eds): Molecular Basis of Biological Degradative Processes. Academic Press, New York, 1980, p 65.
129. Müller-Eberhard HJ, Biro CT: Isolation and description of the fourth component of human complement. J Exp Med 118:447, 1963.
130. Müller-Eberhard HJ, Gotze O: C3 proactivator convertase and its mode of action. J Exp Med 135:1003, 1972.
131. Müller-Eberhard HJ, Polley MJ, Calcott MA: Formation and functional significance of a molecular complex derived from the second and the fourth component of human complement. J Exp Med 125:359, 1967.
132. Müller-Eberhard HJ, Schreiber RD: Molecular biology and chemistry of the alternative pathway of complement. Adv Immunol 29:1, 1980.
133. Naff GB, Byers PH: Complement as a mediator of inflammation in acute gouty arthritis. I. Studies on the reaction between human serum complement and sodium urate crystals. J Lab Clin Med 81:747, 1973.
134. Nagasawa S, Stroud RM: Cleavage of C2 by C1s into the antigenically distinct fragments C2a and C2b: demonstration of binding of C2b to C4b. Proc Natl Acad Sci USA 74:2998, 1977.
135. Nicholson-Weller A, Burge J, Fearon DT, et al: Isolation of human erythrocyte membrane glycoprotein with decay-accelerating activity for C3 convertases of the complement system. J Immunol 129:184, 1982.
136. Norgauer J, Dobos G, Kownatzki E, et al: Complement fragment C3a stimulates Ca^{2+} influx in neutrophils via a pertussis-toxin-sensitive G protein. Eur J Biochem 217:289, 1993.
137. Nussenzweig V: Interaction between complement and immune complexes: role of complement in containing immune complex damage. In Fougerau M, Dausset J (eds): Progress in Immunology. Academic Press, New York, 1980.
138. Pangburn MK, Morrison DC, Schreiber RD, Müller-Eberhard HJ: Activation of the alternative pathway: recognition of surface structures on activators by bound C3b. J Immunol 124:977, 1980.
139. Pangburn MK, Müller-Eberhard HJ: Complement C3 convertase: cell surface restriction of β1H and generation of restriction on neuraminidase-treated cells. Proc Natl Acad Sci USA 75:2416, 1978.
140. Pangburn MK, Müller-Eberhard HJ: Relation of a putative thioester bond in C3 to activation of the alternative pathway and the binding of C3b to biological targets of complement. J Exp Med 152:1102, 1980.
141. Pangburn MK, Meri S: Molecular mechanism of recognition by the alternative pathway of complement and locations of the restriction and sialic acid sites. Complement Inflam 6:383, 1989.
142. Pangburn MK, Schreiber RD, Müller-Eberhard HJ: Deficiency of an erythrocyte membrane protein with complement regulatory activity in paroxysmal nocturnal hemoglobinuria. Proc Natl Acad Sci USA 80:5430, 1983.
143. Pangburn MK, Schreiber RD, Müller-Eberhard HJ: Human complement C3b inactivator: isolation, characterization and demonstration of an absolute requirement for the serum protein β1H for cleavage of C3b and C4b in solution. J Exp Med 146:257, 1977.
144. Pangburn MK, Schreiber RD, Trombold JT, Müller-Eberhard HJ: Paroxysmal nocturnal hemoglobinuria: deficiency in factor H-like functions of the abnormal erythrocytes. J Exp Med 157:1971, 1983.
145. Perlmann P, Perlmann H, Müller-Eberhard HJ: Cytolytic lymphocytic cells with complement receptor in human blood: induction of cytolysis by IgG antibody but not target cell-bound C3. J Exp Med 141:287, 1975.
146. Peerschke EIB, Malhotra R, Ghebrehiwet B, et al: Isolation of a human endothelial cell C1q receptor (C1q-R). J Leukoc Biol 53:179–184, 1993.
147. Peerschke EIB, Reid KBM, Ghebrehiwet B: Identification of a novel 33-kDa C1q binding site on human blood platelets. J Immunol 152:5896, 1994.
148. Perez HD, Goldstein IM, Webster RO, Henson PM: Enhancement of the chemotactic activity of human C5a des Arg by an anionic polypeptide ("cochemotaxin") in normal serum and plasma. J Immunol 126:800, 1981.
149. Petersen BH, Graham JA, Brooks GF: Human deficiency of the eighth component of complement: the requirement of C8 for serum Neisseria gonorrhoeae bactericidal activity. J Clin Invest 57:283, 1976.
150. Platts-Mills, TAI, Ishizaka K: Activation of the alternate pathway of human complement by rabbit cells. J Immunol 113:348, 1974.
151. Plaut AG, Cohen S, Tomasi TB: Immunoglobulin M: fixation of human complement by the Fc fragment. Science 176:55, 1972.
152. Podack ER, Biesecker G, Kolb WP, Müller-Eberhard HJ: The C5b-6 complex: reaction with C7, C8, C9. J Immunol 121:484, 1978.
153. Podack ER, Biesecker G, Müller-Eberhard HJ: Membrane attack complex of complement: generation of high affinity phospholipid binding sites by the fusion of six hydrophilic, plasma proteins. Proc Natl Acad Sci USA 76:897, 1979.
154. Podack ER, Dennert G: Assembly of two types of tubules with putative cytolytic function by cloned natural killer cells. Nature 302:442, 1983.
155. Podack ER, Esser AF, Biesecker G, Müller-Eberhard HJ: Membrane attack complex of complement: a structural analysis of its assembly. J Exp Med 151:301, 1980.
156. Podack ER, Müller-Eberhard HJ: Binding of desoxycholate, phosphatidylcholine vesicles, lipoprotein and of the S protein to complexes of terminal complement components. J Immunol 121:1025, 1978.
157. Podack ER, Müller-Eberhard HJ: Complement mediated injury of tumor cells: release of membrane fragments by C5b-9. Fed Proc 40:359, 1981.
158. Podack ER, Müller-Eberhard HJ, Horst H, Hoppe W: Membrane attack complex of complement (MAC): three dimensional analysis of MAC-phospholipid vesicle recombinants. J Immunol 128:2353, 1982.
159. Podack ER, Stoffel W, Esser AF, Müller-Eberhard HJ: Membrane attack complex of complement: distribution of subunits between hydrocarbon phase of target membranes and water. Proc Natl Acad Sci USA 78:4544, 1981.
160. Podack ER, Tschopp J: Polymerization of the ninth component of complement (C9): formation of poly (C9) with a tubular ultrastructure resembling the membrane attack complex of complement. Proc Natl Acad Sci USA 79:574, 1982.
161. Podack ER, Tschopp J, Müller-Eberhard HJ: Molecular organization of C9 within the membrane attack complex of complement: induction of circular C9 polymerization by the C5b-8 assembly. J Exp Med 156:268, 1982.
162. Porter RR: Structure and activation of the early components of complement. Fed Proc 36:2191, 1977.
163. Porter RR: The proteolytic enzymes of the complement system. Methods Enzymol 80:3, 1981.
164. Rao AG, Howard OMZ, Ng SC, et al: Complementary DNA and derived amino acid sequence of the α subunit of human complement

C8: evidence for the existence of a separate α subunit messenger RNA. Biochemistry 26:3556, 1987.

165. Ratnoff OD, Naff GB: The conversion of C1s to $\overline{C1s}$ by plasmin and trypsin. J Exp Med 125:337, 1967.

166. Ratnoff OD, Pensky D, Ogston D, Naff GB: The inhibition of plasmin, plasma kallikrein, plasma permeability factor and the C1r subcomponent of the first component of complement by serum C1 esterase inhibitor. J Exp Med 129:315, 1969.

167. Reid KBM, Gagnon J, Frampton J: Completion of the amino acid sequences of the A and B chains subcomponent C1q of the first component of human complement. Biochem J 203:559, 1982.

168. Reid KBM, Porter RR: Subunit composition of subcomponent C1q of the first component of human complement. Biochem J 155:19, 1976.

169. Reid KBM, Sim RB, Faiers AP: Inhibition of the reconstitution of the hemolytic activity of the first component of human complement by a pepsin-derived fragment of subcomponent C1q. Biochem J 161:239, 1977.

170. Ross GD, Lambris JD, Cain JA, Newman SL: Generation of three different fragments of bound C3 with purified factor I or serum. I. Requirements for factor H vs. CR_1 cofactor activity. J Immunol 129:2051, 1982.

171. Ruddy S, Carlo J, Conrad J: Mechanism of action of β1H globulin on C3b. J Immunol 120:1794, 1978.

172. Sahu A, Kozel TR, Pangburn MK: Specificity of the thioester-containing reactive site of human-C3 and its significance to complement activation. Biochem J 302:429, 1994.

173. Sastry K, Herman GA, Day L, et al: The human mannose-binding gene. J Exp Med 10:1175, 1989.

174. Schreiber AD, Kaplan AP, Austen KF: Inhibition by $\overline{C1}$ INH of Hageman factor fragment activation of coagulation, fibrinolysis and kinin-generation. J Clin Invest 52:1401, 1973.

175. Schreiber RD: The chemistry and biology of complement receptors. Springer Semin Immunopathol 7:221, 1984.

176. Schreiber RD, Feldman HA: Identification of the activation system for antibody to Toxoplasma as the classical complement pathway. J Infect Dis 141:366, 1980.

177. Schreiber RD, Morrison DC, Podack ER, Müller-Eberhard HJ: Bactericidal activity of the alternative complement pathway generated from eleven isolated plasma proteins. J Exp Med 149:870, 1979.

178. Schreiber RD, Müller-Eberhard HJ: Fourth component of human complement: description of a three polypeptide structure. J Exp Med 140:1324, 1974.

179. Schreiber RD, Pangburn MK, Medicus RG, Müller-Eberhard HJ: Raji cell injury and subsequent lysis by purified cytolytic alternative pathway of human complement. Clin Immunol Immunopathol 15:384, 1980.

180. Sellar GC, Blake DJ, Reid KBM: Characterization and organization of the genes encoding the A-, B-, C-chains of human complement subcomponent C1q. Biochem J 274:481, 1991.

181. Shelton E, Yonemasu K, Stroud RM: Ultrastructure of the human complement component C1q. Proc Natl Acad Sci USA 69:65, 1972.

182. Singer L, Colten HR, Wetsel RA: Complement C3 deficiency: human, animal and experimental models. Pathobiology 62:14, 1994.

183. Smith MA, Kerr MA: The kinin activity generated in C1-INH deficient plasma is not derived from C2 and originates from the kallikrein kininogen pathway. Immunobiology 164:299, 1983.

184. Snyderman R, Durack DT, McCarty GA, et al: Deficiency of the fifth component of complement in human subjects. Am J Med 63:638, 1979.

185. Sobel AT, Bokisch VA: Receptor for C1q on peripheral human lymphocytes and human lymphoblastoid cells. Fed Proc 34:965, 1975.

186. Sontheimer RD, Lieu T-S, Capra JD: The diverse functional repertoire of calreticulin, a new human autoantigen. Immunologist 1:155, 1993.

187. Stanley KK, Kocher HP, Luzio JP, et al: The sequence and topology of human complement component C9. EMBO J 4:374, 1985.

188. Strang CJ, Cholin S, Spragg J, et al: Angioedema induced by a peptide derived from complement component component C2. J Exp Med 168:1685, 1988.

189. Stroud RM, Volanakis JE, Nagasawa S, Lint TF: Biochemistry and biological reactions of complement proteins. In Atassi MZ (ed): Immunochemistry of Proteins. Vol. 3. Plenum, New York, 1979, p 167.

190. Tack BF, Morris SC, Prahl JW: Third component of human complement: structural analysis of the polypeptide chains of C3 and C3b. Biochemistry 18:1497, 1979.

191. Takada F, Seki N, Masuda Y-I, et al: Localization of the genes for the 100-kDa complement activating components of Ra-reactive factor (CRARF and *Crarf*) to human 3q27-q28 and mouse 16B2-B3. Genomics 25:757, 1995.

192. Tenner AJ: Functional aspects of the C1q receptors. Behring Inst Mitt 93:241, 1993.

193. Thiel S: Mannan-binding protein, a complement activating animal lectin. Immunopharmacology 24:91, 1992.

194. Tranum-Jensen J, Bhakdi S, Bhakadi-Lehnen B, et al: Complement lysis: the ultrastructure and orientation of the C5b-9 complex on target sheep erythrocyte membranes. Scand J Immunol 7:45, 1978.

195. Tschopp J, Müller-Eberhard HJ, Podack ER: Formation of transmembrane tubules by spontaneous poymerization of the hydrophilic complement protein C9. Nature 298:1982, 1982.

196. Valet G, Cooper NR: Isolation and characterization of the proenzyme form of the C1s subunit of the first complement component. J Immunol 112:339, 1974

197. Vogt W: Substrate modulation as a control mechanism in the activation of plasma multi-enzyme systems. In Fugii S, Moriya H, Suzuki T (eds): Kinins IIB: Systemic Proteases and Cellular Function. Advances in Experimental Medicine and Biology, Vol 120. Plenum, New York, 1979, p 125.

198. Volanakis JE, Kaplan MH: Interaction of C-reactive protein complexes with the complement system. II. Consumption of guinea pig complement by CRP complexes: requirement for C1q. J Immunol 113:9, 1974.

199. Webster ME, Maling HM, Zweig MH, et al: Urate crystal induced inflammation in the rat: evidence for the combined actions of kinins, histamine and complement. Immunol Commun 1:185, 1972.

200. Weigle WO, Goodman MG, Morgan EL, Hugli TE: Regulation of immune response by components of the complement cascade and their activated fragments. Springer Semin Immunopathol 6:173, 1983.

201. Wetsel RA: Structure, function and cellular expression of complement anaphylatoxin receptors. Curr Opin Immunol 7:48, 1995.

202. Whaley K, Ruddy S: Modulation of the alternative complement pathway by β1H globulin. J Exp Med 144:1147, 1976.

203. Ziccardi RJ: The first component of human complement (C1): activation and control. Springer Semin Immunopathol 6:213, 1983.

204. Ziccardi RJ, Cooper NR: Active disassembly of the first complement component, C1 by C1-inactivator. J Immunol 123:788, 1979.

205. Ziccardi RJ, Cooper NR: The subunit composition and sedimentation properties of human C1. J Immunol 118:2047, 1977.

14 Bradykinin Formation: Plasma and Tissue Pathways

SESHA R. REDDIGARI MICHAEL SILVERBERG ALLEN P. KAPLAN

The plasma kinin–forming system consists of three essential plasma proteins that interact in a complex fashion once bound to certain negatively charged surfaces or macromolecular complexes. These are coagulation Factor XII (Hageman factor or HF), prekallikrein, and high molecular weight kininogen (HK). Once Factor XII is activated to Factor XIIa, it converts plasma prekallikrein to kallikrein and kallikrein digests HK to liberate bradykinin. Factor XIIa also converts coagulation Factor XI to Factor XIa to continue the intrinsic coagulation cascade. The interactions of all four of these proteins to initiate blood clotting is known as contact activation; thus the formation of bradykinin is a cleavage product of the initiating step of this cascade (Fig. 14–1).

PROTEIN CONSTITUENTS

FACTOR XII

Factor XII circulates as a single chain zymogen with no detectable enzymatic activity.[200] It has a molecular weight of 80,000 on SDS gel electrophoresis[174] (Table 14–1), is synthesized in the liver, and circulates in plasma at a concentration of 30 to 35 μg/ml. Its primary sequence has been deduced from cDNA analysis[41, 162] and from direct protein sequence data.[64, 132] The 596 amino acids present account for a molecular weight of 66,915; the remainder (16.8%) is carbohydrate. The protein has distinct domains homologous to fibronectin, plasminogen, and plasminogen activators[31, 41] at its N-terminal end, whereas the C-terminus has the catalytic domain. This latter portion is homologous to serine proteases such as pancreatic trypsin and even more so to the catalytic domain of plasminogen activators.

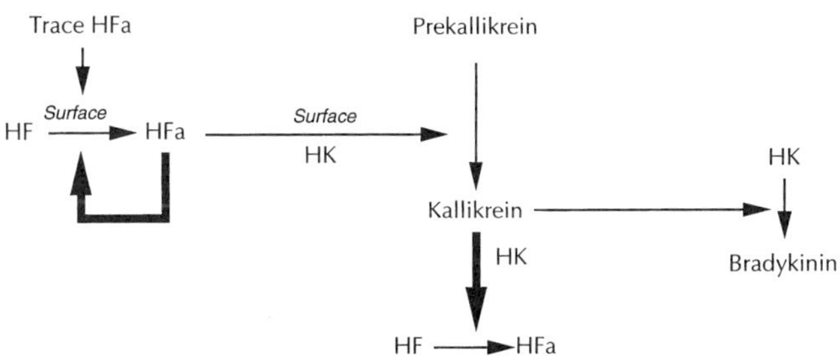

FIGURE 14–1. Pathway for generation of bradykinin in human plasma. Hageman factor (HF) autoactivation is the initiating step. It is followed by conversion of prekallikrein to kallikrein and digestion of HK to release bradykinin. A positive feedback involves HF activation by kallikrein, which is 50- to 100-fold more rapid than autoactivation. Prekallikrein is bound to HK, and the complex attaches to the surface as indicated along the arrow.

Factor XII is unusual because it is capable of autoactivating once bound to initiating surfaces.[199, 213] Thus Factor XII that is bound undergoes a conformational change that renders it a substrate for Factor XIIa.[78] Gradually, all of the bound Factor XII can be converted to Factor XIIa. Whether plasma normally has a trace of Factor XIIa present is unknown, but if so, its concentration is less than 0.01% of Factor XII. The alternative is that the first molecule of Factor XIIa is formed by interaction of two Factor XII zymogen molecules on the surface, but this presumes some minimal activity present in the zymogen. If so, it is below our limits of detection, and we favor the former scenario.[200]

Activation of Factor XII is due to cleavage of the molecule at a critical Arg-Val bond[64] contained within a disulfide bridge such that the resultant Factor XIIa is a two-chain, disulfide-linked 80-kD enzyme consisting of a heavy chain of 50 kD and a light chain of 28 kD.[173] The light chain contains the enzymatic active site[133] and is at the carboxy-terminal end, whereas the heavy chain contains the binding site for the surface and is at the amino-terminal end.[156] Further cleavage can occur at the C-terminal end of the heavy chain to produce a series of fragments of activated Factor XII that retain enzymatic activity.[102, 103] The most prominent of these is a 30-kD species termed Factor XII_f. Careful examination of Factor XII_f on SDS gels under nonreducing conditions reveals a doublet in which the higher band at 30 kD is gradually converted to the lower band that has a molecular weight of 28.5 kD.[54] Reduced gels demonstrate that these species consist of the light chain of Factor XIIa and a very small piece of the original heavy chain. These fragments lack the binding site to the surface and lose much of the ability of Factor XIIa to convert Factor XI to Factor XIa and do not participate in Factor XII autoactivation. However, these fragments remain potent activators of prekallikrein.[102] Thus formation of Factor XII_f allows bradykinin production to continue until the enzyme is inactivated and the reactions can proceed at sites distant from the initiating surface. A diagrammatic representation of

TABLE 14–1
PHYSICAL AND CHEMICAL DATA OF CONTACT ACTIVATION PROTEINS

Protein	Factor XII	Prekallikrein	Factor XI	HK
Molecular weight (kD)	80.4	79.5	140	116.7
Carbohydrate, %	16.8	15	5	40
Isoelectric point	6.3	8.7	9.1	4.7
Extinction coefficient, 280 nm ($E^{1\%}$)	14.2	11.7	13.4	7
Plasma concentration, μg/ml (nM)	30–35 (400)	35–50 (534)	4–6 (36)	70–90 (686)

the cleavages in Factor XII to generate Factor XIIa and Factor XII_f is shown in Figure 14–2.

Once Factor XIIa interacts with prekallikrein, rapid conversion to kallikrein ensues, followed by an important positive feedback in which kallikrein digests surface-bound Factor XII to form Factor XIIa and then Factor XII_f.[36, 55, 133] This reaction is 50- to 100-times more rapid than the autoactivation reaction.[55, 213] Thus quantitatively, most of the Factor XIIa or Factor XII_f activity generated when plasma is activated is a result of kallikrein activation of Factor XII. Yet the autoactivation phenomenon can be demonstrated in plasma that is congenitally deficient in prekallikrein (Fletcher trait) and therefore cannot generate any bradykinin.[178, 232, 237] However, clotting (conversion of Factor XI to Factor XIa by Factor XIIa) does proceed, albeit at a much slower rate, and the partial thromboplastin time (PTT) can be shown to progressively shorten as the time of incubation of the plasma with the surface is increased prior to recalcification. This is probably due to Factor XII autoactivation on the surface. As more and more Factor XIIa forms, the rate of Factor XI activation increases and the PTT approaches normal.

PREKALLIKREIN

Prekallikrein is also a zymogen without detectable proteolytic activity that is converted to kallikrein by cleavage during contact activation.[124] On SDS gels, it has two bands at 88 and 85 kD. The entire amino acid sequence of the protein has been determined by a combination of direct protein sequencing and amino acid sequence prediction from cDNAs isolated from a λgt-11 expression library.[34] A signal peptide of 19 residues (which is cleaved off prior to secretion) is followed by the sequence of the mature plasma prekallikrein, which has 619 amino acids with a calculated molecular weight of 69,710. There is 15% carbohydrate as well. The heterogeneity on SDS gel electrophoresis is not reflected in the amino acid sequence and thus may be due to variation

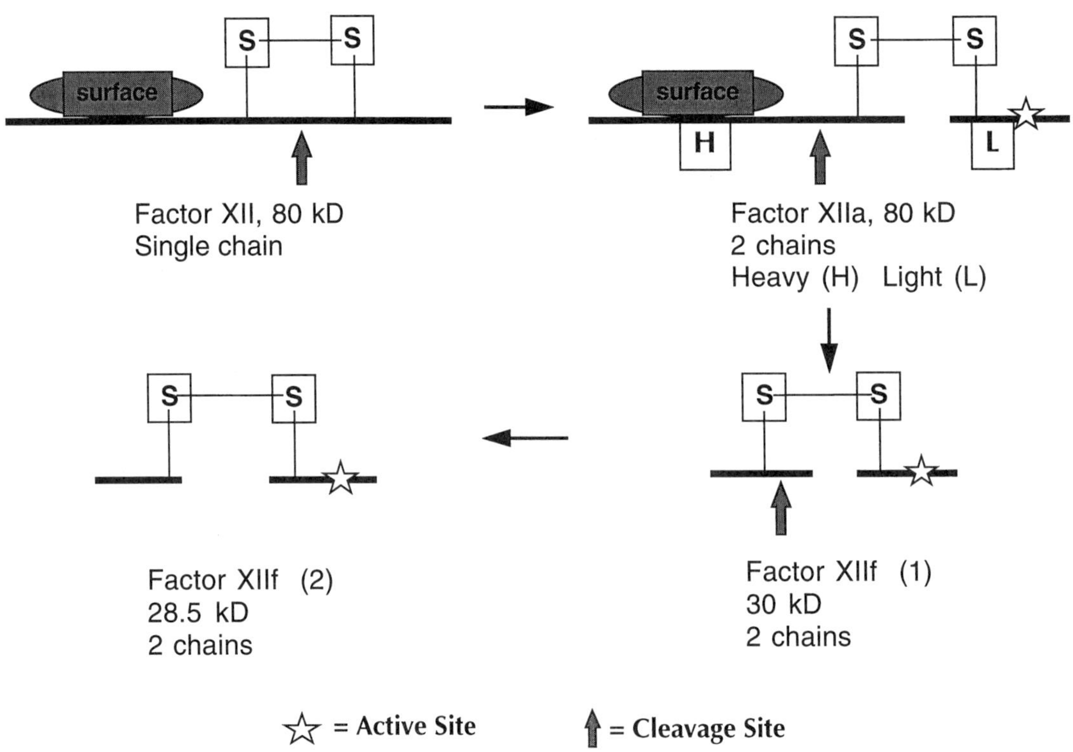

FIGURE 14–2. Schematic representation of cleavages occurring in Factor XII that activate it to Factor XIIa and then further cleave it to the two forms of Factor XII_f.

in glycosylation. Activation of prekallikrein by Factor XIIa or Factor XII_f is due to cleavage of a single Arg-Ile band within a disulfide bridge such that a heavy chain of 56 kD is disulfide linked to a light chain of either 33 or 36 kD, each of which has a DFP-inhibitable active site.[24, 124] This light chain heterogeneity reflects the two forms of the zymogen.

The amino acid sequence of the kallikrein heavy chain is unusual and is homologous only to the corresponding portion of Factor XI. It has four tandem repeats, each of which contains approximately 90 to 91 amino acids. The presence of six cysteines per repeat suggests a repeating structure with three disulfide loops. It is postulated that a gene coding for the ancestor of this repeat sequence duplicated and then the entire segment duplicated again to give the present structure. The light chain, containing the active site, is homologous to many of the catalytic domains of other enzymes of the coagulation cascade.

In contrast to Factor XII, prekallikrein does not circulate as a separate protein. It is bound to HK in a 1:1 bimolecular complex through a site on its heavy chain. The binding is firm, with a dissociation constant of 12 to 15 nM,[20, 123] and this is unchanged upon conversion of prekallikrein to kallikrein. Thus about 80 to 90% of prekallikrein is normally complexed to HK in plasma.[188] It is the prekallikrein-HK complex that binds to surfaces during contact activation and the binding is primarily through HK,[234] although some interaction of prekallikrein with the surface can be inferred.[131] The dissociation of 10 to 20% of the kallikrein that forms from the surface may serve to propagate the formation of bradykinin in the fluid phase and at sites distant from the initiating reaction.[35, 201]

PROKALLIKREIN AND TISSUE KALLIKREINS

Tissue kallikrein is a single chain, acidic glycoprotein that is physicochemically and immunologically distinct from plasma kallikrein. The reported molecular weight ranges from 25 to 43 Kd because of considerable heterogeneity, most of which is due to proteolysis subsequent to secretion. It is produced in abundance by major exocrine organs such as the pancreas and salivary glands, as well as the kidney.[150] It is actually widespread, however, and can be found in the colon,[179] prostate, pituitary gland,[59, 157] brain tissue,[32] and neutrophils.[59]

Within a given species, tissue kallikreins derived from all organs are immunologically identical,[61] and cDNA cloning and subsequent analysis reveal the same amino acid sequence of 238 residues.[8, 65] In rodents, tissue kallikrein is a member of a large multigene family of over 20 members; in humans, it is encoded by no more than two or three closely related genes, but only one yields bonafide tissue kallikrein.[8, 236] Tissue kallikrein is synthesized within these cells (tissues) as a preproenzyme. In some organs, the proenzyme (prokallikrein) predominates intracellularly, where it is converted to tissue kallikrein. Urine for example, contains a mixture of prokallikrein and tissue kallikrein.[210] A multitude of isoelectric forms can be found that reflect microheterogeneity due to variable glycosylation. Intracellular conversion of prokallikrein to kallikrein is mediated by enzymes that are not well characterized. Secreted prokallikrein can be converted to tissue kallikrein extracellularly by either plasmin or plasma kallikrein.[210, 212]

FACTOR XI

Coagulation Factor XI is the second substrate of Factor XIIa (see Fig. 14–1) but has no role in bradykinin formation. Factor XI is unique among the clotting factors because the circulating zymogen consists of two identical chains linked by disulfide bonds.[23, 114] The dimer has an apparent molecular weight of 160 kD on SDS gel electrophoresis but reveals a single 80-kD protein upon reduction. Factor XI activation follows the familiar pattern of cleavage of a single peptide band (Arg-Ile) within a disulfide bridge to yield an amino-terminal heavy chain of 50 kD and a disulfide-linked light chain of 33 kD. Since both subunits can be cleaved by Factor XIIa and each resultant light chain bears a functional active site, Factor XIa is a four-chain protein with two active sites. The concentration in plasma is only 4 to 8 μg/ml, the lowest among the contact proteins, and its heavy chain(s), like that of kallikrein, binds to the light chain of HK. Thus Factor XI and HK also circulate as a complex.[217] The dissociation constant is 70 nM,[209] which is high enough to ensure that virtually all the Factor XI is complexed. The molar ratio of the complex can consist of one or two molecules of HK per Factor XI because of the dimeric nature of Factor XI.[231] The binding site for HK on Factor XI has been localized to the first (N-terminal) tandem repeat.[7] The Factor XI-HK complex binds to the surface, and conversion to Factor XIa must occur on the surface; fluid-phase conversion by Factor XII_f is only 2 to 4% of that of surface-bound Factor XIIa.[103] The primary function of Factor XIa is to activate Factor IX to IXa, which is the first calcium-dependent reaction in the intrinsic coagulation cascade.

The amino acid sequence of human Factor XI has been determined by cDNA analysis.[62] It has a 19 amino acid leader peptide followed by a 60% amino acid sequence for each of the two chains of the mature protein. The amino acid sequence of the heavy chain of Factor XIa, like that of kallikrein, has 4 tandem repeats of about 90 amino acids, with 6 cysteines per repeat implying 3 disulfide bands. Unpaired cysteines in the first and fourth repeats are postulated to form the interchain disulfide bridges between monomers to produce the homodimer. The striking similarity in structure between prekallikrein and Factor XI is shown in Figure 14–3.

HIGH MOLECULAR WEIGHT KININOGEN (HK)

HK circulates in plasma as a 115-kD nonenzymatic glycoprotein at a concentration of 70 to 90 μg/ml.[2, 15, 39, 159, 168] Its apparent molecular weight by gel filtration is aberrant at about 200,000, indicative of a large partial specific volume due to its conformation in solution.[123] HK forms noncovalent complexes with both prekallikrein and Factor XI, with dissociation constants of 15nM[19, 20] and 70 nM,[209, 219] respectively. There is sufficient HK in plasma to theoretically bind both Factor XII substrates, and the excess HK (about 10–20%) circulates uncomplexed. The complexes of HK with prekallikrein or Factor XI are formed with the light chain region of HK; the isolated light chain (after reduction and alkylation) possesses the same binding characteristics as the whole molecule.[218, 219] HK functions as a coagulation cofactor, and this activity resides in the light chain,[218] which consists of a

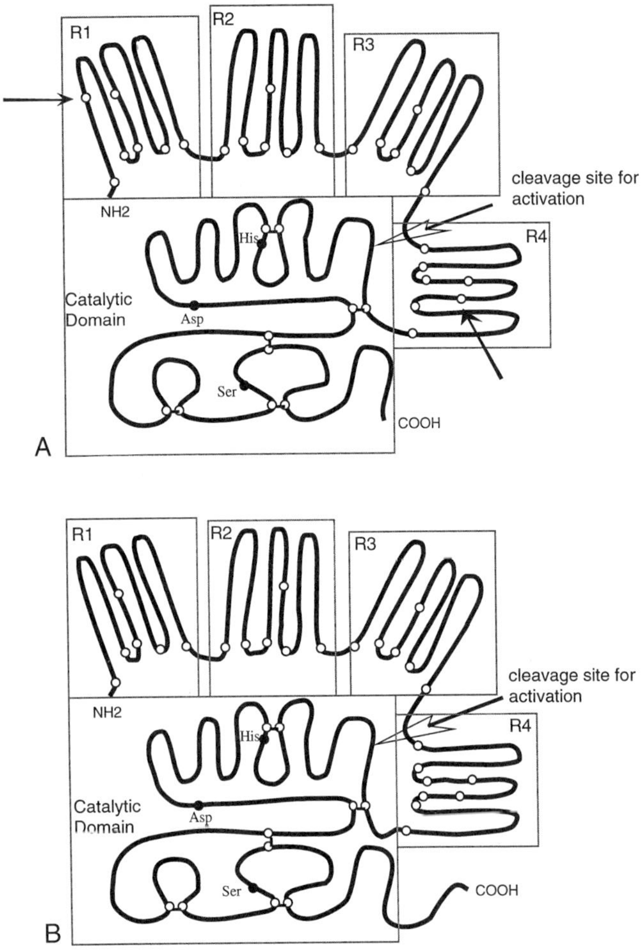

FIGURE 14–3. Schematic diagram of the protein chains of **(A)** Factor XI and **(B)** prekallikrein, showing the structural domains inferred from sequence homologies. The catalytic triad residues are shown by solid circles, half-cystines are indicated by open circles, and the cleavage sites leading to activation by activated Factor XII are marked with open arrows. The solid arrows indicate the unmatched half-cystines that might be involved in interchain disulfide bonds. (Adapted with permission from Fujikawa K, Chung KW, Hendrickson LE, Davie EW: Amino acid sequence of human factor XI: a blood coagulation factor with four tandem repeats that are highly homologous with plasma prekallikrein. Biochemistry 25:2417, 1986. Copyright 1986 American Chemical Society.)

basic (histidine rich) amino-terminal domain that binds to initiating surfaces[95] and a carboxy-terminal domain that binds prekallikrein or Factor XI.[208] The one cysteine in the light chain links it to the heavy chain. The prekallikrein-binding site maps to residues 194 to 224,[208, 209] and the Factor XI site maps to residues 185 to 242.[209] Since these sites overlap, one molecule of HK can only harbor either prekallikrein or Factor XI at a time.

During contact activation, kallikrein cleaves HK at two positions within a disulfide bridge; first at the C-terminal Arg-Ser[139, 140] and then at the N-terminal Lys-Arg to release the nonapeptide bradykinin (Arg-Pro-Pro-Gly-Phe-Ser-Pro-Phe-Arg). A two-chain disulfide-linked kinin-free HK results, consisting of a heavy chain of 65,000 and a light chain variously reported at molecular weights of 56 to 62,000. A subsequent further cleavage of the light chain yields a final product of 46 to 49,000,[19, 139, 140, 169, 182] which retains all light chain functions. Tissue kallikrein can also digest HK to liberate kallidin or Lys-bradykinin, leaving the heavy chain disulfide linked to the 56- to 62-kD light chain; the additional cleavage of the light chain is not made by this enzyme.[169] Tissue kallikrein is immunologically and structurally unrelated to plasma kallikrein. It is secreted by various organs or cells such as the salivary glands, kidney, pancreas, prostate, pituitary gland, and neutrophils and is found in high concentrations in saliva, urine, and prostatic fluid. Tissue kallikrein's primary substrate is low molecular weight kininogen (LK), but it can release kallidin (lysylBK) from either HK or LK. Kallidin is functionally very similar to bradykinin, albeit slightly less potent. A plasma amino peptidase[80] removes the N-terminal Lys to convert it to bradykinin.

The very unusual domain structure of HK is shown in Figure 14–4. Domain 5, the histidine-rich region at the N-terminal end of the light chain, binds to initiating surfaces, whereas the binding of prekallikrein or Factor XI at the C-terminal domain 6 of the light chain accounts for the cofactor function of HK in intrinsic coagulation and kinin generation. The complete amino acid sequence of HK has been determined as translated from the cDNA as well as by direct sequence analysis of the purified protein.[106, 108, 120, 211] HK has 626 amino acids with a calculated molecular weight of 69,896. An unusually high content of carbohydrate accounts for 40% of the observed molecular weight of 115 kD. The heavy chain of 362 residues is derived from the N-terminus. This is followed by the 9 residue bradykinin (domain 4) sequence and then the light chain of 265 residues. The N-terminal end is blocked with pyroglutamic acid (cyclic glutamine). The carbohydrate is distributed via three N-linked glycosidic linkages on the H chain and nine O-linked glycosidic linkages on the L chain. The H chain has three contiguous and homologous apple-type domains consisting of residues 1 to 116, 117 to 238, and 239 to 360 (see Fig. 14–4). There are 17 cysteines, 1 of which is disulfide linked to the L chain and the others form 8 disulfide loops within these domains.[106] The three domains on the heavy chain are homologous to the cystatin family of protease inhibitors and function to inactivate sulfhydryl-containing proteases such as certain cathepsins. Domains 2 and 3 (but not 1) retain this inhibitory function; for example, native HK can bind and inactivate two molecules of papain.[75, 89, 96, 142] Limited proteolysis of the heavy chain can occur at susceptible bonds that separate the domains so that individual domains can be isolated. Cleavage at these sites may occur under certain pathologic conditions.

LOW MOLECULAR WEIGHT KININOGEN (LK) AND KININOGEN GENES

Plasma contains another precursor of bradykinin (68 kD) known as low molecular weight kininogen (LK). Its digestion by tissue kallikrein yields Lys-bradykinin and a kinin-free two-chain molecule consisting of a 65-kD heavy chain disulfide linked to a light chain of only 4 kD.[97, 100, 106, 121, 143] LK is not cleaved by plasma kallikrein. The amino acid sequences of HK and LK are identical starting from the amino terminus through the bradykinin sequence plus the next 12 residues,[143] after which the two sequences diverge. Thus LK does not bind to surfaces or to prekallikrein or Factor XI. The kininogens are produced from a single gene thought to have originated by two successive duplications of a primordial cystatin-like gene.[108] As represented in Figure 14–5,

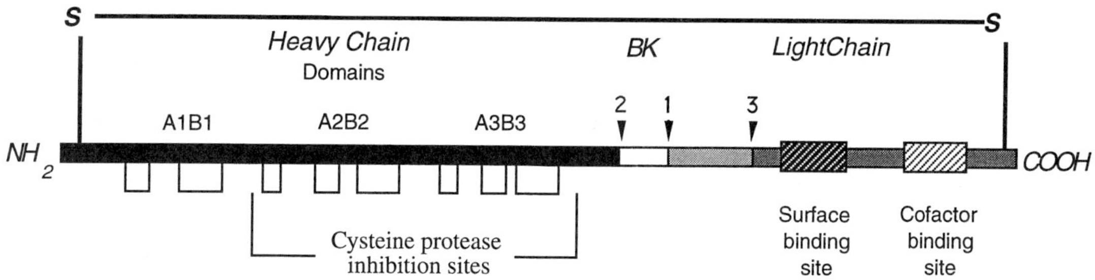

FIGURE 14–4. The structure of high molecular weight (HMW) kininogen. The heavy chain region consists of three homologous domains, A1B1, A2B2, and A3B3, of which the latter two are sulfhydryl protease inhibition sites. The small rectangles under the heavy chain region represent the eight intra–heavy chain disulfide bonds. The light chain region of HMW kininogen, which contains the binding sites for surfaces and prekallikrein or Factor XI, is located toward the C-terminal end of the protein. The heavy and light chains are held together by the ninth disulfide bond. The arrowheads labeled 1, 2, and 3 indicate the sites and the order in which plasma kallikrein cleaves HMW kininogen. BK = bradykinin.

there are 11 exons. The first nine code for the heavy chain, and each of the three domains in this portion of the protein is represented by three exons. The 10th exon codes for bradykinin and the light chain of HK, whereas the light chain of LK is encoded by the 11th exon. The mRNAs for HK and LK are produced by alternative splicing at a point 12 amino acids beyond the bradykinin sequence, thus enabling the two proteins to have different light chains (see Fig. 14–5).

MECHANISMS OF BRADYKININ FORMATION

CONTACT ACTIVATION

Contact activation was initially observed by the interaction of blood with glass surfaces[126]; subsequently, finely divided kaolin was used extensively as an experimental surface and for coagulation assays such as the partial thromboplastin time.[158] Ellagic acid,[165] a tanninlike substance used as a component of many commercial assay systems, was purported to be a soluble initiator but was later shown to form large sedimentable aggregates catalyzed by trace heavy metal ions, so it too is particulate.[21] Dextran sulfate[63, 111] and sulfatide[63] have also been used to study contact activation. Although sulfatide, a galactose sulfate sphingolipid found in nerve tissue, is an activator, it occurs in quantities too small to be an effective activator. When purified, however, it can form highly charged micelles, which are very efficient initiators.[77, 215] Dextran sulfate is a truly soluble activator and a close homologue of naturally occurring sulfated mucopolysaccharides. High molecular weight preparations of 500 kD are typically used,[63, 200, 213] but in a study of Factor XII

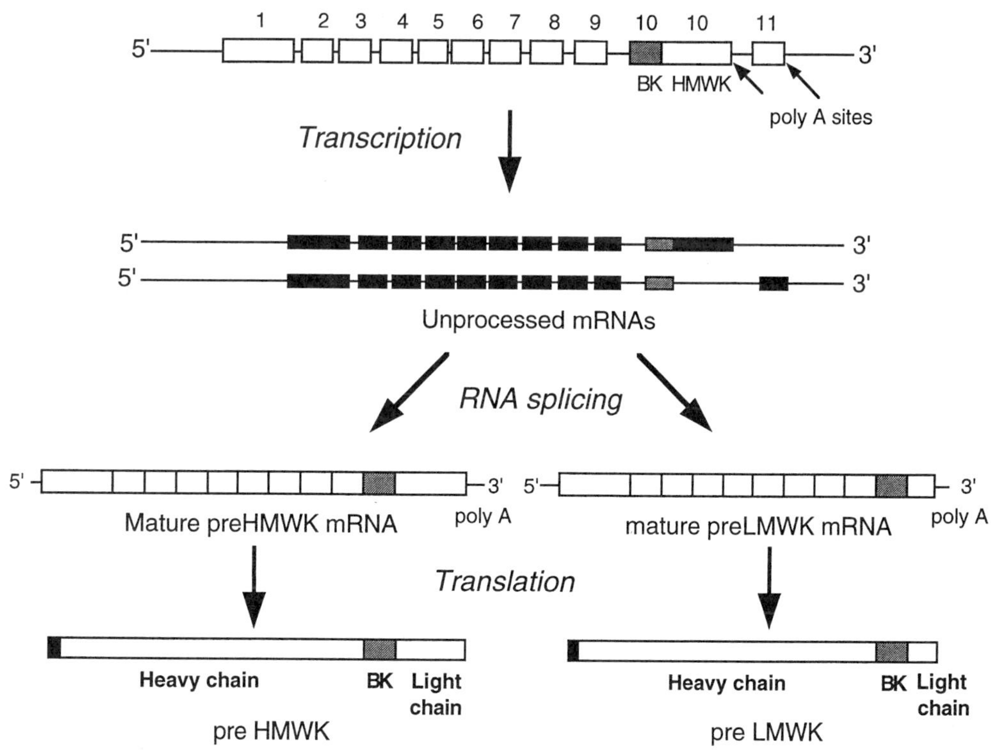

FIGURE 14–5. The gene for high molecular weight kininogen (HK). The boxes labeled 1 to 9 represent the exon coding for the heavy chain of both HK and low molecular weight kininogen (LK). Exon 10 codes for the bradykinin (BK) sequence and the light chain of HK, whereas exon 11 codes for the light chain of LK. The mature mRNAs are assembled by alternative splicing events in which the light chain sequences are attached to the 3′ end of the 12-amino acid common sequence C terminal to BK.

autoactivation,[198] much smaller fractions were effective as low as 5 kD. The rate of Factor XII activation increased markedly with dextran sulfate at 10 kD (or more), where the theoretical number of Factor XII molecules capable of binding per particle increased from one to two, and similar results were seen with heparin. This presumably provides a critical intermolecular interaction required for optimal autoactivation.

Naturally occurring polysaccharides are effective if they are highly sulfated, and these include heparin and chondroitin sulfate E (described in rodent mucosal mast cells).[91] Other mucopolysaccharides known to catalyze Factor XII autoactivation are dermatan sulfate, keratin polysulfate, or chondroitin sulfate C.[26] The basement membrane of endothelial cell matrix may support contact activation, but this has not been demonstrated in vivo. Collagen, long thought to be an initiator, was proven to be ineffective, and the activity reported was possibly due to contaminating matrix proteins. One pathophysiologic substance very likely to initiate contact activation in vivo is endotoxin.[141, 152, 176] There is good reason to believe that the contact cascade is activated in septic shock and that the observed symptoms are due, in part, to the generation of bradykinin.[105, 128] Crystals of uric acid and pyrophosphate can also initiate kinin formation via this pathway.[70, 107]

REGULATION OF CONTACT ACTIVATION

The various interactions of these constituents are shown in Figure 14–6, which includes the steps inhibited by C1 inhibitor (C1-INH). The autoactivation of Factor XII as shown is very slow. However, the reciprocal reactions involving kallikrein contribute to a tremendously fast activation of Factor XII as illustrated by the finding that if one molecule each of FXIIa and kallikrein per milliliter are present in a mixture of Factor XII and prekallikrein at their plasma concentrations, 50% of Factor XII would be activated in 13 seconds.[213] This corresponds to 5×10^{-13}% of active enzyme in the preparations. The in vivo source of the active enzyme is unknown but may be formed by other plasma proteases such as plasmin. In fact, very slow turnover of the cascade may always be occurring[13, 14, 171, 196] and controlled by plasma inhibitors.[233] Introduction of a surface or other polyanionic substance could accelerate many thousand fold the baseline turnover of Factor XII and prekallikrein to ignite the cascade. The addition of the cofactor HK (which was not included in the aforementioned kinetic analysis) accelerates these reactions even further but requires the surface to be present. The surface appears to create a local milieu in the contiguous fluid[77, 79, 197] phase, where the local concentrations of reactants are greatly increased, which increases the rates of the reciprocal interactions. In addition, surface-bound Factor XII undergoes a conformational change that renders it more susceptible to cleavage.[78] The alternative idea[115, 131, 166] that binding of Factor XII induces a conformation change that exposes an active site has essentially been disproved.

Inhibitors such as C1-INH are not bound to the surface; thus the balance between activation and inactivation is upset. The effect of dilution on plasma also diminishes the effect of inhibitors far more than any slowing of enzymatic reaction rates. The net effect is therefore a marked augmentation of reaction rate. Using dextran sulfate, the effect of the surface upon Factor XIIa conversion of prekallikrein to kallikrein increased 70 fold,[213] whereas the effect upon digestion of Factor XII by kallikrein increased as much as 3,000 to 12,000 fold.[177, 213] This latter reaction is about 2,000-fold more rapid than the rate of Factor XII autoactivation, and this kinetic dominance means that prekallikrein must be considered a coagulation factor. As indicated earlier, the PTT of prekallikrein-deficient plasma is much prolonged but does autocorrect as Factor XII autoactivates on the surface. On the other hand, Factor XII–deficient plasma has a markedly abnormal PTT and does not autocorrect and is essentially devoid of intrinsic clotting or kinin formation. Alternatively, purified Factor XII preparations activate when tested with a

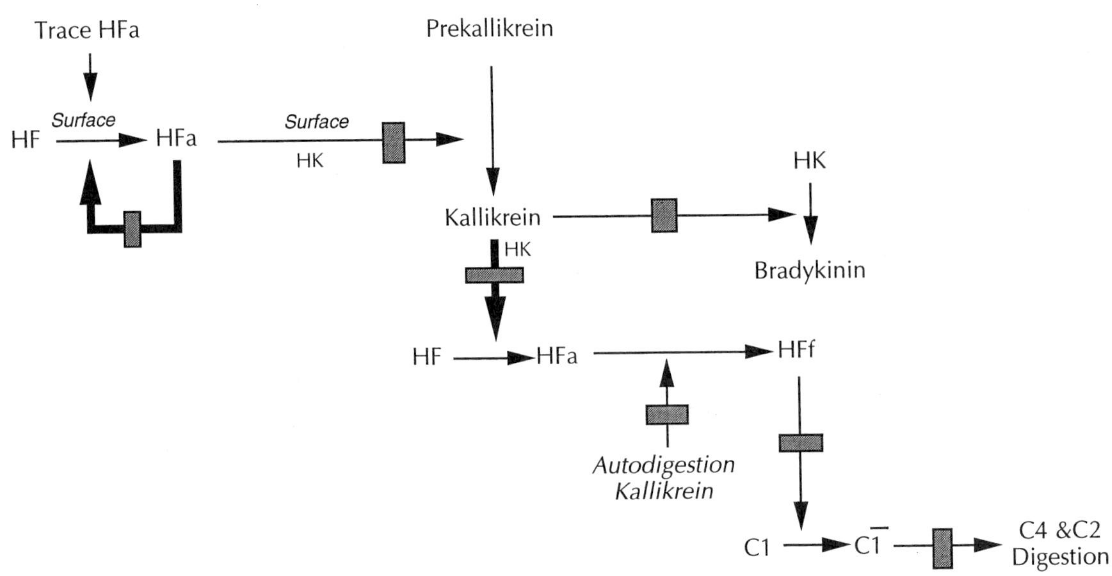

FIGURE 14–6. The plasma kinin-forming cascade depicting the initiating autoactivation step, the positive feedback involving kallikrein, and a linkage to the complement cascade. All steps inhibited by C1 INH are shown.

surface or polyanion under physiologic conditions,[199, 213, 216] whereas prekallikrein does not. Hence, Factor XII is considered absolutely requisite for intrinsic coagulation, whereas prekallikrein acts as an accelerator.

In plasma, the involvement of HK was indicated by the discovery of persons whose plasma had a very prolonged PTT and who generated no bradykinin upon incubation with kaolin but were not deficient in Factor XII or prekallikrein.[38, 52, 238] This phenomenon was explained by the identification of HK as a nonenzymatic cofactor in contact activation. It appeared to accelerate activation of both Factor XII and prekallikrein as well as Factor XI.[79, 133, 173, 234] The discovery that prekallikrein and Factor XII circulate bound to HK provided the mechanistic key to the explanation.[123, 217] One function of HK is to present the substrates of Factor XIIa in a conformation that facilitates their activation. Thus prekallikrein that is bound to a surface in the absence of HK is not subsequently activated by Factor XIIa.[201] A synthetic peptide encompassing the HK-binding site for prekallikrein can interfere with contact activation by competitively interfering with the binding of prekallikrein to the HK light chain.[209] Similarly, a monoclonal antibody to this binding site inhibits coagulation and kinin formation in plasma.[167]

Factor XI activation is almost totally dependent upon the formation of a surface-binding complex with HK. HK also augments the rate of Factor XII activation in plasma,[173, 234] although it does not augment the activity of kallikrein against synthetic substrates. The effect seems to be largely indirect. First, it is required for efficient formation of kallikrein in surface-activated plasma. Second, since kallikrein can dissociate from surface-bound HK, it can interact with surface-bound Factor XII on an adjacent particle, thereby disseminating the reaction.[35, 201, 234] As a result, the effective kallikrein/Factor XII ratio is increased in the presence of HK. Finally, in plasma, HK can displace other adhesive glycoproteins, such as fibrinogen, from binding to the surface.[184] These data indicate that HK must also be considered a coagulation cofactor because it is required for the generation of kallikrein (a Factor XII activator) as well as the activation of Factor XI. HK-deficient plasma has a profoundly prolonged activated PTT that is almost as abnormal as that of Factor XII deficiency,[38, 52, 238] although persons with congenital HK deficiency have no bleeding diathesis.

Regulation of contact activation occurs via plasma protease inhibitors. A summary of the major control proteins of this pathway is given in Table 14–2. C1-INH is a major inhibitor of Factor XIIa or XII_f[46, 60, 155, 187] and is not active against other coagulation enzymes except for a weak inhibition of Factor XIa. The inhibitor is cleaved by the protease and then binds at the active site of the protease in a 1:1 molar covalent complex that completely inactivates the enzyme.[220] Antithrombin III, which is a critical control protein for much of the coagulation cascade, makes a minor contribution to Factor XIIa (f) inactivation.[29, 46, 155, 205] Heparin can augment the inhibition by AT III, although there is some variance reported as to the magnitude of augmentation. Heparin can also function as an activating polyanion for contact activation.[91, 198] Curiously, α_2-macroglobulin, which is an inhibitor of broad reactivity with enzymes, does not significantly inhibit any of the forms of activated Factor XII.

Kallikrein is inhibited by both C1-INH and α_2-macroglobulin,[69, 83, 129] which together account for over 90% of the inhibitory activity of plasma.[181, 222] α_2-Macroglobulin does

TABLE 14–2
PLASMA INHIBITORS OF ENZYMES OF CONTACT ACTIVATION: RELATIVE CONTRIBUTIONS TO INHIBITION IN NORMAL PLASMA

	Enzyme			
	Factors			
Inhibitor	*XIIa*	*XIIf*	*Kallikrein*	*Factor XIa*
C1 inhibitor	91.3	93	52 (84)*	47 (76)‡
Antithrombin III†	1.5	4	nd	5 (18)‡
α_2-Macroglobulin	4.3	—	35 (16)*	—
α_1-Protease inhibitor	—	—	nd	23.5 (2)‡
α_2-Antiplasmin	3.0	3	nd	24.5 (4)‡

*Data obtained from generation of kallikrein in situ.
†Data are for results obtained in the absence of added heparin.
‡In the presence of heparin.
nd = not determined separately.

not bind to the active site but traps the protease within its structure so as to sterically interfere with its ability to cleave large protein substrates.[9] About one third of the enzyme's activity on small synthetic substrates is retained by the complex, whereas the activity on its natural substrates is less than 1%. Although these two inhibitors contribute roughly equally when kallikrein is added to plasma,[84, 181, 222] when a surface such as kaolin is added, 70 to 80% of the kallikrein formed is bound to C1-INH.[84] The reason for this difference is unknown. Conversely, at low temperatures, C1-INH is less effective, and much of the kallikrein inhibition is mediated by α_2-macroglobulin.[84]

Factor XIa is inhibited to a great extent by C1-INH.[239] When purified FXIa was added to plasma and its distribution among various inhibitors was determined, most of the added XIa was found to be complexed to C1-INH followed by FXIa:α_1-antitrypsin and FXIa:α_2-antiplasmin. However, α_1-antitrypsin was found to be the major inhibitor when chromatographic plasma fractions were tested against FXIa.[86, 189] Earlier studies[134, 189] found that C1-INH and AT III were inhibitors of factor XIa. Heparin augments AT III inhibition of all enzymes and C1-INH inhibitional factors XI (see Table 14–2).

Activation on a surface occurs very quickly, whereas inhibition has a slower reaction rate. In plasma of patients with hereditary angioedema (HAE) in which C1-INH is absent or dysfunctional, the amount of surface needed to produce maximal activation is 10- to 20-fold less than that needed to activate normal plasma.[29]

TISSUE PATHWAY OF BRADYKININ FORMATION

The tissue pathway for bradykinin formation is far simpler because only tissue kallikrein is involved, regardless which cell or tissue produces it. Tissue kallikrein[146] digests HK or LK to produce kallidin (lysyl-bradykinin), and a plasma aminopeptidase rapidly converts kallidin to bradykinin.[195] Kallidin and bradykinin possess identical biologic activities and act via the same receptor. However, in most assays, kallidin has 80 to 90% of the potency of bradykinin. The concentration of LK is much greater than that of HK; thus LK is preferentially cleaved. By contrast, plasma kallikrein is quite specific in utilizing HK as substrate.

The regulatory mechanisms of the tissue kallikrein pathway of bradykinin formation are not well known, and it was thought for a long time that none of the inhibitors of the contact pathway are involved in controlling tissue kallikrein. However, Rahman et al[164] have detected tissue kallikrein:α_1-antitrypsin complexes in synovial fluid from rheumatoid arthritis patients. In porcine plasma, exogenously added tissue kallikrein was found, to some extent, to form complexes with α_2-macroglobulin and α_1-antitrypsin.[18] However, tissue kallikrein activity was still present some 12 hours after the addition, suggesting that these macromolecular inhibitors may not provide significant regulation of tissue kallikrein in plasma. Since tissue kallikrein is not a major player in plasma kinin generation, the significance of these studies is unclear. Other kallikrein-binding proteins, which specifically bind and inhibit tissue kallikrein (but not plasma kallikrein), have been identified in rat and human tissues.[17] However, the functional significance of these binding proteins is still unclear (reviewed in 17). Peptide sequences analogous to the C-terminal sequence of kinins (Ac-Ser-*Pro-Phe-Arg*-Ser-Val-Gln-NH2) have been reported to be potent synthetic inhibitors of kallikrein.[28]

BRADYKININ: FUNCTIONS AND CONTROL MECHANISMS

The functions of bradykinin include venular dilatation, increased vascular permeability,[172] constriction of uterine and gastrointestinal smooth muscle, constriction of coronary and pulmonary vasculature, bronchoconstriction, and activation of phospholipase A2 to augment arachidonic acid metabolism. It acts in most tissues via B2 receptors, and selective B2 receptor antagonists have been synthesized. In plasma, bradykinin is first digested by carboxypeptidase N (also known as the anaphylatoxin inactivator or kininase I),[56] which removes the C-terminal Arg, leaving des-Arg^9 bradykinin.[194] This peptide lacks the inflammatory function of bradykinin (vasodilatation, increased permeability) that is evident in skin or smooth muscle but can interact with B1 receptors in the vasculature to cause hypotension. It has been reported that B1 receptors are induced during inflammatory conditions,[172] whereas B2 receptors are synthesized constitutively. However, in cultured bovine pulmonary artery endothelial cells, both B1 and B2 receptors are made constitutively.[1] When serum is examined, the rate of removal of the C-terminal Arg is more rapid than can be attributed to carboxypeptidase N.[195] This may be due to secretion (from cells) or activation of carboxypeptidase U, a newly described exopeptidase.[230] The next cleavage is by angiotensin-converting enzyme, which digests des-Arg^9 bradykinin (Arg-Pro-Pro-Gly-Phe-Ser-Pro-Phe) via its tripeptidase activity[193] (dipeptidase activity converts angiotensin I to angiotensin II) to yield Arg-Pro-Pro-Gly-Phe + Ser-Pro-Phe. These products are inactive on both B1 and B2 receptors. Further slow digestion leads to the final products of Arg-Pro-Pro plus one mole each of the amino acids Gly, Ser, Pro, and Arg and two moles of Phe.[195]

In vivo, kinin degradation occurs rapidly along endothelial cells of the pulmonary vasculature. But here, the predominant enzyme is ACE, which acts as a dipeptidase if the C-terminal Arg is present to remove Phe-Arg. The resultant heptapeptide is cleaved once again at the C-terminal end to liberate Ser Pro, leaving the pentapeptide Arg-Pro-Pro-Gly-Phe.[193] These peptides are further metabolized to Arg-Pro-Pro and free amino acids. The cough and angioedema associated with the use of ACE inhibitors for treatment of heart failure, hypertension, diabetes, or scleroderma may be due to inhibition of kinin inactivation and accumulation of bradykinin as conversion to angiotensin II is prevented.

INTRINSIC FIBRINOLYTIC CASCADE

A Factor XII–dependent pathway leading to the conversion of plasminogen to plasmin was described in the 1960s and early 1970s.[94, 130, 149] A defect in this pathway has been observed in plasmas deficient in Factor XII, prekallikrein, or HK.[38, 52, 178, 232, 237, 238] The Factor XII–dependent fibrinolytic activity is relatively weak and difficult to demonstrate in whole plasma because large quantities of a potent plasminogen activator are not formed. Relatively little plasmin is generated, which is rapidly inactivated by plasma inhibitors (α_2-antiplasmin, α_2-macroglobulin). Most studies have therefore used diluted, acidified plasma[148] or chloroform-treated plasma[149] in which inhibitors of contact activation and plasmin are rendered inactive; euglobulin preparations that concentrate the plasma enzymes and cofactors but limit inhibition[109]; or plasma following addition of organic compounds that destroy α_2-antiplasmin and C1-INH can also be employed.[110, 136, 137] Such measures are not needed to study blood coagulation or the liberation of bradykinin.

Factor XII–dependent activation of plasminogen is accomplished primarily by kallikrein[37] and Factor XIa.[124, 125] When purified preparations are compared, kallikrein and Factor XIa directly activate plasminogen with equal potency.[125] The plasma concentration of prekallikrein, however, is about 10-fold higher than that of Factor XI. In addition, Factor XIIf can readily convert prekallikrein to kallikrein in the fluid phase,[102, 214] whereas it has minimal activity on Factor XI.[103] Additional kallikrein can dissociate from surfaces and act in the fluid phase, whereas Factor XIa cannot. Therefore, kallikrein is more important for this pathway.

Activated Factor XII (XIIa or XIIf) can also convert plasminogen to plasmin,[72] but its activity is only 5% of that of kallikrein. These are all weak reactions in that the potencies of kallikrein and Factor XIa as plasminogen activators are thousands of times lower than the potency of urokinase.[101, 125, 135] Thus it can be argued that plasminogen is not a significant substrate for any of them. Although each of these proteins is capable of converting plasminogen to plasmin, the other blood-clotting enzymes—Factors IXa, Xa, VIIa, and thrombin—have no such activity, which argues against this activity (of contact activation enzymes) as being a nonspecific phenomenon.

Some studies of contact-activated fibrinolysis suggest that kallikrein activates the trace quantity of prourokinase in plasma[85] and that urokinase is the main plasminogen activator of plasma.[93] Inhibition by antiurokinase antisera supports this notion as do zymographic gel studies using plasma euglobulin preparations.[85, 136] Investigators in other studies have suggested a role for plasma urokinase in Factor XII–independent fibrinolysis.[112] Although urokinase is clearly a much more potent plasminogen activator than any of the enzymes associated with contact activation, the quantities of urokinase generated are small. If the effects of α_2-antiplasmin and C1-INH are abrogated by addition of flufenamic acid derivatives, contact activation results in the formation of about 35 ng/mL of plasmin,[137] which represents activation of 0.05% of plasma plasminogen.

However, these studies with whole, diluted, or modified plasma ignore the in vivo situation where platelets and other blood cells are clearly involved in coagulation/fibrinolysis. In this respect, studies suggesting an important role for platelet-bound contact factors in fibrinolysis are noteworthy.[122] They have shown that the contact-dependent intrinsic pathway of fibrinolysis may be mediated by platelets due to the presence of platelet-bound prekallikrein. When prekallikrein was activated by Factor XIIa in a thrombus, local activation of platelet-associated prourokinase occurred, promoting targeted plasminogen activation and fibrinolysis.[81, 122] During cardiopulmonary bypass surgery, the incidence of thrombus formation was reportedly higher in Factor XII–deficient patients than in normals.[27, 138] In a separate study, recurrence of myocardial infarction was found to correlate with lower than normal levels of plasma prekallikrein and Factor XII–dependent fibrinolytic activity.[151] Another study has demonstrated that generation of bradykinin was associated with activation of the fibrinolytic system (a positive correlation was found between plasmin:α_2-antiplasmin complexes and cleaved HK) during acute attacks of angioedema in HAE patients.[44] These observations suggest that the contact system may really be more critical for fibrinolysis than for thrombosis and that studies involving the interaction of contact factors with cells may be more valuable than studies of their interactions in whole plasma.

Studies with a baboon sepsis model also have indicated that Factor XII and the contact system play an important role in both fibrinolysis and complement activation.[98] It was shown that administration of monoclonal anti–Factor XII to baboons suffering from lethal sepsis was accompanied by decreased activation of the complement and fibrinolytic systems.

An alternative interaction between the kallikrein-kinin system and in vivo fibrinolysis is suggested by the observation that bradykinin is a potent stimulator of tPA released from endothelial cells.[203]

REGULATION OF BLOOD PRESSURE

The possible relationship of the contact system to blood pressure regulation is an intriguing issue. As already seen, ACE plays a major role in inactivating the hypotensive effects of bradykinin, and administration of ACE inhibitors causes cough and occasional swelling that may be kinin dependent. An unfortunate circumstance has dramatized the kinin-forming capacity of Factor XIIf; trauma patients given plasma protein fractions as plasma expanders that were contaminated with Factor XIIf showed profound hypotension.[3, 4] The mechanism by which infused Factor XII_f causes hypotension has been demonstrated to involve bradykinin formation rather than prostaglandins.[227] A much more tenuous connection also exists between blood pressure regulation and the contact system in the Factor XII–dependent activation of plasma prorenin. Prorenin is activated to renin by cold treatment of plasma or acidification to pH 3.3. Reneutralization is accompanied by appearance of renin activity, and this is mediated by kallikrein,[47, 191] as is the cold-induced activation.[25] Kallikrein is able to activate purified prorenin, but when added to plasma, it does not cause prorenin activation without an acidification step.[240] Although the acid treatment is supposed to destroy kallikrein inhibitors, prorenin is not activated in plasma deficient in C1-INH or α_2-macroglobulin.[161] Thus some other event must occur on acidification, such as a conformational change in prorenin, to form a kallikrein substrate. The physiologic significance of this reaction is uncertain.

Bradykinin is known to have direct effects on homeostasis.[22] Intravenous administration of bradykinin lowered the systemic blood pressure in a dose-dependent manner in both normotensive and hypertensive subjects. The blood pressure reduction observed in these two groups was not dependent upon changes in sodium metabolism, β-adrenergic receptors, histamine-1 receptors, or prostaglandins. ACE inhibitors such as captopril potentiated the blood-pressure lowering effects of bradykinin approximately 20 to 50 fold. Patients deficient in carboxypeptidase N (kininase I), one of the enzymes responsible for the degradation of bradykinin, were suggested to have elevated bradykinin levels and were hypotensive.[6, 207] Finally, rodent models of hypertension have revealed that the effects of ACE inhibitors are reversed by B2 receptor antagonists, suggesting that prevention of bradykinin degradation by ACE may be important in lowering blood pressure apart from inhibition of angiotensin II formation.[87]

INTERACTION WITH OTHER PLASMA PROTEASES

Factor XIIf has been reported to activate Factor VII[163, 192] and thereby initiate the extrinsic coagulation pathway. This reaction contributes minimally to the kaolin-APTT as usually performed, but it is responsible for the shortened clotting time seen when plasma is exposed to the cold.[71, 116] Factor VII activation is accentuated in women who use oral contraceptives containing estrogen, apparently due to an increased concentration of Factor XII.[73, 74, 99] This might contribute to the increased incidence of thrombosis reported as a complication of oral contraceptive use. Interestingly, there are data suggesting that oral contraceptives also increase the fibrinolytic state in women.[30] An increase in Factor XII and prekallikrein levels as well as α_1-antitrypsin is seen as a result of oral contraceptive use.

Factor XII_f (but not Factor XIIa) can enzymatically activate the first component of complement when it is incubated with purified C1 or added to plasma.[68] C1 activation is due to cleavage of the CIr subcomponent[67] by Factor XIIf. Little complement activation is seen when kaolin is incubated with whole plasma, and significant complement activation may be seen only in conditions that result in substantial conversion of Factor XIIa to Factor XIIf. One such circumstance is HAE in which Factor XII activation may contribute to complement consumption.[49, 58] Kallikrein can also cleave C1 subcomponents, but the net result is destruction rather than activation. On the other hand, kallikrein can activate Factor

B of the alternative complement pathway and thereby substitute for Factor D.[48]

INTERACTIONS WITH CELLS

Kallikrein has been reported to interact with human leukocytes in a variety of ways. It is a chemotactic factor for neutrophils[104] and monocytes[66] and has been shown to cause neutrophil aggregation[180] and release of elastase.[225] In a rabbit model, kallikrein stimulation of chemotaxis appeared to require cleavage of C5 and release of C5a chemotactic factor.[235] Therefore, C5 bound to the surface of neutrophils can possibly be cleaved in the aforementioned reactions. Antikallikrein serum was inhibitory, whereas anti-C5 serum had no effect. The investigators therefore concluded that the effect of kallikrein on human neutrophils is independent of complement. Furthermore, a degraded form of kallikrein (β-kallikrein), in which the heavy chain is partially digested, is enzymatically active on kininogen to form kinin, but its reactivity with neutrophils is markedly attenuated.[40] Factor XIIa has also been shown to stimulate neutrophils; since Factor XIIf did not do this, a requirement for a binding site in the heavy chain was inferred.[226] No studies have demonstrated either a cell surface receptor for these enzymes or required cleavage of surface components. In each instance, the active site of the enzyme is required so that the proenzyme or DFP-treated enzyme is inactive.[104, 180]

The components of the contact activation system also appear to interact with platelets. Apparently, plasma Factor XI and Factor XIa have separate platelet receptors.[202] Platelets also have an intrinsic protein with Factor XI activity, which cross-reacts with plasma Factor XI immunologically but differs from it in molecular weight and isoelectric point. This activity is present in patients who are deficient in plasma Factor XI.[118, 221] Platelet-associated Factor XI can be activated by Factor XII–dependent and Factor XII–independent mechanisms.[229] The membrane of activated platelets may also provide a surface on which Factor XII can be activated in the presence of prekallikrein and HK[229] so that bound Factor XI is then activated. HK has been shown to be present within the alpha granules of platelets.[186] To become available during platelet activation,[185] HK exhibits zinc-dependent[82] binding to the platelet surface[76, 186] and augments binding of Factor XIa.[202]

Despite the demonstrated interactions of contact factors with platelets, platelets clearly are not requisite for contact activation as they are for later steps in coagulation. Thus contact activation proceeds normally in platelet-poor plasma, and the addition of platelets provides little or no augmentation. In fact, evidence exists that platelets may actually inhibit prekallikrein and Factor XII activation by secretion of β-thromboglobulin.[113, 190] Nevertheless, platelet activation in peripheral tissues due to injury or localized thrombosis may possibly contribute to contact activation and local kinin formation. In some circumstances, the platelets may also provide a Factor XII bypass in contact activation.[228]

All the components of the contact activation cascade have been demonstrated to bind to endothelial cells also. Schmaier and colleagues[183] and van Iwaarden and colleagues[223] first described binding of HK to human umbilical vein endothelial cells in a zinc-dependent reaction. This binding subsequently was demonstrated in situ by immunochemical staining of umbilical cord segments following incubation with HK.[145] The HK-HUVEC interaction was saturable, reversible, dependent on 25 to 50 μM zinc (normal plasma concentration), and fulfilling the characteristics of a receptor-mediated interaction. There are 1×10^6 to 1×10^7 binding sites (an unusually large number) with a high affinity ($K_d \approx 40–50$ nM). Binding is seen with either chain of HK (heavy and light chains); thus a complex interaction with subsites within the receptor seems likely.[170] A similar complex interaction has been observed with platelets, although the binding site number is far less. Since prekallikrein and Factor XI circulate bound to HK, these are brought to the endothelial cell surface via HK.[16] There are no separate receptor sites for either prekallikrein or Factor XI. When we examined binding of Factor XII, we found binding characteristics of a receptor that were strikingly similar to those seen with HK, including a requirement for zinc.[171] We then demonstrated that HK and Factor XII can compete for binding at a comparable molar basis, suggesting that they bind to the same receptor.[171] We have identified a zinc-dependent binding protein for HK and Factor XII derived from endothelial cell membranes. It is identical to gC1qR, the receptor for the globular heads of C1q.[115a]

We also demonstrated that Factor XII can slowly autoactivate when bound to endothelial cells[171] and that addition of kallikrein can digest bound HK to liberate bradykinin at a rate proportional to the kallikrein concentration and with a final bradykinin level dependent on the amount of bound HK. Thus activation of the cascade along the endothelial cell surface is likely, as illustrated in Figure 14–7; bradykinin is liberated and then interacts with the B2 receptor to increase permeability. Bradykinin can also stimulate cultured endothelial cells to secrete tissue plasminogen activator,[203] prostaglandin I_2 (prostacyclin), and thromboxane A_2[43, 92] and can thereby modulate platelet function and stimulate local fibrinolysis. Neutrophils also bind HK via the $C3b_i$ (CR3) receptor,[224] which is absent on endothelial cells, and all components of the kinin-forming cascade can interact at the cell surface.[88]

CLINICAL CONSIDERATIONS

KININ FORMATION IN HEREDITARY ANGIOEDEMA

The pathogenesis of HAE suggests liberation of a kinin that has variously been considered to be a product of the second component of complement or produced by contact activation. As shown in Figure 14–6, if C1-INH is either absent (Type I HAE) or dysfunctional (Type II HAE), there is insufficient inhibition of all the activated forms of Factor XII, kallikrein, or activated C1 (specifically C1r and C1s, each of which is inhibited by C1-INH). The production of bradykinin is markedly augmented under these conditions, and it has been shown that addition of dextran sulfate at concentrations insufficient to activate normal plasma leads to complete digestion of HK in HAE plasma within a few minutes.[29] Thus seemingly insignificant trauma or infections may be sufficient to initiate an attack in such patients.

Soon after C1-INH deficiency was shown to be the cause of HAE, evidence was presented to suggest that cleavage of C2[50] or C2b[53] would generate a kinin that was responsible

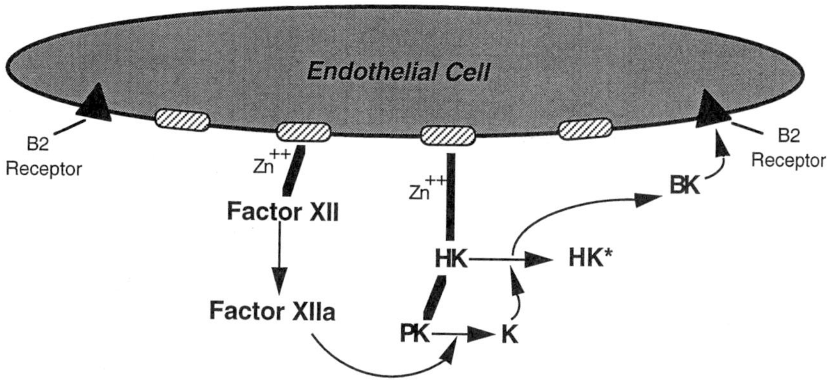

HK=HMW Kininogen; PK=Prekallikrein; K=Kallikrein; HK*=Cleaved HK; BK=Bradykinin

FIGURE 14–7. Assembly of the proteins involved in bradykinin formation along the endothelial cell surface. A common receptor binds Factor XII and HK, requiring zinc ion. Bradykinin, once liberated, acts on the B2 receptor to activate endothelial cells and increase vascular permeability.

for the symptoms. Attempts to produce this kinin by cleavage of C2 or C2b have, in general, been negative,[57] nor has such a kinin been shown to circulate in patients during an attack. On the other hand, synthesis of overlapping peptides within the C2b portion of the molecule revealed a sequence that possessed kinin-like peptides.[206] However, enzymatic cleavage of the protein to release this peptide has not yet been achieved.

Activated kallikrein has been shown to be present in markedly augmented amounts in blister fluids derived from patients, and bradykinin has been reported to be the major kinin found when HAE plasma is activated.[45] The bulk of evidence favors a major role for bradykinin in causing the symptoms of HAE.[57] However, the presence of an additional kinin-like fragment derived from C2 by a mechanism that is not yet understood is possible. If so, synergy between the two kinins might occur. Use of B2 receptor antagonists in such patients, once they are available for human use, should help settle the question.

Complement is nevertheless clearly activated in HAE, and this may be due to the autoactivation of C1r when C1-INH is absent. C4 levels are diminished, presumably due to consumption by C1s in HAE patients even when they are asymptomatic; with attacks of swelling, C4 levels approach zero and C2 levels diminish. As seen in Figure 14–6, this process may be augmented by Factor XII_f (HF_f), which has been shown to enzymatically cleave and activate C1r, and to a lesser degree C1s.[67] Use of androgenic therapeutic agents (Danazol, Stanozolol) may increase synthesis of C1-INH sufficiently to prevent swelling. Levels of C4 and C1-INH increase, although the magnitude may not parallel the clinical effect. Agents that inhibit plasminogen activation (ε-amino caproic acid, tranexamic acid) are also effective therapeutic agents that prevent formation of plasmin; they may also have direct inhibitory effects on C1 activation.[204] Plasmin is also an enzymatic activator of Factor XII[103] and might thereby contribute to HF_f production and bradykinin formation or digest C2b to yield a kinin-like fragment.[206]

CONTACT ACTIVATION IN ALLERGIC DISEASES

By analogy with observations using dextran sulfate, naturally occurring glycosaminoglycans or proteoglycans may be able to induce contact activation. We have tested heparin proteoglycan from the Furth murine mastocytoma for its ability to activate a mixture of Factor XII and prekallikrein. There is progressive conversion of prekallikrein to kallikrein as the concentration of mast cell heparin is increased. The potency of heparin proteoglycan equals that of dextran sulfate, and its activity is inhibited by heparinase I or II but not by heparitinase or chondroitinase ABC. Of the glycosaminoglycans we have tested, heparin, dermatan sulfate, keratin polysulfate, and chondroitin sulfate C are positive in the assay (in that order), whereas heparan sulfate and chondroitin sulfate A are negative. Collagen types I, III, IV, and V, laminin, fibronectin, and vitronectin are also negative. Activation can then occur by release of heparin and/or other mucopolysaccharides secreted by mast cells and basophils upon exposure to plasma proteins and via interaction of these proteins with exposed connective tissue proteoglycans during tissue injury. The proteins of the kinin-forming system have been shown to be present in interstitial fluid of rabbit skin; thus the source may not solely be dependent upon exudation and activation of plasma.

Any aspect of inflammation that leads to dilution of plasma constituents or exclusion of inhibitors will augment contact activation since inhibitory functions are very dependent upon concentration. Thus activation of plasma can be shown to be related directly to dilution. Once levels of C1-INH are less than 25% of normal (a 1:4 dilution), patients with HAE are prone to attacks of swelling.

Activation of the plasma and tissue kinin-forming systems has been observed in allergic reactions in the nose, lungs, and skin, including both the immediate and late phase reactions, although the contributions of the plasma and tissue kallikrein pathways to each aspect of allergic inflammation are likely quite different. Antigen challenge of the nose followed by nasal lavage revealed an increase in TAME esterase activity, which is largely attributable to kallikrein(s).[160] The activation was seen during the immediate response as well as the late phase reaction.[42] Both LK and HK were shown to be present in nasal lavage fluid,[12] and fractionation of nasal washings demonstrated evidence of both tissue kallikrein[10] and plasma kallikrein.[11] Tissue kallikrein can be secreted by glandular tissue as well as by infiltrating cells, such as neutrophils, and will cleave LK to yield kallidin. Plasma kallikrein will digest HK to yield bradykinin directly. HPLC analysis of kinins in nasal washings revealed both kallidin and bradykinin. The latter can be formed from kallidin by aminopeptidase action, although a portion of the bradykinin is also likely the direct result of plasma kallikrein activity. Tissue kallikrein has also been found in bronchoalveolar lavage fluids of asthmatics.[33]

Studies of the allergen-induced late phase reactions in the skin[5] have demonstrated the presence of kallikrein–C1-INH and activated Factor XII–C1-INH complexes in induced blisters observed for an 8-hour period. Elevated levels of these complexes were seen between 3 and 6 hours coincident with the late phase response and were specific for the antigen to which the patient was sensitive.

OTHER DISORDERS

Endotoxic shock is associated with depletion of contact activation proteins,[90, 128, 147, 175] and serial HK levels have prognostic value[90] since a drop to near zero usually indicates a fatal outcome as do lower prekallikrein levels.[147] A monoclonal antibody to Factor XII markedly diminished the mortality by 50% in a baboon monkey model of endotoxic shock.[153, 154] Parameters of disseminated intravascular coagulation (DIC) were unaffected and likely medicated via tissue thromboplastin, although DIC due to endothelial cell injury and/or endotoxemia is associated with diminished levels of Factor XII, prekallikrein, and kallikrein inhibiting activity.[117, 127]

The synovial fluid of patients with rheumatoid arthritis has been shown to contain plasma kallikrein, which can activate stromelysin and convert procollagenase to collagenase.[144] Uric acid and pyrophosphate crystals can act as surfaces for contact activation[70, 107] and may contribute to the inflammation seen in gout or pseudogout. However, at least one case of gout[119] and one of rheumatoid arthritis[51] have been reported in Factor XII–deficient subjects.

Pancreatitis, particularly acute hemorrhagic pancreatitis, is associated with release of large quantities of tissue kallikrein, thus kallidin and/or bradykinin may contribute to the pooling of fluid within the abdominal cavity and hypotension that can result.

REFERENCES

1. Smith J, Webb C, Holford J, et al: Signal transduction pathways for B1 and B2 bradykinin receptors in bovine pulmonary artery endothelial cells. Mol Pharmacol 47:525, 1995.
2. Adam A, Albert A, Calay G, et al: Human kininogens of low and high molecular mass: quantification by radioimmunoassay and determination of reference values. Clin Chem 31:423, 1985.
3. Alving BM, Hojima Y, Pisano JJ, et al: Hypotension associated with prekallikrein activator (Hageman factor fragments) in plasma protein fraction. N Engl J Med 229:66, 1978.
4. Alving BM, Tankersley DL, Mason BL, et al: Contact activation factors: contaminants of immunoglobulin preparations with coagulant and vasoactive properties. J Lab Clin Med 96:334, 1980.
5. Atkins PC, Miragliotta G, Talbot SF, et al: Activation of plasma Hageman factor and kallikrein in ongoing allergic reactions in the skin. J Immunol 139:2744, 1987.
6. Auchincloss JH, Streeten DH, Gilbert R, et al: Dyspnea in patients with hyperbradykininism and excessive venous pooling. Am J Med 81:260, 1986.
7. Baglia FA, Sinha D, Walsh PN: Functional domains in the heavy-chain region of factor XI: a high molecular weight kininogen-binding site and a substrate binding site for factor IX. Blood 74:244, 1989.
8. Baker AR, Shine J: Human kidney kallikrein: cDNA cloning and sequence analysis. DNA 4:445, 1985.
9. Barrett AJ, Starkey PM: The interaction of α_2-macroglobulin with proteinases. Biochem J 133:709, 1973.
10. Baumgarten CR, Nichols RC, Naclerio RM, et al: Plasma kallikrein during experimentally-induced allergic rhinitis: role in kinin formation and contribution to TAME esterase activity in nasal secretions. J Immunol 137:977, 1986.
11. Baumgarten CR, Nichols RC, Naclerio RM, et al: Concentrations of glandular kallikrein in human nasal secretions increase during experimentally-induced allergic rhinitis. J Immunol 137:1323, 1986.
12. Baumgarten CR, Togias AG, Naclerio RM, et al: Influx of kininogens into nasal secretions after antigen challenge of allergic individuals. J Clin Invest 76:191, 1985.
13. Bernardo MM, Day DE, Halvorson HR, et al: Surface-independent acceleration of Factor XII activation by zinc ions. II. Direct binding and fluorescence studies. J Biol Chem 268:12477, 1993.
14. Bernardo MM, Day DE, Olson ST, et al: Surface-independent acceleration of Factor XII activation by zinc ions. I. Kinetic characterization of the metal ion rate enhancement. J Biol Chem 268:12468, 1993.
15. Berrettini M, Lammle B, White T, et al: Detection of in vitro and in vivo cleavage of high molecular weight kininogen in human plasma immunoblotting with monoclonal antibodies. Blood 68:455, 1986.
16. Berrettini M, Schleef RR, Heeb MJ, et al: Assembly and expression of intrinsic factor IX activator complex on the surface of cultured human endothelial cells. J Biol Chem 267:19833, 1992.
17. Bhoola KD, Figueroa CD, Worthy K: Bioregulation of kinins: kallikreins, kininogens, and kininases. Pharmacol Rev 44:1, 1992.
18. Blackberg M: Interactions in vitro and in vivo between porcine tissue kallikrein and porcine plasma proteinase inhibitors. Scand J Clin Lab Invest 54:643, 1994.
19. Bock PE, Shore JD: Protein-protein interaction of blood coagulation. Characterization of a fluoroscein-labeled human high molecular weight kininogen light chain as a probe. J Biol Chem 258:15079, 1983.
20. Bock PE, Shore JD, Tans G, et al: Protein-protein interactions in contact activation of blood coagulation. Binding of high molecular weight kininogen and the 5-(iodoacetamido) fluorescein-labeled kininogen light chain to prekallikrein, kallikrein, and the separated kallikrein heavy and light chains. J Biol Chem 260:12434, 1985.
21. Bock PE, Srinivasan KR, Shore JD: Activation of intrinsic blood coagulation by ellagic acid: insoluble ellagic acid metal ion complexes are the activating species. Biochemistry 20:7258, 1981.
22. Bönner G, Preis S, Schunk U, et al: Hemodynamic effects of bradykinin on systemic and pulmonary circulation in healthy and hypertensive humans. J Cardiovasc Pharmacol 15:S46, 1990.
23. Bouma BN, Griffin JH: Human blood coagulation factor XI: purification, properties, and mechanism of activation by factor XII. J Biol Chem 252:6432, 1977.
24. Bouma BN, Miles LA, Barretta G, et al: Human plasma prekallikrein. Studies of its activation by activated factor XII and of its inactivation by diisopropyl phosphofluoridate. Biochemistry 19:1151, 1980.
25. Brown CF, Osmond DH: Factor XII and prekallikrein-kallikrein-kinin in the cryoactivation of human plasma prorenin. Clin Sci (Colch) 66:533, 1984.
26. Brunnée T, Reddigari SR, Shibayama Y, et al: Activation of the contact system by glycosaminoglycan derived from mast cell proteoglycan. 1995; (submitted).
27. Burman JF, Chung HI, Lane DA, et al: Role of factor XII in thrombin generation and fibrinolysis during cardiopulmonary bypass. Lancet 344:1192, 1994.
28. Burton J, Benetos A: The design of specific inhibitors of tissue kallikrein and their effect on the blood pressure of rat. Adv Exp Med Biol 247B:9, 1989.
29. Cameron CL, Fisslthaler B, Sherman A, et al: Studies on contact activation: effects of surfaces and inhibitors. Med Prog Technol 15:53, 1989.
30. Campbell SJ, Mackie IJ, Robinson GE, et al: Contact factor mediated fibrinolysis is increased by the combined oral contraceptive pill. Br J Obstet Gynaecol 100:79, 1993.

31. Castellino FJ, Beals JM: The genetic relationships between the kringle domains of human plasminogen, prothrombin, tissue plasminogen activator, urokinase, and coagulation factor XII. J Mol Evol 26:358, 1987.
32. Chao J, Woodley-Miller C, Chao L: Identification of tissue kallikrein in brain and in the cell-free translation product encoded by brain mRNA. J Biol Chem 258:15173, 1983.
33. Christiansen SC, Proud D, Cochrane CG: Detection of tissue kallikrein in the bronchoalveolar lavage fluids of asthmatic subjects. J Clin Invest 79:188, 1987.
34. Chung DW, Fujikawa K, McMullen BA, et al: Human plasma prekallikrein, a zymogen to a serine protease that contains four tandem repeats. Biochemistry 25:2410, 1986.
35. Cochrane CG, Revak SD: Dissemination of contact activation in plasma by plasma kallikrein. J Exp Med 152:608, 1980.
36. Cochrane CG, Revak SD, Wuepper KD: Activation of Hageman factor in solid and fluid phases. J Exp Med 138:1564, 1973.
37. Colman RW: Activation of plasminogen by plasma kallikrein. Biochem Biophys Res Commun 351:273, 1969.
38. Colman RW, Bagdasarian A, Talamo RC, et al: Williams trait: human kininogen deficiency with diminished levels of plasminogen proactivator and prekallikrein associated with abnormalities of the Hageman factor dependent pathways. J Clin Invest 56:1650, 1975.
39. Colman RW, Muller-Esterl W: Nomenclature of kininogens. Thromb Haemost 60:340, 1988.
40. Colman RW, Wachtfogel YT, Kucich V, et al: Effect of cleavage of the heavy chain of human plasma kallikrein on its functional properties. Blood 65:311, 1985.
41. Cool DE, Edgell CS, Louie GV, et al: Characterization of human blood coagulation factor XII cDNA. J Biol Chem 25:13666, 1985.
42. Creticos PS, Peters SP, Adkinson NF Jr, et al: Peptide leucotriene release after antigen challenge in patients sensitive to ragweed. N Engl J Med 310:1626, 1984.
43. Crutchly DJ, Ryan JW, Ryan US, et al: Bradykinin induced release of prostacyclin and thromboxanes from bovine pulmonary artery endothelial cells. Biochim Biophys Acta 751:99, 1983.
44. Cugno M, Hack CE, de Boer JP, et al: Generation of plasmin during acute attacks of hereditary angioedema. J Lab Clin Med 121:38, 1993.
45. Curd JG, Prograis LF Jr, Cochrane CG: Detection of active kallikrein in induced blister fluids of hereditary angioedema patients. J Exp Med 152:742, 1980.
46. de Agostini A, Lijnen HR, Pixley RA, et al: Inactivation of factor XII active fragment in normal plasma. Predominent role of C1-inhibitor. J Clin Invest 73:1542, 1984.
47. Derkx FHM, Bouma BN, Schalekamp MPA, et al: An intrinsic factor XII-prekallikrein-dependent pathway activates the human plasma renin-angiotensin system. Nature 280:315, 1979.
48. DiScipio RG: The activation of the alternative pathway C3 convertase by human plasma kallikrein. Immunology 45:587, 1992.
49. Donaldson VH: Mechanism of activation of C1 esterase in hereditary angioneurotic edema in vitro. The role of Hageman factor, a clot promoting agent. J Exp Med 127:411, 1967.
50. Donaldson VH, Ratnoff OD, Dias DaSilva W, et al: Permeability-increasing activity in hereditary angioedema plasma II mechanism of formation and partial characterization. J Clin Invest 48:642, 1969.
51. Donaldson VH, Glueck HI, Fleming T: Rheumatoid arthritis in a patient with Hageman trait. N Engl J Med 386:528, 1972.
52. Donaldson VH, Glueck HI, Miller MA: Kininogen deficiency in Fitzgerald trait: role of high molecular weight kininogen in clotting and fibrinolysis. J Lab Clin Med 89:327, 1976.
53. Donaldson VH, Rosen FS, Bing DH: Role of the second component of complement (C2) and plasmin in kinin release in hereditary angioneurotic edema (H.A.N.E.) plasma. Trans Assoc Am Physicians 40:174, 1977.
54. Dunn JT, Kaplan AP: Formation and structure of human Hageman factor fragments. J Clin Invest 70:627, 1982.
55. Dunn JT, Silverberg M, Kaplan AP: The cleavage and formation of activated Hageman factor by autodigestion and by kallikrein. J Biol Chem 275:1779, 1982.
56. Erdos EG, Sloane GM: An enzyme in human plasma that inactivates bradykinin and kallidins. Biochem Pharmacol 11:585, 1962.
57. Fields T, Ghebrehiwet B, Kaplan AP: Kinin formation in hereditary angioedema plasma: evidence against kinin derivation from C2 and in support of "spontaneous" formation of bradykinin. J Allergy Clin Immunol 72:54, 1983.
58. Fields T, Ghebrehiwet B, Kaplan AP: Kinin formation in hereditary angioedema plasma: evidence against kinin derivation from C2 and in support of "spontaneous" formation of bradykinin. J Allergy Clin Immunol 72:54, 1983.
59. Figueroa C, Maciver AG, Bhoola KD: Identification of a tissue kallikrein in human polymorphonuclear leukocytes. Br J Haematol 72:321, 1989.
60. Forbes CO, Pensky J, Ratnoff OD: Inhibition of activated Hageman factor and activated plasma thromboplastin antecedent by purified C1 inactivator. J Lab Clin Med 76:809, 1970.
61. Fritz H, Fiedler F, Dietl T, et al: On the relationships between porcine pancreatic, submandibular and urinary kallikrein. In Haberland GL, Rohen JW, Suzuki T (eds): Kininogenases:Kallikrein. Schattauer-Verlag, Stuttgart/New York, 1977, p 15.
62. Fujikawa K, Chung DW, Hendrickson LE, et al: Amino acid sequence of human factor XI, a blood coagulation factor with four tandem repeats that are highly homologous with plasma prekallikrein. Biochemistry 25:2417, 1986.
63. Fujikawa K, Heimark RL, Kurachi K, et al: Activation of bovine factor XII (Hageman factor) by plasma kallikrein. Biochemistry 19:1322, 1980.
64. Fujikawa K, McMullen BA: Amino acid sequence of human b-factor XIIa. J Biol Chem 258:10924, 1983.
65. Fukushima D, Kitamura N, Nakanishi S: Nucleotide sequence of cloned cDNA for human pancreatic kallikrein. Biochemistry 24:8037, 1985.
66. Gallin JI, Kaplan AP: Mononuclear cell chemotactic activity of kallikrein and plasminogen activator and its inhibition by C1 INH and $\alpha 2$ macroglobulin. J Immunol 113:1928, 1974.
67. Ghebrehiwet B, Randazzo BP, Dunn JT, et al: Mechanism of activation of the classical pathway of complement by Hageman factor fragment. J Clin Invest 71:1450, 1983.
68. Ghebrehiwet B, Silverberg M, Kaplan AP: Activation of the classical pathway of complement by Hageman factor fragment. J Exp Med 153:665, 1981.
69. Gigli I, Mason JW, Coleman RW, et al: Interaction of plasma kallikrein with the C1 inhibitor. J Immunol 104:574, 1970.
70. Ginsberg M, Jaques B, Cochrane CG, et al: Urate crystal dependent cleavage of Hageman factor in human plasma and synovial fluid. J Lab Clin Med 95:497, 1980.
71. Gjonnaess H: Cold promoting activation of factor VII. I. Evidence for existence of an activation. Thromb Diath Haemorrh 28:155, 1972.
72. Goldsmith G, Saito H, Ratnoff OD: The activation of plasminogen by Hageman factor (factor XII) and Hageman factor fragments. J Clin Invest 12:54, 1978.
73. Gordon EM, Douglas J, Ratnoff OD: Influence of augmented Hageman factor (factor XII) titers on the cryoactivation of plasma prorenin in women using oral contraceptives. J Clin Invest 72:1833, 1983.
74. Gordon EM, Ratnoff OD, Saito H, et al: Rapid fibrinolysis, augmented Hageman factor (factor XII) titers and decreased C1 esterase inhibitor titers in women using oral contraceptives. J Lab Clin Med 96:762, 1980.
75. Gounaris AD, Brown MA, Barrett AJ: Human plasma α_1-cysteine proteinase inhibitor. Purification by affinity chromatography, characterization, and isolation of an active fragment. Biochem J 221:445, 1984.
76. Greengard JS, Griffin JH: Receptor for high molecular kininogen on stimulated washed human platelets. Biochemistry 23:6863, 1984.
77. Griep MA, Fujikawa K, Nelsestuen GL: Binding and activation properties of human factor XII, prekallikrein and derived peptides with acidic lipid vesicles. Biochemistry 24:4124, 1985.
78. Griffin JH: Role of surface in surface-dependent activation of Hageman factor (blood coagulation factor XII). Proc Natl Acad Sci USA 75:1998, 1978.
79. Griffin JH, Cochrane CG: Mechanisms for the involvement of high molecular weight kininogen in surface-dependent reactions of Hageman factor. Proc Natl Acad Sci USA 73:2554, 1976.
80. Guimaraes JA, Borges DR, Prado ES, et al: Kinin converting aminopeptidase from human serum. Biochem Pharmacol 22:403, 1973.
81. Gurewich V, Johnstone M, Loza JP, et al: Pro-urokinase and prekallikrein are both associated with platelets. Implications for the intrinsic pathway of fibrinolysis and for therapeutic thrombolysis. FEBS Lett 318:317, 1993.
82. Gustafson EJ, Schutsky D, Knight LC, et al: High molecular weight kininogen binds to unstimulated platelets. J Clin Invest 78:310, 1986.

83. Harpel PC: Circulatory inhibitors of human plasma kallikrein. In Pisano JJ, Austen KF (eds): Chemistry and Biology of the Kallikrein-Kinin System in Health and Disease. Vol 27. US Government Printing Office, Washington, DC, 1974, p 169.
84. Harpel PC, Lewin MF, Kaplan AP: Distribution of plasma kallikrein between C1 inactivator and α_2-macroglobulin-kallikrein complexes. J Biol Chem 260:4257, 1985.
85. Hauert J, Nicoloso G, Schleuning WD, et al: Plasminogen activators in dextran sulfate-activated euglobulin fractions: a molecular analysis of factor XII- and prekallikrein-dependent fibrinolysis. Blood 73:994, 1989.
86. Heck LW, Kaplan AP: Substrates of Hageman factor: I. Isolation and characterization of human factor XI (PTA) and inhibition of the activated enzyme by α_1-antitrypsin. J Exp Med 140:1615, 1974.
87. Hecker M, Porsti I, Busse R: Mechanisms involved in the angiotensin II-dependent hypotensive action of ACE inhibitors. Braz J Med Biol Res 27:1917, 1994.
88. Henderson LM, Figueroa CD, Müller-Esterl W, et al: Assembly of contact phase factors on the surface of the human neutrophil membrane. Blood 84:474, 1994.
89. Higashiyama S, Ohkubo I, Ishiguro H, et al: Human high molecular weight kininogen as a thiol protease inhibitor: presence of the entire inhibition capacity in the native form of heavy chain. Biochemistry 25:1669, 1986.
90. Hirsh EF, Nakajima T, Oshima G, et al: Kinin-system responses in sepsis after trauma in man. J Surg Res 17:147, 1974.
91. Hojima Y, Cochrane CG, Wiggins RC, et al: In vitro activation of the contact (Hageman factor) system of plasma by heparin and chondroitin sulfate E. Blood 63:1453, 1984.
92. Hong SL: Effect of bradykinin and thrombin on prostacyclin synthesis in endothelial cells from calf and pig aorta and human umbilical cord vein. Thromb Res 18:787, 1980.
93. Huisveld IA, Haspers H, Van Heeswijk GM, et al: Contribution of contact activation factors to urokinase-related fibrinolytic activator in whole plasma. Thromb Haemost 54:102, 1985.
94. Iatridis PG, Ferguson JH: Active Hageman factor. A plasma lysokinase of the human fibrinolytic system. J Clin Invest 41:1277, 1962.
95. Ikari N, Sugo T, Fujii S, et al: The role of bovine high molecular weight kininogen in contact-mediated activation of bovine factor XII: interaction of HMW kininogen with kaolin and plasma prekallikrein. J Biochem (Tokyo) 89:1699, 1981.
96. Ishiguro H, Higashiyama S, Ohkubo I, et al: Mapping of functional domains of human high molecular weight and high molecular weight kininogens using murine monoclonal antibodies. Biochemistry 26:7021, 1987.
97. Jacobsen S, Kritz M: Some data on two purified kininogens from human plasma. Br J Pharmacol 29:25, 1967.
98. Jansen PM, Pixley RA, Chang ACK, et al: Inhibition of factor XII in septic baboons attenuates activation of complement and fibrinolytic systems and reduces the release of neutrophil elastase. Intensive Care Med 20:S2, 1994.
99. Jesperson J, Kluft C: Increased euglobulin potential in women on oral contraceptives low in oestrogen-levels of extrinsic and intrinsic plasminogen activators, prekallikrein, factor XII and C1-inactivator. Thromb Haemost 54:454, 1985.
100. Johnson DA, Salveson G, Brown M, et al: Rapid isolation of human kininogens. Thromb Res 48:187, 1987.
101. Jorg M, Binder BR: Kinetic analysis of plasminogen activation by purified plasma kallikrein. Thromb Res 39:323, 1985.
102. Kaplan AP, Austen KF: A prealbumin activator of prekallikrein. J Immunol 105:802, 1970.
103. Kaplan AP, Austen KF: A prealbumin activator of prekallikrein II: derivation of activators of prekallikrein from active Hageman factor by digestion with plasmin. J Exp Med 133:696, 1971.
104. Kaplan AP, Kay AB, Austen KF: A prealbumin activator of prekallikrein III. Appearance of chemotactic activity for human neutrophils by the conversion of human prekallikrein to kallikrein. J Exp Med 135:81, 1972.
105. Kaufman N, Page JD, Pixley RA, et al: α_2 Macroglobulin-kallikrein complexes detect contact system activation in hereditary angioedema and human sepsis. Blood 77:2660, 1991.
106. Kellermann J, Lottspeich F, Henschen A, et al: Completion of the primary structure of human high molecular weight kininogen. The amino acid sequence of the entire heavy chain and evidence for its evolution by gene triplication. Eur J Biochem 154:471, 1986.
107. Kellermeyer RW, Breckenridge RT: The inflammatory process in acute gouty arthritis, I. Activation of Hageman factor by sodium urate crystals. J Lab Clin Med 63:307, 1965.
108. Kitamura N, Kitagawa H, Fukushima D, et al: Structural organization of the human kininogen gene and a model for its evolution. J Biol Chem 260:8610, 1985.
109. Kluft C: Occurrence of C1-inhibitor and other proteinase inhibitors in euglobulin fractions and their influence on fibrinolytic activity. Haemostasis 5:136, 1976.
110. Kluft C: Elimination of inhibition of euglobulin fibrinolysis by use of flufenamate: involvement of C1-inactivator. Haemostasis 6:351, 1977.
111. Kluft C: Determination of prekallikrein in human plasma: optimal conditions for activating prekallikrein. J Lab Clin Med 91:83, 1978.
112. Kluft C, Wijngaards G, Jie AFH: Intrinsic plasma fibrinolysis: involvement of urokinase-related activity in the factor XII independent plasminogen proactivator pathway. J Lab Clin Med 103:408, 1984.
113. Kodama K, Kato H, Iwanaga S: Isolation of bovine platelet cationic proteins which inhibit the surface-mediated activation of factor XII and prekallikrein. J Biochem (Tokyo) 97:139, 1985.
114. Kurachi K, Davie EW: Activation of human factor XI (plasma thromboplastin antecedent) by factor XIIa (activated Hageman factor). Biochemistry 16:5831, 1977.
115. Kurachi K, Fujikawa K, Davie EW: Mechanism of activation of bovine factor XI by factor XII and factor XII_a. Biochemistry 19:1330, 1980.
115a. Kusuman J, Ghebrehiwet B, Peerschke E, et al: Identification of the zinc-dependent endothelial cell binding protein for high molecular weight kininogen and Factor XII: Identity with the receptor which binds the globular "heads" of C1q (gC1qR). PNAS 93:8552, 1996.
116. Laake K, Vennerod AM, Hargen G, et al: Cold-promoted activation of factor VII in human plasma: studies on the associated acyl-arginine esterase activity. Thromb Res 4:769, 1974.
117. Lämmle B, Tran TH, Ritz R, et al: Plasma prekallikrein, factor XII, antithrombin III, C_1-inhibitor and α_2-macroglobulin in critically ill patients with suspected disseminated intravascular coagulation (DIC). Am J Clin Pathol 82:396, 1984.
118. Lipscomb MS, Walsh PN: Human platelets and factor XI. Localization in platelet membranes of factor XI-like activity and its functional distinction from that of factor XI. J Clin Invest 63:1006, 1979.
119. Londino A, Luparello FJ: Factor XII deficiency in a man with gout and angioimmunoblastic lymphadenopathy. Arch Intern Med 144:1497, 1984.
120. Lottspeich F, Kellermann J, Henschen A, et al: The amino acid sequence of the light chain of human high molecular mass kininogen. Eur J Biochem 152:307, 1985.
121. Lottspeich F, Kellermann J, Henschen A, et al: Human low-molecular-mass kininogen. Amino-acid sequence of the light chain; homology with other protein sequences. Eur J Biochem 142:227, 1984.
122. Loza JP, Gurewich V, Johnstone M, et al: Platelet-bound prekallikrein promotes pro-urokinase-induced clot lysis: a mechanism for targeting the factor XII dependent intrinsic pathway of fibrinolysis. Thromb Haemost 71:347, 1994.
123. Mandle RJ Jr, Colman RW, Kaplan AP: Identification of prekallikrein and HMW-kininogen as a complex in human plasma. Proc Natl Acad Sci USA 73:4179, 1976.
124. Mandle RJJ, Kaplan AP: Hageman factor substrates. II. Human plasma prekallikrein. Mechanism of activation by Hageman factor and participation in Hageman factor-dependent fibrinolysis. J Biol Chem 252:6097, 1977.
125. Mandle RJJ, Kaplan AP: Hageman factor dependent fibrinolysis. Generation of fibrinolytic activity by the interaction of human activated factor XI and plasminogen. Blood 54:850, 1979.
126. Margolis J: Activation of plasma by contact with glass: evidence for a common reaction which releases plasma kinin and initiates coagulation. J Physiol 144:1, 1958.
127. Mason JN, Colman RW: The role of Hageman factor in disseminated intravascular coagulation induced by sepsis, neoplasia, or liver disease. Thromb Diath Haemorrh 26:325, 1971.
128. Mason JW, Kleeberg UR, Dolan P, et al: Plasma kallikrein and Hageman factor in gram-negative bacteremia. Ann Intern Med 73:545, 1970.
129. McConnell DJ: Inhibitors of kallikrein in human plasma. J Clin Invest 51:1611, 1972.
130. McDonagh JS, Ferguson JH: Studies on the participation of Hageman factor in fibrinolysis. Thromb Haemost 24:1, 1970
131. McMillin CR, Saito H, Ratnoff OD, et al: The secondary structure of human Hageman factor (factor XII) and its alteration by activating agents. J Clin Invest 54:1312, 1974.

132. McMullen BA, Fujikawa K: Amino acid sequence of the heavy chain of human a-factor XIIa (activated Hageman factor). J Biol Chem 260:5328, 1985.
133. Meier HL, Pierce JV, Colman RW, et al: Activation and function of human Hageman factor. The role of high molecular kininogen and prekallikrein. J Clin Invest 60:18, 1977.
134. Meijers JC, Vlooswijk RAA, Bouma BN: Inhibition of human blood coagulation factor XIa by C1 inhibitor. Biochemistry 27:959, 1988.
135. Miles LA, Greengard JS, Griffin JH: A comparison of the abilities of plasma kallikrein, factor XIIa, factor XIa, and urokinase to activate plasminogen. Thromb Res 29:407, 1983.
136. Miles LA, Rothschild Z, Griffin JH: Dextran sulfate stimulated fibrinolytic activity in whole human plasma. Dependence on the contact activation system and a urokinase-related antigen. Thromb Haemost 46:211, 1981.
137. Miles LA, Rothschild Z, Griffin JH: Dextran sulfate dependent fibrinolysis in whole human plasma. J Lab Clin Med 101:214, 1983.
138. Moorman RM, Reynolds DS, Comunale ME: Management of cardiopulmonary bypass in a patient with congenital factor XII deficiency. J Cardiothorac Vasc Anesth 7:452, 1993.
139. Mori K, Nagasawa S: Studies on human high molecular weight (HMW) kininogen. II. Structural change in HMW kininogen by the action of human plasma kallikrein. J Biochem 89:1465, 1981.
140. Mori K, Sakamoto W, Nagasawa S: Studies on human high molecular weight (HMW) kininogen III. Cleavage of HMW kininogen by the action human salivary kallikrein. J Biochem 90:503, 1981.
141. Morrison DC, Cochrane CG: Direct evidence for Hageman factor (factor XII) activation by bacterial lipopolysaccharides (endotoxins). J Exp Med 140:797, 1974.
142. Muller-Esterl W, Fritz H, Machleidt IW, et al: Human plasma kininogens are identical with α_2-cysteine protease inhibitors. Evidence from immunological, enzymological, and sequence data. FEBS Lett 182:310, 1985.
143. Muller-Esterl W, Rauth G, Lottspeich F, et al: Limited proteolysis of human low-molecular mass kininogen by tissue kallikrein. Isolation and characterization of the heavy and light chains. Eur J Biochem 149:15, 1985.
144. Nagase H, Cawston JE, DeSilva M, et al: Identification of plasma kallikrein as an activator of latent collagenase in rheumatoid synovial fluid. Biochim Biophys Acta 707:133, 1982.
145. Nishikawa K, Kuna P, Calcaterra E, et al: Generation of the vasoactive peptide bradykinin from human high molecular weight kininogen bound to human umbilical vein endothelial cells. Blood 80:1980, 1992.
146. Nustad K, Orstavik TB, Gautvik KM, et al: Glandular kallikreins. Gen Pharmacol 9:1, 1978.
147. O'Donnell TF, Clowes GHJ, Talamo RC, et al: Kinin activation in the blood of patients with sepsis. Surg Gynecol Obstet 143:539, 1976.
148. Ogston D, Bennett NB, Ogston CM, et al: The assay of a plasma component necessary for the generation of a plasminogen activator in the presence of Hageman factor (Hageman factor cofactor). Br J Haematol 20:209, 1971.
149. Ogston D, Ogston LM, Ratnoff OD, et al: Studies on a complex mechanism for the activation of plasminogen by kaolin and by chloroform. The participation of Hageman factor and additional cofactors. J Clin Invest 48:1786, 1967.
150. Ole-Moiyoi O, Spragg J, Helbert SP: Immunologic reactivity of purified human urinary kallikrein (urokallikrein) with anti-serum directed against human pancreas. J Immunol 118:667, 1977.
151. Pedersen OD, Munkvad S, Gram J, et al: Depression of factor XII-dependent fibrinolytic activity in survivors of acute myocardial infarction at risk of reinfarction. Eur Heart J 14:785, 1993.
152. Pettinger MA, Young R: Endotoxin-induced kinin (bradykinin) formation: activation of Hageman factor and plasma kallikrein in human plasma. Life Sci 9:313, 1970.
153. Pixley RA, De La Cadena RA, Page JD, et al: The contact system contributes to hypotension but not disseminated intravascular coagulation in lethal bacterimia. In vivo use of a monoclonal anti factor XII antibody to block contact activation in baboons. J Clin Invest 92:61, 1993.
154. Pixley RA, De La Cadena RA, Page JD, et al: Activation of the contact system in lethal hypotensive bacteremia in a baboon model. Am J Pathol 140:897, 1992.
155. Pixley RA, Schapira M, Colman RW: The regulation of human factor XII by plasma proteinase inhibitors. J Biol Chem 260:1723, 1985.
156. Pixley RA, Stumpo LG, Birkmeyer K, et al: A monoclonal antibody recognizing an icosapeptide sequence in the heavy chain of human factor XII inhibits surface-catalyzed activation. J Biol Chem 262:10140, 1987.
157. Powers CA, Nasjletti A: A novel kinin generating protease (kininogenase) in the porcine anterior pituitary. J Biol Chem 257:5594, 1982.
158. Proctor RR, Rapaport SJ: The partial thromboplastin time with kaolin: a simple screening test for first stage clotting deficiencies. Am J Clin Pathol 35:212, 1961.
159. Proud D, Pierce JV, Pisano JJ: Radioimmunoassay of human high molecular weight kininogen in normal and deficient plasma. J Lab Clin Med 95:563, 1980.
160. Proud D, Togias AG, Naclerio RM, et al: Kinins are generated in vivo following nasal airway challenge of allergic individuals with allergen. J Clin Invest 72:1678, 1983.
161. Purdon AD, Schapira M, de Agostini A, et al: Prorenin activation by plasma kallikrein in inhibitor deficient plasma. J Lab Clin Med 105:694, 1985.
162. Que BG, Davie EW: Characterization of a cDNA coding for human factor XII (Hageman factor). Biochemistry 8:1525, 1986.
163. Radcliffe R, Bagdassarian B, Colman RW, et al: Activation of factor VII by Hageman factor fragments. Blood 59:611, 1977.
164. Rahman MM, Worthy K, Elson CJ, et al: Inhibitor regulation of tissue kallikrein activity in the synovial fluid of patients with rheumatoid arthritis. Br J Rheumatol 33:215, 1994.
165. Ratnoff OD, Crum JD: Activation of Hageman factor by solutions of ellagic acid. J Lab Clin Med 63:359, 1964.
166. Ratnoff OD, Saito H: Amidolytic properties of single chain activated Hageman factor. Proc Natl Acad Sci USA 76:1461, 1979.
167. Reddigari S, Kaplan AP: Monoclonal antibody to human high molecular weight kininogen recognizes its prekallikrein binding site and inhibits its coagulant activity. Blood 74:695, 1989.
168. Reddigari S, Kaplan AP: Quantification of human high molecular weight kininogen by immunoblotting with a monoclonal anti-light chain antibody. J Immunol Methods 119:19, 1989.
169. Reddigari SR, Kaplan AP: Cleavage of high molecular weight kininogen by purified kallikreins and upon contact activation of plasma. Blood 71:1334, 1988.
170. Reddigari SR, Miragliotta G, Kuna P, et al: Human high molecular weight kininogen binds to human umbilical vein endothelial cells via its heavy and light chains. Blood 81:1306, 1993.
171. Reddigari SR, Shibayama Y, Brunnee T, et al: Human Hageman factor (FXII) and high molecular weight kininogen compete for the same binding site on human umbilical vein endothelial cells. J Biol Chem 268:11982, 1993.
172. Regoli D, Barabe J: Pharmacology of bradykinin and related kinins. Pharmacol Rev 32:1, 1980.
173. Revak SD, Cochrane CG, Griffin JH: The binding and cleavage characteristics of human Hageman factor during contact activation: a comparison of normal plasma with plasma deficient in factor XI, prekallikrein or high molecular weight kininogen. J Clin Invest 58:1167, 1977.
174. Revak SD, Cochrane CG, Johnston AR, et al: Structural changes accompanying enzymatic activation of human Hageman factor. J Clin Invest 54:619, 1974.
175. Robinson JA, Klodynicky ML, Loeb HS, et al: Endotoxin, prekallikrein, complement, and systemic vascular resistances. Sequential measurement in man. Am J Med 59:61, 1975.
176. Roeise O, Bouma BN, Stadaas JO, et al: Dose dependence of endotoxin-induced activation of the plasma contact system: an in vitro study. Circ Shock 26:419, 1988.
177. Rosing J, Tans G, Griffin JH: Surface-dependent activation of human factor XII by kallikrein, and its light chain. Eur J Biochem 151:531, 1985.
178. Saito H, Ratnoff OD, Donaldson VH: Defective activation of clotting, fibrinolytic and permeability-enhancing systems in human Fletcher trait. Circ Res 34:641, 1974.
179. Schachter M, Peret MW, Billing AG, et al: Immunolocalization of protease kallikrein in the colon. J Histochem Cytochem 31:1255, 1983.
180. Schapira M, Despland E, Scott CF, et al: Purified human plasma kallikrein aggregates human blood neutrophils. J Clin Invest 69: 1199, 1982.
181. Schapira M, Scott CF, Colman RW: Contribution of plasma protease inhibitors to the inactivation of kallikrein in plasma. J Clin Invest 69:462, 1982.

182. Schiffman S, Mannhalter C, Tynerk D: Human high molecular weight kininogen. Effects of cleavage by kallikrein on protein structure and procoagulant activity. J Biol Chem 255:6433, 1980.
183. Schmaier AH, Kuo A, Lundberg D, et al: The expression of high molecular weight kininogen on human umbilical vein endothelial cells. J Biol Chem 263:16327, 1988.
184. Schmaier AH, Silver L, Adams AL, et al: The effects of high molecular weight kininogen on surface-adsorbed fibrinogen. Thromb Res 33:51, 1984.
185. Schmaier AH, Smith PM, Purdon AD, et al: High molecular weight kininogen: localization in unstimulated and activated platelets and activation by a platelet calpain(s). Blood 67:119, 1986.
186. Schmaier AH, Zuckerberg A, Silverman C, et al: High molecular weight kininogen: a secreted platelet protein. J Clin Invest 71:1477, 1983.
187. Schreiber RD, Kaplan AP, Austen KF: Inhibition by C1 INH of Hageman factor fragment activation of coagulation, fibrinolysis, and kinin generation. J Clin Invest 52:1402, 1973.
188. Scott CF, Colman RW: Function and immunochemistry of prekallikrein-high molecular weight kininogen complex in plasma. J Clin Invest 65:413, 1980.
189. Scott CF, Schapira M, James HL, et al: Inactivation of factor XIa by plasma protease inhibitors. Predominant role of α_1-protease inhibitor and protective effect of high molecular weight kininogen. J Clin Invest 69:844, 1982.
190. Scully MF, Weerasinghe K, Kakhar VV: Inhibition of contact activation by platelet factor 4. Thromb Res 20:461, 1980.
191. Sealey JE, Atlas SA, Laragh JH, et al: Initiation of plasma prorenin activation by Hageman factor-dependent conversion of plasma prekallikrein to kallikrein. Proc Natl Acad Sci USA 76:5914, 1979.
192. Seligsohn U, Osterud B, Brown JF, et al: Activation of human factor VII by Hageman factor fragments. J Clin Invest 64:1056, 1979.
193. Sheikh IA, Kaplan AP: Studies of the digestion of bradykinin, lysylbradykinin and des-arg9 bradykinin by angiotensin converting enzyme. Biochem Pharmacol 35:1951, 1986.
194. Sheikh IA, Kaplan AP: Studies of the digestion of bradykinin, lysylbradykinin and kinin degradation products by carboxypeptidases A, B and N. Biochem Pharmacol 35:1957, 1986.
195. Sheikh IA, Kaplan AP: The mechanism of digestion of bradykinin and lysylbradykinin (kallidin) in human serum: the role of carboxypeptidase, angiotensin converting enzyme, and determination of final degradation products. Biochem Pharmacol 38:993, 1989.
196. Shibayama Y, Brunnée T, Kaplan AP, et al: Activation of human Hageman factor (factor XII) in the presence of zinc and phosphate ions. Braz J Med Biol Res 27:1817, 1994.
197. Silverberg M, Diehl SV: The activation of the contact system of human plasma by polysaccharide sulfates. Ann NY Acad Sci 516:268, 1987.
198. Silverberg M, Diehl SV: The autoactivation of factor XII (Hageman factor) induced by low Mr heparin and dextran sulphate. Biochem J 248:715, 1987.
199. Silverberg M, Dunn JT, Garen L, et al: Autoactivation of human Hageman factor. J Biol Chem 255:7281, 1980.
200. Silverberg M, Kaplan AP: Enzymatic activities of activated and zymogen forms of human Hageman factor (factor XII). Blood 60:64, 1982.
201. Silverberg M, Nicoll JE, Kaplan AP: The mechanism by which the light chain of cleaved HMW-kininogen augments the activation of prekallikrein, factor XI, and Hageman factor. Thromb Res 20:173, 1980.
202. Sinha D, Seaman FS, Koshy A, et al: Blood coagulation factor XIa binds specifically to a site on activated human platelets distinct from that for factor XI. J Clin Invest 73:1550, 1984.
203. Smith D, Gilbert M, Owen WG: Tissue plasminogen activator release in vivo in response to vasoactive agents. Blood 66:835, 1985.
204. Soter NA, Austen KF, Gigli I: Inhibition by E-aminocaproic acid of the activation of the first component of the complement system. J Immunol 114:928, 1975.
205. Stead N, Kaplan AP, Rosenberg RD: Inhibition of activated factor XII by antithrombin-heparin cofactor. J Biol Chem 251:6481, 1976.
206. Strang CJ, Cholin S, Spragg J, et al: Angioedema induced by a peptide derived from complement component C2. J Exp Med 168:1685, 1988.
207. Streeten DHP, Kerr LP, Prior JC, et al: Hyperbradykinism: a new orthostatic syndrome. Lancet 2:1048, 1972.
208. Tait J, Fujikawa K: Identification of the binding site plasma prekallikrein in human high molecular weight kininogen. J Biol Chem 261:15396, 1986.
209. Tait JF, Fujikawa K: Primary structure requirements for the binding of human high molecular weight kininogen to plasma prekallikrein and factor XI. J Biol Chem 262:11651, 1987.
210. Takada Y, Skidgel RA, Erdos EG: Purification of human urinary prokallikrein. Identification of the site of activation by the metalloproteinase thermolysin. Biochem J 232:851, 1985.
211. Takagaki Y, Kitamura N, Nakanishi S: Cloning and sequence analysis of cDNAs for high molecular weight and low molecular weight prekininogens. J Biol Chem 260:8601, 1985.
212. Takahashi S, Irie A, Katayama Y, et al: N-terminal amino acid sequence of human urinary prokallikrein. J Biochem (Tokyo) 99:989, 1986.
213. Tankersley DL, Finlayson JS: Kinetics of activation and autoactivation of human factor XII. Biochemistry 23:273, 1984.
214. Tankersley DL, Fournel MA, Schroeder DD: Kinetics of activation of prekallikrein by prekallikrein activator. Biochemistry 19:3121, 1980.
215. Tans G, Griffin JH: Properties of sulfatides in factor XII dependent contact activation. Blood 59:69, 1982.
216. Tans G, Rosing J, Griffin JD: Sulfatide dependent autoactivation of human blood coagulation factor XII (Hageman factor). J Biol Chem 258:8215, 1983.
217. Thompson RE, Mandle RJ Jr, Kaplan AP: Association of factor XI and high molecular weight kininogen in human plasma. J Clin Invest 60:1376, 1977.
218. Thompson RE, Mandle RJ, Kaplan AP. Characterization of human high molecular weight kininogen. Procoagulant activity associated with the light chain of kinin-free high molecular weight kininogen. J Exp Med 147:488, 1978.
219. Thompson RE, Mandle RJ, Kaplan AP: Studies of the binding of prekallikrein and factor XI to high molecular weight kininogen and its light chain. Proc Natl Acad Sci USA 76:4862, 1979.
220. Travis J, Salvesen GS: Human plasma proteinase inhibitors. Ann Rev Biochem 52:655, 1983.
221. Tuszynski GP, Bevacona SJ, Schmaier AH, et al: Factor XI antigen and activity in human platelets. Blood 59:1148, 1982.
222. van der Graaf F, Koedam JA, Bouma BN: Inactivation of kallikrein in human plasma. J Clin Invest 71:149, 1983.
223. Van Iwaarden F, deGroot PG, Bouma BN: The binding of high molecular weight kininogen to cultured human endothelial cells. J Biol Chem 263:4698, 1988.
224. Wachtfogel YT, De La Cadena RA, Kunapuli SP, et al: High molecular weight kininogen binds to Mac-1 on neutrophils by its heavy chain (domain 3) and its light chain (domain 5). J Biol Chem 269:19307, 1994.
225. Wachtfogel YT, Kucich U, James HL, et al: Human plasma kallikrein releases neutrophil elastase activity during blood coagulation. J Clin Invest 22:1672, 1983.
226. Wachtfogel YT, Pixley RA, Kucich U, et al: Purified plasma factor XIIa aggregates human neutrophils and causes degranulation. Blood 67:1731, 1986.
227. Waeber G, Schapira M, Waeber B, et al: Hypotensive effect of the active fragment derived from factor XII is mediated by an activation of the plasma kallikrein-kinin system. Circ Shock 26:375, 1988.
228. Walsh PN: The effects of collagen and kaolin on the intrinsic coagulant activity of platelets. Evidence for an alternative pathway in intrinsic coagulation not requiring factor XII. Br J Haematol 22:393, 1972.
229. Walsh PN, Griffin JH: Contributions of human platelets to the proteolytic activation of blood coagulation factors XII and XI. Blood 57:106, 1981.
230. Wang W, Hendriks DK, Scharpé SS: Carboxypeptidase U, a plasma carboxypeptidase with high affinity for plasminogen. J Biol Chem 269:15937, 1994.
231. Warn-Cramer BJ, Bajaj SP: Stoichiometry of binding of high molecular weight kininogen to factor XI/XIa. Biochem Biophys Res Commun 133:417, 1985.
232. Weiss AS, Gallin JI, Kaplan AP: Fletcher factor deficiency. A diminished rate of Hageman factor activation caused by absence of prekallikrein with abnormalities of coagulation, fibrinolysis, chemotactic activity, and kinin generation. J Clin Invest 53:622, 1974.
233. Weiss R, Silverberg M, Kaplan AP: The effect of C1 inhibitor upon Hageman factor autoactivation. Blood 68:239, 1986.
234. Wiggins RC, Bouma BN, Cochrane CG, et al: Role of high molecular weight kininogen in surface-binding and activation of coagulation factor XIa and prekallikrein. Proc Natl Acad Sci USA 77:4636, 1977.
235. Wiggins RC, Giglas PC, Henson PM: Chemotactic activator generated from the fifth component of complement by plasma kallikrein of the rabbit. J Exp Med 153:1391, 1981.
236. Wines DR, Brady JM, Pritchett DB, et al: Organization and expression of the rat kallikrein gene family. J Biol Chem 264:7653, 1989.

237. Wuepper KD: Prekallikrein deficiency in man. J Exp Med 138:1345, 1973.
238. Wuepper KD, Miller DR, LaCombe MJ: Flaujeac trait. Deficiency of human plasma kininogen. J Clin Invest 56:1663, 1975.
238a. Wuillemin WA, Eldering E, Citavella F, et al: Modulation of contact system proteases by glycosaminoglycans. J Biol Chem 271:12913, 1996.
239. Wuillemin WA, Minnema M, Meijers JC, et al: Inactivation of factor XIa in human plasma assessed by measuring factor XIa-protease inhibitor complexes: major role for C1-inhibitor. Blood 85:1517, 1995.
240. Yokosawa N, Takahashi N, Inagami T, et al: Isolation of completely inactive plasma prorenin and its activation by kallikreins. Biochim Biophys Acta 569:211, 1979.

15 Endothelial Cells and Cell Adhesion

BRUCE S. BOCHNER ROBERT P. SCHLEIMER

During inflammatory reactions, tissue-resident cells generate signals that activate cellular and fluid elements in the intravascular compartment, resulting in the initiation of a cascade of events leading to leukocyte recruitment. During this process, the vascular endothelium was initially believed to play only a passive barrier role, the integrity of this barrier becoming altered to allow the influx or leakage of cells and plasma into the site. The concept that the vascular endothelium could itself be actively involved in local inflammation site was initially suggested in the late 1800s by studies that detected histologic changes in endothelial cells at inflammatory sites.[104] Subsequently, animal models of inflammation utilizing techniques such as intravital microscopy revealed that local tissue injury caused circulating cells to rapidly marginate onto the adjacent luminal surface of the vasculature.[11] However, one of the most significant advances in the field of endothelial biology occurred when techniques were developed to isolate and culture vascular endothelial cells from sources such as human umbilical veins[171, 224] and dermal microvascular sites.[580] Analysis of cultured endothelial cells led to dramatic improvements in our understanding of the role of the endothelial cell in a variety of normal and pathologic responses, including angiogenesis, atherogenesis, wound healing, tumor metastasis, coagulation, and leukocyte recruitment during inflammation.

Occurring in parallel with these latter studies were discoveries related to leukocyte surface structures involved in cell migration and attachment. From these investigations emerged novel areas of research focusing on cell adhesion molecules and their role in inflammation. Adhesion molecules are now known to be critical for virtually every step in cell recruitment, including margination, diapedesis, and chemotaxis. Within the past decade, tremendous growth has occurred in our knowledge of these ever-increasing families of molecules. More than 20 adhesion molecules have now been identified and cloned. A variety of adhesion molecule knock-out mice have been created, and adhesion molecule antagonists have been developed that are now being tested in vivo. These and other studies have contributed greatly to our understanding of the biologic importance and relative contributions of these molecules in a variety of immunologic responses.

The goal of this chapter is to summarize the function of endothelial cells and leukocytes during human inflammatory reactions, especially those events mediated by cell-cell contact through adhesion molecules. Many aspects of endothelial cell biology cannot be covered but fortunately have been summarized elsewhere. For example, the embryologic, ultrastructural, and morphologic characteristics of endothelial cells have been the subject of several excellent texts.[348, 434–436, 473] Similarly, the important functions of endothelium in regulating blood flow and coagulation processes have been discussed elsewhere.[313, 434, 498, 534]

This chapter reviews several aspects of human endothelial cell biology and function, beginning with the role of the endothelial cell as a source of inflammatory mediators as well as potential interactions between endothelial cells and adjacent mast cells. This review is followed by a more extensive discussion of leukocyte-endothelial interactions mediated by cell adhesion molecules. Molecular and biologic aspects of adhesion molecule function and expression are considered, and current knowledge regarding in vivo expression and function of these structures is highlighted. Because of their expansive nature, discussions of most of these topics are restricted to those cells and molecules most relevant to allergic inflammation.

REGULATION OF ENDOTHELIAL PERMEABILITY AND PROLIFERATION BY MAST CELLS

The maintenance of vascular integrity is one of the most essential functions of endothelium. Several mast cell–derived mediators, including histamine and arachidonic acid metabolites, can cause increases in vascular permeability,[243] apparently through endothelial cell contraction. The precise mechanisms by which vascular permeability is regulated remain unclear.[166, 348] For histamine, increased permeability is believed to be mediated through an interaction with endothelial H_1 and H_2 cell surface receptors.[472] In addition to its effects on endothelial permeability, histamine rapidly induces the surface expression of the adhesion molecule P-selectin (CD62P), which exists preformed within the Weibel-Palade bodies that also contain von Willebrand factor.[298] Endothelial cells also express neurokinin-1 receptors,[181] which may be responsible for substance P–induced changes in vascular permeability.

The interaction between mast cells and endothelium, however, involves more than the regulation of vascular permeability by mast cell mediators. Several lines of evidence indicate that mast cell heparin can stimulate endothelial cell proliferation and that endothelial cell products can, in turn, stimulate mast cell proliferation. It has clearly been demonstrated that mast cell numbers increase dramatically at sites of angiogenesis such as in solid tumors,[242] and more perivascular mast cells are found in skin biopsy samples of subjects with urticaria.[363] Mast cell heparin stimulates endothelial cell proliferation by physical association with endothelial cell growth factor,[523] increasing the potency of the latter approximately 30-fold.[453] The importance of mast cell heparin in angiogenesis is further suggested by its ability to induce endothelial cell migration.[24] In addition to mast cell–derived substances, other factors, including vascular endothelial growth factor[254] and IL-4,[526] may regulate endothelial migration and proliferation. Mast cells may be a source of cytokines, such as TNF, IL-4, and IL-13,[71, 78, 252, 552] which are capable of activating endothelial adhesion molecule expression.

VASCULAR ENDOTHELIAL CELLS AS ANTIGEN-PRESENTING CELLS

Classically, monocytes and macrophages have been considered the primary cells responsible for antigen presentation, but there is evidence that under certain conditions vascular endothelial cells can perform accessory cell functions. Human umbilical vein and dermal endothelial cells can process and present a variety of soluble antigens to T cells.[106, 403, 545] They can support allogeneic, mitogen-stimulated, and antigen-stimulated T-cell responses.[401] As is the case with macrophages, expression of class II antigens (e.g., HLA-DR and HLA-DS) by endothelial cells can be induced by lymphokines such as gamma interferon.[106] Endothelial cells possess other characteristics of antigen-presenting cells such as the ability to express cell surface receptors for C3b and IgG.[437]

VASCULAR ENDOTHELIAL CELLS AS A SOURCE OF CHEMICAL MEDIATORS AND SOLUBLE PROTEINS

Vascular endothelial cells produce a variety of factors essential to supporting homeostasis throughout the human body.[313, 534] Endothelial cell products important for the maintenance of hemostasis and blood flow include Factor VIII–related antigen,[213] plasminogen activator,[272] thromboplastin,[225] endothelin-1,[534, 535] C1 esterase inhibitor,[452] and angiotensin-converting enzyme.[123] Endothelial cells respond within minutes to stimulation with ionophore, thrombin, bradykinin, histamine, and sulfidopeptide leukotrienes by producing platelet-activating factor (PAF) and prostacyclin, mediators that promote leukocyte activation, vasodilation, and increased vascular permeability.[26, 87, 324, 325, 407, 594] In contrast to the rapid effects of these stimuli on vascular endothelial cells, responses to other agents occur more slowly. For example, IL-1 treatment of vascular endothelial cells leads to the production of PAF (including or exclusively the acyl form) and prostacyclin; but in contrast to the immediate production of these mediators in response to thrombin or histamine, this effect occurs only after a delay of several hours.[79, 426, 530] Activated endothelial cells also produce nitric oxide[388]; matrix proteins, including fibronectin[213]; several cytokines, including IL-1,[497] IL-6,[125, 374] and platelet-derived growth factor[8]; several C-X-C chemokines such as IL-8,[172] groα,[130] and IP-10[308]; several C-C chemokines such as RANTES[314, 494] and MCP-1[420, 468]; and a variety of colony-stimulating factors, including G-CSF, M-CSF, and GM-CSF,[27, 75, 269, 429, 458] which are capable of activating eosinophils[268, 269, 296, 527] as well as endothelial cells themselves.[80, 81] These and potentially other mediators derived from endothelium further illustrate the active role of the vascular endothelium in inflammatory responses.

MOLECULAR ASPECTS OF ADHESION MOLECULES

Many cell surface structures on endothelial cells and leukocytes are capable of mediating adhesion. These molecules are subdivided into families (integrins, immunoglobulin-like structures, selectins, and carbohydrate counterligands for selectins) based on shared structural characteristics and functions. This section describes these structural characteristics on a molecular and biochemical level, as well as various phenotypic and functional aspects of these molecules in vitro. Several additional reviews on these topics have also appeared.[44, 89, 217, 218, 275, 401, 484]

INTEGRINS

The integrin family consists of more than 15 transmembrane, noncovalently associated heterodimers with distinct α and β chains that are responsible for adhesion to other cell surface ligands, complement protein fragments, and extracellular matrix proteins; nearly all have been cloned.[6, 203, 432] These molecules, in addition to mediating adhesion, have important signaling functions.[218, 421, 446, 455] So far, at least 15 α subunits and 8 β subunits have been identified, with 20 heterodimeric pairings documented to date. Although it was initially believed that α and β subunit pairings were restricted according to the β subunits, it is now clear that different α subunits can associate with more than one β subunit.[21]

The structure of a typical integrin is shown schematically in Figure 15–1. The α subunits range in size from 120 to

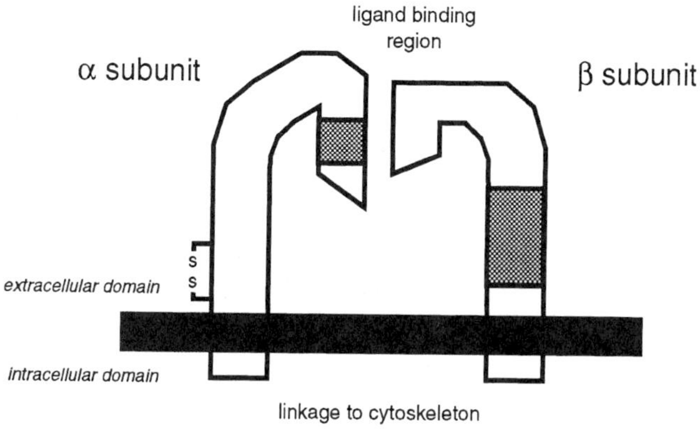

FIGURE 15–1. Basic structure of an integrin heterodimer. The divalent cation binding region on the α subunit and the cysteine-rich repeat region on the β subunit are shown as shaded areas. Some α subunits contain an inserted (I) domain within the ligand binding region located membrane proximal to the cation binding site.

210 kD, and the β subunits range from 90 to 110 kD. Overall, there is a higher degree of homology among β subunits than among α subunits.[247] Characteristic features of the intracytoplasmic domains of these subunits include sites for phosphorylation[85, 96, 208] as well as for attachment to cytoskeletal elements such as talin, vinculin, α-actinin, filamin, and actin.[462, 474] During cell-substratum adhesion, integrins, along with these cytoskeletal proteins, tend to accumulate in patches called focal contacts.[117, 474] A conserved sequence in the cytoplasmic carboxyl terminus of several β subunits, separate from the phosphorylation sites, appears to influence the avidity of binding.[208, 209] Within the extracellular portions of α subunits are three or four domains, each approximately 60 amino acids in length, that resemble calcium-binding sites found in other proteins. By binding divalent cations (typically calcium and magnesium), these domains are believed to contribute to the binding affinity of integrin heterodimers.[135, 210] Another interesting characteristic of some integrins (all of the α chains for the β2 integrins as well as the α1 and α2 chains of β1 integrins) is the presence of an inserted, or I, domain, belonging to a large family of A domain proteins.[107] This site appears to be an important recognition site for integrin-binding activity.[127, 271] A characteristic feature of the extracellular portions of β subunits, unlike α subunits, is the presence of 56 conserved cysteine residues, localized primarily to four tandem domains; their presence is believed to contribute to the rigidity of these molecules.[250]

Umbilical vein endothelial cells express several β1 integrins (α2β1, α3β1, α5β1, α6β1) as well as αvβ3 (Table 15–1)[54]; microvascular endothelial cells may express additional integrins, albeit at relatively low levels.[580] Since integrins can be expressed on both the basal and luminal surfaces of endothelial cells,[7, 109] these receptors are believed to mediate adhesion to substratum as well as to intraluminal ligands. On eosinophils, among the β1 integrins, α4β1 and α6β1 are expressed,[145, 170] whereas basophils and mast cells express α4β1 and α5β1 (Table 15–2).[51, 188, 532] Other integrin subfamilies are restricted to certain cell types. An example of this is the β2 integrins, whose expression is essentially limited to leukocytes.[250] Among different cell types, however, levels of surface expression vary, and the levels of cell surface expression can be altered during hematopoiesis[245, 547] or as a consequence of cellular activation. For example, initial studies of the induction of expression of VLA (very late activation) proteins, a subfamily of integrins now known to represent the β1 integrins, demonstrated that prolonged activation of lymphocytes was required in vitro with mitogens before these structures became expressed.[203]

Other integrins, such as Mac-1 (αMβ2, CD11b/CD18), exist both on the cell surface and in an intracytoplasmic pool of granules, which can rapidly translocate to the cell surface following activation with agents such as chemotactic factors or eosinophil proteins.[349, 459] Whereas chemotactic factors such as fMLP, PAF, and C5a induce up-regulation of Mac-1 on both eosinophils and neutrophils, IL-5 can selectively affect Mac-1 expression on eosinophils.[303, 367, 549] However, in addition to the level of adhesion molecule expression, it is now apparent that conformational changes can occur in integrins,[105] resulting in rapid, reversible changes in binding avidity.[128, 307, 481] These changes occur as a result of ligand binding,[22, 210, 257, 258] occupancy of divalent cation binding sites,[13, 463] or allosteric changes caused by adjacent cell surface structures such as integrin-modulating factor-1[206] or in association with phosphorylation (e.g., via focal adhesion protein-tyrosine kinase) of clustered intracytoplasmic domains of the integrin subunits.[93, 239, 377, 412, 446, 588]

Expression of integrins appears also under transcriptional regulation, and analyses of the promoter sequences of several integrin genes have identified myeloid transcription factors (e.g., PU-1) that influence gene expression.[157, 386, 387, 424, 425] Intracytoplasmic assembly and subsequent expression of integrin heterodimers appear to require an intact β subunit, since genetic mutations in the β2 subunit (especially near the *N*-terminal portion) have been identified in patients with a disorder called leukocyte adhesion deficiency disease type 1, in which leukocyte surface expression of β2 integrins is markedly impaired or totally absent.[16, 21] Indeed, the defect can be corrected by gene transfer.[576]

The functional ligands for integrins expressed on endothelial cells, leukocytes, platelets, and mast cells are listed in Tables 15–1 and 15–2. As a rule, integrins belonging to the β1 family are ligands for extracellular matrix proteins, such as collagen, laminin, and fibronectin, and mediate firm attachment and spreading of cells under static conditions.[464] The integrin α2β1 also functions as a ligand for echovirus.[40, 41] The VLA-4 heterodimer (CD49d/CD29, α4β1) is of particular interest in allergic inflammation.[62] It binds both to the CS-1 (connecting segment-1) portion of the IIICS (type III connecting segment) region of fibronectin (containing the consensus amino acid sequence LDV)[543, 562, 563] and to the regions within the first and fourth domains of VCAM-1 (vascular cell adhesion molecule-1), a molecule expressed on activated endothelial cells (Fig. 15–2).[150, 385, 391, 543, 544]

As with other integrins, expression of VLA-4 is under transcriptional regulation.[422] Several studies suggest that the avidity of VLA-4 for its ligands differs among cell types and can be dramatically altered by cell activation.[94, 95, 211, 318, 410, 441] Other characteristics unique to VLA-4 are its lack of expression on neutrophils, despite broad expression on all other leukocytes,[57, 204] and its ability to mediate adhesion under conditions of shear stress, often referred to as rolling adhesion.[12, 306, 486] This function is usually considered one in which selectins play a more important role. Another β sub-

TABLE 15–1
BIOCHEMICAL AND FUNCTIONAL CHARACTERISTICS OF ENDOTHELIAL ADHESION MOLECULES

Adhesion Molecule	CD	Size (kD)	Expression and/or Inducing Stimuli	Ligands
Integrins				
α2β1 (VLA-2)	CD49b/CD29	160/130	Constitutive	Collagen, laminin, echovirus 1
α3β1 (VLA-3)	CD49c/CD29	150/130	Constitutive	Laminin, fibronectin, collagen
α5β1 (VLA-5)	CD49e/CD29	160/130	Constitutive	Fibronectin
α6β1 (VLA-6)	CD49f/CD29	150/130	Constitutive	Laminin
αVβ3	CD51/CD61	165/105	Constitutive	Vitronectin, fibrinogen, fibronectin, others
Immunoglobulin Gene Superfamily				
ICAM-1	CD54	100	Constitutive, IL-1, TNF, LPS, IFN-γ	CD11a/CD18, CD11b/CD18, rhinovirus
ICAM-2	CD102	60	Constitutive	CD11a/CD18
PECAM-1	CD31	125	Constitutive	CD31
VCAM-1	CD106	100	IL-1, TNF, LPS, IL-4, IL-13	CD49d/CD29 (α4β1) and α4β7
MAdCAM-1*	None	60	Constitutive	α4β7, CD62L (L-selectin)
Selectins				
E-selectin	CD62E	110	IL-1, TNF, LPS	sLe[x], sLe[a], CLA, s-di-Le[x], ESL-1, myeloglycans
P-selectin	CD62P	140	Histamine, thrombin, C5a, peroxides, phorbol esters, ionophores	Le[x], sLe[x], sLe[a], PSGL-1, sulfated glycolipids
Others				
Pgp-1 (Hermes)	CD44	90	Constitutive	Hyaluronate, collagen
VAP-1*	None	90	Constitutive	Unknown lymphocyte structure
L-VAP-2	CD73	70	Constitutive	Unknown lymphocyte structure

*Expressed primarily or exclusively on lymphoid high endothelial venules.

TABLE 15–2
BIOCHEMICAL AND FUNCTIONAL CHARACTERISTICS OF ADHESION MOLECULES ON HUMAN LEUKOCYTES, MAST CELLS, AND PLATELETS

Type	Name (CD)	Size (kD)	Ligands	Cellular Distribution
Integrins				
β1 (VLA) family	α1β1 (CD49a/CD29)	210/130	Laminin, collagen	L
	α2β1 (CD49b/CD29)	160/130	Collagen, laminin	L, M, P
	α3β1 (CD49c/CD29)	150/130	Collagen, laminin, others	L
	α4β1 (CD49d/CD29)	150/130	VCAM-1, fibronectin	L, M, E, B, MC
	α5β1 (CD49e/CD29)	160/130	Fibronectin	L, M, N, B, MC, P
	α6β1 (CD49f/CD29)	150/130	Laminin	L, M, N, E, P
β2 family	LFA-1 (CD11a/CD18)	180/95	ICAM-1, ICAM-2, ICAM-3	L, M, N, E, B
	Mac-1 (CD11b/CD18)	170/95	C3bi, ICAM-1, fibrinogen	L, M, N, E, B
	p150, 95 (CD11c/CD18)	150/95	C3bi, others	L, M, N, E, B, MC*
	αdβ2 (αd/CD18)	125	ICAM-3	L, M, N, E, B
β3 family	αIIbβ3 (CD41/CD61)	120/23/105	Fibrinogen, fibronectin, others	P
	αvβ3 (CD51/Cd61)	163/105	Vitronectin, others	M, MC, P
Other β integrins	α4β7	150/120	MAdCAM-1, VCAM-1, fibronectin	L, M, E, B
	αEβ7	150/25	E-cadherin	L
Immunoglobulin Gene Superfamily				
	ICAM-1 (CD54)	100	LFA-1, Mac-1	L, M, N, B, MC
	ICAM-2 (CD102)	60	LFA-1	L, M, B, MC, P
	ICAM-3 (CD50)	124	LFA-1	L, M, N, E, B, MC
	PECAM-1 (CD31)	125	CD31	L, M, N, E, B, P
	LFA-3 (CD58)	70	CD2	L, M, N, E, B, MC, P
Selectins				
	L-selectin (CD62L)	80	GlyCAM-1, CD34, MAdCAM-1	L, M, N, E, B
	P-selectin (CD62P)	150	PSGL-1, SLe[x]	P
Carbohydrates and Others				
	Lewis[x] (Le[x], CD15)	Unknown	P-selectin	M, N, E
	sLe[x] (CD15s)	Unknown	E-selectin, P-selectin	M, N, E, B
	s-dimeric Le[x]	Unknown	E-selectin	M, N, E, B
	Pgp-1/Hermes (CD44)	90	Hyaluronate, collagen	L, M, N, E, B, MC

*Weakly expressed on uterine mast cells but not mast cells from other tissues.
Abbreviations: L = lymphocytes; M = monocytes; N = neutrophils; E = eosinophils; B = basophils; MC = mast cells; P = platelets.

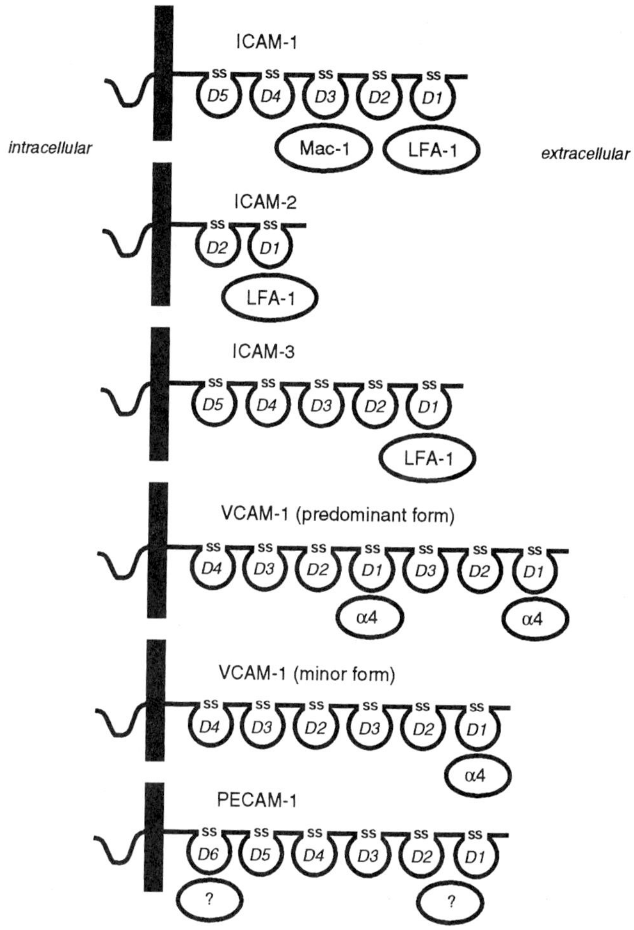

FIGURE 15–2. Basic structures of several immunoglobulin gene superfamily molecules expressed on endothelial cells. Cellular counterligands (ovals) are shown adjacent to the domains (D) containing sequences recognized during binding. The exact counterligands and binding sites on PECAM-1 are unknown. However, mAb that map to domains 1 and 2 block homotypic (PECAM-1 to PECAM-1) adhesion and leukocyte transendothelial migration, and mAb that map to domain 6 block heterotypic adhesion.

unit, β7, can also pair with α4 (α4β7) and, like VLA-4, is capable of binding to fibronectin and VCAM-1.[406, 431] Unlike VLA-4, however, α4β7 binds to another adhesion molecule, MAdCAM-1 (mucosal addressin cell adhesion molecule-1), that appears to be involved in lymphocyte homing to the gut mucosa.[17, 42, 73, 153, 456] Furthermore, β7 can pair with an additional subunit, α^E, which is expressed on lymphocytes (but not granulocytes), where it functions as a ligand for E-cadherin, a molecule found along the basolateral portion of intestinal epithelium.[91, 92]

Ligands for β2 integrins include ICAM-1, ICAM-2, and ICAM-3, as well as fibrinogen, the complement fragment C3bi, and other unidentified structures (see Table 15–2 and Fig. 15–2).[21, 49, 119, 127, 129, 315, 487, 490] For all leukocytes, the processes of firm adhesion, locomotion, and transendothelial migration, as seen in response to stimulation with chemotactic factors, are either partially or completely dependent on β2 integrins. Defects in β2 integrin expression lead to impaired leukocyte recruitment responses, especially in neutrophils.[16, 21]

IMMUNOGLOBULIN GENE SUPERFAMILY

The immunoglobulin gene superfamily of adhesion molecules consists of more than a dozen molecules that have a series of globular domains, formed by disulfide bonds, resembling those found in immunoglobulins.[141] Like integrins, these molecules are responsible for adhesion to other cell surface ligands and have important signaling functions. Members of this family expressed on endothelial cells include ICAM-1, ICAM-2, PECAM-1 (platelet-endothelial cell adhesion molecule-1), VCAM-1, and MAdCAM-1, whereas leukocytes can express ICAM-1, ICAM-2, ICAM-3, PECAM-1, and LFA-3 (CD58) (see Tables 15–1 and 15–2).

The structures of ICAM-1, ICAM-2, ICAM-3, VCAM-1, and PECAM-1 are shown schematically in Figure 15–2; each is discussed in turn. ICAM-1 (CD54) was originally discovered as a ≈90 kD molecule responsible for heterotypic cell adhesion, with a 453 amino acid extracellular domain and putative 24 and 28 amino acid transmembrane and intracytoplasmic domains, respectively.[430, 491] Ligands for the first *N*-terminal domain of ICAM-1 include the β2 integrin LFA-1, fibrinogen, and most serotypes of rhinovirus,[182, 273, 315, 489] whereas the third domain is recognized by the β2 integrin Mac-1.[129] ICAM-1 is constitutively expressed along the luminal, intercellular, and subluminal surfaces of endothelial cells.[383] Various stimuli, including IL-1, TNF, LPS, and IFN-γ, are capable of inducing or enhancing its expression, primarily at the level of transcription (Table 15–3).[142, 546] Unique to IFN-γ is its ability to selectively induce ICAM-1 expression without affecting expression of other adhesion molecules (see Table 15–3).[142, 402] ICAM-1 expression can be induced on several leukocyte types (e.g., eosinophils and basophils)[195, 532] as well as other cells, including respiratory and ocular epithelial cells.[14, 102, 528]

As the name implies, ICAM-2 (CD102) is similar to ICAM-1. It was originally detected as an LFA-1–dependent, ICAM-1–independent 60-kD endothelial ligand with a 202 amino acid extracellular domain and putative transmembrane and intracytoplasmic domains of 26 amino acids each.[120, 490] ICAM-2 has two immunoglobulin-like extracellular domains

TABLE 15–3
EFFECTS OF CYTOKINES ON HUMAN UMBILICAL VEIN ENDOTHELIAL CELL EXPRESSION OF VCAM-1, ICAM-1, AND E-SELECTIN

Endothelial Treatment†	Level of Cell Surface Expression*		
	VCAM-1	*ICAM-1*	*E-Selectin*
None	−	+	−
IFN-γ, 24 hr	−	+ +	−
IL-1, TNF, or LPS, 4–6 hours	+ +	+ + +	+ + + +
IL-1, TNF, or LPS, 24 hours	+ + +	+ + + +	+
IL-4 or IL-13, 4–6 hours	+	+	−
IL-4 or IL-13, 24 hours	+ +	+	−
IL-4 + TNF, 24 hours	+ + + +	+ + +	+/−
IL-4 + TNF (low dose), 24 hours	+ + +	+	−

*Levels of expression, as determined by flow cytometry, are given on a scale of − (absent) to + + + + (maximal). Note that maximal levels of expression differ among these surface structures (ICAM-1>E-selectin>VCAM-1).
†Optimal concentrations for endothelial activation: IFN-γ (10 ng/ml), IL-1 (1 ng/ml), TNF (1 ng/ml or 0.03 ng/ml (low dose)), LPS (bacterial endotoxin, 1 μg/ml), IL-4 (500 units/ml), and IL-13 (10 units/ml).

with 34% homology to the first two domains of ICAM-1.[490] As with ICAM-1, LFA-1–mediated adhesion to ICAM-2 can serve as a costimulatory signal for lymphocyte proliferation.[114] The ligand-binding site for LFA-1 is located in the first *N*-terminal domain in ICAM-1; peptides from this region have been shown to inhibit endothelial cell adhesion.[291] ICAM-2 is constitutively expressed on mononuclear cells, basophils, mast cells, and platelets; endothelial cells, which also express ICAM-2, appear to be the only other cell type that expresses this molecule.[120, 376] ICAM-2 expression is unaffected by cytokines in vitro,[375] although increased levels have been detected in endothelial cells from malignant lymph nodes, suggesting possible regulation of cellular expression in vivo.[414]

ICAM-3 (CD50) also functions as an LFA-1 ligand.[119, 156, 229, 538] It ranges in molecular weight from 116 to 140 kD, depending on the cell type studied, and possesses 48% to 52% homology to ICAM-1 and 31% to 37% homology to ICAM-2.[118, 156, 538] ICAM-3, like ICAM-1, has five immunoglobulin-like extracellular domains (518 amino acids), along with a transmembrane domain of 24 amino acids and an intracytoplasmic domain of 37 amino acids.[118, 156, 538] ICAM-3 is constitutively expressed on all leukocytes and on mast cells; expression on other cell types, including endothelial cells, has not been detected.[119, 156, 532, 538] ICAM-3 appears to act as a signaling molecule, since cross-linking results in calcium mobilization, tyrosine phosphorylation, and adhesion.[101, 230] Following neutrophil activation, the molecule can be proteolytically released from the cell surface.[122]

VCAM-1 (CD106), which is not constitutively expressed on endothelium, was initially identified as a cytokine-inducible structure on endothelial cells that contains six immunoglobulin domains.[384] However, it was later determined that it exists primarily in a seven domain form where there is extensive homology between the three most *N*-terminal domains (labeled domains 1, 2, and 3) and the fourth through sixth domains, suggesting that the molecule developed through gene duplication.[112, 113, 404] In fact, the smaller, six domain form, lacking domain 4, is expressed at very low levels, presumably representing an alternatively spliced form of the molecule.[112, 113, 207, 404] Both the six and seven domain forms have type 1 transmembrane polypeptide anchors consisting of a 22 amino acid transmembrane domain and an intracytoplasmic region of 19 residues.[112, 113, 207, 384, 404] An even smaller glycophosphatidylinositol (GPI)-anchored isoform of VCAM-1 has been detected in murine endothelium.[246, 517] Within the extracellular portions of VCAM-1, domains 1 and 4 are most homologous to each other; these are the domains recognized by VLA-4,[385, 391, 543, 544] although the third domain is needed to stabilize these binding sites.[564]

Although it is usually considered an endothelial cell surface marker, VCAM-1 expression has been detected on other cell types, including macrophages, dendritic cells, astrocytes, and stromal cells in bone marrow.[417, 423] Expression of VCAM-1 on umbilical vein endothelial cells is concentrated on the luminal surface[383] and can be induced de novo within several hours after exposure to interleukin-1 (IL-1), tumor necrosis factor (TNF), or bacterial endotoxin (LPS); expression reaches maximal levels by 24 to 48 hours (see Table 15–3).[117, 384, 416, 573] These treatment conditions lead to increased expression of other endothelial adhesion molecules, including ICAM-1 and E-selectin (see Table 15–3). In contrast, treatment of endothelial cells with IL-4[451, 522] or IL-13[55, 476] leads to selective induction of VCAM-1 expression, and the combination of IL-4 with TNF is synergistic.[316, 521] This effect is due to transcriptional activation and stabilization of VCAM-1 mRNA.[219] Molecular analyses of the VCAM-1 promoter and cell signaling events suggest that NF-κB and protein kinase C are involved in the induction of VCAM-1 expression caused by some cytokines.[121, 368, 467] These patterns of activation may not necessarily be true for other endothelial cell types. For example, human dermal microvascular endothelial cells express VCAM-1 after stimulation with TNF but not after stimulation with either IL-1 or IL-4.[503]

PECAM-1 (platelet-endothelial cell adhesion molecule-1) is a 130-kD molecule with six immunoglobulin-like domains.[124, 351, 370, 499] Unlike other members of this adhesion molecule family, the transmembrane and intracytoplasmic domains are encoded by multiple exons, and several isoforms, due to alternative splicing within these regions, have been identified.[124] As its name implies, PECAM-1 is constitutively expressed on endothelial cells and platelets, although most leukocyte types also express this molecule.[499, 532] The molecule is rapidly shed following activation with chemotactic factors.[499] Both homotypic[9] and heterotypic[352] adhesion via PECAM-1 have been reported, an example of the latter being the interaction of CD31 with sulfated glycosylaminoglycans such as heparan sulfate. Blocking monoclonal antibodies that recognize the second domain are capable of interrupting heterotypic interactions,[124, 351] whereas antibodies to domains 5 and 6, along with antibodies to domains 2 and 3, are required to interrupt homotypic binding, suggesting antiparallel interactions.[155] Cross-linking of PECAM-1 augments avidity of both β1 and β2 integrins.[43, 155, 393, 509]

SELECTINS AND THEIR CARBOHYDRATE LIGANDS

Another family of adhesion molecules is the selectin gene superfamily.[45, 275, 299] The only three known members, E-selectin, L-selectin, and P-selectin, are now referred to as CD62 followed by their respective first letters (CD62E, CD62L, and CD62P). E-selectin (formerly endothelial-leukocyte adhesion molecule-1 or ELAM-1, 115 kD)[48] is expressed exclusively on activated endothelium. P-selectin (formerly GMP-140 or PADGEM, 150 kD),[227] the largest selectin, originally received its name because of its stimulus-induced expression on platelets. It can also be expressed on the surface of endothelial cells. L-selectin is the smallest selectin (formerly TQ1, LECCAM-1, LECAM-1, Leu-8, or LAM-1, 75 kD on lymphocytes, 100 kD on granulocytes, and 110 kD on monocytes)[89, 511] and gets its name because of its restricted expression on leukocytes. It is now believed that the major function of selectins in vivo is to mediate leukocyte-endothelial interactions under conditions of shear stress; L-selectin also functions during lymphocyte trafficking to lymph nodes.[44, 45, 82, 275]

The structures of the selectins are shown schematically in Figure 15–3. Each consists of an *N*-terminal domain of 117 to 120 amino acids possessing calcium-dependent (C type) lectin activity.[137] Proximal to this region is a 32 to 38 amino acid segment with homology to a domain initially discovered

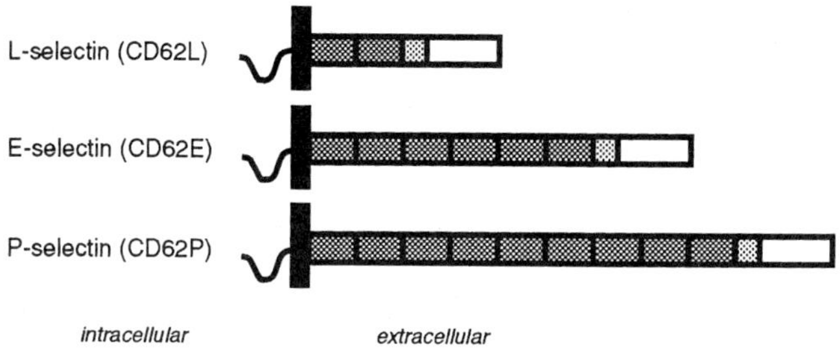

FIGURE 15–3. Basic structures of selectins. The *N*-terminal lectin domains are shown in white, the epidermal growth factor-like domains are shown in light gray, and the complement regulatory-like repeat domains, which vary in number among the different selectins, are shown in dark gray.

in epidermal growth factor, which is referred to as the EGF domain. Proximal to this are two to nine domains of about 60 amino acids in length whose sequences resemble those found in both soluble and membrane-bound complement regulatory (CR) proteins such as CD35 (type 1 complement receptor), decay-accelerating factor (CD55), C1r, C1s, and C4-binding protein.[48, 233] Of note, the genes for selectins are all located on chromosome 1, near the genes for these and other CR proteins.[560] These sequences are then followed by short transmembrane and intracytoplasmic domains of 21 to 35 amino acids each. Although the extracellular domains share significant homology (40–60 overall and 60%–70% within the lectin and EGF domains), little if any homology exists among the transmembrane and intracytoplasmic domains.[275] For P-selectin, two variant forms have been identified: one lacking the transmembrane and intracytoplasmic portions (probably representing a soluble form) and a second alternatively spliced form with eight CR subunits instead of nine.[138, 226] For cell-cell adhesion, the functional portions of all selectins appear to be restricted to the lectin domains, although the presence of the EGF domain may be necessary to confer the appropriate tertiary conformation for binding.[151, 152, 179, 238, 275, 399] For L-selectin, at least, the intracytoplasmic portion of the molecule is also required for adhesive function.[237] Adhesion via selectins or their ligands can alter integrin function as well.[262, 294, 302, 542]

E-selectin is not present on the surface of resting endothelium. Expression of E-selectin is inducible within several hours in cultured endothelial cells, in tissue explants, and/or at injection sites after exposure to various stimuli, including IL-1, TNF, LPS,[16, 234, 379, 470] substance P,[319] IL-3,[74] and uncharacterized substances from platelets.[192] Expression can be potentiated by IFN-γ[284] and inhibited by transforming growth factor β.[164, 165] Once expressed, E-selectin can function as a ligand for leukocytes, including neutrophils,[47, 158, 450] monocytes,[47] eosinophils,[57, 64, 266, 572] basophils,[57, 60] NK cells,[400] and subsets of T lymphocytes.[177, 394, 466] Other cell types, including tumor cells, also recognize E-selectin.[311, 505] Molecular studies of the E-selectin promoter have revealed that transcription is under the control of several transcription factors, including NF-κB.[326, 339] Expression of E-selectin in vitro is relatively transient, with levels approaching those at baseline by 24 hours,[46, 55] although its expression can be prolonged in vitro by incorporating several incompletely defined human plasma-derived factors in the culture.[460] Most of the E-selectin that is expressed is reinternalized and degraded in vitro,[265] but a small amount can be recovered from the culture supernatant, perhaps due to shedding.[283, 371, 398] In vivo, however, E-selectin expression at sites of inflammation is more prolonged,[111, 184] perhaps due to differences in posttranscriptional stability among forms of E-selectin transcripts.[99]

Like E-selectin, P-selectin is not present on the luminal surface of resting endothelium. However, unlike E-selectin, P-selectin exists preformed within granules (the so-called Weibel-Palade bodies)[68, 199, 323, 496] and can be rapidly expressed (within minutes) after stimulation with agents such as histamine, thrombin, phorbol esters, peroxides, and C5a.[159, 167, 389] Expression of P-selectin in vitro is down-regulated as a consequence of endocytosis.[199, 297] P-selectin has been shown to be a ligand for many cell types, including neutrophils, eosinophils, monocytes, and some T lymphocytes.[115, 167, 341, 571] Leukocyte interaction with P-selectin has been shown to alter cellular functions, including superoxide production and integrin-mediated phagocytosis.[110, 531, 578]

The third and smallest member of the selectin family, L-selectin, is found exclusively on leukocytes.[288, 512] It was originally discovered in mice as the peripheral lymph node homing receptor, a molecule responsible for lymphocyte attachment to high endothelial venules.[37, 70, 86, 162, 168, 249, 469, 488] It also functions as an adhesion molecule for vascular endothelium under conditions of shear stress.[35, 253, 306, 482, 483, 541, 542] L-selectin is shed through an undefined proteolytic pathway during leukocyte activation by chemotactic factors, cytokines, and other stimuli.[39, 183, 231, 236, 248, 249, 512]

A great deal of effort has focused on identifying the carbohydrate ligands for selectins.[299, 537] Studies have examined the carbohydrates themselves, the core structures upon which the carbohydrates are expressed, as well as the enzymatic pathways responsible for their synthesis. At first glance, the interactions between selectins and their ligands appear quite similar and difficult to distinguish. In fact, many binding characteristics are shared, including calcium dependence, function at low temperatures and under conditions of shear stress, and sensitivity to treatment with neuraminidase.[255, 261, 275, 276] In addition to the presence of α-2,3–linked terminal sialic acid residues, fucose residues located at specific linkage sites are critical for selectin binding. Under some conditions, all three selectins can bind to carbohydrate structures containing sialylated Lewis X antigen (sLe^x, CD15s) or its isomer, sialyl Lewis A (sLe^a) (Fig. 15–4).[34, 36, 160, 194, 310, 392, 553] On neutrophils and B lymphocytes, these sialylated structures may be carried on CD65, CD66, or additional surface molecules.[263, 405, 500] This is where the similarities end, because a number of important differences exist among ligands for selectins. For example, ligands for P-selectin are protease sensitive and endo–β-galactosidase resistant, whereas E-selectin ligands tend to be protease resistant and endo–β-galactosidase sensitive.[64, 274, 400, 571] This raises the possibility that ligands for P-selectin are sLe^x-containing glycoproteins and ligands for E-selectin are extended-chain forms of sLe^x, such as sialyl-dimeric Le^x (see Fig. 15–4), expressed as protease-resistant glycoproteins and/or glycolipids. For P-selectin, specific glycoprotein ligands have been discovered[340, 342, 372, 438, 590]; one has been named PSGL-1 (P-selectin glycoprotein ligand-1). The search for E-selectin ligands has also revealed several possible structures. Two extended-chain glycoprotein ligands for E-selectin on

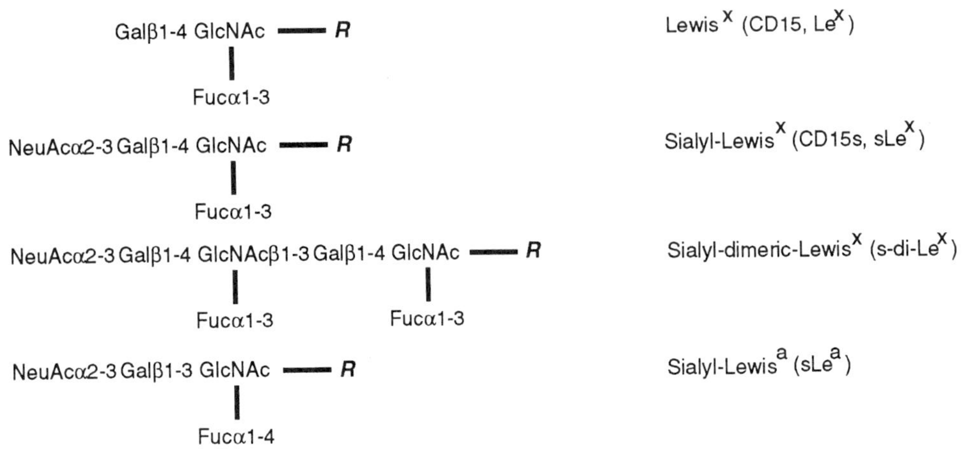

FIGURE 15–4. Chemical structures of several carbohydrate ligands for selectins. Gal = galactose; GlcNAc = *N*-acetyl glucosamine; NeuAc = neuraminic (sialic) acid; Fuc = fucose. R represents additional glycolipid and/or glycoprotein structures to which these terminal sugars may be attached. Note that sLe^x and sLe^a differ only in their galactose and fucose linkages.

the human monocytic cell line U937 were isolated.[390] Using mouse leukocytes, a variant of the fibroblast growth factor receptor was identified as an E-selectin ligand termed ESL-1 (E-selectin ligand-1).[492] Other studies suggest the presence of glycolipid ligands (e.g., sulfated structures such as galactosylceramides) for selectins on leukocytes.[23, 180, 502, 525] For subsets of memory skin-homing lymphocytes, additional sialylated molecules recognized by monoclonal antibodies HECA-452 (the cutaneous lymphocyte antigen) and 2F3 appear to mediate binding to E-selectin but not P-selectin.[38, 379, 394–396, 427] It has also been suggested that carbohydrate structures on L-selectin can interact with E-selectin and P-selectin.[397, 540] For L-selectin, ligands include the sulfated murine molecule glycosylated cell adhesion molecule-1 (GlyCAM-1),[220, 277] CD34,[30] and mucosal addressin cell adhesion molecule-1 (MAdCAM-1),[35] each belonging to the sialomucin family of adhesion molecules[465]; heparin[369, 373]; a sulfoglucuronyl glycolipid ligand that also binds P-selectin but not E-selectin[365]; and an antigen on high endothelial venules from human lymph nodes recognized by monoclonal antibody 2H5.[444]

Studies have begun to define the pathways responsible for synthesis of carbohydrate counterligands for selectins such as sLe^x. Biosynthesis of sLe^x results from the sequential activity of sialyltransferases and fucosyltransferases, particularly α-1,3 fucosyltransferases (Fuc-T) on α-2,3–sialylated lactosamine-type oligosaccharides.[261, 299] To date, five forms of α-1,3 fucosyltransferases have been cloned.[173, 256, 300, 575] One in particular, Fuc-TVII, appears to be especially important for leukocyte synthesis of sLe^x.[364, 443] Interestingly, transfection of this enzyme into cell lines that lacked sLe^x expression resulted in both sLe^x expression and E-selectin binding, although L-selectin binding was not observed.[501] This further highlights the subtle differences in carbohydrate binding specificities for different selectins. In umbilical vein endothelial cells, two α-2,3 sialyltransferases and four α-1,3 fucosyltransferases have been detected. TNF treatment results in increases in fucosyltransferase activity, sLe^x expression, and mRNA levels for Fuc-TVI in association with increased expression of sLe^x.[312] Clearly, additional investigation is needed to identify the specific glycosylated ligands for selectins on normal human cells and to characterize more accurately their affinities for different selectin ligands. Greater understanding is needed of whether there are differences in expression of these enzymes among leukocyte or endothelial subtypes, the regulation of expression and activity of these enzymes, and their specificity for carbohydrates on glycolipid versus glycoprotein substrates.

OTHER ADHESION MOLECULES

Several other adhesion molecules on endothelial cells and/or leukocytes have been identified; some may function during leukocyte recruitment responses. For example, vascular adhesion protein-1 (VAP-1), a 90-kD lymphocyte ligand, has been identified in synovial, mucosal, and peripheral lymph node endothelium and at sites of inflammatory disorders but not on unstimulated or activated umbilical vein endothelium.[439, 440] A similar molecule is L-VAP-2 (lymphocyte-vascular adhesion protein-2), a 70-kD structure constitutively expressed on umbilical vein endothelial cells and some lymphocytes; antibody-blocking studies suggest that it also functions as a lymphocyte ligand.[4] A pulmonary-specific endothelial cell adhesion molecule that participates in metastasis of tumors to the lung has been identified in mice (Lu-ECAM-1),[591, 592] but its counterpart in humans has not been identified. Another molecule, CD44 (formerly Hermes antigen, H-CAM or pgp-1), is found at high levels on most leukocytes, endothelial cells, epithelial cells, and other cell types.[286] Many splice variant forms of differing molecular weights have been identified (85–160 kD, with 90 kD most predominant). This family has been implicated as adhesion molecules for peripheral lymph nodes, hyaluronic acid, and T-cell signaling.[286] CD44 has also been shown to mediate interactions between lymphocytes and airway smooth muscle cells, inducing growth of the latter cell type.[281] The roles of these and other adhesion molecules in allergic inflammation remain to be determined.

PHYSIOLOGY OF CELL ADHESION: A STEPWISE PARADIGM OF CELL MARGINATION, ROLLING, ADHESION, AND TRANSENDOTHELIAL MIGRATION

A sequence of steps is likely involved during the emigration of leukocytes from the intravascular compartment into tissue sites.[3, 10, 83, 178, 485] Under the influence of blood flow, which causes shear forces to be applied to circulating leukocytes, cells undergo a reversible process during which they roll or reversibly attach to the endothelium. Studies employing assays of adhesion under rotational conditions,[253, 483] using flow chambers in vitro,[1, 28, 84, 228, 279, 280, 305, 306, 581] or employing intravital video microscopy in vivo, using tissues such as rat mesentery,[134, 260, 289, 290, 382, 480, 486, 520, 540–542, 593] suggest that these tethering adhesive interactions are mediated primarily by interactions between carbohydrates and their selectin counterligands. However, other studies suggest that the integrin VLA-4 can also participate in cell rolling and arrest for cells expressing this molecule, such as eosinophils, lymphocytes, and monocytes.[12, 228, 305, 306, 486]

The next step requires leukocyte activation, perhaps as a result of their exposure to leukocyte-activating factors produced by and/or displayed on endothelial cells, such as PAF,[298, 595] chemokines, such as IL-8 for neutrophils,[215] and MIP-1β for T cells.[507, 508] Alternatively, contact of leukocytes with endothelial adhesion molecules may activate the cells directly.[294] Associated with these events are increases in both avidity and expression of integrins on the leukocyte surface.[128, 307, 481] Leukocyte rolling and activation are followed by firm leukocyte-endothelial adhesion, mediated by β1 and β2 integrins on leukocytes and VCAM-1, ICAM-1, and E-selectin on cytokine-activated endothelium.[46, 47, 55, 57, 61, 131, 132, 177, 190, 191, 251, 266, 270, 347, 383, 450, 451, 522, 550, 572] Subsequent transendothelial migration (diapedesis), during which the leukocytes emigrate between endothelial cells and penetrate the basement membrane[216] to enter the extravascular space, is mediated by PECAM-1,[124, 351, 353, 536] although integrins, selectins, and their ligands may also participate.[25, 100, 143, 161, 191, 304, 327, 344, 383] Cytokines, chemokines, and other chemotactic factors, by directly activating leukocyte migration responses, can potentiate the process of adhesion and transendothelial migration.[90, 144, 147, 215, 345, 478, 586, 587]

Further support for this paradigm is, in general, provided by studies of patients with genetic defects in human leukocyte β2 integrins (leukocyte adhesion deficiency type 1)[15, 16, 197, 539] and defects in generation of selectin ligands (leukocyte adhesion deficiency type 2)[154, 197, 409, 539] and studies of adhesion molecule knock-out mice (Table 15–4).[20, 77, 189, 267, 322, 477, 513, 577, 579] However, one important exception to this paradigm is seen in the immune response to bacterial infections of the lung. It appears that neutrophil recruitment into the lung is unaffected in P-selectin/ICAM-1 dual knock-out mice,[77] in mice treated with CD18 antibodies,[133] or in patients with leukocyte adhesion deficiency type 1,[15] suggesting the presence of a recruitment pathway that is independent of CD18, ICAM-1, and P-selectin. Whether this pathway is unique to the lung is not known.

Given the significant redundancy in adhesion molecule function, it seems almost certain that preferential recruitment of a given cell type would be the net result of many separate events rather than the effect of a unique cell-specific adhesion molecule pathway for each cell type. This paradigm would predict that a specific leukocyte infiltrate results from a series of relatively selective recruitment events in which overlapping cell adhesion mechanisms and chemotactic factors function in concert. For many cell types, evidence is rapidly accumulating

TABLE 15–4
MANIFESTATIONS OF ADHESION MOLECULE DEFICIENCY STATES IN HUMANS AND KNOCK-OUT MICE

Adhesion Molecule Deficiency	Consequences
Human	
Leukocyte Adhesion Deficiency type I (CD18 deficiency)[15, 16, 197, 539]	Blood neutrophilia with tissue neutropenia, delayed umbilical cord separation, recurrent soft tissue infections, impaired pus formation, and wound healing; pulmonary infections are not usually seen, and eosinophils and mononuclear cells, unlike neutrophils, can be found at sites of soft tissue infections; in vitro or ex vivo: reduced or absent neutrophil adhesion, transendothelial migration, and chemotactic responses are seen, although rolling adhesion is normal
Leukocyte Adhesion Deficiency Type II (Fucose Metabolism Defect)[154, 409, 539]	Severe mental retardation, short stature, distinctive facial appearance, Bombay (hh) blood phenotype, impaired pus formation, recurrent pneumonia, periodontitis, otitis, and cellulitis; neutrophil studies in vitro or ex vivo: reduced or absent sLe^x expression, reduced rolling adhesion, normal firm adhesion and migration in response to chemotactic stimulation
Mouse	
ICAM-1 Knock-out[77, 477, 579]	Impaired leukocyte recruitment to inflamed peritoneum and to sites of contact sensitivity, neutrophilia (≈4–5 × normal), lymphocytosis (≈2 × normal), improved resistance to LPS-induced shock
CD 18 Hypomorphic Mutation[577]	Impaired leukocyte recruitment to inflamed peritoneum and to sites of contact sensitivity, neutrophilia (≈2–3 × normal), lymphocytosis (≈1.5 × normal)
L-Selectin Knock-out[20,513]	Markedly reduced leukocyte rolling and recruitment to inflamed peritoneum and to sites of contact sensitivity, improved resistance to LPS-induced shock, small lymph nodes, splenomegaly, normal antibody production
E-Selectin Knock-out[267]	Normal; profound impairment of PMN recruitment after infusion of P-selectin mAb
P-Selectin Knock-out[77, 322]	Absent leukocyte rolling, neutrophilia (≈2–3 × normal), delayed PMN recruitment to inflamed peritoneum
VCAM-1 Knock-out[189]	Embryonic lethal
Dual ICAM-1/P-Selectin Knock-out[77]	Complete blockade of PMN recruitment during bacterial-induced peritonitis; no inhibition of PMN recruitment during bacterial-induced pneumonitis; blood leukocyte counts similar to ICAM-1 knock-outs

in support of this hypothesis. For example, both in vitro and in vivo studies have identified a number of adhesion-related pathways that may be critical during allergic inflammation.[29, 53, 56, 62, 65, 67, 88, 285, 292, 335, 336, 415, 447, 449, 556, 557]

EOSINOPHIL, BASOPHIL, AND MAST CELL INTERACTIONS VIA SELECTINS, INTEGRINS, AND THEIR COUNTERLIGANDS

In examining mechanisms of allergic inflammation, one useful approach has been to identify processes that activate or mediate eosinophil, basophil, and/or mast cell adhesion responses but not for other leukocyte types (e.g., neutrophils). Such pathways would, in theory, have a much higher likelihood to be of relevance to cellular recruitment responses associated with allergic diseases. For example, in comparing adhesion of eosinophils and neutrophils, it was demonstrated that both cell types can bind to cytokine-activated endothelium under rotational conditions in an L-selectin–dependent manner, although the ability of neutrophils to adhere was much greater than that of eosinophils.[253] However, one L-selectin antibody, LAM 1-11, had an unexpected activity in that it inhibited eosinophil but not neutrophil adhesion under these conditions, raising the possibility that eosinophils utilize an epitope on the L-selectin molecule not used by neutrophils.[253] Basophils also express L-selectin, but no information is available on its function for this cell type. Basophils have been shown to shed this molecule upon activation in vitro or in vivo, although the shedding is less complete compared with other granulocytes.[63, 169]

Eosinophils have been shown to bind at least as well as neutrophils to P-selectin immobilized on plastic surfaces,[531, 571] when expressed on the surface of activated platelets,[244] or in tissue sections from nasal polyps.[504] However, the ability of several enzymes, including proteases, to reduce neutrophil binding was greater than that for eosinophils, suggesting that there may be subtle differences in the level of expression or biochemical composition of P-selectin ligands.[571] Unlike eosinophil adhesion to most other ligands, eosinophils failed to spread on P-selectin and exhibited a reduced capacity to degranulate or produce superoxide anion, suggesting that attachment to P-selectin inhibited eosinophil function.[531] Whether similar functional interactions occur between basophils and P-selectin is not known.

Studies using recombinant E-selectin immobilized on plastic plates confirmed that eosinophils and basophils, like neutrophils, are capable of binding to E-selectin.[64, 66] All three cell types adhered to E-selectin, and their adhesion was dependent on leukocyte surface expression of sialic acid, since neuraminidase treatment and removal of sialic acid abolished essentially all adhesive activity.[64, 66] Interestingly, basophils bound best to E-selectin, followed by neutrophils and eosinophils. This relative rank order of binding efficiency was not directly related to the quantity of sLe^x on the cell surface. Flow cytometric studies using antibodies specific for sLe^x, as well as an extended-chain form of sLe^x (sialyl-dimeric Le^x), revealed that neutrophils had the greatest amount of sLe^x, whereas all three cells had comparable levels of sialyl-dimeric Le^x.[64, 66] That the extended-chain form of sLe^x may be responsible for adhesion to E-selectin was suggested by experiments utilizing endo–β-galactosidase. This enzyme removes the sialyl-dimeric Le^x and almost completely inhibited binding of all three cell types.[64, 66] Thus in spite of the fact that the bulk of sLe^x remained on the surface of neutrophils and basophils after treatment with endo–β-galactosidase, adhesion was dramatically impaired. These same experiments revealed that sialyl-dimeric Le^x is the important and predominant form of sLe^x on the eosinophil surface. Similar conclusions were reached in a study of NK cells.[400] Sialylated, extended-chain glycoprotein ligands for E-selectin have been identified on U937 cells, a human monocyte-like cell line.[390]

Among the earliest studies of cell adhesion were those in which cytokine-activated monolayers of cultured umbilical vein endothelial cells were treated for several hours with IL-1, TNF, or other stimuli, resulting in enhanced adhesion for neutrophils, eosinophils, and basophils.[47, 57, 61, 139, 270, 450] Antibodies to CD18, ICAM-1, and E-selectin inhibited adherence of all three leukocyte types.[57, 61, 266, 270] In contrast, anti–VCAM-1 antibody was extremely effective in inhibiting eosinophil adherence but had no effect on neutrophil adherence, suggesting that eosinophils, unlike neutrophils, recognize VCAM-1.[57] In these studies, basophil adherence was also demonstrated to be partly mediated through VCAM-1, although the inhibitory effect seen with anti–VCAM-1 antibody was less impressive. Furthermore, antibodies to VLA-4 inhibited eosinophil and basophil, but not neutrophil, adhesion to IL-1–stimulated endothelium, corresponding to the expression pattern of the VLA-4 counterligand.[57, 66, 131, 550, 572] The ability of eosinophils and basophils to adhere to VCAM-1 was confirmed by showing that these cells could adhere to an immobilized recombinant form of VCAM-1 and in experiments in which the adhesion was inhibited using VCAM-1 and VLA-4 antibodies.[66, 451, 572]

The finding that VCAM-1/VLA-4–mediated adhesion was different among eosinophils and basophils compared with neutrophils raised the possibility that specific induction of VCAM-1 expression on endothelial cells might promote eosinophil and basophil adherence but not neutrophil adherence. Previous studies suggested that the cytokine IL-4 was capable of selectively inducing VCAM-1 expression in endothelial cells.[522] Incubation of endothelial cells with IL-4 did not influence neutrophil adherence but did induce eosinophil and basophil adherence that was inhibited by more than 70% with either anti–VCAM-1 or anti–VLA-4 antibodies.[451] Similar results have been obtained with IL-13, a cytokine that shares many biologic activities with IL-4.[55] These in vitro findings were consistent with several in vivo murine studies: intraperitoneal or intradermal injection with IL-4 resulted in an eosinophil-rich infiltrate[346]; IL-4 transgenic mice developed tissue eosinophilia and an allergic-like syndrome[515]; mice inoculated with an IL-4 transfected tumor cell line developed local eosinophilia at the tumor site[516]; and anti–IL-4 reduced antigen-induced expression of VCAM-1 in mouse trachea and eosinophil recruitment to the lung.[301, 362] Therefore, IL-4, by selectively promoting VCAM-1 expression, might contribute to the preferential recruitment of eosinophils (and basophils) compared with neutrophils seen during certain inflammatory responses.

The discovery that eosinophils and basophils, but not neutrophils, express $\alpha4\beta7$,[66, 524] a molecule that recognizes both VCAM-1 and MAdCAM-1,[17, 42, 153] suggests that this integrin may also play a role in preferential recruitment responses. However, α4 integrins are expressed on other cell types, including lymphocytes and monocytes.[204] There also are situations in vivo in which acute or chronic eosinophil accumulation occurs without significant endothelial VCAM-1 expression[266, 338, 479] or under conditions in which VCAM-1 is expressed at relatively high levels but little or no eosinophil accumulation is seen.[72, 184, 185] Thus it seems unlikely that the VCAM-1/VLA-4 adhesion pathway is solely responsible for selective eosinophil and basophil recruitment.

Several in vitro studies have begun to analyze the molecular mechanisms regulating eosinophil transendothelial migration. Treatment of endothelial monolayers with IL-1 or TNF increased eosinophil transendothelial migration.[143, 345] Eosinophil transendothelial migration through IL-1–treated endothelium was almost completely inhibited by antibodies to CD18, but CD29 antibody had little or no effect.[143] Antibodies directed against the LFA-1 binding site on ICAM-1 were moderately effective in inhibiting transmigration, although a combination of VCAM-1, ICAM-1, and E-selectin antibodies was more effective than ICAM-1 antibody alone.[143] Cytokines such as GM-CSF or IL-5 will markedly potentiate eosinophil transendothelial migration across unstimulated or cytokine-activated endothelial cell monolayers.[144, 346] In another study, an antibody that activates, rather than inhibits, β1 integrin function dramatically inhibited eosinophil chemotaxis and transendothelial migration, presumably by enhancing adhesion and essentially immobilizing these cells.[264] These data support the hypothesis that transendothelial migration of eosinophils involves the function and expression of adhesion molecules on both the leukocyte and the endothelium and suggest that the mechanisms regulating leukocyte adhesion may differ from those mediating transmigration. Thus far, the role of PECAM-1 in eosinophil transmigration remains unknown, and mechanisms of basophil transendothelial migration have not been examined.

Several stimuli, including cytokines, possess the ability to selectively enhance eosinophil or basophil adhesion-related responses. For example, exposure of eosinophils to IL-3, IL-5, or GM-CSF will promote adhesion molecule function, induce L-selectin shedding and CD11b up-regulation, and facilitate chemoattractant-induced adhesion responses and transendothelial migration.[50, 144, 198, 367, 527, 549, 554, 558, 559] Exposure to the chemokine RANTES, a potent and selective eosinophil activator and chemoattractant in vitro[5, 235, 428, 582] and in vivo,[31, 331] causes eosinophil transendothelial migration.[147] The effects of RANTES on eosinophils were synergistic with IL-5, and both anti-CD18 and anti–VLA-4 antibodies were needed to effectively inhibit RANTES-induced transmigration across IL-1–activated endothelium.[147] Interestingly, eosinophils purified from late-phase reaction bronchoalveolar lavage (BAL) fluids display a similarly potentiated transendothelial migration response.[148] Furthermore, eosinophil-activating cytokines have been detected at sites of allergic inflammation,[140, 193, 241, 317, 343, 380, 381] and both epithelial and endothelial cells have been shown to produce RANTES.[32, 493–495]

Taken together, these data suggest that RANTES and perhaps other C-C chemokines with eosinophil chemotactic activity,[113a, 228a, 376a] especially in the presence of priming cytokines, may play important roles during eosinophil transmigration in vivo. For basophils, IgE-dependent degranulation or treatment with IL-3 will enhance adhesion to endothelial cells in a β2 integrin–dependent manner.[58, 59] Whereas IL-3 and IL-5 are basophil chemoattractants[510]; the C-C chemokines are more potent and have little or no effect on neutrophils.[5a, 49a, 113a, 564a] In each instance, these treatments have little or no effect on neutrophils, and adhesion is mediated primarily through β2 integrins. Preliminary data suggest that β1 integrins on eosinophils exist in a state of partial activation and can be maximally activated for adhesion to VCAM-1 after exposure to certain divalent cations (e.g., Mn^{2+}) or integrin-activating antibodies; these are conditions that do not affect the total cell surface expression of β1 integrins.[320, 574] In contrast, IL-5 prevents cation-induced β1 integrin activation, as did the tyrosine kinase inhibitor tyrphostin.[321, 574] These data suggest that cytokines can cause functional activation of certain adhesion pathways while down-regulating expression and function of other adhesion pathways; the balance determines whether cell adhesion or migration will occur. This occurrence, in fact, has been reported in hematopoietic cell lines.[258]

Once leukocytes enter the extravascular space, migration through the tissue is dependent on their ability to bind to extracellular matrix proteins. Interactions with matrix proteins also appear to be important in mast cell localization within tissues. Since most of the receptors for matrix proteins belong to the β1 integrin family, eosinophils, basophils, and mast cells were examined for their expression of these surface structures.[65, 145, 170, 188, 532, 533] Eosinophils can bind to fibronectin via α4 integrins,[18, 366] although activation of the integrin may be required for binding.[320, 321] Eosinophils can also bind to laminin via α6 integrins.[170] Interestingly, adhesion to fibronectin was shown to activate eosinophil production of superoxide anion,[136] degranulation responses,[366] leukotriene release,[18] and production of IL-3 and GM-CSF, which augmented eosinophil survival in an autocrine fashion.[19] Eosinophil degranulation, aggregation, and cytokine production in response to several stimuli or on various surfaces, including matrix proteins, can be regulated via β2 integrins.[149, 212, 514]

Studies examining expression and function of β1 integrins in human basophils revealed expression of α4 and α5 integrins that are capable of mediating adhesion to VCAM-1 and fibronectin.[65, 66, 333, 532] In addition to α4 and α5 integrins, mast cells also express α3 integrins; the latter mediate adhesion and migration to laminin, whereas all three are capable of mediating fibronectin binding.[108, 116, 518, 519] Mast cell interactions with laminin may be important in tissue localization in vivo.[551] Basophils from asthmatic (but not normal) donors will release histamine upon antibody cross-linking of β1 integrins, whereas IgE-dependent basophil and mast cell mediator release is inhibited.[174, 175, 278] In other studies using rat, mouse, and cultured human mast cells, interactions with fibronectin appeared to enhance IgE-dependent histamine and cytokine release.[333, 411] Adhesion mediated via integrins, or cross-linking of cell surface integrins, can therefore affect a wide range of biologic activities on eosinophils, basophils, and mast cells.

EXPRESSION AND FUNCTION OF ADHESION MOLECULES IN VIVO DURING ALLERGIC AND OTHER INFLAMMATORY RESPONSES IN THE SKIN AND AIRWAYS

One of the first pieces of evidence suggesting the existence of different adhesion-related mechanisms for cell recruitment among granulocyte subtypes was found in patients with leukocyte adhesion deficiency type I, in which eosinophils and mononuclear leukocytes are able to accumulate at sites of infection even though neutrophils are not.[15] These findings suggested that eosinophils, unlike neutrophils, possessed β2 integrin–independent mechanisms for recruitment into tissues probably due, at least in part, to α4 integrins.

The potential role of adhesion molecules in allergic diseases has been the topic of several reviews.[29, 62, 88, 336, 556, 557] Investigators studying this question have taken a number of approaches. One approach has been to attempt to find evidence of endothelial activation at sites of allergic inflammation. The expression of endothelial adhesion molecules has been examined in the skin, nose, and airways following experimental allergen challenge and in allergic and other eosinophilic diseases. Studies using immunohistochemical techniques have demonstrated that intradermal injection of allergic individuals with allergen activates the vascular endothelium to express E-selectin and VCAM-1, and to increase its expression of ICAM-1, in an IgE-dependent manner.[56, 266, 287, 448] Increased expression of VCAM-1 was also observed 24 hours after intranasal allergen challenge, and the numbers of eosinophils infiltrating the tissues correlated, albeit weakly, with the extent and intensity of VCAM-1 staining.[282] Endobronchial allergen challenge resulted in increases in endothelial VCAM-1 staining and epithelial ICAM-1 staining, with a significant correlation between these parameters and eosinophil influx. Allergen challenge of the eye induced ICAM-1 expression on conjunctival epithelium.[102]

There is indirect evidence that endothelial activation also occurs within the human airway following endoscopic intrabronchial allergen challenge, since increased levels of soluble forms of E-selectin, ICAM-1, and VCAM-1 are observed in BAL fluids[169, 506, 589]; in one of these studies, there was a correlation with eosinophil influx and levels of both IL-4 and IL-5.[589] One study found an increase in serum levels of soluble ICAM-1 and E-selectin, but not VCAM-1, in patients admitted for exacerbations of asthma.[337] In nonhuman primates, allergen inhalation resulted in E-selectin expression on the airway vascular endothelium within 6 hours.[186] The pattern of endothelial activation seen during allergic inflammation in vivo suggests that endothelial cells are being exposed to cytokines such as IL-1, TNF, and/or IL-4. Possible cellular sources for IgE-dependent release of these endothelial-activating cytokines are mast cells and basophils. In vitro studies have demonstrated that IgE-dependent stimulation of mast cells results in increased mRNA levels and secretion of a variety of endothelial-activating cytokines, including TNF, IL-4, and IL-13.[69, 71, 78, 146, 163, 176, 552] Basophil production of more impressive quantities of IL-4 has also been clearly demonstrated.[76, 309, 350, 454] Several studies have found evidence that these cytokines may be generated during allergic reactions. For example, IL-1 and IL-4 are released in vivo during experimental allergic reactions,[52, 589] and mRNA has been detected at allergic inflammatory sites for TNF,[585] IL-4,[71, 140, 241, 418, 419, 584] and IL-13.[214]

Especially convincing is the observation that E-selectin expression induced by allergen injection in human skin can be inhibited if the site is immediately biopsied and placed into culture with a mixture of antibodies that neutralize IL-1 and TNF.[287] Eosinophil influx has been observed following injection of IL-1 into the skin of rats[442] or following injection of IL-4 into the skin or peritoneum of mice[346] but not in baboons, despite induction of VCAM-1 expression.[72] In guinea pigs, an IL-1 antagonist inhibited airway hyperreactivity and the development of pulmonary eosinophilia.[561] However, studies in which biopsies were performed after IL-1 or TNF was injected into the skin of humans revealed an intense leukocytic infiltration devoid of eosinophils.[184, 185] Furthermore, it was demonstrated that an IL-1 antagonist could effectively inhibit the human cutaneous late-phase response; yet no significant inhibitory effect on cell influx was seen histologically. It therefore seems likely that other factors, besides nonspecific endothelial activation alone, are required for eosinophil recruitment responses to occur in vivo.[205]

Changes in the expression of cell surface adhesion molecules occur on eosinophils and basophils during their movement from the circulation into tissues, implying an involvement during experimental allergic inflammation. Comparisons of levels of adhesion molecules on granulocytes recovered from blood and either sputum, bronchoalveolar lavage, or nasal lavage post antigen challenge revealed increased expression of CD11b,[29, 169, 196, 259, 457] diminished levels of L-selectin,[29, 169, 328] and little or no change in expression of LFA-1, VLA-4, or sialyl-dimeric Le^x (unpublished observations).[169, 259, 457] Similar phenotypic changes have been observed after eosinophil transendothelial migration in vitro (see Fig. 15–2).[143, 548] Although these data demonstrate dynamic changes in eosinophil and basophil adhesion molecule expression during inflammation, these changes also occur on neutrophils and have been observed on cells obtained from other inflammatory reactions or on those that spontaneously migrate to these sites.[232, 248] Therefore, these events cannot, by themselves, account for selectivity in cell recruitment but instead probably represent a common consequence of cell recruitment.

Several experiments implicating cell adhesion molecules in the pathophysiology of allergic rhinitis and asthma have now appeared. When bronchial mucosal biopsies were obtained from normal subjects and those with mild, stable allergic asthma, immunohistochemical analyses revealed similar levels of endothelial expression of ICAM-1 and E-selectin (VCAM-1 was not studied), despite an increased number of eosinophils in the mucosa of the asthmatic subjects.[338] After 6 weeks of treatment with inhaled budesonide, tissue eosinophilia in the asthmatic subjects was reduced; yet no significant change in the pattern of ICAM-1 and E-selectin expression was observed. A subsequent study compared endothelial adhesion molecule expression in airway biopsies from subjects with allergic and nonallergic asthma as well as normal controls.[33] Constitutive expression of ICAM-1, VCAM-1, and E-selectin was observed in all groups. Endothelial staining for ICAM-1 and E-selectin, but not VCAM-1, was significantly increased in the nonallergic asthmatic group only, whereas epithelial staining for ICAM-1 was increased in both groups of asthmatic subjects.

This is in contrast with another study in which more symptomatic patients with asthma underwent bronchoscopy and biopsy. In this study, strong endothelial staining for VCAM-1, as well as ICAM-1, was observed.[378] Studies of nasal airway tissue from subjects with perennial allergic rhinitis found increased expression of ICAM-1 and VCAM-1, but not E-selectin, compared with tissue from nonallergic

TABLE 15–5
ANTIADHESION TREATMENTS TESTED IN ANIMAL MODELS OF ALLERGIC OR OTHER INFLAMMATORY DISEASES OF THE AIRWAYS OR SKIN

Inflammatory Model	Animal	Treatment*
Airways		
Antigen-induced eosinophil recruitment and airway responsiveness	Monkey	ICAM-1 mAb (iv or inhaled)[568, 569]
Antigen-induced eosinophil recruitment and allergic late-phase responses	Rabbit	VLA-4 mAb, CS-1 peptide[330]
	Sheep	VLA-4 mAb (no efffect on eosinophils)[2]
	Guinea pig	CD18 mAb[332]
		VLA-4 mAb[408]
Antigen-induced T-cell and eosinophil recruitment to trachea	Rat	VLA-4, VCAM-1 mAb[362]
		ICAM-1, CD11a mAb (no effect on eosinophils)[362]
Antigen-induced airway responses and leukocyte recruitment	Rat	CD11a, CD11b, VLA-4 mAb (blocked airway responses but not cell recruitment)[413]
Antigen-induced neutrophil recruitment and allergic late-phase responses	Monkey	E-selectin mAb[186]
		ICAM-1 mAb (no effect)[186]
Chronic eosinophilic airway inflammation	Monkey	ICAM-1 mAb (no effect)[187]
Cobra venom factor-induced, PMN-mediated lung inflammation	Rat	P-selectin mAb[357]
		sLex and derivatives[356]
		L-selectin F(ab')2 mAb[355]
		P-selectin chimera[360]
		L-selectin chimera[360]
		E-selectin chimera (no effect)[360]
IgG immune complexes, PMN-mediated lung inflammation	Rat	E-selectin mAb[359]
		sLex and derivatives[354]
		PECAM-1 mAb[536]
		L-selectin mAb[355]
		L-selectin mAb (iv; not effective it)[358]
		ICAM-1 mAb (iv or it)[358]
		CD11a mAb[361]
		CD11a mAb (iv; not effective it)[358]
		CD11b mAb (not effective)[361]
		CD11b mAb (it; not effective iv)[358]
IgA immune complexes, macrophage-mediated lung inflammation	Rat	ICAM-1 mAb[361]
		CD11a mAb[361]
		CD11b mAb[361]
		VLA-4 mAb[361]
		E-selectin mAb (no effect)[359]
		sLex and derivatives (no effect)[354]
		L-selectin F(ab')2 mAb (no effect)[355]
Bacterial-induced subcutaneous PMN migration	Rabbit	CD18 (no effect)[133, 202]
GM-CSF–induced intrapulmonary PMN sequestration	Monkey	CD18 mAb (small effect)[587]
		CD11b mAb (no effect)[587]
Actinomycetes-induced pneumonitis and fibrosis	Mouse	CD11a[126]
TNF-induced PMN sequestration, pulmonary edema	Guinea pig	ICAM-1, CD11b, CD18 mAb[293]
Skin		
PAF, LTB, and C5a des arg–induced eosinophil influx	Guinea pig	VLA-4 mAb[565]
Delayed-type hypersensitivity	Rat	CD11a mAb[223]
		VLA-4 mAb[222]
		CD11a plus VLA-4 mAb[221]
	Mouse	VLA-4 mAb[98]
		CD11a, ICAM-1 mAb[445]
	Monkey	E-selectin, VCAM-1 mAb[471]
Bacterial-induced subcutaneous PMN migration	Rabbit	P-selectin (no effect)[461]
FMLP-induced PMN infiltration	Rabbit	CD11a, CD18[433]
		CD11b (no effect)[433]
TNF-induced PMN influx into transplanted human skin	SCID mouse	PECAM-1[536]
		E-selectin[583]

*Treatments were effective and given intravenously unless otherwise noted.
Abbreviations: mAb = monoclonal antibody; iv = intravenous; it = intratracheal; PMN = neutrophil.

controls.[334] Seasonal exposure to pollen was associated with a significant increase in nasal epithelial cell expression of ICAM-1 along with increased numbers of eosinophils, neutrophils, and metachromatic cells.[103] Further support for the potential role of VLA-4 VCAM-1–mediated eosinophil recruitment was provided by the demonstration of VCAM-1 staining of blood vessels, without E-selectin staining, in skin biopsies from patients with eosinophilic vasculitis[97] and significant VCAM-1 staining in nasal polyps, tissues in which extensive eosinophilia is seen.[32]

Ultimately, direct proof of adhesion molecule involvement in inflammation of allergic and other diseases will require studies employing specific adhesion molecule antagonists.[201, 529, 566, 570] Although no data have been reported for allergic diseases in humans, humanized antibodies to ICAM-1, CD18, VLA-4, and perhaps others are now available and have been or will be used in other types of clinical trials.[200, 240, 295, 475] These efforts have been motivated in large part by the success in animal studies. Blocking monoclonal antibodies have been infused in vivo in a variety of animal models of allergic and other inflammatory conditions of the lung and skin (Table 15–5).[2, 98, 126, 133, 186, 187, 202, 221–223, 293, 330, 332, 354–362, 408, 413, 433, 445, 461, 471, 536, 565, 568, 569, 583, 587] From several of these studies, however, it became evident that blockade of adhesion molecules might not prevent cell influx yet still have clinical benefit. Examples of this include studies in monkey and sheep models of asthma. In monkeys, antibodies against leukocyte CD11b were given systematically, and the antigen-induced rise in airway responsiveness was inhibited, even though the number of eosinophils recovered by bronchoalveolar lavage was unaffected.[567] Interestingly, eosinophil peroxidase activity in the bronchoalveolar lavage fluids was reduced by antibody treatment, suggesting an effect of the antibody on eosinophil activation and degranulation rather than on recruitment per se. A study using a sheep model also found efficacy of a VLA-4 antibody in preventing late-phase changes in airway function without any significant effect on leukocyte recruitment as assessed by bronchoalveolar lavage.[7] Thus antibodies to cell adhesion molecules may affect cell functions as well as trafficking. Many novel pharmaceutical approaches are being tried in an attempt to prevent cell recruitment responses, and results from additional studies in humans should be forthcoming.[201, 555, 570] Only then will we truly be able to functionally define the role of adhesion molecules and cytokines in human allergic diseases, including rhinitis and asthma.

REFERENCES

1. Abbassi O, Kishimoto TK, Mcintire LV, et al: E-selectin supports neutrophil rolling in vitro under conditions of flow. J Clin Invest 92:2719, 1993.
2. Abraham WM, Sielczak MW, Ahmed A, et al: α_4-integrins mediate antigen-induced late bronchial responses and prolonged airway hyperresponsiveness in sheep. J Clin Invest 93:776, 1994.
3. Adams DH, Shaw S: Leucocyte-endothelial interactions and regulation of leucocyte migration. Lancet 343:831, 1994.
4. Airas L, Salmi M, Jalkanen S: Lymphocyte-vascular adhesion protein-2 is a novel 70-kDa molecule involved in lymphocyte adhesion to vascular endothelium. J Immunol 151:4228, 1993.
5. Alam R, Stafford S, Forsythe P, et al: RANTES is a chemotactic and activating factor for human eosinophils. J Immunol 150:3442, 1993.

5a. Alam R, Forsythe P, Stafford S, et al: Monocyte chemotactic protein-2, monocyte chemotactic protein-3, and fibroblast-induced cytokine—three new chemokines induce chemotaxis and activation of basophils. J Immunol 153:3155, 1994.

6. Albelda SM, Buck CA: Integrins and other cell adhesion molecules. FASEB J 4:2868, 1990.
7. Albelda SM, Daise M, Levine EM, et al: Identification and characterization of cell-substratum adhesion receptors on cultured human endothelial cells. J Clin Invest 83:1992, 1989.
8. Albelda SM, Elias JA, Levine EM, et al: Endotoxin stimulates platelet-derived growth factor production from cultured human pulmonary endothelial cells. Am J Physiol 257:L65, 1989.

Albelda SM, Muller WA, Buck CA, et al: Molecular and cellular properties of PECAM-1 (endoCAM/CD31): a novel vascular cell-cell adhesion molecule. J Cell Biol 114:1059, 1991.

10. Albelda SM, Smith CW, Ward PA: Adhesion molecules and inflammatory injury. FASEB J 8:504, 1994.
11. Allison F, Smith MR, Wood WB: Studies on the pathogenesis of acute inflammation. I. The inflammatory reaction to thermal injury as observed in the rabbit ear chamber. J Exp Med 102:655, 1955.
12. Alon R, Kassner PD, Carr MW, et al: The integrin VLA-4 supports tethering and rolling in flow on VCAM-1. J Cell Biol 128:1243, 1995.
13. Altieri DC: Occupancy of CD11b/CD18 (Mac-1) divalent ion binding site(s) induces leukocyte adhesion. J Immunol 147:1891, 1991.
14. Altman LC, Ayars GH, Baker C, et al: Cytokines and eosinophil-derived cationic proteins upregulate intercellular adhesion molecule-1 on human nasal epithelial cells. J Allergy Clin Immunol 92:527, 1993.
15. Anderson DC, Schmalstieg FC, Finegold MJ, et al: The severe and moderate phenotypes of heritable Mac-1, LFA-1, p150,95 deficiency: their quantitative definition and relation to leukocyte dysfunction and clinical features. J Infect Dis 152:668, 1985.
16. Anderson DC, Springer TA: Leukocyte adhesion deficiency: an inherited defect in the Mac-1, LFA-1, and p150,95 glycoproteins. Annu Rev Med 38:175, 1987.
17. Andrew DP, Berlin C, Honda S, et al: Distinct but overlapping epitopes are involved in $\alpha 4\beta 7$-mediated adhesion to vascular cell adhesion molecule-1, mucosal addressin-1, fibronectin, and lymphocyte aggregation. J Immunol 153:3847, 1994.
18. Anwar ARE, Walsh GM, Cromwell O, et al: Adhesion to fibronectin primes eosinophils via alpha(4)/beta(1) (VLA-4). Immunology 82:222, 1994.
19. Anwar ARF, Moqbel R, Walsh GM, et al: Adhesion to fibronectin prolongs eosinophil survival. J Exp Med 177:839, 1993.
20. Arbones ML, Ord DC, Ley K, et al: Lymphocyte homing and leukocyte rolling and migration are impaired in L-selectin–deficient mice. Immunity 1:247, 1994.
21. Arnaout MA: Structure and function of the leukocyte adhesion molecules CD11/CD18. Blood 75:1037, 1990.
22. Arroyo AG, Sanchez-Mateos P, Campanero MR, et al: Regulation of the VLA integrin ligand interactions through the $\beta 1$ subunit. J Cell Biol 117:659, 1992.
23. Aruffo A, Kolanus W, Walz G, et al: CD62/P-selectin recognition of myeloid and tumor cell sulfatides. Cell 67:35, 1991.
24. Azizkhan RG, Azizkham JC, Zetter BR, et al: Mast cell heparin stimulates migration of capillary endothelial cells in vitro. J Exp Med 152:931, 1980.
25. Babi LFS, Moser R, Soler MTP, et al: Migration of skin-homing T cells across cytokine-activated human endothelial cell layers involves interaction of the cutaneous lymphocyte-associated antigen (CLA), the very late antigen-4 (VLA-4), and the lymphocyte function-associated antigen-1 (LFA-1). J Immunol 154:1543, 1995.
26. Baenziger NL, Fogerty FJ, Mertz LF, et al: Regulation of histamine-mediated prostacyclin synthesis in cultured human vascular endothelial cells. Cell 24:915, 1981.
27. Bagby GC Jr, Dinarello CA, Wallace P, et al: Interleukin 1 stimulates granulocyte macrophage colony-stimulating activity release by vascular endothelial cells. J Clin Invest 78:1316, 1986.
28. Bargatze RF, Kurk S, Butcher EC, et al: Neutrophils roll on adherent neutrophils bound to cytokine-induced endothelial cells via L-selectin on the rolling cells. J Exp Med 180:1785, 1994.
29. Baroody FM, Lee B-J, Lim MC, et al: Implicating adhesion molecules in nasal allergic inflammation. Eur Arch Otorhinolaryngol 252(Suppl 1):S50, 1995.
30. Baumhueter S, Singer MS, Henzel W, et al: Binding of L-selectin to the vascular sialomucin CD34. Science 262:436, 1993.
31. Beck L, Bickel C, Sterbinsky S, et al: Injection of human subjects with RANTES causes dermal infiltration of eosinophils (EOS) and mononuclear cells (MNC). FASEB J 9:A804, 1995.
32. Beck LA, Schall TJ, Beall LD, et al: Detection of the chemokine RANTES and activation of vascular endothelium in nasal polyps. J Allergy Clin Immunol 93:A234, 1994.
33. Bentley AM, Durham SR, Robinson DS, et al: Expression of endothelial and leukocyte adhesion molecules intercellular adhesion molecule-1, E-selectin, and vascular cell adhesion molecule-1 in the bronchial mucosa in steady-state and allergen-induced asthma. J Allergy Clin Immunol 92:857, 1993.
34. Berg EL, Magnani J, Warnock RA, et al: Comparison of L-selectin and E-selectin ligand specificities—the L-selectin can bind the E-selectin

ligands sialyl Le^x and sialyl Le^a. Biochem Biophys Res Commun 184:1048, 1992.
35. Berg EL, McEvoy LM, Berlin C, et al: L-selectin–mediated lymphocyte rolling on MAdCAM- 1. Nature 366:695, 1993.
36. Berg EL, Robinson MK, Mansson O, et al: A carbohydrate domain common to both sialyl Le^a and sialyl Le^x is recognized by the endothelial cell leukocyte adhesion molecule ELAM-1. J Biol Chem 266:14869, 1991.
37. Berg EL, Robinson MK, Warnock RA, et al: The human peripheral lymph node vascular addressin is a ligand for LECAM-1, the peripheral lymph node homing receptor. J Cell Biol 114:343, 1991.
38. Berg EL, Yoshino T, Rott LS, et al: The cutaneous lymphocyte antigen is a skin lymphocyte homing receptor for the vascular lectin endothelial cell-leukocyte adhesion molecule-1. J Exp Med 174:1461, 1991.
39. Berg M, James SP: Human neutrophils release the Leu-8 lymph node homing receptor during cell activation. Blood 76:2381, 1990.
40. Bergelson JM, Chan BMC, Finberg RW, et al: The integrin VLA-2 binds echovirus 1 and extracellular matrix ligands by different mechanisms. J Clin Invest 92:232, 1993.
41. Bergelson JM, Shepley MP, Chan BMC, et al: Identification of the integrin VLA-2 as a receptor for echovirus-1. Science 255:1718, 1992.
42. Berlin C, Berg EL, Briskin MJ, et al: $\alpha 4\beta 7$ integrin mediates lymphocyte binding to the mucosal vascular addressin MAdCAM-1. Cell 74:185, 1993.
43. Berman ME, Muller WA: Ligation of platelet endothelial cell adhesion molecule 1 (PECAM-1/CD31) on monocytes and neutrophils increases binding capacity of leukocyte CR3 (CD11b/CD18). J Immunol 154:299, 1995.
44. Bevilacqua MP: Endothelial-leukocyte adhesion molecules. Annu Rev Immunol 11:767, 1993.
45. Bevilacqua MP, Nelson RM: Selectins. J Clin Invest 91:379, 1993.
46. Bevilacqua MP, Pober JS, Mendrick DL, et al: Identification of an inducible endothelial-leukocyte adhesion molecule. Proc Natl Acad Sci USA 84:9238, 1987.
47. Bevilacqua MP, Pober JS, Wheeler ME, et al: Interleukin 1 acts on cultured human vascular endothelium to increase the adhesion of polymorphonuclear leukocytes, monocytes, and related leukocytic cell lines. J Clin Invest 76:2003, 1985.
48. Bevilacqua MP, Stengelin S, Gimbrone MA Jr, et al: Endothelial leukocyte adhesion molecule 1: an inducible receptor for neutrophils related to complement regulatory proteins and lectins. Science 243:1160, 1989.
49. Bilsland CAG, Diamond MS, Springer TA: The leukocyte integrin p150,95 (CD11C/CD18) as a receptor for iC3b—activation by a heterologous beta subunit and localization of a ligand recognition site to the I domain. J Immunol 152:4582, 1994.
49a. Bischoff SC, Krieger M, Brunner T, et al: RANTES and related chemokines activate human basophil granulocytes through different G-protein–coupled receptors. Eur J Immunol 23:761, 1993.
50. Blom M, Tool ATJ, Kok PTM, et al: Granulocyte-macrophage colony-stimulating factor, interleukin-3 (IL-3), and IL-5 greatly enhance the interaction of human eosinophils with opsonized particles by changing the affinity of complement receptor type 3. Blood 83:2978, 1994.
51. Bochner BS: Basophils. In Frank MM, Austen KF, Claman HN, Unanue ER (eds): Samter's Immunological Diseases, 5th edition. Little, Brown, and Company, Boston, 1994, p 259.
52. Bochner BS, Charlesworth EN, Lichtenstein LM, et al: Interleukin-1 is released at sites of human cutaneous allergic reactions. J Allergy Clin Immunol 86:830, 1990.
53. Bochner BS, Georas SN, Ebisawa M, et al: The role of adhesion molecules in allergic inflammation. In Melillo G, O'Byrne PM, Marone G (eds): Respiratory Allergy—Advances in Clinical Immunology and Pulmonary Medicine. Excerpta Medica, Amsterdam, 1993, p 3.
54. Bochner BS, Klunk D, Sterbinsky SA, et al: Phenotyping of cultured human umbilical vein endothelial cells using the blind panel of monoclonal antibodies. In Schlossman S, Boumsell L, Gilks W, et al (eds): Leukocyte Typing V: White Cell Differentiation Antigens. Oxford University Press, Oxford, 1995, p 1773.
55. Bochner BS, Klunk DA, Sterbinsky SA, et al: Interleukin-13 selectively induces vascular cell adhesion molecule-1 (VCAM-1) expression in human endothelial cells. J Immunol 154:799, 1995.
56. Bochner BS, Lamas AM, Benenati SV, et al: On the central role of vascular endothelium in allergic reactions. In Dorsch R (ed): Late Phase Allergic Reactions. CRC Press, Boca Raton, 1990, p 221.
57. Bochner BS, Luscinskas FW, Gimbrone MA Jr, et al: Adhesion of human basophils, eosinophils, and neutrophils to IL-1-activated human vascular endothelial cells: contributions of endothelial cell adhesion molecules. J Exp Med 173:1553, 1991.
58. Bochner BS, MacGlashan DW Jr, Marcotte GV, et al: IgE-dependent regulation of human basophil adherence to vascular endothelium. J Immunol 142:3180, 1989.
59. Bochner BS, McKelvey AA, Sterbinsky SA, et al: Interleukin-3 augments adhesiveness for endothelium and CD11b expression in human basophils but not neutrophils. J Immunol 145:1832, 1990.
60. Bochner BS, Newman W, McIntyre BW, et al: Counter-receptors for endothelial cell adhesion molecules on human eosinophils and basophils. FASEB J 6:A1435, 1992.
61. Bochner BS, Peachell PT, Brown KE, et al: Adherence of human basophils to cultured umbilical vein vascular endothelial cells. J Clin Invest 81:1355, 1988.
62. Bochner BS, Schleimer RP: The role of adhesion molecules in human eosinophil and basophil recruitment. J Allergy Clin Immunol 94: 427, 1994.
63. Bochner BS, Sterbinsky SA: Altered surface expression of CD11 and Leu-8 during human basophil degranulation. J Immunol 146:2367, 1991.
64. Bochner BS, Sterbinsky SA, Bickel CA, et al: Differences between human eosinophils and neutrophils in the function and expression of sialic acid-containing counterligands for E-selectin. J Immunol 152:774, 1994.
65. Bochner BS, Sterbinsky SA, Knol EF, et al: Function and expression of adhesion molecules on human basophils. J Allergy Clin Immunol 94:1157, 1994.
66. Bochner BS, Newman W, McIntyre BW, et al: Counter-receptors for endothelial cell adhesion molecules on human eosinophils and basophils. FASEB J 6:A1435, 1992.
67. Bochner BS, Undem BJ, Lichtenstein LM: Immunological aspects of allergic asthma. Annu Rev Immunol 12:295, 1994.
68. Bonfanti R, Furie BC, Furie B, et al: PADGEM is a component of Weibel-Palade bodies in endothelial cells. Blood 73:1109, 1989.
69. Borish L, Mascali JJ, Rosenwasser LJ: IgE-dependent cytokine production by human peripheral blood mononuclear phagocytes. J Immunol 146:63, 1991.
70. Bowen BR, Nguyen T, Lasky LA: Characterization of a human homologue of the murine peripheral lymph node homing receptor. J Cell Biol 109:421, 1989.
71. Bradding P, Feather IH, Howarth PH, et al: Interleukin-4 is localized to and released by human mast cells. J Exp Med 176:1381, 1992.
72. Briscoe D, Cotran R, Pober J: Effects of TNF, LPS, and IL-4 on the expression of VCAM-1 in vivo: correlation with CD3+ T cell infiltration. J Immunol 149:2954, 1992.
73. Briskin MJ, McEvoy LM, Butcher EC: MAdCAM-1 has homology to immunoglobulin and mucin-like adhesion receptors and to IgA1. Nature 363:461, 1993.
74. Brizzi MF, Garbarino G, Rossi PR, et al: Interleukin 3 stimulates proliferation and triggers endothelial-leukocyte adhesion molecule 1 gene activation of human endothelial cells. J Clin Invest 91:2887, 1993.
75. Broudy VC, Kaushansky K, Harlan JM, et al: Interleukin 1 stimulates human endothelial cells to produce granulocyte-macrophage colony-stimulating factor and granulocyte colony-stimulating factor. J Immunol 139:464, 1987.
76. Brunner T, Heusser C, Dahinden C: Human peripheral blood basophils primed by interleukin 3 produce IL-4 in response to immunoglobulin E receptor stimulation. J Exp Med 177:605, 1993.
77. Bullard DC, Qin L, Quinlin WM, et al: P-selectin/ICAM-1 double mutant mice: acute emigration of neutrophils into the peritoneum is completely absent but is normal into pulmonary alveoli. J Clin Invest 95:1782, 1995.
78. Burd PR, Thompson WC, Max EE, et al: Activated mast cells produce interleukin-13. J Exp Med 181:1373, 1995.
79. Bussolino F, Breviario F, Tetta C, et al: Interleukin-1 stimulates platelet-activating factor production in cultured human endothelial cells. J Clin Invest 77:2027, 1986.
80. Bussolino F, Wang JM, Defilippi P, et al: Granulocyte–and granulocyte-macrophage–colony stimulating factors induce human endothelial cells to migrate and proliferate. Nature 337:471, 1989.
81. Bussolino F, Ziche M, Wang JM, et al: In vitro and in vivo activation of endothelial cells by colony-stimulating factors. J Clin Invest 87:986, 1991.

82. Butcher EC: Cellular and molecular mechanisms that direct leukocyte traffic. Am J Pathol 136:3, 1990.
83. Butcher EC: Leukocyte-endothelial cell recognition: three (or more) steps to specificity and diversity. Cell 67:1033, 1991.
84. Buttrum SM, Hatton R, Nash GB: Selectin-mediated rolling of neutrophils on immobilized platelets. Blood 82:1165, 1993.
85. Buyon JP, Slade SG, Reibman J, et al: Constitutive and induced phosphorylation of the α- and β-chains of the CD11/CD18 leukocyte integrin family. J Immunol 144:191, 1990.
86. Camerini D, James SP, Stamenkovic I, et al: Leu-8/TQ1 is the human equivalent of the Mel-14 lymph node homing receptor. Nature 342:78, 1989.
87. Camussi G, Aglietta M, Malavasi F, et al: The release of platelet-activating factor from human endothelial cells in culture. J Immunol 131:2397, 1983.
88. Canonica GW, Ciprandi G, Buscaglia S, et al: Adhesion molecules of allergic inflammation—recent insights into their functional roles. Allergy 49:135, 1994.
89. Carlos TM, Harlan JM: Leukocyte-endothelial adhesion molecules. Blood 84:2068, 1994.
90. Casale TB, Erger RA, Little MM: Platelet-activating factor-induced human eosinophil transendothelial migration—evidence for a dynamic role of the endothelium. Am J Respir Cell Mol Biol 8:77, 1993.
91. Cepek KL, Parker CM, Madara JL, et al: Integrin α^E-β7 mediates adhesion of T-lymphocytes to epithelial cells. J Immunol 150:3459, 1993.
92. Cepek KL, Shaw SK, Parker CM, et al: Adhesion between epithelial cells and T lymphocytes mediated by E-cadherin and the $\alpha^E\beta7$ integrin. Nature 372:190, 1994.
93. Chan BM, Kassner PD, Schiro JA, et al: Distinct cellular functions mediated by different VLA integrin alpha-subunit cytoplasmic domains. Cell 68:1051, 1992.
94. Chan BMC, Elices MJ, Murphy E, et al: Adhesion to vascular cell adhesion molecule-1 and fibronectin—comparison of α4β1 (VLA-4) and α4β7 on the human B-cell line JY. J Biol Chem 267:8366, 1992.
95. Chan BMC, Hemler ME: Multiple functional forms of the integrin VLA-2 can be derived from a single alpha(2) cDNA clone—interconversion of forms induced by an anti-beta(1) antibody. J Cell Biol 120:537, 1993.
96. Chatila TA, Geha RS, Arnaout MA: Constitutive and stimulus-induced phosphorylation of CD11/CD18 leukocyte adhesion molecules. J Cell Biol 109:3435, 1989.
97. Chen K-R, Pittelkow MR, Su WPD, et al: Recurrent cutaneous necrotizing eosinophilic vasculitis: a novel eosinophil mediated syndrome. Arch Dermatol 130:1159, 1994.
98. Chisholm PL, Williams CA, Lobb RR: Monoclonal antibodies to the integrin α-4 subunit inhibit the murine contact hypersensitivity response. Eur J Immunol 23:682, 1993.
99. Chu W, Presky DH, Swerlick RA, et al: Alternatively processed human E-selectin transcripts linked to chronic expression of E-selectin in vivo. J Immunol 153:4179, 1994.
100. Chuluyan HE, Issekutz AC: VLA-4 integrin can mediate CD11/CD18-independent transendothelial migration of human monocytes. J Clin Invest 92:2768, 1993.
101. Cid MC, Esparza J, Juan M, et al: Signaling through CD50 (ICAM-3) stimulates T lymphocyte binding to human umbilical vein endothelial cells and extracellular matrix proteins via an increase in β1 and β2 integrin function. Eur J Immunol 24:1377, 1994.
102. Ciprandi G, Buscaglia S, Pesce G, et al: Allergic subjects express ICAM-1 on epithelial cells of conjunctiva after antigen challenge. J Allergy Clin Immunol 91:3783, 1993.
103. Ciprandi G, Pronzato C, Ricca V, et al: Evidence of intercellular adhesion molecule-1 expression on nasal epithelial cells in acute rhinoconjunctivitis caused by pollen exposure. J Allergy Clin Immunol 94:738, 1994.
104. Cohnheim J: Inflammation Lectures in General Pathology. New Sydenham Society, London, 1889, p 242.
105. Coller BS: A new murine monoclonal antibody reports an activation-dependent change in the conformation and/or microenvironment of the platelet glycoprotein IIb/IIIa complex. J Clin Invest 76:101, 1985.
106. Collins T, Kapman AJ, Wake CT, et al: Immune interferon activates multiple class II major histocompatibility complex genes and the associated invariant chain gene in human endothelial cells and dermal fibroblasts. Proc Natl Acad Sci USA 81:4917, 1984.
107. Colombatti A, Bonaldo P: The superfamily of proteins with von Willebrand factor type A-like domains: one theme common to components of extracellular matrix, hemostasis, cellular adhesion and defense mechanisms. Blood 77:2305, 1991.
108. Columbo M, Bochner BS, Marone G: Human skin mast cells express functional β1 integrins that mediate adhesion to extracellular matrix proteins. J Immunol 154:6058, 1995.
109. Conforti G, Dominguez-Jimenez C, Zanetti A, et al: Human endothelial cells express integrin receptors on the luminal aspect of their membrane. Blood 80:437, 1992.
110. Cooper D, Butcher CM, Berndt MC, et al: P-selectin interacts with a β2-integrin to enhance phagocytosis. J Immunol 153:3199, 1994.
111. Cotran RS, Gimbrone MA Jr, Bevilacqua MP, et al: Induction and detection of a human endothelial activation antigen in vivo. J Exp Med 164:661, 1986.
112. Cybulsky MI, Fries JWU, Williams AJ, et al: Alternative splicing of human VCAM-1 in activated vascular endothelium. Am J Pathol 138:815, 1991.
113. Cybulsky MI, Fries JWU, Williams AJ, et al: Gene structure, chromosomal location, and basis for alternative messenger RNA splicing of the human VCAM-1 gene. Proc Natl Acad Sci USA 88:7859, 1991.
113a. Dahinden CA, Geiser T, Brunner T, et al: Monocyte chemotactic protein 3 is a most effective basophil- and eosinophil-activating chemokine. J Exp Med 179:751, 1994.
114. Damle NK, Klussman K, Aruffo A: Intercellular adhesion molecule-2, a second counter-receptor for CD11a/CD18 (leukocyte function-associated antigen-1), provides a costimulatory signal for T-cell receptor-initiated activation of human T-cells. J Immunol 148:665, 1992.
115. Damle NK, Klussman K, Dietsch MT, et al: GMP-140 (P-selectin/CD62) binds to chronically stimulated but not resting CD4+ T-lymphocytes and regulates their production of proinflammatory cytokines. Eur J Immunol 22:1789, 1992.
116. Dastych J, Costa JJ, Thompson HL, et al: Mast cell adhesion to fibronectin. Immunology 73:478, 1991.
117. Davies PF, Robotewskyj A, Griem ML: Endothelial cell adhesion in real time—measurements in vitro by tandem scanning confocal image analysis. J Clin Invest 91:2640, 1993.
118. de Fougerolles AR, Klickstein LB, Springer TA: Cloning and expression of intercellular adhesion molecule 3 reveals strong homology to other immunoglobulin family counter-receptors for lymphocyte function-associated antigen 1. J Exp Med 177:1187, 1993.
119. de Fougerolles AR, Springer TA: Intercellular adhesion molecule 3, a third adhesion counter-receptor for lymphocyte function-associated molecule 1 on resting lymphocytes. J Exp Med 175:185, 1992.
120. de Fougerolles AR, Stacker SA, Schwarting R, et al: Characterization of ICAM-2 and evidence for a third counter-receptor for LFA-1. J Exp Med 174:253, 1991.
121. Deisher TA, Haddix TL, Montgomery KF, et al: The role of protein kinase-C in the induction of VCAM-1 expression on human umbilical vein endothelial cells. FEBS Lett 331:285, 1993.
122. del Pozo MA, Pulido R, Munoz C, et al: Regulation of ICAM-3 (CD50) membrane expression on human neutrophils through a proteolytic shedding mechanism. Eur J Immunol 24:2586, 1994.
123. Del Vecchio PJ, Smith JR: Expression of angiotensin-converting enzyme activity in cultured pulmonary artery endothelial cells. J Cell Physiol 108:337, 1981.
124. DeLisser HM, Newman PJ, Albelda SM: Molecular and functional aspects of PECAM-1/CD31. Immunol Today 15:490, 1994.
125. Delneste Y, Lassalle P, Jeannin P, et al: Histamine induces IL-6 production by human endothelial cells. Clin Exp Immunol 98:344, 1994.
126. Denis M, Bisson D: Blockade of leukocyte function-associated antigen (LFA-1) in a murine model of lung inflammation. Am J Respir Cell Mol Biol 10:481, 1994.
127. Diamond MS, Garcia-Aguilar J, Bickford JK, et al: The I domain is a major recognition site on the leukocyte integrin Mac-1 (CD11b/CD18) for four distinct adhesion ligands. J Cell Biol 120:1031, 1993.
128. Diamond MS, Springer TA: The dynamic regulation of integrin adhesiveness. Curr Biol 4:506, 1994.
129. Diamond MS, Staunton DE, de Fougerolles AR, et al: ICAM-1 (CD54): a counter-receptor for Mac-1 (CD11b/CD18). J Cell Biol 111:3129, 1990.
130. Dixit VM, Green S, Sarma V, et al: Tumor necrosis factor-a induction of novel gene products in human endothelial cells including a macrophage-specific chemotaxin. J Biol Chem 265:2973, 1990.
131. Dobrina A, Menegazzi R, Carlos TM, et al: Mechanisms of eosinophil adherence to cultured vascular endothelial cells: eosinophils bind to

the cytokine-induced endothelial ligand vascular cell adhesion molecule-1 via the very late activation antigen-4 integrin receptor. J Clin Invest 88:20, 1991.
132. Dobrina A, Schwartz BR, Carlos TM, et al: CD11/CD18-independent neutrophil adherence to inducible endothelial-leukocyte adhesion molecules (E-LAM) in vitro. Immunology 67:502, 1989.
133. Doerschuk CM, Winn RK, Coxson HO, et al: CD18-dependent and -independent mechanisms of neutrophil emigration in the pulmonary and systemic microcirculation of rabbits. J Immunol 144:2327, 1990.
134. Dore M, Korthuis RJ, Granger DN, et al: P-selectin mediates spontaneous leukocyte rolling in vivo. Blood 82:1308, 1993.
135. Dransfield I, Cabanas C, Craig A, et al: Divalent cation regulation of the function of the leukocyte integrin LFA-1. J Cell Biol 116:219, 1992.
136. Dri P, Cramer R, Spessotto P, et al: Eosinophil activation on biological surfaces. Production of O_2^- in response to physiologic soluble stimuli is differentially modulated by extracellular matrix components and endothelial cells. J Immunol 147:613, 1991.
137. Drickamer K: Two distinct classes of carbohydrate-recognition domains of animal lectin. J Biol Chem 263:9557, 1988.
138. Dunlop LC, Skinner MP, Bendall LJ, et al: Characterization of GMP-140 (P-selectin) as a circulating plasma protein. J Exp Med 175: 1147, 1992.
139. Dunn CJ, Fleming WE: Increased adhesion of polymorphonuclear leukocytes to vascular endothelium by specific interaction of endogenous (interleukin-1) and exogenous (lipopolysaccharide) substances with endothelial cells "in vitro." Eur J Rheumatol Inflamm 7:80, 1984.
140. Durham SR, Ying S, Varney VA, et al: Cytokine messenger RNA expression for IL-3, IL-4, IL-5, and granulocyte-macrophage colony-stimulating factor in the nasal mucosa after local allergen provocation—relationship to tissue eosinophilia. J Immunol 148: 2390, 1992.
141. Dustin M, Staunton D, Springer T: Supergene families meet in the immune system. Immunol Today 9:213, 1988.
142. Dustin ML, Rothlein R, Bhan AK, et al: Induction by IL 1 and interferon-γ: tissue distribution, biochemistry, and function of a natural adherence molecule (ICAM-1). J Immunol 137:245, 1986.
143. Ebisawa M, Bochner BS, Georas SN, et al: Eosinophil transendothelial migration induced by cytokines. I. Role of endothelial and eosinophil adhesion molecules in IL-1β-induced transendothelial migration. J Immunol 149:4021, 1992.
144. Ebisawa M, Liu MC, Yamada T, et al: Eosinophil transendothelial migration induced by cytokines II. The potentiation of eosinophil transendothelial migration by eosinophil-active cytokines. J Immunol 152:4590, 1994.
145. Ebisawa M, Schleimer RP, Bickel C, et al: Phenotyping of purified human peripheral blood eosinophils using the blind panel of monoclonal antibodies. In Schlossman S, Boumsell L, Gilks W, et al (eds): Leukocyte Typing V: White Cell Differentiation Antigens. Oxford University Press, Oxford, 1995, p 1036.
146. Ebisawa M, Shichijo M, Miura K, et al: Human mast cells produce TNF-α, MIP-1α and IL-5 following activation through FcεRI. J Allergy Clin Immunol 95:219, 1995.
147. Ebisawa M, Yamada T, Bickel C, et al: Eosinophil transendothelial migration induced by cytokines III. Effect of the chemokine RANTES. J Immunol 153:2153, 1994.
148. Ebisawa M, Yamada T, Klunk D, et al: Regulation of eosinophil and neutrophil transendothelial migration by cytokines and chemokines. J Allergy Clin Immunol 91:691, 1993.
149. Egesten A, Gukkberg U, Olsson I, et al: Phorbol ester-induced degranulation in adherent human eosinophil granulocytes is dependent on CD11/CD18 leukocyte integrins. J Leukoc Biol 53:287, 1993.
150. Elices MJ, Osborn L, Takada Y, et al: VCAM-1 on activated endothelium interacts with the leukocyte integrin VLA-4 at a site distinct from the VLA-4/fibronectin binding site. Cell 60:577, 1990.
151. Erbe DV, Watson SR, Presta LG, et al: P-selectin and E-selectin use common sites for carbohydrate ligand recognition and cell adhesion. J Cell Biol 120:1227, 1993.
152. Erbe DV, Wolitzky BA, Presta LG, et al: Identification of an E-selectin region critical for carbohydrate recognition and cell adhesion. J Cell Biol 215, 1992.
153. Erle DJ, Briskin MJ, Butcher EC, et al: Expression and function of the MAdCAM-1 receptor, integrin alpha 4 beta 7, on human leukocytes. J Immunol 153:517, 1994.
154. Etzioni A, Frydman M, Pollack S, et al: Brief report—recurrent severe infections caused by a novel leukocyte adhesion deficiency. N Engl J Med 327:1789, 1992.
155. Fawcett J, Buckley C, Holness CL, et al: Mapping the homotypic binding sites in CD31 and the role of CD31 adhesion in the formation of interendothelial cell contacts. J Cell Biol 128:1229, 1995.
156. Fawcett J, Holness CLL, Needham LA, et al: Molecular cloning of ICAM-3, a third ligand for LFA-1, constitutively expressed on resting leukocytes. Nature 360:481, 1992.
157. Fleming JC, Pahl HL, Gonzalez DA, et al: Structural analysis of the CD11b gene and phylogenetic analysis of the alpha-integrin gene family demonstrate remarkable conservation of genomic organization and suggest early diversification during evolution. J Immunol 150:480, 1993.
158. Fleming WE, Dunn CJ: Interleukin-1 and lipopolysaccharide stimulate delayed PMN-leukocyte adhesion via direct interaction with vascular endothelial cells. Fed Proc 44:1260, 1985.
159. Foreman KE, Vaporciyan AA, Bonish BK, et al: C5a-induced expression of P-selectin in endothelial cells. J Clin Invest 94:1147, 1994.
160. Foxall C, Watson SR, Dowbenko D, et al: The three members of the selectin receptor family recognize a common carbohydrate epitope, the sialyl Lewis oligosaccharide. J Cell Biol 117:895, 1992.
161. Furie MB, Burns MJ, Tancinco MCA, et al: E-selectin (endothelial-leukocyte adhesion molecule-1) is not required for the migration of neutrophils across IL-1-stimulated endothelium in vitro. J Immunol 148:2395, 1992.
162. Gallatin WM, Weissman IL, Butcher EC: A cell-surface molecule involved in organ-specific homing of lymphocytes. Nature 304:30, 1983.
163. Galli SJ: New concepts about the mast cell. N Engl J Med 328:257, 1993.
164. Gamble JR, Khew-Goodall Y, Vadas MA: Transforming growth factor-β inhibits E-selectin expression on human endothelial cells. J Immunol 150:4494, 1993.
165. Gamble JR, Vadas MA: Endothelial adhesiveness for blood neutrophils is inhibited by transforming growth factor-β. Science 242:97, 1988.
166. Garcia JGN, Schaphorst KL: Regulation of endothelial cell gap formation and paracellular permeability. J Invest Med 43:117, 1995.
167. Geng JG, Bevilacqua MP, Moore KL, et al: Rapid neutrophil adhesion to activated endothelium mediated by GMP-140. Nature 343:757, 1990.
168. Geoffroy JS, Rosen SD: Demonstration that a lectin-like receptor ($gp90^{MEL}$) directly mediates adhesion of lymphocytes to high endothelial venules of lymph nodes. J Cell Biol 109:2463, 1989.
169. Georas SN, Liu MC, Newman W, et al: Altered adhesion molecule expression and endothelial activation accompany the recruitment of human granulocytes to the lung following segmental antigen challenge. Am J Respir Cell Mol Biol 7:261, 1992.
170. Georas SN, McIntyre BW, Ebisawa M, et al: Expression of a functional laminin receptor (α6β1, VLA-6) on human eosinophils. Blood 82:2872, 1993.
171. Gimbrone MA Jr: Culture of vascular endothelium. Prog Hematol Thromb 3:1, 1976.
172. Gimbrone MA Jr, Obin MS, Brock AF, et al: Endothelial interleukin-8: a novel inhibitor of leukocyte-endothelial interactions. Science 246:1601, 1989.
173. Goelz SE, Hession C, Goff D, et al: ELFT: a gene that directs the expression of an ELAM-1 ligand. Cell 63:1349, 1990.
174. Goldring K, Lavens SE, Warner JA: Clustering of β1 integrins modifies mediator release from human lung mast cells and basophils: role of actin polymerization. FASEB J 8:A238, 1994.
175. Goldring K, Lavens SE, Warner JA: The effect of RGD and CS-1 peptides on integrin induced histamine release from human basophils. FASEB J 9:A224, 1985.
176. Gordon JR, Galli SJ: Mast cells as a source of both preformed and immunologically inducible TNF-α/cachectin. Nature 346:274, 1990.
177. Graber N, Gopal TV, Wilson D, et al: T cells bind to cytokine-activated endothelial cells via a novel, inducible sialoglycoprotein and endothelial leukocyte adhesion molecule-1. J Immunol 145:819, 1990.
178. Granger DN, Kubes P: The microcirculation and inflammation: modulation of leukocyte-endothelial adhesion. J Leukoc Biol 55:662, 1994.
179. Graves BJ, Crowther RL, Chandran C, et al: Insight into E-selectin/ligand interaction from the crystal structure and mutagenesis of the lec/EGF domains. Nature 367:532, 1994.
180. Green PJ, Tamatani T, Watanabe T, et al: High affinity binding of the leukocyte adhesion molecule L-selectin to 3′-sulphated–Le^a and–Le^x oligosaccharides and the predominance of sulphate in this interaction

demonstrated by binding studies with a series of lipid-linked oligosaccharides. Biochem Biophys Res Commun 188:244, 1992.
181. Greeno EW, Mantyh P, Vercellotti GM, et al: Functional neurokinin 1 receptors for substance P are expressed by human vascular endothelium. J Exp Med 177:1269, 1993.
182. Greve JM, Davis G, Meyer AM, et al: The major human rhinovirus receptor is ICAM-1. Cell 56:839, 1989.
183. Griffin JD, Spertini O, Ernst TJ, et al: Granulocyte-macrophage colony-stimulating factor and other cytokines regulate surface expression of the leukocyte adhesion molecule-1 on human neutrophils, monocytes, and their precursors. J Immunol 145:576, 1990.
184. Groves RW, Allen MH, Ross EL, et al: Tumour necrosis factor alpha is pro-inflammatory in normal human skin and modulates cutaneous adhesion molecule expression. Br J Dermatol 132:345, 1995.
185. Groves RW, Ross E, Barker JNWN, et al: Effect of in vivo interleukin-1 on adhesion molecule expression in normal human skin. J Invest Dermatol 98:384, 1992.
186. Gundel RH, Wegner CD, Torcellini CA, et al: Endothelial leukocyte adhesion molecule-1 mediates antigen-induced acute airway inflammation and late-phase airway obstruction in monkeys. J Clin Invest 88:1407, 1991.
187. Gundel RH, Wegner CD, Torcellini CA, et al: The role of intercellular adhesion molecule-1 in chronic airway inflammation. Clin Exp Allergy 22:569, 1992.
188. Guo CB, Kagey-Sobotka A, Lichtenstein LM, et al: Immunophenotyping and functional analysis of human uterine mast cells. Blood 79:708, 1992.
189. Gurtner GC, Davis V, McCoy MJ, et al: Targeted disruption of murine VCAM1 gene reveals a critical role in fusion of the allantois to the chorion, placental and umbilical cord formation. Genes Dev 9:1, 1995.
190. Hakansson L, Nielsen LS, Teder P: Measurement of neutrophil and eosinophil adhesion to E-selectin, VCAM-1, and ICAM-1 by the use of transfected fibroblast cell lines. J Immunol Methods 176:53, 1994.
191. Hakkert BC, Kuijpers TW, Leeuwenberg JFM, et al: Neutrophil and monocyte adherence to and migration across monolayers of cytokine-activated endothelial cells: the contribution of CD18, ELAM-1, and VLA-4. Blood 78:2721, 1991.
192. Hakomori S, Anderson M: Novel endothelial cell activation factor(s) released from activated platelets which induce E- selectin expression and tumor cell adhesion to endothelial cells: a preliminary note. Biochem Biophys Res Commun 203:1605, 1994.
193. Hamid Q, Azzawi M, Ying S, et al: Expression of mRNA for interleukin-5 in mucosal bronchial biopsies from asthma. J Clin Invest 87:1541, 1991.
194. Handa K, Nudelman ED, Stroud MR, et al: Selectin GMP-140 (CD62; PADGEM) binds to sialosyl-Le^a and sialosyl-Le^x, and sulfated glycans modulate this binding. Biochem Biophys Res Commun 181:1223, 1991.
195. Hansel TT, Braunstein JB, Walker C, et al: Sputum eosinophils from asthmatics express ICAM-1 and HLA-DR. Clin Exp Immunol 86:271, 1991.
196. Hansel TT, Walker C: The migration of eosinophils into the sputum of asthmatics: the role of adhesion molecules. Clin Exp Allergy 22:345, 1992.
197. Harlan JM: Leukocyte adhesion deficiency syndrome—insights into the molecular basis of leukocyte emigration. Clin Immunol Immunopathol 67:S16, 1993.
198. Hartnell A, Kay AB, Wardlaw AJ: Interleukin-3-induced up-regulation of CR3 expression on human eosinophils is inhibited by dexamethasone. Immunology 77:488, 1992.
199. Hattori R, Hamilton KK, Fugate RD, et al: Stimulated secretion of endothelial von Willebrand factor is accompanied by rapid redistribution to the cell surface of the intracellular granule membrane protein GMP-140. J Biol Chem 264:7768, 1989.
200. Haug CE, Colvin RB, Delmonico FL, et al: A phase-I trial of immunosuppression with anti–ICAM-1 (CD54) mAb in renal allograft recipients. Transplantation 55:766, 1993.
201. Hellewell PG: Cell adhesion molecules and potential for pharmacological intervention in lung inflammation. Pulm Pharmacol 6:109, 1993.
202. Hellewell PG, Young SK, Henson PM, et al: Disparate role of the β-integrin CD18 in the local accumulation of neutrophils in pulmonary and cutaneous inflammation in the rabbit. Am J Respir Cell Mol Biol 10:391, 1994.
203. Hemler ME: VLA proteins in the integrin family: structures, functions, and their role on leukocytes. Annu Rev Immunol 8:365, 1990.
204. Hemler ME, Elices MJ, Parker C, et al: Structure of the integrin VLA-4 and its cell-cell and cell-matrix adhesion functions. Immunol Rev 114:45, 1990.
205. Henocq E, Vargaftig BB: Accumulation of eosinophils in response to intracutaneous PAF-acether and allergen in man. Lancet 2:1378, 1986.
206. Hermanowski-Vosatka A, Strijp JAGV, Swiggard WJ, et al: Integrin modulating factor-1: a lipid that alters the function of leukocyte integrins. Cell 68:341, 1992.
207. Hession C, Tizard R, Vassallo C, et al: Cloning of an alternative form of vascular cell adhesion molecule-1 (VCAM-1). J Biol Chem 266:6682, 1991.
208. Hibbs ML, Jakes S, Stacker SA, et al: The cytoplasmic domain of the integrin lymphocyte function-associated antigen-1 beta-subunit—sites required for binding to intercellular adhesion molecule-1 and the phorbol ester stimulated phosphorylation site. J Exp Med 174:1227, 1991.
209. Hibbs ML, Xu H, Stacker SA, et al: Regulation of adhesion to ICAM-1 by the cytoplasmic domain of LFA-1 integrin beta-subunit. Science 251:1611, 1991.
210. Hogg N, Harvey J, Cabanas C, et al: Control of leukocyte integrin activation. Am Rev Respir Dis 148:S55, 1993.
211. Honda S, Campbell JJ, Andrew DP, et al: Ligand-induced adhesion to activated endothelium and to vascular cell adhesion molecule-1 in lymphocytes transfected with *N*-formyl peptide receptor. J Immunol 152:4026, 1994.
212. Horie S, Kita H: CD11b/CD19 (Mac-1) is required for degranulation of human eosinophils induced by human recombinant granulocyte-macrophage colony-stimulating factor and platelet-activating factor. J Immunol 152:5457, 1994.
213. Hormia M, Lehto VP, Virtanen I: Intracellular localization of factor VIII-related antigen and fibronectin in cultured human endothelial cells: evidence for divergent routes of intracellular translocation. Eur J Cell Biol 33:217, 1984.
214. Huang SK, Xiao HQ, Kleine-Tebbe J, et al: Interleukin-13 expression at the sites of allergen challenge in allergic asthmatics. J Allergy Clin Immunol 95:385, 1995.
215. Huber AR, Kunkel SL, Todd RF III, et al: Regulation of transendothelial neutrophil migration by endogenous interleukin-8. Science 254:99, 1991.
216. Huber AR, Weiss SJ: Disruption of the subendothelial basement membrane during neutrophil diapedesis in an in vitro construct of a blood vessel wall. J Clin Invest 83:1122, 1989.
217. Hynes RO: Integrins: a family of cell surface receptors. Cell 48:549, 1987.
218. Hynes RO: Integrins: versatility, modulation, and signaling in cell adhesion. Cell 69:11, 1992.
219. Iademarco MF, Barks JL, Dean DC: Regulation of vascular cell adhesion molecule-1 expression by IL-4 and TNF-alpha in cultured endothelial cells. J Clin Invest 95:264, 1995.
220. Imai Y, Lasky LA, Rosen SD: Sulphation requirement for GlyCAM-1, an endothelial ligand for L-selectin. Nature 361:555, 1993.
221. Issekutz TB: Dual inhibition of VLA-4 and LFA-1 maximally inhibits cutaneous delayed-type hypersensitivity-induced inflammation. Am J Pathol 143:1286, 1993.
222. Issekutz TB: Inhibition of in vivo lymphocyte migration to inflammation and homing to lymphoid tissues by the TA-2 monoclonal antibody—a likely role for VLA-4 in vivo. J Immunol 147:4178, 1991.
223. Issekutz TB: Inhibition of lymphocyte endothelial adhesion and in vivo lymphocyte migration to cutaneous inflammation by TA-3, a new monoclonal antibody to rat LFA-1. J Immunol 149:3394, 1992.
224. Jaffe EA, Nachman RL, Becker CG, et al: Culture of human endothelial cells derived from umbilical veins. Identification by morphologic and immunologic criteria. J Clin Invest 52:2745, 1973.
225. Johnsen ULH, Jyberg T, Galdal KS, et al: Platelets stimulate thromboplastin synthesis in human endothelial cells. Thromb Haemost 49:69, 1983.
226. Johnston GI, Bliss GA, Newman PJ, et al: Structure of the human gene encoding granule membrane protein-140, a member of the selectin family of adhesion receptors for leukocytes. J Biol Chem 265:21381, 1990.
227. Johnston GI, Cook RG, McEver RP: Cloning of GMP-140, a granule membrane protein of platelets and endothelium: sequence similarity to proteins involved in cell adhesion and inflammation. Cell 56:1033, 1989.
228. Jones DA, Mcintire LV, Smith CW, et al: A two-step adhesion cascade

for T cell endothelial cell interactions under flow conditions. J Clin Invest 94:2443, 1994.

228a. Jose PJ, Griffiths-Johnson DA, Collins PD, et al: Eotaxin: a potent eosinophil chemoattractant cytokine detected in a guinea pig model of allergic airways inflammation. J Exp Med 179:881, 1994.

229. Juan M, Vilella R, Mila J, et al: CDw50 and ICAM-3—two names for the same molecule. Eur J Immunol 23:1508, 1993.

230. Juan M, Vinas O, Pinootin MR, et al: CD50 (intercellular adhesion molecule 3) stimulation induces calcium mobilization and tyrosine phosphorylation through p59(fyn) and p56(lck) in Jurkat T cell line. J Exp Med 179:1747, 1994.

231. Jung TM, Dailey MO: Rapid modulation of homing receptors (gpMEL-14) induced by activators of protein kinase C. Receptor shedding due to accelerated proteolytic cleavage at the cell surface. J Immunol 144:3130, 1990.

232. Jutila MA, Rott L, Berg EL, et al: Function and regulation of the neutrophil MEL-14 antigen in vivo: comparison with LFA-1 and MAC-1. J Immunol 143:3318, 1989.

233. Jutila MA, Watts G, Walcheck B, et al: Characterization of a functionally important and evolutionarily well-conserved epitope mapped to the short consensus repeats of E-selectin and L-selectin. J Exp Med 175:1565, 1992.

234. Kaiser J, Bickel C, Bochner BS, et al: The effects of the potent glucocorticoid budesonide on adhesion of eosinophils to human vascular endothelium and on endothelial expression of adhesion molecules. J Pharmacol Exp Ther 267:245, 1993.

235. Kameyoshi Y, Dorschner A, Mallet AI, et al: Cytokine RANTES released by thrombin-stimulated platelets is a potent attractant for human eosinophils. J Exp Med 176:587, 1992.

236. Kanof ME, James SP: Leu-8 antigen expression is diminished during cell activation but does not correlate with effector function of activated T lymphocytes. J Immunol 140:3701, 1988.

237. Kansas GS, Ley K, Munro JM, et al: Regulation of leukocyte rolling and adhesion to high endothelial venules through the cytoplasmic domain of L-selectin. J Exp Med 177:833, 1993.

238. Kansas GS, Spertini O, Stoolman LM, et al: Molecular mapping of functional domains of the leukocyte receptor for endothelium, LAM-1. J Cell Biol 114:351, 1991.

239. Kassner PD, Hemler ME: Interchangeable α chain cytoplasmic domains play a positive role in control of cell adhesion mediated by VLA-4, a β1 integrin. J Exp Med 178:649, 1993.

240. Kavanaugh AF, Davis LS, Nichols LA, et al: Treatment of refractory rheumatoid arthritis with a monoclonal antibody to intercellular adhesion molecule 1. Arthritis Rheum 37:992, 1994.

241. Kay AB, Ying S, Varney SR, et al: Messenger RNA expression of the cytokine gene cluster, interleukin-3 (IL-3), IL-4, IL-5, and granulocyte/macrophage colony-stimulating factor, in allergen-induced late-phase cutaneous reactions in atopic subjects. J Exp Med 173:775, 1991.

242. Kessler DA, Langer RS, Pless NA, et al: Mast cells and tumor angiogenesis. Int J Cancer 18:703, 1976.

243. Killackey JJF, Johnston MG, Movat HZ: Increased permeability of microcarrier-cultured endothelial monolayers in response to histamine and thrombin. Am J Pathol 122:50, 1986.

244. Kim M-K, Brandley BK, Anderson MB, et al: Antagonism of human neutrophil (NEU) and eosinphil (EOS) adhesion by oligosaccharide compounds. J Allergy Clin Immunol 95:220, 1995.

245. Kinashi T, Springer TA: Adhesion molecules in hematopoietic cells. Blood Cells 20:25, 1994.

246. Kinashi T, St Pierre Y, Springer TA: Expression of glycophosphatidylinositol-anchored and –non-anchored isoforms of vascular cell adhesion molecule 1 in murine stromal and endothelial cells. J Leukoc Biol 57:168, 1995.

247. Kishimoto TK, Anderson DC: The role of integrins in inflammation. In Gallin JI, Goldstein IM, Snyderman R (eds): Inflammation: Basic Principles and Clinical Correlates. Raven Press, New York, 1992, p 353.

248. Kishimoto TK, Jutila MA, Berg EL, et al: Neutrophil Mac-1 and MEL-14 adhesion proteins inversely regulated by chemotactic factors. Science 245:1238, 1989.

249. Kishimoto TK, Jutila MA, Butcher EC: Identification of a human peripheral lymph node homing receptor: a rapidly down-regulated adhesion molecule. Proc Natl Acad Sci USA 87:2244, 1990.

250. Kishimoto TK, Larson RS, Corbi AL, et al: The leukocyte integrins. Adv Immunol 46:149, 1989.

251. Kishimoto TK, Warnock RA, Jutila MA, et al: Antibodies against human neutrophil LECAM-1 (LAM-1/Leu-8/DREG-56 antigen) and endothelial cell ELAM-1 inhibit a common CD18-independent adhesion pathway in vitro. Blood 78:805, 1991.

252. Klein LM, Lavker RM, Matis WL, et al: Degranulation of human mast cells induces an endothelial antigen central to leukocyte adhesion. Proc Natl Acad Sci USA 86:8972, 1989.

253. Knol EF, Tackey F, Tedder TF, et al: Comparison of human eosinophil and neutrophil adhesion to endothelial cells under non-static conditions: the role of L-selectin. J Immunol 153:2161, 1994.

254. Koch AE, Harlow LA, Haines GK, et al: Vascular endothelial growth factor. A cytokine modulating endothelial function in rheumatoid arthritis. J Immunol 152:4149, 1994.

255. Kojima N, Handa K, Newman W, et al: Multi-recognition capability of E-selectin in a dynamic flow system, as evidenced by differential effects of sialidases and anti-carbohydrate antibodies on selectin-mediated cell adhesion at low vs. high wall shear stress: a preliminary note. Biochem Biophys Res Commun 189:1686, 1992.

256. Koszdin KL, Bowen BR: The cloning and expression of a human alpha-1,3 fucosyltransferase capable of forming the E-selectin ligand. Biochem Biophys Res Commun 187:152, 1992.

257. Kovach NL, Carlos TM, Yee E, et al: A monoclonal antibody to β1 integrin (CD29) stimulates VLA-dependent adherence of leukocytes to human umbilical vein endothelial cells and matrix components. J Cell Biol 116:499, 1992.

258. Kovach NL, Lin N, Yednock T, et al: Stem cell factor modulates avidity of α4β1 and α5β1 integrins expressed on hematopoietic cell lines. Blood 85:159, 1995.

259. Kroegel C, Liu MC, Hubbard WM, et al: Blood and bronchoalveolar eosinophils in allergic subjects following segmental antigen challenge: surface phenotype , density heterogeneity, and prostanoid production. J Allergy Clin Immunol 93:725, 1994.

260. Kubes P, Kanwar S: Histamine induces leukocyte rolling in post-capillary venules: a P-selectin–mediated event. J Immunol 152:3570, 1994.

261. Kuijpers TW: Terminal glycosyltransferase activity—a selective role in cell adhesion. Blood 81:873, 1993.

262. Kuijpers TW, Hakket BC, Hoogerwerf M, et al: The role of endothelial leukocyte adhesion molecule-1 (ELAM-1) and platelet-activating factor (PAF) in neutrophil adherence to IL-1–prestimulated endothelial cells: ELAM-1–mediated CD18 activation. J Immunol 147:1369, 1991.

263. Kuijpers TW, Hoogerwerf M, Vanderlaan LJW, et al: CD66 nonspecific cross-reacting antigens are involved in neutrophil adherence to cytokine-activated endothelial cells. J Cell Biol 118:457, 1992.

264. Kuijpers TW, Mul EPJ, Blom M, et al: Freezing adhesion molecules in a state of high-avidity binding blocks eosinophil migration. J Exp Med 178:279, 1993.

265. Kuijpers TW, Raleigh M, Kavanagh T, et al: Cytokine-activated endothelial cells internalize E-selectin into a lysosomal compartment of vesiculotubular shape. J Immunol 152:5060, 1994.

266. Kyan-Aung U, Haskard DO, Poston RN, et al: Endothelial leukocyte adhesion molecule-1 and intercellular adhesion molecule-1 mediate the adhesion of eosinophils to endothelial cells in vitro and are expressed by endothelium in allergic cutaneous inflammation in vivo. J Immunol 146:521, 1991.

267. Labow MA, Norton CR, Rumberger JM, et al: Characterization of E-selectin–deficient mice: demonstration of overlapping function of the endothelial selectins. Immunity 1:709, 1994.

268. Lamas AM, Leon OG, Schleimer RP: Glucocorticoids inhibit eosinophil responses to granulocyte-macrophage colony-stimulating factor. J Immunol 147:254, 1991.

269. Lamas AM, Marcotte GV, Schleimer RP: Human endothelial cells prolong eosinophil survival. Regulation by cytokines and glucocorticoids. J Immunol 142:3978, 1989.

270. Lamas AM, Mulroney CR, Schleimer RP: Studies on the adhesive interaction between human eosinophils and cultured vascular endothelial cells. J Immunol 140:1500, 1988.

271. Landis RC, Bennett RI, Hogg N: A novel LFA-1 activation epitope maps to the I domain. J Cell Biol 120:1519, 1993.

272. Lang WE: Secretion of plasminogen activators by cultured bovine endothelial cells: partial purification, characterization, and evidence for multiple forms. Thromb Haemost 45:219, 1981.

273. Languino LR, Plescia J, Duperray A, et al: Fibrinogen mediates leukocyte adhesion to vascular endothelium through an ICAM-1–dependent pathway. Cell 73:1423, 1993.

274. Larsen GR, Sako D, Ahern TJ, et al: P-selectin and E-selectin. Distinct

but overlapping leukocyte ligand specificities. J Biol Chem 267: 11104, 1992.
275. Lasky LA: Selectins—interpreters of cell-specific carbohydrate information during inflammation. Science 258:964, 1992.
276. Lasky LA, Rosen SD: The selectins—carbohydrate-binding adhesion molecules of the immune system. In Gallin JI, Goldstein IM, Snyderman R (eds): Inflammation: Basic Principles and Clinical Correlates. Raven Press, New York, 1992, p 407.
277. Lasky LA, Singer MS, Dowbenko D, et al: An endothelial ligand for L-selectin is a novel mucin-like molecule. Cell 69:927, 1992.
278. Lavens SE, Goldring K, Warner JA: Clustering of β1 integrins modulates histamine release in human basophils: the role of tyrosine kinases. FASEB J 8:A238, 1994.
279. Lawrence MB, Springer TA: Leukocytes roll on a selectin at physiologic flow rates: distinction from and prerequisite for adhesion through integrins. Cell 65:859, 1991.
280. Lawrence MB, Springer TA: Neutrophils roll on E-selectin. J Immunol 151:6338, 1993.
281. Lazaar AL, Albelda SM, Pilewski JM, et al: T lymphocytes adhere to airway smooth muscle cells via integrins and CD44 and induce smooth muscle cell DNA synthesis. J Exp Med 180:807, 1994.
282. Lee B-J, Naclerio RM, Bochner BS, et al: Nasal challenge with allergen upregulates the local expression of vascular endothelial adhesion molecules. J Allergy Clin Immunol 94:1006, 1994.
283. Leeuwenberg JFM, Smeets EF, Neefjes JJ, et al: E-selectin and intercellular adhesion molecule-1 are released by activated human endothelial cells in vitro. Immunology 77:543, 1992.
284. Leeuwenberg JFM, von Asmuth EJU, Jeunhomme TMAA, et al: IFN-γ-regulates the expression of the adhesion molecule ELAM-1 and IL-6 production by human endothelial cells in vitro. J Immunol 145:2110, 1990.
285. Leff AR, Hamann KJ, Wegner CD: Inflammation and cell-cell interactions in airway hyperresponsiveness. Am J Physiol 260:L189, 1991.
286. Lesley JR, Hyman R, Kincade PW: CD44 and its interaction with ECM. Adv Immunol 54:271, 1993.
287. Leung DYM, Pober JS, Cotran RS: Expression of endothelial-leukocyte adhesion molecule-1 in elicited late phase allergic reactions. J Clin Invest 87:1805, 1991.
288. Lewinsohn DM, Bargatze RF, Butcher EC: Leukocyte-endothelial cell recognition: evidence of a common molecular mechanism shared by neutrophils, lymphocytes, and other leukocytes. J Immunol 138:4313, 1987.
289. Ley K, Bullard DC, Arbones ML, et al: Sequential contribution of L- and P-selectin to leukocyte rolling in vivo. J Exp Med 181:669, 1995.
290. Ley K, Gaehtgens P, Fennie C, et al: Lectin-like cell adhesion molecule-1 mediates leukocyte rolling in mesenteric venules in vivo. Blood 77:2553, 1991.
291. Li R, Nortamo P, Valmu L, et al: A peptide from ICAM-2 binds to the leukocyte integrin CD11a/CD18 and inhibits endothelial cell adhesion. J Biol Chem 268:17513, 1993.
292. Lichtenstein LM, Bochner BS: The role of basophils in asthma. Ann N Y Acad Sci 629:48, 1991.
293. Lo SK, Everitt J, Gu J, et al: Tumor necrosis factor mediates experimental pulmonary edema by ICAM-1 and CD18-dependent mechanisms. J Clin Invest 89:981, 1992.
294. Lo SK, Lee S, Ramos RA, et al: Endothelial-leukocyte adhesion molecule-1 stimulates the adhesive activity of leukocyte integrin CR3 (CD11b/CD18, Mac-1, $\alpha_m\beta_2$) on human neutrophils. J Exp Med 173:1493, 1991.
295. Lobb RR, Hemler ME: The pathophysiologic role of α4 integrins in vivo. J Clin Invest 94:1722, 1994.
296. Lopez AF, Williamson DJ, Gamble JR, et al: Recombinant human granulocyte-macrophage colony-stimulating factor stimulates in vitro mature human neutrophil and eosinophil function, surface receptor expression, and survival. J Clin Invest 78:1220, 1986.
297. Lorant DE, Patel KD, Mcintyre TM, et al: Coexpression of GMP-140 and PAF by endothelium stimulated by histamine or thrombin—a juxtacrine system for adhesion and activation of neutrophils. J Cell Biol 115:223, 1991.
298. Lorant DE, Topham MK, Whatley RE, et al: Inflammatory roles of P-selectin. J Clin Invest 92:559, 1993.
299. Lowe JB: Specificity and expression of carbohydrate ligands. In Wegner CD (ed): Adhesion Molecules. Academic Press, London, 1994, p 113.
300. Lowe JB, Stoolman LM, Nair RP, et al: ELAM-1 dependent cell adhesion to vascular endothelium determined by a transfected human fucosyltransferase cDNA. Cell 63:475, 1990.
301. Lukacs NW, Strieter RM, Chensue SW, et al: Interleukin-4-dependent pulmonary eosinophil infiltration in a murine model of asthma. Am J Respir Cell Mol Biol 10:526, 1994.
302. Lund-Johansen F, Olweus J, Horejsi V, et al: Activation of human phagocytes through carbohydrate antigens (CD15, SIALYL-CD15, CDw17, and CDw65). J Immunol 148:3221, 1992.
303. Lundahl J, Hallden G, Hed J: Differences in intracellular pool and receptor-dependent mobilization of the adhesion-promoting glycoprotein Mac-1 between eosinophils and neutrophils. J Leukoc Biol 53:336, 1993.
304. Luscinskas FW, Cybulsky MI, Kiely J-M, et al: Cytokine-activated human endothelial monolayers support enhanced neutrophil transmigration via a mechanism involving both endothelial-leukocyte adhesion molecule-1 and intracellular adhesion molecule-1. J Immunol 146:1617, 1991.
305. Luscinskas FW, Ding H, Lichtman AH: P-selectin and vascular cell adhesion molecule 1 mediate rolling and arrest, respectively, of CD4+ T lymphocytes on tumor necrosis factor alpha-activated vascular endothelium under flow. J Exp Med 181:1179, 1995.
306. Luscinskas FW, Kansas GS, Ding H, et al: Monocyte rolling, arrest and spreading on IL-4–activated vascular endothelium under flow is mediated via sequential action of L-selectin, β1-integrins, and β2-integrins. J Cell Biol 125:1417, 1994.
307. Luscinskas FW, Lawler J: Integrins as dynamic regulators of vascular function. FASEB J 8:929, 1994.
308. Luster AD, Unkeless JC, Ravetch JV: γ-interferon transcriptionally regulates an early-response gene containing homology to platelet proteins. Nature 315:672, 1985.
309. MacGlashan D, White JM, Huang SK, et al: Secretion of IL-4 from human basophils—the relationship between IL-4 mRNA and protein in resting and stimulated basophils. J Immunol 152:3006, 1994.
310. Magnani JL: The tumor markers, sialyl Le[a] and sialyl Le[x] bind ELAM-1. Glycobiology 1:318, 1991.
311. Majuri ML, Mattila P, Renkonen R: Recombinant E-selectin–protein mediates tumor cell adhesion via sialyl-Le[a] and sialyl-Le[x]. Biochem Biophys Res Commun 182:1376, 1992.
312. Majuri ML, Pinola M, Niemela R, et al: α2,3-sialyl and α1,3-fucosyltransferase-dependent synthesis of sialyl Lewis X, an essential oligosaccharide present on L-selectin counterreceptors, in cultured endothelial cells. Eur J Immunol 24:3205, 1994.
313. Mantovani A, Bussolino F, Dejana E: Cytokine regulation of endothelial cell function. FASEB J 6:2591, 1992.
314. Marfaing-Koka A, Devergne O, Gorgone G, et al: Regulation of the production of the RANTES chemokine by endothelial cells—synergistic induction by IFN-γ plus TNF-α and inhibition by IL-4 and IL-13. J Immunol 154:1870, 1995.
315. Marlin SD, Springer TA: Purified intercellular adhesion molecule-1 (ICAM-1) is a ligand for lymphocyte function-associated antigen-1 (LFA-1). Cell 51:813, 1987.
316. Masinovsky B, Urdal D, Gallatin WM: IL-4 acts synergistically with IL-1β to promote lymphocyte adhesion to microvascular endothelium by induction of vascular cell adhesion molecule-1. J Immunol 145:2886, 1990.
317. Massey W, Friedman B, Kato M, et al: Appearance of IL-3 and GM-CSF activity at allergen-challenged cutaneous late-phase reaction sites. J Immunol 150:1084, 1993.
318. Masumoto A, Hemler ME: Multiple activation states of VLA-4. Mechanistic differences between adhesion of CS1/fibronectin and to vascular cell adhesion molecule-1. J Biol Chem 268:228, 1993.
319. Matis WL, Lavker RM, Murphy GF: Substance P induces the expression of an endothelial-leukocyte adhesion molecule by microvascular endothelium. J Invest Dermatol 94:492, 1990.
320. Matsumoto K, Schleimer RP, Bochner BS: Distinct regulation of α4 integrin binding to fibronectin and VCAM-1 in eosinophils and Jurkat cells. J Allergy Clin Immunol 95:338, 1995.
321. Matsumoto K, Zhou D, Schleimer RP, et al: Tyrphostin reduces α4 integrin function in human eosinophils and Jurkat cells. FASEB J 9:A226, 1995.
322. Mayadas TN, Johnson RC, Rayburn H, et al: Leukocyte rolling and extravasation are severely compromised in P selectin-deficient mice. Cell 74:541, 1993.
323. McEver RP, Beckstead JH, Moore KL, et al: GMP-140, a platelet α-granule membrane protein, is also synthesized by vascular endothelial

cells and is localized in Weibel-Palade bodies. J Clin Invest 84:92, 1989.
324. McIntyre TM, Zimmerman GA, Prescott SM: Leukotrienes C_4 and D_4 stimulate human endothelial cells to synthesize platelet-activating factor and bind neutrophils. Proc Natl Acad Sci USA 83:2204, 1986.
325. McIntyre TM, Zimmerman GA, Satoh K, et al: Cultured endothelial cells synthesize both platelet-activating factor and prostacyclin in response to histamine, bradykinin, and adenosine triphosphate. J Clin Invest 76:271, 1985.
326. Meacock S, Pescini-Gobert R, DeLamarter JF, et al: Transcription factor-induced, phased binding of the E-selectin promoter. J Biol Chem 269:31756, 1994.
327. Meerschaert J, Furie MB: Monocytes use either CD11/CD18 or VLA-4 to migrate across human endothelium in vitro. J Immunol 152:1915, 1994.
328. Mengelers HJJ, Maikoe T, Hooibrink B, et al: Down modulation of L-selectin expression on eosinophils recovered from bronchoalveolar lavage fluid after allergen provocation. Clin Exp Allergy 23:196, 1993.
329. Messadi DV, Pober JS, Fiers W, et al: Induction of an activation antigen on postcapillary venular endothelium in human skin organ culture. J Immunol 139:1557, 1987.
330. Metzger WJ, Ridger V, Tollefson V, et al: Anti-VLA-4 antibody and CS-1 peptide inhibitor modifies airway inflammation and bronchial airway hyperresponsiveness (BHR) in the allergic rabbit. J Allergy Clin Immunol 93:183, 1994.
331. Meurer R, Van Riper G, Feeney W, et al: Formation of eosinophilic and monocytic intradermal inflammatory sites in the dog by injection of human RANTES but not human monocyte chemoattractant protein 1, human macrophage inflammatory protein 1α, or human interleukin 8. J Exp Med 178:1913, 1993.
332. Milne AAY, Piper PJ: The effects of two anti-CD18 antibodies on antigen-induced airway hyperresponsiveness and leukocyte accumulation in the guinea pig. Am J Respir Cell Mol Biol 11:337, 1994.
333. Miura K, Ebisawa M, Shichijo M, et al: Adherence of human cord blood derived basophils to fibronectin. J Allergy Clin Immunol 95:293, 1995.
334. Montefort S, Feather IH, Wilson SJ, et al: The expression of leukocyte-endothelial adhesion molecules is increased in perennial allergic rhinitis. Am J Respir Cell Mol Biol 7:393, 1992.
335. Montefort S, Holgate ST: Adhesion molecules and their role in inflammation. Respir Med 85:91, 1991.
336. Montefort S, Holgate ST, Howarth PH: Leucocyte-endothelial adhesion molecules and their role in bronchial asthma and allergic rhinitis. Eur Respir J 6:1044, 1993.
337. Montefort S, Lai CKW, Kapahi P, et al: Circulating adhesion molecules in asthma. Am J Respir Crit Care Med 149:1149, 1994.
338. Montefort S, Roche WR, Howarth PH, et al: Intercellular adhesion molecule-1 (ICAM-1) and endothelial leukocyte adhesion molecule-1 (ELAM-1) expression in the bronchial mucosa of normal and asthmatic subjects. Eur Respir J 5:815, 1992.
339. Montgomery DF, Osborn L, Hession C, et al: Activation of endothelial-leukocyte adhesion molecule1 (ELAM-1) gene transcription. Proc Natl Acad Sci USA 88:6523, 1991.
340. Moore KL, Stults NL, Diaz S, et al: Identification of a specific glycoprotein ligand for P-selectin (CD62) on myeloid cells. J Cell Biol 118:445, 1992.
341. Moore KL, Thompson LF: P-selectin (CD62) binds to subpopulations of human memory lymphocytes-T and natural killer cells. Biochem Biophys Res Commun 186:173, 1992.
342. Moore KL, Varki A, McEver RP: GMP-140 binds to a glycoprotein receptor on human neutrophils: evidence for a lectin-like interaction. J Cell Biol 112:491, 1991.
343. Moqbel R, Hamid Q, Ying S, et al: Expression of messenger RNA and immunoreactivity for the granulocyte/macrophage colony-stimulating factor in activated human eosinophils. J Exp Med 174:749, 1991.
344. Moser R, Fehr J, Bruijnzeel PLB: IL-4 controls the selective endothelium-driven transmigration of eosinophils from allergic individuals. J Immunol 149:1432, 1992.
345. Moser R, Fehr J, Olgiati L, et al: Migration of primed human eosinophils across cytokine-activated endothelial cell monolayers. Blood 79:2937, 1992.
346. Moser R, Groscurth P, Carballido JM, et al: Interleukin-4 induces tissue eosinophilia in mice: correlation with its in vitro capacity to stimulate the endothelial cell–dependent selective transmigration of human eosinophils. J Lab Clin Med 122:567, 1993.
347. Moser R, Schleiffenbaum B, Groscurth P, et al: Interleukin 1 and tumor necrosis factor stimulate human vascular endothelial cells to promote transendothelial neutrophil passage. J Clin Invest 83:444, 1989.
348. Movat HZ. The Inflammatory Reaction. Elsevier, Amsterdam, 1985.
349. Moy JN, Thomas LL, Whisler LC: Eosinophil major basic protein enhances the expression of neutrophil CR3 and p150,95. J Allergy Clin Immunol 92:598, 1993.
350. Mueller R, Heusser CH, Rihs S, et al: Immunolocalization of intracellular interleukin-4 in normal human peripheral blood basophils. Eur J Immunol 24:2935, 1994.
351. Muller WA: The role of PECAM-1 (CD31) in leukocyte emigration: studies in vitro and in vivo. J Leukoc Biol 57:523, 1995.
352. Muller WA, Berman ME, Newman PJ, et al: A heterophilic adhesion mechanism for platelet/endothelial cell adhesion molecule 1 (CD31). J Exp Med 175:1401, 1992.
353. Muller WA, Weigl SA, Deng X, et al: PECAM-1 is required for transendothelial migration of leukocytes. J Exp Med 178:449, 1993.
354. Mulligan MS, Lowe JB, Larsen RD, et al: Protective effects of sialylated oligosaccharides in immune complex-induced acute lung injury. J Exp Med 178:623, 1993.
355. Mulligan MS, Miyasaka M, Tamatani T, et al: Requirements for L-selectin in neutrophil-mediated lung injury in rats. J Immunol 152:832, 1994.
356. Mulligan MS, Paulson JC, Defrees S, et al: Protective effects of oligosaccharides in P-selectin–dependent lung injury. Nature 364:149, 1993.
357. Mulligan MS, Polley MJ, Bayer RJ, et al: Neutrophil-dependent acute lung injury—requirement for P-selectin (GMP-140). J Clin Invest 90:1600, 1992.
358. Mulligan MS, Vaporciyan AA, Warner RL, et al: Compartmentalized roles for leukocytic adhesion molecules in lung inflammatory injury. J Immunol 154:1350, 1995.
359. Mulligan MS, Varani J, Dame MK, et al: Role of endothelial-leukocyte adhesion molecule 1 (ELAM-1) in neutrophil-mediated lung injury in rats. J Clin Invest 88:1396, 1991.
360. Mulligan MS, Watson SR, Fennie C, et al: Protective effects of selectin chimeras in neutrophil-mediated lung injury. J Immunol 151:6410, 1993.
361. Mulligan MS, Wilson GP, Todd RF, et al: Role of β1, β2 integrins and ICAM-1 in lung injury after deposition of IgG and IgA immune complexes. J Immunol 150:2407, 1993.
362. Nakajima H, Sano H, Nishimura T, et al: Role of vascular cell adhesion molecule-1/very late activation antigen-4 and intercellular adhesion molecule-1/lymphocyte function-associated antigen-1 interactions in antigen-induced eosinophil and T-cell recruitment into the tissue. J Exp Med 179:1145, 1994.
363. Natbony SF, Phillips ME, Elias JM, et al: Histologic studies of chronic idiopathic urticaria. J Allergy Clin Immunol 71:177, 1983.
364. Natsuka S, Gersten KM, Zenita K, et al: Molecular cloning of a cDNA encoding a novel human leukocyte α-1,3-fucosyltransferase capable of synthesizing the sialyl Lewis X determinant. J Biol Chem 269:16789, 1994.
365. Needham LK, Schnaar RL: The HNK-1 reactive sulfoglucuronyl glycolipids are ligands for L-selectin and P-selectin but not E-selectin. Proc Natl Acad Sci USA 90:1359, 1993.
366. Neeley SP, Hamann KJ, Dowling TL, et al: Augmentation of stimulated eosinophil degranulation by VLA-4 (CD49d)–mediated adhesion to fibronectin. Am J Respir Cell Mol Biol 11:206, 1994.
367. Neeley SP, Hamann KJ, White SR, et al: Selective regulation of expression of surface adhesion molecules Mac-1, L-selectin, and VLA-4 on human eosinophils and neutrophils. Am J Respir Cell Mol Biol 8:633, 1993.
368. Neish AS, Williams AJ, Palmer HJ, et al: Functional analysis of the human vascular cell adhesion molecule 1 promoter. J Exp Med 176:1583, 1992.
369. Nelson RM, Cecconi O, Roberts WG, et al: Heparin oligosaccharides bind L- and P-selectin and inhibit acute inflammation. Blood 82:3253, 1993.
370. Newman PJ, Berndt MC, Gorski J, et al: PECAM-1 (CD31) cloning and relation to adhesion molecules of the immunoglobulin gene superfamily. Science 247:1219, 1990.
371. Newman W, Beall LD, Carson CW, et al: Soluble E-selectin is found in supernatants of activated endothelial cells and is elevated in the serum of patients with septic shock. J Immunol 150:644, 1993.
372. Norgard KE, Moore KL, Diaz S, et al: Characterization of a specific

ligand for P-selectin on myeloid cells—a minor glycoprotein with sialylated O-linked oligosaccharides. J Biol Chem 268:12764, 1993.
373. Norgard-Sumnicht KE, Varki NM, Varki A: Calcium-dependent heparin-like ligands for L-selectin in nonlymphoid endothelial cells. Science 261:480, 1993.
374. Norioka K, Hara M, Harigai M, et al: Production of B cell stimulatory factor-2/interleukin-6 activity by human endothelial cells. Biochem Biophys Res Commun 153:1045, 1988.
375. Nortamo P, Li R, Renkonen R, et al: The expression of human intercellular adhesion molecule-2 is refractory to inflammatory cytokines. Eur J Immunol 21:2629, 1991.
376. Nortamo P, Salcedo R, Timonen T, et al: A monoclonal antibody to the human leukocyte adhesion molecule intercellular adhesion molecule-2—cellular distribution and molecular characterization of the antigen. J Immunol 146:2530, 1991.
376a. Noso N, Proost P, Van Damme J, et al: Human monocyte chemotactic proteins-2 and 3 (MCP-2 and MCP-3) attract human eosinophils and desensitize the chemotactic responses towards RANTES. Biochem Biophys Res Commun 200:1470, 1994.
377. O'Toole TE, Katagiri Y, Faull RJ, et al: Integrin cytoplasmic domains mediate inside-out signal transduction. J Cell Biol 124:1047, 1994.
378. Ohkawara Y, Yamauchi K, Maruyama N, et al: In situ expression of the cell adhesion molecules in bronchial tissues from asthmatics with air flow limitation: in vivo evidence of VCAM-1/VLA-4 interaction in selective eosinophil infiltration. Am J Respir Cell Mol Biol 12:4, 1995.
379. Ohmori K, Takada A, Ohwaki I, et al: A distinct type of sialyl Lewis X antigen defined by a novel monoclonal antibody is selectively expressed on helper memory T cells. Blood 82:2797, 1993.
380. Ohnishi T, Kita H, Mayeno A, et al: Eosinophil-active cytokines and an inhibitor of cytokine activity in the bronchoalveolar lavage fluids (BALF) of symptomatic patients with asthma. J Allergy Clin Immunol 89:214, 1992.
381. Ohnishi T, Kita H, Weiler D, et al: IL-5 is the predominant eosinophil-active cytokine in the antigen-induced pulmonary late-phase reaction. Am Rev Respir Dis 147:901, 1993.
382. Olofsson AM, Arfors KE, Ramezani L, et al: E-selectin mediates leukocyte rolling in interleukin-1–treated rabbit mesentery venules. Blood 84:2749, 1994.
383. Oppenheimer-Marks N, Davis LS, Bogue DT, et al: Differential utilization of ICAM-1 and VCAM-1 during the adhesion and transendothelial migration of human T lymphocytes. J Immunol 147:2913, 1991.
384. Osborn L, Hession C, Tizard R, et al: Direct expression cloning of vascular cell adhesion molecule 1, a cytokine-induced endothelial protein that binds to lymphocytes. Cell 59:1203, 1989.
385. Osborn L, Vassallo C, Benjamin CD: Activated endothelium binds lymphocytes through a novel binding site in the alternately spliced domain of vascular cell adhesion molecule-1. J Exp Med 176:99, 1992.
386. Pahl HL, Rosmarin AG, Tenen DG: Characterization of the myeloid-specific CD11b promoter. Blood 79:865, 1992.
387. Pahl HL, Scheibe RJ, Zhang DE, et al: The proto-oncogene PU.1 regulates expression of the myeloid-specific CD11b promoter. J Biol Chem 268:5014, 1993.
388. Palmer RMJ, Ashton DS, Moncada S: Vascular endothelial cells synthesize nitric acid from L-arginine. Nature 333:664, 1988.
389. Patel KD, Zimmerman GA, Prescott SM, et al: Oxygen radicals induce human endothelial cells to express GMP-140 and bind neutrophils. J Cell Biol 112:749, 1991.
390. Patel TP, Goelz SE, Lobb RR, et al: Isolation and characterization of natural protein-associated carbohydrate ligands for E-selectin. Biochemistry 33:14815, 1994.
391. Pepinsky B, Hession C, Chen LL, et al: Structure/function studies on vascular cell adhesion molecule-1. J Biol Chem 267:17820, 1992.
392. Phillips ML, Nudelman E, Gaeta FCA, et al: ELAM-1 mediates cell adhesion by recognition of a carbohydrate ligand, sialyl-Le^x. Science 250:1130, 1990.
393. Piali L, Albelda SM, Baldwin HS, et al: Murine platelet endothelial cell adhesion molecule (PECAM-1)/CD31 modulates β2 integrins on lymphokine-activated killer cells. Eur J Immunol 23:2464, 1993.
394. Picker LJ, Kishimoto TK, Smith CW, et al: ELAM-1 is an adhesion molecule for skin-homing T cells. Nature 349:796, 1991.
395. Picker LJ, Michie SA, Rott LS, et al: A unique phenotype of skin-associated lymphocytes in humans. Am J Pathol 136:1053, 1990.
396. Picker LJ, Terstappen LWWW, Rott LS, et al: Differential expression of homing-associated adhesion molecules by T cell subsets in man. J Immunol 145:3247, 1990.
397. Picker LJ, Warnock RA, Burns AR, et al: The neutrophil selectin LECAM-1 presents carbohydrate ligands to the vascular selectins ELAM-1 and GMP-140. Cell 66:921, 1991.
398. Pigott R, Dillon LP, Hemingway IH, et al: Soluble forms of E-selectin, ICAM-1 and VCAM-1 are present in the supernatants of cytokine-activated cultured endothelial cells. Biochem Biophys Res Commun 187:584, 1992.
399. Pigott R, Needham LA, Edwards RM, et al: Structural and functional studies of the endothelial activation antigen endothelial leucocyte adhesion molecule-1 using a panel of monoclonal antibodies. J Immunol 147:130, 1991.
400. Pinola M, Renkonen R, Majuri M-L, et al: Characterization of the E-selectin ligand on NK cells. J Immunol 152:3586, 1994.
401. Pober JS, Cotran RS: The role of endothelial cells in inflammation. Transplantation 50:537, 1990.
402. Pober JS, Gimbrone MA Jr, Lapierre LA, et al: Overlapping patterns of activation of human endothelial cells by interleukin 1, tumor necrosis factor, and immune interferon. J Immunol 137:1893, 1986.
403. Pober JS, Gimbrone J, Cotran RS, et al: Ia expression by vascular endothelium is inducible by activated T cells and by human gamma interferon. J Exp Med 157:1339, 1983.
404. Polte T, Newman W, Raghunathan G, et al: Structural and functional studies of full length vascular cell adhesion molecule-1: internal duplication and homology to several adhesion proteins. DNA Cell Biol 10:349, 1991.
405. Postigo AA, Marazuela M, Sanchez-Madrid F, et al: B lymphocyte binding to E- and P-selectins is mediated through the de novo expression of carbohydrates on in vitro and in vivo activated human B cells. J Clin Invest 94:1585, 1994.
406. Postigo AA, Sanchez-Mateos P, Lazarovits AI, et al: α4β7 integrin mediates B-cell binding to fibronectin and vascular cell adhesion molecule-1—expression and function of α4 integrins on human B-lymphocytes. J Immunol 151:2471, 1993.
407. Prescott SM, Zimmerman GA, McIntyre TM: Human endothelial cells in culture produce platelet-activating factor (1-alkyl-2-acetyl-sn-glycero-3-phosphocholine) when stimulated with thrombin. Proc Natl Acad Sci USA 81:3534, 1984.
408. Pretolani M, Ruffie C, Silva JRLE, et al: Antibody to very late activation antigen 4 prevents antigen-induced bronchial hyperreactivity and cellular infiltration in the guinea pig airways. J Exp Med 180:795, 1994.
409. Price TH, Ochs HD, Gershonibaruch R, et al: In vivo neutrophil and lymphocyte function studies in a patient with leukocyte adhesion deficiency type II. Blood 84:1635, 1994.
410. Pulido R, Elices MJ, Campanero MR, et al: Functional evidence for three distinct and independently inhibitable adhesion activities mediated by the human integrin VLA-4—correlation with distinct alpha4 epitopes. J Biol Chem 266:10241, 1991.
411. Ra CS, Yasuda M, Yagita H, et al: Fibronectin receptor integrins are involved in mast cell activation. J Allergy Clin Immunol 94:625, 1994.
412. Rabb H, Michishita M, Sharma CP, et al: Cytoplasmic tails of human complement receptor Type 3 (CR3, C11b/CD18) regulate ligand avidity and the internalization of occupied receptors. J Immunol 151:990, 1993.
413. Rabb HA, Olivenstein R, Issekutz TB, et al: The role of the leukocyte adhesion molecules VLA-4, LFA-1, and Mac-1 in allergic airway responses in the rat. Am J Respir Crit Care Med 149:1186, 1994.
414. Renkonen R, Paavonen T, Nortamo P, et al: Expression of endothelial adhesion molecules in vivo—increased endothelial ICAM-2 expression in lymphoid malignancies. Am J Pathol 140:763, 1992.
415. Resnick MB, Weller PF: Mechanisms of eosinophil recruitment. Am J Respir Cell Mol Biol 8:349, 1993.
416. Rice GE, Munro JM, Bevilacqua MP: Inducible cell adhesion molecule 110 (INCAM-110) is an endothelial receptor for lymphocytes. A CD11/CD18-independent adhesion mechanism. J Exp Med 171:1369, 1990.
417. Rice GE, Munro JM, Corless C, et al: Vascular and nonvascular expression of INCAM-110. Am J Pathol 138:385, 1991.
418. Robinson D, Hamid Q, Bentley A, et al: Activation of CD4+ T-cells, increased Th2-type cytokine messenger RNA expression, and eosinophil recruitment in bronchoalveolar lavage after allergen inhalation challenge in patients with atopic asthma. J Allergy Clin Immunol 92:313, 1993.
419. Robinson DS, Hamid Q, Ying S, et al: Predominant T_{H2}-like bronchoalveolar T-lymphocyte population in atopic asthma. N Engl J Med 326:298, 1992.

420. Rollins BJ, Pober JS: Interleukin-4 induces the synthesis and secretion of MCP-1/JE by human endothelial cells. Am J Pathol 138:1315, 1991.
421. Rosales C, Juliano RL: Signal transduction by cell adhesion receptors in leukocytes. J Leukoc Biol 57:189, 1995.
422. Rosen GD, Birkenmeier TM, Dean DC: Characterization of the alpha-4 integrin gene promoter. Proc Natl Acad Sci USA 88:4094, 1991.
423. Rosenman SJ, Shrikant P, Dubb L, et al: Cytokine-induced expression of vascular cell adhesion molecule-1 (VCAM-1) by astrocytes and astrocytoma cell lines. J Immunol 154:1888, 1995.
424. Rosmarin AG, Caprio D, Levy R, et al: CD18 (beta(2) leukocyte integrin) promoter requires PU.1 transcription factor for myeloid activity. Proc Natl Acad Sci USA 92:801, 1995.
425. Rosmarin AG, Levy R, Tenen DG: Cloning and analysis of the CD18 promoter. Blood 79:2598, 1992.
426. Rossi V, Breviario F, Ghezzi P, et al: Prostacyclin synthesis induced in vascular cells by interleukin-1. Science 229:174, 1985.
427. Rossiter H, van Reijsen F, Mudde GC, et al: Skin disease–related T cells bind to endothelial selectins—expression of cutaneous lymphocyte antigen (CLA) predicts E-selectin but not P-selectin binding. Eur J Immunol 24:205, 1994.
428. Rot A, Krieger M, Brunner T, et al: RANTES and macrophage inflammatory protein 1α induce the migration and activation of normal human eosinophil granulocytes. J Exp Med 176:1489, 1992.
429. Rothenberg ME, Owen WF Jr, Silberstein DS, et al: Eosinophils cocultured with endothelial cells have increased survival and functional properties. Science 237:645, 1987.
430. Rothlein R, Dustin ML, Marlin SD, et al: A human intercellular adhesion molecule (ICAM-1) distinct from LFA-1. J Immunol 137: 1270, 1986.
431. Ruegg C, Postigo AA, Sikorski EE, et al: Role of integrin α4β7/α4βP in lymphocyte adherence to fibronectin and VCAM-1 and in homotypic cell clustering. J Cell Biol 117:179, 1992.
432. Ruoslahti E: Integrins. J Clin Invest 87:1, 1991.
433. Rutter J, James TJ, Howat D, et al: The in vivo and in vitro effects of antibodies against rabbit β2-integrins. J Immunol 153:3724, 1994.
434. Ryan US:Endothelial Cells. Vol I. CRC Press, Inc, Boca Raton, 1988.
435. Ryan US:Endothelial Cells. Vol II. CRC Press, Inc, Boca Raton, 1988.
436. Ryan US:Endothelial Cells. Vol III. CRC Press, Inc, Boca Raton, 1988.
437. Ryan US, Schultz DR, Ryan JW: Fc and C3b receptors on pulmonary endothelial cells: induction by injury. Science 214:557, 1981.
438. Sako D, Chang X-J, Barone KM, et al: Expression cloning of a functional glycoprotein ligand for P-selectin. Cell 75:1179, 1993.
439. Salmi M, Jalkanen S: A 90-kilodalton endothelial cell molecule mediating lymphocyte binding in humans. Science 257:1407, 1992.
440. Salmi M, Kalimo K, Jalkanen S: Induction and function of vascular adhesion protein-1 at sites of inflammation. J Exp Med 178:2255, 1993.
441. Sanchez-Aparicio P, Ferreira OC, Garcia-Pardo A: 3508α4β1 recognition of the Hep-II domain of fibronectin is constitutive on some hemopoietic cells but requires activation on others. J Immunol 150:3506, 1993.
442. Sanz MJ, Weg VB, Bolanowski MA, et al: IL-1 is a potent inducer of eosinophil accumulation in rat skin—inhibition of response by a platelet-activating factor antagonist and an anti-human IL-8 antibody. J Immunol 154:1364, 1995.
443. Sasaki K, Kurata K, Funayama K, et al: Expression cloning of a novel α-1,3-fucosyltransferase that is involved in biosynthesis of the sialyl Lewis X carbohydrate determinants in leukocytes. J Biol Chem 269:14730, 1994.
444. Sawada M, Takada A, Ohwaki I, et al: Specific expression of a complex sialyl Lewis X antigen on high endothelial venules of human lymph nodes: possible candidate for L-selectin ligand. Biochem Biophys Res Commun 193:337, 1993.
445. Scheynius A, Camp RL, Pure E: Reduced contact sensitivity reactions in mice treated with monoclonal antibodies to leukocyte function-associated molecule-1 and intercellular adhesion molecule-1. J Immunol 150:655, 1993.
446. Schlaepfer DD, Hanks SK, Hunter T, et al: Integrin-mediated signal transduction linked to Ras pathway by GRB2 binding to focal adhesion kinase. Nature 372:786, 1994.
447. Schleimer RP, Benenati SV, Friedman B, et al: Do cytokines play a role in leukocyte recruitment and activation in the lungs? Am Rev Respir Dis 143:1169, 1991.
448. Schleimer RP, Bochner BS: Letter to the editor. J Immunol 147:380, 1991.
449. Schleimer RP, Ebisawa M, Georas SN, et al: The role of adhesion molecules and cytokines in eosinophil recruitment. In Gleich GJ, Kay AB (eds): Eosinophils in Allergy and Inflammation. Marcel Dekker, Inc, New York, 1993, p 99.
450. Schleimer RP, Rutledge BK: Cultured human vascular endothelial cells acquire adhesiveness for leukocytes following stimulation with interleukin-1, endotoxin, and tumor-promoting phorbol esters. J Immunol 136:649, 1986.
451. Schleimer RP, Sterbinsky SA, Kaiser J, et al: Interleukin-4 induces adherence of human eosinophils and basophils but not neutrophils to endothelium: association with expression of VCAM-1. J Immunol 148:1086, 1992.
452. Schmaier AH, Murray SC, Heda GD, et al: Synthesis and expression of C1 inhibitor by human umbilical vein endothelial cells. J Biol Chem 264:18173, 1989.
453. Schreiber AB, Kenney J, Kowalski WJ, et al: Interaction of endothelial cell growth factor with heparin: characterization by receptor and antibody recognition. Proc Natl Acad Sci USA 82:6138, 1985.
454. Schroeder JT, MacGlashan DW, Kagey-Sobotka A, et al: IgE-dependent IL-4 secretion by human basophils—the relationship between cytokine production and histamine release in mixed leukocyte cultures. J Immunol 153:1808, 1994.
455. Schwartz MA: Integrins as signal transducing receptors. In Cheresh DA, Mecham RP (eds): Integrins: Molecular and Biological Responses to the Extracellular Matrix. Academic Press, San Diego, 1994, p 33.
456. Schweighoffer T, Tanaka Y, Tidswell M, et al: Selective expression of integrin α4β7 on a subset of human CD4(+) memory T-cells with hallmarks of gut-trophism. J Immunol 151:717, 1993.
457. Sedgwick JB, Calhoun WJ, Vrtis RF, et al: Comparison of airway and blood eosinophil function after in vivo antigen challenge. J Immunol 149:3710, 1992.
458. Segal GM, McCall E, Stueve T, et al: Interleukin 1 stimulates endothelial cells to release multilineage human colony-stimulating activity. J Immunol 138:1772, 1987.
459. Sengelov H, Kjeldsen L, Diamond MS, et al: Subcellular localization and dynamics of Mac-1 (alpha(m)beta(2)) in human neutrophils. J Clin Invest 92:1467, 1993.
460. Sepp NT, Gille J, Li LJ, et al: A factor in human plasma permits persistent expression of E-selectin by human endothelial cells. J Invest Dermatol 102:445, 1994.
461. Sharar SR, Sasaki SS, Flaherty LC, et al: P-selectin blockade does not impair leukocyte host defense against bacterial peritonitis and soft tissue infection in rabbits. J Immunol 151:4982, 1993.
462. Sharma CP, Ezzell RM, Arnaout MA: Direct interaction of filamin (ABP-280) with the beta 2-integrin subunit CD18. J Immunol 154:3461, 1995.
463. Shimizu Y, Mobley JL: Distinct divalent cation requirements for integrin-mediated CR4+ T-lymphocyte adhesion to ICAM-1, fibronectin, VCAM-1, and invasin. J Immunol 151:4106, 1993.
464. Shimizu Y, Shaw S: Lymphocyte interactions with extracellular matrix. FASEB J 5:2292, 1991.
465. Shimizu Y, Shaw S: Mucins in the mainstream. Nature 366:630, 1993.
466. Shimizu Y, Shaw S, Graber N, et al: Activation-independent binding of human memory T cells to ELAM-1. Nature 349:799, 1991.
467. Shu HB, Agranoff AB, Nabel EG, et al: Differential regulation of vascular cell adhesion molecule 1 gene expression by specific NF-κB subunits in endothelial and epithelial cells. Mol Cell Biol 13:6283, 1993.
468. Sica A, Wang JM, Colotta F, et al: Monocyte chemotactic and activating factor gene expression induced in endothelial cells by IL-1 and tumor necrosis factor. J Immunol 144:3034, 1990.
469. Siegelman MH, Rijn MVD, Weissman IL: Mouse lymph node homing receptor cDNA clone encodes a glycoprotein revealing tandem interaction domains. Science 243:1165, 1989.
470. Silber A, Newman W, Reimann KA, et al: Kinetic expression of endothelial adhesion molecules and relationship to leukocyte recruitment in two cutaneous models of inflammation. Lab Invest 70:163, 1994.
471. Silber A, Newman W, Sasseville VG, et al: Recruitment of lymphocytes during cutaneous delayed hypersensitivity in nonhuman primates is dependent on E-selectin and vascular cell adhesion molecule 1. J Clin Invest 93:1554, 1994.
472. Simionescu N, Heltianu C, Antohe F, et al: Endothelial cell receptors for histamine. Ann NY Acad Sci 401:132, 1982.
473. Simionescu N, Simionescu M: Endothelial Cell Biology in Health and Disease. Plenum Press, New York, 1988, p 1.

474. Simon KO, Burridge K: Interactions between integrins and the cytoskeleton: structure and regulation. In Cheresh DA, Mecham RP (eds): Integrins: Molecular and Biological Responses to the Extracellular Matrix. Academic Press, San Diego, 1994, p 49.
475. Singer II, Kawka DW, Demartino JA, et al: Optimal humanization of 1B4, an anti-CD18 murine monoclonal antibody, is achieved by correct choice of human V-region framework sequences. J Immunol 150:2844, 1993.
476. Sironi M, Sciacca FL, Matteucci C, et al: Regulation of endothelial and mesothelial cell function by interleukin-13: selective induction of vascular cell adhesion molecule-1 and amplification of interleukin-6 production. Blood 84:1913, 1994.
477. Sligh JE, Ballantyne CM, Rich SS, et al: Inflammatory and immune responses are impaired in mice deficient in intercellular adhesion molecule-1. Proc Natl Acad Sci USA 90:8529, 1993.
478. Smart, SJ, Casale TB: Interleukin-8–induced transcellular neutrophil migration is facilitated by endothelial and pulmonary epithelial cells. Am J Respir Cell Mol Biol 9:489, 1993.
479. Smith CH, Barker JNWN, Morris RW, et al: Neuropeptides induce rapid expression of endothelial cell adhesion molecules and elicit granulocytic infiltration in human skin. J Immunol 151:3274, 1993.
480. Smith CW, Kishimoto TK, Abbass O, et al: Chemotactic factors regulate lectin adhesion molecule 1 (LECAM-1)–dependent neutrophil adhesion to cytokine-stimulated endothelial cells in vitro. J Clin Invest 87:609, 1991.
481. Smyth SS, Joneckis CC, Parise LV: Regulation of vascular integrins. Blood 81:2827, 1993.
482. Spertini O, Luscinskas FW, Gimbrone MA, et al: Monocyte attachment to activated human vascular endothelium in vitro is mediated by leukocyte adhesion molecule-1 (L-selectin) under nonstatic conditions. J Exp Med 175:1789, 1992.
483. Spertini O, Luscinskas FW, Kansas GS, et al: Leukocyte adhesion molecule-1 (LAM-1, L-selectin) interacts with an inducible endothelial cell ligand to support leukocyte adhesion. J Immunol 147:2565, 1991.
484. Springer TA: Adhesion receptors of the immune system. Nature 346:425, 1990.
485. Springer TA: Traffic signals for lymphocyte recirculation and leukocyte emigration: the multistep paradigm. Cell 76:301, 1994.
486. Sriramarao P, von Andrian UH, Butcher EC, et al: L-selectin and very late antigen-4 integrin promote eosinophil rolling at physiological shear rates in vivo. J Immunol 153:4238, 1994.
487. Stacker SA, Springer TA: Leukocyte integrin p150,95 (CD11c/CD18) functions as an adhesion molecule binding to a counter-receptor on stimulated endothelium. J Immunol 146:648, 1991.
488. Stamper HB Jr, Woodruff JJ: Lymphocyte homing into lymph nodes: in vitro demonstration of the selective affinity of recirculating lymphocytes for high-endothelial venules. J Exp Med 144:828, 1976.
489. Staunton DE, Dustin ML, Erickson HP, et al: The arrangement of the immunoglobulin-like domains of ICAM-1 and the binding sites for LFA-1 and rhinovirus. Cell 61:243, 1990.
490. Staunton DE, Dustin ML, Springer TA: Functional cloning of ICAM-2, a cell adhesion ligand for LFA-1 homologous to ICAM-1. Nature 339:61, 1989.
491. Staunton DE, Marlin SD, Stratowa C, et al: Primary structure of ICAM-1 demonstrates interaction between members of the immunoglobulin and integrin supergene families. Cell 52:925, 1988.
492. Steegmaier M, Levinovitz A, Isenmann S, et al: The E-selectin ligand ESL-1 is a variant of a receptor for fibroblast growth factor. Nature 373:615, 1995.
493. Stellato C, Beck LA, Gorgone GA, et al: Expression of the chemokine RANTES by a human bronchial epithelial cell line: modulation by cytokines and glucocorticoids. J Immunol 155:410, 1995.
494. Stellato C, Beck LA, Klunk DA, et al: Differential regulation by glucocorticoids (GC) of RANTES production in human epithelial and endothelial cells. J Allergy Clin Immunol 95:299, 1995.
495. Stellato C, Beck LA, Schall TJ, et al: Expression of the chemokine RANTES in human epithelial cells. FASEB J 8:A225, 1994.
496. Stenberg PE, McEver RP, Shuman MA, et al: A platelet alpha granule membrane protein (GMP-140) is expressed on the plasma membrane after activation. J Cell Biol 101:880, 1985.
497. Stern DM, Bank I, Nawroth PP, et al: Self-regulation of procoagulant events on the endothelial cell surface. J Exp Med 162:1223, 1985.
498. Stern DM, Handley DA, Nawroth PP: Endothelium and the regulation of coagulation. In Simionescu N, Simionescu M (eds): Endothelial Cell Biology in Health and Disease. Plenum Press, New York, 1988, p 275.
499. Stockinger H, Gadd SJ, Eher R, et al: Molecular characterization and functional analysis of the leukocyte surface protein CD31. J Immunol 145:3889, 1990.
500. Stocks SC, Kerr MA: Neutrophil NCA-160 (CD66) is the major protein carrier of selectin binding carbohydrate groups Lewis^x and sialyl Lewis^x. Biochem Biophys Res Commun 195:478, 1993.
501. Sueyoshi S, Tsuboi S, Sawada-Hirai R, et al: Expression of distinct fucosylated oligosaccharides and carbohydrate-mediated adhesion efficiency directed by two different α-1,3-fucosyltransferases. Comparison of E- and L-selectin–mediated adhesion. J Biol Chem 269:32342, 1994.
502. Suzuki Y, Toda Y, Tamatani T, et al: Sulfated glycolipids are ligands for a lymphocyte homing receptor, L-selectin (LECAM-1), binding epitope in sulfated sugar chain. Biochem Biophys Res Commun 190:426, 1993.
503. Swerlick RA, Lee KH, Li L, et al: Regulation of vascular cell adhesion molecule 1 on human dermal microvascular endothelial cells. J Immunol 149:698, 1992.
504. Symon FA, Walsh GM, Watson SR, et al: Eosinophil adhesion to nasal polyp endothelium is P-selectin–dependent. J Exp Med 180:371, 1994.
505. Takada A, Ohmori K, Takahashi N, et al: Adhesion of human cancer cells to vascular endothelium mediated by a carbohydrate antigen, sialyl Lewis A. Biochem Biophys Res Commun 179:713, 1991.
506. Takahashi N, Liu MC, Proud D, et al: Soluble intracellular adhesion molecule 1 in bronchoalveolar lavage fluid of allergic subjects following segmental antigen challenge. Am J Respir Crit Care Med 150:704, 1994.
507. Tanaka Y, Adams DH, Hubscher S, et al: T-cell adhesion induced by proteoglycan-immobilized cytokine MIP-1β. Nature 361:79, 1993.
508. Tanaka Y, Adams DH, Shaw S: Proteoglycans on endothelial cells present adhesion-inducing cytokines to leukocytes. Immunol Today 14:111, 1993.
509. Tanaka Y, Albelda SM, Horgan KJ, et al: CD31 expressed on distinctive T-cell subsets is a preferential amplifier of β1 integrin-mediated adhesion. J Exp Med 176:245, 1992.
510. Tanimoto Y, Takahashi K, Kimura I: Effects of cytokines on human basophil chemotaxis. Clin Exp Allergy 22:1020, 1992.
511. Tedder TF, Isaacs CM, Ernst TJ, et al: Isolation and chromosomal localization of cDNAs encoding a novel human lymphocyte cell surface molecule, LAM-1. J Exp Med 170:123, 1989.
512. Tedder TF, Penta AC, Levine HB, et al: Expression of the human leukocyte adhesion molecule, LAM1. Identity with the TQ1 and Leu-8 differentiation antigens. J Immunol 144:532, 1990.
513. Tedder TF, Steeber DA, Pizcueta P: L-selectin deficient mice have impaired leukocyte recruitment into inflammatory sites. J Exp Med 181:2259, 1995.
514. Teixeira MM, Williams TJ, Au B-T, et al: Characterization of eosinophil homotypic aggregation. J Leukoc Biol 57:226, 1995.
515. Tepper RI, Levinson DA, Stanger BZ, et al: IL-4 induces allergic-like inflammatory disease and alters T cell development in transgenic mice. Cell 62:457, 1990.
516. Tepper RI, Pattengale PK, Leder P: Murine interleukin-4 displays potent anti-tumor activity in vivo. Cell 57:503, 1989.
517. Terry RW, Kwee L, Levine JF, et al: Cytokine induction of an alternatively spliced murine vascular cell adhesion molecule (VCAM) messenger RNA encoding a glycosylphosphatidylinositol-anchored VCAM protein. Proc Natl Acad Sci USA 90:5919, 1993.
518. Thompson HL, Burbelo PD, Segui-Real B, et al: Laminin promotes mast cell attachment. J Immunol 143:2323, 1989.
519. Thompson HL, Burbelo PD, Yamada Y, et al: Mast cells chemotax to laminin with enhancement after IgE-mediated activation. J Immunol 143:4188, 1989.
520. Thorlacius H, Raud J, Rosengren-Beezley S, et al: Mast cell activation induces P-selectin–dependent leukocyte rolling and adhesion in postcapillary venules in vivo. Biochem Biophys Res Commun 203:1043, 1994.
521. Thornhill MH, Haskard DO: IL-4 regulates endothelial cell activation by IL-1, tumor necrosis factor, or IFN-γ. J Immunol 145:865, 1990.
522. Thornhill MH, Kyan-Aung U, Haskard DO: IL-4 increases human endothelial cell adhesiveness for T cells but not for neutrophils. J Immunol 144:3060, 1990.
523. Thornton SC, Mueller SN, Levine EM: Human endothelial cells: use of heparin in cloning and long-term serial cultivation. Science 222:623, 1983.

524. Tidswell M, Brown T, Erle D: Characterization of the lymphocyte and eosinophil cell adhesion molecule integrin $\alpha 4\beta 7$. Am Rev Respir Dis 147:A542, 1993.
525. Tiemeyer M, Swiedler SJ, Ishihara M, et al: Carbohydrate ligands for endothelial-leukocyte adhesion molecule 1. Proc Natl Acad Sci USA 88:1138, 1991.
526. Toi M, Harris AL, Bicknell R: Interleukin-4 is a potent mitogen for capillary endothelium. Biochem Biophys Res Commun 174:1287, 1991.
527. Tomioka K, MacGlashan DW Jr, Lichtenstein LM, et al: GM-CSF regulates human eosinophil responses to F-Met peptide and platelet activating factor. J Immunol 151:4989, 1993.
528. Tosi MF, Stark JM, Smith CW, et al: Induction of ICAM-1 expression on human airway epithelial cells by inflammatory cytokines—effects on neutrophil-epithelial cell adhesion. Am J Respir Cell Mol Biol 7:214, 1992.
529. Travis J: Biotech gets a grip on cell adhesion. Science 260:906, 1993.
530. Triggiani M, Schleimer RP, Warner JA, et al: Differential synthesis of 1-acyl-2-acetyl-sn-glycero-3-phosphocholine and platelet-activating factor by human inflammatory cells. J Immunol 147:660, 1991.
531. Vadas MA, Lucas CM, Gamble JR, et al: Regulation of eosinophil function by P-selectin. In Gleich GJ, Kay AB (eds): Eosinophils in Allergy and Inflammation. Marcel Dekker, Inc, New York, 1993, p 69.
532. Valent P: The phenotype of human eosinophils, basophils, and mast cells. J Allergy Clin Immunol 94:1177, 1994.
533. Valent P, Bettelheim P: Cell surface structures on human basophils and mast cells. Biochemical and functional characterization. Adv Immunol 52:333, 1992.
534. Vane JR, Anggard EE, Botting RM: Mechanisms of disease—regulatory functions of the vascular endothelium. N Engl J Med 323:27, 1990.
535. Vanhoutte PM: Endothelin-1. Nature 368:693, 1994.
536. Vaporciyan AA, DeLisser HM, Yan H-C, et al: Involvement of platelet-endothelial cell adhesion molecule-1 in neutrophil recruitment in vivo. Science 262:1580, 1993.
537. Varki A: Selectin ligands. Proc Natl Acad Sci USA 91:7390, 1994.
538. Vazeux R, Hoffman PA, Tomita JK, et al: Cloning and characterization of a new intercellular adhesion molecule ICAM-R. Nature 360:485, 1992.
539. von Andrian UH, Berger EM, Ramezani L, et al: In vivo behavior of neutrophils from two patients with distinct inherited leukocyte adhesion deficiency syndromes. J Clin Invest 91:2893, 1993.
540. von Andrian UH, Chambers JD, Berg EL, et al: L-selectin mediates neutrophil rolling in inflamed venules through sialyl Lewis^x-dependent and Lewis^x-independent recognition pathways. Blood 82:182, 1993.
541. von Andrian UH, Chambers JD, McEvoy LM, et al: Two-step model of leukocyte endothelial cell interaction in inflammation—distinct roles for LECAM-1 and the leukocyte $\beta 2$ integrins in vivo. Proc Natl Acad Sci USA 88:7538, 1991.
542. von Andrian UH, Hansell P, Chambers JD, et al: L-selectin function is required for $\beta 2$-integrin–mediated neutrophil adhesion at physiological shear rates in vivo. Am J Physiol 263:H1034, 1992.
543. Vonderheide RH, Springer TA: Lymphocyte adhesion through very late antigen 4: evidence for a novel binding site in the alternatively spliced domain of vascular cell adhesion molecule 1 and an additional $\alpha 4$ integrin. J Exp Med 175:1433, 1992.
544. Vonderheide RH, Tedder TF, Springer TA, et al: Residues within a conserved amino acid motif of domain-1 and domain-4 of VCAM-1 are required for binding to VLA-4. J Cell Biol 125:215, 1994.
545. Vora M, Yssel H, de Vries JE, et al: Antigen presentation by human dermal microvascular endothelial cells. Immunoregulatory effect of IFN-γ and IL-10. J Immunol 152:5734, 1994.
546. Voraberger G, Schäfer R, Stratowa C: Cloning of the human gene for intercellular adhesion molecule 1 and analysis of its 5′-regulatory region. J Immunol 147:2777, 1991.
547. Wadsworth S, Halvorson MJ, Chang AC, et al: Multiple changes in VLA protein glycosylation, expression, and function occur during mouse T-cell ontogeny. J Immunol 150:847, 1993.
548. Walker C, Rihs S, Braun RK, et al: Increased expression of CD11b and functional changes in eosinophils after migration across endothelial cell monolayers. J Immunol 150:4061, 1993.
549. Walsh GM, Hartnell A, Wardlaw AJ, et al: IL-5 enhances the in vitro adhesion of human eosinophils, but not neutrophils, in a leucocyte integrin (CD11/18)–dependent manner. Immunology 71:258, 1990.
550. Walsh GM, Mermod J, Hartnell A, et al: Human eosinophil, but not neutrophil, adherence to IL-1–stimulated human umbilical vascular endothelial cells is $\alpha 4\beta 1$ (very late antigen-4) dependent. J Immunol 146:3419, 1991.
551. Walsh LJ, Kaminer MS, Lazarus GS, et al: Role of laminin in localization of human dermal mast cells. Lab Invest 65:433, 1991.
552. Walsh LJ, Trinchieri G, Waldorf HA, et al: Human dermal mast cells contain and release tumor necrosis factor α, which induces endothelial leukocyte adhesion molecule 1. Proc Natl Acad Sci USA 88:4220, 1991.
553. Walz G, Aruffo A, Kolanus W, et al: Recognition by ELAM-1 of the sialyl-Le^x determinant on myeloid and tumor cells. Science 250:1132, 1990.
554. Wang JM, Rambaldi A, Biondi A, et al: Recombinant human interleukin 5 is a selective eosinophil chemoattractant. Eur J Immunol 19:701, 1989.
555. Ward PA, Mulligan MS: Blocking of adhesion molecules in vivo as anti-inflammatory therapy. Ther Immunol 1:165, 1994.
556. Wardlaw AJ, Symon FS, Walsh GM: Eosinophil adhesion in allergic inflammation. J Allergy Clin Immunol 94:1163, 1994.
557. Wardlaw AJ, Walsh GM, Symon FA: Mechanisms of eosinophil and basophil migration. Allergy 49:797, 1994.
558. Warringa RAJ, Koenderman L, Kok PTM, et al: Modulation and induction of eosinophil chemotaxis by granulocyte-macrophage colony-stimulating factor and interleukin-3. Blood 77:2694, 1991.
559. Warringa RAJ, Mengelers HJJ, Kuijper PHM, et al: In vivo priming of platelet-activating factor-induced eosinophil chemotaxis in allergic asthmatic individuals. Blood 79:1836, 1992.
560. Watson ML, Kingsmore SF, Johnston GI, et al: Genomic organization of the selectin family of leukocyte adhesion molecules on human and mouse chromosome 1. J Exp Med 172:263, 1990.
561. Watson ML, Smith D, Bourne AD, et al: Cytokines contribute to airway dysfunction in antigen-challenged guinea pigs—inhibition of airway hyperreactivity, pulmonary eosinophil accumulation, and tumor necrosis factor generation by pretreatment with an interleukin-1 receptor antagonist. Am J Respir Cell Mol Biol 8:365, 1993.
562. Wayner EA, Garcia-Pardo A, Humphries MJ, et al: Identification and characterization of the T lymphocyte adhesion receptor for an alternative cell attachment domain (CS-1) in plasma fibronectin. J Cell Biol 109:1321, 1989.
563. Wayner EA, Kovach NL: Activation-dependent recognition by hematopoietic cells of the LDV sequence in the V region of fibronectin. J Cell Biol 116:489, 1992.
564. Webb DL, Marlor CW, Conrad PJ, et al: Role of third N-terminal domain of VCAM-1. Biochem Biophys Res Commun 197:674, 1993.
564a. Weber M, Uguccioni M, Ochensberger B, et al: Monocyte chemotactic protein MCP-2 activates human basophil and eosinophil leukocytes similar to MCP-3. J Immunol 154:4166, 1995.
565. Weg VB, Williams TJ, Lobb RR, et al: A monoclonal antibody recognizing very late activation antigen-4 inhibits eosinophil accumulation in vivo. J Exp Med 177:561, 1993.
566. Wegner CD: Lung inflammation. In Wegner CD (ed): Adhesion Molecules. Academic Press, London, 1994, p 191.
567. Wegner CD, Gundel RH, Letts LG: Expression and probable roles of cell adhesion molecules in lung inflammation. Chest 101:34, 1992.
568. Wegner CD, Gundel RH, Reilly P, et al: Intercellular adhesion molecule-1 (ICAM-1) in the pathogenesis of asthma. Science 247:456, 1990.
569. Wegner CD, Rothlein R, Clarke CC, et al: Inhaled ICAM-1 reduces antigen-induced airway hyperresponsiveness in monkeys. Am Rev Respir Dis 143:A418, 1991.
570. Wein M, Bochner BS: Adhesion molecule antagonists: future therapies for allergic diseases? Eur Respir J 6:1239, 1993.
571. Wein M, Sterbinsky SA, Bickel CA, et al: Comparison of eosinophil and neutrophil ligands for P-selectin: ligands for P-selectin differ from those for E-selectin. Am J Respir Cell Mol Biol 12:315, 1995.
572. Weller PF, Rand TH, Goelz SE, et al: Human eosinophil adherence to vascular endothelium mediated by binding to vascular cell adhesion molecule 1 and endothelial leukocyte adhesion molecule 1. Proc Natl Acad Sci USA 88:7430, 1991.
573. Wellicome SM, Thornhill MH, Pitzalis C, et al: A monoclonal antibody that detects a novel antigen on endothelial cells that is induced by tumor necrosis factor, IL-1, or lipopolysaccharide. J Immunol 144:2558, 1990.
574. Werfel S, Schleimer R, Sterbinsky S, et al: Regulation of $\beta 1$ integrin function on eosinophils (Eos) by Mn^{2+} and IL-5. J Allergy Clin Immunol 95:338, 1995.

575. Weston BW, Smith PL, Kelly RJ, et al: Molecular cloning of a 4th member of a human alpha(1,3)fucosyltransferase gene family—multiple homologous sequences that determine expression of the Lewis X, sialyl Lewis X, and difucosyl sialyl Lewis X epitopes. J Biol Chem 267:24575, 1992.
576. Wilson JM, Ping AJ, Krauss JC, et al: Correction of CD18-deficient lymphocytes by retrovirus-mediated gene transfer. Science 248:1413, 1990.
577. Wilson RW, Ballantyne CM, Smith CW, et al: Gene targeting yields a CD18-mutant mouse for study of inflammation. J Immunol 151:1571, 1993.
578. Wong CS, Gamble JR, Skinner MP, et al: Adhesion protein GMP-140 inhibits superoxide release by human neutrophils. Proc Natl Acad Sci USA 88:2397, 1991.
579. Xu H, Gonzalo JA, St Pierre Y, et al: Leukocytosis and resistance to septic shock in intercellular adhesion molecule 1-deficient mice. J Exp Med 180:95, 1994.
580. Xu YL, Swerlick RA, Sepp N, et al: Characterization of expression and modulation of cell adhesion molecules on an immortalized human dermal microvascular endothelial cell line (HMEC-1). J Invest Dermatol 102:833, 1994.
581. Yago T, Tsukuda M, Yamazaki H, et al: Analysis of an initial step of T cell adhesion to endothelial monolayers under flow conditions. J Immunol 154:1216, 1995.
582. Yamada T, Ebisawa M, MacGlashan J, et al: RANTES is a chemoattractant for human eosinophils. J Allergy Clin Immunol 91:692, 1993.
583. Yan HC, Delisser HM, Pilewski JM, et al: Leukocyte recruitment into human skin transplanted onto severe combined immunodeficient mice induced by TNF-alpha is dependent on E-selectin. J Immunol 152:3053, 1994.
584. Ying S, Durham SR, Jacobson MR, et al: T lymphocytes and mast cells express messenger RNA for interleukin-4 in the nasal mucosa in allergen-induced rhinitis. Immunology 82:200, 1994.
585. Ying S, Robinson DS, Varney V, et al: TNFα mRNA expression in allergic inflammation. Clin Exp Allergy 21:745, 1991.
586. Yong KL, Linch DC: Granulocyte-macrophage–colony-stimulating factor differentially regulates neutrophil migration across IL-1–activated and nonactivated human endothelium. J Immunol 150:2449, 1993.
587. Yong KL, Rowles PM, Patterson KG, et al: Granulocyte-macrophage colony-stimulating factor induces neutrophil adhesion to pulmonary vascular endothelium in vivo—role of β2 integrins. Blood 80:1565, 1992.
588. Zachary I, Rozengurt E: Focal adhesion kinase (p125(FAK))—a point of convergence in the action of neuropeptides, integrins, and oncogenes. Cell 71:891, 1992.
589. Zangrilli JG, Shaver JR, Cirelli RA, et al: sVCAM-1 levels after segmental challenge correlate with eosinophil influx, IL-4 and IL-5 production, and the late phase response. Am J Respir Crit Care Med 151:1346, 1995.
590. Zhou Q, Moore KL, Smith DF, et al: The selectin GMP-140 binds to sialylated, fucosylated lactosaminoglycans on both myeloid and nonmyeloid cells. J Cell Biol 115:557, 1991.
591. Zhu DZ, Cheng CF, Pauli BU: Blocking of lung endothelial cell adhesion molecule-1 (Lu-ECAM-1) inhibits murine melanoma lung metastasis. J Clin Invest 89:1718, 1992.
592. Zhu DZ, Cheng CF, Pauli BU: Mediation of lung metastasis of murine melanomas by a lung-specific endothelial cell adhesion molecule. Proc Natl Acad Sci USA 88:9568, 1991.
593. Zimmerman BZ, Holt JW, Paulson JC, et al: Molecular determinants of lipid mediator-induced leukocyte adherence and emigration in rat mesenteric venules. Am J Physiol 266:H847, 1994.
594. Zimmerman GA, McIntyre TM, Prescott SM: Production of platelet-activating factor by human vascular endothelial cells: evidence for a requirement for specific agonists and modulation by prostacyclin. Circulation 72:718, 1985.
595. Zimmerman GA, Prescott SM, Mcintyre TM: Endothelial cell interactions with granulocytes—tethering and signaling molecules. Immunol Today 13:93, 1992.

16 Chemotactic Molecules and Cellular Activation

NICHOLAS W. LUKACS PETER A. WARD

The movement of leukocytes from the vasculature, through the vessel wall, and into tissue to the site of inflammation is a complex, coordinated, multistep event. Chemotaxis of leukocytes is a central occurrence during immune responses that acts to localize cells to a site of infection or injury. Chemotaxis of leukocytes is initiated by increases in the expression of adhesion molecules on the vascular endothelial cells that allows localization and adherence of leukocyte populations to the area of the inflammatory response. These early adhesion events are induced by a number of early response mediators and cytokines, including histamine, C5a, tumor necrosis factor-alpha (TNF-α), and IL-1. The early response cytokines and mediators up-regulate selectin molecules (E and P) on the endothelial surface and slow the leukocytes from circulatory flow, a phenomenon known as rolling.

After leukocytes have been localized to the inflamed vascular wall, the cells firmly adhere to the endothelium by interaction with adhesion molecules (ICAM-1 and VCAM-1), which allow the spreading of the leukocytes along the endothelial surface.[34, 76] Once firmly adhered to the vascular endothelium, leukocytes can migrate into the tissue, following along chemotactic gradients that not only localize the cells to the site of inflammation but also appear to prime and activate the cells for effector functions. The fate of these cells once in the tissue may be dictated directly by the type of chemotactic signal that motivated the cells to infiltrate.

Numerous molecules in vitro display the ability to be chemokinetic and can induce leukocytes to move indiscriminately. However, the directional movement of cells within tissue must be analyzed carefully before they are referred to as true chemotactic molecules. Molecules such as IL-2, IL-4, and even TNF-α can induce leukocytes to move in a nonspecific (chemokinetic) manner in vitro, yet these molecules are not truly chemotactic. Several molecules appear to have been classified as chemotactic and have demonstrated the ability to induce leukocyte recruitment in vitro and during disease in vivo. The focus of this review is to examine and summarize the classic chemotactic molecules, the specificity of their action, the signals leading to cellular activation, and the evidence for their biologic role in vivo.

CHEMOTACTIC MOLECULES

COMPLEMENT COMPONENTS

One of the immediate events that appears to occur globally during inflammation is the activation of the complement system. The initiation of the complement cascade can be induced by antibody-antigen complexes or bacterial products. Of the complement cascade products, C3a and C5a are some of the most biologically active.[27, 87] C3a is an anaphylatoxin that induces the activation of mast cells and basophils and appears to have direct and indirect effects on vascular permeability. These events may be crucial in allowing easier access of leukocyte populations to migrate through the vascular endothelium and into the inflamed tissue.

C5a is a potent anaphylatoxin that induces mast cell and basophil degranulation, platelet and phagocytic cell activation, and immediate changes in vascular permeability. C5a stimulates smooth muscle contraction and has potent neutrophil chemotactic and activating characteristics that promote directed migration of these leukocytes toward a concentration gradient. C5a stimulates neutrophil oxidative metabolism, granule discharge, and adhesiveness to vascular endothelium, all of which may contribute not only to increasing chemotactic gradients but also to tissue injury. C5a can directly stimulate endothelial cells in a G-protein receptor-dependent fashion to cause signal transduction events, resulting in increased intracellular Ca^{2+}, induction of superoxide (O_2^-), and expression of P-selectin. These events appear to be mediated by engagement of specific C5a receptors. C5a also appears to be a potent eosinophil chemoattractant and activator. Interestingly, C3a has been shown to be preferentially chemotactic for eosinophils but not neutrophils.[17]

Both C3a and C5a have been shown to mediate superoxide production and release of eosinophil cationic protein (ECP) and eosinophil peroxidase at 10^{-7} and 10^{-8} M concentrations, respectively.[82, 91] These attributes may be ultimately important during inflammatory diseases in which multiple activation pathways lead to the accumulation and activation of both neutrophil and eosinophil populations that participate in the pathology to the surrounding tissue. Overall, activation of complement, C3a and C5a, has been shown to play an intricate role in the movement, activation, and degranulation of leukocytes during acute tissue injury and appears to be important in augmentation of chronic inflammatory responses. Evidence for its contribution in disease is discussed in a later section.

LIPID MEDIATORS

Platelet Activating Factor

Platelet activating factor (PAF) is a potent activator of leukocyte chemotaxis and can be released from a variety of cell sources during immune/inflammatory responses. PAF is derived from the biodegradation of arachidonic acids by phospholipase A_2 (Fig. 16–1). PAF has a broad range of specificity in its ability to induce leukocyte chemotaxis, since it induces the recruitment of not only neutrophils but also monocytes, lymphocytes, and eosinophils. During allergic diseases, PAF may have a particular role in augmentation of eosinophil responses. Although PAF is a relatively weak eosinophil chemotactic factor compared with LTB_4[24] or RANTES,[66] PAF does have activating effects on eosinophils, inducing superoxide production and release of ECP, as well as eosinophil peroxidase release.[91] As with all of the eosinophil chemotactic factors, IL-5 enhances the ability of PAF to induce eosinophil chemotaxis.[48]

In addition, PAF also appears to have a significant application for augmenting and directly stimulating cytokine production from leukocyte populations. PAF dose dependently stimulated the production of IL-1 but not TNF-α, in monocyte and macrophage cultures. In addition, PAF has synergistic activating effects on both IL-1 and TNF production when added to LPS-stimulated monocytes/macrophages. Furthermore, PAF-primed neutrophils and monocytes have demonstrated increased superoxide production, elastase release, and endothelial cell lysis in response to phorbol ester or bacterial-derived f-met-leu-phe (FMLP). Not only does PAF have an effect on phagocytic cells, but it also can augment T lymphocyte–derived cytokine production. For example, in vivo infusion of PAF into rats significantly increased the ability to elicit IL-2 from Con A-stimulated spleen cells.[82]

The actions of PAF on endothelial cells indicate that PAF has a direct role in up-regulation of selectin and adhesion molecules and can induce the release of superoxide anion. Instillation of PAF into human, monkey, or guinea pig airways induced an immediate LTC_4-independent bronchoconstrictor response, suggesting a possible role in development of pathophysiology in asthmatic responses. In addition, 3 hours post PAF airway instillation resulted in an accumulation of leukocytes, including macrophages, neutrophils, and eosinophils, accompanied by significant epithelial cell degeneration.[11] Overall, these studies indicate that the signals provided by PAF not only are chemotactic but also can participate in the augmentation of the immune/inflammatory pathway.

Leukotriene B_4 (LTB_4)

Leukotrienes are derived from the oxidative metabolism of arachidonic acid (see Fig. 16–1) that has been produced

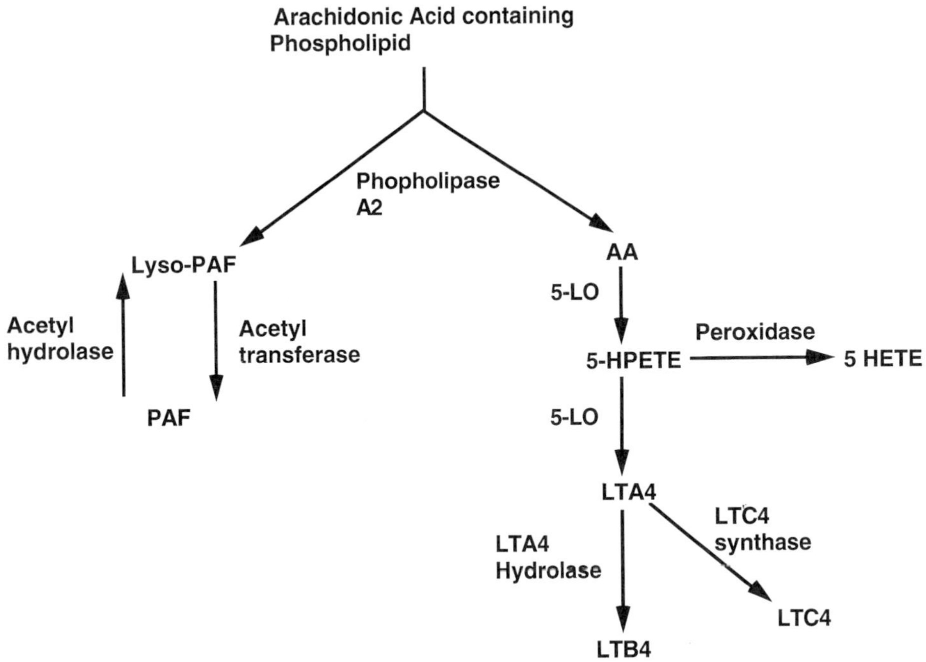

FIGURE 16–1. Arachidonic acid metabolic pathway.

from endogenous sources and released from phospholipids via phospholipases (PLA_2).[65] The production of LTB_4 is dependent upon 5-lipoxygenase (5-LO)–induced conversion of arachidonic acid intermediates, including 5-HPETE and LTA_4, and appears to be the predominant 5-LO metabolite in many cells. Although leukotrienes in general have broad effects on inflammatory responses, LTB_4 is one of the most potent neutrophil chemotactic molecules known and induces superoxide production. However, LTB_4 can also act to recruit other leukocyte populations, such as monocytes and eosinophils. In eosinophil chemotactic assays, LTB_4 is more potent than PAF in the activation and degranulation of eosinophils. LTB_4 has been found in many disease states, including psoriasis, bacterial peritonitis, inflammatory bowel disease, and asthma.

LTB_4 is rapidly synthesized by phagocytic cells (PMNs and macrophages) when stimulated with bacterial LPS or FMLP. PAF is also a potent stimulator of phagocyte-derived LTB_4 and may augment leukocyte migration into tissue via its ability to induce LTB_4 production. Although LTB_4 does not appear to be a direct inducer of IL-1 or TNF-α, it does have the ability to synergistically increase the levels of the cytokines during LPS or muramyl dipeptide stimulation of monocytes. Likewise, in T-cell cytokine responses, production of IL-2 and IFN-γ can be augmented by LTB_4 costimulation. Overall, LTB_4 not only is chemotactic for a number of leukocyte populations but also has the ability to augment inflammatory/immune mediators and therefore has been considered a viable target for therapeutic intervention.

CHEMOKINES

One of the fastest growing areas in inflammation research is the field of chemokine biology. These molecules, unlike complement and lipid mediators, appear to have specificity for inducing chemotactic responses of specific leukocyte populations. Chemokines have avid heparin-binding properties and have been identified in a variety of multiple disease states. Because of the ability of chemokines to bind to heparin and in light of identification of chemokines binding to the heparin-rich proteoglycans, it has been suggested that chemokines operate as a solid phase gradient, together with adhesion molecule expression, to cause leukocytes to home to a site of inflammation. The solid phase–bound chemokines would allow a chemokine gradient to localize the response to a very distinct area without being washed away.

Based upon the first two cysteine residues in their sequence, the chemokines have been divided into two distinct families, the C-X-C (alpha) and the C-C (beta) families.[59, 67] The functional activities of these family members also have distinct properties. The C-X-C family of chemokines is predominantly chemotactic for neutrophils, whereas the C-C family members are chemotactic for mononuclear leukocytes, monocytes, and lymphocytes, as well as differentially chemotactic for eosinophils and basophils, depending on the particular C-C chemokine. These attributes appear to divide the functions between acute (C-X-C) and chronic (C-C) inflammatory events. However, the specificity of biologic activity for chemokines is not completely clear-cut, since multiple studies have identified functions for C-X-C and C-C family members in both neutrophil and mononuclear inflammatory responses.

The C-X-C family includes IL-8, ENA-78, GRO-α, β and γ, CTAP III, NAP-2, MIP-2, PF-4, IP-10, and MIG (Table 16–1). This family can be divided according to the presence of the amino acid motif glutamate-leucine-arginine (ELR), which appears to confer the ability to attract neutrophils and provide an angiogenic signal (endothelial cell growth and migration). IL-8 has also been identified as an eosinophil chemotactic protein during asthmatic responses. The C-C family contains several related proteins: MCP-1,-2,-3, MIP-1α, MIP-1β, eotaxin, and RANTES (see Table 16–1). As discussed previously, these proteins have a role in promoting

TABLE 16–1
HUMAN CHEMOKINE FAMILY MEMBERS

C-X-C Chemokine	C-C Chemokine
ELR containing	
IL-8	MCP-1, 2, 3
ENA-78	MIP-1α
GRO-α, β, γ	MIP-1β
CTAP III	RANTES
NAP-2	Eotaxin
Non-ELR containing	
MIG	
IP-10	
PF-4	

the recruitment of specific leukocyte populations during inflammatory events. Chemokines have the ability to not only specifically recruit particular subsets of leukocytes but also activate the leukocyte populations for effector function, especially neutrophils and eosinophils. Both of these populations have the ability to release oxidants and proteases that damage tissue and disrupt function.

In addition to their ability to recruit specific leukocytes, chemokines also have other functions. IL-8 and the other ELR-containing C-X-C chemokines have potent angiogenic activity, whereas the non-ELR–containing C-X-C members (IP-10, MIG, PF-4) are all angiostatic and inhibit angiogenesis.[81] The C-C chemokine members may have potent effects in augmentation[5] or directional differentiation of T lymphocytes toward TH1 (MIP-1α) or Th2 (MCP-1) phenotypes (Lukacs, unpublished data). These properties suggest that chemokines may play important roles in homeostasis and/or disease progression, inducing events leading to healing.

The production of chemokines can be observed in nearly every cell after stimulation by early response cytokines (IL-1 and TNFα).[80] Chemokine generation results during platelet aggregation, hyperoxia,[49] and cell-to-cell interactions.[44, 45] During an allergic response, mast cells are activated via an IgE-mediated specific antigen stimulation and degranulation. Studies have identified mRNA for both C-X-C (IL-8 and ENA-78) and C-C (MIP-1α, MCP-1, and RANTES) chemokines in human mast cell populations.[69] Mast cells isolated from airway tissue can release multiple C-X-C and C-C chemokines upon activation.[43] The original isolation of marc/fic and TCA-3 proteins (C-C chemokines) from murine mast cells suggests that multiple chemokines are produced and/or stored by these cells. This may provide an initial mechanism for the recruitment and activation of particular leukocyte subsets during allergic inflammation.

C-C chemokines also have activating effects directly on basophil populations.[8, 39, 40] MCP-1 and MCP-3 appear to be the most potent chemokine for activation of basophils, followed by MCP-2, MIP-1α, and RANTES. In addition, these same chemokines have been shown to be chemotactic for mast cells (Taub, personal communication). Therefore, chemokines may play a central role in allergic responses via effects on basophils, mast cells, and eosinophils. The fact that chemokines can directly initiate activation of basophils and eosinophils suggests that this mechanism may be operative during a variety of disease states. Since chemokines are produced by nearly every cell, the cell type, cell location, and level of chemokine produced all influence the directed movement and activation of leukocytes during an inflammatory response. For example, the production of chemokines by type II alveolar epithelial cells in the lung may be necessary to cause initial recruitment of leukocytes into the lung interstitium and subsequently into the airspace. These events probably require the role of multiple chemotaxins expressed at various time points during the inflammatory response.

NOVEL CHEMOATTRACTANTS

Lymphotactin

Lymphotactin, by name, was first identified in 1977 as a thymocyte-derived lymphocyte chemotactic factor with a molecular weight of about 10.5 kD and an isoelectric point of 5.9.[32] It has been cloned from thymocytes and classified as a novel C family chemokine, which appears to have significant homology to the C-C family of chemokines, is produced by $CD8^+$ and double negative thymocytes (but not $CD4^+$ thymocytes), and is chemotactic for lymphocytes (but not monocytes and neutrophils).[37, 38] These properties give lymphotactin a novel characteristic not shared by other chemotactic agents. The location in which lymphotactin is generated, as well as the cells activated by it, suggests that it is possible that lymphotactin is most important in the recruitment of immature lymphocytes ($CD4^-$ and $CD8^-$) to the thymus, where development and maturation occurs. Future studies will determine whether other tissues and cells produce lymphotactin during disease and what function it has during inflammatory events.

Cationic Antimicrobial Protein-37 (CAP37)

CAP37 was originally isolated from azurophilic granules of human neutrophils and is structurally related to the serine protease family, with antibacterial activity sharing significant sequence homology to cathepsin G and elastase. However, no protease activity is contained within CAP37.[61] In addition, CAP37 has potent chemotactic activity that is monocyte specific, increases macrophage survival, induces macrophage differentiation, and, like the chemokines, has a heparin-binding domain. CAP37 is chemotactic for monocytes at concentrations between 1.3×10^{-9} and 10^{-8} M, a range similar to those for FMLP. During bacterial phagocytosis (*Staphylococcus aureus*)-induced degranulation, about 90% of the intracellular CAP37 is released from neutrophils, suggesting that a second wave of inflammatory monocyte/macrophage population could be elicited to the site of inflammation due to CAP37 release. CAP37 and similar proteins found in neutrophilic granules may constitute significant chemotactic signals necessary for successful antigen processing and presentation facilitating specific immune responses, leading to the proper destruction of infectious insults.

RECEPTOR SPECIFICITY AND SIGNALING

Binding of chemoattractants to specific cell surface receptors on leukocyte populations can initiate directed leukocyte

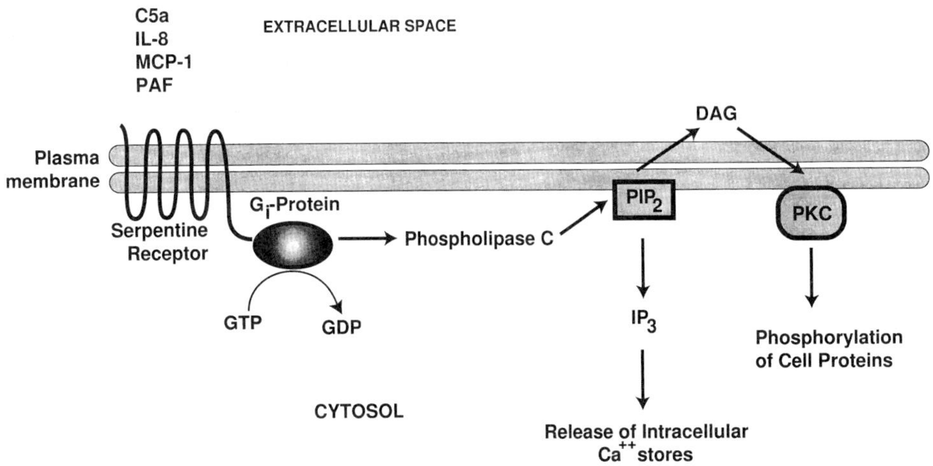

FIGURE 16–2. G protein–coupled receptors.

chemotaxis toward the site of inflammation, as well as a number of other biologic events. The chemoattractant receptors all appear to be coupled to G_i protein–mediated pathways.[9] These pathways utilize the hydrolysis of polyphosphoinositides to initiate Ca^{2+} mobilization and cellular activation (Fig. 16–2). The seven membrane G-protein serpentine receptor coupling induces phospholipase C-mediated hydrolysis of polyphosphoinositols 4,5,-biphosphate (PIP2) to inositol 1,4,5-triphosphate (IP3) and 1,2 sn-diacylglycerol (DAG). Subsequently, these products initiate cell activation by calcium mobilization and protein kinase C (PKC) activation. One technique used to identify G_i protein–coupled activational events involves the use of pertussis toxin, which ADP-ribosylates GTP-binding proteins and abolishes all chemoattractant mediated events, including Ca^{2+} mobilization and PKC activation.

One of the first G protein–coupled receptors to be characterized was the FMLP receptor. Similar to the FMLP receptor, nearly all of the known chemotactic factors appear to operate via the G_i protein–coupled receptor, including C5a, PAF, and LTB_4, as well as C-C and C-X-C chemokines. In neutrophils, the coupling of chemoattractant receptors, such as the FMLP receptor, has been shown to induce superoxide production and lysosomal enzyme release in addition to mediating directional migration of the cells. The activation of the leukocyte by chemoattractant receptors may play a crucial role not only in movement of the cell to the site of inflammation but also as a method to activate and/or modulate the function of the cell. One of the characteristic events that occurs immediately (within seconds) after coupling of a specific chemotactic receptor is polymerization of cytoskeletal actin proteins that, like Ca^{2+} mobilization, can be blocked by addition of pertussis toxin. This latter response is perhaps a better indication of cellular activation for movement of a cell toward a chemotactic factor than are increases in Ca^{+2} mobilization. However, both techniques appear to indicate receptor occupancy and cellular activation.

C5a RECEPTORS

The first G protein–linked chemotactic receptors to be isolated were the FMLP and C5a receptors. The FMLP and C5a receptors appear to have similar origins since both map to chromosome 19.[6] Both of these receptors have been identified on neutrophils and eosinophils, as well as on mononuclear cell populations. However, these two receptors have different signaling pathways, since desensitization studies indicate that PKC-mediated phosphorylation leads to desensitization of C5a but not FMLP receptors.[3] In both monocytes and neutrophils, FMLP and C5a receptors were differentially regulated. However, only FMLP receptors are readily available for reexpression from intracellular pools.[85] The activation of cells via either the FMLP or C5a receptor up-regulates type II adenylate cyclase[84] and induces superoxide (O_2^-) generation.[38a] Productions of both of these products can drastically influence the response of inflammatory cells. Overall, the C5a receptor, although closely related to other G_i protein–linked receptors, appears to have distinctive regulatory and functional characteristics that separate its function from the closely linked FMLP receptor.

PAF RECEPTORS

PAF is a potent stimulant of multiple cell populations, including platelets, PMNs, eosinophils, basophils, monocytes/macrophages, lymphocytes, endothelial cells, smooth muscle cells, fibroblasts, and nerve cells.[48] The specific binding of PAF via G protein–coupled 40-kD receptors induces the activation of serine/threonine and protein kinases, as well as Ca^{2+} mobilization, but adenylate cyclase is inhibited. It appears that the PAF receptor may signal through multiple G proteins as use of pertussis toxin–inhibited activation of phospholipase C but not phospholipase A2. PAF receptors are found on nearly every cell type and appear to transduce a signal upon exposure to PAF. A study of PAF receptor expression on leukocytes demonstrated expression of functional PAF receptors on monocytes and granulocytes but not on resting or activated T and B lymphocytes.[73]

One interesting observation is that endotoxin (LPS) appears to bind to the PAF receptor and transduce an appropriate signal to induce phospholipase C and Ca^{2+} flux.[55] Although rather high levels of LPS were required to stimulate PAF receptor, this finding may represent a possible event during endotoxemia. However, use of a PAF receptor antagonist does not decrease LPS-mediated TNF-α production. Studies of PAF receptor expression and distribution within the tissues and cells of the body have identified two different PAF receptor transcripts. One of the receptor transcripts was observed in every cell type examined (including leukocytes, heart, lung, and so forth), whereas the second was found in lung, spleen, and kidney, but not in circulating leukocyte populations.[71] These two different transcripts may play a role in surface receptor expression, stability of the transcript, or even the signaling intensity to PAF.

CHEMOKINE RECEPTORS

Much attention has been focused on the receptors and their specific ligands and the activational cascade that results from chemokine interactions with leukocytes. It appears that the receptors for both the C-X-C and C-C chemokines are promiscuous in nature, since they have the ability to bind multiple chemokines within their own subfamily (C-X-C or C-C) but not within the other subfamily (Table 16–2). Initially, C-X-C and C-C chemokine family members were clearly shown to have different receptors. All of the known receptors are seven membrane serpentine receptors and G_i protein linked, with signal transduction events following a similar pathway of activation as previously described.

IL-8 RECEPTORS A AND B

Since the original cloning of the IL-8 receptor genes A and B,[31, 54, 83] a great deal of investigation has gone into which cells possess the various receptors and what function they play. The IL-8 A receptor binds IL-8 with high affinity (kD = 2 nm) but binds the other C-X-C family members, MGSA (GRO-α) and NAP-2, with much lower affinity (kD = 500 nm). In contrast, the IL-8 B receptor binds all three C-X-C chemokines with high affinity (kD = 2 nm) and is therefore considered more promiscuous in nature.[12, 41, 42] The two receptors can independently induce G_i protein–dependent activation of neutrophils, characterized by Ca^{2+} flux and chemotaxis.

Regulation of the IL-8 A and B receptor expression on human neutrophils is consistent with the binding studies since IL-8 down-regulated more than 90% of both the A and B receptors, whereas MSGA down-regulated B but not A receptors.[15] In this same study, it was observed that the A receptor fully recovered on the surface of neutrophils, whereas the B receptor only recovered to about 40% of the original density. These latter findings may have important implications in disease in which neutrophils appear to become desensitized and no longer migrate, even in the presence of high tissue concentrations of C-X-C chemokines. The distribution of these two C-X-C receptors, A and B, on various leukocyte populations may be important for directing the movement of these cells during disease progression. Interestingly, the type B receptor has been identified on nonhematopoietic cells and could undergo phosphorylation of serine residues in a dose- and time-dependent fashion after cell contact with MSGA, suggesting that the type B receptors may have a significant activational role for nonhematopoietic cells.[52] This finding has been supported by the fact that the ELR-containing C-X-C chemokines have been shown to be angiogenic and to induce endothelial cell growth.[81]

TABLE 16–2
CHEMOKINE RECEPTORS (HUMAN)

Receptor	Specificity	Cells Expressing
IL-8 A	IL-8	Leukocytes only
IL-8 B	All ELR-containing C-X-C chemokines	Leukocytes, stromal cells
CC-CKR-1	MIP-1α, MIP-1β, MCP-3, RANTES	Leukocytes, ?
CC-CKR-2	MCP-1, MCP-3	Leukocytes, ?
CC-CKR-3	Eotaxin, RANTES, MCP-3	Eosinophils
CC-CKR-4	MIP-1α, RANTES, MCP-1	Basophils
CC-CKR-5	MIP-1α, MIP-1β, RANTES	Leukocytes
DARC	C-X-C and C-C chemokines	RBC, postcapillary endothelial cells

C-C CHEMOKINE RECEPTORS

The initial experiments examining the expression and function of C-C chemokine receptors utilized Ca^{2+} flux desensitization experiments. Using human monocytes, it was demonstrated that MIP-1α and RANTES share receptors, whereas MCP-1 reacts with its own receptor. Molecular cloning of a human C-C chemokine receptor 1 (CC-CKR-1) identified specificity for MIP-1α and RANTES, moderate binding of MIP-1β, and little or no binding of MCP-1.[58] It also binds MCP-3.[6a, 27a] Interestingly, the CC-CKR-1 receptor showed a high degree of specificity to a protein encoded by the cytomegalovirus (CMV), offering a possible unique evasion technique for the virus due to scavenging of the C-C chemokines by this virally encoded protein. A second human C-C chemokine receptor, CC-CKR-2, was cloned that shows exquisite specificity for MCP-1, moderate specificity for MCP-3, and little or no binding of RANTES, MIP-1α, or MIP-1β.[14] The nature of these two receptor binding patterns follows the original desensitization pattern exhibited in Ca^{2+} flux experiments in monocytes. Three more β chemokine receptors have been cloned. CC-CKR-3[15a] has specificity for chemokines active on eosinophils.[23a] CC-CKR-4[62a] is present on basophils and, therefore, is responsive to histamine releasing factors (see Chapter 6). CC-CKR-5[66a] is a co-receptor on mononuclear cells for HIV binding and ingestion.[21a]

In the murine system, two different C-C receptors have been cloned in eosinophils isolated from IL-5 transgenic mice.[62] The mouse CC-CKR-1 has binding specificities that resemble those found with the human CC-CKR-1, with binding competition studies demonstrating that MIP-1α, RANTES, and MIP-1β all appear to bind to the CC-CKR-1 receptor, whereas JE (MCP-1), TCA-3, KC, or MCP-3 did not compete for MIP-1α binding. A second C-C chemokine specific receptor (CC-CKR-3) was identified in eosinophils isolated from similar IL-5 transgenic mice. This chemokine receptor appears to bind MIP-1α and MIP-1β but not RANTES or MCP-1, suggesting a novel receptor with a different specificity when compared with CC-CKR-1. The isolation of two C-C chemokine receptors on eosinophils that bind MIP-1α with high affinity would suggest that MIP-1α may play an important role in recruitment of eosinophils during murine allergic responses. This latter aspect has been verified using a murine model of allergic airway inflammation in which passive immunization of mice with an anti–MIP-1α antibody decreased airway eosinophilia by more than 50%.[46] The specificity of chemokine responses on particular cell populations appears to vary between species.

Duffy Antigen Receptor for Chemokines (DARC)

Observations have identified the ability of red blood cells (RBC) to bind chemokines.[57] Radiolabeled C-X-C and C-C chemokines reversibly bind to RBC surfaces, demonstrating specific receptor sites numbering 1,000 to 9,000 sites per cell. The chemokine binding on RBC utilizes a Duffy antigen, which is a serpentine seven membrane receptor. DARC represents the only chemokine receptor type that has the ability to bind both C-X-C and C-C chemokines. Interestingly, DARC is also the receptor used by the malarial parasite for entry into the RBC and appears to be absent on some individuals in endemic malarial areas. However, individuals without DARC on RBC express DARC on postcapillary venular endothelial cells, as well as within various regions of the CNS. In contrast to RBC, DARC transfected into nucleated cells allows internalization of bound chemokine, suggesting DARC can signal cells that are expressing this novel receptor.[60] The specific role of this receptor has not yet been defined. However, it may play a significant function in clearance of chemokines from circulation by absorption to RBC, as well as by promoting chemotaxis on postcapillary endothelial cells. The examination of DARC has yielded little information as to whether it has a role in chemotaxis or cellular activation.

FUNCTION OF CHEMOATTRACTANTS IN VIVO

The role of various chemoattractants during disease progression has been analyzed using multiple animal models of inflammation and within human disease. Studies in models such as endotoxemia, as well as allergic models of inflammation, have provided much of our knowledge regarding the specific functions of chemotactic molecules in vivo (Tables 16–3, 16–4). These models have been useful for defining the mechanisms of action of specific chemoattractants, as well as identifying useful antagonists for use in human diseases with similar symptomatic phenotypes.

C5a

The utilization of rodent models of endotoxemia has been key to the identification of multiple molecules that may be beneficial to target for therapeutic intervention. Bacterial-induced sepsis has profound effects in the induction of complement activation and its activation products, C5a in particular. Plasma levels of C5a have been correlated with the number of neutrophils accumulating in the lungs in rabbits during septicemia.[7] A specific complement inhibitor (soluble complement receptor, sCR1), which interferes with assembly of C3 and C5 convertases, significantly reduces neutrophil recruitment, adherence, and degranulation, thus blocking much of the damage induced in septic shock models.[10] Likewise, in ischemia/reperfusion injury, sCR1 blocks pulmonary permeability and edema.[30] In both cases, the inhibition of the complement cascade decreases the degree of tissue accumulation of neutrophils and the subsequent tissue damage. Similar results have also been observed employing an IgG immune complex–induced lung injury. In a rat model, pretreatment with sCR1 attenuated pulmonary damage by decreasing neutrophil influx.[53]

Complement activation and the following chemotactic responses may have a significant role in allergic disease. In atopic asthmatics, an increase in complement activation after allergen challenge leads to an increase in histamine levels, suggesting an exaggerated mediator release due to complement activation products.[63] The expression of complement receptors, CR1 and CR3, is significantly increased on the surface of granulocytes after allergen challenge, but not following histamine or methacholine administration, neither of which induces significant leukocyte recruitment.[4] Treatment of asthmatics with corticosteroids is a very successful clinical approach, resulting in a variety of effects, including the down-regulation of complement receptors on monocytes. However, in corticosteroid-resistant asthmatics, no down-regulation of complement receptors occurs, perhaps suggesting a defect in the regulation of complement receptor expression.[36] During allergic responses, such as those observed in asthmatics, complement appears to function in the augmentation of leukocyte recruitment and local inflammation.

TABLE 16–3
CHEMOATTRACTANTS IN ANIMAL MODELS OF SEPSIS

Chemoattractant	Disease Participation	Effectiveness of Specific Therapeutics
C5a	Neutrophil recruitment and activation, induction of vascular permeability	Blocks neutrophil adherence, neutrophil degranulation, and pulmonary edema
PAF	Alters hemodynamics	Reduces mortality, maintains hemodynamics
LTB_4	Neutrophil accumulation, superoxide release	Blocks leukocyte accumulation, decreases systemic arterial hypotension, arterial hypoxemia, pulmonary arterial hypertension, and pulmonary edema
MIP-2 (IL-8 homologue)	Neutrophil accumulation	Decreases neutrophil accumulation and mortality
MIP-1α, RANTES	Mononuclear cell and neutrophil accumulation	Decreases leukocyte accumulation

TABLE 16–4
CHEMOATTRACTANTS IN ANIMAL MODELS OF ALLERGIC AIRWAY INFLAMMATION

Chemoattractant	Role in Disease	Effectiveness of Specific Therapeutics
C5a	Augments histamine release, increases vascular permeability	No data
PAF	Worsens gas exchange, increased hyperreactivity and histamine release	Inhibits bronchoconstriction, eosinophil accumulation, bronchial hyperreactivity, and lung edema
LTB_4	Leukocyte recruitment, bronchoconstriction, airway hyperreactivity	Inhibits eosinophil accumulation, blocks bronchoconstriction and hyperreactivity
MIP-1α, RANTES, eotaxin	Eosinophil recruitment	Inhibits eosinophil accumulation

PAF

The ability of PAF to recruit various cell populations, as well as augment inflammatory cytokine production, would suggest that it may have significant effects during disease syndromes. In human disease, PAF levels have been identified in patients with sepsis. In patients with adult respiratory distress syndrome, a significant elevation in PAF has been observed in bronchoalveolar lavage fluid samples, correlating with the severity of the disease.[47] In a separate study, PAF serum levels and half-life are increased and prolonged in patients with severe septic responses.[28] Because of this correlation between PAF levels and clinical severity during septicemia, specific PAF antagonists have been used as experimental therapy. In a staphylococcal septicemia model in rabbits, PAF antagonist administration significantly improved survival and demonstrated the ability to maintain the hemodynamic state of the animals.[23] PAF in a multicenter clinical trial has demonstrated safe and effective outcomes in patients at all phases of septicemia. In these studies, there appeared to be a 50% reduction in mortality rates in septic patients receiving PAF antagonist, or compared with a group of patients receiving a placebo.[22] These data support the usefulness of PAF antagonists in clinical settings of septicemia.

PAF may have a role during allergic responses. PAF appears to be released during airway allergen challenges in animal models, as well as within patient populations. Administration of PAF in vivo has demonstrated a general worsening of blood gas exchange in mild asthmatics,[25] whereas administration of PAF to allergic guinea pig models has demonstrated a significant increase in histamine-induced airway hyperreactivity.[51] PAF antagonists in animal models have demonstrated effectiveness by blocking PAF in vivo during asthmatic-like responses. PAF antagonists inhibit allergen-induced bronchoconstriction, airway eosinophil accumulation, lung edema, late-phase responses, and bronchial hyperreactivity. These antagonists likely block both direct and indirect pathways of activation as other mediators, such as leukotrienes, thromboxanes, and histamine release, are inhibited.[29] The fact that PAF antagonists appear to affect a number of mediator release pathways may suggest that they will be potentially potent therapeutic reagents. Clinical trials of PAF antagonists in human asthma, however, have been less promising than leukotriene or lipoxygenase antagonists.

LTB_4

The role of lipid mediators during inflammatory responses has been well established. LTB_4 production in patients at risk for ARDS is increased, correlating directly with the intensity of leukocyte infiltration, superoxide levels, tissue damage, and severity of the clinical picture.[64, 79] Furthermore, LTB_4 levels are significantly elevated preceding pulmonary failure in critically ill patients.[20] In animal models, similar correlations have been observed in endotoxemia and endotoxic shock syndromes. Specific LTB_4 antagonists have demonstrated a significant reduction in endotoxin-induced damage, as determined by decreases in systemic arterial hypotension, pulmonary arterial hypertension, arterial hypoxemia, and pulmonary edema and by neutrophil accumulation.[26, 89]

The release of LTB_4, a 5-LO–induced arachidonic acid metabolite, during allergic responses likely contributes to the overall responsiveness of the airway. Measurement of LTB_4 in asthma patients indicated increased production by alveolar macrophage populations.[88] LTB_4 production is diminished by nedocromil sodium, correlating with decreased leukocyte recruitment.[18] Moreover, a significant rise in arterial blood LTB_4 levels was detected in asthmatic patients during wheezing attacks,[72] further demonstrating increased levels of LTB_4 with these symptoms.

In animal models of allergic airway inflammation, inhibition of LTB_4 generation by specific 5-LO inhibitors has demonstrated decreased leukocyte accumulation within the airways (particularly eosinophils), as well as decreased bronchoconstriction and airway hyperresponsiveness.[1, 13] In human studies, the use of 5-LO inhibitors has not provided similar outcomes. A study using zileuton in asthmatics after allergen challenge showed no significant change either in the late asthmatic response or in airway responsiveness to methacholine.[33] A new 5-LO inhibitor failed to show any beneficial effect in asthmatics after allergen challenge.[56] Overall, even though significant effects were obtained in allergic models by blocking 5-LO function, human clinical studies have been less convincing. Leukotriene antagonists directed to the LTD_4 receptor appear more promising (see Chapter 12).

CHEMOKINES

Chemokines appear to play a central role in recruitment of specific leukocyte populations during multiple diseases. The ability of C-X-C and C-C chemokines to differentially stimulate certain leukocyte populations may reflect the severity and progression or the resolution of an inflammatory response. In a bacterial LPS mouse model of endotoxemia, a C-X-C chemokine, MIP-2 (an IL-8 homologue), was shown to play an important role in the recruitment of neutrophils into the lung and liver in LPS-treated animals. Inhibition of MIP-2 with antibody demonstrated significant reductions in neutrophil accumulation in the lung and decreased mortality, suggesting that this neutrophil-specific chemokine plays a role in the septic response via its ability to specifically recruit neutrophil populations.[78]

In addition to C-X-C chemokines, C-C chemokines MIP-1α and RANTES have also been shown to play a role in LPS models of sepsis in mice.[70, 77, 86, 90] The in vivo blockage of either of these two C-C chemokines significantly reduced lethality but did not abrogate it. The fact that multiple chemotactic factors appear to a play significant part in the progression of the septic response may not be surprising. However, it is clear that an effective therapeutic strategy for treatment of bacterial sepsis should inhibit the influx of inflammatory cells into tissue but without interfering with microbial clearance mechanisms.

During allergic inflammation, the production of chemokines likely contributes to both the recruitment of leukocytes and the activation of surrounding cell populations. The expression and cell source of the chemokines may be very important to the recruitment of leukocytes to the lung. The production of chemokines during asthmatic responses in humans may contribute to the influx of eosinophils. Eosinophils have been implicated as a major effector cell inducing airway injury and subsequent late-phase reactivity in asthmatics.[16, 21] A number of the C-C chemokines appear to preferentially recruit eosinophils in vitro, including RANTES, MIP-1α, MCP-3, and eotaxin.[2, 50, 66, 75] IL-8 also appears to have some activity in eosinophil recruitment.[68] Several chemokines have been found during asthmatic responses in humans. Increased MCP-1 expression is observed in the bronchial tissue of asthmatics (as compared with nonasthmatics). Strong expression of MCP-1 occurs in bronchial epithelial cells.[74] In addition, IL-8 and RANTES expression are increased in asthmatics and down-regulated during corticosteroid treatment.[19]

Through the use of animal models, a more in-depth understanding of the role of C-C chemokines in allergic response has been achieved. The measurement of MIP-1α[46] and RANTES (unpublished data) protein in lung homogenates or BAL fluids in a murine model of allergic airway inflammation has demonstrated increased production of both chemokines during the development of an eosinophilic response. MIP-1α was localized in macrophages and bronchial epithelial cells, whereas RANTES was localized primarily in type II alveolar epithelial cells. This pattern of eosinophil-specific chemokines may help to guide the eosinophil through the multiple cell layers within the lung and airway. When either chemokine was neutralized in vivo, a significant decrease in airway eosinophilia was observed with both anti–MIP-1α ($>$50%)[36] and anti-RANTES ($>$60%) antibody administration. A combination of both antibody therapies in vivo did not further decrease the eosinophil levels significantly, suggesting that other chemoattractants also play a role, such as PAF, MCP-3, and/or eotaxin. Interestingly, passive immunization with anti–MCP-1 did not reduce the influx of eosinophils into the airway, following the original chemokine specificity for the response.

MIP-1α and RANTES appear to have a specific effect on eosinophils since mononuclear cell accumulation within the lung is not decreased when these two chemokines were neutralized. In contrast, neutralization of MCP-1 significantly attenuates recruitment of lymphocytes into the lung and airway (unpublished data). The participation of these specific chemokines for eosinophil recruitment appears to follow the binding patterns of chemokine receptors CC-CKR-1 and CC-CKR-3, which have been isolated.[62] In a guinea pig model of allergic airway inflammation, the isolation and characterization of eotaxin (a novel C-C chemokine) may represent the most potent eosinophil-specific chemokine.[35] The relative potency and effectiveness of eotaxin in other animal models and within human disease have yet to be assessed; however, human eotaxin has been identified. Animal models will begin to outline the specific role that C-C chemokines play in allergic airway inflammation, leading to lymphocyte and eosinophil recruitment.

SUMMARY

The chemotaxis of leukocytes during inflammatory/immune reactions requires multiple steps and participation by many chemotactic factors. The use of specific chemoattractants during various phases of disease progression can dictate not only the type of cell to be recruited but also the outcome on the surrounding cells in the areas of recruitment. Chemotactic molecules may provide significant activation of cell populations, thus augmenting the response. The specific inhibition of particular chemoattractant molecules during inflammatory events may provide beneficial therapeutic outcomes, although it is likely that during any inflammatory response multiple mediators are involved, and the inhibition of a single chemoattractant molecule may not offer complete control of the response. Future studies should outline the role of particular chemoattractants during various diseases and the effectiveness of particular therapeutics designed to inhibit the various chemoattractants.

REFERENCES

1. Abraham WM, Ahmed A, Cortes A, et al: The 5-lipoxygenase inhibitor zileuton blocks antigen-induced late airway responses, inflammation and airway hyperresponsiveness in allergic sheep. Eur J Pharmacol 217:119–126, 1992.
2. Alam R, Stafford S, Forsythe P, et al: RANTES is a chemotactic and activating factor for human eosinophils. J Immunol 150:3442–3448, 1993.
3. Ali H, Richardson RM, Tomhave ED, et al: Differences in phosphorylation of formylpeptide and C5a chemoattractant receptors correlate with differences in desensitization. J Biol Chem 268:24247–24254, 1993.
4. Arm JP, Walport MJ, Lee TH: Expression of complement receptors type 1 (CR1) and type 3 (CR3) on circulating granulocytes in experimentally provoked asthma. J Allergy Clin Immunol 83(3):649–655, 1989.
5. Bacon KB, Premack BA, Gardner P, Schall TJ: Activation of dual T cell signaling pathways by the chemokine RANTES. Science 269:1727–1730, 1995.
6. Bao L, Gerard NP, Eddy RL, et al: Mapping of genes for the human C5a receptor (C5AR), human FMLP receptor (FPR), and two FMLP receptor homologue orphan receptors (FPRH1, FPRH2) to chromosome 19. Genomics 13:437–440, 1992.
6a. Ben-Baruch A, Xu L, Young PR, et al: Monocyte Chemotactic protein-3 (MCP3) interacts with multiple leukocyte receptors. J Biol Chem 270:22123, 1995.
7. Bergh K, Olsen PO, Halgunset J, Iversen OJ: Complement activation and pulmonary dysfunction in experimental *Escherichia coli* septicemia. Acta Anaestheiol Scand 35:267–274, 1991.

8. Bischoff SC, Krieger M, Brunner T, et al: RANTES and related chemokines activate human basophil granulocytes through different G protein-coupled receptors. Eur J Immunol 23:761–767, 1993.
9. Bokoch GM: Chemoattractant signaling and leukocyte activation. Blood 86:1649–1660, 1995.
10. Bone RC: Inhibitors of complement and neutrophils: a critical evaluation of their role in the treatment of sepsis. Crit Care Med 20:891–898, 1992.
11. Camussi G, Aglietta M, Malavasi F, et al: The release of platelet-activating factor from human endothelial cells in culture. J Immunol 131(5):2397–2403, 1983.
12. Ceretti DP, Kozlosky CJ, Vanden Bos T, et al: Molecular characteristics of receptors for human interleukin-8, GRO/melanoma growth-stimulatory activity and neutrophil activating peptide-2. Mol Immunol 30:359–367, 1993.
13. Chabot-Fletcher MC, Underwood DC, Breton JJ, et al: Pharmacological characterization of SB 202235, a potent and selective 5-lipoxygenase inhibitor; effects in models of allergic asthma. J Pharmacol Exp Ther 273:1147–1155, 1995.
14. Charo IF, Myers SJ, Herman A, et al: Molecular cloning and functional expression of two monocyte chemoattractant protein-1 receptors reveals alternative splicing of the carboxyl-terminal tails. Proc Natl Acad Sci USA 91:2752–2761, 1994.
15. Chuntharapai A, Kim KJ: Regulation of the IL-8 receptor A/B by IL-8: possible functions of each receptor. J Immunol 155:2587–2594, 1995.
15a. Combadiero C, Ahuja SK, Murphy PM: Cloning and functional expression of a human eosinophil CC chemokine receptor. J Biol Chem 270:16491, 1995.
16. Corrigan CJ, Kay AB: T cells and eosinophils in the pathogenesis of asthma. Immunol Today 13:501–507, 1992.
17. Daffern PJ, Pfeifer PH, Ember JA, Hugli TE: C3a is a chemotaxin for human eosinophils but not for neutrophils. I. C3a stimulation of neutrophils is secondary to eosinophil activation. J Exp Med 181(6):2119–2127, 1995.
18. Damon M, Chavis C, Daures JP, et al: Increased generation of the arachidonic metabolites LTB4 and 5-HETE by human alveolar macrophages in patients with asthma: effect in vitro of nedocromil sodium. Eur Respir J 2:202–209, 1989.
19. Davies RJ, Wang JH, Trigg CJ, Devalia JL: Expression of granulocyte/macrophage-colony-stimulating factor, interleukin-8 and RANTES in the bronchial epithelium of mild asthmatics is down-regulated by inhaled beclomethasone dipropionate. Int Arch Allergy Immunol 107:428–429, 1995.
20. Davis JM, Meyer JD, Barie PS, et al: Elevated production of neutrophil leukotriene B_4 precedes pulmonary failure in critically ill surgical patients. Surg Gynecol Obstet 170:495–500, 1990.
21. Del Prete G: Human Th1 and Th2 lymphocytes: their role in the pathophysiology of atopy. Allergy 47:450–455, 1992.
21a. Deng H-K, Liu R, Ellmeier W, et al: Identification of a major co-receptor for primary isolates of HIV-1. Nature 381:661, 1996.
22. Dhainaut JF, Tenaillon A, Le Tulzo Y, et al: Platelet-activating factor receptor antagonist BN 52021 in the treatment of severe sepsis: a randomized, double blind, placebo-controlled, multicenter clinical trial. BN 52201 sepsis study group. Crit Care Med 22:1720–1728, 1994.
23. Dirkes KBH, Harris RJ, Connolly SD, et al: Platelet activating factor-antagonist improves survival in experimental staphylococcal septicemia. J Pediatr Surg 29:1055–1058, 1994.
23a. Daugherty BL, Siciliano SJ, DeMartino JA, et al: Cloning, expression, and characterization of the human eosinophil eotaxin receptor. J Exp Med 183:2349, 1996.
24. Erger RA, Casale TB: Comparative studies indicate that platelet-activating factor is a relatively weak eosinophilotactic factor. Am J Respir Cell Mol Biol 12:65–70, 1995.
25. Felez MA, Roca J, Barbera JA, et al: Inhaled platelet-activating factor worsens gas exchange in mild asthma. Am J Respir Crit Care Med 150:369–373, 1994.
26. Fink MP, O'Sullivan BP, Menconi MJ, et al: A novel leukotriene B_4-receptor antagonist in endotoxin shock: a prospective, controlled trial in a porcine model. Crit Care Med 21:1825–1837, 1993.
27. Foreman KE, Vaporciyan AA, Bonish BK, et al: C5a-induced expression of P-selectin in endothelial cells. J Clin Invest 94:1147–1155, 1994.
27a. Franci C, Wong LM, Damme JV, et al: Monocyte chemotactic protein-3 but not monocyte chemotatic protein-2 is a functional ligand of the human monocyte chemoattractant protein-1 receptor. J Immunol 154:6511-6517, 1995.
28. Graham RM, Stephens CJ, Silvester W, et al: Plasma degradation of platelet-activating factor in severely ill patients with clinical sepsis. Crit Care Med 22:204–212, 1994.
29. Heuer HO: The effects of hetrazepine PAF antagonists in preclinical models of asthma. Agents Actions Suppl 34:229–245, 1991.
30. Hill J, Lindsay TF, Oritz F, et al: Soluble complement receptor type 1 ameliorates the local and remote organ injury after intestinal ischemia-reperfusion in the rat. J Immunol 149:1723–1728, 1992.
31. Holmes WE, Lee J, Kuang WJ, et al: Structure and functional expression of a human interleukin-8 receptor. Science 253:1278–1280, 1991.
32. Houck JC, Chang CM: The purification and characterization of a lymphokine chemotactic for lymphocytes—lymphotactin. Inflammation 2:105–113, 1977.
33. Hui KP, Taylor IK, Taylor GW, et al: Effect of a 5-lipoxygenase inhibitor on leukotriene generation and airway responses after allergen challenge in asthmatic patients. Thorax 46:184–189, 1991.
34. Imhof BA, Dunon D: Leukocyte migration and adhesion. Adv Immunol 58:345–416, 1995.
35. Jose PJ, Griffiths-Johnson DA, Collins PD, et al: Eotaxin: a potent eosinophil chemoattractant cytokine detected in a guinea pig model of allergic airways inflammation. J Exp Med 179:881–887, 1994.
36. Kay AB, Diaz P, Carmicheal J, Grant IW: Corticosteroid-resistant chronic asthma and monocyte complement receptors. Clin Exp Immunol 44(3):576–580, 1981.
37. Kelner GS, Kennedy J, Bacon KB, et al: Lymphotactin: a cytokine that represents a new class of chemokine. Science 266:1395–1399, 1994.
38. Kennedy J, Kelner GS, Kleyensteuber S, et al: Molecular cloning and functional characterization of human lymphotactin. J Immunol 155:203–209, 1995.
38a. Kocan GP, Partis RA, Mueller RA, et al: Contrasting effects of two arachidonate 5-lipoxygenase inhibitors on formyl-methionyl-leucyl-phenylalanine (fMLP) and complement fragment 5a induced human neutrophil superoxide generation. Biochem Pharmacol 47:1029–1037, 1994.
39. Kuna P, Reddigari SR, Rucinski D, et al: Monocyte chemotactic and activating factor is a potent histamine-releasing factor for human basophils. J Exp Med 175:489–493, 1992.
40. Kuna P, Reddigari SR, Schall TJ, et al: Characterization of the human basophil response to cytokines, growth factors, and histamine releasing factors of the intercrine/chemokine family. J Immunol 150:1932–1943, 1993.
41. Lee J, Kuang W-J, Rince GC, Wood WI: Characterization of complementary DNA clones encoding the rabbit IL-8 receptor. J Immunol 148:1261–1269, 1992.
42. Loetscher P, Seitz M, Clark-Lewis I, et al: Both interleukin-8 receptors independently mediate chemotaxis. Jurkat cells transfected with IL-8R1 or IL-8R2 migrate in response to IL-8, GRO-alpha and NAP-2. FEBS Lett 341:187–192, 1994.
43. Lukacs NW, Strieter RM, Chensue SW, Kunkel SL: Activation and regulation of chemokines in allergic airway inflammation. J Leukoc Biol 59:13–18, 1996.
44. Lukacs NW, Strieter RM, Elner VM, et al: Intracellular adhesion molecule-1 mediates the expression of monocyte-derived MIP-1a during monocyte-endothelial cell interactions. Blood 83:1174, 1994.
45. Lukacs NW, Strieter RM, Elner V, et al: Monocyte-endothelial cell interactions induce chemokine production, IL-8 and MCP-1. Blood 86:2767–2773, 1995.
46. Lukacs NW, Strieter RM, Shaklee CL, et al: Macrophage inflammatory protein-1 α influences eosinophil recruitment in antigen-specific airway inflammation. Eur J Immunol 25:245–251, 1995.
47. Matsumoto K, Taki F, Kondoh Y, et al: Platelet-activating factor in bronchoalveolar lavage fluid of patients with adult respiratory distress syndrome. Clin Exp Pharmacol Physiol 19:509–515, 1992.
48. McCall CE, O'Flaherty JT: Platelet-activating factor and lung. In Phan SH, Thrall RS (eds): Pulmonary Fibrosis. Marcel Dekker, New York, 1995, pp 675–695.
49. Metinko AP, Kunkel SL, Standiford TJ, Strieter RM: Anoxia-hyperoxia induces monocyte-derived interleukin-8. J Clin Invest 90:791–798, 1992.
50. Meurer R, Van Riper G, Feeney W, et al: Formation of eosinophilic and monocytic intradermal inflammatory sites in the dog by injection of human RANTES but not monocyte chemoattractant protein 1, human macrophage inflammatory protein 1 alpha, or human interleukin 8. J Exp Med 178:1913–1921, 1993.
51. Morooka S, Uchida M, Imanishi N: Platelet-activating factor (PAF) plays

an important role in the immediate asthmatic response in guinea-pig by augmenting the response to histamine. Br J Pharmacol 105:756–762, 1992.

52. Mueller SG, Schraw WP, Richmond A: Melanoma growth stimulatory activity enhances the phosphorylation of the class II interleukin-8 receptor in non-hematopoietic cells. J Biol Chem 269:1973–1980, 1994.
53. Mulligan MS, Yeh CG, Rudolph AR, Ward PA: Protective effects of soluble CR1 in complement- and neutrophil-mediated tissue injury. J Immunol 148:1479–1485, 1992.
54. Murphy PH, Tiffany HL: Cloning of complementary DNA encoding a functional human interleukin-8 receptor. Science 253:1280–1283, 1991.
55. Nakamura M, Honda Z, Waga I, et al: Endotoxin induces Ca^{2+} signaling via platelet-activating factor receptor. FEBS Lett 314:125–129, 1992.
56. Nasser SM, Bell GS, Hawksworth RJ, et al: Effect of the 5-lipoxygenase inhibitor on allergen-induced early and late asthmatic responses. Thorax 49:743–748, 1994.
57. Neote K, Darbonne W, Ogez J, et al: Identification of a promiscuous inflammatory peptide receptor on the surface of red blood cells. J Biol Chem 268:12247–12249, 1993.
58. Neote K, DiGregorio D, Mak JY, et al: Molecular cloning, functional expression, and signaling characteristics of a C-C chemokine receptor. Cell 72:415–425, 1993.
59. Oppenheim JJ, Zachariae COC, Mukaida N, Matsushima K: Properties of the novel proinflammatory "intercrine" cytokine family. Annu Rev Immunol 9:617, 1991.
60. Peiper SC, Wang ZX, Neote K, et al: The Duffy antigen/receptor for chemokines (DARC) is expressed in endothelial cell of Duffy negative individuals who lack the erythrocyte receptor. J Exp Med 181:1311–1317, 1995.
61. Pereira HA: CAP37, a neutrophil-derived multifunctional inflammatory mediator. J Leukoc Biol 57:805–812, 1995.
62. Post TW, Bozic CR, Rothenberg ME, et al: Molecular characterization of two murine eosinophil b chemokine receptors. J Immunol 155:5299–5305, 1995.
62a. Power CA, Meyers A, Nemeth K, et al: Molecular cloning and functional expression of a novel CC chemokine receptor cDNA from a human basophil cell line. J Biol Chem 270: 19495, 1995.
63. Radermecker M, Maldague MP, Gustin M, et al: Increased complement-mediated leukocytic histamine release in atopics. Int Arch Allergy Appl Immunol 68(4):365–370, 1982.
64. Rivkind AI, Siegel JH, Guadalupi P, Littleton M: Sequential patterns of eicosanoid, platelet, and neutrophil interactions in the evolution of the fulminant post-traumatic adult respiratory distress syndrome. Ann Surg 210:372–373, 1989.
65. Rola-Peszczynski M: LTB4 and PAF in the cytokine network. In Wong PY-K, Serhan CN (eds): Cell-Cell Interactions in the Release of Inflammatory Mediators. Plenum Press, New York, 1992.
66. Rot A, Krieger M, Brunner T, et al: RANTES and macrophage inflammatory protein 1α induce the migration and activation of normal human eosinophil granulocytes. J Exp Med 176:1489–1495, 1992.
66a. Samson M, Labbe Q, Mollereau C, et al: Molecular cloning and functional expression of a new human CC-chemokine receptor gene. Biochemistry 35:3362, 1996.
67. Schall TJ: Biology of the RANTES/SIS cytokine family. Cytokine 3:165–183, 1991.
68. Schweizer RC, Welmers BAC, Raaijmakers JAM, et al: RANTES- and interleukin-8–induced responses in normal human eosinophils: effects of priming with interleukin-5. Blood 83:3697–3704, 1994.
69. Selvan RS, Butterfield JH, Krangel MS: Expression of multiple chemokine genes by a human mast cell leukemia. J Biol Chem 269:13893–13898, 1994.
70. Shanley TP, Schmal H, Friedl HP, et al: Role of macrophage inflammatory protein-1 alpha (MIP-1 alpha) in acute lung injury in rats. J Immunol 154(9):4793–4802, 1994.
71. Shimizu T, Mutoh H, Waga I, et al: Structure and function of platelet-activating factor receptor. In Navarro J (ed): Molecular Basis of Inflammation. Ares-Serono Symposia Publications, Rome, 1994.
72. Shindo K, Matsumoto Y, Hirai Y, et al: Measurement of leukotriene B_4 in arterial blood of asthmatic patients during wheezing attacks. J Intern Med 228:91–96, 1990.
73. Simon HU, Tsao PW, Siminovitch KA, et al: Functional platelet-activating factor receptors are expressed by monocytes and granulocytes but not by resting or activated T and B lymphocytes from normal individuals or patients with asthma. J Immunol 153(1):364–377, 1994.
74. Sousa AR, Lane SJ, Nakhosteen JA, et al: Increased expression of the monocyte chemoattractant protein-1 in bronchial tissue from asthmatic subjects. Am J Respir Cell Mol Biol 10:142–147, 1994.
75. Sozzani S, Zhou D, Locati M, et al: Receptors and transduction pathways for monocyte chemotactic protein-2 and monocyte chemotactic protein-3: similarities and differences with MCP-1. J Immunol 152:3615–3622, 1994.
76. Springer TA, Dustin ML, Kishimoto TK, Martin SD: The lymphocyte function-associated LFA-1, CD2, and LFA-3 molecules: cell adhesion receptors of the immune system. Annu Rev Immunol 5:223, 1987.
77. Standiford TJ, Kunkel SL, Lukacs NW, et al: Macrophage inflammatory protein-1a mediates lung leukocyte recruitment, lung capillary leak, and early mortality in murine endotoxemia. J Immunol 155:1515–1524, 1995.
78. Standiford TJ, Strieter RM, Lukacs NW, Kunkel SL: Neutralization of IL-10 increases lethality in endotoxemia: cooperative effects of macrophage inflammatory protein-2 and tumor necrosis factor. J Immunol 155: 2222–2229, 1995.
79. Stephenson AH, Lonigro AJ, Hyers TM, et al: Increased concentrations of leukotrienes in bronchoalveolar lavage fluid of patients with ARDS or at risk for ARDS. Am Rev Respir Dis 138:714–719, 1988.
80. Strieter RM, Kunkel SL, Bone RC: Role of tumor necrosis factor-alpha in disease states and inflammation. Crit Care Med 21(10 suppl):S447–463, 1993.
81. Strieter RM, Polverini PJ, Arenberg DA, et al: Role of C-X-C chemokines as regulators of angiogenesis in lung cancer. J Leukoc Biol 57:752–762, 1995.
82. Takafuji S, Tadokoro K, Ito K, Dahinden CA: Degranulation from human eosinophils stimulated with C3a and C5a. Int Arch Allergy Immunol 104(suppl 1) 1:27–29, 1994.
83. Thomas KM, Taylor L, Navarro J: The interleukin-8 receptor is encoded by a neutrophil-specific cDNA clone, F3R. J Biol Chem 266:14839–14841, 1991.
84. Tsu RC, Allen RA, Wong YH: Stimulation of type II adenyl cyclase by chemoattractant formyl peptide and C5a receptors. Mol Pharmacol 47:835–841, 1995.
85. Van Epps DE, Simpson SJ, Chenoweth DE: C5a and formyl peptide receptor regulation on human monocytes. J Leuk Biol 51:393–399, 1992.
86. VanOtteren GM, Strieter RM, Kunkel SL, et al: Compartmentalized expression of RANTES in a murine model of endotoxemia. J Immunol 154:1900–1908, 1995.
87. Ward PA: Biological activities of the complement system. Ann Allergy 30(6):307–314, 1972.
88. Wardlaw AJ, Hay H, Cromwell O, et al: Leukotrienes, LTC4 and LTB4, in bronchoalveolar lavage in bronchial asthma and other respiratory diseases. J Allergy Clin Immunol 84:19–24, 1989.
89. Woolert PS, Menconi MJ, O'Sullivan BP, et al: LY255283, a novel leukotriene B_4 receptor antagonist, limits activation of neutrophils and prevents acute lung injury induced by endotoxin in pigs. Surgery 114:191–198, 1993.
90. Xing Z, Jordana M, Kirpalani H, et al: Cytokine expression by neutrophils and macrophages in vivo: endotoxin induces tumor necrosis factor-a, macrophage inflammatory protein-2, interleukin-1b, and interleukin-6 but not RANTES or transforming growth factor-b1 mRNA expression in acute lung inflammation. Am J Respir Cell Mol Biol 10:148–156, 1994.
91. Zeck-Kapp G, Kroegel C, Riede UN, Kapp A: Mechanisms of human eosinophil activation by complement protein C5a and platelet-activating factor: similar functional responses are accompanied by different morphologic alterations. Allergy 50(1):34–47, 1995.

17 Late Allergic Responses

STEPHEN R. DURHAM A. BARRY KAY

Local provocation with allergen in sensitive subjects results in a characteristic early response with a time course that is maximal at 15 to 30 minutes, resolving within 1 to 2 hours. This is evident in the skin as a classic wheal and flare reaction; in the nose as itch, sneezing, watery discharge, and obstruction; and in the bronchi as wheezing, coughing, and chest tightness. Depending on the level of allergen sensitivity of the subject and the dose of allergen administered, a late allergic response occurs at 6 to 12 hours, generally resolving within 24 to 48 hours (Fig. 17–1). The clinical relevance and pathophysiology of late responses have been extensively reviewed.[48, 50, 77, 94, 102, 114]

With the exception of occupational-type exposures, the late response is rarely used for diagnostic purposes. However, the late response has been used widely as a clinical model for the investigation of basic mechanisms of human allergic disease and in the evaluation of potential new therapeutic agents.[49, 94, 114]

The clinical relevance (and limitations) of late responses is reviewed here in the context of provocation testing of the bronchi, skin, and nose. An overview of pathophysiologic mechanisms includes an evaluation of mediators, cells, and cytokines. Based on controlled studies of blood, lavage, and tissue biopsy samples, a hypothesis is presented regarding the role of mediators, cells, and cytokines in the development of late responses. The practical implications of these findings and their relevance to future therapeutic strategies are considered.

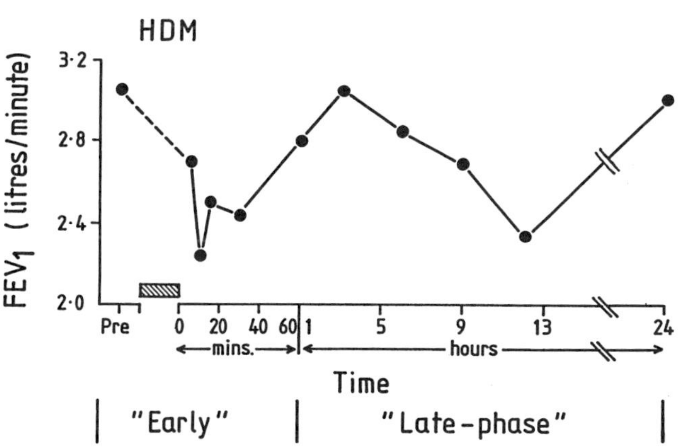

FIGURE 17–1. Time course of changes in forced expiratory volume in 1 second (FEV_1) in a patient who developed a dual asthmatic response after inhalation challenge with house dust mite (HDM).

CLINICAL FEATURES

LATE ASTHMATIC RESPONSES

Allergen provocation in the laboratory is artificial when compared with natural exposure. Inhalation challenge involves inhalation of high concentrations of allergen in solution over a short period, which is in contrast to natural exposure to low concentrations of particulate allergen over months or years. However, there are no satisfactory animal models of asthma, and provocation testing allows controlled exposure of the target organ in humans in order to test mechanisms and evaluate new drugs.

Methods

The two most commonly used methods for inhalation testing involve the tidal breathing method and the dosimeter method.[28, 37, 134] Both involve stepwise incremental inhalations of allergen at 15-minute intervals, the end point being a 20% fall in FEV_1. It is essential to standardize methodology, including use of standardized allergen extracts, calibration of nebulizer output, and duration of inhalation.[82] Patients should be free of allergen exposure, recent infection, and any medication standardized in relation to repeated test measurements. Despite these precautions the reproducibility of the late response after challenge is poorly documented.[25] In one study, the coefficient of repeatability was 23% with a bias of less than 3%.[149] In another study, the variability of the late response was less than 50% in only 7 of 10 subjects on repeat testing.[35] Further reproducibility studies are required.

Prevalence

The end point for provocation testing in the majority of studies has been arbitrarily defined as a 20% fall in FEV_1. In adults so tested,[16, 131] approximately 50% develop a single early asthmatic response (see Fig. 17–1) and 50% develop a

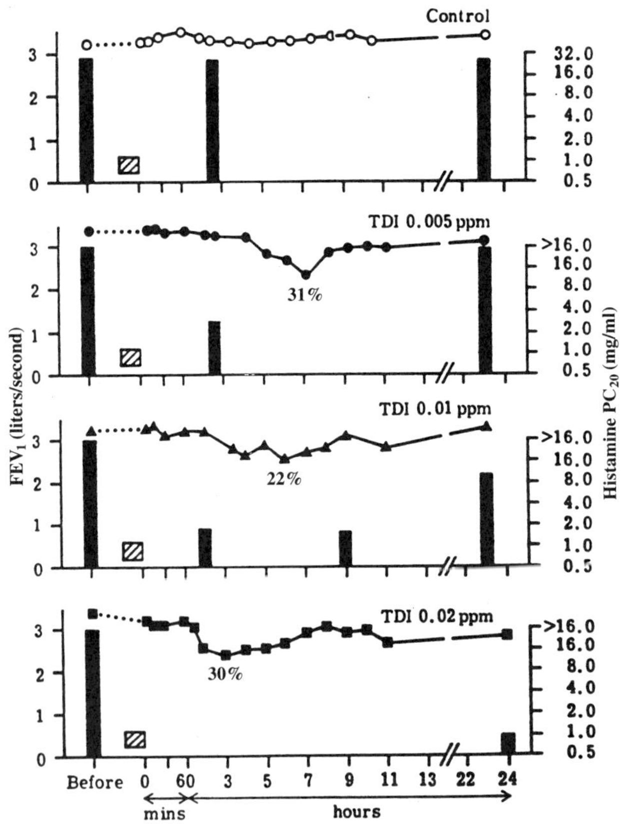

FIGURE 17–2. Increases in airway responsiveness and late asthmatic responses. Occupational-type bronchial provocation in a subject exposed to varnish containing increased amounts of toluene diisocyanate resulted in isolated late asthmatic responses (circle, triangle, square) associated with increased airway responsiveness (decreases in histamine PC_{20}) at 3 and 24 hours. PC_{20} = provocation concentration of inhaled histamine that caused a 20% decrease in FEV_1 (vertical bar). TDI ppm = air concentrations of toluene diisocyanate in exposure chamber (parts per million). (From Durham SR, Graneek BJ, Hawkins R, et al: The temporal relationship between increases in airway responsiveness to histamine and late asthmatic responses induced by occupational agents. J Allergy Clin Immunol 79:398–406, 1987.)

dual or isolated late response, although one study reported a prevalence of 24%.[121] In children, the prevalence of late responses is somewhat higher, approximately 70%.[127, 159] However, the late response is allergen dose dependent. In subjects who underwent repeated allergen challenge at 1-week intervals, isolated late responses became evident at lower doses of allergen than did the immediate response in the majority of subjects.[79] Similarly, isolated late responses may commonly occur after occupational-type exposure to sensitizers encountered in the workplace (Fig. 17–2).[124] The occurrence of definite late responses after nonspecific challenges such as exercise or fog challenge (with ultrasonically nebulized distilled water) is controversial.[20, 21, 26, 55, 68, 80, 83, 101, 140, 141, 156, 166] If they do occur independently of any diurnal change in lung function, they are uncommon and do not result in increased bronchial responsiveness, the hallmark of late responses after specific (allergen) challenge.

Physiology

Late asthmatic responses are generally recorded 3 to 9 hours after challenge. However, studies that followed patients throughout a 24-hour period suggest that peak airway narrowing during late responses occurs at approximately 15 hours.[89, 104] Furthermore, late responses are more marked (compared with a control day) when the timing of allergen challenge is in the evening rather than the morning.[89, 105]

The site of air flow obstruction during late responses has not been clearly defined. In a study of children sensitive to house dust mite, the late response was associated with a disproportionate increase in residual volume/thoracic gas volume ratio compared with the early response for a comparable decrease in peak expiratory flow.[159] By use of helium oxygen flow-volume loop studies before and after challenge, the density dependency of airflow was markedly decreased during early responses but not during late responses,[103] compatible with small airway obstruction during late responses. In the same study, the severity of the late response (measured by changes in FEV_1) was closely related to changes in mid-expiratory flow rates (Vmax 50). One study identified that the perception of breathlessness during the late response was much less than that experienced during the early response after allergen inhalation.[147] These features, unlike the early response, are more in keeping with day-to-day clinical asthma (Table 17–1).

Increased Airway Responsiveness

Cockcroft originally described an increase in bronchial responsiveness to histamine 24 hours after allergen challenge following the late response.[38] Cartier subsequently showed that this increase in responsiveness was commonly associated (although not always[98]) only with those patients who developed late responses after inhalation challenge with allergen. These increases in responsiveness were observed to persist for several days or occasionally even weeks after a single allergen exposure.[27] Subsequent studies showed that late responses were accompanied by an increase in airway histamine responsiveness at 3 hours,[14, 52, 53, 157] that is, before the onset of the late response (see Fig. 17–2). This early increase in responsiveness correlated with the magnitude of the subsequent late response[52] and accompanying changes in blood eosinophil counts.[39] These observations suggested that the tissue events that underlie the late response may occur before the late response is clinically apparent. The results supported the view that airway inflammatory events after allergen exposure may occur in a matter of hours even in the absence of airflow obstruction. This increase in responsiveness predisposes to reactions to nonspecific irritants such as cold air and exercise and lowers the threshold to subsequent allergen exposure, thereby, as suggested by Cockcroft,[33] inducing a vicious cycle of bronchial hyperresponsiveness to both allergic and nonspecific stimuli.

TABLE 17–1
CLINICAL RELEVANCE OF LATE ASTHMATIC RESPONSES

- More prolonged than early responses
- Associated with lung hyperinflation and small airways involvement
- Associated with increases in airway responsiveness
- Inhibitable by anti-inflammatory drugs and immunotherapy

TABLE 17–2
EFFECT OF DRUGS GIVEN IMMEDIATELY BEFORE CHALLENGE ON ALLERGEN-INDUCED ASTHMA

	Early Response	Late Response
Corticosteroids	No effect	Inhibit
Cromolyn sodium	Inhibits	Inhibits
Nedocromil	Inhibits	Inhibits
β-Sympathomimetics	Inhibit	Partial reversal only
Theophylline	Inhibits	Partial/no effect
Antihistamine	Partial	No effect
Antileukotrienes	Inhibit	Inhibit
Cyclosporin A	No effect	Inhibits

Influence of Drugs

The effect of drugs taken immediately before challenge on allergen-induced early and late asthmatic responses is summarized in Table 17–2. β-Sympathomimetic drugs inhibit the early response but have at best only a partial effect on the late response,[60, 72, 117, 150] which may be attributable to either functional antagonism or possibly mast cell stabilization. Although one study suggested that the long-acting β-agonist salmeterol may inhibit the late response,[148] reappraisal of the data suggests that any inhibition may have been due to prolonged bronchodilation. Subsequent studies demonstrated that salmeterol, at least in vivo, was not associated with anti-inflammatory effects.[145] Disodium cromoglycate[17, 100, 123] (and nedocrimal sodium) inhibits both early and late responses. Corticosteroids taken immediately before challenge do not inhibit the early response[17, 34, 35, 116, 123] but have a profound effect on the late response. Both corticosteroids and disodium cromoglycate inhibit associated increases in airway histamine responsiveness.[35] Atropine was without effect on late responses after toluene diisocyanate challenge.[115]

The effect of theophylline on late responses is controversial.[36, 40, 119, 167] A recent study has demonstrated that even low-dose theophylline may have anti-inflammatory properties, although further studies are required.[143] Inhaled furosemide has been shown to inhibit the late response without modifying associated increases in airway methacholine responsiveness.[15] In contrast, nonsteroidal anti-inflammatory drugs (indomethacin) inhibited induced increases in responsiveness but did not alter the late response.[85] Antihistamines, in general, have not shown an inhibitory effect on the late response,[31] although one study involving intramuscular mepyramine resulted in a partial inhibition of the late response.[17] Azelastine was also effective in inhibiting early and late asthmatic responses after allergen challenge,[128] presumably by mechanisms independent of histamine antagonism. One study showed that a PAF antagonist was effective,[131] although this was not subsequently confirmed.[91] Another study demonstrated that a leukotriene C_4 antagonist[10] was effective in inhibiting early and late responses.

Immunosuppressive agents have also been shown to antagonize late asthmatic responses. Methotrexate was effective in inhibiting late responses in a guinea pig model.[69] In a double-blind trial, more than a 50% inhibition of the late response, but not the early response, was observed in allergic asthmatics after pretreatment with cyclosporin A.[137] Cyclosporin A has been previously shown to be effective in patients with severe steroid-dependent asthma. In both rodent and primate models of the late response, antibodies directed against intercellular adhesion molecule-1 (ICAM-1) inhibited the late response and associated eosinophilia and increased bronchial responsiveness.

In general, those drugs that inhibit late responses may have anti-inflammatory properties and be of value in asthma prophylaxis. The use of the late response is limited by the variability of the test, even in skilled hands, and false positives may occur. For example, implementation of a fish oil diet inhibited late responses after allergen challenge,[4] whereas two double-blind, placebo-controlled trials of a fish oil diet in mild and moderately severe asthma were ineffective in improving symptoms or lung function tests.[3, 87] In general, treatments that do not inhibit the late response are unlikely to have prophylactic value in asthma, whereas those that do inhibit the late response may be effective.

Influence of Immunotherapy

Warner examined the influence of hyposensitization treatment on late asthmatic responses in mite-sensitive children.[160] Patients were challenged with house dust mite extract by inhalation before and after 12 months of subcutaneous injections. The occurrence of late responses in the placebo group was unchanged. In contrast, in children who showed symptomatic improvement following immunotherapy, the late response was inhibited following a repeat allergen challenge. This effect of immunotherapy in suppressing late responses has been confirmed in several studies in the lung and skin.[61, 113, 118, 151, 152]

Predictive Factors

Factors predicting late responses are not entirely clear. As mentioned previously, allergen dose is important.[79, 93] Another factor seems to be the level of allergen sensitivity of the subject. For example, Boulet demonstrated that those subjects who developed a late cutaneous response following a small dose of intradermal allergen were more likely to develop a late asthmatic response after allergen inhalation challenge.[19] The occurrence and size of late responses may vary according to the timing of the challenge, with larger late responses occurring compared with the corresponding clock time on a control day when challenge is performed in the evening compared with a morning inhalation challenge.[89, 105] The magnitude of the early response is largely predictable on the basis of the level of airway responsiveness to histamine and allergen sensitivity as determined by skin prick testing or IgE concentrations in serum.[37] No such simple relationship exists for the late response.

In multiple regression analysis, one study suggested that allergen dose, the size of the early response, the level of IgE in serum, and the level of bronchial responsiveness account for the variability of the late response.[42] The late response may occur entirely independently of an early response and at lower allergen concentrations. One study suggested that endogenous cortisol responses may be important,[112] although others have not confirmed this.[55] Thus it is not possible to predict the occurrence of late responses in individual subjects. Paradoxically, patients with hyperresponsive airways (after histamine or methacholine challenge) may be less likely to develop a late response after allergen because of restriction of the dose of allergen that can be given owing to the occurrence of an early response at lower allergen concentrations. In two studies where the early response was inhibited by antihistamines or β-antagonists that enabled higher doses of allergen to be administered, late responses appeared in previous single early responders following allergen challenge.[92, 93]

The traditional view has been that late responses occur as an all-or-nothing event. However, studies have indicated that both within and between subjects development of late responses occurs as a spectrum. It seems likely that all sensitive subjects would eventually develop late responses after high doses of allergen. Late asthmatic responses have also been reported following nonspecific challenges such as exercise[68, 156] and inhalation of nebulized distilled water.[26, 101] However, their occurrence is controversial.[21, 83, 166] Documented late responses after exercise that are not attributable to diurnal variability are infrequent and not associated with increased airway responsiveness.[18]

LATE SKIN RESPONSES

Following intradermal challenge, the time course of early and late skin responses is comparable with that observed in the lung. However, there are two major differences. Whereas dual responses in the lung are biphasic, the immediate wheal and flare in the skin merges imperceptibly into the edema, induration, and erythema that characterize the late skin response.[62] Second, the dose that may be given to the skin (under controlled conditions) is not so restricted on grounds of safety, and at higher doses of allergen a very high proportion of patients will develop a late cutaneous response.[19]

LATE NASAL RESPONSES

Immediate nasal responses are evident as itch, sneezing, watery nasal discharge, and nasal obstruction. Itch and sneezing occur within seconds, whereas mucus discharge and obstruction occur at 5 to 30 minutes. In contrast with the skin and bronchi, late responses in the nose are more difficult to quantify, appear to occur less commonly, and are manifest mainly as nasal obstruction.[71, 155] Late nasal responses are similarly inhibitable by topical corticosteroids and immunotherapy.

PATHOPHYSIOLOGY

The IgE-dependent release of mediators of hypersensitivity from mast cells and basophils characterizes the immediate response to allergen challenge. Although late responses are IgE dependent,[47, 86, 136, 139] these delayed responses are characterized by a different profile of mediators and the activation and recruitment of T lymphocytes, basophils, and eosinophils. The emergence of novel techniques for measuring cells and their activation status and production of cytokines in tissue and biologic fluids and the identification of cytokines with properties that appear to be specific for the allergic inflammatory process have identified a number of potential therapeutic targets. Late responses in the skin, bronchi, and nose have yielded considerable information regarding these processes.

SKIN

The late cutaneous response is IgE dependent. This was originally demonstrated by intradermal injection of $F(ab')_2$ anti-IgE, which resulted in the development of late responses (as well as early responses) clinically and microscopically identical to those occurring after intradermal allergen challenge in atopic subjects.[47] Further evidence came from passive transfer of the late response using serum from an allergic donor injected directly into the skin prior to intradermal allergen challenge.[139] When the donor serum was treated in various ways to remove IgE, the ability of the serum to transfer the late response passively was lost.

Inhalation of a sheep antihuman-IgE resulted in the development of late asthmatic responses.[86, 136] Skin window techniques have identified a delayed influx of eosinophils and basophils during late responses.[139] The use of skin chambers overlying the sites of late cutaneous responses has enabled the identification of mediators of hypersensitivity and cytokines and established the time course of cellular influx.[5, 6, 29, 125, 158] Late cutaneous responses and the associated cell influx were inhibitable by corticosteroids,[30] immunotherapy,[61, 113, 118, 154] and a prostaglandin E analogue,[2] but not by an antihistamine.[153] A study showed that the late cutaneous response was inhibited by soluble IL-1 receptor.[109]

By use of cutaneous biopsies and immunohistologic techniques, the late skin response was associated with increases in $CD4^+$ T lymphocytes, the appearance of activated IL-2 receptor ($CD25^+$)–bearing cells (presumed T cells), and the recruitment and activation of eosinophils.[63] The time course of appearance of these cells paralleled the late response. By use of in situ hybridization, the late response was associated with increases in IL-4, IL-5, and IL-3 and granulocyte-macrophage colony-stimulating factor (GM-CSF), whereas no changes in IL-2 or interferon-γ (IFN-γ) were observed 24 hours after challenge.[84] This profile of cytokines was compatible with a TH2-type response as originally defined in murine studies.[108] TH2 responses have subsequently emerged as characteristic of allergic and parasitic infections in humans.

Findings in allergen-induced late cutaneous responses were in contrast with those following tuberculin injection (classic delayed-type hypersensitivity).[65] In the latter, there was a delayed response that peaked at 24 to 48 hours, which was characterized by T-lymphocyte rather than eosinophil infiltration.[146] Prior treatment with prednisolone (but not cetirizine) inhibited the allergen-induced late response and associated eosinophil recruitment and production of TH2-type cytokines.[144] Successful grass pollen immunotherapy resulted in a similar inhibition of $CD4^+$ T-lymphocyte recruitment and eosinophil numbers. In contrast, however, immunotherapy did not inhibit the late appearance of TH2-type cytokines.[154] After immunotherapy, significant increases in TH1-type cytokines (IL-2 and IFN-γ) were observed in more than half of the patients studied.

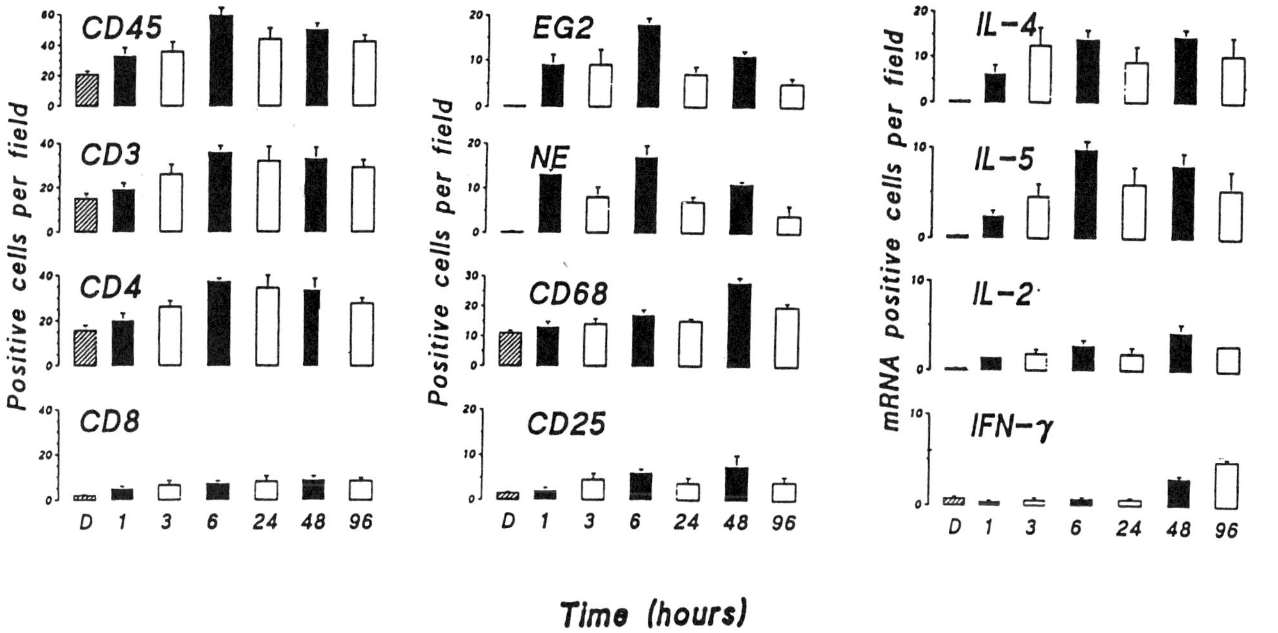

FIGURE 17–3. Time course of allergen-induced cutaneous changes in cells and cytokines up to 48 hours after challenge in two separate groups of six (filled bars, open bars). The size of the clinical late response peaked at 6–24 hours. (From Tsicopoulos A, Hamid Q, Jacobson MR, et al: Kinetics of cell infiltration and cytokine messenger RNA expression after intradermal challenge with allergen and tuberculin in the same atopic individuals. J Allergy Clin Immunol 94:764–772, 1994.)

These results suggest that late cutaneous responses represent a specialized form of cell-mediated hypersensitivity, with recruitment and activation of $CD4^+$ T lymphocytes and production of TH2 cytokines as early as 3 to 6 hours after challenge. The biologic properties of these cytokines are pertinent to the development of late responses. For example, IL-4 is a major cofactor (with IL-13) responsible for B-cell switching in favor of IgE synthesis.[44] IL-3 and GM-CSF result in differentiation and maturation of eosinophils from bone marrow precursors.[32, 96, 133] IL-5 is selective for eosinophils[96] and is the major cofactor responsible for terminal differentiation of eosinophils from bone marrow precursors. In another study, the appearance of cells and cytokines during human late responses was carefully documented and related to the size of the late response (Fig. 17–3). The characteristic finding was a prominent TH2 response with appearance of IL-4 and IL-5 early (6 hours) compared with the tuberculin response, which was characterized by a TH1 response that peaked at 24 to 48 hours.[146]

LATE BRONCHIAL RESPONSES

The late asthmatic response has been associated with the release of inflammatory mediators,[56, 81, 111, 133] activation of peripheral blood leukocytes,[51] alterations in peripheral blood T-cell subsets,[66] and peripheral blood[39, 54, 57, 67, 135] and bronchoalveolar[45] eosinophilia. We and others subsequently showed that changes in blood[39, 67] and bronchoalveolar lavage (BAL) fluid eosinophils[45, 132, 135] correlated closely with the development of the late response and the appearance of increased airway responsiveness. These earlier observations suggested that inflammatory events occurring in the bronchi may account for day-to-day changes in airway caliber.

By use of fiberoptic bronchoscopy after allergen inhalation challenge, a number of groups have shown an increase in bronchoalveolar neutrophils[138] and eosinophils[46, 73, 162] 6 to 48 hours after challenge. Increases in basophil numbers have also been observed.[73] Following local segmental allergen challenge, increases in $CD4^+$ T cells, eosinophils, and basophils were observed after 19 hours.[95] In one study, subjects who developed isolated early asthmatic responses demonstrated an increase of $CD8^+$ T lymphocytes in BAL, whereas this was not observed in subjects who developed late responses.[70] Thus local recruitment of $CD8^+$ cells was considered to afford protection against the development of late responses. In one study involving a limited number of subjects, bronchial biopsies demonstrated an increase in total leukocytes.[9] Increased immunoreactivity for GM-CSF was observed following local allergen challenge.[24]

In a further study of patients with mild atopic asthma and sensitivity to house dust mite, grass pollen, or cats, fiberoptic bronchoscopy was performed 24 hours after allergen challenge and following a control challenge, with each subject acting as his or her own control. Immunostaining of bronchial biopsies revealed 24-hour increases in activated eosinophils (using EG2 monoclonal antibody, which recognizes the cleaved activated form of eosinophil cationic protein [ECP]) (see Fig. 17–3).[13] Similarly, increases in $CD25^+$ (IL-2 R^+) cells were observed. Double immunostaining demonstrated that the majority of these $CD25^+$ cells were indeed T cells.[75] In this study (in contrast with previous findings),[43] no difference in mast cell numbers was observed after challenge. In both bronchoalveolar lavage and bronchial biopsies, in situ hybridization demonstrated significant increases in cells expressing mRNA for IL-5 and GM-CSF, with a trend for increases in IL-4–producing cells.[13]

As previously mentioned, we and others identified late bronchoalveolar eosinophilia after allergen inhalation challenge. A close correlation was observed between the numbers

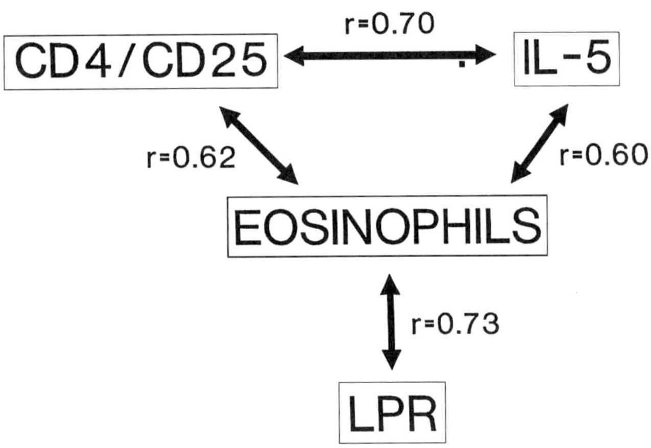

FIGURE 17–4. Associations among activated T lymphocytes, IL-5 mRNA+ cells, and eosinophils in bronchoalveolar lavage fluid at 24 hours after allergen: relationship to size of late response.

of activated IL-2 $R^+/CD4^+$ T lymphocytes as determined by two-color flow cytometry, the number of IL-5 $mRNA^+$ cells, and the number of eosinophils. A correlation was also observed between the eosinophils and the size of the late asthmatic response (Fig. 17–4). Studies involving segmental allergen[78, 142] bronchial provocation have also confirmed BAL eosinophilia. By use of polymerase chain reaction, comparable increases in TH2-type cytokines, including IL-13, were observed by use of in situ hybridization of BAL cells[132] and bronchial biopsies after challenge.[13] The identification of immunoreactivity for GM-CSF[24] lent further support to the view that increased production of eosinophil-modifying cytokines characterized the late asthmatic response.

In our studies, the T lymphocyte appeared to be the major cell expressing mRNA for IL-4 and IL-5[165] (accounting for approximately 80% of cells expressing TH2-type cytokines), whereas other studies from our own and other groups confirm the mast cell[23] as an alternative source of these cytokines in the bronchial mucosa in asthma. Mast cells also express TNF-α.[23] Eosinophils have also been shown to express proinflammatory cytokines, including IL-3, GM-CSF,[88, 106] and IL-6.[23] Another study has shown that eosinophils may also express IL-4 at the gene and protein level.[107] Thus a range of cells may express cytokines during late responses. The cytokine profile is characteristic of a TH2-type T-lymphocyte response, but mast cells, basophils,[97] and possibly eosinophils also represent alternative sources of these cytokines during late responses.

Leukocyte recruitment to the bronchi is dependent on adhesion to the vascular endothelium prior to diapedesis and migration to the respiratory epithelium. There is increased expression of ICAM-1 in asthma and, at 24 hours after allergen, increases in immunostaining for bronchial mucosal VCAM-1, which correlated with tissue eosinophilia and the size of the late response.[11] Further, in a primate model of late responses, an antibody directed against ICAM-1 was effective in inhibiting the late response and associated bronchoalveolar eosinophilia and increased airway responsiveness.[161]

LATE NASAL RESPONSES

The nose is a more accessible organ for study of late responses. As previously mentioned, however, the clinical late response in the nose is less well characterized and in the majority of subjects is evident mainly as nasal obstruction, which is difficult to quantify. Using a nasal lavage technique, Naclerio and colleagues demonstrated that early and late nasal responses were accompanied by increases in histamine, TAME-esterase, and kinins in nasal lavage fluid, whereas increases in mast cell–specific prostaglandin D_2 (PGD_2) were evident only during the early response. This suggested that the late increase in histamine may be secreted by infiltrating basophils.[110] Both eosinophils and basophils are characteristic infiltrating cells during late nasal responses.[7, 8, 122] The late release of mediators[126] and the inflammatory cell influx were inhibitable by corticosteroids.[7, 8] Similarly, ragweed immunotherapy resulted in decreases in the late response and associated release of mediators of hypersensitivity[41] and eosinophil influx.[64]

We used nasal biopsy to investigate tissue events during late nasal responses and the influence of treatment. An advantage of biopsy of the nasal mucosa is that high-quality tissue with intact respiratory epithelium is obtainable. Immunohistology demonstrated activated T lymphocytes and eosinophils during the late response.[155] T lymphocytes compartmentalize to tissue (rather than lavage) during the late nasal response. Biopsies taken during the pollen season in patients sensitive to grass pollen demonstrate an increase in epithelial mast cells (tryptase-only positive mucosal type),[12] whereas this was not observed over the time course of the late response following experimental grass pollen challenge.

In situ hybridization studies demonstrated that the late nasal response was associated with changes identical with those observed during late responses occurring in the skin and bronchus. Thus increases in IL-3, GM-CSF, IL-4, and IL-5 were predominant,[58] with no changes in IL-2 or IFN-γ. The cell sources of IL-4[164] and IL-5[163] were identified principally as T lymphocytes, with a contribution from mast cells[22] and eosinophils.

The influence of treatment was investigated in two large double-blind, placebo-controlled trials. In one study, 48 patients with summer hay fever and lone grass pollen allergy were treated with topical corticosteroids (fluticasone propionate) or matched placebo. A marked decrease in T lymphocytes and eosinophils was observed,[129] particularly in the nasal epithelium. In situ hybridization demonstrated a marked reduction in IL-4 $mRNA^+$ cells after allergen challenge.[99]

In a separate study, 40 adult patients with severe summer hay fever unresponsive to antiallergic drugs were treated for 12 months with immunotherapy using a biologically standardized depot (aluminium hydroxide adsorbed) grass pollen extract or matched placebo subcutaneous injections containing histamine. Inhibition of the late nasal response was accompanied by a decrease in tissue recruitment of $CD4^+$ T lymphocytes and eosinophils.[59] In contrast with the effect of topical corticosteroids, immunotherapy did not inhibit the number of cells expressing mRNA for TH2-type cytokines. Increases in IL-4 and IL-5, as well as IL-3 and GM-CSF, were virtually identical in both immunotherapy- and placebo-treated patients despite virtual complete inhibition of early and late nasal responses after allergen challenge. In contrast, a marked increase in cells expressing IFN-γ was observed. The increase in IFN-γ $mRNA^+$ cells correlated with clinical improvement, as reflected by seasonal symptom

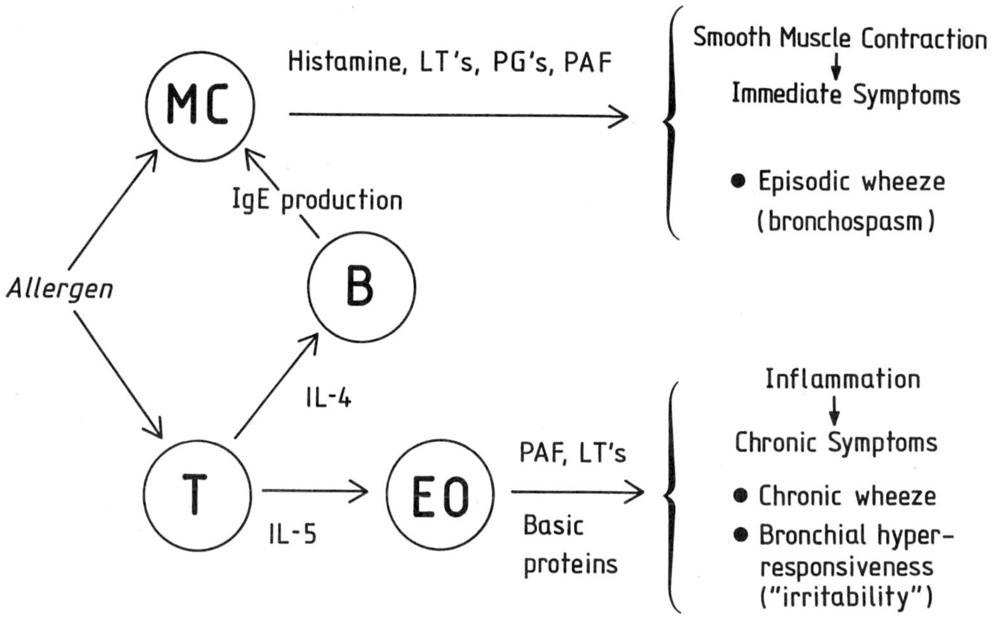

FIGURE 17–5. Hypothesis of the mechanism of human allergic late responses.

scores and medication requirements during the pollen season, only in the immunotherapy-treated group.[59] Studies in the skin demonstrated that the cytokine IL-12 may be the dominant cytokine inducing these preferential TH1 responses after successful immunotherapy.[76]

SUMMARY

A hypothesis relating to the development of late responses in the skin, nose, and lung is summarized in Figure 17–5. Whereas the early response is characterized by IgE-depen-

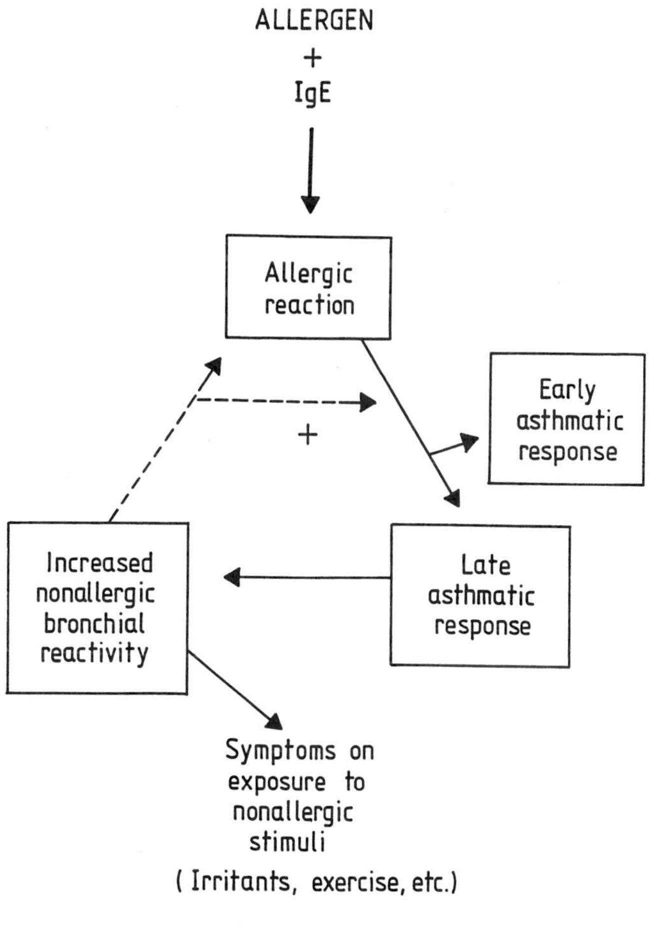

FIGURE 17–6. Mechanism of perennial allergic asthma. (From Cockcroft DW: Mechanism of perennial allergic asthma. Lancet 2:253–256, 1983. © by The Lancet Ltd. 1983.)

dent mast cell activation, the late response additionally may involve recruitment and activation of T lymphocytes. The recruited T lymphocytes (and possibly other cells, including mast cells and eosinophils) synthesize TH2-type cytokines with biologic properties consistent with increases in local IgE and the recruitment and activation of eosinophils, which contribute to late responses.

True late responses (e.g., late asthmatic responses with associated increased airway responsiveness) involve immunologic mechanisms (i.e., previous exposure with induction of memory B and T cells) and so reflect specific sensitization as opposed to occasional late responses that have been reported after nonspecific triggers. Late responses and increased responsiveness result in a lower threshold for further allergic stimulation and exaggerated responses to irritant triggers, setting up, as suggested by Cockcroft,[33] a vicious cycle of ongoing bronchial inflammation (Fig. 17–6).

Treatment options include removal of the allergen, modification of the T-lymphocyte response following allergen by use of immunotherapy, the use of specific pharmacologic antagonists, and strategies directed against specific cytokines. The use of anti–IL-4 or anti–IL-5 or competitive antagonists will be of interest, as will a trial of IFN-γ or IL-12, if feasible, prior to allergen challenge and during naturally occurring allergic disease.

ACKNOWLEDGMENTS

The authors would like to acknowledge Drs. Anthony J. Frew, Andrew M. Bentley, Douglas S. Robinson, Veronica A. Varney, Mina Gaga, Anne Tsicopoulos, Sun Ying, Mikila Jacobson, Sabina Rak, Keisuke Masuyama, Luis Taborda-Barata, and others within the division of Allergy and Immunology, Imperial College School of Medicine at the National Heart and Lung Institute, London. Our special thanks are due to Q. Hamid, Meakins-Christie Laboratories, McGill University, Montreal, Canada, who directed the in situ hybridization studies.

REFERENCES

1. Aalbers R, Kauffman HF, Groen H, et al: The effect of nedocromil sodium on the early and late reaction and allergen-induced bronchial hyperresponsiveness. J Allergy Clin Immunol 87:993–1001, 1991.
2. Alam R, Derjarnatt A, Stafford S, et al: Selective inhibition of the cutaneous late but not immediate allergic response to antigens by misoprostol, a PGE analogue. Results of a double-blind, placebo-controlled randomised study. Am Rev Respir Dis 148:1066–1070, 1983.
3. Arm JP, Horton CE, Mencia Huerta JM, et al: Effect of dietary supplementation with fish oil lipids on mild asthma. Thorax 43:84–92, 1988.
4. Arm JP, Horton CE, Spur BW, et al: The effects of dietary supplementation with fish oil lipids on the airway response to inhaled allergen in bronchial asthma. Am Rev Respir Dis 139:1395–1400, 1989.
5. Atkins PC: Cutaneous late phase responses—an allergic inflammatory response. Allergy Proc 10:417–421, 1989.
6. Atkins PC, Zweiman B: The IgE-mediated late-phase skin response—unravelling the enigma. J Allergy Clin Immunol 79:12–15, 1987.
7. Bascom R, Pipkorn U, Lichtenstein LM, et al: The influx of inflammatory cells into nasal washings during the late response to antigen challenge. Effect of systemic steroid pretreatment. Am Rev Respir Dis 138:406–412, 1988.
8. Bascom R, Wachs M, Naclerio RM, et al: Basophil influx occurs after nasal antigen challenge: effects of topical corticosteroid pretreatment. J Allergy Clin Immunol 81:580–589, 1988.
9. Beasley R, Roche WR, Roberts JA, et al: Cellular events in the bronchi in mild asthma and after bronchial provocation. Am Rev Respir Dis 139:806–817, 1989.
10. Bel EH, Timmers MC, Dijkman JH, et al: The effect of an inhaled leukotriene antagonist, L-648, 051, on early and late asthmatic reactions and subsequent increase in airway responsiveness in man. J Allergy Clin Immunol 85:1067–1075, 1990.
11. Bentley AM, Durham SR, Robinson DS, et al: Expression of endothelial and leukocyte adhesion molecules intercellular adhesion molecule-1, E-selectin, and vascular cell adhesion molecule-1 in the bronchial mucosa in steady state and allergen-induced asthma. J Allergy Clin Immunol 92:857–868, 1993.
12. Bentley AM, Jacobson MR, Cumberworth V, et al: Immunohistology of the nasal mucosa in seasonal allergic rhinitis: increases in activated eosinophils and epithelial mast cells. J Allergy Clin Immunol 89:821–829, 1992.
13. Bentley AM, Qui Meng, Robinson DS, et al: Increases in activated T lymphocytes, eosinophils, and cytokine mRNA expression for IL-5 and GM-CSF in bronchial biopsies after allergen inhalation challenge in atopic asthmatics. Am J Respir Cell Mol Biol 8:35–42, 1993.
14. Bernstein DI, Ploysongsang Y, Mittman RJ, et al: The relationship between airway responsiveness measured before and after the allergen-induced late asthmatic response. Chest 101:437–441, 1992.
15. Bianco S, Pieroni MG, Refini RM, et al: Protective effect of inhaled furosemide on allergen-induced early and late asthmatic reactions. N Engl J Med 321:1069–1073, 1989.
16. Booij-Nord H, De Vries K, Sluiter HJ, et al: Late bronchial obstructive reaction to experimental inhalation of house dust extract. Clin Allergy 2:43–61, 1972.
17. Booij-Nord H, Orie NGM, De Vries K: Immediate and late bronchial obstructive reactions to inhalation of house dust and protective effects of disodium cromoglycate and prednisolone. J Allergy Clin Immunol 48:344–354, 1971.
18. Boner AL, Vallone G, Chiesa M, et al: Reproducibility of late phase pulmonary response to exercise and its relationship to bronchial hyperreactivity in children with chronic asthma. Pediatr Pulmonol 14:156–159, 1992.
19. Boulet LP, Roberts RS, Dolovich J, et al: Prediction of late asthmatic responses to inhaled allergen. Clin Allergy 14:379–385, 1984.
20. Boulet LP, Legris C, Turcotte H, et al: Prevalence and characteristics of late asthmatic responses to exercise. J Allergy Clin Immunol 80:655–662, 1987.
21. Boulet LP, Turcotte H: Re-examination of the late asthmatic response to exercise. Am Rev Respir Dis 138:748–749, 1988.
22. Bradding P, Feather I, Howarth P, et al: Interleukin-4 is localised to and released by human mast cells. J Exp Med 176:1381–1386, 1992.
23. Bradding P, Roberts JA, Britten KM, et al: Interleukin-4, 5, 6 and TNFa in normal and asthmatic airways: evidence for the human mast cell as a source of these cytokines. Am J Respir Cell Mol Biol 10:471–480, 1994.
24. Broide DH, Firestein GS: Endobronchial allergen challenge in asthma. Demonstration of cellular source of granulocyte macrophage colony-stimulating factor by in-situ hybridization. J Clin Invest 88:1048–1053, 1991.
25. Bundgaard A, Boudet L: Reproducibility of late asthmatic response. Eur J Respir Dis 143(suppl):41–43, 1986.
26. Bussieres S, Turcotte H, Boulet LP: Hyperosmolarity-induced increases in airway responsiveness and late asthmatic responses. Eur Respir J 4:290–295, 1991.
27. Cartier A, Thomson NC, Frith PA, et al: Allergen-induced increase in bronchial responsiveness to histamine: relationship to the late asthmatic response and change in airway caliber. J Allergy Clin Immunol 70:170–177, 1982.
28. Chai H, Farr RS, Froehlich LA, et al: Standardisation of bronchial challenge procedures. J Allergy Clin Immunol 56:323, 1975.
29. Charlesworth EN, Hood AF, Soter NA, et al: Cutaneous late phase response to allergen. Mediator release and inflammatory cell infiltration. J Clin Invest 83:1519–1526, 1989.
30. Charlesworth EN, Kagey-Sobotka A, Schleimer RP, et al: Prednisone inhibits the appearance of inflammatory mediators and the influx of eosinophils and basophils associated with the cutaneous late-phase response to allergen. J Immunol 146:671–676, 1991.
31. Charlesworth EN, Massey WA, Kagey-Sobotka A, et al: Effect of H1

receptor blockade on the early and late response to cutaneous allergen challenge. J Pharmacol Exp Ther 262:964–970, 1992.
32. Clutterbuck EJ, Hirst EMA, Sanderson CJ: Human interleukin-5 (IL-5) regulates the production of eosinophils in human bone marrow cultures: comparison and interaction with IL-1, IL-3, IL-6 and GMCSF. Blood 73:1504, 1989.
33. Cockcroft DW: Mechanism of perennial allergic asthma. Lancet 2:253–256, 1983.
34. Cockcroft DW, McParland CP, O'Byrne PM, et al: Beclomethasone given after the early asthmatic response inhibits the late response and the increased methacholine responsiveness and cromolyn does not. J Allergy Clin Immunol 91:1163–1168, 1993.
35. Cockcroft DW, Murdock KY: Comparative effects of inhaled salbutamol, sodium cromoglycate, and beclomethasone dipropionate on allergen-induced early asthmatic responses, late asthmatic responses, and increased bronchial responsiveness to histamine. J Allergy Clin Immunol 79:734–740, 1987.
36. Cockcroft DW, Murdock KY, Gore BP, et al: Theophylline does not inhibit allergen-induced increase in airway responsiveness to methacholine. J Allergy Clin Immunol 83:913–920, 1989.
37. Cockcroft DW, Murdock KY, Kirby J, et al: Prediction of airway responsiveness to allergen from skin sensitivity to allergen and airway responsiveness to histamine. Am Rev Respir Dis 135:264–267, 1987.
38. Cockcroft DW, Ruffin RE, Dolovich S, et al: Allergen induced increase in non-allergic bronchial reactivity. Clin Allergy 7:503–513, 1977.
39. Cookson WOCM, Craddock CF, Benson MK, et al: Falls in peripheral eosinophil counts parallel the late asthmatic response. Am Rev Respir Dis 139:458–462, 1989.
40. Cresioli S, Spinazzi A, Plebani M, et al: Theophylline inhibits early and late asthmatic reactions induced by allergens in asthmatic subjects. Ann Allergy 66:245–251, 1991.
41. Creticos PS, Franklin Adkinson N Jr, Kagey-Sobotka A, et al: Nasal challenge with ragweed in hayfever patients. Effects of immunotherapy. J Clin Invest 76:2247–2253, 1985.
42. Crimi E, Brusasco V, Losurdo E, Crimi P: Predictive accuracy of late asthmatic reaction to *Dermatophagoides pteronyssinus*. J Allergy Clin Immunol 78:908–913, 1986.
43. Crimi E, Chiaramondia M, Milanese M, et al: Increased numbers of mast cells in bronchial mucosa after the late-phase asthmatic response to allergen. Am Rev Respir Dis 144:1282–1286, 1991.
44. Del Prete GF, Maggi E, Parronchi P, et al: IL-4 is an essential factor for the IgE synthesis induced in vitro by human T cell clones and their supernatants. J Immunol 140:4193, 1988.
45. De Monchy JGR, Kauffman HF, Venge P, et al: Bronchoalveolar eosinophilia during allergen-induced late asthmatic reactions. Am Rev Respir Dis 131:373–376, 1985.
46. Diaz PC, Gonzalez MC, Galleguilos FR, et al: Leukocytes and mediators in bronchoalveolar lavage during allergen-induced late-phase asthmatic reactions. Am Rev Respir Dis 139:1383–1389, 1989.
47. Dolovich J, Hargreave FE, Chalmers R, et al: Late cutaneous allergic responses in isolated IgE-dependent reactions. J Allergy Clin Immunol 52:38–48, 1973.
48. Durham SR: Late asthmatic responses. Respir Med 84:263–268, 1990.
49. Durham SR: Late onset reactions. In Morley J (ed): Academic Press, Harcourt Brace Jovanovich, London, 1991, pp 131–140.
50. Durham SR: The significance of late responses in asthma. Clin Exp Allergy 21:3–7, 1991.
51. Durham SR, Carroll M, Walsh GM, et al: Leukocyte activation during allergen-induced late-phase asthmatic reactions. N Engl J Med 311:1398–1402, 1984.
52. Durham SR, Craddock CF, Cookson WO, et al: Increases in airway responsiveness to histamine precede allergen-induced late asthmatic responses. J Allergy Clin Immunol 82:764–770, 1988.
53. Durham SR, Graneek BJ, Hawkins R, et al: The temporal relationship between increases in airway responsiveness to histamine and late asthmatic responses induced by occupational agents. J Allergy Clin Immunol 79:398–406, 1987.
54. Durham SR, Kay AB: Eosinophils, bronchial hyperreactivity and late-phase asthmatic reactions. Clin Allergy 15:411–418, 1985.
55. Durham SR, Keenan J, Cookson WOCM, et al: Diurnal variation in serum cortisol concentrations in asthmatic subjects after allergen inhalation. Thorax 44:582–585, 1989.
56. Durham SR, Lee TH, Cromwell O, et al: Immunologic studies in allergen-induced late-phase asthmatic reactions. J Allergy Clin Immunol 74:49–60, 1984.
57. Durham SR, Loegering DA, Dunnette S, et al: Blood eosinophils and eosinophil-derived proteins in allergic asthma. J Allergy Clin Immunol 84:931–936, 1989.
58. Durham SR, Ying S, Varney V, et al: Cytokine messenger RNA expression for interleukin-3 (IL-3), IL-4, IL-5 and granulocyte/macrophage colony stimulating factor (GM-CSF), in the nasal mucosa after local allergen provocation: relationship to tissue eosinophilia. J Immunol 148:2390–2394, 1992.
59. Durham SR, Ying S, Varney VA, et al: Grass pollen immunotherapy inhibits allergen-induced infiltration of CD4+ T lymphocytes and eosinophils in the nasal mucosa and increases the number of cells expressing messenger RNA for interferon-gamma. J Allergy Clin Immunol. 97:1356, 1996.
60. Eiser N: The effect of a beta 2-adrenergic agonist and a histamine H1-receptor antagonist on the late asthmatic response to inhaled antigen. Respir Med 85:393–399, 1991.
61. Fling JA, Ruff ME, Parker WA, et al: Suppression of the late cutaneous response by immunotherapy. J Allergy Clin Immunol 83:101–109, 1989.
62. Frew AJ, Kay AB: The pattern of human late-phase skin reactions to extracts of aeroallergens. J Allergy Clin Immunol 81:1117–1129, 1988.
63. Frew AJ, Kay AB: The relationship between infiltrating CD4+ lymphocytes, activated eosinophils and the magnitude of the allergen-induced late-phase cutaneous reaction in man. J Immunol 141:4158–4164, 1988.
64. Furin MJ, Norman PS, Creticos PS, et al: Immunotherapy decreases antigen-induced eosinophil migration into the nasal cavity. J Allergy Clin Immunol 88:27–32, 1991.
65. Gaga M, Frew AJ, Varney V, et al: Eosinophil activation and T lymphocyte infiltration in allergen-induced late phase reactions and classical delayed-type hypersensitivity in man. J Immunol 147:816–822, 1991.
66. Gerblich AA, Campbell AE, Schuyler MR, et al: Changes in T lymphocyte sub-populations after antigenic bronchial challenge in asthmatics. N Engl J Med 310:1349–1352, 1984.
67. Gibson PG, Manning PJ, O'Byrne PM: Allergen induced asthmatic responses. Relationship between increases in airways responsiveness and increases in circulating eosinophils, basophils and their progenitors. Am Rev Respir Dis 143:331–335, 1991.
68. Godfrey S: Late response to exercise-induced asthma. J Allergy Clin Immunol 76:876, 1985.
69. Gonokami Y, Konno SI, Kurokawa M, et al: Effect of methotrexate on asthmatic reaction in sensitized guinea pigs. Int Arch Allergy Immunol 106:410–415, 1995.
70. Gonzalez MC, Diaz P, Galleguillos FR, et al: Allergen-induced recruitment of bronchoalveolar helper (OKT4) and suppressor (OKT8) T cells in asthma: relative increases in OKT8 cells in single early responders compared with those in late-phase responders. Am Rev Respir Dis 136:600–604, 1987.
71. Gronborg H, Bisgaard H, Romeling F, et al: Early and late nasal symptom response to allergen challenge. The effect of pretreatment with a glucocorticosteroid spray. Allergy 48:87–93, 1993.
72. Gronnenberg R, Zetterstrom O: Inhibition of anti-IgE induced skin response in normals by formoterol, a new beta 2-adrenoceptor agonist, and terbutaline. 2. Effect on the late phase reaction. Allergy 45:340–346, 1990.
73. Guo CB, Liu MC, Galli SJ, et al: Identification of IgE-bearing cells in the late phase response to antigen in the lung as basophils. Am J Respir Cell Mol Biol 10:384–390, 1994.
74. Hamid Q, Barkans J, Abrams J, et al: Human eosinophils synthesise and secrete interleukin-6, in vitro. Blood 80:1496–1501, 1992.
75. Hamid Q, Barkans J, Robinson DS, et al: Co-expression of CD25 and CD3 in atopic allergy and asthma. Immunology 75:659–663, 1992.
76. Hamid QA, Schotman E, Jacobson MR, et al: Increases in interleukin-12 (IL-12) messenger RNA+ (mRNA+) cells accompany inhibition of allergen induced late skin responses following successful grass pollen immunotherapy. J Allergy Clin Immunol. In press.
77. Hargreave FE: Late phase asthmatic responses and airway inflammation. J Allergy Clin Immunol 83:525–527, 1989.
78. Huang SK, Xiao HQ, Kleine-Tebbe J, et al: Interleukin 13 (IL-13) expression at the sites of allergen challenge in allergic asthmatics. J Allergy Clin Immunol 95:385, 1995. Abstract.
79. Ihre E, Axelsson IGK, Zetterstrom O: Late asthmatic reactions and bronchial variability after challenge with low doses of allergen. Clin Allergy 18:557–568, 1988.
80. Iikura Y, Inui H, Nagakura T, et al: Factors predisposing to exercise-

induced late asthmatic responses. J Allergy Clin Immunol 75:285–289, 1985.

81. Iwamoto I, Ra C, Sato T, et al: Thromboxane A2 production in allergen-induced immediate and late asthmatic responses. Its possible role in inducing the late response. J Asthma 25:117–124, 1988.
82. Juniper EF, Cockcroft DW, Hargreave FE: Histamine and methacholine inhalation tests: tidal breathing method. Laboratory procedure and standardization. Astra Draco AB, Lund, Sweden, 1994.
83. Karjalainen J: Exercise response in 404 young men with asthma: no evidence for a late asthmatic reaction. Thorax 46:100–104, 1991.
84. Kay AB, Sun Ying, Varney V, et al: Messenger RNA expression of the cytokine gene cluster, interleukin-3 (IL-3), IL-4, IL-5 and GM-CSF in allergen-induced late-phase cutaneous reactions in atopic subjects. J Exp Med 173:775, 1991.
85. Kirby JG, Hargreave FE, O'Byrne PM: Indomethacin inhibits allergen-induced airway hyper-responsiveness but not allergen-induced asthmatic responses. Am Rev Respir Dis 135(suppl):312A, 1987. Abstract.
86. Kirby JG, Robertson DG, Hargreave FE, et al: Asthmatic responses to inhalation of anti-IgE. Clin Allergy 16:191–194, 1986.
87. Kirsch CM, Payan DG, Wong MYS, et al: Effect of eicosapentaenoic acid in asthma. Clin Allergy 18:177–188, 1988.
88. Kita H, Ohnishi T, Okubo Y, et al: Interleukin 3 release from human peripheral blood eosinophils and neutrophils. J Exp Med 174:743, 1991.
89. Kondo S: Circadian variation of bronchial caliber and antigen-induced late asthmatic response. Chest 104:801–805, 1993.
90. Kopferschmitt-Kubler MC, Hutt N, Bigot H, et al: Protective effect of nedocromil sodium on the dual asthmatic response to bronchial antigen challenge. Respir Med 60:21–26, 1993.
91. Kuitert LM, Hui KP, Uthayarkumar S, et al: Effect of the platelet-activating factor antagonist UK-74, 505 on the early and late response to allergen. Am Rev Respir Dis 147:82–86, 1993.
92. Lai CK, Beasley R, Holgate ST: The effect of an increase in inhaled allergen dose after terfenadine on the occurrence and magnitude of the late asthmatic response. Clin Exp Allergy 19:209–216, 1989.
93. Lai CK, Twentyman OP, Holgate ST: The effect of an increase in inhaled allergen dose after rimiterol hydrobromide on the occurrence and magnitude of the late asthmatic response and the associated change in non-specific bronchial responsiveness. Am Rev Respir Dis 140:917–923, 1989.
94. Lichtenstein LM: The nasal late-phase response—an in vivo model. Hosp Pract (Off Ed) 23(1):119–126, 135–139, 142, 1988.
95. Liu MC, Hubbard WC, Proud D, et al: Immediate and late inflammatory responses to ragweed antigen challenge of the peripheral airways in allergic asthmatics. Cellular, mediator, and permeability changes. Am Rev Respir Dis 144:51–58, 1991.
96. Lopez AF, Sanderson CJ, Gamble JR, et al: Recombinant human interleukin-5 is a selective activator of human eosinophil function. J Exp Med 167:219, 1988.
97. MacGlashan DW Jr, White JM, Huang SK, et al: Secretion of IL-4 from human basophils. The relationship between IL-4 mRNA and protein in resting and stimulated basophils. J Immunol 152:3006–3016, 1994.
98. Malo JL, Ghezzo H, L'Archeveque J, et al: Late asthmatic reactions to occupational sensitizing agents: frequency of changes in non-specific bronchial responsiveness and of response to inhaled beta 2-adrenergic agent. J Allergy Clin Immunol 85:834–842, 1990.
99. Masuyama K, Jacobson MR, Rak S, et al: Topical glucocorticosteroid (fluticasone propionate) inhibits cytokine mRNA expression for interleukin-4 (IL-4) in the nasal mucosa in allergic rhinitis. Immunology 82:192–199, 1994.
100. Mattoli S, Foresi A, Corbo GM, et al: Effects of two doses of cromolyn on allergen-induced late asthmatic response and increased responsiveness. J Allergy Clin Immunol 79:747–754, 1987.
101. Mattoli S, Foresi A, Corbo GM, et al: Increase in bronchial responsiveness to methacholine and late asthmatic response after the inhalation of ultrasonically nebulized distilled water. Chest 90:726–732, 1986.
102. Metzger WJ, Hunninghake GW, et al: Late asthmatic responses: inquiry into mechanisms and significance. Clin Rev Allergy 3(2):145–165, 1985.
103. Metzger WJ, Nugent K, Richerson HB: Site of airflow obstruction during early and late phase asthmatic responses to allergen bronchoprovocation. Chest 88:369–375, 1985.
104. Metzger WJ, Richerson HB, Wasserman SI: Generation and partial characterization of eosinophil chemotactic activity and neutrophil chemotactic activity during early and late-phase asthmatic response. J Allergy Clin Immunol 78:282–290, 1986.
105. Mohiuddin AA, Martin RJ: Circadian basis of the late asthmatic response. Am Rev Respir Dis 142:1153–1157, 1990.
106. Moqbel R, Hamid Q, Ying S, et al: Expression of mRNA for the granulocyte/macrophage colony-stimulating factor (GM-CSF) in activated human eosinophils. J Exp Med 174:749, 1991.
107. Moqbel R, Ying S, Barkans J, et al: Identification of mRNA for interleukin-4 in human eosinophils with granule localization and release of the translated product. J Immunol 155:4939–4947, 1995.
108. Mosmann TR, Coffman RL: Two types of mouse helper T cell clones. Implications for immune regulation. Immunol Today 8:223, 1987.
109. Mullarkey MF, Leiferman KM, Peters MS, et al: Human cutaneous allergic late-phase response is inhibited by soluble IL-1 receptor. J Immunol 152:2033–2041, 1994.
110. Naclerio RM, Proud D, Togias AG, et al: Inflammatory mediators in late antigen-induced rhinitis. N Engl J Med 313:65–70, 1985.
111. Nakamura T, Morita Y, Kuriyama M, et al: Platelet-activating factor in late asthmatic response. Int Arch Allergy Appl Immunol 82:57–61, 1987.
112. Nakazawa T, Matsui S, Saitoh A, et al: Pituitary and adrenal functions during late asthmatic responses. Ann Allergy 60:355–356, 1988.
113. Nish WA, Charlesworth EN, Davis TL, et al: The effect of immunotherapy on the cutaneous late phase response to antigen. J Allergy Clin Immunol 93:484–493, 1994.
114. O'Byrne PM, Dolovich J, Hargreave FE: Late asthmatic responses. Am Rev Respir Dis 136(3):740–751, 1987.
115. Paggiaro P, Bacci E, Talini D, et al: Atropine does not inhibit late asthmatic responses induced by toluene-diisocyanate in sensitized subjects. Am Rev Respir Dis 136:1237–1241, 1987.
116. Paggiaro PL, Dente FL, Morelli MC, et al: Post-allergen inhaled budesonide reduces late asthmatic response and inhibits the associated increase of airway responsiveness to methacholine in asthmatics. Am J Respir Crit Care Med 149:1447–1451, 1994.
117. Paggiaro PL, Dente FL, Vagaggini B, et al: Salbutamol plus beclomethasone dipropionate, but not salbutamol alone, completely prevent early and late asthmatic responses to allergen. Respir Med 85:401–406, 1991.
118. Parker WA Jr, Whisman BA, Apaliski SJ, et al: The relationships between late cutaneous responses and specific antibody responses with outcome of immunotherapy for seasonal allergic rhinitis. J Allergy Clin Immunol 84:667–677, 1989.
119. Pauwels R: Theophylline activity in late asthmatic response. Drug Intell Clin Pharm 21:755, 1987.
120. Pelikan Z, Knottnerus I: Inhibition of the late asthmatic response by nedocromil sodium administered more than two hours after allergen challenge. J Allergy Clin Immunol 92:19–28, 1993.
121. Pelikan Z, Pelikan-Filipek M: The late asthmatic response to allergen challenge—part I. Ann Allergy 56:414–420, 1986.
122. Pelikan Z, Pelikan-Filipek M: Cytologic changes in the nasal secretions during the late nasal response. J Allergy Clin Immunol 83:1068–1079, 1989.
123. Pepys J, Davies RJ, Breslin ABX, et al: The effect of inhaled beclomethasone dipropionate (Becotide) and sodium cromoglycate on asthmatic reactions to provocation tests. Clin Allergy 4:13–24, 1974.
124. Pepys J, Hutchcroft BJ: Bronchial provocation tests in etiologic diagnosis and analysis of asthma. Am Rev Respir Dis 112:829–859, 1975.
125. Pienkowski MM, Adkinson NF Jr, Plaut M, et al: Prostaglandin D2 and histamine during the immediate and the late-phase components of allergic cutaneous responses. J Allergy Clin Immunol 82:95–100, 1988.
126. Pipkorn U, Proud D, Lichtenstein LM, et al: Inhibition of mediator release in allergic rhinitis by pretreatment with topical glucocorticosteroids. N Engl J Med 316:1506, 1987.
127. Price JF, Hey EN, Soothill JF: Antigen provocation to the skin, nose and lung in children with asthma, immediate and dual hypersensitivity reactions. Clin Exp Immunol 47:587–594, 1982.
128. Rafferty P, Ng WH, Phillips G, et al: The inhibitory actions of azelastine hydrochloride on the early and late bronchoconstrictor responses to inhaled allergen in atopic asthma. J Allergy Clin Immunol 84:649–657, 1989.
129. Rak S, Jacobson MR, Sudderick RM, et al: Influence of prolonged treatment with topical corticosteroid (fluticasone propionate) on early and late phase nasal responses and cellular infiltration in the nasal mucosa after allergen challenge. Clin Exp Allergy 24:930–939, 1994.

130. Roberts NM, Page CP, Chung KF, et al: Effect of a PAF antagonist, BN52063, on antigen-induced acute, and late-onset cutaneous responses in atopic subjects. J Allergy Clin Immunol 82:236–241, 1988.
131. Robertson DG, Kerigan AT, Hargreave FE, et al: Late asthmatic responses induced by ragweed pollen allergen. J Allergy Clin Immunol 54:244–254, 1974.
132. Robinson DS, Hamid Q, Bentley AM, et al: Activation of CD4+ T cells, increased TH2-type cytokine mRNA expression, and eosinophil recruitment in bronchoalveolar lavage after allergen inhalation challenge in atopic asthmatics. J Allergy Clin Immunol 92:313–324, 1993.
133. Rothenberg ME, Petersen J, Stevens RL, et al: IL-5 dependent conversion of normodense human eosinophils to the hypodense phenotype uses 3T3 fibroblasts for enhanced viability, accelerated hypodensity, and sustained antibody-dependent cytoxicity. J Immunol 143:2311, 1989.
134. Ryan G, Dolovich MB, Roberts RS, et al: Standardisation of inhalation provocation tests: two techniques of aerosol generation and inhalation compared. Am Rev Respir Dis 123:195, 1981.
135. Schmekel B, Venge P: Markers for eosinophils and T-lymphocytes as predictors of late asthmatic response. Allergy 48(suppl 17):94–97 (discussion 110–111), 1993.
136. Shampain MP, Behrens BL, Larsen GL, et al: An animal model of late pulmonary responses to Alternaria challenge. Am Rev Respir Dis 126:493–498, 1982.
137. Sihra BS, Walker SM, Kon OM, et al: Inhibition of the allergen-induced late phase asthmatic reaction by oral cyclosporin A (CsA). J Allergy Clin Immunol 97:242, 1996.
138. Smith HR, Larsen GL, Cherniack RM, et al: Inflammatory cells and eicosanoid mediators in subjects with late asthmatic responses and increases in airway responsiveness. J Allergy Clin Immunol 89:1076–1084, 1992.
139. Solley GP, Gleich GJ, Jordan RE, et al: Late phase of the immediate weal and flare skin reaction: its dependence on IgE antibodies. J Clin Invest 58:408–420, 1976.
140. Speelberg B, Panis EA, Bijl D, et al: Late asthmatic responses after exercise challenge are reproducible. J Allergy Clin Immunol 87:1128–1137, 1991.
141. Speelberg B, van den Berg NJ, Oosthoek CH, et al: Immediate and late asthmatic responses induced by exercise in patients with reversible airflow limitation. Eur Respir J 2:402–408, 1989.
142. Su S, Krishnaswarmy G, Liu M, et al: Quantitation of cytokine mRNA's in asthma. J Allergy Clin Immunol 91:347, 1993. Abstract.
143. Sullivan P, Bekir S, Jaffar Z, et al: Anti-inflammatory effects of low-dose oral theophylline in atopic asthma. Lancet 343:1006–1008, 1994.
144. Taborda Barata L, Jacobson M, Walker S, et al: Effect of cetirizine and prednisolone on cellular infiltration and cytokine mRNA expression during allergen-induced late cutaneous responses. Clin Exp Allergy 26:68–78, 1996.
145. Taylor IK, O'Shaughnessy KM, Choudry NB, et al: A comparative study in atopic subjects with asthma of the effects of salmeterol and salbutamol on allergen-induced bronchoconstriction, increase in airway reactivity, and increase in urinary leukotriene E_4 excretion. J Allergy Clin Immunol 89:575–583, 1992.
146. Tsicopoulos A, Hamid Q, Jacobson MR, et al: Kinetics of cell infiltration and cytokine messenger RNA expression after intradermal challenge with allergen and tuberculin in the same atopic individuals. J Allergy Clin Immunol 94:764–772, 1994.
147. Turcotte H, Boulet LP: Perception of breathlessness during early and late asthmatic responses. Am Rev Respir Dis 148:514–518, 1993.
148. Twentyman OP, Finnerty JP, Harris A, et al: Protection against allergen-induced asthma by salmeterol. Lancet 336:1338–1342, 1990.
149. Twentyman O, Holgate ST: Reproducibility of the late asthmatic reaction: comparisons with the histamine bronchoprovocation test. Thorax 44:867, 1989.
150. Twentyman OP, Holgate ST: Reversibility of the allergen-provoked late asthmatic response by an inhaled beta 2-adrenoceptor agonist. Clin Exp Allergy 24:245–249, 1994.
151. Van Bever HP, Stevens WJ: Suppression of the late asthmatic reaction by hyposensitization in asthmatic children allergic to house dust mite *Dermatophagoides pteronyssinus*. Clin Exp Allergy 19:399–405, 1989.
152. Varney V, Gaga M, Frew AJ, et al: Usefulness of immunotherapy in patients with severe summer hay fever uncontrolled by antiallergic drugs. Br Med J 302:265–269, 1991.
153. Varney VA, Gaga M, Frew AJ, et al: The effect of a single oral dose of prednisolone or cetirizine on inflammatory cells infiltrating allergen-induced cutaneous late-phase reactions in atopic subjects. Clin Exp Allergy 22:43–50, 1992.
154. Varney VA, Hamid QA, Gaga M, et al: Influence of grass pollen immunotherapy on cellular infiltration and cytokine mRNA expression during allergen-induced late-phase cutaneous responses. J Clin Invest 92:644–651, 1993.
155. Varney VA, Jacobson MR, Sudderick RM, et al: Immunohistology of the nasal mucosa following allergen-induced rhinitis: identification of activated T lymphocytes, eosinophils and neutrophils. Am Rev Respir Dis 146:170–176, 1992.
156. Verhoeff NP, Speelberg B, Van den Berg NJ, et al: Real and pseudo late asthmatic reactions after submaximal exercise challenge in patients with bronchial asthma. A new definition for late asthmatic responses after exercise challenge. Chest 98:1194–1199, 1990.
157. Violante B, Pellegrino R, Crimi E, et al: Increase in airway responsiveness and effect of deep inhalation on airway caliber in allergen-induced asthma. Relationship to the late-phase response. Am Rev Respir Dis 146:127–131, 1992.
158. Warner JA, Pienkowski MM, Plaut M, et al: Identification of histamine releasing factor(s) in the late-phase of cutaneous IgE-mediated reactions. J Immunol 136:2583–2587, 1986.
159. Warner JO: Significance of late reactions after bronchial challenge with house dust mite. Arch Dis Child 51:905–910, 1976.
160. Warner JO, Price JF, Hey EN, et al: Controlled trial of hyposensitisation to *Dermatophagoides pteronyssinus* in children with asthma. Lancet 2:912–915, 1978.
161. Wegner CD, Gundel RH, Reilly N, et al: Intercellular adhesion molecule-1 (ICAM-1) in the pathogenesis of asthma. Science 247:456–459, 1990.
162. Woolley KL, Adelroth E, Woolley MJ, et al: Effects of allergen challenge on eosinophils, eosinophil cationic protein, and granulocyte-macrophage colony-stimulating factor in mild asthma. Am J Respir Crit Care Med 151:1915–1924, 1995.
163. Ying S, Durham SR, Barkans J, et al: T cells are the principal source of interleukin-5 mRNA in allergen-induced rhinitis. Am J Respir Cell Mol Biol 9:356, 1993.
164. Ying S, Durham SR, Jacobson MR, et al: T lymphocytes and mast cells express messenger for the interleukin-4 in the nasal mucosa in allergen-induced rhinitis. Immunology 82:200–206, 1994.
165. Ying S, Hamid QA, Durham SR, et al: Phenotype of cells expressing mRNA for interleukin-4 and interleukin-5 in atopic asthma. Am J Respir Crit Care Med 149:A953, 1994.
166. Zawadski DK, Lenner KA, McFadden ER Jr: Re-examination of the late asthmatic response to exercise. Am Rev Respir Dis 137:837–841, 1988.
167. Zunich KM, Nelson HS, Patel A, et al: The effect of theophylline and enprofylline on the late cutaneous response to antigen and compound 48/80. J Allergy Clin Immunol 83:428–434, 1989.

18 The Autonomic Nervous System, Neuropeptides, and Allergy

THOMAS B. CASALE JAMES N. BARANIUK

Sensory, parasympathetic, and sympathetic nerves regulate epithelial, vascular, glandular, and smooth muscle functions that protect the nasal, pharyngeal, laryngeal, tracheal, and bronchial airways from injury due to inhaled factors, microbial colonization, and infection.[9, 20, 29, 30] Sensory nerves sense the conditions of the mucosal microenvironment. Through synapses with the central nervous system, local parasympathetic ganglia, and local axon response mechanisms, these nerves recruit systemic parasympathetic and sympathetic reflexes, local parasympathetic responses, and local neuropeptide-induced neurogenic inflammation. Each separate population of sensory, parasympathetic, and sympathetic nerves contains a unique combination of classic neurotransmitters (e.g., acetylcholine, norepinephrine) and neuropeptides (Table 18–1). Nociceptive neurons may contain substance P (SP), neurokinin A (NKA), calcitonin gene-related peptide (CGRP), and other peptides. Parasympathetic neurons usually contain acetylcholine (ACh), vasoactive intestinal peptide (VIP), and related peptides. Sympathetic neurons contain norepinephrine and neuropeptide Y (NPY). In a single neuron, depolarization releases the same combination of neurotransmitters from all peripheral (mucosal) and central neurosecretory sites (CNS) (Dale principle).[83, 98] Because coreleased peptides and other transmitters may have synergistic, antagonistic, or autoregulatory effects, it is misleading to ascribe the functions of nerve populations to individual neurotransmitters.

Pharmacologic studies with adrenergic and cholinergic antagonists have provided a physiologic classification of neural functions: adrenergic (bronchodilator), cholinergic (bronchoconstrictor), inhibitory nonadrenergic noncholinergic bronchodilator (i-NANC), and excitatory nonadrenergic noncholinergic bronchoconstrictor (e-NANC).[24, 26] Pharmacologically defined NANC actions were once thought to define a new system of nerves; it is now appreciated that existing anatomically defined sensory, parasympathetic, and sympathetic neural systems contain heterogenous populations of nerve fibers with various combinations of classic neurotransmitters and neuropeptides that collectively lead to the pharmacologically defined cholinergic, adrenergic, i-NANC, and e-NANC effects (Table 18–2).

This chapter will first review the innervation of the upper and lower airways and describe the location and functions of the neurotransmitters and neuropeptides important to the respiratory nervous system. The second part of this chapter will focus on the role of the nervous system in controlling normal airway functions and the putative contribution of abnormal neural function in mediating airway diseases, especially rhinitis and asthma.

NOCICEPTIVE SENSORY NERVES

INNERVATION

Nasal sensory nerves originate in the trigeminal ganglion and innervate the nose via ethmoidal and posterior nasal nerves.[265, 328] These highly branched neurons innervate vessels, glands, and the epithelium where they extend between basal cells. Some endings have fine terminal extensions that reach up between epithelial cells to the region of the tight junctions. Nociceptive (pain message) nerves are unmyelinated bare fibers (type C) that do not have specialized sensory organs. The turbinate, septal, and sinus mucosa do not appear to have other specialized sensory organs like the skin or tendons. The olfactory mucosa, which covers the superior portion of the nasal cavity, is innervated by the first cranial nerves. The nervus terminalis also innervates this region.[88] In the CNS, trigeminal nociceptive neurons enter the pons through the sensory root and turn caudally in the trigeminal spinal tract to terminate in the pars caudalis of the nucleus of the spinal tract in the lower medulla and upper three cervical segments of the spinal cord.[39] Pars caudalis interneurons cross the midline to enter the trigeminothalamic tract and terminate in the medial part of the ventral posterior thalamic nucleus (arcuate or semilunar nucleus). Painful and strong thermal stimuli are appreciated at the thalamic level. Tertiary neural relays to the lower third of parietal cortical somesthetic areas provide greater localization of painful stimuli.

The dorsal part of the trigeminal spinal tract includes a small bundle of thermosensitive and nociceptive neurons from the facial, glossopharyngeal, and vagal nerves.[39] The glossopharyngeal nerve innervates the posterior third of the tongue, upper pharynx, tonsils, eustachian tube, and middle ear. Glossopharyngeal afferents from the carotid sinus baroreceptors and carotid body chemoreceptors assist in the regulation of arterial blood pressure and oxygen tension/ventilatory

TABLE 18–1
NEUROTRANSMITTERS AND ADDITIONAL PEPTIDES

Trigeminal Sensory Neurons	
Tachykinins: Substance P	SP
Neurokinin A	NKA
Neuropeptide K	
Neurokinin B	NKB
Calcitonin gene-related peptide	CGRP
Gastrin-releasing peptide	GRP
Postganglionic Parasympathetic Neurons	
Acetylcholine	ACh
Vasoactive intestinal peptide	VIP
Peptide with histidine at the N-terminal and methionine at the C-terminal	PHM
Peptide with histidine at the N-terminal and isoleucine at the C-terminal	PHI
Peptide with histidine at the N-terminal and valine at the C-terminal	PHV
Helodermin	
Postganglionic Sympathetic Neurons	
Norepinephrine	
Neuropeptide tyrosine (Y)	NPY
Other Neuropeptides That May Occur in Respiratory Mucosa	
Galanin	GAL
Atrial natriuretic peptide	ANP
Neurotensin	NT
Enkephalins	ENK
Dynorphin	DYN
Cholecystokinin octapeptide	CCK-8
Pituitary adenylate cyclase–activating peptide	PACAP PACAP-27
Somatostatin	SOM
Calcitonin	CALC
Endothelin I, II, and III	ET_1, ET_2, ET_3
Proteolytic Peptide Products From Plasma and Mucosal Proteins	
Bradykinin	BK
Kallidin (lysyl-bradykinin)	Lys-BK
Complement fragments	C3a, C5a

function, respectively. Vagal afferents with cell bodies in the small superior or nodose vagal ganglia innervate the lower pharynx, epiglottis, larynx (recurrent laryngeal nerve), trachea, main stem and subsegmental bronchi, and esophagus, whereas the vagal auricular branch innervates a portion of the external ear, auditory canal, tympanic membrane, middle ear, and eustachian tube. Central glossopharyngeal and vagal afferents descend in the medullary solitary tract and end in the more caudal part of its nucleus. From these nuclei, interneuron connections are made with the dorsal motor neurons of the vagus nerve, reticular visceral centers, and subsequently hypothalamic nuclei. The neurotransmitters of these interneurons are not known. However, SP receptors in the ventrolateral medulla regulate ventilatory responses,[72] suggesting that tachykinins are candidate neurotransmitters.

Fibers transmitting data for touch from the posterior tongue, pharynx, and larynx may terminate in the nucleus of either the trigeminal spinal tract or the solitary tract. These serve as the afferent limbs of the gag reflex.[39] The efferent limb of the gag reflex involves activation of the nucleus ambiguus and hypoglossal nucleus and stimulation of the striated muscle of the soft palate, pharynx, larynx, and upper esophagus. The motor division of the accessory nerve innervating these structures could be thought of as a division of the vagal motor nerve, but common convention does not support this contrary view. Connections between the afferent interneurons of the nuclei of the trigeminal spinal tract and the solitary tract with the nucleus ambiguus establish the reflexes for sneezing, coughing, gagging, and vomiting that have critical functions in protecting the integrity and patency of the nasal, pharyngeal, and laryngeal airways. These connections also regulate parasympathetically mediated glandular secretion in the nose (superior salivatory nucleus and facial nerve) and bronchial glandular and smooth muscle function in trachea and bronchi (dorsal motor nuclei of the vagal nerve). Parasympathetic function is described later.

NOCICEPTION

Two types of nerve fibers mediate nociceptive functions. A_{delta} fibers convey initial sharp pain, which is followed by the delayed transmission of dull, more prolonged pain sensations conveyed by unmyelinated C fibers. C fibers have bare neural endings that appear to be the most evolutionarily primitive sensory apparatus. These chemosensitive and mechanothermal sensitive neurons can be stimulated by in-

TABLE 18–2
MAJOR MUCOSAL FUNCTIONS THAT ARE REGULATED BY NEURAL PATHWAYS

Function	Mechanism	Mediators
Tracheobronchial air flow		
Bronchoconstriction	Smooth muscle contraction	Parasympathetic (ACh m_3), sensory (NKA>SP, CGRP) endothelin
Bronchorelaxation	Smooth muscle relaxation	NO?, VIP?, prostaglandins?, β_2-adrenergic stimuli
Nasal airflow resistance determined by mucosal thickness (sinusoidal filling)	Vasodilation	Sensory (SP, CGRP), parasympathetic (ACh, VIP), bradykinin
	Vasoconstriction	Sympathetic (norepinephrine, NPY), endothelin?
Vascular permeability	Endothelial cell contraction and plasma extravasation	Sensory (SP)
	Vasoconstriction	Sympathetic (norepinephrine, NPY)
Glandular secretion of antimicrobial defense factors, mucins, and other products	Exocytosis and expulsion	Sensory (SP, GRP), parasympathetic (muscarinic M_3, possibly M_1, VIP), sympathetic (α-adrenergic), endothelin

flammatory mediators such as histamine, bradykinin, serotonin, K^+, and H^+ that are released following mucosal injury or mast cell degranulation after allergen exposure.[9, 69] Prostaglandins and peptidoleukotrienes modulate sensory nerve function by altering the threshold to depolarization, making it easier to stimulate these nerves.[220] Other inhaled agents such as SO_2, O_3, formaldehyde, nicotine, cigarette smoke, and capsaicin can also stimulate these nerves.

Depolarization of the peripheral nociceptive nerve ending generates a wave of depolarization that extends throughout the entire length of the nerve axon and all the extensively branched rami. The wave of depolarization releases colocalized combinations of neuropeptides from neurosecretory swellings (varicosities) that are found near glands and vessels. The neuropeptides, including CGRP, gastrin-releasing peptide (GRP), the tachykinins SP and NKA, and possibly other unidentified neuropeptides.[9, 20, 29, 30, 69] The varicosities are strung like beads on a string along the extensively branched peripheral sensory nerve. The same combination of neuropeptides is packaged in vesicles in all the varicosities and released from all the central and peripheral varicosities of a single neuron (Dale principle).[83, 98] Sensory neuropeptides act upon specific receptors on target cells to initiate and amplify inflammatory responses to mucosal injury. This axon response mechanism mediates cutaneous wheal and flare reactions,[12] and in the respiratory tract initiates and amplifies local mucosal vasodilation, vascular permeability, and glandular exocytosis and may facilitate vascular wall leukocyte adhesion.[143, 222] SP likely plays a central role in this inflammatory process since ^{125}I-SP–binding sites are widely distributed, and SP stimulates many proinflammatory effects in various models in vivo and in vitro.[16, 65] CGRP may be an important long-acting vasodilator and contribute to filling of venous sinusoids.[14] Sensory nerve stimulation and central reception of nociceptive nerve impulses in the brain stem and higher centers lead to the appreciation of sensations of itch, burning, and congestion and the initiation of important central reflexes such as sneeze, cough, and parasympathetic secretory reflexes.[265, 266]

Neuropeptide actions are limited by enzymes such as neutral endopeptidase (NEP)[50, 240, 275] and angiotensin-converting enzyme (ACE).[247] It is thought that all cells bearing peptide receptors also express NEP. Destruction of NEP activity may lead to prolonged, unopposed inflammatory effects of neuropeptides and may contribute to respiratory hyperresponsiveness that can develop in some inflammatory rhinitic conditions and asthma.

When used as antihypertensives, ACE inhibitors have been found to produce cough that may be associated with increased airway hyperreactivity.[58, 193] It has been postulated that the cough and airway hyperreactivity associated with the use of ACE inhibitors are mediated by kinins. However, the role of kinins has not been clearly defined.[93] ACE inhibitors have also been shown to augment both spontaneous and antigen-induced histamine release from lung and skin and to potentiate antigen-induced cutaneous responses.[194] These data suggest that ACE inhibitors might also contribute to neurogenic inflammation.

PARASYMPATHETIC NERVES

INNERVATION

Nociceptive sensory nerve stimulation leads to central recruitment of parasympathetic reflexes. This is possibly the most important function of nociceptive nerves in the human respiratory tract. Parasympathetic efferent connections in the nasal cavity, ethmoid sinuses, and anterior nasopharynx are derived from preganglionic seventh nerve motor fibers from the superior salivatory nucleus that synapse in the sphenopalatine ganglion.[173] Vagal efferent fibers originating in the dorsal motor nucleus innervate laryngeal and tracheobronchial parasympathetic ganglia. The brainstem parasympathetic nuclei appear capable of regulating independent nasal, laryngeal, and tracheobronchial efferent responses to irritant stimulation in each respiratory tract location, a response that contrasts with the generalized all-or-nothing response of the sympathetic nervous system.

Postganglionic fibers innervate glands and some vessels in the nasal, pharyngeal, laryngeal, and tracheobronchial mucosa. Additional glossopharyngeal, vagal, and spinal accessory motor neurons innervate pharyngeal, laryngeal, and upper esophageal striated muscle and participate in the gag reflex that serves to protect the laryngonasal airway and clear obstructions from this critical passage.

Preganglionic parasympathetic nerves release acetylcholine (ACh) and possibly other neurotransmitters that act upon nicotinic receptor/ion channels on postganglionic neurons in airway walls. Postganglionic neurons may act as electrical filters by assessing various stimulatory and inhibitory inputs before being triggered to depolarize. Stimulation of excitatory autoreceptors by SP or other tachykinins may increase the likelihood of postganglionic cell depolarization.[28] Stimulation of inhibitory autoreceptors such as muscarinic M_2, NPY, $GABA_B$, histamine H_3, α_2- and β_2-adrenergic, μ-opioid,[273] and other receptors may decrease postganglionic cell depolarization (Table 18–3).

Postganglionic parasympathetic secretory neurons release ACh, VIP,[27] and other VIP-related peptides.[328] The cholinergic component of parasympathetic reflexes is the predominant stimulus for mucus secretion in allergic rhinitis and perhaps other respiratory diseases.[207] Nitric oxide has been proposed

TABLE 18–3
PUTATIVE AUTORECEPTOR FUNCTIONS OF VARIOUS MEDIATORS ON NEURAL DEPOLARIZATION

Depolarize Neurons	Enhance Depolarization	Inhibit Depolarization
Thermal stimuli	Prostaglandins	μ-opioid
Mechanical stimuli	Leukotrienes	β_2-adrenergic
Capsaicin (ruthenium red sensitive)	Substance P	α_2-adrenergic
Bradykinin (B_2) and electrical field stimulation (w-conotoxin sensitive) (voltage gated Ca^{2+} channel)	Neurokinin A	NPY
H^+, K^+		5-HT_3
SO_2, O_3		$GABA_B$
Histamine (H_1)		M_2 muscarinic
Serotonin (5-HT)		Histamine H_3
PAF		
Peroxides, free radicals, TDI (toluene diisocyanate)		
Neurotensin, CCK_8, $GABA_A$		
IL-1, IL-8?		
Nicotine		
Formaldehyde		
Cigarette smoke		

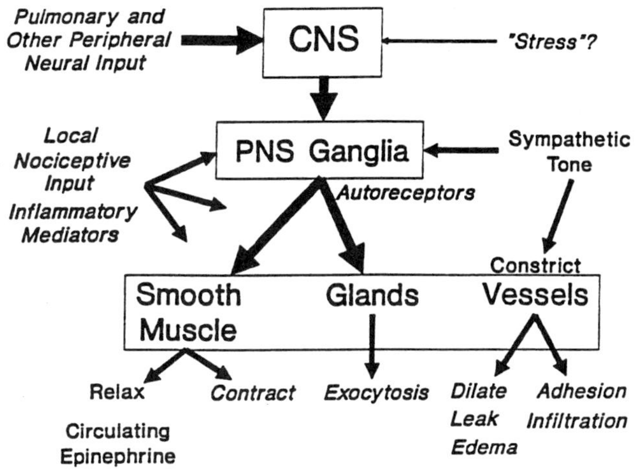

FIGURE 18–1. Airway effects of parasympathetic nervous system. Brainstem stimuli cause central nervous system (CNS) activation of vagal efferent pathways innervating the airways. These pathways are regulated by peripheral nervous system (PNS) ganglia and ultimately lead to effector functions on the target organs, smooth muscle, glands, and blood vessels. The ganglionic and postganglionic effects are influenced by nociceptive input, mediators, autoreceptors, and sympathetic tone.

as a postganglionic transmitter since constitutively expressed nitric oxide synthetase-immunoreactive material has been detected in airway nerves, but functional evidence has been mixed.[102, 174, 177, 339] A summary of parasympathetically mediated effects in the airways is illustrated in Figure 18–1.

MUSCARINIC RECEPTORS

At least five muscarinic receptor genes (m1–m5) have been cloned.[190] However, since there are partially selective pharmacologic ligands for only three receptors (M_1–M_3),[33] it is not known with certainty which of these receptor subtypes mediates ACh's actions in vivo.[27, 95] The M_3-receptor appears to be the preeminent functional subtype on cells in human nasal and bronchial mucosa and to be responsible for smooth muscle contraction and glandular secretion.[214, 248] Sensory nerve stimulation and parasympathetic reflexes likely contribute to the pathology of inflammatory conditions such as allergic rhinitis, vasomotor rhinitis, infectious rhinitis (common cold), chronic bronchitis, asthma, and infectious bronchitis.[9] Anticholinergics and muscarinic mechanisms are discussed later.[99]

SYMPATHETIC NERVES

Sympathetic reflexes have been poorly studied yet probably play a crucial role in the normal homeostasis of nasal mucosa and the responses to exercise and other stresses that require a patent nasal and bronchial airway.[10, 173, 271] Preganglionic sympathetic nerve fibers originate in the intermediolateral cell column of thoracic spinal segments.[39] Those destined to regulate respiratory vascular functions in the head synapse with postganglionic cells in the superior cervical ganglion, whereas those regulating thoracic functions synapse predominantly in the superior, middle, and lower cervical ganglia and the upper five thoracic ganglia. Sympathetic reflexes induce vasoconstriction in respiratory mucosa and may stimulate some glandular secretion in the trachea and bronchi. In the lower respiratory tract, sympathetic neural reflexes do not appear to contribute to bronchodilation. Adrenal release of epinephrine may be of greater significance in controlling bronchospasm.[25]

Sympathetic nerves contain either norepinephrine or norepinephrine plus N4P[10, 179, 180, 259]; both are potent vasoconstrictors. Agonists of α_1- and α_2-adrenergic receptors are popular nasal decongestants that effectively reduce mucosal thickness in vivo, whereas β_2-adrenergic agonists are the mainstay of bronchodilator therapy. The adrenergic receptor system is becoming more complex, as multiple α_1-receptors ($\alpha_{1a/d}$, α_{1b}, α_{1c}), α_2-receptors (α_{2c10}, α_{2c2}, α_{2c4}), and β-receptors (β_1, β_2, β_3) have been cloned.[62] The receptor mRNAs expressed in the respiratory tract are still being defined. Abnormalities of the adrenergic system that may contribute to asthma and hyperresponsiveness are discussed later.

TACHYKININS

Stimulation of nociceptive sensory nerves leads to the release of the tachykinins SP and NKA, as well as the release of CGRP and probably GRP.

TACHYKININ GENES

SP and NKA are the products of the preprotachykinin A (PPT-I) gene.[140, 243] The PPT-I gene contains seven exons. SP is coded by exon 3, and NKA by exon 6. PPT-I generates three distinct mRNAs: alpha–PPT-I lacks exon 6 and codes for SP alone; beta–PPT-I contains all the exons and codes for both NKA and SP; and gamma–PPT-I mRNA excludes exon 4 and codes for SP, NKA, and neuropeptide gamma. Nerve growth factor and noxious stimuli may up-regulate PPT-I transcription, whereas glucocorticoids may down-regulate transcription.[140, 168, 195, 196, 209] In rats, the delta-PPT gene codes for a theoretical, novel tachykinin called NP-delta.[132] NKB is produced from the PPT-II gene but has not yet been described in peripheral mammalian tissue.[140]

TACHYKININ RECEPTORS

Three tachykinin receptors, NK_1, NK_2, and NK_3, have been cloned.[120, 246, 319, 347] SP is the preferred ligand for NK_1-receptors, whereas NKA is the preferred ligand for NK_2-receptors. NKB binds preferentially to NK_3-receptors. Pharmacologic data suggest that there may be additional SP receptors and that there may be additional subtypes of NKA-preferring receptors.[5, 256] Each of the three receptors stimulates phosphoinositol metabolism when activated.

Tachykinin receptors belong to the seven transmembrane region, rhodopsin-like receptor gene superfamily.[334] Over 100 structurally and evolutionarily related G protein–associated receptors have been cloned, including α- and β-adrenergic, muscarinic, tachykinin, dopamine, serotonin, histamine, bradykinin, GRP, NPY, ANP, CCK, IL_8, odorant, and light receptors. These proteins have a glycosylated extracellular NH_2-terminal, seven transmembrane regions (Tm_1–Tm_7), three extracellular loops (E_1–E_3), three intracellular or cytoplasmic loops (C_1–C_3), and an intracellular C-terminal tail.[105] The transmembrane regions stack parallel to each other in the membrane. Specific amino acid side chains of the extracellular domains and upper portions of the transmembrane regions form the ligand binding pocket and determine the specificity and avidity of ligand binding. The third intracellular loop binds to specific G proteins that are stimulated when the ligand binds the receptor and transduce that signal into the cytoplasm.[52] The C-terminal tails contain phosphorylation sites that regulate the binding of G proteins, and so the activity of the receptor. Phosphorylation of this tail after receptor binding may be one mechanism of receptor tachyphylaxis. The nature of the G proteins associated with each receptor is under intense scrutiny but is beyond the scope of this review.[46]

SUBSTANCE P

The distribution of NK_1-receptors has been suggested by autoradiographic studies of ^{125}I-SP–binding sites.[16, 65] ^{125}I-SP binds to epithelium, vessels, glands, and smooth muscle in the upper and lower respiratory tracts (Tables 18–4 and 18–5). This distribution is consistent with the known ability of SP to induce vasodilation, vascular permeability, glandular secretion, epithelial goblet cell exocytosis, and tracheobronchial smooth muscle contraction in vivo and in vitro.[26, 204, 291, 297, 324] SP may also increase cholinergic neural responses by potentiating postganglionic parasympathetic activity.[42, 131]

In normal and mildly asthmatic humans, neither intravenous nor inhaled SP cause significant bronchoconstriction.[112, 167] Degradation of SP by NEP or ACE may explain this lack of effect. Such a hypothesis is supported by animal studies that showed enhanced SP-induced airway contraction and mucus secretion with use of specific NEP inhibitors or epithelial stripping.[242] Furthermore, in more severe asthmatics, inhaled SP did cause a dose-related decrease in FEV_1, which was blocked by nedocromil.[80] Either increased nonspecific bronchial hyperreactivity or a relative deficiency of NEP due to the increased airway epithelial damage associated with moderate to severe asthma may explain these findings.

SP nasal provocation apparently has minimal effects in normal subjects but induces albumin secretion and obstructs nasal air flow in allergic rhinitis subjects.[55, 90] Responses appear to be greater in subjects with established inflammatory syndromes such as allergic rhinitis or asthma, suggesting that neurogenic inflammatory mechanisms play a role in these diseases or airway hyperresponsiveness. The effects of neutral endopeptidase on tachykinins and neurogenic inflammation are discussed later.

SP induces serous and mucus glandular secretion from human nasal mucosal explants in vitro.[16] In pig nasal mucosa, SP increases nasal blood flow and the thickness of the mucosa.[313] SP-immunoreactive material can be collected in nasal lavage fluid[232] and bronchoalveolar lavage fluid[245] from allergic subjects after allergen challenge, suggesting that SP is released during this process. It is most likely that nociceptive nerves are the source of this SP, although other sources such as inflammatory cells have been suggested in the past.[254]

Probably more important than bronchoconstriction is the effect of SP on bronchovascular permeability and blood flow. SP and, to a lesser extent, NKA are potent inducers of bronchovascular permeability.[204] In addition, SP, NKA, and CGRP all cause vasodilation and thereby may increase fluid exudation by increasing bronchial blood flow.[112, 183] SP-induced vasodilation and plasma extravasation could be due to stimulation of endothelial cell nitric oxide (NO) production.[60]

SP can directly modulate the functions of immune/inflammatory cells. SP causes T lymphocytes to proliferate,[253] activation of macrophages,[136] enhanced macrophage and neutrophil phagocytosis,[38] chemotaxis,[63, 217] and enhanced production of IgA and IgM by B lymphocytes.[306] SP has also been shown to degranulate guinea pig eosinophils, although not via classic NK receptors.[176] Although able to induce skin mast cell degranulation in mice and humans, SP is unable to cause human lung mast cells or basophils to release histamine.[188, 221] SP can, however, stimulate human blood monocytes to release IL-1, IL-6, and TNF-α.[199] SP can stimulate endothelial cell proliferation in vitro.[350] SP and NKA may modulate human B lymphocyte maturation.[187] Thus

TABLE 18–4
RADIOLIGAND BINDING SITES FOR VARIOUS MEDIATORS IN HUMAN NASAL MUCOSA

	Sensory				Parasympathetic				Sympathetic			Inflammatory		
	SP	*NKA*	*CGRP*	*GRP*	*VIP*	*M_1*	*M_2*	*M_3*	α	β	*NPY*	*BK*	*Histamine*	*ET_1*
Epithelium	+	0	0	+ +	+	+	0	+*	?	?	0	0	0	0
Serous cells	+	0	0	+ +	+	+	0	+	?	?	0	0	0	0**
Mucous cells	+	0	0	+ +	+	+	0	+	?	?	0	0	0	0**
Vessels														
Resistance (artery, AVA)	+	+	+ +	0	+	+	0	+	?	?	+ +	+ +	+	+
Capacitance (sinusoids)	+	0	±	0	0	+	0	+	?	?	0	+ +	+	+
Permeable (postcapillary venules)	+	0	±	0	0	+	0	+	?	?	0	+ +	+	±

? Not reported.
0 Not present.
± Weak binding suggesting low density of binding sites.
\+ Binding sites present.
\+ + Dense binding suggesting high density of binding sites.
* M3 autoradiography results confirmed by in situ hybridization for m3 receptor mRNA.
** Myoepithelial cell binding sites appear to be present.

TABLE 18–5
RADIOLIGAND BINDING SITES FOR NEUROTRANSMITTERS IN HUMAN TRACHEOBRONCHIAL MUCOSA

	Sensory				Parasympathetic					
	SP	*NKA*	*CGRP*	*GRP*	*VIP*	*m1**	*m2**	*m3**	*m4**	*m5**
Epithelium	+	?	0	+	+	0	0	+	0	0
Glands	+	?	0	+	+	0	0	+	0	0
Vessels	+ +	?	+	0	+	0	0	+	0	0
Smooth muscle										
Large a/w	+	+ +	0	±	+	0	+	+	0	0
Small a/w	+	+	0	?	0	0	+	+	0	0
Alveoli	+	?	+	?	±	+	0	0	0	0

? Not reported.
0 Not present.
± Weak binding suggesting low density of binding sites.
\+ Binding sites present.
\+ + Dense binding suggesting high density of binding sites.
* Muscarinic receptor binding sites demonstrated by in situ hybridization.

tachykinins may contribute to the pathogenesis of asthma through numerous proinflammatory properties.

SP is present, along with VIP, in human eosinophils[4] and rat basophilic leukemia cells (a model mast cell).[123]

NEUROKININ A

NKA is probably the dominant tachykinin inducing bronchoconstriction in human airways,[1, 5] although SP may have activity in some other species. Moreover, whereas NK_1-receptors have greater affinity for SP, NK_2-receptors have greater affinity for NKA. Tachykinin-induced bronchoconstriction may play a role in the maturation of neural responses in the developing airway.[321]

NKA is colocalized with SP, and capsaicin depletes both of these neuropeptides from sensory afferent nerves.[203, 205] However, NKA-immunoreactive nerves are more prominently localized to bronchial smooth muscle.[327] The relative contribution of NK_2-receptors is greater than that of NK_1-receptors for bronchoconstriction.[210, 211] NKA and NK_2-receptor–mediated airway actions likely result from both direct effects on airway smooth muscle and facilitated postganglionic cholinergic activity.[131] NK_2-receptors are believed to be located on small airway smooth muscle, cholinergic neurons and ganglia, and inflammatory cells (see Tables 18–4 and 18–5). Consistent with the localization of NKA-immunoreactive nerves, NKA is a potent bronchoconstrictor, both in vitro and in vivo.[244, 327] Unlike SP, both intravenous and inhaled NKA caused dose-dependent bronchoconstriction in mild asthmatics,[167] suggesting a more important role for NKA in regulating airway tone.

TACHYKININS AND INFLAMMATION

Capsaicin, the hot, spicy essence of chili peppers,[144] specifically stimulates and depolarizes nociceptive sensory nerves and induces the sensation of burning pain. Capsaicin has proved invaluable for the investigation of these nerves in the respiratory tract.[110] Capsaicin has been used to estimate the magnitude of the axon response in pig nasal mucosa,[313] where it stimulates an increase in nasal blood flow and mucosal volume. The effect is ablated by ganglion-blocking drugs, indicating that recruited parasympathetic reflexes mediate most of the vascular reaction induced by capsaicin. When higher doses of capsaicin are combined with ganglion blockade, the axon response can be detected as a small increase in superficial blood flow. This indicates that in higher animals the axon response mechanism exists but that the major effect of sensory nerve stimulation is recruitment of parasympathetic nerves. The effects of axon responses on glandular secretion are suggested but have not been definitively shown. Evaluation of the precise role of SP and other neuropeptides in the axon response and respiratory inflammation will require the use of SP-specific antagonists.[1, 210, 267, 338] The magnitude of tracheobronchial axon responses in humans in vivo continues to be a subject of debate.

In guinea pigs, the tachykinin antagonist CP 96345 markedly inhibits SP-induced decreases in R_L and blood pressure but has no effect in allergen-induced bronchial changes, suggesting that SP has no role in the acute allergen-induced bronchoconstriction.[279] FK-888 is also effective against SP and capsaicin-induced plasma extravasation in vivo and bronchial smooth muscle contraction in vitro.[237]

Cigarette smoke has been used to stimulate neurogenic inflammation with plasma extravasation and goblet cell exocystosis in guinea pig and rat trachea in vivo. These effects are antagonized by the tripeptide SP antagonist FR 113680 and FK 224, implicating SP in cigarette smoke–induced neurogenic inflammation.[231] Dry gas hyperpnea in guinea pigs induces bronchoconstriction that can be blocked by NK_1 antagonists, indicating that irritant-induced neurogenic inflammation can lead to bronchoconstriction in vivo.[296] Nociceptive sensory neuropeptides appear capable of stimulating bronchoconstriction in vivo, but this neurogenic effect is a minor component of allergen-induced bronchoconstriction,[92] where mast cell–derived mediators are of much greater importance.

Effects of tachykinins and other neuropeptides on immune responses and inflammatory cells have been suggested. The SP antagonist spantide reduced cutaneous inflammation induced by tuberculin (delayed-type hypersensitivity) and benzoic acid–induced contact urticaria but not inflammation induced by benzalkonium chloride (irritant-delayed reaction) or UV_B irradiation.[337]

TACHYKININ ANTAGONISTS

The specificity of the SP binding to NK_1-receptors appears to reside in the positively charged N-terminal region of the peptide and interactions with the second and third extracellular loops of the receptor.[105] Cross-reactivity between tachykinin peptides is likely to be determined by the shared C-terminal regions, whereas specificity is determined by the vastly different N-terminal regions. An epitope near the sixth transmembrane region, however, may be critical for SP or NKA binding.[121] Interactions with residue 290 of the seventh transmembrane region account for difference in rat and human receptor binding.[276]

The molecular actions of tachykinin antagonists[260, 338] have been elegantly demonstrated by kinetic binding studies using chimeric receptors and the nonpeptide antagonist CP 96345.[103, 121] CP 96345 appears to bind to His[197] of the NK_1-receptor located at the junction of the second extracytoplasmic loop and the extracellular side of the fifth transmembrane region. This amino acid does not appear to be necessary for SP binding to the receptor or for the activation of associated G proteins. Binding of CP 96345 to His[197] and surrounding moieties appears to fill the well that is formed between the seven transmembranous loops of the receptor and prohibits SP docking into that well. By blocking access, CP 96345 denies SP the opportunity to interact with its receptor and activate its associated G protein. These antagonistic actions of CP 96345 are probably prototypic of other receptor antagonists.[338] However, CP 96345 and its nonantagonistic stereoisomer have calcium channel antagonist properties that may also cause effects in experimental systems. Hence, both stereoisomers should be tested to ensure NK_1-receptor specificity. Other drugs that may have tachykinin antagonist properties include imipramine,[160] actinomycin-D,[109] lithium,[335] and sodium cromoglycate.[81]

Modification of these antagonist compounds very likely will lead to the development of receptor subtype–specific antagonists that will be of great use for defining pharmacologic events and likely have utility as very specific treatments for neurotransmitter-mediated conditions.[332, 342, 343] The explosion in the number of nonpeptide receptor agonists and antagonists is in stark contrast with recent opinions that the complexity of the peptide-binding sites could demand unique peptide derivatives that could be difficult and expensive to produce and be subject to proteolysis. The lipophilicity of the nonpeptide antagonist compounds suggests that they may readily pass through the blood-brain barrier and be active in the central nervous system. These drugs may unlock many of the mysteries of the human psyche, the actions of peripheral and central nerves, neurotransmitters, and other inflammatory mediators that bind to seven transmembrane–type receptors.

In addition to interactions with NK_1-receptors and possible cross-reactivity on NK_2-receptors, some of SP's remarkable effects may be mediated by nonspecific biophysical interactions with membranes or membrane components.[268] The SP N-terminal is strongly anionic, whereas its tail is hydrophobic. The N-terminal may interact with membrane phospholipids by binding to cationic phosphate groups through hydrostatic forces while the hydrophobic C-terminal tail inserts itself between membrane lipids. This unique interaction may explain some of SP's profuse phenomenology.

SUMMARY

These data suggest that SP released from nociceptive sensory nerves may induce vasodilation, vascular permeability, and glandular secretion in respiratory mucosa but that tachykinin effects may be more prominent during inflammation. NKA released from the same neurons may be more potent than SP for induction of bronchoconstriction. The most important effects of tachykinins may be their actions on interneurons in the brain stem, spinal cord, and local parasympathetic ganglia that lead to the recruitment of systemic and parasympathetic reflexes and the supratentorial appreciation of pain (Table 18–6).

CALCITONIN GENE-RELATED PEPTIDE

Calcitonin gene-related peptide (CGRP) is also colocalized with tachykinins in sensory afferent nerves (see Table 18–1) and released by similar stimuli.[203, 205] CGRP is 37 amino acid residues long and produced in two forms: CGRP-I (CGRP-α, A-CGRP) and CGRP-II (CGPR-β, B-CGRP), which differ by three amino acids. Both forms are vasodilators. CGRP is produced by alternative processing from the same genes as calcitonin,[307] but CGRP is the predominant gene product in neural tissue. CGRP is produced along with calcitonin in tracheobronchial neuroendocrine cells.[302]

In the fetal human, CGRP is present in trigeminal ganglion cells either alone or colocalized with SP. The percentage of ganglion cells staining for CGRP or SP reaches adult levels in the immediate preterm period.[302] The roles of these neurons during development of the airways are not known. CGRP has been reported to be present in rat stomach lamina propria mononuclear cells[163] and rat tracheal epithelial serous cells[8] and may play a role in epithelial cell proliferation.

CGRP Receptors

CGRP receptor genes have not been characterized as yet, but two or possibly three receptor subtypes that are linked to G_s and stimulate adenylyl cyclase have been suggested by pharmacologic studies using the $CGRP_1$-selective agonist CGRP (8–37), the $CGRP_2$-selective agonist [Cys(acetamidomethyl)^{2,7}]-hCGRP-α, and amylin, a CGRP-like peptide with about 50% sequence homology to CGRP-α and CGRP-β.[74] Studies of CGRP receptor subtypes may prove difficult since CGRP and CGRP-related peptides may also interact with tachykinin and CCK receptors. Further pharmacologic studies and receptor cloning are required to evaluate these possibilities.

CGRP Functions

In the adult human nasal mucosa, CGRP-containing nerve fibers densely innervate arterial vessels but also innervate venous vessels and some gland acini and extend into the epithelium.[14, 328] CGRP appears to be colocalized with SP in tracheobronchial nerves.[148] ^{125}I-CGRP–binding sites are concentrated on arterioles in nasal and bronchial mucosa (see Tables 18–4 and 18–5).[14, 213] These distributions of

TABLE 18–6
PUTATIVE ACTIONS OF NEUROTRANSMITTERS

System	Transmitter	Receptor	Actions
Sensory	SP > NKA	NK_1	Arterial dilation, vascular permeability, mucus secretion, leukocyte infiltration
	NKA > SP	NK_2	Bronchoconstriction
	CGRP	CGRP	Arterial dilation
	GRP	GRP	Serous secretion, mucus secretion, trophic factor
Parasympathetic	ACh	M_1	Glandular secretion
		M_2	Inhibitory autoreceptor
		M_3	Glandular secretion, vasodilation, smooth muscle contraction
		M_4	?
		M_5	?
	VIP	VIP	Arterial dilation, bronchodilation, gland secretion
	Nitric oxide?	Guanylate cyclase	Bronchodilation, vasodilation
Sympathetic	Norepinephrine	α_1, α_2	Vasoconstriction, bronchoconstriction (α_1, weak)
	Epinephrine*	$\beta_2 > \beta_1$	Bronchodilate, vasodilate
	NPY	Y_1	Postsynaptic receptors stimulate vasoconstriction
		Y_2	Presynaptic receptors inhibit neurotransmitter release

*Adrenal origin.

CGRP nerve fibers and binding sites are consistent with the physiologic role of CGRP as a long-acting and potent arterial vasodilator.[183]

CGRP is a very potent vasodilator with a relatively slow onset in action but very prolonged duration of action.[53, 54] CGRP does not induce vascular permeability on its own but can synergistically interact with other vasomotor agents to increase blood flow[53, 54, 114] and augment the vascular permeability effects of SP and other peptides (see Tables 18–2 and 18–6). CGRP agonists may have some utility as arterial dilators in the treatment of congestive heart failure,[118, 287, 312] cardiac arrhythmias,[348, 349] Raynaud's disease,[286] and erectile dysfunction[94, 309] and the salvage of traumatic tissue flaps with compromised blood supply.[165] CGRP antagonists could act as decongestants of CGRP-induced arterial dilation.

In vitro, biologic effects of CGRP include bronchoconstriction, vasodilation, and mucus secretion. These effects appear to be mediated by specific receptors linked to adenylate cyclase.[30] Although CGRP-immunoreactive nerves are found near ganglia, blood vessels, tracheobronchial smooth muscle, and respiratory epithelium, CGRP receptors are localized predominantly to airway blood vessels.[213, 290] Therefore, in concert with SP and NKA, CGRP may contribute to airway edema through potent and prolonged vasodilation and increased blood flow.[280] Moreover, both CGRP and SP may contribute to increased airway secretions via effects on submucosal glands, glycoprotein secretion, goblet cells, and epithelial ion transport.[37, 264, 272, 324] Indirect evidence supporting a role for CGRP in airway disease includes increased levels of tissue CGRP after aeroallergen challenge and chronic smoke exposure.[200]

CGRP-binding sites have not been found on glandular cells.[14] In short-term explant cultures of human nasal mucosa, CGRP failed to stimulate mucus release.[14] Although CGRP-immunoreactive nerve fibers are present in gland acini, the release of CGRP from nerves in glands probably does not lead to exocytosis since there are no CGRP-binding sites on those cells. In contrast, CGRP stimulated nasal glandular secretion from guinea pig nasal mucosa,[116] indicating that there are significant differences in the responses to peptides in different species, and that conclusion drawn from animal experiments may not be representative or extrapolated to human conditions.

CGRP and its degradation products may be chemotactic for eosinophils.[138] In contrast to SP, however, CGRP may also have anti-inflammatory properties, such as inhibition of hydrogen peroxide production and antigen presentation by macrophages.[85]

GASTRIN-RELEASING PEPTIDE

Gastrin-releasing peptide (GRP) is a 27 amino acid peptide that shares sequence homology with GRP_{10} (GRP [18–27] or neuromedin C) and bombesin (14 amino acid amphibian peptide).[317] Related peptides include neuromedin B (NMB) and NMB_{10} and the amphibian peptides ranatensin, litorin, and phyllolitorin. Mammalian and amphibian GRP and NMB are derived from genes having three exons, whereas it is thought that amphibian bombesin, ranatensin, and phyllolitorin are derived from genes with only a single exon. Mammalian equivalents of bombesin, ranatensin, and phyllolitorin have not yet been identified.

The GRP bombesin peptides share a common aminated heptapeptide C-terminal sequence (WAVGHLM-NH_2) that is the active part of the peptide.[206, 317, 340] Bombesin-immunoreactive peptides are expressed by normal human bronchial epithelial neuroendocrine cells[325] and can be detected in bronchoalveolar lavage fluids.[3] Bombesin-reactive antiserum recognizes GRP, GRP_{10}, bombesin, and possibly other peptides.

GRP gene transcripts are processed differently in endocrine and neural tissues,[300, 301] suggesting that mRNA splicing may contribute to the diversity of bombesin-immunoreactive peptides. Three prepro-GRP mRNAs have been identified that code for an N-terminal signal peptide, GRP_{27}, and a C-terminal extension peptide (CTEP). Each of the three mRNAs codes for a different CTEP. Functions for the signal peptides and CTEPs have not been determined. GRP and related peptides are NEP substrates; some of the diversity of peptides detected by HPLC may represent proteolytic digestion in vivo.

Three receptors have been cloned for bombesin family peptides.[40, 79, 101, 336] GRP receptors preferentially bind GRP, neuromedin C, and bombesin, whereas NMB receptors prefer neuromedin B and bombesin over GRP. Bombesin receptor subtype 3 (BRS-3) has been cloned, but the endogenous peptide ligand has not been identified. The distributions of each receptor subtype in normal respiratory mucosa have not been fully determined. Since these receptors may play autocrine, trophic roles in small cell carcinoma in vitro,[317] it is possible that GRP, NMB, or other related peptides have trophic properties in respiratory mucosa in vivo.

In human nasal mucosa, GRP nerve fibers are present in the walls of arterial and venous vessels and around glandular acini.[15] Their distribution is very similar to that of CGRP and NKA and suggests, but does not prove, that GRP is colocalized in the same trigeminal sensory neurons. ^{125}I-GRP–binding sites are localized to the epithelium and submucosal glands of human nasal and tracheal mucosa (see Tables 18–4 and 18–5).[15] In vitro, GRP induces both serous and mucous cell exocytosis from human nasal mucosa. In vivo, bombesin stimulates mucous glycoconjugate and lysozyme secretion from human nasal mucosa but does not stimulate albumin secretion,[23] suggesting an effect on submucosal (and possibly goblet cell) secretion without increases in vascular permeability. The C-terminal region is essential for function since GRP, bombesin, and GRP (20–27) stimulate secretion in human nasal and feline tracheal mucosa in vitro and guinea pig nasal mucosa in vivo, whereas GRP (1 16), an N-terminal fragment, is inactive.[15, 115, 206] Bombesin is a bronchoconstrictor in guinea pig tracheal smooth muscle in vitro and in vivo.[43]

GRP-containing neuroendocrine cells are rare in normal, nonsmoking adults but as much as 10 times more common in cigarette smokers and in hamsters exposed to cigarette smoke.[3] GRP and NMB and their receptors are present in small cell carcinomas and cell lines derived from these tumors and are proliferation factors for these cells.[117] GRP and related peptides may also stimulate proliferation of nonneoplastic cells in inflammatory conditions such as asthma and bronchopulmonary dysplasia, suggesting that autocrine release of GRP may play a role in many bronchial disorders.

These varied effects suggest that GRP or related peptides may be released from trigeminal sensory nerves and bronchial neuroendocrine cells and may act as a serous and mucous cell secretagogue, a bronchoconstrictor, and potential growth factors in human respiratory mucosa (see Tables 18–2 and 18–6).

NEUTRAL ENDOPEPTIDASE

The actions of neuropeptides are limited by their degradation by neutral endopeptidase E.C.3.4.24.11 (NEP),[50, 241, 275] with contributions by other enzymes such as angiotensin converting enzyme,[247] aminopeptidase M, carboxypeptidase M,[89] and others in various systems. NEP is active upon SP, NKA, CGRP, GRP, bombesin, enkephalins, endothelin, atrial natriuretic peptide (ANP), bradykinin, and many other peptides. NEP is postulated to be present on all cells that possess peptide receptors.[241, 275]

The NEP gene of 24 exons codes for a 749 amino acid long membrane-bound protein.[82, 293] Alternative mRNA splicing generates several different-size mRNA's, including one with a deletion of exon 16 that yields a nonfunctional protein[152] and a hypothetical product with a deletion of exons 5 through 18.[197]

The inhibition of NEP enzyme activity with phosphoramidon or thiorphan augments many peptide-induced effects, including epithelial cell ciliary beat frequency; goblet cell secretion; mucus secretion from ferret and feline tracheas; airway microvascular leak induced by tachykinins, bradykinin, depolarization of the vagal nerve, electrical field stimulation, and capsaicin; and neutrophil adhesion to the endothelial surface of vessels.[50, 241, 257, 275] These functional data indicate that NEP activity is present on epithelial, glandular, vascular, and smooth muscle cells. The distributions of NEP-immunoreactive material and mRNA are consistent with these activities. In situ hybridization of NEP mRNA and immunohistochemistry of NEP-immunoreactive material have revealed NEP in epithelium, glands, and vessels of human nasal mucosa[18] as well as tracheobronchial smooth muscle cells.[17] As already shown, these cells are innervated by neuropeptide-containing nerves and possess neuropeptide-binding sites. These data are consistent with the hypothesis that NEP is present in all cells that bear neuropeptide receptors and that NEP plays a role in regulating neuropeptide-mediated responses.

NEP may have many diverse functions in vivo. Jejunal mucosal NEP may digest peptides.[59] A limited amount of longitudinal and circular intestinal muscle also expresses NEP mRNA, but vessels in the lamina propria and ganglion cells have been negative. Renal proximal tubule brush border contains abundant NEP that may degrade urinary filtrate peptides so that their amino acids can be absorbed. NEP may also help regulate renal blood flow by actions on atrial natriuretic peptide (ANP), renin, bradykinin, or other vasoactive peptides. NEP may play a role in vascular remodeling in rats exposed to chronic hypoxia[341] and regulate other vascular events through actions on arterial and venous endothelial cells.[198] NEP may play a regulatory role in the developing human fetal lung since it is expressed at the growing front of airway epithelium.[316]

There has been intense speculation regarding the role of NEP in neurogenic inflammation. Inhibition of neutral endopeptidase potentiates inflammation and bronchial smooth muscle contraction induced by SP, capsaicin, and vagal nerve stimulation, suggesting that tachykinins and/or other NEP substrate peptides can cause neurogenic inflammation and that their effects are regulated by NEP.[145, 329] Decreases in NEP activity may underlie the increased responses of respiratory mucosa to neurogenic inflammation and some agonists (hyperresponsiveness) found during and after viral and *Mycoplasma* infections[162, 223, 257] and after exposure to cigarette smoke,[97] ozone,[345] and hypochlorous acid.[185, 238] The release of peptides into areas with reduced NEP activity could lead to enhanced peptide-induced epithelial cell function, glandular secretion, vascular permeability, and smooth muscle contraction. Cell surface NEP activity may also be modulated by rapid internalization and proteolytic degradation as occurs in human neutrophils, which are activated by phorbol ester or diacylglycerol.[100] Although alterations of NEP activity or expression in human diseases have yet to be demonstrated in vivo, inhalation of thiorphan, an NEP inhibitor, permits inhaled NKA to exert a mild bronchoconstrictor effect in nonasthmatic subjects who otherwise do not respond to inhaled NKA.[73] This suggests that tonic peptide and NEP activities exist in the normal airway and that the balance between the two influences can be altered to produce bronchoconstriction in an otherwise normal airway.

Glucocorticoid treatment, on the other hand, has been shown to increase NEP mRNA and enzyme activity in a cultured, SV-40 transformed human epithelial cell line[51] and Calu-1 cells (human lung epidermoid carcinoma cell line).[185] This enhancement of NEP expression may explain the beneficial effects of glucocorticoids on neurogenic plasma extravasation in virus-infected rat trachea.[223, 257] Glucocorticoid treatment also alters the size of NEP mRNA transcripts,[51] suggesting complex regulation at the level of mRNA transcription and/or pretranslational processing. NEP expression by lung fibroblasts in culture can be increased by incubation with cytokines such as IL-1α, TNF-α, transforming growth factor, IL-6, and GM-CSF.[175] Cyclic nucleotide and prostaglandin-dependent mechanisms may mediate these effects. These cytokines may play a role in the induction of NEP in perivascular cells of synovial vessels from rheumatoid arthritis and osteoarthritis patients.[216] Synovium from normal joints demonstrates no immunohistochemical staining, indicating that some aspect of the disease state can induce NEP immunoreactivity. Induction or suppression of NEP would be expected to alter the responses of cells to other peptides and could represent a very efficient method of autoregulation.[308] Contrary reports, however, show that glucocorticoids have no effect on NEP expression in some cultured human epithelial cell lines[263] and that no changes in NEP activity have been detected in asthma or other chronic respiratory conditions.[274]

Although these investigations of NEP and its complex regulation continue to direct speculations regarding the significance of neurogenic inflammation in human disease, there is still a need to continue to measure actual NEP activities in vivo in human tissues in order to clearly define whether NEP or reductions in its activity play any significant pathogenic role in human disease.

VASOACTIVE INTESTINAL PEPTIDE

Vasoactive intestinal peptide (VIP) is colocalized with ACh in parasympathetic neurons in the bronchi and nose (see Table 18–1).[19, 91, 181] Parasympathetic ganglia may be able to alter their repertoire of neuropeptide expression and neurotransmitter phenotype since heart-lung transplant can lead to the expression of NPY by these cells.[304] It remains undetermined if there are analogous changes during airway inflammatory diseases such as asthma. VIP may also be present in some subsets of sensory nerves.[135]

The VIP gene complex has been cloned and demonstrates that posttranslational modification of prepro-VIP[346] yields VIP plus PHM (polypeptide with histidine at the N-terminal and methionine at the C-terminal). PHM is the human form of PHI (isoleucine at the C-terminal), which was previously described in porcine neural tissues.[75] Other VIP-like peptides have also been described, including PHV (peptide with histidine at the N-terminal and valine at the C-terminal), helodermin, helospectin, pituitary adenylate cyclase–activating peptide (PACAP and PACAP-27), extendin-3, growth hormone–releasing factor, and secretin.[29] These peptides share sequence homology, may interact with VIP receptors, and have similar vasodilatory, bronchodilatory, and secretomotor effects. Separate VIP-preferring[157, 305] and secretin-preferring[156] receptors have been cloned, and it is likely that additional PACAP and extendin-3 receptors will also be discovered. In general, VIP and these related peptides are thought to stimulate adenylyl cyclase to increase cAMP levels through receptor-mediated activation of G_s. VIP is a neutral endopeptidase substrate.[124]

Standard autoradiographic receptor localization studies with ^{125}I-VIP have identified VIP-binding sites on nasal epithelium, glands, and vessels (see Table 18–4).[19] In the lung, VIP-binding sites are found on epithelium, submucosal glands, vessels, and smooth muscle of large airways (see Table 18–5).[64] VIP receptor density appears to decrease as airways become smaller. This may be related to a decrease in the parasympathetic innervation in these smaller bronchi. Some VIP-binding sites are also present on alveolar cells, but their functions, and the alveolar source of VIP in vivo, are unclear.

Both VIP and PHM are potent large airway relaxants (see Tables 18–2 and 18–6).[202] In vitro, VIP is approximately 50 times more potent than isoproterenol.[251] Thus both the localization and physiologic effects of VIP and PHM on larger airways suggest that these neuropeptides antagonize the bronchoconstrictor effects of ACh. The mechanism of this antagonism appears to involve direct bronchodilatory effects on airway smooth muscle and cholinergic inhibition at the level of both ganglia and ACh release.[219, 284, 315] VIP has been touted as a major NANC bronchodilator, that is, a bronchodilating neurotransmitter released after vagal nerve stimulation in the presence of adrenergic and cholinergic blockade, but this contention is controversial.[102, 339] As will be discussed elsewhere in this text, it is likely that nitric oxide (NO) released from parasympathetic and/or other nerve populations or stimulated end organs that express the constitutive NO-synthetase have more potent bronchodilating effects.[102]

VIP dilates both resistance and capacitance vessels in nasal mucosa.[215] In vitro, VIP stimulates serous cell exocytosis of lactoferrin and mucin-immunoreactive material from human nasal mucosal explants.[236] VIP and ACh did not have additive effects in this system. VIP increases mucus secretion from cat trachea[292] and epithelial cell secretion in dog and ferret trachea.[270] In contrast, VIP may inhibit mucus secretion from human bronchial explants.[77] Anti-VIP antibodies may play a pathologic role in some cases of chronic bronchitis.[218] In vivo, VIP may be more active as a vasodilator than as a secretagogue since atropine blocks essentially all gland secretion but only partially blocks neurogenically induced blood flow.[186, 201, 215] Effective VIP antagonists will be required to determine the relative importance of ACh and VIP in parasympathetically mediated secretion.

VIP also has a variety of anti-inflammatory actions. VIP inhibits natural killer cell activity, lymphocyte traffic and proliferation, IL-2 release, and mast cell degranulation.[330] VIP may act as a free radical scavenger.[277] Conversely, mast cell mediators, such as tryptase and chymase, are capable of degrading VIP.[71, 104] Indeed, the limited bronchodilatory potency of VIP in several human in vivo studies may be related to rapid enzymatic degradation of the peptide.[33, 230, 320] Thus interactions between VIP and inflammatory cells may significantly affect lung function.

VIP is also present along with SP in human eosinophils[4] and rat basophilic leukemia cells,[124] indicating that these neuropeptides may act as inflammatory mediators.

Evaluation of the full range of VIP-related effects will result from the use of peptide and nonpeptide VIP antagonists.[260] VIP agonists may be developed as clinically useful vasodilating agents. They would be of value as bronchodilators in asthma only if peptidase-resistant agonists were found that could be effectively inhaled or injected, if their effects were synergistic with β_2-adrenergic agonist bronchodilator drugs, and if hypotension did not limit their effective dose. Treatment of hypertension is an alternative application.

Abnormalities of VIP have been postulated to contribute to bronchial hyperreactivity, asthma, and other chronic lung diseases. Although supporting data are sparse, these abnormalities may include a deficiency in inhibitory NANC neuron density, altered release or corelease of neurotransmitters, receptor deficiencies, and depressed postreceptor responses. Airway VIP receptor number may be reduced in cystic fibrosis but not in asthma.[285] An absence of VIP-immunoreactive nerve fibers has been reported in cystic fibrosis[139] that could contribute to a decrease in VIP-induced serous cell secretion and formation of thick, mucoid secretions. More important, however, may be the effect of inflammatory mediators, such as mast cell tryptase and chymase, on VIP degradation. Pretreatment with a protease inhibitor abolished antigen-induced dysfunction of inhibitory NANC activity in a cat model.[229] A loss of VIP from human pulmonary nerve fibers has also been demonstrated in severe, but not mild, asthma. Ollerenshaw and colleagues did not find immunoreactive VIP in any lung sections from asthmatics dying of status asthmaticus but found them within nerves in more than 92% of lung sections from nonasthmatics, including smokers.[250]

Increased VIP nerve fiber density has been demonstrated in vasomotor rhinitis (chronic cholinergic rhinitis).[178] Increased glandular secretion and vasodilation may contribute to chronic vascular congestion and hypersecretion.

The rate of nerve depolarization may vary the amounts of ACh, VIP, and PHM released from parasympathetic nerves.[142] At low rates, ACh is released, whereas at high rates, acetylcholine plus VIP is released. VIP may augment the postsynaptic ACh-induced secretory response in glands (e.g., cat salivary glands)[201] but may also have presynaptic inhibitory effects, which act to limit neuropeptide release. This mechanism would conserve the amount of stored peptide since there are no reuptake mechanisms, and peptides can only be resupplied by axonal transport from the neural cell body.

NITRIC OXIDE

Increasing evidence suggests that nitric oxide (NO) may also be an important inhibitory NANC neurotransmitter in human airways (see Table 18–2).[44, 191] Nitric oxide synthetase is constitutively expressed in airway parasympathetic ganglia.[177] Low levels of inhaled NO or NO-releasing agents have been shown to be potent bronchodilators in guinea pigs.[96] Inhibition of NO synthesis in both human and guinea pig trachea blocks nonadrenergic bronchodilation and enhances cholinergic neurotransmission.[44, 326] Thus, like VIP, NO may act as both a direct bronchodilator and an antagonist of cholinergic responses.

NEUROPEPTIDE TYROSINE

Neuropeptide tyrosine (NPY) is present with norepinephrine in a population of sympathetic neurons and shares many of the same properties (see Tables 18–1 and 18–2).[179, 255, 259] NPY-induced vasoconstriction is slower in onset but longer in duration than that of norepinephrine. The walls of nasal arterioles and arteriovenous anastomoses are very densely innervated by NPY nerve fibers.[21, 328] Individual fibers are also located in venous vessels. A few fibers are present in glandular acini. NPY has no direct effect on tracheobronchial smooth muscle contraction.[191, 314]

NPY may occur in some cholinergic neurons[180, 189, 289] and a small population of VIP containing sphenopalatine neurons that innervate nasal glands.[180] The functions of colocalized neuropeptides such as NPY plus VIP are difficult to predict since complex synergistic and antagonistic interactions can occur when mixtures of peptides are released.[172]

^{125}I-NPY–binding sites have been localized by autoradiography on the smooth muscle of arterioles and the arteriolar portion of anteriovenous anastomoses, with less dense representation on the adjacent venous portions.[21] There is a strong correlation between the locations of NPY nerve fibers, NPY-binding sites on vessels, and the vasoconstrictor function of this peptide. Exogenous administration of NPY to the human nasal mucosa in vivo reduces nasal air flow resistance and albumin exudation without stimulating submucosal gland secretion, suggesting that NPY agonists may be useful for the treatment of mucosal diseases characterized by vasodilation, vascular permeability, and plasma exudation. Because NPY is a long-acting vasoconstrictor, NPY agonists may offer advantages over α-agonists for the treatment of chronic vascular congestion.

NPY receptor subtypes have been suggested (see Table 18–6). Postsynaptic Y_1-receptors may be linked to phosphatidylinositol hydrolysis[130, 141] and may potentiate the postjunctional effects of norepinephrine.[259] Prejunctional Y_2-receptors are coupled to adenylate cyclase inhibition.[130] Prejunctional Y_2-receptors on sympathetic nerves may inhibit norepinephrine release and serve to prevent depletion of these neurotransmitters. NPY inhibits cholinergic transmission in guinea pig trachea by a direct effect upon NPY receptors on postganglionic cholinergic nerves or other unresolved presynaptic sites.[314] Conceivably, adrenergic nerves could inhibit cholinergic neurotransmission by norepinephrine and NPY acting on a_2- and Y_2-receptors, respectively. Relevance to human lung physiology remains unclear, however, because NPY has no effect on either airway tone or cholinergic neurotransmission in human airways in vitro.[28]

BRADYKININ

Bradykinin (BK) and Lys-BK are generated in the respiratory tract during all forms of allergic, nonallergic, and viral inflammation from high and low molecular weight kininogens, respectively (see Table 18–1).[261] Nasal BK receptor distribution is shown in Table 18–4. BK is a potent bronchoconstrictor in asthmatic patients and also induces coughing and a sensation of chest tightness, which closely mimics a naturally occurring asthma attack.[111] Yet BK is a weak constrictor of human airways in vitro, suggesting that its potent constrictor effect is mediated indirectly. BK is a potent activator of bronchial C fibers in dogs[171] and releases sensory neuropeptides from perfused rodent lungs[282] and heart.[119] In guinea pigs, BK instilled into the airways causes bronchoconstriction, which is reduced significantly by a cholinergic antagonist (as in asthmatic patients) and by capsaicin pretreatment.[30] This indicates that BK activates sensory nerves in the airways and that part of the bronchoconstrictor response is mediated by release of constrictor peptides from capsaicin-sensitive nerves (see Table 18–3).

A component of the BK-induced bronchoconstriction seen in asthmatic patients is due to sensory neuropeptide release since specific tachykinin antagonists, cromolyn sodium, and nedocromil sodium reduce the airway changes.[111, 150] BK nasal provocation induces vascular permeability and albumin secretion by direct actions upon vascular BK receptors[13, 21] and stimulates pharyngeal discomfort by stimulating sensory nerves.[262] BK-induced responses are greater in perennial allergic rhinitis subjects than normal subjects.[20] BK-induced glandular secretion in vitro is mediated by arachidonic acid metabolites.[22] BK may be an important stimulant of combined plasma extravasation/edema and nociceptive neural reflex-mediated effects in upper and lower airways and may contribute significantly to the sensations associated with airway inflammation.

ENDOTHELIN

Endothelins are potent bronchoconstrictors. Three endothelins have been described: ET_1, ET_2, and ET_3.[48, 154, 155, 159] They have internal disulfide bonds and similar C-terminal regions. They are processed from separate genes into prepro-endothelins (big endothelins) and finally released as 27 amino acid peptides. Endothelins are generated by bronchial neuroendocrine, endothelial, and epithelial cells of asthmatics[303] and nasal epithelium and endothelium[235] and are also present in dorsal root ganglia, where they may act as neurotransmitters.[122]

Two G protein–related receptors have been cloned.[146, 147, 278] ET-receptors bind ET_1 and ET_2 more than ET_3, whereas ET_B-receptors bind all three with equal affinity. ET_B-receptors account for about 80% of airway smooth muscle endothelin-binding sites and appear to be responsible for ET-mediated contraction in human bronchus.[125] ET_A-receptors on submucosal gland myoepithelial cells stimulate contraction of these cells and extrusion of mucus exocytosed from submucosal gland cells through ducts to the mucosal surface (see Table 18–4). ET_A-receptors also are present on epithelial cells and contribute to epithelial proliferation.[166] Although endothelins are potent bronchoconstrictors and secretagogues, their true significance in asthma awaits the development of potent endothelin antagonists for human use.[76]

ADRENERGIC (SYMPATHETIC) SYSTEM

The relatively sparse sympathetic innervation of tracheobronchial airways is concentrated around parasympathetic ganglia and mucosal vessels, with minimal sympathetic innervation of airway smooth muscle.[24] Despite the lack of adrenergic innervation, there are significant numbers of both α- and β-receptors in human lung, indicating that adrenergic influences are important in determining airway tone. Quantitatively, there is a much higher density of β-receptors than α-receptors. Overall, β_2-receptors outnumber β_1-receptors approximately three to one, with airway smooth muscle, epithelial cells, and mast cells having exclusively β_2-adrenoceptors.[66, 298] Although norepinephrine is the neurotransmitter of sympathetic nerves, circulating epinephrine secreted from the adrenal medulla probably plays a more important role in lung physiology, since physiologic epinephrine concentrations induce potent bronchodilation in both normal and asthmatic subjects.[45] Abnormalities in β-receptors, α-receptors, and catecholamine secretion have been proposed to contribute to the pathogenesis of asthma.

BETA-ADRENERGIC ABNORMALITIES

The beneficial effects of β-agonists and detrimental effects of β-antagonists have justifiably suggested a role for β-adrenergic dysfunction in bronchial asthma. Well-known effects of β_2-receptor stimulation include bronchodilation, decreased mast cell degranulation, and increased mucus and water secretion.[69] Furthermore, stimulation of β_2-receptors inhibits both cholinergic and noncholinergic excitatory neurotransmission, and blockade of these receptors may mediate β-antagonist–induced bronchospasm in asthmatics.[127, 153, 269]

The β-adrenergic theory of asthma was first proposed by Szentivanyi over 30 years ago, and a comprehensive theory was published in 1968.[318] Szentivanyi's theory was based in part on a model involving injection of living or killed Bordetella pertussis organisms into certain strains of rodents, which led to features reminiscent of human asthma. These features included hypersensitivity to mediators such as histamine and BK and nonspecific stimuli such as cold air and respiratory irritants and hyposensitivity to catecholamines, with a reversal of normal adrenergic metabolic activity. Enhanced reagin-like antibody production and marked eosinophilia were also associated with these abnormalities. Szentivanyi believed that adrenergic abnormalities similar to those associated with the pertussis-induced hypersensitive state might account for both the pharmacologic and immunologic abnormalities associated with asthma.

Early support for Szentivanyi's theory came from in vivo observations demonstrating a decreased rise in blood sugar, lactate, pyruvate, cAMP, and pulse pressure in response to β-adrenergic stimulation in allergic asthmatic patients compared with normal individuals. The β-antagonist propranolol caused acute bronchoconstriction in asthmatic subjects but had no effect on airway responses of normal subjects to histamine or cholinergic aerosols.[67] Subsequent in vivo studies by Kaliner and colleagues, measuring pulse pressure and cAMP responses to isoproterenol, concluded that intrinsic β-adrenergic hyporeactivity exists in asthmatic subjects unrelated to previous adrenergic drug administration.[169] Interestingly, a comparable degree of β-adrenergic hyporesponsiveness was observed in nonasthmatic allergic subjects as well.

Spina and colleagues compared the distribution, density,

and function of β-receptors in postmortem lung samples from asthmatic and normal subjects.[298] They found attenuated in vitro responsiveness to β-agonists, but there was no reduction in β-receptor density in asthmatic lung samples.

Since analysis of lung β-receptors in living subjects has not been possible, surrogate studies have examined β-receptors on peripheral blood leukocytes. Lymphocytes of asthmatic patients have a lower density of β-receptors[57, 170] and generate less cAMP in response to β-agonists.[87, 252, 283] Other groups, however, have found reduced leukocyte β-receptor number and cAMP generation only after continuous treatment with β-agonists.[78, 113] Sano and colleagues found lower β-receptor density in mononuclear but not polymorphonuclear leukocytes of asthmatics not taking medications.[281] Interpretation of these studies is difficult because drug use can clearly affect β-receptor density on peripheral blood leukocytes. β-Agonists can decrease whereas corticosteroids can increase β-receptor density.[56, 311] Furthermore, the results may differ depending on whether mononuclear or polymorphonuclear cells are studied. One study found that treatment with terbutaline had no effect on human lung β-receptors, whereas a 57% decline was measured in the number of β-receptors on peripheral mononuclear cells of the same patients.[49] Thus it is very difficult to extrapolate results from studies of circulating leukocytes to the assessment of pulmonary β-receptors. Since in vitro autoradiography has not substantiated a decrease in β-receptor density in the airways of asthmatics and since neither β-antagonists nor adrenalectomy causes asthma in normal subjects, it is unlikely that a fundamental defect in the β-receptor system is solely responsible for the development of asthma and bronchial hyperreactivity.

Some of these β-receptor abnormalities may actually represent the consequence of the active disease state. Meurs and colleagues found a reduction in human lymphocyte β-receptor density and responsiveness only after an allergen-induced asthmatic reaction.[226] They also demonstrated a disparity between the reduction in β-receptor density (about 20%) and the loss of agonist-induced adenylate cyclase activity. They postulated that this discrepancy may indicate an uncoupling of the receptor from the adenylate cyclase complex. It has been suggested that postreceptor mechanisms include alteration of G proteins or possibly an activation of protein kinase C.[225]

Airway inflammation may lead to β-receptor dysfunction. Busse demonstrated that viral respiratory infections can lead to airway inflammation, airway hyperreactivity, and concomitant neutrophil β-adrenergic hyporesponsiveness.[61] In vitro incubation of neutrophils with rhinovirus-16 significantly decreased responses to isoproterenol.[61] Inflammatory mediators, such as platelet-activating factor (PAF), may contribute to β-adrenergic hyporesponsiveness by down-regulation of β-receptors.[2] Activation of phospholipase A_2, in addition to initiating PAF synthesis, may also stimulate a decrease in the number of β-adrenergic receptors coincident with an increase in α_1-receptors.[137]

Autoantibodies to β-receptors occur in 10% to 15% of allergic individuals and 5% of asthmatic children.[47, 333] However, since they are also found in a similar percentage of normal individuals, β-receptor autoantibodies are of doubtful pathogenic significance.[133]

In summary, although there is ample evidence of β-adrenergic dysfunction in asthmatics, it remains unclear whether this is a primary abnormality, secondary to therapy, or a consequence of inflammatory processes. The latter two possibilities are most tenable. Since most asthmatics respond very well to β-agonists and normal subjects do not become asthmatic when treated with β-antagonists, any abnormality is likely to play a minor role in asthma pathogenesis.

ALPHA-ADRENERGIC ABNORMALITIES

In comparison with β-receptors, there are relatively few α-receptors in the lung. Their role in regulating airway function is not clear. α-Receptor subtypes include postjunctional excitatory α_1-receptors and prejunctional inhibitory α_2-receptors. The subtypes of α_1- and α_2-adrenoceptors involved have not been identified. Stimulation of α_1-receptors produces modest airway constriction, increased mucus production, and enhanced mast cell degranulation.[69] Moreover, by decreasing bronchial blood flow, α_1-receptor stimulation may indirectly contribute to bronchoconstriction by facilitating airway cooling.[24]

Conversely, α_2-receptors may play a protective role in asthma. Stimulation of α_2-receptors, presumably on parasympathetic ganglia and/or postganglionic fibers, has been shown to inhibit both cholinergic and noncholinergic excitatory transmission.[128, 129] The role of prejunctional α_2-receptors on airway sympathetic nerves, however, has not been defined because the airway effects mediated by sympathetic nerves, such as bronchial blood flow and mucus secretion, are more difficult to measure.[28] Nonetheless, abnormalities of the α-adrenergic system, such as up-regulation of α_1-mediated vasoconstriction or down-regulation of α_2-mediated effects, might be expected to contribute to the pathogenesis of asthma.

Early in vivo studies by Kaliner and colleagues suggested generalized α-adrenergic hyperresponsiveness in asthmatics.[169] α-Adrenergic responsiveness, as measured by pupillary dilation and reduction in cutaneous blood flow in response to phenylephrine, was significantly greater in allergic asthmatics compared with both normal controls and allergic rhinitis subjects. Subsequent studies by Davis both confirmed these results and correlated pupillary responses with airway reactivity as measured by methacholine challenge.[86]

Using a guinea pig model of asthma, Barnes and colleagues reported a doubling in the numbers of α-receptors of lung homogenates of sensitized animals chronically exposed to ovalbumin aerosol.[34] The number of β-receptors was marginally decreased such that the ratio of α- to β-receptors nearly tripled. This alteration in this ratio was proposed as an explanation for altered adrenergic sensitivity in asthma. Other investigators, however, failed to detect a change in α_1-receptor density 24 hours after aeroallergen challenge of sensitized guinea pigs, despite a decrease in β-receptor density and exaggerated airway responsiveness to histamine.[233]

Asthmatic and normal human lung contain very low levels of α_1-receptors, and phenylephrine fails to induce significant increases in bronchial tone in vitro.[299] Thomson and colleagues demonstrated that phenylephrine was unable to induce bronchoconstriction in asthmatics.[323] In a study of nine asthmatics, inhaled prazosin, a potent and selective α_1-

antagonist, failed to alter air flow when compared with placebo.[35]

In contrast, methoxamine, another nonspecific α-agonist, did cause bronchoconstriction in asthmatic but not normal subjects.[295] Several in vitro studies suggested that α-adrenergically mediated airway constriction may only occur in inflamed lung tissue.[68] α-Antagonists have been shown to partially inhibit both histamine- and exercise-induced bronchoconstriction in asthmatic subjects.[41, 164]

In summary, there is no direct sympathetic innervation of airway smooth muscle, and the effects of α-agonists and α_1-antagonists on bronchoconstriction and bronchodilation, respectively, are weak. Therefore, it is doubtful that airway smooth muscle α_1-receptors play a significant role in airway hyperreactivity. It remains possible, however, that α_1-mediated decreases in bronchial blood flow may partially contribute to exercise-induced asthma.[24] It is also possible that dysfunction of inhibitory α_2-receptors may predispose subjects toward bronchospasm. As previously mentioned, stimulation of α_2-receptors can inhibit both cholinergic and excitatory NANC neurotransmission. Selective α_2-agonists can attenuate excitatory NANC neurotransmission in a dose-dependent manner.[161] Inhaled clonidine, an α_2-agonist, can block aeroallergen-induced bronchoconstriction in allergic asthmatics.[192] Oral clonidine, however, increased bronchial hyperreactivity to histamine.[344] These results may be explained by the reduction in overall sympathetic tone caused by CNS α_2-receptor stimulation. Overall, it appears that α-adrenergic function has minimal effects on regulation of airway function in normal or asthmatic lung.

CIRCULATING CATECHOLAMINES

In human airways, electrical field stimulation shows no evidence of adrenergic bronchodilator responses in vitro.[28] However, since β-antagonists precipitate bronchospasm in many asthmatics, this suggests an increase in bronchial adrenergic drive. Circulating catecholamines are probably responsible for this effect. Although norepinephrine is normally present in the highest plasma concentrations, norepinephrine infusions have no effect on airway caliber in asthmatics.[45] Epinephrine, however, is a potent bronchodilator, even at low doses. Since the adrenal medulla is the sole source of epinephrine, and surgical adrenalectomy can potentiate histamine-induced bronchoconstriction, the increased adrenergic drive of asthmatics is most likely provided by circulating epinephrine.[25]

Although plasma catecholamine levels are similar in stable asthmatics and normal subjects, there is evidence of a blunted rise in both epinephrine and cAMP during exercise-induced bronchoconstriction.[32, 134] Therefore, an abnormality in either epinephrine secretion or clearance may be present in some asthmatic patients. Since clearance of epinephrine does not appear to be increased, these patients may well have a defect in epinephrine secretion. This defect appears to be selective for exercise-induced bronchoconstriction, however, since both insulin-induced hypoglycemia and histamine infusion stimulate a normal rise in plasma epinephrine in asthmatics. Although this potential abnormality in catecholamine response may potentiate bronchoconstriction, it is unlikely to be a primary defect since neither adrenalectomy nor chronic β-antagonist therapy causes asthma in normal subjects.[25]

SUMMARY OF ADRENERGIC EFFECTS

Adrenergic mechanisms appear to influence cholinergic and noncholinergic excitatory activity, airway smooth muscle, mast cells, submucosal glands, and bronchial vasculature. Numerous studies have implicated abnormal adrenergic activity in the pathogenesis of asthma. Most attention has focused on mechanisms of reduced β_2-mediated effects, and these may, in part, be secondary to inflammation and/or medications rather than primary abnormalities. Current knowledge suggests only a minor role for α_1-mediated effects in normal or diseased lung, although decreased α_2-mediated inhibitory effects on both cholinergic and noncholinergic excitatory activity may be important. Although a defect in epinephrine secretion may partially contribute to exercise-induced bronchoconstriction, this is unlikely to represent a fundamental abnormality.

CHOLINERGIC (PARASYMPATHETIC) SYSTEM

The cholinergic nervous system is responsible for maintaining resting bronchial tone and, in large part, mediating acute bronchospastic responses. Cholinergic innervation also provides a major stimulus for mucus secretion from submucosal glands and goblet cells.[36, 207] The density of muscarinic receptors is greatest in larger proximal airways and least in the smaller peripheral airways, consistent with the pattern of vagal-mediated airway constriction.[31] Vagal-mediated bronchoconstriction is blocked by atropine and potentiated by acetylcholinesterase inhibitors, indicating that the effect is produced by the neurotransmitter ACh acting on muscarinic receptors.[68]

Because the cholinergic system plays an important role in maintaining resting smooth muscle tone, producing airway smooth muscle contraction, and regulating airway mucus secretion, many potential abnormalities may contribute to asthma pathophysiology. These abnormalities would be expected to either increase ACh release from cholineric nerve terminals or increase the responsiveness of target tissues. Potential mechanisms include enhanced vagal output from the CNS, enhanced cholinergic reflex activity, increased ACh release, alterations in muscarinic receptors, and enhanced airway smooth muscle responsiveness. Airway inflammation and inflammatory mediators may contribute significantly to several of these mechanisms.

ENHANCED VAGAL OUTPUT FROM CNS

Psychogenic factors have long been suspected to play some role in precipitating asthma attacks. Evidence exists that psychogenic factors can influence airway tone through vagal efferent pathways. For example, in response to inhaled saline, McFadden and colleagues demonstrated a decrease in specific airway conductance in asthmatics who were led to believe they were inhaling bronchospastic agents.[224] Furthermore, this effect was inhibited by atropine, suggesting that cholinergic pathways were involved. Moreover, enhanced vagal cardiac tone has been demonstrated in asthmatics, which indirectly suggests that asthmatics have an increase in central vagal drive. An increase in sinus arrhythmia corresponding to nocturnal bronchoconstriction has also been demonstrated.[258] Thus enhanced vagal output from the CNS may partially contribute to asthmatic bronchoconstriction.

ENHANCED CHOLINERGIC REFLEX ACTIVITY

Enhanced cholinergic reflex activity was initially postulated as a mechanism for bronchial hyperresponsiveness because it was observed that many stimuli that produce bronchoconstriction in asthmatics, such as sulfur dioxide and histamine, also stimulate vagal sensory nerve endings. Furthermore, cholinergic antagonists can inhibit the bronchoconstrictive responses to these same stimuli.[294] In addition, other inflammatory mediators, such as serotonin, prostaglandin $F_{2\alpha}$, and BK, may stimulate afferent sensory nerves, leading to bronchoconstriction.[28] Airway epithelial damage probably increases the exposure of these sensory nerve endings, thereby enhancing reflex activity due to any stimulus. This may trigger not only a reflex increase in efferent cholinergic activity but also the antidromic release of tachykinins and calcitonin gene-related peptide via a short-circuited local reflex loop.[26]

INCREASED ACETYLCHOLINE RELEASE

Efferent cholinergic discharge of ACh may be modulated at the level of postganglionic nerves or ganglia. Inflammatory mediators, such as serotonin, SP, $PGF_{2\alpha}$, TxA_2 and PAF (in the presence of platelets), may augment ACh release by prejunctional mechanisms.[84, 158] Other mediators, such as PGE_2, PGI_2, and surprisingly histamine, have the opposite effect. Histamine can inhibit vagally mediated airway contraction via H_3-receptors, although its effect is relatively weak.[149, 151] Evidence suggests that both β_2- and α_2-agonists can also inhibit cholinergic neurotransmission. Furthermore, feedback inhibition of cholinergic neurotransmission by ACh acting on M_2-autoreceptors is discussed later in this chapter. Lung parasympathetic ganglia, which are located in airway walls and surrounded by mast cells, may also be a site of neuromodulation by inflammatory mediators.[28] Once released, reduced degradation by acetylcholinesterase could potentially increase local ACh concentrations, but there is no direct evidence that this occurs. Thus modulation of cholinergic neurotransmission and ACh release is complex and involves both inflammatory mediators and neural mechanisms. Since many inflammatory mediators postulated to be important in asthma can increase ACh release, the inflammatory response noted in asthma might contribute to airway hyperresponsiveness via their effects on vagal pathways.

ALTERATIONS IN MUSCARINIC RECEPTORS

Although there are at least five muscarinic receptor genes (m_1–m_5), only three pharmacologically defined muscarinic receptor subtypes (M_1–M_3) have been identified in the human lung (Tables 18–7 and 18–8). Autoradiographic studies have revealed dense muscarinic receptor labeling over submucosal glands and airway ganglia in addition to moderate labeling of airway smooth muscle in humans.[214] The muscarinic receptors of human airway smooth muscle were entirely of the M_3 subtype, whereas bronchial submucosal glands contained both M_3- and M_1-receptors in a 2:1 ratio. These findings were confirmed by in situ hybridization techniques (see Table 18–5).[212] Airway parasympathetic ganglia are believed to contain predominantly M_1-receptors, which act to facilitate vagal transmission that classically occurs through nicotinic receptors. The M_2-receptor subtype is felt to be a presynaptic inhibitory autoreceptor on cholinergic nerves. However, mRNA for M_2-receptors is also present in human airway smooth muscle. Airway smooth muscle contraction, mucus secretion, and vasodilation are mediated predominantly by M_3-receptors. Therefore, increases (M_1, M_3) or decreases (M_2) in numbers and/or affinity of muscarinic receptors have been postulated to contribute to asthma pathophysiology.

Lammers and colleagues have shown that pirenzepine, a specific M_1-receptor antagonist, inhibits reflex bronchoconstriction due to SO_2 inhalation in humans.[184] Therefore, they hypothesized that abnormally responsive M_1-receptors in ganglia may enhance vagal reflexes in asthma by facilitating nicotinic ganglionic neurotransmission. Using nonspecific ligands, numbers of muscarinic receptors have been shown to increase slightly in guinea pigs following prolonged sensitization to ovalbumin.[228] However, Casale found no changes in muscarinic receptor number or agonist/antagonist affinity following in vitro human lung anaphylaxis.[70] Therefore, there does not appear to be generalized qualitative or quantitative muscarinic receptor alterations in acute allergic lung responses, although changes accompanying chronic allergic inflammation cannot be ruled out.

However, there are data to support down-regulation of

TABLE 18–7
PHARMACOLOGY OF MUSCARINIC RECEPTORS

Receptor	Ligands	G Protein	G-Protein Effect
M_1	Pirenzepine, telenzepine	G_q	Stimulate PLC, release IP_3 and DAG
M_2	AF DX-116, gallamine, methoctramine, himbascine, AQRA741 (pilocarpine is an agonist)	G_i	Inhibit adenyl cyclase
M_3	4-DAMP, p-F-HHSiD, zamifenacin	G_q	Stimulate PLC, release IP_3 and DAG
M_4	Himbascine	G_i	Inhibit adenyl cyclase
M_5	Not defined	G_q	Stimulate PLC

TABLE 18–8
AUTORADIOGRAPHIC LOCALIZATION OF MUSCARINIC RECEPTORS IN HUMAN NASAL AND TRACHEOBRONCHIAL AIRWAYS

Subtype	Localization	Function
M_1	Parasympathetic ganglia	Facilitate neurotransmission
	Nasal submucosal glands	Exocytosis?
	Alveolar walls	?
M_2	Postganglionic cholinergic nerves	Inhibit ACh release
	Airway smooth muscle	Inhibit adenylyl cylase, antagonize adrenergic bronchodilation
	Sympathetic nerves	Inhibit norepinephrine release
M_3	Airway smooth muscle	Contraction
	Submucosal glands	Exocytosis
	Goblet cells?	Exocytosis
	Epithelial cells	Increased ciliary beat frequency?
	Endothelial cells	Release of nitric oxide and vasodilation
M_4	Alveolar walls*	?
	Airway smooth muscle*	?
	Postganglionic cholinergic nerves	Inhibit ACh release

*Rabbit only.

inhibitory M_2-autoreceptors in asthmatics. For example, low doses of ipratropium can potentiate, rather than block, vagally induced bronchoconstriction in guinea pigs.[107] Furthermore, both antigen challenge of sensitized guinea pigs and parainfluenza virus infection can alter neuronal M_2-receptors so that they no longer function to inhibit ACh release.[106, 108] Human data also indirectly support a role for M_2-receptor dysfunction in asthma. Minette and colleagues found that, in normals, pilocarpine (an M_2-agonist) inhibited cholinergic reflex bronchoconstriction induced by inhaled SO_2.[227] Similarly, Ayala and Ahmed showed that methacholine pretreatment suppressed histamine-induced bronchoconstriction in normals.[6] In both studies, however, asthmatic subjects were not protected by such cholinergic agonists. These studies clearly suggest the possibility of M_2-receptor dysfunction in asthma. Barnes has suggested that such a defect might explain the paradoxical bronchoconstriction seen with low doses of anticholinergics as well as contribute to β-blocker–induced asthma. The loss of M_2-receptor–mediated and blockade of β-receptor–mediated inhibitory activity might allow unchecked cholinergic responses in these asthmatics.[27]

The mechanism of M_2-autoreceptor dysfunction may be related to airway inflammation. Fryer suggested that neuraminidase released from inflammatory cells may cleave critical sialic acid residues from M_2-receptors and thereby weaken agonist binding.[106] The same mechanism might account for postviral airway hyperreactivity. Eosinophil-derived major basic protein may bind M_2-receptors and make them dysfunctional. Furthermore, oxygen-derived free radicals generated by inflammatory cells may have a similar effect.[28]

M_2-receptors on smooth muscle cells may also contribute to bronchoconstriction. M_2-receptors inhibit cAMP formation. M_2 stimulation would be expected to antagonize the effects of β_2-adrenoceptor stimulation by inhibiting adenylate cyclase activity and cAMP formation.[99] Combined stimulation of M_2- and M_3-receptors on bronchial smooth muscle during periods of high vagal tone could overcome the bronchodilatory effects of circulating epinephrine or inhaled β_2-agonists. However, the predominate smooth muscle effects mediated by muscarinic receptor subtypes are those attributable to M_3-receptors (see Table 18–6).

ENHANCED AIRWAY SMOOTH MUSCLE RESPONSIVENESS

Bai showed that tracheal smooth muscle obtained from asthmatics who died during severe asthma attacks had increased in vitro cholinergic- and histamine-induced responsiveness.[7] Others, however, have failed to show increased airway smooth muscle responsiveness to cholinergic agonists in vitro.[126] Thus it remains unclear whether enhanced airway smooth muscle responsiveness contributes to asthma pathogenesis.

Other potential mechanisms of bronchial hyperresponsiveness may include decreases in either internal or external loads on airway smooth muscle. For example, Stephens and colleagues demonstrated that an internal resistance to shortening is markedly decreased in the airway smooth muscle of allergic dogs.[310] Moreover, in vivo, geometric factors related to airway thickening and edema may uncouple airway-parenchyma interdependence and result in exaggerated bronchoconstriction in response to any particular stimulus.[208] Therefore, compared with normals, the airways of asthmatics may narrow proportionately more in response to equivalent bronchoconstricting stimuli.

MUSCARINIC REFLEXES AND NASAL PATHOLOGY

Parasympathetically released ACh is paramount in stimulating submucosal gland secretion in human nasal mucosa.[248, 265, 331] About 55% of the muscarinic receptors are of the M_3 type, and the remainder are M_1 (see Table 18–4).[248] M_1-binding sites are present on epithelium and submucosal glands. M_3-receptors and M_3 mRNA have been identified by autoradiography and in situ hybridization,[11] respectively, on the epithelium, submucosal glands, and endothelium. M_2-binding sites are apparently not present in human nasal mucosa. M_4 sites were not examined.

Methacholine stimulates both serous and mucous cell exocytosis, an effect that is inhibited by M_3 antagonists and weakly inhibited by M_1 antagonists.[234, 236] In vivo, cholinergic

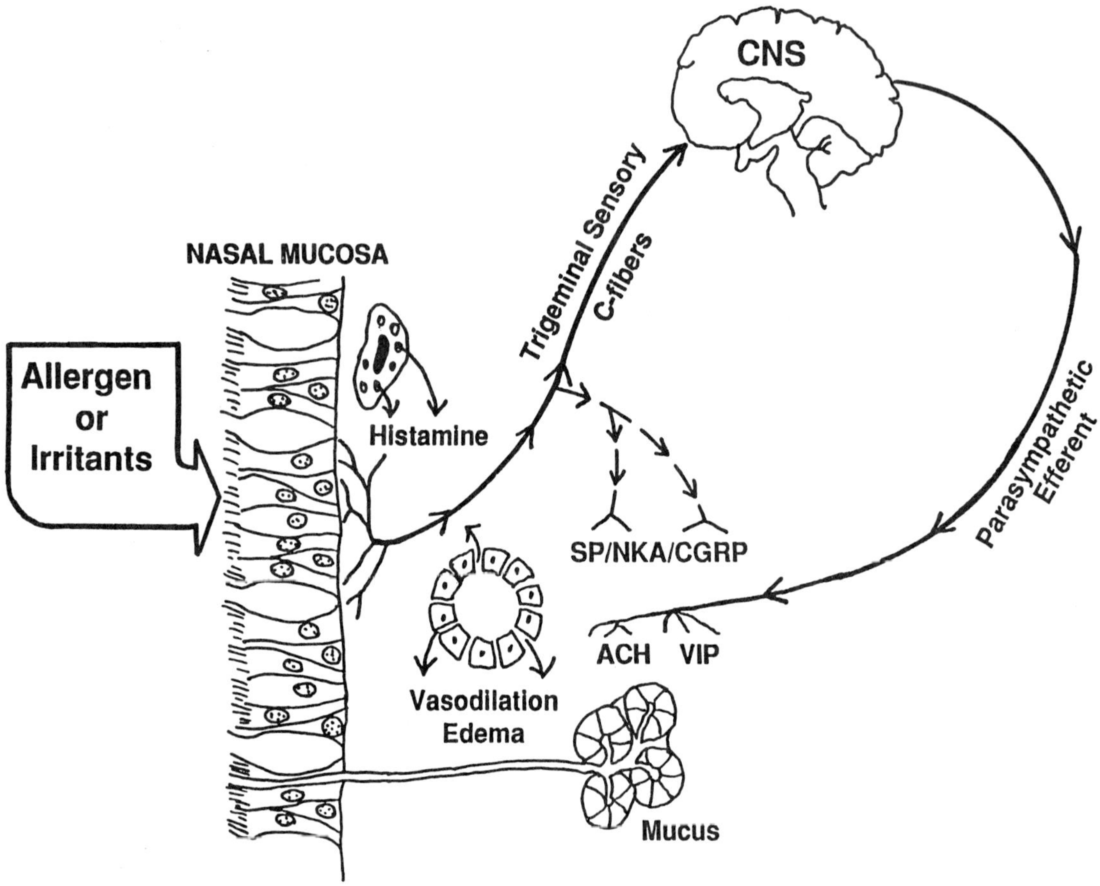

FIGURE 18–2. Schematic diagram of the neuropeptide-containing neural pathways likely to play a role in the pathogenesis of rhinitis. Inhaled allergen stimulates the release of histamine. Inhaled irritants and released histamine activate trigeminal sensory C-fibers in the nasal mucosa. This evokes release of acetylcholine (ACh) and VIP from parasympathetic efferents via a central reflex and release of SP, NKA, and CGRP from the peripheral ends of sensory fibers via a local axon reflex. These neuropeptides (and ACh) can cause vasodilation and edema and stimulate mucus production. (From Casale TB, Little MM: Neuropeptides and allergic diseases. In Middleton E Jr et al (eds): Allergy: Principles and Practice, 3rd edition (update series #2). C.V. Mosby, St. Louis, MO, 1989.)

reflexes act upon resistance vessels to increase superficial blood flow, but there is little effect on capacitance vessels (sinusoids) that control mucosal thickness or postcapillary venules that are the site of vascular permeability.

Stimulation of nasal nociceptive sensory nerves by cold dry air, capsaicin, histamine, BK, or allergic reactions recruits parasympathetic reflexes.[240, 265, 313] These reflexes are the most important mechanism regulating glandular serous and mucous cell exocytosis, a finding clearly demonstrated in unilateral provocation models (Fig. 18–2). For example, unilateral histamine provocation leads to the direct activation of H_1-receptors on vessels to stimulate arterial dilation, sinusoidal filling with obstruction to nasal air flow, and vascular permeability with the secretion of a fluid enriched by albumin, IgG, and other plasma proteins.[265] Nociceptive sensory nerves are stimulated to transmit sensations of itch and trigger protective reflexes, including sneezing. Bilateral, cholinergic reflexes stimulate glandular secretion of mucous cell mucoglycoproteins and serous cell lysozyme, lactoferrin, secretory IgA, and other enzymes. The noncholinergic component of the reflex-mediated nasal obstruction has not been well quantitated.

The muscarinic antagonists atropine and ipratropium bromide effectively reduce glandular secretion and dry the mucosa but have no effect on sneezing or vascular congestion.[239] Selective M_3-receptor antagonists may have clinical utility in rhinitis, in which parasympathetic glandular secretion is a significant cause of patient discomfort. However, reductions in glandular secretion volume could reduce the amounts of serous cell–derived antimicrobial and lubricating proteins on the mucosal surface and lead to drying of the surface, irritation, and sensory nerve stimulation. Use of cholinergic antagonists in asthma is discussed elsewhere in this text.

SUMMARY OF CHOLINERGIC MECHANISMS IN HYPERRESPONSIVENESS

A variety of mechanisms, including increased cholinergic reflex activity, increased ACh release, and M_2-autoreceptor dysfunction, could contribute to the pathogenesis of asthma. Some of these abnormalities may reflect the effects of inflammatory mediators on vagal pathways.

M_3- and M_2-receptors appear to predominate in the human respiratory tract. M_1 mRNA is present in unidentified alveolar cells but not in bronchi.[212] M_3 mRNA is found in bronchial epithelium, endothelium, glands, and smooth muscle. M_2 mRNA is found in smooth muscle and ganglion cells, whereas M_4 and M_5 mRNA are not detectable. M_3-receptor activation is the major tonically active stimulus for smooth muscle contraction and glandular exocytosis. M_3 antagonists may be beneficial, selective inhibitors of glandular secretion and vasodilation in human nasal mucosa and bronchoconstriction in human bronchi that may be free of side effects caused by actions on M_2-receptors and other subtype receptors. M_2-receptors appear to be critical for the regulation of parasympathetic ganglion function since M_2-autoreceptor stimulation may reduce ACh release. On smooth muscle, M_2 agonists may enhance cholinergically induced contraction by antagonizing cAMP formation and the relaxant effects of β_2-adrenergic agonists. These M_2-autoreceptor events may be at odds with each other, since ganglionic effects would promote bronchodilation and reduce cholinergically induced glandular secretion, whereas smooth muscle effects would promote bronchoconstriction. These issues will be resolved by clinical studies as new selective muscarinic receptor agonists and antagonists are developed. Inhibitors of cholinergic pathways in the lower airways are shown schematically in Figure 18–3. Future use of agents such as those shown might ultimately prove useful for the therapy of asthma.

NONADRENERGIC NONCHOLINERGIC (NANC) EFFECTS

NOCICEPTIVE NEURONS

As with the other autonomic systems, a variety of altered noncholinergic excitatory nerve mechanisms have been proposed in asthmatics. Potential abnormalities include increased afferent nerve density and/or accessibility to stimuli, increased synthesis/release of tachykinins and CGRP, decreased local proteolytic degradation, increased receptor density and/or affinity, and increased postreceptor responses. There are data to support some of these abnormalities, although direct evidence is lacking. Moreover, since inhaled capsaicin caused equal bronchoconstriction in asthmatic and normal subjects, a fundamental abnormality in noncholinergic excitatory activity in asthmatics is less likely.[110]

The simplest mechanism for increasing noncholinergic excitatory activity is increased stimulation of sensory afferent nerves. For example, allergic inflammation involves release of mast cell mediators, such as histamine and BK, which are known to activate sensory nerves. Inflammatory mediators may also sensitize afferent nerve endings, leading to hyperalgesia of inflamed airways.[85] Furthermore, the epithelial dam-

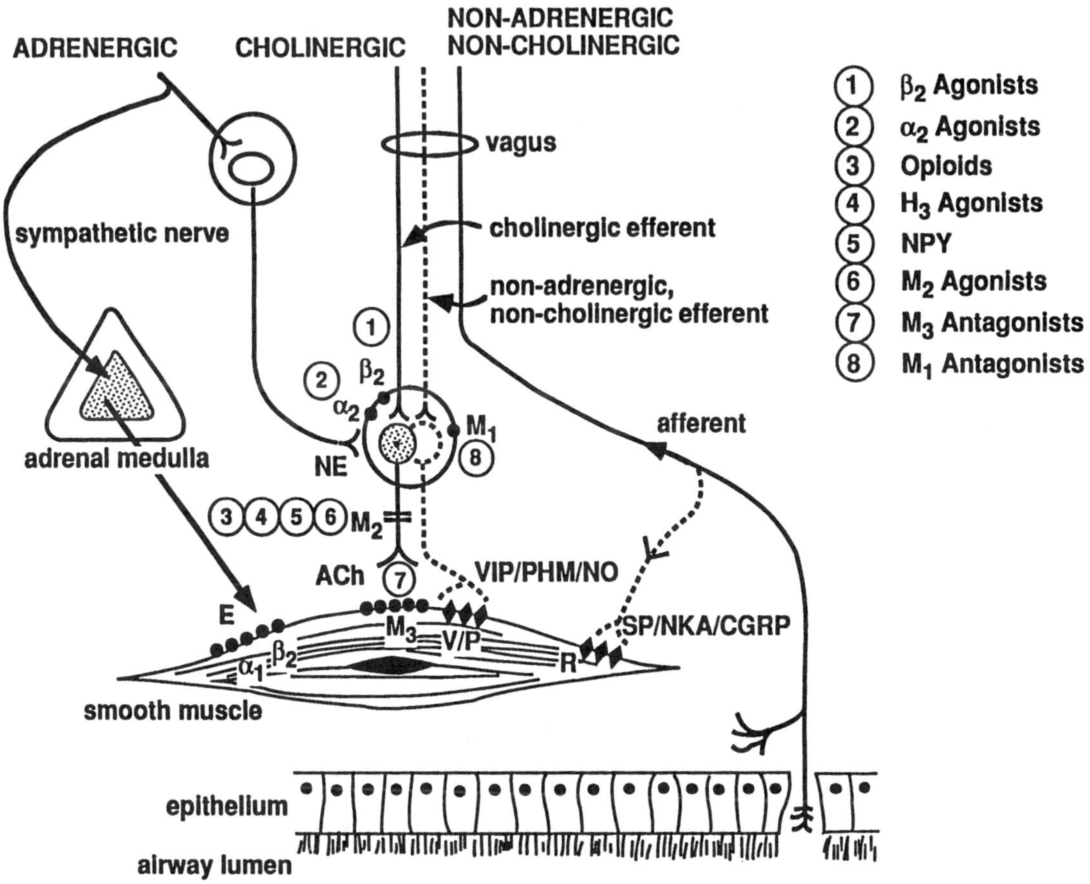

FIGURE 18–3. Inhibitors of cholinergic activity. The adrenergic and cholinergic nervous systems (solid lines) and the nonadrenergic and noncholinergic nervous systems (dashed lines) are shown schematically in the lower airways. Release of neurotransmitters epinephrine (E) and acetylcholine (ACh) stimulates specific α, β, and muscarinic M receptors. Nonadrenergic inhibitory nerves running in the vagus likely release NO and VIP and PHM, which stimulate specific airway receptors (V and P, respectively). Stimulation of collateral branches of sensory afferent nerves causes the antidromic release of SP, NK, and CGRP, which also stimulate specific airway receptors (R). NE is norepinephrine. Specific inhibitors of the cholinergic efferent pathway are listed on the right with their sites of action shown in the diagram.

age characteristic of asthma would be expected to increase accessibility of sensory nerve endings to both inhaled stimuli and locally released mediators. Ollerenshaw and colleagues have described an increase in SP-immunoreactive nerves in asthmatic compared with nonasthmatic airways.[249] Although chronic inflammation may lead to structural changes in innervation, these results may also be explained by increased neuropeptide synthesis. Alterations in local production or release of nerve growth factor may affect both of these possibilities.[195] Whether antigenic stimulation or airway inflammation can alter neuropeptide gene transcription awaits the development of specific antagonists and molecular studies.[85]

Evidence suggests that reduced degradation of tachykinins by NEP may also lead to increased noncholinergic excitatory activity, presumably by increasing local concentrations and prolonging the half-life of these neuropeptides. For example, inhibitors of NEP, such as phosphoramidon, have been shown in guinea pigs to augment airway responsiveness to both SP and capsaicin, but not ACh.[322] Neurogenic inflammation in rat trachea is also enhanced after treatment with NEP inhibitors.[329] Moreover, Sheppard and colleagues found that toluene diisocyanate–induced bronchoconstriction in guinea pigs occurs largely through inhibition of airway NEP.[288] Cigarette smoke and viral infections have also been shown to decrease NEP activity while increasing airway hyperresponsiveness.[97, 162] In vitro, removal of airway epithelium exaggerates responses to tachykinins.[244] Therefore, loss of NEP as a consequence of the in vivo epithelial denudation seen in asthma and viral infections may well facilitate tachykinin-induced proasthmatic effects.

Although alterations in neuropeptide receptors or postreceptor mechanisms may theoretically augment noncholinergic excitatory responses, evidence is not available to support this possibility. Potential abnormalities include alterations in neuron densities, neuropeptide release and degradation, regulation of cotransmitter release, neuropeptide receptors, and postreceptor responses (see Table 18–3).

Inhibitors of noncholinergic excitatory activity in the lower airways are schematically shown in Figure 18–4. Some of these agents are already in use for asthma or are undergoing clinical trials.

NONADRENERGIC NONCHOLINERGIC INHIBITORY SYSTEM

The nonadrenergic inhibitory system, currently thought to consist of VIP, VIP-related peptides, or NO, is thought to be the only known bronchodilatory neural pathway in human lung, since direct sympathetic innervation is lacking.[182, 191, 251] The i-NANC system is postulated to have an antiasthmatic effect by inducing bronchodilation, cholinergic antagonism, decreased mucus secretion, and anti-inflammatory actions. Abnormalities of this system have been postulated to contribute to the development of bronchial hyperreactivity, asthma,

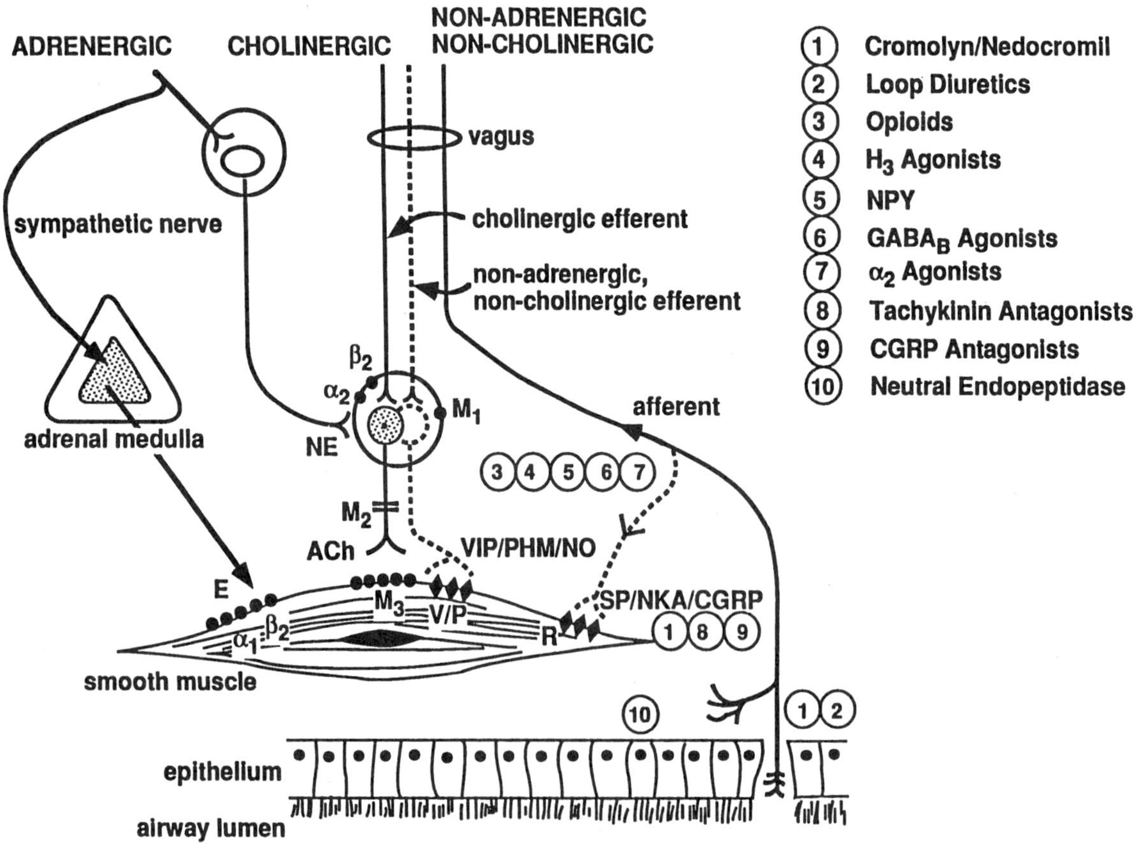

FIGURE 18–4. Inhibitors of noncholinergic excitatory activity. See Figure 18–2 legend for explanation regarding the diagram. Inhibitory sites include activation of afferent nerves (1 and 2), release of neuropeptides (3–7), antagonism of neuropeptide action (1, 8, and 9), and degradation of neuropeptides (10).

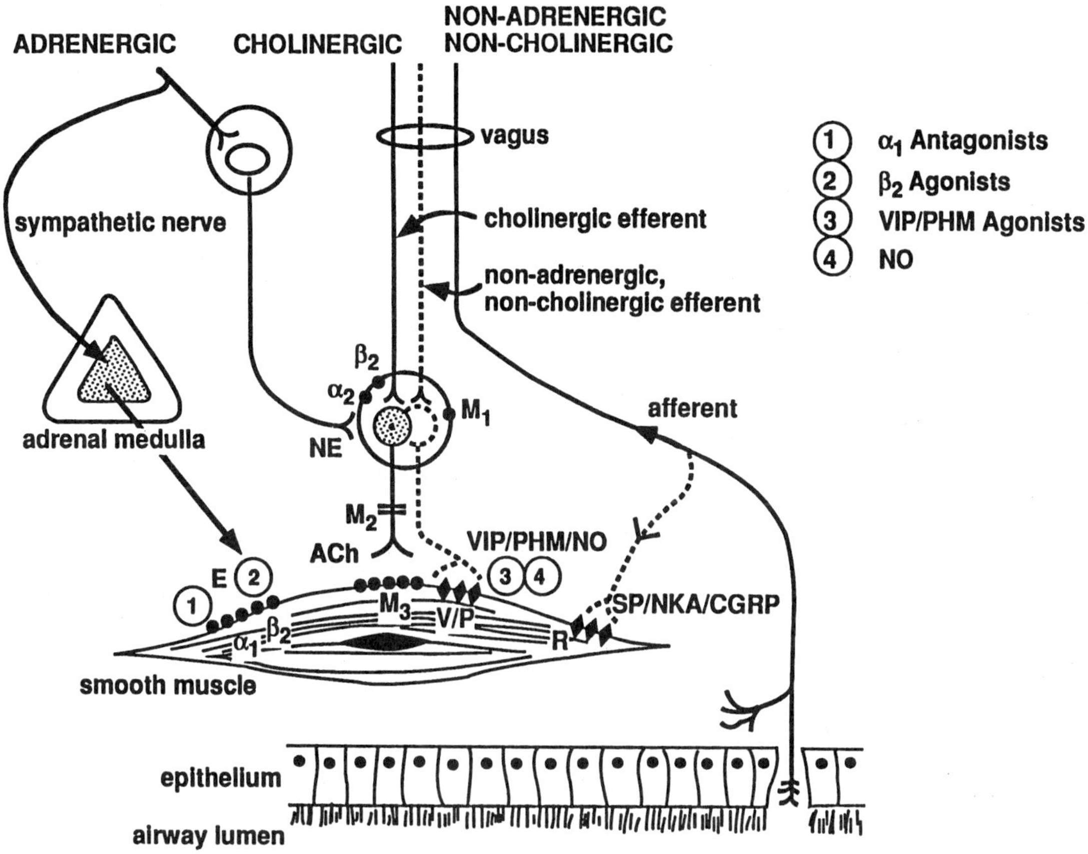

FIGURE 18–5. Modulators of adrenergic and nonadrenergic inhibitory systems. See Figure 18–2 legend for explanation regarding the diagram. Specific modulators are listed on the right with their sites of action shown in the diagram.

and other chronic lung diseases. Although supporting data are sparse, these abnormalities could include a deficiency in inhibitory NANC neuron density, altered release or corelease of neurotransmitters, receptor deficiencies, and depressed postreceptor responses. An absence of VIP-immunoreactive nerve fibers has been reported in cystic fibrosis[139] that could contribute to a decrease in VIP-induced serous cell secretion and formation of thick, mucoid secretions. A loss of VIP from human pulmonary nerve fibers has also been demonstrated in asthmatics in some, but not all, studies examining this issue.

In a study by Ollerenshaw and colleagues, immunoreactive VIP was not seen within any lung sections from asthmatics but was identified within nerves in more than 92% of lung sections from nonasthmatics, including smokers.[250] Loss of actual neurons, reduced synthesis within neurons, or excessive degradation by proteases are all potential explanations. Whether the absence of VIP-immunoreactive nerves is a primary event or secondary to the active disease process remains unknown. Airway VIP receptor number may be reduced in cystic fibrosis but not in asthma.[285] Inflammatory mediators, such as mast cell tryptase and chymase, may degrade VIP, whereas superoxide can degrade NO. Pretreatment with a protease inhibitor abolished antigen-induced dysfunction of inhibitory NANC activity in a cat model.[229] The mediators, function, and significance of the i-NANC system in human airway disease remain speculative.

Modulators of adrenergic and nonadrenergic inhibitory systems that might prove useful for asthma therapy are shown in Figure 18–5. β_2-Agonists are the mainstay of asthma treatment, and α_1-antagonists[41, 164] have had limited success. Whether VIP and PHM agonists and stimulation of NO synthetase might prove useful remains to be determined.

NPY

As mentioned previously, NPY may act in conjunction with norepinephrine to stimulate parasympathetic ganglion cell Y_2- and α_2-receptors, respectively, to reduce ACh release and hence permit bronchorelaxation. However, NPY has no effect on either airway tone or cholinergic neurotransmission in human airways in vitro.[28] Hence, NPY may not contribute to i-NANC bronchodilation.

SUMMARY

Sensory nerves detect the conditions of inspired air and respond to inhaled noxious agents and mucosal injury. Different forms of insults may generate a wide variety of mediators, including H^+, K^+, prostaglandins, leukotrienes, BK, and histamine, that may stimulate or modulate nociceptive sensory nerves by acting upon specific receptors, ion channels, or other macromolecules in nerves. These mediators may also act directly upon vessels to induce vascular permeability and venous sinusoidal filling. Release of sensory neuropeptides such as SP, NKA, CGRP, GRP, and others causes the local axon response. The magnitude of the axon response may be subtle in large animals, as demonstrated by the modest increase in superficial blood flow found in the pig, and less potent than the effects found in rodent airways.

The most important effects of sensory nerve stimulation in the nose are the recruitment of parasympathetic and other central reflexes and the induction of the sensation of pain. These lead to sneezing and other avoidance behaviors that attempt to rapidly clear the upper airway of offending agents while protecting the lower airways. Parasympathetic reflexes cause rapid and copious secretion of submucosal gland mucus and vasodilation, which increases nasal air flow resistance. Muscarinic M_3-receptors, and possibly M_1-receptors, most likely mediate glandular secretion. The sensory nerve–parasympathetic reflex arc is of paramount importance in the normal nose and contributes significantly to the pathology of allergic, infectious, and other nonallergic rhinitis. Thus nociceptive sensory nerves and the recruitment of parasympathetic reflexes are potent proinflammatory mechanisms in the nasal mucosa.

Nociceptive sensory nerve stimulation in the tracheobronchial tree may induce bronchospasm, vasodilation, vascular permeability, and glandular secretion and contribute to the hyperresponsiveness characteristic of asthma and rhinitis. However, in allergen-induced bronchoconstriction, this nociceptive neural component has only a minor contribution compared with the overwhelming effects of mast cell mediators.[29, 167] Substantial evidence supports the existence of NANC pathways in human lung. VIP and NO are the likely inhibitory NANC neurotransmitters, while SP, NKA, and CGRP are the likely excitatory NANC neurotransmitters. Bronchoconstrictor effects appear to be primarily mediated by NKA, whereas mucus hypersecretion and airway edema are primarily mediated by SP and CGRP. Inflammation is probably the major contributing factor to defects of these pathways as well. Both increased degradation of VIP and NO, secondary to proteases and oxygen radicals, and decreased degradation of tachykinins, secondary to loss of epithelial-associated NEP, are likely to contribute to asthma pathogenesis. Indeed, initial lung inflammatory responses may lead to neurogenic inflammation, setting in motion a vicious cycle.

The cholinergic nervous system, acting through M_3-receptors, provides the main bronchoconstrictor and glandular secretory pathways. Increased cholinergic responses probably result from both prejunctional facilitation of ACh release and vagal reflex stimulation by inflammatory mediators. Dysfunctional M_2-autoreceptors may contribute to enhanced cholinergic activity.

Circulating epinephrine is an important bronchodilator by directly relaxing smooth muscle in human airways. α- and β-adrenoceptors on ganglion cells may modulate cholinergic tone. The nasal sympathetic nervous system acts to reduce mucosal blood flow, sinusoidal filling, and mucosal thickness and so induces restoration of nasal air flow and nasal patency. Short-acting norepinephrine and long-acting NPY are potent vasoconstrictors. Loss of sympathetic influences may contribute to some chronic, nonallergic rhinopathies.

Neutral endopeptidase may also act in an anti-inflammatory fashion by degrading neuropeptides and so limiting the durations of their actions in vivo. Destruction or downregulation of NEP may contribute to the hyperresponsiveness of this mucosa that can occur after infection or exposure to cigarette smoke or other toxic gases. Restoration of NEP activity may be a beneficial effect of glucocorticoid use.

Sensory, parasympathetic, and sympathetic nerves play key, coordinated roles in respiratory homeostasis and in pathologic situations. Drugs based upon neurotransmitters, such as the α- and β-adrenergic agonists and anticholinergic agents, have been among the most successful medications. Further investigations with neuropeptide analogues, such as tachykinin antagonists, will reveal additional information about the roles of these nerves and their neurotransmitters in health and disease.

ACKNOWLEDGMENTS

James N. Baraniuk has been awarded the Tobacco Council for Research Scholar Award. Thomas B. Casale is the recipient of a Clinical Investigation Award from the Department of Veterans Affairs.

REFERENCES

1. Advenier C, Naline E, Toty L, et al: Effects on the isolated human bronchus of SR 48968, a potent and selective nonpeptide antagonist of the neurokinin A (NK_2 receptors. Am Rev Respir Dis 146:1177, 1992.
2. Agrawal DK, Townley RG: Effect of platelet-activating factor on beta-adrenoceptors in human lung. Biochem Biophys Res Commun 143:1, 1987.
3. Aguayo SM, Kane MA, King TE Jr, et al: Increased levels of bombesin-like peptides in the lower respiratory tract of asymptomatic cigarette smokers. J Clin Invest 84:1105, 1989.
4. Aliakbari J, Sreedharan SP, Turck CW, et al: Selective localization of vasoactive intestinal polypeptide and substance P in human eosinophils. Biochem Biophys Res Commun 148:1440, 1987.
5. Astolfi M, Meini S, Treggiara S, et al: Characterization of the NK-2 receptor which mediates the motor response to tachykinins in human isolated bronchi. Neuropeptides 24:189A, 1993.
6. Ayala LE, Ahmed T: Is there loss of protective muscarinic receptor mechanism in asthma? Chest 96:1285, 1989.
7. Bai TR: Abnormalities in airway smooth muscle in fatal asthma. Am Rev Respir Dis 141:552, 1990.
8. Baluk P, Nadel JA, McDonald DM: Calcitonin gene related peptide in secretory granules of serous cells in the rat tracheal epithelium. Am J Respir Cell Mol Biol 8:446, 1993.
9. Baraniuk JN: Neural control of human nasal secretion. Pulm Pharmacol 4:20, 1991.
10. Baraniuk JN, Castellino S, Goff J, et al: Neuropeptide Y (NPY) in human nasal mucosa. Am J Respir Cell Mol Biol 3:165, 1990.
11. Baraniuk JN, Kaliner MA, Barnes PJ: Muscarinic M3 receptor mRNA in situ hybridization in human nasal mucosa. Am J Rhinol 6:145, 1992.
12. Baraniuk JN, Kowalski M, Kaliner M: Neuropeptides in the skin. In Bos JD (ed): Skin Immune System (SIS), CRC Press, Boca Raton, FL, 1990, p 307.
13. Baraniuk JN, Lundgren JD, Mizoguchi H, et al: Bradykinin and respiratory mucous membranes: analysis of bradykinin binding site distribution and secretory responses in vitro and in vivo. Am Rev Respir Dis 141:706, 1990.
14. Baraniuk JN, Lundgren JD, Goff J, et al: Calcitonin gene related peptide in human nasal mucosa. Am J Physiol 258:L81, 1990.
15. Baraniuk JN, Lundgren JD, Goff J, et al: Gastrin releasing peptide in human nasal mucosa. J Clin Invest 85:998, 1990.
16. Baraniuk JN, Lundgren JD, Okayama M, et al: Substance P and neurokinin A in human nasal mucosa. Am J Respir Cell Mol Biol 4:228, 1991.
17. Baraniuk JN, Mak J, Letarte M, et al: Neutral endopeptidase mRNA expression in airways. Am Rev Respir Dis 143:A40, 1991.
18. Baraniuk JN, Ohkubo K, Kwon OJ, et al: Identification of neutral endopeptidase mRNA in human nasal mucosa. J Appl Physiol 74:272, 1993.
19. Baraniuk JN, Lundgren JD, Okayama M, et al: Vasoactive intestinal peptide in human nasal mucosa. J Clin Invest 86:825, 1990.

20. Baraniuk JN, Silver PB, Kaliner MA, Barnes PJ: Perennial rhinitis subjects have altered vascular, glandular, and neural responses to bradykinin nasal provocation. Int Arch Allergy Immunol 103:202, 1994.
21. Baraniuk JN, Silver PB, Kaliner MA, et al: Neuropeptide Y is a vasoconstrictor in human nasal mucosa. J Appl Physiol 73:1867, 1992.
22. Baraniuk JN, Silver PB, Kaliner MA, et al: Ibuprofen augments bradykinin-induced glycoconjugate secretion by human nasal mucosa in vivo. J Allergy Clin Immunol 89:1032, 1992.
23. Baraniuk JN, Silver PB, Lundgren JD, et al: Bombesin stimulates human nasal mucous and serous cell secretion in vivo. Am J Physiol 262:L48, 1992.
24. Barnes PJ: Neural control of human airways in health and disease. Am Rev Respir Dis 134:1289, 1986.
25. Barnes PJ: Endogenous catecholamines and asthma. J Allergy Clin Immunol 77:791, 1986.
26. Barnes PJ: Asthma as an axon reflex. Lancet 1:242, 1986.
27. Barnes PJ: Muscarinic receptor subtypes: implications for lung disease. Thorax 44:161, 1989.
28. Barnes PJ: Modulation of neurotransmission in airways. Physiol Rev 72:699, 1992.
29. Barnes PJ, Baraniuk JN, Belvisi MG: Neuropeptides in the respiratory tract. Part 1. Am Rev Respir Dis 144:1187, 1991.
30. Barnes PJ, Baraniuk JN, Belvisi MG: Neuropeptides in the respiratory tract. Part 2. Am Rev Respir Dis 144:1391, 1991.
31. Barnes PJ, Basbaum CB, Nadel JA: Autoradiographic localization of autonomic receptors in airway smooth muscle marked differences between large and small airways. Am Rev Respir Dis 127:758, 1983.
32. Barnes PJ, Brown MJ, Silverman M, et al: Circulating catecholamines in exercise and hyperventilation induced asthma. Thorax 36:435, 1981.
33. Barnes PJ, Dixon CMS: The effect of inhaled vasoactive intestinal peptide on bronchial reactivity to histamine in humans. Am Rev Respir Dis 130:162, 1984.
34. Barnes PJ, Dollery CT, MacDermot J: Increased pulmonary alpha-adrenergic and reduced beta-adrenergic receptors in experimental asthma. Nature 285:569, 1980.
35. Barnes PJ, Ind PW, Dollery CT: Inhaled prazosin in asthma. Thorax 36:378, 1981.
36. Barnes PJ, Kuo HP, Rogers DF, et al: Effect of vagus nerve stimulation on goblet-cell secretion in guinea-pig trachea in vivo. J Physiol 422:99P, 1990.
37. Barnes PJ, Kuo HP, Rogers DF, et al: Effects of sensory neuropeptides on goblet-cell secretion in guinea-pig trachea in vivo. J Physiol 422:100P, 1990.
38. Bar-Shavit Z, Goldman R, Stabinsky Y, et al: Enhancement of phagocytosis—a newly found activity of substance P residing in its N-terminal tetrapeptide sequence. Biochem Biophys Res Commun 94:1445, 1980.
39. Barr ML: The Human Nervous System, 2nd edition. Harper & Row, Hagerstown, MD, 1974.
40. Battey JF, Way JM, Corjay MH, et al: Molecular cloning of the bombesin/gastrin-releasing peptide receptor from Swiss 3T3 cells. Proc Natl Acad Sci USA 8:395, 1991.
41. Beil M, de Kock MA: Role of alpha-adrenergic receptors in exercise-induced bronchoconstriction. In Herzog H (ed): Respiration. S. Karger, Basel, Switzerland, 1978, p 78.
42. Belvisi MG, Patacchini R, Barnes PJ, et al: Facilitory effects of selective agonists for tachykinin receptors on cholinergic neurotransmission—evidence for species differences. Br J Pharmacol 111:103, 1994.
43. Belvisi MG, Stretton CD, Barnes PJ: Bombesin-induced bronchoconstriction in the guinea pig: mode of action. J Pharmacol Exp Ther 258:36, 1991.
44. Belvisi MG, Stretton D, Barnes PJ: Nitric oxide as an endogenous modulator of cholinergic neurotransmission in guinea-pig airways. Eur J Pharmacol 198:219, 1991.
45. Berkin KE, Inglis GC, Ball SG, et al: Effect of low dose adrenaline and noradrenaline infusions on airway calibre in asthmatic patients. Clin Sci 70:347, 1986.
46. Birnbaumer L, Brown AM: G proteins and the mechanism of action of hormones, neurotransmitters, and autocrine and paracrine regulatory factors. Am Rev Respir Dis 141:S106, 1990.
47. Blecher M, Lewis S, Hicks JM, et al: Beta-blocking autoantibodies in pediatric bronchial asthma. J Allergy Clin Immunol 74:246, 1984.
48. Bloch KD, Friedrich SP, Lee ME, et al: Structural organization and chromosomal assignment of the gene encoding endothelin. J Biol Chem 264:10851, 1989.
49. Böhm M, Gengenbach S, Hauck RW, et al: Beta-adrenergic receptors and m-cholinergic receptors in human lung: findings following in vivo and in vitro exposure to the beta-adrenergic receptor agonist, terbutaline. Chest 100:1246, 1991.
50. Borson DB: Roles of neutral endopeptidase in airways. Am J Physiol 260:L212, 1991.
51. Borson DB, Gruenert DC: Glucocorticoids induce neutral endopeptidase in transformed human trachea epithelial cells. Am J Physiol 260:L83, 1991.
52. Boyd ND, MacDonald SG, Kage R, et al: Substance P receptor. Biochemical characterization and interactions with G proteins. Ann NY Acad Sci 632:79, 1991.
53. Brain SD, Williams TJ: Inflammatory oedema induced by synergism between calcitonin gene-related peptide (CGRP) and mediators of increased vascular permeability. Br J Pharmacol 86:855, 1985.
54. Brain SD, Williams TJ: Substance P regulates the vasodilator activity of calcitonin gene related peptide. Nature 335:73, 1988.
55. Braunstein G, Fajac I, Lacronique J, et al: Clinical and inflammatory responses to exogenous tachykinins in allergic rhinitis. Am Rev Respir Dis 144:630, 1991 [Published erratum appears in Am Rev Respir Dis 148:following 1700, 1993.]
56. Brodde OE, Howell U, Egerszegi S, et al: Effect of prednisolone and ketotifen on β2-adrenoreceptors in asthmatic patients receiving β2-bronchodilators. Eur J Clin Pharmacol 34:145, 1988.
57. Brooks SM, McGowan K, Bernstein IL, et al: Relationship between numbers of beta adrenergic receptors in lymphocytes and disease severity in asthma. J Allergy Clin Immunol 63:401, 1979.
58. Bucknall CE, Neilly JB, Carter R, et al: Bronchial hyperreactivity in patients who cough after receiving angiotensin converting enzyme inhibitors. Br Med J 296:86, 1988.
59. Bunnett NW, Collins SM, Payan D, et al: Downregulation of neutral endopeptidase (EC 3.4.24.11) in the inflamed rat intestine. Am J Physiol 264(pt 1):G735, 1993.
60. Busija DW, Chen J: Effects of trigeminal neurotransmitters on piglet pial arterioles. J Dev Physiol 18:67, 1992.
61. Busse WW: Respiratory infections: their role in airway responsiveness and the pathogenesis of asthma. J Allergy Clin Immunol 85:671, 1990.
62. Bylund DB, Eikenberg DC, Hieble JP, et al: International Union of Pharmacology. Nomenclature of adrenoceptors. Pharmacol Rev 46:121, 1994.
63. Carolan EJ, Casale TB: Effects of neuropeptides on neutrophil migration through noncellular and endothelial barriers. J Allergy Clin Immunol 92:589, 1993.
64. Carstairs JR, Barnes PJ: Visualization of vasoactive intestinal peptide receptors in human and guinea pig lung. J Pharmacol Exp Ther 239:249, 1986.
65. Carstairs JR, Barnes PJ: Autoradiographic mapping of substance P receptors in lung. Eur J Pharmacol 127:295, 1986.
66. Carstairs JR, Nimmo AJ, Barnes PJ: Autoradiographic visualization of beta-adrenoceptor subtypes in human lung. Am Rev Respir Dis 132:541, 1985.
67. Casale TB: The role of the autonomic nervous system in allergic disease. Ann Allergy 51:423, 1983.
68. Casale TB: Neuromechanisms of asthma. Ann Allergy 59:391, 1987.
69. Casale TB: Neurogenic control of inflammation and airway function. In Middleton E, Jr, Reed CE, Ellis EF, et al (eds): Allergy: Principles and Practice, 4th edition. Mosby-Yearbook Co, St. Louis, MO, 1993, p 650.
70. Casale TB: Acute Effects of in vitro mast cell degranulation on human lung muscarinic receptors. Am Rev Respir Dis 147:940, 1993.
71. Caughey GH, Leidig F, Viro NF, et al: Substance P and vasoactive intestinal peptide degradation by mast cell tryptase and chymase. J Pharmacol Exp Ther 244:133, 1988.
72. Chen Z, Hedner J, Hedner T: Substance P in the ventrolateral medulla regulation in oblongata regulates ventilatory responses. J Appl Physiol 68:2631, 1990.
73. Cheung D, Bel EH, Den Hartigh J, et al: The effect of an inhaled neutral endopeptidase inhibitor, thiorphan, on airway responsiveness to neurokinin A in normal humans in vivo. Am Rev Respir Dis 145:1275, 1992.
74. Chin SY, Hall JM, Brain SD, et al: Do amylin and CGRP interact with similar receptors in the perfused rat isolated kidney? Neuropeptides 24:207, 1993.

75. Christolfides ND, Polak JM, Bloom SR: Studies on the distribution of PHI in mammals. Peptides 5:261, 1984.
76. Clozel M, Breu V, Burri K, et al: Pathophysiological role of endothelin revealed by the first orally active endothelin receptor antagonist. Nature 365:759, 1993.
77. Coles SJ, Said SI, Reid LM: Inhibition by vasoactive intestinal peptides of glycoconjugate and lysozyme secretion by human airways in vitro. Am Rev Respir Dis 124:531, 1981.
78. Conolly ME, Greenacre JK: The lymphocyte β-adrenoceptor in normal subjects and patients with bronchial asthma: the effect of different forms of treatment on receptor function. J Clin Invest 58:1307, 1976.
79. Corjay MH, Dobrzanski DJ, Way JM, et al: Two distinct bombesin receptor subtypes are expressed and functional in human lung carcinoma cells. J Biol Chem 266:18771, 1991.
80. Crimi N, Palermo F, Oliveri R, et al: Effect of nedocromil on bronchospasm induced by inhalation of substance P in asthmatic subjects. Clin Allergy 18:375, 1988.
81. Crossman DC, Dashwood MR, Taylor GW, et al: Sodium cromoglycate: evidence of tachykinin antagonist activity in the human skin. J Appl Physiol 75:167, 1993.
82. D'Adamio L, Shipp MA, Masteller EL, et al: Organization of the gene encoding common acute lymphoblastic leukemia antigen (neutral endopeptidase 24.11): multiple miniexons and separate 5′ untranslated regions. Proc Natl Acad Sci USA 86:7103, 1989.
83. Dale HH: Pharmacology and nerve endings. Proc R Soc Med 68:319, 1935.
84. Daniel EE, O'Byrne P: Effect of inflammatory mediators on airway nerves and muscle. Am Rev Respir Dis 143:S3, 1991.
85. Daniele RP, Barnes PJ, Goetzl EJ, et al: NHLBI Workshop Summaries. Neuroimmune interactions in the lung. Am Rev Respir Dis 145:1230, 1992.
86. Davis PB: Pupillary responses and airway reactivity in asthma. J Allergy Clin Immunol 77:667, 1986.
87. Davis PB, Simpson DM, Paget GL, et al: Beta-adrenergic responses in drug-free subjects with asthma. J Allergy Clin Immunol 77:871, 1986.
88. Demski LS, Schwanzel-Fukuda M (eds): The terminal nerve (nervus terminalis): structure, function, and evolution. Introduction. Ann NY Acad Sci 519:ix, 1987.
89. Desmazes N, Lockhart A, Lacroix A, et al: Carboxypeptidase M-like enzyme modulates the noncholinergic bronchoconstrictor response in guinea pig. Am J Respir Cell Mol Biol 7:477, 1992.
90. Devillier P, Dessanges JF, Rakatosihanaka F, et al: Nasal response to substance P and methacholine in subjects with and without allergic rhinitis. Eur Respir J 1:356, 1988.
91. Dey RD, Shannon WA Jr, Said SI: Localization of VIP-immunoreactive nerves in airways and pulmonary vessels of dogs, cat, and human subjects. Cell Tissue Res 220:231, 1981.
92. Didier A, Kowalski ML, Jay J, et al: Neurogenic inflammation, vascular permeability, and mast cells. Capsaicin desensitization fails to influence IgE-anti-DNP-induced vascular permeability in rat airways. Am Rev Respir Dis 141:398, 1990.
93. Dixon CMS, Fuller RW, Barnes PJ: The effect of an angiotensin converting enzyme inhibitor, ramipril, on bronchial responses to inhaled histamine and bradykinin in asthmatic subjects. Br J Clin Pharmacol 23:91, 1987.
94. Djamilian M, Stief CG, Kuczyk M, et al: Follow-up results of a combination of calcitonin gene related peptide and prostaglandin E1 in the treatment of erectile dysfunction. J Urol 149:1296, 1993.
95. Dorje F, Wess J, Lambrecht G, et al: Antagonist binding profiles of five cloned human muscarinic receptor subtypes. J Pharmacol Exp Ther 256:727, 1991.
96. Dupuy PM, Shore SA, Drazen JM, et al: Bronchodilator action of inhaled nitric oxide in guinea pigs. J Clin Invest 90:421, 1992.
97. Dusser DJ, Djoric TD, Borson DB, et al: Cigarette smoke induces bronchoconstrictor hyperresponsiveness to substance P and inactivates airway neutral endopeptidase in the guinea pig. J Clin Invest 84:900, 1989.
98. Eccles JC: Chemical transmission and Dale's principle. Prog Brain Res 68:3, 1986.
99. Eglen RM, Reddy H, Watson N, et al: Muscarinic acetylcholine receptor subtypes in smooth muscle. Trends Pharmacol Sci 15:114, 1994.
100. Erdos EG, Wagner B, Harbury CB, et al: Down-regulation and inactivation of neutral endopeptidase 24.11 (enkephalinase) in human neutrophils. J Biol Chem 264:14519, 1989.
101. Fathi Z, Corjay MH, Shapira H, et al: BRS-3: a novel bombesin receptor subtype selectively expressed in testis and lung carcinoma cells. J Biol Chem 268:5979, 1993.
102. Fisher JT, Anderson JW, Waldron MA: Nonadrenergic noncholinergic neurotransmitter of feline trachealis: VIP or nitric oxide? J Appl Physiol 74:31, 1993.
103. Fong TM, Cascieri MA, Yu H, et al: Amino-aromatic interaction between histidine 197 of the neurokinin-1 receptor and CP 96345. Nature 362:350, 1993.
104. Franconi GM, Graf PD, Lazarus SC, et al: Mast cell trytase and chymase reverse airway smooth muscle relaxation induced by vasoactive intestinal peptide in the ferret. J Pharmacol Exp Ther 248:947, 1989.
105. Fraser CM, Lee NH: Molecular characterization of autonomic and neuropeptide receptors. In Kaliner MA, Barnes PJ, Kunkel GHH, et al (eds): Neuropeptides in Respiratory Medicine. Marcel-Dekker, New York, 1994, p 225.
106. Fryer AD, Jacoby DB: Parainfluenza virus infection damages inhibitory M_2 muscarinic receptors on pulmonary parasympathetic nerves in the guinea-pig. Br J Pharmacol 102:267, 1991.
107. Fryer AD, Maclagan J: Ipratropium bromide potentiates bronchoconstriction induced by vagal nerve stimulation in the guinea-pig. Eur J Pharmacol 139:187, 1987.
108. Fryer AD, Wills-Karp M: Dysfunction of M2-muscarinic receptors in pulmonary parasympathetic nerves after antigen challenge. J Appl Physiol 71:2255, 1991.
109. Fujii T, Murai M, Morimoto H, et al: Effects of actinomycin-D on airway constriction induced by tachykinins and capsaicin in guinea pigs. Eur J Pharmacol 194:183, 1991.
110. Fuller RW, Dixon CMS, Barnes PJ: Bronchoconstrictor response to inhaled capsaicin in humans. J Appl Physiol 58:1080, 1985.
111. Fuller RW, Dixon CMS, Cuss FM, et al: Bradykinin-induced bronchoconstriction in humans. Mode of action. Am Rev Respir Dis 135:176, 1987.
112. Fuller RW, Maxwell DL, Dixon CMS, et al. Effect of substance P on cardiovascular and respiratory function in subjects. J Appl Physiol 62:1473, 1987.
113. Galant SP, Duriseti L, Underwood S, et al: Beta adrenergic receptors of polymorphonuclear particulates in bronchial asthma. J Clin Invest 65:577, 1980.
114. Gamse R, Saria A: Potentiation of tachykinin induced plasma protein extravasation by calcitonin gene related peptide. Eur J Pharmacol 114:61, 1985.
115. Gawin A, Baraniuk JN, Lundgren JD, et al: Effects of gastrin-releasing peptide and analogues on guinea pig nasal mucosal secretion. Am J Physiol 264:L345, 1993.
116. Gawin A, Baraniuk JN, Kaliner M: Effects of substance P and calcitonin gene related peptide (CGRP) on guinea pig nasal mucosal secretion in vivo. Acta Otolaryngol (Stockh) 113:533, 1993.
117. Gazdar AF, Carbone DP: The Biology and Molecular Genetics of Lung Cancer. R.G. Landes Co, Austin, TX, 1994.
118. Gennari C, Nami R, Agnusdei D, et al: Improved cardiac performance with human calcitonin gene related peptide in patients with congestive heart failure. Cardiovasc Res 24:239, 1990.
119. Geppetti P, Maggi CA, Perretti F, et al: Simultaneous release by bradykinin of substance P- and calcitonin gene-related peptide immunoreactivities from capsaicin-sensitive structures in guinea-pig heart. Br J Pharmacol 94:288, 1988.
120. Gerard NP, Eddy RL Jr., Shows TB, et al: The human neurokinin A (substance K) receptor. Molecular cloning of the gene, chromosome localization, and isolation of cDNA from tracheal and gastric tissues. J Biol Chem 266:1354, 1991.
121. Gether U, Yokata Y, Emonds-Alt X, et al: Two nonpeptide tachykinin antagonists act through epitopes on corresponding segments of the NK1 and NK2 receptors. Proc Natl Acad Sci USA 90:6194, 1993.
122. Giaid A, Gibson SJ, Ibrahim BN, et al: Endothelin 1, an endothelium-derived peptide, is expressed in neurons of the human spinal cord and dorsal root ganglia. Proc Natl Acad Sci USA 86:7634, 1989.
123. Goetzl EJ, Sreedharan SP, Turck CW: Structurally distinctive vasoactive intestinal peptides from rat basophilic leukemia cells. J Biol Chem 263:9083, 1988.
124. Goetzl EJ, Sreedharan SP, Turck CW, et al: Preferential cleavage of amino- and carboxy-terminal oligopeptides from vasoactive intestinal polypeptide by human recombinant enkephalinase (neutral endopeptidase, ED 3.4.24.11). Biochem Biophys Res Commun 158:850, 1989.
125. Goldie RG, Henry PJ, Self GJ, et al: Endothelin receptor subtype

distribution, density, and function in human isolated asthmatic and non-diseased bronchus. Am J Respir Crit Care Med 149:A472, 1994.
126. Goldie RG, Spina D, Henry PJ, et al: In vitro responsiveness of human asthmatic bronchus to carbachol, histamine, β-adrenoceptor agonists, and theophylline. Br J Clin Pharmacol 22:669, 1986.
127. Grieco MH, Pierson RN Jr: Mechanism of bronchoconstriction due to beta adrenergic blockade. Studies with practolol, propranolol, and atropine. J Allergy Clin Immunol 48:143, 1971.
128. Grundström N, Andersson RGG: Inhibition of the cholinergic neurotransmission in human airways via prejunctional α_2-adrenoceptors. Acta Physiol Scand 125:513, 1985.
129. Grundström N, Andersson RGG, Wikberg JES: Inhibition of the excitatory non-adrenergic, non-cholinergic neurotransmission in the guinea pig tracheo-bronchial tree mediated by α_2-adrenoceptors. Acta Pharmacol Toxicol 54:8, 1984.
130. Håkanson R, Wahlestedt C: Neuropeptide Y acts via prejunctional (Y_2) and postjunctional (Y_1) receptors. Neuroscience 22:S679, 1987.
131. Hall AK, Barnes PJ, Meldrum LA, et al: Facilitation by tachykinins of neurotransmission in guinea-pig pulmonary parasympathetic nerves. Br J Pharmacol 97:274, 1989.
132. Harmar AJ, Hyde V, Chapman C: Identification and cDNA of delta-preprotachykinin, a fourth splicing variant of the rat substance P precursor. FEBS Lett 275:22, 1990.
133. Harrison LC, Callaghan J, Venter JC, et al: Atopy, autonomic function and β-adrenergic receptor autoantibodies. In: Receptors, Antibodies, and Disease. Pitman. (Ciba Foundation Symposium), London, 1982, p 248.
134. Hartley JPR, Davies CJ, Charles TJ, et al: Plasma cyclic nucleotide levels in exercise-induced asthma. Thorax 36:823, 1981.
135. Hartschuh W, Weihe E, Reinecke M: Peptidergic (neurotensin, VIP, substance P) nerve fibres in the skin. Immunohistochemical evidence of an involvement of neuropeptides in nociception, pruritus, and inflammation. Br J Dermatol 109(suppl):25:14, 1983.
136. Hartung HP, Wolters K, Toyka KV: Substance P: binding properties and studies on cellular responses in guinea pig macrophages. J Immunol 136:3856, 1986.
137. Hayashi K, Taki F, Sugiyama S, et al: Mechanism responsible for alterations in numbers of autonomic nerve receptors in experimental asthma. Int Arch Allergy Appl Immunol 86:170, 1988.
138. Haynes LW, Manley C: Chemotactic responses of guinea-pig eosinophil polymorphonucleocytes in vitro to rat calcitonin gene-related peptide (rCGRP-I) and proteolytic fragments. J Physiol 422:79P, 1988.
139. Heinz-Erian P, Dey RD, Flux M, et al: Deficient vasoactive intestinal peptide innervation in the sweat glands of cystic fibrosis patients. Science 229:1407, 1985.
140. Helke CJ, Krause JE, Mantyh PW, et al: Diversity in mammalian tachykinin peptidergic neurons: multiple peptides, receptors, and regulatory mechanisms. FASEB J 4:1606, 1990.
141. Hinson J, Rauh C, Coupet J: Neuropeptide Y stimulates inositol phopholipid hydrolysis in rat brain miniprisms. Brain Res 446:379, 1988.
142. Hokfelt T, Fuxe K, Pernow B: Coexistence of neuronal messengers: a new principle in chemical transmission. Prog Brain Res 68:1, 1987.
143. Holzer P: Local effector functions of capsaicin-sensitive sensory nerve endings: involvement of tachykinins, calcitonin gene related peptide and other neuropeptides. Neuroscience 24:739, 1988.
144. Holzer P: Capsaicin: cellular targets, mechanisms of action, and selectivity for thin sensory neurons. Pharmacol Rev 43:143, 1991.
145. Honda I, Kohrogi H, Yamaguchi T, et al: Enkephalinase inhibitor potentiates substance P- and capsaicin-induced bronchial smooth muscle contractions in humans. Am Rev Respir Dis 143:1416, 1991.
146. Hori S, Komatsu Y, Shigemoto R, et al: Distinct tissue distribution and cellular localization of two messenger ribonucleic acids encoding different subtypes of rat endothelin receptors. Endocrinology 130:1885, 1992.
147. Hosoda K, Nakoa K, Arai H, et al: Cloning and expression of human endothelin-1 receptor cDNA. FEBS Lett 287:23, 1991.
148. Hua XY: Tachykinins and calcitonin gene related peptide in relation to peripheral functions of capsaicin-sensitive sensory nerves. Acta Physiol Scand Suppl 551:1, 1986.
149. Ichinose M, Barnes PJ: Histamine H_3 receptors modulate antigen-induced bronchoconstriction in guinea pigs. J Allergy Clin Immunol 86:491, 1990.
150. Ichinose M, Nakajima N, Takahashi T, et al: Neurokinin-receptor antagonist inhibits bradykinin-induced bronchoconstriction and cough in asthmatic patients. Am Rev Respir Dis 147:A298, 1993.
151. Ichinose M, Stretton CD, Schwartz JC, et al: Histamine H_3-receptors inhibit cholinergic neurotransmission in guinea-pig airways. Br J Pharmacol 97:13, 1989.
152. Iijima H, Gerard NP, Squassoni C, et al: Exon 16 del: a novel form of human neutral endopeptidase (CALLA). Am J Physiol 262(Lung Cell Mol Physiol 6):L725, 1992.
153. Ind PW, Dixon CMS, Fuller RW, et al: Anticholinergic blockade of beta-blocker-induced bronchoconstriction. Am Rev Respir Dis 193:1390, 1989.
154. Inoue A, Yanagisawa M, Kimura S, et al: The human endothelin family: three structurally and pharmacologially distinct isopeptides predicted by three separate genes. Proc Natl Acad Sci USA 86:2863, 1989.
155. Inoue A, Yanagisawa M, Takuwa Y, et al: The human preproendothelin-1 gene complete nucleotide sequence and regulation of expression. J Biol Chem 264:14954, 1989.
156. Ishihara T, Nakamura S, Kaziro Y, et al: Molecular cloning and expression of a cDNA encoding the secretin receptor. EMBO J 10:1635, 1991.
157. Ishihara T, Shigemoto R, Mori K, et al: Functional expression and tissue distribution of a novel receptor for vasoactive intestinal polypeptide. Neuron 8:811, 1992.
158. Ito Y: Prejunctional control of excitatory neuroeffector transmission by prostaglandins in the airway smooth muscle tissue. Am Rev Respir Dis 143:S6, 1991.
159. Itoh Y, Yanagisawa M, Ohkubo S, et al: Cloning and sequence analysis of cDNA encoding the precursor of a human endothelium-derived vasoconstrictor peptide, endothelin: identity of human and porcine endothelin. FEBS Lett 231:440, 1988.
160. Iwashita T, Shimizu T: Imipramine inhibits intrathecal substance P-induced behavior and blocks spinal substance P receptors in mice. Brain Res 581:59, 1992.
161. Jacobsson L, Grundström N, Andersson RG: Influence of some α2-receptor agonists and antagonists on the excitatory non-adrenergic, non-cholinergic neurotransmission in the airways of guinea-pigs in vivo. Acta Physiol Scand 142:91, 1991.
162. Jacoby DB, Tamaoki J, Borson DB, et al: Influenza infection causes airway hyperresponsiveness by decreasing enkephalinase. J Appl Physiol 64:2653, 1988.
163. Jakab G, Webster HD, Salamon I, et al: Neural and non-neural origin of calcitonin gene related peptide (CGRP) in the gastric mucosa. Neuropeptides 24:117, 1993.
164. Jenkins C, Breslin ABX, Marlin GE: The role of alpha and beta adrenoceptors in airway hyperresponsiveness to histamine. J Allergy Clin Immunol 75:364, 1985.
165. Jernbeck J, Dalsgaard CJ: Calcitonin gene related peptide treatment of flaps with compromised circulation in humans. Plast Reconstr Surg 91:236, 1993.
166. Johnson CW, Rieves RD, Logun C, et al: Endothelin-1 stimulates secretion of respiratory glycoprotein from human airways in vitro. Am Rev Respir Dis 143:A138, 1991.
167. Joos G, Pauwels R, Van Der Straeten M: Effect of inhaled substance P and neurokinin A on the airways of normal and asthmatic subjects. Thorax 42:779, 1987.
168. Kageyama R, Sasai Y, Nakanishi S: Molecular characterization of transcription factors that bind to the cAMP responsive region of the substance P precursor gene: cDNA cloning of a novel C/EBP-related factor. J Biol Chem 266:15525, 1991.
169. Kaliner M, Shelhamer JH, Davis PB, et al: Autonomic nervous system abnormalities and allergy. Ann Intern Med 96:349, 1982.
170. Kariman K: β-adrenergic receptor binding in lymphocytes from patients with asthma. Lung 158:41, 1980.
171. Kaufman MP, Coleridge HM, Coleridge JCG, et al: Bradykinin stimulates afferent vagal C-fibres in intrapulmonary airways of dogs. J Appl Physiol 48:511, 1980.
172. Khalil Z, Andrews PV, Helme RD: VIP modulates substance P-induced plasma extravasation in vivo. Eur J Pharmacol 151:281, 1988.
173. Klaassen AB, van Megen YJ, Kuijpers W, et al: Autonomic innervation of the nasal mucosa. J Oto-Rhinolaryngol 50:32, 1988.
174. Kobzik L, Bredt DS, Lowenstein CJ, et al: Nitric oxide synthase in human and rat lung: immunocytochemical and histochemical localization. Am J Respir Cell Mol Biol 9:371, 1993.
175. Kondepudi A, Johnson A: Cytokines increase neutral endopeptidase activity in lung fibroblasts. Am J Respir Cell Mol Biol 8:43, 1993.
176. Kroegel C, Yukawa T, Barnes PJ: Substance P induces degranulation of eosinophils. Am Rev Respir Dis 139:A238, 1989.

177. Kummer W, Fischer A, Lang RE, et al: Nitric oxide and guanylyl cyclases: correlation with neuropeptides. In Kaliner MA, Barnes PJ, Kunkel GHH, et al (eds): Neuropeptides in Respiratory Medicine. Marcel-Dekker, New York, 1994, p 641.
178. Kurian SS, Blank MA, Sheppard MN: Vasoactive intestinal polypeptide (VIP) in vasomotor rhinitis. Clin Biochem 11:425, 1983.
179. Lacroix JS: Adrenergic and non-adrenergic mechanisms in sympathetic vascular control of the nasal mucosa. Acta Physiol Scand 136(suppl 581):1–49, 1989.
180. Lacroix JS, Ångård A, Hökfelt T, et al: Neuropeptide Y: presence in sympathetic and parasympathetic innervation of the nasal mucosa. Cell Tissue Res 259:119, 1990.
181. Laitinen A, Partanen M, Hervonen A, et al: VIP like immunoreactive nerves in human respiratory tract. Light and electron microscopic study. Histochemistry 82:313, 1985.
182. Laitinen LA, Laitinen A: Innervation of airway smooth muscle. Am Rev Respir Dis 136:S38, 1987.
183. Laitinen LA, Laitinen A, Salonen RO, et al: Vascular actions of airway neuropeptides. Am Rev Respir Dis 136:S59, 1987.
184. Lammers JWJ, Minettle P, McCusker M, et al: The role of pirenzepine-sensitive (M_1) muscarinic receptors in vagally mediated bronchoconstriction in humans. Am Rev Respir Dis 139:446, 1989.
185. Lang Z, Murlas CG: Neutral endopeptidase of a human airway epithelial cell line recovers after hypochlorous acid exposure: dexamethasone accelerates this by stimulating neutral endopeptidase mRNA synthesis. Am J Respir Cell Mol Biol 7:300, 1992.
186. Larsson O, Duner-Engstrom M, Lundberg JM, et al: Effects of VIP, PHM and substance P on blood vessels and secretory elements of the human submandibular gland. Regul Pept 13:319, 1986.
187. Laurenzi MA, Persson MA, Dalsgaard CJ, et al: Stimulation of human B lymphocyte differentiation by the neuropeptides substance P and neurokinin A. Scand J Immunol 30:695, 1989.
188. Lawrence ID, Warner JA, Cohan VL, et al: Purification and characterization of human skin mast cells. Evidence for human mast cell heterogeneity. J Immunol 139:3062, 1987.
189. Lehmann J: Neuropeptide Y: an overview. Drug Devel Res 19:329, 1990.
190. Levine RR, Birdsall NJM, North RA, et al: Subtypes of muscarinic receptors III. Trends Pharmacol Sci 9(suppl):1, 1991.
191. Li CG, Rand MJ: Evidence that part of the NANC relaxant response of guinea-pig trachea to electrical field stimulation is mediated by nitric oxide. Br J Pharmacol 102:91, 1991.
192. Lindgren BR, Ekström T, Andersson RGG: The effect of inhaled clonidine in patients with asthma. Am Rev Respir Dis 134:266, 1986.
193. Lindgren BR, Persson K, Kihlström JE, et al: ACE-inhibitor-induced enhancement of spontaneous and IgE-mediated histamine release from mast cells and basophilic leukocytes and the modulatory effect of capsaicin sensitive nerves. Pharmacol Toxicol 64:159, 1989.
194. Lindgren BR, Rosenquist U, Ekström T, et al: Increased bronchial reactivity and potentiated skin responses in hypertensive subjects suffering from coughs during ACE-inhibitor therapy. Chest 95:1225, 1989.
195. Lindsay RM, Harmar AJ: Nerve growth factor regulates expression of neuropeptide genes in adult sensory neurons. Nature 337:362, 1989.
196. Lindsay RM, Lockett C, Sternberg J, et al: Neuropeptide expression in cultures of adult sensory neurons: modulation of substance P and calcitonin gene related peptide levels by nerve growth factor. Neuroscience 33:53, 1989.
197. Llorens-Cortes C, Giros B, Schwartz JC: A novel potential metallopeptidase derived from the enkephalinase gene by alternative splicing. J Neurochem 55:2146, 1990.
198. Llorens-Cortes C, Huang H, Vicart P, et al: Identification and characterization of neutral endopeptidase in endothelial cells from venous or arterial origins. J Biol Chem 267:140112, 1992.
199. Lotz M, Vaughan JH, Carson DA: Effect of neuropeptides on production of inflammatory cytokines by human monocytes. Science 241:1218, 1988.
200. Lundberg JM, Alving K, Karlsson JA, et al: Sensory neuropeptide involvement in animal models of airway irritation and of allergen-evoked asthma. Am Rev Respir Dis 143:1429, 1991.
201. Lundberg JM, Angaard A, Fahrenkrug J: Complementary role of vasoactive intestinal peptide (VIP) and acetylcholine for cat submandibular gland blood flow and secretion. Acta Physiol Scand 113:329, 1981.
202. Lundberg JM, Fahrenkrug J, Hökfelt T, et al: Co-existence of peptide HI (PHI) and VIP in nerves regulating blood flow and bronchial smooth muscle tone in various mammals including man. Peptides 5:593, 1984.
203. Lundberg JM, Lundblad L, Martling CR, et al: Coexistence of multiple peptides and classic transmitters in airway neurons: functional and pathophysiologic aspects. Am Rev Respir Dis 136:S16, 1987.
204. Lundberg JM, Saria A, Brodin E, et al: A substance P antagonist inhibits vagally induced increase in vascular permeability and bronchial smooth muscle contraction in the guinea pig. Proc Natl Acad Sci USA 80:1120, 1983.
205. Lundberg JM, Saria A, Theodorsson-Norheim E, et al: Multiple tachykinins in capsaicin-sensitive afferents: occurrence, release, and biological effects with special reference to irritation of the airways. In Håkanson R, Sundler F (eds): Tachykinin Antagonists. Elsevier Science Publishers BV (Biomedical Division), Amsterdam, 1985, p 159.
206. Lundgren J, Baraniuk JN, Ostrowski N, et al: Gastrin-releasing peptide stimulates glycoconjugate release from feline trachea. Am J Physiol 258:L68, 1990.
207. Lundgren JD, Shelhamer JH: Pathogenesis of airway mucus hypersecretion. J Allergy Clin Immunol 85:399, 1990.
208. Macklem PT: Factors determining bronchial smooth muscle shortening. Am Rev Respir Dis 143:S47, 1991.
209. MacLean DB, Bennett B, Morris M, et al: Differential regulation of calcitonin gene related peptide and substance P in cultured neonatal rat vagal sensory neurons. Brain Res 478:349, 1989.
210. Maggi CA, Patacchini R, Astolfi M, et al: NK2-receptor agonists and antagonists. Ann NY Acad Sci 632:184, 1991.
211. Maggi CA, Patacchini R, Rovero P, et al: Tachykinin receptors and noncholinergic bronchoconstriction in the guinea-pig isolated bronchi. Am Rev Respir Dis 144:363, 1991.
212. Mak JC, Baraniuk JN, Barnes PJ: Localization of muscarinic receptor subtype mRNAs in human lung. Am J Respir Cell Mol Biol 7:344, 1992.
213. Mak JCW, Barnes PJ: Autoradiographic localization of calcitonin gene-related peptide (CGRP) binding sites in human and guinea pig lung. Peptides 9:957, 1988.
214. Mak JC, Barnes PJ: Autoradiographic visualization of muscarinic receptor subtypes in human and guinea pig lung. Am Rev Respir Dis 141:1559, 1990.
215. Malm L, Sundler F, Uddman R: Effects of vasoactive intestinal peptide on resistance and capacitance vessels in nasal mucosa. Acta Otolaryngol (Stockh) 90:304, 1980.
216. Mapp PI, Walsh DA, Kidd BL, et al: Localization of the enzyme neutral endopeptidase to the human synovium. J Rheumatol 19:1838, 1992.
217. Marasco WA, Showell HJ, Becker EL: Substance P binds to the formylpeptide chemotaxis receptor on the rabbit neutrophil. Biochem Biophys Res Commun 99:1065, 1981.
218. Marom ZM, Goswami SK: Respiratory mucus hypersecretion (bronchorrea): a case discussion—possible mechanism(s) and treatment. J Allergy Clin Immunol 87:1050, 1991.
219. Martin JG, Wang A, Zacour M, et al: The effects of vasoactive intestinal polypeptide on cholinergic neurotransmission in an isolated innervated guinea pig tracheal preparation. Respir Physiol 79:111, 1990.
220. Martins MA, Shore SA, Drazen JM: Release of tachykinins by histamine, methacholine, PAF, LTD4, and substance P from guinea pig lungs. Am J Physiol 261:L449, 1991.
221. Matsuda H, Kawakita K, Kiso Y, et al: Substance P induces granulocyte infiltration through degranulation of mast cells. J Immunol 142:927, 1989.
222. McDonald DM: Neurogenic inflammation in the rat trachea. I. Changes in venules, leukocytes and epithelial cells. J Neurocytol 17:605, 1988.
223. McDonald DM: Infections intensify neurogenic plasma extravasation in the airway mucosa. Am Rev Respir Dis 146:S40, 1992.
224. McFadden ER Jr, Luparello T, Lyons HA, et al: The mechanism of action of suggestion in the induction of acute asthma attacks. Psychosom Med 31:134, 1969.
225. Meurs H, Kauffman HF, Koëter GH, et al: Regulation of the beta-receptor-adenylate cyclase system in lymphocytes of allergic patients with asthma: possible role for protein kinase C in allergen-induced nonspecific refractoriness of adenylate cyclase. J Allergy Clin Immunol 80:326, 1987.
226. Meurs H, Koëter GH, de Vries K, et al: The beta-adrenergic system and allergic bronchial asthma: changes in lymphocyte beta-adrenergic receptor number and adenylate cyclase activity after an allergen-induced asthmatic attack. J Allergy Clin Immunol 70:272, 1982.

227. Minette PAH, Lammers JWJ, Dixon CMS, et al: A muscarinic agonist inhibits reflex bronchoconstriction in normal but not in asthmatic subjects. J Appl Physiol 67:2461, 1989.
228. Mita H, Yui Y, Yasueda H, et al: Changes of alpha-1- and beta-adrenergic and cholinergic muscarinic receptors in guinea pig lung sensitized with ovalbumin. Int Arch Allergy Appl Immunol 70:225, 1983.
229. Miura M, Ichinose M, Kimura K, et al: Dysfunction of nonadrenergic noncholinergic inhibitory system after antigen inhalation in actively sensitized cat airways. Am Rev Respir Dis 145:70, 1992.
230. Morice AH, Sever PS: Vasoactive intestinal peptide as a bronchodilator in severe asthma. Peptides 7:279, 1986.
231. Morimoto H, Yamashita M, Matsuda A, et al: Effects of FR113680 and FK 224, novel tachykinin receptor antagonists, on cigarette smoke-induced rat tracheal plasma extravasation. Eur J Pharmacol 224:1, 1992.
232. Mosimann BL, White MV, Hohman RJ, et al: Substance P, calcitonin gene related peptide, and vasoactive intestinal peptide increase in nasal secretions after allergen challenge in atopic patients. J Allergy Clin Immunol 92:95, 1993.
233. Motojima S, Yukawa T, Fukuda T, et al: Changes in airway responsiveness and β- and α-1-adrenergic receptors in the lungs of guinea pigs with experimental asthma. Allergy 44:66, 1989.
234. Mullol J, Baraniuk JN, Logun C, et al: M1 and M3 muscarinic antagonists inhibit human nasal glandular secretion in vitro. J Appl Physiol 73:2069, 1992.
235. Mullol J, Chowdhury BA, White MV, et al: Endothelin in human nasal mucosa. Am J Respir Cell Mol Biol 8:393, 1993.
236. Mullol J, Rieves RD, Baraniuk JN, et al: The effects of neuropeptides on mucous glycoprotein secretion from human nasal mucosa in vitro. Neuropeptides 21:231, 1992.
237. Murai M, Maeda Y, Hagiwara D, et al: Effects of an NK1 receptor antagonist, FK888, on constriction and plasma extravasation induced in guinea pig airway by neurokinins and capsaicin. Eur J Pharmacol 236:7, 1993.
238. Murlas CG, Murphy TP, Lang Z: HOCl causes airway substance P hyperresponsiveness and neutral endopeptidase hypoactivity. Am J Physiol 258:L361, 1990.
239. Mygind N, Borum P: Anticholinergic treatment of water rhinorrhea. Am J Rhinol 4:1, 1990.
240. Naclerio RM: Allergic rhinitis. N Engl J Med 325:860, 1991.
241. Nadel JA: Decreased neutral endopeptidases: possible role in inflammatory diseases of airways. Lung 168(suppl):123, 1990.
242. Nadel JA, Borson DB: Modulation of neurogenic inflammation by neutral endopeptidase. Am Rev Respir Dis 143:S33, 1991.
243. Nakanishi S: Substance P precursor and kininogen: their structures, gene organizations, and regulation. Physiol Rev 67:1117, 1987.
244. Naline E, Devillier P, Drapeau G, et al: Characterization of neurokinin effects and receptor selectivity in human isolated bronchi. Am Rev Respir Dis 140:679, 1989.
245. Nieber K, Baumgartern CR, Rathsack R, et al: Substance P and β-endorphin-like immunoreactivity in lavage fluids of subjects with and without allergic asthma. J Allergy Clin Immunol 90:646, 1992.
246. Ohkubo H, Nakanishi S: Molecular characterization of the three tachykinin receptors. Ann NY Acad Sci 632:53, 1991.
247. Ohkubo K, Lee CH, Baraniuk JN, et al: Angiotensin-converting enzyme in the human nasal mucosa. Am J Respir Cell Mol Biol 11:173, 1994.
248. Okayama M, Mullol J, Baraniuk JN, et al: Muscarinic receptor subtypes in human nasal mucosa: characterization, autoradiographic localization and function in vitro. Am J Respir Cell Mol Biol 8:176, 1993.
249. Ollerenshaw SL, Jarvis DL, Woolcock AJ: Substance P immunoreactive nerves in airways from asthmatics and nonasthmatics. Eur Respir J 4:673, 1991.
250. Ollerenshaw S, Jarvis D, Woolcock A, et al: Absence of immunoreactive vasoactive intestinal polypeptide in tissue from the lungs of patients with asthma. N Engl J Med 320:1244, 1989.
251. Palmer JB, Cuss FMC, Barnes PJ: VIP and PHM and their role in nonadrenergic inhibitory responses in isolated human airways. J Appl Physiol 61:1322, 1986.
252. Parker C, Smith JW: Alterations in cyclic adenosine monophosphate metabolism in human bronchial asthma. I. Leukocyte responsiveness to beta-adrenergic agents. J Clin Invest 52:48, 1973.
253. Payan DG, Brewster DR, Goetzl EJ: Specific stimulation of human T lymphocytes by substance P. J Immunol 131:1613, 1983.
254. Payan DG, Levine JD, Goetzl EJ: Modulation of immunity and hypersensitivity by sensory neuropeptides. J Immunol 132:1601, 1984.
255. Pernow J: Co-release and functional interactions of neuropeptide Y and noradrenaline in peripheral sympathetic vascular control. Acta Physiol Scand Suppl 568:1, 1988.
256. Petitet F, Saffroy M, Torrens Y, et al: Possible existence of a new tachykinin receptor subtype in the guinea pig ileum. Peptides 13:383, 1992.
257. Piedemonte G, McDonald DM, Nadel JA: Glucocorticoids inhibit neurogenic plasma extravasation and prevent virus-potentiated extravasation in the rat trachea. J Clin Invest 86:1409, 1990.
258. Postma DS, Keyzer JJ, Koeter GA, et al: Influence of the parasympathetic and sympathetic nervous systems on nocturnal bronchial obstruction. Clin Sci 69:251, 1985.
259. Potter EK: Neuropeptide Y as an autonomic neurotransmitter. Pharmacol Ther 37:251, 1988.
260. Presti ME, Gardner JD: Receptor antagonists for gastrointestinal peptides. Am J Physiol 264:G399, 1993.
261. Proud D, Kaplan AP: Kinin formation: mechanisms and role in inflammatory disorders. Annu Rev Immunol 6:49, 1988.
262. Proud D, Reynolds CJ, Lacapra S, et al: Nasal provocation with bradykinin induces symptoms of rhinitis and a sore throat. Am Rev Respir Dis 137:613, 1988.
263. Proud D, Subauste MC, Ward PE: Glucocorticoids do not alter peptidase expression on a human bronchial epithelial cell line. Am J Respir Cell Mol Biol 11:57, 1994.
264. Rangachari PK, McWade D: Effects of tachykinins on the electrical activity of isolated canine tracheal epithelium: an exploratory study. Regul Pept 12:9, 1985.
265. Raphael GD, Baraniuk JN, Kaliner MA: How and why the nose runs. J Allergy Clin Immunol 87:457, 1991.
266. Raphael GD, Igarashi Y, White MV, et al: The pathophysiology of rhinitis. V. Sources of protein in allergen-induced nasal secretions. J Allergy Clin Immunol 88:33, 1991.
267. Regoli D, Nantel F, Tousidgnant C, et al: Neurokinin agonists and antagonists. Ann NY Acad Sci 632:170, 1991.
268. Repke H, Bienert M: Structural requirements for mast cell triggering by substance P-like peptides. Agents Actions 23:207, 1988.
269. Rhoden KJ, Meldrum LA, Barnes PJ: Inhibition of cholinergic neurotransmission in human airways by β_2-adrenoreceptors. J Appl Physiol 65:700, 1988.
270. Richardson PS, Webber SE: The control of mucous secretion in the airways by peptidergic mechanisms. Am Rev Respir Dis 136:S72, 1987.
271. Richerson HB, Seebohm PM: Nasal airway response to exercise. J Allergy 41:269, 1968.
272. Rogers DF, Aursudkij B, Barnes PJ: Effects of tachykinins on mucus secretion in human bronchi in vitro. Eur J Pharmacol 174:283, 1989.
273. Rogers DF, Barnes PJ: Opioid inhibitions of neurally mediated mucus secretion in human bronchi. Lancet 1:930, 1989.
274. Roisman GL, Lacronique J, Carre C, et al: Neutral endopeptidase and kininase II activities in bronchial mucosa in asthmatic and normal subjects. Am J Respir Crit Care Med 149:A956, 1994.
275. Roques BP, Noble F, Dauge V, et al: Neutral endopeptidase 24.11: structure, inhibition, and experimental and clinical pharmacology. Pharmacol Rev 45:87, 1993.
276. Sachais BS, Snider RM, Lowe JA, III, et al: Molecular basis for the species selectivity of the substance P antagonist CP-96,345. J Biol Chem 268:2319, 1993.
277. Said SI: VIP as a modulator of lung inflammation and airway constriction. Am Rev Respir Dis 143:S22, 1991.
278. Sakamoto A, Yanagisawa M, Sakurai T, et al: Cloning and functional expression of human cDNA for the ET_B endothelin receptor. Biochem Biophys Res Commun 178:656, 1991.
279. Sakamoto T, Barnes PJ, Chung KF: Effect of CP-96,345, a non-peptide NK1 receptor antagonist, against substance P-, bradykinin-, and allergen-induced airway microvascular leakage and bronchoconstriction in the guinea pig. Eur J Pharmacol 231:31, 1993.
280. Salonen RO, Webber SE, Widdicombe JG: Effects of neuropeptides and capsaicin on the canine tracheal vasculature in vivo. Br J Pharmacol 95:1262, 1988.
281. Sano Y, Watt G, Townley RG: Decreased mononuclear cell beta-adrenergic receptors in bronchial asthma: parallel studies of lymphocyte and granulocyte desensitization. J Allergy Clin Immunol 72:495, 1983.

282. Saria A, Martling CR, Yan Z: Release of multiple tachykinins from capsaicin-sensitive sensory nerves in the lung by bradykinin, histamine, dimethylphenyl piperazinium, and vagal nerve stimulation. Am Rev Respir Dis 137:1330, 1988.
283. Sato T, Bewtra AK, Hopp RJ, et al: Alpha- and beta-adrenergic-receptor systems in bronchial asthma and in subjects without asthma: reduced mononuclear cell beta-receptors in bronchial asthma. J Allergy Clin Immunol 86:839, 1990.
284. Sekizawa K, Tamaoki J, Graf P, et al: Modulation of cholinergic transmission by vasoactive intestinal peptide in ferret trachea. J Appl Physiol 69:2433, 1988.
285. Sharma RK, Jeffery PK: Airway VIP receptor number is reduced in cystic fibrosis but not asthma. Am Rev Respir Dis 141:A726, 1990.
286. Shawket S, Dickerson C, Hazleman B, et al: Prolonged effect on CGRP in Raynaud's patients: a double-blind randomized comparison with prostacyclin. Br J Clin Pharmacol 32:209, 1991.
287. Shekhar YC, Anand IS, Sarma R, et al: Effects of prolonged infusion of human α-calcitonin gene-related peptide on hemodynamics, renal blood flow and hormone levels in congestive heart failure. Am J Cardiol 67:732, 1991.
288. Sheppard D, Thompson JE, Scypinski L, et al: Toluene diisocyanate increases airway responsiveness to substance P and decreases airway neutral endopeptidase. J Clin Invest 81:1111, 1988.
289. Sheppard MN, Polak JM, Allen JM, et al: Neuropeptide tyrosine (NPY): a newly discovered peptide is present in the mammalian respiratory tract. Thorax 39:326, 1984.
290. Shimosegawa T, Said SI: Pulmonary calcitonin gene-related peptide immunoreactivity: nerve-endocrine cell interrelationships. Am J Respir Cell Mol Biol 4:126, 1991.
291. Shimura S, Sasaki T, Ikeda K, et al: Neuropeptides and airway submucosal gland secretion. Am Rev Respir Dis 143:S25, 1991.
292. Shimura S, Sasaki T, Ikeda K, et al: VIP augments cholinergic-induced glycoconjugate secretion in tracheal submucosal glands. J Appl Physiol 65:2537, 1988.
293. Shipp MA, Richardson NE, Sayre PH, et al: Molecular cloning of the common acute lymphoblastic leukemia antigen (CALLA) identifies a type II integral membrane protein. Proc Natl Acad Sci USA 85:4819, 1988.
294. Simonsson BG, Jacobs FM, Nadel JA: Role of the autonomic nervous system and the cough reflex in the increased responsiveness of airways in patients with obstructive airway disease. J Clin Invest 46:1812, 1967.
295. Snashall PD, Boother FA, Sterling GM: The effect of α-adrenoreceptor stimulation on the airways of normal and asthmatic man. Clin Sci Mol Med 54:283, 1978.
296. Solway J, Koa BM, Jordan JE, et al: Tachykinin receptor antagonists inhibit hyperpnea-induced bronchoconstriction in guinea pigs. J Clin Invest 92:315, 1993.
297. Solway J, Leff AR: Sensory neuropeptides and airway function. J Appl Physiol 71:2077, 1991.
298. Spina D, Rigby PJ, Paterson JW, et al: Autoradiographic localization of beta-adrenoceptors in asthmatic human lung. Am Rev Respir Dis 140:1410, 1989.
299. Spina D, Rigby PJ, Paterson JW, et al: α_1-adrenoceptor function and autoradiographic distribution in human asthmatic lung. Br J Pharmacol 97:701, 1989.
300. Spindel ER, Sunday ME, Hofler H: Transient elevation of messenger RNA encoding gastrin releasing peptide (GRP), a putative pulmonary growth factor in human fetal lung. J Clin Invest 80:1172, 1987.
301. Spindel ER, Zilberberg MD, Chin WW: Analysis of the gene and multiple messenger ribonucleic acids (mRNAs) encoding human gastrin releasing peptide: alternate RNA splicing occurs in neural and endocrine tissue. Mol Endocrinol 1:224, 1987.
302. Springall DR, Collins G, Barer G, et al: Increased intracellular levels of calcitonin gene related peptide-like immunoreactivity in pulmonary endocrine cells of hypoxic rats. J Pathol 155:259, 1988.
303. Springall DR, Howarth PH, Counihan H, et al: Endothelin immunoreactivity of airway epithelium in asthmatic patients. Lancet 337:697, 1991.
304. Springall DR, Polak JM, Howard L: Persistence of intrinsic neurones and possible phenotypic changes after extrinsic denervation of human respiratory tract by heart-lung transplantation. Am Rev Respir Dis 141:1538, 1990.
305. Sreedharan RP, Patel DR, Huang JX, et al: Cloning and functional expression of a human neuroendocrine vasoactive intestinal peptide receptor. Biochem Biophys Res Commun 193:546, 1993.
306. Stanisz AM, Befus D, Bienenstock J: Differential effects of vasoactive intestinal peptide, substance P, and somatostatin on immunoglobulin synthesis and proliferations by lymphocytes from Peyer's patches, mesenteric lymph nodes, and spleen. J Immunol 136:152, 1986.
307. Steenbergh PH, Hoppener JW, Zandberg J, et al: Structure and expression of the human calcitonin/CGRP genes. FEBS Lett 209:97, 1986.
308. Stefano GB, Paemen LR, Hughes TK Jr: Autoimmunoregulation: differential modulation of CD10/neutral endopeptidase 24.11 by tumor necrosis factor and neuropeptides. J Neuroimmunol 41:9, 1992.
309. Stief CG, Wetterauer U, Schaebsdau FH, et al: Calcitonin-gene-related peptide: a possible role in human penile erection and its therapeutic application in impotent patients. J Urol 146:1010, 1991.
310. Stephens NL, Seow CY, Kong SK: Mechanical properties of sensitized airway smooth muscle shortening capacity. Am Rev Respir Dis 143:S13, 1991.
311. Stern L, Kunos G: Synergistic regulation of pulmonary β-adrenergic receptors by glucocorticoids and interleukin-1. J Biol Chem 263:15876, 1988.
312. Stevenson RN, Roberts RH, Timmins AD: Calcitonin gene related peptide: a haemodynamic study of a novel vasodilator in patients with severe chronic heart failure. Int J Cardiol 37:407, 1992.
313. Stjarne P, Lacroix JS, Anggard A, et al: Compartment analysis of vascular effects of neuropeptides and capsaicin in the pig nasal mucosa. Acta Physiol Scand 141:335, 1991.
314. Stretton CD, Belvisi MG, Barnes PJ: Neuropeptide Y modulates nonadrenergic, non-cholinergic neural bronchoconstriction in vivo and in vitro. Neuropeptides 17:163, 1990.
315. Stretton CD, Belvisi MG, Barnes PJ: Modulation of neural bronchoconstrictor responses in the guinea-pig respiratory tract by vasoactive intestinal peptide. Neuropeptides 18:149, 1991.
316. Sunday ME, Hua J, Torday JS, et al: CD10/neutral endopeptidase 24.11 in developing human fetal lung patterns of expression and modulation of peptide-mediated proliferation. J Clin Invest 90:2517, 1992.
317. Sunday ME, Kaplan LM, Motoyama E, et al: Gastrin releasing peptide (mammalian bombesin) gene expression in health and disease. Lab Invest 59:5, 1988.
318. Szentivanyi A: The beta adrenergic theory of the atopic abnormality in bronchial asthma. J Allergy 42:203, 1968.
319. Takahashi K, Tanaka A, Hara M, et al: The primary structure and gene organization of human substance P and neuromedin K receptors. Eur J Biochem 204:1025, 1992.
320. Tam EK, Franconi GM, Nadel JA, et al: Protease inhibitors potentiate smooth muscle relaxation induced by vasoactive intestinal peptide in isolated human bronchi. Am J Respir Cell Mol Biol 2:449, 1990.
321. Tanaka DT, Grunstein MM: Maturation of neuromodulatory effect of substance P in rabbit airways. J Clin Invest 85:345, 1990.
322. Thompson JE, Sheppard D: Phosphoramidon potentiates the increase in lung resistance mediated by tachykinins in guinea pigs. Am Rev Respir Dis 137:337, 1988.
323. Thomson NC, Daniel EE, Hargreave FE: Role of smooth muscle $alpha_1$-receptors in nonspecific bronchial responsiveness in asthma. Am Rev Respir Dis 126:521, 1982.
324. Tokuyama K, Kuo HP, Rohde JA, et al: Neural control of goblet cell secretion in guinea pig airways. Am J Physiol 259:L108, 1990.
325. Tsutsumi Y: Immunohistochemical localization of gastrin releasing peptide in normal and diseased human lung. Ann NY Acad Sci 547:336, 1988.
326. Tucker JF, Brave SR, Charalambous L, et al: L-N^G-nitro arginine inhibits non-adrenergic, non-cholinergic relaxations of guinea-pig isolated tracheal smooth muscle. Br J Pharmacol 100:663, 1990.
327. Uchida Y, Nomura A, Ohtsuka M, et al: Neurokinin A as a potent bronchoconstrictor. Am Rev Respir Dis 136:718, 1987.
328. Uddman R, Sundler F: Innervation of the upper airways. Clin Chest Med 7:201, 1986.
329. Umeno E, Nadel JA, Huang HT, et al: Inhibition of neutral endopeptidase potentiates neurogenic inflammation in the rat trachea. J Appl Physiol 66:2647, 1989.
330. Undem BJ, Dick EC, Buckner CK: Inhibition by vasoactive intestinal peptide of antigen-induced histamine release from guinea-pig minced lung. Eur J Pharmacol 88:247, 1983.
331. van Megen YJB, Klaassen ABM, Rodrigues de Miranda JF, et al: Alterations of muscarinic acetylcholine receptors in the nasal mucosa of allergic patients in comparison with nonallergic individuals. J Allergy Clin Immunol 87:521, 1991.
332. Venepalli BR, Aimone LD, Appell KC, et al: Synthesis and substance

P receptor binding activity of androstanol[3,2-b]pyrimido[1,2-a]benzimidazoles. J Med Chem 35:374, 1992.

333. Venter SC: Autoantibodies to the beta-adrenergic receptor. In Kaliner M (moderator): Autonomic Nervous System Abnormalities and Allergy. Ann Intern Med 96:349, 1982.

334. Venter JC, Di Porzio U, Robinson DA, et al: Evolution of neurotransmitter receptor systems. Prog Neurobiol 30:105, 1988.

335. Vincent MB: Lithium inhibits substance P and vasoactive intestinal peptide-induced relaxations on isolated porcine ophthalmic artery. Headache 32:335, 1992.

336. Wada E, Way J, Shapira H, et al: cDNA cloning, characterization and brain region-specific expression of a neuromedin-B-preferring bombesin receptor. Neuron 6:421, 1991.

337. Wallengren J: Substance P antagonist inhibits immediate and delayed type cutaneous hypersensitivity reactions. Br J Dermatol 124:324, 1991.

338. Watling KJ: Nonpeptide antagonists herald new era in tachykinin research. Trends Pharmacol Sci 13:266, 1992.

339. Watson N, MacLagan J, Barnes PJ: Vagal control of guinea pig tracheal smooth muscle: lack of involvement of VIP or nitric oxide. J Appl Physiol 74:1964, 1993.

340. Willey JC, Lechner JF, Harris CC: Bombesin and the C-terminal tetradecapeptide of gastrin-releasing peptide are growth factors for normal human bronchial epithelial cells. Exp Cell Res 153:245, 1984.

341. Winter RJD, Zhao L, Krausz T, et al: Neutral endopeptidase 24.11 inhibition reduces pulmonary vascular remodeling in rats exposed to chronic hypoxia. Am Rev Respir Dis 144:1342, 1991.

342. Wong SM, Kullnig R, Dedinas J, et al: Anthrotainin, an inhibitor of substance P binding produced by *Gliocladium catenulatum*. J Antibiot (Tokyo) 46:214, 1993.

343. Wong SM, Musza LL, Kydd GC, et al: Fiscalins: new substance P inhibitors produced by the fungus *Neosartorya fischeri*. Taxonomy, fermentation, structures, and biological properties. J Antibiot (Tokyo) 46:545, 1993.

344. Xuan ATD, Regnard J, Matran R, et al: Effects of clonidine on bronchial responses to histamine in normal and asthmatic subjects. Eur Respir J 1:345, 1988.

345. Yeadon M, Wilkinson D, Payne AN: Ozone induces bronchial hyperreactivity to inhaled substance P by functional inhibition of enkephalinase. Br J Pharmacol 99:191, 1990.

346. Yiangou Y, Requejo F, Polak JM, et al: Characterization of a novel prepro VIP derived peptide. Biochem Biophys Res Commun 139:1142, 1986.

347. Yokata Y, Sasai Y, Tanaka K: Molecular characterization of a functional cDNA for rat substance P receptor. J Biol Chem 264:17649, 1989.

348. Zhang JF, Lui J, Lui XZ: Stabilization of cardiac rhythm in subsequently fatal ventricular tachycardia and fibrillation by calcitonin gene related peptide. Int J Cardiol 34:101, 1992.

349. Zhang JF, Lui J, Lui XZ, et al: The effect of calcitonin gene related peptide on arrhythmia caused by adenosine diphosphate and desacetyldigilanide-C in rats. Int J Cardiol 33:43, 1991.

350. Ziche M, Morbidelli L, Pacini M: Substance P stimulates neovascularization in vivo and proliferation of cultured endothelial cells. Microvasc Res 40:264, 1990.

II Assessment of Allergic Diseases

19 Diagnostic Testing: SKIN TESTS, IgE QUANTITATION

JOHN W. YUNGINGER

Diagnostic tests for suspected allergic disease may be conveniently divided into in vivo and in vitro categories. In vivo tests include the skin test and various mucosal provocation tests; inhalation challenge tests for asthma are discussed elsewhere in this volume. In vitro diagnostic tests include the measurement of total serum IgE protein and allergen-specific IgE antibody. These various tests are discussed individually in sections of this chapter.

The selection of appropriate diagnostic tests is wholly dependent on the clinical history presented by the patient. It therefore follows that diagnostic tests should be ordered only after a careful history and physical examination have been obtained. The use of screening batteries of tests or excessive use of routine tests as a substitute for careful history taking is intellectually lazy and often expensive and should be condemned.

SKIN TESTS

Direct skin testing is the most commonly used diagnostic test for allergy. The ability to reproduce a specific allergic reaction by this in vivo localized challenge test is the most sensitive technique for demonstrating the presence of immediate hypersensitivity.

Generalized allergic reactions after skin testing are unusual,[31, 52] but their possible occurrence should be appreciated. Skin test facilities should be equipped with tourniquets, an oxygen supply, and resuscitation equipment and medications for treatment of cardiovascular collapse.[1] Syringes containing epinephrine and diphenhydramine already drawn up in appropriate doses should be immediately available.

ALLERGENIC EXTRACTS

In most cases, allergenic extracts are crude complex mixtures of allergens, pigments, enzymes, toxins, nonallergenic proteins, and/or sugars. In only a few cases have the active allergenic materials been isolated and characterized with respect to their physicochemical, biochemical, and immunochemical properties.

Source Materials

Pollen extracts are prepared from pollens that have been cleaned by sieving, dried to low residual moisture, and defatted. Most fungal extracts are prepared from both spores and mycelial mats, although some commercial extracts also contain metabolic antigens isolated from dialyzed, lyophilized synthetic culture medium.[51] Most mammalian extracts are prepared from animal pelts, although commercial cat extracts are now available as either pelt or hair/dander extracts; the latter extracts contain lower quantities of cat serum albumin. House dust mite extracts marketed in the United States are prepared from whole mites that have been removed from their culture medium,[12] whereas in Europe, whole mite culture extracts are available in which the spent medium and living mites are collectively extracted.[29] Honey bee venom is obtained by electrical stimulation, whereas vespid venoms are obtained by extracting extirpated venom sacs from yellow jackets, hornets, and wasps. Food extracts are usually prepared from fresh, lyophilized foods, with or without defatting.

Extraction

Source materials may be extracted in distilled water, sodium bicarbonate, ammonium bicarbonate, sodium chloride, or 50% glycerin. The final form of the extract (aqueous, glycerinated, or lyophilized) usually dictates the extraction buffer used. Extracts are clarified by centrifugation or coarse-membrane filtration and then sterilized by filtration through 0.2 μm membranes. Extracts packaged in multiple-dose containers contain phenol, at a concentration of 0.4%, and/or 50% glycerin to inhibit microbial growth.

Stability

When shipped by the manufacturer, aqueous extracts are given a 12- to 18-month label dating, whereas glycerinated extracts and lyophilized extracts are given a 3-year label dating. The potency of allergenic extracts decreases gradually during storage. The most important variables affecting loss of potency include temperature, the presence of proteases in the crude extract, and the adsorption of allergen to the inner wall of the container. The stability of allergenic extracts is enhanced by lyophilizing, packaging in 50% glycerin, or incorporating human serum albumin into the diluent.[40, 43]

Labeling

For decades, allergenic extracts marketed in the United States have been labeled in weight:volume units (w:v) or in protein nitrogen units (PNU); one PNU equals 10^{-5} mg of protein. The w:v system merely tells how the extract was prepared. For example, a 1:10 w:v extract is prepared by extracting 1 gram of source material in 10 ml of appropriate buffer. Because all allergens are proteins, a measurement of the total protein in an allergenic extract might be expected to correlate with its biologic potency. However, both allergenic and nonallergenic proteins are included in this quantitation.

A method of measuring the biologic activity of an extract involves intradermal skin testing of several sensitive persons with serial threefold dilutions of both test and reference allergenic extracts,[59] the latter having been assigned previously a potency in allergy units (AU). In the United States, house dust mite extracts are required to be marketed with AU labeling.

Because it is desirable to have one unit of a pollen extract biologically equivalent to one unit of a mite extract, and so forth, the Food and Drug Administration has introduced the bioequivalent allergy unit (BAU). At present, only cat extracts are available in the United States with BAU labeling,[42] but several grass pollen extracts will be required to have BAU labeling.

Standardization

In the United States, standardized allergenic extracts are available for short ragweed pollen, Hymenoptera venoms, cat pelt, cat hair/dander, and *Dermatophagoides pteronyssinus* and *D. farinae* house dust mite extracts. Although they are more expensive than the unstandardized extracts with w:v or PNU labeling, standardized extracts offer several advantages.[69] First, standardized extracts are less variable from lot to lot. Second, standardized extracts provide more quantitative and meaningful schedules for diagnostic testing or immunotherapy. Third, standardized extracts permit a safer, more orderly, more efficient, and less expensive transfer of immunotherapy from one allergist's office to another when patients move from one part of the country to another.

SKIN TEST PROCEDURES

Skin testing is usually performed by either the puncture or intradermal technique. Puncture tests may be done on the forearm or the back. The patient's skin is wiped with 70% ethanol and allowed to dry, after which the sites for testing are marked with a pen. The sites should be at least 7 cm apart to allow accurate measurement of the resulting wheal-and-flare reactions. Unstandardized extracts for puncture testing are usually supplied as 1:10 to 1:20 (w:v) or 10,000 to 20,000 PNU/ml solutions in 50% glycerine. Standardized cat or house dust mite extracts are usually tested at 10,000 BAU/ml or 10,000 to 30,000 AU/ml, respectively. A drop of each test extract is placed on the skin using a dropper or glass applicator, after which the skin is punctured with a sterile lancet. To help avoid carryover of allergen from one test site to another, a separate lancet may be employed for each test extract. However, some individuals use the same lancet for all tests, wiping it briefly on a sterile gauze between tests. The puncture should be deep enough to penetrate the epidermis but not so deep as to draw blood. After the puncture is made, the drop of the allergen may be left on the skin or wiped away after a minute or two. The diameters of the resulting wheal-and-flare reactions are recorded 10 to 15 minutes later. The size of the reactions is dependent to some degree upon the particular device used for the puncture and the anatomic location of the test sites.[41]

Intradermal tests are usually performed on the arm. The test sites are prepared and marked as for puncture tests. The procedure described by Norman is used by many allergists.[44] Using sterile, disposable tuberculin syringes fitted with 26- or 27-gauge needles, sufficient extract is injected intracutaneously so as to raise an initial 3 mm wheal; this quantity is approximately 0.02 ml. The resulting wheal-and-flare reaction is read in 15 minutes. Tests are graded on a semiquantitative scale from 0 to 4+ (Table 19–1). Care must be taken to evacuate all air bubbles from the syringe and needle prior to placing the test. If air is inadvertently injected with the extract, the precision of the test is reduced. Extracts for

TABLE 19–1
GRADING SYSTEM FOR INTRADERMAL SKIN TESTS

Grade	Wheal (mm)	Erythema (mm)
0	<4	<5
+−	5–10	5–10
1+	5–10	11–20
2+	5–10	21–30
3+	10–15*	31–40
4+	>15†	>40

*Or with pseudopods.
†Or with many pseudopods.
From Norman PS: Skin testing. In Rose NR, Conway de Macario E, Fahey JL, et al (eds): Manual of Clinical Laboratory Immunology, 4th edition. American Society for Microbiology, Washington, DC, 1992, p 685.

intradermal testing are usually nonglycerinated and are 100- to 1,000-fold more dilute than those used for puncture testing. Typical intradermal test concentrations are 1:100 to 1:1,000 w:v, or 200 to 1,000 PNU/ml (for unstandardized pollen, epidermal, or mold extracts); 1 ng/ml to 1 μg/ml (for Hymenoptera venoms); 100 BAU/ml (for cat extracts); and 30 to 300 AU/ml (for house dust mite extracts). Intradermal injection of glycerinated extracts is painful; moreover, intradermal injection of extracts containing 6% or more glycerine may cause nonspecific irritant–positive reactions.[30]

A more quantitative estimate of the patient's reactivity may be obtained using end point skin test titrations. Rather than using a single, arbitrary allergen test concentration, 3- to 10-fold dilutions of the test allergens are placed beginning with the most dilute solutions.[59] If a negative test is produced, the patient is tested with successively more concentrated solutions until a positive reaction is produced or until the most concentrated solution is tested. The most dilute solution required to produce a 1+ or 2+ reaction is considered the end point. This titration system can be used for either puncture tests or intradermal tests.

CONTROLS

Positive and negative control tests with histamine phosphate and diluent, respectively, should always be done whenever a patient undergoes skin testing. For puncture tests, a histamine solution of 1 to 10 mg/ml in 50% glycerine is used, whereas for intradermal tests, a histamine solution of 0.01 to 0.15 mg/ml is sufficient. Concomitant ingestion of medications such as antihistamines, hydroxyzine, or tricyclic antidepressants by the patient suppresses skin test reactivity,[10] which is evident by the diminished skin test response to the histamine control test. Some individuals exhibit dermographism or react nonspecifically to the minor skin trauma associated with testing; the negative control test may aid in identifying such patients.

INTERPRETATION

It must be appreciated that a positive test reaction can be produced in any person, allergic or nonallergic, if the test materials are sufficiently concentrated. Such irritant reactions are not usually a problem with extracts in common use, in which any high incidence of positive reactions soon alerts the practitioner to their occurrence, but are more likely to occur with less commonly used materials.

Positive skin test reactions may not always indicate current clinical sensitivity to the allergen being tested. Middle-aged adults with a history of autumn hay fever during childhood frequently continue to exhibit positive skin tests to weed pollens despite having outgrown their rhinitis. Conversely, a positive skin test may be a harbinger of future sensitivity. In a study of more than 600 college students, Hagy and Settipane found that clinically asymptomatic freshmen with positive pollen skin tests were 10 times more likely to develop clinical hay fever by their senior year than were asymptomatic freshmen whose initial skin tests were negative.[18]

OTHER IN VIVO TESTS

Passive transfer (P-K) skin testing involves the sensitization of skin sites in a nonallergic recipient by aseptically injecting serum from a sensitized donor.[50] After 48 hours, both the passively sensitized areas and nonsensitized sites are challenged with various test allergens. This procedure is time consuming, is not as sensitive as direct skin testing, and carries the risk of transfer of hepatitis or human immunodeficiency viruses. For these reasons, the P-K test is rarely used.

Mucosal challenge tests, in which allergenic extracts are applied to the conjunctival sac or nasal mucosa, may also serve as diagnostic procedures. Compared with direct skin testing, however, these mucosal tests are time consuming and imprecise, and they are considered research procedures for the most part. A monograph provides a comprehensive review of these procedures.[58]

TOTAL IgE LEVELS

METHODS

Total serum IgE levels are measured by immunoassay; immunodiffusion techniques are not sufficiently sensitive to detect IgE in normal sera. A polyclonal or monoclonal anti-IgE antibody coupled covalently to a solid phase is incubated with standard or test sera, after which the bound IgE is detected by addition of a radiolabeled or enzyme-labeled polyclonal or monoclonal second antibody to human IgE. The concentration of IgE in serum is calculated by comparison with a standard curve. IgE concentrations are reported in international units (IU) per milliliter, kU per liter, or μg per liter; 1 IU equals 2.4 ng.[2]

NORMAL VALUES

Several studies have been reported on serum IgE concentrations in healthy subjects.[15, 25, 27, 45] Different analytic techniques have yielded somewhat different results in adults and children. Data from one study of older children and adults are shown in Table 19–2. The frequency distribution of IgE concentrations in adults is skewed, with wide 95th percentile limits and a disproportionate number of low IgE values. Accordingly, when calculating the 95th percentile limits,

TABLE 19–2
TOTAL SERUM IgE LEVELS IN SKIN TEST NEGATIVE OLDER CHILDREN AND ADULTS

Age (years)	No.	Sex	Geometric Mean (IU/ml)	Geometric Mean ± 2 SD (IU/ml)
6–14	69	M	40.9	2.0—824.1
	71	F	40.7	3.4—452.9
15–34	213	M	23.3	0.9—635.3
	201	F	16.5	0.8—349.1
35–54	145	M	20.4	0.9—443.6
	154	F	14.6	0.7—286.4
55–74	224	M	19.8	0.8—484.2
	348	F	10.7	0.6—198.6
75+	61	M	17.8	0.8—387.3
	83	F	8.9	0.4—208.9

From Klink M, Cline MG, Halonen M, et al: Problems in defining normal limits for serum IgE. J Allergy Clin Immunol 85:440, 1990.

most investigators have treated their data by logarithmic transformation, thus yielding upper limits of normal that are seemingly high when compared with the arithmetic mean. These high upper limits of normal serve to diminish the diagnostic sensitivity of the serum IgE level as a test for clinical allergy.

Serum IgE concentrations in infants and younger children are shown in Table 19–3. Although the human fetus can synthesize IgE as early as the 11th week of gestation,[38] cord serum contains very little IgE protein. The concentrations of IgE in maternal sera and in cord sera are not correlated,[24, 37] indicating that there is no appreciable placental transfer of maternal IgE. Moreover, the finding of specific IgE antibodies to cow's milk in cord sera but not in maternal sera indicates that intrauterine sensitization probably does occur and supports the conclusion that the IgE protein detected in cord serum is of fetal origin.[37]

FACTORS INFLUENCING IgE LEVELS

In addition to age-related factors, serum IgE levels are influenced by a variety of genetic, racial, and seasonal factors. Early data from studies of monozygous and dizygous twins by Bazaral and colleagues suggested that levels of serum IgE were in large part genetically determined, as the IgE levels were much more closely correlated in monozygous than in dizygous twin pairs.[3] Moreover, estimates of heritability were higher for child twins (79%) than for adult twins (59%).[3] Marsh and Bias originally postulated the existence of a single major regulator gene locus for basal serum IgE level.[32] They assumed that inheritance of low IgE phenotype (R) was dominant over the high IgE phenotype (r). When this hypothesis was tested in studies involving 30 families with 118 offspring, the observed and expected numbers of offspring with high IgE levels (rr) were very close to one another. These findings were subsequently confirmed by Gerrard and colleagues in a larger study of 173 families.[13]

In a study involving 170 individuals from 11 Amish families, Marsh and colleagues obtained evidence for linkage of five markers in chromosome 5q31.1, especially the IL-4 gene, with a gene-controlling total serum IgE concentration.[34] No linkage was found between these markers and specific IgE antibody concentrations, suggesting that IL-4 or a nearby gene in 5q31.1 regulates IgE production in a nonantigen-specific fashion.

Racial factors also influence serum IgE levels. Orgel and colleagues studied 27 Filipino and 24 Caucasian children born and raised in the United States.[47] In the Filipino children, both the incidence of atopic disease (48% versus 25%) and the geometric mean IgE level (227 IU/ml versus 69 IU/ml) were significantly higher than in the Caucasian group. These data suggest that races that have evolved in tropical and subtropical regions where parasitic diseases are prevalent tend to have a higher genetic capacity to produce IgE, and this is perhaps associated with an enhanced capacity to resist parasitic infestation. When parasitic disease is reduced or eliminated, an inherited capacity to synthesize IgE may result in a high incidence of atopy. Other investigators have reported higher serum IgE levels among blacks[66] and South American Indians.[23]

Patients with seasonal allergic rhinitis due to spring or summer pollens[4] or ragweed pollen[68] have shown seasonal changes in serum IgE levels. Peak levels are usually reached about 4 to 6 weeks after the peak pollination period.

TABLE 19–3
SERUM IgE LEVELS IN INFANTS AND YOUNGER CHILDREN

Age	No.	Geometric Mean (ng/ml)	95th Percentile Limits (ng/ml)
Cord blood	24	0.53	0.1–3.1
6 Weeks	17	1.67	0.2–15
3 Months	15	1.98	0.4–9.1
6 Months	15	6.49	1.0–39
9 Months	16	5.71	1.8–18
1 Year	12	8.45	1.9–37
2 Years	18	7.33	0.8–71
3 Years	6	4.36	0.5–41
4 Years	7	20.8	2.6–167
7 Years	18	31.2	2.5–390

From Kjellman N-IM, Johansson SGO, Roth A: Serum IgE levels in healthy children quantified by a sandwich technique (PRIST). Clin Allergy 6:51, 1976.

INTERPRETATION

Although total serum IgE levels are elevated in most individuals with allergic (IgE mediated) disease, this is not the case with all patients. In a study of adults attending an allergy clinic, Henderson and colleagues found elevations of serum IgE in only 30 of 48 patients with IgE-mediated rhinitis (62%) and only 23 of 30 patients with IgE-mediated asthma (76%).[19] Marsh and colleagues measured total serum IgE levels in a primarily Caucasian population that had been characterized with respect to presence or absence of allergic disease.[33] Although maximum discrimination between the allergic and nonallergic groups was seen at an IgE level of 100 IU/ml, approximately 20% of each of the two populations had total IgE levels atypical of their allergy phenotype.

Many nonallergic diseases may be associated with elevations in serum IgE (Table 19–4), including parasitic, infectious, immunologic, neoplastic, or cutaneous diseases. The elevations measured have ranged from moderate (500–2,000 IU/ml), in the case of certain viral infections, to extreme

TABLE 19–4
NONALLERGIC DISEASES ASSOCIATED WITH ELEVATED SERUM IgE LEVELS

Parasitic Diseases
- Ascariasis
- Capillariasis
- Echinococcosis
- Fascioliasis
- Filariasis
- Hookworm
- Onchocerciasis
- Paragonimiasis
- Schistosomiasis
- Strongyloidiasis
- Trichinosis
- Visceral larval migrans

Infections
- Allergic bronchopulmonary aspergillosis
- Cytomegalovirus mononucleosis
- Epstein-Barr virus
- Leprosy
- Respiratory syncytial virus bronchiolitis
- Systemic candidiasis

Others
- Burns
- Cystic fibrosis
- Drug-induced interstitial nephritis
- Guillain-Barré syndrome
- Infantile polyarteritis nodosa
- Kawasaki syndrome
- Nephrotic syndrome
- Primary pulmonary hemosiderosis
- Rheumatoid arthritis

Immunologic Diseases
- Acquired immunodeficiency syndrome
- Graft-versus-host disease
- Job-Buckley syndrome
- Malignant lymphogranulomatosis
- Nezelof syndrome
- Selective IgA deficiency
- Thymic alymphoplasia
- Wiskott-Aldrich syndrome

Neoplastic Diseases
- Bronchial carcinoma
- Hodgkin's disease
- IgE myeloma
- Post–bone marrow transplantation

Cutaneous Diseases
- Bullous pemphigoid
- Chronic acral dermatitis
- Streptococcal erythema nodosum
- Other dermatoses

Modified from Yunginger JW: Clinical significance of IgE. In Middleton E Jr, Reed CE, Ellis EF, et al (eds): Allergy Principles and Practice, 3rd edition. Vol II. CV Mosby Co, St Louis, 1988, p 854.

(>50,000 IU/ml), as seen in some cases of atopic dermatitis, parasitic infestation, or hyper-IgE syndrome.

Low levels of serum IgE are frequently seen in immunodeficiency diseases such as hypogammaglobulinemia[35] or ataxia telangiectasia.[6] However, otherwise healthy individuals may have an isolated serum IgE deficiency.[28]

INDICATIONS

Although some authorities advocate quantitation of serum IgE as a routine test for all persons suspected of having allergic disease,[22] the nonspecificity of the test has limited its usefulness. As noted previously, a substantial proportion of individuals with well-documented allergic rhinitis or IgE-mediated asthma have normal serum IgE levels. A conservative listing of indications for quantitation of serum IgE is shown in Table 19–5.

TABLE 19–5
CLINICAL INDICATIONS FOR SERUM IgE QUANTITATION

1. To predict the development of allergic disease in infants
2. To evaluate immunodeficient patients
3. To screen for infestation with tissue-invading parasites
4. To aid in diagnosis and follow-up of patients with allergic bronchopulmonary aspergillosis

In a prospective study involving 34 infants, Orgel and colleagues measured sequential serum IgE levels during the first year of life.[46] In 12 infants whose serum IgE rose significantly (to >20 IU/ml), nearly all were classified as definitely or possibly atopic on clinical grounds by 12 months of age (Fig. 19–1). A few were evident by as early as 5 to 6 months. The rise in serum IgE frequently preceded the clinical manifestations of atopic disease. Similar findings were observed in subsequent studies of Scandinavian[24] and French[37] infants and children.

Serum IgE levels may be useful for evaluating immunodeficient persons. Low IgE levels are usually seen in congenital or acquired hypogammaglobulinemia and in ataxia telangiectasia, whereas elevated levels are seen in the Wiskott-Aldrich[63] and Job-Buckley[9] syndromes.

Parasitic diseases are likely to produce elevations in serum IgE levels only when body tissues are invaded by the parasite. Infestations that are confined to the gastrointestinal tract of the host (e.g., pinworms) do not usually produce elevations in serum IgE.

Measurement of serum IgE provides useful information in patients with allergic bronchopulmonary aspergillosis at the time of diagnosis and for follow-up. A rise in serum IgE may herald a relapse in these individuals.[64]

ALLERGEN-SPECIFIC IgE ANTIBODY LEVELS

In contrast to the nonspecificity of total serum IgE measurements, procedures that identify allergen-specific IgE anti-

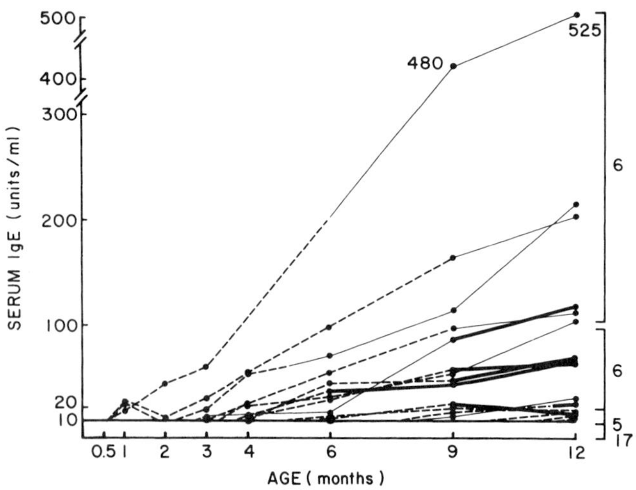

FIGURE 19–1. Serum IgE levels of 34 infants from 2 weeks to 1 year of age. Seventeen babies had a serum IgE that remained under 10 IU/ml throughout their first year, whereas five others were 10–20 IU/ml and 12 exceeded 20 IU/ml. Heavy line = definite atopy; lighter line = possible atopy; dashed line = normal. (From Orgel HA, Hamburger RN, Bazaral M, et al: Development of IgE and allergy in infancy. J Allergy Clin Immunol 56:296, 1975.)

bodies are of greater benefit to the clinician. The most widely used of these are solid-phase immunoassays.

METHODS

Solid-phase immunoassays are multistage assays analogous in principle to the indirect Coombs test. Sera to be tested for specific IgE antibodies are reacted with allergen coupled to a solid-phase support material. After an initial incubation, nonantibody serum components are washed away. During the second stage, the allergen solid-phase conjugate is incubated with radiolabeled[65] or enzyme-labeled[56] affinity chromatography-purified polyclonal (or monoclonal) antibody to human IgE. In the case of radiolabeled anti-IgE, the allergen solid-phase conjugate is washed again and counted in a gamma spectrometer. In the case of enzyme-labeled anti-IgE, the allergen solid-phase conjugate is washed again and incubated with a chromogenic substrate for the enzyme, after which the intensity of the color produced is measured in a spectrophotometer or colorimeter. Enzyme immunoassays permit avoidance of handling, storage, and disposal of radioactive waste.

Immunochemiluminometric assays for allergen-specific IgE antibodies use antihuman IgE antibodies labeled with horseradish peroxidase[8] or with acridinium ester[26] in the second stage of the assay. After incubation and washing steps, the light reactions of the samples are detected in a chemiluminometer by addition of enzyme substrate and hydrogen peroxide and determination of photoemissions.

As originally described,[65] specific IgE antibody assays employed allergens coupled covalently to Sephadex beads. A variety of other particulates have been used, including microcrystalline cellulose particles, agarose beads, or polyacrylamide beads. Other assay systems use allergens coupled to filter paper disks or cellulose caps or allergens adsorbed onto the wells of plastic microtiter plates, plastic cylinders, or paramagnetic particles. The use of these solid-phase carriers avoids the need for centrifugation, which is required for the particulate assays. Ideally, any solid-phase allergen reagent should contain all the allergenic constituents in the fluid allergenic extract, preferably in the same proportions found in the original allergenic extract. However, most published studies have not shown that all relevant protein allergens have been coupled in different allergen systems.

For screening purposes, solid-phase reagents have been developed that contain mixtures of several common inhalant allergens[36, 48] or mixtures of inhalant and food allergens.[62] Results of these screening assays are usually scored as positive or negative; positive sera are retested using single allergen immunoassays.

In another type of immunoassay for specific IgE antibodies, fluid-phase allergens are attached by means of their NH_2, OH, COOH, or SH groups to a soluble polymer matrix labeled with biotin.[61] A tube also coated with biotin serves as the reaction vessel for the initial reaction between IgE in the test serum and the fluid-phase allergen-biotin–labeled matrix. After a short incubation, avidin is added to link the allergen-biotin–labeled matrix/IgE complex to the biotin-coated tube. The second stage of the assay proceeds as described for the solid-phase immunoassays.

SCORING

The actual concentrations of IgE antibodies may not be reported in mass units. In sera from many allergic individuals, the concentrations of IgE antibodies exceed the binding capacity of the allergen solid-phase conjugates, and the first-stage incubation supernatants contain residual quantities of specific IgE antibodies.[17] Thus the final binding reflects both the quantity and the affinity of the antibodies present. Nevertheless, over a limited range of concentrations, the radioactive counts bound or the color produced does increase in a linear fashion with the concentration of IgE antibodies. This relationship has been exploited to measure specific IgE antibodies quantitatively by reference to a calibrated dose-response curve.[16, 55, 70]

Assay results for IgE antibodies are reported in a variety of ways by different laboratories. One method uses a scoring system with semiquantitative grading (grade 0 to 4) by comparison with a reference dose-response curve. Other laboratories report results in terms of the absolute number of radioactive counts bound to the allergen conjugate, or the percentage of total radioactive counts bound, or as a ratio of the binding produced by a test serum divided by the binding produced by a serum pool from nonatopic individuals.

A modified RAST and scoring system have been advocated by some individuals to increase the sensitivity of the IgE antibody assay.[39] In this assay, the radioactive binding produced by the binding of IgE antibodies to allergen disks is compared with the radioactive binding of a standard serum containing 25 IU IgE/ml to an anti-IgE disk. Results are expressed in semiquantitative terms (class 0–6). However, the cutoff point for positivity in the modified RAST assay may be set too low, because positive results have been obtained with non–IgE-containing fluids (e.g., 5% human serum albumin) in as many as 30% of assays, depending on the allergen system being tested.[54]

FACTORS INFLUENCING IgE ANTIBODY LEVELS

Many technical factors influence IgE antibody levels. One of the most important is the cutoff point used to differentiate positive and negative results, as previously discussed. Another important technical factor is the variability of the test itself. Depending on the allergen being tested and the method of scoring results, the intra-assay coefficient of variation may range from 7% to 30%.[11] In the face of such variability, the assay should be performed in replicate. Likewise, the interassay coefficient of variation is sufficiently great that if one wishes to examine longitudinal changes in IgE antibody in a given patient, the sequential serum specimens should be tested together in the same assay.

In some assay systems, sera with markedly elevated levels of IgE protein yield weakly positive results with every allergen conjugate, presumably owing to increased nonspecific binding of IgE.[20] This phenomenon is not usually seen unless the IgE concentration exceeds 1,000 IU/ml, which may often occur in patients with atopic dermatitis and multiple allergic diseases. The specificity or nonspecificity of IgE antibody results can be tested by attempting to inhibit binding to the allergen solid-phase conjugate with addition of free allergen in the first stage of the assay. If addition of free allergen does not reduce radioactive binding or color development, the IgE antibody results should be considered falsely positive.

Inhibition of binding of IgE antibodies occurs in some analytic systems as a result of competition for allergen binding sites by specific IgG antibodies.[71] These IgG antibodies may be present in microgram per milliliter quantities in patients who have undergone high-dose immunotherapy. This interference can be eliminated by increasing the relative quantity of solid-phase allergen.

Some nontechnical factors influencing allergen-specific IgE antibody levels include age and allergen exposure. IgE antibody levels are generally highest in school-age children and young adults; lower values are usually seen in adults over age 50. IgE antibody levels also vary seasonally in patients with pollen allergies, reaching a zenith about 4 weeks after the pollen season and a nadir just prior to the onset of the next pollen season.[67] Likewise, IgE antibodies to insect venoms are elevated in many individuals after an uneventful sting, but in the absence of future stings, the antibody levels usually decrease to normal or background levels after several weeks or months.[72]

CORRELATIONS BETWEEN IgE ANTIBODY LEVELS AND IN VIVO PROVOCATION TESTS

In patients with allergic respiratory disease, there is usually a good correlation between results of IgE antibody tests and results of inhalation provocation tests.[5, 65] The best agreement has been noted in patients with moderate to severe disease. Very few false-positive IgE antibody results are noted in patients with negative provocation tests. The correlation between skin test results and IgE antibody results has been better with pollen allergens or purified allergens than with mold or dander allergens.

In patients with food allergy, the results of IgE antibody assays are most specific in cases of anaphylactic sensitivity to foods such as fish, legumes, or nuts.[14] Unlike the situation with pollen allergies, elevated IgE antibodies to foods are frequently seen in patients who have negative feeding challenges to the same foods.[53] Skin tests may be useful when selecting foods for challenge feedings, however.[7]

In patients with suspected insect sting allergy, skin testing with insect venom is a more sensitive procedure than measurement of venom-specific IgE antibodies.[57] However, neither procedure is particularly specific, as up to 75% of untreated individuals with histories of sting anaphylaxis and either positive skin tests or elevated IgE antibodies do not react to deliberate insect sting challenges.[21, 49, 60]

INDICATIONS

Measurements of IgE antibody are appropriate whenever skin testing is judged to be impossible, inappropriate, or dangerous. Examples of the former include the unavailability of appropriate skin test materials (e.g., a patient with anaphylactic sensitivity to some exotic food), the inability of a patient to discontinue such medications as antihistamines or hydroxyzine, or the patient with widespread dermatitis or dermographism. A possible example of inappropriate skin testing is that of an infant or toddler who requires testing with multiple allergens. In such a case, obtaining a venipuncture may be less traumatic and time consuming than placing multiple skin tests. Skin testing may be dangerous in a person with a history of extreme sensitivity to a food, such as fish or nuts. In vitro measurement of IgE antibodies may be preferred in such an individual.

ACKNOWLEDGMENTS

This work was supported by the Mayo Foundation. The secretarial assistance of Marian Bortolon is greatly appreciated.

REFERENCES

1. American Academy of Allergy and Immunology Executive Committee: Personnel and equipment to treat systemic reactions caused by immunotherapy with allergenic extracts. J Allergy Clin Immunol 77:271, 1986.
2. Bazaral M, Hamburger RN: Standardization and stability of immunoglobulin E (IgE). J Allergy Clin Immunol 49:189, 1972.
3. Bazaral M, Orgel HA, Hamburger RN: Genetics of IgE and allergy: serum IgE levels in twins. J Allergy Clin Immunol 54:288, 1974.
4. Berg T, Johansson SGO: IgE concentrations in children with atopic diseases: a clinical study. Int Arch Allergy Appl Immunol 36:219, 1969.
5. Berg TLO, Johansson SGO: Allergy diagnosis with the radioallergosorbent test: a comparison with the results of skin and provocation tests in an unselected group of children with asthma and hay fever. J Allergy Clin Immunol 54:209, 1974.
6. Biggar D, Lapointe N, Ishizaka K, et al: IgE in ataxia-telangiectasia and family members. Lancet 2:1089, 1970.
7. Bock SA: Food sensitivity: a critical review and practical approach. Am J Dis Child 134:973, 1980.
8. Brown CR, Higgins KW, Frazer K, et al: Simultaneous determination of total IgE and allergen-specific IgE in serum by the MAST chemiluminescent assay system. Clin Chem 31:1500, 1985.
9. Buckley RH, Wray BB, Belmaker EZ: Extreme hyperimmunoglobulinemia E and undue susceptibility to infection. Pediatrics 49:59, 1972.
10. Cook TJ, MacQueen DM, Wittig HJ, et al: Degree and duration of skin test suppression and side effects with antihistamines. J Allergy Clin Immunol 51:71, 1973.
11. Evans R III: Variability in the measurement of specific immunoglobulin E antibody by the RAST procedure. J Allergy Clin Immunol 69:245, 1982.
12. Ford A, Seagroatt V, Platts-Mills TAE, et al: A collaborative study on the first international standard of *Dermatophagoides pteronyssinus* (house dust mite) extract. J Allergy Clin Immunol 75:676, 1985.
13. Gerrard JW, Rao DC, Morton NE: A genetic study of immunoglobulin E. Am J Hum Genet 30:46, 1978.
14. Gillespie DN, Nakajima S, Gleich GJ: Detection of allergy to nuts by the radioallergosorbent test. J Allergy Clin Immunol 57:302, 1976.
15. Gleich GJ, Averbeck AK, Swedlund HA: Measurement of IgE in normal and allergic serum by radioimmunoassay. J Lab Clin Med 77:690, 1971.
16. Gleich GJ, Jacob GL, Yunginger JW, et al: Measurement of the absolute levels of IgE antibodies in patients with ragweed hay fever. J Allergy Clin Immunol 60:188, 1977.
17. Gleich GJ, Jones RT: Measurement of IgE antibodies by the radioallergosorbent test. II. Analyses of quantitative relationships in the test. J Allergy Clin Immunol 55:346, 1976.
18. Hagy GW, Settipane GA: Prognosis of positive allergy skin tests in an asymptomatic population: a three year follow-up of college students. J Allergy Clin Immunol 48:200, 1971.
19. Henderson LL, Swedlund HA, Van Dellen RG, et al: Evaluation of IgE tests in an allergy practice. J Allergy Clin Immunol 48:361, 1971.
20. Hoffman DR: Comparison of methods of performing the radioallergosorbent test: Phadebas, Fadal-Nalebuff and Hoffman protocols. Ann Allergy 45:343, 1980.
21. Hunt KJ, Valentine MD, Sobotka AK, et al: A controlled trial of immunotherapy in insect hypersensitivity. N Engl J Med 299:157, 1978.

22. Johansson SGO, Bennich HH: The clinical impact of the discovery of IgE. Ann Allergy 48:325, 1982.
23. Kaplan JE, Larrick JW, Yost JA: Hyperimmunoglobulinemia E in the Waorani, an isolated Amerindian population. Am J Trop Med Hyg 29:1012, 1980.
24. Kjellman N-IM: Predictive value of high IgE levels in children. Acta Paediatr Scand 65:465, 1976.
25. Kjellman N-IM, Johansson SGO, Roth A: Serum IgE levels in healthy children quantified by a sandwich technique (PRIST). Clin Allergy 6:51, 1976.
26. Kleine-Tebbe J, Eickholt M, Gätjen M, et al: Comparison between MAGIC LITE®- and CAP®-system: two automated specific IgE antibody assays. Clin Exp Allergy 22:475, 1992.
27. Klink M, Cline MG, Halonen M, et al: Problems in defining normal limits for serum IgE. J Allergy Clin Immunol 85:440, 1990.
28. Levy DA, Chen J: Healthy IgE-deficient person. N Engl J Med 283:541, 1970.
29. Lind P: Standardization of mite extracts: qualitative and quantitative investigations of three kinds of preparations with CRIE and RAST. Allergy 35:227, 1980.
30. Lindblad JH, Farr RS: The incidence of positive intradermal reactions and the demonstration of skin sensitizing antibody to extracts of ragweed and dust in humans without history of rhinitis or asthma. J Allergy 32:392, 1961.
31. Lockey RF, Benedict LM, Turkeltaub PC, et al: Fatalities from immunotherapy (IT) and skin testing (ST). J Allergy Clin Immunol 79:660, 1987.
32. Marsh DG, Bias WB: The genetics of atopic allergy. In Samter M (ed): Immunological Diseases, 3rd edition. Vol II. Little Brown, Boston, 1978, p 819.
33. Marsh DG, Bias WB, Ishizaka K: Genetic control of basal serum immunoglobulin E level and its effect on specific reaginic sensitivity. Proc Natl Acad Sci USA 71:3588, 1974.
34. Marsh DG, Neely JD, Breazeale DR, et al: Linkage analysis of IL4 and other chromosome 5q31.1 markers and total serum immunoglobulin E concentrations. Science 264:1152, 1994.
35. McLaughlan P, Stanworth DR, Webster ADB, et al: Serum IgE in immune deficiency disorders. Clin Exp Immunol 16:375, 1974.
36. Merrett J, Merrett TG: Phadiatop—a novel IgE antibody screening test. Clin Allergy 17:409, 1987.
37. Michel FB, Bousquet J, Greillier P, et al: Comparison of cord blood immunoglobulin E concentrations and maternal allergy for the prediction of atopic diseases in infancy. J Allergy Clin Immunol 65:422, 1980.
38. Miller DL, Hirvonen T, Gitlin D: Synthesis of IgE by the human conceptus. J Allergy Clin Immunol 52:182, 1973.
39. Nalebuff DJ, Fadal RG, Ali M: IgE in investigation and management of atopic disorders: recent advances. J Cont Educ ORL Allergy 40:47, 1978.
40. Nelson HS: The effect of preservatives and dilution on the deterioration of Russian thistle (Salsola pestifer): a pollen extract. J Allergy Clin Immunol 63:417, 1979.
41. Nelson HS, Rosloniec DM, McCall LI, et al: Comparative performance of five commercial prick skin test devices. J Allergy Clin Immunol 92:750, 1993.
42. Nightengale SN: Alert on changes in standardized cat allergen extract products. JAMA 268:2491, 1992.
43. Norman PS, Marsh DG: Human serum albumin and Tween 80 as stabilizers of allergen solutions. J Allergy Clin Immunol 62:314, 1978.
44. Norman PS: Skin testing. In Rose NR, Conway de Macario E, Fahey JL, et al (eds): Manual of Clinical Laboratory Immunology, 4th edition. American Society for Microbiology, Washington, DC, 1992, p 685.
45. Nye L, Merrett TG, Landon J, et al: A detailed investigation of circulating IgE levels in a normal population. Clin Allergy 5:13, 1975.
46. Orgel HA, Hamburger RN, Bazaral M, et al: Development of IgE and allergy in infancy. J Allergy Clin Immunol 56:296, 1975.
47. Orgel HA, Lenoir MA, Bazaral M: Serum IgG, IgA, IgM, and IgE levels and allergy in Filipino children in the United States. J Allergy Clin Immunol 53:213, 1974.
48. Ownby DR, Anderson JA, Jacobs GL, et al: Development and comparative evaluation of a multi-antigen RAST as a screening test for inhalant allergy. J Allergy Clin Immunol 73:466, 1984.
49. Parker JL, Santrach PJ, Dahlberg MJE, et al: Evaluation of Hymenoptera-sting sensitivity with deliberate sting challenges: inadequacy of present diagnostic methods. J Allergy Clin Immunol 69:200, 1982.
50. Prausnitz C, Kustner H: Studiem uber ueberempfindlichkeit. Zentralbl Bakteriol 86:160, 1921.
51. Prince HE: Molds and bacteria in the etiology of respiratory allergic diseases. XXI. Studies with mold extracts produced from cultures grown in modified synthetic media: a preliminary report. Ann Allergy 19:259, 1961.
52. Reid MJ, Lockey RF, Turkeltaub PC, et al: Survey of fatalities from skin testing and immunotherapy 1985–1989. J Allergy Clin Immunol 92:6, 1993.
53. Sampson HA: Eczema and food hypersensitivity. In Metcalfe DD, Sampson HA, Simon RA (eds): Food Allergy: Adverse Reactions to Foods and Food Additives. Blackwell Scientific Publications, Cambridge, MA, 1991, p 113.
54. Santrach PJ, Parker JL, Jones RT, et al: Diagnostic and therapeutic applications of a modified radioallergosorbent test and comparison with the conventional radioallergosorbent test. J Allergy Clin Immunol 67:97, 1981.
55. Schellenberg RR, Adkinson NF Jr: Measurement of absolute amounts of antigen-specific human IgE by a radioallergosorbent test (RAST) elution technique. J Immunol 115:1577, 1975.
56. Schroder H, Kober A, Yman L: New developments in specific IgE antibody measurement—phadezym RAST. Correlation between RIA and EIA (phadebas RAST). Allergol Immunopathol (Madr) 9(suppl):46, 1981.
57. Sobotka AK, Adkinson NF Jr, Valentine MD, et al: Allergy to insect stings. IV. Diagnosis by radioallergosorbent test (RAST). J Immunol 121:2477, 1978.
58. Spector SL (ed): Provocation Testing in Clinical Practice. Marcel Dekker, Inc, New York, 1995.
59. Turkeltaub PC, Rastogi SC, Baer H, et al: A standardized quantitative skin-test assay of allergen potency and stability; studies of the allergen dose-response curve and effect of wheal, erythema, and patient selection on assay results. J Allergy Clin Immunol 70:343, 1982.
60. van der Linden PW, Hack CE, Struyvenberg A, et al: Insect-sting challenge in 324 subjects with a previous anaphylactic reaction: current criteria for insect-venom hypersensitivity do not predict the occurrence and the severity of anaphylaxis. J Allergy Clin Immunol 94:151, 1994.
61. van Houte AJ, Bartels PCM: Comparative evaluation of the Pharmacia CAP system and the DPC AlaSTAT system for in vitro detection of allergen-specific IgE with the skin prick test. Eur J Clin Chem Clin Biochem 30:101, 1992.
62. van Toorenenbergen AW, Oranje AP, Vermeulen AM, et al: IgE antibody screening in children. Evaluation of the Phadiatop Paediatric. Allergy 46:180, 1991.
63. Waldmann TA, Polmar SH, Balestra ST, et al: Immunoglobulin E in immunologic deficiency diseases. II. Serum IgE concentration of patients with acquired hypogammaglobulinemia, thymoma and hypogammaglobulinemia, myotonic dystrophy, intestinal lymphangiectasia, and Wiskott-Aldrich syndrome. J Immunol 109:304, 1972.
64. Wang JLF, Patterson R, Roberts M, et al: The management of allergic bronchopulmonary aspergillosis. Am Rev Respir Dis 120:87, 1979.
65. Wide L, Bennich H, Johansson SGO: Diagnosis of allergy by an in-vitro test for allergen antibodies. Lancet 2:1105, 1967.
66. Wittig HJ, Belloit J, DeFillippi I, et al: Age-related serum immunoglobulin E levels in healthy subjects and in patients with allergic disease. J Allergy Clin Immunol 66:305, 1980.
67. Yunginger JW, Gleich GJ: Seasonal changes in IgE antibodies and their relationship to IgG antibodies during immunotherapy for ragweed hay fever. J Clin Invest 52:1268, 1973.
68. Yunginger JW, Gleich GJ: Seasonal changes in serum and nasal IgE concentrations. J Allergy Clin Immunol 51:174, 1973.
69. Yunginger JW: Standardization of allergenic extracts. Ann Allergy 66:107, 1991.
70. Zeiss CR, Pruzansky JJ, Patterson R, et al: A solid phase radioimmunoassay for the quantitation of human reaginic antibody against ragweed antigen E. J Immunol 110:414, 1973.
71. Zimmermann EM, Yunginger JW, Gleich GJ: Interference in ragweed pollen and honeybee venom radioallergosorbent tests. J Allergy Clin Immunol 66:386, 1980.
72. Zora JA, Swanson MC, Yunginger JW: A study of the prevalence and clinical significance of venom-specific IgE. J Allergy Clin Immunol 81:77, 1988.

20 Respiratory Physiology in Asthma: PULMONARY FUNCTION TESTING, BRONCHOPROVOCATION, AND MUCOCILIARY CLEARANCE

GERALD C. SMALDONE

In terms of pulmonary mechanics, asthma can be viewed primarily as a disorder of airways with reduced air flow due to reversible increases in airway resistance. The cellular diathesis in asthma is complex and only partially understood. Airway function is affected in terms of smooth muscle constriction as well as infiltration by inflammatory cells and secretion of mucus. Clinically, patients complain of air flow limitation (shortness of breath) and airway hyperreactivity (cough, sensitivity to cold air, sensitivity to inhaled particulates). In addition to the history and physical examination, objective assessment of airway function is an important part of the diagnostic evaluation and measure of response to various forms of therapy.

Abnormalities in airway resistance are not specific to asthma. In addition, other factors besides bronchial smooth muscle and airway secretions can affect airway function. The purpose of this chapter is to review the basic principles of lung and chest wall mechanics leading to a physiologic definition of asthma. The fundamentals of this model are developed from generally accepted sources in the literature and provide a basis for a rational approach to clinical diagnosis and assessment of response to therapy. Current and more controversial concepts are identified and used to illustrate trends in asthma research.

LUNG VOLUMES

When visualizing an intact thorax (a chest wall containing a lung) in a relaxed normal individual between tidal breaths, the respiratory muscles are inactive and there is no movement of gas into or out of the lung. Because the thorax is not moving, the forces acting on it must be balanced, or in equilibrium. The pleural space is virtual, and the volume of gas in the lung and chest wall is the same (Fig. 20–1A).

The forces acting within the thorax can be visualized by an experiment that upsets chest wall–lung interaction. Figure 20–1B demonstrates a pneumothorax in which air enters the pleural space (the muscles of respiration have been paralyzed). In this configuration, the lung and chest wall can independently attain their own equilibrium volumes. The lung collapses to a much smaller volume (minimal volume [MV]) at which all the elastic elements (tissue and surface forces) in the lung are no longer stretched. The chest wall behaves in the opposite manner. It expands during the pneumothorax to its equilibrium volume, which is about 1 L above the equilibrium position of the intact thorax. Therefore, the volume of the intact chest wall–lung system at end expiration is determined by the sum of two opposing forces: the outward expanding force of the chest wall and the inward recoil force of the lung. This equilibrium volume is defined as the functional residual capacity (FRC). The above summary of the factors determining FRC in the normal subject illustrates a fundamental principle in pulmonary function: volume is a result of the interaction between the chest wall and the lung.[24] FRC in the normal subject is a unique volume in that the respiratory muscles are not involved.

In order to synthesize chest wall–lung interaction, the individual behavior of these components should be studied. If the lung is removed from the thorax and the trachea attached to a piston pump, the pressure-volume characteristics of lung can be measured. Figure 20–2 demonstrates a typical relationship; the lung inflates from minimal volume at zero airway pressure smoothly to a plateau at approximately 30 cm H_2O.[30] These pressures represent the forces of elastic recoil in the lung (PEL). Pressure-volume hysteresis is not discussed in this review. The simplified curve in Figure 20–2 represents a deflation pressure-volume curve that most closely approximates the in vivo situation.[18, 29] In addition to the actual data, the pressure-volume diagram demonstrates the concept of transmural pressure. In Figure 20–2, the actual forces responsible for inflation of the lung are the intraluminal and surrounding pressures.

Because the lung is excised and the surrounding pressure is atmospheric (0 cm H_2O), physiologists frequently relate

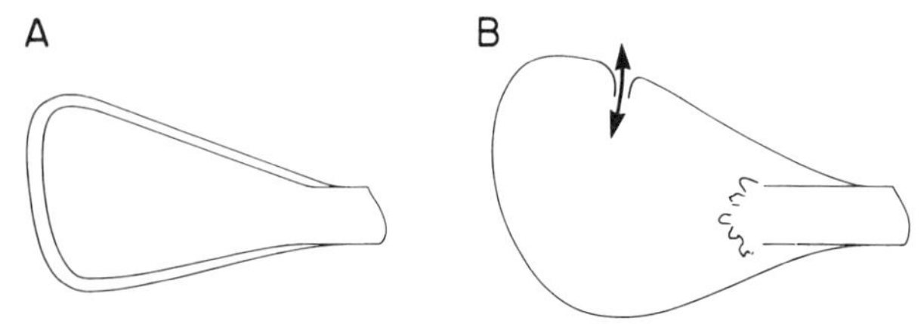

FIGURE 20–1. **(A)** Model of an intact thorax. The chest wall and lung are connected in parallel at FRC. **(B)** Pneumothorax induced by penetration through the chest wall. The lung has collapsed to minimal volume, and the chest wall is inflated to its equilibrium volume.

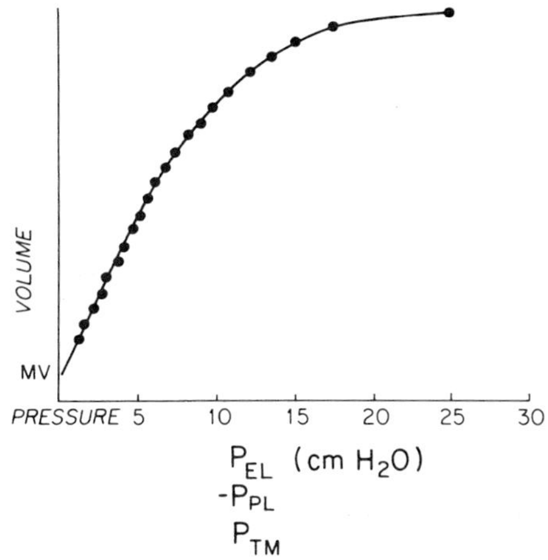

FIGURE 20–2. Pressure–volume curve of an excised human lung. Volume (on the ordinate) is related to pressure (on the abscissa).

the expansion of a distensible viscus to the changing intraluminal pressure (PEL). This does not diminish the importance of the surrounding pressure, and volume should always be related to the difference between intraluminal and surrounding pressures. By convention, transmural pressure (PTM) is defined as

$$P_{TM} = P_{intraluminal} - P_{surrounding} \quad [1]$$

From equation 1, if the piston pump was removed and the lung inflated by making the surrounding pressure negative with respect to atmospheric pressure, the curve would be unchanged if the x-axis was labeled $-P_{surrounding}$ because intraluminal pressure is now zero. In the intact thorax, $P_{surrounding}$ would be equal to the pleural pressure (PPL); in any experimental configuration, the x-axis can be labeled PTM.

In Figure 20–3, the pressure-volume curve for the lung is again represented, and the chest wall is studied. In a "thought experiment," the lungs are removed from the thorax, and the chest wall is repaired and attached to a pump via the thoracic outlet. At a PTM of zero, the isolated chest wall is at its equilibrium volume, which is considerably larger than that of the lung. A positive pressure applied to the thorax results in further expansion without a significant plateau in the pressure range shown in Figure 20–3. To reduce chest wall volume below equilibrium, the piston pump must exert progressively negative pressures, approaching a plateau at a volume somewhat above MV. If the chest wall–lung system returns to its intact state and its pressure-volume behavior is measured, the piston pump would exert pressures along a curve that represents the sum of the component pressures. The pump would not have to generate any pressure to maintain FRC, as the expansile forces of the chest wall are balanced by the retractile forces of the lung. Further expansion of the intact thorax by the pump is assisted by the tendency of the chest wall to expand until the equilibrium position of the chest wall is reached. Beyond this point, the piston must work against both the chest wall and the lung. Deflation below FRC is aided by the lung, which always tends to empty to MV, but progressively negative pressures are required owing to the contribution of the chest wall.

The pump is removed, and power is restored to the respiratory muscles. Increasing inspiratory effort results in expansion of the thorax along the thoracic pressure-volume curve until maximal effort is reached on the plateau somewhat beyond 30 cm H_2O. This volume is defined as total lung capacity (TLC). With normal muscles, TLC is determined primarily by the lung (see Fig. 20–3). Relaxation of the inspiratory muscles returns the system to equilibrium (FRC). Further expiration beyond FRC requires use of the expiratory muscles, and the system follows the thoracic curve until maximal effort, where the curve closely approximates the chest wall plateau, at residual volume (RV). Thus the limits of voluntary ventilation are determined by muscle effort and the mechanical properties of the thorax. The respirable volume between these limits is the vital capacity (VC).

AIR FLOW, EFFORT, AND VOLUME

The preceding paragraphs describe measurements made in the absence of air flow (statics); that is, the pressure-volume relationships represent the forces necessary to overcome elastic recoil. Additional pressure is needed during active breathing to overcome the resistance of the airways (dynamics). A convenient way to illustrate the air flow capability of the lung is presented in Figure 20–4. Inspiratory and expiratory flows are plotted against lung volume. By

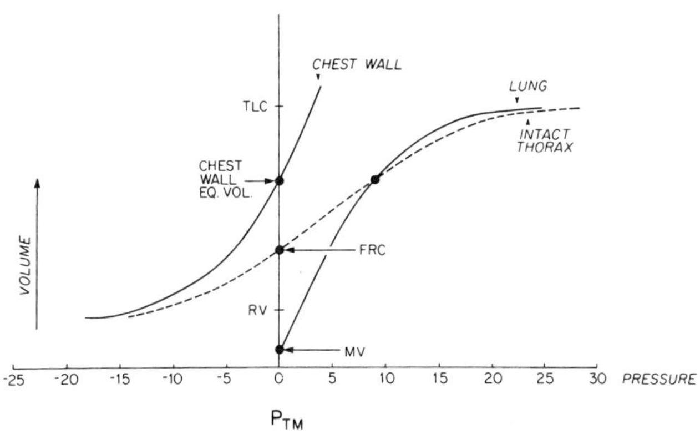

FIGURE 20–3. The pressure–volume relationship for the intact thorax and its components, the chest wall and the lung.

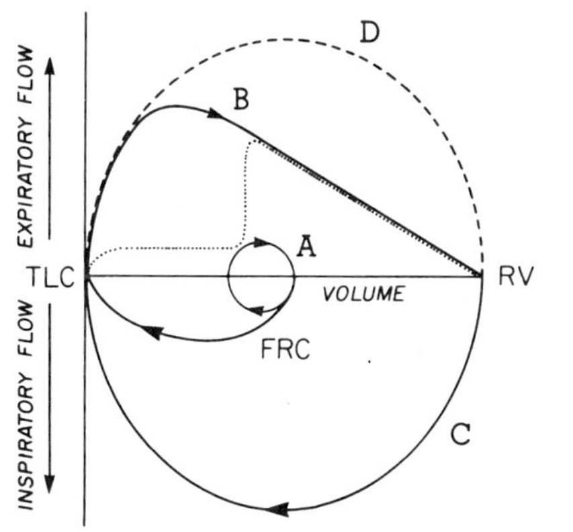

FIGURE 20–4. Maximal flow–volume curve related to the tidal loop and submaximal inspiratory and expiratory efforts.

convention, the extremes of the VC are arranged with TLC on the left and RV on the right. During quiet breathing, a normal subject begins an inhalation from FRC. A complete tidal breath describes the relatively symmetrical loop A in Figure 20–4.

Slow inspiration to TLC is indicated, followed by a maximal expiration from TLC to RV. This relationship (curve B in Fig. 20–4) defines the maximal expiratory flow volume (MEFV) curve. Similarly, a maximal inspiratory effort results in the maximal inspiratory curve C in Figure 20–4. There are important differences between inspiration and expiration. The inspiratory flows peak at mid lung volume and are very dependent on effort. The more effort, the higher the flow; maximal inspiratory flows are clearly related to maximal inspiratory effort. Expiratory flow peaks near TLC and decreases smoothly as RV is approached. In addition, maximal expiratory flows are independent of effort. For example, a slow expiration from TLC is shown in Figure 20–4 (dotted line). Near FRC, the subject increases effort; flow increases to curve B, but no further. If conditions within the lung during expiration were identical to those during inspiration, the expiratory muscles should raise expiratory flows beyond curve D (the mirror image of C), as the expiratory muscles are stronger than those of inspiration. In fact, at levels of effort far below maximal, expiratory flows cannot be increased. In summary, Figure 20–4 demonstrates that after exceeding a threshold of minimal effort, maximal expiratory flow is essentially a function of lung volume.[11]

The factors that govern maximum expiratory flow ($\dot{V}max$) are illustrated in Figure 20–5. Flow in any tube can be related to the pressure gradient along the tube by

$$\dot{V} = (P_1 - P_2)/R \qquad [2]$$

R, the resistance to flow, is a complex function of tube diameter and length and the type of flow, such as laminar or turbulent. In the lung, for expiratory flow, P_1 is alveolar pressure (P_{ALV}) and P_2 is pressure at the downstream end of the airway, mouth pressure (P_M). Thus equation 2 becomes

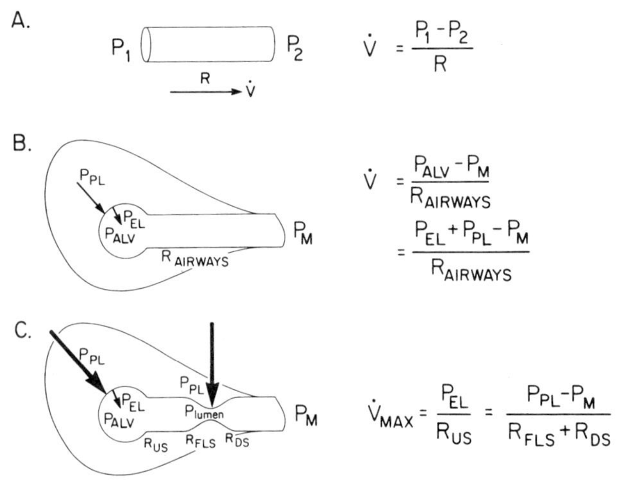

FIGURE 20–5. Models of expiratory flow. **(A)** A simple tube. **(B)** A lung at fixed volume during a submaximal expiration (pleural pressures are below threshold). **(C)** The same lung, at the same volume, during a maximal expiration (pleural pressures are high); the FLS has formed in the central airways.

$$\dot{V} = (P_{ALV} - P_M)/R_{airways} \qquad [3]$$

Because flow is a function of volume (see Fig. 20–4), our image of the lung must be frozen at constant volume during an expiration before further analysis. This has been done in Figure 20–5B. At a fixed lung volume, alveoli have been added to the tube (airways), and the chest wall has been attached. The pressure within alveoli is composed of the recoil forces in the lung (P_{EL}) and the pleural pressure (P_{PL}) that presses on alveoli during a forced expiration. The components of alveolar pressure can be included in equation 3

$$\dot{V} = (P_{EL} + P_{PL} - P_M)/R_{airways} \qquad [4]$$

The resistance term in equation 4 defines R as the resistance along the entire airway. When pleural pressure is increased by the action of the respiratory muscles, the driving pressure and flow increase, as shown in equation 4. However, pleural pressure also acts on intrathoracic airways. If P_{PL} exceeds the pressure within the lumen of the airway, the airway is compressed and its diameter decreases. There are several approaches toward analysis of this problem that are not detailed here. All analyses lead to a common result: the dynamic compression of intrathoracic airways causes a reduced airway diameter and concomitant increase in resistance.[10] Once the airways are compressed, the pleural component of the alveolar driving pressure is effectively cancelled by the same pleural pressure pressing on the airways. Therefore, the effects of added expiratory effort in raising pleural pressure are dissipated by an adjustable resistor, a flow-limiting segment (FLS) that forms at the site of dynamic compression.[30] Under these unique conditions, equation 4 can be modified to

$$\dot{V}_{MAX} = P_{EL}/R_{US} \qquad [5]$$

where R_{US} is the upstream resistance, that is, the resistance of airways between alveoli and FLS with flow in the expiratory direction, the upstream segment.[30]

This equation reflects several major changes; the absence of P_{PL} and P_M as variables, and the statement that the only pertinent resistance determining maximum flow is that of the upstream airways.[19] It is beyond the scope of this chapter to rigorously prove equation 5. Indeed, equation 5 grossly oversimplifies what is currently known about flow limitation, but for clinical purposes it is quite adequate. The elimination of P_{PL}, P_M, and part of R can be qualitatively explained by referring to Figure 20–5C. The airway can be divided into three serial sections: upstream, or peripheral, airways; the FLS; and the downstream, or central, airways. If we propose that the FLS forms when P_{PL} just exceeds P_{lumen}, as a first approximation we can equate the two pressures

$$P_{PL} \sim P_{lumen} \text{ at FLS} \qquad [6]$$

From equations 2 and 6, flow through the FLS and downstream airways (DS) can be described

$$\dot{V}_{MAX} = (P_{PL} - P_M)/(R_{FLS} + R_{DS}) \qquad [7]$$

Increasing P_{PL} with increased expiratory effort causes a matching increase in the adjustable resistance, R_{FLS}, such that V̇MAX remains constant.[30] Equations 5 and 7 are both equal to V̇MAX because the pertinent resistances are serial components of $R_{airways}$. However, only equation 5 *determines* V̇MAX because its components are independent of the FLS.[19, 26] Equation 5 illustrates the dependence of V̇MAX on lung volume, as the recoil pressure (PEL) is a strict function of volume (see Fig. 20–2). In summary, after minimal expiratory effort, expiratory flow is a function of factors intrinsic to the lung; lung recoil (PEL) and resistance of the upstream airways. With inspiration, on the other hand, the lung is free of flow-limiting segments because PPL during inspiration is always less than P_{lumen} and dynamic compression of intrathoracic airways does not occur. Thus inspiratory flow does not reflect parameters intrinsic only to the lung and intrathoracic airways but can be influenced by pleural pressure and conditions in the extrathoracic airways.

ASTHMATIC ATTACK

The normal tidal loop and MEFV curve are replotted in Figure 20–6. From a mechanical point of view, the initial event in a clinical asthmatic attack is an increase in the resistance of relatively small upstream airways. Equation 5 predicts a decrease in maximum expiratory flow, which is observed in the measured curve (dashed line) in Figure 20–6. The illustrated attack is a mild one and does not interfere with the tidal loop. There are other more subtle changes, however. As stated in the discussion on static lung volumes, RV is determined primarily by the resistance of the chest wall to further compression below its equilibrium volume. In the normal young adult, these static interactions are not influenced by air flow.[14] In acute asthma, the increase in RUS combined with the normal decrease in PEL at the small volumes (below FRC) markedly reduce V̇MAX to such an extent that the patient cannot exhale long enough to reach the static RV. The sensation of dyspnea forces the patient to inhale at a volume larger than true RV, e.g., RV′. Thus aberrations in lung dynamics can influence the measurement of normally static parameters. This increase in RV is also found in other types of obstructive lung disease as well as with age in the normal subject. A more severe increase in RUS can reduce the MEFV curve to the point where RV′ is at a volume above FRC (dotted curve, Fig. 20–6). Under these circumstances, the patient cannot ventilate at all near the static equilibrium position of the chest wall and the lung.[13] Indeed, in order to maintain tidal breathing at the original flow, the patient must always ventilate at volumes above FRC and therefore can never relax the muscles of inspiration. Techniques to measure FRC (helium dilution and plethysmography) use the end expiratory position of the tidal loop to define FRC. In asthma, this volume is not necessarily the equilibrium FRC but can be a significantly larger volume (FRC′, Fig. 20–6) determined, like RV′, by the dynamic forces of flow limitation.

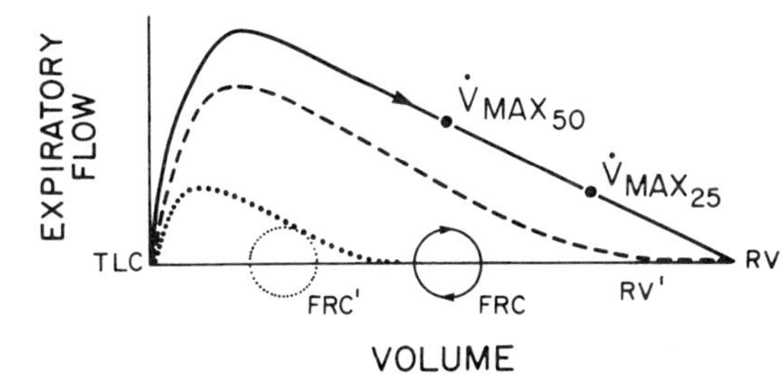

FIGURE 20–6. Maximal expiratory flow–volume relationship. $\dot{V}MAX_{50}$ and $\dot{V}MAX_{25}$ are values of maximal flow measured at 50 and 25%, respectively, of the absolute vital capacity. They are frequently used in clinical studies to represent the MEFV curve. Solid line = normal; dashed line = mild asthmatic attacks; dotted line = severe attacks.

The elevation of the apparent FRC and RV above the static values is often termed air trapping. Further increases in upstream resistance force the patient to breathe at progressively larger volumes to maintain tidal flow. This increase in trapped air reduces the vital capacity and clearly cannot progress further beyond the point where FRC′ equals TLC. At this limiting volume, ventilation can continue only if TLC somehow increases. There is some evidence that this can occur. Clinically, the chest x-ray film obtained at TLC frequently demonstrates elevated volume.[8] Measurement of FRC by helium dilution and plethysmography has indicated values of FRC′ above the original TLC.[41] However, these measurements are difficult to perform in severely ill patients, and induced bronchospasm in the laboratory can introduce artifacts that have been shown to falsely increase measured volumes.[37] In addition, TLC is largely determined by the static pressure-volume characteristics of the lung, and at first glance, these do not seem to be easily changed. However, the pressure-volume curve may be altered pharmacologically with infusion of agents that act on smooth muscle presumably located in very small airways or alveolar ducts.[15] Furthermore, the single-breath diffusing capacity of carbon monoxide (DLCO), which is measured at TLC and clinically is a function of lung (alveolar) volume and capillary blood volume, is significantly elevated in acute asthma.[21]

Parallel to these changes in lung mechanics are ventilation-perfusion abnormalities that lead to arterial hypoxia and hypocapnia.[40] The ability to increase lung volume and maintain ventilation and gas exchange may be compromised in asthmatic patients with associated diseases of the chest wall. Patients with kyphoscoliosis, obesity, neuromuscular disorders, and severe muscle fatigue may fail to elevate lung volume sufficiently to maintain adequate ventilation at degrees of bronchospasm usually tolerated by asthmatic subjects who are otherwise normal. Hypercapnia can result, and these patients may need mechanical ventilation.

The MEFV curve and static lung volumes are parameters frequently measured in the clinical laboratory. Another common practice is to relate expired volume to time (spirometry). These measurements require less sophisticated equipment and reveal similar clinical information. For example, Figure 20–7 shows spirograms corresponding to the MEFV curves that were discussed in Figure 20–6. The normal spirogram (solid line) reveals a rapid expiration of most of the VC in 1.0 sec (forced expiratory volume [FEV_1]). The remaining volume is exhaled in a few seconds, and the curve approaches a plateau. The entire exhaled volume (VC) is often called the forced vital capacity (FVC). As depicted in Figure 20–7, the FEV_1 and FVC are reduced as the attack progresses. Early in the attack, with mild bronchospasm, the FEV_1 is reduced out of proportion to the FVC. This measure of obstruction is expressed clinically as the ratio FEV_1/FVC or FEV_1%. This ratio is not useful in severe attacks because the FVC is markedly reduced and the ratio can improve. In

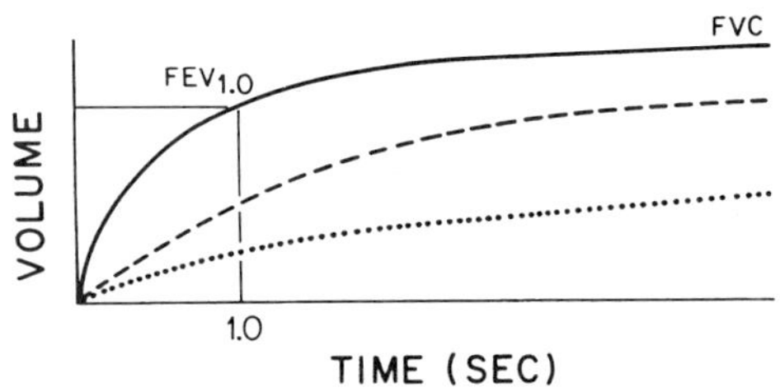

FIGURE 20–7. Spirograms (exhaled volume versus time) corresponding to the MEFV curves illustrated in Figure 20–6.

this situation, without independent measurement of lung volumes (FRC and RV), the diagnosis of restrictive rather than obstructive disease might be made. Conversely, as the patient improves and the small airways begin to dilate, the FVC frequently is the most affected parameter and the ratio worsens.

DIFFERENTIAL DIAGNOSIS

Equation 5 demonstrates that reduced expiratory flow can occur without changes in airway resistance. For example, in emphysema, loss of elastic recoil reduces $\dot{V}_{MAX}$ as effectively as an increase in R_{US}. TLC and FRC clearly increase in emphysema, as the disease can be defined mechanically as a shift in the static recoil curve of the lung upward and to the left of the normal curve. In addition to these static changes, the reduction in $\dot{V}_{MAX}$ elevates RV and FRC by the same dynamic mechanisms as those described for asthma. Thus with reduced flows and elevated lung volumes, the MEFV curve and spirogram of emphysema and asthma can be identical. The underlying pathology is obviously different, and the differential diagnosis requires a test that assesses the integrity of the lung parenchyma. As stated previously, the single-breath DLCO is a function of alveolar membrane surface area and capillary blood volume. The destruction of lung parenchyma in emphysema reduces both components of the DLCO, and therefore this test is key in separating these diagnoses. In classic emphysema, it can be markedly reduced, whereas in asthma, the DLCO is above normal.

The use of the diffusing capacity can be more helpful than the other common differential tool used to evaluate patients with obstructive disease, that is, reversibility. Asthma is certainly a reversible disorder, and patients with reduced flows frequently respond immediately with increased flow following inhalation of a bronchodilator. However, some patients with asthma do not. As discussed previously, the mechanical definition used for asthma is a reversible increase in airway resistance. Smooth muscle is not the only factor that can affect airways and increase resistance. Generalized inflammation and derangements in mucociliary clearance are also involved in asthma, probably more so in severe, chronically ill patients. It has been observed for a long time that some patients with asthma, usually during an exacerbation, expectorate mucus plugs, and plugs have been found in the autopsied lungs of patients dying in status. Clinicians are also aware of the frequent association of asthma with infection and the marked response patients have to steroid therapy. The individual contributions of derangements in the mucociliary apparatus, direct mechanical impairments of mucociliary and cough clearance (e.g., diminished air flow during cough, damage to the airway epithelium), and generalized airway edema are not known, and these areas are being intensively investigated. Of clinical importance is the observation that improvement may not be observed for several days and full improvement not noted for weeks following initiation of intensive therapy with bronchodilators and steroids. A patient with obstructive disease, elevated lung volumes, and a preserved or an elevated DLCO without a significant, immediate response to an inhaled bronchodilator should be treated for a prolonged period before a diagnosis of irreversible disease is made.

AIRWAY MECHANICS, PARTICLE DEPOSITION, AND BRONCHOPROVOCATION TESTING

Bronchoprovocation testing with inhaled histamine and methacholine is commonly used in both clinical practice and asthma research. It is based on the rationale that airways of asthmatics are intrinsically more responsive to lower doses of inhaled bronchoprovocation agents than are normal subjects.[4, 38] The cause of the increased responsiveness is not known precisely, but it is likely to be multifactorial, as in vitro sensitivity to histamine does not correlate with in vivo bronchoprovocation response.[2, 39] Most investigators consider the presence of hyperresponsiveness a hallmark of the asthmatic syndrome and believe that it should be incorporated into its definition. Therefore, hyperresponsiveness can be used as a diagnostic test in the evaluation of a patient thought to have asthma. As an extension of this logic, because hyperresponsiveness is an important component of clinical asthma, changes in hyperresponsiveness may be useful in assessing the response to therapeutic agents.

The details of the various methods for bronchoprovocation testing with aerosols are described elsewhere in extensive reviews.[9, 36] Briefly, using methacholine as an example, aerosolized particles of drug are inhaled by the patient in such a way that some assessment of the dose is documented and a measure of airway function is made as an assessment of response.

DOSE

Only a few investigators have actually measured the dose of an inhaled bronchoprovocation agent in the lungs. Using tracer dyes and relatively complex filter techniques, it has been shown that measurable changes in airway function can be observed in asthmatics to approximately one tenth of the deposited dose compared with normal subjects.[5, 12, 17] These differences are so great that modern screening tests that are used to clinically define the degree of airway responsiveness make no attempt to measure airway dose but simply quantify the amount inhaled by the test subject.[28] Differences in the amount exhaled between test subjects, although considerable, are much smaller than the threshold dose required to induce measurable airway constriction.

The exquisite reactivity of the asthmatic airway to inhaled methacholine also allows for considerable variation in efficiency of drug delivery between devices designed for bronchoprovocation testing. Although attempts have been made to standardize technique,[6] gravimetric testing of delivery systems can fail to detect important differences between nebulizers.[33] Again, these differences appear to be relatively insignificant in establishing the presence of clinically significant hyperreactivity.

SITES OF DEPOSITION

The local dose to the airway of an aerosolized drug will obviously depend on the actual sites of particle deposition. It has been suspected that a significant component of reactivity in asthma may be related to differences between sites of deposition in normal subjects and those with increased hyperreactivity. This hypothesis can be synthesized from the fact that central airways are thought to be more responsive[27] and patients with airway obstruction are known to deposit particles in more proximal airways.[25] Studies designed to test this hypothesis have been difficult because of an inherent circular logic that applies when the patient population consists of asthmatics. That is, as the bronchoprovocating agent deposits and airways constrict, it is known that deposition sites will become more central. Thus it is uncertain whether the increased reactivity measured is related to central deposition or vice versa, that is, the central deposition is caused by bronchoconstriction secondary to increased reactivity.

A different approach to testing this hypothesis involved a study in which the deposition pattern during bronchoprovocation with methacholine was measured in both normal subjects and asthmatic patients.[23] When aerosolized methacholine is inhaled from a nebulizer, patients with mild asthma and normal pulmonary function exhibit similar deposition patterns in the lung to those of normal subjects inhaling the same particles. As illustrated in Figure 20–8, the

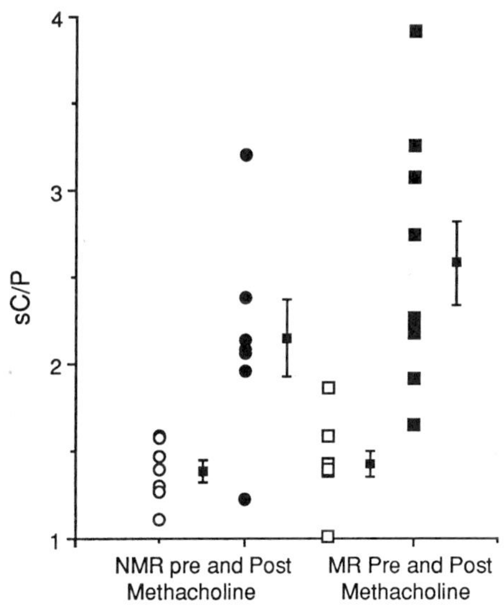

FIGURE 20–8. Deposition patterns of individual subjects before and after methacholine inhalation. Mean ± SE are also shown. PC_{20} = methacholine concentration required to produce a 20% reduction in FEV_1%; MR = subjects achieving a PC_{20}; NMR = subjects not achieving a PC_{20}; sC/P = deposition pattern, measured before (pre) and after (post) methacholine inhalation. (From O'Riordan TG, Walser L, Smaldone GC: Changing patterns of aerosol deposition during methacholine bronchoprovocation. Chest 103:1387, 1993.)

ratio of radiolabeled particles deposited in central airways versus peripheral airways (sC/P ratio, measured by gamma camera) is indistinguishable between subjects who are reactive to methacholine (methacholine reactive [MR]) and subjects who are not reactive to methacholine (NMR). However, as the methacholine test continues, the asthmatics exhibit a decrease in FEV_1 of 20% or greater.

In Figure 20–8, particle deposition then shifts from the more peripheral airways (sC/P ratio approximately 1.5) to decidedly central airways (sC/P ratio approximately 2.5). This response was expected and has been described by several groups of investigators. However, the nonreactive subjects, by definition, do not have significant changes in FEV_1. After inhaling similar amounts of methacholine to those inhaled by asthmatics, the normal subjects also demonstrated major shifts in sites of particle deposition to the same central airways. This shift was not expected in the nonasthmatic individuals. Although they are clinically designated as having normal airway responsiveness, it is clear that the airways do react, as evidenced by the changes in sites of deposition. Yet their response as assessed by FEV_1 was much different than those of individuals thought to have asthma. These data illustrate that the differences in responsiveness between asthmatic individuals with increased reactivity to methacholine and normal subjects are not secondary to differences in sites of deposition. These data again support the basic observation that the syndrome of asthma is associated with an intrinsic hyperresponsiveness that is not explained by technical factors such as lung dose or sites of aerosol deposition.

RESPONSE

The response to inhaled methacholine is usually assessed in two ways: by measurement of airway resistance utilizing body plethysmography and by means of spirometry. Results from the former are expressed as RAW (airway resistance), or, the inverse, airway conductance (GAW), whereas the latter technique yields the FEV_1 and FVC (see Fig. 20–7). Physiologic interpretation of changes in these parameters is complex, and reconciliation of results from studies using different techniques can often be impossible, primarily because they are measuring different airway events.[16] During a forced expiration, as outlined in the earlier parts of this chapter, flow-limiting segments form in central airways, and maximum expiratory flow reflects changes in elastic recoil and the resistance of small airways between alveoli and sites of FLS (see Fig. 20–5, equation 5). From a practical point of view, this model illustrates the fact that measurements of forced expiration (FEV_1, FVC), which are measured along the MEFV curve, primarily reflect events that occur within intrathoracic airways. On the other hand, during the panting maneuver (the breathing pattern characteristic of measurement of airway resistance in the plethysmograph), changes in airway resistance can represent events that occur anywhere in the tracheobronchial tree from alveoli to the mouth.

From earlier studies utilizing retrograde catheters, the airway resistance estimated by plethysmographic measurement frequently measures events along the upper airways (from 2 mm airways to the mouth), which may be more indicative of hay fever rather than asthma. Conversely, patients with clinically evident lung disease may have flow-limiting segments operative even during tidal breathing (see Fig. 20–6). In these patients, plethysmographic measurement of airway resistance reflects changes that include peripheral airways, sites of flow limitation, and upper airways. Thus the reversible nature of bronchospasm in asthma can make it difficult to interpret changes in airway resistance because the site of the pertinent resister can be obscure. Measurements of forced expiration tend to avoid this difficulty. Therefore, in studies employing bronchoprovocation testing, the choice of the measure of response may affect overall conclusions regarding reactivity in certain groups of subjects. For example, patients with a history of hay fever, but not asthma, have been reported to respond significantly to inhaled allergens with respect to airway resistance measurements, but not to measurements of forced expiration.[7]

DIAGNOSTIC IMPLICATIONS OF THE UNCERTAINTIES IN BRONCHOPROVOCATION TESTING

This chapter has focused on three general aspects of bronchoprovocation testing that are related primarily to airway physiology: the technical issues regarding local airway dose, that is, the failure to measure airway dose in most studies of bronchoprovocation and the uncertainties regarding sites of deposition; the vagaries of nebulizer function; and the differences in techniques for measuring response. The impact that these considerations have on clinical studies of hyperresponsiveness is best determined by first clarifying the clinical issue to be studied.

Diagnosis

Because hyperresponsiveness is often incorporated in the definition of asthma, its presence can be utilized as a diagnostic tool. To be useful, the conditions for testing must be specified. Logically, the patient should not be sick at the time of testing. If there are clinical signs and symptoms typical of asthma, the diagnosis can be made independently, without bronchoprovocation testing. For example, a patient with moderate or severe obstruction as evidenced by spirometry, air trapping by measurement of lung volumes, and an elevated diffusion capacity has asthma. However, an individual with normal pulmonary function but a history consistent with reversible changes in airway function and/or chronic undiagnosed cough, nocturnal symptoms, and other signs also may have asthma, and the clinical diagnosis can be enhanced by detection of bronchial hyperreactivity. Under those circumstances the vagaries of the bronchoprovocation test are not important. The points discussed previously emphasize that in individuals with normal pulmonary function undergoing methacholine testing during tidal breathing maneuvers, the dose and site of methacholine in the lung do not appear to be important in defining the presence of the disease. Although laboratories should endeavor to standardize their aerosol delivery technique, the utility of bronchoprovocation testing in diagnosis must, in retrospect, reflect the relative unimportance of these variables in establishing the presence of the disease.

Changes in Hyperresponsiveness as a Result of Therapy

Changes in airway reactivity are often utilized as an estimate of efficacy to therapeutic agents. The growing dependence of clinical investigators on this technique is related to the fact that newer drugs, such as aerosolized steroids, often do not result in immediate effects. Bronchodilators, on the other hand, respond relatively instantaneously, and the dose-versus-response relationship can be assessed clinically quite easily. However, almost all other classes of drugs are delayed in action. A major challenge in clinical pharmacology is the assessment of the response to agents that do not have immediate effects on airway caliber.[35] For example, anti-inflammatory drugs utilized in patients with relatively normal pulmonary function may have no measurable effect on spirometric values or airway resistance. In those patients, daily diaries and a measure of airway reactivity are critical in assessing the response to therapy. However, these drugs are often utilized in patients who have chronic obstruction. As the drugs become effective, the degree of obstruction can change, thus altering their overall mechanical state. Changes in airway caliber may affect the measurement of airway reactivity without affecting intrinsic responsiveness. Any drug that affects airway geometry will affect sites of deposition and possibly total dose of deposited methacholine. In any event, it is certain that the local airway dose will change after therapy.

Whereas the diagnosis of bronchial hyperresponsiveness is easy to make because of the large differences in reactivity between asthmatics and normal subjects, the changes in hyperresponsiveness as evidenced by changes in reactivity before and after therapy are much more difficult to interpret. It is absolutely critical in such studies that the aerosol delivery systems and methods of assessing airway function be rigidly standardized. Until studies in which the dose and response of the local airway can be more directly estimated, changes in reactivity, while being indicative of clinical improvement, may not be reflective of changes in bronchial hyperresponsiveness per se. Techniques have been developed for measuring the dose and site of aerosolized agents, and these measurements have been related to clinical response.[32, 34] However, these studies have not been performed for tests of airway reactivity.

DEPOSITION AND CLEARANCE OF PARTICLES IN ASTHMA: MEASURES OF RESPONSE TO THERAPY

Invasive techniques utilizing bronchoalveolar lavage and airway epithelial biopsy have revealed persistent inflammation in mild asthma and strengthened the link between the pathophysiology of the disease and derangements in mechanisms of inflammation. Because the deposition of particles is sensitive to local airway geometry, test aerosols can be used as probes of peripheral airway function independent of and complementary to standard pulmonary function testing. In a given patient with a standardized breathing pattern, a test aerosol may provide important insights as to changes in small airway function before and after a given therapeutic regimen. For example, the change in deposition site during methacholine bronchoprovocation may complicate the as-

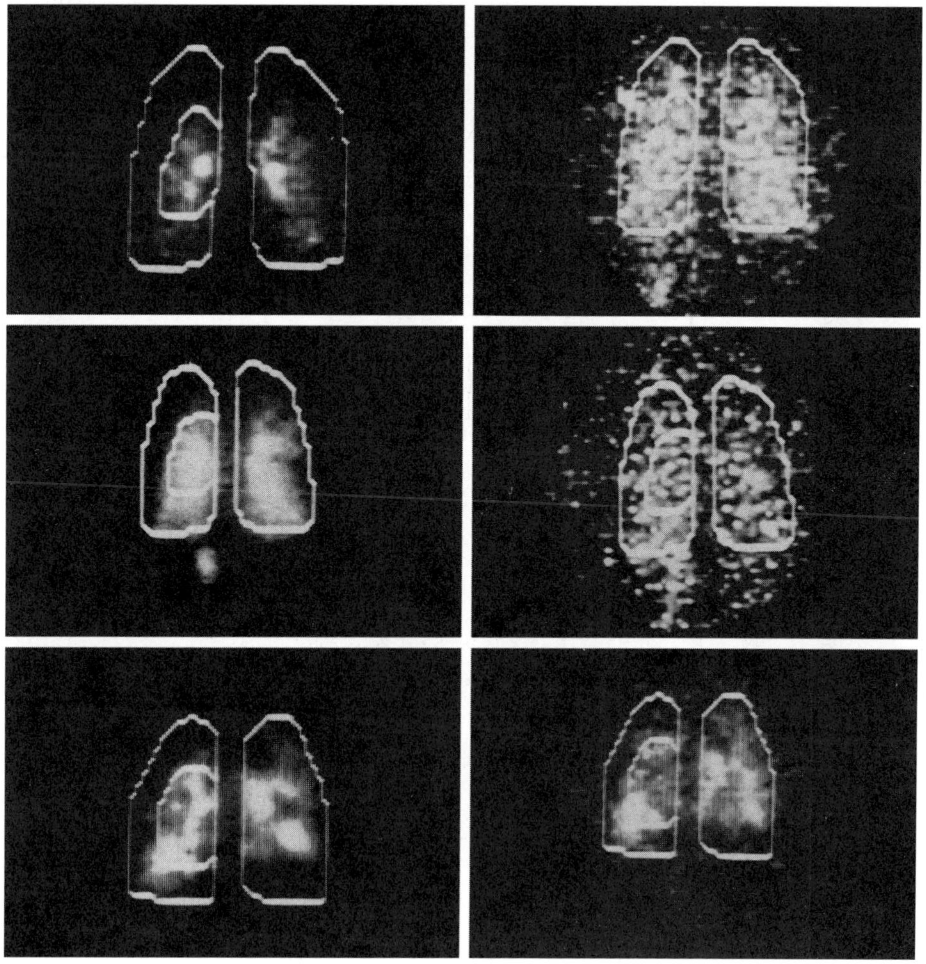

FIGURE 20–9. Gamma camera images at zero time immediately after aerosol deposition (left) and at 24 hours (right). Normal subject is in upper panels, mild asthmatic patient in middle panels, and severe asthmatic patient in lower panels. Only the flow-limited, severe asthmatic patient retains significant aerosol in central airways at 24 hours. (From Smaldone GC, Perry RJ, Bennett WD, et al: Interpretation of '24 hour lung retention' in studies of mucociliary clearance. J Aerosol Med 1:18, 1988.)

sessment of that test, but the change in site of a test aerosol may be indicative of peripheral airway effects of drugs that may not be detected by spirometry alone.

Besides the pattern of deposition, the clearance of radiolabeled test aerosols from the same airways may also be an index of overall epithelial function. For various reasons, the mucociliary apparatus is thought to be affected in different lung diseases, such as changes in the rheology of secretions (cystic fibrosis), ciliary ineffectiveness in the ciliary dyskinesias,[3] and inflammatory damage to the airway epithelium (asthma). Airway biopsies in patients with asthma suggest that the epithelium is abnormal even in subjects with mild disease.

In asthma, mucociliary clearance abnormalities in central airways have been described 24 hours after the deposition of an inhaled aerosol.[31] As shown in Figure 20–9, gamma camera images in subjects with severe asthma can retain particles in central airways over 24 hours, an interval of time previously thought long enough to allow for 100% clearance from ciliated airways.

In order to further quantify the importance of these observations and link this incidental observation to clinical exacerbations, mucociliary clearance has been measured in hospitalized asthmatics who present in status. Those data are shown in Figure 20–10. When a radioactive test aerosol is deposited in the lung, mucociliary clearance can be estimated by measuring residual radioactivity in the lung over time. These data are expressed as retention, the percentage of the initial amount of radioactivity in the lung at the beginning of the study, versus time. As demonstrated in Figure 20–10, asthmatic patients in the hospital retain all the deposited radiolabel over the first 2 hours of study, consistent with autopsy studies that have clearly shown small airway obstruction with mucus plugs at the time of death. The data in Figure 20–10 confirm noninvasively that the mucociliary apparatus is indeed deranged in these very sick patients.[20] Following full therapy, including intravenous steroids as well as nebulized and systemic bronchodilators, an improvement in mucociliary clearance in all patients was seen after discharge as evidenced by decreased retention over time.

The fact that this hospitalized population recovered considerable mucociliary function after discharge indicates that, although inflamed, the outpatient asthmatic airway has a functioning respiratory epithelium. However, there is a question as to whether the epithelium is functioning normally. In another group of closely followed asthmatic subjects with a wide range of airway function, changes in mucociliary clearance can be readily distinguished from inpatients with an exacerbation (Figure 20–11). When compared with normal subjects, however, mild stable asthmatics may have normal to enhanced mucociliary clearance (Fig. 20–12).[22]

SUMMARY

A pattern is emerging indicating that mucociliary function measured by radioaerosol may be an accurate and precise

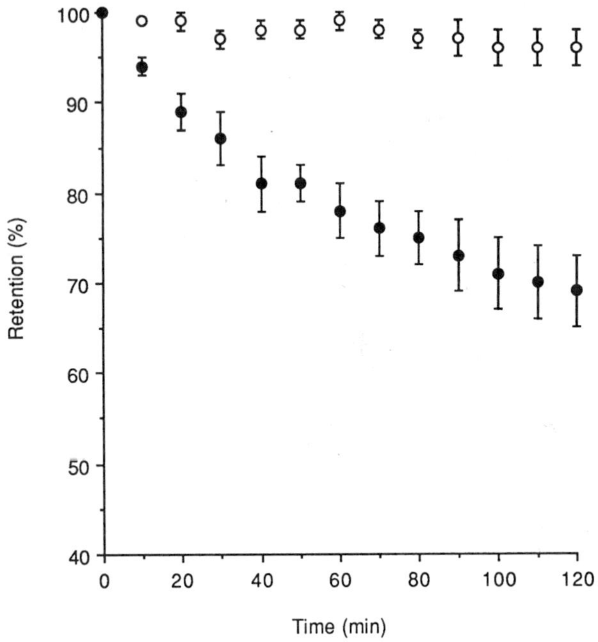

FIGURE 20–10. Whole lung retention versus time in acute asthma. Patients hospitalized with severe asthma (open circles, mean ±SE, n=5) retain almost all the deposited activity over 2 hours. After discharge (closed circles), mucociliary clearance in the same patients is much improved. (From Messina MS, O'Riordan TG, Smaldone GC: Changes in mucociliary clearance during acute exacerbations of asthma. Am Rev Respir Dis 143:995, 1991.)

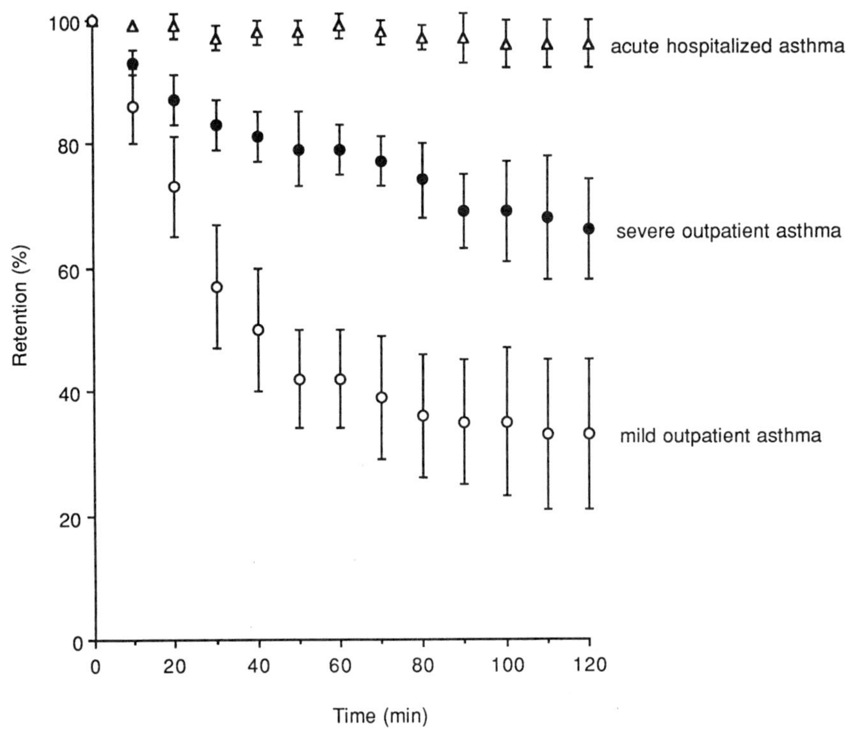

FIGURE 20–11. Whole lung data from hospitalized patients with acute asthma, outpatients with chronic severe airway obstruction (results from Messina MS, O'Riordan TG, Smaldone GC: Changes in mucociliary clearance during acute exacerbations of asthma. Am Rev Respir Dis 143:993, 1991) and outpatients with mild disease corresponding to those from studies utilizing BAL and biopsy (modified from O'Riordan TG, Zwang J, Smaldone GC: Mucociliary clearance in adult asthma. Am Rev Respir Dis 146:601, 1992).

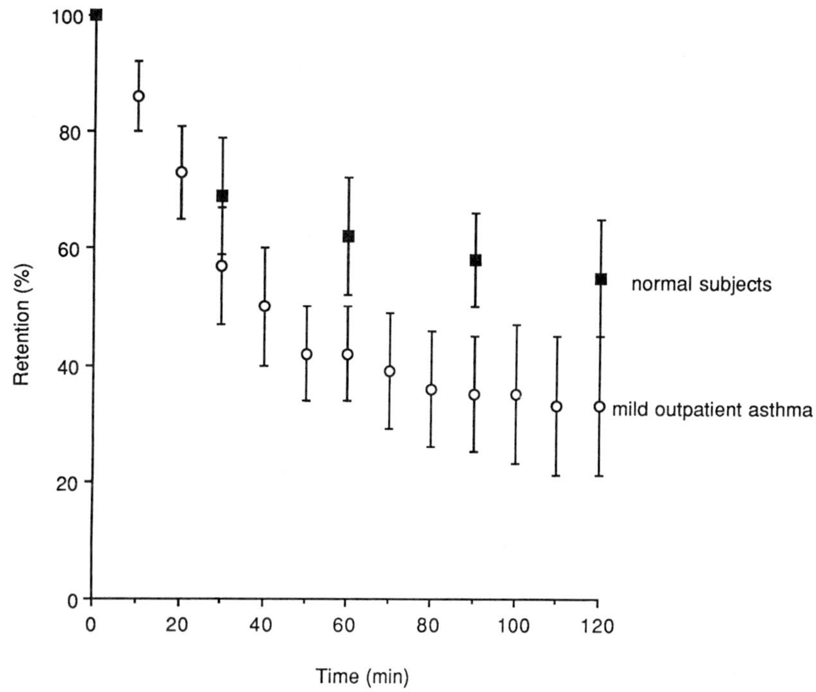

FIGURE 20–12. Mucociliary clearance measured in patients with mild asthma compared with that of normal subjects. (Data from O'Riordan TG, Zwang J, Smaldone GC: Mucociliary clearance in adult asthma. Am Rev Respir Dis 146:598, 1992.)

noninvasive test of epithelial function in the airways of patients affected by asthma. In addition to the studies illustrated here, which measured retention of material in the whole lung, others have measured definite increases in clearance following steroid therapy in peripheral airways.[1] Thus as newer drugs with delayed responses are being developed, the combination of changes in responsiveness to bronchoprovocation, changes in the sites of deposition of test aerosols, and changes in mucociliary clearance may provide a more sensitive and specific assessment of airway integrity and act as better predictors of clinical control to a given therapeutic regimen.

REFERENCES

1. Agnew JE, Bateman JRM, Pavia D, Clarke SW: Peripheral airways mucus clearance in stable asthma is improved by oral corticosteroid therapy. Bull Eur Physiopathol Respir 20:295, 1984.
2. Armour CL, Lazar N, Schellenberg R, et al: A comparison of in vivo and in vitro human airway reactivity to histamine. Am Rev Respir Dis 129:907, 1984.
3. Camner P, Mossberg B: Mucociliary disorders: a review. J Aerosol Med 1:21, 1988.
4. Cockcroft D, Hargreave F: Airway hyperresponsiveness: relevance of random population data to clinical usefulness. Am Rev Respir Dis 142:497, 1990.
5. Donna E, Danta I, Kim CS, Wanner A: Relationship between deposition of and responsiveness to inhaled methacholine in normal and asymptomatic subjects. J Allergy Clin Immunol 83:456, 1989.
6. Dolovich MB: Technical factors influencing response to challenge aerosols. In Hargreave FE, Woolcock AJ (eds): Airway Responsiveness Measurement and Interpretation. Astra Pharmaceuticals Canada Ltd, Mississauga, Ontario, 1985, p 9.
7. Fish JE, Kelly JF: Measurement of responsiveness in bronchoprovocation testing. J Allergy Clin Immunol 64:592, 1979.
8. Fraser RG, Pare JAP: Diagnosis of Diseases of the Chest, 2nd edition. Saunders, Philadelphia, 1977.
9. Hargreave FE, Woolcock AJ (eds): Airway Responsiveness Measurement and Interpretation. Astra Pharmaceuticals Canada Ltd, Mississauga, Ontario, 1985.
10. Hyatt RE: Expiratory flow limitation. J Appl Physiol 55:1–7, 1983.
11. Hyatt RE, Schilder DP, Fry DL: Relationship between maximum expiratory flow and degree of lung inflation. J Appl Physiol 13:331, 1958.
12. Itkin IH, Anand S, Yau M, Middlebrook G: Quantitative inhalation challenge in allergic asthma. J Allergy 34:97, 1963.
13. Kimball WR, Leith DE, Robins AG: Dynamic hyperinflation and ventilation dependence in chronic obstructive pulmonary disease. Am Rev Respir Dis 126:991, 1982.
14. Leith DE, Mead J: Mechanisms determining residual volume of the lungs in normal subjects. J Appl Physiol 23:221, 1967.
15. Macklem PT: Respiratory mechanics. Am Rev Physiol 40:157, 1978.
16. Macklem PT: The interpretation of lung function tests. In Hargreave FE, Woolcock AJ (eds): Airway Responsiveness Measurement and Interpretation. Astra Pharmaceuticals Canada Ltd, Mississauga, Ontario, 1985, p 69.
17. Makino S: Clinical significance of bronchial sensitivity to acetylcholine and histamine in bronchial asthma. J Allergy 38:127, 1966.
18. Mead J: Mechanical properties of lungs. Physiol Rev 41:281, 1961.
19. Mead J, Turner MM, Macklem P, Little JB: Significance of the relationship between lung recoil and maximum expiratory flow. J Appl Physiol 22:95, 1967.
20. Messina MS, O'Riordan TG, Smaldone GC: Changes in mucociliary clearance during acute exacerbations of asthma. Am Rev Respir Dis 143:993, 1991.
21. Ohrnan JL, Schmidt-Nowara W, Lawrence M, et al: The diffusing capacity in asthma. Am Rev Respir Dis 107:932, 1973.
22. O'Riordan TG, Zwang J, Smaldone GC: Mucociliary clearance in adult asthma. Am Rev Respir Dis 146:598, 1992.
23. O'Riordan TG, Walser L, Smaldone GC: Changing patterns of aerosol deposition during methacholine bronchoprovocation. Chest 103:1385, 1993.
24. Otis AB: The work of breathing. In Fenn WD, Rahn H (eds): Handbook of Physiology. Sect 3: Respiration. Vol I. American Physiological Society, Washington, DC, 1964, p 463.
25. Pavia D, Thomson ML, Clarke SW, Shannon HS: Effect of lung function and mode of inhalation on penetration of aerosol in the human lung. Thorax 32:194, 1977.
26. Pride NB, Permutt S, Riley RL, Bromberger-Barnea B: Determinants of maximal expiratory flow from the lungs. J Appl Physiol 23:646, 1967.
27. Ruffin RE, Dolovich MB, Wolff RK, Newhouse MT: The effects of preferential deposition of histamine in the human airway. Am Rev Respir Dis 117:485, 1978.
28. Rosenthal RR: Methodologies of aerosol delivery. In Spector SL (ed): Provocation Testing in Clinical Practice. Vol 5. Marcel Dekker, Inc, New York, 1995, p 215.

29. Saibene F, Mead J: Frequency dependence of pulmonary quasi-static hysteresis. J Appl Physiol 26:732, 1969.
30. Smaldone GC: Delineation of flow-limiting segment and predicted airway resistance by movable catheter. J Appl Physiol 40:943, 1976.
31. Smaldone GC, Perry RJ, Bennett WD, et al: Interpretation of '24 hour lung retention' in studies of mucociliary clearance. J Aerosol Med 1:11, 1988.
32. Smaldone GC, Dickinson G, Marcial E, et al: Deposition of aerosolized pentamidine and failure of pneumocystis prophylaxis. Chest 101:82, 1991.
33. Smaldone GC: Drug delivery by nebulization: Reality testing. J Aerosol Med 7:213, 1994. Editorial.
34. Smaldone GC: Regional analysis of deposition of aerosolized drugs in disease. In Byron PR, Dahlby RN, Farr SJ (eds): Respiratory Drug Delivery IV. Interpharm Press, Buffalo Grove, IL, 1994, p 163.
35. Smaldone GC: Determinants of dose and response to inhaled therapeutic agents in asthma. In Schleimer R, Busse W, O'Bryne P (eds): Topical Glucocorticoids in Asthma-Mechanisms and Clinical Actions. Marcel Dekker, Inc, New York, NY. In press.
36. Spector SL (ed): Provocation Testing in Clinical Practice. Vol 5. Marcel Dekker, Inc, New York, 1995.
37. Staneseu DC, Rodenstein D, Cauberghs M, Van de Woestijne KP: Failure of body plethysmography in bronchial asthma. J Appl Physiol 52:939, 1982.
38. Tattersfield AE: Measurement of bronchial reactivity: a question of interpretation. Thorax 36:561, 1981.
39. Vincenc KS, Black J, Yan K, et al: Comparison of in vivo and in vitro responses to histamine in the human airways. Am Rev Respir Dis 128:875, 1983.
40. West JB: Obstructive diseases. In West JB (ed): Pulmonary Pathophysiology. Williams & Wilkins, Baltimore, MD, 1977, p 87.
41. Woolcock AJ, Rebuck AS, Code JF, Read J: Lung volume changes in asthma measured concurrently by two methods. Am Rev Respir Dis 104:703, 1971.

21 Airborne Allergens

WILLIAM R. SOLOMON MARY L. JELKS

Windborne agents are familiar factors in allergic disease, often producing seasons or spatial patterns of morbidity that suggest specific offenders. Carriers of airborne atopic allergens include pollens, fungus and possibly slime mold particles, insect and arachnid (e.g., mite) debris, animal emanations, algae, and a variety of other materials. Additional windborne agents such as actinomycetes and protozoa are implicated in allergic alveolitis, and still others may provoke contact dermatitis; these are discussed in Chapters 32 and 36, respectively. Considering the profusion of common airborne allergens (aeroallergens), it is not surprising that many natural exposures are qualitatively complex. Notable health effects may reflect one or more allergens, microbial products, direct chemical or physical irritants, and additional modulators of target organ function.

Immunochemical studies continue to clarify the molecular characteristics of major biogenic allergens, some of which have been cloned and produced in suitable expression vectors. Typical sensitizing materials (e.g., specific pollens) often have shown more than one active substance, the components differing in amount and sensitizing potency but generally comprising proteins of 10 to 60 kilodaltons (kD). Designation of these molecules now conforms to international rules, reflecting their source and place in an order of description.[93] With this approach, a biogenic allergen acquires the first three letters of its source's (Latin) generic name and the first letter of its species epithet. For short ragweed (*Ambrosia artemisiifolia*) pollen, then, all allergens are designated Amb a. An Arabic number follows, indicating where in the sequence of *A. artemisiifolia* allergens this agent was characterized. For short ragweed pollen, Amb a 1, the principal and first described allergen was previously known as antigen E. Based on these conventions, additional Amb a allergens are Amb a 2, 3, 4, 5, and so forth. These and some other characterized agents are shown in Table 21–1 with prior designations.

As complex proteins, defined allergens often comprise several molecular domains (epitopes) that elicit specific reactivity by an individual's B or T lymphocytes. To the extent that such responses are finely cell subset–specific, it may be possible to manipulate the immune responses to complex allergens. In addition to familiar natural allergens, IgE-mediated responses to highly reactive small molecular species, such as chloroplatinates,[42] phthalic and trimellitic anhydrides,[17] and phenylglycine,[87] have determined instances of occupational asthma.

Well-known vectors of allergenic activity, such as pollen and spores, are solid aerosols, generally 2 to 60 μm in size, and often distinctive microscopically. Additional natural dusts, including seed pomaces, animal danders, and much arthropod debris, lack defined morphology or characteristic particle size and may be distinctly smaller. Aerosols in this

TABLE 21–1
SOME INHALANT ALLERGENS WITH DEFINED SEQUENCES

Source	Allergen	Prior Designation	Molecular Weight (kD)
Rye grass *(Lolium perenne)*	Lol p 1	Group I	27–28
	Lol p 2	Group II	11
	Lol p 3	Group III	11
	Lol p 5		31
	Lol p 9	Lol p Ib	31–34
June (blue) grass *(Poa pratensis)*	Poa p 1	Group I	33
	Poa p 9		32–34
Timothy *(Phleum pratense)*	Phl p 1		
	Phlp 5	Ag 25	32
Bermuda grass *(Cynodon dactylon)*	Cyn d 1		32
Eur. birch *(Betula verrucosa)*	Bet v 1		17
	Bet v 2		15
Eur. alder *(Alnus glutinosa)*	Aln g 1		17
Eur. hazel *(Corylus avellana)*	Cor a 1		17
Sugi *(Cryptomeria japonica)*	Cry j 1		41–45
Short ragweed *(Ambrosia artemisiifolia)*	Amb a 1	Antigen E	38
	Amb a 2	Antigen K	38
	Amb a 3	Ra 3	11
	Amb a 5	Ra 5	5
	Amb a 6	Ra 6	10–11
Giant ragweed *(Ambrosia trifida)*	Amb t 5	Ra 5G	4–5
Cat *(Felis domesticus)*	Fel d 1	Cat 1	38
Rat *(Rattus norvegicus)* urine	Rat n 1		17
Mouse *(Mus musculus)* urine	Mus m 1	MUP	19
Aspergillus fumigatus	Asp f 1		18
Alternaria alternata	Alt a 1		28–30
Mite *(Dermatophagoides pteronyssinus)*	Der p 1	Ag P_1	25
	Der p 2		14
Mite *(Dermatophagoides farinae)*	Der f 1		25
	Der f 2		14

micronic range are readily dispersed by ambient air currents, although transport beyond 1 km is not assured. Once suspended, particles are variably removed by gravitational fallout, impaction on obstructions, and rainfall, especially the relatively small drops of steady frontal rain. The effectiveness of each of these air-cleansing processes rises as increasingly larger aerosols are considered; similarly, deposition in the respiratory tract is particle size dependent. During nasal respiration, the uppermost airway captures most units 10 μm and larger, whereas 50% of 6 to 7 μm spherical particles escape nasal deposition.[124] Mouth breathing affords only slightly less efficient particle removal. With either respiratory mode, theory predicts minimal penetration of pollen-sized (≥15 μm) aerosols beyond the carina. Such exclusion generally has been confirmed in practice,[216] although contradictory results have also been obtained.

Because, at most, few larger particles reach intrapulmonary airways, it has been difficult to attribute allergic asthma to such deposition. For pollens studied in vitro, allergen activity often is released rapidly in aqueous media, suggesting that bloodborne allergens might challenge the bronchi following elution on moist mucosal surfaces.[81] Distant immunologic effects of mucosally applied allergens have been shown.[99] However, efforts to determine whether the nasal mucosa of the atopic subject is abnormally permeable have yielded conflicting results.[26, 99]

A compatible alternative view that pollen and possibly other allergens might be airborne in quite small aerosol fractions is supported by data for ragweed and grass and suggested for some tree emanations.[71, 98, 182] The sources and magnitude of such activity remain speculative but may involve transport of anther fragments or vegetative debris bearing allergenic determinants. In the case of grass pollen, dispersion of allergen-coated starch granules from osmotically lysed grains has been especially suggested.[98] Dissolved materials eluted on moist surfaces might be dispersed in allergen-rich jet droplets produced by bursting bubbles and impactions on fluid films.[159] The relative contribution to inhaled allergen burdens of such paucimicronic aerosols remains uncertain. However, it is clear that immunochemical indexes of total airborne allergen provide useful correlates for interpreting more traditional prevalence estimators (viz., direct tallies of particles or microbial colonies).[4]

In addition to potent sensitizers and favorable size, clinically prominent aeroallergens must be abundant in the human microenvironment. Circumstances of dispersion and transport differ among particle types and may change continuously. However, all ultimately inhaled units first must be mobilized by substrate movement, scavenging air currents or actively discharged as shown for ascospores and basidiospores (ballistospores). Once airborne, particles are mixed by vertical and horizontal vectors, turbulent eddies, and gravitational settling. Such forces, as well as interception by vegetation, can rapidly deplete aerosol concentrations, which often decline as the fourth power of distance from a discrete source.[70] However, such formulations provide only limited predictors of human exposure.

In nature, allergens generally arise from multiple points or large area sources rather than single sites, and transport is complex. Furthermore, especially near the ground, obstructions modify air flow, creating poorly ventilated stagnation points upwind and, at times, downwind eddies that concentrate suspended particles.[148] Differential heating of terrain varies the extent of thermals (rising columns of heated air). In addition, the higher mean temperatures of cities limit the subsidence (downward movement) of air over municipalities compared with surrounding vegetated areas.[70] These factors, as well as the lapse rate (change in air temperature with altitude), at any instant help determine the volume in which particle dispersion can occur. On sunny days, a deep mixing layer can dilute particles originating at the surface. In addition, allergens often are carried upward as solar heating proceeds and descend as parcels of air cool after sundown. Wherever air temperature rises locally with altitude, a limit is placed on the depth of the subjacent mixing volume. Such a temperature inversion occurs especially when a warm air mass has overrun a cooler (and denser) one or (often at night) when radiational cooling of the surface has been prominent. The shallow mixing layers that result serve to confine dispersed particles to air near the ground and are typical of calm, overcast periods.

Weather conditions that affect transport potential and the depth of mixing layers also determine factors (e.g., temperature, humidity, and solar input) that control the availability of allergens (e.g., pollens and spores) for dispersion. The interrelationships among these variables are sufficiently complex to discourage predictions of allergen prevalence based on individual weather components, such as temperature or wind speed.

Whether mediated by low-level winds, playing children, or earthquakes, disturbance regularly promotes the primary dispersion or reflotation of allergens. Visible particle clouds generated by agricultural activities dramatically illustrate this effect; however, lesser perturbations also suffice. Human activity is an especially important dispersive factor in otherwise calm domestic and occupational settings. Indoor situations often house distinctive aerosol sources, such as dust mites, pets, and fungi with simple nutritional needs. In addition, particles originating in nature readily penetrate closed structures and move by bulk flow through open doors and windows.[141] Therefore, it cannot be assumed safely that allergens recovered indoors necessarily indicate interior sources. A further concern is that particles infiltrating enclosed spaces often show prevalence peak hours or days after maximal levels have occurred in nature.[141] Whatever their sources, deposited particles may be mobilized by later human activity, resulting in anomalous symptom or particle collection patterns. Yet, indoor allergen sources may have minimal health impact if they are undisturbed and effectively sequestered from free air circulation.

ALLERGEN EXPOSURE AND SYMPTOM SEVERITY

Allergens, such as those of pollens, elute readily from native particles, facilitating reaction with sensitized cells at mucosal sites and possible bloodborne transport.[99] The mean allergen doses required to elicit or sustain clinical symptoms are poorly known and appear to vary, often widely, among sensitive subjects. However, exposure levels of mite and roach allergens at which sensitization of atopic persons can be expected have been proposed. Empirical correlations of clinical and air sampling data have indicated that daily mean grass pollen levels of 50 grains/m^3 suffice to elicit symptoms in all affected subjects in and around London, England.[44] It is not certain how many of these persons experienced pollinosis at lower concentrations or what effect preceding days of increasing pollen exposure may have produced. However, comparisons of pollen prevalence and pollinosis severity suggest that dose-response relationships vary with exposure history; that is, preceding exposure serves to facilitate subsequent response. A decreasing threshold for nasal allergic responses has been described as daily challenges with dry defatted ragweed pollen proceeded.[40] This acquired, heightened reactivity was not allergen specific and also affects responses to reflex and direct pharmacologic stimuli. Such a priming effect has been confirmed in numerous studies using allergen extracts and vasoactive agents.

EVALUATING EXPOSURE TO ALLERGENS

Environmental exposures often rapidly provoke clinical events that indict causal allergens, as in immediate responses to foods, animals, clouds of fungus spores, or commercially reared insects. Similarly, the circannual timing of hay fever seasons with cycles of local floral activity has implicated otherwise unobtrusive sources of offending pollens. However, field observations alone provide an incomplete view of aeroallergen exposure. Many sources, such as common fungi, algae, and house dust mites, are quite inapparent to even painstaking gross examination. Higher plants, especially numerous or showy types, such as roses and goldenrods, may claim attention despite negligible pollen output for wind dispersion, whereas less apparent but highly productive sources are overlooked. Furthermore, allergen occurrence shows marked short-period weather effects and can vary strikingly among both outdoor and indoor sites, as well as over surprisingly short distances in nature. These limitations of field-based observations led quite naturally to direct sampling and analysis of air as a complementary index of exposure.

TECHNIQUES FOR STUDYING AEROALLERGEN PREVALENCE

In considering aerometric (air quality measuring) techniques, the clinician confronts a group of relatively simple but unfamiliar devices with occasionally overlapping applications. This diversity is partly the legacy of technical evolution but reflects more the different collection capabilities required to monitor a variety of airborne agents. Methodological relationships are understood best by recognizing that each approach involves both a *collection* and an *analysis* function. The collection function is implicit, as all current methods require the harvesting of atmospheric particles, usually by depositing them on specialized surfaces. Deposition may be effected by several strategies and ideally results in samples that are volumetric (derived from known volumes of processed air). Particle size (and shape) is probably the most important single factor influencing the effectiveness of various collection techniques.

Deposited materials may admit analysis by one or more approaches. Units of certain fungi, algae, actinomycetes, and bacteria, for example, form identifiable colonial growth on laboratory media, permitting analysis by culture. In addition, some particles exhibiting growth potential, and many types without it, are sufficiently distinctive in form to be identified and enumerated microscopically. Pollen grains and many larger fungus spores are easily recognized and tallied in this way. However, small spores, such as those of species of *Aspergillus* and *Penicillium*, are mutually indistinguishable in most cases (and are readily confused even with ash spheres and oil droplets formed in burning pulverized fuels); for these, culture currently is essential, although nongrowing spores will be overlooked.

The limitations of analysis in culture are often ignored but can strongly bias data resulting from viable collection. For a distinctive colony to result, factors that include absolute viability, substrate demands, physical conditions of culture, and relations with neighboring growth must be favorable. Because these requirements often are unmet, only a fraction of microbial types are monitored well by cultural methods; for these, colony counts tend to greatly underestimate prevalence when compared with direct particle enumeration.[28] Clearly, analysis in culture is desirable where particles can germinate and grow, but microscopic recognition is infeasible, such as with many small-spored imperfect fungi, bacteria, actinomycetes, and algae. For some additional particle types, such as fungal hyphae, cultural analysis also may offer relative advantages.

Many allergenic agents defy enumeration by either microscopy or propagation in culture. This group, which includes animal allergens, food residues, arthropod debris, and several simple chemical sensitizers, traditionally has lent itself only to source recognition. Antibodies to defined allergen epitopes have raised hopes that immunochemical staining might define such materials in particle deposits.[163] More immediately useful are methods to assess the allergen present in bulk collections by using their eluates to inhibit binding to solid-phase immunosorbents in assays such as the radioallergosorbent test (RAST) and enzyme-linked immunosorbent assay (ELISA).[4] Because this approach offers a reflection of total allergen, regardless of carrier attributes, it is also applicable to agents such as pollens and fungus particles. Neither the value nor the limitations of this approach have been defined fully, yet it is applicable to complex mixtures and offers an innovative tool for atmospheric aerosol analysis.[143]

BEHAVIOR OF SUSPENDED PARTICLES

The interaction of moving particles with sampling units, which determines the latter's collection efficiency, is substantially determined by particle size. This effect is best appreciated, however, by reference to a condition rare in nature: the behavior of aerosol units in totally still air (Fig. 21–1). Falling particles in this situation progressively accelerate due to gravity, finally reaching a speed that remains constant. At this terminal fall rate, or Stokes' settling velocity (S_f), gravity's pull is just balanced by two opposing forces: the particle's buoyancy and its drag coefficient, which reflects frictional interaction with surrounding gas molecules. For smooth, spherical, micronic particles, S_f may be estimated using simple parameters:

$$S_f = \frac{gd^2(\rho \text{ part.} - \rho \text{ air})}{18 \text{ u}}$$

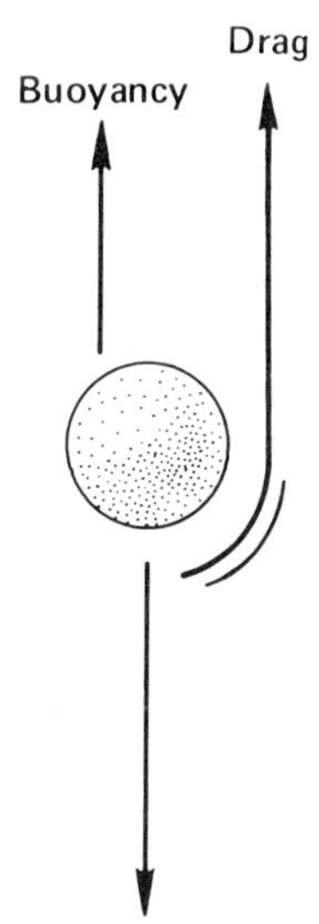

FIGURE 21–1. Forces that act on a particle falling in still air. The acceleration of gravity is opposed by buoyancy and drag. When these forces reach equilibrium, the particle settles at a fixed terminal velocity.

where g is the acceleration of gravity on unit mass, d is the effective particle diameter, u is the viscosity of ambient air, and ρ part. and ρ air are the respective densities of the particle and ambient air.

This equation emphasizes the dominant (exponential) influence of particle size on fall speed. Thus two spheres with respective diameters of 2 and 20 μm will differ by a factor of 100, i.e. $\left(\frac{20}{2}\right)^2$, in their tendencies to deposit on an intercepting surface. This profound particle size–dependence governs all recoveries based on fallout and determines the underrepresentation of smaller aerosol units on horizontal slides and open culture plates. Additional correlates of S_f also are noteworthy. The probability that a particle will strike any barrier in its path, rather than follow the diverging lines of air flow around it, rises with S_f and therefore exponentially with size. Conversely, small aerosols (with low S_f values) are relatively more responsive to drag forces, tending to flow around barriers and respond faithfully to rapid changes in direction of the entraining air stream. Such aerosols enter suction devices, such as spore traps and filter samplers, far more predictably than do larger units.

Although defined for smooth spheres, the relationships of S_f also are adaptable to many micronic particles that are neither smooth nor spherical. In practice, aerosol units may be described and compared in terms of equivalent aerodynamic diameter (EAD) after empirical determination of S_f. EAD is the diameter of that unit density sphere having the same S_f as the particle type in question. EAD may be surprisingly low for elongated aerosols that often align their principal axes to lines of air flow and are problematic for asymmetric types that tend to yaw and tumble during fallout.

GRAVITATIONAL COLLECTION

Particle collection on greased microslides and open culture dishes maintained a deceptive simplicity for clinicians until recent years. This approach was bolstered in 1946 when Durham described a standard sampling device. The Durham sampler provided support for a 1 × 3-inch microslide beneath a 9-inch diameter rain shield. Commonly, slides were lightly coated with soft glycerin jelly, petrolatum, or a silicone grease and passively exposed during 24-hour periods. Examination by transmitted light required mounting portions of the deposit with an aqueous medium, such as Calberla's solution,* containing fuchsin or other basic dyes. Because deposits resulting from fallout tended to be relatively sparse, counting large areas was required to reduce sampling error.

The simple and durable Durham sampler produced great masses of data, prompting a popular assumption that gravity slide collections accurately described prevalence. However, both theoretic concerns and practical comparisons have made this view untenable. Reservations arise from three principal points: (a) the volume of air providing particles to any collection is undefined, making comparisons between samples tenuous, even for single particle types; (b) size-dependent bias in recovery precludes valid estimates of relative prevalence for unlike-sized aerosol types; and (c) high

*Calberla's solution usually is prepared as 5 ml glycerin, 10 ml 95% ethanol, 15 ml distilled water, and 1 to 3 drops of a saturated aqueous solution of basic fuchsin.

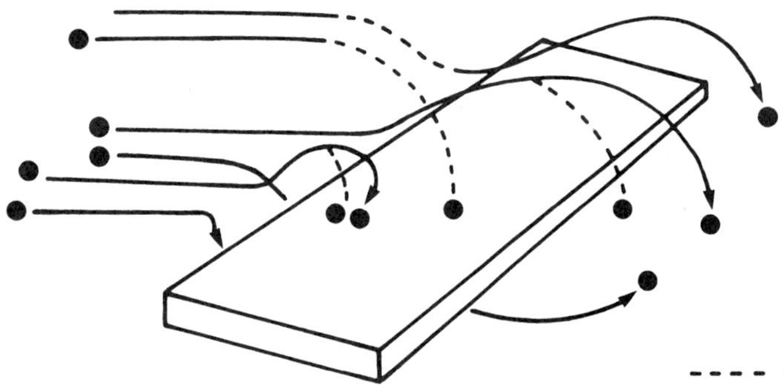

FIGURE 21–2. Eddying air flow around a horizontal slide. Deposition is influenced strongly by wind and slide orientation as the form and extent of eddies produced rapidly change.

levels of sampling error affect the counts, especially for smaller and less common particle categories.

With its rain shield in place, simple fallout on a gravity slide is possible only from the overlying 3-inch-deep layer of air, so that under unusually calm conditions, very few particles deposit. In fact, most recoveries reflect horizontal air flow with particles delivered by turbulent eddies. As shown in Figure 21–2, the size of these oscillations and their varying patterns around the microslide strongly affect collection probabilities. The changing impact of air flow on particle deposition predicted the failure of any empirically derived conversion factors to reliably transform gravity slide counts into particles per unit volume of air. Gravity collections do provide insight into trends for comparatively large and abundant particles. However, more exacting requirements demand the volumetric data available from rotating-arm impactors and suction devices.

ROTATING-ARM IMPACTORS

Narrow filaments and rods intercept particles from moving air with surprising effectiveness. Studies using thin vertical cylinders have shown that their collection efficiency varies with air speed, as well as particle S_f, and falls as increasingly broad obstructions are tested.[70] For use as samplers, however, such rods must be wind oriented, and the volume of passing air flow determined. One practical approach is to move a narrow collection surface through air along a circular path and at a speed that generally exceeds ambient flow. Of several devices employing this principle, only the Rotorod line of samplers has remained available commercially. Rotorod instruments collect particles on paired, grease-coated, angular, lucite rods that are rotated through air at 2,400 rpm. Because impactor surfaces often become measurably overloaded in only 30 minutes of rotation, operation during 24-hour periods must be intermittent. A Rotorod unit powered by alternating current and designed to operate for 1 out of every 10 minutes is marketed (Fig. 21–3). The device uses rods that spring into sampling position centrifugally during rotation and are shielded by a broad crosspiece between operating intervals; adventitious particle pickup is nil.

Rotating-arm impactors offer volumetric potential since the volume of air processed in any sampling period may be calculated. For the intermittent Rotorod, each (paired) sampling surface is effectively 2.3 cm long and 0.159 cm wide and revolves at 2,400 rpm through a circle of 27 cm perimeter (8.6 cm distance between rods (diameter) $\times$ π). In a single rotation, 0.73 cm^2 $\times$ 27 cm, or 19.7 cm^3, is swept out, and this value $\times$ 2,400 $\times$ total minutes of operation is the volume of air contributing relevant particles.

Rotorod recoveries facilitate particle identification by direct microscopy. A Lucite stage support grooved to position pairs of rods is commonly used, rod surfaces are gently flooded with a suitable mounting medium, and a cover slip is applied. The resulting (temporary) preparations have good optical properties but adapt poorly to storage for reexamination. Prepared but unmounted rods, both before and after exposure, may be kept for extended periods in dust proof, field carriers.

Because impactors (and other samplers under most conditions) cannot deliver 100% efficiency, actual prevalence levels (per cubic meter of ambient air) cannot be derived simply by dividing particles recovered by volume of air processed; additional factors are required. Collection efficiency has two components: (a) an expression (impaction efficiency) of the probability that a particle in the rod's path will, in fact, be

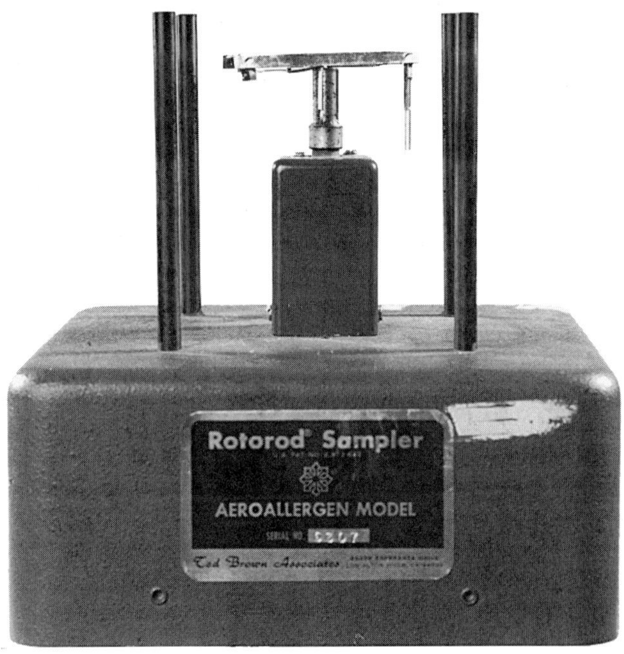

FIGURE 21–3. Intermittent (ac-powered) Rotorod. For illustration purposes, the right-hand rod is shown deployed for collection. Its mate (not shown) is retracted in the crosspiece.

struck and (b) the percent (adhesive efficiency) of intercepted particles that will adhere. Theoretic impaction efficiency varies with particle S_f from a few percent for the smallest micronic particles to over 90% for most pollens. Adhesive efficiency per se has not been estimated, although coatings such as silicone grease, petrolatum, and Lubriseal are useful. In addition, it is clear that adhesive competence decreases, often severely, as particle loading proceeds; this decrement varies with total prevailing atmospheric aerosol. However, the one easily manipulated variable is total operating time. For Midwestern stations, a limit of 20 to 30 minutes per sample has allowed stable adhesive performance.[180]

Collection capabilities of rotating-arm impactors fall substantially with aerosol size, although estimates are possible even for small-particle classes. These realities have prompted use of impactors primarily for recognizable allergens over 10 to 15 μm. For all types, the lack of absolute estimates of efficiency precludes statements of actual prevalence levels. Instead, it is practical to use standardized sampling protocols and express results as particles recovered per unit volume of air processed.

SUCTION SAMPLERS

Devices that recover allergens from measured volumes of aspirated air are varied and offer special advantages for the collection of relatively small particles. In general, two groups of samplers rely on suction sources: filtration units and impingers (including spore traps). Although these devices exploit rather different strategies of collection, they share certain requirements for correct operation. When used in moving air, the entrance efficiency of all suction devices depends on how faithfully they are aligned with the prevailing air stream. Variances of a few degrees may have discernible effects, and orifices at right angles to the wind will be severely disadvantaged.[70] Deficiencies in collection due to improper wind orientation increase with wind speed and the size of particles considered. Although losses of small particles occur, their more faithful response to the drag of entering air lessens their probability of loss.

In addition to the need for wind orientation, optimal entrance efficiency requires equivalent air speed within the entrance orifice and in the immediately surrounding free stream. In this situation of equality, termed isokinetic, lines of air flow enter the sampler without deviation. Because isokinetic conditions are almost impossible to sustain without complex equipment, it is fortunate that errors resulting from their absence normally are relatively low for many airborne allergens.[212] Again, particle size is a factor, with recoveries of the largest and smallest units being most distorted, whereas sampling of 15 to 20 μm particles tends to be least affected when sampling is anisokinetic (not isokinetic).[212]

These considerations suggest basic guidelines for the use of filters and other suction devices. To operate these samplers in freely moving (outdoor) air requires substantial wind vanes, as well as low-friction bearings. However, in relatively still conditions, particle losses due to directional variances are far lower, permitting orifices to be upright (or otherwise arbitrarily directed).

Filters, especially membrane filters, offer low cost and relatively simple volumetric potential. Retention of intercepted particles by intact filters can be essentially complete, and this barrier function extends to aerosols sized well below the rated pore size of the membrane. Compact filter supports facilitate sampling in confined places where air flow is sluggish and wind orientation is not a concern (Fig. 21–4A). The resulting collections may be examined microscopically after clearing the filters with immersion oil or other compatible fluids; specific stains may be applied first. Alternatively, filters exposed with aseptic precautions may be floated on liquid culture media, allowing nutrients to percolate upward through the matrix and support colonial growth.

Membrane filters of various sizes also provide deposits for analysis of specific allergen content. Immunochemical assays for airborne agents have relied on large (e.g., 20 × 25 cm) fiberglass filters exposed for 24-hour periods in high-volume samplers (see Fig. 21–4B).[4] These units are fundamentally large vacuum cleaners rated for continuous operation and adapted for filter supports. High-volume samplers were developed to study total suspended particulates, most of which are between 0.1 and 2 μm. The devices are operated traditionally with filter surfaces directed upward. In rapidly moving air, this approach must be expected to impair collection, at least of relatively large particles, without wind orientation. However, where air speed is quite low, high-volume samplers

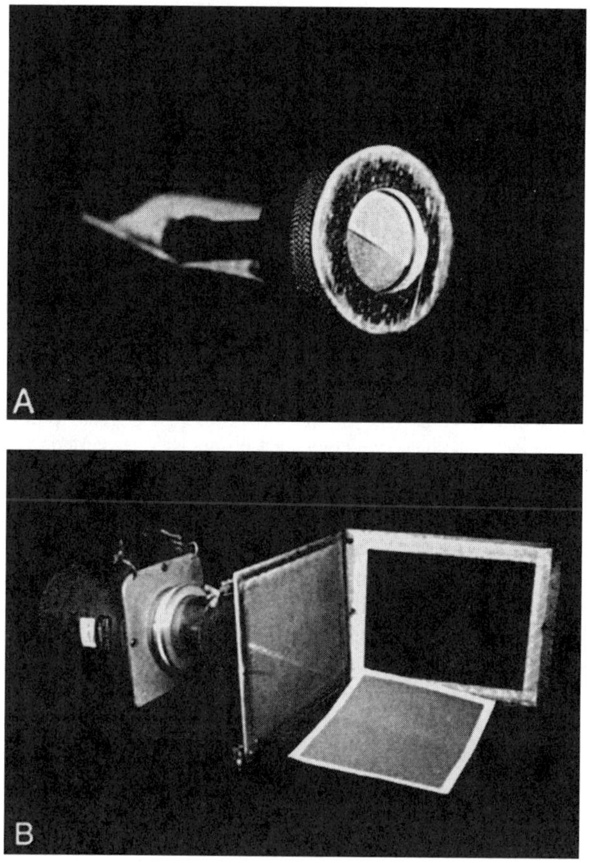

FIGURE 21–4. Two types of sampler that employ the principle of filtration. **(A)** Open-faced filter assembly, with the molecular membrane filter cut away to show supporting grid. **(B)** High-volume sampler partially disassembled to show (exposed) the 8 × 10-inch fiberglass filter.

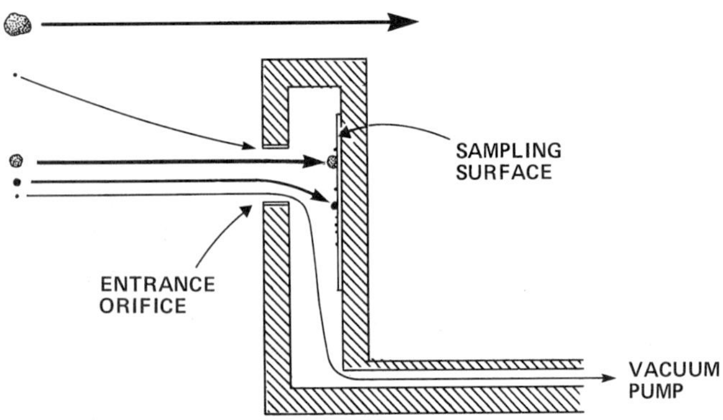

FIGURE 21–5. Inertial deposition by a suction trap. A sharp bend in the flow channel creates the setting for deposition. The greater probability that smaller particles will enter such a sampler is suggested.

provide large amounts of extractable material with reasonable collection efficiency.

Suction traps (inertial suction samplers, impingers) are a diverse group of collectors for biogenic agents. Like filters, these devices need briskly responsive wind orientation and show collection bias when conditions are grossly anisokinetic. Like filters also, suction traps are especially efficient in gathering small micronic particles; therefore, their assets complement (and partially match) those of rotating-arm impactors. All share an operating mode in which particles are aspirated into a flow channel, accelerated, and then forced to negotiate a very sharp bend (Fig. 21–5). Because the ability to change direction varies roughly with $1/S_f$, larger particles are least nimble in this respect and tend to strike (impinge on) the walls of the flow channel. By placing collecting surfaces at impingement points, particle deposits are obtained. The acceleration imparted to a particle helps determine its probability of collection. If particles are raised in stages to progressively higher levels of momentum, as by passage through nozzles of decreasing caliber, progressively small particle fractions tend to impinge at channel bends. This principle is applied directly in cascade impactors, which provide deposits for microscopy, and in sieve impingers, such as the Andersen sampler, which deposit particles in size-specific fractions directly on growth media. However, because the sizing of an aerosol has limited importance for allergists, methods yielding one or two integrated collections receive primary attention.

Perhaps the simplest of practically useful suction samplers are those all-glass devices in which aerosol is accelerated and strikes an obstruction beneath the surface of a fluid volume (Fig. 21–6).[70] The intercepted particles become suspended and, after subsequent filtration, may be grown in culture (or examined microscopically). Considering its relative simplicity (although a pump is required), this approach should be well suited to studying comparatively still interior air. Its appeal, however, is principally cost effectiveness, as other hardware can achieve comparable or better recoveries with fewer steps. Of these, the Andersen sieve impinger continues to provide a standard for volumetric culture collectors. Models designed to separate aerosol into several size-related fractions are widely employed, and single culture plates may be used to telescope collections. Additional volumetric devices facilitate one-plate culture collections during operation in a fixed upright position or can be used as a wand through battery power. A few samplers also provide time-related recoveries by moving the single culture dish with a revolving turntable. Specifications and sources for samplers and air movers have been serially reviewed.[5]

Their value as viable collectors notwithstanding, suction traps function principally to provide volumetric particle deposits for microscopy. This precedence reflects almost exclusively the utility of one device, the Burkard version of the Hirst spore trap. This unit aspirates air at 10 L per minute through a 14 × 2-mm slit, impinging the particles on an adhesive-coated, tape-wound drum. A large integrated vane provides brisk wind responsiveness, and a key-wound clock mechanism allows sampling for 6 or 7 days between drum changes. Intake flow usually is well maintained but should be checked weekly using a specially adapted flowmeter. Various adhesives have been proffered, including silicone greases, petrolatum, and 90% petrolatum and 10% mineral oil. Similarly, diverse materials, including Permount and polyvinyl alcohol-based formulas, are used to mount previously exposed tape segments for microscopy.

We found a combination of Lubriseal grease and hard glycerin jelly mounting medium (prepared by mixing 40 g gelatin, 4 g phenol, 40 ml H_2O, and 195 ml glycerin, with moderate warming in a water bath) to provide optically clear preparations with excellent shelf lives; cover slips of 60 mm

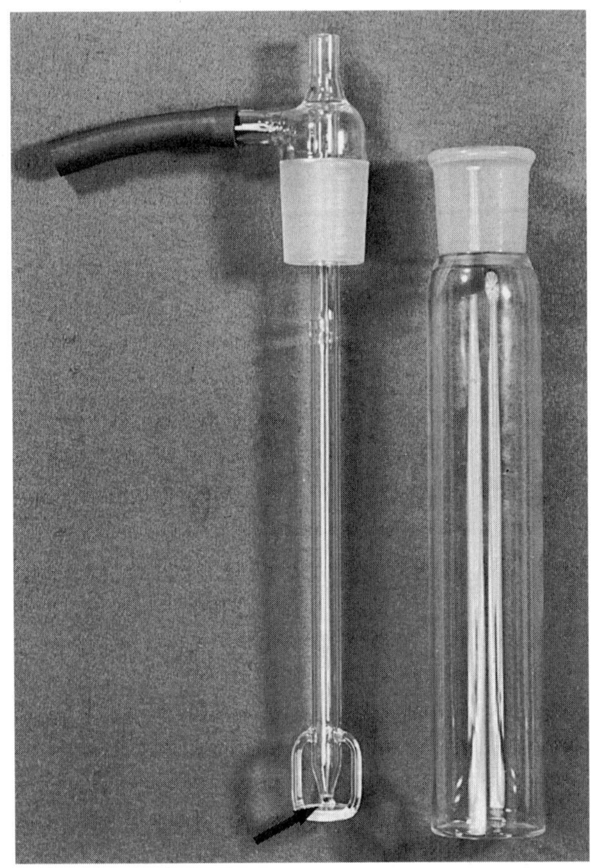

FIGURE 21–6. All-glass impinger. For operation, the impinger tube (left) is partially immersed in fluid contained in the outer cylinder (right). The impinger nozzle and subjacent baffle are shown at the arrow. Air enters the system through the open tube (top) when suction is applied to the rubber tubing (top left).

length are preferred. Deposits may be scanned longitudinally to yield average counts during 24 hours; alternatively, transverse traverses (reflecting specified times) are counted. In either case, the diameter of the microscopic field used and the rate of tape advance must be determined precisely. Assuming a 10 L per minute throughput, a 450 μm field, and a 2 mm (2,000 μm) per hour advance, particles from 600 liters are deposited in 1 hour over a 14 mm band, 2,000 μm in width. One transverse scan, using a 450 μm field, reveals particles derived from 450/2,000 of the 600 L (135 L). As 135 L is 0.135 m^3, direct counts would be divided by 0.135 to derive data per cubic meter, a preferred volumetric unit of reference.

Deposition across the 14 mm band may vary nonrandomly. Therefore, to avoid systematic bias, fields counted during longitudinal scans should be staggered laterally rather than counted in tandem. Only a few estimates of overall efficiency for specific particles exist, but these suggest values exceeding 50% for most expected wind speeds.[70] Unlike most impactors, suction traps show high efficiency for particles 5 to 10 μm and below, although pollen recoveries by the Burkard trap and intermittent Rotorod have been essentially comparable.[177] Additional devices more or less resembling the Burkard trap have been introduced, including the LPPS trap. The performance of the less costly Kramer-Collins trap, which produces particle deposits in discrete time-specific bands, is subject to confirmation but appears fully adequate outdoors.[101] By contrast, samplers without wind orientation are best confined to indoor uses; these include the Burkard 7-day indoor and personal devices, the latter providing a single, discrete collection band on an ordinary microslide. For viable recoveries, the RCS (centrifugal) unit and handheld SAS unit powered by direct current provide integrated collections but do not equal the efficiency of the Andersen sampler.

SELECTING A SAMPLING POINT

Proper siting of collection devices is essential to any aeroallergen sampling effort. Unobstructed access to air flow and an absence of unrecognized sources are paramount. The atmosphere shows a limited capacity for time-dependent mixing, especially near the surface. As a result, sampling may define a series of variably communicating functional mixing volumes, ranging from highly circumscribed interior compartments to extensive air masses at moderate elevations in which homogeneous background levels of natural aerosol prevail. Traditional collections at urban rooftop sites are primarily intended to sample the latter mode but are readily influenced by nearby plantings and other productive sources at the surface. Unimpeded horizontal air flow is especially desirable for rooftop sites. Closely adjacent walls or installation in cul-de-sacs ensures distorted lateral air movement if not flow stagnation. Similar concerns argue against placement of samplers on porches and balconies, where air flow is often predominantly vertical.

Closer to the ground, important opportunities exist for defining patients' exposure hazards both indoors and outdoors using small portable collectors, such as Rotorods powered by direct current and all-glass impingers. Membrane filters and miniaturized pumps, effective as personal samplers in industrial settings, are easily adaptable to particulate allergens. Indoor samples often are essential to identify restricted interior sources, although, as noted previously, the resulting recoveries cannot be assumed to originate within the enclosure studied. To minimize such concerns, studies targeted to indoor sources should be done (where possible) when extramural particulate levels are lowest; in addition, concurrent outdoor allergen levels should be determined.[173] Because even subtle disturbances may substantially elevate local allergen levels, sampling protocols should control for this, recalling that air movers and traffic by technical personnel can effectively promote particle takeoff.

ANALYSIS OF COLLECTIONS

Regardless of their mode of recovery, mixed biogenic aerosols are analyzed by one of three techniques: direct microscopy, culture, or immunoassay. Of these approaches, immunochemical analysis following elution offers an analytic approach to materials without growth potential or defined form, such as animal allergens, seed pomaces, and arthropod debris. Pollen allergens in oligomicron or submicron aerosols have been assayed similarly in bulk samples.[4, 71]

Microscopic identification of distinctive particles is an approach validated by years of increasingly revealing aerometric observations. Correlations between numbers of particles, such as specific pollen grains, and levels of related, assayable allergen, although positive, remain to be precisely defined. However, it is clear that microscopic counts, where feasible, can eliminate viability as one source of low prevalence estimates. Furthermore, a variety of distinctive particles—including many basidiospores and ascospores, plus additional spore emanations of rusts, smuts, and downy and powdery mildews, as well as those of primitive green plants—fail entirely to grow on most laboratory media. Limitations of particle recognition are also easily cited. Generic assignments for hyphal fragments, for example, are effectively speculative, and a host of small spheroidal spores, mutually indistinguishable, often dominate situations, especially indoors. Furthermore, many ascospores and basidiospores lack distinctive features, and spores of some imperfect fungi may vary sufficiently (among species and developmental stages) to blur the best diagnostic criteria. Particle analysis by microscopy, despite its overriding value, requires acceptance of a substantial unknown category.

Approaches to enumerating small-spored imperfect fungi, as well as algae, actinomycetes, and bacteria, all rely on growth in culture. Such viable collections require materials, space, sterile precautions, and painstaking sequential observations, often with microscopy of primary isolates or subcultures. At best, cultures tend to understate levels of prevalence.[28] At worst, numerous airborne types, such as *Botrytis, Helminthosporium*, and *Stemphylium* species, often grow only casually on the most useful multipurpose media, such as malt extract agar and potato dextrose agar.[30] Faulty views of prevalence also may result if a spore of one life cycle stage produces a different growth form of the same species in culture. For example, certain common ascospores (sexual spores) may germinate on agar to produce only reproductive stages bearing abundant asexual spores, although the latter spores seldom occur in free air. In this scenario, the actual

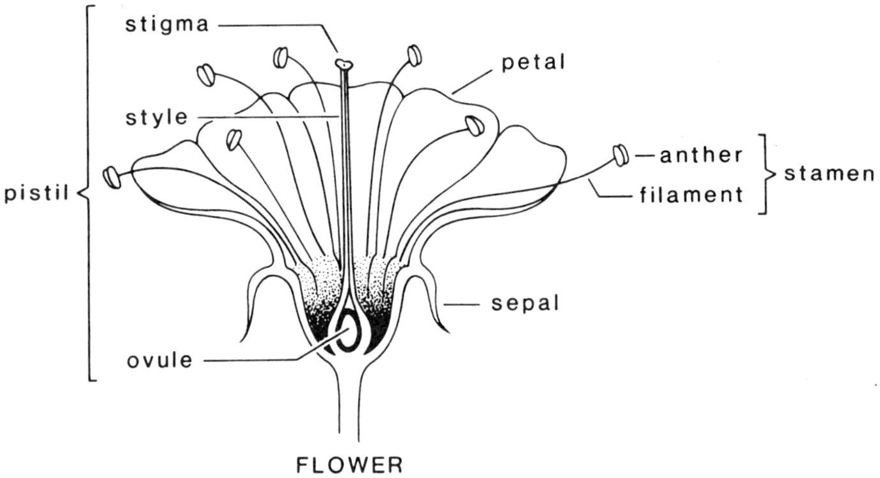

FIGURE 21–7. Parts of a "perfect" flower, in cross section.

vectors of exposure may be overlooked unless nonviable samples also are examined. Overall, culture remains a necessity for many small-spored taxa but generally is not preferred for types readily identified by direct microscopy.

ALLERGENIC POLLENS AND THEIR SOURCES

Flowering plants can be classified according to their mode of pollination. Anemophilous plants disperse pollens by wind, entemophilous species are insect pollinated, and amphiphilous types utilize both wind and insect or other self-propelled vectors. Wind-dispersed pollens tend to be abundant, small, and relatively smooth walled, whereas entemophily promotes fewer grains that are sticky and often deeply sculptured. Wind-pollinated flowers, lacking insect attractants, have inconspicuous petals and sepals, whereas, among entemophilous plants, these are typically large and brightly colored and enclose nectar-producing glands (Fig. 21–7). The flowers of anemophilous plants are often unisexual (imperfect), in contrast to the usually perfect flowers of insect-pollinated types, in which stamens and pistils occur together.

In some species, termed "dioecious," individual plants have exclusively pollen-producing or pollen-receiving organs. Other species are monoecious, having separate staminate and pistillate flowers present on the same plant, as in *Ambrosia* (ragweeds). Important allergenic pollen sources are primarily anemophilous, the ragweeds being good examples. However, a few of the amphiphilous plants, such as willow and linden, also share limited importance. In addition, some entemophilous species that are cropped extensively or overplanted in the urban landscape may become locally significant.

Wind dispersal of genetic material is an ancient strategy. Spores of ferns and fungi spread in this way, as do pollens of the relatively primitive gymnosperms (conifers and their allies). In the middle Mesozoic Era (perhaps 150 million years ago), the angiosperms (including most familiar flowering plants except conifers) appeared, coevolving with insect vectors. Later, some angiosperms readapted to wind pollination, and about 10% of species are anemophilous today.

FUNCTIONAL ANATOMY OF POLLENS

Pollen functions ultimately to carry male genes to the ovule, permitting fertilization. However, this outcome first requires transfer of suitable grains to the stigma, the most accessible portion of the pistil. Grains develop in cavities of the anther in a medium of tapetal fluid, undergo reduction division following pollination, and produce haploid (unpaired chromosome-bearing, reproductive nuclei (Fig. 21–8).

The pollen wall has two principal components: an outer, highly durable, exine (secreted by the tapetum) and, within it, the intine contributed by the developing protoplast (Fig. 21–9). The exine has two layers: the sexine, with a sculptured layer of tiny rods called baculae, and the more continuous inner nexine. The rods, which can be fused, often support a roof (tectum) that is smooth or ornamented with verrucae (warts) or spines. Except for an innermost layer (nexine-2), the exine stains well with basic dyes, such as fuchsin.

The featureless intine of microfibrillar cellulose is not readily stained but contains acid phosphatase, ribonuclease, nonspecific esterase, amylases, and proteases.[76] These enzymes are concentrated at apertures (when present), where the pollen tube is most apt to emerge during germination (Fig. 21–10). The exine has storage areas for soluble substances secreted by tapetal cells, including potential allergens. After the pollen grain contacts a stigma, this surface material provides signals recognizable by a compatible female organ.[76] The secretions of a receptive stigma hydrate the grain, releasing enzymes that dissolve a path for the pollen tube as it grows down through stigmatic tissue to the ovule. Bousquet and Michel[22] found that the enzyme content of certain pollens parallels their allergen potency, although this correlation is not universal. However, a role in pollen-stigma recognition processes is strongly suspected for several major pollen allergens. Whether additional sensitizers are localized to intine remains to be established.

Some differences among pollen allergens of even closely related plant species may be assumed, even when grains are indistinguishable morphologically. Therefore, pollen recoveries from air are best correlated with community surveys of prevalent anemophilous plants and clinical symptom patterns. Several illustrated references provide help in gaining

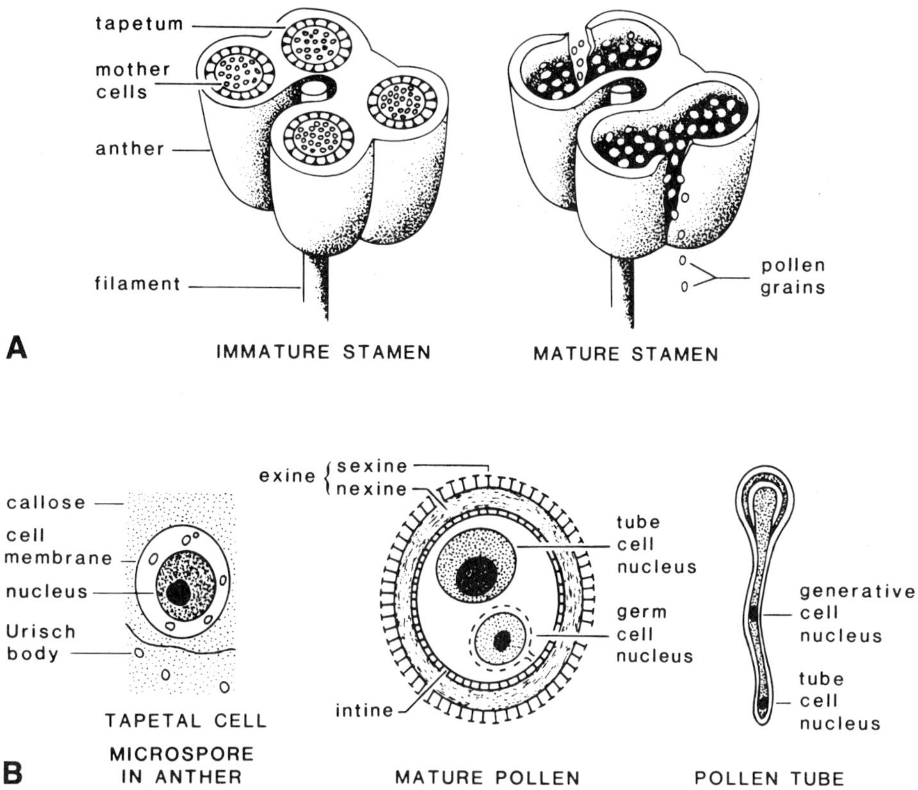

FIGURE 21–8. (A) Pollen grain development occurs in the anther sacs of stamens from generative (mother) cells. A nutritive cell layer (tapetum) lines these cavities. Anther breakdown (right) leads to liberation of pollen. **(B)** Three stages in the life cycle of a pollen grain. A developing grain, or microspore, is nurtured by tapetal cells (at left). In some species, tiny spheres of exine substance (Übisch bodies) also are formed and released. At center, a mature (multicellular) pollen grain is shown. On a receptive stigma, viable grains will germinate (at right) to form a pollen tube, which facilitates penetration of the ovary and fertilization.

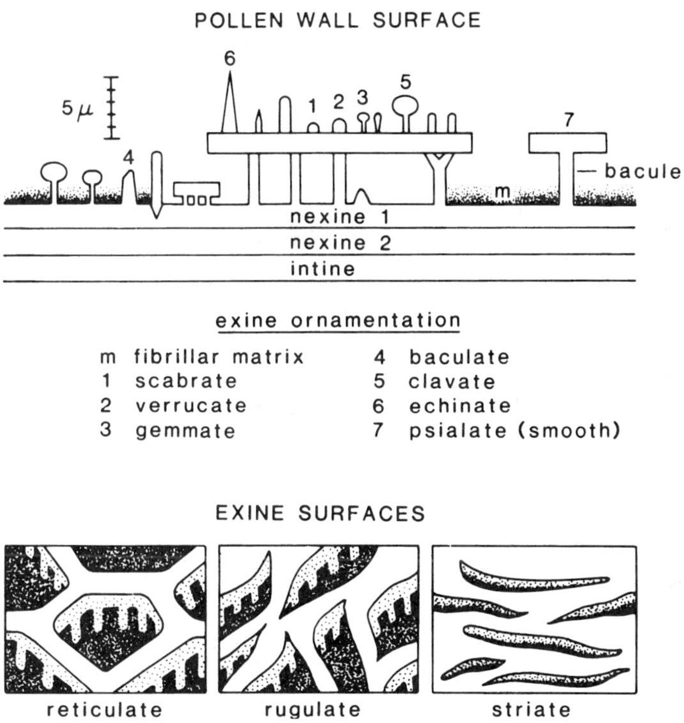

FIGURE 21–9. Features of the pollen grain surface. The diagram at top shows a cross section of the wall layers. Numbered surface features and descriptive designations correspond.

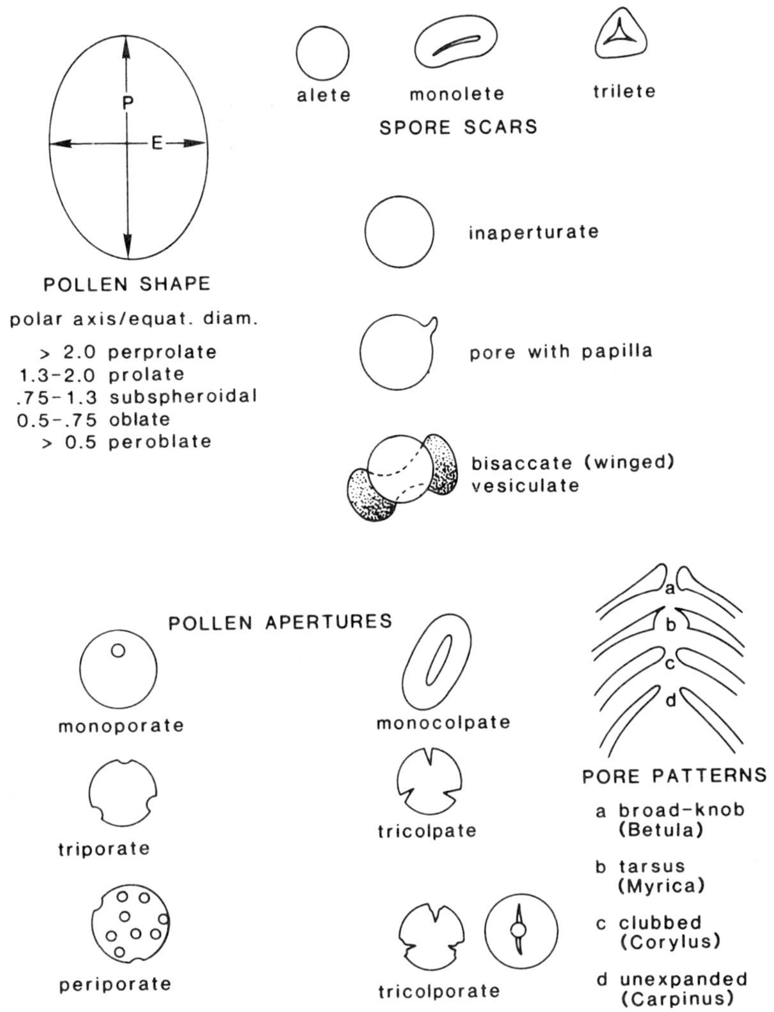

FIGURE 21–10. Terminology of pollen shape, apertures, and other features. E = equatorial diameter; P = polar diameter.

familiarity with pollen sources.[16, 53, 67, 85, 97, 125, 199, 218] In addition, the *Popular Series* of the Southwest Parks and Monuments Association in Tuscon, AZ, provides insight into plants of that region.

CRITERIA FOR POLLEN IDENTIFICATION

Although authenticated known specimens (appropriately mounted and stained) best illustrate the distinctions among pollen types, published manuals also provide assistance.[15, 82, 109, 135, 172] Most pollen types recovered from air prove to be single grains. A few exist as tetrads *(Typha)* or polyads *(Acacia)*, and others are vesiculate (have air bladders), such as those of *Pinus* and *Podocarpus*. With hydration, most types assume a more or less spherical shape designated according to the polar axis/equatorial diameter index. The poles are areas at the ends of one or more furrows or the regions farthest from the centers of a (frequent) meridian of pores, termed the equator. See Figure 21–10 for designations of pollen shape and examples of various scar, pore, and furrow characteristics. Pollen grains are described in terms of their sizes, shapes, apertures (pores or furrows), and surface textures—smooth, verrucate, echinulate, reticulate, rugulate, or striate (see Fig. 21–9). The pores may be capped by a disc of exine (operculum), or there may be a refractile transparent collar (aspis) beneath the stained exine or a surface ring of thickened exine (annulus) around the pore.

ECOLOGY OF POLLEN PREVALENCE

A single anemophilous plant may produce millions of pollen grains. Rupture of the ripe anthers occurs when proper conditions of light, temperature, and relative humidity exist. Once the pollen dries following release, it is dispersed readily by wind, but long-range transport is the exception. In ragweeds, for example, over 95% is lost, chiefly by fallout, within 1 km of the plant. The shape, size, and weight of a pollen grain are important factors affecting its potential for both fallout and significant transport. In addition, buildings and trees may intercept pollens, and fallout may rise modestly with high humidity, thereby lowering atmospheric prevalence.

A fraction of aerodynamically small particles may be transported great distances by wind. Pollens of birches and pines have been recovered on ships 35 to 55 km from land, and over the mid-Atlantic, 0.7 to 1.4 pollen grains/100 cubic meters have been found.[70] Such long-range transport is opposed by size-dependent deposition tendencies. At equilibrium, a spherical 20 μm unit density grain falls at 4.8 cm/second; one of 30 μm falls at 10.9 cm/second. An average-sized (25 μm) pollen grain would travel 67 meters while falling at 7.5 cm/second from the height of 1 meter in a steady wind of 10 knots. However, other factors affect particle transport, most notably downwind, crosswind, and vertical velocity components, which may aid or oppose fallout.

Upward air currents carry particles emitted near the surface to higher levels. The extent of vertical movement depends on the stability of the lower atmosphere; this in turn is governed by the lapse rate (rate of vertical temperature decrease). If the lapse rate exceeds 1°C per 100 meters, there will be relative instability, active upward motion, and good mixing in a relative deep atmospheric layer. By contrast, in a stable atmosphere, where cooling with height is less, particles (and pollutants) may travel long distances with minimal vertical motion, and the mixing layer often is relatively shallow. The stability of the lowest kilometer of the atmosphere undergoes continuous variation, often changing sharply with passage of weather fronts. During the night, there is radiative cooling of the earth's surface, which promotes stability as the normal fall of temperature with altitude is reversed. After sunrise, progressive solar heating of the earth's surface leads to instability and active vertical movement.

Environmental conditions strongly influence pollen shedding (anthesis). Among many grasses, the start of the flowering period demands critical levels of cumulative temperature, and anthesis requires sunshine and is inhibited by overcast conditions. However, a rapid decrease in light intensity can cause a burst of anthesis by rye flowers that are ready to open, an effect that can occur naturally from the passing of clouds. Ragweeds are stimulated to develop flower clusters with increasing night length (negative photoperiodism), and their typical pollen shedding shortly after sunrise requires rising temperatures and decreasing relative humidity.[48]

For the ragweeds, Reiss[151] noted abundant pollen in a season after the temperature had stayed above 60°F from early May through mid-June and a mid- to late-spring period of rainfall appeared to increase the pollen yield. Most short ragweed seeds germinate in May, so that favorable conditions early allow a longer growth period before anthesis. In temperate regions, trees form flower bud primordia (for the following spring) during the summer months. If it is especially hot and dry, the stress stimulates increased production of these structures and potentially the next year's pollen output.

At the beginning of a flowering period for any species, sexual parts are maturing progressively, and there is a large store of pollen-filled stamens awaiting favorable (generally warm and dry) weather conditions. Toward the end of that season, however, nearly all stamens have been discharged, and, even with favorable weather conditions, progressively less pollen is released.

Ironically, where the natural flora is most altered, selective factors often favor plants producing especially allergenic pollens. At the edges of cultivated fields, the ragweeds, as well as *Amaranthus* and *Chenopodium* species, grow well, and as fields are abandoned (or harvested), these plants quickly take over. Silted soil in waterways is preferred by giant ragweed, Johnson grass, nettles, amaranths, and chenopods. The latter two groups, along with plantain and Bermuda grass, also thrive where soil is compacted by foot traffic that may have destroyed less resilient native species. The cultivation of hemp *(Cannabis)* for fiber in the Midwestern United States during the 1940s introduced an aggressive weed that is still abundant. Similarly, the southwestern deserts were a refuge for pollinosis sufferers until the population grew, bringing development, cultivation, and irrigation, with rapid invasion and growth of wind-pollinated plants.

SOURCES OF ALLERGENIC PLANT PARTICLES

CLUB MOSSES AND FERNS (DIVISION PTERIDOPHYTA)

Pteridophytes are plants with specialized vascular channels that reproduce by spores rather than flowers and seeds. Club mosses (*Lycopodium* species) often carpet northern woodlands, sporulating from midsummer onward. The highly flammable spores are used in fireworks and stage lighting and formerly provided an inert powder for pharmaceuticals. Sporadic reports of occupational allergic symptoms from these materials have appeared. The spores average 33 μm and are somewhat triangular, with a reticulate outer coating and a triradiate (trilete) scar (see Fig. 21–10). Ferns are related plants with similar spores (often containing chlorophyll), which occasionally are found on air sampling in natural areas. Clinical sensitivity to these has been described, especially in Southeast Asia, but their impact remains unclear.

GYMNOSPERMS

Gymnosperms are relatively ancient plants, with some contemporary types also prominent in fossil deposits, e.g., Cycadales (sago palm and comfort root) and ginkgo. In this group of naked seed-bearing plants are the conifers, such as pines, firs, and larches, and the Gnetales (desert and tropical plants), including *Ephedra*, the source for ephedrine.

The ginkgo (maidenhair tree) is a dioecious tree with small, broad fan-shaped leaves. Mature male specimens shed moderate amounts of lightweight pollen, which like that of the palms is boat shaped and 27 to 32 μm long, with a single, longitudinal furrow. Its allergenic activity remains to be assessed.

The pines *(Pinus)*, spruces *(Picea)*, and firs *(Abies)* have two sizable air bladders on each pollen grain for added buoyancy and are woody evergreens with linear leaves (Fig. 21–11). The familiar pines have long needles in discrete bundles with staminate cones clustered at the base of each new year's growth. Their grains range from 44 to 65 μm exclusive of the bladders, which are 20 μm or larger. Pollen is shed copiously and may be transported great distances. However, it has been reported only rarely to cause overt allergy. The clinical significance of spruce and fir pollens is equally uncertain. Kalliel and Settipane[86] found that 10% of seasonal rhinitis patients were positive to a white pine pollen extract, whereas 6% were positive among those with perennial symptoms.

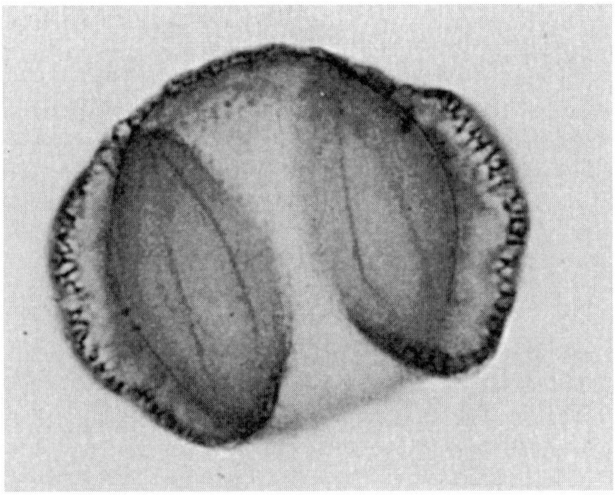

FIGURE 21–11. Pine pollen. The large central grain and two ventrolateral bladders are characteristic of pine, spruce, and fir pollens.

Spruces have separate, four-angled leaves distributed evenly around the stems. The pollens resemble those of pines but are larger, averaging 68 to 91 μm exclusive of the two bladders. The white and red spruces are common in colder parts of the eastern United States, whereas the Engelmann, Colorado blue, and Sitka spruces are familiar evergreens of the northwest. Firs, with flattened evergreen needles that are two ranked, produce the largest bladdered pollen grains of the conifers, ranging from 78 to over 100 μm.

The hemlocks *(Tsuga)* are tall pyramidal trees. *T. canadensis* and *T. heterophylla* pollens have no evident bladders and are 60 to 85 μm and 50 to 55 μm, respectively. Hemlock pollen is locally abundant and may contribute briefly to allergic symptoms.

The Cupressaceae is a grouping of woody plants with reduced, scale-like leaves and very small pistillate cones. Their pollens are 20 to 40 μm and spheroidal, with a thick intine that can swell to rupture and cast off the fragile exine (Fig. 21–12). Immunologic cross-reactivity patterns among cypress *(Cupressus)*, arbor vitae *(Thuja)*, incense cedar *(Libocedrus)*, and juniper *(Juniperus)* species have been verified.[223] The coast redwood *(Sequoia)*, Japanese cedar *(Cryptomeria)*, and bald cypress *(Taxodium)* appear to have different antigenic affinities, as seen by double diffusion and direct allergenic skin testing.[223] *Cryptomeria japonica* (Sugi) is the most important tree pollen allergen source in Japan, causing major morbidity.[222] *Taxodium distichum* is a common tree of southeastern swamps with deciduous leaves; the larches *(Larix)* also are leafless in winter. Bucholtz and colleagues[25] reported the occurrence of respiratory allergy to bald cypress pollen in Florida.

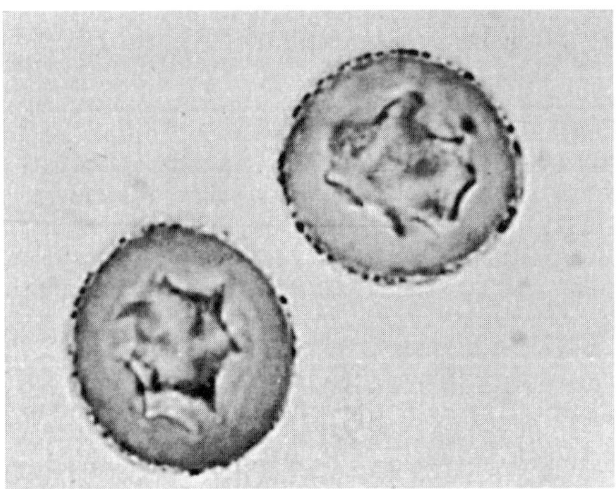

FIGURE 21–12. Juniper pollen. The star-shaped (central) protoplast and thick surrounding intine are typical of many species of the Cupressaceae, the juniper–cypress family.

Juniperus ashei (mountain cedar) probably is the principal hay fever plant among the gymnosperms. *J. virginiana* (eastern red cedar), *J. communis*, and related species are similar but lesser pollen producers. In milder climates, including much of the American southwest, *J. ashei* pollen is shed in midwinter. Elsewhere, pollination by other species can occur in the fall or more commonly in early spring. These small shrubs and trees are dioecious, with tiny staminate cones producing, in the third year after pollination, a berry-like fruit that is blue, blue-black, brown, or red. *J. ashei (syn. J. mexicana, J. sabinoides)* has become a dominant species in parts of west Texas and nearby areas where overgrazing has depleted the natural grasses. The allergenic activity of mountain cedar pollen may be concentrated in a single carbohydrate-rich glycoprotein.[147] Patients with isolated reactivity to mountain cedar pollen are not rare, whereas others show additional sensitivities. A pronounced negative correlation between HLA-DR4 and *J. ashei*–specific IgE responses has been described.[150] Pollen of the Japanese cedar *(Cryptomeria japonica)* contains a glycoprotein allergen of 40,000 kD that may resemble a component of mountain cedar[222] although this view is not uniformly held.[223] A 43 kD major (glycoprotein) allergen of *Cupressus arizonica* pollen also has been described, which appears to show marked lability during extraction.[47]

ANGIOSPERMS

Conventional flowering plants (angiosperms) comprise two subclasses, the Monocotyledonae and Dicotyledonae; members of both groups produce pollen allergens. Features of typical Monocotyledonae include discrete vascular bundles scattered throughout the stems, parallel leaf venation, and flowering parts, such as petals, sepals, and anthers, arranged in threes or its multiples. By contrast, Dicotyledonae tend to show rings (cylinders) of vascular elements, freely branching venation, and flowering parts usually in multiples of fours and fives.

Monocotyledons

The grasses (Gramineae), with usually perfect flowers, comprise the largest grouping of contemporary anemophilous plants. Of approximately 4,500 species worldwide and 1,100 native to North America, however, only a fraction are important allergenically. Some grasses are self-fertile, and the majority cross-pollinate; most shed relatively small amounts of pollen. Many grasses bloom during 3- to 6-week seasons that overlap partially, but, in milder climates, some species pollinate nearly throughout the year. Grass pollen, although

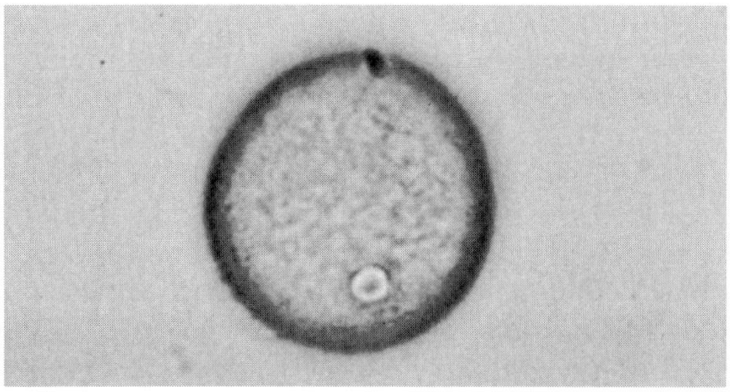

FIGURE 21–13. Grass pollen. The single pore and central operculum are typical.

probably the leading plant-derived allergen in most of Europe, is second in importance to ragweed in North America. People who reactive exclusively to grass pollen are not rare, and Bousquet[21] has suggested that these people may show different IgE-dependent amplification mechanisms from those with diverse pollen sensitivities and more favorable responses to immunotherapy. An association of adverse reactivity to certain foods, especially tomato, has been described in grass pollen sensitivity; however, neither the basis nor the overall impact of this has been defined.[138]

The grass pollens all are fairly similar in appearance, having a finely granular, thin exine and a single germinal pore with a central operculum (Fig. 21–13). Although the mean pollen sizes of various grasses may differ characteristically, most grains cannot be assigned to source species microscopically.

Grass pollen allergens comprise several groups that differ among species and may be absent selectively from some taxa. Among cool temperate zone grasses, group I and V allergens appear to be especially important, whereas groups II, III, IV, and VI and profilins seem less significant.[1] Multiple IgE-reactive epitopes are present on at least some allergens, as shown for Phl p 5a of timothy grass.[27] The occurrence of grass pollen allergens in multiple isoforms over a pH range from 4 to 9 further increases their complexity.

Sweet vernal *(Anthoxanthum odoratum)* is a fragrant grass that blooms from the first week of May to mid-June in the northern tier of states and adjacent Canada. Orchard grass *(Dactylis glomerata)*, which grows in moist areas with cool climates, often follows, with pollen from late May to late June. The June (blue) grasses are important early summer species of northern states. Kentucky blue grass *(Poa pratensis)* reaches 1 to 3 feet, is widespread, and blooms from early May to late June. A shorter relative, *Poa annua*, also is common but emits very little airborne pollen. *Poa compressa* is a more productive, related pollinator in the northern United States and Canada, flowering from June to August.

Timothy *(Phleum pratense)* is a widely utilized, temperate zone hay and pasture grass with a weedy potential. It blooms in June and July and has a compact terminal spike of tiny flowers (florets). During the same season, red top grass *(Agrostis alba)* is locally important. This species often reaches 2 to 4 feet in height and has a branched arrangement (panicle) of florets from June to July in northern states, and earlier at lower latitudes. As seeds mature, the floral parts take on a distinctive, deep maroon color.

Bermuda grass *(Cynodon dactylon)* is a principal pollen source in southern and southwestern states, blooming essentially throughout the year in frost-free areas. It is also widely distributed throughout the Eastern Hemisphere and in warmer regions worldwide. Little or no cross-reactivity of Bermuda grass pollen with those of previously mentioned types is recognized, requiring them to be treated as separate entities for purposes of skin testing and immunotherapy. Chang and colleagues[36] described 11 isoforms of Cyn d 1, including both acidic and basic types. The basic isoform, Cyn d 1-J (33 kD), may be especially necessary, along with acidic isoforms, for testing and treatment.

Johnson grass *(Sorghum halepense)* is a robust perennial that produces a large, open, purplish panicle from July to September in southern states. Its pollen size (40–46 μm) generally exceeds those of previously mentioned species. A taller relative, Sudan grass *(Sorghum vulgare* var. *sudanense)*, is an annual with greenish flower clusters; both add variably to the (Bermuda) grass pollen allergen load.

Perennial rye grass *(Lolium perenne)* is present in most of North America and Europe and seems especially important on the Pacific coast. The pollen is shed principally in July and early August and has two well-characterized allergens, Lol p 1 (27 kD) and Lol p 2 (11 kD).[64] Reaction rates to Lol p 1 have been 85% to 90% among subjects sensitive to rye grass pollen, whereas half this number respond to Lol p 2. Although these allergens lack cross-reactivity, responses to both molecules may reflect common genetic control elements.

Fescues, including *Festuca elatior*, a 2- to 5-foot species, and the shorter *F. rubra*, bloom during June and July in cooler parts of North America and are prominent pasture grasses, often used to cover shady ground. The related *Festuca ovina* (sheep fescue) is another common eastern species. All are grass pollen sources of limited importance.

A host of additional less generous sources, which might produce pollinosis owing to local abundance, may be cited. Quack grass *(Agropyron repens)* is widespread and blooms from July to September. Western June grass *(Koeleria cristata)* is especially prevalent in Oregon and Wyoming. Velvet grass *(Holcus lanatus)* flowers from June to August in the Pacific Northwest and British Columbia. Beach grass *(Ammophila spp.)* grows on dunes and in wetlands from North Carolina to Newfoundland and along the Great Lakes, flowering from June to September. Salt grass *(Distichlis spicata)* is conspicuous all along the eastern and gulf coastlines, whereas *Bromus rigidus* and *B. mollis* shed pollen on the Pacific coast from May to July. Pollen of *Secale cereale* (cultivated rye) is large (53–57 μm) and is said to be more common as an allergen in Europe. St. Augustine grass *(Stenotaphrum secundatum)*, a common lawn grass of the south with a dense web of runners, sheds little pollen but contributes much aerial *Helminthosporium* contamination from its thatch, especially when mowed. *Paspalum notatum* is widespread in Florida and Texas, eliciting positive skin reactions in exposed allergic children (M. L. Jelks, unpublished data), a finding noted elsewhere by Hensel and Griffith.[73] Pollen of *Zea mays* (corn), which is among the largest windborne grains (80 to well over 100 μm), generally falls out too rapidly to cause pollinosis at any distance from plants in tassel.

Although turf cutting facilitates exposure to grass pollen, other previously deposited pollens, arthropod fragments and abundant fungus particles also are dispersed. Patients sensitive to fungus often report symptoms when cutting grass or performing other turf care activities.

Less important grass allies include the sedges (Cyperaceae), which flower in wetlands from April through July. The pollen is distinctively pear shaped and averages 38 μm in its longest dimension. Members of the Juncaceae, especially the wood rush, *Juncoides (Luzula) campestre*, have pollen grains in tetrads (fixed groupings of four), but these rarely are recovered away from woodlands. The cattails (Typhaceae) have grass-like pollens with coarsely granular surfaces. Pollen grains of *Typha latifolia* also are dispersed in tetrads, whereas those of *T. angustifolia* occur singly. The flowers of both species form solitary spikes of densely crowded stamens above the pistils. Pollens of both sedges and cattails show definite allergenic differences from pollens of familiar grasses.[179]

Leiferman and Gleich[105] studied grass pollen allergens and found strong similarities among those of June, fescue, orchard, and perennial rye. Partial cross-reactivity of timothy pollen with those of many other northern grasses is suggested, although distinctive features of timothy also are recognized. Osterballe[139] demonstrated that whole timothy pollen allergen extract provided superior immunotherapy to a purified pollen allergen that contained only 2 other components of a 20-component grass extract. Martin and colleagues[117] found that timothy, June, fescue, red top, and perennial rye, which shared group I rye grass allergens, also contained some allergens of brome grasses. The grasses with prominent group II allergens—brome, sweet vernal, and paspalum—lacked some group I components. Pollens of group III affinity—quack, salt, and Bermuda grasses—shared activity but were only minimally related to groups I and II. Pollen reactivity of western wheat grasses was most unlike that of group I allergens, and Johnson and grama grasses were also quite distinctive. These relationships may have substantial practical importance in planning immunotherapy. In addition, Turkeltaub[197] emphasized the potential dangers of administering irrelevant allergens with conversion to positive skin tests in nonatopics after grass allergoid injections, one subject developing clinical symptoms on subsequent natural exposure.

Palms (Palmaceae) vary in allergenicity, with coconut palm pollen tenuously implicated in tropical areas; most are probably minor offenders at best. All palm pollens are elongated, with a single furrow when dry, and subspherical when expanded in aqueous media. The date palms *(Phoenix)* are mainly anemophilous and may cause pollinosis locally, whereas the queen palm, *Syagrus romanzoffianum* (syn. *Arecastrum r., Cocos plumosus*) is partially insect pollinated; both have commercial skin test extracts. *Paurotis wrightii* (or *Acoelorrhaphe wrightii*) is a wind-pollinated native of the Florida everglades. However, *Sabal palmetto* is definitely insect pollinated, as are the saw palmetto *(Serenoa repens)* and the widely planted royal palm.

Dicotyledons

Salicaceae (willows and poplars). Many willows are mainly insect pollinated but also contribute windborne pollen in small amounts. Willow grains are small and easily dispersed; upright male and female catkins are produced on separate

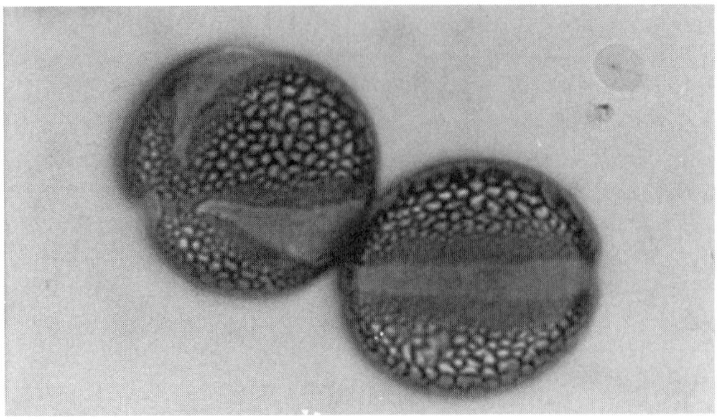

FIGURE 21–14. Willow pollen. The somewhat elongated (prolate) grains with a reticulum that becomes finer close to the three furrows identify this type.

trees. In some species, such as *Salix purpurea*, the catkins (elongated, densely packed flower clusters) appear before the leaves; others flower as the leaves expand. *Salix nigra*, a common eastern willow, grows along streams and has linear leaves with finely toothed margins; the leaves are lustrous green above and paler on the underside. Pollination occurs from March to early July, depending on the location. As a sensitizer, willow pollen is of modest importance in many areas. The grains are 18 to 20 μm and prolate, with three parallel furrows and a prominently reticulate exine (Fig. 21–14). Although unrelated, tamarisk *(Tamarix)* species have morphologically similar pollen grains, produced in summer, especially in southwestern states.

The poplars, aspens, and cottonwoods (genus *Populus*) are entirely wind-pollinated dioecious trees. Both staminate and pistillate catkins are pendulous, typically appearing just before the leaves in early spring. *Populus* pollen is spheroidal and 27 to 34 μm in diameter with a thin, granular, unsculptured exine and a thick hyaline intine; no obvious apertures are present. *Populus deltoides*, reaching 100 feet in eastern North America, has triangular leaves and commonly grows in moist situations. The seeds of the many poplars and cottonwoods have cottony tufts that are highly visible and cause these trees to be blamed, usually erroneously, for allergic symptoms in summer, long after the pollen is gone. *Populus alba, P. nigra* (black or Lombardy poplar), and *P. canadensis* (Carolina poplar, a sterile hybrid producing little or no pollen) are used widely as windbreaks. *P. tremuloides* (quaking aspen) is common in cooler portions of North America where a relative, *P. grandidentata*, also occurs; both are rapid-growing colonizers where climax growth has been removed.

Betulaceae (birches, alders, hornbeams, hazels). Members of this woody family shed large amounts of windborne pollen. Birch pollen is a principal allergen in Scandinavia and is widespread in colder, temperate regions.[83] The trees are monoecious, with pendulous, unisexual catkins opening in spring just as the leaves expand. Birches often are pioneer species in fire scars and are prominent under maturing pines in forests of the southeast. The paper birch of Canada and the northeastern United States and the river birch often grow up to 100 feet. Birch pollens appear in April and May and closely resemble those of *Celtis* (hackberry), *Comptonia* (sweet fern), *Myrica* (bayberry), and *Casuarina* (Australian pine), which are plants of unrelated families. Grains are 25 to 30 μm in diameter and have a smooth exine and three protruding pores with underlying appendages (aspides).

In the Pacific Northwest, the alders *(Alnus)*, especially red alder *(A. rubra)*, are important pollen producers. Alders often are the first trees in a locality to bloom. In southern states, pollen may appear in January; in northern areas, March or April is more typical. The pollens are 19 to 27 μm and have four or usually five pores that protrude and are connected by curved bands of thickened exine (arci). *Alnus* species are especially prominent within 50 km of the seacoasts of North America.

Carpinus caroliniana (American hornbeam) grows mainly east of the Mississippi River and blooms briefly in April and May. The pollen is three-pored and close to 26 μm in diameter; a close relative, *Ostrya virginiana* (ironwood, hophornbeam), flowering concurrently, has similar pollen. *Corylus americana* (hazel) blooms very early in the year with pollen that is superficially similar to birch but more triangular in outline. Many pollen allergens of the Betulaceae cross-react with or resemble components of common foods. Breiteneder and colleagues[24] showed binding of sera from appropriately sensitive subjects to natural Aln g 1 *(Alnus glutinosa)* protein, as well as recombinant proteins rAln g 1 and rBet v 1. The major pollen allergens of European birch, *Betula verrucosa* (Bet v 1), alder (Aln g 1), hazel (Cor a 1), and hornbeam (Car a 1) are homologous at the nucleic acid and amino acid level. In fact, Valenta and colleagues[201] have suggested that Bet v 1–rich extracts should be sufficient to deal with sensitivity to European birch, alder, hazel, and hornbeam, both diagnostically and therapeutically. Hirschwehr and collegues[78] found a 14 kD protein of hazel pollen and hazelnut (per se) belonging to the profilins, which also resembled birch profilin (Bet v 2). They described an 18 kD allergen in hazelnut extract that shared epitopes with European hazel pollen and birch pollen. These determinants were present also in many fruits and vegetables and may help to explain increased food intolerance observed among affected pollinosis patients.[138] A report by Gall and colleagues,[65] describing 22 patients with kiwi fruit allergy and serum antibodies that cross-reacted with birch pollen, provides the latest addition to a food list, including apple, carrot, potato, hazelnut, and several stone fruits, to which birch pollinosis patients more often are intolerant. On the other hand, Pastorello and colleagues[140] described an oral allergy syndrome with ingestion of fruits of the Prunoideae, such as apples and cherries, having a common 13 kD allergen unrelated to grass or birch pollen components.

Fagaceae (beech, oak, chestnut, chinquapins). Fagus grandifolia (American beech) is a deciduous tree reaching 60 to 100 feet with globular staminate heads that shed pollen as the leaves open. In February or March in the Gulf States and later in the North, the 40 μm spherical grains with three tapered furrows may reach moderate levels locally. Beech pollen has received little attention in North America but a European species is regarded as a regionally important aeroallergen.

Oaks (the genus *Quercus*), both deciduous (leafless in winter) and evergreen, contribute one of the most abundant and familiar pollen types in wooded areas. The 25 to 32 μm grains have three furrows and coarsely granular exines (Fig. 21–15). There are approximately 275 major varieties of oaks in North America, including Mexico, with special abundance in eastern forests. Four groupings of oaks are described: black oaks, willow oaks, white oaks, and chestnut oaks. Of the black oaks, *Quercus velutina* and *Q. rubra* in the east, with deeply lobed leaves, and *Q. nigra* in the southeast, with almost smooth margins, are especially prominent; all are deciduous. The willow oaks have lance-shaped leaves and some, such as *Quercus phellos*, are semievergreen in the south. The white oaks comprise the largest division of the family and overall are most abundant. *Quercus alba* dominates this group in the eastern states and has smoothly rounded leaf lobes. Live oak *(Quercus virginiana)*, a large coastal tree, is evergreen, with thick, leathery leaves falling off just as new leaves appear. There are smaller evergreen oaks of the white oak group that are scrubby, such as *Q. minima* and *Q. geminata*, as well as scrub oaks, including the bur oak *(Q. macrocarpa)*, Gambel's oak, and others. Additional scrub oaks belong to the black oak group, along with the northern red. The chestnut oaks, such as *Q. prinus*, have coarsely toothed leaves, grow in rocky areas, and are least often implicated as hay fever plants.

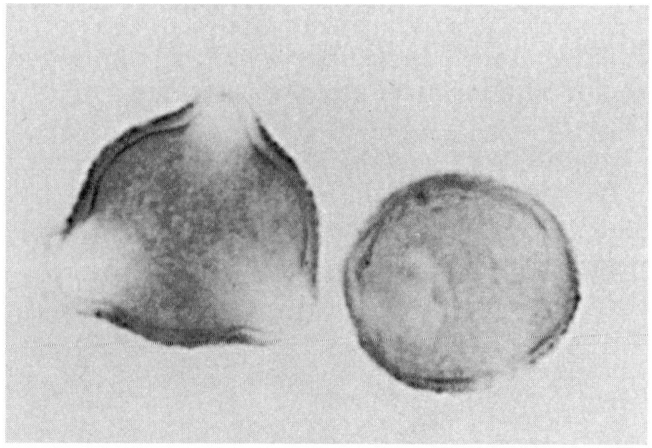

FIGURE 21–15. Oak pollen. The grain at left is seen in a polar view; that to the right shows one furrow in an equatorial view.

In general, the oaks are major sources of tree pollinosis and skin reactivity where this has been examined. Flowering periods commonly overlap those of early grasses. Although broad cross-reactivity has been implied, species-specific allergens may differ substantially; further study should focus on regionally more common species. Tree pollens in general and oaks specifically are more important allergenically than is often recognized. However, chestnuts, chinquapins, and tan bark oaks are substantially insect pollinated.

Urticaceae (hackberry, mulberry, hemp, nettle family) and Ulmaceae (elms). In temperate regions, the most clinically important members of the Ulmaceae historically have been the elms *(Ulmus)*, with perfect flowers opening before the leaves. The pollen is abundant and allergenically potent. Elm grains are oblately flattened and 29 to 43 μm in diameter, with four to six (usually five) pores defining an equator (Fig. 21–16). These pores are not prominent but often give the grain a pentagonal outline. The American elm *(Ulmus americana)* is now almost confined to urban areas, where spraying has delayed its elimination by Dutch elm disease, a fungus

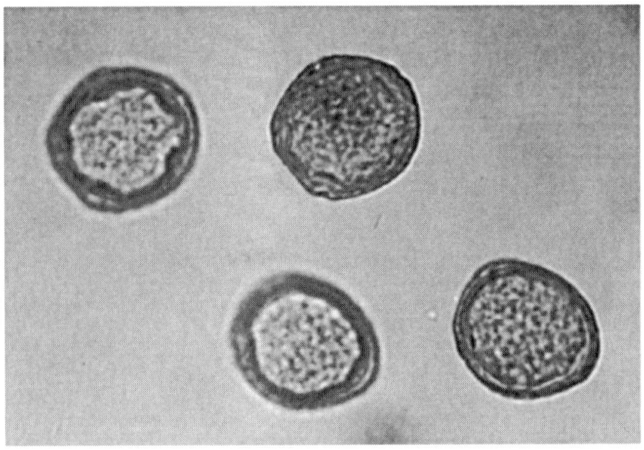

FIGURE 21–16. Elm pollen. The undulating surface and pentagonal aspect in a polar view are helpful points.

blight. The smaller slippery elm, *U. fulva*, is common in the Great Plains and east, and *U. pumila* is a hardy smaller elm of cool western regions; all flower in spring. In the south, there are a number of fall-blooming elms, including *U. crassifolia* and *U. serotina*. In California, *U. parvifolia* sheds pollen from August to October.

The hackberries or nettle trees *(Celtis)* are widespread temperate species, often encountered in eastern and gulf coast states. They have wind-pollinated, perfect flowers and bloom briefly from April to May in Tennessee and February to March in Texas and Louisiana, where they are especially abundant. The pollen grains are three-pored, average 32 μm, and microscopically resemble those of birches, bayberry, osage orange, hemp, and hop.

In the genus *Morus*, red mulberry *(Morus rubra)* of the Midwest and white mulberry *(M. alba)* of southwestern states are common and shed abundant pollen grains, 16 to 20 μm in diameter with two or three pores. These species flower in April and May and can create substantial pollen exposures, even from a single, mature, highly productive tree.

Broussonetia papyrifera (paper mulberry) is a small ornamental tree, related to the true mulberries, with flowers that forcibly eject their pollen. The grains are quite small, averaging 13.4 μm, have two eccentric pores, and are potent sensitizers locally throughout the warmer parts of North America.

Maclura pomifera, a native of the southern Great Plains, is planted often as a hedge and blooms in June. The two- or three-pored grains, 20 μm in diameter, are said to be allergenically related to *Morus* and *Broussonetia*.

Nettles *(Urtica)* of several species are prickly herbs, widespread in damp situations, and shed their moderately reactive pollen abundantly usually just before ragweed pollen appears. Grains are rarely recovered by fallout methods, as they are only 15 μm or less in diameter. Except that their three pores do not protrude, these grains look much like tiny birch pollens. Among fall pollinosis patients, roughly one third react to *Urtica* pollen in the Midwest. *Parietaria officinalis* (pellitory), a related, nonwoody species, is second only to grass as a pollinosis source in southern Europe. The pollen is microscopically indistinguishable from *Urtica* but appears to be unrelated allergenically.[77] Crifo and Iannetti[41] found 10 antigens that gave skin reactions in the crude extract of *P. officinalis*, and additional Mediterranean species, such as *P. judaica*, require study. *Parietaria floridana* is a common plant of waste places in Florida, blooming from January to May, but of unproven clinical significance. Although *P. officinalis* has been observed, its clinical significance anywhere in North American remains speculative.

Cannabis sativa (hemp) is dioecious and entirely anemophilous, producing much buoyant, airborne pollen. Hemp has palmately divided leaves, and the spikes of staminate flowers above them open from July to September. It was planted in the Midwest during the 1940s as a source of fiber for cordage but has escaped and is prevalent especially in southwestern Minnesota and surrounding areas. Marijuana and hashish are obtained from the pistillate (female) flower clusters of specific strains. Hemp pollen is 25 μm in diameter and three pored. *Humulus lupulus* (hops) is grown especially in the northwestern United States, where it produces pollen essentially indistinguishable from hemp grains and blooms in July and August.

Oleaceae (ashes and olive). Of the 20 genera comprising this family, most are insect pollinated, but the ashes and olive are anemophilous and clinically potent. Olive *(Olea europaea)* sheds pollen during April and May in California and Arizona from abundant, pale, imperfect flowers. The grains average 22 μm and have three furrows and a coarse intervening surface reticulum. The privets, including *Ligustrum lucidum* and *L. vulgare*, have larger but similar pollen that is almost exclusively insect borne.

Of native eastern species, the common white ash *(Fraxinus americana)* is a tall dioecious forest tree that sheds large amounts of pollen in the spring; *F. pennsylvania* is smaller, and both are also widely planted in cities. *F. velutina* is common in Arizona, New Mexico, and Texas, where it flowers from February to March. *F. oregona*, of the northwest, is also considered an important allergen source, blooming in April and May. Ash pollen is 20 to 25 μm and has four furrows, conferring a frequently squarish appearance, and a finely reticulate exine. The antigenic differences among ash, olive, and privet pollens are said to be fewer than those among the various grass species.[20]

Juglandaceae (hickory, walnut, pecan). The pecans and black walnuts are the most important wind-pollinated trees of this family. The pecans *(Carya pecan, C. texana,* and *C. illinoensis)* are prevalent in southern states, especially Georgia and Texas. *Carya pecan* pollen averages 44 μm, has three uncollared pores, and is shed from late March to May. Pecan pollens are confirmed clinical allergens, and hickories, such as shellbark *(C. ovata)* and mockernut *(C. glabra)*, are believed to elicit symptoms in cooler regions also.

In April and May, the California and eastern black walnuts *(Juglans spp.)* shed allergenically potent pollen. Grains average 34 to 42 μm in diameter and have an oblately spheroidal shape and bulging pores, usually 12 in number, which are arranged around the equator and on one half of the grain surface.

When dry (collapsed), hickory pollens appear like saucers, and walnut grains are cup-like, with that half without pores invaginated. Definite differences between pollen allergens of *Carya* and *Juglans* species have been noted.

Myricaceae (sweet gale family). Wax myrtle or bayberry

(Myrica cerifera) is a robust, evergreen, coastal shrub found from New Jersey to Florida and along the gulf to Texas; *M. californica* grows from British Columbia to southern California. Both species have male and female flowers on separate plants and, along with a larger relative *(M. pensylvanica)*, are wind pollinated. These shrubs and juniper are winter hay fever plants of limited importance in Bermuda. In addition, bayberry pollen is thought to cause pollinosis in Florida, where 15% of 400 atopic subjects showed skin reactivity to it,[84] and northward along the east coast. *Myrica* pollen is shed from March to April and more or less resembles the grains of birch, hackberry, hemp, and hazelnut, all being three-pored, 25 μm grains. Sweet fern *(Comptonia peregrina)* is a related, small inland shrub, native to the northeastern states and Canada, where it blooms in April and May. The pollens of sweet fern, Australian pine, ironwood, hornbeam, and filbert pollens also are similarly three pored but are closer to 28 μm in diameter.

Platanaceae (sycamores). *Platanus occidentalis* (sycamore) is a native tree of eastern and midwestern states, where it is a canopy species (growing to 100 feet) of river bottoms. The trunk is mottled with flaking bark in patches of buff to gray-green, and leaves are large and lobed palmately (like a human hand). The pollen is windborne and 18 to 20 μm in diameter, with three or four furrows and a finely reticulate exine. Sycamores shed pollen in the south during March and April and in the north in May. *P. racemosa* of California and *P. acerifolia* (London plane tree) are additional common trees of variable importance as allergen sources. The latter, a cultivated form of uncertain origin, is the sycamore, common as a street tree in eastern cities.

Hamamelidaceae (witch hazel family). Sweet gum *(Liquidambar styraciflua)* is a large shade tree present in the eastern United States with star-shaped leaves and separate male and female flower clusters. The pollen is large (often 38 μm), appears in March and April, and features 12 to 20 irregularly shaped and sized (4–8 μm) pores that bulge out from the grain surface. Other familiar members of this family are strictly insect pollinated.

Aceraceae (maples). *Acer negundo* (box elder) is the most productive and wholly anemophilous member of this family. It is common in the Midwest and locally throughout the United States east of the Cascades. Box elder has staminate and pistillate flowers on separate trees, and the highly potent pollen has a thin, faintly granular exine. Most other familiar maples combine insect and wind pollination, have perfect flowers, and produce pollen with distinct striae on the exine. Pollen of the red maple *(A. rubrum)* is seen in January and February in southern areas and later in the north. February and March see minor shedding by the silver maple *(A. saccharinum)*. In April and May, *A. saccharum* (sugar maple) pollinates in cooler localities. *A. negundo*, common in the Midwest, blooms in April before its compound leaves, comprising three leaflets, appear. Maple pollens all display three furrows and are 30 to 50 μm, with those of box elder occupying the lower end of this range. Clinical attention has been directed increasingly to sugar maple in New England and red maple in middle Atlantic states.

Tiliaceae (lindens). The native *(Tilia americana)* is primarily insect pollinated and of little allergenic importance in North America, despite the mounting popularity of cultivated forms as street trees. In Germany, lindens may be clinically important pollinosis sources, although aerometric data are inconclusive. The oblate, triangular grains of lindens are among the most distinctive pollens microscopically.

Leguminosae (pea family). Airborne pollen produced by members of this large, essentially entemophilous family is recovered in small amounts, perhaps due to spillage by foraging insects. *Prosopis juliflora* (mesquite), which is believed to cause pollinosis in western states and Hawaii, blooms from May to July. The pollen is spheroidal to triangular and 22 to 32 μm in diameter, with three furrows. Positive skin responses to mesquite extracts also may reflect sensitivity to antigens of other legumes, resulting in higher than expected but species-nonspecific reactivity patterns.[133]

Various acacias, including *Acacia farnesiana*, (huisache) *A. greggi, A tortuoso,* and *A. longifolia*, may be minor causes of allergy in California although they are substantially insect pollinated. Acacia pollen typically is a compound unit with 16 flattened grains and often measures 50 μm in diameter. All species bloom in the spring.

Carob *(Ceratonia siliqua)* is another legume of warmer regions that can grow as a small tree in southern Florida and California. Its pollen is reported to cause symptoms in the Middle East and Mediterranean areas during October and November.

Casuarinaceae (Australian pines). The Australian pines *(Casuarina spp.)* are not true pines but beefwoods from the South Pacific, which are planted in southern Florida and California; there are no close relatives. Copious airborne pollen is produced from the tips of slim green branchlets, which appear much like pine needles. The true leaves are reduced to closely applied scales that encircle these structures. *C. equisetifolia* flowers in spring and again in November but also sporadically all summer. It is planted prominently in coastal Florida, being tolerant to salt but not cold. *C. glauca*, by contrast, thrives inland and flowers earlier in spring and fall, along with *C. cunninghamiana*, a locally introduced west coast species. The pollens are 27 to 32 μm and have three protruding pores with collars, making them similar to those of birch and bayberry but slightly larger (Fig. 21–17). *Casuarina* competes aggressively in warm areas but fails rapidly above the frost line.

Plantaginaceae (plantains). In North America, English plantain *(Plantago lanceolata)* is the principal, albeit modest, pollen source of this family. Although widespread, *P. major* and *P. rugelii* are far less productive. Perfect flowers, borne on a short spike, bloom from the base upward with the anthers protruded on long filaments. Anthesis begins in May and June but may continue until frost. The pollen is 25 to 40 μm in diameter and has 4 to 14 pores, each resembling the single pore of grass pollen (Fig. 21–18). *P. psyllium* furnishes the medicinal psyllium seed, which also has caused allergic symptoms on ingestion and increasingly is recognized as an inhalant allergen for health care personnel.[9]

Compositae (composite family). The composites (Fig. 21–19) form a large and variously classified grouping. When

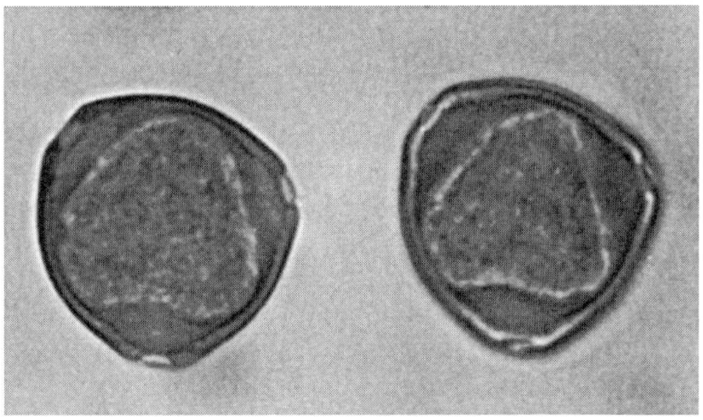

FIGURE 21–17. *Casuarina* pollen. The triporate grains with slightly collared pores, each with an aspis, somewhat resemble those of members of the birch and bayberry families.

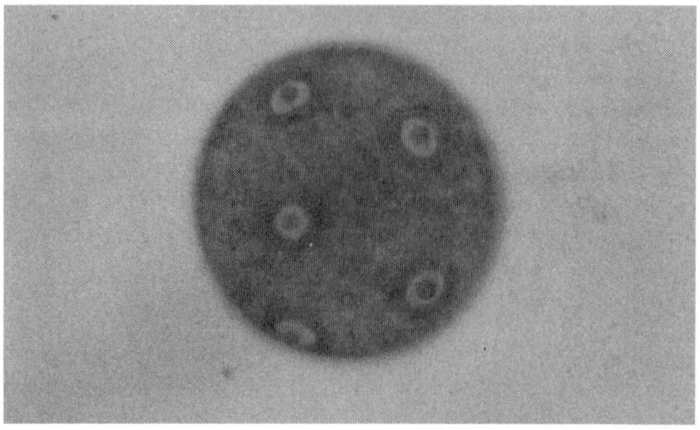

FIGURE 21–18. Plantain pollen. Five to 12 pores, each with a distinct operculum, are typical.

considering aeroallergen sources, it seems best to recognize one huge family (Compositae) with several tribes or subfamilies, notably the Ambrosieae (ragweeds), Anthemideae (sages), and other sections accommodating the sunflowers, asters, and additional types.

Ambrosieae. The ragweeds (Fig. 21–20A) are monoecious, with staminate terminal spikes and groups of single, pistillate florets just below, in the axils of the upper leaves. Pollen of short ragweed develops as nights lengthen to a critical point, a phenomenon termed negative photoperiodism. When weather conditions are properly dry and warm, male florets elongate before dawn, with protrusion of the five fused anthers; these dry further after sunrise, split, and release their pollens.[48] A final sweeping out of remaining pollen may be effected by the rapid growth of the pistillodium, a central structure in each floret (see Fig. 21–20B–F). If the temperature is less than 10°C or relative humidity over 70%, substantial pollen emission is unlikely. Pollen initially falls in moist aggregates on the underlying leaves, where it dries and is dispersed, even by light breezes. After fertilization, each pistil becomes an achene, a small, hardy seed that often still can germinate after being buried for 40 years or longer. This stored generative potential allows ragweeds quickly to take possession of freshly disturbed soils. However, after a few years of growth without further disturbance, competing perennials such as grasses tend to reclaim a site, thereby eliminating ragweeds. Before land was cleared, ragweeds were restricted to river banks, flood plains, and other areas of repeated natural disturbance. Overturning of soil for cultivation of field crops now is a major factor promoting the success of ragweeds. In addition, each building site and new mile of highway seems to foster ragweed pollen sources. All species of *Ambrosia* are wind pollinated. Short, giant, west-

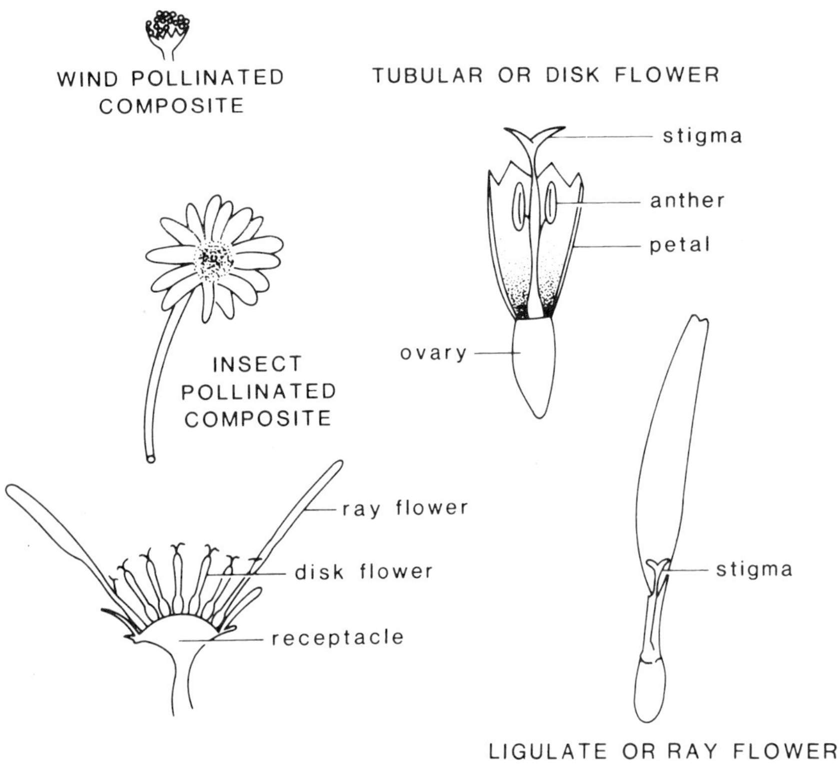

FIGURE 21–19. Composite flowers. Flower heads of composite family members are large groups of minute flowers on the end of a stalk broadened to form a receptacle. The outer (ray) flowers can be pistillate or neuter (in which case they serve only to attract insects). The central tubular (disk) flowers may be perfect or staminate. Wind-pollinated composites usually lack ray flowers.

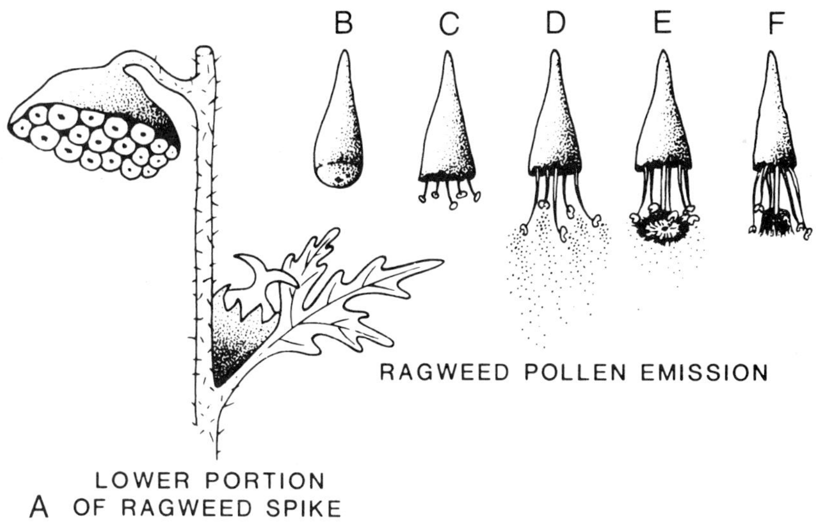

FIGURE 21–20. **(A)** Lower portion of a spike of short ragweed flowers, showing the most inferior male composite flower cluster (above) and an axillary female flower (below). **(B–F)** Ragweed pollen emission. **(B)** One of the male flowers enlarges in the hours after midnight. **(C)** Stamen filaments grow rapidly, and five anthers force open the perianth. **(D)** Sun dries and cracks the anthers; pollen escapes 1 to 3 hours after sunrise. **(E)** The pistillodium sweeps out the final grains of pollen. **(F)** The dried pistillodium hangs limply before retracting, and the floret begins to close.

ern, and southern ragweeds are most abundant in North America. Municipal ragweed clearance programs have not substantially decreased airborne pollen levels,[209] although removal of ragweeds around patients' homes certainly is justified. Away from North America, ragweed pollinosis is distinctly uncommon, although sites in Eastern France, the Balkans, and areas around the Black Sea are recognized.

Pollen allergens of short ragweed *(Ambrosia artemisiifolia)* have been better studied clinically and immunochemically than those of any other species. Rodent antisera recognize many antigens in ragweed pollen extracts, several of which also appear to sensitize atopic humans; at least eight have been distinguished and partly characterized. Of recognized allergenic components, Amb a 1 has gained special attention as the most widely reactive factor in skin test surveys of ragweed-sensitive groups. Amb a 1 also is the most concentrated allergen in aqueous extracts, although it comprises only 6% of extractable pollen proteins. At least five additional allergens of lesser sensitizing potential have been described and named using accepted international guidelines.[93] Reactivity to these varies among patients, and individual sensitivity to still other components may occur. Broad cross-reactivity among species of ragweeds and bur ragweeds (previously classified as *Franseria* species) denotes a sharing of Amb a 1.[106] However, pollens of related genera, the sages *(Artemisia)* and *Iva* species, appear to lack Amb a 1, despite recognized *Ambrosia*-like potency, suggesting additional shared components.

A. artemisiifolia (formerly *A. elatior*) is the principal offender in this group. It is essentially never taller than 4 feet but blooms at heights of a few inches in mowed lawns or very poor soil. In favorable situations, it is a many-branched, drought-resistant plant with finely divided leaves covered with delicate hairs. The pollen is 18 to 21 μm in diameter and has blunt spines and pores that fill three very short furrows (Fig. 21–21). It is shed from July to October in much of eastern North America.

Ambrosia trifida (giant ragweed) grows in richer soils and flood plains, reaches heights of 10 to 20 feet, and has large leaves that are oval or 2 or 3 lobed. It is especially abundant from the Appalachians to the Great Plains, each plant producing many more pollen grains than the smaller but more numerous short ragweeds. *A. trifida* pollen grains average 17.7 μm and have spines slightly larger and further apart than those of short ragweed; however, distinction by light microscopy is impractical.

Ambrosia bidentata (southern ragweed) is a smaller (1–3 feet) species with variably lobed, lance-shaped leaves that are very hairy and essentially lack stems. It is found from southern Illinois to Louisiana and west to Kansas and Oklahoma, with a preference for pastures and fallow fields.

Ambrosia psilostachya (western ragweed) is a perennial with a creeping rootstock. The plant has hairy, finely divided leaves. The pollen resembles those of other ragweeds but is somewhat larger (22–27 μm) and has definite furrows and pores. The plants also flower from July to October and are widespread over the western Great Plains and Canada.

Ambrosia hispida (seashore ragweed) is a small, relatively hairy plant similar to short ragweed. However, its pollen is 23 to 28 μm, with spines 3 to 4 μm apart, and many grains have four furrows. The seashore ragweed blooms throughout the year and is prevalent in Florida and the West Indies.

Ambrosia (Franseria) tenuifolia, slender ragweed of the

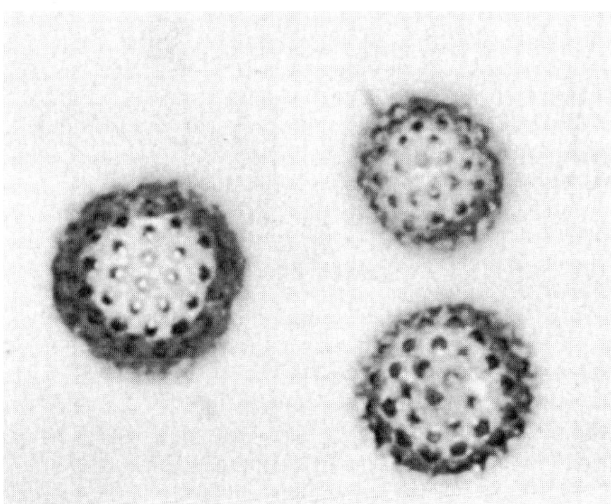

FIGURE 21–21. Ragweed pollen. The 18 to 22 μm grains with short conical spines constitute an important and widespread type. The three pores are often difficult to discern.

western Great Plains and Great Basin, resembles western ragweed and has pollen typical of ragweeds but is southern in distribution. *A. (F.) acanthicarpa* also is similar but concentrated in higher latitudes of the west. These species bloom from May to November and August to December, respectively. Plants previously classified as *Franseria* have prominent spines on the mature pistillate head but are typical ragweeds in other respects.

Cyclachaena (Iva) xanthifolia (burweed marsh elder or prairie ragweed) is a sturdy species recalling giant ragweed but has a branching flower cluster and numerous axillary spikes of florets. The leaves are large and not as deeply cleft as in giant ragweed. The pollen averages 18 μm and has small, relatively blunt spines, with definite furrows enclosing the pores. The plant is western in distribution and blooms from July to late August.

Iva ciliata (rough marsh elder), a coarse ragweed-like species with long flowering spikes, grows in moist soils of the midsouthern United States and blooms from August to September. The pollen measures 21 μm and has well-defined spines that are 4 μm apart. *I. frutescens* (high-tide bush) is a salt marsh shrub of the east, and *I. axillaris* (poverty weed) grows in alkaline soil in the far west; their pollens are similar to those of rough marsh elder.

Xanthium spinosum, like other cocklebur species, is a coarse weed in barren soils and has triangular leaves and pistillate flowers that form a definite bur. The pollen is at least 25 μm in diameter and has short, blunt spines and pores that fill three very short furrows. It is shed sparsely from late July to October in much of eastern and central North America.

Anthemideae. Members of the mayweed family are mostly insect pollinated, with chrysanthemums, chamomiles, yarrows, tansy, and pyrethrum as familiar representatives. Sagebrush, mugworts, and wormwoods are the wind-pollinated family members and important allergen sources. However, they do not appear generally to share major pollen allergens, such as Amb a 1, with their relatives, the ragweeds.[106, 224] Most mayweed family members have typical daisy-like composite clusters with central disk flowers and peripheral, usually sterile, ray flowers, the latter usually missing in wind-pollinated species (see Fig. 21–19).

Artemisia tridentata (sagebrush) is a gnarled shrub, 3 to 12 feet high, with wedge-shaped, alternate leaves that are three toothed at the apex and covered with silvery gray hairs. The clustered flower heads are yellow-green, and the perfect tubular flowers produce much pollen from July to late September. It is a western United States species that is abundant in Utah and Nevada and, like other *Artemisia* species, is strongly aromatic. *A. campestris* and *A. frigida* (field sageworts) are smaller relatives that grow as far north as the Yukon and are favored by overgrazing. *A. ludoviciana* and *A. californica* are also prevalent in western states, reaching Arizona and New Mexico and have a more linear leaf form. Wodehouse[218] described antigenic similarities among *Artemisia* pollens.

Artemisia vulgaris (mugwort) is increasingly widespread in the eastern states and becoming a major allergen source. *A. annua* and *A. biennis* are also locally recognized hay fever plants. The pollen grains of sages are spheroidal and 18 to 28 μm in diameter and have three furrows. The exine has a very faintly pebbled surface, and in optical sections, columellae are prominent within the exine wall (Fig. 21–22). *Artemisia spp.* pollens share some secondary ragweed-type allergens, and cross-reactivity with other composite pollens is established.

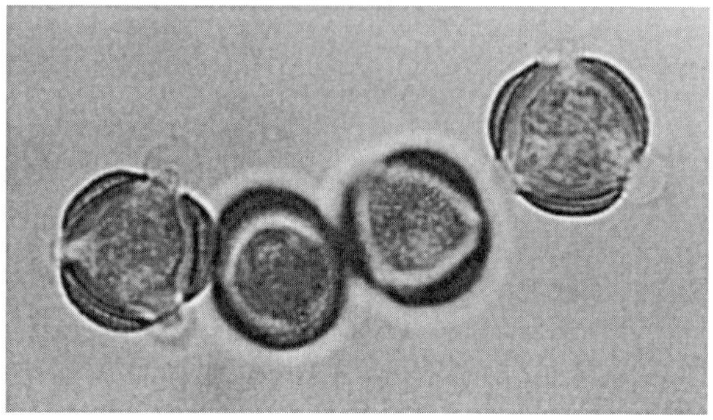

FIGURE 21–22. Sage pollen. In a polar view, the three pores and radiating exine elements (bacula) create a distinctive appearance.

Some entemophilous composites produce excessive pollen, and during dry, windy weather, incidental aerial dispersion occurs. *Eupatorium capillifolium* (dog fennel) and *Baccharis halmifolia* (groundsel bush), both of the southeastern states, display this effect. Both bloom from September to December and have pollen grains of 17 to 25 μm with fine conical spines and three furrows. *B. sarothroides* (desert broom) of the west behaves similarly, and a variety of asters, goldenrods, and other plants may contribute small spiney grains in modest numbers. Among these, American feverfew (*Parthenium hysterophorus*) of the Gulf Coast has received particular attention.[214] It flowers in late summer, shares some pollen allergens with ragweeds, and is implicated as both an inhalant and contact sensitizer in India at sites of introduction.

Chenopodiaceae. The chenopods are a large family of somewhat fleshy annual or perennial herbs with inconspicuous green flowers that are usually wind pollinated. Like members of the closely related amaranth family (Amaranthaceae), the pollen grains are covered with many small pores, recalling tiny golf balls.

Chenopodium album (lamb's quarters) is an abundant semisucculent pleomorphic herb with mealy appearing leaves and very small dusty-white clusters of five-sepaled flowers. It blooms from July to September, and the pollen is spheroidal, averaging 28 μm in diameter, with 2.5 μm pores that are regularly arranged and 5.4 μm apart. Pollens of chenopods and amaranths are similar enough that, usually, one can only guess at the source of single grains by light microscopy (Fig. 21–23). However, average values for grain and pore diameters, as well as pore spacing, have been defined for individual species. *Chenopodium ambrosioides* (Mexican tea) is an erect annual with a vivid green appearance and disagreeable odor. Both of these chenopods are widespread in North America. Mexican tea blooms from August to October, and its grains average 22.8 μm and have smaller, more numerous pores than those of *C. album*.

Salsola pestifer (Russian thistle) has abundantly produced, strongly antigenic pollen and is a dominant tumbleweed in western states and in poor sandy or saline soils locally to the

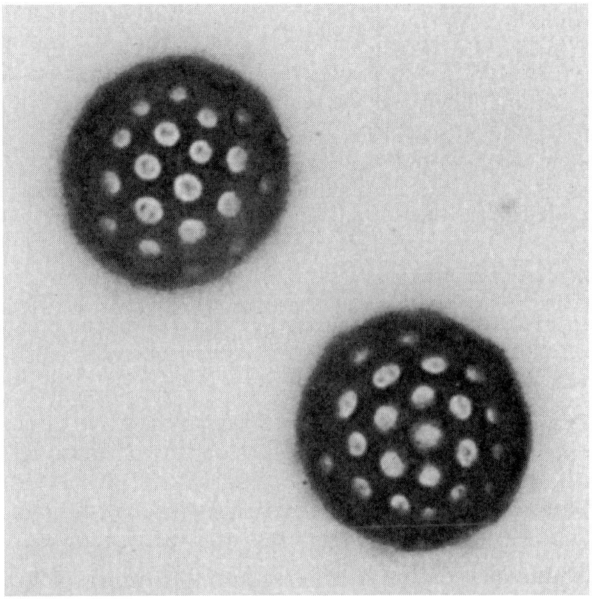

FIGURE 21–23. Chenopod–amaranth pollen. Periporate grains like these are typical of members of the large chenopod and amaranth families. In any locality, the most important sources of such pollen are best determined by careful field observations.

east. The brittle stems are numerous, ascending, and branched, with rigid linear leaves and tiny, greenish axillary flowers, each with two small bracts. Typical chenoped pollen averages 27 μm in diameter and is shed from June to late September.

Kochia scoparia (Mexican fireweed or burning bush) is a sometimes cultivated Eurasian species, widespread through the west and steadily extending its range eastward. It has many branched stems with simple, linear 1- to 2-inch leaves. Perfect small green flowers develop in the upper leaf axils and in small panicles at the branch tips. Many specimens turn a brilliant magenta during fall, becoming quite showy. The spheroidal pollen is 29 to 34 μm and has broadly spaced 2.9 μm pores. In many areas east of the Mississippi, this has become the most prolific source of chenopod (amaranth) pollen.

Other related chenopods include greasewood (*Sarcobatus vermiculatus*), which grows in arid, saline soils of the west and flowers in late summer. The pollen (24–30 μm) has more widely spaced (10.8 μm) pores than any other grain of this type. Sea blite (*Suaeda suffrutescens*) also is widespread in southwestern states, and *Beta vulgaris* (sugar beet) is grown in Arizona, New Mexico, and western Texas. Sugar beet grains are small (19–20 μm) and have notably few pores.

Atriplex wrightii (annual saltbush) is a 3- to 4-foot tall herb with imperfect flowers, the staminate in long terminal panicles, and the pistillate in the upper leaf axils. Pollination occurs from June to November in New Mexico and Arizona, where the species is widely abundant. *Atriplex patula* (spearscale) is present in many North American saline soils and marshes and blooms in late summer. *Atriplex arenaria* (seabeach atriplex) grows from Maine to Florida and produces limited pollen. Wingscale (*Atriplex canescens*), lenscale (*A. lentiformis*), shadscale (*A. confertifolia*), and allscale (*A. polycarpa*) are southwestern desert saltbushes or oraches that shed abundantly from May to September. Although potent antigenically, much pollen is confined to areas of low population.

Amaranthaceae. Amaranthus retroflexus (redroot pigweed) is a coarse weed of medium height, reported to be common throughout North America but apparently rare or absent south of the Carolinas in southeastern states. Although a familiar species, it is not as prolific a pollen producer as other amaranths, including *A. palmeri* and *A. hybridus*, which are more widespread in western regions. Long terminal and axillary flower spikes with pointed scales surrounding each flower are typical of amaranths. In *A. spinosus*, the flowers are distinctive, with sterile slender spikes above and the fertile members below in globular axillary clusters. *Acnida altissima* (waterhemp) is a dioecious species having the male plants more prostrate in growth form. Like those of chenopods, amaranth pollens are periporate and variable (22–32 μm) in diameter. In most localities, one or more species are in bloom from June to October. However, amaranth pollen appears to reach substantial levels primarily on the Great Plains.

The allergens of chenopods and amaranths appear to cross-react broadly, both within and between groups. Weber and colleagues' study[213] suggested that *Salsola* had the most potent antigens, with *Chenopodium album* closely related. *Kochia* and *Bassia hyssopifolia* (smotherweed) shared antigens with *Salsola*, and pigweeds and water hemp reacted similarly.

Polygonaceae. Rumex acetosella (sheep sorrel) is a low, perennial dioecious plant with halberd-shaped leaves and erect clusters of flowers. It is present throughout the United States and southern Canada and generally blooms from May to early July. *R. crispus*, as well as other docks, may contribute limited pollen in that season; buckwheat is a related, cultivated species apparently without clinical impact. *Rumex* pollen is spheroidal (22–24 μm) and has four slit-like furrows and central germ pores. The exine is pitted, and interior starch granules are prominent. A number of patients with positive skin tests have reacted to nasal challenge with *Rumex* pollen, suggesting a clinical potential.[174]

In areas of intense monoculture, even largely entemophilous crops may cause localized pollinosis. This role has been claimed most convincingly for cashew (*Anacardium occidentale*) in India[58] and suggested for rapeseed (grown for its oil) in Europe and North America.

DOMESTIC DUST AND ARTHROPOD ALLERGENS

During the early 1920s, Cooke defined house dust allergy as a clinical entity of unspecified but distinctive origin. Domestic dust has been found to contain bacteria and their toxins, indigenous mites, animal emanations, human skin (desquamated cells), fungi (especially *Aspergillus, Cladosporium,* and *Penicillium* species, insect debris, decaying plant fibers, and algae in varying associations. Its reactivity differs from that of soil particles and reflects no specific pollen allergens. In 1964, Voorhorst and Spieksma[208] described (pyroglyphid) dust mites as the principal allergen source of house dust, and confirmation swiftly followed (Fig. 21–24).

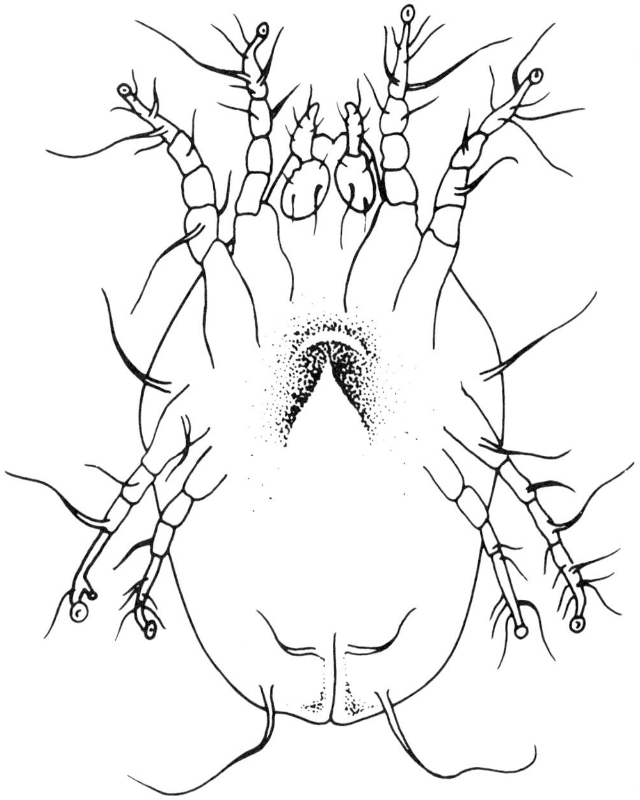

FIGURE 21–24. *Dermatophagoides pteronyssinus* (shown) is the most cosmopolitan pyroglyphid, but *D. farinae* is more common in North America. The adult mite is 170 to 500 μm long. They are common in carpets, upholstery, bird and animal nests, cereals, flour, animal feeds, and yeast products. Familiar pyroglyphids have five life stages—egg, larva, protonymph, tritonymph, and adult—and the life cycle averages 23 to 30 days. House dust mites feed on human skin scales, which are abundant, as the average human sheds 0.7 to 1.4 gm of scales per day. They grow optimally at 22° to 27°C and when the relative humidity is 70% to 80%. Mites are rare at elevations higher than 1,500 meters above sea level.

Regional surveys suggest that *Dermatophagoides pteronyssinus (D.p.)* is most prevalent in Eurasia, with either this species or *D. farinae (D.f.)* predominating in North American homes. There is partial antigenic cross-reactivity between the two *Dermatophagoides* species.[43] Tovey[195] described mite feces as a major allergen reservoir and suggested that gut enzymes were major sources. In fact, the major mite allergens, Der p 1 and Der f 1, are cysteine proteases, whereas Der p 3 and Der f 3 are serine proteases. In addition, a 60 kD mite amylase has been shown to elicit skin reactivity in 25% of children and 46% of adults clinically allergic to dust mites.[103]

House dust mites proliferate best at temperatures above 25°C and at a relative humidity over 70%; dry surroundings are tolerated poorly. The percent weight of mites per gram of house dust and concentration of mites in samples have varied inversely with altitude, probably reflecting indoor relative humidity. Warm and humid coastal regions harbor especially high interior mite populations.

Other mites, such as *Blomia tropicalis*, are prevalent in warmer regions of the Americas and elsewhere. Allergenic cross-reactivity with *Dermatophagoides* species appears to be minimal.[145] Studies in Tampa (Fla) have shown that *Blomia* are especially abundant in summer, with skin reactivity demonstrable in one third of 118 allergic rhinitis patients and twice that number sensitive to *D.p.* and *D.f.*[187] The favored foodstuff of house dust mites seems to be desquamated skin scales, although cereal dusts and fungal particles are preferred by some species, and fungi, especially aspergilli, may predigest some nutrients. However, regardless of location, tight, generously humidified modern homes, with most surfaces carpeted, offer excellent growth conditions. Tovey and colleagues[195] studied the major allergen of the house dust mite, *D. pteronyssinus*. They found that mite feces contained 99% of the recoverable Der p 1 activity, previously characterized by Chapman,[37] whereas whole mite body provided only 0.6 percent. The separated cuticles supplied 0.4% of activity, the eggs none. Mite fecal pellets have a mean diameter of 24 μm, and 95% of these particles settle to the floor within 5 minutes after a disturbance, such as dusting or house cleaning, or shortly thereafter.[143]

How far these (mite) particles penetrate into the human respiratory tract is not clear. However, exposure levels of major *Dermatophagoides* allergens in excess of 2.0 μm per gram of dust seem to be required for specific IgE synthesis by most genetically predisposed persons.[37]

In Ohio homes, Arlian and colleagues[8] found mites concentrated on carpeted floors and in upholstered furniture but somewhat less in mattresses, where previous studies in Europe and Asia have shown great numbers. In these homes, fitted sheets seem to have prevented skin scales from penetrating to the mattresses. Repeated vacuuming and cleaning of fabric-covered surfaces did not decrease the mite population, contrary to popular belief. During the winter, these workers found viable, desiccation-resistant protonymphs (larval forms), which could supply stock for repleting mite populations in the spring. Murray and Zuk[129] found that mite numbers in Vancouver, British Columbia, varied with relative humidity and peaked from July to October, a seasonal pattern confirmed in other North American studies[196] and by van der Heide and colleagues[204] in the Netherlands.

By history, house dust sensitivity should be suspected with perennial symptoms, especially if these become worse while sweeping, vacuuming, making beds, or shaking blankets; improvement on going outside also is suggestive.[128] Forced air heating and other disturbances that disperse dust increase symptoms in cold weather. Murray and Ferguson's[127] finding that asthmatics sensitive to house dust responded favorably to environmental control, including elimination of carpets and plastic encasing of upholstery and bedding, has been repeatedly confirmed when antidust measures are rigorously applied.

Despite the importance of mites, it seems clear that allergens of mites and house dust cannot be equated perfectly, especially in areas with cold, dry winters. Because of this, many believe that both house dust and defined mite extracts are desirable for skin testing of individuals potentially sensitive to dust. Regardless of one's approach, it is evident that allergens from sources other than mites, pets, and fungi elicit symptoms in some persons sensitive to dust. Cockroach and rat emanations often appear to be implicated.

Cockroach allergen was described as a cause of perennial symptoms by Bernton and Brown in 1964, but it was Kang and coworkers[88] who focused the attention of clinicians on this offender. In patients who developed nonpollen asthma after moving from rural areas to urban housing in Durban,

South Africa, Fraser[63] found 80% with house dust or dust mite sensitivity and 30% reactive to cockroach allergens. The latter have been variably separated, and several components have been described.[35, 221, 226] Principal allergen sources appear to be the insect gut and Malpighian vessels, which function to excrete fluid.[226] Major species-specific allergens in aqueous whole body extracts of American *(Periplanata americana)* and German *(Blatella germanica)* cockroaches were found to be cross-reactive by Schou and colleagues.[162] Pollart and colleagues[144] described the major allergens, Bla g 1 and Bla g 2, mainly in feces or secretions of German cockroaches. Using RAST, Musmand and colleagues[131] confirmed these as major allergens in testing 37 asthmatics specifically sensitive to cockroaches. However, other allergens were recognized by 20% of cockroach-reactive patients. In dose-response studies, 2 U/gm, or more of Bla g 2 in house dust correlated with sensitization of exposed susceptible individuals.[160] The kitchen generally has been the principal site of domestic cockroach antigens. Useful avoidance measures include removal of food and water sources, sealing of access and entry points, use of bait stations, and application of hormonal/chemical pesticides, emphasizing the least toxic materials that provide control. Low-income, inner-city housing carries special risks of exposure. However, even here, cockroach allergen levels are considerably lower in dwellings with resident cats than in other interiors.[66]

Poorly maintained urban dwellings also commonly contain rodent allergens in widely variable amounts. In homes, airborne Der p 1 was not detected without dust disturbance, although following activity, levels of 5 to 100 ng/m^3 were recorded.[143] In rodent care facilities, however, suspended rat allergen was always detectable (baseline = 3–18 ng/m^3). This increased to 1,800 to 6,000 ng/m^3 on shaking the bedding, with half of this activity present in 5 to 10 μm particle fractions.

NONDOMESTIC ARTHROPOD ALLERGENS

Arthropod inhalant allergens have been recognized in work areas and related situations involving respiratory exposure to honeybees, fruit flies,[183] beetles,[164] grasshoppers,[181] locusts,[61] weevils,[217] box elder beetles,[130] and mushroom flies.[92] Anecdotal reports implicating other types abound.

Kino and Oshima[95] described 50 asthmatic patients sensitive to the silkworm moth *(Bombyx mori)*. Others have reported allergy to sericin, a natural gelatinous substance that binds silk fibers together. A strong sensitizer, unwashed silk can be a hazard to sensitive subjects but is seldom encountered today.

Stevenson and Mathews[188] reported inhalant allergy from bee moth *(Galleria mellonella)* larvae (waxworms) reared for fish bait. Occupational inhalant allergy to chironomid larvae and their major allergen (Chi t 1) also is recognized in fish food workers.[192] In addition, anglers and bait handlers clinically reactive to green bottle *(Lucilia caesar)* larvae and mealworm *(Tenebrio molitor)* have been well described.[169] Related use of crickets also has resulted in allergic rhinitis.[12]

The mayfly group (Ephemeridae) has produced a sporadic inhalant allergy problem, especially at the western end of Lake Erie and surrounding areas.[165] When molting to its short-lived adult stage, these insects shed a pellicle that fragments, forming the main allergen source. Although sensitive patients still suffer in June and July, mayfly populations have varied in response to industrial pollution and cleanup of lake habitats. The caddis fly has a related life history and allergenic potential but prefers clear, moving streams at the eastern end of Lake Erie. Exposure is imposed by innumerable minute hairs that the insects shed during swarming periods from June to August.[165] Similar events appear to have provoked epidemics of respiratory allergy in North African populations due to the periodic abundance of a nonbiting midge.[90]

Atopic persons often show many strongly positive reactions to other locally prevalent insects. Kino and colleagues[94] confirmed this experience in Japanese asthmatics using extracts of moth, butterfly, caddis fly, and chironomid. In addition, they found particles bearing these insect allergens in aerosol fractions below 10 micra with spring and fall prevalence peaks. However, the impact of such casual exposure remains speculative.

The gypsy moth *(Porthetria (Lymantria) dispar)* has caused allergic rhinitis in New England during major infestation years and probably will continue to do so.[55] Coghlan and colleagues[39] have suggested that different moth species are likely to contain unique as well as cross-reactive allergens, and Shulman[168] summarized initial immunochemical data for selected insect allergens. It seems likely that additional arthropod allergen sources will be recognized as this phylum is further investigated clinically, although documentation of exposure remains problematic.

OTHER INHALANT ALLERGENS

KAPOK

Seed hair from the tropical kapok tree *(Ceiba pentandra)* is used to stuff throw pillows and employed in sleeping bags, life jackets, and boat cushions. As a component of bedding, it has been replaced by synthetic fibers. Kapok appears to become more allergenic with aging, perhaps by oxidative degradation but more probably through invasion by mites or microbial contaminants.

COTTONSEED

Water-soluble proteins of cottonseed are such potent allergens that skin testing by any but an epidermal (prick) approach can be perilous. Cottonseed allergen may be present incidentally in upholstery, mattresses, and cushions and occurs regularly as a meal (pomace) in animal feeds and fertilizers and less predictably in baked goods. Cottonseed and other vegetable oils are unlikely to contain allergenic protein because of the denaturing effects of processing them at 400°C.

FLAXSEED

Flaxseed also is a very potent allergen, occurring in animal feeds, hair preparations, and patent leather and potentially present in insulating materials, rugs, and cloth (linen) containing flax fibers. Cereals, such as Roman Meal, Uncle Sam's Breakfast foods, and Malt-O-Meal, as well as flours and baked goods, provide inhalant or ingestant sources.

CASTOR BEAN AND SOYBEAN

Both castor bean of the spurge family and soy, a pea family member, have strong sensitizing potential. Castor bean's many uses include laxatives, linoleum, and lubricants. The pulp and hulls provide high nitrogen fertilizers, and the associated dust has caused both dermatitis in agricultural workers and community outbreaks of asthma. Sacks previously used to ship castor beans have produced allergic symptoms when reused to ship green coffee, although coffee bean dust also contains distinctive allergens. Soybean meal is encountered in fertilizers, animal foods, adhesives, water-based paints, paper sizing, firefighting foam, and waterproof materials.

VEGETABLE GUMS

Vegetable gums are plant derivatives used where viscosity, gloss, or marketable bulk is desired. Ongoing exposure to these ubiquitous additives often is inapparent. Karaya, tragacanth, acacia (gum arabic), and quince seed gums have been used for decades. Carob, carrageenan, chicle, algin, agar, bassora, gelatin, ghatti, gum guar, mesquite, and pectin have gained increasing favor. Gums are used as fillers or emulsifiers in foods, hair preparations, denture adhesives and powders, cosmetics, and cloth sizing, as well as in printing and paper making. Cross-reactions among gums seem minor, making them difficult inhalants to suspect. Workers with rhinitis and asthma due to inhalation of dry carob bean flour used in confiture preparation and guar gum as a dye fixative emphasize a potential for occupational sensitization.[203]

ORRIS ROOT AND DERRIS ROOT

The root of the orris plant (iris family) has a gentle fragrance and has been used, finely ground, in powders and cosmetics, even though it frequently caused respiratory allergy. Orris root generally is absent from today's domestic cosmetics, especially hypoallergenic products, but may still occur in imported preparations.

Derris root is used to make an insecticide and fish poison, rotenone, which has low toxicity for warm-blooded animals. Allergic reactions to the crude plant product occasionally are reported in both domestic and occupational settings.

PYRETHRUM

Pyrethrum is a genus of old world composite plants (ragweed related) with flowering heads that are dried and extracted for use in popular insecticides. The resulting preparations have low human toxicity but, especially in the past, have caused severe inhalant allergy, as well as allergic eczematous contact dermatitis. Although contemporary processing has reduced these risks, especially the latter, an increasing array of garden sprays and over-the-counter scabicides contain pyrethrum derivatives as active ingredients. Visitors to the tropics may note symptoms from pyrethrum volatilized for indoor mosquito control.

GLUE

Fish-based glues have provided inhalant allergens, and some household glues or foreign postage stamps may still use these adhesives. Cooking odors (osmyls) arising from fish and seafood preparation are associated with airborne food molecules that can cause intense respiratory symptoms in the most highly sensitive individuals.[56] Similar mechanisms may have been responsible for 35 cases of occupational asthma among 313 workers in snow crab processing plants reported by Cartier and colleagues.[34]

ENZYMES

Papain is encountered in pharmaceuticals, laboratory reagents, meat tenderizers, and beer processing. The enzyme is a respiratory irritant, but Dolovich and colleagues[50] reported sensitization by this route as well. A large proportion of detergent workers and some consumers exposed to enzymes of *Bacillus subtilis* have developed similar sensitivity, although improved processing has largely curtailed this problem. Pancreatin inhalant allergy has been reported, and Pineau and colleagues[142] have reported occupational asthma due to pepsin. Aspergillus-derived enzymes (amylase, cellulase, hemicellulase, and glucoamylase) are used in commercial bread making to hasten and economize the process. Encountered as fine powders, these enzymes have become common occupational allergens.[146] Merget and colleagues[121] have summarized techniques helpful in identifying allergy to enzymes.

ALGAE

Algae from both aquatic and terrestrial niches can become airborne and sensitize some atopic persons.[18, 119] Components of one green organism *(Chlorella)* were found in three different commercial house dust extracts and elicited positive skin reactions in 60% of atopic patients.[18] Mittal and colleagues[122] found fewer positive skin tests in atopics using 10 locally common airborne algae; primarily irritation was not a factor. The more reactive agents in this Indian population were *Lyngbya, Phormidium, Anabaena, Sytoema,* and *Chlorella* species.[122] The potential for dissemination of algae from water and soil, as well as their size and sensitizing properties, mandates their further investigation. Emissions from aquariums in homes and other fluid reservoirs containing algae raise a question of resulting, unanticipated health effects.[159]

One of several red tide organisms *(Ptychodiscus brevis)* is a recognized bronchitis-producing and asthmogenic agent along sea coasts; effects are not limited to atopic subjects. The neurotoxin of this species stimulates axon sodium channels with release of acetylcholine at postganglionic nerve endings in the tracheobronchial tree.[166]

MISCELLANEOUS PLANT-DERIVED AGENTS

Jute from *Corchorus* and from hemp is used for burlap, rope, and rug matrix. Like kapok, these fibers may have primary allergens, although suspected reactions probably reflect microbial contaminants. Twiggs and colleagues[198] reported allergy to the dust of dried baby's breath plants (*Gypsophila paniculata*) among florists. Garlic dust inhalation has been described as a cause of asthma,[113] although the mechanism of response is not clear. Some reported adverse reactions to kiwi fruit may reflect allergy to actinidin, a proteolytic enzyme.[59] Reported associations with pollen and latex allergy are under study.[65, 115]

Tobacco smoke aggravates asthma in smokers and in passively exposed children and adults, although claims of true allergy remain controversial. O'Connell and Logan[134] reported a 90% improvement in asthma among 20 children after exposure to tobacco smoke was stopped, whereas only 27% of those with continuing exposure were better. Menon and colleagues[120] documented increased bronchial reactivity in asthmatics and some asymptomatic persons exposed to sidestream smoke. Ferguson and colleagues[57] suggested that an increase in parental smoking of five cigarettes per day resulted in a 2.5- to 3.5-fold increase in the incidence of lower respiratory illnesses among exposed children. Persistent middle ear effusions also were greatly increased by parental smoking.[100]

Although true tobacco sensitivity may exist, sensitization to unrelated inhalants may be promoted by smoking-induced impairment of pulmonary clearance. Respiratory distress due to marijuana smoking is common, although atopic sensitivity to this material is not suggested.[108]

Warren and colleagues[211] found elevated IgE levels in smokers without specificity for any allergen or component of tobacco smoke. The observation that maternal smoking during pregnancy is associated with a threefold elevation of cord serum IgE is probably related.[114] Affected infants also have a distinctly increased risk of atopic manifestations by the age of 18 months. In metropolitan regions with unsatisfactory air quality, as much as twice the expected incidence of wheal and flare skin responses has been noted. Takafuji and colleagues[190] suggested that inhaled diesel exhaust particles could act as an adjuvant for IgE production in mice, and evidence for related human effects is increasingly persuasive. Possible adjuvant and sensitizing properties of airborne 2 to 10 μm particles derived from the wear of rubber tires have also been emphasized.[215]

ANIMAL ALLERGENS (DANDERS)

The use of animals as companions and sources of food and raw materials has ensured the persistence of species-specific sensitivities. In examining this clinical problem, a narrow (conventional) definition of dander as minute epidermal scales or scurf is insufficient. Rather, adverse responses occur to proteins of several dispersible emanations, including epidermal squames, hair, urine, and fecal materials, as well as lacrimal and salivary secretions. Rates of exposure to horses and livestock appear to have lessened, whereas contact with dogs, cats, rodents, and other small mammals in homes and laboratories has risen sharply.

Animal (dander) sensitivities are among the most potent sources of allergic morbidity, leading at times to airway responses, urticaria, flares of eczema, or rarely even anaphylaxis on exposure to specific offenders. Although tractable asthma and rhinitis most commonly result, prolonged disabling symptoms provoked by a single housepet is a situation familiar to clinicians. Assessing exposure to danders may be simple and straightforward. However, animal hair present in clothing, bedding, toys, and other items, especially imported articles with unlabeled components, is easily overlooked. Danders from discrete sources may also contaminate the complex ventilation systems of buildings containing laboratories or housing multiple family units.

In addition, the physician must recognize the reticence of many patients to admit exposure to animals or resulting symptoms for fear of separation from a beloved pet. Related problems of evaluation and management arise with patients, such as veterinarians, ranchers, and biomedical investigators, whose careers or educational advancement demand work with other species. However, sensitive persons who rigidly exclude animals from their homes and workplaces still may suffer while visiting others who keep pets.

Although rates of clinical reactivity to specific mammalian species, using extracts of defined potency, are unknown and clearly vary with exposure intensity, the overall problem is large. Positive skin test frequencies, using crude dander extracts, have been estimated at 8% to 20% for horses, 5% to 30% for dogs, and 9% to 26% for cats.[60, 155] As with other materials, not all test responders experience symptoms in natural challenge situations, although cat exposure seems especially potent clinically.

Epidermal debris apparently is the principal source of species-specific allergens from cats, dogs, horses, and cows.[111] Because dander exposures often reflect discrete, manipulable sources, defining these may be feasible and facilitate management. Commercial dust masks or respirators can reduce the symptoms of some persons during finite (and preferably brief) animal contacts. Prophylactic use of antihistamines, bronchodilators, or cromolyn/nedocromil also is worthy of trial. Removal of offending species and animal products from the patient's environment offers more certain benefit but requires a firm etiologic diagnosis and recognition that substantial relief will not be prompt.

Disturbances, such as bed making or vacuuming a room, further increase levels of indoor bioaerosols. Cat and rodent allergens remain high, even in undisturbed rooms, and show substantial wall deposition.[220] In homes where a cat had never been kept, van der Brempt and colleagues[202] found levels of the major feline allergen, Fel d 1, of 1.4 μg/gm of mattress dust, whereas in homes with resident cats, an average of 21.9 μm/gm of mattress dust was recovered. Where cats had been removed within the previous 5 years, the mean Fel d 1 level was 14 μg/gm of mattress dust; absence for more than 5 years resulted in a mean of 3.1 μg/gm.

These data confirm that cat allergens are pervasive and remain long after a cat leaves and, incidentally, that cats spend ample time on and around beds. It follows that brief trials of pet removal cannot assess the effectiveness of more extended animal avoidance, especially exclusion of cats. If the priorities of the patient or family make removing an offending pet difficult, it may be helpful to remove carpets and reduce upholstered furniture, exclude the cat from the patient's bedroom, and use vacuums with double thickness bags and perhaps a HEPA room air cleaner.[45] The value of regularly washing cats has not been established.[96] Even with personal avoidance effort, cat allergen may be encountered passively in schools and public places in amounts sufficient to elicit symptoms.[52]

When avoidance of danders is not a practical possibility, despite excessive allergic symptoms, specific immunotherapy may be considered. Van Metre and colleagues[206] confirmed earlier reports by showing efficacy in treating asthmatics with extracts unstandardized for Fel d 1 content. Alvarez-Cuesta and colleagues[7] showed a good response without significant side effects in a blinded study using a dose of 13.2 μg of standardized Fel d 1 antigen. Characterization of Fel d 1 B-cell epitopes has facilitated their recognition in other felines, suggesting that current treatment methods and materials may benefit symptomatic handlers of larger cat species.[200]

The continuing popularity of dogs, especially of cold-intolerant breeds maintained in small domestic interiors, has enhanced their importance as allergen sources. In a study of pet owners' homes in Japan, Sakaguchi and colleagues[156] found airborne allergens of dog and cat at levels 100 times higher than those of dust mites. IgE-reactive components have been shown in dog serum (especially canine IgG), urine, and saliva, as well as skin. The major allergen, Can f 1, to which 70% of dog-sensitive subjects react, was characterized by Schou and colleagues[161] and is present in especially large amounts in canine saliva.[46]

Allergenic differences among major canine breeds were suggested several decades ago[80] and have been supported by IgE-based in vitro techniques,[19, 23, 123] although unique breed-specific allergens have not been demonstrated.[19] Variations in the responses of sensitive persons tested with various dog extracts may reflect inequalities between breeds in shared components or artifact due to the limited size of samples representing breeds. In any case, rates of reactivity to the dander, urine, and serum of several dog breeds have significantly exceeded those of a single mixed dog epithelial preparation.[112]

Interest in human sensitivity to cats reflects their growing popularity as pets and the isolation of the potent major allergen Fel d 1, a 36 kD protein.[107] Levels of this component exceeding 10 μg/gm of house dust strongly determine symptoms in sensitive subjects.[205] School children in Sweden were shown to encounter levels of Fel d 1 and Can f 1 in school rooms sufficient to induce perennial asthma, even when there was no pet at home.[126] Additional cat allergens, including feline serum albumin, appear to be less clinically significant. Fel d 1 is present in parotid tissue and may be transferred to skin in part through the grooming process. It is substantially absent from serum and urine but present primarily in feline sebaceous glands.[137] Possible differences among major cat breeds in Fel d 1 or other allergens have not been defined. However, Fel d 1 content has been strongly correlated with the dissimilar potency levels noted for various commercial cat extracts as test reagents. Cross reactions between the epithelia[19, 23] and sera[19, 136] of dogs and cats seem to reflect shared components of uncertain nature, although similarities in serum albumins may contribute.[184] Dog and cat emanations regularly help confer allergenic activity on house dusts, and horse and cow epithelia also may occur in some interiors. Historically, allergens of these larger species have been derived from hair products present in mattresses, upholstery, and pads for carpeting, but these risks seem minimal today. The impress of local factors is important, especially in rural and farm situations or anywhere that outdoor perils require pets to remain indoors.[185] Because IgE antibodies may recognize epithelial derivatives, serum components, or both, dander-sensitive subjects may or may not tolerate therapeutically administered horse serum.

Of the many other species, including primates, with allergenic danders, rodents and rabbits (lagomorphs) have a specially prominent impact on laboratory personnel. In one study of 238 persons with frequent occupational exposure to laboratory animals, over 10% developed clinically evident symptoms.[110] Surveys focused on workers with rodents have reported approximately 30% with related allergic problems. Rodents, especially hamsters, gerbils, and guinea pigs, also have become popular cage pets in homes and elementary school classrooms. In addition, rat populations in poor urban housing, storage facilities, and sewers may create exposure hazards. For guinea pigs, rats and mice, the most important allergens are derived from urine, making optimal containment of these fluids a priority, especially in the laboratory setting.[69, 193]

The use of goat (as cashmere and mohair), camel, alpaca, and vicuna hair in fabrics is seldom a source of symptoms referable to dander sensitivities. Similarly, the view that sheep wool is an important allergen source remains unsubstantiated. The acknowledged tendency of wool fibers to irritate sensitive or xerotic skin is often misinterpreted by patients as allergy. Extracts of commercial wool have been shown to contain house dust activity, human dander, and other acquired components. If raw wool does harbor specific ovine allergen, substantial reduction in its activity might be expected to occur in commercial processing, but specific components have not been recorded.

Symptoms on exposure to feathers, especially chicken feathers, are widely recorded. The down and flight feathers of ducks, geese, and other species are less often implicated as allergens. Significantly, the aging process produces material increasingly active in skin and respiratory tests, whereas freshly plucked feathers and their extracts usually elicit little response. This suggests that feathers may be degraded or invaded by external agents, thereby acquiring activity; possible associations with both fungi and mites have been suggested.[207] Plucked feathers also tend to fragment in time, producing a fine dust with irritant properties that may also sensitize. The scope of feather allergens remains obscure, although clinical sensitivity seems evident, and differences from house dust components have been emphasized.

Experience suggests that persons with skin test or respiratory reactivity to feathers have no greater risk of mishap on eating cooked meat or egg of the corresponding species than do random atopic persons. Similarly, egg-grown vaccines appear to pose no excessive threat to feather-sensitive persons, despite expressed implications to the contrary.

LATEX

Recognition of IgE-mediated reactions to rubber latex has increased steadily, soaring with the adoption of universal precautions in the late 1980s. Adverse responses may vary from mild contact urtication to fatal anaphylaxis; at least 15 deaths were reported from 1989 to 1993.[170] The risk group is dominated by biomedical workers and persons having frequent latex contact with tissues or mucosal surfaces, such as children with spina bifida or urogenital defects. Among the former, respiratory exposure to aerosolized latex allergens (largely from powdered gloves) producing rhinitis and asthma is encountered increasingly. Carriage of latex allergens by cornstarch particles has been confirmed, allowing partial abatement of this factor.[194]

Multiple latex (protein) allergens exist, but testing still has required the use of moist latex film, crude extracts, or suboptimally sensitive in vitro assays. Latex allergy is correlated with sensitivity to certain foods, such as banana, chestnut, avocado, and kiwi fruit, but the clinical impact of this association still is unclear.[115] Avoidance of topical and inhalant exposure remains essential, since masks offer limited protection.

ALLERGENIC FUNGI

Human sensitivity to fungi was first recognized over 60 years ago as bronchospastic responses among farm workers exposed to clouds of spores from heavily parasitized crops. Since then, evidence has grown that rhinitis, conjunctivitis, and asthma, as well as allergic alveolitis, may result from fungus emanations. In approaching the fungi, established references treat points of technique,[171] taxonomy,[6, 72, 91] and identification[10, 13, 14, 54, 135, 172] in some detail. However, dose-response formulations for fungi remain unexplored, and relatively few types are accepted as clinically important allergens with complete certainty.

Although allergic respiratory illness produced by airborne fungi remains a foremost concern, other avenues of clinical impact have been suggested. An association between urticaria and ingestion of food yeasts or intestinal *Candida albicans* growth has been proposed but never rigorously confirmed. Even less evidence exists for a chronic candida sensitivity syndrome (CCSS) in which a universe of morbid effects are attributed to intestinal or other carriage of *C. albicans*. However, the view that IgE-mediated reaction to this organism may favor some instances of intractable *Candida* vaginitis now has provisional support, and trials of high-dose injection immunotherapy have suggested benefit, although further study is indicated.[152, 153]

Possible links between atopic dermatitis activity and cutaneous or gut *C. albicans* carriage have not emerged. However, many affected eczematous patients have shown strong IgE reactivity to a lipophilic commensal yeast, *Pityrosporum ovale*, a normal inhabitant of human sebaceous structures and skin surfaces.[132] Improvement in some eczematous persons given antifungal therapy has stimulated further interest in this association.[49]

Studies, especially by Ward and associates,[210] have reawakened interest in possible associations of respiratory allergy and superficial fungus infections. These workers have identified a small subset of asthmatic patients with strong skin and respiratory sensitivity to *Trichophyton tonsurans*, a common dermatophyte. Some of these patients lacked any additional IgE specificities, appearing by all other criteria as intrinsic asthmatics, and have benefited from antifungal therapy. Although allergen absorption from cutaneous foci is assumed, inhalation of fungus-laden squames may impose additional exposure burdens. However, it still seems that extrinsic determinants of fungus exposure far outweigh sources on or in the body.

Although only a minority of fungi produce widespread aerial contamination, their variety is so large that atmospheric burdens at any point usually comprise many types. In addition, the spectrum of airborne fungi often changes rapidly with weather events or disturbance of substrates. Differences in air spora between sites also are prominent, with distinctive species patterns in many interiors, although these too change with time. Resulting exposures are complex and may overlap pollen seasons and perennial allergen burdens, such as dust and animal emanation. As subjects with multiple skin and clinical sensitivities are commonplace, it is often difficult to assign symptoms to fungus inhalants or weigh the health effects of specific offenders.

Major problems in documenting fungus exposure also remain. Sources of most inhaled fungal materials are microscopic, confounding even careful field observation. Concepts of occurrence have required direct sampling of air, and the collection methods employed have shaped our notions of fungus prevalence. For example, reliance on gravity fallout techniques effectively concealed the abundance of ascospores and basidiospores, as well as other smaller forms, until the advent of suction samplers. Similarly, monitoring programs based on agar cultures select bioaerosols with compatible growth potential and fail completely to represent parasites and fastidious saprophytes, however abundant.

STRUCTURAL BASIS OF FUNGUS LIFESTYLES

Fungi comprise a galaxy of organisms that are neither plants nor animals but form a separate kingdom of ancient and still obscure origin.[91] In adapting to most natural and manmade niches, fungi have evolved models of physical organization from single cells to forms with large and complex organs, usually for reproduction. The latter types often are designated fleshy fungi, and those lacking macroscopic organs often are thought of as molds. Diversity has been achieved with just two basic structural units (Fig. 21–25). A heterogeneous minority of taxa (yeasts) grow as single cells and reproduce by fission or budding to produce two daughter cells, or more if budding is multicentric. In culture, yeasts appear as glossy or mucinous bacteria-like colonies, with individual cells generally appearing discrete at high-dry magnification (unlike bacteria). However, most fungi comprise branching threads termed hyphae, which are usually 3 to 10 μm wide. Hyphal filaments have well-defined cell walls, containing chitin or cellulose, and true nuclei, visualized only by special processing. In aggregate, hyphal strands form a mycelium that expands as individual fibers grow and branch. Hyphae often are modified to bear or form the simple reproductive units of molds and are the structural substance of fleshy fruiting bodies, such as mushrooms, puffballs, and rust pustules.

Hyphae of most organisms have cross walls dividing the strands, although perforations allow protoplasmic continuity. The resulting segments may change with age, showing pig-

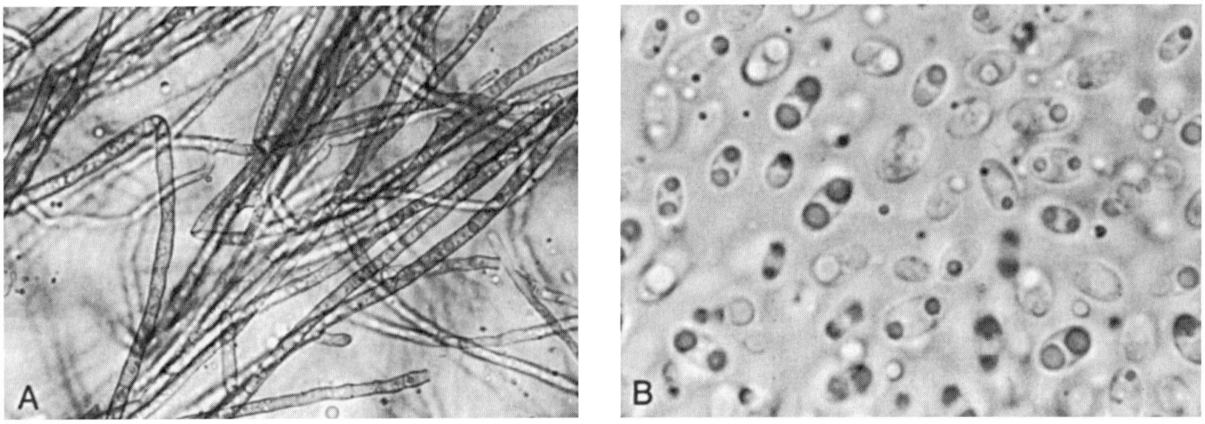

FIGURE 21–25. Basic structural units of fungi. (A) Interlacing hyphal filaments from a colony of a *Dreschslera* species. (B) Discrete yeast cells of a *Rhodotorula* species.

mentation or varying wall thickness and often accumulating metabolic debris. In a minority of types with coenocytic hyphae, cross walls are few or absent, and protoplasm streams unimpeded. Coenocytic hyphae, which tend to be broader than septate types, are a feature of many bread and sugar molds (Zygomycetes) and the downy mildews (Oömycetes).

SPORE FEATURES AND FORMATION

Spores comprise the bulk of recognizable airborne fungus materials, and their mode of formation facilitates classification of organisms. Fungi reproduce by sexual or asexual spores; dispersed hyphal fragments further provide colony-forming units (CFU). Ascospores and basidiospores are widely prevalent sexual spore categories that may include important aeroallergens. Asexual spores of two major types are recognized: sporangiospores, which originate in closed sacs (sporangia) and conidia, which are borne on exposed hyphal structures. Both types include recognized human sensitizers. In addition, many fungi produce thick-walled, resistant chlamydospores by the rounding up and condensation of intercalary hyphal segments. Although some conidia are produced as arthrospores by simple segmentation of vegetative hyphae, most conidia originate at the tips of specialized filaments (conidiophores) (Fig. 21–26). Differences in the process of spore production distinguish organisms producing morphologically similar conidia. In addition, color, size, shape, and surface texture are features that aid identification. Designations based on spore septation are also common; categories include no septa (amerospores), a single septum (didymospores), two or more parallel septa (phragmospores), and both transverse and longitudinal septa (dictyospores).

SPORES AND RELATIONSHIPS AMONG FUNGI

Fungus life cycles may be quite simple but often involve production of both sexual and asexual spores from morphologically distinctive stages termed perfect and imperfect, respectively. These reproductive forms often occur at separate times, and, under unfavorable growth conditions, either or both may be suppressed indefinitely. As a result, fungus life histories generally are pieced together from widely separated observations rather than being revealed in a rapid and orderly sequence. The description of individual fungus stages as separate, named organisms has been an understandable result of this process when true biologic relationships were obscure. The ascomycete, *Neurospora sitophila*, for example, which produces sexual spores (ascospores) widely studied by microbial geneticists, also has a separately designated asexual (imperfect) stage, *Monilia sitophila* (the red bread mold), with distinctively formed conidia. Similarly, many *Aspergillus* types now are recognized as imperfect stages of separately named ascomycetes, and under favorable culture conditions, conidia and ascospores may coexist.

Organisms assigned to different genera because of distinctive perfect stages may have strikingly similar conidial forms. Efforts to group these asexual stages on morphologic grounds alone therefore have often united organisms lacking close, natural evolutionary ties. Such categories, defined largely by similarities of conidial structure, are termed form genera. These somewhat artificial groupings comprise the large and

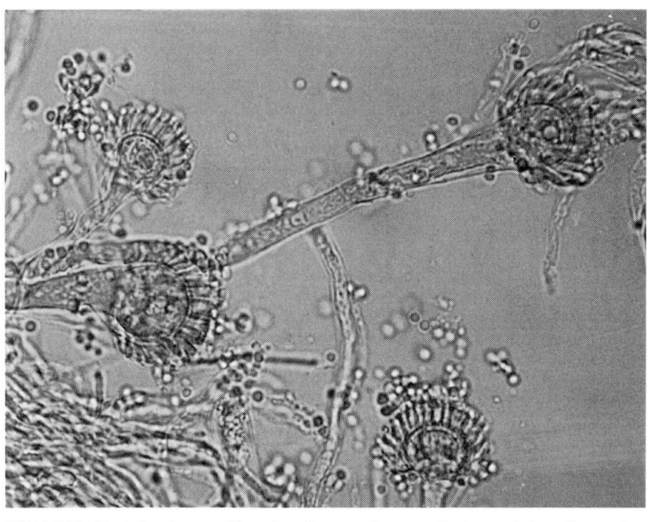

FIGURE 21–26. *Aspergillus fumigatus*. Spore chains arising from the swollen terminal vesicle of a conidiophore are a principal feature of this form genus.

diverse form class Deuteromycetes or Fungi Imperfecti. As perfect stages of these organisms are identified, reclassification occurs, although familiar deuteromycete designations often persist. Furthermore, it appears that certain imperfect fungi may totally lack perfect stages that might serve as more reliable taxonomic criteria.

Form genera do bestow a superficial order on fungi that produce asexual spores. However, because these categories often do not reflect natural affinities, there is little reason to expect uniformity of allergens among their component form species.

DETERMINANTS OF AIRBORNE FUNGUS LOADS

The pressures of colonizing almost every conceivable natural setting have produced a remarkable diversity of fungus lifestyles. Many live and reproduce entirely in aquatic niches; others are dispersed by specific vectors, such as insects. Many terrestrial fungi occupy sequestered sites from which only limited travel of reproductive units is possible. However, at least five major orders have representatives that achieve substantial free atmospheric dispersion: the Oömycetes, Zygomycetes, Ascomycetes, Basidiomycetes, and Deuteromycetes. Features of these distinctive groups will be summarized; in addition, certain commonalities are noteworthy.

Familiar fungi all require oxygen during active growth, unlike some bacteria and actinomycetes. Furthermore, traces of formed carbohydrate generally are essential, although inorganic nitrogen sources usually suffice. Carbohydrate-rich media often promote florid hyphal growth but may, in fact, discourage reproductive structures. By contrast, optimal amounts of B vitamins, yeast extract, and additional factors, including exposure to specific ultraviolet (UV) bands, may stimulate spore formation by otherwise sterile colonies. The addition of undefined natural components, such as V8 juice, hay, animal dung, sawdust, and fruit pulp, may foster the aerometric recovery or sporulation of certain fastidious saprophytes. However, these media are only modestly successful as supplements to malt extract or potato dextrose agar for surveillance sampling and do not replace the latter multipurpose substrates (culture media) for routine use.

Vegetative hyphae of most familiar fungi grow best between 15° and 25°C, a mesophilic range, although individual types may have narrower preferences. Dormancy occurs commonly at subfreezing temperatures, except for certain cryophilic forms that may sporulate between 0° and −5°C. Storage at −45° to −60°C or lower is widely successful for maintaining prolonged viability, unmodified characteristics, and freedom from contamination.

Although factors such as substrate nutrients, water, and tonicity can modify tolerance to extremes of temperature, most fungi succumb at 71°C. A few thermophilic organisms will grow only above limits of 45° to 65°C. In addition, many thermotolerant types, including several aspergilli, flourish in ranges favoring both mesophilic and thermophilic forms.

Environmental moisture strongly influences the development, as well as the dispersion and deposition, of fungus emanations. Many types survive prolonged dryness in a dormant state but require available water for active growth. Often, however, fungi stressed by low moisture or marginal amounts of carbohydrate respond with augmented spore production. When substrates are notably dry, relative humidity levels in surrounding air of 70% or more may support growth. However, microenvironmental conditions are not well reflected by discrete, fixed sensors. High humidities may prevail along discrete drainage paths or adjacent to shaded soil or leaf surfaces, especially when air mixing is sluggish. Chilled surfaces, such as outer walls in winter, also may allow condensation, even when the main volume of warmer interior air is palpably dry.

The reproductive units of many fungi are dispersed by direct wind-scouring or wind-driven agitation of substrates. Such dry spore dissemination is optimal with brisk winds and low relative humidities, conditions typical of sunny, hot, breezy afternoon periods. At these times, spores of form species of *Alternaria, Cladosporium, Epicoccum, Helminthosporium-Drechslera, Stemphylium,* and *Pithomyces*, as well as those of smuts, rusts, and certain oomycete genera, such as *Peronospora*, often become abundant (Fig. 21–27). A similar process governs spore takeoff in some *Aspergillus, Penicillium,* and *Rhizopus* species, which may predominate indoors. Generally, dry spore dispersion falls in still, muggy air and is markedly suppressed by dew formation or active rainfall.

Although dry spore types decline in rainy weather, total fungus levels actually may rise, reflecting forms dispersed by moisture-dependent mechanisms. Ascospores and basidiospores often dominate the wet weather air spora (Fig. 21–28). Both groups produce spores, termed ballistospores, that are shot actively from their points of development by mechanisms requiring free water. Ballistospores may be recovered continuously during a local growing season but reach abundance peaks especially with rainfall and fog, as well as after dark, when falling temperatures favor humid conditions. Spores produced in slimy masses also are readily dispersed by the impact of rainfall or dew, as spore-rich aggregates imbibe water and fracture into microdroplets. This sequence determines the wet weather prominence of genera including *Fusarium, Cephalosporium, Phoma,* and *Trichoderma*, as well as diverse yeast taxa.

Circadian trends in temperature, humidity, wind speed, and solar input often interact to foster a diurnal air spora with dark deuteromycetes (especially *Cladosporium*), rusts,

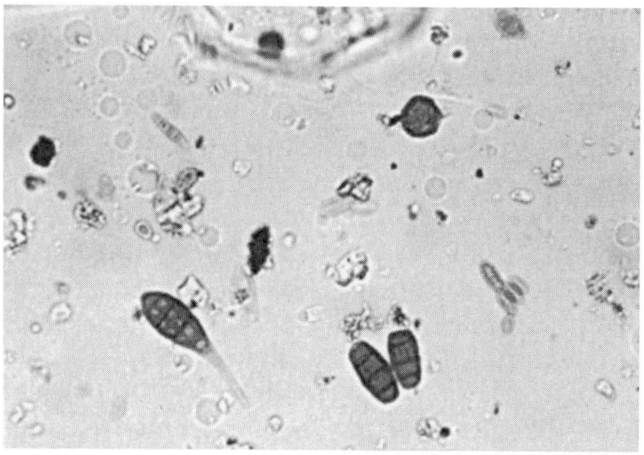

FIGURE 21–27. Typical dark spore recoveries during warm, dry weather. Upper right: round, warty spore of *Epicoccum*. Lower left: tadpole-shaped *Alternaria* spore. Lower and right of center: two barrel-shaped spores of *Pithomyces chartarum*. To their right: five spores of a *Cladosporium* species.

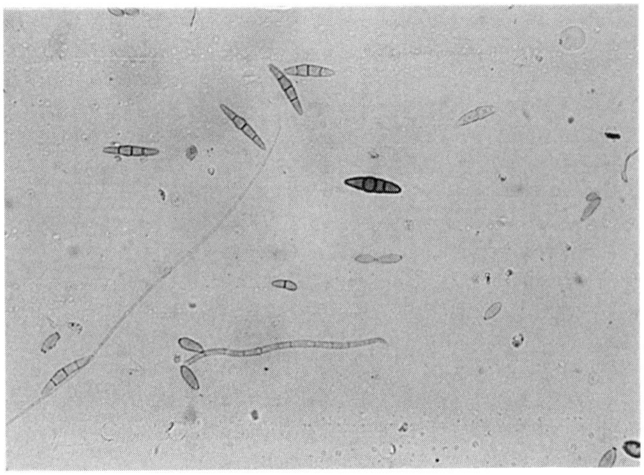

FIGURE 21–28. Spore recoveries characteristic of humid or rainy weather. Most are variously shaped ascospores. Occasional basidiospores also are seen, as are some spores *(Cladosporium)* more typical of dry periods.

and smuts and a nocturnal array dominated by ballistospores. Effects of light intensity and duration also are recognized on spore development and germination. In addition, UV irradiation may substantially lower the growth potential even of darkly pigmented spores, leading to substantial underestimates of prevalence when data are based on culture alone.[102]

ASPECTS OF CLINICAL ALLERGY TO AIRBORNE FUNGI

The ability of fungi to produce allergic airway responses is established and may be modeled, albeit imperfectly, by laboratory provocation. Impressions that clinical allergic responses to natural spore clouds tend to be unusually long or associated with laryngitis or bacterial superinfection have not been critically examined. If ultimately confirmed, they might reflect associated exposure to bacteria or endotoxins also present in implicated dusts.[51, 154]

IgE reactivity to fungi underlies most observed skin and respiratory responses. Antibodies of other isotypes, especially IgG, also develop after natural exposure or immunotherapy. The probability that such factors contribute to tissue changes in allergic bronchopulmonary aspergillosis and candidiasis (see Chapter 31) has suggested possible roles for fungus-specific IgG in atopy. To date, only tenuous evidence links late asthmatic responses with IgG levels to particular fungi. However, further study, especially of prolonged responses at skin test and immunotherapy sites, may prove fruitful.[149]

Efforts to define immunologic cross-reactivity among fungi, although strengthened by the description of a few major allergens, still largely rely on RAST and ELISA inhibition. Species of *Alternaria* and *Stemphylium*, plus *Curvularia* and *Stachybotrys* (W. R. Solomon, unpublished data), show strong similarities in these assays, and between the first two, sharing of the allergen Alt-1 has been confirmed.[3] Whether concordant skin reactivity described for extracts of *Alternaria* and *Phoma* species is similarly based remains to be seen. The same assay systems, as well as differential skin testing, have repeatedly suggested qualitative or quantitative allergen differences among members of deuteromycete form genera, notably *Alternaria*,[29] *Aspergillus*,[89] and *Cladosporium* (W. R. Solomon, unpublished data). Variations between batches in the activity of extracts based on single strains must be overcome to pursue these studies. Furthermore, for a single organism, such as *Alternaria alternata*, extracts derived from separated spores, spore-free mycelium, or filtered fluid culture medium have shown differences in allergenic activity.[79, 178] These observations dictate caution in appraising differential relationships of fungi and their derivatives. Efforts to define major allergens still are preliminary, and standards for reagent preparation have yet to emerge, although approaches have been suggested.[2] With so many uncertainties, it seems prudent to consider most fungus organisms allergenically distinctive until similarities are clearly shown.

PATTERNS OF AIRBORNE FUNGUS PREVALENCE

Numbers of outdoor, airborne fungi vary seasonally in patterns that follow vegetation cycles. Cool temperate regions experience their lowest levels with local snow cover, and prevalence rises to peaks from midsummer to autumn. In frost-free areas of North America, perennial fungus occurrence is typical, with lesser peak-to-trough concentration differences. With few exceptions, local fungus burdens parallel the dominant occurrence of *Cladosporium*, such as *C. herbarum* and *C. cladosporioides*, form species. Other taxa exhibit different, usually shorter, prevalence periods. In the Great Lakes region, for example, brief waves of specific ascospores appear from early spring to midsummer, whereas others persist throughout the growing season, along with basidiospores of *Coprinus* and *Ganoderma*. Ballistospores of other gilled and bracket mushrooms are recovered primarily during late summer and autumn, when the mirror yeasts, principally *Sporobolomyces* species, also are abundant. Deuteromycete form genera with summer and fall peaks include *Stemphylium, Helminthosporium-Drechslera, Curvularia, Pithomyces*, and *Epicoccum*. In many areas, form species of *Penicillium* show little annual variation, whereas peak recoveries of aspergilli, including *A. fumigatus*, have occurred unpredictably from August to April. Specific prevalence periods for other fungus taxa occur in temperate areas and probably also in tropical regions, where the abundance of airborne fungi is year long.

Because periods of mold prevalence are prolonged and variable, reflect multiple contributors, and overlap local pollen seasons, annual patterns of morbidity offer limited help in identifying clinical fungus sensitivity. Affected persons often report symptoms throughout the local growing season, with heightened severity from midsummer onward. Symptoms may appear during late winter thaws and often persist after a local killing frost (−3°C or lower at ground level). Furthermore, with fungus-induced rhinitis and asthma often prominent at midsummer, multiply sensitive persons tend to find no respite in symptoms between periods of local grass and ragweed pollinosis.

Reports of symptoms on ingesting mold-containing foods are of unproven value in identifying subjects reactive to airborne fungi. Intense allergic events provoked by various food mushrooms (basidiomycete fruiting bodies) or truffles or morels (ascomycete fruiting bodies) are seldom encountered. Many foods contain or are prepared using brewers' or bakers' yeast (*Saccharomyces cereviseae*); however, it is not clear that intolerance to these predicts sensitivity to unrelated, especially filamentous, fungi. Similar reservations surround reputed associations between mold sensitivity and adverse reactivity to beers and wines. These nondistilled beverages do acquire microbial components. Unfortunately, adverse reactions on imbibing also may be due to the volume consumed, carbon dioxide, ethanol, and other components that may include high levels of histamine[189] or additives, such as sulfites or rarely egg white and soy.

Correlation of allergic symptoms with situations imposing heavy, short-term fungus exposures provides more valid diagnostic clues than do seasonal or gastronomic histories. Disturbance of natural or cultivated plant growth can increase respiratory burdens by primary liberation, as well as reflotation, of fungus particles; both processes are fostered when substrates are relatively dry. This effect has been most evident in overgrown old field situations, where levels of smut and dark deuteromycete spores 10- to 20-fold or more above background have been measured around an adult hiker.[118] Particle liberation by similar activity was progressively lower on mowed lawns and especially within wood lots.[118] Exposure risks rise predictably with less subtle disturbance, so that field cutting, threshing, and baling may create spore clouds, even from relatively healthy crops. Similar hazards result during work with silage, mulches, and compost heaps. Lawn cutting and collection of clippings often provoke symptoms in fungus-sensitive persons during any season, although algae, arthropod fragments, and refloated pollens also may contribute. Adverse responses to dry soil particles and garage dusts may affect such persons, but lake shores and marshy areas seem to be no more problematic than upland situations.

Fungi readily colonize interior substrates, including many that are marginal nutritionally, producing potential sources of perennial exposure. Especially during periods without snow, many fungi recovered indoors have originated in nature and penetrated structures secondarily; however, mold growth is familiar in damp home or work environments. These indigenous populations usually comprise small-spored deuteromycetes, with *Penicillium, Aspergillus*, yeasts, and occasionally zygomycetes, such as *Rhizopus* and *Mucor*, preponderant. On rare occasions, indoor sources of *Cladosporium* or *Aureobasidium* predominate. However, interior growth of *Alternaria* and other dark-spored imperfect taxa has been rare, unless crude plant materials are present.

Familiar factors promote indoor fungus growth: substrate moisture, local humidity, tolerable temperature, acceptable physical and chemical conditions, and minimal nutritive requirements for metabolism. Food storage areas, garbage containers, and soiled upholstery often support domestic mold growth. In addition, animal hair products are colonized readily, and fungal cellulases promote utilization of cotton, kapok, and conventional wallpaper. The porosity of foam rubber and its tendency to retain moisture favor mold contamination, a risk shared by synthetic foams. Other nutritionally marginal surfaces also are colonized if water is available, including basement or cold outside walls, window moldings, shower curtains, plumbing fixtures, and refrigerator drip trays.

Poorly maintained cold mist vaporizers have been shown to emit dense fungus aerosols, although boiler-type units have not been similarly implicated.[175] Viable microbial outputs by ultrasonic units have been reported, although their extent and determinants remain obscure.[167] Console and centrally installed humidifiers harbor large fungus populations less frequently.[31] Plant-derived materials, including burlap, wicker, bark, and stored firewood, afford substrates for microfungi, unless absolutely dry. In addition, healthy living plants and soils can contribute indoor fungi but, like other substrates, usually require physical disturbance or active air motion for spore dispersal. Direct sampling has not suggested that a few undisturbed houseplants significantly raise indoor fungus levels,[32] although greenhouse conditions should be avoided and soils can harbor both allergens and potential pathogens.[186]

EVALUATING AIRBORNE FUNGUS PREVALENCE

The variations in air spora among sites in nature and frequently distinctive mycoflora of specific enclosures seriously limit predictions of personal exposure based on average conditions. Direct air sampling by continuous monitoring or brief spot checks can provide clinically instructive data for specific situations.

The challenge of collecting diverse fungal particle sizes with limited bias has been reviewed, and overriding merits of volumetric recoveries have been emphasized. Despite traditional emphasis on agar cultures, direct microscopy of particle deposits, when usable, offers more accurate prevalence estimates, since growth potential is not a prerequisite. Many fungal particles, including ascospores and basidiospores, as well as selected spores of smuts, rusts, oömycetes, and parasitic deuteromycetes, may be recognized morphologically but fail to grow on available laboratory media. Particle deposits have special merit in monitoring outdoor air, with spore traps facilitating the broadest range of recoveries and Rotorods usually reserved for larger units (8–10 μm). Collections generally are examined unstained in aqueous media, although small hyaline spores first may be stained with phenosaffranin or cotton blue. Unfortunately, authenticated spore samples are difficult to obtain. Although no comprehensive manual of identification exists, illustrations in several references are helpful.[10, 13, 14, 54, 70, 135, 172]

The limitations of visual identification for small, nondescript spores mandate culture-based techniques as part of any comprehensive sampling effort. Viable recoveries are key within enclosures and wherever yeasts, zygomycetes, and nonpigmented deuteromycetes, such as *Penicillium, Aspergillus, Trichoderma, Verticillium, Beauveria*, and *Paecilomyces* species, may be prominent. Because few minute spores fall on horizontal surfaces, little confidence can be attached to data from open culture dishes.[173] Slit samplers and sieve impingers best accomplish home surveys. However, membrane filters and liquid impingers also are useful volumetric collectors in relatively still air.

Of several general-purpose media, including Sabouraud's and potato dextrose agars, commercially prepared malt ex-

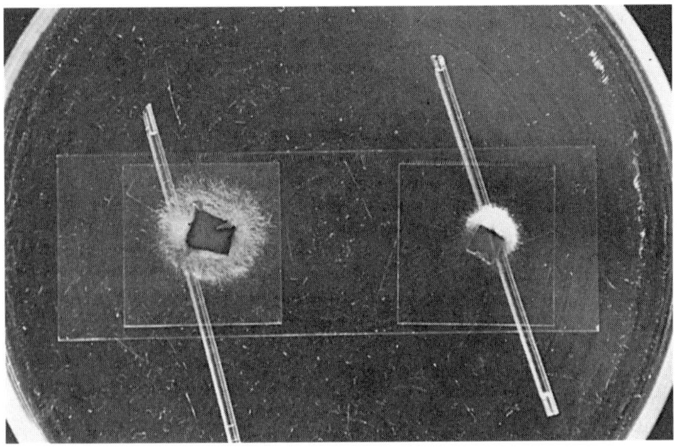

FIGURE 21–29. Technique of slide culture, which allows delicate fungus structures to be viewed intact microscopically. Glass rods support the slides in moist chambers.

tract agar promotes identifiable growth of an especially broad variety of microfungi. However, some previously favored substrates, such as malt salt and Mehrlich's media, have been found to recover many fewer types.[30] Subculture on substrates such as tap water agar, corn meal agar, or V8 agar occasionally promotes sporulation, and near-UV irradiation may induce fruiting by previously sterile hyphal growth.

Developing colonies often can be identified to the level of form genus by gross appearance, although many determinations require microscopy at scanning or higher power. Structural details are easily observed using thin agar squares placed on sterile glass microslides and maintained under cover slips after inoculation. These slide cultures may be viewed unmounted or as preparations in fluid media, such as lactophenol or Meltzer's reagent (Fig. 21–29). Lactophenol is prepared by combining 10 gm phenol, 10 gm lactic acid syrup, 20 gm glycerol, and 10 ml distilled water; with the addition of 50 mg cotton blue to each deciliter of medium, it is possible to stain many fungal structures, including hyaline spores. Meltzer's reagent is especially useful in restoring the turgor and natural appearance of dried-out materials and is prepared by mixing 1.5 gm potassium iodide, 0.5 gm iodine, and 2.2 gm chloral hydrate in 20 ml of water.

FUNGI IMPLICATED IN INHALANT ALLERGY

Members of five fungal classes have been implicated as sources of aeroallergens on more or less compelling evidence; however, the clinical impact of many familiar types has remained speculative. This section surveys categories of air spora reputed to have allergenic impact under realistic exposure conditions.

DEUTEROMYCETES (FUNGI IMPERFECTI)

The form class Deuteromycetes comprises most microfungi designated molds in the literature on human hypersensitivity. By definition, its members do not produce sexual spores, although many have separately described ascomycete or basidiomycete perfect stages. Four form orders are recognized, of which two, the Melanconiales and Mycelia Sterilia, remain to be implicated convincingly as allergen sources; members of both groups are important plant pathogens. Mycelia Sterilia comprises a few taxa that appear to lack any true spores, with dispersion by hyphal fragments or specialized appendages. These fungi must be distinguished from organisms that simply fail to sporulate on specific media despite vegetative growth. Most of the latter (sterile) isolates seem to originate from ascospores or basidiospores, and the term Mycelia Sterilia should be restricted to members of that specific deuteromycete group, such as *Pythium* and *Rhizoctonia*.

The form order Sphaeropsidales unites imperfect fungi that bear flask-shaped fruiting bodies (pycnidia) in which conidia form on short hyphae (Fig. 21–30). Spores are extruded in mucinous masses when mature and are commonly splash dispersed. Pycnidia often are evident macroscopically and superficially resemble the fruiting structures (perithecia) of certain ascomycetes; airborne spores of both groups are prominent in wet weather. During autumn rains, levels of *Phoma* species may reach, but rarely exceed, 200 CFU per cubic meter in the upper Midwest.

The form order Moniliales is the largest division of the Deuteromycetes and includes those fungi most familiar to clinicians. A few especially prominent groupings are described to emphasize their characteristic relationships and human impact.

Cladosporium

The characteristic ovoid, pigmented spores of *Cladosporium* form species are widespread in areas lacking permanent snow cover, commonly outnumbering all other biologic particles (see Fig. 21–27). A few types of *Cladosporium* have ascomycetous perfect stages, such as *Venturia* and *Mycosphaerella*, and several are costly parasites of bananas, spinach, and other crops. A tomato pathogen and reputed aeroallergen previously described as *C. fulvum* has been reclassified as *Fulvia sp.*[54] Its allergenic relationships, if any, remain to be defined. Two form species, *C. herbarum* and *C. cladosporioides*, are widespread dominants in temperate areas, with average levels exceeding 5,000 spores/m^3. Both these and

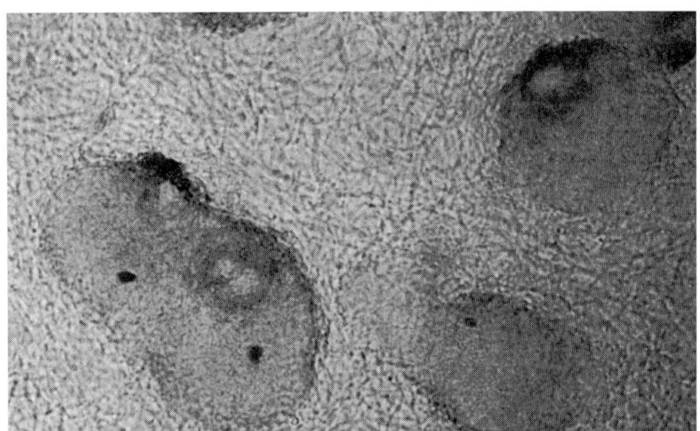

FIGURE 21–30. Sphaeropsid of the genus *Phoma*. Two of the typical pycnidia are shown. Single-celled spores are extruded in slimy masses through the light-colored openings.

less abundant form species, such as *C. macrocarpum* and *C. sphaerospermum*, reach peak prevalence in midsummer during warm, dry diurnal periods. Hot spots of local spore profusion are produced when standing or composting vegetation, including grass clippings, are disturbed. At least one major allergen of *C. herbarum* has been described partially.[11] However, interspecies allergen patterns are unclear. The generic name *Hormodendrum* is an obsolete term still used at times to denote *Cladosporium*.

Alternaria and Other Dictyospore Producers

Several form genera produce smokey green colonies and elongated spores with both transverse and longitudinal septa. In North America, however, such fungi most often are *Alternaria* form species (see Fig. 21–27), which reach notable abundance especially in grain-growing areas. Daily *Alternaria* spore levels averaging 500 to 1,000/m^3 are common during late summer and fall peaks in the Great Lakes area. A majority of these, on cultural isolation, have proved to be *A. tenuissima* and *A. alternata* (Fr.) Keissler (= *A. tenuis* C. G. Nees); however, additional form species, including obligate parasites, are recovered. Extracts of *Alternaria* cultures, generally *A. alternata*, have elicited the highest reactivity rates among atopic North Americans skin tested with multiple fungus eluates. This potency has been attributed to Alt a 1, a carbohydrate-rich protein (30,000 kD) characterized as a major allergen of *A. alternata*.[225] However, additional reactive components have been described in extracts of this organism.[33] Allergenic complexity also might be predicted from variable patterns of skin and immunosorbent reactivity among individual subjects tested with *A. alternata, A. tenuissima, A. longissima,* and *A. brassicae* extracts.[29]

Form species of *Stemphylium* and *Pithomyces chartarum* contribute lower levels of dark dictyospores that lack the strongly beaked appearance of *Alternaria* (see Fig. 21–27). Spores of *Sporidesmium, Ulocladium,* and some ascomycetes also must be distinguished. *Stemphylium botryosum* has a known ascomycete perfect stage, *Pleospora herbarum*, with asci also producing dictyospores. Despite fundamental differences in sporogenesis—spores of *Alternaria* are produced in chains and those of *Stemphylium* develop singly—species of both taxa share the major allergen, Alt a 1.[3]

Helminthosporium/Drechslera

Of deuteromycetes producing dark, elongated spores with prominent septa or pseudosepta, *Helminthosporium/Drechslera* species are most familiar (Fig. 21–31). Typical phragmospores may be 50 to 100 μm or more long and produce extremely dark, low colonies. In North America, *H. solani* and *H. velutinum* are common, and epidemic plant infections, especially of corn and potatoes, may boost local spore levels. Long, brown phragmospores characterize additional deuteromycete form genera, and a few ascospores and rust teliospores also must be distinguished. Spores of *Curvularia* form species have three to five transverse septa but are strongly curved and have an enlarged central cell. Rates of skin reactivity to common species of these form genera often equal or exceed those to *Alternaria* extracts in atopic midwesterners.

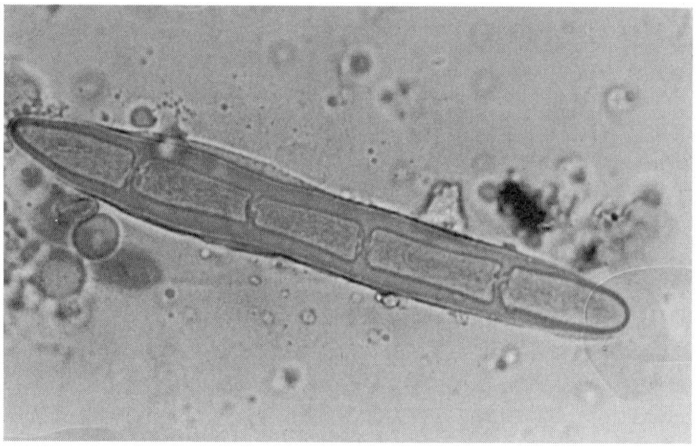

FIGURE 21–31. Multicelled phragmospore of *Helminthosporium* species.

Epicoccum

The taxon *Epicoccum* is widely encountered as a single form species, *E. purpurascens*, prevalent especially in grasslands and field crops; textiles and foodstuffs also may be colonized. The brown, warty, multiseptate conidia arise in masses on hyphal cushions (sporodochia), which appear grossly as black dots in culture (Fig. 21–32). Agricultural sites in North America commonly see background spore levels averaging 100 to 200/m^3 in late summer and fall, although disturbance of standing and fallen vegetation can magnify these. The production of orange or rust-colored, diffusible pigments in agar culture is a helpful but not unique trait of *E. purpurascens*. On most substrates, near-UV irradiation promotes spore production. Although varied estimates of skin reactivity to *Epicoccum* extracts have been reported in North America, attention probably is warranted where prevalence is high.

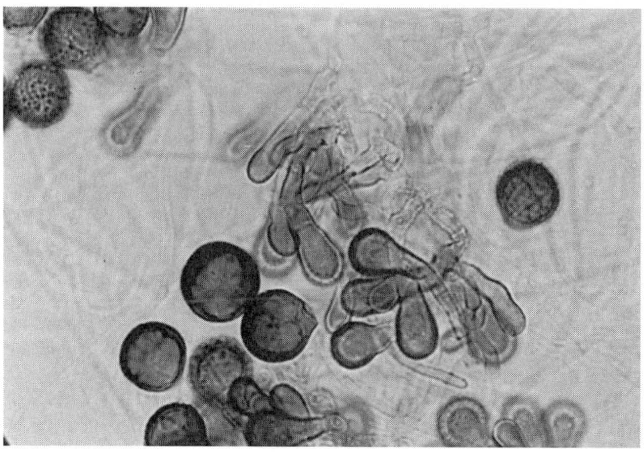

FIGURE 21–32. Portion of a slide culture of *Epicoccum purpurascens*. Several stages in the development of the rough-surfaced, brown, multiseptate spores are shown.

Fusarium

Like *Epicoccum, Fusarium* is identified with a form family (Tuberculariaceae) producing sporodochia. However, *Fusarium* spores form mucinous masses, facilitating splash dispersal. More than a dozen form species are recognized, both saprophytes and serious crop pathogens. *F. nivale*, which grows beneath snow cover on plant debris, appears early in spring; other form species typically are prevalent later.

Fusarium isolates often secrete soluble (red or violet) pigments and may form large, hyaline, curved, fusiform, multiseptate macroconidia; small, ovoid or comma-shaped, single-celled microconidia may occur instead, or both may occur together. Fusiform ascospores frequently are confused with *Fusarium* macrospores in particle deposits. Because *Fusarium* spores are strictly hyaline, distinctions involving lightly colored ascospores are easily resolved. Furthermore, on close scrutiny, each *Fusarium* macroconidium shows one end cell distinctly elongated, producing a minutely asymmetrical spore.

Several *Fusarium* form species have ascomycete sexual stages, such as *Gibberella, Nectria,* and *Calonectria*, producing abundant airborne spores, and it is likely that many *Fusarium* colonies result from ascospore germination. Extracts of several form species, especially *F. vasinfectum*, show reactivity in atopic groups, although relevant ascospore preparations have not been compared.

Pullularia/Aureobasidium

Changes in the name of this form genus have created periodic confusion; hence, both generic designations are given. It accommodates a single pleomorphic organism, *P./A. pullulans*, which is widely distributed but rarely achieves prevalence levels above several hundred units per cubic meter in free air. Indoors, this fungus readily defaces paper, lumber, and painted finishes and colonizes plastic and ceramic bathroom surfaces. In agar culture, *P/A. pullulans* generates numerous tiny subhyaline blastopores, and, with age, the hyphae develop into rows of dark, thick-walled chlamydospores. Grossly, this change transforms cream-colored, mucinous colonies into black leathery discs. Despite the ubiquity of *P/A. pullulans*, positive skin tests are elicited in no more than 8% to 12% of atopic midwesterners.

Aspergillus

Aspergillus comprises many widely prevalent spoilage organisms and several thermotolerant forms, some of which, such as *A. fumigatus* and *A. flavus*, are recognized human pathogens. In addition, the production of soy sauce, saki, and certain enzymes reflects the metabolic repertoire of *A. oryzae*. Other aspergilli synthesize commercial organic chemicals, such as citric and oxalic acids. Spores of *Aspergillus* form species are individually small and nondescript. However, their origin in chains, from specialized structures (sterigmata) borne on the swollen end (vesicle) of a conidiophore, is quite distinctive (see Fig. 21–26). These arrangements, with characteristic colony colors, may be observed in culture. Occasional ascocarps confirm specific form species as ascomycete imperfect stages.

Aspergilli often are common in outdoor air, with prominent differences in prevalent taxa among sites.[116] Seasonal patterns vary, with annual peaks at least as often in summer as in colder periods.[176] Aspergilli also are abundant in many interiors. Differential inhibition studies, as well as skin tests, have shown allergenic differences among common form species. Overall levels of reactivity are well below those of *Alternaria* form species, with *A. niger* often producing the lowest reaction rates.

Penicillium

The form genus *Penicillium* presents vast size and complexity, its members showing broad distribution, wide commercial exploitation, and frequent abundance in enclosed spaces. Penicillia are widely evident spoilage microbes, and specific taxa (*P. roquefortii* and *P. camembertii*) are regularly ingested in their respective cheese products. Neither symptoms following ingestion of these fermented foods nor skin reactivity to other penicillia predicts adverse reactivity to therapeutic penicillins or other beta lactam drugs.

Penicillium form species are moderately variable, and the identification of strains is tedious; as a result, few surveys have attempted infrageneric distinctions. Limited data suggest that, in temperate regions, any of almost two dozen taxa may be widely prevalent. Individual form species may reach selective abundance in specific interiors sampled directly. Recoveries occasionally are dominated by related form genera, including *Gliocladium*, especially from humidifier sources, and *Paecilomyces*.

Less Familiar Deuteromycetes

Spores of additional filamentous deuteromycetes occur often enough to constitute possible aeroallergens. The frequent prevalence of *Polythrincium trifolii*, an obligate parasite of clover and other legumes, as well as taxa, such as *Cercospora, Torula*, and *Periconia* spp., which grow poorly or not at all on laboratory media, invites study. Spores of *Botrytis* species, especially *B. cinerea*, also are represented poorly in culture, despite abundance outdoors in summer and within plant-propagating facilities at any season. Certain small-spored taxa, including form species of *Wallemia, Sporothrix, Tritirachium*, and *Cephalosporium*, grow well in culture, appearing almost exclusively in volumetric collections. An additional type, *Monilia (Neurospora) sitophila* (the red bread mold), is prominent in tropical areas but favors bakeries and flour mills in cooler regions. Still other hyphal imperfect fungi are commonly recovered and may reach clinically significant levels in brief seasons or discrete situations, including species of *Arthrinium, Coniosporium, Cylindrocarpon, Gliocladium, Nigrospora, Scopulariopsis, Spondylocladium, Trichoderma, Trichothecium*, and *Verticillium*.

YEASTS

Fungi of unicellular growth form (yeasts) have diverse affinities, so that allergenic uniformity within this group should not be expected. In general, these organisms form gelatinous, bacteria-like colonies on laboratory media, with their cells discernible as discrete units (unlike many bacteria) at high-dry power (see Fig. 21–25B). Bakers' (brewers') yeast *(Saccharomyces cerevisiae)* forms ascospores, whereas other familiar types, such as *Rhodotorula* and *Cryptococcus* species, replicate as deuteromycetes by budding and rarely fission. Additional genera, notably *Sporobolomyces* and *Bullera*, form bean-shaped ballistospores on peg-like sterigmata, which are discharged actively much like basidiospores.

Yeast cells are readily splash dispersed and form a prominent part of the nocturnal and wet weather air spora. In central North America, peak recoveries from air occur during autumn rains; orchards are exceptionally strong sources. Spectacular levels of airborne *Sporobolomyces roseus* occur during late summer in England and Wales, where they may produce widespread respiratory allergy. Although this organism also occurs in North America, its prevalence and clinical impact seem lower.

Notable tolerance to acid or hypertonic conditions allows some yeasts access to specialized domestic and industrial niches. Indoor colonization by *Rhodotorula* species is especially prominent and commonly centers in fluid reservoirs, such as those of console and cold-mist humidifiers.[175] Food yeasts, primarily *S. cerevisiae*, may heighten the allergen load of some atopic persons but seem rarely to evoke symptoms.

Candida species are widespread in nature and form branching chains of adherent cells (pseudohyphae) from which groups of spores (blastospores) are budded. Special interest surrounds a possible role for *C. albicans* in respiratory allergy, since human IgE and precipitin, as well as cell-mediated, responses to it are well documented. However, the frequent presence of this organism in the flora of the skin, gut, mouth, and vagina may better explain such reactivity. *C. albicans* is seldom recovered from air away from the human microenvironment, although additional species occasionally occur.

ZYGOMYCETES

The grouping Zygomycetes, also termed Phycomycetes, comprises genera of familiar saprophytes, such as *Absidia, Mucor*, and *Rhizopus*. Many species form rapidly spreading high-pile mycelia of broad, coenocytic hyphae liberally sprinkled with sporangia (Fig. 21–33). Although uncommon in most well-mixed free air, sporangiospores are often abundant near leaf litter and in interiors where soil water or storage of plant materials is a factor. Skin reactivity to cosmopolitan Zygomycetes, such as *Rhizopus nigricans* and *Mucor racemosus*, occurs in a distinct minority of fungus-sensitive North American subjects.

OÖMYCETES

Members of the Oömycetes, especially the downy mildews (Peronosporaceae), are widespread and often devastating plant parasites. Extensive infections of grasses and crops, including grapes, potatoes, and onions, still shake regional economies and produce moderate atmospheric levels of the ovoid, almost featureless spores. Human sensitivity to downy mildews has not been evaluated, although occupational allergy to a related Oömycete has been described.[158]

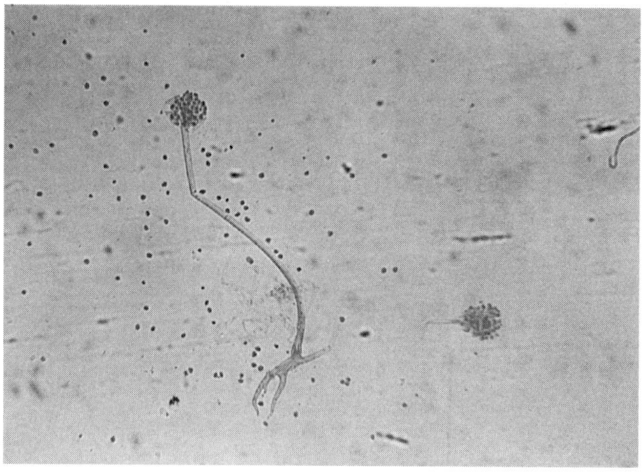

FIGURE 21–33. Slide culture of *Rhizopus* species. The broad hyphae with few septa and the sporangium shown are noteworthy features of the Zygomycetes.

ASCOMYCETES

The Ascomycetes form a huge, structurally diverse class, with its common feature a sac-like cell, the ascus, in which unattached ascospores mature in a fluid matrix. Commonly, eight spores develop per ascus and are actively discharged; however, exceptions are frequent. Asci may be single or multiple and may be borne exposed or in specialized fruiting bodies (ascocarps). The latter structures include truffles, morels, and cup fungi, but most are visible only as minute dots on stem and leaf surfaces and easily overlooked. Many ascomycete life cycles include asexual spores, identifiable with and often named as deuteromycete form taxa, such as *Aspergillus, Stemphylium,* and *Fusarium*.

During humid periods, thousands of ascospores per cubic meter typically dominate the air spora of tropical and temperate areas (see Fig. 21–28). Many particle types are distinctive, but others defy precise identification. Efforts to harvest spores from minute ascocarps have proved remarkably tedious. Despite these difficulties, reactivity to a few accessible spore types has been demonstrated, especially by British workers[62, 75]; reactivity to *Chaetomium* was described many years ago. In central North America, the multiseptate ascospores of *Leptosphaeria* species are especially prominent. Other common types are derived from species of *Nectria, Xylaria, Daldinia*, and *Ophiobolus*, as well as other taxa.

Conidial forms of some ascomycetes may be easily recognized on agar media. In addition, the powdery mildews are leaf surface parasites that produce dense mycelial mats bearing conidia, as well as minute ascocarps, which incidentally facilitate overwintering. The relatively large, hyaline, somewhat box-shaped spores are released in clouds with substrate disturbance, such as during lawn care. Skin sensitivity to conidia of a powdery mildew, *Microsphaera alni*, has been described, but the clinical significance of these common fungi remains to be clarified.

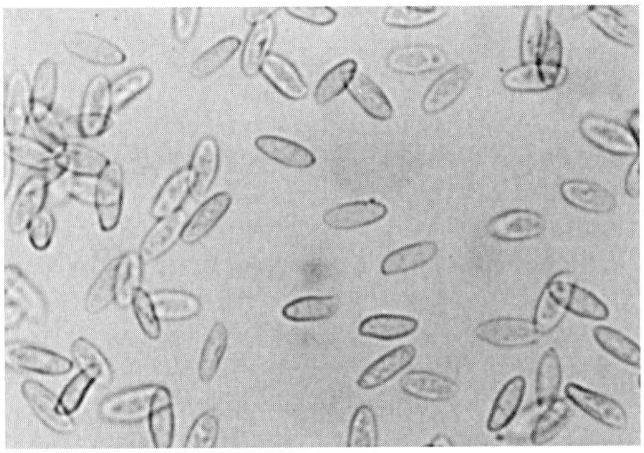

FIGURE 21–34. Basidiospores of a gilled fungus. On close examination, each is seen to have a projection (apiculus) marking its former point of attachment to the basidium.

BASIDIOMYCETES

Among the class Basidiomycetes are mushrooms, puffballs, jelly fungi, rusts, and smuts, a diverse array of parasites and saprophytes, including forms with multistage life cycles. Unifying this group is the basidium, a specialized structure on which usually four basidiospores develop and from which they are forcefully discharged (Fig. 21–34). Basidiospores are often bilaterally symmetrical, with a short eccentric projection (the apiculus) marking former attachment to the basidium. In addition, the hyphae of these fungi often show sharply curved clamp connections that bridge the septa of adjacent segments.

Basidiomycetes comprises two major divisions with distinctive lifestyles. Mushrooms and puffballs form basidiospores almost exclusively, although imperfect stages producing arthrospores also occur. Their emanations usually peak in forested areas and during periods of darkness and rainfall. Both hyaline and colored basidiospore levels rise during late summer and fall, with maximum variety at this time. However, spores of bracket fungi, such as *Ganoderma* species, may maintain daily levels of several hundred spores per cubic meter, except in winter. The dark, barrel-shaped spores of *Coprinus* species (the inky caps) are prevalent throughout the growing season in Europe and North America, except during drought. Although spores of many fleshy basidiomycetes are easily collected, studies of their clinical potential still are limited. Skin and mucus test positively to spore extracts of agarics, such as *Agaricus, Armillarea, Coprinus*, and *Hypholoma* species, and bracket fungi, such as *Ganoderma, Merulius*, and *Polyporus*, were noted by British workers.[74, 75] Respiratory allergy induced indoors by *Merulius lacrymans* (dry rot) spores also is documented. However, among unselected, exposed atopics, no more than 15% have shown immediate skin reactivity to extracts of the related *Ganoderma applanatum*.[191] Higher response rates have been reported in other small groups with or without prominent, isolated late reactions.[68, 157] Almost one third of atopic subjects studied by Lehrer and colleagues[104] showed skin test responses to regionally prominent basidiospores.

A second division of Basidiomycetes is best known for the rusts (Uredinales) and smuts (Ustilaginales). These largely parasitic forms often are important crop pathogens, many with several hosts and spore-bearing stages. Respiratory illness in farm workers massively exposed to rust spores drew attention to fungus-induced allergy. Thereafter, sensitivity to rusts and smuts stimulated brief, intense interest. However, it is not clear that these are often important clinically, except close to agricultural sources. Rusts having both short and multistage life cycles tend to produce urediospores most abundantly (Fig. 21–35), so that field exposures generally emphasize these particles. However, urban levels in the Midwest only rarely exceed 100/m^3. In addition, during late summer, low numbers of dark teliospores (teleutospores)

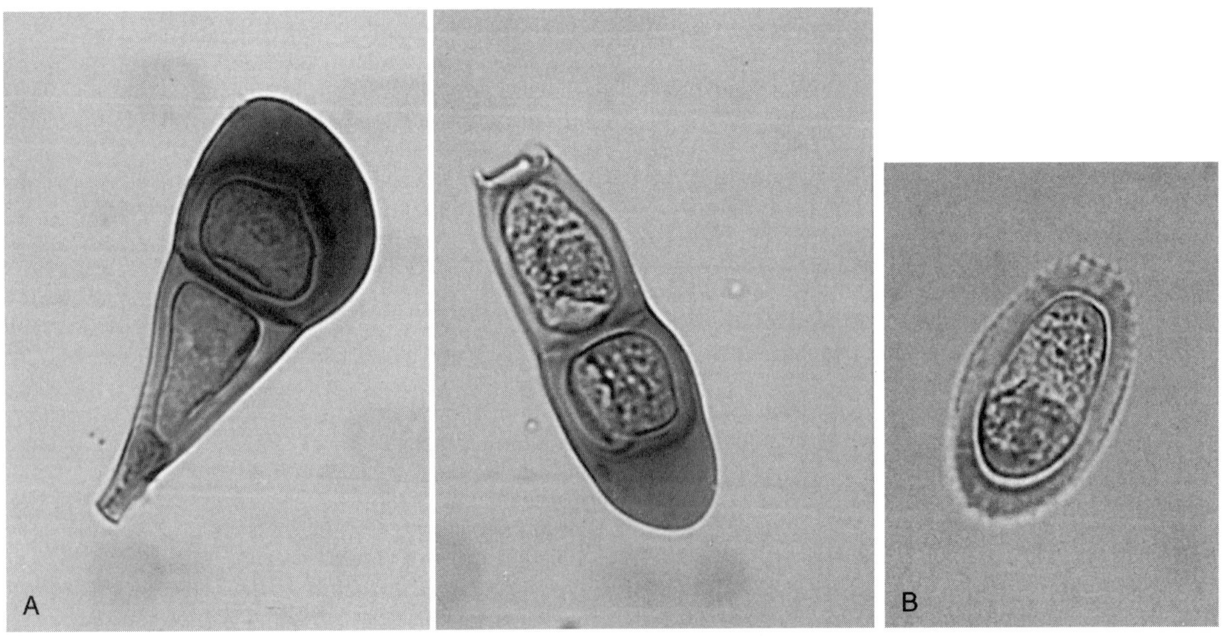

FIGURE 21–35. **(A)** Teliospores typical of the rust *Puccinia*, which allow the fungus to overwinter. **(B)** Characteristic, usually golden-colored rust ureidospore (urediospore).

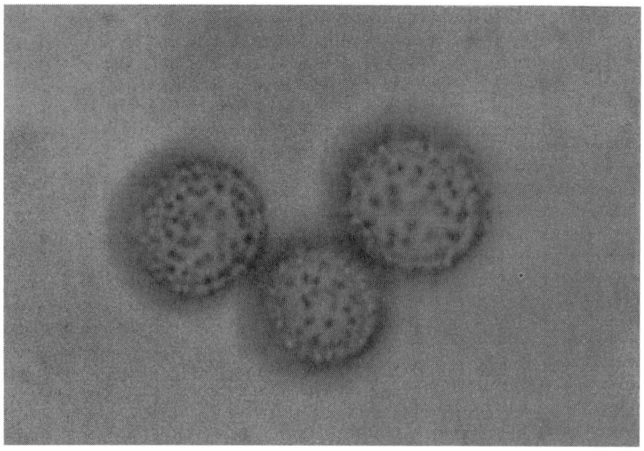

FIGURE 21–36. Brown warty spores of corn smut *(Ustilago maydis)*.

appear during dry periods. These units are distinctive for specific rust genera, unlike urediospores and basidiospores.

Spores of smuts are widespread, even in urban air, but especially abundant near infected grain and wild grasses (Fig. 21–36). Most North American recoveries represent the genus *Ustilago*. These particles often average below 10 μm, with spines uniformly distributed (corn smut) or confined to one hemisphere (the oat smut type). Visible clouds of spores that arise when smutted grain is cut can produce respiratory irritation directly. Less often, allergic responses seem to result, but their frequency in both rural and especially adventitiously exposed urban populations remains speculative. Skin reactivity to common smuts is demonstrable in no more than 10% of Midwestern clinic populations, although rates in farm workers may average higher.

REFERENCES

1. Aasmul-Olsen S, Lombardero M, Løwenstein H, Ipsen H: Characterization of group I and 2/3 allergens from eleven grasses. J Allergy Clin Immunol 95:307, 1995. Abstract.
2. Agarwal MK, Jones RT, Yunginger JW: Immunochemical and physicochemical characterization of commercial Alternaria extracts: a model for standardization of mold allergen extracts. J Allergy Clin Immunol 70:432, 1982.
3. Agarwal MK, Jones RT, Yunginger JW: Shared allergenic and antigenic determinants in Alternaria and Stemphylium extracts. J Allergy Clin Immunol 70:437, 1982.
4. Agarwal MK, Yunginger JW, Swanson MC, et al: An immunochemical method to measure atmospheric allergens. J Allergy Clin Immunol 68:194, 1981.
5. American Conference of Governmental Industrial Hygienists: Air Sampling Instruments for Evaluation of Atmospheric Contaminants, 7th edition. NIOSH, Cincinnati, 1989.
6. Alexopoulos CJ: Introductory Mycology, 3rd edition. Wiley, New York, 1979.
7. Alvarez-Cuesta E, Cuesta-Herranz J, Puyana-Ruiz J, et al: Monoclonal antibody-standardized cat extract immunotherapy: risk-benefit effects from a double-blind placebo study. J Allergy Clin Immunol 93:556, 1994.
8. Arlian LG, Bernstein IL, Gallagher JS: The prevalence of house dust mites (Dermatophagoides sp.) and associated environmental conditions in homes in Ohio. J Allergy Clin Immunol 69:527, 1982.
9. Arlian LG, Vyszenski-Moher DL, Lawrence AT, et al: Antigenic and allergenic analysis of psyllium seed components. J Allergy Clin Immunol 89:866, 1992.
10. Arx JA von: The Genera of Fungi Sporulating in Pure Culture, 3rd edition. Lubrecht & Cramer, Monticello, NY, 1981.
11. Aukrust L, Broch S: Partial purification and characterization of two Cladosporium herbarum allergens. Int Arch Allergy Appl Immunol 69:68, 1979.
12. Bagenstose AH, Mathews KP, Homburger HH: Inhalant allergy due to crickets. J Allergy Clin Immunol 65:71, 1980.
13. Barnett HL, Hunter BB: Illustrated Genera of Imperfect Fungi, 3rd edition. Burgess, Minneapolis, 1972.
14. Barron GL: The Genera of Hyphomycetes from Soil. Krieger, Melbourne, 1977.
15. Bassett IJ, Crompton CW, Parmelee JA: An Atlas of Airborne Pollen Grains and Common Fungus Spores of Canada. Monograph 18. Canada Department of Agriculture. Thorn Press, Ottawa, 1978.
16. Batson WT: Genera of the Eastern Plants, 3rd edition. Wiley, New York, 1975.
17. Bernstein DI, Patterson R, Zeiss CR: Clinical and immunologic evaluation of trimellitic anhydride and phthalic anhydride exposed workers using a questionnaire with comparative analysis of enzyme linked immunosorbent and radioimmunoasssy studies. J Allergy Clin Immunol 69:311, 1982.
18. Bernstein IL, Safferman RS: Sensitivity of skin and bronchial mucosa to green algae. J Allergy 38:166, 1966.
19. Blands J, Løwenstein H, Weeke B: Characterization of extract of dog hair and dandruff from six different dog breeds by quantitative immunoelectrophoresis identification of allergens by crossed radioimmunoelectrophoresis (CRIE). Acta Allergol 32:147, 1977.
20. Bousquet J, Guerin B, Dhivert H, et al: Cross allergenicity among Oleaceae pollens. J Allergy Clin Immunol 69:145, 1982.
21. Bousquet J, Hejjaoui A, Becker WM, et al: Clinical and immunologic reactivity of patients allergic to grass pollens and to multiple pollen species. I. Clinical and immunologic characteristics. J Allergy Clin Immunol 87:737, 1991; Bousquet J, Becker WM, Hejjaoui A, et al: Efficacy of a double-blind, placebo-controlled, specific immunotherapy with standardized extracts. J Allergy Clin Immunol 88:43, 1991.
22. Bousquet J, Michel FB: Enzyme des Pollens. Les Pollinoses. Lab. Fison, Montpellier, France, 1979.
23. Brandt R, Yman L: Dog dander allergens: specificity studies based on radioallergosorbent technique. Int Arch Allergy Appl Immunol 61:361, 1980.
24. Breiteneder H, Ferreira F, Reikerstorfer A, et al: Complementary DNA cloning and expression in *Escherichia coli* of *Aln g* I, the major allergen in pollen of alder *(Alnus glutinosa)*. J Allergy Clin Immunol 90:909, 1992.
25. Bucholtz G, Lockey R, Binford L, Serbausek D: Allergenicity of the bald cypress tree (Taxodium distichum). J Allergy Clin Immunol 71:96, 1983.
26. Buckle FG, Cohen AB: Nasal mucosal hyperpermeability to macromolecules in atopic rhinitis and extrinsic asthma. J Allergy Clin Immunol 55:213, 1975.
27. Bufe A, Becker W-M, Schramm G, et al: Major allergen Phl p Va (timothy grass) bears at least two different IgE-reactive epitopes. J Allergy Clin Immunol 94:173, 1994.
28. Burge HP, Boise JR, Rutherford JA, Solomon WR: Comparative recoveries of airborne spores by viable and non-viable modes of volumetric collection. Mycopathologia 61:27, 1977.
29. Burge HP, Muilenberg ML, Solomon WR: Alternaria allergens at the species level. J Allergy Clin Immunol 67:69, 1981. Abstract.
30. Burge HP, Solomon WR, Boise JR: Comparative merits of eight popular media in aerometric studies of fungi. J Allergy Clin Immunol 60:199, 1977.
31. Burge HA, Solomon WR, Boise JR: Microbiol prevalence in domestic humidifiers. Appl Environ Microbiol 39:840, 1980.
32. Burge HA, Solomon WR, Muilenberg ML: Evaluation of indoor plantings as allergen exposure sources. J Allergy Clin Immunol 70:101, 1982.
33. Bush RK, Voss MJ, Bashirian S: Detection of Alternaria allergens by crossed radioimmunoelectrophoresis. J Allergy Clin Immunol 71:239, 1983.
34. Cartier A, Lafrance M, Pineau L, et al: Occupational asthma in crab-processing workers. J Allergy Clin Immunol 71:159, 1983.
35. Chang JL, Johnson J, Kang BS: Characterization of cockroach antigen. J Allergy Clin Immunol 71:161, 1983.
36. Chang Z-N, Liu C-C, Tam MF, et al: Characterization of the isoforms of the group I allergen of *Cynodon dactylon*. J Allergy Clin Immunol 93:1206, 1995.
37. Chapman MD, Heymann PW, Wilkins SR, et al: Monoclonal immuno-

assays for major dust mite *(Dermatophagoides)* allergens, *Der p* I and *Der* f 1, and quantitative analysis of the allergen content of mite and house dust extracts. J Allergy Clin Immunol 80:184, 1987.

38. Charpin C, Mata P, Charpin D, et al: Fel d I allergen distribution in cat fur and skin. J Allergy Clin Immunol 88:77, 1991.
39. Coghlan TH, Vinson SB, Paull BR: Moth scale allergy. J Allergy Clin Immunol 71:159, 1983.
40. Connell JT: Quantitative intranasal pollen challenges. III. The priming effect in allergic rhinitis. J Allergy 43:33, 1969.
41. Crifo S, Iannetti G: Antigens of Parietaria off. pollen (Urticaceae), separated by discontinuous electrophoresis in polyacrylamide gel. Acta Allergol 24:294, 1969.
42. Cromwell O, Pepys J, Parish WE, Hughes EG: Specific IgE antibodies to platinum salts in sensitized workers. Clin Allergy 9:109, 1979.
43. Daily F, Stier R, Featherstone L: Incomplete cross reactivity between the mites, Dermatophagoides farinae and D. pteronyssinus. J Allergy Clin Immunol 69:127, 1982. Abstract.
44. Davies RR, Smith LP: Forecasting the start and severity of the hay fever season. Clin Allergy 3:263, 1973.
45. deBlay F, Chapman MD, Platts-Mills TAE: Indoor environmental control techniques for reducing airborne cat allergen (Fel d 1). J Allergy Clin Immunol 87 (pt 2):169, 1991.
46. deGroot H, Goei KGH, vanSwieten P, Aalberse RC: Affinity purification of a major and a minor allergen from dog extract: serologic activity of affinity-purified Can f 1 and of Can f 1-depleted extract. J Allergy Clin Immunol 87:1056, 1991.
47. DiFelice G, Caiaffa MF, Bariletto G, et al: Allergens of Arizona cypress *(Cupressus arizonica)* pollen: characterization of the pollen extract and identification of the allergenic components. J Allergy Clin Immunol 94:547, 1994.
48. Dingle AN, Gill GC, Wagner WH Jr, Hewson EW: The emission, dispersion, and deposition of ragweed pollen. Adv Geophys 6:367, 1959.
49. Doekes G, vanIeperen-vanDijk AG: Allergens of *Pityrosporum ovale* and *Candida albicans* and atopic dermatitis. Clin Exp Allergy 48:394, 1993.
50. Dolovich J, Shaikh W, Tarlo S, et al: Human exposure and sensitization to airborne papain. Ann Allergy 38:382, 1977. Abstract.
51. Do Pico GA, Glaherty D, Bhansali P, Chavaje N: Grain fever syndrome induced by inhalation of airborne grain dust. J Allergy Clin Immunol 69:435, 1982.
52. Dreborg SKG, Munir MD, Einarrson R: The level of *Fel d* I in school dust is sufficiently high to induce symptoms in asthmatics! J Allergy Clin Immunol 87(pt 2):169, 1991.
53. Elias TS: The Complete Trees of North America, 2nd edition. Gramercy Pub Co, New York, 1987.
54. Ellis MB: Dematiaceous Hyphomycetes. Commonwealth Mycology Institute, Surrey, UK, 1971.
55. Farnham JE, Beaucher WN: Gypsy moth infestation: effects on an allergic population. J Allergy Clin Immunol 69:113, 1982.
56. Feinberg SM, Aries PL: Asthma from food odors. JAMA 98:2280, 1932.
57. Ferguson DM, Harwood LJ, Shannon FT, Taylor B: Parental smoking and lower respiratory illness in the first 3 years of life. J Epidemiol Community Health 35:180, 1981.
58. Fernandes L, Mesquita AM: *Anacardium occidentale* (cashew) pollen allergy in patients with allergic bronchial asthma. J Allergy Clin Immunol 95:501, 1995.
59. Fine A: Hypersensitivity reaction to kiwi fruit (Chinese gooseberry, Actinidia chinensis). J Allergy Clin Immunol 68:235, 1981.
60. Fontana VJ, Wittig H, Hold LE Jr: Observations on the specificity of the skin test: the incidence of positive skin tests in allergic and nonallergic children. J Allergy 34:348, 1963.
61. Frankland AW: Locust sensitivity. Ann Allergy 11:445, 1953.
62. Frankland AW, Gregory PH: Allergenic and agricultural implications of airborne ascospore concentrations from a fungus, *Didymella exitialis*. Nature 245:336, 1973.
63. Fraser BN: Cockroaches in relation to bronchial asthma in the Durban area. S Afr Med J 55:637, 1979.
64. Freidhoff LR, Ehrlich-Kautzky E, Grant JH, et al: A study of the human immune response to *Lolium perenne* (rye) pollen and its components. Lol p I and Lol p II (rye I and rye II). I. Prevalence of reactivity to the allergens and correlations among skin test, IgE antibody and IgG antibody data. J Allergy Clin Immunol 78:1190, 1968.
65. Gall H, Kalveram K-J, Forck G, Sterry W: Kiwi fruit allergy: a new birch pollen-associated food allergy. J Allergy Clin Immunol 94:70, 1994.
66. Gelber L, Selzer L, Pollart S, et al: Specific IgE ab and exposure to cat and cockroach allergens as risk factor for acute asthma. J Allergy Clin Immunol 87(pt 2):233, 1991. Abstract.
67. Godfrey MA: A Sierra Club Naturalist's Guide—The Piedmont. Sierra Books, San Francisco, 1980.
68. Gold BL, Burge HA, Muilenberg ML, Solomon WR: Epidermal reactivity to basidiospore extracts. J Allergy Clin Immunol 73:113, 1984. Abstract.
69. Gordon S, Tee RD, Newman Taylor AJ: Analysis of rat urine proteins and allergens by sodium dodecyl sulfate-polyacrylamide gel electrophoresis and immunoblotting. J Allergy Clin Immunol 92:298, 1993.
70. Gregory PH: The Microbiology of the Atmosphere, 2nd edition. Wiley, New York, 1973.
71. Habenicht HA, Burge HA, Muilenberg ML, Solomon WR: Allergen carriage by atmospheric aerosol. II. Ragweed-pollen determinants in submicronic atmospheric fractions. J Allergy Clin Immunol 74:64, 1984.
72. Hawksworth DL, Kirsop E (eds): Filamentous fungi (Living Resources for Biotechnology Ser.) Cambridge Univ Press, Cambridge, 1988.
73. Hensel AE, Griffith RC: Clinical experiences with Paspalum notatum (Bahia grass), a new grass antigen. South Med J 65:690, 1972.
74. Herxheimer H, Hyde HA, Williams DA: Allergic asthma caused by basidiospores. Lancet 2:131, 1969.
75. Herxheimer H, Hyde HA, Williams DA: Allergic asthma caused by fungal spores. Lancet 1:572, 1966.
76. Heslop-Harrison J: The physiology of the pollen grain surfaces. Proc R Soc Lond B Biol Sci 190:275, 1975.
77. Hewitt B, Bousquet J, Guerin B, Michel FB: Cross allergenicity among Urticaceae pollens. J Allergy Clin Immunol 71:105, 1983. Abstract.
78. Hirschwehr R, Valenta R, Ebner C, et al: Identification of common allergenic structures in hazel pollen and hazelnuts: a possible explanation for sensitivity to hazelnuts in patients allergic to tree pollen. J Allergy Clin Immunol 90:928, 1992.
79. Hoffman DR, Cummins LH, Kozak PP, et al: Isolation of spore allergens from Alternaria. Ann Allergy 46:310, 1981.
80. Hooker SB: Qualitative differences among canine danders. Ann Allergy 2:281, 1944.
81. Hussain R, Norman PS, Marsh DG: Rapidly released allergens from short ragweed pollen. II. Identification and partial purification. J Allergy Clin Immunol 67:217, 1981.
82. Hyde HA, Adams KF: An Atlas of Airborne Pollen Grains. St. Martin's Press, New York, 1958.
83. Ipsen H, Løwenstein H: Immunochemical characteristics of the major allergen from birch pollen (Betula verrucosa) and its relation to alder and hazel. Int Arch Allergy Appl Immunol 69:127, 1982.
84. Jacinto CM, Nelson RP, Bucholtz GA, et al: Nasal and bronchial provocation challenges with bayberry *(Myrica cerifera)* pollen extract. J Allergy Clin Immunol 90:312, 1992.
85. Jelks M: Allergy Plants (That Cause Sneezing and Wheezing.) World-Wide Printing, Tampa, FL, 1986.
86. Kalliel JN, Settipane GA: Eastern pine sensitivity in New England. New Engl Region Allergy Proc 9:223, 1988.
87. Kammermeyer JK, Mathews KP: Hypersensitivity to phenylglycine acid chloride. J Allergy Clin Immunol 52:73, 1973.
88. Kang B, Vellody D, Homburger HA, Yunginger JW: Cockroach cause of allergic asthma: its specificity and immunologic profile. J Allergy Clin Immunol 63:80, 1979.
89. Karr RM, Lehrer SB, Butcher BT, et al: Analysis of antigenic relationships among species of Aspergillus. J Allergy Clin Immunol 63:213, 1979.
90. Kay AB, MacLean U, Wilkinson AH, Gad El Rab MO: The prevalence of asthma and rhinitis in a Sudanese community seasonally exposed to a potent airborne allergen (the "green nimitti" midge, *Cladotanytarsus lewisi*). J Allergy Clin Immunol 71:345, 1983.
91. Kendrick B: The Fifth Kingdom. Mycologue Publications, Waterloo, Ontario, 1985.
92. Kern RA: Asthma due to sensitivity to mushroom fly (Aphiochaeti agarici). J Allergy 9:604, 1938.
93. King TP, Hoffman D, Løwenstein H, et al: Allergen nomenclature. Int Arch Allergy Immunol 105:224, 1994.
94. Kino T, Chihara J, Fukuda K, et al: Allergy to insects in Japan. III. High frequency of IgE antibody responses to insects (moth, butterfly, caddis fly, and chironomid) in patients with bronchial asthma and immunochemical quantitation of the insect-related airborne particles smaller than 10 μm in diameter. J Allergy Clin Immunol 79:857, 1987.

95. Kino T, Oshima S: Allergy to insects in Japan II. The reaginic sensitivity to silkworm moth in patients with bronchial asthma. J Allergy Clin Immunol 64:131, 1979.
96. Klucka CV, Ownby DR, Green J, Zoratti E: Cat shedding of *Fel d* I is not reduced by washings, Allerpet-C spray, or acepromazine. J Allergy Clin Immunol 95:1164, 1995.
97. Knobel E: Field Guide to the Grasses, Sedges and Rushes of the United States. Dover, New York, 1977.
98. Knox RB: Grass pollen, thunderstorms and asthma. Clin Exp Allergy 23:354, 1993.
99. Kontou-Karakitsos K, Salvaggio JE, Mathews KP: Comparative nasal absorption of allergens in atopic and nonatopic subjects. J Allergy Clin Immunol 55:241, 1975.
100. Kraemer MJ, Richardson MA, Weiss NS, et al: Risk factors for persistent middle ear effusions. Otitis media, catarrh, cigarette smoke exposure and atopy. JAMA 249:1022, 1983.
101. Kramer CL, Pady SM: A new 24-hour spore sampler. Phytopathology 56:517, 1966.
102. Kramer CL, Pady SM: Viability of airborne spores. Phytopathology 60:448, 1968.
103. Lake FR, Ward LD, Simpson RJ, et al: House dust mite-derived amylase: allergenicity and physicochemical characterization. J Allergy Clin Immunol 87:1035, 1994.
104. Lehrer SB, Lopez M, Butcher BT, et al: Basidiomycete mycelia and spore-allergen extracts: skin reactivity in adults with symptoms of respiratory allergy. J Allergy Clin Immunol 78:478, 1986.
105. Leiferman KM, Gleich GJ: The cross reactivity of IgE antibodies with pollen allergens. I. Analysis of various species of grass pollens. J Allergy Clin Immunol 58:129, 1976.
106. Leiferman KM, Gleich GJ, Jones RT: The crossreactivity of IgE antibodies with pollen allergens. II. Analysis of various species of ragweed and other fall weed pollens. J Allergy Clin Immunol 58:140, 1976.
107. Leiferman K, Ohman HL: Cat allergen 1: biological, antigenic, and allergenic properties. J Allergy Clin Immunol 74:147, 1984.
108. Lewis CR, Slavin RG: Allergy to marijuana: a clinical and skin testing study. J Allergy 55:131, 1975.
109. Lewis WH, Vinay P, Zenger VE: Airborne and Allergenic Pollen of North America. Johns Hopkins Univ Press, Baltimore, 1983.
110. Lincoln TA, Bolton NE, Garrett AS: Occupational allergy to animal dander and sera. J Occup Med 16:465, 1974.
111. Løwenstein H, Gravesen S, Larsen L, et al: Indoor allergens. J Allergy Clin Immunol 78:1035, 1986.
112. Lutsky I, Fink JN, Arkins JA, et al: Skin test reactivity to dog-derived antigens. Clin Allergy 10:331, 1980.
113. Lybarger JA, Gallagher JS, Pulver DW, et al: Occupational asthma induced by inhalation and ingestion of garlic. J Allergy Clin Immunol 69:448, 1982.
114. Magnusson CGM: Maternal smoking influences cord serum IgE and IgD levels and increases the risk for subsequent infant allergy. J Allergy Clin Immunol 78:898, 1986.
115. Makinen-Kiljunen S: Banana allergy in patients with immediate type hypersensitivity to natural rubber latex: characterization of cross-reacting antibodies and allergens. J Allergy Clin Immunol 93:990, 1994.
116. Mallea M, Murray IG, Segretain G, et al: Census of Aspergillus colonies in the air: comparison between London, Paris, Lyon, Marseilles. Acta Allergol 27:273, 1972.
117. Martin BG, Mansfield LE, Nelson HS: Patterns of cross allergenicity among grasses. J Allergy Clin Immunol 65:229, 1980.
118. McDonald JL, Solomon WR: Effect of outdoor activity on aeroallergens in the human microenvironment. J Allergy Clin Immunol 55:89, 1975. Abstract.
119. McElhenny TR, McGovern JP: Possible new inhalant allergens. Ann Allergy 10:467, 1970.
120. Menon P, Rando RJ, Stankus RP et al: Passive cigarette smoke-challenge studies: increase in bronchial hyperreactivity. J Allergy Clin Immunol 89:560, 1992.
121. Merget R, Stollfuss J, Wiewrodt R, et al: Diagnostic tests in enzyme allergy. J Allergy Clin Immunol 92:264, 1993.
122. Mittal A, Agarwal MK, Shivpuri DN: Respiratory allergy to algae: clinical aspects. Ann Allergy 42:253, 1979.
123. Moore BS, Hyde JS: Breed-specific dog hypersensitivity in humans. J Allergy Clin Immunol 66:198, 1980.
124. Morrow PE: Aerosol characterization and deposition. Am Rev Resp Dis 110 (pt 2):88, 1974.
125. Muenscher WC: Weeds, 2nd edition. Comstock, Ithaca, NY, 1980.
126. Munir AKM, Einarsson R, Schou C, Dreborg SKG: Allergens in school dust. I. The amount of the major cat (Fel d I) and dog (Can f I) allergens in dust from Swedish schools is high enough to probably cause perennial symptoms in most children with asthma who are sensitized to cat and dog. J Allergy Clin Immunol 91:1067, 1993.
127. Murray AB, Ferguson AC: Dust free bedrooms in the treatment of asthmatic children with house dust or house dust mite allergy, a controlled study. Pediatrics 71:418, 1983.
128. Murray AB, Ferguson AC, Morrison BJ: Diagnosis of house dust mite allergy in asthmatic children: what constitutes a positive history? J Allergy Clin Immunol 71:21, 1983.
129. Murray AB, Zuk P: The seasonal variation in a population of house dust mites in a North American city. J Allergy Clin Immunol 64:266, 1979.
130. Murray FJ, Brown H, Bernton HS: A case of asthma caused by box elder beetle. J Allergy 45:103, 1970.
131. Musmand JJ, Horner WE, Lopez M, Lehrer SB: Identification of important allergens in German cockroach extracts by sodium dodecylsulfate-polyacrylamide gel electrophoresis and Western blot analysis. J Allergy Clin Immunol 95:877, 1995.
132. Nordvall SL, Scheynius A: Pityrosporum ovale and atopic eczema. Allergy 48:391, 1993.
133. Novey HS, Roth M, Wells ID: Mesquite pollen—an aeroallergen in asthma and allergic rhinitis. J Allergy Clin Immunol 59:359, 1977.
134. O'Connell EJ, Logan GB: Parental smoking in childhood asthma. Ann Allergy 32:142, 1974.
135. Ogden EC, Raynor GS, Hayes JV, et al: Manual for Sampling Airborne Pollen. Hafner Press, New York, 1974.
136. Ohman JL, Bloch KJ, Kendall S, Lowell FC: Allergens of mammalian origin. IV. Evidence for common allergens in cat and dog serum. J Allergy Clin Immunol 57:560, 1976.
137. Ohman JL Jr, Lowell FC, Bloch KJ: Allergens of mammalian origin. III. Properties of a major feline allergen. J Immunol 113:1668, 1974.
138. Ortolani C, Ispana M, Pastorello E, et al: The oral allergy syndrome. Ann Allergy 61:47, 1988.
139. Osterballe O, Ibsen H, Weeke B, Løwenstein H: Specific IgE response toward allergenic molecules during perennial hyposensitization: a three year prospective double blind study. J Allergy Clin Immunol 71:40, 1983.
140. Pastorello EA, Ortolani C, Farioli L, et al: Allergenic cross-reactivity among peach, apricot, plum, and cherry in patients with oral allergy syndrome: an in vivo and in vitro study. J Allergy Clin Immunol 94:699, 1994.
141. Petersen J: Estimating air infiltration into houses: an analytical approach. ASHRAE J 21:60, 1979.
142. Pineau L, Cartier A, Malo JL, et al: Occupational asthma due to pepsin. J Allergy Clin Immunol 71:158, 1983.
143. Platts-Mills TAE, Longbottom JL, Wilkins SR: Airborne allergens associated with asthma: comparison of dust mite and rat urinary allergens. J Allergy Clin Immunol 71:157, 1983.
144. Pollart SM, Mullins DE, Vailes LD, et al: Identification, quantitation, and purification of coackroach allergens using monoclonal antibodies. J Allergy Clin Immunol 87:511, 1991.
145. Puerta Llerena L, Fernandez-Caldas E, Caraballa LR, Lockey RF: Sensitization to *Blomia tropicalis* and *Lepidoglyphus destructor* in *Dermatophagoides spp.* allergic individuals. J Allergy Clin Immunol 88:943, 1991.
146. Quirce S, Cuevas M, Diez-Gomez ML, et al: Respiratory allergy to Aspergillus-derived enzymes in bakers' asthma. J Allergy Clin Immunol 90:970, 1992.
147. Ramirez DA: The natural history of mountain cedar pollinosis. J Allergy Clin Immunol 73:88, 1984.
148. Raynor GS, Ogden EC, Hayes JV: Enhancement of particulate concentrations downwind of vegetative barriers. Agricult Meterol 13:181, 188, 1974.
149. Reed CE, Busse W, Crandall M: Adverse reactions to immunotherapy with Alternaria. J Allergy Clin Immunol 51:84, 1973. Abstract.
150. Reid MJ, Nish WA, Whisman BA, et al: HLA-DR4-associated nonresponsiveness to mountain-cedar allergen. J Allergy Clin Immunol 89:593, 1992.
151. Reiss NM, Kostic SR: Pollen season severity and meteorological parameters in central New Jersey. J Allergy Clin Immunol 57:609, 1975.
152. Regúlez P, Garcia Fernández JF, Moragues MD, et al: Detection of anti-*Candida albicans* IgE antibodies in vaginal washes from patients with acute vulvo-vaginal candidiasis. Gynecol Obstet Invest 37:110, 1994.

153. Rosedale N, Brown K: Hyposensitization in the management of recurring vaginal candidiasis. Ann Allergy 43:250, 1979.
154. Rylander R, Morey P: Airborne endotoxin in industries processing vegetable fibres. Am Ind Hyg Assoc J 43:811, 1982.
155. Rynes SE: A critical analysis of animal dander reactions. J Allergy 8:470, 1937.
156. Sakaguchi M, Inouye S, Irie T, et al: Airborne cat (*Fel d* I), dog (*Can f* I), and mite (*Der I* and *Der II*) allergen levels in the homes of Japan. J Allergy Clin Immunol 92:797, 1993.
157. Santilli J, Rockwell WJ, Collins RP: The significance of the spores of the Basidiomycetes (mushrooms and their allies) in bronchial asthma and allergic rhinitis. Ann Allergy 55:469, 1985.
158. Schaubschläger WW, Becker W-M, Mazur G, Gödde M: Occupational sensitivity to *Plasmopara viticola*. J Allergy Clin Immunol 93:457, 1994.
159. Schlichting HE: Ejections of microalgae into the air via bursting bubbles. J Allergy Clin Immunol 53:185, 1974.
160. Schou C, Fernandez-Caldas E, Lockey RF, Løwenstein H: Environmental assay for cockroach allergens. J Allergy Clin Immunol 85:828, 1991.
161. Schou C, Svendsen UG, Løwenstein H: Purification and characterization of the major dog allergen *Can f* I. Clin Exp Allergy 21:321, 1991.
162. Schou C, Lind P, Fernandez-Caldas E, et al: Identification and purification of an important cross-reactive allergen from American (*Periplaneta americana*) and German (*Blattella germanica*) cockroach. J Allergy Clin Immunol 86:935, 1990.
163. Schumacher MJ, Griffith RD, O'Rourke MK: Recognition of pollen and other particulate aeroantigens by immunoblot microscopy. J Allergy Clin Immunol 82:608, 1988.
164. Sheldon JM, Johnston JH: Hypersensitivity to beetles (Coleoptera). J Allergy 12:493, 1941.
165. Sheldon JM, Lovell RG, Mathews KP: A Manual of Clinical Allergy. Saunders, Philadelphia, 1967.
166. Shimoda T, Krzanowski J, Lockey R, et al: Lower airway smooth muscle contraction induced by *Ptychodiscus brevis* (red tide) toxin. J Allergy Clin Immunol 79:899, 1987.
167. Shiue ST, Scherzer HH, DeGraff AC Jr, Cole SR: Hypersensitivity pneumonitis associated with the use of ultrasonic humidifiers. New York State J Med 90:263, 1990.
168. Shulman S: Insect allergy: biochemical and immunological analyses of the allergens. Prog Allergy 12:246, 1968.
169. Siracusa A, Bettini P, Bacoccoli R, et al: Asthma caused by live fish bait. J Allergy Clin Immunol 93:424, 1994.
170. Slater JE: Latex allergy. J Allergy Clin Immunol 94:138, 1994.
171. Smith D, Onions HS: Preservation & Maintenance of Living Fungi. Labrecht & Cramer, Forestburgh, NY, 1983.
172. Smith EG: Sampling and Identifying Allergenic Pollens and Molds. Blewstone Press, San Antonio, 1990.
173. Solomon WR: Assessing fungus prevalence in domestic interiors. J Allergy Clin Immunol 56:235, 1975.
174. Solomon WR: An appraisal of Rumex pollen as an aeroallergen. J Allergy 44:25, 1969.
175. Solomon WR: Fungus aerosols arising from cold mist vaporizers. J Allergy Clin Immunol 54:222, 1975.
176. Solomon WR, Burge HA, Boise JR: Airborne Aspergillus fumigatus outside and within a large clinical center. J Allergy Clin Immunol 62:56, 1978.
177. Solomon WR, Burge HA, Boise JR, Becker M: Comparative particle recoveries by the retracting rotorod, rotoslide and Burkard spore trap sampling in a compact array. Int J Biometeorol 24:107, 1980.
178. Solomon WR, Burge HA, Muilenberg ML: Allergenic properties of Alternaria spore, mycelial and "metabolic" extracts. J Allergy Clin Immunol 65:229, 1980. Abstract.
179. Solomon WR, Burge HP, Muilenberg ML: Pollens of grass allies as potential allergens. J Allergy Clin Immunol 65:56, 1981. Abstract.
180. Solomon WR, Cathey J: Collection deficits due to particle loading by rotating arm samplers. J Allergy Clin Immunology 87:169, 1991. Abstract.
181. Soparkar GR, Patel PC, Cockcroft DW: Inhalant atopic sensitivity to grasshoppers in research laboratories. J Allergy Clin Immunol 92:61, 1993.
182. Spieksma FThM, Kramps JA, vanDer Linden AC, et al: Evidence of grass-pollen allergenic activity in the smaller micronic atmospheric aerosol fraction. Clin Exp Allergy 20:273, 1990.
183. Spieksma FThM, Vooren PH, Kramps JA, Dijkman JH: Respiratory allergy to laboratory fruit flies (*Drosophila melanogaster*). J Allergy Clin Immunol 77:108, 1986.
184. Spitzauer S, Schweiger C, Sperr WR, et al: Molecular characterization of dog albumin as a cross-reactive allergen. J Allergy Clin Immunol 93:614, 1994.
185. Sporik R, Rose G, Honsinger R, et al: Sensitization to dog allergen (*Can f 1*) as a risk factor for asthma in New Mexico: relationship to allergen exposure in houses. J Allergy Clin Immunol 93:229, 1994. Abstract.
186. Staib F: Pathogenic fungi in human dwellings. Mycoses 35:289, 1992.
187. Stanaland BE, Fernandez-Caldas E, Jacinto CM, et al: Sensitization to *Blomia tropicalis*: skin test and cross-reactivity studies. J Allergy Clin Immunol 94:452, 1994.
188. Stevenson DD, Mathews KP: Occupational asthma following inhalation of moth particles. J Allergy 39:274, 1967.
189. Styler HR: Significance of histamine content of alcoholic beverages. J Allergy 43:160, 1969. Abstract.
190. Takafuji S, Suzuki S, Koizumi K, et al: Diesel-exhaust particulates inoculated by the intranasal route have an adjuvant activity for IgE production in mice. J Allergy Clin Immunol 79:639, 1987.
191. Tarlo SM, Bill B, Srinivasan J, et al: Human sensitization to Ganoderma antigen. J Allergy Clin Immunol 64:43, 1979.
192. Tautz C, Rihs H-P, Thiele A, et al: Association of class II sequences encoding DR1 and DQ5 specificities with hypersensitivity to chironomid allergen *Chi t* I. J Allergy Clin Immunol 93:918, 1994.
193. Taylor AM, Longbottom JL, Pepys J: Respiratory allergy to urinary proteins of rats and mice. Lancet 2:847, 1977.
194. Tomazic VJ, Shampaine EL, Lamanna A, et al: Cornstarch powder on latex products is an allergen carrier. J Allergy Clin Immunol 93:75, 1994.
195. Tovey ER, Chapman MD, Platts-Mills TAE: Mite feces are a major source of house dust allergens. Nature 289:592, 1981.
196. Tovey ER, Chapman MD, Wells CW, Platts-Mills TAE: The distribution of dust mite allergen in the houses of patients with asthma. Am Rev Respir Dis 124:630, 1981.
197. Turkeltaub PC, Marsh DG, Lichtenstein LM, Norman PS: Development of long-lasting immediate hypersensitivity in non-atopic volunteers parenterally immunized with a purified grass pollen extract. J Allergy Clin Immunol 61:171, 1978.
198. Twiggs JT, Yunginger JW, Agarwal MK, Reed CE: Occupational asthma in a florist caused by the dried plant, baby's breath. J Allergy Clin Immunol 69:474, 1982.
199. US Department of Agriculture, Agricultural Research Service: Common Weeds of the United States. Dover, New York, 1971.
200. Vailes LD, Li Y, Bao Y, et al: Fine specificity of B-cell epitopes on *Felis domesticus* allergen I (*Fel d* I): effect of reduction and alkylation or deglycosylation on *Fel d* I structure and antibody binding. J Allergy Clin Immunol 93:22, 1994.
201. Valenta R, Breiteneder H, Pettenburger K, et al: Homology of the major birch-pollen allergen, Bet v I, with the major pollen allergens of alder, hazel, and hornbeam at the nucleic acid level as determined by cross-hybridization. J Allergy Clin Immunol 87:677, 1991.
202. van der Brempt X, Charpin D, Haddi E, et al: Cat removal and *Fel d* I levels in mattresses. J Allergy Clin Immunol 87:596, 1991.
203. van der Brempt X, Ledent C, Mairesse M: Rhinitis and asthma caused by occupational exposure to carob bean flour. J Allergy Clin Immunol 90:1008, 1992.
204. van derHeide S, deMonchy JGR, deVries K, et al: Seasonal variation in airway hyperresponsiveness and natural exposure to house dust mite allergens in patients with asthma. J Allergy Clin Immunol 93:470, 1994.
205. Van Metre TE, Marsh DG, Adkinson NF, et al: Dose of cat (*Felis domesticus*) allergen (Fel d I) that induces asthma. J Allergy Clin Immunol 78:62, 1986.
206. Van Metre TE, Marsh DG, Adkinson NF, et al: Immunotherapy for cat asthma. J Allergy Clin Immunol 79:125, 1987.
207. Voorhorst R, Spieksma FTM, Varekamp H: House-Dust Atopy and the House Dust Mite. Staflen's Scientific, Leiden, Netherlands, 1969.
208. Voorhorst R, Spieksma FTM, Varekamp H, et al: The house dust mite (Dermatophagoides pteronyssinus) and the allergens it produces: identity with the house-dust allergen. J Allergy 39:325, 1967.
209. Walzer M, Siegel BB: The effectiveness of the ragweed eradication campaigns in New York City: a 9 year study (1946–1954). J Allergy 27:113, 1956.
210. Ward GW, Rose G, Karlsson G, Platts-Mills TAE: Trichophyton asthma:

sensitization of bronchi and upper airways to dermatophyte antigen. Lancet i:859, 1989.
211. Warren CPW, Holford-Stevens V, Wong C, Manfreda J: The relationship between smoking and total immunoglobulin E levels. J Allergy Clin Immunol 69:370, 1982.
212. Watson HH: Errors due to anisokinetic sampling of aerosols. Am Ind Hyg Assoc Q 15:21, 1954.
213. Weber R, Mansfield LE, Nelson HS: Cross reactivity among weeds of the amaranth and chenopod families. J Allergy Clin Immunol 61:172, 1978. Abstract.
214. Wedner JH, Wilson P, Lewis WH: Allergic reactivity to *Parthenium hysterophorus* pollen: an ELISA study of 582 sera from the United States Gulf Coast. J Allergy Clin Immunol 84:263, 1989.
215. Williams PB, Buhr MP, Weber RW, et al: Latex allergen in respirable particulate air pollution. J Allergy Clin Immunol 95:88, 1995.
216. Wilson AF, Novey HS, Berke RA, Suprenant EL: Deposition of inhaled pollen and pollen extract in human airways. N Engl J Med 288:1056, 1973.
217. Wittich FW: Allergic rhinitis and asthma due to sensitization to Mexican bean weevil (Zabrotes subfasciatus). J Allergy 12:42, 1940.
218. Wodehouse RP: Hayfever Plants. Their Appearance, Distribution, Time of Flowering and Their Role in Hayfever, 2nd edition (revised). Hafner, New York, 1971.
219. Wodehouse RP: Pollen Grains. Hafner, New York, 1971.
220. Wood RA, Mudd KE, Eggleston PA: The distribution of cat and dust mite allergens on wall surfaces. J Allergy Clin Immunol 89:126, 1992.
221. Wu CH, Lan J-L: Cockroach hypersensitivity: isolation and partial characterization of major allergens. J Allergy Clin Immunol 82:727, 1988.
222. Yasueda H, Yui Y, Shima T, Shida T: Isolation and partial characterization of the major allergen from Japanese cedar *(Cryptomeria japonica)* pollen. J Allergy Clin Immunol 71:77, 1983.
223. Yoo TJ, Spitz E, McGerity JL: Conifer pollen allergy; studies of immunogenicity and cross antigenicity of conifer pollens in rabbit and man. Ann Allergy 38:87, 1975.
224. Yunginger JW, Gleich GJ: Measurement of ragweed antigen E by double antibody radioimmunoassay. J Allergy Clin Immunol 50:326, 1972.
225. Yunginger JW, Jones RT, Nesheim ME, Geller M: Studies on Alternaria allergens. III. Isolation of a major allergenic fraction (ALT-1). J Allergy Clin Immunol 66:138, 1980.
226. Zwick H, Popp W, Serti K, et al: Allergenic structures in cockroach hypersensitivity. J Allergy Clin Immunol 87:626, 1991.

22 Structure and Function of the Upper Airway; Rhinoscopy

MICHAEL REDMAN ROBERT M. NACLERIO

Whereas the majority of this book focuses on mechanisms and treatment of diseases or components of the inflammatory response, this chapter focuses on structure and function of the upper airway. Since function often follows structure, these are presented together. Clinical applications of structure and function are highlighted to emphasize their importance. The last part of the chapter deals with endoscopy of the upper airway. The application of fiberoptic technology to instrumentation that can be easily passed through the upper airway provides unparalleled viewing and understanding of the region in health and disease. Other methods to assess the upper airway, such as imaging studies, are discussed in other chapters.

STRUCTURE AND FUNCTION OF THE UPPER AIRWAY

NOSE

The external nose is a pyramidal structure located in the midface, with its base on the facial skeleton and its apex projecting anteriorly. It is formed by the paired nasal bones superiorly and two sets of paired cartilage inferiorly. The paired upper lateral cartilages provide the shape of the middle third of the nose and support for the nasal valve area, an important air flow–limiting segment. The paired lower lateral cartilages, formed by the medial and lateral crura, are horseshoe shaped. The medial crus forms the columella, and the lateral crus defines the shape of the nasal alae and maintains the patency of the underlying nasal vestibule. Internally, the nasal pyramid is supported by the nasal septum.[33] Because of its prominent location, the nose is subject to trauma. Observing abnormalities in the normal external structure suggest that traumatic or congenital abnormalities may contribute to air flow obstruction.

Small muscle groups overlying the bony and cartilaginous framework contribute to the function of the external nose. The nasalis muscle extends laterally from the alae and functions to depress the nares. The anterior and posterior naris, depressor septi, and levator labii superioris nasi all function to dilate the nostrils and thus decrease resistance.[70] During periods of increased nasal breathing, such as exercise or respiratory distress, an increase in the activity of the dilating muscles occurs and increases nasal airway patency.[29] These muscles are innervated by the buccal branch of the facial nerve.

The vestibule or entrance to the nose is the first part of the respiratory tract to contact inhaled air. Thick hairs called vibrissae function to filter out large particulate matter.[21] The epithelium of the mucous membranes begins as stratified squamous anteriorly and then becomes transitional and, finally, pseudostratified columnar in the main part of the nasal cavity. Anterior nasal glands, located near the junction of the squamous and respiratory epithelium, secrete serous mucus. Forced inspiration, as in sniffing, atomizes these secretions. The vestibule also contains thermoreceptors, which upon stimulation lead to changes in nasal airway resistance.[58] Inspiring warm air leads to a decrease in nasal resistance, whereas inspiring cold air leads to the opposite effect.[37, 106] The vestibule is the most important area for sensing nasal air flow.[24, 25]

The nasal valve, a slitlike structure located just posterior to the nasal vestibule, causes about half of the total resistance to inspired air flow from ambient air to the pulmonary alveolus.[92] This area is bounded laterally by the caudal end of the upper lateral cartilages, medially by the septum, and inferiorly by the lower rim of the pyriform aperture.[116] The total cross-sectional area of the nasal valve is 40 mm^2.[28] This cross-sectional area of the nasal valve can be increased by the contraction of the dilator naris muscle, leading to an increase in air flow.[70] This contraction manifests itself as nasal flaring, as seen in periods of respiratory exertion. Rhythmic increases in tone of the dilator naris muscle occur just prior to the onset of inspiration, preceding diaphragmatic activation.[114] Abnormalities in the area of the nasal valve, such as anterior deviation of the nasal septum or edema of the mucosa, lead to major problems with nasal airway obstruction. Alteration of the nasal valve during cosmetic rhinoplasty, such as partial resection of the upper lateral cartilages or low lateral osteotomies beginning at the lower lateral portion of the pyriform aperture, can weaken or narrow the nasal valve, leading to nasal obstruction.

The nasal septum, about 10 to 14 cm in length, divides the nasal cavity into two separate compartments, thereby increasing the total mucosal surface area. It consists of an anterior cartilaginous portion, which provides support for the nasal tip, and a posterior bony plate formed by the perpendicular plate of the ethmoid and the vomer. Structural deviations of the septum affect nasal airway resistance. Small anterior deviations at the level of the nasal valve can lead to significant nasal airway obstruction, whereas deviations in the posterior portion of the nasal cavity may have no effect on air flow resistance.[46] Structural deviations of the septum can also contribute to sinus infections or the inability to introduce intranasal medications.[46] Aging cartilage loses its strength and weakens support to the nasal tip and nasal valve, thus compromising air flow.[46]

The turbinates are three, occasionally four, scroll-like projections from the lateral nasal wall (Fig. 22–1). The inferior and middle turbinates are the lower two turbinates and are most functionally significant. Each turbinate consists of a bony framework covered with pseudostratified columnar epithelium, similar to the lining of the rest of the nasal cavities and tracheobronchial tree.[83] Like the nasal septum, the turbinates aid in increasing the mucosal surface area of the nasal cavity to approximately 100 to 200 cm^2.[115] The turbinates also function to regulate air flow. An increase in turbinate size reduces air flow and vice versa.

The nasal lining consists of a mucosal epithelial layer with an underlying submucosa. The mucosa consists of pseudostratified columnar epithelium containing goblet cells, nonciliated and ciliated columnar cells with microvilli, and occasionally intraepithelial mast cells, eosinophils, and lymphocytes.[55] The latter change in the presence of disease. Epithelial goblet cells produce secretions that contribute to the mucous blanket.[118] These cells also provide a protective barrier and produce inflammatory substances and the secretory portion of IgA.[67, 82]

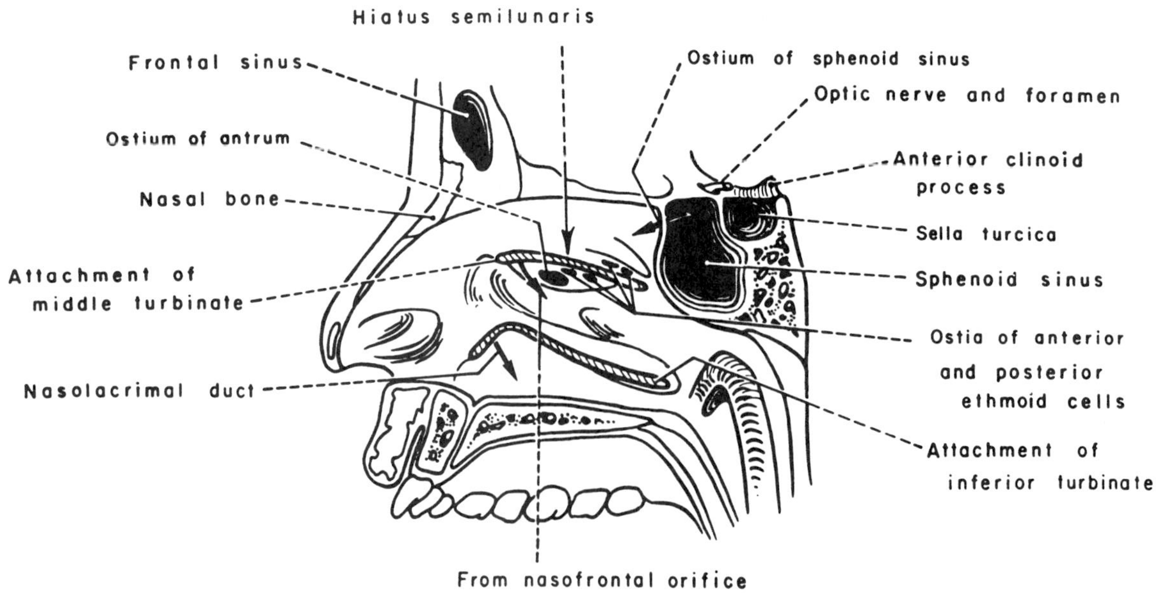

FIGURE 22–1. Sagittal view of the lateral nasal wall with the inferior and middle turbinate partially removed. The relationships of the sinus ostia and eustachian tubes are depicted. (From Montgomery WW: Surgery of the Upper Respiratory System. Vol 1. Lea & Febiger, Philadelphia, PA, 1971.)

The submucosa is separated from the epithelial layer by a basement membrane and contains nerves, blood vessels, and nasal glands. The submucosal nasal glands produce the greatest proportion of nasal secretions. Three major types of nasal glands exist: anterior serous glands, seromucous glands, and Bowman's glands. The anterior nasal glands can be found near the nasal vestibule and aid in moisturizing the nasal mucosa as these thin secretions are spread by the inspired air. Seromucous glands account for the largest proportion of nasal secretions. They are located throughout the nasal cavity, but the highest concentration may be found in the anterior nasal cavity. Depending on the cell type, these glands produce either a serous or mucous secretion. Secretion from these glands is probably controlled by both neural input and local mediators. Bowman's glands are serous glands in the olfactory region that aid in smell. Unlike the gut and the bronchial submucosa, the nasal submucosa does not contain lymphoid aggregates, although numerous T and B lymphocytes and antigen-presenting cells exist there and more can be recruited.

Blood flow contributes greatly to the functioning of the nose. Both the internal and external carotid circulations donate to the arterial supply of the nasal cavity.[21] The anterior and posterior ethmoid arteries, branches of the ophthalmic artery, enter the nose after passing through the orbit and lamina papyracea. The sphenopalatine artery, a terminal branch of the external carotid artery, enters the nose through the posterior lateral inferior wall. These vessels anastomose with branches of the facial artery, a branch of the external carotid artery, in the cartilaginous septum of the vestibule. This area is referred to as either Kiesselbach's or Little's area and is the most common site of epistaxis. The veins of the nasal cavity are valveless and run adjacent to the arteries, draining into the pterygoid and ophthalmic venous plexi. Some of the venous drainage subsequently passes intracranially into the cavernous sinus, a potential route for the spread of infection.[21]

The arteries supplying the subepithelial and glandular zones arise from the perichondrial and periosteal arteries. They ascend toward the surface, giving branches to the cavernous plexi before forming a subepithelial network of fenestrated capillaries.[22] The fenestrations face the respiratory surface and are believed by Cauna and Hinderer to be the major source of fluid for humidification.[22]

Alteration in blood flow into the cavernous sinusoids of the inferior and middle turbinate and the septum regulates nasal air flow.[21] The tone of the vessels in the arteriovenous anastomosis and venous drainage regulate the amount of blood in this valveless plexus. Changes in the size of the cavernous sinusoids occur while recumbent,[94] with elevated levels of inspired carbon dioxide,[73] and with changes in inspired air temperature.[37, 48] Vascular engorgement within the sinusoids presents clinically as nasal congestion.

Evidence for alpha, beta, cholinergic, histaminic, and hormonal receptors on blood vessels has come from pharmacologic studies. Alpha-adrenergic agents cause vasoconstriction in both arteries and cavernous plexus.[50, 74] Alpha 2–adrenergic agents cause vasoconstriction in both the capillary and cavernous plexus,[50, 74] whereas alpha 1 receptor agonists primarily affect the capillary plexus. Nasal administration of beta agonists causes vasodilatation.[50] Parasympathomimetics, such as methacholine, induce vasodilatation,[40] which is not blocked by atropine. Topically administered histamine causes vasodilatation and an increase in vasopermeability.[14] Premedication with H_1 antagonists blocks the increased permeability associated with histamine stimulation, but not the nasal congestion, which appears to be partially blocked by the addition of an H_2 antagonist.[107] The nasal vasculature appears to be four times more sensitive to circulating epinephrine than does the heart.[69] Changes in the levels of circulating hormones during pregnancy can cause rhinitis, which usually clears postpartum.[81] Sexual excitement,[117] hypothyroidism,[93] and emotional stress[52] also affect the nasal vasculature. Drugs demonstrating effects on these receptors should be considered in the differential diagnosis of nasal congestion.

Lymphatic vessels from the nasal vestibule and preturbinate area drain toward the external nose and then along the facial vessels to the submandibular lymph node group, whereas lymphatic vessels of the nasal fossae drain toward the nasopharynx. Two main collecting trunks, one high in the nasal vault and the other located inferiorly, drain toward and around the eustachian tube orifice and into the first echelon nodal group, the lateral retropharyngeal lymph nodes.[102] These lymph nodes are situated along the bodies of the vertebrae and thus cannot be palpated. This pattern of flow explains the rare observation of palpable lymphadenopathy with rhinosinusitis.

Neuronal control plays a major role in the local regulation of air flow, blood flow, and glandular secretion. Reflexes originating within the nose have distal effects, such as sneezing. After irritation of sensory receptor, the sneeze propagates one or more spasmodic inspirations. The glottis and velopharyngeal aperture close, allowing an increase in lower airway pressure. These structures suddenly open, allowing a blast of air to escape through the nose and mouth, in an attempt to clear the nasal passage.[19] This reflex can be initiated by viral infections,[49] exposure to allergens,[84] and in some individuals, following exposure to bright light.[41] The latter demonstrates afferent sensory innervation into the nasal cavity.

Neuronal stimulation originating within the nose can affect function elsewhere. Mucosal irritation can initiate the submersion reflex, marked by apnea, glottic closure, bradycardia, and vasocontriction,[7, 11, 34] in an attempt to protect the heart and brain by redistributing blood flow to these vital organs.[30] In contrast, nasal vasocontriction can be initiated by cooling of the skin.[37]

A nasopulmonary reflex has been suggested to explain a relationship between events occurring in the upper and lower airways. Sercer hypothesized the existence of such a reflex after he observed that blowing air into one nostril of laryngectomized patients induced expansion of the ipsilateral hemithorax.[110] In a separate study, bronchoconstriction occurred in individuals who had silica dust blown into their nose.[60] In one subject who had previously undergone a unilateral trigeminal nerve resection, bronchoconstriction occurred only when dust was blown through the neurologically intact side.[59] However, other investigators have been unable to confirm this nasopulmonary reflex.[108, 112] The nasopulmonary reflex is postulated to be responsible for the hypoxia and hypercapnia seen with posterior nasal packing.

Sensory innervation to the nose and nasal cavity, other than the olfactory nerves, comes from both the ophthalmic and maxillary divisions of the trigeminal nerve. So far, only mechanical (touch, pressure) and pain receptors have been identified in the nasal mucosa.[23] The parasympathetic and sympathetic nervous systems also supply innervation to the nose. These fibers enter the nose through the sphenopalatine foramina. The parasympathetic fibers originate in the superior salivary nucleus of the midbrain and then travel with the fibers of the seventh cranial nerve. At the geniculate ganglion in the temporal bone, these fibers separate to form the greater superficial petrosal nerve. These fibers traverse the floor of the anterior cranial fossa and the pterygomaxillary space and synapse in the sphenopalatine ganglion. From this point, parasympathetic fibers distribute to mucosal and submucosal appendages via the vidian nerve.[39] Stimulation of the parasympathetic nerves induces primarily glandular secretions and some vasodilatation, effects that occur following nasal challenge with cholinergic agents.[17] Sympathetic fibers originate in the hypothalamus. These fibers synapse in the superior cervical ganglion and then travel with the carotid plexus until they join the parasympathetic fibers in the vidian nerve.[16] The sympathetic fibers, in contrast to the parasympathetic, do not synapse in the sphenopalatine ganglion. Stimulation of the sympathetic system causes vasoconstriction with an associated decrease in nasal airway resistance.[6] Exercise stimulates the sympathetic system, causing an increase in nasal air flow, which can be blocked by an anesthetic injection into the superior cervical ganglion.[95]

In addition to the classic cholinergic and adrenergic innervation, the nerve supply to the nose also consists of a nonadrenergic, noncholinergic (NANC) system. NANC nerves, first described in the gastrointestinal tract, have been found in the upper respiratory system.[10] The neurotransmitters of the NANC system include neuropeptides, such as vasoactive intestinal peptide (VIP); substance P; neurokinins; or calcitonin gene-related peptide. An increase in VIP immunoreactive nerves has been reported in the nasal mucosa of patients with vasomotor rhinitis.[65, 119] Although the pathophysiologic role of this system is unclear, further understanding may lead to specific therapeutic advances.

Nasal Air Flow

The nasal valve directs inspired air upward past the middle turbinate, where inspiratory velocity of air reaches 12 to 18 m/sec. More posteriorly, air flow assumes a horizontal course through the main portion of the nasal cavity. Here, air flow slows to 2 to 3 m/sec.[27, 115] The nose is capable of handling 20 to 30 liters of air flow per minute. Higher volumes require oral breathing to supplement nasal breathing. Laminar air flow occurs at the nasal valve, but this pattern is lost as air passes posteriorly into the nasal cavity. If laminar air flow was maintained in the nasal cavity, effective heat and water exchange between the nasal mucosa and the inspired air would be less efficient, as the central air column would not be modified during its passage through the nasal cavity.[26]

After inspired air passes through the nasal valve area, fast laminar flow is lost and slower turbulent flow begins. This slower turbulent flow allows inspired air maximal contact with the warmer, moist nasal mucosa. This contact allows ambient air to be warmed to 31°C before it reaches the pharynx. This same mechanism humidifies inspired air so that the relative humidity approaches 100% as inspired air reaches the larynx. Since evaporation cools the mucosa, the now cooler mucosa reclaims some of the heat and moisture lost during inspiration during the low-flow portion of expiration into the nasal cavity.

A preference for nasal breathing begins in newborns, who are obligate nose breathers until the age of 5 to 6 months, and persists into adult life, with about 85% of adults breathing by nose. The physiologic disturbances associated with bilateral choanal atresia, a cause of total posterior nasal obstruction in the newborn, exemplifies this point.[80] When these occur at birth, prompt intervention is required. In adults, nasal airway obstruction may induce obstructive sleep apnea.[75]

Nasal Cycle

Changes in the blood content of the highly vascular turbinates occur reciprocally and rhythmically, resulting in alternating volume reductions in the lumen of the two nasal cavities. This phenomenon, termed the nasal cycle, was first described by Kayser in 1895 using clinical observation.[61] More objective assessments, such as rhinomanometry, have only served to confirm the original observation. The nasal cycle occurs in approximately 80% of adult volunteers. The duration of one cycle varies between 50 minutes and 4 hours. Most individuals are unaware of this cycling. It is absent in subjects with laryngectomies and is interrupted by the vasoconstrictive effects of medication or exercise, which markedly reduce the total nasal air flow resistance.[51] Kennedy and colleagues observed the nasal cycle using T2-weighted magnetic resonance imaging (MRI) by demonstrating an alternating increase and decrease in signal intensity and turbinate size over time (see Fig. 23–12).[62] This observation is important not because it demonstrated the nasal cycle with a highly sophisticated piece of equipment but because the nasal cycle may inadvertently be diagnosed as sinus disease. The adult pattern of nasal cycling begins to emerge between the ages of 7 and 10 years.[77] Patients with nasal congestion often describe alternating nasal obstruction, which most likely represents an exaggeration of the nasal cycle. Patients with anatomic obstructions, such as septal deviations, describe fixed obstructions.

Mucus

A mucous blanket, 10 to 15 microns deep, composed of secretions from the goblet cells, submucosal glands, and fluid transported across the epithelium, covers the entire nasal cavity.[121] This mucous layer consists of a sol phase, which is the watery periciliary layer, and a gel phase, which is the portion closest to air. Soluble materials like droplets, formaldehyde, and CO_2 dissolve in the periciliary layer after impaction of the air stream. Thus the mucus effectively filters and removes nearly 100% of particles greater than 4 microns in diameter. In addition to its filtering ability, the mucous blanket serves important protective functions. It is the first line of defense against bacterial and viral infections. Submucosally produced IgA is the major immunoglobulin in nasal secretions, and it can prevent pathogens from adhering to the nasal mucosa and thus prevent their entry.[13] The mucous blanket also provides water for humidification. Estimates of daily mucus production range from 1 to 2 liters, the majority being water. Most of the mucus is produced by the submucosal glands, in which serous glands outnumber mucous glands eight to one.[117, 118] One of the glandular products, mucin, is an extremely large molecular weight (2.3×10^6 daltons) glycoprotein. Mucin gives mucus its unique attributes of viscosity. Mucin consists of a polypeptide backbone with oligosaccharide side chains.[15, 101] Many other components have been identified in mucus.[12, 20, 42, 54, 68, 84, 98, 99, 120] Increased mucus production is a common response to nasal stimulation regardless of the cause.

Mucociliary Transport

Mucociliary transport is the mechanism by which the nasal cavity clears itself of secretions and debris. Since a primary function of the nose is to filter air, this system is extremely important to health. Abnormalities of this system, such as immotile cilia syndrome, present challenging clinical problems because they affect the entire nasal, sinus, ear, and pulmonary mucosa.

The cilia, 5-micron cellular projections, are composed of a shaft covered by a cell membrane. The shaft, or axoneme, consists of microtubules arranged as nine peripheral doublets surrounding two central singlets. Nexin links connect adjacent pairs of doublets, and each doublet is connected to the central tubules by spokes. Each doublet has two dynein arms that contain the ATPase, providing the energy of motion.[100]

The mucus and ciliated epithelial cells function together in this process. Mucociliary transport moves mucus and its contents toward the nasopharynx with the exception of the anterior portion of the inferior turbinates, where transport is anteriorly. Cilia can transport particles an average of 6 mm per minute, with a range of 1 to 20 mm per minute; thus this transport can clear inhaled particles from the nasal cavity in 10 to 20 minutes.[4] Sniffing, sneezing, and nose blowing aid in clearance.[53]

Cilia beat in a fixed direction that is determined by the orientation of the basal feet of the cilia in which all cilia have similar orientation.[113] There is a two-stroke pattern to their beat: an effector stroke, in which the cilia straighten, contact the gel phase, and move the mucus, and a recovery stroke, in which the cilia bend and move in the watery sol phase. It is unknown how movement is coordinated and synchronized. Ciliary beat frequency is approximately 1,000 beats per minute.[100] Cilia and mucociliary transport also occurs within the sinus cavities.

Disorders of mucociliary transport present clinically with pooled secretions along the floor of the nasal cavity. In immotile cilia syndrome, there is a defect in the ciliary structure that prevents movement.[2] Common cold viruses can lead to impaired mucociliary transport for up to 2 weeks by decreasing the number of ciliated cells.[89, 104] In chronic sinusitis, nasal secretion clearance may be prolonged because of an increase in the viscosity of the secretions.[105] In cystic fibrosis, abnormal mucus is produced. The defect is located at the epithelial cell surface, where there is altered sodium and chloride ion transport, leading to thick, tenacious mucus production. Destruction of cells and the release of DNA also contribute to the viscosity of mucus in cystic fibrosis. In all of the preceding disorders, stasis of secretions occurs and can lead to the development of chronic rhinosinusitis.

Mucociliary clearance functions over a wide range of environmental conditions. The nose transforms inspired air to nearly 100% relative humidity by the time it reaches the nasopharynx. Despite both heat and water loss during inspiration, the two components are recovered during expiration, and the mucociliary clearance is not affected.[3] Therapeutic interventions to improve mucociliary transport have been proposed, but little evidence supports their effectiveness in improving mucociliary transport or clinical outcome.

Olfaction

The olfactory mucosa, located in the roof of the nasal cavity, has a surface area of about 200 to 400 mm^2. This airway (1–2 mm wide) lies above the middle turbinate just inferior to the cribriform plate between the septum and the lateral nasal wall. It is poorly ventilated, as most of the inhaled air passes through the lower aspect of the nasal cavity. Sniffing helps to bring inspired air into this part of the nasal cavity. The olfactory epithelium contains bipolar neurons that form the first cranial (olfactory) nerve.[55] Similar to the nasal mucosa, the olfactory epithelium is covered by a layer of mucus containing IgA, IgM, lactoferrin, and lysozyme, which may aid in preventing intracranial entry of pathogens through the cribriform plate.[76] The ophthalmic and maxillary divisions of the fifth cranial nerve participate in olfaction by mediating a common chemical sense. This system has little ability for odor identification but can detect irritants such as ammonia.[111]

Little is known about the mechanisms of odor recognition and differentiation. Odorant-binding proteins have been identified that act as specific receptors for odorant molecules.[94] These binding proteins help transport the lipophilic odorant molecules through the hydrophilic mucus to the olfactory epithelium and may aid in odorant transport to the olfactory receptors faster than by simple diffusion.[90] The initial step in olfactory processing occurs when the odorant molecules contact the cilia of the receptor cells, whose axons pass through the cribriform plate and into the central nervous system to synapse in the olfactory bulb. From there, projections travel to the piriform cortex, anterior olfactory nucleus, amygdala, entorhinal cortex, hippocampus, hypothalamus, and thalamus.[63] Although the sense of smell is better developed in lower mammals, humans use the sense of smell to perceive taste, warn of impending hazards, and enhance social interactions. Olfactory disturbances may arise from inflammatory causes, such as rhinosinusitis or nasal polyposis; trauma, such as foreign bodies, nasal or skull base surgery, or closed head injury; congenital or developmental causes, such as choanal atresia, adenoidal hypertrophy, or Turner's syndrome; metabolic disorders, such as vitamin A or thiamine deficiency; or neoplasms of the nasal or cranial cavity.[63]

PARANASAL SINUSES

The paranasal sinuses consist of four paired cavities that open into the nasal cavity. The ethmoid sinuses are the first

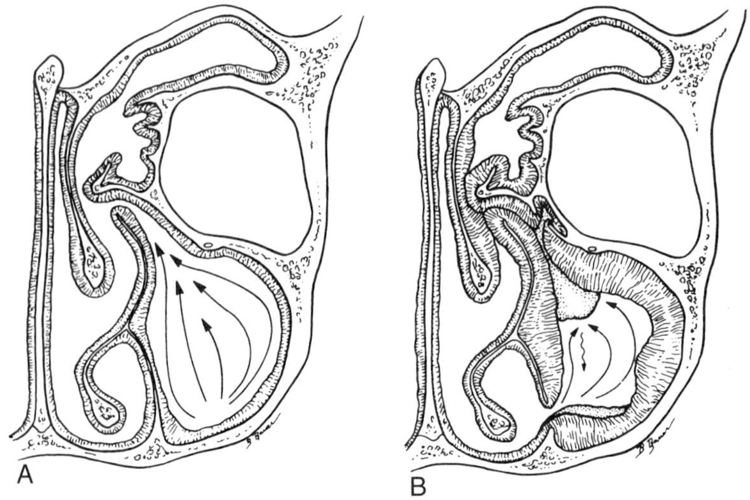

FIGURE 22–2. (A) Diagrammatic representation of normal maxillary mucociliary clearance (arrows) (after Hilding). Mucociliary flow passes laterally to the uncinate process through the narrow ethmoid infundibulum before reaching the middle meatus. **(B)** Diagrammatic representation of mucociliary clearance where there is residual osteomeatal disease following nasal antral window. The mucosa is swollen, and the infundibulum is obstructed. Mucus is cleared toward the infundibulum where it collects. Eventually some mucus may fall to the floor of the sinus by gravity. From the floor of the sinus, some mucus is again circulated toward the ostium, although some may pass into the nose through antrostomy. (From Stammberger H: Functional Endoscopic Sinus Surgery. Philadelphia, BC Decker, 1991.)

to develop and form a honeycomb of cells that are located lateral and posterior to the middle turbinate.[71] The lamina papyracea, their lateral borders, forms part of the medial wall of the orbit, and the roof is the floor of the anterior cranial fossa. The paranasal sinuses are divided into anterior and posterior air cells by the grand lamella. The anterior ethmoid air cells open into the semilunar hiatus, which is situated under the middle turbinate, also known as the middle meatus. This area, which coincides with the spot where air flow changes from the upward to the horizontal directions, is the major point for impaction of environmental particles. Besides physiologic studies, this concept is supported by the observation that adenocarcinomas in hardwood workers begin here.[1] It is believed that this area of marked turbulence is the origin of most cases of sinusitis,[79] because in addition to the ethmoid, the frontal and the maxillary sinuses drain near this anatomic site.[86] Posterior ethmoid cells have their ostia in the superior meatus. The frontal sinuses vary considerably in size between sides and between individuals. Their development begins above the superior orbital rim at age 6 and finishes during early adolescence.

The maxillary sinuses are the largest in size, each having a volume of about 15 ml. They are pyramidal in shape, with their apex lying at the root of the zygomatic process of the maxilla and the base facing toward the lateral surface of the nasal cavity. The roof of the maxillary sinus is separated from the orbit by a thin plate of bone that is traversed by the infraorbital branch of the maxillary nerve, which is incased in a thin-walled or partly dehiscent canal. As stated previously, the maxillary sinus opens into the nasal cavity in close proximity to the openings of the frontal and anterior ethmoid sinuses.[9] The sphenoid sinuses are located just inferior to the sella turcica and medial to the cavernous sinus. They open into the posterior medial aspect of the nasal cavity. Knowing the anatomic relationship of the paranasal sinuses is essential for understanding their role and appreciating potential complications in disease.

The function of the sinuses under normal, healthy conditions remains to be elucidated. The following speculations regarding their function have been made: (1) supply resonance to the voice; (2) protect the ear from one's own speech; (3) aid in the air conditioning of inspired air by supplying already warm and humid air; (4) equalize pressure during inspiration and expiration as well as under more extreme situations, such as sneezing or rapid changes in altitude; (5) aid in olfaction; (6) reduce the weight of the skull; (7) protect intracranial structures from trauma; and (8) provide heat insulation for the skull and orbit.[38] In healthy individuals, the sinuses are hollow spaces lined by a thin, ciliated epithelium with a few goblet cells and glands.[66]

Like the nasal cavity, the sinuses are cleared by mucociliary transport. Carbon particles placed anywhere in the maxillary antrum will be moved toward the natural ostia, located in the superior medial aspect of the cavity (Fig. 22–2). The direction of mucociliary clearance does not change with surgery, as evidenced by a similar direction after healing of the maxillary sinus following a Caldwell-Luc operation. The lymphatics of the sinuses exit through their natural ostia to join the lymphatics of the nasal cavity. These then drain to the lateral pharyngeal wall lymph nodes.[78]

PHARYNX

The pharynx is a collapsible muscular tube that is anatomically divided into three sections: nasopharynx, oropharynx, and hypopharynx. The hypopharynx and oropharynx are lined with squamous epithelium, and the nasopharynx is lined with pseudostratified columnar epithelium. The pharynx functions as a conduit for gases, liquids, and solids from the external to the internal environment. With respect to air, and occasionally to liquids and solids, the reverse movement is equally important.

The patency of the pharynx to air is maintained by the actions of 22 muscles.[91] The mandible and other parts of the skull directly and indirectly help to support many of the pharyngeal muscles. An example of the interplay between muscle and bone is shown by the electromyographic studies displaying that the genioglossus and the styloglossus stabilize the larynx during inspiration.[5] Equally important is the coordination of the neurons controlling muscular activity. Activation of the recurrent laryngeal nerve precedes activation of the phrenic nerve, and activation of the laryngeal abductors occurs during expiration.[47, 85] If partial obstruction occurs in any segment of the upper airway during inspiration, decreased inspiratory pressure below the site of obstruction increases the tendency of the muscular tube to collapse, limiting flow even further.[91] For example, nasal obstruction increases the tendency of the pharynx to collapse. This concept may be important in the understanding of obstructive sleep apnea. Jan and colleagues showed (in awake individuals) that lying in comparison with sitting is associated with a smaller cross-sectional area.[57] Neck extension, as often seen in sleeping children with large tonsils, increases the pharyngeal airway.

Irritation of neurons within the pharynx can induce vagal reflexes similar to those following laryngeal stimulation. These vagal reflexes can be exhibited as dysrhythmia, bradycardia, coronary angiospasm, laryngospasm, bronchospasm, prolonged apnea, and hiccups. Gastroesophageal reflux may be a frequent irritant initiating such a reflex.[31]

Major abnormalities of the posterior nasal cavity, such as adenoidal hypertrophy, may compromise nasal air flow.[28] After exiting the posterior choanae of the nasal cavity, inspired air is forced caudal toward the glottis by the adenoid pad (nasopalatine tonsil) located on the posterior wall. Adenoidal hypertrophy is a major cause of nasal obstruction in children. Each eustachian tube orifice may be found just lateral to the adenoids. The superior constrictor muscle lies underneath these structures. Contraction of this muscle propels secretions toward the stomach. Beginning with this muscle, mucus transport proceeds by muscular contraction instead of ciliary movement.

Mucus located in the nasopharynx and in other parts of the upper airway is not sterile. The normal flora of the nasopharynx consists of *Haemophilus influenzae, Streptococcus pneumoniae,* and β-hemolytic streptococcus, making interpretation of nasopharyngeal cultures difficult.[122]

Chronic nasal obstruction by adenoidal hypertrophy or other mechanisms forces oral breathing. Continuous oral breathing during growth prevents the tongue from modeling the hard palate and leads to a high arched palate, prominent maxilla, and detrimental effects on dentition. The term given to this developmental abnormality is adenoid faces.

Just inferior to the posterior choana of the nose on the anterior wall of the nasal pharynx sits the muscular soft palate. This structure functions to direct the flow of air and food between the oropharynx and nasopharynx. During swallowing, the soft palate is elevated, preventing the reflux of fluid into the nose. During quiet respiration, the oropharynx is occluded, directing inspired air through the nose.[97, 115] During forceful expiration, the soft palate is moved toward the nasopharynx, directing air through the oral cavity.[96] During speech, the soft palate directs air between both the nose and the mouth, with air escaping normally through the nose only with the formation of the *ng, n,* and *m* sounds.[32] Excessive or limited air flow through the nose leads to abnormal speech patterns, like those seen in subjects with cleft palate deformities.

The oropharynx is covered with squamous epithelium. The middle constrictor muscle underlies the majority of the posterior and lateral surfaces and functions during deglutition. The palatopharyngeal and palatoglossus muscles form the posterior and anterior tonsillar pillars, respectively. Similar to the rest of the pharynx, the muscles of the oropharynx are innervated by branches of the glossopharyngeal and vagus nerves. Like the adenoids (nasopalatine), the palatine tonsils are composed of lymphoid tissue. This tissue may be the site of acute or recurrent infections, and their enlargement may contribute to airway obstruction, particularly in children.

The hypopharynx controls the distribution of food and air to their appropriate organs, with the epiglottis being primarily responsible for this phenomenon. During swallowing, the glottic chink is closed, the larynx elevated, and the epiglottis pulled over the laryngeal inlet, directing food into the piriform sinuses. The opposite sequence allows air to enter the trachea and lungs. The cricopharyngeal sphincter, another hypopharyngeal structure, controls the passage of the food bolus into the cervical esophagus.[8, 35] Most hypopharyngeal activity is involuntarily controlled.[18, 36, 56]

The lingual tonsils are lymphoid aggregates located on the tongue base within the hypopharynx. Enlargement of this tissue can result in difficulty in swallowing or even a choking sensation. The hypopharynx also contains numerous submucosal glands, termed minor salivary glands. These glands can be stimulated by parasympathetic input to contribute to airway secretions.[43]

The larynx, the gate keeper of the airway, primarily functions to prevent aspiration. The production of voice, however, is the function most appreciated. Visualization of the larynx can differentiate hoarseness from a localized *Candida* overgrowth secondary to the use of inhaled steroids from the laryngitis associated with seasonal allergen exposure. Vocal cord dysfunction, characterized by upper airway obstruction with varying degrees of stridor and wheezing, is typically misidentified as bronchial asthma. The symptoms, which can be quite severe, fail to respond to bronchodilators or steroids, sometimes leading to emergency airway intervention. This condition represents a psychiatric disorder. The episodic and variable wheezing of this disorder helps to differentiate it from tracheal tumors, stenosis, and other anatomic airway obstructions.

EAR

The ear functions in hearing and balance. The middle ear cleft shares mucosal similarities with the nasal mucosa. The eustachian tube (ET) develops as an outpouching of the first pharyngeal pouch and connects the middle ear with the nasopharynx. The distal portion expands to become the tympanic cavity, whereas the proximal part becomes the ET. From its opening in the torus tuborum, the ET extends backward and upward toward the middle ear cleft. The ET primarily functions to allow equilibration of air pressure on both sides of the tympanic membrane. This equilibration permits maximum resonance of the tympanic membrane. Popping of the ears, often described by patients with allergic rhinitis, represents exaggerated opening of the ET. Other functions of the ET include drainage of secretions produced by the middle ear mucosa and the prevention of reflux of nasopharyngeal secretions. The latter function is accomplished passively, since the normal ET is collapsed until actively opened by the tensor veli palatini muscle with contributions from the levator palatini and salpingopharyngeus.

The middle ear cleft is lined by a delicate epithelium and enclosed in a bony vault, except for the tympanic membrane. Its primary function is the conversion of sound to mechanical vibration.[64] Immunologically, the middle ear mucosa can respond to disease similarly to the nose.

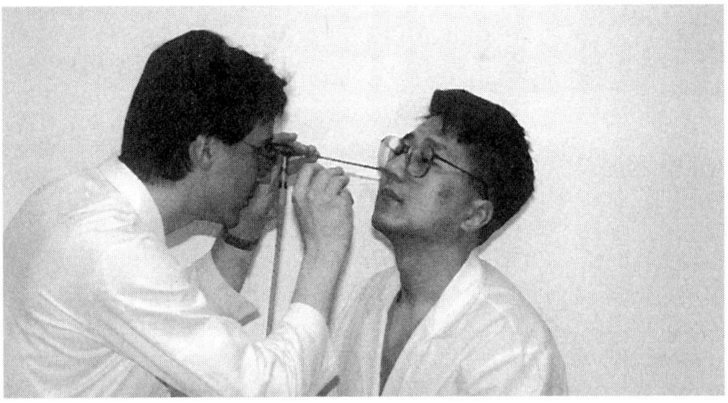

FIGURE 22–3. Demonstration of the use of a rigid telescope to obtain a culture.

ORAL CAVITY

Between the lips and the anterior arch of the soft palate lies the oral cavity. This anatomic area functions in speech, mastication, and breathing. The dental arches, composed of the hard palate superiorly and the mandible inferiorly, contain teeth.[45, 109] The maxillary molars and premolars lie inferior to the maxillary sinus. The roots of these teeth are separated by only millimeters of bone from the antral mucosa. Thus infected teeth can precipitate sinusitis.

The genioglossus muscle, innervated by the hypoglossal nerve, forms the bulk of the tongue. Its mobility is reflected in its role in articulation and swallowing. Afferent inputs for touch come from the third division of the fifth cranial nerve, whereas taste follows a different pathway. In the anterior two thirds of the tongue, afferent taste fibers travel with the chorda tympani nerve, which eventually joins the seventh cranial nerve, whereas input from taste receptors in the posterior one third travel with the ninth cranial nerve. The sensations of bitter, sweet, sour, and salty arise from the special sensory receptors located in the tongue.[72] However, most of what normal individuals describe as taste relates to the sense of olfaction.

The oral cavity also functions in oronasal breathing. As the requirement for oxygen increases, an individual must increase the air flow. However, the nose has a maximum obtainable air flow. Therefore, at a certain point during exertion, an individual must supplement nasal air flow with oral air flow.[87, 88, 103] When an exercising individual's ventilatory volume reaches 90 liters per minute, one third of the air flow passes through the nose. During oronasal breathing, the tongue forms a passage between itself and the palate. This slit provides contact between air and mucosa, allowing for heating and humidification. Some of the moisture comes from goblet cells and minor salivary glands. The remainder comes from the major salivary glands: the parotid, submandibular, and sublingual glands.[43]

RHINOSCOPY

Rhinoscopy implies inspection of the nasal cavity and is usually designated anterior or posterior. The terms used to describe these procedures vary, but this chapter refers to a clinical procedure usually performed after the application of a decongestant and local anesthetic. A principle for all endoscopy is that the light visualized represents reflected light. Thus the greater the amount of light entering the nasal cavity and the larger the viewing device, the greater the visualization.

Anterior rhinoscopy with a speculum or nasal adapter for an otoscope permits visualization of the vestibule, anterior septum, anterior portion of the inferior turbinate, and occasionally the anterior tip of the middle turbinate. Treating the nasal mucosa with a decongestant improves visualization but at best permits visualization of the anterior third of the nose. Posterior rhinoscopy refers to the visualization of the nasopharynx from the oropharynx. Light reflected from a mirror or a right-angled telescope can permit visualization of the eustachian tube orifice, adenoids, and posterior choanae.

Anterior and posterior rhinoscopy does not visualize the middle of the nasal cavity. This area that contains the drainage pathways of the sinuses can be easily visualized with a rigid or flexible endoscope. The use of these instruments has been a major advance in the diagnostic and therapeutic armamentarium. The endoscopes can be divided into rigid and flexible scopes. The rigid scopes provide the best optics, particularly for photography. The rigid scopes can be held with one hand, while the other hand can be used for manipulating instruments (Fig. 22–3). For example, a culture can be obtained from purulent secretions draining from the middle meatus (Fig. 22–4).

The rigid scopes come in a variety of sizes and viewing angles. The standard scopes are 4 mm in diameter, whereas the smaller 2.7 mm scopes are useful when dealing with narrow nasal cavities, such as those in children (Fig. 22–5).

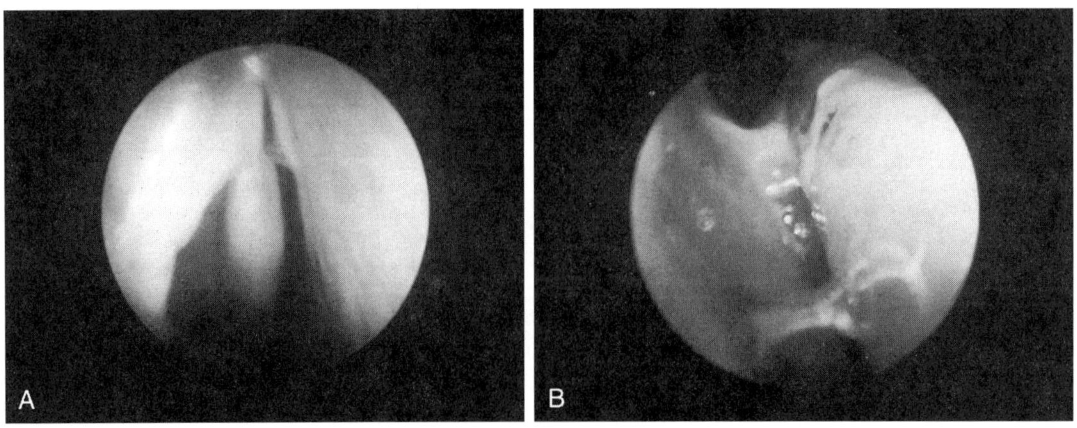

FIGURE 22–4. **(A)** Endoscopic view of the middle meatus. **(B)** Advancing endoscope shows purulent drainage from the hiatus semilunaris.

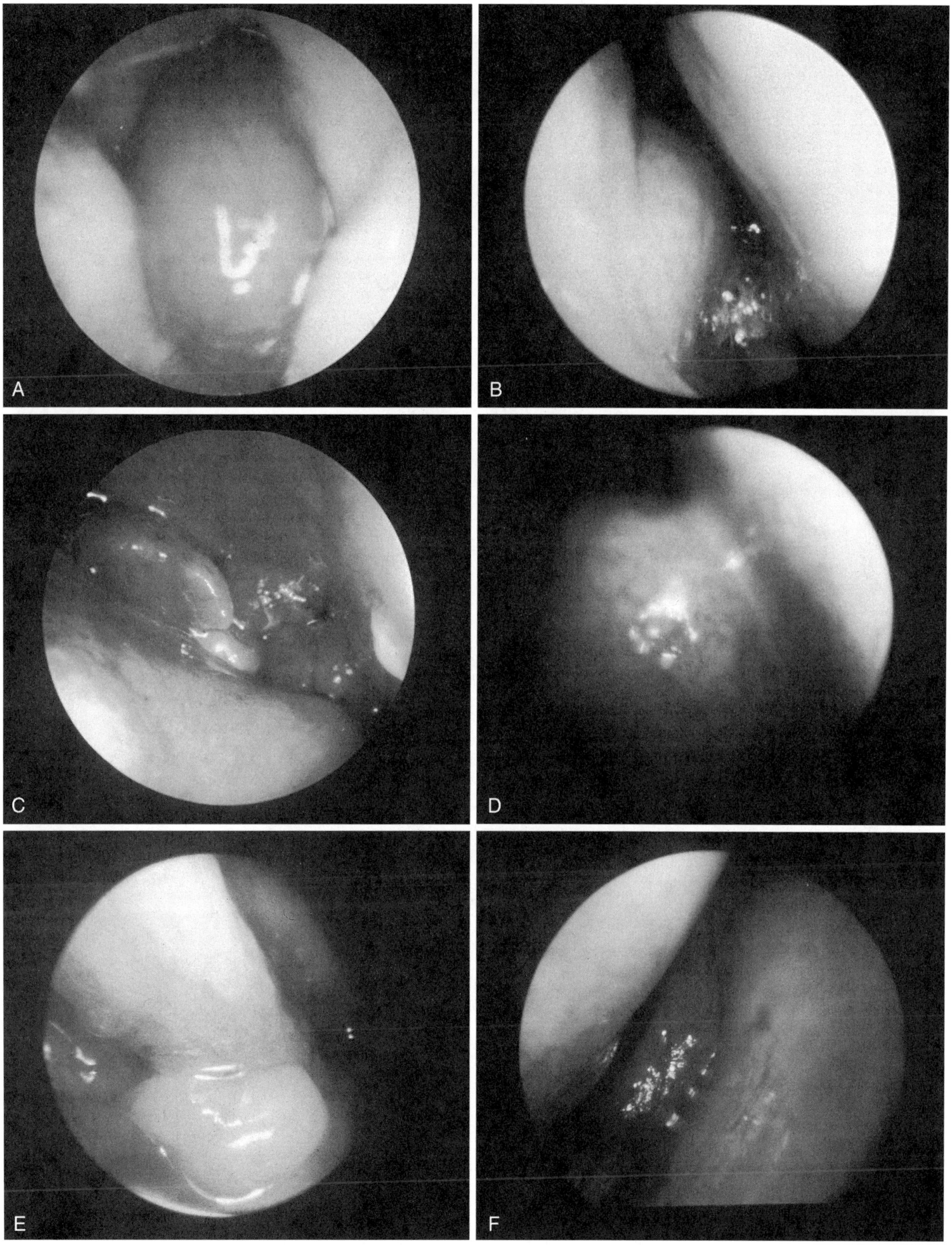

FIGURE 22–5. Endoscopic views of the nasal cavity showing different pathologic entities. **(A)** Large nasal polyp. **(B)** Mucus pooling on the floor of the nose suggestive of total nasal obstruction or immotile ciliary syndrome. **(C)** Multiple small polyps originating from the osteomeatal region. **(D)** Concha bullosa of the middle turbinate touching the lateral wall of the nasal cavity. **(E)** Antrochoanal polyp originating from an ostium in the posterior fontanel of the maxillary sinus. **(F)** Inflamed paradoxical middle turbinate during an episode of acute sinusitis.

Because of their smaller size, these scopes provide less viewing power. The lens at the front can be angled at 0° for straight ahead viewing or 30°, 70°, and 120° for angled viewing. The lens is a fish eye. These lenses provide a panoramic view that magnifies objects up close and shrinks objects at a distance. The scopes are attached to a light source whose costs vary greatly. Unfortunately, the more expensive xenon light sources provide superior light. Fortunately, these are not necessary for routine diagnostics. The light at the lens is cool, so the patient does not feel warmth from the insertion of the instrument.

The alternative endoscopes for viewing are the flexible scopes. Although the optics are inferior to the rigid scope, they are more than adequate for diagnostic purposes. The use of these scopes is easily learned. The flexibility provides less risk to the patient when the scope is manipulated by a novice technician. Besides visualizing the nasal cavity, endoscopes can be advanced into the nasopharynx and rotated inferiorly to view the larynx. Adenoidal hypertrophy in children and laryngeal disturbances in adults can be diagnosed.

The advantages of endoscopy and its marked superiority over other alternatives may cause some to ask why endoscopy is not performed on everyone who has a nasal complaint. The answer is simply cost. The instrumentation is expensive, and the cost must be transferred to the patient. To scope every patient with a nasal complaint would be an enormous financial burden on our health care system. The American Academy of Allergy and Immunology Upper Airway Allergy Committee endorsed its use in all patients with rhinitis except those with uncomplicated allergic rhinitis who respond to treatment.[44] The need for endoscopy increases with the complexity of the case and probably is more frequent in an otolaryngologist's office than in a generalist's office.

REFERENCES

1. Acheson ED, Dowdell RN, Hadfield E, et al: Nasal cancer in woodcutters in the furniture industry. BMJ 1:587, 1968.
2. Afzelius B: The immotile cilia syndrome and other ciliary diseases. Int Rev Exp Pathol 19:1, 1979.
3. Anderson I, Lundqvist G, Jensen PL, et al: Human response after 78 hours' exposure to dry air. Arch Environ Health 29:319, 1974.
4. Anderson I, Lundqvist G, Jensen PL, et al: Human response to controlled levels of sulfur dioxide. Arch Environ Health 28:31, 1974.
5. Andrew BL: The respiratory displacement of the larynx: a study of the innervation of accessory respiratory muscles. J Physiol 130:474, 1955.
6. Angaard A, Denset O: Adrenergic innervation of the nasal mucosa in the cat. Acta Otolaryngol (Stockh) 78:232, 1974.
7. Angell-Jumes JE, Daly MB: Nasal reflexes. Proc R Soc Med 62:1287, 1969.
8. Atkinson M, Kramer P, Wyman SM, et al: The dynamics of swallowing. I. Normal pharyngeal mechanism. J Clin Invest 36:581, 1957.
9. Aust RR, Drettner B: The patency of the maxillary ostium in relation to body posture. Acta Otolaryngol (Stockh) 80:443, 1975.
10. Barnes PJ: Neuropeptides in the lung: localization, function, and pathophysiology implications. J Allergy Clin Immunol 78:285, 1987.
11. Barrow CS, Alarie Y, Stock MF: Sensory irritation and incapacitation evoked by thermal decomposition products of polymers and comparisons with known sensory irritants. Arch Environ Health 33:79, 1978.
12. Baumgarten CR, Togias AG, Naclerio RM, et al: Influx of kininogens into nasal secretions following antigen challenge of allergic individuals. J Clin Invest 76:191, 1985.
13. Bellanti JA, Artenstein MS, Beuscher EL: Characterization of virus-neutralizing antibodies in human serum and nasal secretions. J Immunol 94:344, 1965.
14. Bentley AJ, Jackson RT: Changes in the patency of the upper nasal passage induced by histamine and antihistamine. Laryngoscope 80:1859, 1970.
15. Boat TF, Cheng PW, Iyer RN, et al: Human respiratory tract secretion. Mucous glycoproteins of nonpurulent tracheobronchial secretions and sputum of patients with bronchitis and cystic fibrosis. Arch Biochem Biophys 177:95, 1976.
16. Boles R: Neuroanatomy for the otolaryngologist. In Paparella M, Shumrick D (eds): Otolaryngology. WB Saunders Co, Philadelphia, 1980, pp 166–170.
17. Borum P: Nasal methacholine challenge. A test for the measurement of nasal reactivity. J Allergy Clin Immunol 63:253, 1979.
18. Boushey HA, Richardson PS, Widdicombe JG, et al: The response of laryngeal afferent fibers to mechanical and chemical stimuli. J Physiol 240:153, 1974.
19. Brubaker A: The physiology of sneezing. JAMA 73:585, 1919.
20. Butler WT, Rossen RD, Waldmann TA: Mechanism of appearance of immunoglobulin A in nasal secretions in man. J Clin Invest 46:1883, 1967.
21. Cauna N: Blood and nerve supply of the nasal lining. In Proctor DF, Anderson IB (eds): The Nose. Elsevier Biomedical Press, Amsterdam, 1982, pp 45–70.
22. Cauna N, Hinderer KH: Fine structure of blood vessels of the human nasal respiratory mucosa. Ann Otol Rhinol Laryngol 78:865, 1969.
23. Cauna N, Hinderer KH, Wentges RT: Sensory receptor organs of the human nasal respiratory mucosa. Am J Anat 124:187, 1969.
24. Clarke RW, Jones AS: Nasal airflow receptors: the relative importance of temperature and tactile stimulation. Clin Otolaryngol 17:388, 1992.
25. Clarke RW, Jones AS, Charters P, et al: The role of mucosal receptors in the nasal sensation of airflow. Clin Otolaryngol 17:383, 1991.
26. Cole P: Upper respiratory airflow. In Proctor DF, Anderson IB (eds): The Nose—Upper Airway Physiology and the Atmospheric Environment. Elsevier Science Publishing Company, New York, 1982, pp 163–189.
27. Cole P: Nasal and oral airflow resistors. Arch Otolaryngol Head Neck Surg 118:790, 1992.
28. Cole P, Chaban R, Naito K, et al: The obstructive nasal septum. Arch Otolaryngol Head Neck Surg 114:410, 1988.
29. Connel DC, Fregosi RF: Influence of nasal airflow and resistance on nasal dilator muscle activities during exercise. J Appl Physiol 74: 2529, 1993.
30. Craig AB: Underwater swimming and loss of consciousness. JAMA 176:255, 1961.
31. Cunningham ET, Ravich WJ, Jones B, et al: Vagal reflexes referred from the upper aerodigestive tract: an infrequently recognized cause of common cardiorespiratory responses. Ann Intern Med 116:575, 1992.
32. Dale PS: Language Development—Structure and Function. Dryden Press, Philadelphia, 1972.
33. Dion MC, Jafek BW, Tobin CJ: The anatomy of the nose: external support. Arch Otolaryngol 104:145, 1978.
34. Dixon WE, Brodie TG: Contributions to the physiology of the lungs. J Physiol 29:97, 1903.
35. Donner M: Radiologic evaluation of swallowing. Am Rev Respir Dis 131(suppl):S20, 1985.
36. Doty RW: Neural organization of deglutition. Am Physiol Soc Hdbk Physiol 4:1861, 1968.
37. Drettner B: Vascular reactions of the human nasal mucosa on exposure to cold. Acta Otolaryngol Suppl (Stockh) 166:1, 1961.
38. Drettner B: The paranasal sinuses. In Proctor DF, Anderson IB (eds): The Nose—Upper Airway Physiology and the Atmospheric Environment. Elsevier Biomedical Press BV, Amsterdam, 1982.
39. Eccles R: Neurological and pharmacological consideration. In Proctor DF, Anderson IB (eds): The Nose—Upper Airway Physiology and the Atmospheric Environment. Elsevier Biomedical Press BV, Amsterdam, 1982.
40. Eccles R, Wilson H: The parasympathetic secretory nerves of the nose of the cat. J Physiol 230:213, 1973.
41. Evert HC: Sneezing in response to light. Neurology 14:483, 1964.
42. Fleming A: On a remarkable bacteriolytic element found in tissues and secretions in normal subjects. Proc R Soc Lond B Biol Sci 93:306, 1922.
43. Gates GA, Johns ME: Embryology and anatomy of the salivary glands. In Paparella M, Shumrick D (eds): Otolaryngology. WB Saunders, Philadelphia, 1980.
44. Georgitis J, Druce H, Goldstein S, et al: Rhinopharyngolaryngoscopy. J Allergy Clin Immunol 91:956, 1993.

45. Graber TM: Orthodontics, Principles and Practice. WB Saunders, Philadelphia, 1972.
46. Gray L: Deviated nasal septum. III. Its influence on the physiology and disease of the nose and ears. J Laryngol 81:953, 1967.
47. Green JH, Neil E: The respiratory function of the laryngeal muscles. J Physiol 129:134, 1955.
48. Gsic B, Krajina Z, Lakic L, et al: Damage of the respiratory mucous membranes of rats exposed to cold. Acta Otolaryngol (Stockh), 57:342, 1964.
49. Gwaltney JM Jr: The common cold. In Mandell GL, Douglas RG Jr, Bennett JE (eds): Principles and Practice of Infectious Disease. John Wiley and Sons, New York, 1979, pp 429–434.
50. Hall LJ, Jackson RT: Effects of alpha and beta adrenergic agonists on nasal blood flow. Ann Otol Rhinol Laryngol 77:1120, 1968.
51. Hasegawa M, Kern EB: The human cycle. Mayo Clin Proc 52:28, 1977.
52. Holmes TH, Goddell H, Wolf S, et al: The Nose: An Experimental Study of Reactions Within the Nose in Human Subjects During Varying Life Experiences. Charles C Thomas, Springfield, IL, 1950.
53. Hounam RF: The removal of particles from the nasopharyngeal (NP) compartment of the respiratory tract by nose blowing and swabbing. Health Phys 28:743, 1975.
54. Ishizaka K, Newcomb RM: Presence of IgE in nasal washes and sputum from asthmatic patients. J Allergy 46:197, 1970.
55. Jafek BW: Ultrastructure of the human nasal mucosa. Laryngoscope 93:1576, 1983.
56. Jammes Y, Mei N: Assessment of the pulmonary origin of bronchoconstrictor vagal tone. J Physiol (Lond) 291:305, 1976.
57. Jan M, Marshall I, Douglas N: Effect of posture on upper airway dimensions in normal human. Am J Respir Crit Care Med 149:145, 1994.
58. Jones AS, Wight RG, Durham LH: The distribution of thermoreceptors within the nasal cavity. Clin Otolaryngol 14:235, 1989.
59. Kaufman J, Chen JC, Wright GW: The effect of trigeminal resection on reflex bronchoconstriction after nasal and nasopharyngeal irritation in man. Am Rev Respir Dis 101:768, 1970.
60. Kaufman J, Wright GW: The effect of nasal and nasopharyngeal irritation on airway resistance in man. Am Rev Respir Dis 100:626, 1969.
61. Kayser R: Messung der Luftdurchgangigkeit der Nose. Arch Laryngol 3:101, 1895.
62. Kennedy DW, Zinreich SJ, Kumar AJ, et al: Physiologic mucosal changes within the nose and ethmoid sinus: imaging of the nasal cycle by MRI. Laryngoscope 98:928, 1988.
63. Kimmelman CP: Clinical review of olfaction. Am J Otolaryngol 14:227, 1993.
64. Krikae I: Physiology of the middle ear including eustachian tube. In Paparella M, Shumrick D (eds): Otolaryngology. WB Saunders, Philadelphia, 1980.
65. Kurrian SS, Blank MA, Sheppard MN, et al: Vasoactive intestinal peptide (VIP) in vasomotor rhinitis. IRCS Med Sci 11:425, 1983.
66. Latta JS, Schall RF: The histology of the epithelium of the paranasal sinuses under various conditions. Ann Otol Rhinol Laryngol 43:945, 1934.
67. Leikauf GD, Veki IF, Nadel JA: Bradykinin stimulates chloride secretion and prostaglandin E2 release by canine tracheal epithelium. Am J Physiol 258:F48, 1985.
68. Lorin MI, Gaerlan PF, Mandel ID: Quantitative composition of nasal secretions in normal subjects. J Lab Clin Med 1980:275, 1972.
69. Malcolmson KG: The vasomotor activites of the nasal mucous membrane. J Laryngol Otol 73:73, 1959.
70. Mann DG, Sasaki CT, Suzuki M, et al: Dilator naris muscle. Arch Otolaryngol 86:362, 1977.
71. Maresh MM: Paranasal sinuses from birth to late adolescence. Am J Dis Child 60:55, 1940.
72. McBurney D, Gent J: On the nature of taste qualities. Psychol Bull 86:151, 1979.
73. McCaffrey TV, Kern EB: Response of nasal airway resistance to hypercapnia and hypoxia in man. Ann Otol Rhinol Laryngol 88:247, 1979.
74. McLaurin JW, Shipman WF, Rosedale R Jr: Oral decongestants. Laryngoscope 71:54, 1961.
75. McNichols WT, Tarlo S, Cole P, et al: Obstructive apneas during sleep in patients with seasonal allergic rhinitis. Am Rev Respir Dis 126:625, 1982.
76. Mellert TK, Getchell ML, Sparks L, et al: Characterization of the immune barrier in human olfactory mucosa. Otolaryngol Head Neck Surg 106:181, 1992.
77. Mennella JA, Beauchamp GK: Developmental changes in nasal airflow patterns. Acta Otolaryngol (Stockh) 112:1025, 1992.
78. Messerkliner W: Uber die drainage der menschlichen Nasennebenhohlen unter normalen und pathologischen Bendingungen. Monatsschr Ohrenheilkd 101:313, 1967.
79. Messerkliner W: Endoscopy of the nose. Urban & Schwarzenberg, Baltimore, 1978.
80. Meyer CM, Cotton RT: Nasal obstruction in the pediatric patient. Pediatrics 72:766, 1983.
81. Mohun M: Incidence of vasomotor rhinitis during pregnancy. Arch Otolaryngol 37:699, 1943.
82. Mostov KE, Blobel G: A transmembrane precursor of secretory component. The receptor for transport of polymeric immunoglobulins. J Biol Chem 257:11816, 1982.
83. Mygind N, Pedersen M, Nielsen M: Morphology of the upper airway epithelium. In Proctor DF, Anderson IB (eds): The Nose—Upper Airway Physiology and the Atmospheric Environment. Elsevier Biomedical Press BV, Amsterdam, 1982, pp 71–98.
84. Naclerio RM, Meier HL, Kagey-Sobotka A, et al: Mediator release after airway challenge with antigen. Am Rev Respir Dis 128:597, 1983.
85. Nakamura F, Ukeda Y, Sonoda Y: Electromyographic study of respiratory movements of the intrinsic laryngeal muscles. Laryngoscope 68:109, 1958.
86. Negus VE: The comparative anatomy and physiology of the nose and paranasal sinuses. E & S Livingston, Edinburgh, 1958.
87. Niinimaa V, Cole P, Mintz S, et al: A head-out body plethysmograph. J Appl Physiol 47:1336, 1979.
88. Patrick GA, Sharp GR: Oronasal distribution of inspiratory flow during various activities. J Physiol 206:22P, 1970.
89. Pederson M, Sakakura Y, Winther B, et al: Nasal mucociliary transport, number of ciliated cells and beating patterns in naturally occurring colds. Eur J Respir Dis Suppl 128:355, 1983.
90. Pevsner J, Reed RR, Feinstein PG, et al: Molecular cloning of odorant binding protein: member of a ligand carrying family. Science 241:336, 1988.
91. Proctor DF: The naso-oro-pharyngo-laryngeal airway. Eur J Respir Dis Suppl 128 64:89, 1983.
92. Proctor DF, Adams GK: Physiology and pharmacology of nasal function and mucus secretion. Pharmacol Ther 2B:492, 1976.
93. Proetz AW: Further observations of the effects of thyroid insufficiency on the nasal mucosa. Laryngoscope 60:627, 1950.
94. Rao SS, Potdar A: Nasal airflow with body in various positions. J Appl Physiol 28:162, 1970.
95. Richardson HB, Seebohm PM: Nasal airway response to exercise. J Allergy 41:269, 1968.
96. Rodenstein DO, Stanescu DC: Absence of nasal airflow during pursed lips breathing, the soft palate mechanisms. Am Rev Respir Dis 128:716, 1983.
97. Rodenstein DO, Stanescu DC: Soft palate and orofacial development. J Appl Physiol 57:651, 1984.
98. Rossen RD, Alford RH, Butler WT, et al: The separation and characterization of proteins intrinsic to nasal secretions. J Immunol 97:369, 1966.
99. Rossen RD, Schade AL, Butler WT, et al: The proteins in nasal secretions: a longitudinal study of IgA, IgG, albumin, siderphilin, and total protein concentrations in nasal washes from adult male volunteers. J Clin Invest 45:768, 1966.
100. Rossmann CM, Lee R, Forrest JB, et al: Nasal ciliary ultrastructure and function in patients with primary ciliary dyskinesia compared with that in normal subjects and in subjects with various respiratory diseases. Am Rev Respir Dis 129:161, 1984.
101. Roussel P, Degand P, Lamblin G, et al: Biochemical definition of human tracheobronchial mucus. Lung 154:241, 1978.
102. Rouviere H: Anatomy of the Human Lymphatic System. A Compendium. Edward Brothers, Ann Arbor, MI, 1938.
103. Saibene F, Mognoni P, Lafortuna CL, et al: Oronasal breathing during exercise. Pflugers Arch 1978;378:65.
104. Sakakura Y: Changes of mucociliary function during colds. Eur J Respir Dis Suppl 128:348, 1983.
105. Sakakura Y, Ukai K, Majima Y, et al: Nasal mucociliary clearance under various conditions. Acta Otolaryngol (Stockh) 96:167, 1983.
106. Salman SD, Proctor DF, Swift DL, et al: Nasal resistance: description of a method and effect of temperature and humidity changes. Ann Otol Rhinol Laryngol 80:736, 1971.
107. Secher C, Kirkegaard J, Mygind N: Significance of H1 and H2 recep-

tors in the human nose. Potential for clinical use of combined preparations. Clin Allergy 70:211, 1982.
108. Sedee GA: Relation between the functions of nose and lung on the same side of the body. Int Rhinol 7:7, 1969.
109. Seltzer S: Endodontology. McGraw-Hill, New York, 1971.
110. Sercer A: Investigations sur l'influence réflectorisée de la cavité nasale sur le poumon du même côté. Acta Otolaryngol (Stockh) 14:82, 1930.
111. Silver NL, Finger TE: The trigeminal system. In Getchell TV, Bartolshuck LM, Doty RL, et al (eds): Smell and Taste in Health and Disease. Raven Press, New York, 1991, pp 97–108.
112. Silverstein EB, Lewis JT, Quenelle DJ: Study of the physiologic relationship of lower and upper airways with Xenon-133. Ann Otol Rhinol Laryngol 89:62, 1980.
113. Sleigh MA: The nature and action of respiratory tract cilia. In Brain JD, Proctor DF, Reid LM (eds): Respiratory Defense Mechanisms. Marcel Dekker, Inc, New York, 1977, 247–288.
114. Strohl KP, Hensley MJ, Hallet M, et al: Activation of the upper airway muscle before onset of inspiration in normal humans. J Appl Physiol 49:638, 1980.
115. Swift DL, Proctor DF: Access of air to the respiratory tract. In Brain JD, Proctor DF, Reid LM (eds): Respiratory Defense Mechanisms. Marcel Dekker, Inc, New York, 1977, pp 63–93.
116. Tarabichi M, Fanous N: Finite element analysis of airflow in the nasal valve. Otolaryngol Head Neck Surg 119:638, 1993.
117. Taylor M: The origin and function of nasal mucus. Laryngoscope 84:612, 1974.
118. Tos M: Goblet cell and glands in the nose and paranasal sinuses. In Proctor DF, Anderson IB (eds): The Nose—Upper Airway Physiology and the Atmospheric Environment. Elsevier Biomedical Press BV, Amsterdam, 1982, pp 99–144.
119. Uddman R, Sundler F: Vasoactive intestinal peptide nerves in human upper respiratory tract. Oto Rhino Laryngol 41:221, 1979.
120. Watson ED, Hoffmann NJ, Simmens RW, et al: Aerobic and anaerobic bacterial counts of nasal washings: presence of organisms resembling *Corynebacterium acnes*. J Bacteriol 83:144, 1962.
121. Wilson WR, Allansmith MR: Rapid, atraumatic method for obtaining nasal mucus samples. Ann Otol Rhinol Laryngol 85:391, 1976.
122. Winther FO, Horthe K, Lystad A, et al: Pathogenic bacterial flora in the upper respiratory tract of healthy students. Prevalence and relationship to nasopharyngeal inflammatory symptoms. J Laryngol Otol 88:407, 1974.

23 Imaging Techniques in Nasal Allergy and Sinusitis

HOWARD M. DRUCE DAVID S. MARTIN DAVID LOWRY

Imaging tests are only rarely required for the diagnosis of nasal allergy. Nevertheless, patients with atypical syndromes or whose symptoms are chronic and sometimes resistant to conventional medication are candidates for imaging tests. Multiple syndromes may coexist and require appropriate therapy. Since sinusitis is part of the differential diagnosis of many of these syndromes, an imaging test is frequently helpful. In chronic disease where there is a high degree of suspicion of sinusitis, the imaging test should follow an adequate medical therapeutic trial. The choice of imaging test depends on the patterns of symptoms. Computed tomography (CT) scans, magnetic resonance imaging (MRI), and direct observation with the aid of endoscopes have largely supplanted plain radiography.

IMAGING IN NASAL ALLERGY

Seasonal allergic rhinitis and viral upper respiratory tract infections are primarily mucosal processes, and imaging is not usually required. Differential diagnoses are more readily resolved by tests such as nasal cell smears and allergy skin tests. Classic presentations of chronic syndromes, such as perennial allergic rhinitis, also do not usually require an imaging test. When symptoms are vague, atypical, or resistant to optimal medical management, an imaging test may prove valuable.

INDICATIONS

A patient with typical nasal allergy who presents with sneezing, itching, rhinorrhea, and nasal obstruction does not need an imaging test as part of the routine work-up (Fig. 23–1). The nasal mucosa should be viewed by anterior rhinoscopy using an otoscope with a large diameter nasal head. This should be combined with a topical decongestant with 1% phenylephrine to shrink the mucosa. This will allow examination of the middle turbinates and give an indication of the maximal nasal patency that might be obtained after therapeutic decongestion. To view more of the surface area of the nasal mucosa, a flexible or rigid endoscope is used. A summary of clinical indications to obtain an imaging test is listed in Table 23–1. The tests commonly used are listed in Table 23–2.

The most common syndromes requiring imaging usually

Nasal Allergy	☛	**No need for imaging**
⇓		
Recalcitrant Nasal Obstruction	☛	**Assess need for screening image**
⇓		
Polyps/Sinusitis	☛	**Assess need for imaging**
⇓		
Unusual Symptoms	☛	**Probable need for imaging**

FIGURE 23–1. Simplified flow chart for imaging in suspected chronic or recurrent sinusitis.

include the symptom of nasal obstruction. These include nasal polyposis, deviated nasal septum, and sinusitis. These are discussed under the differential diagnosis of sinusitis. Unilateral nasal obstruction may be a manifestation of the nasal cycle. If fixed, the age of the patient is relevant. Children frequently place foreign objects in the nose, and these may become epithelialized, producing obstruction rather than discharge.

IMAGING IN SINUSITIS

The diagnosis of sinusitis is frequently made incorrectly, especially when no imaging test is obtained. A classification of sinusitis is given in Table 23–3. Acute sinusitis is usually an acute bacterial infection following an unresolved viral upper respiratory infection. Symptoms have usually been present for less than 2 weeks. The symptoms are those of a severe head cold: nasal congestion, purulent rhinorrhea and postnasal drip, headache, and fever. Radiographic findings include characteristic air-fluid levels, opacification, and mucoperiosteal thickening of the affected sinus (Figs. 23–2 and 23–3). Other causes of acute sinusitis include barotrauma, direct trauma, and nosocomial infection.

An imaging test allows one to document the syndrome. When positive, an imaging test differentiates sinusitis from purulent rhinitis. This may not always be a necessary step. A plain sinus radiograph is not needed for the management of uncomplicated acute sinusitis. Table 23–4 presents arguments for and against obtaining a radiograph. Alternative approaches are detailed in Table 23–5.

Recurrent acute sinusitis may be defined as repetitive episodes of symptoms of sinus infection occurring at the same time as abnormal radiographic findings. Microbiologic cultures would show evidence of infection, but not necessarily with the same organisms each time. Radiographs, or other imaging tests, obtained between attacks show no abnormality but are rarely obtained to confirm that resolution has occurred. Subacute sinusitis is a term used to indicate the presence of symptoms lasting from 2 weeks to 3 months but has not gained wide acceptance.[13] The time course of chronic sinusitis is considered to be 3 months or more. In chronic sinusitis, both symptoms and abnormal images persist. Acute-on-chronic disease (or exacerbation of chronic disease) may be characterized by reappearance of infectious symptoms, such as purulent discharge, on a background of chronic symptoms (see Table 23–3). The background may be clear or intermittent colored nasal discharge or may be another sinus-related symptom, such as head pressure or congestion.

TABLE 23–1
INDICATIONS FOR IMAGING TESTS IN PATIENTS WITH CHRONIC NASAL SYMPTOMS

- Recalcitrant nasal obstruction
- Unilateral nasal symptoms
- Severe or recalcitrant nasal pain
- Unexplained bleeding
- Concomitant deformity or congenital abnormality

TABLE 23–2
IMAGING TESTS

- Plain radiography
- A-mode ultrasound
- Computed tomography
- Magnetic resonance imaging
- Fiberoptic endoscopy

SINUS-RELATED SYMPTOMS

Sinus-related syndromes include isolated vacuum (or pressure)-type headaches referred to the sinuses in the absence of demonstrable pathology. Other possible symptoms that may occur in isolation or in combinations are listed in Table 23–6.

One report described sinusitis as a disease characterized by inflammation of the paranasal sinuses and associated with obstruction of the sinus ostia, retention of secretions, and infection.[36] Patients enrolled in this study were considered to have chronic sinusitis based on history, roentgenographic appearance, or physical examination. The elements in the history required for a positive diagnosis were not enumerated in the methods section. Thus a normal radiograph would be compatible with the diagnosis. The authors developed a scoring system for CT abnormalities. Chronic cases were patients defined as having symptoms for more than 3 months, as opposed to acute sinusitis, defined by signs and symptoms of an upper respiratory infection persisting between 7 and 10 days or longer. The pattern of observed symptoms described in the results is typical of similar studies. Relying on abnormal CT data as indicating the presence of sinus pathology without excluding the presence of a common cold needs caution in the light of data showing that coronal CT abnormalities could occur after a common cold.[23]

TABLE 23–3
CLASSIFICATION OF SINUSITIS SYNDROMES

- Acute sinusitis
- Recurrent or relapsing acute sinusitis
- Chronic sinusitis
- Acute-on-chronic (or exacerbation of chronic) sinusitis
- Sinus-related headaches or nasal symptoms

From Druce HM: Diagnosis and management of chronic sinusitis and its complications. Immunol Allergy Clin North Am 7:117–132, 1987.

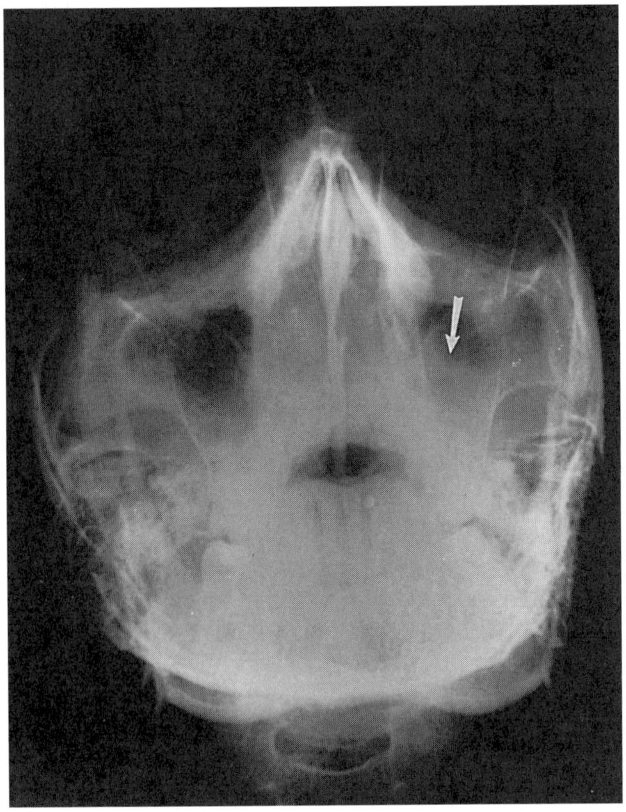

FIGURE 23–2. Waters view of a patient with an air-fluid level in the maxillary sinus (arrow).

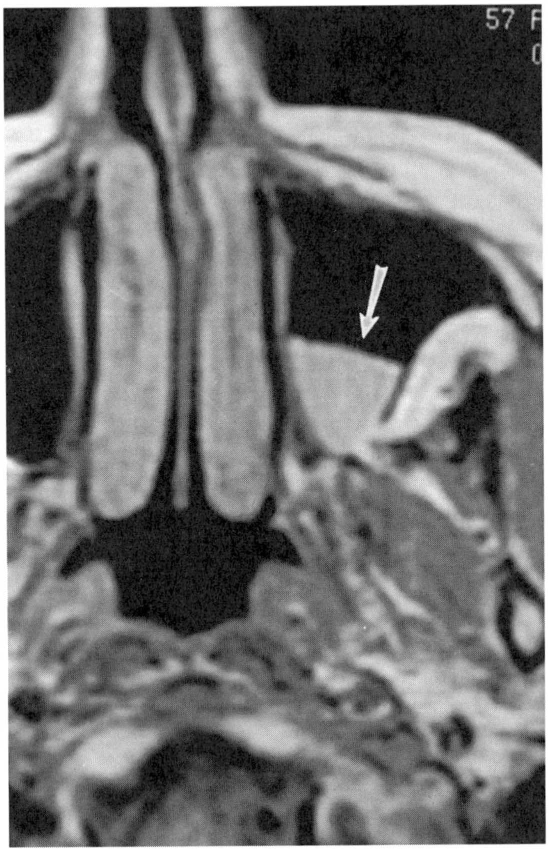

FIGURE 23–3. Proton density axial MRI shows an air-fluid level in the left maxillary sinus (arrow).

TABLE 23–4
ARGUMENTS ON OBTAINING PLAIN RADIOGRAPHS IN SUSPECTED ACUTE SINUSITIS

For
- Prescription of antibiotics in view of a normal radiograph may be wasteful
- Establishes baseline to compare with later improvement or deterioration
- Rough idea of extent and location of pathology may aid in prognosis

Against
- Characteristic appearance will not influence management
- Unnecessary radiation
- Insensitive technique for localization of disease, especially with ethmoid involvement
- Should obtain follow-up film after treatment to ensure resolution of pathology

Williams and colleagues[53] attempted to identify the most useful clinical examination findings for the diagnosis of acute and subacute sinusitis. The authors discussed the overlap in symptoms between acute sinusitis and rhinitis but did not produce a definition. They accepted an abnormal radiograph as indicating the presence of sinusitis, as opposed to rhinitis. The patients in the study presented with nasal discharge of any quality, facial pain unrelated to trauma, or self-suspected sinusitis.

Wald and colleagues[51] proposed arbitrary temporal modifiers for sinusitis based on discussions at a closed conference.[4] Acute was defined as onset to 2 to 4 weeks; subacute was 2 to 4 weeks to 2 to 3 months, and chronic was more than 2 to 3 months. It has been documented that the radiographic findings of paranasal sinus opacification and mucosal thickening, the hallmarks of sinusitis, can also be found in children free of symptoms.[1, 46] Dohlman and colleagues[13] defined subacute sinusitis symptoms as mucoid nasal drainage, cough, or poorly controlled asthma for more than 3 weeks but less than 3 months with radiographic evidence of sinusitis, that is, mucosal thickening of more than 6 mm of the maxillary sinuses or more than 33% loss of airspace volume within the maxillary sinuses and/or opacification or air-fluid levels of any of the paranasal sinuses.

DIFFERENTIAL DIAGNOSIS (Table 23–7)

Diagnosis is difficult because the sinus mucosa is hidden. Even the most sensitive imaging technique provides an indi-

TABLE 23–5
ALTERNATIVE APPROACHES TO REGULARLY OBTAINING SINUS RADIOGRAPHS

- Obtain plain films only for a first episode
- Obtain a film only for atypical symptoms
- Obtain a baseline coronal CT scan for atypical symptoms
- Use A-mode ultrasound to document the presence of fluid in the maxillary sinuses if the major differential diagnosis is acute sinusitis
- Use empiric therapeutic trials followed by imaging tests (usually coronal CT) to document residual rather than untreated disease

TABLE 23–6
SINUS-ASSOCIATED SYMPTOMS

Local	***Systemic***
• Facial pain/pressure	• Fever
• Head congestion/stuffiness	• Malaise
• Purulent nasal discharge	
• Headache	
• Bad breath	
• Toothache (upper jaw)	
• Facial swelling	
• Sore throat	
• Fullness, pain, or popping of ears	

rect method of proving the presence of disease. There are few studies of mucosal pathology in chronic sinusitis, and no consistent pathologic finding has been described that would merit the inconvenience of routine diagnostic biopsy.[37] Beyond imaging techniques, direct visualization of the ostiomeatal area has been enhanced by introduction of fiberoptic rhinoscopy with the flexible endoscope.[45] This enables pathology that may lead to sinus ostial obstruction to be seen. Pus draining from the ostia may also be seen, but the sinus ostia cannot be cannulated to visualize the sinus cavities. The short rigid endoscope may be used to define ostiomeatal anatomy.[26]

Antral aspiration has been used in both acute and chronic sinusitis to obtain cultures for microbiologic analysis. Its place in chronic sinusitis syndromes in which inflammatory changes are more likely is undetermined. Unless characteristic ultrastructural observations can be identified that correlate well with symptoms, diagnosis will continue to be inferential.

Chronic sinusitis is frequently incorrectly diagnosed when there is no sinus pathology. This underscores the importance of demonstrating pathology within the sinus cavities in contrast to symptoms that could refer to the sinuses or adjacent structures. For example, both chronic sinusitis and nonallergic rhinitis may present with only postnasal drip or mucous pooling in the back of the throat at night, leading to cough. An imaging test that concentrates on the ethmoid sinuses could provide inferential evidence to make this distinction (Fig. 23–4). Nonallergic rhinitis may present with nasal obstruction and intermittent symptom expression referable to the sinuses, leading to confusion with true chronic sinusitis.[14, 16]

Structural rhinitis may be caused by a marked nasal septal deflection, concha bullosa, nasal septal erosion, ulcer, or perforation (Fig. 23–5). The symptoms of obstruction and rhinorrhea may mimic chronic sinusitis or nonallergic rhinitis. Allergic rhinitis usually presents a distinct pattern with sneezing paroxysms and clear rhinorrhea. However, nasal obstruction may present as the only symptom. Coronal CT examination has shown that sinus-related symptoms can occur when the sinus ostia are blocked. In some cases, this occurs without infection or inflammation in the sinus cavi-

TABLE 23–7
DIFFERENTIAL DIAGNOSIS OF CHRONIC SINUSITIS

- Idiopathic/vasomotor rhinitis/perennial nonallergic rhinitis
- Structural rhinitis
- Allergic rhinitis
- Sinus ostial obstruction
- Nasal polyposis
- Aspirin/NSAID sensitivity
- Foreign body
- Dental abscess
- Chronic headache
- Abnormal visual refraction
- Malignancy

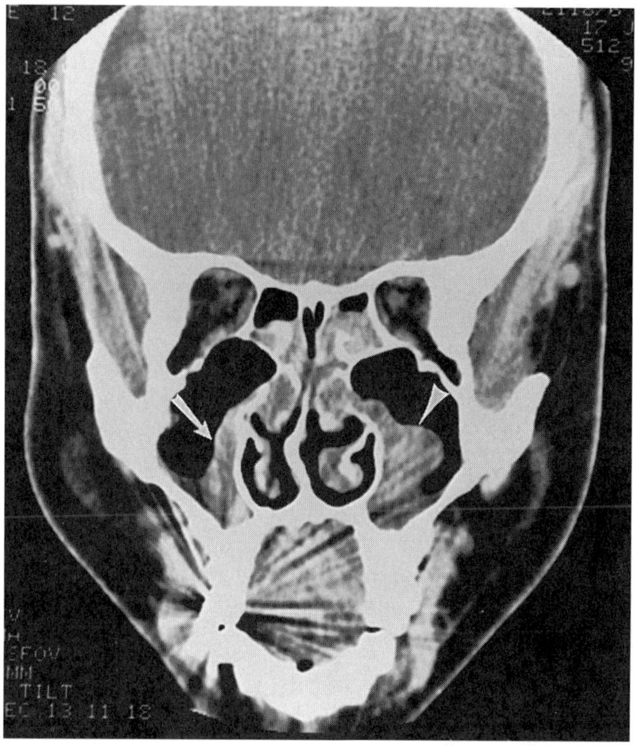

FIGURE 23–4. Coronal CT in a patient with chronic sinusitis. There is polypoid mucosal thickening on the right (arrowhead) and smooth mucosal thickening on the left (arrow). The ethmoid sinuses are also partially opacified.

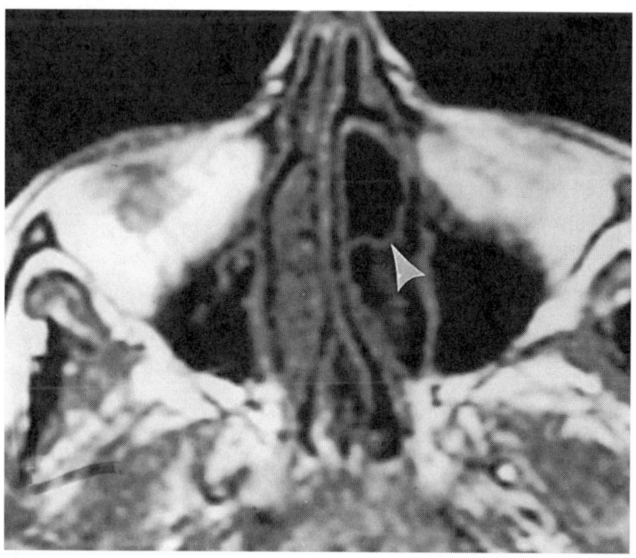

FIGURE 23–5. Axial T1-weighted MRI of a pneumatized middle turbinate (concha bullosa), which is dark because it is air filled (arrowhead).

ties. This may be due to anatomic variation or intranasal inflammation.

Nasal obstruction in polyposis may be unilateral or bilateral, progressive or intermittent, and associated with anosmia (Fig. 23–6). If no obvious cause for nasal obstruction is seen on inspection of the anterior part of the nose, the next logical step is to view the nose directly. The first step should be decongestion of the nasal mucosa. If no obvious cause is seen, flexible endoscopy (rhinolaryngeal pharyngoscopy) should be performed.

Sensitivity to aspirin or nonsteroidal anti-inflammatory drugs (NSAIDs) presents with one of two major syndromes: chronic urticaria and rhinosinusitis. It may not be appreciated that chronic sinusitis can be due to repetitive ingestion of these drugs. Patients may not consider these analgesics as drugs when giving their medication history.

Dental abscess in the upper jaw produces intermittent or chronic pain that can mimic maxillary sinusitis. Pressure on the affected tooth may precipitate symptoms. Patients who complain of chronic upper facial pain should be examined for abnormal visual refraction. Although tumors of the sinuses are rare, they present late. Any suspicion of a space-occupying or bleeding lesion should prompt urgent referral and evaluation (Fig. 23–7). Nasal obstruction is the major symptom and a differential diagnosis is given in Table 23–8.

TABLE 23–8
DIFFERENTIAL DIAGNOSIS OF NASAL OBSTRUCTION

- Nasal polyposis
- Sinusitis
- Deviated nasal septum
- Foreign body
- Tumors
- Hypertrophy of nasal turbinate mucosa (allergic, nonallergic)
- Atrophic rhinitis
- Trauma (e.g., nasal fracture)

MANAGEMENT OF SUSPECTED CHRONIC SINUSITIS

The place for a medical therapeutic trial depends on the likelihood of reaching a diagnosis of sinusitis. If the clinician is confident of the diagnosis from the history and physical examination (Fig. 23–8A), it is reasonable to proceed to a medical therapeutic trial before obtaining an imaging test. The imaging tests may then be used to define residual disease after optimal medical treatment. This strategy is not always appropriate for acute symptoms and should not be considered if the acute symptoms are very severe.

If the trial is successful, no further investigation is needed. Patients may be maintained on empiric medication, such as nasal steroids and decongestants, for selected symptoms. Partial success, such as relief of some symptoms, should point directly to the medications that need to be continued. Complete relief, which lasts only for a limited duration, may indicate any of the factors described in Table 23–9.

If the differential diagnosis is still unclear and the suspicion of sinusitis is weaker, tests to visualize the area may be done sooner (see Fig. 23–8B). It is hard to justify the expense of a complete CT scan for an uncertain diagnosis; thus, a screening CT may be considered. Failure of a medical therapeutic trial undertaken without evidence of sinus-related pathology should prompt a more intensive search for alternative diagnoses. Diagnoses of exclusion, such as nonallergic perennial rhinitis or tension headache, should not be applied as a label for untreatable symptoms without appropriate consideration of a differential diagnosis and testing.

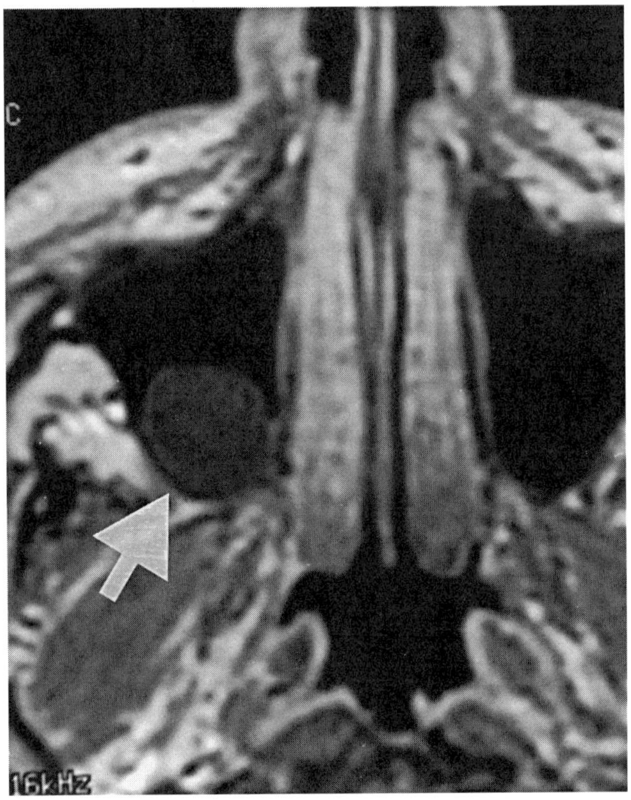

FIGURE 23–6. Axial T1-weighted MRI of a polyp or retention cyst in the maxillary sinus (arrow). It is relatively dark on this sequence and would appear relatively bright on T2-weighted images.

LATE RECURRENT OR PERSISTENT DISCHARGE OR POSTNASAL DRIP AFTER SINUS SURGERY

CT scans before and after surgery should be reviewed. Comparable cuts should be taken. If there is no evidence of disease on the imaging test, endoscopy and microbial cultures should be obtained. Aerobic and anaerobic bacterial and fungal cultures may be appropriate. Antibiotic treatment should be selected accordingly if cultures suggest the pres-

TABLE 23–9
FACTORS IMPLICATED IN TREATMENT FAILURE

- Is the diagnosis correct?
- Is there a need for multimodal therapy?
- Is the organism sensitive to the antibiotic chosen?
- Is the dose of therapy sufficient?
- Is the duration of treatment adequate?
- Is the patient compliant with the medication regimen?
- Is the cause of the symptoms environmental?
- Excess mucus may be physiologic

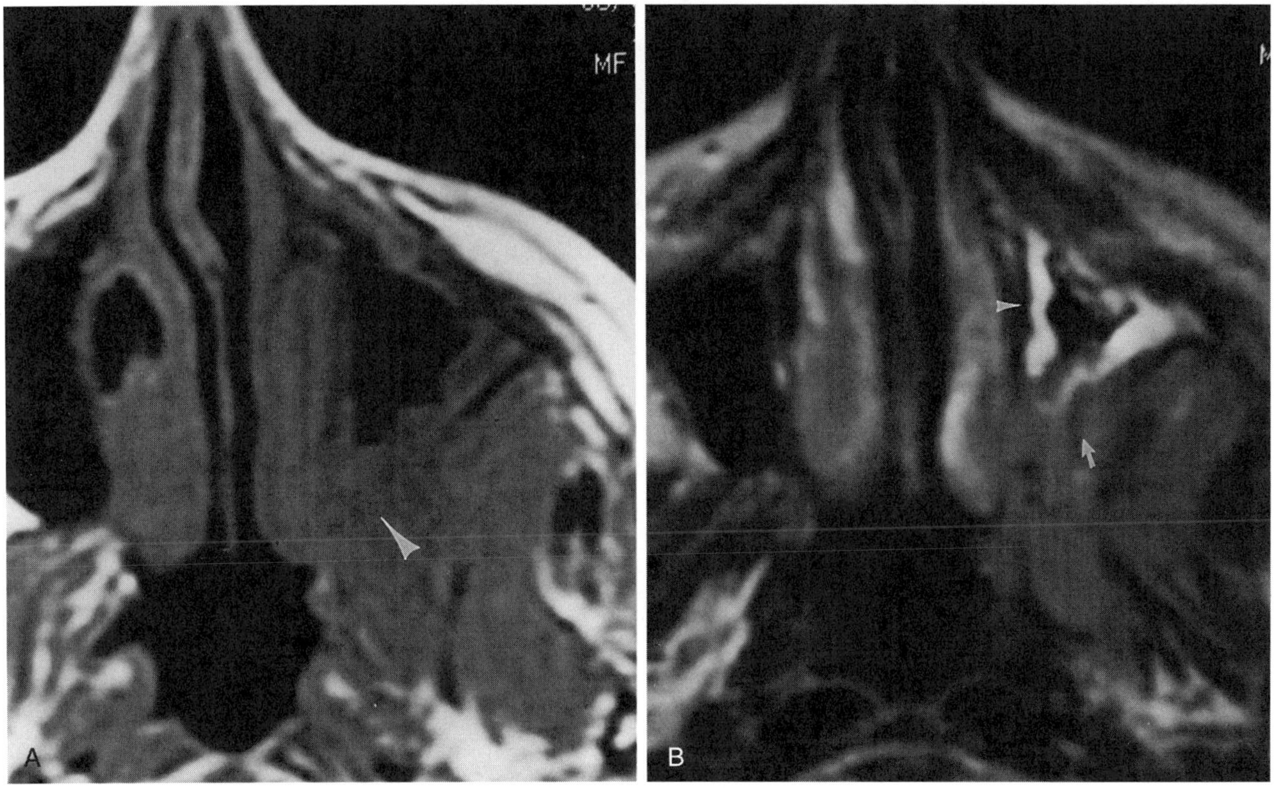

FIGURE 23–7. (A) Noncontrast axial T1-weighted image through the mid maxillary sinus in a patient with sinus lymphoma. Note that the tumor is isointense to muscle (arrowhead). **(B)** Noncontrast axial T2-weighted image at the same level shows that the tumor is still isointense to muscle (arrow). Note that the sinus mucosa is edematous and thickened and thus is bright (arrowhead).

ence of an organism that might be producing the symptoms. It is important to realize which organisms may be commensals or colonizing the postsurgical site. Symptomatic treatment should be combined with antibiotics, or used without antibiotics if the cultures are negative, or if symptoms persist after an adequate antibiotic course. Such therapy can include lavage, steam and saline instillation, Alkylol nasal spray, topical antibiotics and antiseptics, pharmacotherapy such as the expectorant guaifenesin and decongestant combinations, and the use of empiric antibiotics known to decrease mucus viscosity, such as erythromycin or clarithromycin. Failure of these therapies should lead to further consideration of revision surgery.

Symptoms occurring immediately postoperatively include adhesions and the failure to eradicate key ethmoid air cells. Multiple factors need to be considered when treatment failure occurs (see Table 23–9).

IMAGING MODALITIES

STANDARD RADIOGRAPHY

Various tests have been used to image the sinuses or locate the pathology from which sinus-related symptoms arise. Standard radiography is no longer the accepted standard for diagnosis of chronic sinusitis, despite widespread use. The likelihood of detecting the presence of antral fluid increases with the number of views obtained.[1] In screening for chronic sinusitis in which fluid is frequently absent, two or three projections are usually obtained.[18] The occipitomental view (Waters' projection) gives the best image of the maxillary sinuses, and the occipitofrontal view (Caldwell's projection) shows the frontal and ethmoid sinuses.[28] Studies have compared radiographic abnormalities with the occurrence of fluid in the maxillary antra and recovery of bacteria from antral punctures.[1] Some of these studies have specifically addressed acute sinusitis, and others have not distinguished patients with acute and chronic syndromes. In chronic sinusitis, there is no good correlation between symptoms, signs, and the prediction of an abnormal radiograph. Moreover, patients with minimal mucosal thickening alone, who on Evans' and colleagues'[18] data would not be expected to have a bacterial infection, respond only to antibiotic therapy.

The significant incidence of abnormal radiographic findings in asymptomatic patients makes the continued use of plain radiographs tenuous. In a study of children undergoing sinus radiography for reasons unrelated to respiratory infection, Kovatch and colleagues[28] found a 53% incidence of abnormal radiographs in children above the age of 1. These studies discounted the suggestion that opacification or sinus fluid can be produced by crying. A similar proportion of abnormal sinus images occurs using other techniques.

ULTRASOUND

The advantages of ultrasound include absence of ionizing radiation, rapid test time, and patient convenience. Repetitive studies can be done on the same individual to assess re-

Clinical Diagnosis

(Strong Suspicion)

↓

Medical Therapeutic Trial

↓

(Fail)

↓

CT and/or Endoscopy

↓

A **Surgical Evaluation**

Clinical Diagnosis

(Weak Suspicion)

↓

Screening CT and/or Endoscopy

↓

Medical Therapeutic Trial

↓

(Fail)

↓

Selective Symptomatic Medical Management

↓

Re-consider Differential Diagnosis

(e.g. Nonallergic Perennial Rhinitis,

B **Tension Headache)**

FIGURE 23–8. (A, B) Management of suspected sinusitis.

sponse to treatment. Initial studies from Finland[40, 41] and Germany[33] reported a high correlation between positive echoes on A-mode ultrasound and the presence of fluid on maxillary antral puncture. Experience in the United States with two commercially available instruments has been mixed. Besides case reports,[29] two series were reported. Shapiro and colleagues[45] found a poor correlation between ultrasound and radiographic findings in a mixed population of children and adults, whereas the data of Rohr and associates[42] suggested a better correlation. Poor correlation between ultrasound findings and the presence of pus in the antra was noted in a Swedish study.[2]

No longitudinal data have been presented on patients with chronic sinusitis. Two major problems arise with ultrasound. First, only the maxillary and frontal sinuses may be examined. Second, most patients with chronic sinusitis do not have fluid in the sinuses but have mucosal thickening. No reported study has examined this systematically. Our data suggested a poor correlation between ultrasonographic criteria for mucosal thickening and its detection on plain radiographs.[15] We suggested that another parameter needs to be correlated with the ultrasound for it to have any relevance. These data are not available, and ultrasound should be reserved as a screening method to detect the presence of maxillary antral fluid. This may be especially useful when the maxillary antra are opacified after sinus surgery. Enthusiasm for ultrasound in the United States has declined.

COMPUTED TOMOGRAPHY

CT produces greater definition of the contents and anatomy of the sinus cavities.[5, 7] In patients who have had surgery, the technique may be useful to distinguish fluid from fibrosis or mucoperiosteal thickening.[6] CT is especially useful if sphenoid sinusitis,[31] ethmoid sinusitis,[48, 49] malignancy,[27] or other complications, such as orbital cellulitis, are suspected (Fig. 23–9). CT has supplanted multidirectional tomography[43] and plain radiography to some extent. Coronal view CT without contrast is favored as the most reliable test to detect inflammatory sinus disease. Screening protocols involving fewer cuts, and therefore less time and expense, have been introduced. Examples of procedures include screening protocols (5 to 12 coronal slices, 5 mm thick every 7 mm), limited protocols (24 to 30 coronal slices, thin cuts

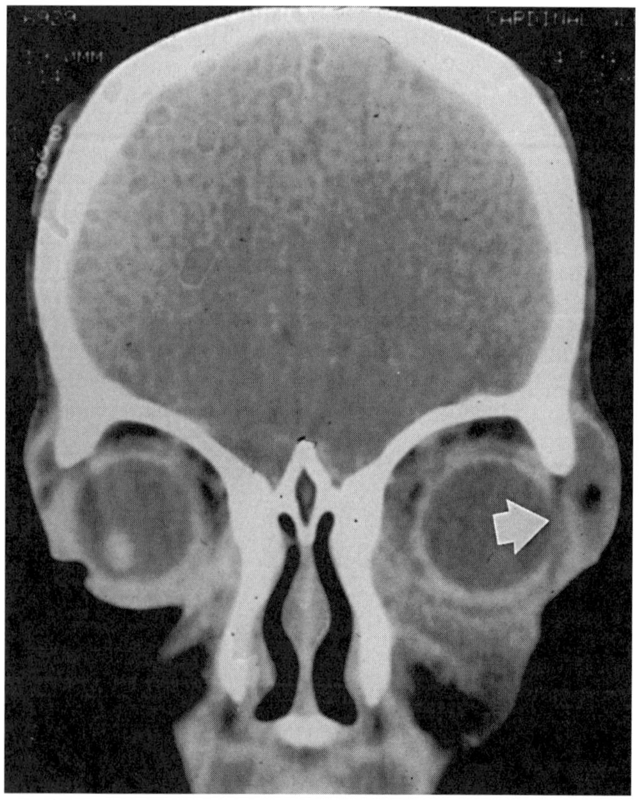

FIGURE 23–9. Coronal CT through the mid orbit in a patient with orbital cellulitis. Note the soft tissue swelling, hypodense fluid collection, and central gas collection in the abscess (arrow).

through the ostiomeatal complex, and 5-mm cuts elsewhere), and complete protocols (50 axial and coronal slices, axial 5 mm thick every 5 mm, coronal 3 mm thick every 3 mm through the ostiomeatal complex and 5 mm thick every 5 mm elsewhere). Approximate costs of $135, $250, and $450 compare favorably with $100 for a three-view plain radiograph series.

CT has led to widespread acceptance of functional endoscopic sinus surgical procedures on the ostiomeatal complex. Most otolaryngologists prefer a complete CT examination before surgery and would not accept a screening protocol (defined as one that shows only the ostiomeatal complex area) as adequate. Timing of the CT scan in relation to the presence of symptoms is critical. Data have shown that common colds can cause abnormalities to appear on the CT scan.[23] Thus CT scans should be obtained only in the context of chronic symptoms and after an adequate therapeutic trial to allow demonstration of residual disease.

Modern CT has high resolution and speed. Slice thickness can be as small as 1 mm. Slice acquisition time for routine scanning is 2 seconds. The improved resolution provides greater anatomic detail, and the superior speed affords greater convenience and comfort. Complete imaging of the paranasal sinuses is performed in axial and coronal planes. For axial slices, the patient lies supine on the scanning couch with the head in a holder. For direct coronal series, the patient is either prone or supine with the neck extended. Slice locations are prescribed from a lateral digital radiograph.

The complete series consists of images in both axial and coronal planes. A coronal slice set is prescribed from the anterior aspect of the frontal sinus to the posterior limit of the sphenoid sinus. An axial set consists of slices between the superior limit of the frontal sinus and the superior alveolar ridge of the maxilla. Slice thickness varies from 3 to 5 mm.[21]

The limited or screening sinus CT scan is a subset of the complete series[21, 22, 52] (Fig. 23–10). It is useful as an inexpensive alternative to the relatively insensitive plain sinus film series and the relatively expensive complete sinus CT examination. The screening examination can detect sinus inflammatory disease with a reasonable sensitivity yet maintain low cost. It is not designed for preoperative planning. Our screening sinus examination consists of four noncontiguous 3- to 5-mm coronal slices using a scout radiograph made by the CT machine. One coronal slice is made through the central portion of each of the paired paranasal sinuses. Slices from sinus CT examinations are filmed at wide and narrow window settings (window widths 300 HU and 250 HU, respectively; window level 250 HU and 10 HU, respectively) and placed side by side on a 4 × 3 film matrix.

NUCLEAR MAGNETIC RESONANCE

MRI has superb contrast resolution with better depiction of soft tissue anatomy than CT. It easily detects change in soft tissue water content and is thus extremely sensitive to edema in mucous membranes. It can be used to distinguish tumor from inflammatory disease by differences in signal patterns (Fig. 23–11).[30] CT is not able to detect such subtle differences and relies on the presence of bone destruction to suggest the presence of aggressive pathology. MRI has additional advantages, such as not using ionizing radiation. One can perform multiplanar imaging without changing the patient's position. MRI is the only imaging modality that can obtain direct sagittal images on live patients.

MRI also has some definite disadvantages. It is twice as expensive and takes three times as long to perform compared with a CT scan of the same area. MRI images are easily degraded by patient motion. MRI can be fatal to those with intracranial aneurysm clips and can blind those with metal fragments in their eyes. It is also capable of causing malfunctions in life support equipment and pacemakers. It is further limited by its inability to display bony landmarks. The small bore of most superconducting and high field strength mag-

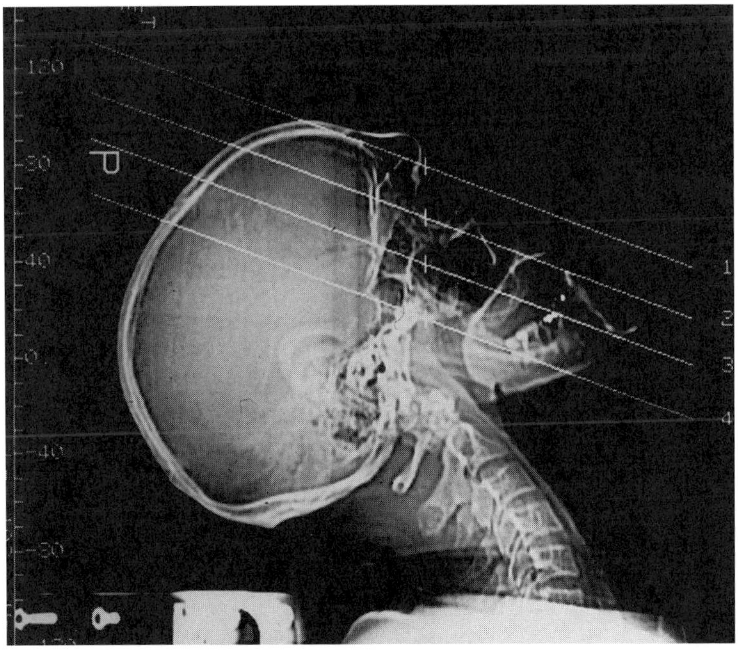

FIGURE 23–10. Lateral digital radiograph with the four direct coronal slice locations identified for a screening CT of the sinuses.

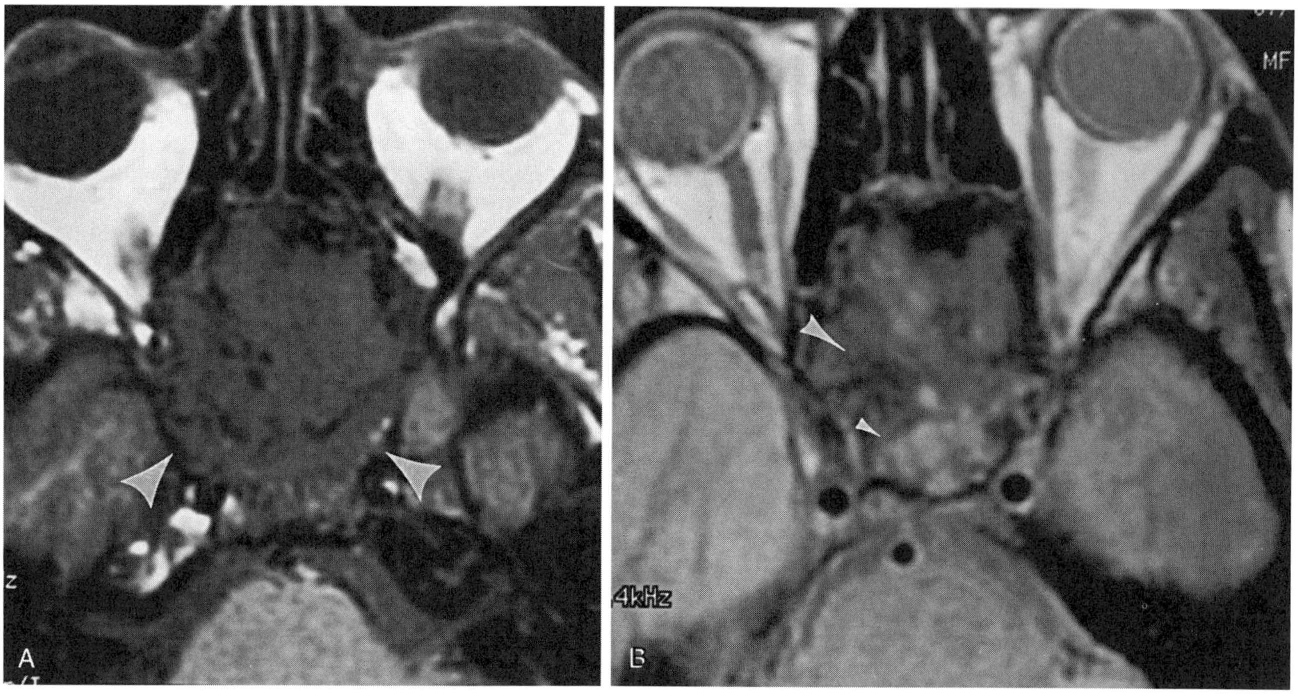

FIGURE 23–11. (A) Noncontrast axial T1-weighted MRI in a patient with inflammatory pseudotumor. A homogeneous, expansile, isointense mass fills the sphenoid sinus (arrowheads). **(B)** Proton density image shows the inhomogeneity of signal with some relatively bright (small arrowhead) and dark (large arrowhead) areas.

nets limits monitoring and observation of patients and causes claustrophobia in a small percentage. Since calcification may lack MRI signal, a densely calcified fungus ball in a sinus may mimic aeration of the sinus.[47]

CT is sufficient for imaging of most inflammatory disease of the paranasal sinuses. MRI is useful when inflammatory sinus disease is complicated by nasal or nasopharyngeal extension because direct sagittal and coronal images provide valuable supplementary information.[50] MRI is very important when inflammatory sinus disease is secondary to an obstructing primary or secondary neoplasm. When an encephalocele mimics inflammatory sinus disease, MRI may be essential in preoperative evaluation. Contrast can be administered during MRI examinations. MRI increases the signal of areas with increased vascularity, such as infections and neoplasms.

Our technique for MRI of the paranasal sinuses has the patient placed supine with the head in a standard head coil. The sinuses and adjacent structures are identified on a preliminary sagittal image. T1- and T2-weighted sequences are then obtained in axial and coronal planes. The slice thickness is usually 3 to 5 mm. If contrast is used, both precontrast and postcontrast series are obtained using T1-weighted sequences.

Incidental sinus abnormalities occur on both CT and MRI. Minimal mucosal thickening in the sinuses may have no clinical significance.[11, 12, 17, 34, 39] Therefore, images must be correlated with the clinical history and physical and laboratory test values.

In one study, MRI was administered to 272 patients as part of a neurologic evaluation.[8] As with CT, a high incidence of abnormal images was detected. Sixty out of 272 patients (22%) had abnormal findings. Solitary maxillary disease was found in 37%, and combined maxillary and ethmoid disease occurred in 42%. Two patients had isolated ethmoiditis, two had sphenoiditis, and one had combined ethmoid and sphenoid disease. Data such as these make assertions that ethmoid and frontal sinusitis are always associated with maxillary disease less tenable.[32] In another study, MRI was administered to 1,120 patients as part of a neurologic evaluation. As with CT, a high incidence of abnormal images was detected, with 13% having abnormal findings.[9] MRI is considered the imaging test of choice to detect fungal disease or cancer in the sinus cavities.

FLEXIBLE ENDOSCOPY

The introduction of flexible endoscopes with a small diameter (3 to 4 mm) and light bending radius permits detailed examination of the upper nasal cavities and posterior nasopharynx. A variety of pathologic processes may be identified.[44] Use of the endoscope involves administration of a topical local anesthetic and decongestant to the nasal mucosa, but this should not replace use of the head mirror and posterior pharyngoscopy in those patients who can tolerate it. We use endoscopy for atypical and recalcitrant symptoms and to identify structural abnormalities high in the nasal vault. Endoscopy is useful for detecting rostral septal deviations, ethmoid polyps, and residual adenoid tissue in adolescents. Skill is required not only in passing the endoscope but also in differentiating variations in normal anatomy from pathologic lesions. Guidelines for the use of the flexible endoscopes have been proposed. Even the fiberoptic scope does not readily reveal the maxillary sinus ostia. Rigid endoscopy, after more extensive topical anesthesia, is well suited for this purpose.[35]

RIGID ENDOSCOPY

When there is questionable pathology in the area of the ostiomeatal complex, flexible endoscopes do not give an adequate view. The rigid endoscope can provide a superior image in this area. The rigid endoscope should not be handled by the casual user. Considerable skill and training are needed to identify structures through any scope other than with the 0° viewing angle. Endoscopes of 30° and 120° are used largely by otolaryngologists.

MAXILLARY ANTRAL ASPIRATION

Puncture of the maxillary antrum is an office procedure that may be used for diagnostic aspiration or therapeutic lavage. It is more commonly used in Europe than in the United States. Approaches may be made intranasally through the maxillary antrum or through the canine fossa.[10] Therapeutic lavage can be performed in acute sinusitis to relieve pressure symptoms. No systematic data are available to document its efficacy. Its role in chronic disease is undetermined. Diagnostic lavage should be considered in patients with resistant air-fluid levels or when there is a high probability of recovering unusual organisms, such as in immunocompromised patients or malignancy.

OTHER INDIRECT IMAGING MODALITIES

Although not studied systematically, thermography[3, 38] and positron emission tomography have potential to show active inflammation in the sinus cavities. Radionuclides such as ^{67}Ga cannot be currently localized with the precision required to differentiate sinus disease from intranasal pathology. Xenon-enhanced dynamic CT may allow assessment of sinus ventilation.[24]

STAGING

Staging techniques to quantify the extent of disease identified within a sinus cavity have been proposed by several authors, including Friedman and colleagues[19, 20] and Kennedy,[25] and clinical staging was proposed by Newman and colleagues.[36] However, these are more appropriate for baseline evaluation and/or follow-up of cases intended for surgery.

RESEARCH APPLICATIONS

Most clinical trials of new antibiotics have focused on the maxillary sinuses as the target location for the presence of pathology. The air-fluid level in the presence of typical symptoms is a reliable indicator of acute sinusitis but frequently is not seen. Thus some arbitrary amount of mucosal thickening or sinus cavity opacification is taken as a surrogate clinical marker. Care should be taken, as positioning of the patient may affect the test result, and reliability of serial images is highly dependent on operator consistency. Serial images may be desirable to document progression or resolution of disease but expose the patient to increased radiation. Serial images may enhance image quality and allow for recognition of smaller increments of change in disease bulk but are subject to high costs and potential logistic difficulties in patient scheduling.

TABLE 23–10
RESEARCH APPLICATIONS OF NASAL AND SINUS IMAGING

- Clinical trials
- Nasal cross-sectional area
- Nasal patency
- Mucosal bulk assessment

To accelerate patient accrual for some clinical trials, the presence of an abnormal image alone has been considered as a surrogate marker. However, this is unreliable unless there is a clinical correlation with symptoms. Since residual disease may be confined to the ethmoid sinuses, the presence or absence of ethmoid disease at patient entry is an important determinant of prognosis. Tests of adjunctive agents, such as decongestants and nasal steroids, will also require an appropriate imaging test as a surrogate marker for clinical studies.

Imaging tests are not usually selected as end points for clinical trials. However, images photographed through the nasal endoscope may be standardized to obtain an assessment of a nasal cavity cross-sectional area. Imaging may be required to quantify a nasal cross-sectional area and nasal patency and indirectly to obtain an estimate of mucosal bulk. For these, standardized planes are necessary (Table 23–10). Such studies have shown that turbinate asymmetry may be due to the nasal cycle and not necessarily to a fixed structural lesion (Fig. 23–12).[54]

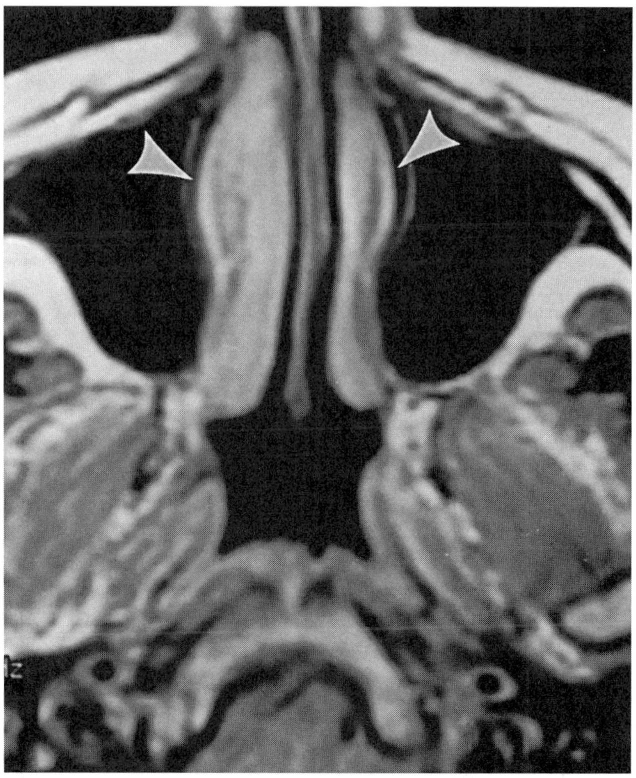

FIGURE 23–12. Axial T1-weighted MRI through the nose demonstrating normal asymmetry of the soft tissue of the turbinates (arrowheads) as part of the nasal cycle.

REFERENCES

1. Axelsson A, Grebelius N, Chidekel N, Jensen C: The correlation between the radiologic examination and the irrigation findings in maxillary sinusitis. Acta Otolaryngol (Stockh) 69:302–306, 1970.
2. Berg O, Carenfelt C: Etiological diagnosis in sinusitis: ultrasonography as clinical component. Laryngoscope 95:851–853, 1985.
3. Berman SZ, Mathison DA, Stevenson DD, et al: Maxillary sinusitis and bronchial asthma: correlation of roentgenograms, cultures, and thermograms. J Allergy Clin Immunol 53:311–317, 1974.
4. Bluestone CB: The diagnosis and management of sinusitis in children: proceedings of a closed conference. Pediatr Infect Dis 6(suppl):S49–81, 1985.
5. Brant-Zawadki MN, Minagi H, Federle MP: High resolution CT with image reformation in maxillofacial pathology. Am J Radiol 138:477–483, 1982.
6. Cable HR, Jeans WD, Cullen RJ, et al: Computerized tomography of the Caldwell-Luc cavity. J Laryngol Otol 95:775–783, 1981.
7. Carter BL, Bankoff MS, Fisk JD: Computed tomographic detection of sinusitis responsible for intracranial and extracranial infections. Radiology 147:739–742, 1983.
8. Conner BL, Phillips K, Roach ES, et al: Nuclear magnetic resonance (NMR) imaging of paranasal sinuses: frequency of abnormalities. J Allergy Clin Immunol 77:139, 1986. Abstract.
9. Conner BL, Roach ES, Laster W, Georgitis JW: Magnetic resonance imaging of the paranasal sinuses: frequency and type of abnormalities. Ann Allergy 62:457–460, 1989.
10. DeWeese DD, Saunders WH: Acute and chronic sinusitis. In: Textbook of Otolaryngology, 6th edition. Mosby, St. Louis, 1982, pp 223–237.
11. Diament MJ, Senac MO Jr, Gilsanz V, et al: Prevalence of incidental paranasal sinuses opacification in pediatric patients: a CT study. J Comput Assist Tomogr 11:426–431, 1987.
12. Digre KB, Maxner CE, Crawford S, Yuh WTC: Significance of CT and MR findings in sphenoid sinus disease. Am J Neuroradiol 10:603–606, 1989.
13. Dohlman AW, Hemstreet MPB, Odrezin GT, Bartolucci AA: Subacute sinusitis: are antimicrobials necessary? J Allergy Clin Immunol 91:1015–1023, 1993.
14. Druce HM: Chronic sinusitis and nonallergic rhinitis. Am J Rhinol 2:163–168, 1988.
15. Druce HM, Heiberg E, Rutledge J: Imaging in chronic sinusitis: disparity between radiographic and ultrasound interpretation. Am J Rhinol 2:61–64, 1988.
16. Druce HM, Rutledge JL: Chronic sinusitis and rhinitis. Am J Rhinol 3:163–166, 1989.
17. Duvoisin B, Agrifoglio A: Prevalence of ethmoid sinus abnormalities on brain CT of asymptomatic adults. Am J Neuroradiol 10:599–601, 1989.
18. Evans FO, Sydnor JB, Moore WEC, et al: Sinusitis of the maxillary antrum. N Engl J Med 293:735–739, 1975.
19. Friedman WH, Katsantonis GP: Staging systems for chronic sinus disease. ENT J 73:480–484, 1994.
20. Friedman WH, Katsantonis GP, Sivore M, Kay S: Computed tomography staging of the paranasal sinuses in chronic hyperplastic rhinosinusitis. Laryngoscope 100:1161–1165, 1990.
21. Goodman G, Martin DS, Klein J, et al: A comparison of a screening versus a conventional coronal sinus CT series for the evaluation of nonsurgical patients with presumptive sinusitis. Ann Allergy. In press.
22. Gross GW, McGeady SJ, Kerut T, Ehrlich SM: Limited-slice CT in the evaluation of paranasal sinus disease in children. Am J Radiol 156:367–369, 1991.
23. Gwaltney JM Jr, Phillips CD, Miller RD, Riker DK: Computed tomographic study of the common cold. N Engl J Med 330:25–30, 1994.
24. Kalender WA, Rettinger G, Suess C: Measurement of paranasal sinus ventilation by xenon-enhanced dynamic computed tomography. J Comput Assist Tomogr 9:524–529, 1985.
25. Kennedy DW: Prognostic factors, outcomes, and staging in ethmoid sinus surgery. Laryngoscope 102(pt 2):1–18, 1992.
26. Kennedy DW, Zinreich SJ, Rosenbaum AE, et al: Functional endoscopic sinus surgery. Arch Otolaryngol 111:576–582, 1985.
27. Kondo M, Horiuchi M, Shiga H, et al: Computed tomography of malignant tumors of the nasal cavity and paranasal sinuses. Cancer 50:226–231, 1982.
28. Kovatch AL, Wald ER, Ledesman-Medina J, et al: Maxillary sinus radiographs in children with non-respiratory complaints. Pediatrics 73:306–308, 1984.
29. Landman MD: Ultrasound screening for sinus disease. Otolaryngol Head Neck Surg 94:157–164, 1986.
30. Lanzieri CF, Shah M, Krauss D, Lavertu P: Use of gadolinium-enhanced MR imaging for differentiating mucoceles from neoplasms in the paranasal sinuses. Radiology 178:425–428, 1991.
31. Lew D, Southwick FS, Montgomery WW, et al: Sphenoid sinusitis: a review of 30 cases. N Engl J Med 309:1149–1154, 1983.
32. Ludman H: Paranasal sinus diseases. Br Med J 282:1054–1058, 1981.
33. Mann W, Beck C, Apostolidis T: Liability of ultrasound in maxillary sinus disease. Arch Oto-Rhino-Laryngol 215:67–74, 1977.
34. McAlister WH, Lusk R, Muntz HR: Comparison of plain radiographs and coronal CT scans in infants and children with recurrent sinusitis. Am J Radiol 153:1259–1264, 1989.
35. Messerklinger W: Endoscopy of the Nose. Urban & Schwartzenberg, Baltimore, 1978.
36. Newman L, Platts-Mills TAE, Phillips CD, et al: Chronic sinusitis: relation of computed tomographic findings to allergy, asthma, and eosinophilia. JAMA 271:363–367, 1994.
37. Ohashi Y, Nakai Y: Functional and morphological pathology of chronic sinusitis mucous membrane. Acta Otolaryngol Suppl (Stockh) 397:11–48, 1983.
38. Phipatankul CS, Slavin RG: Use of thermography in clinical allergy. J Allergy Clin Immunol 50:264–275, 1972.
39. Rak KM, Newell JD, Yakes WF, et al: Paranasal sinuses on MR images of the brain: significance of mucosal thickening. Am J Neuroradiol 11:1211–1214, 1990.
40. Revonta M: Ultrasound in the diagnosis of maxillary and frontal sinusitis. Acta Otolaryngol Suppl (Stockh) 370:1–54, 1980.
41. Revonta M, Suonpaa J: Diagnosis and follow-up of ultrasonographical sinus changes in children. Int J Pediatr Otorhinolaryngol 4:301–308, 1982.
42. Rohr AS, Spector SL, Siegel SC: Correlation between A-mode ultrasound and radiography in the diagnosis of maxillary sinusitis. J Allergy Clin Immunol 78:58–61, 1986.
43. Schneider G, Sager WD, Lepuschutz H: Multidirectional tomography and high resolution CT in lesions of the paranasal sinuses and the pharyngeal cavity. Acta Radiol Diagnosis 23:63–69, 1982.
44. Selner JC, Koepke JW: Rhinolaryngoscopy in the allergy office. Ann Allergy 54:479–482, 1985.
45. Shapiro GG, Furukawa CT, Pierson WE, et al: Blinded comparison of maxillary sinus radiography and ultrasound for diagnosis of sinusitis. J Allergy Clin Immunol 77:59–64, 1986.
46. Shopfner CE, Rossi JO: Roentgen evaluation of the paranasal sinuses in children. Am J Radiol 118:176–186, 1973.
47. Som PM, Dillon WP, Curtin HD, et al: Hypointense paranasal sinus foci: differential diagnosis with MR imaging and relation to CT findings. Radiology 176:777–781, 1990.
48. Som PM, Lawson W, Biller HF, et al: Ethmoid sinus disease: CT evaluation in 400 cases. Part 1. Nonsurgical patients. Radiology 159:591–597, 1986.
49. Som PM, Lawson W, Biller HF, et al: Ethmoid sinus disease: CT evaluation in 400 cases. Part II. Postoperative findings. Radiology 159:599–604, 1986.
50. Som PM, Shapiro MD, Biller HF, et al: Sinonasal tumors and inflammatory tissues: differentiation with MR imaging. Radiology 167:803–808, 1988.
51. Wald ER, Byers C, Guerra N, et al: Subacute sinusitis in children. J Pediatr 115:28–32, 1989.
52. White PS, Robinson JM, Stewart IA, Doyle T: Computerized tomography mini-series: an alternative to standard paranasal sinus radiographs. Aust NZ J Surg 60:25–29, 1990.
53. Williams JW, Simel DL, Roberts L, Samsa GP: Clinical evaluation for sinusitis: making the diagnosis by history and physical examination. Ann Intern Med 117:705–710, 1992.
54. Zinreich SJ, Kennedy DW, Kumar AJ, et al: MR imaging of normal nasal cycle: comparison with sinus pathology. J Comput Assist Tomogr 12:1014–1019, 1988.

III Allergic Diseases

24 Epidemiology and Genetics of Asthma and Allergy

MALCOLM N. BLUMENTHAL

Asthma and allergies are conditions that involve genetic and environmental factors. The epidemiology of these conditions is the science that deals with their etiology, relationships between the various factors that determine their frequency and distribution, and control. It involves the understanding of the interaction between the host, the disease-causing agents, and the environment that ultimately results in allergy and asthma. The etiology of these conditions is multifactorial, depending on the interaction, in genetically susceptible individuals, between time and environmental factors, such as the amount of allergen exposure and the presence of nonspecific adjuvant factors, including air pollution.

One of the problems studying the epidemiology of these conditions is the definition of the disease under study. In addition to problems of definition, the clinical manifestations or phenotypes of these conditions may depend on many variables, such as age and sex, as well as a multitude of environmental factors, such as time and amount of exposure to allergens, infections, air pollution, and smoke.

DEFINITIONS

Epidemiologists have been using working definitions because it has often been difficult to obtain disease-defining laboratory evidence of the allergic condition under study. During the 20th century, more objective measures of allergy-related phenotypes have been developed, which are now available for study. These include assays of total serum and antigen/allergen-specific immunoglobulin levels, skin test reactivity, and cytokines, as well as parameters of bronchial hyperreactivity.

ALLERGY

The immune system and the presence of humoral antibodies were only thought of in terms of body defense systems, such as the response to infection, up to the beginning of the 20th century. At that time, through the work of Arthus, von Pirquet, and Schick, it was demonstrated that although the immune system protects the body, other immune reactions, including those involving humoral antibodies, could mediate adverse reactions.[4, 81, 103, 127, 140, 141] This resulted in the development of the term allergy by von Pirquet,[140] referring to adverse immune reactions. This term, although initially used to describe humoral or antibody-mediated reactions, has also been used for cellular adverse reactions, such as the tuberculin reaction.[127] In this chapter, allergy is defined as an adverse immune reaction.

ATOPY

In 1923, Coca and Cooke[33] proposed the term atopy to identify a subgroup of clinical allergies that involved reaginic

Supported in part by NIH Grant 5U01 HL49609.

or skin-sensitizing antibodies and are subject to hereditary influence. Atopy, derived from the Greek work meaning out of place or strange disease, is a term that has been redefined by many investigators. Some have used atopy to refer to allergic phenomena regardless of whether an antibody could be demonstrated, whereas others believe it refers to the occurrence of an allergen-specific skin-sensitizing reaginic or IgE antibody. In this chapter, atopy is defined as adverse immune reactions involving IgE antibodies.

ASTHMA

The term asthma is derived from a Greek word that means panting and was described in ancient times. The first valid description of asthma was by Aretaeus in A.D. 81. Asthma was then further classified by Hippocrates, Galen, and Celsus. Environmental factors were noted to be associated with the development of asthma by Cardan in 1545, who diagnosed asthma triggered by feathers. Attacks of asthma caused by house dust and by eating fish fried in oil were described by van Helmont in the 17th century. Von Pirquet noted patients who developed urticaria and asthma after horse serum therapy.[82, 127] In 1910, Meltzer[89] made the connection between asthma and a hypersensitivity state or reaction in the immunologic sense.

Since the early descriptions of asthma, many definitions have been suggested; these have ranged from defining every condition that causes wheezing as asthma to defining asthma as a specific condition caused by specific pathways resulting in a very specific clinical picture. There is consensus that asthma is a condition characterized by paroxysmal symptoms of wheezing, shortness of breath, and cough associated with evidence of airway hyperreactivity and/or reversibility.[3]

RHINITIS

Allergic rhinitis may be defined as inflammation of the nasal mucous membrane that is characterized by periods of nasal discharge, sneezing, and congestion, which involves an IgE mechanism. In the 6th century, Rhazes' dissertation on the cause of the coryza that occurs in the spring when the "roses give forth their scent" gave the first known description of hay fever. In 1819, Bostock described a syndrome from which he suffered that he termed hay fever.[81, 82, 127] The identification of pollen as a cause of this disease was reported by Wyman,[150] who also noted a family predisposition. Blackley performed a systematic study to evaluate causative agents of hay fever and asthma, stressing the importance of pollen.[13, 81] Wolff-Eisner[148] demonstrated the connection between allergic rhinitis and the immune system in 1906.

ANAPHYLAXIS

Anaphylaxis is considered an IgE-mediated, allergen-induced reaction in animals characterized by systemic manifestations involving various tissues of the body, including the cardiovascular and gastrointestinal systems, as well as the respiratory tract and skin.[113] The death of Menes (2641 B.C.) was reported to have resulted from an anaphylactic reaction to venom. Animal models of what we now call anaphylaxis were described by Magendi in 1839, followed by Flexner and Smith.[82, 127] The classic description of anaphylaxis was reported by Portier and Richet in 1902.[103] Clinical reports of anaphylaxis were initially ascribed to horse serum used for administration of diphtheria and tetanus antitoxins. In the early 20th century, Rosenau and Anderson[113] reported cases of anaphylaxis after horse serum, which at times led to death.[81] Subsequently, many foreign materials, especially drugs and stinging insects, have been reported to cause anaphylaxis.[84]

URTICARIA AND ANGIOEDEMA

Urticaria is defined as a cutaneous elevation that typically appears as a wheal with erythema and that blanches with pressure. It is frequently associated with itching. Angioedema is thought to involve a similar process but involves the deep dermal and subcutaneous tissue. Hippocratic writings reported urticaria from mosquito bites and from gastrointestinal disturbances. Sydenham in 1685 described urticaria as similar to the stinging of nettles. Quincke[106] was credited to have given the first description of angioedema in 1882, although Bray states that Stolpertus first described it in 1778.[67] Urticaria and angioedema are conditions resulting from a multitude of mechanisms, with allergy being only one of many factors that may be involved.

ECZEMA/ATOPIC DERMATITIS

There has been controversy about the proper definition of eczema or atopic dermatitis. The term eczema comes from a Greek root meaning to bubble, boil, or burst forth. Eczema, although described since ancient times, has never been satisfactorily defined clinically.[102, 137] Atopic dermatitis has been defined as a chronic, heritable, especially pruritic form of eczema (dermatitis) that possesses distinctive features with respect to localization of the lesion and is frequently associated with asthma and allergic rhinitis.[59, 60, 137] In addition, most, but not all, atopic dermatitis patients have elevated IgE levels. A variety of clinical manifestations of atopic dermatitis can be seen in infants, teens, and adults. Hanifin and Rajka[60] published diagnostic features of atopic dermatitis that have been useful to investigators as well as practitioners. Seymour and colleagues[122] further defined atopic dermatitis in children below the age of 5, especially in infants.

Through the years, allergic conditions, such as asthma, hay fever, atopic dermatitis, and anaphylaxis, have been difficult to define. There is general agreement that there is no agreement on many of these definitions. It has not been shown whether many of these conditions called allergy, such as asthma, atopy, and eczema, are a single disease involving a common pathway regulated by particular genes, a group of similar-appearing diseases involving common pathways regulated by a variety of genes, or groups of conditions with similar clinical pictures that are a result of a variety of different mechanisms regulated by a variety of genes. We do not know whether asthma involves one phenotype or multiple phenotypes. The study of the epidemiology of these conditions (including genetic and environmental factors) using working definitions, as well as the more objective measurements, should resolve these questions.

FREQUENCY, INCIDENCE, PREVALENCE, RISK FACTORS, AND TRENDS

The frequency, incidence, and prevalence of allergy and asthma are difficult to investigate in view of the problems of definition and the influence of multiple variables, such as age, sex, and environmental factors (including pollution, smoke, allergen exposure, and infections) on the ultimate clinical picture or phenotype. Despite these problems, researchers have studied allergy and specific allergy-related conditions, such as asthma, rhinitis, urticaria/angioedema, anaphylaxis, and atopic dermatitis, as well as components involved in these conditions, such as total serum IgE, specific IgE as measured by skin testing, or serum-specific IgE assays, and measures of bronchial hyperactivity. The majority of the epidemiologic studies of allergy and specific allergy-related conditions have been performed using questionnaires without many objective measures of the biology specific for the disease process under study. Frequency refers to how common the disease or condition under study occurs in a population. The incidence of a disease is the rate at which new cases occur in a given population. The prevalence of a disease refers to the number of cases of a condition per unit of population at one point in time. The prevalence rate will depend on the definition, incidence, and duration of the condition under study, as well as the population surveyed.

ALLERGY/ATOPY

It has been mentioned that allergies occur in approximately one of every six Americans. Of these, 41% are due to hay fever, 25% to asthma, and the remainder to other allergies, such as atopic dermatitis, urticaria, angioedema, and food reactions.[27] These figures, however, are based on little well-defined data. The perception of allergies may be greater than their actual occurrence.

ASTHMA

Although most individuals believe that they can easily recognize asthma, the exact definition used for studies has been difficult to determine. Most investigations have been based on questionnaire data stressing symptoms and physicians' diagnoses. The majority of investigations do not have the advantage of definitions using pulmonary function or other more objective data.

Of the few studies of the actual incidence of asthma, it appears that asthma varies with age. The incidence of asthma has been estimated to be between 2 and 5 people per 1,000 each year for all age groups, with the highest incidence among children under the age of 5 years.[25, 145]

The prevalence rates reported vary. Geographic location appears to play a role. The prevalence rates range in the world literature between 0.2% and 25%, depending on definition, methodology, and geographic location.[27, 48, 49] Using the American Thoracic Society's definition, the prevalence rates have ranged from 3% to 10.5% in the United States.[145] Most studies during childhood demonstrated that the prevalence rate for asthma is higher in boys than in girls.

There has been a lack of longitudinal prospective investigations regarding asthma. These types of studies are needed to understand the natural history of asthma. Although all age groups have been noted to have asthma, investigators have divided asthma into two major groups: those beginning during childhood and those beginning in adulthood. Childhood asthma has been suggested to be associated with atopy, whereas this association is less common in adults. Several studies have evaluated wheezing in infants and its association with viral infections.[27, 32, 48, 49, 145] It appears that such infants with acute viral respiratory infections are liable to continue to wheeze for a few more years and have some bronchial reactivity. Long-term cohort studies suggest that childhood asthma often remits for several years and then recurs later. The prevalence of active asthma is highest during childhood. Settipane and colleagues,[120] however, reported on a group of college-age students who were followed over a period of time and found that the frequency of asthma and allergic rhinitis increased as the individuals became older. In their study, allergic rhinitis and positive allergy skin tests are significant risk factors for developing new asthma.[120]

There are few data on trends in incidence. One study indicated that the annual age- and sex-adjusted incidence of definite plus probable asthma increased from 1.8 to 2.8 per 1,000 people over a 20-year period.[152] This was found only in children 1 to 14 years of age. Asthma prevalence appears to be increasing in the United States, Sweden, Finland, and Australia, with rates of increase ranging from 3.2 to 4.3 per 100 in the United States to .29 to 1.79 per 100 in Finland.[27, 48, 49, 145] In addition, mortality and morbidity from this condition are also increasing, as measured by ambulatory care visits, hospitalization, and mortality rates.[48, 49, 145]

RHINITIS

Prevalence rates for allergic rhinitis vary from country to country.[48, 125] Studies in the United States tend to show the highest rates, with a range of 3% to 19% and there is some evidence that the prevalence of allergic rhinitis has increased.[25] Most patients with allergic rhinitis develop their symptoms prior to the age of 20. The peak incidence is seen in adolescents aged 10 to 15 years, and the incidence declines with increasing age. An additional 20% of children and young adults complain of chronic rhinitis that is not considered to be allergic. There appears to be no difference in the sex distribution for allergic rhinitis. The great majority of nasal polyps occur after the age of 40, and nasal polyps are rare under the age of 10. Few studies have been performed regarding the incidence of allergic rhinitis. A study by Broder and colleagues[25] reported that the incidence rate for allergic rhinitis ranged from 2.8 to 7.9 in males and 1.9 to 6.0 in females.

The natural history of allergic rhinitis has not been adequately studied. One study reported that the overall remission rate was 10% per year for males and 5% per year for females.

URTICARIA AND ANGIOEDEMA

The relative frequency, prevalence, and incidence of the different types of urticaria and angioedema in the general population is unknown and depends on the definitions and sampling population.[101, 117] In general, urticaria has been reported to have a cumulative prevalence rate between 0.05% and 35%. Reports of frequency have ranged from 0.05% in the Faroe Island population study to 16.3% in children and 35% in adults in a physician's office setting. Newer studies report prevalence rates in the general population between 1% and 5%. These rates vary greatly depending on the definition, geographic location, and type of urticaria. Current concepts of pathogenesis indicate a need to separate acute urticaria due to allergen exposure (foods, drugs, insect bites or stings) from physically induced hives, chronic urticaria (possibly autoimmune), and other types.[67]

ATOPIC DERMATITIS

The reported frequency rates of atopic dermatitis have varied from less than 1.4% to over 20%.[48, 72] Studies in general from Finland, the United States, and Sweden revealed prevalence rates between 1.4% and 3%. The prevalence varies with age and is highest among children under the age of 5 and low in adults, with an estimated prevalence of 0.7%.

Atopic dermatitis usually begins during infancy and early childhood, becoming much less frequent after the age of 20.[108] The majority of cases occur in infants age 6 months or younger. There is recovery in 5 years following the start of the affliction in 90% of cases. Only 5% to 10% of cases persist to adulthood. From 10% to 20% of individuals with atopic dermatitis have been reported to develop asthma, and presumably a higher percentage develop allergic rhinoconjunctivitis later in life.[72]

The estimated frequency measured as the cumulative incidence rate has increased throughout the last decades in the industrialized world. At least 10% to 12% of children are expected to suffer from atopic dermatitis. In one survey, the prevalence in the United States was estimated to be between 7% and 24%. Females outnumber males in the order of 1.4 to 1.0.[72] Another study reports that the cumulative incidence rate (up to 7 years) of atopic dermatitis increased significantly from 0.06 for the birth cohort 1965–1969 to 0.12 for the birth cohort 1975–1979.[133] It appears that the frequency of atopic dermatitis is still increasing, suggesting that environmental factors are operating in genetically susceptible persons.

ANAPHYLAXIS

Data on the overall incidence or prevalence of anaphylaxis, or attempts to ascertain the risk of anaphylaxis to a given antigen, are generally unavailable. Orange and Donsky[98] estimated the rate of fatal anaphylaxis from any cause to be 0.4 cases per million people per year in Ontario. Rates of 0.002% of fatal anaphylaxis to penicillin and 0.00002% caused by Hymenoptera stings have been reported.[96, 144] The risk of nonfatal anaphylaxis is more difficult to determine. It has been estimated to range from 0.7% to 10% for penicillin. Anaphylaxis to the stinging insects of the order Hymenoptera has been estimated to occur in 0.4% of the population.

SKIN TEST REACTIVITY

Skin test reactivity depends on the allergen used, its concentration, the method of administration, the definition of a significant reaction, and recording of the results. Significant skin reactivity has been reported in asymptomatic populations to be as high as 45%.[10, 26, 145] In the United States, the rate of any positive skin test in the general population was reported to be 20.2%.[145] There is some evidence that the prevalence of positive skin tests may be increasing.[11] Cross-sectional studies show that the prevalence of positive skin tests reaches a peak in young adult life, followed by a decline that is gradual at first and then more steep. Although a few studies have suggested that these reactions are predictive of later manifestations of clinical atopic disease, it has not been well established.[120] Some investigations suggest that certain atopic conditions, such as asthma, are particularly associated with sensitivities to certain allergens, such as mites.[11]

SERUM IgE LEVELS

Elevated serum IgE levels are found in many conditions in addition to atopic allergies, such as asthma and allergic rhinitis.[151] Mean serum IgE levels in nonatopic people are reported to be 14 to 22 IU/ml, compared with 60 to 107 IU/ml in the atopic population. There is a great deal of overlap in serum IgE levels between atopic and nonatopic populations; 60% of atopic people fall in the range of 30 to 100 IU/ml, and 30% of nonatopic people fall in this range. Values less than 20 IU/ml or greater than 200 IU/ml occur in less than 5% of atopic and nonatopic populations, respectively. Serum IgE levels are elevated in individuals with atopic dermatitis. A number of nonatopic diseases are also associated with increased IgE levels, such as immunodeficiencies, neoplastic diseases, and parasitic and viral infections. It appears that serum IgE levels peak in early adulthood and decrease after the age of 40 to 50.[6, 128]

BRONCHIAL HYPERREACTIVITY

Whereas asthmatics usually express abnormal bronchial provocation responses to nonspecific challenges (histamine, methacholine), so do a significant proportion of subjects with allergic rhinitis and even normal individuals. It has been suggested that airway hyperreactivity is a prerequisite to asthma. In general, the prevalence of bronchial hyperreactivity is twofold to threefold higher than the prevalence of asthma. A prevalence of increased bronchial responsiveness between 11% and 29.9% has been reported in random populations studied. From 20% to 50% of subjects with increased airway responsiveness have no symptoms. Nonasthmatic, nonatopic individuals with family histories of asthma were found to have bronchial hyperreactivity more often than were nonasthmatic individuals from nonatopic families. It is apparent that increased bronchial responsiveness and asthma are not the same.[14, 147]

Clifford and colleagues[31] have shown that there is a significant association between atopy and bronchial hyperreactivity to methacholine, independent of symptoms.[31] The prevalence of asthma and bronchial hyperreactivity is higher in atopic subjects than in nonatopics.[14] Reactivity to methacholine has also been reported to occur in 30% of individuals with allergic rhinitis. Bronchial reactivity appears to be less associated with allergy after 65 than in the younger subject. An association between serum IgE levels and bronchial hyperreactivity has been reported.[104] However, the importance of allergen exposure as a cause of bronchial reactivity is controversial. It is suggested that the major role of pollen or dust mite allergen in asthma is that it may be a cause of bronchial reactivity, as well as a triggering factor for an acute attack. Normal subjects will have increases in airway reactivity after certain viral infections and exposure to cigarette smoke.[147]

GENETICS OF ALLERGY AND ASTHMA

Early anecdotal and the more systematic studies of Cooke and VanderVeer[39] and others in the first half of the 20th century indicated a familial if not genetic basis of asthma and allergies. However, progress in our understanding in this area has been hampered by many problems, such as inadequate knowledge of the biology of asthma, definition of the phenotype, parameters to be measured, study design, selection of subjects, and methods of statistical analysis. Developing an understanding of asthma and allergy has been difficult; it is impossible to fully understand their biology without identifying the genes involved, and it is impossible to identify the genes without detailed knowledge of the biology.

Advances in several fields are making it possible to begin understanding the genetics of complex diseases, such as asthma and allergies.[38, 42, 44] A better definition of the pathogenesis of atopic conditions is allowing us to characterize their phenotype. Determination of the role of IgE antibody, T cells, and cytokines in particular disorders has been critical. Other advances have been those made in molecular genetics, such as the discovery of recombinant DNA, the cloning of DNA fragments, the demonstration that DNA fragments could be separated by electrophoresis, and the development of the polymerase chain reaction, which allows the rapid amplification of short regions of DNA with great ease. Statistical methods have improved, permitting the analysis of the genetics of complex diseases such as allergy. Studies to define the genetics of asthma can be performed using such methods as associations and disequilibrium studies, determinations of heritability and risk to relatives, segregation analysis, and linkage analysis and mapping.

TOOLS FOR INVESTIGATING THE GENETICS OF ASTHMA AND ALLERGIES

The understanding of the genetics of complex diseases, such as asthma and allergies, involves the determination of their heritability, their mode of inheritance, and the characteristics of the genes involved. To do this, one has to know everything about the gene: its chromosomal location, its DNA sequence, how its expression is controlled, and what its product does. For a given disease, there are several routes to characterizing the genes involved. The main routes used are forward genetics and reverse or positional genetics, and the candidate gene approach.[38, 42, 44]

Forward Genetics

Forward genetics has been one of the initial methods to study the genetics of human disease. Examples of forward genetics are the studies of hemoglobinopathies and inborn errors of metabolism, in which the defective gene has been identified and characterized. For asthma, studies of the transcriptional control of airway inflammation may provide the necessary information to evaluate its forward genetics. The genes of the cell adhesion molecules and, in turn, the gene products that control them are candidates for abnormal expression in inflammation. If the defective factor is known, forward genetics can be performed by first identifying the DNA and then the gene sequence and ultimately its location.

Reverse or Positional Genetics

Positional genetics is a method used for many diseases, such as asthma and allergies, where the underlying defect is not known. Identification of any single gene of unknown function is a complex problem. The human genome comprises approximately 3×10^9 base pairs; thus any specific gene represents only a very small fraction of the total DNA. The first step is to identify the gene location. We are therefore mapping the chromosomal location of the gene and cloning the gene knowing nothing else about it except for its location. Once this is done, we can then determine the gene sequence, its DNA structure, and ultimately the gene product that results in the production of the disease. This has been called positional or reverse genetics.

Candidate Gene Approach

Another approach is that of the candidate gene. Using this method, one identifies a gene or group of genes that appear to be important in the development of the phenotype under study. An example would be the phenotype for IgE, which appears to be influenced by several genes already identified, such as IL-4, IL-5, and IL-9. Therefore, studies are set up to evaluate the relationships between these candidate genes, which are on chromosome 5, to IgE levels.

Positional genetics and the candidate gene approach are being used for the study of complex diseases, such as asthma and allergies, which are multifactorial in origin and appear to be genetically heterogeneous. Using molecular biologic methods, we are now able to define the basis of these diseases. We will be able not only to obtain information that will give us a blueprint for the causation of these disorders but also to have substances available that will allow us to treat the disease once it develops and potentially to correct the errant DNA that causes it. Using these new methodologies, many genetic studies have been undertaken, making many claims and there have been counterclaims but few triumphs.

RATIONALE FOR ASTHMA AND ALLERGY GENETIC STUDIES

Asthma and allergies are good models for studying the genetics of complex diseases because they are caused by the interaction of genetic and environmental factors, they are common conditions, the clinical picture has been well defined, the causative allergen can usually be identified and characterized, the immune response (such as an IgE response) can be defined, and a suggested pathogenesis is available to use as a model.[1, 15, 130]

Model for Asthma and Allergy

Multiple cell types and numerous cellular control mechanisms influence the development of the clinical picture of asthma and allergies and their response to treatment. Our hypothesis is that asthma and allergies are genetically determined diseases in which the underlying pathophysiology is caused by a chronic inflammatory process that is driven by cytokines derived from activated CD4$^+$ T cells. T lymphocytes are thought to play an essential role in the pathogenesis of allergies by migrating into the tissue involved, becoming activated, and releasing cytokines, which results in the recruitment and activation of a variety of cells, resulting in an inflammatory process. An important step in the development of this inflammatory process is the passage of inflammatory cells from the blood vessels into the tissue involved. Adhesion molecules play a key role in this process. According to current understanding, the following model is being used for the investigation of the epidemiology of asthma and allergy.

SENSITIZATION

Exposure to the allergen (antigen) occurs, which is then taken up by an antigen-presenting cell (APC), such as a dendritic or B cell. Through intracellular processing, the allergen (antigen) will be broken down into a specific peptide, which becomes associated with a class II major histocompatibility complex (MHC) molecule selected from an MHC library. The allergen (antigen) peptide–MHC complex then moves to the surface of the APC complex, where it can interact with a subset of T cells designated CD4$^+$ cells, which have T-cell receptors (TCR) specific for the class II peptide complex chosen from a TCR library. These CD4$^+$ cells may differentiate into either cells called T helper (Th) 1, which produce largely the cytokine interferon-γ, or cells called Th2, which produce mainly IL-4 and a set of associated molecules as the main cytokines.

IL-4 appears to be necessary for IgE production and is important in all forms of antibody production. Interferon-γ is a principal regulator of cellular immunity and is associated with a decrease in IgE production. In atopic individuals, there appears to be the preferential development of a disproportionate number of Th2 as opposed to Th1 cells that interact with the allergen (antigen). B-cell clones possessing surface immunoglobulin react with the specific allergen, make contact with the CD4$^+$ cells, and are stimulated by locally produced cytokines derived from these cells as well as the APC. This complex interaction results in signals for the B cells to differentiate and produce antigen-specific antibodies whose Ig has been chosen from a V(h) library based on its ability to bind the allergen (antigen). This step may result in B cells maturing to plasma cells. In the allergen-specific response, isotope switching occurs, followed by the production of allergen-specific IgE. After the specific IgE is formed, it will interact with a cell containing an IgE receptor.

REEXPOSURE

Upon reexposure, the allergen (antigen) will interact with allergen-specific IgE on the surfaces of cells, which will initiate the release of inflammatory mediators. These mediators will act on the end organ, whose response will result in the acute symptoms. Stimuli for cell priming, up-regulation of endothelial cell adhesion molecules, and release of chemotactic substances lead to the late-phase inflammatory reaction, which results in the persistence of symptoms.

It is evident that each of these activities must be coordinated to produce asthma and allergy. In addition, there are a multitude of steps in which the process can be enhanced or attenuated. Many of these steps are under genetic control and involve environmental interactions. By studying this proposed mechanism, we should be able to further define the biology of asthma and allergies and develop an understanding of the genetics involved. This will enable us to approach the management of these conditions in a more rational manner.

GENETIC STUDIES OF ASTHMA, ALLERGIES, AND RELATED CONDITIONS

Evidence of a hereditary factor in the development of asthma and allergies has been suggested in early reports.[15, 18, 104] The definition of the phenotype to be studied has proved to be difficult. Researchers have attempted to define phenotypes clinically, biochemically, and genetically. In view of the problem of pleiotropism (multiple effects of a single mutant gene) and genetic heterogeneity, investigators studying the genetics of asthma have tended to belong in two traditional groups: lumpers and splitters. Initially, the lumpers were common. Complex phenotypes were used to study the genetics of asthma and allergies. Because of this complexity and lack of agreement regarding the definition of the complex phenotypes, many investigators became splitters and used the less complex asthma-associated or intermediate phenotypes (the specific immune response, IgE regulators, and mediator release, as well as end organ response), based on the hypothesis of how asthma develops, to study this condition.

INTERMEDIATE ASTHMA AND ALLERGY-ASSOCIATED PHENOTYPES

Specific Immune Response

The overall mechanism of the specific immune response has been studied and defined.[1, 15, 87, 130] Adequate studies involve using an allergen that is well defined with regard to size, structure, sequence, epitopes, and binding capacity to T- and B-cell sites. The smaller the allergen and the fewer the epitopes, the better it is to study. Ragweed has been used as one of the models to study the immune response in atopic conditions. It contains at least 55 allergens, of which approximately 22 have been reported to be important clinically and to bind to IgE. *Amb a* I is one of the major purified allergens of short ragweed, with a molecular weight of 35,000. *Amb a* V, the smallest ragweed allergen identified, has been used to characterize the specific immune response. It has a molecular weight of 4500 and has been sequenced and shown to have 45 amino acids. Its structure is known.

At least three epitopes have been identified that bind to immunoglobulins. The binding affinity or association constant (K_{ass}) for *Amb a* V IgE antibodies range from 0.9×10^{-10} M to 26×10^{-10} M, compared with 1×10^{-7} M for anti–*Amb a* V IgG. It has also been demonstrated that in the same individual, different epitopes can bind to different immunoglobulin groups; that is, the epitope for binding IgE may be different from that for IgG in the same individual.[68] Using the ragweed system, early studies by Levine and colleagues demonstrated that the response to *Amb a* I was associated with the HLA system.[74] Work in our laboratory showed that *Amb a* I was linked with the class II molecules of the HLA system.[17] Because of its large size and multiple epitopes, *Amb a* V was then studied. It has been noted to be strongly associated with HLA DR2 *1500.[20, 43, 85–87] The β chain of the HLA restriction element appears to be needed for presentation to T cells.[153] It also has been shown that each *Amb a* V from short, giant, and false ragweed was associated with HLA DR2, although they were immunologically different.[85] When the deduced amino acid sequences of the respective class II β and α polypeptides were compared in *Amb a* V–sensitive and *Amb a* V–nonsensitive DR2-positive individuals by Zwollo and colleagues[153] and our own laboratory, no differences were noted. This suggests that *Amb a* V responders have no unique sequences within the HLA DR2 loci.

An increasing number of purified allergens are being found to be associated with HLA class II molecules.[85] These include those of olive (*Ole* 1), giant ragweed (*Amb t* V), and rye grass (*Lol p* I).[86] There is growing evidence that the specific immune response is on chromosome 6 associated with the HLA system, specifically the DR region. The presence of a particular DR-associated class II molecule appears to provide a necessary, but not the only, condition for responsiveness to a particular epitope.

A subsequent step in the immune response involves the interaction of the HLA class II allergen complex of the APC with the TCR. The arrangement of TCR-binding domains for allergen (hypervariable regions) on the α and β chains appears to determine the antigen specificity of the T cell. Renz and colleagues[110] demonstrated in mice that specific Vβ-expressing T-cell subpopulations are involved in the stimulation of IgE/IgG1 production and increased airway responsiveness. In humans, a genetic linkage of the TCR α/δ complex to the specific IgE responses has been suggested by Moffatt and colleagues.[91] Their study suggests that chromosome 14 may be important in the specific atopic response.

IgE Regulation

IgE regulation is another phenotype investigated genetically. It appears that the up-regulation of IgE synthesis in atopy is due to the induction of IgE isotype utilization at the DNA level in B cells. IgE synthesis appears to involve signals following direct T cell–B cell interaction. One is delivered by an IgE-promoting cytokine provided by the activated CD4 T cell, that is, Th2 cell-derived IL-4. Others are the cognate signals delivered by $CD4^+$ T cells. These involve TCR, CD4 and class II MHC molecules, CD40 and CD40 ligand, and CD23. IgE synthesis appears to be down-regulated by certain cytokines (e.g., interferon-γ, interferon-α).[130]

Concordance rates in monozygotic twins have been reported to be from 0.36 to 0.88, compared with 0.16 to 0.63 in dizygotic twins. Heritability between 50% and 60% has been reported in families.[19, 61]

In general, serum IgE level heritability has been demonstrated in twins, families, and population studies. A major gene appears to be involved. The mode of inheritance and location of the gene have not been well delineated. Dominant, codominant, and recessive models have all been suggested.[19, 21, 56, 61]

Evidence that suggests that one of the genes involved in the synthesis of IgE regulation is located on 5q 31.1 has been presented in studies by Marsh and colleagues[88] and Meyers and colleagues.[90] Marsh and colleagues suggest that the locus is at the IL-4 gene locus, whereas Meyers' best evidence for linkage was not found to be at the IL-4 locus but in a nearby region. Work performed in our laboratories could not confirm these findings.[22] No HLA associations with serum IgE levels have been adequately demonstrated.

Receptors

The genetics of the IgE receptors has been studied. High-affinity receptors on basophils and mast cells and low-affinity receptors on eosinophils and lymphocytes have been identified and characterized. Sandford and colleagues[116] and Shirakawa and colleagues[123] from the same group reported that the gene regulating the β chain of the high-affinity receptor for IgE (FcεRIβ) is on chromosome 11q. A variant of the receptor (Leu181) was observed that segregated with atopy when maternally inherited. Further polymorphisms of FcεRIβ are being found by these investigators. These findings have not been confirmed by other groups.

Allergen/IgE/Receptor Interaction and Mediator Release

The genetic control of the release of mediators or cytokines subsequent to allergen interaction with cell-bound IgE has not been extensively examined. A variety of mast cell mediators have been investigated, including secretory granule preformed mediators (histamine, heparin, tryptase), cytokines (IL-4, IL-5, IL-6), and lipid mediators (leukotriene B4, leukotriene C4, prostaglandin D2). The phenotype of histamine release following the anti-IgE challenge of peripheral blood basophils has been noted to have heritability in a twin study by Marone and colleagues[83] and a nuclear family study by Roitman-Johnson and colleagues.[112]

End Organ Response

The pathogenesis of bronchial hyperreactivity is complex and not fully understood.[14, 34] Two abnormalities have been reported to be found in asthma: hypersensitivity to stimuli, such as histamine or methacholine, and an increase in maximal airway narrowing. There is evidence that the two abnormalities are controlled by partly independent mechanisms. It appears that many steps are needed to develop airway hyperresponsiveness in asthma. These steps include the agonist-receptor interactions leading to smooth muscle activation; shortening of muscle; and luminal narrowing further dependent on submucosal swelling due to inflammation, intraluminal secretions, and geometric factors related to airway caliber. Each of these steps may be under separate control and probably are influenced by genetic factors. As a result, bronchial hyperreactivity has been poorly defined genetically. Many population studies show a unimodal distribution of responsiveness with a great deal of overlap between asthmatic and nonasthmatic individuals. Familial factors have been reported to be involved in the development of bronchial hyperresponsiveness, defined principally as the bronchial response to methacholine and histamine inhalation challenge. Although many studies have provided evidence of heritability of bronchial hyperreactivity, there is distinct heterogeneity.[14, 64] A study by Postma and colleagues[104] reported that regions of 5q31–33 are important in the regulation of bronchial hyperreactivity in asthma.

Studies of the genetic polymorphism of the β2-adrenergic receptors have shown no evidence of a genetic defect of these receptors in asthma.[5, 109] These investigators did find that mutations of the β-adrenergic receptor may act to modulate the severity of symptoms. For example, an arginine-16 mutant receptor significantly increased the degree of agonist-promoted down-regulation of receptor expression and was seen more often in subjects who had severe asthma, as well as those with nocturnal asthma.

Inflammation

The mechanisms involved in the inflammatory response in asthma and its genetics are just being studied. New factors influencing inflammation, such as cytokines, chemokines, and cell adhesion molecules, as well as other mediators of the inflammatory response (e.g., heat shock proteins), have been identified, characterized, and localized to specific chromosomal regions. The activation of transcription factors, as well as the role of TGF-β; growth factors such as EGF, ICAM's, CD-23 (low-affinity IgE receptor), HLA DR, IL-1, and TNF-α; and Th2-associated cytokines such as IL-4, IL-5, and IL-10 are a few of the many areas that may be involved in the development of asthma that are being studied.[73]

SUMMARY

It appears that the development of asthma and allergy-associated phenotypes is complex and involves many different processes influenced by genetic factors. The specific immune response to certain aeroallergens is genetically influenced by genes located on chromosome 6 at the DR loci. The TCR may play a role in the specific IgE response. One report relates it to be on chromosome 14. IgE regulation is heritable and probably due to a major gene; its mode of inheritance and the characterization of the genes involved are under intense study, especially on chromosome 5q. The FcεRIβ chain has been suggested in one study to be under genetic control due to a gene on chromosome 11q and related to the development of atopy. Histamine release and bronchial hyperreactivity appear to have heritability, but whether there is a major gene for each and the location of that gene are not well established. One study has noted that the gene for bronchial hyperreactivity is on chromosome 5q near the gene suggested to be responsible for IgE levels. Phenotypes of the inflammatory processes in asthma are currently being studied.

COMPLEX PHENOTYPES

Investigators emphasized the familial nature of the complex phenotypes of asthma and atopic diseases and provided evidence of a genetic predisposition. The first serious modern study of the heritability of asthma and hay fever was undertaken by Cooke and VanderVeer in 1916.[39] As many as 40% to 80% of patients with allergic rhinitis or bronchial asthma have been noted to have a positive family history of allergy, as opposed to 20% or less of the nonallergic subjects. There is strong evidence that there is heritability of asthma and allergic rhinitis. Heritability has been reported in the range of 0.5% to 1.0%. Studies also suggest that the incidence of allergic disease in children roughly doubles with each parent who is allergic or has asthma. The problems of definition of phenotypes as well as the methodology in these early studies are apparent. Investigators have been attempting to study the complex phenotypes of diseases, such as atopy and asthma, using updated parameters and more sophisticated molecular genetic and statistical approaches.[19]

Atopy

A variety of different parameters, including those of IgE responses, have been used to define atopy. Cookson and colleagues[40] studied the genetics of atopy, which was defined as an elevated serum IgE level and/or an elevated specific IgE as measured by a radioallergosorbent or skin test. Using this definition, they suggested that atopy is inherited as an autosomal dominant trait and linked to chromosome 11q. Similar linkage was noted by Collee and colleagues,[36] Shirakawa and colleagues,[124] and Hizawa and colleagues.[62] Rich and colleagues[111] investigated the same complex phenotype of atopy with respect to its genetics and environmental determinants. Using the phenotype of Cookson and colleagues, as well as several other phenotypes, no evidence for linkage was found in three large pedigrees using the dominant mode of inheritance. Lympany and colleagues,[78, 79] Hizawa and colleagues,[63] Brereton and colleagues,[24] and Amelung and colleagues[2] also could not confirm Cookson and colleagues' observations. Cookson and colleagues[41] suggested that the 11q13-linked atopy gene is inherited preferentially from the maternal side, possibly due to either paternal genetic imprinting or maternal modification of the infants' IgE responses through the placenta or breast milk. These studies have not been confirmed by other groups. Association of atopy with genes regulating immunoglobulins has been suggested.[50, 142]

Asthma

The complex phenotypes of asthma have been investigated with regard to their genetics and relationship to known genetic markers. One of the major problems of studying asthma in this manner is determining the definition of the phenotype used. Most phenotypes of asthma have consisted of symptoms such as coughing, wheezing, and shortness of breath, as well as evidence of bronchial hyperreactivity as demonstrated by reversibility and/or a bronchial challenge with an agent such as histamine or methacholine. Others have suggested using IgE responsiveness as a parameter. Asthma has been defined by Morton[94] as a disorder characterized by wheezing and bronchial hyperresponsiveness, for which atopy is the major cause. Atopy is defined as a condition characterized by a heritable and persistent IgE response to protein allergens. Using these definitions, the two traits are correlated and multivariate, including total and specific IgE titer, skin prick tests, medical history, and tests of bronchial reactivity. Burrows and colleagues[28] and Sears and colleagues[121] have stressed the relationship between IgE levels and asthma, whether the latter is defined as atopic or idiopathic (intrinsic). They have presented evidence that there may be a major gene for asthma that is different from the gene for IgE.

Epidemiologic studies of asthma suggest that many factors, both genetic and environmental, are involved with the development of asthma.[11, 49] Asthma clusters in families. Although this is suggestive of a genetic basis of asthma, it is not proof, as common environmental factors, as well as a high prevalence of asthma, could possibly account for this familial aggregation. The presence of atopy, exposure to smoke, pollution, home dampness and molds, poverty, viral infections, prematurity with low birth weight, and exposure to cats, dogs, and mites during childhood are a few of the many factors that have been reported to be associated with the development of asthma. It appears that the ultimate clinical picture of asthma is due to a multitude of risk factors, both genetic and nongenetic.

The relative risk for asthma, defined as the prevalence of asthma in the first-degree relatives of an affected individual (proband) divided by the prevalence in the general population, has been estimated to be between 3 and 6. Twin studies demonstrate a concordance rate for asthma in monozygotic twins between 12% and 89% and between 4.8% and 33% in dizygotic twins. Heritability in twins ranges between 36% and 72%. Family studies also suggest heritability. Although it appears that asthma has heritability, its mode of inheritance and characterization of the genes involved are not yet known.[19, 49, 55]

Investigation of markers on the C6 chromosome has yielded conflicting results regarding the location of the gene regulating asthma.[45, 46] An increase in HLA B8 associated with asthma was reported by Thorsby and associates,[134] Morris,[92] and Turner.[135] On the other hand, Rachelefsky and colleagues[107] found an increase in HLA A2 but a decrease in HLA B8 in patients with bronchial asthma. No changes in the B8 frequencies in asthma could be found by Geerts and associates.[53] These studies stress the importance of having a well-defined phenotype. In view of the problems of defining asthma, investigators directed their attention to phenotypes involving known triggers of asthma.

The phenotype of mite-sensitive allergic asthma has been investigated in relationship to HLA antigens. HLA segregation was studied in 20 families with allergic asthma and *Dermatophagoides farinae* sensitivity and 8 families with intrinsic or nonallergic asthma by Caraballo and Hernandez.[29] Genetic analysis using the affected sib pair method suggests the existence of an HLA-linked recessive gene controlling the IgE immune responsiveness to mite allergens and conferring susceptibility to allergic asthma. Hsieh and colleagues[65] found an association of house dust mite reactivity to HLA-DQw2. Association of other specific triggers, such as aspirin-induced asthma, with the HLA system was reported by Mullarkey and colleagues[95] but was not confirmed in a study by Lympany and colleagues.[77] Responsiveness to isothiocyanates has been reported to be associated with antigens of the HLA system.[8]

Extended HLA haplotypes, which include group I, II, and III (complotype) antigens, have been associated with the general expression of certain diseases. Different extended haplotypes may contain different patterns of chromosomal deletions and insertions, some of which may influence the level of gene expression. Therefore, certain combinations of alleles, especially of the D/DR and complement loci, are highly associated with particular diseases. We have studied the association of ragweed allergic rhinitis and bronchial asthma with the extended HLA haplotype.[20] Total serum IgE concentrations and titers of IgE-specific anti–*Amb a* V were measured in 144 patients with ragweed pollen allergy. MHC haplotypes were determined for 50 of these patients and 28 nonatopic controls.

Unimodally distributed total IgE levels were found in all study groups. The levels were higher in the atopic subjects in general compared with the nonatopic subjects. Although anti–*Amb a* V IgE levels were all low in the nonatopic subjects, a group within the atopic subjects had high levels of IgE *Amb a* V. Those with asthma had distinctly higher levels than those with rhinitis only or the nonatopic population. The frequencies of HLA-DR2 and the extended MHC haplotype B7, SC31, DR2 were significantly increased among the patients with asthma and high titers of IgE anti-*Amb a* V. Conversely, this group had decreased frequencies of HLA-DR3 and the extended haplotype HLA B8, SC01, DR3 compared with patients with only rhinitis; the latter group had an increased number of individuals with the extended haplotype HLA B8, SC01, DR3 and lower levels of IgE anti–*Amb a* V. These findings are consistent with a dominant MHC-linked gene or genes on HLA B7, SC31, DR2 controlling the IgE immune response to *Amb a* V and predisposing to asthma.

There is evidence that TNF-α may be important in the pathogenesis of asthma.[139] The gene for TNF-α is within the class III region of the MHC on chromosome 6p, and polymorphism within the class III MHC may be associated with asthma.[93]

Other genetic markers have also been studied in relationship with asthma. Because chromosome 5q contains many genes implicated in allergic inflammation, the candidate gene approach has been used to study the relationship of asthma to loci on 5q. Investigations by Postma and colleagues[104] suggest that the region of 5q31–33 is important in the regulation of bronchial hyperreactivity. Rosenwasser and colleagues[114] suggest that a polymorphism within the IL-4 promoter may be associated with biologic alterations in asthma.

Several studies have suggested that gene variants on chromosome 14 for α_1-antitrypsin may be associated with asthma. Children with more severe and steroid-dependent asthma had more Z heterozygotes than did nonsteroid-dependent and less severe asthmatics. Other associations with α-antitrypsin genotypes have also been noted, but there has been a lack of adequate confirmation of these observations.[37, 51, 76, 105] Associations of asthma and bronchial hyperresponsiveness have been reported with heterozygosity for cystic fibrosis on chromosome C7, whereas others suggest that heterozygosity may give protection.[58, 119, 143] Allotypes on C14 (immunoglobulin heavy chain) have been suggested to be associated with asthma.[50, 99] A possible protection against asthma was also suggested to occur in heterozygotes for familial Mediterranean fever.[23]

Allergic Rhinitis/Hay Fever

Allergic rhinitis has been reported to have a hereditary diathesis by many early investigators, including Bostock, Elliotson, Wyman, and Mackenzie, as well as Cooke and VanderVeer.[16, 34, 81, 82] Factors that have been reported to influence the development of allergic rhinitis are family history, birth date, and birth order.[11, 125] Allergic rhinitis has been correlated with a positive family history. In addition, allergic rhinitis in response to allergens is associated with exposure to these allergens during the first year of life. This has been suggested in reports with mite and animal exposures, as well as the allergens in the air at the month of birth. A British study reported that the risk of hay fever at age 23 declined as the number of older siblings in the family increased.[132] Another study suggested that the prevalence of hay fever was higher in the first-born child.[129] Others have not been able to confirm these results. Maternal age at conception, maternal and paternal smoking, birth weight, and breast feeding have all been suggested, but not confirmed, as risk factors. There have been few studies of the genetics of allergic rhinitis using newer methodology. The HLA system has been studied without any definite consistent findings. Kitano and colleagues[69] noted that subjects with *D. farinae* and allergic rhinitis showed a positive association with HLA-DQ3 and a negative association with HLA-A2. HLA-DQB1*0303 was increased in the patients with mite allergy.

Urticaria and Angioedema

A variety of complex cellular and humoral factors are involved in the pathogenesis of urticaria and angioedema. Although many etiologic factors have been suggested, the majority are without a definite known etiology. Risk factors and trends are difficult to determine in view of the heterogeneity of the condition. Several familial if not hereditary syndromes of urticaria and angioedema have been reported. Angioedema was reported in the last part of the 19th century to have a hereditary factor, according to reports by Quincke, Dinkelacher, Valentin, Strubing, and Osler.[16, 67, 97, 136, 149] Hereditary angioedema, probably the best defined of these genetic syndromes, is associated with an autosomal-dominant deficiency of C1 esterase inhibitor activity.[97, 126, 138] The C1 INH gene is located on human chromosome 11 region q11–q13. It is comprised of seven exons and at least seven introns. The C1 INH gene also contains several copies of Alu sequences that are highly repetitive DNA sequences dispersed throughout the human genome.

Two subtypes of HAE have been defined on the basis of apparent protein abnormalities. HAE type I, comprising about 85% of patients with HAE, is characterized by a decreased level of functionally normal C1 INH in plasma. The underlying molecular event is the apparent lack of function of one C1 INH allele in the genome. Genomic sequence analysis indicates partial deletions or insertions within the C1 INH gene. However, a polymorphism is not seen in 80 to 85% of type I HAE patients. In these cases, it is suggested that small mutations are present in regions of the C1 INH gene that are required for either proper transcription or translation. Type II HAE accounts for 15% of the cases of HAE and is characterized by normal or increased levels of C1 INH, but the protein has reduced functional activity. The underlying molecular changes responsible for the functional defects are of two types: mutation within and outside of the reactive site of C1 INH. C1 INH cleavage by C1s or C1r takes place between C1 INH residues Arg and Thr. Thus binding and cleavage of C1 INH by the target proteases require an intact Arg-Thr peptide bond and the proper folding of the C1 INH reactive loop. Point mutations affecting the nucleotides that code for Arg are responsible for about 70% of all cases of type II HAE. Random point mutation of the P1 Arg (CGC) could potentially give rise to six different substitutions. A less well defined syndrome is familial cold urticaria, which is thought to be an autosomal-dominant syndrome.[67] Other defined hereditary syndromes include hereditary vibratory angioedema[67] and urticaria and deafness associated with amyloidosis,[12] both of which appear to be autosomal-dominant conditions.

Eczema/Atopic Dermatitis

Despite the many definitions, there is a family history of allergy in patients with atopic dermatitis; however, 10% of patients without such a history have been reported to have atopic dermatitis.[72, 136] Thus the presence of a family history of atopic dermatitis is a risk factor for atopic dermatitis. Frequent wheezing and abnormal spirometry in childhood and early onset of asthma are associated with poorer outcome of atopic dermatitis. It has been reported that the detection of food allergy in a child presenting with atopic dermatitis is likely to indicate a prognosis of severe atopic dermatitis and also may be a predictor of respiratory symptoms. Other risk factors are contact with house dust mites and air pollution. Genetic factors have been strongly associated with the development of atopic dermatitis. The pairwise concordance rate was 0.72 in monozygotic and 0.23 in dizygotic twin pairs. Children whose parents had atopic dermatitis have a high risk for atopic dermatitis compared with children whose parents had asthma or allergic rhinitis.

Associations between atopic dermatitis and the HLA system have also been reported.[46] Ozawa and colleagues[100] noted that patients with atopic dermatitis, bronchial asthma, and allergic rhinitis had an increase in HLA-B12 and B40, but there was no difference in the HLA antigen frequencies in patients with atopic dermatitis alone. Svejgaard and colleagues[131] noted that the frequency of HLA-DR7 was decreased in patients with atopic dermatitis when uncorrected, but there was no negative association when corrected for multiple variables. Scholz and colleagues[118] noted an association of the HLA system with atopic dermatitis in 19 families studied. Goundemand and colleagues[57] showed an increased BW35 among 27 patients. Saeki and colleagues[115] also found associations with HLA antigens, but none remained significant after p values were corrected. Others have found no associations with the HLA system.[46] Kuwata and colleagues[71] studied the polymorphism of transporter associated with antigen-processing genes in atopic dermatitis. They reported that the gene frequency of TAP1 637Asp exhibited a tendency to increase in the patients with atopic dermatitis. They suggested that this may contribute to the pathogenesis of atopic dermatitis in combination with HLA-DRB1*1302DQ B1*0604. In view of the studies suggesting that atopy was associated with chromosome site 11q13, this region was studied in regard to atopic dermatitis. Coleman and colleagues[35] found no evidence of linkage of atopic dermatitis with markers on 11q13.

Allergic Contact Dermatitis

Allergic contact dermatitis is a result of sensitization to a wide variety of potential contactant materials usually considered to be mediated by a cellular nonatopic mechanism. The immunogens or contactants are simple substances (haptens) that form covalent derivatives with skin proteins. They are taken in by the antigen-presenting cells, where they combine with MHC molecules. These molecules interact with the T cells (primarily $CD4^+$ Th1 cells), which sets in motion the release of mediators, ultimately resulting in contact dermatitis.[7, 52, 70] Contact dermatitis appears to result from common antigens such as poison ivy, metals such as nickel, and cosmetics, as well as medications.[80] Genetic factors are probably involved, as shown in the guinea pig by Chase[30] and Geczy and de Weck.[52] Association between the contact dermatitis and the HLA system has been suggested.[47, 66, 75] There does not appear to be more allergic contact dermatitis in atopic compared with nonatopic populations.

ENVIRONMENTAL FACTORS IN ASTHMA AND ALLERGY

Although the genetic composition of the subject is probably the most important factor determining the development of asthma and allergy, interaction with environmental factors, almost by definition, are needed.[11, 146] Environmental factors play a major role in the development of asthma and allergies; however, the mechanisms involved are still largely unknown. Sensitization to allergens are essential for the development of an allergy. It appears that the age of exposure (allergen exposure in early life), type of allergen (mites, cockroaches, dogs, and cats being associated with asthma), allergen load (low levels more likely than high levels to produce specific IgE production), and month of birth are a few of the environmental factors that influence the expression of the allergy. Infections may also influence the various clinical phenotypes of allergy. Parasitic infections will increase IgE levels, yet there appears to be an inverse relationship between parasitic disease and high IgE levels with asthma and allergies in nonwesternized countries. IgE levels are also elevated at times by viral infections, especially infectious mononucleosis and cytomegalovirus infections. The relationship between rhinovirus and asthma is not clear. Factors such as age, sex, and air pollution, including tobacco smoke, and psychological factors all appear to influence the various phenotypes of allergies and asthma. It is possible that environmental factors may modulate the genetic factors, as well as the resulting clinical picture.

BENEFITS OF EPIDEMIOLOGIC AND GENETIC STUDIES OF ASTHMA AND ALLERGY

Many questions can now be answered as a result of a better understanding of the epidemiology and genetics of asthma and allergies, but this area of investigation is in its infancy. In the future, we will be able to understand their biology and redefine them in terms of their genetic basis. The diagnostic armamentarium will increase greatly. Accurate diagnosis is important and will be enhanced by chromosomal and biochemical methods. Asthma and allergies, as we diagnose them today, are most likely diseases of many different phenotypes based on different genetic mechanisms and pathways.

Risk estimates can be obtained regarding the occurrence of asthma and allergies, as well as their severity, based on the proper characterization of each disease. Ideally, we will be able to predict in advance whether a person may suffer from these conditions, as well as how severe it will be. Although in principle this should occur, much controversy has developed over the benefits of genetic studies. Many do not agree that human beings are constructed from blueprints that we can learn to read. It has been stated that we cannot make predictions, as we do not know enough. This is because development is dialectical and not linear. What happens to a person all along the way, and what that person makes happen, may continuously affect her or his biologic, psychological, and social growth, as well as the development of conditions such as asthma. Although this information provides a benefit, it is not without a cost. The question of a threat to civil liberties has been considered. Will this information be used against the individual? Will it prevent a person from becoming insured? Elmer-Dewitt[54] has stated that "Genetic privacy will be the major constitutional issue of the next generation."

New regimes of management of asthma and allergies can be developed. These may involve prevention, such as gene manipulation, as well as interference with pathways activated by the environmental-genetic interaction. This type of treatment has generated a great deal of discussion. Although most people may be in favor of this approach to treatment, many believe altering human genes and their actions is against the will of God. Many ethical questions will arise. It has been suggested that equating genetic prediction with prevention at this time may not be possible.[9, 54]

Despite arguments against genetic studies, this knowledge is providing needed information to understand asthma and allergies and manage individuals in a rational way using methods of prevention and active treatment. Prevention may involve genetic counseling and ultimately gene therapy, as well as avoidance of known high-risk environmental factors, in individuals at high risk. Identification of the genes, gene products, and pathways involved should allow us to prevent, modulate, or reverse the disease progress. Once individuals have the information, how they wish to deal with it becomes a personal decision.

REFERENCES

1. Abbas A, Lichtman AH, Pober JS: Cellular and Molecular Immunology. WB Saunders, Philadelphia, 1991, pp 186–203.
2. Amelung PJ, Panhuysen CIM, Postma DS, et al: Atopy and bronchial hyperresponsiveness: exclusion of linkage to markers on chromosomes 11q and 6q. Clin Exp Allergy 22:1077–1084, 1992.
3. American Thoracic Society Committee on Diagnostic Standards for Non-Tubercular Respiratory Disease: Definitions and classification of chronic bronchitis, asthma and pulmonary emphysema. Am Rev Respir Dis 85:762–768, 1962.
4. Arthus M: Injections repetees de serum de cheval chez le pain. C R Seances Soc Biol Fil 55:817, 1903.
5. Bai TR, Zhou D, Aubent J, et al: Expression of β 2 adrenergic receptor mRNA in peripheral lung in asthma and chronic obstructive pulmonary disease. Am J Respir Cell Mol Biol 8:325, 1993.
6. Barbee R, Halonen M, Haltenborn W, et al: A longitudinal study of serum IgE in a community cohort: correlation with age, sex, smoking and atopic status. J Allergy Clin Immunol 29:919–927, 1982.
7. Becker D, Neiss U, Neiss S, et al: Contact allergens modulate the expression of MHC class II molecules on murine epidermal Langerhans cells by endocytotic mechanisms. J Invest Dermatol 98:700–705, 1992.
8. Bignon J, Aron Y, Jo L, et al: HLA class II alleles in isocyanate-induced asthma. Am J Respir Crit Care Med 149:7–15, 1994.
9. Biotechnology and genetics. The Economist 334:3–18, 1995.
10. Björkstén B: Clinical methods to study the immune system. In Blumenthal MN, Björkstén B (eds): Genetics of Allergy and Asthma: Methods for Investigative Studies. Marcel Dekker, New York. In press.
11. Björkstén B: Epidemiology of risk factors. In Blumenthal MN, Björkstén B (eds): Genetics of Allergy and Asthma: Methods for Investigative Studies. Marcel Dekker, New York. In press.
12. Black JT: Amyloidosis, deafness, urticaria, and limb pain: a hereditary syndrome. Ann Intern Med 70:989–994, 1969.
13. Blackley CH: Experimental Researches on the Causes and Nature of Catarrhus Aestivus (Hay Fever or Hay Asthma). Bailliere, Tindall and Cox, London, 1873.
14. Bleecker E, Meyers D: Bronchial hyperreactivity. In Blumenthal MN, Björkstén B (eds): Genetics of Allergy and Asthma: Methods for Investigative Studies. Marcel Dekker, New York. In press.
15. Blumenthal MN: Family, twin and population studies of allergic responsiveness. In Marsh DG, Lockhart A, Holgate ST (eds): The Genetics of Asthma. Blackwell Scientific Publications, Oxford, 1993, pp 133–141.
16. Blumenthal MN: Historical perspectives. In Blumenthal MN, Björkstén B. (eds): Genetics of Allergy and Asthma: Methods for Investigative Studies. Marcel Dekker, New York. In press.
17. Blumenthal MN, Amos D, Noreen H, et al: Genetic mapping of Ir locus in man: linkage to the second locus of HLA. Science 181:1201, 1974.
18. Blumenthal MN, Björkstén B (eds): Genetics of Allergy and Asthma: Methods for Investigative Studies. Marcel Dekker, New York. In press.
19. Blumenthal MN, Bonini S: Immunogenetics of specific immune responses to allergens in twins and families. In Marsh DG, Blumenthal MN (eds): Genetic and Environmental Factors in Clinical Allergy. University of Minnesota Press, Minneapolis, 1990, pp 132–142.
20. Blumenthal MN, Marcus-Bagley D, Adweh Z, et al: Extended major: HLA-DR2, [HLA-B7, SC31, DR2] and [HLA-B8, SC01, DR3] haplotypes distinguish subjects with asthma from those with only rhinitis in ragweed pollen allergy. J Immunol 148:411–416, 1992.
21. Blumenthal MN, Namboodiri M, Gleich G, et al: Genetic transmission of serum IgE levels. Am J Genet 10:219–228, 1981.
22. Blumenthal MN, Wang Z, Weber J, Rich SS: Absence of linkage between 5q markers and serum IgE levels in four large atopic families. Clin Exp Allergy. In press.
23. Brenner-Ullman A, Melzer-Ofin H, Daniels M, Shohat M: Possible protection against asthma in heterozygotes for familial Mediterranean fever. Am J Med Genet 53: 172–175, 1994.
24. Brereton HM, Ruffin RW, Thompson PJ, Turner DR: Familial atopy in Australian pedigrees: adventitious linkage to chromosome 8 is not confirmed nor is there evidence of linkage to high-affinity IgE receptor. Clin Exp Allergy 24:868–877, 1994.
25. Broder I, Higgins M, Mathews K, Keller J: Epidemiology of asthma and allergic rhinitis in a total community, Tecumseh, Michigan. IV. Natural history. J Allergy Clin Immunol 54:100–110, 1974.
26. Burr M: Introduction. In Burr M (ed): Epidemiology of Clinical Allergy. Monographs in Allergy 31. S Karger, Basel, New York, 1993, pp 1–8.
27. Burr M: Epidemiology of asthma. In Burr M (ed): Epidemiology of Clinical Allergy. Monographs in Allergy 31. S Karger, Basel, New York, 1993, pp 80–102.
28. Burrows B, Martinez F, Halonen, et al: Association of asthma with serum IgE level and skin test reactivity to allergens. N Engl J Med 320:271, 1989.
29. Caraballo LR, Hernandez M: HLA haplotype segregation in families with allergic asthma. Tissue Antigens 35:182–186, 1990.
30. Chase MW: Inheritance in guinea pigs of the susceptibility to skin sensitization with simple chemical compounds. J Exp Med 73:711–726, 1941.
31. Clifford RD, Howell J, Radford M, Holgate S: Associations between respiratory symptoms, bronchial response to methacholine and atopy in two age groups of schoolchildren. Arch Dis Child 64:1133–1139, 1989.
32. Clough J, Holgate S: Episodes of respiratory morbidity in children with cough and wheeze. Am J Respir Crit Care Med 150:48–53, 1994.
33. Coca AF, Cooke RA: On the classification of the phenomena of hypersensitiveness. J Immunol 8:163–182, 1923.
34. Cockcroft DW, O'Byrne PM: Mechanisms of airway hyperresponsiveness. In Weiss EB, Stein M (eds): Bronchial Asthma, 3rd edition. Little, Brown and Co., Boston, Toronto, London, 1993, pp 32–42.
35. Coleman R, Trembath RC, Harper JI: Chromosome 11q13 and atopy underlying atopic eczema. Lancet 341:1121–1122, 1993.
36. Collee JM, ten Kate LP, de Vries HG, et al: Allele sharing on chromosome 11q in sibs with asthma and atopy. Lancet 342:936, 1993.
37. Colp C, Lieberman J: Asthma and α-1 antitrypsin. In Weiss E, Stein M (eds): Bronchial Asthma, 3rd edition. Little, Brown and Co, New York, 1993, pp 1185–1187.
38. Connor JM, Ferguson-Smith MA: Essential Medical Genetics, 3rd edition. Blackwell Scientific Publications, Oxford, 1991.
39. Cooke RA, VanderVeer A: Human sensitization. J Immunol 1:201–305, 1916.
40. Cookson WO, Sharp PA, Faux JA, Hopkin JM: Linkage between immunoglobulin E responses underlying asthma and rhinitis and chromosome 11q. Lancet 1:1292–1295, 1989.
41. Cookson WOCM, Young RP, Sandford AJ, et al: Maternal inheritance of atopic responsiveness on chromosome 11q. Lancet 340:381–384, 1992.
42. Cooper ND, Schmidtke J: Molecular genetic approaches to the analysis and diagnosis of human inherited disease: an overview. Ann Med 24:29–42, 1992.
43. Coulter KM, Dorval G, Goodfriend L: Genetic control of IgE antibody responses in humans: the Amb V (Ra 5) model. In Marsh DG, Blumenthal MN (eds): Genetic and Environmental Factors in Clinical Allergy. University of Minnesota Press, Minneapolis, 1990, pp 124–131.
44. Davies KE, Read AP, eds: Molecular Basis of Inherited Diseases, 2nd edition. IRL Press, Oxford, Washington, DC, 1988.
45. de Weck AL, Blumenthal MN: HLA and Allergy. Monographs in Allergy 11. S Karger, Basel, 1977.
46. de Weck A, Blumenthal MN, Yunis E, Jeannet M: HLA in allergy. In Dausset J, Svejgaard A (eds): HLA and Disease. Williams and Wilkins, Copenhagen, Munksgaard, Baltimore, 1977, pp 196–211.

47. Emtestam L, Zetterquist H, Olerup O: HLA-DR, -DQ and -DP alleles in nickel, chromium, and/or cobalt-sensitive individuals: genomic analysis based on restriction fragment length polymorphisms. J Invest Dermatol 100:271–274, 1993.
48. Evans R: Epidemiology and natural history of asthma, allergic rhinitis and atopic dermatitis (eczema). In Middleton E, Reed CE, Ellis EF, et al (eds): Allergy Principles and Practice, 4th edition. CV Mosby, St Louis, 1993, pp 1109–1136.
49. Freidhoff L: Epidemiology of atopic allergy. In Marsh DG, Blumenthal MN (eds): Genetic and Environmental Factors in Clinical Allergy. University of Minnesota Press, Minneapolis, 1990, pp 53–72.
50. Fujii H, Kondo N, Agata H, et al: Genetic analysis of IgE and the IGHE, IGHEP1 and IGEHEP2 in atopic families. Int Arch Immunol 106:62–68, 1995.
51. Gaillard M, Zwi S, Nogueira C, et al: Ethnic difference in the occurrence of the M1 (ala 213) haplotype of alpha 1 antitrypsin in asthmatic and non asthmatic black and white South Africans. Clin Genet 45:122–127, 1994.
52. Geczy A, de Weck AL: Genetic control of sensitization to chemically defined antigens and its relationship to histocompatibility antigens in guinea pigs. In Parker D, Truk JL (eds): Contact Hypersensitivity in Experimental Animals. S Karger, Basel, 1974, pp 83–88.
53. Geerts SJ, Pöttgens H, Limburg M, van Rood JJ: Predisposition for atopy or allergy linked to HLA. Lancet I(7904):461, 1975.
54. Elmer-Dewitt P: The genetic revolution. Time 143:46–57, 1994.
55. Gerrard JW, Blumenthal MN: Genetic factors. In Weiss EB, Stein M (eds): Bronchial Asthma, 3rd edition. Little, Brown and Co, Boston, Toronto, London, 1993, pp 26–31.
56. Gerrard JW, Rao DC, Morton NE: A genetic study of immunoglobulin E. Am J Hum Genet 30:46–58, 1978.
57. Goundemand J, Defrenne C, Desmons F: HLA antigens and atopic dermatitis. In de Weck AL, Blumenthal MN (eds): HLA and Allergy. Monographs in Allergy 11. S Karger, Basel, New York, 1977, pp 24–29.
58. Gyokovits K, Markus V, Bittern I: Cystic fibrosis heterozygosity in childhood bronchial asthma. Lancet 1:203, 1977.
59. Hanifin JM: Atopic dermatitis. In Middleton E, Reed C, Ellis E, et al (eds): Allergy Principles and Practice, 4th edition. Vol II. CV Mosby, St. Louis, 1988, pp 1581–1604.
60. Hanifin JM, Rajka G: Diagnostic features of atopic dermatitis. Acta Derm Venereol Suppl (Stockh) 92:44–47, 1980.
61. Hanson B, McGue M, Roitman-Johnson B, et al: Atopic disease and immunoglobulin E in twins reared apart and together. Am J Hum Genet 48:873–879, 1991.
62. Hizawa N, Yamaguchi E, Furuya K, et al: Association between high serum total IgE level and D11595 of chromosome 11q13 in Japanese subjects. J Med Genet 32:363–369, 1995.
63. Hizawa N, Yamaguchi E, Ohe M, et al: Lack of linkage between atopy and locus 11q13. Clin Exp Allergy 22:1065–1069, 1992.
64. Hopp RJ, Nair NM, Bewtra AK, Townley RG: Genetic aspects of bronchial hyperreactivity. In Marsh DG, Blumenthal MN (eds): Genetic and Environmental Factors in Clinical Allergy. University of Minnesota Press, Minneapolis, 1990, pp 143–152.
65. Hsieh KH, Shien CC, Hsieh RP, Liu WJ: Association of HLA-DQW2 with Chinese childhood asthma. Tissue Antigens 38:181–182, 1991.
66. Jovanovic M, Poljacki M, Milakov J, et al: Phenotyping: personal contribution to research on increased susceptibility of individual HLA phenotype combinations in predisposition to contact allergies. Med Pregl 46:221–224, 1993.
67. Vaughn W, Black NH: Practice of Allergy, 3rd edition. CV Mosby, St Louis, 1048, 1954
68. Kim KE, Rosenberg A, Roberts S, Blumenthal MN: Affinity of allergen-specific IgE and the competition between IgE and IgG for the allergen in Amb a V-sensitive individuals. Mol Immunol 33:873–880, 1996.
69. Kitano V, Sadanaga Y, Ishikawa T: Genetic regulation of allergic rhinitis. Acta Paediatr Jpn 29:654–657, 1985.
70. Kohler J, Martin S, Pflugfelder U, et al: Cross-reactive trinitrophenylated peptides as antigens for class II major histocompatibility complex-restricted T cells and inducers of contact sensitivity in mice: limited T cell receptor repertoire. Eur J Immunol 25:92–101, 1995.
71. Kuwata S, Yanagisawa M, Saeki H, et al: Polymorphisms of transporter associated with antigen processing genes in atopic dermatitis. J Allergy Clin Immunol 94:565–574, 1994.
72. Larson FS: The epidemiology of atopic dermatitis. In Burr M (ed): Epidemiology of Clinical Allergy. Monographs in Allergy 31. S Karger, Basel, New York, 1993.
73. Lee T, Lympany PA: Inflammation. In Blumenthal MN, Björkstén B (eds): Approaches to the Study of the Genetics of Allergy and Asthma. Marcel Dekker, New York. In press.
74. Levine B, Stember R, Fotino M: Ragweed hayfever: genetic control and linkage to HLA haplotypes. Science 178:1201, 1972.
75. Liden S, Beckman L, Cedergren B, et al: HLA antigens in allergic contact dermatitis. Acta Derm Venereol Suppl (Stockh) 58:53–56, 1978.
76. Lindmark B: Asthma and heterozygous $\alpha 1$ antitrypsin deficiency: prevalence and clinical spectrum in asthmatic children. Allergy 45:197–203, 1990.
77. Lympany P, Welsh KI, Christie PE, et al: An analysis with sequence-specific oligonucleotide probes of the association between aspirin-induced asthma and antigens of the HLA system. J Allergy Clin Immunol 92:114–123, 1993.
78. Lympany P, Welsh KI, Cochrane GM, et al: Genetic analysis of the linkage between chromosome 11q and atopy. Clin Exp Allergy 22(12):1085–1092, 1992.
79. Lympany P, Welsh K, MacCochrane G, et al: Genetic analysis using DNA polymorphism of the linkage between chromosome 11q13 and atopy and bronchial hyperresponsiveness to methacholine. J Allergy Clin Immunol 89:619–628, 1992.
80. Maibach HI, Epstein E, Lahti A: Contact skin allergy. In Middleton E, Reed CE, Ellis EF, et al (eds): Allergy Principles and Practice, 3rd edition. Vol II. CV Mosby, St Louis, 1988, pp 1429–1468.
81. Major RH: A History of Medicine. Vol 2. CC Thomas, Springfield, IL, 1954.
82. Major RH: Classic Descriptions of Disease, 3rd edition. CC Thomas, Springfield, IL, 1955.
83. Marone G, Poto S, Celestino D, Bonini S: Human basophil releasability. III. Genetic controls of the human basophil releasability. J Immunol 137:3588–3592, 1986.
84. Marquardt DL, Wasserman SI: Anaphylaxis. In Middleton E, Reed C, Ellis E, et al (eds): Allergy Principles and Practice, 3rd edition. Vol II. CV Mosby, St Louis, 1988, pp 1365–1376.
85. Marsh DG: Immunogenetic and immunochemical factors determining immune responsiveness to allergens: studies in unrelated subjects. In Marsh DG, Blumenthal MN (eds): Genetic and Environmental Factors in Clinical Allergy. University of Minnesota Press, Minneapolis, 1990, pp 97–123.
86. Marsh DG, Blumenthal MN, Ishikawa T, et al: HLA and specific immune responsiveness to allergens. In Tsuji K, Aizawa M, Sasazuki T (eds): HLA 1991: Proceedings of the 11th International Histocompatibility Workshop. Oxford University Press, New York, 1992, pp 765–771.
87. Marsh DG, Meyers DA, Freidhoff LR, et al: HLA-Dw2: a genetic marker for human immune response to short ragweed pollen allergen Ra5. II. Response after ragweed immunotherapy. J Exp Med 155:1452–1463, 1982.
88. Marsh DG, Neely JD, Breazeale DR, et al: Linkage analysis of IL-4 and other chromosome 5q31.1 markers and total serum immunoglobulin E concentrations. Science 264:1152–1156, 1994.
89. Meltzer SJ: Bronchial asthma as a phenomenon of anaphylaxis. JAMA 55:1021–1024, 1910.
90. Meyers DA, Postma DS, Panhuysen CIM, et al: Evidence for a locus regulating total serum IgE levels mapping to chromosome 5. Genomics 23:464–470, 1994.
91. Moffatt MF, Hill MR, Cornelis F, et al: Genetic linkage of T-cell receptors and α/δ complex to specific IgE response. Lancet 343:1597–1600, 1994.
92. Morris MJ, Vaughan H, Lane DJ, Morris PJ: HLA in asthma. In de Weck AL, Blumenthal MN (eds.): HLA and Allergy. Monographs in Allergy 11. S Karger, Basel, New York, 1977.
93. Morrison J: Class III MHC polymorphisms and asthma. In Genetics of Asthma. The Wellcome Trust, Presented at Broadway. Worcestershire, UK, 1995, p 47.
94. Morton N: Statistical methods. In Blumenthal MN, Björkstén B (eds.): Genetics of Allergy and Asthma: Methods for Investigative Studies. Marcel Dekker, New York, In press.
95. Mullarkey M, Thomas P, Hansen J, et al: Association of aspirin-sensitive asthma with HLA-DQW2. Am Rev Respir Dis 133:261–263, 1986.
96. Müller V: Epidemiology of insect sting allergy. In Burr M (ed): Epidemiology of Clinical Allergy. Monographs in Allergy 31. S Karger, Basel, New York, 1993, pp 131–146.
97. Oltvai ZN, Wong E, Atkinson J, Tung K: C-1 inhibitor deficiency: molecular and immunologic basis of hereditary and acquired angioedema. Lab Invest 65:381–388, 1991.

98. Orange RP, Donsky GJ: Anaphylaxis. In Middleton E, Reed CE, Ellis EF (eds.): Allergy Principles and Practice, 1st edition. Vol II. CV Mosby, St Louis, 1978.
99. Oxelus VA, Hultquist C, Husby S: GM allotype as indicators of non-atopic bronchial asthma. Int Arch Allergy Immunol 101:66–71, 1993.
100. Ozawa A, Ohkido M, Tsuji S: Some recent advances in HLA and skin disease. J Am Dermat 205–230, 1981.
101. Paul E, Greilich K, Dominante G: Epidemiology of urticaria. In Schlumberger HD (ed): Monographs in Allergy 21. S Karger, Basel, 1987, pp 87–117.
102. Pillsbury DM, Shelley W, Kligman A: Dermatitis and eczema. In: Dermatology. WB Saunders, Philadelphia, 1965, pp 363–458.
103. Portier P, Richet C: Chapter de l'action anaphylactique de certains benins. C R Seances Soc Biol Fil 54:170, 1902.
104. Postma DS, Bleecker ER, Amelung PJ, et al: Genetic susceptibility to asthma—bronchial hyperresponsiveness coinherited with a major gene for atopy. N Engl J Med 333:894–900, 1995.
105. Prados M, Montseirin F, Carranco M, et al: Phenotype of alpha 1 antitrypsin in intrinsic asthma and ASA triad patients. Allergol Immunopathol (Madr) 23:24–28, 1995.
106. Quincke H: Über akutes umschreibenes H-autoderm. Monatschrift Für Praktische Dermatologie 1:129–131, 1882.
107. Rachelefsky GS, Terasaki PI, Katz RM, Siegel SC: B lymphocyte and histocompatibility antigens in extrinsic asthma. In de Weck AL, Blumenthal MN (eds): HLA and Allergy. Monographs in Allergy 11. S Karger, Basel, New York, 1977, p 35.
108. Rajka G: Essential Aspects of Atopic Dermatitis. Springer, Berlin, 1989.
109. Reihsaus E, Innis M, MacIntyre N, Ligget S: Mutation in the gene encoding for the β 2 adrenergic receptor in normal and asthma subjects. Am J Respir Cell Mol Biol 8:334, 1993.
110. Renz H, Saloga J, Bradley KL, et al: Specific V β T cell subsets mediate the immediate hypersensitivity response to ragweed allergy. J Immunol 151:1907–1917, 1993.
111. Rich SS, Roitman-Johnson B, Greenberg B, et al: Genetic analysis of atopy in three large kindreds: no evidence of linkage to D11S97. Clin Exp Allergy 22:1070–1076, 1992.
112. Roitman-Johnson B, Blumenthal MN: Family analysis of histamine release. J Allergy Clin Immunol 81:232, 1988.
113. Rosenau M, Anderson JG: Hypersusceptibility. JAMA 42:1007–1010, 1906. Abstract.
114. Rosenwasser L, Klemm DJ, Dresback JK, et al: Promoter polymorphisms in the chromosome 5 gene cluster in asthma and atopy. Clin Exp Allergy 25:74–78, 1995.
115. Saeki H, Kuwata S, Nakagawa H, et al: HLA and atopic dermatitis with high serum IgE levels. J Allergy Clin Immunol 94:575–583, 1994.
116. Sandford AO, Shirakawa TS, Moffatt MF, et al: Localization of atopy and the β sub unit of the high-affinity immunoglobulin E receptor (FcεR1) on chromosome 11q. Lancet 341:332–334, 1993.
117. Schaefer T, Ring J: Epidemiology of urticaria. In Burr M (ed): Epidemiology of Clinical Allergy. Monographs in Allergy 31. S Karger, Basel, 1993, pp 49–60.
118. Scholz S, Ziegler E, Wüstner H, et al: HLA family studies in patients with atopic dermatitis. In de Weck AL, Blumenthal MN (eds): HLA and Allergy. Monographs in Allergy 11. S Karger, Basel, New York, 1977, p 44.
119. Schroeder SA, Gaughan DM, Swift M: Protection against bronchial asthma by CFTR-δ 508 mutation: a heterozygote advantage in cystic fibrosis. Nature Med 1:703–705, 1995.
120. Settipane R, Hagy G, Settipane GA: Long term risk factors for developing asthma and allergic rhinitis: a 23-year follow-up study of college students. Allergy Proc 15:21–25, 1994.
121. Sears M, Burrows B, Flannery G, et al: Relationship between airway responsiveness and serum IgE in children with asthma and in apparently normal children. N Engl J Med 325:1067, 1991.
122. Seymour JL, Keswick BH, Hanifin JM, et al: Clinical effects of diaper types on the skin of normal infants and infants with atopic dermatitis. J Am Acad Dermatol 17:988–997, 1987.
123. Shirakawa T, Airong L, Dubowitz M, et al: Association between atopy and variants of the β sub unit of the high-affinity immunoglobulin E receptor. Nat Genet 7(2):125–129, 1994.
124. Shirakawa T, Hashimoto T, Furuyama J, Morimoto K: Linkage between severe atopy and chromosome 11q13 in Japanese families. Clin Genet 46:228–232, 1994.
125. Sibbald B: Epidemiology of allergic rhinitis. In Burr M (ed): Epidemiology of Clinical Allergy. Monographs in Allergy 31. S Karger, Basel, 1993, pp 61–79.
126. Siddique Z, McPhaden AR, Whaley K: Characterisation of nucleotide sequence variants and disease-specific mutations involving the 3′ end of the C1-inhibitor gene in hereditary angio-oedema. Hum Hered 45:98–102, 1995.
127. Silverstein M: A History of Immunology. Academic Press, San Diego, 1989.
128. Stoy P, Roitman-Johnson B, Walsh G, et al: Aging and serum IgE levels. J Allergy Clin Immunol 68:421, 1981.
129. Strachan DP: Hayfever, hygiene and household size. Br Med J 299:1259–1266, 1989.
130. Sutton BJ, Gould HJ: The human IgE network. Nature 366:421–428, 1993.
131. Svejgaard E, Jakobsen B, Svejgaard A: Studies of HLA-ABC and DR antigens in pure atopic dermatitis and atopic dermatitis combined with allergic respiratory disease. Acta Derm Venereol Suppl (Stockh) 114:72–76, 1985.
132. Taylor B, Wadsworth J, Golding J, Butler N: Breastfeeding, eczema, asthma, and hayfever. J Epidemiol Community Health 37:97–99, 1983.
133. Taylor B, Wadsworth M, Wadsworth J, Pelzham C: Changes in the reported prevalence of childhood eczema since the 1939–45 war. Lancet ii:1255–1258, 1984.
134. Thorsby E, Engeset A, Lie SO: HLA antigens and susceptibility to disease: a study of patients with acute lymphoblastic leukemia, Hodgkins disease, and childhood asthma. Transplant Proc 1(3):147–152, 1971.
135. Turner MN, Brostoff J, Wells SR, Soothill JF: Histocompatibility antigens in atopy with special reference to eczema and hayfever. In de Weck AL, Blumenthal MN (eds): HLA and Allergy. Monographs in Allergy 11. S Karger, Basel, New York, 1977.
136. Vaughan WT: Practice of Allergy, 3rd edition. CV Mosby, St Louis, 1957.
137. Vaughan WT, Black JJH: Skin diseases. In Vaughan WT (ed): Practice of Allergy, 3rd edition. CV Mosby, St Louis, 1954.
138. Verpy E, Couture-Tosi E, Eldering E, et al: Crucial residues in the carboxy-terminal end of C1 inhibitor revealed by pathogenic mutants impaired in secretion or function. J Clin Invest 95:350–359, 1995.
139. Virchow JC, Walker C, Hafner D, et al: T cells and cytokines in bronchoalveolar lavage fluid after segmented allergen provocation in atopic asthma. Am J Respir Crit Care Med 151:960–968, 1995.
140. Von Pirquet C, Clemens M: Med Wochenschr 53:1457, 1906. [Prausnitz C, trans: Gell PGH. In Coombs RRA (ed): Clinical Aspects of Immunology. FA Davis Company, Philadelphia, 1963.]
141. Von Pirquet C, Schick B: Die serum Krankheit. Deuticke, Vienna, 1906. [English trans. Serum sickness. Williams and Wilkins, Baltimore, 1951.]
142. Walter MA, Chambers C, Zimmerman B, Cox D: A multigene deletion in the immunoglobulin heavy chain region in a highly atopic individual. Hum Genet 85:643–647, 1990.
143. Warner JO, Norman A, Soothill J: Cystic fibrosis heterozygosity in the pathogenesis of allergy. Lancet 1:990–991, 1976.
144. Wasserman SI, Marquardt DL: Anaphylaxis. In Middleton E, Reed CE, Ellis EF, et al (eds): Allergy Principles and Practice, 3rd edition. CV Mosby, St Louis, 1988, pp 1365–1376.
145. Weiss K, Gergen P: The epidemiology of asthma: risk factors, rates and trends. In Blumenthal MN, Björkstén B (eds): Genetics of Allergy and Asthma: Methods for Investigative Studies. Marcel Dekker, New York. In press.
146. Weiss K, Gergen P: Epidemiology of atopic disease. In Blumenthal MN, Björkstén B (eds): Genetics of Allergy and Asthma: Methods for Investigative Studies. Marcel Dekker, New York. In press.
147. Weiss S, Speizer F: Epidemiology and natural history. In Weiss EB, Stein M (eds): Bronchial Asthma, 3rd edition. Little, Brown, and Co, Boston, 1993.
148. Wolff-Eisner A: Das heufieber: sein wesen und seine behandlung. Munich, 1906.
149. Wolffler W: Hereditary angioedema. Am J Med Sci 95:362, 1888.
150. Wyman M: Autumnal catarrh. Hurd and Houghton, New York, 1872.
151. Yunginger JW: Clinical significance of IgE. In Middleton E, Reed CE, Ellis EF, et al (eds): Allergy Principles and Practice, 3rd edition. CV Mosby, St Louis, 1988, pp 849–860.
152. Yunginger J, Reed C, O'Connell E, et al: A community-based study of asthma. I. Incidence rates 1964–84. Am Rev Respir Dis 146:888–894, 1992.
153. Zwollo P, Ehrlich-Kautzky E, Scharf S, et al: Sequencing of HLA-D in responders and nonresponders to short ragweed allergen Amb a V. Immunogenetics 33:141–151, 1991.

25 Allergic Rhinitis, Nonallergic Rhinitis, and Ocular Allergy

KARALASINGAM RAJAKULASINGAM DAVID F. ANDERSON
STEPHEN T. HOLGATE

RHINITIS

NASAL PHYSIOLOGY AND FUNCTIONAL ANATOMY

The nasal air passages are the first part of the respiratory tract and serve an important protective role for the lower airways. Air passing through the nose is filtered, warmed, and humidified. To achieve this with maximum efficiency, the air stream through the nasal passages is turbulent, and rapid changes are induced in nasal patency, nasal secretions, and nasal blood flow. In allergic and nonallergic forms of rhinopathy, disordered or inappropriate alterations in this regulation occur, leading to nasal obstruction and excessive nasal secretions as part of the symptom complex in these disorders. An appreciation of the approach to the relief or prevention of these symptoms is dependent on an understanding of the normal nasal physiology and its derangement in pathologic states.

The two nasal air passages are separated medially by the nasal septum and laterally by a compliant nasal vestibule anteriorly and a bony cavum posteriorly. The lateral wall of the bony component is lined by the turbinates. During nasal breathing, the nose contributes up to two thirds of the total respiratory resistance. The major site of airway resistance is approximately 3 cm into the nostrils at the anterior end of the inferior turbinate (Fig. 25–1).[133] This flow-limiting site is termed the nasal valve and is critically dependent on the state of engorgement of the venous sinusoids within the inferior turbinates. At this site, the air flow changes from laminar to turbulent. Turbulent air flow facilitates the mixing, warming, and humidification of the inspired air and also assists with particle deposition by inertial impaction.

Impacted particles stick to the nasal epithelial mucus layer and are transported in the mucus by coordinated ciliary movement backward to the oropharynx. The nasal epithelium is rich in mucus glands and goblet cells. The submucosa is richly vascularized, being supplied by the sphenopalatine and anterior ethmoidal arteries. The nasal vasculature is complex and characterized by the presence of an extensive sinusoidal network of large capacitance vessels deep in the mucosa and arteriovenous anastomoses, particularly in the respiratory mucosa (Fig. 25–2).[72, 102, 290] It can be divided into four subgroups: capacitance vessels (venous sinusoids), exchange vessels (capillaries), resistance vessels (precapillary sphincters and arterioles), and postcapillary venules. There are also arteriovenous anastomoses diverting blood directly from the arterial to the venous system. It has been estimated that 60% of the total nasal blood flow is shunted through the arteriovenous anastomoses.

Regulation of the capacitance vessels, which alter the nasal air flow and nasal airway resistance, is primarily autonomic, with a prominent sympathetic innervation. The superficial capillaries are fenestrated and can allow rapid exudation of protein-rich fluid into the nasal cavity, thereby contributing

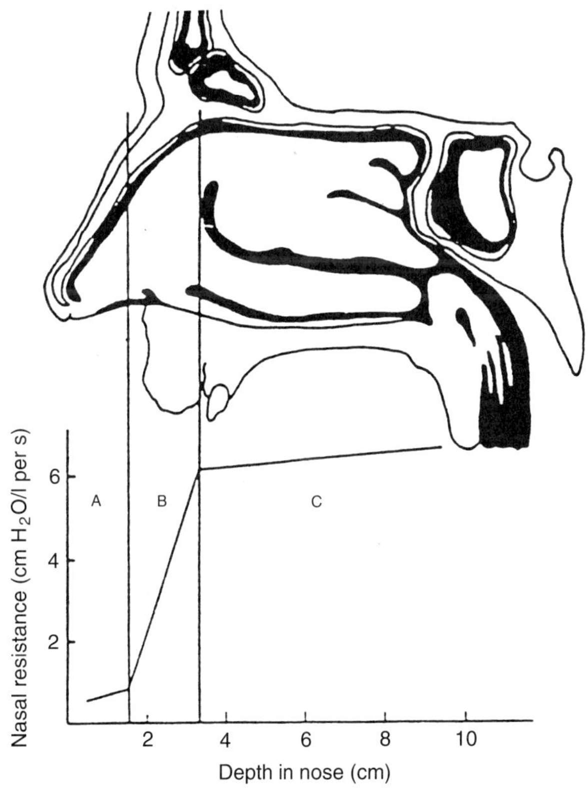

FIGURE 25–1. Changes in resistance to air flow along the nasal passage. Nasal resistance can be divided into the three components illustrated. A = nasal vestibule; B = nasal valve; C = nasal turbinates. (From Mackay I (ed): Rhinitis: Mechanisms and Management. Royal Society of Medicine Services Ltd, London, 1989, p 54.)

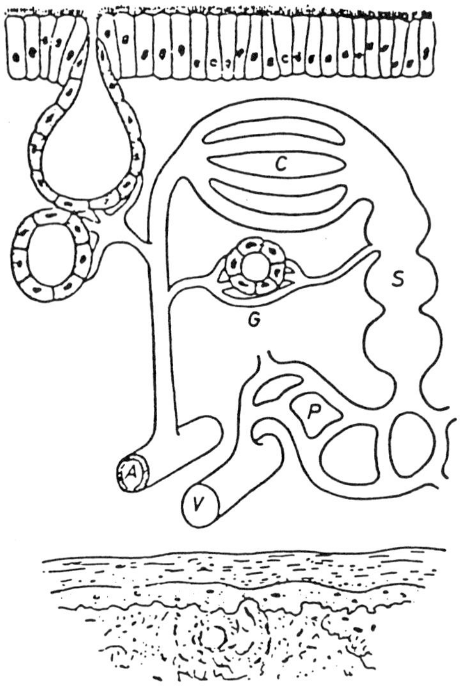

FIGURE 25–2. Simplified diagram showing arrangement of blood vessels in nasal mucosa. A = artery; V = vein; S = venous sinusoids; C = arteriole; P = venular plexus; G = capillary. (From Brown S: Diseases of the Ear, Nose and Throat, 4th edition. Butterworth-Heinemann Ltd, Oxford, 1984.)

to nasal secretions. The cavernous sinusoids, which comprise a plexi of venous capacitance vessels, are in their densest concentration in the mucosa of the inferior and middle turbinates. Their capacitance volume is under neural regulation, with an intrinsic neural tone limiting the sinusoidal capacity. Changes in the venous capacitance volume alter the nasal air flow and nasal airway resistance due to the effect on turbinate size.

DEFINITION OF RHINITIS

There are no widely agreed upon criteria for the diagnosis or classification of rhinitis. Theoretically, rhinitis means an inflammation of the nasal mucosa. Rhinitis is a common yet sometimes surprisingly complex condition. It is a heterogeneous disease process set into motion by multiple triggering factors (Table 25–1). The difficulty lies in distinguishing rhinitic from normal subjects, since the characteristic symptoms of rhinitis may occur occasionally in all individuals. Clinical definitions therefore focus on the identification of people whose symptoms are severe enough to warrant treatment. Although allergy is a common cause of rhinitis, it is by no means the only one, as inflammation may arise from a multitude of factors. This condition can be broadly divided into four main groups: allergic, infective, structural, and amorphous (see Table 25–1).

The allergic type can be seasonal or perennial. Infective rhinitis may be acute or chronic. Acute infective rhinitis is usually viral and self-limiting. Chronic infection may occur due to infections with bacteria, fungi, and specific organisms, such as leishmaniasis, or may be associated with host defense deficiency, which may be local (ciliary dyskinesia) or systemic (immune deficiency, including AIDS). Structural and other amorphous or miscellaneous types are mentioned in Table 25–1. Rhinitis also occurs as part of systemic diseases, such as cystic fibrosis, sarcoidosis, connective disease disorders, and Wegener's granulomatosis, and due to hematopoietic diseases. This chapter will focus mainly on allergic rhinitis and other types of rhinitis that simulate it. Infections of the nose are not discussed, except for their role in differential diagnosis.

Allergic Rhinitis

Allergic rhinitis is characterized by cell accumulation and cell activation within the nasal mucosa, along with enhanced plasma vascular permeability. It is the most common form of allergic disease, affecting about 10% to 20% of the general population,[213] and its incidence seems to be increasing.[9, 187] Allergic rhinitis can be specifically precipitated by exposure to seasonal airborne allergens, such as pollens and mold spores, and to perennial allergens, such as house dust mite, animal proteins, and insect-related allergens. Patients with seasonal and perennial allergic rhinitis present with similar symptoms, characterized by itching, sneezing, nasal blockage, excess lacrimation, and runny nose. Less commonly, itching of the palate, throat, or ears occurs. Some patients can present with nonspecific symptoms, such as

TABLE 25–1
CAUSES OF RHINITIS

Allergic
Pollen
Dust mites
Animal proteins
Insect-related allergens
Nonallergic
Infections
Acute (viral, bacterial)
Chronic (fungal, leishmaniasis, rhinoscleroma, immune deficiency)
Structural
Septal deviation
Adenoidal hypertrophy
Meningocele/encephalocele
Congenital choanal atresia
Foreign body
Tumors of the nasopharynx
Cerebrospinal fluid leak
Atrophic rhinitis
Amorphous
Vasomotor rhinitis
Eosinophilic (nonallergic rhinitis with eosinophilia)
Cold air
Irritants (environmental)
Noninflammatory
Rhinitis medicamentosa
Hormonal (pregnancy, puberty, menopause, hypothyroidism, acromegaly)
Reflux induced
Drugs

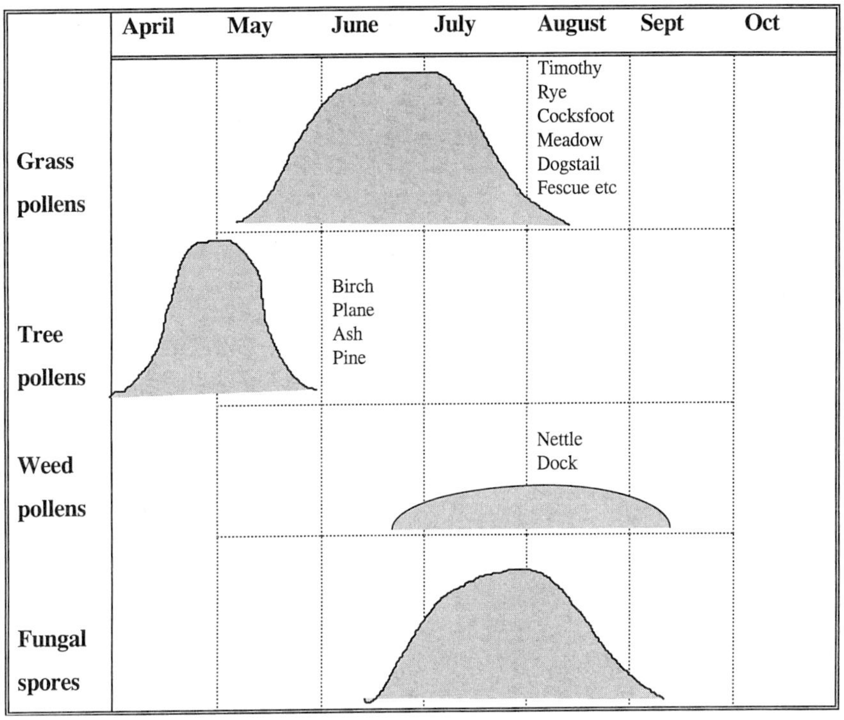

FIGURE 25–3. Distribution of pollens in the United Kingdom.

fatigue, mild headache or facial discomfort, mild sore throat, partial anosmia, and some sensation of ear plugging.

Seasonal Allergic Rhinitis

Pollen is the major cause of this disease, which usually presents the least trouble in diagnosis. A variety of aeroallergens also give rise to seasonal allergic symptoms (Fig. 25–3). The grass pollen season in the Northern Hemisphere extends from mid May through early August, peaking in June and early July. The tree pollen season extends from late February to the end of April. Mold spores are also known to cause rhinitis and are found in warm, damp places. The most common mold allergens present in largest amounts between May and October. Weed pollens, such as dock and nettle, are prominent in England and Northern Europe from July to mid September. Ragweed, pigweed, and marsh elder are seen in the United States and Canada from mid August through September. This condition is characterized by a history of nasal itch, sneezing, nasal blockage, and watery nose recurring during summer months. Here the history is usually diagnostic, and skin prick testing with grass pollen allergens for evidence of immediate hypersensitivity can be considered only confirmatory rather than mandatory to the diagnosis.

Perennial Allergic Rhinitis

This condition is characterized by inflammation of the nasal mucosa occurring chronically or recurring throughout the year, and the diagnosis is often more difficult to make. Patients with perennial rhinitis are also known to present with symptoms such as headaches, decrease or loss of taste and smell, postnasal drip, loss of hearing, earaches, and sleep apnea, with or without sneezing, pruritus, and nasal blockage.

All conditions, however, share two general features. First, there is invasion of the nasal mucosa by inflammatory cells, such as eosinophils, lymphocytes, neutrophils, basophils, and mast cells, and the release of inflammatory and immunologic mediators. Second, the mediators act directly and indirectly on the target systems in the nose, nasal vasculature, and submucosal mucus glands.

Epidemiology of Rhinitis

Unlike bronchial asthma, there is no objective test to diagnose rhinitis. The diagnosis of this condition must be based on questionnaires, interviews, examinations, and additional laboratory tests. Much of the epidemiology of rhinitis presently derives from studies of self- or physician-diagnosed disease, subject to considerable bias in the estimation of prevalence. An undetermined number of rhinitics do not consult their physician, and thus relatively little is known about the prevalence or distribution of rhinitis. However, it is estimated that the prevalence of seasonal allergic rhinitis in different countries varies between 0.5% and 28% in children and between 0.5% and 15% in adults.[195] This significant variation between countries is mainly due to the criteria used to make the diagnosis and the nature of the sample population.

Using standardized, although crude, criteria, studies have shown variation in the prevalence of hay fever within countries. For example, in Britain, the prevalence of the disease was greater in the south than in the north of the country.[111, 124] A similar regional variation for eczema has also been reported in the same populations. This regional variation is thought to be due to a combination of inter-regional migration and differing allergen loads during the critical period of sensitization. Similarly, a National Health Survey in Australia showed that there was an increase in self-reported cases of hay fever in southern and western states.[22] This difference was attributed to variations in aeroallergen burden inland.[64] Regional variations in the United States are dictated by differences in allergen prevalence (e.g., ragweed, western ragweed) and climatic conditions in different parts of the country.

The prevalence of atopy is highest among patients with seasonal symptoms alone (>75%) and lower in those with perennial symptoms alone (50%).[249] Sneezing and nasal pruritus are common among subjects with seasonal allergic rhinitis, and nasal blockage is more commonly associated with perennial allergic rhinitis. Dust, pollen, fumes, and animal proteins have been identified as major provoking factors in atopics. In contrast, infection has been identified as the most common provoking factor in nonatopic individuals.[250] Few community-based studies have been carried out. A study in London showed that the prevalence of all forms of rhinitis was 24%.[249] About 3% had symptoms of seasonal allergic rhinitis, and 78% of them were found to be atopic by skin prick testing. Thirteen percent of this population had perennial nasal symptoms, and 50% of them were found to be atopic by skin prick testing. Eight percent of this population had perennial nasal symptoms with seasonal exacerbations, and 68% of them were found to be atopic. However, this study was limited to London and does not necessarily apply elsewhere. Furthermore, many of the limited studies in rhinitis relate to seasonal allergic rhinitis, and the true prevalence of rhinitis in general is not known.

Population surveys identify positive relationships between specific allergen sensitivity and the development of rhinitis. In patients with perennial rhinitis, positive skin prick tests to mite allergen have been found in 40% of patients compared with less than 10% of a control population. Epidemiologic studies suggest that perennial rhinitis due to mite sensitivity is much less common at higher altitudes.

Pathogenesis

Sensitization of atopic subjects occurs following exposure to a relevant allergen. On reexposure to the particular allergen, soluble antigens are eluted from the pollen by nasal secretions and pass through the mucosa to react with IgE bound to mast cells. This is followed by mast cell degranulation and release of chemical mediators, which then result in immediate symptoms of rhinorrhea, itch, sneezing, and nasal congestion (Fig. 25–4). Continual allergen exposure results in invasion of the nasal mucosa by migratory cells, such as eosinophils, lymphocytes, neutrophils, and mast cells, and release of inflammatory and immunologic mediators (see Fig. 25–4). The released mediators act both directly and indirectly on target cells in the nose, the nasal vasculature, nerves, and submucosal glands.

VASCULAR PATHOPHYSIOLOGY

Many of the functional attributes of the nasal mucosa result from the properties of the complex vascular system. The physiologic advantage of the capacitance system is that it contributes to the air-conditioning function of the nose.[84] However, in pathologic conditions, their distension plays a major role in inducing nasal blockage. As mentioned earlier, the major site of nasal resistance lies at the anterior end of the inferior turbinate,[133] and the nasal mucosa at these sites are known to have erectile properties.[133] As a consequence, the tissue at these sites can congest to completely obstruct

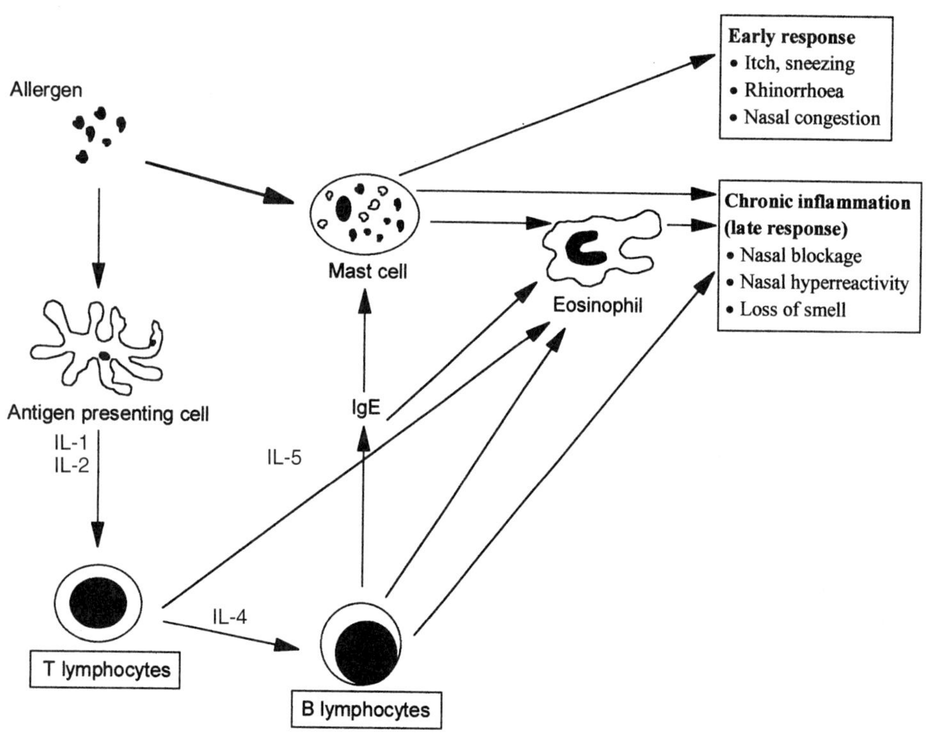

FIGURE 25–4. Schematic diagram of development of nasal symptoms and involvement of inflammatory cells and their products following provocation of nasal airways with allergen.

the nasal airway. The level of congestion is primarily under the influence of neural reflex control.[290]

In normal subjects, nasal resistance to air flow is primarily regulated by sympathetic activity, which determines the state of engorgement of the venous erectile tissue, with release of noradrenaline and neuropeptide Y as cotransmitters. Consistent with this, immunohistochemistry studies have identified the presence of noradrenaline and neuropeptide Y in the nasal mucosal nerves,[274, 275] and nasal administration of these agents causes vasoconstriction. Therefore, a reduction in sympathetic activity results in nasal congestion. In contrast, the parasympathetic nervous system in the nose functions as a vasodilator, with acetylcholine and neuropeptides such as vasoactive intestinal polypeptide as cotransmitters.[176, 275] In support of this, acetylcholinesterase and vasoactive intestinal polypeptide have been identified in the nasal mucosal nerves. The cholinergic nervous system plays a relatively minor role in maintaining nasal vascular tone or vascular permeability. Thus histologic studies have demonstrated the presence of only sparse cholinergic innervation of the capacitance vessels.[205] While recognizing the importance of neuroeffector mechanisms in maintaining nasal patency, the relative balance of the autonomic motor neurotransmitters on different components of the nasal vasculature is not clearly understood.

Axon reflexes also play an important role in inducing vascular changes in the nasal mucosa.[175, 176] Activation of these afferent neurones by irritants and locally released inflammatory mediators causes vasodilatation and microvascular leakage.[175, 176] The neurotransmitters involved in the axon reflex include the sensory neuropeptides, substance P, neurokinin A (NKA), and calcitonin gene–related peptide (CGRP).[274, 275] Activation of the sensory nerves also influences the neural vascular control through an action on the nerve cell bodies in the trigeminal and sphenopalatine ganglia. The reflexes seem to be mainly vasodilatory, causing nasal blockage. Studies in humans have demonstrated the presence of receptors for substance P, NKA, and CGRP in the nasal epithelium, venous blood vessels, arterial blood vessels, glands, and neural ganglia of the nasal mucosa.[33, 34] Substance P has been found in increased amounts in nasal lavage fluid following nasal allergen challenge,[202] and nasal challenge with substance P has been shown to induce nasal blockage.[91] The axon reflex vasodilatation has been shown to be inhibited by local anesthetics and by depleting the sensory nerves of their neuropeptides by repeated pretreatment with capsaicin.

The nasal vasculature is also known to be affected by a large number of inflammatory and immunologic mediators.[178] As might be expected, the action of inflammatory mediators on nasal blood vessels is complex. Mediators such as noradrenaline, neuropeptide Y, and prostaglandin $F_{2\alpha}$ ($PGF_{2\alpha}$) cause vasoconstriction.[140] In contrast, mediators such as histamine, bradykinin, prostaglandin D_2 (PGD_2), and platelet-activating factor (PAF) cause vasodilatation.[140, 224]

NASAL SECRETION

Nasal secretions comprise a mixture of fluids from the secretory glands, goblet cells, and blood vessels due to an increase in microvascular permeability. Mucus secretion in the nose is derived from epithelial goblet and serous cells, submucosal submucous glands, and anterolateral deep glands in the nose.[163, 287, 291] The secretions that originate from serous cells contain immunoglobulins, lactoferrin, and lysozyme; hence these glands may play an important role in both nasal allergy and infection. Mucosal exudation of plasma and plasma-derived factors has been implicated as a major respiratory defense mechanism.[215]

GLANDULAR SECRETION

Parasympathetic cholinergic nerves play a crucial role in controlling nasal glandular secretions. Thus nasal challenge with methacholine, a selective cholinergic agonist, produces hypersecretion in both normal subjects and subjects with allergic or nonallergic rhinitis.[55, 96] Pretreatment with atropine or ipratropium bromide significantly inhibits methacholine-induced nasal secretions.[54] Unilateral nasal challenge with histamine induces bilateral nasal hypersecretion due to stimulation of afferent sensory nerves and reflex parasympathetic stimulation to the contralateral nasal glands.[199] It follows that unilateral transection of cholinergic fibers to the nose (vidian neurectomy) results in the reduction of nasal secretions after ipsilateral stimulation.[164] These studies suggest that stimulation of cholinergic receptors plays an important role in augmenting glandular secretion. Axon reflexes and substance P also increase glandular secretion in the nose,[216] adding to the view that sensory neuropeptides play a key role in regulating both the output and composition of the secretions. A number of mediators and neurotransmitters affect nasal secretion.[44, 224, 266, 287] Neurotransmitters such as acetylcholine and substance P and inflammatory mediators such as histamine, bradykinin, 5-hydroxytryptamine, leukotrienes, and prostaglandins are known to increase nasal secretions.

MICROVASCULAR LEAKAGE AND PLASMA PROTEIN TRANSUDATION

Plasma exudation has long been known to be a cardinal factor in inflammation. A role for exuded plasma proteins and peptides in rhinitis is supported by data indicating that plasma exudation is a better correlate of disease activity than is the presence of individual inflammatory mediators.[214] Inflammatory mucosal provocation produces exudative responses without disrupting the epithelial lining and without increasing the airway tissue penetration of luminal substances.[106, 130, 179] It seems likely that this exudative response serves as a primary mucosal defense mechanism to permit immunoglobulins, kinins, coagulation peptides, complement components, and other proteins to operate at the mucosal surface of the nasal airway. If this becomes exaggerated, then symptomatic rhinitis results.

The increase in vascular permeability is restricted to venules, especially postcapillary venules. On mucosal provocation with inflammatory stimuli, the venules respond promptly with extravasation of plasma. Exudated plasma then distributes in the submucosal interstitial spaces of the airway and is then slowly cleared by the lymphatic system, although some reabsorption into the airway microvessels also occurs. A more important route for the clearance of extravasated plasma is across the epithelial lining, where admixtures with the mucosal secretions occur. The mechanism of exudation is due to gaps that form in the endothelium. The gaps are thought to result from an active change in the configuration of endothelial cells.[154, 182–184] Plasma extravasation into the interstitial space increases the hydrostatic pressure, and this exerts a compressive effect on the epithelial cells. This results in transient separation of tight junctions, allowing lumenal entry of exudate along a pressure gradient.

Postcapillary venules have a superficial location in the mucosa and, apart from being somewhat larger, are morphologically similar to capillaries. Studies undertaken in rats show that postcapillary venules have a continuous endothelium ensheathed by a continuous basal lamina. Fenestrations have been found in some of the endothelial cells. Adjacent endothelial cells are joined by tight junctions consisting of discontinuous strands[35] that are susceptible to the effects of inflammatory mediators. Furthermore, the nerves in the nasal mucosa act differently on the postcapillary venules in order to facilitate plasma exudation.[190] The permeability of venules in nasal mucosa is increased by irritants acting via sensory neurones.[177] This effect may be produced either through a central neural reflex, associated with efferent parasympathetic cholinergic neurotransmission, or via antidromic release of neuropeptides from sensory neurons, although this axonal pathway has not been clearly demonstrated in humans.

The role of sensory nerves in causing plasma exudation has been clearly documented in several animal studies. In rats, nasal challenge with capsaicin induces plasma exudation mediated via type C fibers.[176] This is believed to be due to the release of sensory neuropeptides, such as substance P, neurokinins, and CGRP. In contrast, nasal challenge with capsaicin in humans has no vascular effects, indicating that capsaicin-sensitive nerve fibers do not play a role in causing plasma leakage.[226] In animal models, nasal challenge with substance P induced plasma leakage that was inhibited by pretreatment with capsaicin or substance P antagonist.[176] Consistent with this, studies undertaken in humans have demonstrated the presence of receptors for substance P, NKA, and CGRP in the nasal mucosa.[33, 34] Substance P has also been recovered in increased amounts in nasal lavage fluid following nasal allergen challenge.[202] Thus the role of neural pathways in causing plasma leakage in allergic rhinitis remains unclear.

Like histamine, other inflammatory mediators, such as bradykinin, PAF, and leukotrienes, can also increase microvascular permeability to macromolecules in the nose. The acute response to these mediators has been shown to involve interendothelial gap formation in postcapillary venules. In animals, mediator antagonists inhibit antigen-induced airway microvascular leakage. With inhalation of ovalbumin in sensitized guinea pigs, A-63162, a selective 5-lipoxygenase inhibitor, has been shown to inhibit airway microvascular leakage to a greater extent than air flow obstruction.[143] However, other than antihistamines, mediator antagonists have not proven to be effective at inhibiting plasma leakage in allergic rhinitis.

MEDIATORS

Identification of Mediators in the Upper Airways. In atopic subjects, nasal allergen challenge induces immediate itching, sneezing, and rhinorrhea, with nasal blockage developing a few minutes after challenge and persisting for up to 2 hours, depending on the strength of the allergen signal. During this immediate nasal response, release of mediators such as histamine, bradykinin, PGD_2, leukotriene C_4 (LTC_4) and leukotriene B_4 (LTB_4) has been demonstrated in nasal lavage fluid.[87, 200] These mediators are also found in increased amounts in lavage fluids in naturally occurring allergic rhinitis.[260] Increased recovery of bradykinin and histamine has also been demonstrated in the late phase of allergen-induced rhinitis.[201]

Mediator Relevance in Vivo. It is possible to explain many of the features of rhinitis on the basis of mast cell mediator release, in particular histamine, which is an important mediator in the pathogenesis of allergic rhinitis. The identification of histamine in nasal lavage following allergen challenge and the proven efficacy of oral antihistamines are strong evidence supporting a primary role for histamine in allergic rhinitis. Histamine has both direct and indirect nasal effects, inducing itching, sneezing, rhinorrhea, and transient nasal blockage following nasal insufflation. Like histamine, mediators such as bradykinin, PGD_2, and LTC_4 are also known to cause symptoms and signs of rhinitis[95, 135, 193] (Fig. 25–5). The involvement of nonhistamine mediators is strengthened by the incomplete therapeutic effect of antihistamines on nasal blockage in naturally occurring disease.[140]

MUCOSAL INFLAMMATION AND ALLERGIC RHINITIS

Allergic rhinitis is characterized by mucosal inflammation. Nasal biopsy studies in both seasonal and perennial allergic rhinitis identify a specific leukocytic accumulation within the nasal mucosa.

Immediate symptoms of rhinitis occur as a consequence of the IgE-dependent activation of nasal mucosal mast cells. Mast cell degranulation has been observed in nasal biopsies following local allergen challenge, and there is an increase in tryptase-containing mast cells within the nasal epithelium.[41, 104, 105, 218] There also occurs an increase in the number of metachromatic cells observed in nasal smears with features characteristic of basophils rather than mast cells.[209] It is the release of preformed and newly generated mediators from these cell populations, along with cell activation, that leads to the classic symptoms of nasal itch, sneeze, rhinorrhea, and nasal blockage, through an interaction with neural and vascular elements within the nose.[140]

With more severe and chronic disease, the mucosal swelling results in loss of sense of smell, impaired taste, impaired drainage of the sinuses predisposing to sinusitis, headache and a posterior nasal discharge, impairment of eustachian tube function, and in some individuals, sleep apnea. A further characteristic feature of allergic rhinitis is local eosinophilia, which is evident in both nasal lavage[36] and mucosal biopsies.[280] Although the precise mechanism of tissue eosinophilia is not clearly understood, it most likely results from a combination of increased eosinophil vascular adhesion and chemotaxis, increased bone marrow production, and prolonged survival.

In seasonal rhinitis, tissue eosinophilia is associated with local up-regulation of vascular cell adhesion molecule 1 (VCAM-1) expression in the endothelium. VCAM-1 binds to

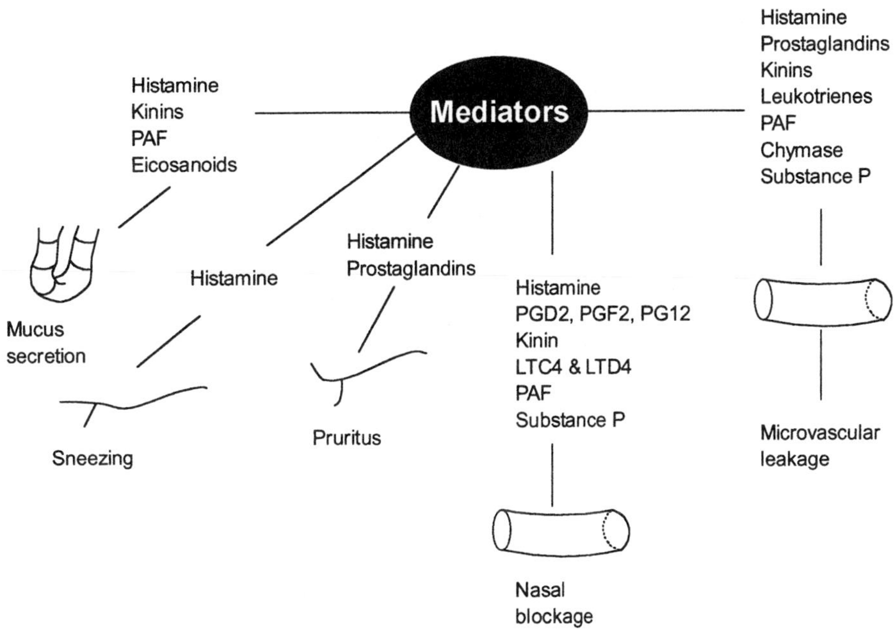

FIGURE 25–5. Interaction between mediators and neural and vascular structures in rhinitis. (From Busse WW, Holgate ST (eds): Asthma and Rhinitis. Blackwell Scientific Publications, Boston, 1995, p 1249. Reprinted by permission of Blackwell Science, Inc.)

the β_1 integrin ligand VLA-4 (CD49d/CD29) on eosinophils, as well as on basophils and lymphocytes, and is required for their transendothelial migration into tissues. Although eosinophils are also present in perennial allergic disease, in this form, there is more of a mixed leukocyte population, including neutrophils, expressing the cell surface marker, lymphocyte function–associated antigen 1 (LFA-1), within the tissues.[194] In addition to VCAM-1 up-regulation, there is also enhanced expression of the constitutively expressed cell adhesion molecule (CAM), intercellular adhesion molecule 1 (ICAM-1).[194] ICAM-1 binds to LFA-1 or MAC-1 expressed on the surface of the leukocytes. The expression of the endothelial adhesion molecules is regulated by the local synthesis and release of cytokines, in particular tumor necrosis factor-α (TNF-α) and interleukin 4 (IL-4).[235] Studies have colocalized these cytokines in a preformed state to tissue mast cells.[61] The activation of mast cells, by the cross-linkage of cell surface IgE following allergen exposure in a sensitized individual, not only leads to the release of the classic granule-associated preformed mediators, including histamine, tryptase, and heparin, and the newly formed eicosonoids, but also several cytokines. There is direct evidence for immunologic IL-4 release from purified human mast cells in vitro[61] and indirect evidence for TNF-α release from nasal mast cells.[63] Furthermore, in situ hybridization studies demonstrated preferential mRNA expression for IL-4 and IL-5 during the late phase at 24 h. following nasal allergen challenge,[98] supporting a role for Th2-type cytokines in the pathogenesis of allergic rhinitis.

DIAGNOSIS

History. The diagnosis of allergic rhinitis is based on a thorough history of exposure to allergens and symptoms related to this exposure. It is one disease in which identification of specific triggering factors, coupled with appropriate environmental manipulation, can have a dramatic impact. It is necessary for a physician seeing many patients to know not only the nature of the allergic disease but also the distribution of allergens in the environment and the methods used for investigation of particular allergen exposure. Although much is known about the seasonal variation in aerobiology, the local distribution of allergens must be known for each region separately to understand local factors that may be important in causing nasal allergies. Questionnaires have been found to be useful when taking a history. About 75% of children whose parents both suffer from the same allergic disease become allergic before school age.[159] Heredity is therefore of importance for predicting whether rhinitic symptoms are of allergic origin. History of other allergic diseases is also a predictor of allergy as a cause of rhinitis.

LABORATORY TESTS

Peripheral Blood Count. A moderate eosinophilia (> 10%) may be present, especially during the offending pollen season. But marked allergic symptoms can occur in its absence.

Total Serum IgE. A measurement of total serum IgE by radioimmunosorbent methods or enzyme methods (ELISA) may help to differentiate allergic from nonallergic rhinitis in questionable cases.

Skin Prick Test. Skin prick tests remain the most useful method of establishing specific causative allergens. This test is less helpful before the age of 3 because skin reactivity is reduced in very young children.

Radioallergosorbent Test. Methods of measuring specific IgE antibodies against a large number of allergens are available. The correlation of the findings of radioallergosorbent tests (RAST) with those of skin prick tests for pollens is approximately 80%. The main advantages of this method are the lack of any risk to the patient, lack of dependence on skin reactivity, and stability of antigen in the solid-phase state. The present drawbacks include lack of immediate available results, increased expense, and reduced sensitivity compared with that of skin prick testing. They can be helpful in patients with severe atopic dermatitis, poor skin reactivity, or enhanced skin reactivity (dermographism) or in patients being treated with long-acting antihistamines.

Nasal Provocation Test. Nasal provocation tests involve direct application of allergen to the nasal mucosa and observing the patient for signs and symptoms of rhinitis. This method is occasionally helpful when skin prick tests do not correlate with the history of rhinitis. Unlike bronchial challenge, there is no standardized protocol for nasal challenge, and outcome is measured by a variety of techniques. Allergen can be delivered using a dosimeter or a hand-held pump spray. In general, patients record their symptoms of itching, sneezing, rhinorrhea, pain, and nasal blockage during challenge period on separate rating scales. Objectively, changes in nasal airway resistance or airway caliber can also be measured.[224]

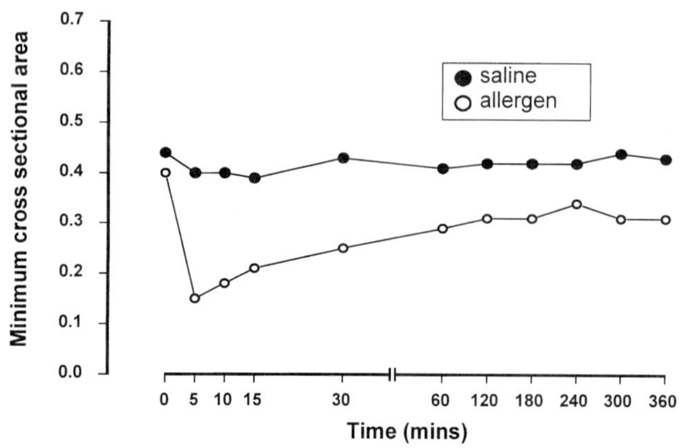

FIGURE 25–6. Changes in nasal airway caliber following allergen and saline challenge in subjects with seasonal allergic rhinitis. This illustration shows significant decrease in nasal airway caliber 5 to 10 minutes postchallenge (early response) and continuation of this response up to 6 hours.

Nasal Airway Resistance. In view of physiologic variation between both nostrils due to the nasal cycle, it is advisable to undertake bilateral nasal challenge using allergen and matched placebo on two occasions separated by at least 2 weeks. Nasal airway resistance (NAR) is measured before and after each challenge, at the time points indicated, by active posterior rhinomanometry using a rhinomanometer. Nasal resistance to air flow is calculated from measurements of nasal air flow and transnasal pressure (resistance = pressure/flow). There is one pressure gradient across the nose that generates the air flows through the two nasal passages. In the nose, the relationship between pressure and flow is complex due to turbulent air flow, and a plot of pressure against flow is curvilinear. It is therefore necessary to define the point on the curve where resistance is measured, which is usually 75 pascal (Pa) for posterior rhinomanometry. NAR may be automatically computed by an on-line microprocessor from simultaneous measurement of air flow through the nose and the transnasal pressure over four nasal cycles employing measurement of flow at a constant 75 Pa transnasal pressure differential. For this measurement, subjects sit with a clear airtight plastic face mask held over the nose and mouth. The face mask is attached to a pneumotachograph to monitor nasal air flow while breathing quietly through the nose with the mouth closed. The transnasal pressure is derived from measurement of pressure external to the nostrils and pressure within the oropharynx through a fine bore silicon tube placed over the tongue and held through sealed lips. This method of measurement of NAR has a coefficient of variation of repeated measurements of about 10.7% if done in trained subjects.[224]

Nasal Airway Caliber. Acoustic rhinometry is a newly introduced method to assess the geometry of the nasal cavity. It is based on sound reflection analysis to provide an estimate of the cross-sectional area of the nasal cavity as a function of the distance from the nostril. The cross-sectional area at the inferior turbinates and the total volume of the nasal cavities can be measured sequentially to study the effect of nasal antigen challenge on nasal airway caliber. This instrument is sensitive enough to measure both early and continued nasal airway narrowing after allergen challenge (Fig. 25–6).

Nasal Lavage. Nasal lavage is used to collect fluid from the lining of the nose.[224] Subjects are instructed to tilt their neck backward about 30° from the vertical while in the sitting position, hold their breath, and refrain from swallowing. Two and a half ml of 0.15 M prewarmed saline is then instilled into each nostril. After 10 seconds, the subjects are asked to flex their necks and expel the mixture of mucus and saline into a collection vessel. Samples are immediately sieved to remove mucus and stored on ice until the conclusion of the experiments, when they can be used immediately or frozen at −70°C to await further analysis. The fluid can be used to analyze for the presence of several agents, including mediators, proteins, and cells.

Management

PATIENT EDUCATION

Perhaps the most crucial component of any patient therapeutic plan is the one most often neglected—patient education. It is important that patient educators spend some time with patients to review the plan of action, including discussion about the nature of their disease, proper use of medications, and potential side effects. Discussing these issues is important to improve patient compliance.

ALLERGEN AVOIDANCE

A great deal of knowledge has been gained regarding aeroallergens and their relationship to rhinitis. This is dealt with in more detail in a separate chapter, but it is helpful to highlight some basic aspects about aeroallergens in order to understand the rationale and methods to avoid these agents. Allergen avoidance is the preferred mode of management for allergic rhinitis caused by single agents, such as animal danders, localized insect debris, seeds, and vegetable gums. Although other allergens cannot be avoided completely, attempts can be made to reduce their exposure.

Indoor exposure to pollen and some fungal spores can be substantially reduced by keeping the windows and doors shut. In summer months, this is tolerable with the aid of an air conditioner. Since an air conditioner also creates a draft, some patients with vasomotor rhinitis may complain of worsening of their symptoms. If rhinitic patients wish to ascertain whether symptoms improve with air conditioning, spending several hours in an air-conditioned public building may help with the decision about buying this equipment for their home. Electrostatic filters have been found to be effective in removing pollen and larger fungal spores. Therefore, installing both an air conditioner and an electrostatic filter would be an effective way of minimizing pollens and large fungal spores inside the house. These measures, however, are not effective against house dust and indigenous fungi.

Another possible approach is to remove the patient from sources of exposure to causative allergens. This is particularly valuable in cases of occupational-related rhinitis, such as animal homes and zoos. In case of seasonal rhinitis, one other option would be to move away from the area of high pollen exposure to another geographic location where the pollen count is lower. However, sensitization to allergens in a new area is likely. Although temporarily effective, this option is not often practicable. Apart from avoiding specific allergens, it is also desirable to avoid irritants such as fumes, smoke, and certain perfumes, as these agents are known to induce nonspecific irritation of the inflamed nasal mucosa and thereby aggravate symptoms.

House Dust Mite Avoidance. Dust mites of the genus *Dermatophagoides* are the most important indoor allergens found worldwide in domestic dust samples.[145] Although there are about 10 species of the dust mite family Pyroglyphidae, four species have been identified to be important in causing dust allergy:[220] *Dermatophagoides pteronyssinus (Der p), Dermatophagoides farinae (Der f), Dermatophagoides microceras (Der m),* and *Euroglyphus maynei*. Most studies on dust mite allergy have concentrated on *Der p* since this is the most prevalent. The allergenic components of *Der p* (of which at least 12 have been identified) reside in the fecal particles, which are about 10 to 30 μm in diameter.[261] These large particles tend to settle rapidly following a disturbance[221] after being airborne for minutes only. However, once in contact with a moist mucosal surface, dust mite allergens are leached out within 30 seconds.[145] The amount of dust allergens needed for sensitization to induce rhinitis is not known. It also is not clear whether measurement of airborne or surface-settled allergens is more appropriate. Sensitization of the mucosa is probably enhanced by the proteolytic enzymatic properties of the major allergens *Der pI–Der pIV.*

Airborne levels are difficult to measure, being at the limit of detection by assays, unless carried out after a disturbance, such as vacuum cleaning. To implement measures to reduce dust mites, it is important to understand the distribution and biology of the domestic mites. The highest concentration of mites and their allergens is found in mattresses and bedding, carpets, and soft furnishings, as they feed on shed human skin scales.[220] Optimal growth of dust mites requires a warm humid atmosphere, with replication optimally occurring at 25 to 30°C and a relative humidity of 75% to 80%.[19] It takes about 4 weeks for an egg to mature to an adult mite, and each adult lives for about 6 weeks. During this period, a female mite lays 40 to 80 eggs. It has been estimated that each dust mite produces about 20 fecal pellets per day, and each pellet contains about 100 pg of *Der pI*.[267] Standardized methods to measure mite allergen exposure are essential for the assessment of exposure-response relationships in the sensitization and provocation of rhinitic symptoms. The most widely used methods are assays that detect *Der pI* allergen (ELISA).

Methods of Allergen Avoidance. Many studies and substantive data support an association between sensitization to dust mite allergens and bronchial asthma. A prospective study by Sporik and colleagues[255] has shown that exposure to more than 10 μg of mite allergen per gram of dust in early childhood is an important predictor for the development of asthma by the age of 11 years. However, there are no solid data regarding the correlation of specific mite levels with symptoms of rhinitis. Since the highest concentration of mites and their allergens is found in bedding and carpets, these represent the main targets for specific allergen reduction measures. Two studies have reported improvement in rhinitic symptoms with dust mite reduction measures. The first has shown that the use of a semipermeable bedding barrier system (Intervent) over the mattress, duvet, and pillows resulted in a 42% reduction in symptoms of rhinitis over a period of 6 weeks.[142] A second study has shown that the use of a benzyl benzoate acaricidal spray (Acarosan) treatment of soft furniture and carpets in all rooms resulted in a 30% reduction in rhinitic symptoms over a 52-week period.[161] Table 25–2 presents current strategies for reducing house dust mite exposure in the domestic environment.

Animal Allergen. Animal allergens are another important cause of allergic rhinitis in the domestic environment. A study by Wood and colleagues[297] has shown that about 40% of an asthmatic population had skin tests positive to cat and dog allergens, which were found in household dust from almost every home sampled. Other than cats and dogs, guinea pigs, hamsters, rabbits, rats, and mice are also kept as pets in homes, schools, and pediatric hospitals. Several major allergens have now been defined for cats *(Fel dI)*, dogs (multiple antigens), rats *(Rat nI, nII)*, mice *(Mus mI)*, and horses *(Equ cI, cII, cIII)*. For cats and dogs, the allergens are most localized to the saliva and pelt. For rats and mice, the allergenic component is found in the urine, and in horses it is in the pelt.

Immediate sensitivity to cats is well recognized among atopic patients. The major cat allergen *(Fel dI)* from skin and saliva is deposited on animal fur during grooming and

TABLE 25–2
CONTROL OF DUST MITES AT HOME

- Use house dust mite impermeable bedding system (Intervent or plastic cover) to encase mattress, duvet, and pillows.
- Remove carpets from bedrooms.
- Remove upholstered furniture from bedrooms.
- Wash bed linen every week at temperature of > 55° C.
- Vacuum carpets, curtains, and upholstered furniture at least twice a week.
- Control humidity (relative humidity < 50%). Keep bathroom windows open. Use a dehumidifier if necessary.

becomes airborne after drying. As the particle size of *Fel dI* is less than 5 μm,[174] unlike dust mite allergens, *Fel dI* remains airborne for several hours and adheres to walls, clothing, and other surfaces.[298] Patients typically allergic to cats report a rapid onset of symptoms after exposure. The most obvious technique to reduce airborne animal allergens is to remove them completely or keep them outdoors. It may take about 6 months or longer to totally remove *Fel dI* from the domestic environment.[296] It is also important to note that passive transfer of cat allergen into a house on the clothing of occupants or visitors can produce significant levels of allergens. If a pet cannot be removed, then the allergen exposure may be limited by confining the animal to one room or one part of the house, which should be accomplished by removing the carpet and soft furnishing in that particular area.[90] Washing a cat weekly also may be of benefit.[123] Clinical trials are needed to confirm the effectiveness of avoidance measures in reducing the symptoms of pet allergic rhinitis.

Cockroach. Cockroaches have now become a source of indoor allergen in areas of inner-city dwellings, especially in the United States and Africa. There are more than 50 species of cockroach, about 8 of which are associated with indoor allergy. At least two allergens have been identified and defined *(Bla gI* and *Bla gII)*.[223] There is now convincing evidence to support a role for cockroach allergy in asthma, but there are no similar studies in rhinitis. Moreover, no environmental control studies for cockroach allergens have been published, and thus no clear guidelines established for cockroach eradication. Despite the use of pesticides, reinfestation often occurs.

Other Allergens. Many other indoor allergens (feathers, other mites, fungi, various insects, other mammals) could contribute to rhinitis. The difficulty in interpretation of skin prick test results and the lack of standardized good quality allergen extracts make it difficult to study the allergic diseases induced by these agents. The importance of these allergens may be relevant in an individual case, but their relative importance in rhinitis remains to be assessed.

PHARMACOTHERAPY

Allergen avoidance, especially of house dust mite, does not totally abolish nasal symptoms, and best measures may only achieve about 30% to 40% reduction in nasal symptoms. As a consequence, one has to turn to medical treatment. This treatment is based on the understanding that allergic rhinitis is characterized by the release of inflammatory mediators causing early and late symptoms (see Fig. 25–4). In rhinitis, treatment can be directed at a number of targets. It can be directed to reduce the tissue response nonspecifically at the end organ, including vasoconstriction with α-agonists and blocking the end-organ effects of locally released inflammatory or neuronal mediators at specific receptors, such as histamine, leukotrienes, and acetylcholine. Treatment also can be directed against differing aspects of mucosal cell infiltration and cell activation, such as cytokine synthesis, receptor inhibitors, or cell adhesion molecule expression.

Vasoconstrictors (End-Organ Directed Treatment). Adrenergic decongestant drugs are used to lessen nasal blood flow, reduce capillary and venular pressures, and thereby reduce nasal blockage.[185] Both α_1 and α_2 receptors are involved in the mediation of these responses. Drugs belonging to this class can be administered either topically or systemically and are efficacious by both routes.[286] Although both groups of drugs reduce vascular engorgement, α_2-agonists reduce nasal mucosal blood flow by about 40%, whereas α_1-agonists have little effect on nasal mucosal blood flow.[16, 39] It follows that selective α_1-agonists would be appropriate as decongestant agents since they constrict sinusoids but minimally affect mucosal blood flow. Comparative studies using the two groups of α-agonists reveal that the duration of action of α_1-agonists is much reduced in the nose.[38, 39] The imidazole group of α_2-agonists (e.g., oxymetazoline) has been widely used, despite the potential local side effects. However, this group of drugs is not recommended for prolonged topical regular use since these drugs may in turn lead to rhinitis medicamentosa and do not relieve the symptoms of itch, rhinorrhea, and sneeze. Topical decongestants are often used either intermittently to facilitate sleep during rhinitic exacerbations or as a regular treatment on a short-term basis to reduce nasal congestion and permit the introduction of other topical therapy, such as nasal corticosteroids.

Antihistamines (Specific Receptor Antagonism). Antihistamines are discussed in greater detail in a separate chapter. Since histamine is considered the predominant nasal mediator in rhinitis, H_1 antihistamines are the major oral therapy, particularly with the advent of the newer nonsedating H_1-receptor antagonists, such as terfenadine, astemizole, loratadine, and cetirizine. The new generation of antihistamines has largely replaced the more traditional sedative antihistamines, such as chlorpheniramine maleate. When compared with placebo, regular treatment with H_1-receptor antagonists, such as terfenadine 60 mg twice daily or 120 mg daily, astemizole 10 mg daily, or cetirizine 10 mg daily, significantly reduces nasal symptoms, particularly sneezing, itching, and excessive nasal secretion.[67, 141, 229, 293] The effect of oral antihistamines on nasal blockage is less marked and variable. Several comparative studies between these differing antihistamines show comparable clinical efficacy at standard clinical doses.[66, 170, 301] In general, subjects with perennial rhinitis exhibit a slow response to treatment when compared with those with seasonal allergic rhinitis. This has been attributed to the chronicity of the disease process in the perennial form of allergic rhinitis.

Somnolence is a major complaint in many patients taking oral antihistamines. Other side effects include nervousness, excitation, insomnia, dizziness, tinnitus, and blurred vision. Gastrointestinal symptoms of nausea, vomiting, and constipation are also recognized. Sedation was a common side effect of the first generation of antihistamines. However, the newer drugs not only are more selective but also do not cross the blood-brain barrier and therefore are less sedative. There have been reported cases of serious cardiac arrhythmias with overdose of terfenadine and astemizole, especially when taken together with drugs that interfere with hepatic metabolism.[138] These antihistamines are safe when taken at standard clinical doses and without such interacting drugs as erythromycin or fluconazole.

This group of drugs is not effective in relieving nasal blockage, which is not unexpected since mediators such as kinins, PGD_2, and leukotrienes C_4 and D_4 are also known to increase nasal airway resistance and on a molar basis bradykinin and PGD_2 are more potent than histamine in inducing vascular changes in the nose.[95, 225] There are no specific PGD_2 receptor or kinin receptor antagonists available for use in clinical practice, although new drugs are in clinical trials. A single dose of the LTD_4 receptor antagonist (ICI 204, 219) has been reported to reduce acute seasonal ragweed pollen exposure-induced nasal blockage, sneezing, and rhinorrhea.[93] Specific inhibition of rhinorrhea can be achieved with the antimuscarinic agent ipratropium bromide, but this drug has no effect on nasal blockage or sneezing.[56]

Studies have also been undertaken with the H_1 antihistamines azelastine and levocabastine administered topically. Administered in this way, antihistamines are also effective against nasal pruritus, sneezing, and rhinorrhea, and these effects are comparable to those of oral antihistamines and topical steroid budesonide.[277] However, in common with oral route, they are not particularly effective against nasal blockage. Since antihistamines have little effect on nasal blockage, clinical studies have been undertaken using combinations of decongestants such as pseudoephedrine with antihistamines. Some of these studies have shown improvement in nasal air flow following treatment.[136, 257] The main disadvantage of using this approach is the side effects of pseudoephedrine, which cause insomnia and restlessness in up to 30% of patients.[136]

Anti-Inflammatory Treatment. Inhibition of cell influx or mediator release would be expected to provide a greater symptomatic relief than does antagonism of the end-organ effects of a single mediator; future options for this may include specific targeting against cell adhesion molecules or cytokines. Three classes of drug treatment can be considered under this heading: sodium cromoglycate and nedocromil sodium, corticosteroids, and immunotherapy. Although β-agonists effectively inhibit immunologically stimulated human mast cell degranulation,[75] in clinical practice their intranasal administration in rhinitis achieves little benefit. This may relate to their vasodilator property limiting efficacy by increasing nasal resistance, to the predominant presence of basophilic cells in nasal scrapings that are unresponsive to β-agonists, or to down regulation of β_2-receptor responsiveness on nasal mast cells in rhinitis.[75] As sodium cromoglycate is also ineffective in limiting immunologically stimulated basophil degranulation[288] but is partially effective in relieving nasal symptoms, including nasal blockage, the lack of a therapeutic response to β-agonists is probably not related to mediator release from basophils.

Responsiveness of the rhinitic airways to sodium cromoglycate in rhinitis varies and is more efficacious in patients who fulfill the following criteria: (1) nasal eosinophilia, (2) obvious allergic etiology, (3) predominant symptoms of rhinorrhea and sneezing, (4) young age, (5) shorter duration of disease, and (6) absence of nasal polyps.[198] Nedocromil sodium, a drug reported to be more potent than sodium cromoglycate on inflammatory cell activation in vitro, has also been assessed in the treatment of seasonal rhinitis and found to be comparable to cromoglycate. Regular treatment with sodium cromoglycate compares favorably with H_1 antihistamines,[206] and one study revealed benefits similar to those of immunotherapy.[17] One drawback of the antiallergic drugs is the necessity to administer them four times daily. However, this group of drugs causes very few mild local adverse effects, with sneezing, stinging, burning, and irritation reported by less than 10% of patients.

Corticosteroids are the most potent pharmacologic medication available for the treatment of allergic rhinitis. In the case of perennial allergic rhinitis, this medication is the single most effective and acceptable medication for long-term therapy. Oral, subcutaneous, and topical corticosteroids are effective in relieving all the nasal symptoms of rhinitis, including nasal blockage. The potential adverse effects of prolonged systemic administration of corticosteroids and the limited morbidity of allergic rhinitis dictate that topical administration is the preferred route of administration. The principal use of oral corticosteroids is in patients with total nasal obstruction where oral decongestants or antihistamines are not effective and in whom topical corticosteroids cannot be applied effectively. The development of a range of topical corticosteroids has dramatically reduced the need for systemic corticosteroid treatment. When compared with placebo, several topical corticosteroid preparations, including betamethasone, dexamethasone, beclomethasone dipropionate, flunisolide, budesonide, triamcinolone, and fluticasone propionate, have been found to offer considerable benefit. Used on a regular basis, the clinical efficacy of topical corticosteroid therapy exceeds that of antihistamines, decongestants, or sodium cromoglycate.[134, 156, 288]

When given as a regular treatment, corticosteroids are known to inhibit the migration of mast cells into the nasal mucosa and the appearance of basophilic cells in nasal secretions,[127, 208] reduce nasal mucosal eosinophil numbers,[57, 156] inhibit basophil-histamine release,[242] and modulate arachidonic acid metabolism in basophils and eosinophils.[47] Topical corticosteroids have also been shown to reduce mediator release in allergic rhinitis via reducing the number of mast cells in nasal mucosal epithelium.[219] After symptom control is attained, the maintenance dosage can usually be reduced. The main adverse effects are local and include sneezing, stinging, and burning. Epistaxis occurs in less than 5% of patients. Localized infections of the nose and pharynx with *Candida albicans* or ulceration of the nasal mucosa occurs rarely. Systemic steroid effects are not reported when recommended doses are used.

Immunotherapy. The first prophylactic treatment for allergic rhinitis was specific immunotherapy, which has been shown to be effective in optimal conditions.[59, 60] This mode of therapy appears to be valuable in patients with severe rhinitis who have not responded well to other treatments.[279] Although the safety of immunotherapy has been questioned and led to a reduction in its use in the United Kingdom,[85] if used under well-defined and safe conditions, this mode of therapy has been effective in pollen-induced rhinitis and has cellular effects comparable to those of corticosteroids. Immunotherapy reduces mast cell numbers in nasal epithelial brushings and eosinophils in nasal washings,[87, 97, 117, 210] and it also modifies the T-lymphocyte response following allergen inhalation.[97, 234]

RECOMMENDATIONS FOR IMMUNOTHERAPY

- Allergen immunotherapy should be used on a routine

basis only in patients with seasonal allergic rhinitis who have failed to respond adequately to antiallergic drug.

- Immunotherapy should be administered only in hospitals or specialized offices or clinics with easy access to resuscitation facilities. Patients should be kept under observation for 60 minutes after each injection.
- The use of immunotherapy in children requires specialist assessment since the disease shows a natural tendency toward improvement as children grow older.

Prognosis

Seasonal allergic rhinitis is a chronic, recurring condition. The expression of symptoms depends both on environmental exposure and intrinsic host responsiveness. Symptom patterns fluctuate throughout life; childhood symptoms often diminish during puberty and might return in the third or fourth decade. Pregnancy is often associated with a period of quiescence, and symptoms can be aggravated by menopause. Asthma with varying severity can develop in about 3% to 10% of patients with hay fever.

Summary

With the improved understanding of the pathogenesis of allergic rhinitis, it should be possible to apply a rational treatment approach to achieve symptom control in patients suffering with either seasonal or perennial allergic rhinitis in whom there is no nasal structural abnormality.

NONALLERGIC RHINITIS

Since there is no distinct boundary between health and disease, a considerable overlap exists between healthy subjects and symptomatic rhinitic patients. It also has been difficult to develop methods to discriminate the nonallergic rhinitic from normal healthy subjects. Subjects with chronic and perennial nasal symptoms are included in this category (see Table 25–1). It is estimated, however, that about 5% to 10% of the general population suffers from nonallergic rhinitis, many of whom have symptoms daily, with no seasonal pattern. In comparison to allergic rhinitis, the majority of patients with the nonallergic form develop this condition in adulthood.[263] On the other hand, only about 8% of patients under the age of 20 years have nonallergic chronic rhinitis. The term vasomotor rhinitis has been commonly used to describe nonallergic chronic rhinitis. It is now recognized that this term was misleading, as there are several conditions that might fit into this group of patients.

Symptoms

Symptoms of nonallergic rhinitis are similar to those of its allergic perennial counterpart—nasal symptoms on exposure to everyday stimuli and provoked by abrupt changes in the environment, including chemical irritants, tobacco smoke, perfumes, food, wine, cold air, spices, or sexual excitement. Many patients who experience nasal symptoms on exposure to these stimuli do not necessarily present with those symptoms, highlighting the overlap between healthy and symptomatic patients.

Diagnosis

The diagnosis of this condition is based on the exclusion of an allergic etiology. The best way to differentiate between nonallergic and allergic rhinitis is to perform specific skin and RAST tests. A good history is also invaluable in the diagnosis of this condition. In contrast with patients with perennial allergic rhinitis, the majority of subjects with nonallergic rhinitis are not able to identify specific stimuli responsible for their symptoms; even those who can will blame nonspecific stimuli, such as those mentioned previously. Patients with nonallergic rhinitis most frequently present with symptoms for the first time in adulthood. These patients have less association with other atopic diseases, such as asthma and eczema, and have a history of one or more episodes of sinusitis. Some patients with negative skin prick tests also may have allergy to allergens that cannot be tested by available techniques. Nasal challenge with histamine, methacholine, and capsaicin has been performed in order to discriminate between healthy persons and those with nonallergic rhinitis.[55, 81, 256] These studies do not clearly differentiate the two groups and therefore are not reliable in clinical practice. Further development of tests that can discriminate between these two conditions is needed.

Neoplasms, anatomic abnormalities, and rhinitis induced by excessive use of decongestants manifest with severe nasal obstruction and can be diagnosed by history and with the aid of nasal endoscopy. In cases with unilateral severe nasal obstruction, nasal neoplasm should always be included in the differential diagnosis. Table 25–3 lists some guidelines for differentiating between allergic and nonallergic types of rhinitis. Since 20% of the population at large is atopic, it is also possible to have a nonallergic form of rhinitis in someone with a positive family history of allergy. Even more difficult to diagnose with certainty is a nonallergic rhinitis together with a seasonal allergic rhinitis in the same person. Table 25–1 lists some of the causes of nonallergic rhinitis.

Pathogenesis

The pathogenesis of nonallergic rhinitis is not clearly understood. Mechanisms have mainly been sought in cases in

TABLE 25–3
DIFFERENTIATION OF ALLERGIC AND NONALLERGIC RHINITIS

	Allergic Rhinitis	Nonallergic Rhinitis
Patterns of symptoms	Seasonal or perennial	Perennial
Cause of symptoms	Specific allergen	Nonspecific agents
Age of onset	Younger (< 20 years)	Older (> 20 years)
Atopy	Present	Absent
Family history	Present	Absent
Specific tests		
IgE	Frequently raised	Normal
RAST	Positive for specific allergen	Negative

which the perennial symptoms are induced by a well-defined stimulus, including cold air, hot food, and drugs such as aspirin. Togias and colleagues[264] demonstrated that nasal challenge with cold, dry air induces release of histamine and PGD_2 in nasal lavage fluid, suggesting a mast cell–mediated mechanism of action. This stimulus also produced a late response characterized by the further release of histamine and TAME esterase activity. This model resembles allergen challenge in atopic subjects. In contrast with allergen challenge in atopics, pretreatment with a topical tricyclic antihistamine did not inhibit cold, dry air-induced nasal symptoms and the release of mediators; the reason is unclear. It is also not known whether mediator release occurs with natural exposure to cold air. Eating spicy foods may also induce rhinorrhea, a reaction that is neurogenic and inhibited by pretreatment with atropine or ipratropium bromide, pointing to a cholinergic mechanism.[228] Aspirin-sensitive patients show increased leukotrienes in nasal lavage following oral aspirin challenge.[108] This is explained by excessive generation of sulfidopeptide leukotrienes mediated by shifting the arachidonate metabolism to the 5-lipoxygenase pathway. The reasons for this are under intense investigation but are possibly related to inhibition of a down-regulating prostanoid, such as PGE_2.

Exposure to air pollutants may manifest as chronic rhinitis. On the other hand, pollen-induced rhinitis is characteristically seasonal in presentation. Air pollution research has focused principally on the lungs, and the nose was considered relatively unimportant. However, it is now known that the properties of the nose protect the lungs from air pollution, making the nose a potential target for pollution-induced damage. Exposure to air pollutants causes irritation, nasal blockage, and inflammation. Furthermore, preexisting disease may also affect an individual's response to pollutants, although this has not been studied in depth. Several agents are known to cause air pollution, and there is a particular interest in the relationship of ozone to respiratory diseases. Epidemiologic studies have not addressed the effects of ozone on the nose, indicating the need for more research as to whether air pollutants contribute to common nasal diseases. At least two thirds of patients with chronic rhinitis do not have a specific etiology, and air pollution may well have a role in their symptomatology. Table 25–4 outlines some of the common air pollutants.

It is not clearly understood whether nasal hyperreactivity exists in nonallergic rhinitis. Several studies have investigated the nasal response to various nonspecific stimuli.[55, 109, 256] Attempts to discriminate between patients and healthy subjects have led to conflicting results. As these investigations differ markedly in the provocation technique used, the methods used for assessing symptoms, and the selection of patients, comparison of studies is almost impossible. In conclusion, unlike allergic rhinitis, differentiation between nonallergic rhinitics and healthy subjects is not clear cut. Only in cases in which the symptoms are reproducible by a relevant stimulus in an experimental setting can specific pathophysiologic information be obtained.

TABLE 25–4
COMMON CAUSES OF AIR POLLUTION AND THEIR SOURCES

Common Air Pollutants	Source
Ozone	Secondary outdoor air pollutants, photocopiers, and electrical devices
Allergens	Dust mites, cats, rodents, and cockroaches
Sulfur dioxide	Coal-fired power plants
Tobacco smoke	Smoking
Formaldehyde	Glues and furnishings
Volatile organic products	Cleaning solutions and building materials (sick building syndrome)
Nitrogen oxides	Gas stoves and automobile exhaust
Bioaerosols	Buildings with water leaks and moist ventilation systems
Wood smoke	Wood stoves

Treatment

Since there is a general lack of knowledge regarding the pathogenesis of nonallergic rhinitis, treatment is mostly nonspecific and, in many cases, not very effective. Patients with a history of a predominant symptom of sneezing may benefit from antihistamine therapy.[294] The mechanism of this is unknown, as it is not understood how histamine release occurs in this group of patients. Patients with a history of a predominant symptom of nasal blockage may benefit from nasal decongestants, but these drugs are not recommended for prolonged use in view of local complications. Patients with excessive rhinorrhea have benefited from a topical anticholinergic agent, such as ipratropium bromide.[92, 162] This agent is also beneficial in a large number of elderly patients with nonatopic rhinorrhea. Vidian neurectomy is also useful in dealing with excessive rhinorrhea.[125]

Although the disease is nonallergic in origin, topical corticosteroids have been beneficial in this group of patients.[186, 189] However, in one comparative trial between atopic and nonatopic rhinitic subjects, it has been demonstrated that the majority of those responding to topical corticosteroids belonged to the atopic group.[251] Those patients who responded to topical steroids in the nonatopic group probably had underlying inflammation, whereas those who did not respond had other mechanisms to account for their symptoms. Nasal smears or secretions can be used to diagnose underlying inflammation. In this respect, the presence of eosinophilia is useful, especially as a favorable factor for the efficacy of topical nasal steroids.[251] Patients with the NARES syndrome, consisting of a nonallergic rhinitis with eosinophilia, are included in this group.

Several other agents also hold promise as therapeutic agents targeted against neural components. Capsaicin, an extract of red hot pepper, is known to inhibit sensory nerve activity. Repeated capsaicin pretreatment has been shown to inhibit airway vascular responses to mediator challenge in animal models.[175, 176] One study has demonstrated beneficial effects following repeated nasal capsaicin application in patients with severe chronic rhinitis.[167] Capsaicin is unpleasant to take, and ablation of sensory neurones may not be totally innocuous, since the long-term effects remain to be demonstrated. Alternative therapies might include peptide derivatives of neuropeptide Y or topical opioids, since both approaches may modulate cholinergic neurotransmission.[258] It could also be speculated that antagonists of substance P or CGRP may reduce glandular and vascular reactions secondary to sensory neural stimulation and local axon reflexes.

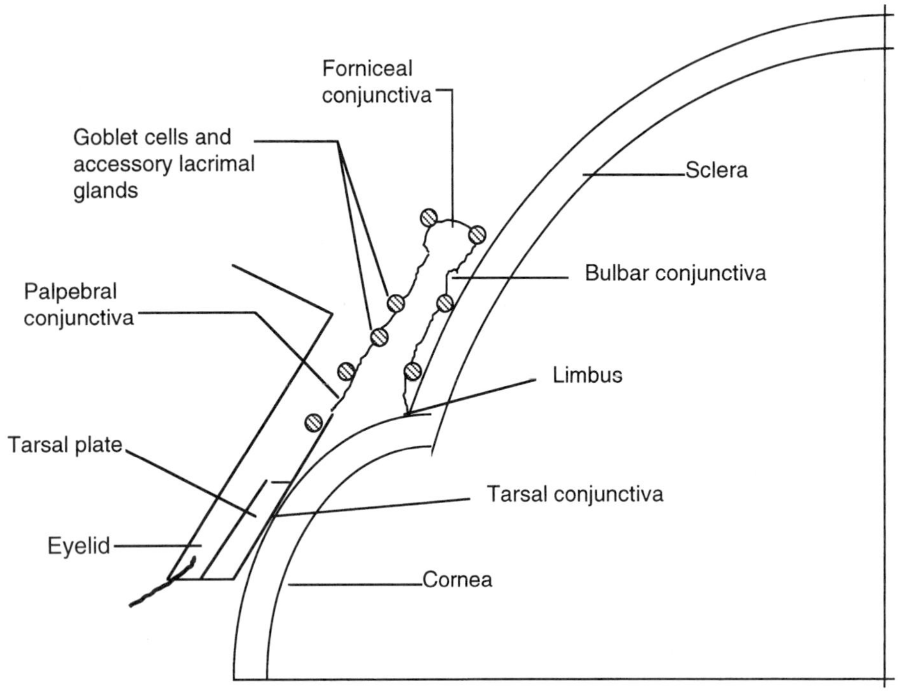

FIGURE 25–7. Schematic diagram to show the relations of the conjunctiva. (From Kanski JJ: Clinical Ophthalmology: Systematic Approach, 3rd edition. Butterworth-Heinemann Ltd, Oxford, 1994, p 72.)

Summary

Nonallergic rhinitis is a common condition, and there is considerable overlap between healthy subjects and patients. The etiology is not known in the majority of patients, and nonallergic rhinitis is diagnosed by exclusion of allergic rhinitis. The treatment options are limited in this condition and should be chosen based on the type of symptomatology. Topical corticosteroids are effective in cases in which nasal cytology shows eosinophilia. Overall, more research is required to discover new ways of treating what is often a very distressing condition.

OCULAR ALLERGY

Inflammation of the mucous membrane of the eye in response to airborne allergen is the basis of allergic conjunctivitis. The mast cell and its secreted products are central effectors in the inflammatory response, but the broad spectrum of disease is testament to the contribution of multiple factors. Symptoms of allergic conjunctivitis were first attributed to pollen exposure by Charles Blackley in 1873.[46] Subsequent disease classifications have been based solely upon clinical criteria. A history of atopy and signs of mild conjunctival injection, edema, and papillary hypertrophy are characteristic presentations. The spectrum of disease ranges from the common hay fever conjunctivitis, in which symptoms may be unpleasant but the signs are minimal or absent, to the less prevalent forms of allergic eye disease, atopic and vernal keratoconjunctivitis, which may threaten sight through corneal involvement. An appreciation of the normal conjunctival anatomy and histology are required before the pathophysiology of the disease state is understood.

ANATOMY

The conjunctiva is a mucous membrane that lines the undersurface of the eyelids. The tarsal portion overlies the tarsal plate, continues as the palpebral conjunctiva, and is reflected forward in the conjunctival fornices to cover the globe of the eye where it becomes the bulbar conjunctiva (Fig. 25–7). Anteriorly, the conjunctiva is continuous with the stratified squamous epithelium of the cornea. Posteriorly, it is continuous with the skin of the eyelid margin at the posterior border of the meibomian gland openings. Fibrous septa adhere the tarsal conjunctiva to the tarsal plate, restricting the conjunctival mobility at this site. The remaining conjunctiva is less firmly attached to the underlying tissue that allows for movement with the eyelids and eyeball. The tear film bathes the entire conjunctival and corneal surface, lubricating and protecting these structures but also exposing this large surface area to dissolved allergen. The inflamed conjunctiva may release cytotoxic mediators into the tears, where prolonged contact with the cornea may eventually result in scarring and visual loss.

Blood Supply

The blood supply to the conjunctiva is derived from the anterior and posterior conjunctival arteries arising from the anterior ciliary arteries and the palpebral arches of the eyelids. The conjunctival veins accompany the arteries and drain into the palpebral veins or the superior and inferior ophthalmic veins.

Lymphatic Drainage

The lymphatic drainage of the lateral conjunctiva is provided by the superficial parotid nodes. The medial conjunctiva drains to the submandibular nodes.

Nerve Supply

Sensory innervation of the conjunctiva is provided mainly by the nasociliary, frontal, and lacrimal branches of the ophthalmic division of the trigeminal nerve. The infraorbital branch of the maxillary division innervates a small area of the inferior fornix and palpebral conjunctiva.

Histology

The stratified columnar conjunctival epithelium (two to five cells thick) rests on a loose substantia propria of connective tissue that invests blood vessels, nerves, and smooth muscle. Goblet cells are commonly found lining crypts within the superficial epithelium and are more numerous at the caruncle and in the bulbar conjunctiva. Goblet cells secrete mucus directly onto the epithelial microvilli, reducing the surface adherence of potential pathogens and the surface tension of the precorneal tear film, which results in greater stability at the hydrophobic corneal interface. The accessory lacrimal glands are concentrated in the substantia propria of the forniceal conjunctiva, where they augment the tear production of the main lacrimal gland.

PATHOGENESIS OF ALLERGIC CONJUNCTIVITIS

An appreciation of the biology of the mast cell is central to the understanding of allergic eye disease. Activation of the mast cell leads to the release of both preformed and newly generated lipid-derived mediators of inflammation.[118] This response may be modulated by both mast cell location and phenotype, the latter defined by the neutral protease content. The mast cell acts in concert with the other cellular constituents of the conjunctival epithelium and substantia propria.

Mast Cell Activation and Conjunctival Hypersensitivity

Mast cell activation is dealt with more fully in an earlier chapter of this book. Briefly, multivalent antigen ligates cell surface IgE bound to the high-affinity IgE receptor FcϵR1. The resultant physical approximation of adjacent FcϵR1 receptors triggers exocytosis. Less commonly, mast cells may be activated through direct ligand binding to receptors at sites distinct from the FcϵR1.[78] This has been demonstrated for vasoactive intestinal polypeptide and somatostatin.[172] Coca and Cooke in 1922[82] first used the term atopy to describe individuals in whom this type of hypersensitivity reaction occurred in response to common allergens.

In addition to the immediate allergic response, also termed the early-phase response, several workers have described an IgE-mediated late-phase response in the skin,[253] nose,[212] and eye.[52] The conjunctival late-phase response appears clinically 6 to 12 hours after allergen exposure and is manifest as ocular discomfort and hyperemia. When provoked by allergen challenge, the response appears to be dose dependent.[52]

Inflammatory Mediators

HISTAMINE

Histamine is the central mediator of ocular allergic inflammation. Histamine bound to heparin is released with the newly generated products of membrane phospholipid metabolism, as well as a spectrum of cytokines upon activation of the mast cell. Histamine rapidly dissociates from heparin to act on cellular and tissue H_1, H_2, and H_3 receptors.[7, 289] Ligation of H_1 and H_2 receptors on blood vessels and capillaries leads to vasodilation and increased capillary permeability.[129] This is manifest in the eye by chemosis and hyperemia[2, 53, 79] reproducible by direct application of histamine to the conjunctiva.

Allergen challenge of atopic patients results in an increase in tear histamine and tryptase levels[70] in vernal keratoconjunctivitis (VKC). Histamine levels are not elevated in giant papillary conjunctivitis (GPC). The bimodal rise of histamine after allergen challenge suggests that histamine may play a part in the conjunctival late-phase response. This extends the scope of histamine activity to include participation in ongoing conjunctival inflammation. The absence of tryptase at this time implies involvement of cells other than mast cells, such as eosinophils and basophils, in the late-phase reaction.[25] Histamine activity is rapidly terminated by histaminase, which is found in the extracellular space and has also been detected in the tears of patients with VKC.[3]

PRODUCTS OF ARACHIDONATE METABOLISM

The cyclooxygenase pathway appears to be the principle route for metabolism of arachidonate liberated by phospholipase A_2 from cell membrane phospholipids in human mast cells. The products include PGD_2, PGE_2, and $PGF_2\alpha$, of which PGD_2 is produced in the greatest quantity. The topical application of PGD_2 to the eye leads to the signs of acute inflammation,[6] although the small quantities released relative to histamine imply that PGD_2 serves to augment the vasodilatory action of histamine. Metabolism of arachidonic acid by lipoxygenase yields the leukotrienes comprising the dihydroxy metabolite LTB_4 and the sulfidopeptide product LTC_4. Once released, LTC_4 is further modified extracellularly to form LTD_4 and LTE_4, which together with the parent molecule LTC_4 were formally known as the slow reacting substance of anaphylaxis (SRS-A).

Topical application of LTD_4 and LTC_4 increases microvascular permeability in hamster conjunctiva,[299] whereas LTB_4, LTC_4, LTD_4, and LTE_4 are chemotactic for eosinophils[254] and neutrophils[268] in human and rat conjunctiva, respectively. The sulfidopeptide leukotrienes have been demonstrated in the tears of patients who underwent conjunctival allergen challenge[43] and may play an important role in the recruitment of effector cells to the area of conjunctival inflammation.

PAF is a membrane-derived phospholipid released from mast cells, basophils, eosinophils, neutrophils, and endothelial cells. PAF is reported to be among the most potent eosinophil chemotactic factors isolated. Secretion of PAF from eosinophils in response to IgE implicates its participation in eosinophil-mediated inflammation. PAF is a potent mediator of vascular leakage, vasodilatation, and platelet aggregation. Topical conjunctival application of PAF in animals and some human studies reliably reproduced the clinical signs of allergic conjunctivitis.[121]

CYTOKINES—INTERCELLULAR MESSENGERS

T cells are an important source of multifunctional cytokines.[131, 158] The Th2 subset in particular[211, 292] may play an important role in conjunctival inflammation by releasing a selective panel of cytokines.[217] Interleukin-3 (IL-3), IL-4, and IL-10, act synergistically[18, 29] to promote mast cell growth; IL-4, IL-5, and IL-6 promote B-cell growth; IL-4 and IL-13 promote activation and isotype switching from IgG1 to IgE production; and IL-3 and IL-5 promote eosinophil growth, differentiation, and survival.[83] Th2 lymphocytes have been shown to accumulate in the conjunctiva of patients with VKC,[181] where significant increases in the tryptase only mast cells (MC_T) population are noted.[146]

The discovery that mast cells undergo IgE-dependent[150, 222] and IgE-independent[51] release of these mediators provides an alternative mechanism for a rapid, localized response to allergic inflammation prior to T-cell ingress. Il-4, Il-5, Il-6,[61, 62] TNF-α,[128, 284] GM-CSF,[295] and stem cell factor[171] have all been localized to human mast cells. TNF-α produced by skin mast cells induces the expression of E-selectin on vascular endothelial cells[160] and thus may contribute to the late-phase reaction by enhancing granulocyte, monocyte, and memory T-cell binding to activated endothelium.[42] Human mast cells have also been shown to induce IgE production in B cells,[120] providing an elegant positive feedback mechanism for the early induction and maintenance of the allergic response. Finally, release of chemokines (MCP-1, MCP-3, RANTES) may contribute to the late-phase accumulation of basophils, eosinophils, and mononuclear cells.

Neutral Proteases and Mast Cell Heterogeneity

Although proteases form the main secretory product of mast cells by weight,[282] little is known about their role in human allergic reactions. The three proteases isolated from human mast cells are tryptase,[245] chymase,[240] and carboxypeptidase A.[126, 148] A cathepsin G–like protease has also been localized to human mast cells.[241] All of the proteases are stored in a fully active form bound to proteoglycans within the mast cell granules. Tryptase, a tetrameric serine endoprotease, appears to be unique to mast cells[244] and forms the majority of the protease content. Tryptase may drive the inflammatory response by up-regulating ICAM-1 expression and Il-8 release from epithelial cells[166, 285] and indirectly recruit other cells. Tryptase has kininogenase activity, and the generation of bradykinin releases a powerful mediator of increased vascular permeability.[283] The ability of tryptase to cleave at Arg:Lys bonds confers a predicted ability to degrade the small neuropeptides vasointerstitial peptide and calcitonin gene-related peptide, providing a potential role in peptide regulation.

Chymase is a monomeric endoprotease bound to heparin within the mast cell granule. When injected intracutaneously in humans, it has been shown to induce a weal and flare response[132] and to produce vascular leakage when injected into rat skin.[247] These actions may synergize with those of histamine, bradykinin, and PAF to produce the marked vascular leakage that characterizes some ocular allergic states. Carboxypeptidase A is a matrix metalloproteinase bound to proteoglycan complexed with chymase. The pericellular metalloproteinases are known to play an important role in the regulation of cytokine receptors and adhesion molecules at the cell surface. Whether carboxypeptidase plays a part in immunoregulation alone or in concert with other proteases is unknown.

Cathepsin G is found in neutrophils and monocytes and has been demonstrated by dual immunohistochemistry in mast cells of the (MC_{TC}) type.[241] This serine protease may modulate the conjunctival inflammatory response by its ability to cleave IL-4, TNF-α,[273] and lymphotoxin[238] and may contribute to tissue destruction by degrading elastin[58] and fibronectin.[165]

Neutral proteases bestow phenotypic heterogeneity upon mast cells, although the biologic significance of this remains incompletely understood. Tryptase is common to all mast cells.[149] The additional presence of chymase, carboxypeptidase, and cathepsin G phenotypically distinguishes two distinct subtypes of mast cells. Those mast cells containing all four proteases (MC_{TC}) predominate in connective tissue and skin, whereas those containing tryptase alone (MC_T) prevail at mucosal surfaces.[149]

Conjunctival biopsies obtained from normal individuals and from patients with VKC, GPC, seasonal allergic conjunctivitis (SAC),[27] and atopic keratoconjunctivitis (AKC) show a predominance of the MC_{TC} phenotype, although the numbers of MC_T increase significantly in SAC, perennial allergic conjunctivitis (PAC), and AKC when compared with normal controls.[52] Phenotypic heterogeneity between mast cells may be associated with functional diversity, but multiple other factors also contribute to this.[119] For example, MC_{TC} from human skin and lung release a different spectrum and quantity of eicosanoids in response to stimulation with anti-IgE.[233] MC_{TC} from skin demonstrate secretory activity when stimulated by substance P and other neuropeptides, whereas MC_{TC} from intestinal mucosa do not.[76] When tarsal and bulbar biopsy specimens from the same eye are compared, the population of mast cells show different neutral protease expression independent of the disease state.[168] These observations support the view that the cellular microenvironment influences both the phenotypic and functional heterogeneity of the mast cell.

In vitro, cell coculture experiments with 3T3 fibroblasts[147, 168, 169] and stem cell factor produced by fibroblasts and other constitutive cells[23, 204] have demonstrated that immature mast cells can be induced to switch phenotype from MC_T to MC_{TC}. Whether this process occurs in vivo at tissue level or whether phenotypically committed progenitor cells are selectively stimulated to expand is unclear.

Other Cellular Constituents of the Ocular Allergic Response

Dendritic cells and small numbers of neutrophils and lymphocytes are found in the normal conjunctival epithelium. Mast cells are found in the submucosa, often associated with blood vessels and lash follicles.[196] Aggregates of lymphocytes, predominantly T cells, in the substantia propria cause small, discrete elevations of the conjunctiva that macroscopically resemble sago rice grains. These lymphoid follicles constitute the ocular mucosal-associated lymphoid tissue (MALT), are acquired from approximately 3 months after birth, and are found mainly in the lower fornix. The normal conjunctiva is devoid of eosinophils and basophils.[12] The presence of large numbers of eosinophils, particularly in the epithelium, is pathognomonic of VKC.[15, 116] Plasma cells in the substantia propria secrete dimeric IgA associated with a single J chain that stabilizes the molecule.[265] The polymeric Ig receptor mediates the transcytosis of this complex through the cytoplasm of the epithelial cells.[252] Enzymatic cleavage at the apical surface releases the IgA dimer bound to the secretory component of the receptor. IgA protects mucosal surfaces by preventing bacterial, viral, and toxin adherence. Unique protective functions within the epithelium and substantia propria have also been proposed.[188]

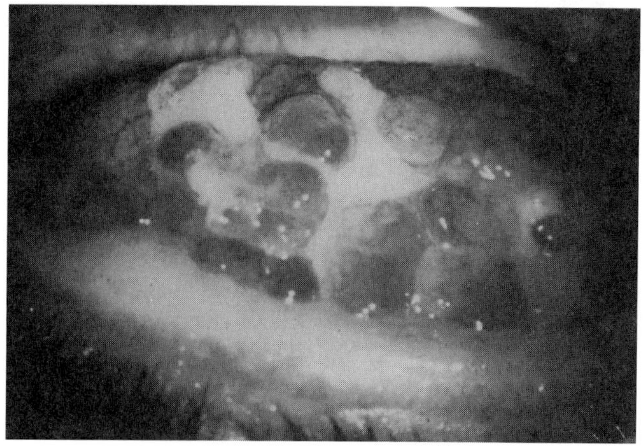

FIGURE 25–8. Giant papillae on the upper tarsal conjunctiva. (Courtesy of JI McGill.)

CLINICAL PRESENTATION OF ALLERGIC EYE DISEASE

Although the clinical manifestations of allergic conjunctivitis are protean, the cardinal symptoms of itch and mucus discharge and the presence of milky conjunctival edema and papillae are characteristic. Although the features are typically bilateral, they may be asymmetrical, reflecting the local nature of the response to conjunctival allergen. Airborne, wind-dispersed pollens are ubiquitous, and symptoms coincide with the release of particular pollen classes throughout the summer. Patients often have identified an antigenic source. Although less common, perennial symptoms reflect continual exposure to antigen and typify perennial allergic conjunctivitis and the atopic states of VKC and AKC. A comprehensive history should be taken, including a personal and family history of allergy and all current or prior treatment. The use of a detailed questionnaire to augment the history has been advocated by some centers.[74] The majority of diagnoses are arrived at after examination of the patient, although ancillary tests are occasionally required. Conjunctival biopsy and tear mediator assay remain principally in the domain of research, but skin prick testing and examination of conjunctival cytology are easily performed in the office and often yield significant results.

Examination of the patient should include a systemic review, with particular focus on eliciting other signs of atopy, such as dermatitis and asthma. The visual acuity should be determined first. A bright pen torch or the equivalent is essential for the ocular examination. A glass rod or equivalent should be available to evert the upper eyelid. The use of a slit lamp biomicroscope is advantageous, as it enables manipulation of the light source and allows for up to ×40 magnification of the image, which is particularly useful when examining the cornea. Examination of the eyelids may reveal swelling, eczema, or blepharitis, a common cause of ocular irritation, particularly in AKC. Small quantities of thin, clear mucus in the lower conjunctival fornix are not abnormal, but variations from this should be noted. A healthy lid margin tear strip is of particular importance, as patients with dry eye syndrome often experience more marked symptomatology. Conjunctival follicles are usually present, particularly in the lower fornix, but the presence of large numbers of follicles are pathologic and often indicate an infective process. Papillae may be present but should be smaller than 0.3 mm in diameter. Those between 0.3 mm and 1.0 mm are macropapillae. Those greater than 1.0 mm in diameter are termed giant papillae and are typical of VKC and GPC (Fig. 25–8).

The cornea should be examined carefully before the use of any topical preparations, as these often have transient mild toxic effects that alter the corneal surface characteristics. Fluoroscein 1% drops highlight defects in the surface epithelium when viewed through either the cobalt blue filter of the slit lamp or a separate filter attached to the pen torch. The principal types of allergic conjunctivitis are SAC, PAC, VKC, AKC, and GPC.

SEASONAL AND PERENNIAL ALLERGIC CONJUNCTIVITIS

Pollen is the sensitizing allergen in seasonal (hay fever) allergic conjunctivitis. Produced in large amounts in the summer first by trees and then by grass, ragweed, and fungi, grains of pollen are blown onto the conjunctiva, where they dissolve into the tear film. The transmucosal presentation of this allergen by professional antigen-presenting cells (dendritic cells) to T helper cells is particularly adept at eliciting IgE production by B lymphocytes, sensitizing the individual. Subsequent diffusion of pollen across the epithelium to bind to the surface IgE of mucosal mast cells leads to a classic type I hypersensitivity reaction, first described by Coombs and Gell[86] and recognized clinically as the early-phase response.[144] This same mechanism is responsible for the milder symptoms of perennial allergic conjunctivitis triggered by chronic exposure to the house dust mite, *D. pteronyssinus, D. farinae,* or animal dander. Tear levels of allergen-specific IgE[13] exceed those in plasma.[88] Further evidence for a localized type I reaction forming the basis of allergic conjunctivitis came from the reproducibility of the response when serum from an affected individual was transferred to a nonaffected individual subsequently challenged with allergen.[13] The demonstration of eosinophils in conjunctival scrapings[8] and in the epithelium and substantia propria of conjunctival biopsy specimens taken from affected patients[26] provides histologic support for this mechanism.

A reliable model of allergic conjunctivitis has been produced by the conjunctival allergen challenge studies of Abelson.[5] This technique has been used to investigate the conjunctival late-phase response. Atopic patients have elevated concentrations of histamine and eosinophil cationic protein in their tears 6 hours after challenge with allergen, with a corresponding cellular infiltrate of mast cells, eosinophils, and neutrophils on conjunctival biopsy.[25] This initial work suggests that this process may explain the transition from acute type I reactions seen in allergic conjunctivitis to the chronic inflammation seen in vernal and seasonal atopic disease.

Clinical Features

The cardinal symptom of allergic conjunctivitis is itch, with tearing usually minimal. The common association with allergic rhinitis leads to use of the term rhinoconjunctivitis. Exacerbation of symptoms occurs with peaks of pollen release and in locations with high pollen counts and high atmospheric pollution.[278] Signs are usually bilateral. The eyelids may be swollen, but marked edema is atypical and usually reflects digital rubbing or, less commonly, the presence of animal dander within the conjunctival sac. Hyperemia of the conjunctival vessels leads to a pink rather than red appearance, with the latter more suggestive of an infective etiology. Eversion of the upper eyelid may reveal a mild papillary reaction; if excess mucus has been produced, this is present as a thin stringy mass in the lower fornix.

Diagnosis

The diagnosis is often made on the history alone, as signs may be subtle or absent. Ancillary tests are not usually required, although skin prick tests may confirm sensitization to *D. pteronyssinus* or *D. farinae*. Patients with seasonal allergy may test positive to several pollen subtypes.[279] Conjunctival scrapings represent a convenient method to examine the conjunctival cytology for eosinophils, although a negative test result does not rule out the diagnosis.[8]

Management

The avoidance of allergen is the single most effective strategy to reduce symptoms. Warm, dry days with bright sunshine stimulate pollen release, and this pollen tends to accumulate in grassy open spaces or parks, particularly when the wind speed is low. Sunglasses offer some protection against wind-blown allergen, although inevitably variable quantities will deposit in the tear film. Conjunctival allergen can be washed out by using lubricating eye drops as required.

Topical vasoconstrictors may be used to relieve mild symptoms, although rebound vasodilation and limited efficacy necessitate their combination with other agents. Many patients progress to the use of mast cell stabilizing agents. In the United Kingdom, topical cromolyn sodium 2% or 4% is widely prescribed by both family practitioners[248] and ophthalmologists for use in SAC and PAC. The principal action of cromolyn sodium is thought to be prevention of mast cell degranulation. When comparisons are made between mast cells of different phenotype or tissue origin, however, this response is highly variable.[77] Other studies have demonstrated the ability of cromolyn sodium to block the activation of neutrophils, eosinophils, and monocytes[157] and to prevent the release of neuropeptides from nerve terminals,[112] which may contribute to a dampening of both the early- and late-phase response. Clinically, the drug has been shown to be highly effective in reducing symptoms,[14] particularly when used regularly rather than as required.[155] Response to treatment, however, often takes several days.

Newer mast cell stabilizing agents are gaining prominence. Lodoxamide 0.1% ophthalmic solution has been shown to be effective and safe in the treatment of VKC, AKC, and GPC. Further trials are awaited to determine the efficacy and safety of lodoxamide in SAC and PAC, although early work has yielded encouraging results.[73] The potent ability to block conjunctival mast cell mediator release in animal experiments[153, 300] and experience of safe, effective use in VKC, AKC, and GPC suggest that lodoxamide may become an important addition to the first-line treatment options for allergic conjunctivitis.

Nedocromil sodium is a pyranoquinoline and has been demonstrated to reduce mast cell, eosinophil, and neutrophil activation in the lung.[65] The twice daily application of nedocromil sodium 2% has produced significant improvements in both objective and subjective measures of SAC with minimal adverse effects.[49, 192] Although ocular H_2 receptors have been demonstrated,[7] no benefit from their manipulation has been described.

The efficacy of topical H_1 antagonists, however, has been demonstrated. Levocabastine 0.05% has a rapid mode of onset and has been shown to be as effective as cromolyn sodium[80] and in some cases superior to cromolyn sodium[24, 89, 151] in alleviating the symptoms of SAC. Levocabastine appears to be safe and well tolerated[151] in the treatment of SAC and to lack central effects, principally drowsiness.[20] Abelson[1] noted decreased hyperemia, suggesting the possible location of H_1 receptors on conjunctival blood vessels.

Oral antihistamines may be effective in the treatment of rhinoconjunctivitis, but systemic adverse effects, particularly drowsiness, tend to limit their use. Topical corticosteroids are linked with raised intraocular pressure, cataract formation, immunosuppression, and delayed wound healing. For these reasons, their use for the essentially self-limiting condition of allergic conjunctivitis is strongly discouraged. The effectiveness of topical corticosteroids in the management of other allergic eye disease has been partly responsible for stimulating the interest in developing nonsteroidal anti-inflammatory agents for the topical treatment of allergic conjunctivitis. Ketorolac tromethamine blocks the cyclooxygenase arm of the arachidonate metabolism pathway, reducing the production of prostaglandins. Ketorolac tromethamine 0.5% ophthalmic solution used four times daily for 1 week significantly improved conjunctival inflammation and itch in SAC[262] and proved superior to placebo for overall therapeutic effect.[30] Other nonsteroidal agents under investigation include flurbiprofen.[45]

VERNAL KERATOCONJUNCTIVITIS

Markedly different characteristics of VKC predominate with geographic variation. In the Western Hemisphere, the condition is rare and strongly associated with other atopic disease. In the Mediterranean, Middle East, and North Africa, the incidence is higher, with limbal inflammation more common and blinding corneal complications rare.[271] Onset usually occurs in the first decade of life,[37, 69] and the condition is usually bilateral. Boys are affected more frequently than are girls, although this bias is reduced with a later age of onset. The peak in incidence between April and August led Saemisch in 1872[236] to name the condition spring catarrh. The definitive clinical finding is that of raised, flat-topped cobblestone papillae on the upper tarsal plate. Visual loss occurs through corneal scarring.

Histopathologically, VKC is characterized by the presence of increased numbers of mast cells, eosinophils, basophils,[11] and Th2 lymphocytes[181] in the substantia propria. The MC_{TC} phenotype predominates, and a large proportion of these cells have been observed to be degranulated,[149] with both mast cell and eosinophil granules found free in the intercellular matrix.[270] The localization of mast cells, basophils, and eosinophils to a hyperplastic conjunctival epithelium occurs in VKC, but not in normal controls.[11] This correlates with the finding of increased levels of IgE,[32] IgG,[31] eosinophil major basic protein (EMBP),[276] eosinophil cationic protein (ECP),[237] and histamine[3] in the tears. The superficial location of these cells can be detected clinically by the presence of eosinophils in conjunctival scrapings.[181] These findings suggest that mast cells, eosinophils, and T cells are central effectors in the pathology of VKC. Activated Th2 cells and mast cells produce a variety of cytokines capable of stimulating mast cell and eosinophil proliferation and degranulation.

The transition from an acute to a chronic inflammatory response leads to the deposition of collagen and large amounts of hyaline fibrous tissue to form the characteristic flat-topped papillae of the tarsal plate.[173] VKC is sight threatening because corneal inflammation and the formation of a vernal plaque, particularly in the presence of superimposed bacterial, viral, or fungal infection, may lead to irreversible scarring. Initial damage to corneal epithelial cells leads to microerosions, which may coalesce to form an ulcer. The deposition of fibrin-like material[231] can lead to the formation of the vernal plaque. The cationic products of eosinophil degranulation have been implicated as instrumental in this process and in contributing to a second wave of mast cell degranulation, prolonging the inflammatory response. EMBP demonstrates a dose-related cytotoxicity for human respiratory and intestinal epithelial cells[122] and delays corneal epithelial wound healing in vitro.[269] ECP has also been shown to be toxic to epithelium.[281] Both EMBP and eosinophil peroxidase stimulate secretion of histamine from rat mast cells.[110, 137]

Clinical Features

The intense itching associated with VKC can be both distressing and disabling. Photophobia and blepharospasm result from corneal involvement, and the production of a viscid, tenacious mucus may combine to impair lid opening in the morning. Conjunctival vasodilation lends a pink rather than red hue to the eye. Eversion of the upper eyelid reveals the characteristic flat-topped cobblestone papillae. Chronic disease rarely leads to conjunctival cicatrization, although if present, fine reticular scarring indicates the subepithelial fibrosis. The corneal changes have been reclassified by Buckley[69] (Table 25–5).

TABLE 25–5
CLASSIFICATION OF THE CORNEAL CHANGES SEEN IN VERNAL KERATOCONJUNCTIVITIS

1. Punctate epithelial keratitis
2. Epithelial macroerosion
3. Vernal plaque
4. Subepithelial scarring
5. Peripheral corneal deposits (pseudogerontoxon)

From Buckley RJ: Vernal keratopathy and its management. Trans Ophthal Soc UK 101:234–238, 1981.

The progression from microcorneal erosions to shield ulcer formation is associated with the deposition of inflammatory material, resulting in the vernal plaque (Fig. 25–9). The anterior surface of the plaque is hydrophobic, which disrupts the tear film. The posterior surface initially sits on and then coalesces with Bowman's membrane, so that lamellar dissection from the cornea after this stage leaves a ring-shaped scar. The toxic constituents of the plaque prevent reepithelialization of the cornea and are resistant to removal by nonsurgical means. Plaques usually form in the upper pole of the cornea from contact with the inflamed upper tarsal conjunctiva. This location spares the visual axis, and a surprisingly high visual acuity can often be maintained.

Inflammation at the limbal conjunctiva results in regional hyperemia. Gelatinous swellings known as vegetations may occur at any meridian and, although usually discrete, may blend to form an arc or ring associated with limbal papillae. The accumulation of eosinophils and their products in chalky white marks at the limbus are known as Trantas' dots and are seen in both VKC and AKC.

Management

Prophylactic treatment consists of avoiding locations with high pollen counts and animals. A clean air-conditioned

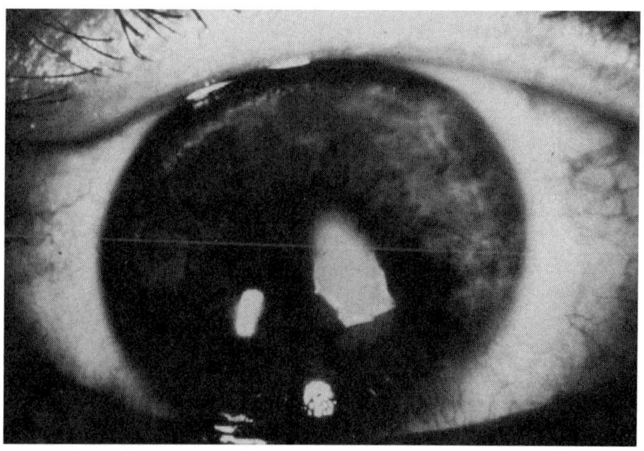

FIGURE 25–9. Corneal shield ulcer with overlying plaque characteristic of vernal disease. (Courtesy of JI McGill.)

environment is ideal. Patients whose condition warrants their admission to the hospital often improve markedly for this reason alone. Lubricant eye drops can be used to wash out allergen and to supplement the tear film in cases of vernal plaque. Cromolyn sodium 2% or 4% has been used for many years with significant therapeutic efficacy in the treatment of mild or moderate VKC. Adverse effects are mild and uncommon, and corticosteroid requirements are reduced.[100, 103, 114] Lodoxamide 0.1% has been shown to be equal or superior to cromolyn sodium in relieving the primary symptoms of VKC[71] to improve corneal epithelial disease.[239] Nedocromil sodium 2% has been shown to be more effective than placebo in the treatment of VKC, including reducing the number of inflammatory cells obtained from the tears of patients after treatment.[50] The majority of patients, however, will require topical corticosteroids at some stage to control episodes of severe ocular inflammation or as an adjunct to surgical intervention.

Corticosteroid use is usually confined to high-dose pulse regimens, as adverse effects include cataracts, glaucoma, and exacerbation of corneal herpes virus or bacterial infection. To avoid these effects, steroid-sparing agents are under trial. Cyclosporine is an immunomodulator that prevents the clonal expansion of T cells by blocking Il-2 synthesis.[243] Topical cyclosporine 2% has been used successfully in the short-term treatment of severe VKC. Significant reductions in both symptoms and signs, including keratopathy, were observed, with no detectable systemic absorption of the drug or effect on renal or hepatic function.[40, 48, 246] Nonsteroidal anti-inflammatory agents have also shown promise. For example, suprofen administered topically[68] and aspirin are effective adjuncts for therapy.[4] Medical treatment of vernal plaque is unsatisfactory, and delay in resolution may result in stimulus deprivation amblyopia in young children. Lamellar dissection of the plaque is usually carried out under general anesthesia and promotes more rapid corneal reepithelialization than does medical treatment alone.[69]

TABLE 25–6
COMPARISON BETWEEN VKC AND AKC

VKC	AKC
Onset in first decade of life	Adult onset
Spontaneous remission not uncommon	Chronic disorder; spontaneous resolution rare
Usually the first manifestation of atopic disease	Often follows other atopic diatheses, such as atopic dermatitis and asthma
Peak onset in the spring	Perennial symptoms with no pattern of seasonal onset
Bilateral ocular involvement	Also bilateral
Characterized by the production of thick mucus	Tenacious mucus combines with xerosis to disrupt the tear film
Giant cobblestone papillae present on upper tarsal conjunctiva rare	Less pronounced papillary hypertrophy affecting inferior palpebral conjunctiva
Fine reticular scarring of upper tarsal conjunctiva rare	Conjunctival scarring and foreshortening of the inferior fornix; disease progression leads to fibrous band formation between the tarsal and bulbar conjunctivae
Vernal shield ulcer formation on the cornea	Corneal ulceration often complicated by superimposed infection
Cataract formation may result from topical steroid use	Cataract formation may arise de novo prior to iatrogenic causes
Raised specific IgE in tears	Raised specific IgE in serum
Conjunctival biopsies demonstrate raised numbers of mast cells and eosinophils in the epithelium and substantia propria; raised T-lymphocyte count in substantia propria	Raised mast cells, T cells, macrophages, and antigen-presenting cell count in the epithelium; increased mast cell, B-cell, T-cell, and macrophage counts in the substantia propria

ATOPIC KERATOCONJUNCTIVITIS

AKC is an uncommon, symmetrically bilateral disease that usually manifests in the second decade of life and tends to run a protracted course (Table 25–6). Symptoms are perennial, with exacerbations unconfined to particular seasons. AKC represents the ocular manifestation of atopic disease and usually develops after the onset of one of a number of other atopic diatheses, such as allergic asthma, hay fever, or rhinitis. The presence of atopic dermatitis is required to form the clinical triad of chronic conjunctivitis, keratitis, and dermatitis first described by Hogan[139] to establish the diagnosis. Corneal involvement in the inflammatory process may be markedly worsened by infection, particularly reactivation of herpes simplex keratitis, which may eventually result in loss of sight.

Histopathologic evidence suggests the contribution of both type I (immediate) and type IV (delayed) hypersensitivity reactions to the inflammatory process in AKC. Total serum IgE and total and pollen-specific tear IgE levels are elevated in AKC when compared with controls, but reported symptoms and clinical signs appear to have no relationship to tear IgE concentration.[272] The normal conjunctival epithelium is devoid of mast cells, eosinophils, activated T cells ($CD25^+$), and Th2 cells; their presence in association with increased numbers of antigen-presenting macrophages and dendritic cells[115] is a striking feature of AKC. The inflammatory cell infiltrate in the substantia propria comprises Th2 cells, cytotoxic T cells, B cells, and large numbers of mast cells.[115, 197] The latter are predominantly of the MC_{TC} phenotype,[52] and many are degranulated.

The recruitment of eosinophils to trigger a second wave of mediator release is a disease mechanism common to both AKC and VKC. A major difference, however, is the subepithelial fibrosis and resultant conjunctival foreshortening seen in the former disorder, which is similar to that seen in ocular pemphigus[230] and implicates fibroblast activation. The keratitis produced in AKC is often complicated by superinfection, particularly with herpes simplex virus.[99] With time, vascularization of the corneal stroma may result in the deposition of lipid to produce a lipid keratopathy.

The hereditary nature of the condition, strong association with other atopic disease, and cellular profile described previously implicate a genetically determined abnormality of T-cell regulation as the underlying pathologic abnormality of AKC. The emerging role of the mast cell in the local regulation of conjunctival inflammation and deficiencies in our understanding of the pathways of cellular communication serve to emphasize the complexities of this disease process.

Clinical Features

The typical AKC sufferer is an adult male with a strong family and personal history of atopy.[152] Tuft and colleagues[272] reported that 95% of AKC patients in their study had eczema and 87% had asthma, and the association with atopic dermatitis is well documented.[232] Patients complain of ocular itch, foreign body sensation, and mucus discharge. Symptoms may be attributed to a variety of allergens, including animal dander, dust, and food. The presence of a keratitis leads to more intense ocular discomfort and photophobia. Examination of the eyelids may reveal eczema. More commonly, lid margin blepharitis is present, with collarettes of skin squames around the lash bases, loss and misdirection of the lashes, and irregularities of the lid margin.

A papillary conjunctivitis predominantly affects the lower tarsal plate. The upper tarsal giant papillae of VKC are not seen, but fine reticular scarring may be visible in both the upper and lower tarsal conjunctiva. Inflammation of the limbal conjunctiva and Trantas' dots are present less frequently than in VKC. The most significant finding of conjunctival foreshortening usually affects the lower fornix and may be associated with adhesion of the tarsal to the bulbar conjunctiva known as symblepharon.[113, 207] The resultant loss of goblet cells and accessory lacrimal glands exacerbates corneal disease by leading to xerosis and tear film instability. Paradoxically, displacement of the lacrimal punctum produces epiphora. Other corneal findings, including keratoconus and neovascularization, may contribute to visual loss. Cataracts may form as a result of corticosteroid treatment, but the characteristic anterior subcapsular shield cataract is typical of AKC and occurs independently of corticosteroid use (Fig. 25–10).

Treatment

Control of environmental factors to reduce allergen exposure is as important as in vernal disease. Lid margin blepharitis should be treated by regular cleansing, supplemented by topical antibiotic if necessary. Long-term treatment with a systemic tetracycline is helpful in resistant cases. Lubricant eye drops ameliorate the tear film disruption caused by blepharitis and serve as replacement therapy in cicatrization of the conjunctiva. The role of eye drops in irrigating allergen has been previously discussed. The use of cromolyn sodium 2% and 4% regularly has been shown to be effective in reducing both subjective and objective scores of disease activity.[152, 207] Lodoxamide 0.1% has also been demonstrated to be efficacious and safe in early studies.[107] Oral antihistamines are commonly prescribed, particularly when the patient is symptomatic from dermatitis.

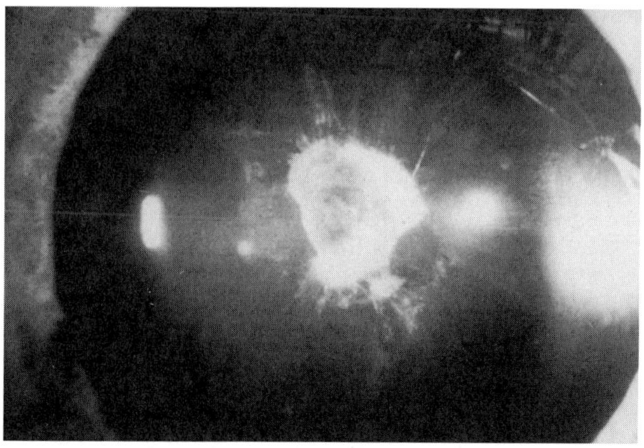

FIGURE 25–10. Anterior subcapsular shield cataract of atopic keratoconjunctivitis. (Courtesy of Annette Bacon.)

Topical corticosteroids are best administered by high-frequency pulse therapy. If prolonged treatment is necessary, care must be taken to detect and treat adverse effects. The use of topical corticosteroids should be reserved for the ophthalmologist, as reactivation of herpes simplex keratitis or local immunosuppression leading to superadded bacterial infection may lead to permanent corneal scarring and potentially loss of the eye.

Cyclosporine has been used as a steroid-sparing immunomodulator in VKC with promising results, but use in AKC remains anecdotal.[113] The systemic nature of atopic disease is highlighted by the hyperimmunoglobulinemia E syndrome, in which patients with defective neutrophil chemotaxis, chronic atopic dermatitis, and keratoconjunctivitis often prove resistant to both topical and oral corticosteroids. Two such patients underwent a trial of plasmapheresis[21] and showed dramatic improvement. The potential adverse effects of the treatment, however, weigh heavily against its use in less aggressive disease. Prompt recognition of herpes simplex and bacterial keratitis is essential so that treatment is not delayed after cultures have been obtained. Many patients, however, will not escape stromal scarring from complications or the primary disease process. These patients and a proportion of patients with keratoconus may require corneal transplantation, although vascularization or infective keratitis greatly reduces the surgical success rate.

GIANT PAPILLARY CONJUNCTIVITIS

GPC affects patients whose ocular surface is disrupted by the presence of a foreign body. The condition usually occurs in contact lens wearers[10] but has also been described in patients with corneal sutures[203, 259] and ocular prostheses.[180] GPC is not sight threatening but is increasing in frequency as contact lens wear becomes more commonplace. Contact lens intolerance may eventually become absolute, which has profound implications for individuals who lack an intraocular lens, as spectacle wear produces marked optical distortion. A mixture of chronic trauma and mucus adherence to the lens surface are likely etiologic agents in GPC. Lens polymers themselves appear to be inert. Biopsies of the upper tarsal conjunctiva performed by Allansmith and colleagues[11] revealed an influx of mast cells and to a lesser degree eosinophils in the conjunctival epithelium and increased numbers of neutrophils, mast cells, basophils, and eosinophils in the substantia propria compared with normals. These findings were less marked than those found in biopsies obtained from patients with VKC but support an immunologic mechanism as the basis of the disease pathophysiology. Other similarities between the two conditions include the deposition of EMBP in the upper tarsal conjunctiva[270] and the recovery of Charcot-Leyden crystal protein and IgG and IgE from the tears of patients with both conditions.[31, 32, 34] The levels of tear Charcot-Leyden crystal protein in GPC were low compared with VKC, where levels correlated with disease activity,[276] but both conditions appear to share eosinophil degranulation as a common characteristic. The most striking dissimilarity between VKC and GPC is the absence of corneal damage and thus blinding sequelae in GPC, which fundamentally reduces the disease morbidity.

Clinical Features

Ocular discomfort, itch, and pronounced mucus discharge are commonly reported by patients with GPC. Blurred vision usually occurs with excess mucus deposition on the contact lens surface; otherwise patients are visually asymptomatic. Symptoms may be relieved by removal of the lens, although this may exacerbate itching. There may be hyperemia of the bulbar and less commonly the limbal conjunctiva. A fine papillary reaction at both the upper and lower tarsal sites is common. Macropapillae precede the formation of giant papillae, which displace the former and are characteristically found on the upper tarsal plate.[10]

Management

Meticulous daily lens cleaning with the use of preservative-free reagents and regular papain protein digestion are primary strategies. Patients may benefit from changing to a different lens design or composition or using disposable lenses but ultimately may have to discontinue lens use altogether. Offending corneal sutures should be removed if possible. Preservative-free lubricant eye drops may be used to irrigate the eye. Trials are awaited to demonstrate the efficacy of cromolyn sodium, although preliminary work suggests a favorable response.[194] Nedocromil sodium 2% has been shown to decrease itch and upper tarsal mucus deposition when compared with placebo, although the response to treatment lost statistical significance after 4 weeks.[28] The use of topical corticosteroids is reserved for the rare patient who develops GPC from an ocular prosthesis. The troublesome but ultimately benign nature of the condition does not warrant the use of a potentially blinding drug.

FUTURE DIRECTIONS

Key areas for investigation include a more comprehensive understanding of mast cell gene regulation and cytokine expression in the normal and allergic state. Ultimately, the ability to regulate specific cytokine production should enable clinicians to interrupt the allergic process prior to the onset of damaging ocular sequelae, particularly in the case of VKC and AKC.

Topical immunomodulation with cyclosporine and other corticosteroid-sparing agents promises to reduce the high complication rates that accompany both short- and long-term corticosteroid use. Immunotherapy may complement the treatment of patients with a spectrum of allergic conjunctivitis. The low incidence of generalized anaphylaxis necessitates that this form of therapy be carried out in specialized centers with appropriate patient observation.[279] The infrequency of adverse effects and efficacy of both primary and booster therapy in atopic patients, however,[101, 227] suggests a promising future role of immunotherapy in the treatment of allergic conjunctivitis.

REFERENCES

1. Abelson MB, George MA, Schaefer K, et al: Evaluation of the new ophthalmic antihistamine, 0.05% levocabastine, in the clinical allergen challenge model of allergic conjunctivitis. J Allergy Clin Immunol 94(3):458–464, 1994.
2. Abelson MB, Allansmith MR: Histamine and the Eye. In Silverstein AM, O'Connor GR (eds): Proceedings of the 2nd International Symposium on the Immunology and Immunopathology of the Eye. Masson Publishing, New York, 1979, pp 362–364.
3. Abelson MB, Baird RS, Allansmith MR: Tear histamine levels in vernal conjunctivitis and other ocular inflammations. Ophthalmology 87:812–814, 1980.
4. Abelson MB, Butrus SI, Weston BA: Aspirin therapy in vernal conjunctivitis. Am J Ophthalmol 95:502–505, 1983.
5. Abelson MB, Chambers WA, Smith LM: Conjunctival allergen challenge: a clinical approach to studying allergic conjunctivitis. Arch Ophthalmol 108:84–88, 1990.
6. Abelson MB, Madiwale NA, Weston JH: The role of prostaglandin D_2 in allergic ocular disease. In O'Connor GR, Chandler JW (eds): Advances in Immunology and Immunopathology of the Eye. Masson, New York, 1995.
7. Abelson MB, Udell IJ: H_2-receptors in the human ocular surface. Arch Ophthalmol 99:302–304, 1981.
8. Abelson MB, Udell IJ, Weston JH: Conjunctival eosinophils in allergic ocular disease. Arch Ophthalmol 101:631, 1983.
9. Aberg N: Asthma and allergic rhinitis in Swedish conscripts. Clin Exp Allergy 19:59–63, 1989.
10. Allansmith MR, Korb DR, Greiner JV, et al: Giant papillary conjunctivitis in contact lens wearers. Am J Ophthalmol 83(5):697–708, 1977.
11. Allansmith MA, Baird RS, Greiner JV: Vernal conjunctivitis and contact lens-associated giant papillary conjunctivitis compared and contrasted. Am J Ophthalmol 87:544–555, 1979.
12. Allansmith MR, Greiner JV, Baird RS: Number of inflammatory cells in the normal conjunctiva. Am J Ophthalmol 86:250–259, 1978.
13. Allansmith MR, O'Connor GR: Immunoglobulins: structure, function and relation to the eye. Surv Ophthalmol 14:367–402, 1970.
14. Allansmith MR, Ross RN: Ocular allergy and mast cell stabilizers. Surv Ophthalmol 30(4):229–244, 1986.
15. Allansmith MR, Ross RN: Ocular allergy. Clin Allergy 18:1–13, 1988.
16. Anderson KE, Bende M: Adrenoceptors in the control of human nasal mucosal blood flow. Ann Otol Rhinol Laryngol 93:179–182, 1984.
17. Anderson NH, Jeppeson F, Schioler T, Osterballe O: Treatment of hay fever with sodium cromoglycate, hyposensitisation, or a combination. Allergy 42:343–351, 1987.
18. Arai K, Lee F, Miyajima A, et al: Cytokines: coordinators of immune and inflammatory responses. Annu Rev Biochem 59:783, 1990.
19. Arilan LG: Biology and ecology of house dust mites *Dermatophagoides* species and *Euroglyphus* species. Immunol Allergy Clin N Am 9:339–356, 1989.
20. Arriaga F, Rombaut N: Absence of central effects with levocabastine eye drops. Allergy 45(7):552–554, 1990.
21. Aswad MI, Tauber J, Baum J: Plasmapheresis treatment in patients with severe atopic keratoconjunctivitis. Ophthalmology 95(4):444–447, 1988.
22. Australian Bureau of Statistics: 1989–90. National Health Survey. Asthma and other respiratory conditions, Australia. Catalogue no. 4373. Commonwealth of Australia, Canberra, 1991.
23. Aye MT, Hashemi S, Leclair B, et al: Expression of stem cell factor and c-kit mRNA in cultured endothelial cells, monocytes and cloned human bone marrow stromal cells (CFU-RF). Exp Haematol 20(4):523–527, 1992.
24. Azevedo M, Castel-Branco MG, Oliveira JF, et al: Double-blind comparison of levocabastine eye drops with sodium cromoglycate and placebo in the treatment of seasonal allergic conjunctivitis. Clin Exp Allergy 21(6):689–694, 1991.
25. Bacon AS, Baddeley SM, Walters C, et al: The cellular infiltrate and tear inflammatory mediators of the conjunctival late phase response. Submitted.

26. Baddeley SM: Cellular Mechanisms in Allergic Eye Disease. University of Southampton, United Kingdom, 1994. Thesis.
27. Baddeley SM, Bacon AS, McGill JI, et al: Mast cell distribution and neutral protease expression in acute and chronic allergic conjunctivitis. Clin Exp Allergy 25:41–50, 1995.
28. Bailey CS, Buckley RJ: Nedocromil sodium in contact-lens-associated-papillary conjunctivitis. Eye 7(suppl 3):29–33, 1993.
29. Balkwill FR, Burke F: The cytokine network. Immunol Today 10(9):299–304, 1989.
30. Ballas Z, Blumenthal M, Tinkelman DG, et al: Clinical evaluation of ketorolac tromethamine 0.5% ophthalmic solution for the treatment of seasonal allergic conjunctivitis. Surv Ophthalmol 38(suppl):141–148, 1993.
31. Ballow M, Donshik PC, Mendelson L, et al: IgG specific antibodies to rye grass and ragweed pollen antigens in the tear secretions of patients with vernal conjunctivitis. Am J Ophthalmol 95(2):161–168, 1983.
32. Ballow M, Mendelson L: Specific immunoglobulin E antibodies in tear secretions of patients with vernal conjunctivitis. J Allergy Clin Immunol 66(2):112–118, 1980.
33. Baraniuk JN, Lundgren JD, Goff J, et al: Calcitonin gene related peptide (CGRP) in human nasal mucosa. Am J Physiol 258:L81–L88, 1990.
34. Baraniuk JN, Lundgren JD, Okayama M, et al: Substance P and neurokinin A (NKA) in human nasal mucosa. Am J Respir Cell Mol Biol 4:228–236, 1991.
35. Bartels H: Open junctions in the venular plexuses of the bronchial microcirculation. J Submicrosc Cytol 14:93–97, 1982.
36. Bascom R, Pipkorn U, Lichtenstein LM, Naclerio R: The influx of inflammatory cells into nasal washings during the late response to antigen challenge: effect of corticosteroid treatment. Am Rev Respir Dis 81:580–589, 1988.
37. Beigelman MN: Dystrophy of the corneal epithelium in vernal catarrh. Am J Ophthalmol 15(2):95–103, 1932.
38. Bende M, Anderson KE, Johansson CJ, et al: Vascular effects of phenylpropanolamine on human nasal mucosa. Rhinology 23:43–48, 1985.
39. Bende M, Loth S: Vascular effects of topical oxymetazoline on human nasal mucosa. J Laryngol Otol 100:285–288, 1986.
40. BenEzra D, Pe'er J, Brodsky M, Cohen E: Cyclosporine eyedrops for the treatment of severe vernal keratoconjunctivitis. Am J Ophthalmol 101:278–282, 1986.
41. Bentley AM, Jacobson MR, Cumberworth V, et al: Immunohistology of the nasal mucosa in seasonal allergic rhinitis: increases in activated eosinophils and epithelial mast cells. J Allergy Clin Immunol 89:821–829, 1992.
42. Bevilacqua MP: Endothelial-leukocyte adhesion molecules. Annu Rev Immunol 11:767–804, 1993.
43. Bisgaard H, Ford-Hutchinson AW, Charleson S, Taudorf E: Production of leukotrienes in human skin and conjunctival mucosa after specific allergen challenge. Allergy 40:417–423, 1985.
44. Bisgaard H, Romeling R, Mygind N, et al: Measurement of LTC_4 and histamine in nasal lavage fluid. In Mygind N, Pipkorn U (eds): Allergic and Vasomotor Rhinitis: Pathophysiological Aspects. Munskgaard, Copenhagen, 1987, pp 189–197.
45. Bishop K, Abelton NB, Cheetham J, et al: Evaluation of flurbiprofen in the treatment of antigen-induced allergic conjunctivitis. Invest Ophthalmol Vis Sci 31(suppl):487, 1990.
46. Blackley CH: Experimental researches on the causes and cure of Catarrhus Aestivus (hayfever or hay asthma). Ballieri, (ed). Tindall and Cox Ltd, 1873.
47. Blackwell GJ, Carmiccio R, Di Rossa M, et al: Macrocortin: a polypeptide causing the anti-phospholipase effect of glucocorticoids. Nature 287:147–149, 1980.
48. Bleik JH, Tabbara KF: Topical cyclosporine in vernal keratoconjunctivitis. Ophthalmol 98:1679–1684, 1991.
49. Blumenthal M, Casale T, Dockham R, et al: Efficacy and safety of nedocromil sodium ophthalmic solution in the treatment of seasonal allergic conjunctivitis. Am J Ophthalmol 113(113):56–63, 1992.
50. Bonini S, Barney NP, Schiavone M, et al: Effectiveness of nedocromil sodium 2% eyedrops on clinical symptoms and tear fluid cytology of patients with vernal conjunctivitis. Eye 6(6):648–652, 1992.
51. Bonini S, Bonini S: IgE and non-IgE mechanisms in ocular allergy. Ann Allergy 71:296–299, 1993.
52. Bonini S, Bonini S, Bucci MG, et al: Allergen dose response and late symptoms in a human model of allergy. J Allergy Clin Immunol 86:869–876, 1990.
53. Bonini S, Schiavone M, Centofanti M, et al: Conjunctival hyperresponsiveness to ocular histamine challenge in patients with vernal conjuncivitis. J Allergy Clin Immunol 89(1):103–107, 1992.
54. Borum P: Intranasal ipratropium: inhibition of methacholine induced hypersecretion. Rhinology xvi:225–233, 1978.
55. Borum P: Nasal methacholine challenge. J Allergy Clin Immunol 63:253–257, 1979.
56. Borum P, Mygind N, Drettner B, Malmberg H: Anticholinergic agents. In Mygind N, Weeke B (eds): Allergic and Vasomotor Rhinitis: Clinical Aspects. Munksgaard, Copenhagen, 1985, pp 151–158.
57. Boscomb R, Wachs M, Naclerio RM, et al: Basophil influx occurs after nasal antigen challenge: effects of topical corticosteroid pretreatment. J Allergy Clin Immunol 81:580–589, 1988.
58. Boudier C, Holle C, Bieth JG: Stimulation of the elastolytic activity of leukocyte elastase by leukocyte cathepsin G. J Biol Chem 256:10256–10258, 1981.
59. Bousquet J, Guerin B, Dotte A, et al: Comparison between rush immunotherapy with a standardized allergen and an alum aduved pyridine extracted material in grass pollen allergy. Clin Allergy 15:179–193, 1985.
60. Bousquet J, Maasch HJ, Hejjaoui A, et al: Double-blind, placebo-controlled immunotherapy with mixed grass pollen allergoids. III. Efficacy and safety of unfractionated and high molecular weight preparations in rhinoconjunctivitis and asthma. J Allergy Clin Immunol 84:546–556, 1989.
61. Bradding P, Feather IH, Howarth PH, et al: Interleukin-4 is localized to and released by human mast cells. J Exp Med 176:1381–1386, 1992.
62. Bradding P, Feather IH, Wilson S, et al: Immunolocalisation of cytokines in the nasal mucosa of normal and perennial rhinitic subjects. J Immunol 151(7):3853–3865, 1993.
63. Bradding P, Mediwake R, Feather IH, et al: TNFα is localised to nasal mucosal mast cells and is released in acute allergic rhinitis. Clin Exp Allergy 25(5):406–415, 1995.
64. Britton WJ, Woolcock AJ, Peat JK, Prevalence of bronchial hyperresponsiveness in children: the relationship between asthma and skin reactivity to allergens in two communities. Int J Epidemiol 15:202–209, 1986.
65. Brogden RN, Sorkin EM: Nedocromil sodium: an updated review of its pharmacological properties and therapeutic efficacy in asthma. Drugs 45(5):693–715, 1993.
66. Bruttman G, Arendt C, Bernheim J: Double-blind, placebo controlled comparison of cetirizine 2HCl and terfenadine in the treatment of perennial allergic rhinitis. Acta Therapeutica 15:99–109, 1989.
67. Bruttman G, Charpin D, Germonty J, et al: Evaluation of the efficacy and safety of loratadine in perennial allergic rhinitis. J Allergy Clin Immunol 83:411–416, 1989.
68. Buckley DC, Caldwell DR, Reaves TA Jr: Treatment of vernal conjunctivitis with suprofen, a non-steroidal anti-inflammatory agent. Invest Ophthalmol Vis Sci 27(suppl):29, 1986.
69. Buckley RJ: Vernal keratopathy and its management. Trans Ophthal Soc UK 101:234–238, 1981.
70. Butrus SI, Ochsner KI, Abelson MB, et al: The level of tryptase in human tears. Ophthalmology 97:1678–1683, 1990.
71. Caldwell DR, Verin P, Hartwich-Young R, et al: Efficacy and safety of lodoxamide 0.1% vs cromolyn sodium 4% in patients with vernal keratoconjunctivitis. Am J Ophthalmol 113:632–637, 1992.
72. Cauna N: Blood and nerve supply to the nasal lining. In Proctor DF, Andersen IB (eds): The Nose: Upper Airway Physiology and the Atmospheric Environment. Elsevier Biomedical Press BV, Amsterdam, 1982, pp 45–69.
73. Cerquerti PM, Ricca V, Tosca MA, et al: Lodoxamide treatment of allergic conjunctivitis. Int Arch Allergy Immunol 105:185–189, 1994.
74. Christiansen SC: Evaluation and treatment of the allergic patient. Int Ophthalmol Clin 28:283–293, 1988.
75. Church MK: Modulation of mast cell mediator secretion by drugs used in the treatment of allergic disease. In Holgate ST (ed): Mast cells, mediators and disease. Holgate Kluwer Academic Publishers, Amsterdam, 1988, pp 259–279.
76. Church MK, Benyon RC, Rees PH, et al: Functional heterogeneity of human mast cells. In Galli SJ, Austen KF (eds): Mast Cell and Basophil Differentiation and Function in Health and Disease. Raven Press, New York, 1989, p 161.
77. Church MK, Caulfield JP: Mast cell and basophil functions. In Holgate ST, Church MK (eds): Allergy. Raven Press Ltd, New York, 1993, pp 5–11.

78. Church MK, Lowman MA, Rees PH, Benyon RC: Plenary lecture. Mast cells, neuropeptides and inflammation. Agents Actions 27:8–16, 1989.
79. Ciprandi G, Buscaglia S, Pesce GP, et al: Ocular challenge and hyperresponsiveness to histamine in patients with allergic conjunctivitis. J Allergy Clin Immunol 91(6):1227–1230, 1993.
80. Ciprandi G, Cerqueti PM, Sacca S, et al: Levocabastine versus cromolyn sodium in the treatment of pollen-induced conjunctivitis. Ann Allergy 65(2):156–158, 1990.
81. Clement PAR, Stoop AP, Kaufmann L. Histamine threshold and nasal hyperreactivity in non-specific allergic rhinopathy. Rhinology 23:35–42, 1985.
82. Coca AF, Cooke RA: On the classification of the phenomena of hypersensitiveness. J Immunol 8(3):163–182, 1922.
83. Coffman RL, Carty J: A T cell activity that enhances polyclonal IgE production and its inhibition by interferon-gamma. J Immunol 136:949–954, 1986.
84. Cole P: Modification of inspired air. In Proctor DR, Andersen IB (eds): The Nose: Upper Airway Physiology and the Atmospheric Environment. Elsevier, Amsterdam, 1982, pp 351–375.
85. Committee on Safety of Medicine: Desensitization vaccines. Br Med J 293:948, 1986.
86. Coombs RRA, Gell PGH: Classification of allergic reaction responsible for clinical hypersensitivity and disease. In Gell C, Lachmann PJ (eds): Clinical Aspects of Immunology. Blackwell, Oxford, 1975, pp 761–782.
87. Creticos PS, Adkinson FN Jr, Sobotka AK, et al: Nasal challenge with ragweed in hayfever patients: effect of immunotherapy. J Clin Invest 76:2247–2253, 1985.
88. Dart JKG, Monnickendan M, Prasad J: Perennial allergic conjunctivitis: definition, clinical characteristics and prevalence. Trans Ophthalmol Soc UK 105:513–520, 1986.
89. Davies BH, Mullins J: Topical levocabastine is more effective than sodium cromoglycate for the prophylaxis and treatment of seasonal allergic conjunctivitis. Allergy 48(7):519–524, 1993.
90. DeBlay F, Chapman MD, Platts-Mills TAE: Airborne cat allergen (Fel dI): environmental control with the cat in situ. Am Rev Respir Dis 143:1334–1339, 1991.
91. Devillier P, Dessanges JF, Rakotosihanaka F, et al: Nasal response to substance P and methacholine in subjects with and without allergic rhinitis. Eur Res J 1:356–361, 1988.
92. Dolovich J, Mukherjee J, Salvatori VA: Intranasal ipratropium bromide to control the hypersecretion of vasomotor rhinitis: a dose response study. Am J Rhinology 3:221–224, 1989.
93. Donnelly A, Glass M, Muller B, et al: Leukotriene D_4 (LTD_4) antagonist ICI 204, 219 relieves ragweed allergic rhinitis symptoms. J Allergy Clin Immunol 91(1 pt 2):A474, 1993.
94. Donshik PC, Ballow M: Tear immunoglobulins in giant papillary conjunctivitis induced by contact lenses. Am J Ophthalmol 96(4):460–466, 1983.
95. Doyle WJ, Boehm BS, Skoner DP: Physiologic responses to intranasal dose-response challenges with histamine, methacholine, bradykinin and prostaglandin in adult volunteers with and without nasal allergy. J Allergy Clin Immunol 86:924–935, 1990.
96. Druce HM, Wright RH, Kossof D, Kaliner MA: Cholinergic nasal hyperreactivity in atopic subjects. J Allergy Clin Immunol 76:445–452, 1985.
97. Durham SR, Varney VA, Jacobson MR, et al: Effect of grass pollen immunotherapy on allergen-induced early and late nasal responses. J Allergy Clin Immunol 91:299, 1993.
98. Durham SR, Ying S, Varney VA, et al: Cytokine messenger RNA expression for IL-3, IL-4, IL-5 and granulocyte/macrophage-colony-stimulating factor in the nasal mucosa after local allergen provocation: relationship to tissue eosinophilia. J Immunol 148:2390–2394, 1992.
99. Easty D, Entwistle C, Funk A, Witcher J: Herpes simplex keratitis and keratoconus in the atopic patient: a clinical and immunological study. Trans Ophthalmol Soc UK 95:267–276, 1975.
100. Easty DL, Rice NSC, Jones BR: Clinical trial of topical disodium cromoglycate in vernal kerato-conjunctivitis. Clin Allergy 2:99–107, 1972.
101. Ebner C, Kraft D, Ebner H: Booster immunotherapy (BIT). Allergy 49:38–42, 1994.
102. Eccles R, Bend M, Widdicombe JG: Nasal blood vessels. In Mygind N, Pipkorn U (eds): Allergic and Vasomotor Rhinitis: Pathophysiological Aspects. Munksgaard, Copenhagen, 1987, pp 63–76.
103. El Hennawi M: Clinical trial with 2% sodium cromoglycate (Opticrom) in vernal keratoconjuncticitis. Br J Ophthalmol 64:483–486, 1980.
104. Enerback L, Pipkorn U, Granerus G: Intraepithelial migration of nasal mucosal mast cells in hay fever. Int Arch Allergy Appl Immunol 80:44–51, pp 1986.
105. Enerback L, Pipkorn U, Olafsson A: Intraepithelial migration of mucosal mast cells in hay fever: ultrastructural observations. Int Arch Allergy Appl Immunol 81:289–297, 1986.
106. Erjefalt I, Persson CGA: Allergen, bradykinin and capsaicin increase outward but not inward macromolecular permeability of guinea pig tracheobronchial mucosa. Clin Exp Allergy 21:217–224, 1991.
107. Fahy G: Double masked efficacy and safety evaluation of lodoxamide 0.1% ophthalmic solution versus Opticrom 2%: a multicentre study. In Ferraz de Oliviera LN (ed): Ophthalmology Today. Elsevier Science, Amsterdam, 1988, pp 341–342.
108. Ferrer NR, Howland WC, Stevenson DD, et al: Release of leukotrienes, prostaglandins, and histamine into nasal secretions of aspirin-sensitive asthmatics during reaction to aspirin. Am Rev Respir Dis 137:847–854, 1988.
109. Filiaci F, Zambetti G: A specific nasal reactivity in allergic and non-allergic rhinopathy. Rhinology 21:329–234, 1983.
110. Filley WV, Holley KE, Cephart GM, et al: Identification by immunofluorescence of eosinophil granule major basic protein in lung tissues of patients with bronchial asthma. Lancet 2:11–16, 1982.
111. Fleming DM, Crombie DL: Geographical variations in person consulting rates in general practice in England and Wales. Health Trends 21:51–55, 1989.
112. Foreman JC: Substance P and calcitonin gene-regulated peptide: effects on mast cells and in human skin. Int Arch Allergy Appl Immunol 82:366, 1987.
113. Foster CS, Calonge M: Atopic keratoconjunctivitis. Ophthalmology 97:992–1000, 1990.
114. Foster CS, Duncan J: Randomized clinical trial of topically administered cromolyn sodium for vernal keratoconjunctivitis. Am J Ophthalmol 90:175–181, 1980.
115. Foster CS, Rice CA, Dutt JE: Immunopathology of atopic keratoconjunctivitis. Ophthalmology 98:1190–1196, 1991.
116. Friedlaender MH, Okumoto M, Kelley J: Diagnosis of allergic conjunctivitis. Arch Ophthalmol 102:1198–1199, 1984.
117. Furin MJ, Norman PS, Creticos PS, et al: Immunotherapy decreases antigen-induced eosinophil migration into the nasal cavity. J Allergy Clin Immunol 88:27–32, 1991.
118. Galli SJ: New concepts about the mast cell. New Engl J Med 328:257–265, 1993.
119. Galli SJ: Biology of disease. New insights into "the riddle of the mast cells": microenvironmental regulation of mast cell development and phenotypic heterogeneity. Lab Invest 62(1):5–33, 1990.
120. Gauchat JF, Henchoz S, Mazzei G, et al: Induction of human IgE synthesis in B cells by mast cells and basophils. Nature 365:340–343, 1993.
121. George MA, Smith LM, Berdy GJ, et al: Platelet activating factor induced inflammation following topical ocular challenge. Invest Ophthalmol Vis Sci 31(suppl):63, 1990.
122. Gleich GJ, Frigas E, Loegering DA, et al: Cytotoxic properties of the eosinophil granule major basic protein. J Immunol 123(6):2925–2927, 1979.
123. Glinert R, Wilson P, Wedner HJ: Fel dI is markedly reduced following sequential washing of cats. J Allergy Clin Immunol 85:225A, 1990.
124. Golding J, Peters T: Eczema and hayfever. In Butler N, Golding J (eds): From Birth to Five. A Study of the Health and Behaviour of Britain's Five Year-Olds. Pergamon Press, Oxford, 1986, pp 171–186.
125. Golding-Wood PH: Petrosal and vidian neurectory in chronic vasomotor rhinitis. J Laryngol 75:232–247, 1961.
126. Goldstein SM, Kaempfer CE, Kealey JT, Wintroub BU: Human mast cell carboxypeptidase. Purification and characterisation. J Clin Invest 83:1630–1636, 1989.
127. Gomez E, Clague JE, Gatland D, Davis RJ: Effect of topical corticosteroids on seasonally induced increases in nasal mast cells. Br Med J 296:1572–1573, 1988.
128. Gordon JR, Galli SJ: Mast cells as a source of both preformed and immunologically inducible TNF-α/cachectin. Nature 346:274–276, 1990.
129. Greaves MW, Marks R, and Robertson I: Receptors for histamine in human blood vessels. A review. Br J Dermatol 92:225–228, 1977.
130. Greiff L, Wollmer P, Pipkorn U, Persson CGA: Absorption of ^{51}Cr-EDTA across the human nasal airway barriers in the presence of topical histamine. Thorax 46:630–632, 1991.

131. Groopman JE, Molina JM, Scadden DT: Haematopoietic growth factors: biology and clinical applications. N Engl J Med 321:1449–1459, 1989.
132. Hagermark O, Rajka G, Berqvist U: Experimental itch in human skin elicited by rat mast cell chymase. Acta Derm Venereol (Stockh) 52:125–128, 1972.
133. Haight JSJ, Cole P: The site and function of the nasal valve. Laryngoscope 93:49–55, 1983.
134. Harding SM, Heath S: Intranasal steroid aerosol in perennial rhinitis: comparison with an antihistamine compound. Clin Allergy 6:369–372, 1976.
135. Harrison K, Robinson C, Brewster H, Howarth PH: Comparative effects of prostaglandin D_2, 9a 11B PGF_2 and histamine on nasal airflow. In Samuellson B (ed): Prostaglandins and Related Compounds. 7th International Conference Proceedings. Raven Press, New York, 1990, p 323.
136. Henauer S, Seppey M, Huguenot C, Pecond A: Effects of terfenadine and pseudoephedrine alone and in combination in a nasal provocation test and in perennial rhinitis. Eur J Clin Pharmacol 41:321–324, 1991.
137. Henderson WR, Chi EY, Klebanoff SJ: Eosinophil peroxidase-induced mast cell secretion. J Exp Med 152:265–279, 1980.
138. Hibbert J, Howarth PH: Anti-histamines and cardiac arrhythmias. Prescribers Journal. In press.
139. Hogan MJ: Atopic keratoconjunctivitis. Am J Ophthalmol 36:937–947, 1953.
140. Howarth PH: Allergic rhinitis: a rational choice of treatment. Respir Med 83:179–188, 1989.
141. Howarth PH, Holgate ST: Comparative trial of two non-sedative H_1-antihistamines, terfenadine and astemizole, for hay fever. Thorax 39:668–672, 1984.
142. Howarth PH, Lunn A, Tomkins S: Bedding barrier intervention in house dust mite respiratory allergy. Clin Exp Allergy 22:140A, 1992.
143. Hui KP, Lotvall J, Chung KF, Barnes PJ: Attenuation of inhaled allergen-induced microvascular leakage and airflow obstruction in guinea pigs by a 5-lipoxygenase inhibitor. Am Rev Respir Dis 143:1015–1019, 1991.
144. Iliopoulos O, Proud D, Adkinson NF, et al: Relationship between the early, late and rechallenge reaction to nasal challenge with antigen: observations on the role of inflammatory mediators and cells. J Allergy Clin Immunol 86:851–861, 1990.
145. International Workshop Report: Dust mite allergens and asthma—a worldwide problem. J Allergy Clin Immunol 83:416–427, 1989.
146. Irani AA, Butrus SI, Tabbara KF, Schwartz LB: Human conjunctival mast cells: distribution of MCT and MCTC in vernal conjunctivitis and giant papillary conjunctivitis. J Allergy Clin Immunol 86:34–39, 1990.
147. Irani AA, Craig SS, Nilsson G, et al: Characterisation of human mast cells developed in vitro from fetal liver cells cocultured with murine 3T3 fibroblasts. Immunology 77:136–143, 1992.
148. Irani AA, Sanford MG, Wintroub BU, et al: Human mast cell carboxypeptidase. Selective localisation to MCTC Cells. J Immunol 147(1):247–253, 1991.
149. Irani AA, Schechter NM, Craig SS, et al: Two types of human mast cells that have distinct neutral protease compositions. Proc Natl Acad Sci USA 83:4464–4468, 1986.
150. Ishizaka T: Mechanisms of IgE-mediated hypersensitivity. In Middleton JE Jr, Reed CE, Ellis EF, et al (eds): Allergy. Principles and Practice. The CV Mosby Co, St Louis, 1988.
151. Janessen M, Blockhuys S: Tolerability of levocabastine eye drops. Doc Ophthalmol 84(2):111–118, 1993.
152. Jay JL: Clinical features and diagnosis of adult atopic keratoconjunctivitis and the effect of treatment with sodium cromoglycate. Br J Ophthalmol 65:335–340, 1981.
153. Johnson HG, VanHout CA, Wright JB: Inhibition of allergic reactions by cromoglycate and by a new antiallergy drug U-42,585E. II. Activity in primates against aerosolized *Ascaris suum* antigen. Int Arch Allergy Appl Immunol 56:481, 1978.
154. Joris I, Majno G, Ryan GB: Endothelial contraction in vivo: a study of the rat mesentery. Virchows Arch B Cell Pathol 12:73–83, 1972.
155. Juniper EF, Guyatt GH, Ferrie PJ, King DR: Sodium cromoglycate eye drops: regular versus "as needed" use in the treatment of seasonal allergic conjunctivitis. J Allergy Clin Immunol 94(1):36–43, 1994.
156. Juniper EF, Kline PA, Hargreave FE, Dolovich J: Comparison of beclomethasone dipropionate aqueous nasal spray, astemizole, and the combination in the prophylactic treatment of ragweed pollen-induced rhinoconjunctivitis. J Allergy Clin Immunol 83:627–633, 1989.
157. Kay AB, Walsh GM, Moqbel R: Disodium cromoglycate inhibits activation of human inflammatory cells in vitro. J Allergy Clin Immunol 80:1, 1987.
158. Kay AB, Ying S, Varney V, et al: Messenger RNA expression of the cytokine gene cluster, interleukin 3 (IL-3), IL-4, IL-5, and granulocyte/macrophage colony-stimulating factor, in allergen-induced late-phase cutaneous reactions in atopic subjects. J Exp Med 173:775–778, 1991.
159. Kjellman NIM: Atopic disease in seven-year old children. Acta Paediatr Scand 22:465–471, 1977.
160. Klein LM, Lavker RM, Matis WL, Murphy GF: Degranulation of human mast cells induces an endothelial antigen central to leukocyte adhesion. Proc Natl Acad Sci USA 86:8972–8976, 1989.
161. Kneist FM, Young E, Van praag MCG, et al: Clinical evaluation of a double-blind dust-mite avoidance trial with mite-allergic rhinitic patients. Clin Exp Allergy 21:39–47, 1991.
162. Knight A, Kazim F, Salvatori VA: A trial of intranasal atrovent versus placebo in the treatment of vasomotor rhinitis. Ann Allergy 57:348–354, 1986.
163. Knowles M, Clark CE, Fisher ND, et al: Nasal secretions: role of epithelial ion transport. In Mygind N, Pipkorn U (eds): Allergic and Vasomotor Rhinitis: Pathophysiological Aspects. Munksgaard, Copenhagen, 1987, pp 77–90.
164. Konno A, Togawa K: Role of the vidian nerve in nasal allergy. Ann Otol Rhinol Laryngol 88:258–266, 1979.
165. Kubes P, Smith R, Grisham MD, Granger DN: Neutrophil mediated proteolysis. Differential roles for cathepsin G and elastase. Inflammation 17:321–332, 1993.
166. Kunkel SL, Standiford T, Kasahara K, Strieter RM: Interleukin 8 (IL-8): the major neutrophil chemotactic factor in the lung. Exp Lung Res 17:17, 1991.
167. Lacroix JS, Buvelot JM, Polla BS, Lundberg JM: Improvement of symptoms of non-allergic chronic rhinitis by local treatment with capsaicin. Clin Exp Allergy 21:595–600, 1991.
168. Levi-Schaffer F, Rubinchik E: Mast cell/fibroblast interactions. Clin Exp Allergy 24:1016–1021, 1994.
169. Levi-Schaffer F, Segal V, Shalit M: Effects of interleukins on connective tissue type mast cells co-cultured with fibroblasts. Immunology 72:174–180, 1991.
170. Lobaton P, Moreno P, Coulie P: Comparison of cetirizine with astemizole in the treatment of perennial allergic rhinitis and study of the concomitant effect of histamine and allergen-induced wheal responses. Ann Allergy 65:401–405, 1990.
171. Longley BJ, Morganroth GS, Tyrell L, et al: Altered metabolism of mast cell growth factor (c-kit ligand) in cutaneous mastocytosis. N Engl J Med 328(18):1302–1307, 1993.
172. Lowman MA, Benyon C, Church MK: Characterisation of neuropeptide-induced histamine release from human dispersed skin mast cells. Br J Pharmacol 95:121–130, 1988.
173. Lucus DR: The conjunctiva, cornea, and sclera. In Lucas DR (ed): Greer's Ocular Pathology. Blackwell Scientific Publications, Oxford, 1989, pp 56–57.
174. Luczynska CM, Li Y, Chapman MD, Platts-Mills TAE: Airborne concentrations and particle size distribution of allergen derived from domestic cats. Am Rev Respir Dis 141:361–367, 1990.
175. Lunblad L, Lundberg JM, Anggard A: Local and systemic capsaicin pretreatment inhibits sneezing and the increase in nasal vascular permeability induced by certain chemical irritants. Naunyn Schmiedeberg Arch Pharmacol 326:254–261, 1984.
176. Lunblad L, Saria A, Lundberg JM, Anggard A: Increased vascular permeability in rat nasal mucosa induced by substance P and stimulation of capsaicin sensitive trigeminal neurons. Acta Otolaryngol (Stockh) 96:479–484, 1983.
177. Lundberg JM, Saria A: Capsaicin-induced desensitization of airway mucosa to cigarette smoke, mechanical and chemical irritants. Nature 302:251–253, 1983.
178. Lung MA, Phipps RC, Wang JJC, Widdicombe JG: Control of nasal vasculature and airflow resistance in the dog. J Physiol 349:535–551, 1984.
179. Luts A, Sundler F, Erjefalt I, Persson CGA: The airway epithelial lining in guinea pigs is intact promptly after the mucosal crossing of a large amount of plasma exudate. Int Arch Allergy Appl Immunol 91:385–388, 1990.
180. Mackie IA, Wright P: Giant papillary conjunctivitis (secondary vernal) in association with contact lens wear. Trans Ophthalmol Soc UK 98(1):3–9, 1978.
181. Maggi E, Biswas P, Del Prete G, et al: Accumulation of Th2-like helper T cells in the conjunctiva of patients with vernal conjunctivitis. J Immunol 146:1169–1174, 1991.

182. Majno G, Gilmore V, Leventhal M: On the mechanism of vascular leakage caused by histamine type mediators. Circ Res 21:833–847, 1967.
183. Majno G, Leventhal M: Pathogenesis of histamine type vascular leakage. Lancet 8:99–100, 1967.
184. Majno G, Shea SM, Leventhal M: Endothelial contraction induced by histamine type mediators. J Cell Biol 42:647–672, 1969.
185. Malm L, Druce HM, Holgate ST: Vasoconstrictors and antihistamines. In Mygind N, Weeke B (eds): Allergic and Vasomotor Rhinitis: Clinical Aspects. Munksgaard, Copenhagen, 1985, pp 140–150.
186. Malm L, Wihl J: Inta-nasal beclomethasone dipropionate in vasomotor rhinitis. Acta Allergol 31:245–253, 1976.
187. Malmberg H: Symptoms of chronic and allergic rhinitis and occurrence of nasal secretion granulocytes in university students, school children and infants. Allergy 34:389–395, 1979.
188. Mazanec MB, Nedrud JG, Kaetzel CS, Lamm ME: A three-tiered view of the role of IgA in mucosal defense. Immunol Today 14(9):431–435, 1993.
189. McAllen MK, Ingman MJS: A controlled trial of dexamethasone snuff in chronic perennial rhinitis. Lancet 1:968–971, 1969.
190. McDonald DM, Mitchell RA, Gabella G, Haskell A: Neurogenic inflammation in the rat trachea. Identity and distribution of nerves mediating the increase in vascular permeability. J Neurocytol 17:605–628, 1988.
191. Meisler DM, Berzins UJ, Krachmer JH, et al: Cromolyn treatment of giant papillary conjunctivitis. Arch Ophthalmol 100:1608–1610, 1982.
192. Melamed J, et al: Evaluation of nedocromil sodium 2% ophthalmic solution for the treatment of seasonal allergic conjunctivitis. Ann Allergy 73:57–66, 1994.
193. Miadonna A, Tedeschi A, Leggiere E, et al: Behaviour and clinical relevance of histamine and lecotrienes C_4 and B_4 in grass pollen-induced rhinitis. Am Rev Respir Dis 136:357–362, 1987.
194. Montefort S, Feather IH, Wilson SJ, et al: The expression of leukocyte-endothelial adhesion molecules is increased in perennial allergic rhinitis. Am J Respir Cell Mol Biol 7:393–398, 1992.
195. Montgomery Smith J: Epidemiology and natural history of asthma, allergic rhinitis, and atopic dermatitis (eczema). In Middleton E, Reed CE, Ellis EF, et al (eds): Allergy. Principle and Practice. CV Mosby, St Louis, 1983, pp 771–803.
196. Morgan SJ, Williams JH, Walls AF, et al: Mast cell numbers and staining characteristics in the normal and allergic human conjunctiva. J Allergy Clin Immunol 87:111–116, 1991.
197. Morgan SJ, Williams JH, Walls AF, Holgate ST: Mast cell hyperplasia in atopic keratoconjunctivitis. Eye 5:729–735, 1991.
198. Mygind N: Nasal Allergy. Blackwell Publications, Oxford, 1979.
199. Mygind N, Secher C, Kirkegaard J: Role of histamine and antihistamines in the nose. Eur J Res Dis Suppl 64(128):16–20, 1983.
200. Naclerio RM, Meier HL, Sobotka AK, et al: Mediator release after nasal airway challenge with allergen. Am Rev Respir Dis 128:597–602, 1983.
201. Naclerio RM, Proud D, Togias AG, et al: Inflammatory mediators in late antigen-induced rhinitis. N Engl J Med 313:65–70, 1985.
202. Nieber K, Rathsack R, Henning R, et al: Substance P in bronchoalveolar lavage and nasal lavage fluids after allergen provocation in patients with asthma. Allergologie 12:60, 1990.
203. Nirankari VS, Karesh JW, Richards RD: Complications of exposed monofilament sutures. Am J Ophthalmol 95:515–519, 1983.
204. Nocka K, Buck J, Levi E, Besmer P: Candidate ligand for the c-kit transmembrane kinase receptor: KL, a fibroblast derived growth factor stimulates mast cells and erythroid progenitors. Eur Mol Biol Organ J 9:3287, 1990.
205. Nomura Y, Matsuura T: Distribution and clinical significance of the autonomic nervous system in the human nasal mucosa. Acta Otolaryngol (Stockh) 73:493–501, 1972.
206. Orgel HA, Meltzer EO, Kemp JP, et al: Comparison of intranasal cromolyn sodium, 4% and oral terfenadine for allergic rhinitis: symptoms, nasal cytology, nasal ciliary clearance and rhinometry. Ann Allergy 66:237–244, 1991.
207. Ostler HB, Martin RG, Dawson CR: The use of disodium cromoglycate in the treatment of atopic ocular disease. In Leopoid JH, Burns RD (eds): Symposium on Ocular Therapy. John Wiley, New York, 1977, pp 99–108.
208. Otsuka H, Denburg JA, Befus AD, et al: Effect of beclomethasone dipropionate on nasal metachromatic cell sub-populations. Clin Allergy 16:589–595, 1986.
209. Otsuka H, Denburg JA, Dolovich J, et al: Heterogeneity of metachromatic cells in human nose: significance of mucosal mast cells. J Allergy Clin Immunol 76:695–702, 1985.
210. Otsuka H, Mezawa A, Ohnishi M, et al: Changes in nasal metachromatic cells during allergen immunotherapy. Clin Exp Allergy 21:115–120, 1991.
211. Parronchi P, Macchia D, Piccinni MP, et al: Allergen and bacterial component T cell clones established from atopic donors show a different profile of cytokine production. Proc Natl Acad Sci USA 88:4538–4542, 1991.
212. Pelikan Z: Late and delayed responses of the nasal mucosa to allergen challenge. Ann Allergy 41:37–47, 1978.
213. Perki JM: Allergy in general practice. Practitioner 208:776–783, 1972.
214. Persson CGA: Plasma exudation and asthma. Lung 166:1–23, 1988.
215. Persson CGA, Erjefalt I, Alkner U, et al: Plasma exudation as a first line respiratory mucosal defence. Clin Exp Allergy 21:17–24, 1991.
216. Petersson G, Malm L, Ekman R, Hakanson R: Capsaicin evokes secretion of nasal fluid and depletes substance P and calcitonin gene-related peptide from the nasal mucosa in the rat. Br J Pharmacol 98:930–936, 1989.
217. Petz G: A role for CD4+ T cell subsets producing a selective pattern of lymphokines in the pathogenesis of human chronic inflammatory and allergic diseases. Immunol Rev 123:23–35, 1991.
218. Pipkorn U, Karlsson G, Enerback L: The cellular response of human allergic mucosa to natural allergen exposure. J Allergy Clin Immunol 82:414–418, 1988.
219. Pipkorn U, Proud D, Lichtenstein LM, et al: Inhibition of mediator release in allergic rhinitis by pretreatment with topical glucocorticosteroids. N Engl J Med 316:1506–1510, 1987.
220. Platts-Mills TAE, Heyden ML, Chapman MD, Wilkins SR: Seasonal variation in dust mite and grass pollen allergens in dust from houses of patients with asthma. J Allergy Clin Immunol 79:781–791, 1987.
221. Platts-Mills TAE, Heyman PW, Longbottom JL, Wilkins SR: Airborne allergens associated with asthma: particle sizes carrying dust mite and rat allergens measured with a cascade impactor. J Allergy Clin Immunol 77:850–857, 1986.
222. Plaut M, Pierce JH, Watson CJ, et al: Mast cell lines produce lymphokines in response to cross-linkage of FCεR1 or to calcium ionophores. Nature 339:64–67, 1989.
223. Pollart SM, Mullins DE, Vailes LD, et al: Identification, quantification and purification of cockroach allergens using monoclonal antibodies. J Allergy Clin Immunol 87:511–521, 1991.
224. Rajakulasingam K, Polosa R, Church MK, et al: Kinins and rhinitis. Clin Exp Allergy 22:734–740, 1992.
225. Rajakulasingam K, Polosa R, Lau LCK, et al: Comparative nasal effects of bradykinin and histamine: influence on nasal airways resistance and plasma protein exudation. Thorax 48:324–329, 1993.
226. Rajakulasingam K, Polosa R, Lau LCK, et al: Nasal effects of bradykinin and capsaicin: influence on plasma protein exudation and role of sensory neurones. J Appl Physiol 72(4):1418–1424, 1992.
227. Rak S, Hakanson L, Venge P: Immunotherapy abrogates the generation of eosinophil and neutrophil chemotactic activity during pollen season. J Allergy Clin Immunol 86:706–713, 1990.
228. Raphel GD, Hauptschein-Raphel M, Kaliner MA: Gustatory rhinitis. Am J Rhinol 3:145–149, 1989.
229. Renton R, Fidder C, Rosenberg R: Multicentre, crossover study of the efficacy and tolerability of terfenadine 120 mg, versus cetirizine 10 mg in perennial allergic rhinitis. Ann Allergy 67:416–420, 1991.
230. Rice BA, Foster CS: Immunopathology of cicatricial pemphigoid affecting the conjunctiva. Ophthalmology 97:1476–1483, 1990.
231. Rice NSC, Easty D, Garner A, et al: Vernal keratoconjunctivitis and its management. Trans Ophthalmol Soc UK 91:483–489, 1971.
232. Rich LF, Hanifin JM: Ocular complications of atopic dermatitis and other eczemas. Int Ophthalmol Clin 25:61–76, 1985.
233. Robinson C, Benyon C, Holgate ST, Church MK: The IgE and calcium-dependant release of eicosanoids and histamine from human purified cutaneous mast cells. J Invest Dermatol 93:397–404, 1989.
234. Rocklin RE, Sheffer AL, Greineder DR, Melmon KL: Generation of antigen specific suppressor cells during allergy desensitisation. New Engl J Med 302:1213–1219, 1980.
235. Rothlein R, Czajkowski M, O'Neill M, et al: Induction of ICM-1 on primary and continuous cell lines by pro-inflammatory cytokines. J Immunol 141:1665–1669, 1988.
236. Saemisch T, Brockhaus C: Ueber den Fruhjahrskatarrh der Conjuntiva. In: Inaug.-Diss. Bonn, 1872.

237. Saiga T, Ueno N, Shimizu Y: Deposition of eosinophil cationic protein in conjunctival tissues and tears in vernal keratoconjunctivitis. Invest Ophth Vis Sci 32:682, 1991.
238. Sanderi P, Nez PA, Duerr ML, et al: Cathepsin G and leukocyte elastase inactivate human tumor necrosis factor and lymphotoxin. Cell Immunol 135:299–313, 1991.
239. Santos CI, Huang AJ, Abelson MB, et al: Efficacy of lodoxamide 0.1% ophthalmic solution in resolving corneal epitheliopathy associated with vernal keratoconjunctivitis. Am J Ophthalmol 117:488–497, 1994.
240. Schechter NM, Choi JK, Slavin DA, et al: Identification of a chymotrypsin-like proteinase in human mast cells. J Immunol 137(3):962–970, 1986.
241. Schechter NM, Irani AA, Sprows JL, et al: Identification of a cathepsin G-like proteinase in the MCTC type of human mast cell. J Immunol 145:2652–2661, 1990.
242. Schleimer RP, Lichtenstein LM, Gillespie E: Inhibition of basophil histamine release by anti-inflammatory steroids. Nature 292:454–455, 1981.
243. Schreiber SL, Crabtree GR: The mechanism of action of cyclosporin A and FK506. Immunol Today 13:136, 1992.
244. Schwartz LB, Irani AA, Roller K, et al: Quantification of histamine, tryptase, and chymase in dispersed human T and TC mast cells. J Immunol 138(8):2611–2615, 1987.
245. Schwartz LB, Lewis RA, Austen KF: Tryptase from human pulmonary mast cells. Purification and characterisation. J Biol Chem 256:11939–11943, 1981.
246. Secchi AG, Tognon S, Leonardi A: Topical use of cyclosporine in the treatment of vernal keratoconjunctivitis. Am J Ophthalmol 110:641–645, 1990.
247. Seppa H: The role of chymotypsin-like protease of rat mast cells in inflammatory vasopermeability and fibrinolysis. Inflammation 4:1–8, 1980.
248. Sheldrick JH, Wilson AD, Vernon SA, Sheldrick CM: Management of ophthalmic disease in general practice. Br J Gen Pract 43(376):459–462, 1993.
249. Sibbald B: Epidemiology of allergic rhinitis. In Burr ML (ed): Monograph on epidemiology of allergic disease. S Karger, Basel, 1993, pp 61–79.
250. Sibbald B, Rink E: The labelling of rhinitis and hayfever by doctors. Thorax 46:378–381, 1991.
251. Small P, Black M, Frenkiel S: Effects of treatment with beclomethasone dipropionate in subpopulations of perennial rhinitis patients. J Allergy Clin Immunol 70:178–182, 1982.
252. Solari R, Kraehenbuhl JP: The biosynthesis of secretory component and its role in the transepithelial transport of IgA dimer. Immunol Today 6(1):17–20, 1985.
253. Solley GO, Gleich GJ, Jordan RE, Schroder AL: The late phase of the immediate wheal and flare skin reaction: its dependence upon IgE antibodies. J Clin Immunol 58:408–420, 1976.
254. Spada CS, Woodward DF, Hawley SB, Nieves AL: Leukotrienes cause eosinophil emigration into conjunctival tissue. Prostaglandins 31:795–809, 1986.
255. Sporik R, Holgate ST, Plats-Mills TAE, Cogswell J: Exposure to dust mite allergen (Der pI) and the development of asthma in childhood: a prospective study. N Engl J Med 323:502–507, 1990.
256. Stjarne P, Lundblad L, Lundberg JM, Anggard A: Capsaicin and nicotine—sensitive afferent neurones and nasal secretion in healthy human volunteers and in patients with vasomotor rhinitis. Br J Pharmacol 96:693–701, 1989.
257. Storms WW, Stephen FB, Nathan A, et al: SCH 434: a new antihistamine/decongestant for seasonal allergic rhinitis. J Allergy Clin Immunol 83:1083–1090, 1989.
258. Stretton CD, Barnes PJ: Modulation of cholinergic transmission in guinea pig trachea by neuropeptide Y. Br J Pharmacol 93:672–678, 1988.
259. Sugar A, Meyer RF: Giant papillary conjunctivitis after keratoplasty. Am J Ophthalmol 91(2):239–242, 1981.
260. Svensson C, Andersson M, Persson CGA, et al: Albumin, bradykinin and eosinophil cationic protein on the nasal mucosal surface in patients with hay fever during natural allergen exposure. J Allergy Clin Immunol 85:828–833, 1990.
261. Thomas B, Heap P, Carswell F: Ultrastructural localisation of the allergen Der pI in the gut of the house dust mite *Dermatophagoides pteronyssinus*. Int Arch Allergy Appl Immunol 94:365–367, 1991.
262. Tinkelman DG, Rupp G, Kaufman H, et al: Double-masked, paired-comparison clinical study of ketorolac tromethamine 0.5% ophthalmic solution compared with placebo eyedrops in the treatment of seasonal allergic conjunctivitis. Surv Ophthalmol 38(suppl):133–140, 1993.
263. Togias A: Age relationships and clinical features of non-allergic rhinitis. J Allergy Clin Immunol 85:182, 1990.
264. Togias AG, Naclerio RM, Proud D, et al: Nasal challenge with cold, dry air results in release of inflammatory mediators. Possible mast cell involvement. J Clin Invest 76:1374–1381, 1985.
265. Tomasi TB, Grey HM: The structure and function of immunoglobulin A. Prog Allergy 16:81–213, 1972.
266. Tonnesen P: Serotonin in nasal secretion. In Mygind N, Pipkorn U (eds): Allergic and Vasomotor Rhinitis: Pathophysiological Aspects. Munskgaard, Copenhagen, 1987, pp 208–213.
267. Tovey ER, Chapman MD, Platts-Mills TAE: Mite faeces are a major source of house dust mite allergens. Nature 289:592–593, 1981.
268. Trocme SD, Gilbert CM, Allansmith MR, et al: Characteristics of the cellular response of the rat conjunctiva to topically applied leukotriene B_4. Ophthalmic Res 21:297–302, 1989.
269. Trocme SD, Gleich GJ, Zieske JD: Eosinophil granule major basic protein inhibits corneal epithelial wound healing in vitro. Invest Ophthalmol Vis Sci 35:3051–3056, 1994.
270. Trocme SD, Kephart GM, Allansmith MR, et al: Conjunctival deposition of eosinophil granule major basic protein in vernal keratoconjunctivitis and contact lens-associated giant papillary conjunctivitis. Am J Ophthalmol 108:57–63, 1989.
271. Tuft SJ, Dart JKG, Kemeny M: Limbal vernal keratoconjunctivitis: clinical characteristics and immunoglobulin E expression compared with palpebral vernal. Eye 3:420–427, 1989.
272. Tuft SJ, Kemeny DM, Dart JKG, Buckley RJ: Clinical features of atopic keratoconjunctivitis. Ophthalmology 98:150–158, 1991.
273. Tunon de Lara JM, Okayama Y, McEuen AR, et al: Release and inactivation of interleukin 4 by mast cells. Ann NY Acad Sci. In press.
274. Uddman R, Anggard A, Widdicombe JG: Nerves and neurotransmitters in the nose. In Mygind N, Pipkorn U (eds): Allergic and Vasomotor Rhinitis: Pathophysiological Aspects. Munksgaard, Copenhagen, 1987, pp 50–62.
275. Uddman R, Sundler F: Innervation of the upper airways. Clin Chest Med 7:201–209, 1966.
276. Udell IJ, Gleich GJ, Allansmith MR, et al: Eosinophil granule major basic protein and Charcot-Leyden crystal protein in human tears. Am J Ophthalmol 92:824–828, 1981.
277. Van de Heyning PH, van Hesendonck J, Creten W, Rombaut N: Effect of topical levocabastine on allergic and non-allergic perennial rhinitis: a double-blind study, levocabastine versus placebo, followed by an open, prospective, single-blind study on beclomethasone. Allergy 43:386–391, 1988.
278. Varney V: Hay fever in the United Kingdom. Clin Exp Allergy 21:757–762, 1991.
279. Varney VA, Gaga M, Frew AJ, et al: Usefulness of immunotherapy in patients with severe summer hayfever uncontrolled by anti-allergic drugs. BMJ 302:265–269, 1991.
280. Varney VA, Jacobson MR, Sudderick RM, et al: Immunohistology of the nasal mucosa following allergen-induced rhinitis. Am Rev Respir Dis 146:170–176, 1992.
281. Venge P, Dahl R, Fredens K, et al: Epithelial injury by human eosinophils. Am Rev Respir Dis 138:S54–57, 1988.
282. Walls AF: The roles of neutral proteases in asthma and rhinitis. In Busse WW, Holgate ST (eds): Asthma and Rhinitis. Blackwell Scientific Publications, Boston, 1995, pp 801–824.
283. Walls AF, Bennett AR, Suieras-Diaz J, Olsson H: The kininogenase activity of human mast cell tryptase. Biochem Soc Trans 20:260S, 1992.
284. Walsh LJ, Trinchieri G, Waldorf HA, et al: Human dermal mast cells contain and release tumor necrosis factor α, which induces endothelial leukocyte adhesion molecule 1. Proc Natl Acad Sci USA 88:4220–4224, 1991.
285. Warringa RAJ, Schweizer RC, Maikoe T, et al: Modulation of eosinophil chemotaxis by interleukin-5. Am J Respir Cell Mol Biol 7:631–636, 1992.
286. Weiner N: Norepinephrine, epinephrine and the sympathomimetic amines. In Gilman AG, Goodman LS, Rall TW, Murad F (eds): Goodman and Gilman's the Pharmacological Basis of Therapeutics, 7th edition. Macmillan, New York, 1985, pp 145–180.
287. Wells U, Widdicombe JG: Lateral nasal gland secretion in the anaesthetized dog. J Physiol 374:359–374, 1986.

288. Welsh PW, Stricker WE, Chu CP, et al: Efficacy of beclomethasone nasal solution, flunisolide, and cromolyn in relieving symptoms of ragweed allergy. Mayo Clin Proc 62:125–134, 1987.
289. Weston JH, Udell IJ, Abelson MB: H_1 receptors in the human ocular surface. Invest Ophthalmol Vis Sci 20(suppl):32, 1981.
290. Widdicombe JG: The physiology of the nose. Clin Chest Med 7:159–170, 1986.
291. Widdicombe JG, Wells UM: Airway secretions. In Proctor DF, Andersen IB (eds): The Nose: Upper Airway Physiology and the Atmospheric Environment. Elsevier, Amsterdam, 1982, pp 215–244.
292. Wierenga EA, Snoek M, de Groot C, et al: Evidence for compartmentalisation of functional subsets of CD4 T lymphocytes in atopic patients. J Immunol 144:4651–4656, 1990.
293. Wihl JA, Nuchel-Peterson B, Nuchel-Peterson L, et al: Effect of the non-sedative H1-receptor antagonist astemizole in perennial allergic and non-allergic rhinitis. J Allergy Clin Immunol 75:720–727, 1985.
294. Wihl JA, Petersen BN, Mygind N: The role of histamine in non-allergic perennial rhinitis. Acta Otolaryngol (Stockh) 214:99–102, 1984.
295. Wodnar-Filipowicz A, Heusser CH, Moroni C: Production of the haemopoietic growth factors GM-CSF and interleukin-3 by mast cells in response to IgE receptor-mediated activation. Nature 339:150–152, 1989.
296. Wood RA, Chapman MD, Adkinson Jr NF, Eggleston PA: The effect of cat removal on allergen content in household dust samples. J Allergy Clin Immunol 83:730–734, 1989.
297. Wood RA, Eggleston PA, Lind BA: Antigenic analysis of household dust samples. Am Rev Respir Dis 137:358–363, 1988.
298. Wood RA, Mudd KE, Eggleston PA: The distribution of cat and dust mite allergens on wall surfaces. J Allergy Clin Immunol 89:126–130, 1992.
299. Woodward DF, Ledgard SE: Comparison of leukotrienes as conjunctival microvascular permeability factors. Ophthalmic Res 17:318–320, 1985.
300. Yanni JM, Weimer LK, Glaser RL, et al: Effect of lodoxamide on in vitro and in vivo conjunctival immediate hypersensitivity responses in rats. Int Arch Allergy Immunol 101(1):102–106, 1993.
301. Zetterstorm E, Holopainen E, Johnson C: Efficacy and tolerability of cetirizine and terfenadine in the treatment of perennial allergic rhinitis. Allergy 47:179, 1992.

26 Nasal Polyps and Sinusitis

RAYMOND G. SLAVIN

NASAL POLYPS

First described more than 3,000 years ago, nasal polyps are the most common group of mass lesions found in the nose. Despite their frequent occurrence and long history, many questions still exist in regard to incidence, pathogenesis, and treatment.

CHARACTERISTICS

Nasal polyps are typically smooth, gelatinous, semitranslucent, round or pear-shaped, and pale and appear to be outgrowths of the nasal mucosa (Fig. 26–1). Most polyps are located in the middle meatus along the lateral wall of the nose and originate from the ethmoid sinuses. Histologically, the mass of a nasal polyp is chiefly made up of edema fluid with sparse fibrous cells and a few mucous glands. Surface epithelium is pseudostratified, and the supporting structure is interspersed with masses of lymphocytes, plasma cells, eosinophils, and a few mast cells. Histochemical stains of nasal polyps and adjacent normal respiratory mucosa reveal the same characteristics.[94] However, studies utilizing immunocytochemical techniques demonstrate more $CD8^+$ (suppressor/cytotoxic) than $CD4^+$ (helper/inducer) cells in nasal polyps in contrast with normal nasal tissue.[91] Eosinophils were found in moderate to large numbers in 77% of patients, with neutrophils being present in 35%. Mast cells and plasma cells were detected in moderate numbers. Nasal

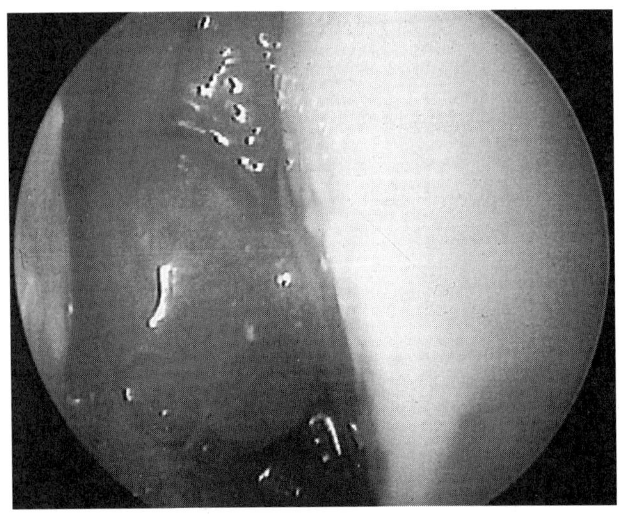

FIGURE 26–1. Nasal polyps visible through nasoscope.

polyp fluid contains concentrations of IgA, IgE, IgG, and IgM that are greater than one would expect from passive filtration.[12, 94]

It has been generally thought that no matter what the cause or associated condition, there is marked uniformity in the histologic pattern of nasal polyps. This may not be so. One study looking at nasal polyps of cystic fibrosis patients reported a triad of a barely visible basement membrane, a lack of eosinophils, and a preponderance of acid mucin.[64] In contrast, nasal polyps from atopic patients showed a thickened basement membrane, numerous eosinophils, and a neutral mucin.

Histamine content in nasal polyps is higher than in normal mucosa, as are norepinephrine levels in the base of polyps.[7] Whereas in general there were no differences in the levels of histamine, serotonin, and norepinephrine in the polyps of atopic and nonatopic patients, polyps of patients with the aspirin triad (nasal polyps, aspirin sensitivity, and asthma) have much lower histamine concentrations than do nasal polyps of other patients.

INCIDENCE

The majority of nasal polyps appear in individuals aged 40 years or more, and nasal polyps are twice as likely to occur in men.[59] Nasal polyps are rare under the age of 10. When they do occur in that age group, thought should be given to cystic fibrosis. In one large series, nasal polyps were present in 26% of 605 patients with cystic fibrosis.[88] Adult patients with cystic fibrosis have an incidence of nasal polyposis of 48%.[14] Table 26–1 shows the frequency of nasal polyps in various medical conditions.[77]

PATHOGENESIS

A number of mechanisms for the formation of nasal polyps have been suggested, but the pathogenesis is not known. The two most frequently mentioned theories are allergic and infectious.

The major features pointing to an allergic cause of nasal polyps are the clinical complaints of profuse rhinorrhea, sneezing and itching, degranulated mast cells in polyps, marked tissue eosinophilia, elevated histamine and IgE in extracellular polyp fluid, and association with asthma. However, many studies cast great doubt on the importance of allergy in the etiology of nasal polyps.[84] In a group of 3,000 atopic patients, only 0.5% had nasal polyps.[10] The incidence of nasal polyps is significantly higher in patients with nonatopic asthma and rhinitis than in those with atopic asthma and rhinitis (see Table 26–1). Drake-Lee and Pitcher-Wilmott[17] found no evidence of an increased incidence of allergic disorders in 200 consecutive patients admitted for polypectomy. In another study comparing children who had both cystic fibrosis and polyps with children who had cystic fibrosis alone, there was no evidence on history, skin tests, or IgE levels that the patients with polyps were more allergic.[17]

Drake-Lee and colleagues[19] point out that there are many causes of eosinophilia, elevated histamine levels, and mast cell degranulation other than those that are IgE mediated and that the presenting symptoms of patients with nasal polyps are similar to those with allergic rhinitis. In other studies, Drake-Lee[18] found no difference in polyp histamine levels in patients with positive skin tests and allergic rhinitis compared with patients with negative skin tests and no allergic rhinitis symptoms. This same author found that only a minority of patients have a positive radioallergosorbent test (RAST) to inhalant allergens in polyp fluid and positive in vitro challenge of polyp tissue with allergen extracts or anti-IgE. In summary, it is apparent that allergic reactions occur infrequently in patients with nasal polyps. Backing this up is the finding that epithelial mast cells in nasal polyps are equally elevated in nonallergic and allergic patients.[72] Mast cells are more frequent in the stroma or submucosa than in the epithelium of nasal polyps, indicating that inhalant-induced IgE-mediated degranulation of mast cells is a doubtful causal factor.[20]

In a prospective study comparing patients requiring surgery for polyposis with patients requiring nasal surgery for other reasons, atopy did not differentiate between patients with or without polyposis.[17] Blood eosinophilia was present in patients with polyps, possibly due to increased granulocyte macrophage–colony stimulating factor (GM-CSF) production by affected epithelial cells and fibroblasts.[101]

Although a single etiologic factor for the formation of nasal polyps is unlikely, there might be a final common pathway. Edema secondary to an allergic, inflammatory, or irritant reaction may induce enough swelling of nasal mucosa to pinch off eventually with the help of gravity.[22] The combination of mucosal injury, interference with sinus drainage, and decrease in ciliary action will then create a static environment susceptible to bacterial invasion, resulting in sinusitis. More venous status and mucosal edema occurs, which leads to further enlargement of polyps. Histamine has also been invoked as a common final pathway.[18] The elevated histamine levels in nasal polyps could cause cells to separate and leak electrolyte-rich fluid into the mucosal interstitium by its effects on H_1 receptors on capillary endothelial cells and tissue on nasal turbinate bones or in ethmoid sinuses. The sheer mass of extracapillary fluid within tissue that is constricted into the nasopharynx could potentiate polyp formation. The lack of smooth muscle in the area prevents backflow of fluid into capillaries and venules.

TABLE 26–1
FREQUENCY OF NASAL POLYPS IN VARIOUS CONDITIONS

Diagnosis	Frequency, (%)
Aspirin intolerance	36.0
Adult asthma	7.0
Intrinsic	13.0
Atopic	5.0
Chronic rhinitis	2.0
Nonallergic	5.0
Allergic	1.5
Childhood asthma/rhinitis	0.1
Cystic fibrosis	20.0

From Settipane GA: Nasal polyps. Immunol Allerg Clin North Am 7:105, 1987.

CLINICAL FEATURES

Most patients with nasal polyps have a long history of perennial rhinitis. In a large series of patients admitted for polypectomy,[19] all patients had nasal blockage and 75% had hyposmia. Rhinorrhea was present in 60%, sneezing in 60%, postnasal drainage in 65%, facial pain in 35%, and ocular itching in 25%. Symptoms were frequently exacerbated by irritative stimuli, such as temperature changes, fumes, odors, dusts, and chemicals. One third of these patients had evidence of sinusitis, and 5.5% were aspirin sensitive. On physical examination, polyps appear round or pear-shaped and translucent. They are soft, gelatinous, mobile, and insensitive to manipulation and do not readily bleed.

The association of nasal polyps with asthma has been known since the time of Hippocrates. One large series of patients with nasal polyposis found an asthma incidence of 20%. In this same study, 32% of asthmatic patients had nasal polyps.[59] Settipane and associates[75] analyzed 5,000 patients with asthma or allergic rhinitis. Of the 211 patients with nasal polyps, 70% had asthma. Looking at the total number of patients with asthma, 16.7% had polyps. In another study of 200 consecutive patients admitted for polypectomy, 30% had a history of asthma.[19]

Several reports have demonstrated evidence of bronchial hyperreactivity in patients with nasal polyps and no history of asthma.[41, 47] This was especially true in nonatopic patients.[57] A long-term follow-up confirmed that the incidence of subsequent clinically significant bronchial asthma was much higher than in the general population.[47]

The morphologic similarity of pathologic changes occurring in the nasal mucous membrane and bronchial mucosa has been described. In a series of 30 patients with nasal polyps, all showed epithelial damage in nasal polyps similar to that seen in the bronchial mucosa of asthmatic individuals.[100]

An association between nasal polyps and mediators of asthma was shown by Kaliner and coworkers.[42] Polyps from patients with allergic rhinitis released histamine, slow-reacting substance (leukotrienes), and eosinophil chemotactic factors when stimulated with the appropriate antigen. When polyps of patients with chronic sinusitis were passively sensitized with IgE and then challenged with antigen, there was a greater release of the leukotrienes than of histamine.

Moloney and Oliver[60] have tissue typed patients with nasal polyps with and without asthma. They showed a significant increase in haplotype HLA-A1 and HLA-B8 in patients with both polyps and asthma. This suggests that tissue typing may be of some use in predicting which patients with nasal polyps are likely to develop asthma. It may also mean that an abnormality of the immune response is associated with the pathogenesis of both nasal polyps and asthma.

A subpopulation of asthmatic patients with aspirin sensitivity has an especially high incidence of nasal polyps, on the order of 49%.[76] The association of nasal polyps, bronchial asthma, and aspirin sensitivity has been well described. Vasomotor rhinitis associated with profuse rhinorrhea generally occurs first in these patients. Intense nasal congestion follows, with the subsequent development of nasal polyps, bronchial asthma, and finally aspirin sensitivity. It has been shown that 8% of patients with nasal polyps, who were unaware of being sensitive to aspirin, are sensitive on appropriate challenge.[76]

DIFFERENTIAL DIAGNOSIS

The most common condition confused with nasal polyps is hypertrophied or polypoid nasal turbinates. One distinguishing characteristic is that nasal polyps are insensitive to pain on direct manipulation. Tumors and neoplasms, including squamous cell carcinoma, sarcoma, angiofibroma, encephalocele, and inverting papilloma, may also be mistaken for nasal polyps. Features that should alert the physician to refer to the otolaryngologist include unilateral presence, friability, firmness, and bleeding spontaneously or with manipulation.

COMPLICATIONS

The major complication of nasal polyps is sinusitis. Infection can also occur in the nose, surrounding bone, orbit, and even central nervous system. Nasal polyps may grow so large as to expand the nasal bones and broaden the nasal bridge.

MANAGEMENT

The management of nasal polyps may include both medical and surgical approaches. Antihistamines, decongestants, and cromolyn sodium are of little benefit. Appropriate antibiotics are useful in superimposed bacterial infection. Immunotherapy is helpful in treatment of allergic rhinitis but generally does not affect existing nasal polyps.

Corticosteroids are extremely effective in reducing polyp size and can be administered by aerosol, by direct injection into the polyp, or systemically. Significant improvement in 80% of patients with moderate to severe polyposis has been reported in well-controlled studies using a variety of intranasal preparations.[62, 73] In addition to decreasing polyp size and increasing airway conductance, there is also a decrease in eosinophils in the nasal smear, with a decrease in albumin, IgG, and IgE in the secretions.[73]

Although the technique of direct injection of corticosteroids into the polyp is widely used, there are well-documented reports of unilateral visual loss following intranasal steroid injection.[34] The mechanism for visual loss is thought to be both vasospastic and embolic, with particulate material reaching the ophthalmic artery through anastomosis with the superficial temporal artery. These reports have prompted the Food and Drug Administration not to approve the use of steroids for this procedure.

A fundamental effect of corticosteroids in inhibiting protein synthesis at the cellular level has led to fears that protracted use of intranasal steroids might lead to atrophic changes, as seen in the skin with protracted use of topical steroids. Examination of nasal polyp biopsies after 5 years of local beclomethasone treatment showed no change from pseudostratified to squamous metaplasia of surface epithelium that would be indicative of atrophic rhinitis. This is probably because of the rapid removal of beclomethasone from mucous membranes. The mucous membrane half-life of beclomethasone is 30 minutes, in contrast to 6 to 10 hours in the skin.[77]

A number of reasons might explain the failure of intranasal steroids to manage nasal polyps. One reason would be total blockage of the nasal airway, which would preclude the entrance of the drug. Systemic steroids should be given first in this instance to reduce polyp size. Another reason would be concomitant infection of the nasal mucous membranes or the sinuses, in which case an antibiotic must be added.

In the case of marked mechanical obstruction, particularly with associated sinusitis, polypectomy may have to be performed. Once radiographic changes have occurred, it is rare for polyps and sinusitis to resolve without surgical intervention.

The aim of polypectomy is to excise the polyps as completely as possible, improve nasal aeration, and drain infected sinuses. Preoperative systemic steroids are frequently administered to reduce the recurrence rate of polyps and to prevent serious sequelae, including asthma. There is some evidence that postpolypectomy, treatment with inhaled corticosteroids decreases the recurrence of nasal polyps.[21]

The extraordinary recurrence rate of polyps following simple polypectomy is well known.[77] More lasting surgical relief is obtained with procedures that remove the tissue source of the polyps. Functional endoscopic surgery (FESS) has been reported to result in a far smaller recurrence rate of polyps.[50]

In one study, surgical removal of nasal polyps was compared with the use of systemic steroids. After initial treatment with either surgery or systemic steroids, both groups of patients were given topical steroids and followed for 1 year. Both groups experienced a similar increase in nasal expiratory peak flow and sense of smell with a statistically significant increase in benefit from medication. The two major conclusions of the authors, who were otolaryngologists, were that (1) the continued postoperative use of topical steroids postpones or even prevents nasal polyps and (2) surgical removal should be reserved for those few cases in which the presence of residual or recurrent polyps justifies the inherent risks and discomfort for the patient.[51] Based on these and other studies, a reasonable medical approach to the management of nasal polyps would be a 10- to 14-day course of oral prednisone followed by intranasal corticosteroids (Table 26–2).

There has been controversy as to the safety of surgical removal of nasal polyps in patients with asthma, particularly those with intolerance to aspirin. Several older reviews claimed worsening of asthma after polypectomy.[29, 85] However, controlled studies have shown polypectomy to be safe and to have little effect on the development of asthma or on bronchial reactivity and the severity of asthma once established.[4, 74] It is of course important to control the asthmatic condition preoperatively in those patients undergoing polypectomy who also have asthma.

SINUSITIS

STRUCTURE AND FUNCTION OF THE PARANASAL SINUSES

In order to better understand the pathogenesis of sinusitis, it is important to review the structural anatomy of the upper airway. The paranasal sinuses are four paired bony structures surrounding the nasal cavities. Each sinus has an opening or ostium on the lateral side of the nose through which drainage occurs. The maxillary sinus is located in the general area of the cheek. The floor of the sinus is part of the tooth-bearing area of the maxilla and in adults is below the floor of the nasal cavity. This is particularly important in terms of pathogenesis, as will be discussed later. The roof of the maxillary sinus is the base of the orbit. The maxillary sinus ostium opens into the middle meatus between the middle and inferior turbinates. The frontal sinus forms the middle portion of the roof of the orbit and is within the frontal bone. Its ostium opens into the anterior part of the middle meatus. The ethmoidal sinus lines the medial wall of the orbit in close proximity to the cranial cavity, from which it is separated by the cribriform plate. Bony septa divide the ethmoid sinuses into anterior, middle, and posterior sections. The posterior ethmoidal cells drain into the superior meatus, whereas the anterior sinus cells drain into the upper posterior aspect of the medial meatus. The sphenoidal sinus empties into the sphenoethmoidal recess above the superior turbinate. Its roof is the pituitary fossa, and its lateral aspect is formed by the cavernous venous sinuses.

TABLE 26–2
MANAGEMENT OF NASAL POLYPS

A 12-day tapering course of oral prednisone beginning with 20 mg three times a day and decreasing by 5 mg each day
On the third day, begin administering a topical nasal corticosteroid
Reserve polypectomy for medically resistant cases

Developmentally, the maxillary and ethmoid sinuses are present at birth and evident by radiography in infancy. The frontal sinuses become recognizable anatomically by the 6th to 12th month and appear radiographically between the 3rd and 7th years. The sphenoid sinuses develop by the third year of life but do not appear radiographically until the ninth year. There is great variation in shape and size of the sinuses at all ages, particularly the frontal sinuses.

The paranasal sinuses form as invaginations of the mucous membrane of the nasal cavity. It therefore follows that the mucosal lining of the sinuses should be similar to the mucosal lining of the nasal cavity, that is, ciliated pseudostratified columnar epithelium with goblet cells.[69] The precise functions of the paranasal sinuses are not clear. However, some suggestions have included roles in olfaction, voice response, production of protective mucus, dampening of sudden pressure changes in the nose during respiration, and lessening of skull weight.

PATHOGENESIS

Protection against infection of the paranasal sinuses is largely provided by the mucociliary apparatus. Microorganisms, pollutants, irritants, and other foreign particles that escape the filtering apparatus of the nose are trapped in the mucus of the sinuses and then removed through the draining ostia by constant movement of the mucus blanket propelled by the underlying cilia. When this self-cleansing mechanism is impaired, bacterial infection occurs.

Several factors may result in retention of secretions in the paranasal sinuses: swelling of the mucus membrane, leading to reduced patency of ostia; reduced transport capacity related to abnormalities of the cilia, including quantitative reduction, retardation of movement, and insufficient coordination of movement; and overproduction of secretions.[68]

Of these factors, patency of the ostia is the most important in the development of sinusitis.[69] The ostia functions primarily for drainage of secretions and for gas exchange. Obstruction of the ostium leads to retention of secretions and a low oxygen content in the sinuses, both of which favor increased bacterial growth and purulence. Mucociliary activity of the sinuses is of extreme importance in protection against sinusitis because spontaneous drainage of the maxillary sinus is nearly impossible for two reasons. First, the maxillary ostium is not simply an opening of 1 to 2 mm in diameter, but rather a circuitous channel 6 mm in length that connects the maxillary antrum to the middle meatus. This is referred to as the osteomeatal complex. Second, as stated before, the floor of the maxillary sinus is below the floor of the nasal cavity, thus placing the maxillary ostium in the superior portion of the maxillary antrum. Therefore, for spontaneous drainage to occur into the nose in the upright position, the antrum must be completely filled before the contents can spill over, or ciliary action must move secretions in a cephalad direction against the force of gravity. For these reasons, the maxillary sinus is by far the most common site of sinusitis, followed in decreasing order of incidence by the ethmoid, frontal, and sphenoid sinuses. With this information on pathophysiology, we can determine the factors that predispose to the development of sinusitis (Table 26–3).

Although systemic factors, particularly hypogammaglobulinemia, may play some role, far and away the most common factors predisposing to sinusitis are local. Heading the list are viral upper respiratory infections and allergic rhinitis, in which the mechanism for the development of sinusitis would appear to be similar. Acute rhinitis of either infectious or allergic etiology results in edematous obstruction of the nasal ostia, decreased paranasal sinus ciliary action, and increased mucus production. With the subsequent accumulation of mucus in the sinus, the stage is set for secondary bacterial infection and the conversion of mucus to mucopus. Mucopus further impairs ciliary function and increases swelling around ostia when it discharges into the nose, creating a vicious cycle.

MICROBIOLOGY OF SINUSITIS

Normal sinuses do not yield any bacteria.[46] Nasal smears and cultures give an inaccurate picture of the organisms responsible for sinusitis because of contamination with other organisms. The only true microbiologic picture of sinusitis comes from sinus aspirates obtained by direct antral puncture or by sampling directly from the involved sinus during surgery.

Cultures from both adults[24] and children[94] with acute sinusitis grow predominantly aerobic organisms, with the heaviest yield being *Streptococcus pneumoniae, Haemophilus influenzae,* and *Moraxella* (formerly *Branhamella*) *catarrhalis.*

Poor drainage of the chronically infected maxillary sinus reduces antral PO_2 and pH, which would in turn be expected to encourage the growth of anaerobic bacteria by providing them with the optimal oxidation reduction potential. In one report, anaerobic organisms, predominantly cocci and *Bacteroides* species, were found in 88% of adults with chronic maxillary sinusitis. Forty-four percent of the *Bacteroides* were β-lactamase producers.[3]

Chronic sinusitis in childhood has been thought to be caused by the same organisms that cause chronic sinus disease in adults, but this may not be true. Wald and colleagues[95] studied 40 nonallergic children with chronic sinusitis. Sinus aspirates were positive in 58%, with the predominant bacteria being *S. pneumoniae, H. influenzae,* and *M. catarrhalis.* No anaerobes were isolated. In a study of chronic sinusitis in children with respiratory allergies, similar results were shown.[31] *Moraxella* was the most common pathogen, with anaerobic organisms being rare. Maxillary antral cultures from patients with cystic fibrosis are somewhat different, with *Pseudomonas aeruginosa* being the most common, followed by *H. influenzae, Streptococcus* species, and anaerobes.[78]

Fungal infection of the paranasal sinuses may occur in both immunocompromised and immunocompetent individuals. *Aspergillus fumigatus* is the most common fungus found in both groups.[61] Other fungi causing sinusitis include actinomycetes, *Nocardia, Mucor, Candida, Sporothrix schenkii, Alternaria,* and *Bipolaris* species. It has been suggested that mycoses of the paranasal sinuses occur more frequently than has been assumed.[87] Improved diagnostic techniques make it possible to more readily recognize mycoses, whereas factors that predispose to fungus infections, such as radiation therapy, cytostatic and immunosuppressive treatment, and long-term cortisone and antibiotic regimens, are increasingly common. It should be emphasized, however, that mycoses of the paranasal sinuses can develop in people who are otherwise healthy.

Paranasal sinus infections with *Aspergillus* may take the form of one of four distinct syndromes: indolent or localized invasive aspergillosis,[38] invasive or fulminant aspergillosis, aspergilloma or mycetoma, and allergic *Aspergillus* sinusitis.[80] The histologic picture in allergic *Aspergillus* sinusitis is one of a distinct mucinous material containing eosinophils, Charcot-Leyden crystals, and fungal hyphae. Katzenstein and colleagues[43] have commented that the pathologic finding in allergic *Aspergillus* sinusitis is indistinguishable from the appearance of mucoid impaction of the bronchi associated with allergic bronchopulmonary aspergillosis. Patients with this syndrome are generally young adults with asthma, chronic nasal polyps, recurrent sinusitis, and radiographically opacified sinuses. None has shown pulmonary manifestations of allergic bronchopulmonary aspergillosis.

Several cases of allergic fungal sinusitis have been reported as being caused by *Bipolaris spicifera,* a dematiaceous saprophytic mold similar to *Curvularia* and *Alternaria.*[33]

TABLE 26–3
FACTORS PREDISPOSING TO SINUSITIS

Local	Swimming and diving
Upper respiratory infection	Cigarette smoke
Allergic rhinitis	Barotrauma
Nonallergic rhinitis	Dental extraction/injections
Overuse of topical decongestants	***Systemic***
Hypertrophied adenoids	Immune deficiency
Deviated nasal septum	Bronchiectasis
Bone spurs	Dysmotile cilia syndrome
Nasal polyps	Cystic fibrosis
Tumors	
Foreign bodies	

DIAGNOSIS

History and Physical Examination

The most important clinical clue to the diagnosis of acute sinusitis is the failure of symptoms to clear after a typical cold. The previously clear nasal discharge becomes yellow or green. Fever persists, chills may develop, and pain is often felt in the cheek, which may be referred to the forehead. The discomfort is often worse on bending or straining. Pain may be felt in the teeth if the ostium of the maxillary sinus is blocked. On physical examination, thick purulent green or yellow secretions may be seen in the middle meatus, the site of drainage of the maxillary sinus. The technique of fiberoptic nasopharyngoscopy affords a better opportunity for visualization of the draining ostia of infected sinusitis.[70] Frequently, a streak of pus may be seen along the lateral wall of the oropharynx.

If mucopus is not evacuated, acute sinusitis may enter a subacute or chronic phase. Persistent chronic infection of the upper sinuses is invariably associated with infection in the lower air cells. Chronic maxillary sinusitis may exist alone, but chronic ethmoid and frontal sinusitis is generally associated with maxillary antral infection. The general lack of pain or systemic symptoms makes chronic sinusitis difficult to diagnose on history alone. The patient with chronic sinusitis generally presents with persistent and sometimes unilateral nasal stuffiness, hyposmia, purulent nasal and postnasal secretions, sore throat, fetid breath, and malaise. The secretions often pool in the hypopharynx at night, and the patient complains of increasing postnasal drainage, with resultant cough and sometimes wheezing. Coexistent otitis media is frequently present in children.[40] In a series of 48 children with sinusitis and reactive airway disease, 94% had sore throat, 63% had nasal discharge, and 56% had earache. Headache was present in only 21%, as was fever, 6% had tooth pain, and 6% had facial pain.[67] The subtle clinical presentation of chronic sinusitis requires a high degree of diagnostic index of suspicion on the part of the clinician. On physical examination, the patient with chronic sinusitis may display an edematous and hyperemic nasal mucosa bathed in mucopus. In fungal sinusitis, the sinus exudate is generally thick, of a peanut butter–like consistency. Direct sinus tenderness on percussion is rarely present in chronic sinusitis.

In one study, chronic sinusitis was found to be more common in allergic individuals than in controls. Extensive disease of the sinuses correlated with asthma, specific IgE antibodies, and in particular, eosinophilia. Eighty-seven percent of patients with peripheral eosinophilia had extensive disease of the sinuses.[63]

Nasal Smear and Sinus Culture

As stated earlier, nasal culture does not give an adequate picture of the organisms responsible for sinusitis. Microscopic examination of nasal secretions, however, may be of great diagnostic value. In instances of sinusitis, one sees sheets of polymorphonuclear neutrophils and bacteria. This is unlike viral upper respiratory infections, in which polymorphonuclear neutrophils are scanty, or allergic rhinitis, in which a high percentage of eosinophils may be seen. Antral puncture gives a true specimen of the microbiology of the sinus cavity and is generally performed by an otolaryngologist. Newer devices make intranasal puncture easier to perform and less painful.

Transillumination

A carefully controlled study has shown that transillumination of the sinuses is of limited usefulness in the diagnosis of sinusitis.[86] Although the technique is reasonably accurate in detecting frontal sinusitis, it is very poor in diagnosing maxillary disease. Transillumination perhaps has some use in screening patients, such as those who are pregnant.

Ultrasonography

This technique, also termed ultrasound, is rapid and painless and utilizes nonionizing radiation. In one study in adults, it was shown to be particularly useful in predicting the presence of fluid in patients whose sinus radiographs showed partial or complete opacification.[52] Wald and colleagues[95] reported that in children who had totally opaque sinuses radiographically, all had abnormal ultrasound patterns. However, some patients with mucosal thickening on radiographs and a positive aspirate culture had no sonographic abnormality. In another study, Shapiro and colleagues,[79] comparing ultrasound with radiography in both children and adults, showed a false-positive rate of 39% to 45% and a false-negative rate of 42% to 56% using ultrasound. They concluded that ultrasound is not sufficiently accurate to be used as a substitute for radiography in diagnosing sinusitis.

Radiology (See Chapter 23)

Radiographic views have long been considered the most reliable adjunct in the clinical diagnosis of sinusitis. The occipitomental or Waters' view best demonstrates the maxillary sinus. The head is tilted back so that the dense petrous bone does not occlude the lower part of the maxillary antra. The occipitofrontal or Caldwell's view demonstrates both the ethmoid and frontal sinus. The sphenoid sinus is seen on a lateral view.

The correlation, or lack thereof, of radiologic evidence of sinusitis and positive antral culture along with clinical evidence of sinusitis has been the subject of many publications. Earlier studies reported radiographic evidence of maxillary sinus abnormality in 26% of asymptomatic normal subjects[25] and 52% of asthmatic subjects.[89] The latter study reported only a 20% positive bacterial growth in antral cultures in association with positive radiographs. This discrepancy in contrast with later studies is due to the fact that the roentgenographic diagnosis of sinusitis was made on the basis of only minor degrees of mucosal thickening (1–5 mm). Mild mucosal edema of this degree may be seen in a patient with edema of the nasal mucosa from any cause. In a study of adults with sinusitis, Evans and colleagues[24] reported abnormal sinus aspirates in 17 of 18 patients with radiographic opacity of the sinus and abnormal aspirates in all subjects with air-fluid levels or mucosal thickening of greater than 8 mm. This same degree of correlation of sinus radiographic abnormalities with results of sinus aspirates has also been reported in children.[95]

It thus would appear that in adults, radiographic evidence of mucosal thickening of 6 to 8 mm or greater (Fig. 26–2),

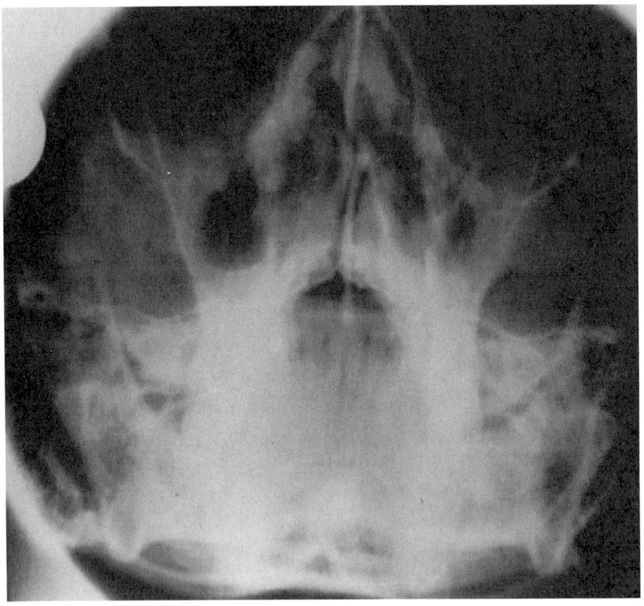

FIGURE 26–2. Plain film showing marked mucoperiosteal thickening of both maxillary sinuses.

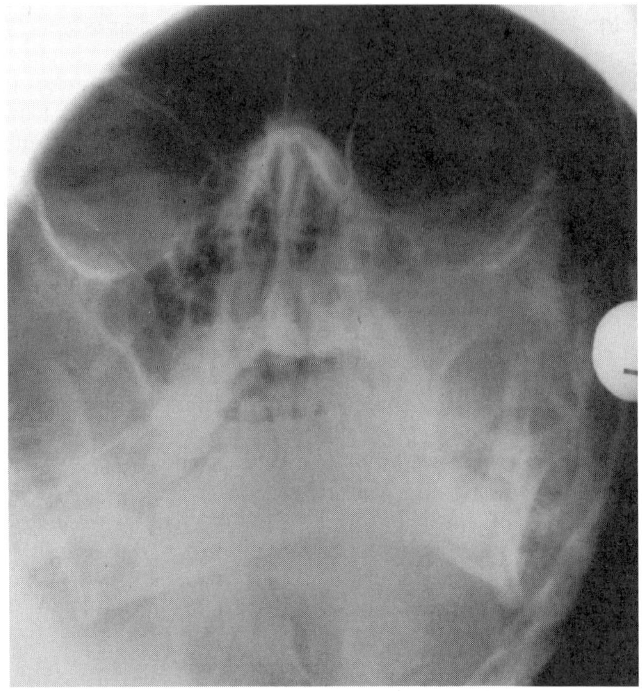

FIGURE 26–4. Total opacification of the left maxillary sinus.

air-fluid levels (Fig. 26–3), or opacification (Fig. 26–4) indicates bacterial infection of the sinuses. In children, mucosal thickening of 4 mm correlates with positive antral puncture.[71, 95]

It has been generally thought that sinus radiographs are of little use in children, in that redundant sinus mucosa or even tears could result in an opaque radiographic appearance.[19] In addition, some have cautioned that asymmetry in facial bone or sinus development, overlying soft tissue swelling, or both can produce differences in apparent aeration of the maxillary sinuses,[19] leading to misinterpretation of radiographs. In a report on a true control group of children without signs or symptoms of respiratory inflammation, sinus radiographs appear to be of limited utility in infants before their first birthday.[48] However, beyond the age of 1 year, abnormal maxillary sinus radiographs are infrequent and generally related to inflammation of the upper respiratory tract. The data suggest that crying alone is distinctly not a cause of abnormal maxillary sinus radiographs in children more than 1 year of age.

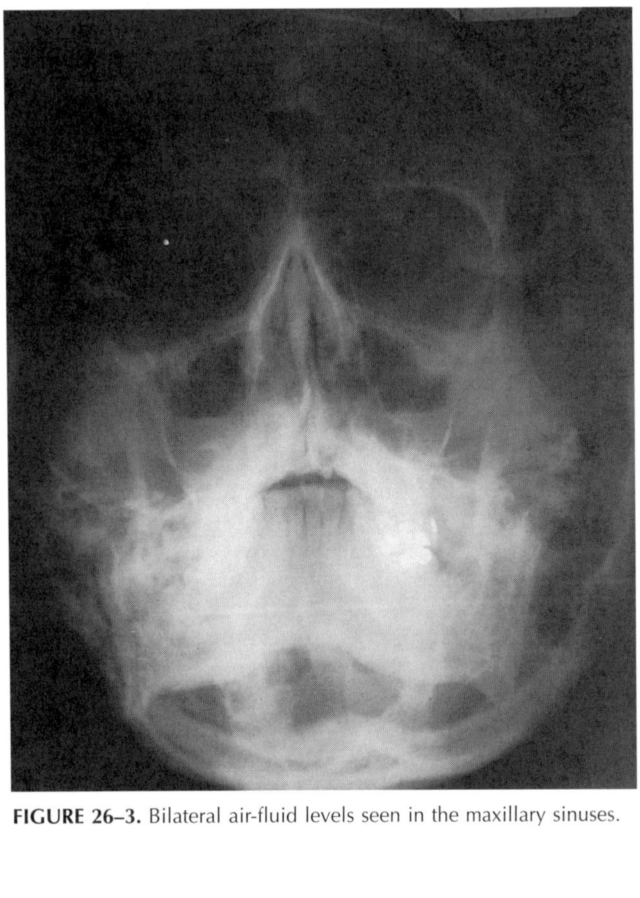

FIGURE 26–3. Bilateral air-fluid levels seen in the maxillary sinuses.

Computed Tomography

A major development in the diagnosis of sinusitis is the application of computed tomographic (CT) scans. Pluridirectional tomography can delineate sinus disease more clearly than do plain radiographs, revealing the extent of disease and bone destruction and distinguishing opacification from membrane thickening.[11] Coronal CT scans demonstrate the osteomeatal complex and detect subtle disease not shown on plain radiographs (Fig. 26–5). In a study comparing plain radiographs with coronal CT scans in 70 infants and children with recurrent sinusitis, 80% of the CT scans were abnormal. In 75% of patients, plain radiographs did not correlate with CT. Forty-five percent of patients had normal findings on radiographs of at least one sinus with abnormality of that sinus on CT. Thirty-five percent had what was interpreted as abnormality of at least one sinus on plain radiographs, but that sinus was normal on CT. The authors concluded that sinusitis in infants and children is often underdiagnosed or overdiagnosed on the basis of plain x-rays, and this error

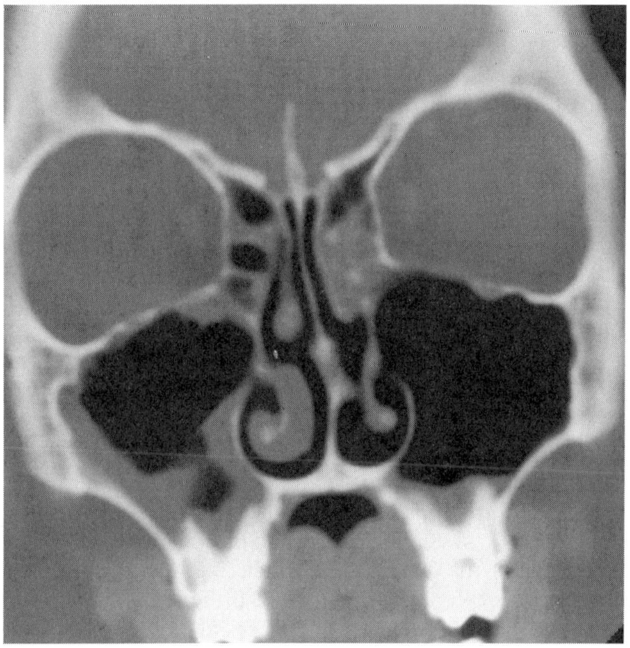

FIGURE 26–5. CT scan of the sinuses showing mucoperiosteal thickening of the right maxillary sinus, opacification of most of the left ethmoid sinus, and scattered opacification of the right ethmoid sinus. (Courtesy of David S. Martin, St. Louis University School of Medicine, St. Louis, MO.)

cannot be used to determine the need for or to guide endoscopic surgery on sinuses.[53]

CT may also be of great help in interpreting postoperative sinus films. One third of post–Caldwell-Luc operative x-rays are opaque. The antral lumen can be reduced by fibrosis or true bony thickening. CT has been shown to be the best method of differentiating components of opacification seen on plain films or ordinary tomography. More details of mucosal changes and bone defects are seen with CT.[8] Another advantage of CT is in diagnosis of fungal sinusitis, which reveals high-intensity material within the sinus cavity. On magnetic resonance imaging, fungal sinusitis can be isointense to hypointense compared with normal mucosa due to iron and manganese within the fungus.[102]

It has been suggested that a limited four-slice coronal CT scan of the sinuses provides excellent imaging of the sinuses, osteomeatal complex, and other nasal structures at a reasonable cost.[13] One group of investigators has developed a scoring system for CT scans to quantitate the extent of disease. Points are based on the degree of obstruction in the nasal passages and each of the two osteomeatal complex units and on the maximal single-wall mucosal thickening of each of seven sinus areas (two frontal, two maxillary, two ethmoid, and one sphenoid). A total of 30 points is possible, with limited disease ranging from 0 to 11 points and extensive disease being more than 12 points.[63]

Positive CT scans of the sinuses are not specific for bacterial or fungal sinusitis. In a group of adults with naturally acquired common colds, the vast majority had osteomeatal and sinus abnormalities.[35]

Ancillary Laboratory Tests

For resistant chronic sinusitis, other diagnostic tests must be considered. Immune deficiency can be diagnosed by quantitation of serum immunoglobulins, antibody responses to specific antigens, such as pneumococcus, diphtheria, and tetanus, and IgG subclasses.[65, 89] Underlying allergy can be determined by a careful history and appropriate skin testing.

COMPLICATIONS

Complications of sinusitis have shown some increase caused by the evolution of drug-resistant bacteria and by immunosuppression secondary to chemotherapy. The most commonly seen complications are orbital and include cellulitis, abscess, and cavernous sinus thrombosis.[80] The second most common complication is an intracranial extension of infection that may include epidural or subdural abscess. A third complication is mucocele formation, and a fourth is osteomyelitis. Another possible complication of sinusitis is bronchial asthma, which will be discussed later.

WEGENER'S GRANULOMATOSIS

(See Chapter 52)

In any adult with particularly severe and resistant sinusitis, thought should be given to Wegener's granulomatosis. This is a disease of unknown cause characterized by necrotizing granulomatous vasculitis. Seventy-five percent of patients have nasopharyngeal involvement, and 90% have paranasal sinus disease. The lesion frequently is destructive and may cause erosion of adjacent bone, nasal septal perforation, and saddle-nose deformity. In addition to upper respiratory tract involvement, the patient may have lower respiratory tract disease, glomerulonephritis, and disseminated small vessel vasculitis.[26] The similarity of Wegener's granulomatosis to other vasculitides of known immunologic mediation strongly suggests that an immunologic phenomenon may play a predominant pathogenetic role.[27]

The patient with Wegener's granulomatosis typically presents with severe upper respiratory tract complaints, including persistent rhinorrhea or a purulent nasal discharge. What appears to be a cold or an attack of sinusitis persists far longer than the usual expectation. Sinus x-rays are generally abnormal. In the early stages, mucosal thickening of maxillary antra is seen that progresses to complete opacification or air-fluid levels usually in association with secondary infection. The organism most frequently encountered is *S. aureus.*

Dramatic therapeutic results with long-term remissions have been seen with the use of cytotoxic agents, particularly cyclophosphamide.[28]

MANAGEMENT

Medical Treatment

Sinusitis should be thought of as an abscess, that is, an infection within a closed anatomic space. In addition to appropriate antibiotics, every effort should be made to remove infected contents from the sinus cavity. When purulent secretions are removed, one sees an increase of sinus pO_2, a decrease in sinus pCO_2, and a decrease in lactate content, all of which lead to a milieu that is unfavorable to anaerobic organisms. There is also a decrease in proteolytic enzymes, which are so damaging to the sinus mucosa, as well as an increase in ciliary movement, which leads to a more rapid and complete return to normal sinus physiology. The overall medical treatment approach to sinusitis is seen in Table 26–4.

Saline nasal spray or douches are useful to liquify secretions, prevent crusting, and decrease nasal blood flow, with a resultant decongestant effect. Topical decongestants may be helpful in promoting sinus drainage but should be used for only a few days to avoid the vasodilating rebound phenomenon. Oral phenylpropanolamine has been shown to increase the functional diameter of the maxillary ostium.[55]

In cases of hyperplastic rhinosinusitis, particularly in association with nasal polyps, a short course of systemic corticosteroids is indicated. One study indicates that intranasal flunisolide spray is a useful adjunct to antibiotic therapy for sinusitis.[56] Compared with placebo spray, the corticosteroid spray improved global evaluations, improved symptoms, decreased inflammatory cells in nasal cytograms, normalized ultrasound scans, and aided in regression of radiographic abnormalities.

There is no controlled study demonstrating the efficacy of mucoevacuants in treating sinusitis. However, it seems reasonable that thinning secretions would promote drainage and removal of purulent material from the sinuses.

The antibiotic of choice for treatment of sinusitis is ampicillin or amoxicillin because the organisms responsible are sensitive to these drugs, and there is good evidence that adequate mucosal and even sinus fluid levels of these antibiotics are obtained.[23] In one report dealing with children, amoxicillin or cefaclor appeared to be of comparable efficacy.[97] When amoxicillin or cefaclor fails, erythromycin with sulfisoxazole is appropriate.[96] In the case of penicillin sensitivity, trimethoprim with sulfamethoxazole is an adequate alternative, as is erythromycin.

Increasing numbers of bacteria responsible for sinusitis have become resistant to penicillin and cephalosporins by producing β-lactamase enzymes that destroy the β-lactam nucleus of these antibiotics. Clavulanic acid, an inhibitor of the β-lactamases, has been introduced in combination with amoxicillin for treatment of β-lactamase–producing organisms.[98] Other antibiotics useful in treatment of resistant sinusitis include cefuroxime and cefprozil.[93] The duration of treatment is as important as the choice of antibiotics. Ten to 14 days of antibiotic therapy is generally adequate for acute sinusitis, with chronic sinusitis requiring 3 to 4 weeks or longer.

The management of invasive fungal sinusitis includes extensive debridement and parenteral antifungal drugs. The allergic form of fungal sinusitis most commonly caused by *Aspergillus* or *Bipolaris* is treated by debridement and systemic steroids.[81]

The effects of aspirin desensitization on aspirin-sensitive patients with rhinosinusitis and asthma have been reported. Patients desensitized with aspirin and then maintained on daily aspirin experienced significant improvement in sense of smell, nasal symptoms, and numbers of episodes of upper respiratory infections and sinusitis per year, with impressive declines in nasal polypectomies and sinus operations.[92]

If allergic rhinitis underlies chronic sinusitis, appropriate medical therapy is needed, including symptomatic measures, such as antihistamines, decongestants, intranasal cromolyn, and topical or systemic corticosteroids. Environmental control involving the avoidance of offending allergens and immunotherapy can also be beneficial. If there is no significant clinical and radiographic improvement after appropriate and vigorous medical therapy, the patient should be referred to an otolaryngologist.

TABLE 26–4
MEDICAL TREATMENT OF SINUSITIS

Steam and saline
Decongestants
  Topical: oxymetazoline, phenylephrine
  Oral: pseudoephedrine, phenylpropanolamine
Corticosteroids
  Topical: beclomethasone, flunisolide, triamcinolone, budesonide
  Oral: prednisone
Mucoevacuants: guaifenesin (glyceryl guaiacolate)
Antibiotics: ampicillin or amoxicillin
  trimethoprim with sulfamethoxazole
    (in case of penicillin sensitivity)
  amoxicillin–clavulanate
  cefuroxime
  cefprozil

Surgical Treatment

Persistent or recurrent episodes of sinusitis that occur despite appropriate medical therapy necessitate consideration of surgical intervention. The tasks of the otolaryngologist are to relieve the obstruction of the ostia, resect inflamed or infected tissues, and provide an airway with drainage for all nasal and sinus compartments.[81] A variety of surgical procedures have been utilized for the treatment of sinusitis, but functional endoscopic surgery has emerged as the technique of choice in most instances. Reestablishment of ventilation and mucociliary clearance of the sinuses is accomplished by the endoscopic removal of diseased tissue from the key areas of the anterior ethmoid sinus, middle turbinate, and middle meatus. The objective is to remove, in a limited resection, the inflammatory and anatomic defects that interfere with normal mucociliary clearance and produce the resistant inflammation. Advantages are minimal trauma to normal nasal and sinus structures and conservative removal of diseased tissue. A return to the natural physiology and mucociliary clearance and function of the sinuses is thus made possible.[45] The availability of endoscopes with a variety of angles of view has greatly expanded the usefulness of this technique.

RELATIONSHIP OF SINUSITIS TO ASTHMA

The frequent association of nasal and paranasal sinus disease with bronchial asthma has been appreciated for many years.[6, 32, 99] One group observed an abnormal finding in sinus radiographs of 87% of patients with exacerbation of asthma.[71] A large number of studies performed both in experimental animals and humans have demonstrated that reflex bronchoconstriction can result from stimulation of receptors in the nose and nasopharynx. In 1870, Kratchmer[49] showed that a variety of irritants, such as ether, sulfur dioxide, and cigarette smoke, applied to the nasal mucous membrane of cats and rabbits resulted in bronchoconstriction. Other investigators later showed that the bronchoconstriction caused by mechanical or electric stimulation of the nasal mucosa could be abolished by vagus nerve resection.[15] Kaufman and Wright[44] exposed the nose and nasopharynx of subjects with no evidence of pulmonary disease to silica particles. This resulted in a significant increase in lower airway resistance that could be abolished by pretreatment with atropine.

The clinical association of sinusitis and asthma has been revived.[66, 67, 82] One study indicates that the association between chronic sinusitis and asthma was strong only in the group with extensive disease.[63]

There is no doubt that sinusitis and asthma coexist. However, the overriding question is whether sinusitis and asthma are manifestations of the same disease process in different parts of the respiratory tract or whether sinusitis triggers bronchial asthma. Convincing evidence from prospective, double-blind, placebo-controlled trials is lacking.[54] Nevertheless, data indicating that patients with refractory asthma show improvement when concurrent sinusitis is appropriately managed strongly suggest a contributory role for sinusitis in lower airway disease.

Several studies in children with combined sinusitis and hyperreactive airway disease have shown that management of sinusitis results in significant improvement in asthma.[30, 85] Rachelefsky and colleagues[67] found that 76% of 48 such children could discontinue bronchodilators once the sinusitis resolved. Further, 67% of those with pretreatment abnormalities in pulmonary function had normal test results after therapy.

The same improvement in the asthmatic state following definitive nasosinus surgery has also been seen in adults.[58, 66] A 5-year follow-up in patients who underwent bilateral intranasal sphenoethmoidectomy revealed that those who showed improvement within 2 years of surgery were likely to continue improving throughout the entire observation period. Sixty percent showed an improvement in asthma with a corresponding decrease in corticosteroid use.[58] Similar results have been reported following functional endoscopic surgery.[39]

Several mechanisms have been proposed to explain the relationship between sinusitis and asthma.[83] In a rabbit model, sterile sinusitis induced by chemotactic complement fragment C5a des arg increased lower airway responsiveness to histamine. The most likely mechanism based on positioning of the animal is postnasal dripping of cells or cell products into the lower airway.[5] Others have pointed out that extrapolation of data to suggest that postnasal dripping of cells or cell products causes increases in airway resistance in humans appears uncertain because of interspecies differences.[1] Indeed, the draining of sinus contents directly into the lung seems unlikely, since a study utilizing isotope labeling failed to show pulmonary aspiration of sinus contents in patients with asthma and sinusitis.[2]

It has been suggested that the eosinophil, which plays an important role in causing injury to the bronchial epithelium in asthmatics, might cause inflammation in the paranasal epithelium. Sinus tissue from patients with chronic asthma was extensively infiltrated with eosinophils, whereas patients with chronic sinusitis alone had few if any eosinophils.[37] One study demonstrated that the marked tissue eosinophilia associated with chronic hyperplastic sinusitis is strongly correlated with local cytokine production, particularly GM-CSF and IL-3. Interestingly, IL-5 mRNA expression was not a prominent feature.[36] Another mechanism involves local stimulation of irritant receptors, causing reflex bronchospasm. Levels of sulfidopeptide leukotrienes, prostaglandin D2, and histamine in maxillary sinus lavage fluid are significantly higher than nasal lavage fluid in the range associated with local inflammation and irritant receptor stimulation.[90]

REFERENCES

1. Bardin PG, Joubert JR: Increased lower airway responsiveness associated with sinusitis in a rabbit model. Am Rev Respir Dis 148:821, 1993.
2. Bardin PG, Van Heerden BB, Jourbert JR: Absence of pulmonary aspiration of sinus contents in patients with asthma and sinusitis. J Allergy Clin Immunol 86:82, 1990.
3. Brook I: Bacteriology of chronic maxillary sinusitis in adults. Ann Otol Rhinol Laryngol 98:426, 1989.
4. Brown BL, Harner SG, VanDellen RG: Nasal polypectomy in patients with asthma and sensitivity to aspirin. Arch Otolaryngol 105:413, 1979.
5. Brugman SM, Larsen GL, Henson PM, et al: Increased lower airways responsiveness associated with sinusitis in a rabbit model. Am Rev Respir Dis 147:314, 1993.
6. Bullen SS: Incidence of asthma in 400 cases of chronic sinusitis. J Allergy 4:402, 1932.
7. Bumstead RH, el-Ackad T, Smith JM, et al: Histamine, norepinephrine and serotonin content of nasal polyps. Laryngoscope 89:832, 1984.
8. Cable HR, Jeans WD, Cullen RJ, et al: Computerized tomography of the Caldwell-Luc cavity. J Laryngol Otol 95:775, 1981.
9. Caffey J: Pediatric X-Ray Diagnosis, 6th edition. Yearbook, Chicago, 1972.
10. Caplin I, Haynes TJ, Sphahn J: Are nasal polyps an allergic phenomenon? Ann Allergy 29:63, 1971.
11. Carter BL, Bankoff MS, Fisk JD: Computed tomographic detection of sinusitis responsible for intracranial and extracranial infections. Radiology 147:739, 1983.
12. Chandra RK, Abol BM: Immunopathology of nasal polypi. J Laryngol Otol 88:1019, 1974.
13. Davidson TM, Brahme FJ, Gallagher ME: Radiographic evaluation for nasal dysfunction: computed tomography versus plain films. Head Neck 11:405, 1989.
14. DiSant' Agnese PA, Davis PB: Cystic fibrosis in adults: 75 cases and a review of 232 cases in the literature. Am J Med 66:121, 1979.
15. Dixon WE, Brodie TG: The bronchial muscles: their innervation and the action of drugs upon them. J Physiol (Lond) 29:93, 1993.
16. Dolovich J, Jeffery P, Kawabori S, et al: Cellular infiltration in nasal polyps does not correlate with blood counts or the allergic state. J Allergy Clin Immunol 83:308, 1989.
17. Drake-Lee AB, Pitcher-Wilmott RW: The clinical and laboratory correlates of nasal polyps in cystic fibrosis. Int J Pediatr Otorhinolaryngol 4:209, 1982.
18. Drake-Lee AB: Histamine and its release from nasal polyps: preliminary communication. J R Soc Med 77:120, 1984.
19. Drake-Lee AB, Lowe D, Swanston A, et al: Clinical profile and recurrence of nasal polyps. J Laryngol Otol 98:783, 1984.
20. Drake-Lee AB, Chevreton E, Lowe D: The effect of different fixations on the distribution and numbers of mast cells in patients with nasal polyps. J Laryngol Otol 102:1099, 1988.
21. Drettner B, Ebbesen A, Nilsson M: Prophylactic treatment with flunisolide after polypectomy. Rhinology 20:149, 1982.
22. Eichel B: Ethmoiditis: pathophysiology and medical management. Otolaryngol Clin North Am 18:43, 1985.
23. Eneroth CM, Lundberg C: The antibacterial effect of antibiotics in treatment of maxillary sinusitis. Arch Otolaryngol 81:475, 1976.
24. Evans FO Jr, Syndnor JB, Moore WE, et al: Sinusitis of the maxillary antrum. N Engl J Med 293:735, 1975.

25. Fascenelli FW: Maxillary sinus abnormalities: radiographic evidence in an asymptomatic patient. Arch Otolaryngol 90:98, 1969.
26. Fauci AS, Wolff SM: Wegener's granulomatosis: studies in eighteen patients and a review of the literature. Medicine 52:535, 1973.
27. Fauci AS, Wolff SM: Immunological features of Wegener's granulomatosis. Lancet 1:688, 1974.
28. Fauci AS: Granulomatous vasculitides: distinct but related. Ann Intern Med 87:782, 1977.
29. Francis C: The prognosis of operation for removal of nasal polypi in cases of asthma. Practitioner 123:272, 1929.
30. Friedman R, Ackerman M, Wald E, et al: Asthma and bacterial sinusitis in children. J Allergy Clin Immunol 74:185, 1984.
31. Goldenhersh MJ, Rachelefsky GS, Dudley J, et al: The microbiology of chronic sinus disease in children with respiratory allergy. J Allergy Clin Immunol 85:1030, 1990.
32. Gottlieb MS: Relation of intranasal sinus disease in the production of asthma. JAMA 85:105, 1925.
33. Gourley DS, Whisman BA, Jorgensen NL, et al: Allergic *Bipolaris* sinusitis: clinical and immunopathic characteristics. J Allergy Clin Immunol 85:583, 1990.
34. Guntert VG: A serious complication (blindness) after intranasal injection of hydrocortisone. HNO 11:77, 1963.
35. Gwaltney JM Jr, Phillips CD, Miller RD, et al: Computed tomographic study of the common cold. N Engl J Med 330:25, 1994.
36. Hamilos DL, Leung DYM, Wood R, et al: Chronic hyperplastic sinusitis: association of tissue eosinophilia with mRNA expression of granulocyte-macrophage colony-stimulating factor and interleukin-3. J Allergy Clin Immunol 92:39, 1993.
37. Harlin BL, Ansel DG, Lane SR, et al: A clinical and pathologic study of chronic sinusitis: the role of the eosinophil. J Allergy Clin Immunol 81:867, 1988.
38. Hora J: Primary aspergillosis of paranasal sinuses and associated areas. Laryngoscope 75:768, 1965.
39. Hosemann W, Michelson A, Weindler J, et al: The effect of endonasal paranasal sinus surgery on lung function of patients with bronchial asthma. Laryngorhinootologie 69:521, 1990.
40. Hoshaw TC, Nickman NJ: Sinusitis and otitis in children. Arch Otolaryngol 100:94, 1974.
41. Jacobs RL, Freda AJ, Culver WG: Primary nasal polyposis. Ann Allergy 51:500, 1983.
42. Kaliner M, Wasserman SI, Austen KF: Immunologic release of chemical mediators from human nasal polyps. N Engl J Med 289:277, 1973.
43. Katzenstein AL, Sale SR, Greenburger PA: Allergic aspergillus sinusitis: a newly recognized form of sinusitis. J Allergy Clin Immunol 72:89, 1983.
44. Kaufman J, Wright GW: The effect of nasal and nasopharyngeal irritation on airway resistance in man. Am Rev Respir Dis 100:626, 1969.
45. Kennedy DW: Functional endoscopic sinus surgery technique. Arch Otolaryngol 3:643, 1985.
46. Kern EB: Sinusitis. J Allergy Clin Immunol 73:25, 1984.
47. Kordash TR, Gleich G, Kern EB: Evidence for increased risk of development of asthma in patients with nasal polyps. J Allergy Clin Immunol 61:138, 1975.
48. Kovatch AL, Wald ER, Ledesma-Medina J, et al: Maxillary sinus radiographs in children with non-respiratory complaints. Pediatrics 73:306, 1984.
49. Kratchmer I: Cited by: A Kiyoshi: Physiologic relationship between nasal breathing and pulmonary function. Laryngoscope 76:30, 1966.
50. Lanza DC, Kennedy DW: Current concepts in the surgical management of nasal polyposis. J Allergy Clin Immunol 90:543, 1992.
51. Lildholdt T, Fogstrup J, Gammelgoard N, et al: Surgical versus medical treatment of nasal polyps. Acta Otolaryngol (Stockh) 105:140, 1988.
52. Mann W, Beck C, Apostolides T: Liability of ultrasound in maxillary sinus disease. Arch Otorhinolaryngol 215:67, 1977.
53. McAlister WH, Lusk R, Muntz HR: Comparison of plain radiographs and coronal CT scans in infants and children with recurrent sinusitis. Am J Roentgenol 153:1259, 1989.
54. McFadden ER Jr: Nasal-sinus-pulmonary reflexes and asthma. J Allergy Clin Immunol 78:1, 1986.
55. Meln I, Friberg B, Andreasson L, et al: Effects of phenylpropanolamine on ostial and nasal patency with patients treated for chronic maxillary sinusitis. Acta Otolaryngol (Stockh) 101:494, 1986.
56. Meltzer EO, Orgel HA, Bockhaus JW, et al: Intranasal flunisolide spray as an adjunct to oral antibiotic therapy for sinusitis. J Allergy Clin Immunol 92:812, 1993.
57. Miles-Lawrence R, Kaplan M, Cheng K: Methacholine sensitivity in nasal polyposis and the effects of polypectomy. J Allergy Clin Immunol 69:102, 1982.
58. Mings R, Friedman WH, Slavin RG, et al: Five year follow-up of the effects of bilateral intranasal sphenoethmoidectomy in patients with sinusitis and asthma. Am J Rhinol 71:123, 1988.
59. Moloney JR: Nasal polyps, nasal polypectomy, asthma and aspirin sensitivity: their association in 445 cases of nasal polyps. J Laryngol Otol 91:837, 1977.
60. Moloney JR, Oliver RTD: HLA antigens, nasal polyps and asthma. Clin Otolaryngol 5:183, 1980.
61. Morgan MA, Wilson WR, Neel HB III, et al: Fungal sinusitis in healthy and immunocompromised individuals. Am J Clin Pathol 82:597, 1984.
62. Mygind N, Pedersen DB, Prytz S, et al: Treatment of nasal polyps with intranasal beclomethasone dipropionate aerosol. Clin Allergy 5:159, 1975.
63. Newman LJ, Platts-Mills TAE, Phillips CD, et al: Chronic sinusitis: relationship of computed tomography findings in allergy, asthma and eosinophilia. JAMA 271:363, 1994.
64. Oppenheimer EH, Rosenstein BJ: Differential pathology of nasal polyps in cystic fibrosis and atopy. Lab Invest 40:445, 1979.
65. Oxelius V, Laurel A, Lindquist B, et al: IgG subclasses in selective IgA deficiency. N Engl J Med 304:1476, 1981.
66. Phipatanakul CS, Slavin RG: Bronchial asthma produced by paranasal sinusitis. Arch Otolaryngol 100:109, 1974.
67. Rachelefsky GS, Katz RM, Siegel SC: Chronic sinus disease with associated reactive airway disease in children. Pediatrics 73:526, 1984.
68. Reiner A, von Mecklenburg C, Toremalm NG: The mucociliary activity of the upper respiratory tract. III. A functional and morphologic study on human and animal material with special reference to the maxillary sinus diseases. Acta Otolaryngol Suppl (Stockh) 355:1, 1978.
69. Rohr AS, Spector SL: Paranasal sinus anatomy and pathophysiology. Clin Rev Allergy 2:387, 1984.
70. Rohr A, Hassner A, Saxon A: Rhinopharyngoscopy for the evaluation of allergic immunologic disorders. Ann Allergy 50:380, 1983.
71. Rossi OVJ, Pirila T, Laitinen J, et al: Sinus aspirates and radiographic abnormalities in severe attacks of asthma. Int Arch Allergy Immunol 103:209, 1994.
72. Ruhno J, Howee K, Anderson M, et al: The increased number of epithelial mast cells in nasal polyps and adjacent turbinate is not allergy-dependent. Allergy 45:370, 1990.
73. Ruhno J, Anderson B, Denburg J, et al: A double-blind comparison of intranasal budesonide with placebo for nasal polyposis. J Allergy Clin Immunol 86:946, 1990.
74. Schenck NL: Nasal polypectomy in the aspirin sensitive asthmatic. Trans Am Acad Ophthalmol Otolaryngol 78:109, 1974.
75. Settipane GA, Chaffee FH, Klein DE: Aspirin intolerance: a prospective study in an atopic and normal population. J Allergy Clin Immunol 53:200, 1974.
76. Settipane GA, Chaffee FH, Klein DE: A critical evaluation of aspirin challenge in patients with nasal polyps. J Allergy Clin Immunol 69:148, 1982.
77. Settipane GA: Nasal polyps. Immunol Allerg Clin North Am 7:105, 1987.
78. Shapiro ED, Milmoe GJ, Wald ER, et al: Bacteriology of the maxillary sinuses in patients with cystic fibrosis. J Infect Dis 146:589, 1982.
79. Shapiro G, Furukawa CT, Pierson WE, et al: Blinded comparison of maxillary sinus radiograph and ultrasound for diagnosis of sinusitis. J Allergy Clin Immunol 77:59, 1986.
80. Sheffield RW, Cassisi NJ, Karlan MS: Complications of sinusitis: what to watch for. Postgrad Med 63:93, 1978.
81. Slavin RG, Cannon RE, Friedman WH, et al: Sinusitis and bronchial asthma. J Allergy Clin Immunol 66:250, 1980.
82. Slavin RG: Relationship of nasal disease and sinusitis to bronchial asthma. Ann Allergy 49:76, 1982.
83. Slavin RG, Pipkorn U, McFadden ER Jr: Pathophysiology interaction of the upper and lower airway. J Respir Dis 12:5991, 1991.
84. Slavin RG: Allergy is not a significant cause of nasal polyps. Arch Otolaryngol Head Neck Surg 118:771, 1992.
85. Snyder RD, Siegel GL: An asthma triad. Ann Allergy 25:377, 1967.
86. Spector SL, Lotan A, English G, et al: Comparison between transillumination and the roentgenogram in diagnosing paranasal sinus disease. J Allergy Clin Immunol 67:22, 1981.
87. Stammberger H: Endoscopic surgery for mycotic and chronic recurring sinusitis. Ann Otol Rhinol Laryngol Suppl 94:1, 1985.

88. Stern RC, Boat TF, Wood RE, et al: Treatment and prognosis of nasal polyps in cystic fibrosis. Am J Dis Child 136:1067, 1982.
89. Stiehm ER: Immunodeficiency disorders—general considerations. In Stiehm ER, Fulginiti VA (eds): Immunologic Disorders in Infants and Children. WB Saunders, Philadelphia, 1989.
90. Stone BD, Georgitis JW, Matthews B: Inflammatory mediators in sinus lavage fluid. J Allergy Clin Immunol 85:222, 1990.
91. Stoop AE, van der Heyden HAMD, Breivenga J, et al: Lymphocyte and non-lymphoid cells in human nasal polyps. J Allergy Clin Immunol 87:470, 1991.
92. Sweet JM, Stevenson DD, Simon RS, et al: Long-term effects of aspirin desensitization-treatment for aspirin sensitive rhinosinusitis-asthma. J Allergy Clin Immunol 85:59, 1990.
93. Sydnor AJ, Gwaltney JM Jr, Coccheto DM, et al: Comparative evaluation of cefuroxime axatil and cefaclor for treatment of acute bacterial maxillary sinusitis. Arch Otolaryngol Head Neck Surg 115:1430, 1989.
94. Taylor M: Histochemical studies of nasal polypi. J Laryngol Otol 77:326, 1973.
95. Wald ER, Milmoe GJ, Bowen A, et al: Acute maxillary sinusitis in children. N Engl J Med 304:749, 1981.
96. Wald ER, Byers C, Guerra N, et al: Subacute sinusitis in children. J Pediatr 115:28, 1989.
97. Wald ER, Reilly JS, Casselbrant M, et al: Treatment of acute maxillary sinusitis in childhood: a comparative study of amoxicillin and cefaclor. J Pediatr 104:297, 1984.
98. Wald ER, Chiponis D, Ledesma-Medina J: Comparative effectiveness of amoxicillin and amoxicillin-clavulanate potassium in acute paranasal sinus infections in children: a double-blind, placebo-controlled trial. Pediatrics 77:795, 1986.
99. Weille FL: Studies in asthma. XIX. The nose and throat in 500 cases of asthma. N Engl J Med 215:235, 1936.
100. Wladislavosky-Waserman P, Kern EB, Holley KE, et al: Epithelial damage in nasal polyps. Clin Allergy 14:241, 1984.
101. Wong D, Jordana G, Denburg J, et al: Blood eosinophilia and nasal polyps. Am J Rhinol 6:195, 1992.
102. Zinreich SJ, Kennedy DW, Malat J, et al: Fungal sinusitis: diagnosis with CT and MR imaging. Radiology 169:439, 1988.

27 *Asthma in Infants and Children*

JEFFREY R. STOKES MARY K. SCHROTH ROBERT F. LEMANSKE, Jr.*

Asthma in infancy and childhood may mean different things to different people. To the child, asthma means episodes of wheezing, shortness of breath, and chest tightness that can interfere with daily activities and sleep. To the parent, it may mean administering multiple medications episodically or on a regular basis and the institution of environmental control measures that may be a hardship both monetarily and emotionally (e.g., removal of a pet). To the clinician, it means developing a therapeutic plan that will maximize both compliance and disease control while minimizing any potential side effects. To the pathologist, asthma is the presence of bronchial smooth muscle hypertrophy, mucus hypersecretion, and airway inflammation. To the physiologist, it is the presence of airway hyperresponsiveness to a range of chemical (methacholine), microbiologic (viruses), physical (exercise), and immunologic (allergens) stimuli that influence patterns of disease and therapeutic responses both acutely and chronically. Perhaps as a result of these variable views, many pseudonyms have been used to describe childhood asthma, including reactive airway disease, asthmatic bronchitis, wheezy bronchitis, and chronic bronchitis with bronchospasm. Further, some have chosen to divide asthma into two categories: extrinsic, in which an external triggering factor can be identified (e.g., allergens), or intrinsic, in which no known external allergic cause is demonstrable.[126]

In an attempt to provide a framework upon which proper diagnostic and therapeutic decisions can be made, a National Asthma Education Program Expert Panel was formed in the early 1990s. Members of the panel suggested that asthma be defined as a lung disease with reversible airway obstruction (not completely in some patients) either spontaneously or with treatment, airway inflammation, and increased airway responsiveness (hyperresponsiveness) to a variety of stimuli.[105] One potential problem with this definition is that its primary focus is the pathophysiologic abnormalities that are found in asthma, while not addressing the clinical manifestations of wheeze, cough, chest tightness, and dyspnea that are perceived as being more important to the patient and/or their parents.[138] However, since multiple other lung diseases can present with some or all of these clinical findings, the concepts of airway obstruction, reversibility, and hyperresponsiveness are more meaningful as differentiating features.

EPIDEMIOLOGY

Asthma is the most common chronic respiratory illness of childhood, affecting an estimated 2 to 5 million children in

*Supported by National Institutes of Health grants number AI34891, AI00995, and HL51843.

the United States.[37] Morbidity from asthma reflects several factors. The National Health Interview Survey in 1988 questioned over 17,000 families with children and found that asthmatic children missed 10.1 million days of school and had 200,000 hospitalizations that resulted in 1.9 million days of inpatient care.[162] Asthmatic children were also noted to have a 1.7 times increased risk of learning disabilities, especially those in fair to poor health, when compared with their nonasthmatic peers.[43]

PREVALENCE

Asthma during childhood has shown a worldwide consistent pattern of increasing prevalence over the last several decades,[17] estimated at 5% to 15% for the entire pediatric population.[107] This increase may be due to either an actual increase in the number of children with the disease or an increased recognition of the disease so that pseudonyms such as wheezy bronchitis may be more properly replaced with diagnoses of asthma. From 1976 to 1980, the 2nd National Health and Nutrition Examination Surveys found that 6.7% of U.S. children 3 to 17 years old had asthma. The prevalence in African-American children was greater than in Caucasian children, 9.4% and 6.2%, respectively, as was that in males (7.8%) compared with females (5.5%).[48] During the 1980s, Weitzman and colleagues[178] found that the prevalence of asthma increased 3.1% to 4.3%. Interestingly, these trends were predominantly due to increases in the Caucasian (2.7–4.1%) rather than the African-American population of children (5.3–5.1%), even though the latter group had the highest prevalence rate. When evaluated over 19 years (1965–1984), the prevalence rate of asthma in children 6 to 11 years of age was found to be even more substantially increased (50%).[37]

INCIDENCE

Only a few studies have looked at the incidence of childhood asthma.[25] In several different studies, boys were noted to have an overall increased incidence, regardless of age group or study location (United Kingdom, Australia, or the United States). In Australia, the incidence was found to be greater in 8 year olds compared with 12 year olds. In the United States, however, the 0–4 age group had the greatest incidence compared with the 5–9 and 10–14 age ranges.

SEVERITY

During the 1980s, children with asthma had better overall health as assessed by decreases in school absenteeism, bedridden days, decreased hospital admissions in the previous year, and fewer extreme behavioral problems.[178] Of all children with asthma, only 10% had severe asthma, but this small subset accounted for 27% of school days missed, 35% of hospitalizations, and 77% of inpatient days. Almost 30% of asthmatic children have some limitations in activity, compared with 5% of children without asthma. African-American children seem to have more severe functional limitations and more hospitalizations than their Caucasian counterparts.[162]

RISK FACTORS

Asthma affects 5% to 30% of infants less than 1 year old; of these, 50% develop symptoms by the age of 2, and 80% by the time they start school.[32, 107] Under the age of 2 and perhaps related, at least in part, to airway geometry, several viruses can produce episodes of wheezing (e.g., respiratory syncytial virus), making diagnostic differentiation of asthma from bronchiolitis challenging. Many asthma experts will diagnose asthma if more than two such episodes accompany upper respiratory tract infections, particularly if the clinical manifestations respond to bronchodilator and/or anti-inflammatory therapy.

In children, it has been well established that viruses are the predominant microorganism associated with infection-induced wheezing.[30] In children with diagnosed asthma, respiratory infections tend to be more prevalent than in their nonasthmatic counterparts, further increasing the risk for wheezing during viral infections.[176] A predilection toward wheezing with viral illness may be related to a diminution in airway size, perhaps being a greater risk factor in girls compared with boys despite the incidence of asthma being greater in boys.[90]

In addition to airway size and exposure to respiratory viruses, a number of other factors, including family history of asthma, serum IgE levels, and exposure to passive smoking, may place a child at increased risk of manifesting asthmatic symptoms. In a study evaluating over 1,000 children prospectively, Martinez and colleagues[91] noted a number of important relationships among these variables and transient versus persistent wheezing. Children who had transient wheezing (wheezing before age 3 but not at age 6) were more likely to have mothers who smoked but not mothers with asthma. They have normal serum IgE levels, no skin-test reactivity, and diminished lung functions at 1 and 6 years of age. Those children who wheezed persistently (wheezing before age 3 and at age 6) were more likely to have a mother with a history of asthma, elevated serum IgE, and normal lung function in the first year of life but diminished lung function at age 6. Children with late-onset wheezing (no wheezing before age 3 but wheezing at age 6) were associated with a maternal history of asthma and rhinitis in the first year of life.

With increasing age, the prevalence of asthma continues to be higher in boys than girls, reaching a peak by midchildhood.[32] The risk of developing asthma in boys less than 10 years old is almost double the risk in girls.[176] By the age of 14, boys are four times more likely to develop chronic asthma and twice as likely to be hospitalized. During and after adolescence, however, the male predominance begins to decrease. Indeed, postpubertal females are at a slightly greater risk of developing asthma and up to three times more likely to be hospitalized. These gender shifts may be related to as yet undefined hormonal or biochemical alterations that affect immunologic or biologic pathways relevant to asthma pathogenesis.[127, 147] Other risks for the development of childhood asthma, in addition to male gender, include African-American race, tobacco smoke exposure, and low socioeconomic class.[100]

Low socioeconomic class and its inherent living conditions are particularly problematic in relationship to asthma. Children living in poverty are more likely to use neighborhood health centers or hospital clinics than physicians' offices. Moreover, when these children are acutely symptomatic, they are four times more likely to use an emergency room as a primary care source than are children from higher socioeconomic environments.[61] Further, asthmatic children with family incomes less than $20,000 are twice as likely to be held behind in school than are their nonasthmatic counterparts.[43] Finally, allergen sensitization to house dust mite or cockroach allergen is more prevalent in inner-city children, with house dust mite sensitivity present in up to 80% of this population.[19, 171] Chronic exposure to these environmental allergens may perpetuate ongoing inflammation in the airway, resulting in more labile disease control over time.[84, 85]

HOSPITALIZATION

During the early 1980s, increased rates of hospitalization occurred, especially in the African-American population.[150] Over a 19-year period (1965–1983), asthma hospitalizations increased over 200% for children, with rates for non-Caucasians compared with Caucasians increasing 150% during this same time.[37] Children up to 4 years old seemed to have the greatest increase in hospitalizations compared with children 5 to 17 years old. African-American children up to 4 years old had nearly a twofold greater increase than did Caucasian children, with an average increase of 6.8% per year.[49] Whereas the number of admissions has increased, the average length of stay for asthmatic children has decreased by 26%.[60] The peak and trough for asthma hospitalizations are September through November and June through August, respectively; these trends may be related to an increase in viral exacerbations during certain months.[25]

MORTALITY

The death rate for children and infants due to asthma is relatively low. In the 1980s, however, the mortality rate for individuals 5 to 34 years old was increasing,[150] with the rate in the African-American population fivefold greater than that in Caucasians. The rates for children 5 to 14 years old increased significantly faster than the rates for adolescents and young adults 15 to 34 years old.[175] In addition to age and race, several other risk factors for increasing asthma mortality have been identified.[144] Asthmatic patients with a previous history of intubation or respiratory acidosis not requiring intubation are considered high risk. Patients who have had more than two admissions for status asthmaticus despite long-term oral corticosteroid treatments, who are inadequately treated for their asthma, who overuse beta-agonists and underuse anti-inflammatory drugs, who are depressed, or who have poor access to medical care are at increased risk of morbidity and mortality from their disease. Misconceptions regarding disease severity may also be problematic. Robertson and colleagues[129] found that in a review of 51 deaths of patients younger than 20 years old due to asthma, 33% were considered to have mild or trivial asthma premortem. Unfortunately, 39% of the patients had potentially preventable elements to their disease severity, such as inadequate treatment, poor compliance, or delays in seeking medical care.

HISTOPATHOLOGY

In asthma, air flow obstruction is produced by a combination of pathogenic abnormalities. The precise contribution of each of these abnormalities varies among asthmatic patients and no doubt affects the diversity in clinical manifestations, such as triggering factors, the chronicity and severity of the disease, and the therapeutic response to various medications. It is unknown at what age or stage of lung development relevant changes specific to asthma develop or precisely how these histopathologic abnormalities fluctuate over time, either spontaneously or in response to therapy.

FACTORS CONTRIBUTING TO THE AIRWAY OBSTRUCTION IN ASTHMA

Airway Smooth Muscle Spasm

The ability to produce symptomatic improvement with bronchodilators and the remarkable airway hyperresponsiveness to a wide variety of stimuli seen in asthmatic patients have indicated that bronchial smooth muscle spasm contributes significantly to airway obstruction. These features would suggest that either the quantity or the function of bronchial smooth muscle in asthma is abnormal. Autopsy specimens obtained from asthmatic patients dying of their disease have demonstrated both hypertrophy and hyperplasia of airway smooth muscle, with variable distribution of these abnormalities within the airway.[36] When examined in vitro, some, but not all, investigators have demonstrated a greater maximal response to contractile agonists and an impaired relaxation to beta-agonists and theophylline.[7, 8] The airway contains a number of resident cells (mast cells, alveolar macrophages, airway epithelium and endothelium), as well as immigrating inflammatory cells (eosinophils, lymphocytes, neutrophils, basophils, platelets), that are capable of generating a wide variety of mediators that can induce bronchospasm (histamine, platelet activating factor, and a number of derivatives of the arachidonic acid cascade, such as prostaglandin D_2, and leukotrienes C_4, D_4, and E_4, slow-reacting substances of anaphylaxis). Direct interactions of inflammatory cells and airway smooth muscle have also been reported. T lymphocytes have been demonstrated to adhere to airway smooth muscle cells via integrins and are capable of inducing smooth muscle DNA synthesis.[80] These interactions of airway smooth muscle and lymphocytes may have effects on lymphocyte activation and function, as well as airway smooth muscle cell growth and reactivity.

Edema of the Airway Mucosa

Edema of the airway mucosa is due to increased capillary permeability, with leakage of serum proteins into interstitial areas. A number of cell-derived mediators are capable of inducing edema formation, including histamine, prostaglandin E, leukotrienes C_4 (LTC_4) and D_4 (LTD_4), platelet activating factor (PAF), and bradykinin. Although the precise contribution of edema to the episodic airway obstruction seen in asthma is unknown, it has been demonstrated that one of the striking immediate features of local airway allergen challenge is extensive mucosal edema.[97] Further, increased bronchovascular permeability occurs after local allergen exposure in sensitive asthmatic patients.[44] Finally, using mathematical modeling, it has been shown that both edema and cellular inflammation result in an increased airway wall thickness in patients that contributes to the mechanics of airway narrowing in asthma.[68, 179]

Alterations in Respiratory Secretions With Mucus Plugging of Smaller Airways

One of the characteristic pathologic features seen in status asthmaticus is the formation of tenacious mucus plugs within the airways. Increased mucus secretion contributes to both hyperinflation and focal atelectasis and may be the result of both hyperplasia and metaplasia of goblet cells lining the airway. The pathogenesis of mucus hypersecretion is complex, with multiple mediators and cells capable of influencing this particular aspect of the airway obstruction in asthma. Factors important in this regard have been extensively reviewed by Lundgren and Schelhamer.[87]

Inflammation

Airway inflammation has long been recognized to be a major feature of the histopathologic findings in many patients dying in status asthmaticus.[94] Significant findings include denudation of the airway epithelium, mucus plugging of segmental bronchi and bronchioles, so-called thickening of the epithelial basement membrane (actually collagen deposition beneath it), edema of the submucosa, infiltration by polymorphonuclear leukocytes (predominantly eosinophils), and smooth muscle hypertrophy. These findings differ in some respects from those seen in other forms of chronic lung disease, such as cystic fibrosis in both children and adults or chronic bronchitis in adults, in which significant airway neutrophilia is more characteristic,[132] whereas eosinophil degranulation[78] and plasma cell infiltration of the lamina propria and thickening of the basement membrane[132] are more characteristic of asthma. However, in nonatopic nonasthmatic children with recurrent bronchitis, epithelial cell damage, epithelial edema, and lymphocyte epithelial infiltration have been reported.[46] Moreover, since sudden-onset fatal asthmatic episodes can be characterized histologically by few eosinophils and relatively more neutrophils in the airway submucosa, the specificity of various histologic abnormalities to asthma still remains to be established.[157]

Of equally important clinical relevance, however, has been the observation that significant tissue inflammation can be noted in bronchial biopsy specimens even in patients whose symptoms can be readily controlled clinically with intermittent bronchodilator therapy. Cutz and colleagues[27] were one of the first groups to observe these changes in their evaluation of lung biopsies from two children with bronchial asthma in remission compared with two children dying in status asthmaticus. Bronchial changes, such as goblet cell hyperplasia, mucus plugging, and increased collagen deposition beneath the epithelial basement membrane, were comparable in the two groups. Interestingly, the only differences were the presence of a larger number of submucosal eosinophils and more extensive denudation of the epithelium in fatal asthma.

Since these early observations, various procedures (bronchoalveolar lavage, bronchial biopsy, and analysis of induced sputum) and techniques (immunohistochemistry, in situ hybridization, and polymerase chain reactions) to analyze airway inflammation have been aggressively applied to the asthmatic population. Indeed, a virtual explosion of publications has appeared that has evaluated the presence and participation of a number of resident (e.g., mast cells, epithelial cells, alveolar macrophages) and inflammatory (eosinophils, lymphocytes, neutrophils, basophils) cells, mediators, cytokines, and adhesion molecules.[94, 180] Although not observed uniformly, the following changes have been reported in mild to moderate asthmatic patients: denudation of the airway epithelium, collagen deposition beneath the basement membrane, mast cell degranulation, and lymphocyte and eosinophil infiltration and activation. Many of the cells present in the airway appear to be in an activated state (e.g., lymphocytes, eosinophils, epithelial cells), supporting a direct role for them in asthma pathogenesis through the release of various preformed or generated mediators.

The presence of various cytokines, such as tumor necrosis factor (TNF), interleukin 1β (IL–1β), interleukin 5 (IL-5), interleukin 6 (IL-6), granulocyte-macrophage colony-stimulating factor (GM-CSF),[15] and endothelin,[170] in bronchoalveolar lavage fluid or the demonstration of intracellular mRNA coding for them have provided further evidence for an ongoing inflammatory response in the asthmatic airway (see Chapters 17, 18, and 28). Since these cytokines are elaborated by, and can have multiple effects on, a number of resident and inflammatory cells, the variety of autocrine, paracrine, and endocrine cytokine networks is obviously complex and in many cases redundant. The ability of cytokines to induce the expression of various adhesion molecules, such as intracellular adhesion molecule (ICAM), vascular cell adhesion molecule (VCAM), and endothelial-leukocyte adhesion molecule (ELAM), no doubt provides a mechanism for inflammatory cell adhesion and migration from the circulation into the lamina propria, the epithelium, and in many cases, the airway lumen itself.[82]

Because of obvious ethical issues, information regarding asthmatic inflammation is not as abundant in children as in adults. However, numbers of BAL eosinophils and mast cells obtained from the lungs of children with chronic asthma have been demonstrated to correlate with bronchial responsiveness to histamine.[41] Data obtained from leukocytes isolated from the peripheral blood of asthmatic children would further support the concept that the activation state of eosinophils may contribute to bronchial hyperresponsiveness and relative disease activity over time.[13, 135, 136, 186]

Although the recognition that inflammation is present even in mild to moderate asthma has influenced our traditional therapeutic approach to asthma management, much remains to be learned. It is unclear when this inflammatory process starts and how the characteristics of it may change over time in response to various triggering mechanisms or to therapeutic intervention. Since many lung diseases are characterized by airway inflammation, cell migration patterns, cell location, cell activation patterns, cytokine elaboration, and adhesion molecule expression that are specific and/or pathognomonic of asthma need to be established. Finally, the relationships of these immunohistopathologic alterations to airway physiologic changes, such as airway hyperresponsiveness, need further exploration and definition.

DIAGNOSIS

The diagnosis of asthma in infants and children begins with an initial suspicion based on history and clinical presentation (recurrent wheezing, shortness of breath, dyspnea, chronic cough, particularly at night), associations (rhinitis, atopy, perennial exacerbation), precipitating factors (allergen exposure, viruses, exercise, environmental irritants, aspirin, gastroesophageal reflux), or documented response to asthma medications (bronchodilators, mast cell stabilizers, corticosteroids). Since asthmatic symptoms are characteristically episodic, it is possible that physical examination of the lungs may be normal, particularly in mild and moderate disease.

In children less than 5 years of age, pulmonary function testing is usually not possible due to the patient's inability to physically coordinate a reproducible expiratory maneuver. In this age group, history and response to bronchodilator and/or anti-inflammatory therapy become essential to making a proper diagnosis. In some research hospitals, infant pulmonary function testing may be performed to assess the degree of airway obstruction and/or response to therapeutic intervention.[90] Chest radiographs demonstrating peribronchial inflammatory changes and hyperinflation would provide additional diagnostic information in this age group. In general, however, the lack of specificity of the radiographic findings in asthma makes this laboratory test of questionable benefit either diagnostically or therapeutically.[130]

In older children and adolescents, peak expiratory flow measurements at home or spirometry in a clinic setting can document baseline air flow obstruction and the extent to which this obstruction is reversible using bronchodilators acutely or inhaled or oral glucocorticosteroid therapy on a more chronic basis. Obstructive disease can show reduced or normal forced vital capacity (FVC), reduced forced expiratory flow in 1 second (FEV_1), a reduced ratio of FEV_1/FVC (normal is approximately 80%), a decreased forced expiratory flow between 25% and 75% of FVC (FEF_{25-75}), or reduced peak expiratory flow (PEF) measurement. It is important to remember that expiratory flow rates are effort dependent and therefore can be influenced by a number of factors, including age (inability to comprehend or cooperate with the procedure), technical malfunction (broken peak flow meter), or psychosocial issues (purposely decreasing flow rates to manipulate a particular family situation).

When baseline spirometry is normal but the diagnosis of asthma is highly suspect, bronchoprovocation can be performed using methacholine (or histamine) or exercise. A positive methacholine test (decrease of $FEV_1 \geq 15\%$ from baseline) is indicative of airway hyperresponsiveness but is not a diagnostic test for asthma.[83] Many individuals with acute (viral infections or irritant exposures) and chronic respiratory tract conditions (allergic rhinitis, cystic fibrosis, bronchitis) will demonstrate an enhanced bronchial response to methacholine inhalation. As a group, asthmatic patients may be the most sensitive, but the threshold of reactivity may fluctuate over time based on exposure to recent triggering factors or concurrent medication use. Exercise bronchoprovocation may be less sensitive than methacholine in demonstrating airway hyperresponsiveness, but a positive response is more specific for asthma.[83] Since a positive response to methacholine is almost always demonstrable in asthmatic patients, a negative methacholine challenge test can be useful in potentially eliminating asthma from further diagnostic or therapeutic consideration.

DIFFERENTIAL DIAGNOSIS

The differential diagnosis for the two most common symptoms of asthma, coughing and wheezing, is extensive in children. Patients and their parents can describe the same sound in different ways, and on physical examination, the transmission of upper airway noise to the lower airway can also pose challenges in locating the source of the abnormality and thereby correctly and expeditiously addressing the problem. Once accomplished, proper location of the problem within the airway is a useful starting point in developing the differential diagnosis (Table 27–1).[105, 169]

UPPER RESPIRATORY TRACT

In the upper respiratory tract, allergic rhinitis, infectious rhinitis, sinusitis, choanal atresia, adenoidal/tonsillar hypertrophy, and other structural abnormalities can produce variable coughing and abnormal inspiratory and expiratory sounds that parents may variably describe as wheezing, whistling, or rattling. Since antigen-specific IgE antibody responses do not develop to aeroallergens (e.g., house dust mites, pollens, molds, animal danders) until after the first 2

TABLE 27–1
DIFFERENTIAL DIAGNOSIS OF COUGH AND WHEEZE IN INFANTS AND CHILDREN

Upper Respiratory Tract	Middle Respiratory Tract	Lower Respiratory Tract
Allergic rhinitis	Laryngeal webs	Asthma
Infectious rhinitis	Laryngomalacia	Viral bronchiolitis
Sinusitis	Tracheomalacia	Cystic fibrosis
Choanal atresia	Tracheoesophageal fistula	Bronchopulmonary dysplasia
Adenoidal/tonsillar hypertrophy	Tracheostenosis	Foreign body
Foreign body	Bronchiostenosis	Gastroesophageal reflux
	Vascular rings	Chronic aspiration
	Enlarged lymph nodes	Bronchiectasis
	Tumor	$Alpha_1$-antitrypsin deficiency
	Foreign body	Löffler's syndrome
	Pertussis	Pulmonary hemosiderosis
	Epiglottitis	Pulmonary interstitial emphysema
	Laryngotracheobronchitis	Chlamydia trachomatis
	Toxic inhalation	Obliterative bronchiolitis
	Vocal cord dysfunction	Toxic inhalation
		Pulmonary edema
		Mitral valve prolapse
		Tumor
		Hyperventilation syndrome

to 3 years of life, allergic disease would be an unusual etiology for any airway problem in this age group. Foods rarely may induce attacks of asthma, but airway symptoms are almost always accompanied by cutaneous or gastrointestinal manifestations concomitantly. In older children and adolescents, however, allergic disease of the respiratory tract (allergic rhinitis and/or asthma) tends to be a very common cause of airway symptomatology.

MIDDLE RESPIRATORY TRACT

Middle respiratory tract problems that may occasionally mimic asthma include congenital structural abnormalities that may produce turbulent air flow in the large airways, such as laryngeal webs, laryngomalacia, tracheomalacia, tracheoesophageal fistula, tracheostenosis, bronchiostenosis, and vascular rings. Space-occupying lesions that cause either internal or external compromise or compression of the airway (e.g., enlarged lymph nodes or tumors) also produce adventitious sounds that may be mistaken for asthma. Other confounding problems may arise from infectious etiologies (epiglottitis, laryngotracheobronchitis, pertussis), toxic etiologies (inhalation of dust, gas, or talc), or dysfunction of the vocal cords or larynx from neurologic and/or psychologic factors.

Abnormalities of vocal cord function have been recognized with increasing frequency in children and adolescents who have recurrent asthmatic airway symptoms that do not respond to conventional medical therapy. Since the incidence of these problems seems to be increasing, they deserve special consideration.[21, 53] Vocal cord dysfunction (VCD) can exist as an isolated abnormality or be present concomitantly with asthma, the combination being particularly challenging to proper diagnosis and medical management.[96] In the acute situation, these patients commonly present with signs and symptoms of significant airway obstruction accompanied by normal arterial blood gases. In more chronic situations, the symptoms can be perceived as severe enough to warrant chronic corticosteroid therapy.

Unfortunately, the variability of clinical presentations and psychodynamics of VCD make recognition and appropriate management difficult, especially when asthma is also present. Diagnostic studies that may be useful include methacholine bronchoprovocation (to evaluate airway hyperresponsiveness as a factor),[140] flow volume loops (as inspiratory and expiratory flow are both limited in VCD),[53] and when indicated, direct visualization of the larynx. A skilled speech pathologist can often have patients reproduce their symptoms during direct vocal cord visualization while simultaneously teaching them proper vocal cord relaxation techniques to attenuate or abrogate the problem. Finally, since many of these patients have a significant psychologic triggering mechanism, proper evaluation and management may require psychiatric evaluation by individuals familiar with the complex nature of the problem and its acute and chronic management.[140]

LOWER RESPIRATORY TRACT

Lower respiratory tract causes of wheezing and coughing are the most difficult to differentiate from asthma, since asthma initially affects small airways. Children with a history of prematurity and mechanical ventilation are at risk for the development of bronchopulmonary dysplasia or pulmonary interstitial emphysema. Many of these children eventually develop severe chronic obstructive lung disease, which is indistinguishable from asthma in many instances. Cystic fibrosis may also present with recurrent asthmatic-like symptoms, and many children with cystic fibrosis can also have asthma and/or allergic rhinitis. Digital clubbing is rarely seen in asthma but is invariably present in cystic fibrosis. Finally, although nasal polyps affect the upper respiratory tract, their presence demands that a sweat test be performed to eliminate cystic fibrosis, the most common coexisting disease.

Viral bronchiolitis is one of the most difficult entities to differentiate from asthma in very young children, since wheezing and abnormalities of gas exchange are significant alterations found in both, and viruses are a major triggering factor of asthma in this age group. Viruses such as respiratory syncytial virus may provoke isolated episodes of wheezing in children. When wheezing occurs repetitively with colds, however, asthma should be considered as the underlying cause producing the symptoms. Foreign body aspiration can produce both acute and chronic wheezing (both unilateral and bilateral) and coughing typically in children less than 2 years old. Gastroesophageal reflux, in addition to periodically worsening asthma, can cause wheezing and coughing by itself. In physically impaired children with dysfunctional swallowing mechanisms, chronic aspiration may contribute to airway abnormalities that can either mimic asthma or exacerbate it in children who have it. Finally, less common causes such as alpha$_1$-antitrypsin deficiency, bronchiectasis, hypersensitivity lung diseases (molds, fibers), pulmonary eosinophilia (Löffler's syndrome), pulmonary hemosiderosis, chlamydia trachomatis, obliterative bronchiolitis, pulmonary edema, and mitral valve prolapse have occasionally produced diagnostic challenges to clinicians evaluating children and young adults for asthma.

TRIGGERS

ALLERGENS

The fundamental elements to produce an immediate hypersensitivity skin test response (IgE antibody on the surface of cutaneous mast cells, integrity of mast cell mediator release, and dermal response to the mediator effects) are present at about 1 month of age. The formation of antigen-specific IgE antibody to aeroallergens (e.g., mites, trees, grasses, animal dander) does not usually occur until 2 to 3 years of life. Thus aeroallergen-induced asthma is uncommon during the first year of life, begins to increase in prevalence during later childhood and adolescence, and peaks in the second decade of life. Once established in genetically predisposed individuals, however, IgE-mediated reactions are a major contributor to both chronic airway inflammation and acute asthmatic symptoms. Indeed, sensitization to either indoor (dust mites, pets, molds) or outdoor (pollens, molds) allergens should be considered when evaluating children or adolescents with asthma, especially those with moderate to severe disease.[114]

Chronic low-level exposure to indoor allergens, particularly dust mite and cat proteins, may play a major role in both asthma pathogenesis and triggering chronic and recurrent symptoms.[34] Removing offending pets from the home, or limiting exposure to dust mite or mold proteins, may result in dramatic relief from asthma and rhinitis symptoms and reductions in airway hyperresponsiveness over time.[121] Aeroallergen-induced asthma typically has a well-defined seasonal incidence[128] and is usually mild to moderate in severity. In contrast with most aeroallergens, alternaria may produce particularly severe acute asthmatic symptoms, as sensitivity to alternaria has been implicated as a risk factor for sudden respiratory arrest in adolescents and young adults with asthma.[117]

Although food allergy may produce bronchospasm along with skin and/or gastrointestinal symptoms, it is very unusual for food allergy to produce an isolated respiratory reaction.[69] When an allergic reaction to food does produce asthma, symptoms typically appear soon after the offending food is eaten, and the reactions tend to occur consistently each time after eating that particular food protein.

INFECTION

Viral upper respiratory tract infections (URIs) are one of the major triggers for asthmatic symptoms in children. In an early prospective study, inpatients 1 to 5 years of age with moderate to severe asthma were followed over a 2-year period; 42% of their wheezing episodes were associated with a viral URI.[95] Respiratory syncytial virus (RSV) was the most common virus isolated.[95] In outpatient asthmatic children ages 3 to 11, asthmatic exacerbations (61 total) were frequently associated with viral URI.[95] In this age group, rhinovirus was the most prevalent isolate.[98] In both of these studies, bacterial infections were not associated with increased asthma symptoms.[95, 98] In a study conducted in the University of Virginia Emergency Room, viruses were detected by either culture or immunofluorescence from 31% of children more than 2 years of age and 70% of children less than 2 years of age.[35]

Age appears to be a factor in determining the type of virus that provokes asthmatic exacerbations. Rhinovirus strains are detected most often in older children, whereas RSV isolates are found most often in those less than 2 years of age.[28, 35, 119] Studies utilizing the more sensitive polymerase chain reaction indicate that rhinovirus infections may be responsible for an even greater number of asthma exacerbations in both children[70] and adults[112] than had been realized. Other infectious agents associated with wheezing episodes include parainfluenza, influenza A and B, coronavirus, adenovirus, *Mycoplasma pneumoniae,* enterovirus, and chlamydia.[28, 35, 112, 119] One confounding epidemiologic variable is that some viral respiratory infections can cause wheezing in children without asthma. RSV is the most frequent culprit, but parainfluenza, adenovirus, and *Mycoplasma pneumoniae* have also been indicated, especially in children less than 2 years of age.[63]

Persistent adenovirus infection has been associated with severe asthma in children that is refractory to bronchodilator and corticosteroid treatment.[88] Mycoplasma infections may cause airway obstruction and wheezing in children,[75, 131] but prospective studies have generally found that asthmatic exacerbations are not frequently associated with mycoplasma infection.[81, 119] Sinus infections may also aggravate asthmatic symptoms in children, and antibiotic treatment can lead to improvement in asthma control.[124] The mechanisms by which sinusitis and viral URIs exacerbate asthma are unknown.

EXERCISE

Exercise-induced asthma (EIA) is the development of lower airway obstruction that occurs during or following exercise. A history of asthmatic symptoms is helpful in making a diagnosis of EIA, but as many as one half of children with EIA have no previous history of asthma.[77] Children and adolescents with EIA may develop wheezing, coughing, and shortness of breath related to activities as diverse as riding a tricycle and playing competitive sports. Complaints of chest pain in this age group can also be a symptom of EIA.[115] Young athletes with asthma may be reluctant to admit to such symptoms for fear of being different and often present with an inability to keep up with peers, despite good conditioning. This is an especially important feature of EIA that is often overlooked by patients, trainers, and physicians, who otherwise attribute breathlessness to poor physical conditioning.

The diagnosis of EIA is often apparent after taking a careful history, and a therapeutic trial may provide confirmatory evidence. Objective data, obtained by using a peak flow meter in the field or generated in a pulmonary function lab during a formal exercise tolerance test, can also be very helpful when the history is uncertain or therapeutic trials have met with limited success. A drop in FEV_1 or PEF of 15% or more is compatible with EIA, although other disorders, such as vocal cord dysfunction, must also be considered.

Air flow obstruction severe enough to warrant hospitalization or death due to exercise alone is exceedingly rare. With this knowledge, parents and teachers should not discourage children with asthma from participating in athletic activities. Physicians should likewise not unnecessarily exclude patients with asthma from participating in various sports. Although many children with asthma are not physically fit,[155] withdrawing from physical activities may foster poor self-image and reduce self-esteem in a child with asthma.[154] To date, several studies have evaluated the potential benefits of exercise on the overall management of asthma. Although aerobic conditioning programs may not change bronchial hyperresponsiveness,[113] regular exercise may attenuate exercise-induced reductions in FEV_1 or PEF, improve self-confidence, and reduce the frequency of asthma attacks, use of medications, and school absenteeism.[4, 59, 159] In addition, an almost universal feature of exercise programs is improved physical fitness.

TOBACCO SMOKE

Numerous investigators have demonstrated that the lung function of children is affected by passive, secondhand smoke. Cigarette smoke contains certain toxins, including carbon monoxide, ammonia, nicotine, hydrogen cyanide, and formaldehyde,[23] that can be irritating to a child's airways.

In most studies, one interesting finding is that maternal smoking tends to be more detrimental than paternal smoking, perhaps related to the fact that mothers spend more time at home with their children, especially during infancy. Most evaluations have had difficulty in separating the effects of prenatal and postnatal maternal smoking on infants, since mothers who smoke during pregnancy are also likely to smoke once the baby is born.

Tobacco smoke exposure may be associated with an increasing incidence of asthma, even in infants. One study done with infants found that airway responsiveness was increased in infants exposed to parental smoke and in children with a family history of asthma.[184] In another study of over 4,000 children, an increased incidence of diagnosed asthma or the use of asthma medications in the first year of life was seen if the mother smoked more than a half pack of cigarettes a day.[177] Others found that the combination of less than 12 years of education and smoking more than one pack of cigarettes per day increased the risk of asthma 2.5-fold.[89] Interestingly, in those mothers who smoked but had more than 12 years of education, no association of increased asthma was seen in their children. In a study comparing a rural and urban smoking environment, an increased risk of asthma and an increased prevalence of symptomatic asthma were seen in both rural and urban children whose mothers smoked.[55] This study concluded that 18% to 34% of asthma reported in these samples was due to maternal smoking.

Children already diagnosed with asthma seem to show a greater negative effect when exposed to passive smoke. Parents have reported that when their asthmatic children were exposed to cigarette smoke, their asthma worsened, and elimination of smoking led to improvement of their symptoms.[116] In addition to more symptoms, asthmatic children have worse pulmonary function tests and increased bronchial responsiveness if they are exposed to maternal cigarette smoke, with increasing age and male gender increasing relative risk rates.[102, 104] Climatic conditions may also affect response to tobacco smoke.[103] Asthmatic children whose mothers smoked were found to have worsening pulmonary functions only when evaluated during cold and wet seasons. These changes may have been related to more prolonged time spent indoors because of poor weather conditions.

GASTROESOPHAGEAL REFLUX

Gastroesophageal reflux (GER) in children has been associated with certain respiratory diseases, such as apnea, recurrent pneumonia, recurrent bronchitis, near-miss SIDS, bronchiectasis, and asthma.[108] It has been estimated that most adult asthmatics have GER, with 80% in one study.[151] In asthmatics 6 to 20 years old, the prevalence of pathologic reflux has been demonstrated to be 60%.[57]

Initially, the mechanism believed to cause asthmatic symptoms in those with reflux was microaspiration of gastric contents, especially at night.[108] However, Gustafsson and colleagues[57] found that worsening of symptoms due to reflux in children and young adults was usually caused by exposure of the distal esophagus to acid; they therefore hypothesized that asthmatic symptoms related to GER may be due to a vagal reflux, as opposed to aspiration.

Nocturnal reflux produces more prolonged acid exposure (supine position, decreased saliva and swallowing). Children with prominent nocturnal asthmatic symptoms, such as cough, are more likely to have GER.[118] One adult study found that asthmatics compared with nonasthmatics have decreased lower esophageal sphincter pressures, greater esophageal acid exposure time, more frequent episodes, and longer acid clearance rates.[151]

Evidence of the effect of intraesophageal acid on air flow in adults has been conflicting.[64, 161] Wilson and colleagues[181] found that over 25% of children with reflux and moderate to severe asthma had increased bronchial responsiveness to intraesophageal acid. All of those children also had consequential nocturnal symptoms. Davis and colleagues[31] exposed asthmatic children to either acid or saline in the lower esophagus at midnight and at 4 to 5 a.m. Only those children who were symptomatic with their reflux (heartburn) had wheezing and bronchoconstriction with the 4 to 5 a.m. dose of intraesophageal acid; interestingly, they did not respond to it at midnight.

In asthmatic children with pathologic reflux, 30% demonstrate improvement of their nocturnal asthmatic symptoms and their degree of reflux when treated with ranitidine.[58] However, treatment with antacids and positioning may not be efficacious in children who are steroid dependent.[142]

Certain asthma medications, such as beta-agonists and theophylline, can relax lower esophageal sphincter tone, thereby promoting reflux. In patients who need theophylline and have nocturnal asthmatic symptoms or documented GER, treatment with ranitidine may be preferred to cimetidine due to cimetidine's interaction with theophylline.[54]

MEDICATIONS

Certain medications or food additives are associated with either the development of acute asthmatic symptoms or the exacerbation of chronic symptoms in children with asthma. In studies with children who have moderate to severe asthma, up to 28% may experience significant airway obstruction after aspirin ingestion.[123, 165] In addition to aspirin, children with chronic asthma have also been shown to develop significant bronchoconstriction to the food preservative sodium metabisulfite.[165] Children with asthma and aspirin sensitivity may also be more prone to developing sinusitis and nasal polyposis.[123, 173, 185]

The effects of aspirin and other nonsteroidal anti-inflammatory drugs (NSAIDs) appear to be proportional to their inhibition of cyclooxygenase[158] and increased bronchial sensitivity to leukotrienes,[5] especially LTE_4. Drugs that have weak effects on cyclooxygenase, such as acetaminophen, sodium salicylate, and choline salicylate, are safe for the majority of aspirin-sensitive individuals.[18, 42]

Beta-adrenergic blockers, such as propranolol, may also cause symptoms in children with asthma or may unmask previously unrecognized asthma.[67] Bronchospasm triggered by beta blockers may be refractory to treatment with beta-adrenergic agonists or epinephrine but may respond to anticholinergic medications, such as inhaled ipratropium.

TREATMENT

Although nothing unique about the pathogenesis of asthma in children has been identified, the treatment of asthma in this age group can be very challenging. The cognitive and social development of the child greatly influences asthma therapy, including the choice of the drug delivery system, determining who has the responsibility for medication administration, and compliance with doctor's orders. Asthma education, a cornerstone of any treatment plan, must include not only the patient and parent but also teachers and coaches. Asthma treatment plans, which should include environmental control of relevant allergens, self-monitoring guidelines, medication prescriptions, and an emergency care plan, should be provided in writing to the patient, parents, schools, and any other caretakers. The National Heart, Lung, and Blood Institute[106] has published a clinician's guide containing many valuable educational materials, including asthma treatment plan work sheets, that are designed for duplication and office use. The overall goals of therapy include maintaining normal activity levels at home and school, maintaining optimal pulmonary function, preventing chronic symptoms (e.g., coughing or breathlessness in the night, early morning, and after exertion), preventing recurrent exacerbations of asthma, and avoiding adverse effects from asthma medications.

MONITORING ASTHMA

Children with asthma, like adults, have a limited ability to perceive the degree of obstruction in their own airways.[148] Peak flow meters provide a reasonably accurate and portable means of obtaining objective pulmonary function measurements. These devices measure PEF, which is the greatest flow velocity (liters per second) that is generated during forced expiration. This measurement correlates well with FEV_1 and provides an accurate measurement of airway obstruction. These values, when combined with clinical information, such as symptoms and medication requirements, can be used by the patient, parent, and physician to make intelligent decisions pertaining to asthma therapy.[105] Use of a peak flow meter may also have psychologic benefits for children and adolescents, as it allows them to effectively manage most asthmatic exacerbations, providing positive feedback for the asthma treatment plan and increasing feelings of self-control over their chronic disease. Peak flow meters may also be useful in evaluating the possibility of asthma in a patient who has suggestive symptoms at night or after exercise yet has normal pulmonary function in the clinic.

A useful protocol for using peak flow meters in managing asthma is outlined in the Guidelines for the Diagnosis and Management of Asthma published by the U.S. Department of Health and Human Services (Table 27–2).[105] The first goal is to ascertain the patient's personal best peak flow rate, which requires the appropriate use of medications to maximize pulmonary function. Once this value has been established, the calculation of green (80–100% of personal best), yellow (50–80% of personal best), and red (<50% of personal best) zones can be accomplished. Peak flow rates in the green zone indicate stable disease activity, provided that no other warning signs are present (nocturnal awakenings

TABLE 27–2
POSSIBLE APPLICATIONS OF PEAK EXPIRATORY FLOW RATE MEASUREMENT

Clinician's Office (Chronic Asthma and Acute Episodes)	Clinician's Office/ Emergency Department (Acute Episode)	Hospital	Home	School	Workplace
1. Classify severity of patient's asthma	1. Assess severity of episode on arrival	1. Follow course of asthma episode and therapy	1. Self-monitor asthma to increase or decrease therapy	1. Guide decisions by school personnel when student has acute episodes of asthma at school	1. Detect occupational exposures inducing or exacerbating asthma
2. Follow trends in patients (seasonal episodes, increase or decrease medications, effect of new medication)	2. Measure response to therapy	2. Predict hospital discharge	2. Detect increases in circadian variation in PEF that predict instability of asthma	2. Identify exercise-induced asthma	
3. Exercise testing to determine exercise-induced asthma	3. Assess the need for hospitalization		3. Detect decreases in PEF that indicate early deterioration of asthma	3. Increase sports participation by using PEF to determine need to increase treatment	
4. Utilize objective information to guide therapy over telephone			4. Identify triggers of asthma (e.g., seasons, environmental exposures, viral infections, exercise)	4. Detect asthma that is not under control	
			5. Report changes in PEF to physician for guidance over the phone		

From National Asthma Education Program, National Heart, Lung, and Blood Institute, National Institutes of Health: Guidelines for the Diagnosis and Management of Asthma. NIH Publication No 91-3042. US Department of Health and Human Services, Bethesda, MD, 1991.

due to asthma, exercise intolerance, etc.). If the patient's peak flow rate is in the yellow zone and the administration of a beta-agonist does not result in bringing the peak flow value back into the green zone, many asthma specialists would recommend doubling the maintenance dose of anti-inflammatory therapy until peak flow rates are consistently back in the green zone. If peak flow rates continue to deteriorate while in the yellow zone or if they are in the red zone, oral corticosteroid therapy should be initiated, and the patient should contact a physician as soon as possible.

PEF readings, especially those obtained at home, should be interpreted with an understanding that there are many causes of falsely low or high readings. Peak flow meters can malfunction, as children may subject these instruments to conditions unforeseen by the engineers that designed them. It is also important to remember that results obtained with a peak flow meter depend on both effort and technique. Thus PEF values may be manipulated by some children in order to avoid school attendance or participation in physical education classes.

CONTROL OF ENVIRONMENTAL ALLERGENS

As discussed previously and in other chapters, there is overwhelming evidence that respiratory allergies are a major factor in the pathogenesis of asthma in children. Furthermore, limiting exposure to relevant indoor allergens may lead to reductions in asthma symptoms, bronchial hyperresponsiveness, and use of asthma medications.[34] Therefore, children with significant asthma should be evaluated for respiratory allergies, and the asthma treatment plan should always include detailed instructions to the child and family to help minimize exposure to relevant allergens. Recommendations for reductions in various environmental allergens and pollutants have been reviewed.[121, 153, 183]

MEDICATIONS

When considering pharmacotherapy for children and adolescents with asthma, special consideration must be given to potential side effects of medications and also to the method of drug delivery. Adverse effects on either growth or behavior are particularly undesirable during this period of rapid physical and intellectual development.

DRUG DELIVERY SYSTEMS

Aerosol delivery of medications would seem to be ideally suited for asthma therapy since drug delivery to the small airway is maximized while systemic effects of medications, which are generally undesirable, are minimized. Although there are definite theoretic advantages to drug delivery via inhalation, clinical responses to aerosol medications vary widely. The principal reason for these inconsistent responses is the many variables that determine the amount of medicine that actually reaches the target tissues, including the particle size generated by the delivery system and the mechanics of breathing (e.g., inspiratory flow and duration of breath holding).[111] Thus it is of primary importance to understand the various delivery systems and to teach the patient to use them correctly.

Inhaled medications are usually administered by either nebulizer or pressurized metered-dose inhaler (MDI), although an increasing number of dry powder inhalers are available in response to a demand for chlorofluorocarbon-free alternatives. The optimum particle size for lower airway deposition is 1 to 5 μm, and larger droplets are likely to impact in the upper airway.[101] MDIs generate relatively more small respirable particles compared with nebulizers, which may account for why nebulizer doses of beta-agonists must be 3 to 10 times larger to achieve the same degree of bronchodilation.[109] MDIs have the additional advantages of being more portable and quicker to use and costing 50 to 75% less per treatment compared with nebulizers.[12, 156] Although nebulizers have traditionally been used in medical facilities for treatment of acute asthma, MDIs provide bronchodilation that is faster and of equal or greater magnitude but may require larger than standard doses.[73, 110]

Unfortunately, children and adolescents may not be able to use MDIs correctly and thus may not derive full benefit from the medications contained within them. Spacer devices can improve the efficacy of inhaled medications in those patients who are unable to master correct inhaler technique.[26, 164] These devices work by trapping most of the large aerosol droplets, while the smaller particles are held in a reservoir until they are inhaled. Some brands of spacers, such as the Aerochamber, may be equipped with either mouthpieces or variable-size masks, which are suitable for use by children under 3 years of age. For older children, spacers equipped with mouthpieces are preferred since the nose may filter out particles that would otherwise be deposited in the lung. In addition to improving drug delivery to the lower airways, the use of a spacer with inhaled corticosteroids may also reduce the incidence of side effects, such as oral candidiasis and hoarse voice.[133]

BETA-ADRENERGIC AGONISTS

Beta-adrenergic drugs are the most potent and rapidly acting bronchodilators in clinical use.[50] Their availability in multiple forms (short, intermediate, and long acting) and delivery systems (MDIs, nebulizer solutions, oral liquids and tablets, respirable powders) gives them wide clinical versatility. Paradoxically, the rapid onset of action and potent bronchodilator activity may lead to deterioration of asthma disease control if the patient uses beta-agonists to the exclusion of anti-inflammatory medications, which do not produce any immediate positive feedback. Therefore, increasing frequency of beta-agonist use should be considered as an indicator of inadequate disease control, signaling the need for a medical evaluation. Side effects of selective $beta_2$-agonists include tremor, tachycardia, and increased anxiety, but these effects are minimal when beta-agonists are administered via inhalation.

For acute rescue management of asthma exacerbations, intermediate-acting beta-agonists (albuterol, terbutaline, pirbuterol, metaproterenol) may be used every 4 to 6 hours either orally or by aerosolized delivery devices (metered-dose inhalers or nebulizers). A need for more frequent administration than every 4 hours, more than eight inhalations from a metered-dose inhaler per day, or more than one inhaler per month should alert the treating physician that the child's underlying disease process (inflammation) needs more aggressive and appropriate intervention. Intermediate-acting beta-agonists are also very effective for prophylaxis of allergen-[22, 66] or exercise-induced[149] asthma. The long-acting beta-agonist salmeterol is also effective for these types of exposures.[56, 166]

The potential for the development of tolerance, coupled with the ability of beta-agonists to be potent and rapid symptom relievers, has led to concern regarding the safety of beta-agonists as chronic maintenance therapeutic agents for asthma. Indeed, studies in adult patients suggest that their regular use in asthma may be associated with increased morbidity[139] or even mortality.[152] Not all clinicians have considered these observations to be demonstrable of a true cause-and-effect relationship, however, and the issue remains controversial.[93] Interestingly, clinical trials evaluating the long-acting beta-agonist salmeterol have not demonstrated any loss of bronchodilator potency over time[120] or any increases in airway inflammation.[47]

THEOPHYLLINE

Theophylline is an old medication that continues to be useful in the treatment of asthma in children and adolescents. Theophylline is a methylxanthine bronchodilator with extrapulmonary effects, including enhancement of respiratory muscle contractility. Theophylline is easily administered to children, as it is available in liquid, beaded capsule, and tablet formulations; sustained-release formulations may be given at 8- to 24-hour intervals.

Serum levels of theophylline, which is extensively metabolized by the liver, may be markedly affected by a number of variables, including age, diet, disease states, and drug interactions, all of which contribute to the complexity of using this medication.[62, 174] For example, tobacco and marijuana smoking increases theophylline metabolism, whereas febrile illnesses and high carbohydrate diets significantly decrease theophylline metabolism. In addition, drug interactions must be considered, and the theophylline dose adjusted accordingly. Phenytoin, phenobarbital, carbamazepine, and rifampin increase theophylline clearance by more than 25%, whereas macrolide antibiotics, cimetidine, ciprofloxacin, and oral contraceptives decrease theophylline clearance by 10% to 25%.[62, 71] Due to the variability of theophylline metabolism, as well as a narrow therapeutic index, children using theophylline must have serum levels monitored periodically.

Theophylline is an effective bronchodilator at serum concentrations of 5 to 20 μg/mL. Other beneficial effects of theophylline include attenuation of the early- and late-phase response to allergen, steroid-sparing effects, and improved exercise tolerance.[174] When compared with beta$_2$-agonists, theophylline has a slower onset of action and a lower peak effect, making it less suitable for acute therapy.

Unfortunately, theophylline may produce a number of dose-related side effects. Gastrointestinal symptoms may be intolerable to some patients, even well within the usual therapeutic drug levels. Of greatest concern to parents and teachers is that theophylline might adversely affect school performance,[45, 125] although studies have not substantiated this association. Lindgren and colleagues[86] surveyed the records of 255 asthmatic children and found no difference in scholastic achievement test scores related to theophylline use. Bender and colleagues[10, 11] conducted two studies of asthmatic children whose parents had reported theophylline-related behavioral problems. In an open-label trial, children treated with theophylline had improved attention spans, but their parents reported increased conduct problems and hyperactivity. In a second study with a double-blind, placebo-controlled, crossover design, treatment-related improvement in attention was again documented, but parents were unable to detect any theophylline-related behavioral effects. However, theophylline-treated children exhibited mild increases in anxiety and hand tremor that resembled a caffeine-like effect. In light of these findings, it seems prudent to avoid prescribing theophylline to children with preexisting behavioral and/or school difficulties.

CROMOLYN AND NEDOCROMIL

Cromolyn sodium (Intal) and nedocromil sodium (Tilade) are two structurally different anti-inflammatory medications for the treatment of chronic asthma that have similar properties. They are rapidly absorbed from the lungs and impressively safe. Both medications inhibit inflammatory cell activation and mediator release, early and late allergen-induced bronchoconstriction, and airway hyperresponsiveness. They are effective in attenuating exercise-induced bronchospasm and have an onset of action of minutes for prophylaxis. The mechanism of action is not well understood. They do not have direct bronchodilating effects. Cromolyn sodium is available in both an MDI form and a form for nebulization and has been studied and approved for use in children of all ages. Nedocromil sodium is available as an MDI only and has been studied and approved for use in children 12 years and older.

Clinical studies evaluating the efficacy of cromolyn sodium in children and adolescents determined that use of a spinhaler or nebulized cromolyn sodium provided benefit, with reduction in respiratory symptoms over placebo.[65, 99] Similarly, in a double-blind, placebo-controlled study of nedocromil sodium, Armenio and colleagues[6] found that over 12 weeks of treatment, children treated with nedocromil sodium had improved symptom scores, peak expiratory flow measurements, and decreased inhaled bronchodilator use. Comparative studies of nedocromil sodium and cromolyn sodium suggest that nedocromil sodium may be more effective in treating reversible airway obstruction and at lower doses than cromolyn sodium.[33, 79] In some adult studies, concurrent use of nedocromil sodium with corticosteroids allowed for decreased oral and inhaled corticosteroid dosing. In one study with children and adolescents, nebulized cromolyn sodium had similar symptom control effectiveness compared with triamcinolone acetonide MDI.[143] These studies support the clinical usefulness of cromolyn sodium and nedocromil sodium in the treatment of mild to moderate chronic asthma.

Reported adverse effects for cromolyn sodium include increased cough and wheeze, dermatitis, myositis, and gastroenteritis.[141] The adverse effects reported for nedocromil sodium include nausea, vomiting, sore throat, throat irritation, cough, and headache.[14] Unpleasant taste is reported much more frequently in adult than pediatric literature.[6]

GLUCOCORTICOSTEROIDS

Glucocorticosteroids (GCS) are the most potent anti-inflammatory agents available for the treatment of asthma.[137] Their efficacy is related to many factors, including a diminution in inflammatory cell function and activation, stabilization of vascular leakage, a decrease in mucus production, and an increase in beta-adrenergic response.

Unfortunately, chronic administration of GCS can result in multiple adverse effects, including hypothalamic pituitary adrenal (HPA) axis suppression, osteoporosis, posterior subcapsular cataracts, hyperglycemia, hypertension, dermal thinning and striae, and the potential for growth retardation.[1, 76, 122] The rank propensity of various cortcosteroid regimens to produce these changes is as follows: high dose daily oral>low dose daily oral>high dose alternate day oral>low dose alternate day oral>high dose inhaled>moderate dose inhaled>low dose inhaled.

Fortunately, since inhaled corticosteroids (ICS) are efficacious in children and young adults, the need for oral corticosteroid regimens has diminished substantially.[24, 168] Although ICS have minimal adverse effects when used in recommended doses (with the exception of oral candidiasis when oral hygiene is suboptimal), studies have rekindled concern about the long-term effects of these compounds on growth in children.[163, 182] The issue of growth in children who are atopic[40] and/or have asthma[9] is further complicated by the fact that both conditions appear to delay the onset of puberty, an effect that can confound any analysis of the effects of GCS on growth. The relative importance of corticosteroid therapy on growth in children with asthma has been evaluated by meta-analysis.[1] When attained heights were compared with expected heights of asthmatic children treated with inhaled beclomethasone dipropionate (BDP) therapy, no significant association between BDP use and the adverse effect of diminished stature could be demonstrated. Indeed, there was no statistical evidence for BDP therapy to be associated with growth impairment at higher doses, for longer durations, or among patients with more severe asthma. The authors cautioned, however, that the effects on growth of doses of BDP greater than 800 μg/day needed to be more comprehensively evaluated.

On a microgram per microgram basis, there are no convincing data that any one formulation of ICS available in the United States (e.g., beclomethasone dipropionate, triamcinolone acetonide, flunisolide) is clinically more potent or less likely to produce side effects. As a general rule, doses below 400 μg/day are usually safe for use in children and doses of 400 to 800 μg/day are reasonably safe. Once doses above 800 μg/day are needed, the potential for significant effects on linear bone growth and adrenal suppression is substantially increased. It should be emphasized, however, that individual tolerances of corticosteroid doses vary considerably. Therefore, all children requiring ICS doses above 400 μg/day, or prolonged oral corticosteroids at any dose, should be measured carefully at routine intervals.

In addition to growth, one additional complication of GCS therapy in children deserves mentioning. Although single case reports of fatal varicella infection in children with asthma receiving systemic steroids suggest a potential danger,[74, 145] some studies conclude that systemic steroids do not contribute to the morbidity or mortality rates associated with varicella in asthmatic patients.[39, 52, 172] Perhaps as a result of these disparate reports, the U.S. Food and Drug Administration requested in 1991 that all manufacturers of oral, injectable, and inhaled corticosteroids make labeling changes indicating these potential risks. Unfortunately, since there has been no definite link between inhaled corticosteroid use and disseminated varicella infections, there is concern among asthma specialists that such labeling may create a steroid phobia that could interfere with the use of these agents in children and adolescents who could markedly benefit from such therapy. As a result, a position statement was formulated by the American Academy of Allergy and Immunology to address these concerns.[38]

ASTHMA TREATMENT GUIDELINES IN CHILDREN

The pharmacologic treatment of asthma can be viewed in terms of both the frequency (intermittent versus chronic) (Fig. 27–1) and intensity (mild, moderate, severe) of symptoms. A classification by frequency will involve the identification of various triggering factors (exercise, allergen, infection). Stratification by disease intensity will further influence the types of medications initially prescribed, as well as guiding adjustments in maintenance asthma therapy depending on each patient's fluctuations in symptoms over time.

INTERMITTENT THERAPY

Exercise-Induced Asthma

Exercise-induced asthma (EIA) in children is best treated with a combination of nonpharmacologic and pharmacologic therapeutic modalities. Nonpharmacologic strategies involve inducing a refractory period and selecting climatic conditions for exercise that are less likely to provoke EIA.[29] Forty to fifty percent of patients develop a refractory period after EIA, and a second exercise challenge in these subjects produces less than half of the initial response. This can be used to their advantage, as the incorporation of exercise warm-ups (e.g., wind sprints), which may provoke mild episodes of EIA, could be performed just prior to more competitive activities (e.g., mile run). The likelihood of EIA can also be reduced by choosing sports that tend to minimize heat and water loss (e.g., swimming) or having younger children wear a protective mask or scarf when playing outside in colder weather. Pharmacologic strategies for EIA involve premedication with either an intermediate-acting beta$_2$-agonist (e.g., albuterol, metaproterenol, terbutaline) or cromolyn or nedocromil 5 to 10 minutes before exercise.[29] In patients with moderate or moderate to severe asthma, the use of anti-inflammatory therapy (inhaled corticosteroids) and/or theophylline may be beneficial in decreasing overall airway hyperresponsiveness and improving baseline bronchodilation, respectively.[29] The use of long-acting beta-agonists has

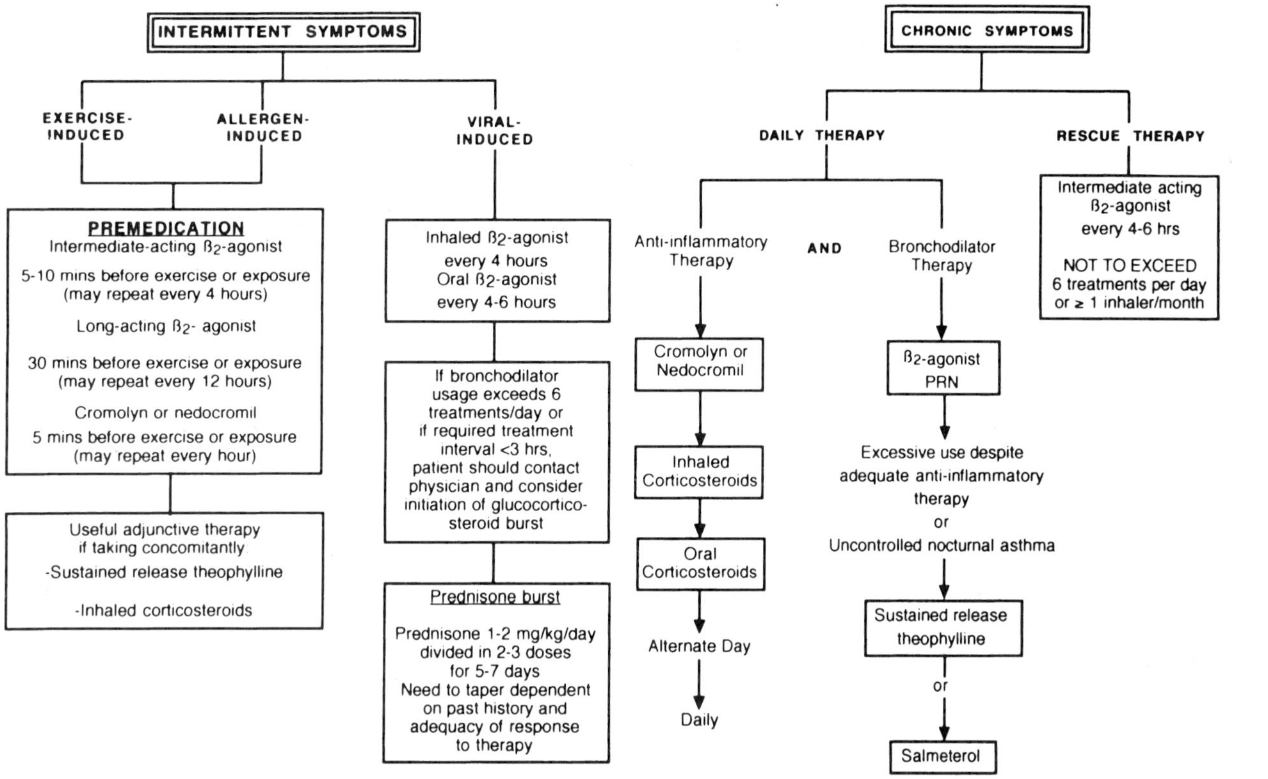

FIGURE 27–1. Asthma treatment in children based on frequency of symptoms. (From Lemanske RF Jr, Gern JE: Childhood asthma. In Lichtenstein L, Fauci A (eds). Current Therapy in Allergy, Immunology, and Rheumatology. Mosby-Year Book, Inc, St. Louis, 1996.)

also been shown to be beneficial in the prevention of EIA.[56, 146]

Virus-Induced Asthma

Infections are a common precipitant of asthma in children. Since viruses are the predominant etiologic agents, treatment with antibiotics is not usually helpful unless the asthmatic episode is accompanied by otitis media and/or sinusitis. In mild cases of wheezing and/or cough associated with rhinorrhea and low-grade fever, initial treatment with a beta-agonist may be tried. Symptoms unresponsive to bronchodilator therapy may respond to oral prednisone or prednisolone (1–2 mg/kg/day, maximum 40 mg in most cases) for 5 to 7 days.

Allergen-Induced Asthma

The development of asthmatic symptoms resulting from exposure to relevant allergens in sensitized patients can best be treated by avoidance. In the case of animal sensitivity, the issues pertaining to avoidance and/or removal are challenging once patients and/or other family members have bonded to their pets. In situations when avoidance cannot be accomplished (holiday visitations to relatives), premedication with a beta$_2$-agonist every 4 hours during exposure and/or cromolyn or nedocromil every 2 hours can be useful.

OVERVIEW OF CHRONIC THERAPY

Once bronchodilators are used for more than exercise prophylaxis, for allergen exposure, or for burst therapy during viral respiratory infections, the introduction of daily anti-inflammatory therapy should be considered (Fig. 27–1 to 27–4). Because of proven efficacy and a paucity of side effects, cromolyn and nedocromil are the preferred first-line anti-inflammatory medications in children with moderate asthma.[105] If the response to these medications is not satisfactory, theophylline can be added to the regimen, or inhaled corticosteroids may be substituted. Most asthma specialists recommend using doses of oral and/or inhaled corticosteroids that maximize lung function, as assessed by objective parameters, such as peak flow rates or spirometry, in older children, or based on symptom control and rescue beta-agonist usage in younger children. Once stability is achieved, periodic reductions in dosages should be attempted to establish the minimum amount of GCS needed to maintain acceptable symptom control.

Children with moderate to severe asthma who are receiving maintenance anti-inflammatory therapy rely on rapid-onset inhaled beta$_2$-agonists as rescue medicines to relieve acute symptoms. Children using the long-acting beta-agonist salmeterol, which has a delayed onset of action (10–20 minutes), to help treat chronic symptoms also require a rapid-onset beta$_2$-agonist as a rescue medication. Unresponsiveness to the regimens described should prompt a review of exposure to triggers (allergens, tobacco smoke, sinusitis), inhaler technique, compliance, and other possible diagnoses

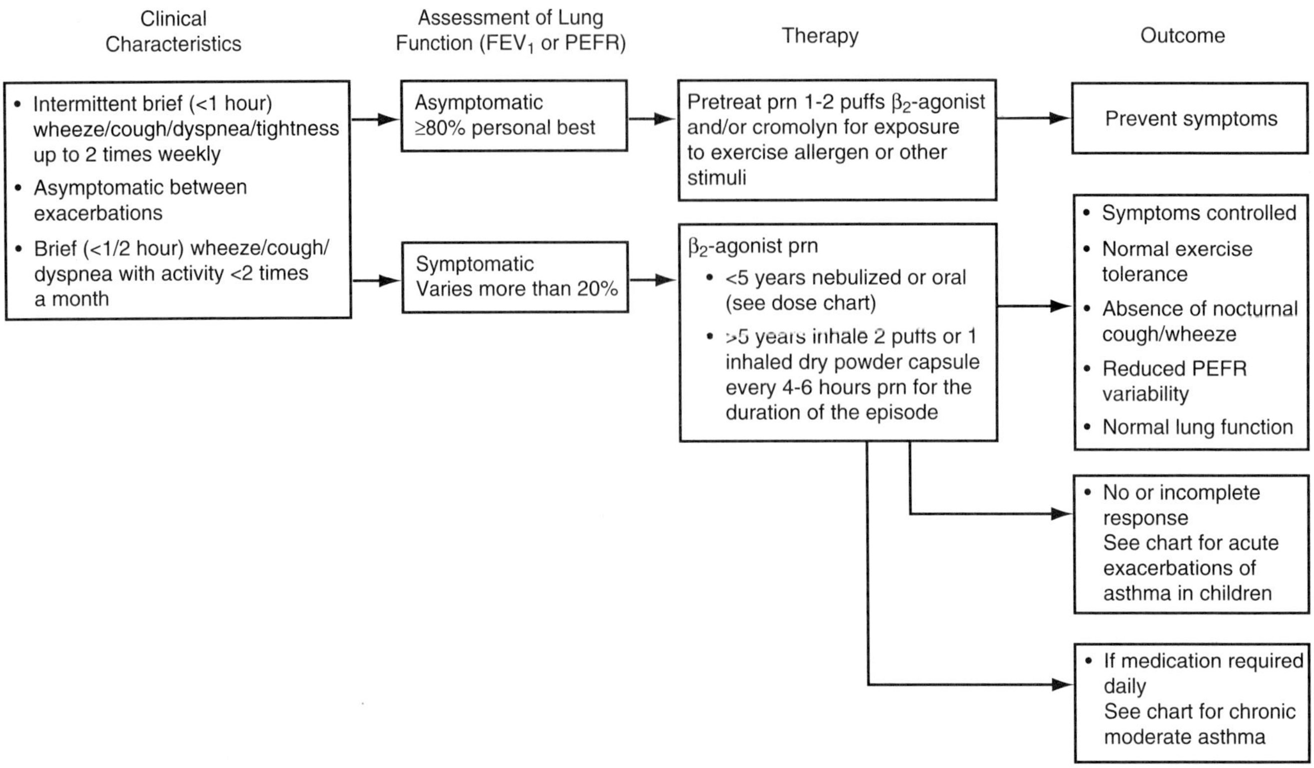

FIGURE 27–2. Medical management of chronic mild asthma in children. (From National Asthma Education Program, National Institutes of Health: Guidelines for the Diagnosis and Management of Asthma. NIH publication #91-3042. US Department of Health and Human Services, Bethesda, MD, 1991.)

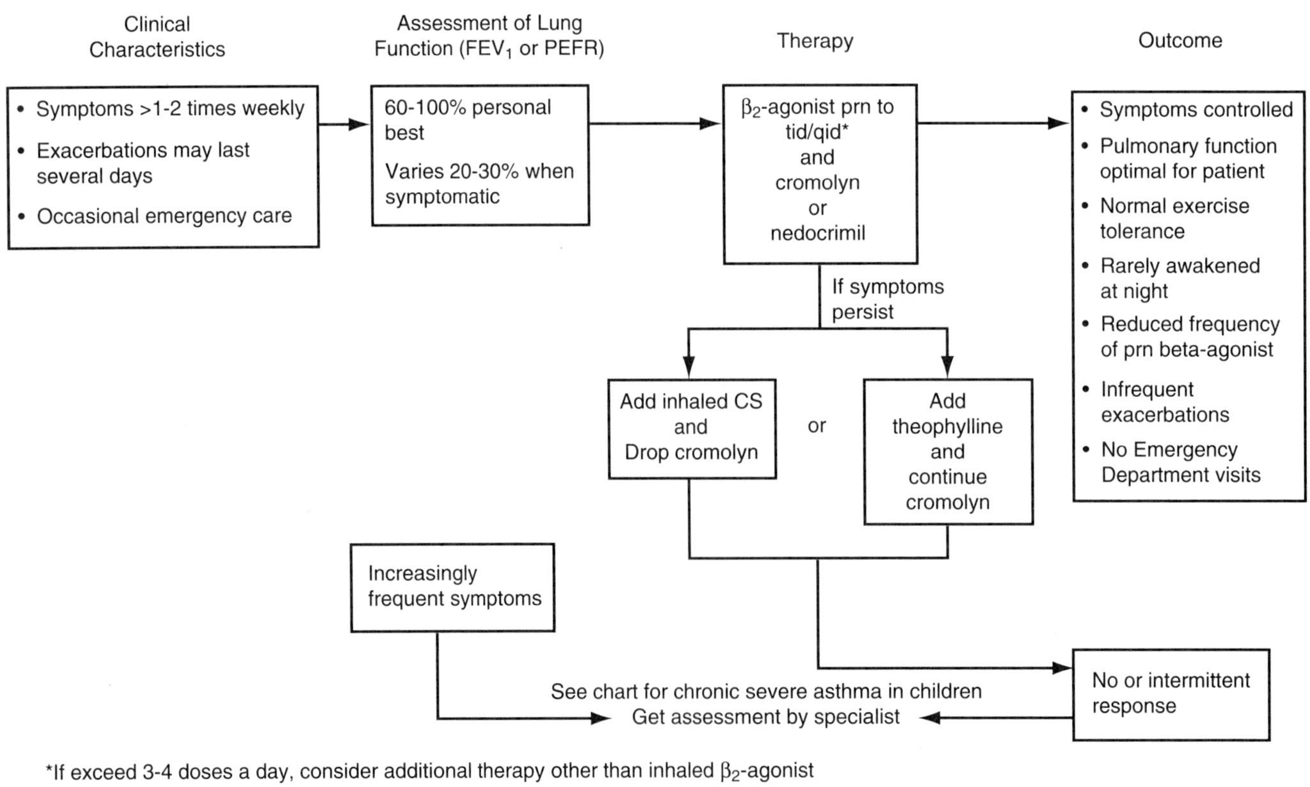

FIGURE 27–3. Medical management of chronic moderate asthma. (From National Asthma Education Program, National Institutes of Health: Guidelines for the Diagnosis and Management of Asthma. NIH publication #91-3042. US Department of Health and Human Services, Bethesda, MD, 1991.)

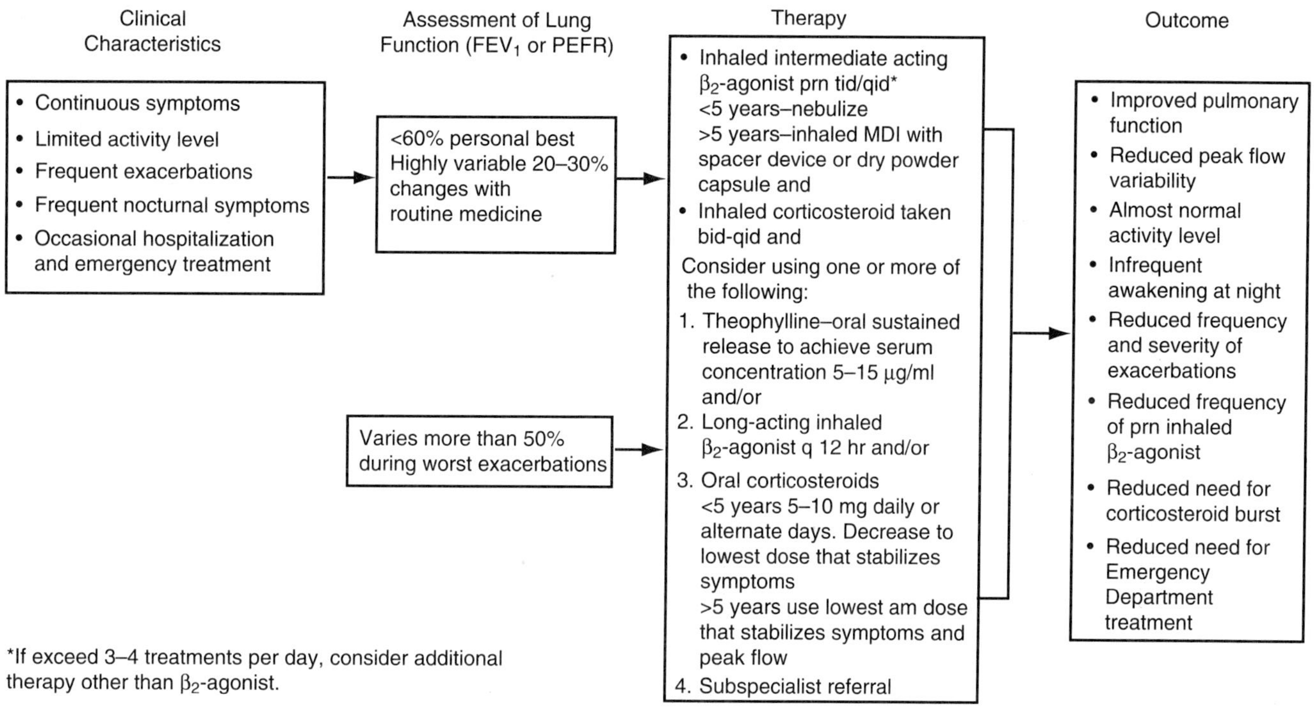

FIGURE 27–4. Medical management of chronic severe asthma in children. (From National Asthma Education Program, National Institutes of Health: Guidelines for the Diagnosis and Management of Asthma. NIH publication #91-3042. US Department of Health and Human Services, Bethesda, MD, 1991.)

(cystic fibrosis, VCD) before oral GCS are prescribed. The National Asthma Education Program[105] has developed algorithms to aid in the management of children with mild, moderate, and severe asthma. The dosages for medications used for maintenance therapy in childhood asthma are shown in Table 27–3.

TREATMENT OF ACUTE ASTHMA

There is no question that inhaled rapid-onset beta$_2$-agonists (albuterol, metaproterenol, pirbuterol, terbutaline) are first-line drugs for rescue treatment of acute asthmatic symptoms in patients of all ages. Because of the potential for the development of progressive life-threatening symptoms if treatment of acute exacerbations of asthma is delayed, an expert panel from the American Academy of Allergy and Immunology[2] recommends that children with asthma who have sufficient maturity to control the use of inhaled medications be permitted to carry their beta$_2$-agonist inhalers with them at school and use them as needed.

As in other age groups, the treatment of acute exacerbations of asthma in children and adolescents will depend on the severity of air flow obstruction, as assessed by objective measurements (peak flow rates, spirometry, pulse oximetry, physical findings) and the initial response to bronchodilator therapy (Table 27–4). Additional algorithms based on the same principles have been established for managing acute asthma at home and in the hospital setting (Fig. 27–5).[105] Several studies have demonstrated that oral or parenteral GCS may be useful for the treatment of acute exacerbations of asthma that respond poorly to bronchodilator therapy.[20, 134, 160] The overall goal of asthma therapy should be to eliminate, or at least significantly reduce, acute asthmatic exacerbations that require emergency room treatment or hospitalizations (Table 27–5).

PROGNOSIS

REMISSION

It is clear that not all children diagnosed with asthma will have asthma as adults. Coultas and colleagues[25] reviewed 7 studies and found that 30 to 70% of asthmatic children had improved or were asymptomatic by adolescence or early adulthood. They tried to identify predictors of asthmatic remissions. Gender and age of diagnosis were found not to be consistent predictors of outcome, but duration of symptoms was. In children 14 years old who had frequent wheezing, 68% still had asthma by 28 years of age.[16] Atopy, or eczema beyond childhood cradle cap, tended to be associated with asthma lasting into adulthood.[72] Sensitization to *Dermatophagoides pteronyssinus*, especially in infancy, was a strong predictor of recurrent wheezing.[167] Family history of asthma or atopy also was seen more commonly in those children with persistent asthma. Mazon and colleagues[92] found that perennial symptoms (sensitization to house dust mites, molds, pollen, or milk protein) were associated with persistence of asthma. Severity of wheezing, or reduced FEV$_1$ in childhood, may predict wheezing into adulthood, but not asthma severity.[51] In a study of over 8,000 children, a mother's age at the time of her child's birth was shown to be a predictor of asthma remission, with children of younger mothers more likely to have persistent asthma.[3] Exposure to tobacco smoke is also associated with airway obstruction into adulthood.[32]

TABLE 27–3
DOSAGE FOR MAINTENANCE THERAPY IN CHILDHOOD ASTHMA

Bronchodilators

Beta-Agonists

Inhaled
- Examples: albuterol, metaproterenol, terbutaline, pirbuterol, bitolterol
- Mode of administration
  - Metered dose inhaler, 2 puffs q 4–6 hrs
  - Powder inhaler device, 1 capsule q 4–6 hrs (albuterol)
- Nebulizer solution
  - Albuterol 5 mg/ml, 0.1–0.15 mg/kg in 2 ml saline q 4–6 hrs, maximum 5.0 mg
  - Metaproterenol 50 mg/ml, 0.25–0.50 mg/kg in 2 ml of saline q 4–6 hrs, maximum 15.0 mg

Oral
- Liquids
  - Albuterol, 0.1–0.15 mg/kg q 4–6 hrs (maximum 4 mg)
  - Metaproterenol, 0.3–0.5 mg/kg q 4–6 hrs (maximum 10 mg)
- Tablets
  - Albuterol, 2–4 mg q 4–6 hrs, 4 or 8 mg sustained release albuterol q 12 hrs
  - Metaproterenol, 10–20 mg q 4–6 hrs
  - Terbutaline, 2.5–5.0 mg q 4–6 hrs

Theophylline

(Dosage is based on serum level. Dosage to achieve serum concentration of 5–15 μg/ml)
- Liquids
- Tablets, capsules (caution–pharmacokinetics of different brands may vary considerably)
- Sustained release tablets, capsules [dosing interval (q day vs BID vs TID) will depend on product formulation and rate of metabolism]

Ipratropium Bromide

Metered dose inhaler (18 μg/puff) 2 puffs QID
Nebulizer solution (250 μg/ml)
- Ages 3–12 yrs 100–500 μg 8 hrs
- > 12 yrs 250–500 μg q 8 hrs

Anti-Inflammatory Agents

Antiallergic Compounds

Cromolyn sodium
- MDI, 1.0 mg/puff, 2 puffs BID-QID
- Nebulizer solution, 20 mg/2 ml ampule, 1 ampule BID-QID

Nedocromil sodium
- MDI, 1.75 mg/puff, 2 puffs BID-QID

Glucocorticoids

Glucocorticoid	mcg per inhalation	Usually starting dose and interval	Maximum dose (puff/day) Ages 6–12	Ages > 12
Beclomethasone dipropionate	42	2–4 puffs BID-QID	10	20
Triamcinolone acetonide	100	2–4 puffs BID-QID	12	16
Flunisolide	250	2–4 puffs BID	4	8

Oral†
- Liquids
  - Prednisone, 5 mg/5 ml
  - Prednisolone
    - 5 mg/5 ml
    - 15 mg/5 ml
- Tablets
  - Prednisone, 1, 5, 10, 20, 50 mg
  - Methylprednisolone 2, 4, 8, 16, 24, 32 mg

*200 μg per actuation, but 100 μg retained in spacer.
†Burst therapy 1–2/mg/kg/day split BID–TID 5–7 days. Maintenance therapy lowest daily dose, alternate day whenever possible.
From Lemanske RH Jr, Gern JE: Childhood asthma. In Lichtenstein L, Fauci A (eds): Current Therapy in Allergy, Immunology, and Rheumatology. Mosby-Year Book, Inc, St. Louis, 1996.

TABLE 27–4
ESTIMATION OF SEVERITY OF ACUTE EXACERBATIONS OF ASTHMA IN CHILDREN*

Sign/Symptom	Mild	Moderate	Severe
Respiratory rate	Normal to <1 standard deviation from the norm (S.D.) for age	Normal to <2 S.D. for age	Normal to >2 S.D. for age
Alertness	Normal	Normal	May be decreased
Dyspnea†	Absent or mild; speaks in complete sentences	Moderate; speaks in phrases or partial sentences	Severe; speaks only in single words or short phrases
Pulsus paradoxus	<10 mmHg	10–20 mmHg	20–40 mmHg
Accessory muscle use	No intercostal to mild retractions	Moderate intercostal retraction with tracheosternal retractions; use of sternocleidomastoid muscles	Severe intercostal retractions; tracheosternal retractions with nasal flairing
Color	Good	Pale	Possibly cyanotic
Auscultation	End respiratory wheeze only	Wheeze during entire expiration and inspiration	Breath sounds becoming inaudible
Oxygen saturation	>95%	90–95%	<90%
PCO_2	<35	<40	>40
PEF	70–80% predicted or personal best	50–70% predicted or personal best	<50% predicted or personal best

*Within each category, the presence of several parameters, but not necessarily all, indicates the general classification of the exacerbation.
†Parent's or physician's impression of degree of child's breathlessness.
From National Asthma Education Program, National Heart, Lung, and Blood Institute, National Institutes of Health: Guidelines for the Diagnosis and Management of Asthma. NIH Publication No 91–3042. US Department of Health and Human Services, Bethesda, MD, 1991.

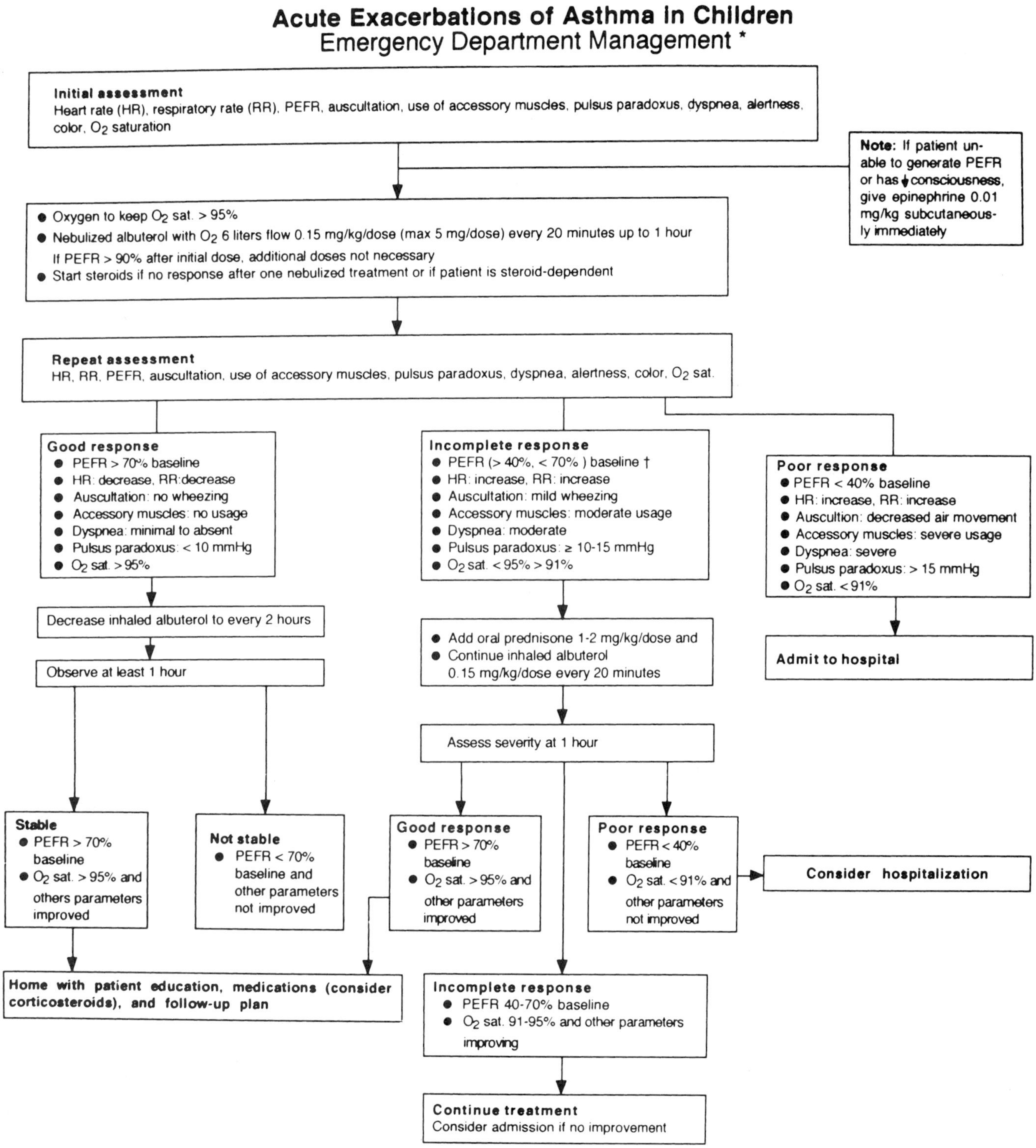

* Therapies are often available in a physician's office. However, most acutely severe exacerbations of asthma require a complete course of therapy in an Emergency Department.

† PEFR % baseline refers to the norm for the individual, established by the clinician. This may be % predicted based on standardized norms or patient's personal best.

FIGURE 27–5. Emergency room management of acute exacerbations of asthma in children. (From Lemanske RF Jr, Gern JE: Childhood asthma. In Lichtenstein L, Fauci A (eds). Current Therapy in Allergy, Immunology, and Rheumatology. Mosby-Year Book, Inc, St. Louis, 1996.)

TABLE 27–5
DOSAGES OF DRUGS IN ACUTE EXACERBATIONS OF ASTHMA IN CHILDREN

Drug	Available Form	Dosage	Comment
Inhaled Beta$_2$-Agonist			
Albuterol			
Metered-dose inhaler	90 μg/puff	Two inhalations every 5 minutes for total of 12 puffs, with monitoring of PEFR or FEV_1 to document response	If not improved, switch to nebulizer. If improved, decrease to 4 puffs every hour.
Nebulizer solution	0.5% (5 mg/mL)	0.1–0.15 mg/kg/dose up to 5 mg every 20 minutes for 1–2 hours (minimum dose 1.25 mg/dose)	If improved, decrease to 1–2 hours. If not improved, use by continuous inhalation.
Metaproterenol			
Metered-dose inhaler	650 μg/puff	Two inhalations	Frequent high-dose administration has not been evaluated. Metaproterenol is not interchangeable with albuterol.
Nebulizer solution	5% (50 mg/mL) 0.6% unit dose vial of 2.5 mL (15 mg)	0.1–0.3 cc (5–15 mg). Do not exceed 15 mg. As above 5–15 mg. Do not exceed 15 mg.	
Systemic Beta-Agonist			
Epinephrine HCl	1:1000 (1 mg/mL)	0.01 mg/kg up to 0.3 mg subcutaneously every 20 minutes for 3 doses.	Inhaled beta$_2$-agonist preferred.
Terbutaline	(0.1%) 1 mg/mL solutions for injection in 0.9% NaCl.	Subcutaneous 0.01 mg/kg up to 0.3 mg every 2–6 hours as needed. Intravenous 10 μg/kg over 10 minutes loading dose. Maintenance: 0.4 μg/kg/minute. Increase as necessary by 0.2 μg/kg/minute and expect to use 3–6 μg/kg/minute.	Inhaled beta$_2$-agonist preferred.
Corticosteroids			
Outpatients	Oral prednisone, prednisolone, or methylprednisolone	1–2 mg/kg/day in single or divided doses (maximum 40–60 mg/day)	Reassess at 3 days, as only a short burst may be needed. No need to taper dose in most instances.
Emergency department or hospitalized patients	Methylprednisolone I.V. or P.O.	1–2 mg/kg/dose every 6 hrs for 24 hrs then 1–2 mg/kg/day in divided doses q 8–12 hours	Length depends on response. May need only a few days. Need to taper based on characteristic of current and previous exacerbations.
Methylxanthines			
Theophylline	Aminophylline (80% anhydrous theophylline)	Loading dose:* If theophylline concentration known: every 1 mg/kg aminophylline will give 2 μg/mL increase in concentration. Loading dose: *If theophylline concentration is unknown: —No previous theophylline: 6 mg/kg aminophylline —Previous theophylline: 3 mg/kg aminophylline Constant infusion rates:* Infusion rates to obtain a mean steady-state concentration of 15 μg/mL: Age 1–6 months 0.5 mg/kg/hr aminophylline 6 mo–1 year 1.0 mg/kg/hr aminophylline 1–9 years 1.5 mg/kg/hr aminophylline 10–16 years 1.2 mg/kg/hr aminophylline	Not first-line therapy. Use in acute setting usually does not provide any additional benefit beyond that seen with adequate therapy with beta-agonist.

*Check serum concentration at approximately 1, 12, and 24 hours after starting the infusion.
From National Asthma Education Program, National Heart, Lung, and Blood Institute, National Institutes of Health: Guidelines for the Diagnosis and Management of Asthma. NIH Publication No 91–3042. US Department of Health and Human Services, Bethesda, MD, 1991.

REFERENCES

1. Allen DB, Mullen M, Mullen B: A meta-analysis of the effect of oral and inhaled corticosteroids on growth. J Allergy Clin Immunol 93:967–976, 1994.
2. American Academy of Allergy and Immunology: Position statement. The use of inhaled medications in school by students with asthma. J Allergy Clin Immunol 84:400–402, 1989.
3. Anderson HR, Bland JM, Patel S, et al: The natural history of asthma in childhood. J Epidemiol Community Health 40:121–129, 1986.
4. Arborelius M Jr, Svenonius E: Decrease of exercise-induced asthma after physical training. Eur J Respir Dis Suppl 65(136):25–31, 1984.
5. Arm JP, O'Hickey SP, Spur BW, et al: Airway responsiveness to histamine and leukotriene in subjects with aspirin-induced asthma. Am Rev Respir Dis 140:148–153, 1989.
6. Armenio L, Baldini G, Bardare M, et al: Double-blind, placebo con-

trolled study of nedocromil sodium in asthma. Arch Dis Child 193–197, 1993.
7. Bai TR: Abnormalities in airway smooth muscle in fatal asthma. Am Rev Respir Dis 141:552–557, 1990.
8. Bai TR, Mak JCW, Barnes PJ: A comparison of beta-adrenergic receptors and in vitro relaxant responses to isoproterenol in asthmatic airway smooth muscle. Am J Respir Cell Mol Biol 6:647–651, 1992.
9. Balfour-Lynn L: Growth and childhood asthma. Arch Dis Child 61:1049–1055, 1986.
10. Bender B, Milgrom H: Theophylline-induced behavior change in children: an objective measure of parents' perceptions. JAMA 2621–2624, 1992.
11. Bender BG, Lerner JA, Ikle D, et al: Psychological change associated with theophylline treatment of asthmatic children: a 6-month study. Pediatr Pulmonol 233–244, 1991.
12. Berenberg MJ, Baigelman W, Cupples LA, et al: Comparison of metered-dose inhaler attached to an aerochamber with updraft nebulizer for the administration of metaproteranol in hospitalized patients. J Asthma 22:87–92, 1985.
13. Berends C, Hoekstra MO, Dijkhuizen B, et al: Expression of CD35 (CR1) and CD11b (CR3) on circulating neutrophils and eosinophils from allergic asthmatic children. Clin Exp Allergy 23:926–933, 1993.
14. Brogden RN, Sorkin EM: Nedocromil sodium. An updated review of its pharmacologic properties and therapeutic efficacy in asthma. Drugs 45:693–715, 1993.
15. Broide DH, Lotz M, Cuomo AJ, et al: Cytokines in symptomatic asthma airways. J Allergy Clin Immunol 89:958–967, 1992.
16. Burney PGJ: Epidemiology. In Clark TJH, Godfrey S, Lee TH (eds): Asthma, 3rd edition. Chapman & Hall Medical, London, 1992, pp 254–307.
17. Burr ML: Epidemiology of childhood asthma. Allerg Immunol (Paris) 23:348–350, 1991. Abstract.
18. Bush RK, Asbury D: Aspirin-sensitive asthma. In Busse WW, Holgate ST (eds): Asthma and Rhinitis. Blackwell Scientific Publications, Boston, 1995, pp 1429–1439.
19. Call RS, Smith TF, Morris E, et al: Risk factors for asthma in inner city children. J Pediatr 121:862–866, 1992.
20. Chapman KR, Verbeek PR, White JG, et al: Effect of a short course of prednisone in the prevention of early relapse after the emergency room treatment of acute asthma. N Engl J Med 324:788–794, 1991.
21. Christopher KL, Wood RP, Eckert RC, et al: Vocal-cord dysfunction presenting as asthma. N Engl J Med 308:1566–1570, 1983.
22. Cockcroft DW, Murdock KY: Comparative effects of inhaled salbutamol, sodium cromoglycate, and beclomethasone dipropionate on allergen-induced early asthmatic responses, and increased bronchial responsiveness to histamine. J Allergy Clin Immunol 79:734–740, 1987.
23. Committee on Environmental Hazards: Involuntary smoking—a hazard to children. Pediatrics 77:755–757, 1986.
24. Connett G, Lenney W: Prevention of viral induced asthma attacks using inhaled budesonide. Arch Dis Child 68:85–87, 1993.
25. Coultas DB, Samet JM: Epidemiology and natural history of childhood asthma. In Tinkelman DG, Naspitz CK (eds): Childhood Asthma: Pathophysiology and Treatment, 2nd edition. Marcel Dekker, Inc, New York, 1993, pp 71–114.
26. Cunningham SJ, Crain EF: Reduction of morbidity in asthmatic children given a spacer device. Chest 106:753–757, 1994.
27. Cutz E, Levison H, Cooper DM: Ultrastructure of airways in children with asthma. Histopathology 2:407–421, 1978.
28. Cypcar D, Busse WW: Role of viral infections in asthma. Immunol Allergy Clin North Am 13:745–766, 1993.
29. Cypcar D, Lemanske RF Jr: Asthma and exercise. In Weisman IM, Zeballos RJ (eds): Clinics in Chest Medicine. WB Saunders Co, Philadelphia, 1994, pp 351–368.
30. Cypcar D, Stark J, Lemanske RF Jr: The impact of respiratory infections on asthma. In Stempel DA, Szefler SJ (eds): Pediatric Clinics of North America. WB Saunders Co, Philadelphia, 1992, pp 1259–1276.
31. Davis RS, Larsen GL, Grunstein MM: Respiratory response to intraesophageal acid infusion in asthmatic children during sleep. J Allergy Clin Immunol 72:393–398, 1983.
32. deBenedictis FM, Canny GJ, Levison H: The progressive nature of childhood asthma. Lung 278–285, 1990.
33. del Bono L, Dente FK, Patalano F, et al: Protective effect of nedocromil sodium and sodium cromoglycate on bronchospasm induced by cold air. Eur J Respir Dis 268–270, 1986.
34. Duff AL, Platts-Mills TAE: Allergens and asthma. Pediatr Clin North Am 39:1277–1291, 1992.
35. Duff AL, Pomeranz ES, Gelber LE, et al: Risk factors for acute wheezing in infants and children: viruses, passive smoke, and IgE antibodies to inhalant allergens. Pediatrics 92:535–540, 1993.
36. Ebina M, Takahashi T, Chiba T, et al: Cellular hypertrophy and hyperplasia of airway smooth muscles underlying bronchial asthma. Am Rev Respir Dis 148:720–726, 1993.
37. Evans R, Mullally DI, Wilson RW, et al: National trends in the morbidity and mortality of asthma in the US. Chest 91:65S–74S, 1987.
38. Executive Committee AA: Position statement: inhaled corticosteroids and severe viral infections. J Allergy Clin Immunol 92:223–225, 1993.
39. Falliers CJ, Ellis EF: Corticosteroids and varicella. Arch Dis Child 40:593–599, 1965.
40. Ferguson AC, Murray AB, Tze W: Short stature and delayed skeletal maturation in children with allergic disease. J Allergy Clin Immunol 69:461–466, 1982.
41. Ferguson AC, Whitelaw M, Brown H: Correlation of bronchial eosinophil and mast cell activation with bronchial hyperresponsiveness in children with asthma. J Allergy Clin Immunol 90:609–613, 1992.
42. Fischer TJ, Guilfoile TD, Kesarwala HH, et al: Adverse pulmonary responses to aspirin and acetaminophen in chronic childhood asthma. Pediatrics 71:313–318, 1983.
43. Fowler MG, Davenport MG, Garg R: School functioning of US children with asthma. Pediatrics 90:939–944, 1992.
44. Frick RB, Metzger WJ, Richerson HB, et al: Increased bronchovascular permeability after allergen exposure in sensitive asthmatics. J Appl Physiol 63:1147–1155, 1987.
45. Furukawa CT, Shapiro GG, Bierman CW, et al: A double-blind study comparing the effectiveness of cromolyn sodium and sustained-release theophylline in childhood asthma. Pediatrics 453–459, 1984.
46. Gaillard D, Jouet J, Egreteau L, et al: Airway epithelial damage and inflammation in children with recurrent bronchitis. Am J Respir Crit Care Med 150:810–817, 1994.
47. Gardiner PV, Ward C, Booth H, et al: Effect of eight weeks of treatment with salmeterol on bronchoalveolar lavage inflammatory indices in asthmatics. Am J Respir Crit Care Med 150:1006–1011, 1994.
48. Gergen PJ, Mullally DI, Evans R: National Survey of Prevalence of Asthma Among Children in the United States, 1976 to 1980. Pediatrics 81:1–7, 1988.
49. Gergen PJ, Weiss KB: Changing patterns of asthma hospitalization among children: 1979 to 1987. JAMA 264:1688–1692, 1990.
50. Gern JE, Lemanske RF Jr: Beta-adrenergic agonist therapy. In Bush RK (ed): Immunology and Allergy Clinics of North America. WB Saunders Co, Philadelphia, 1993, pp 839–860.
51. Gerritsen J, Koeter GH, Postma DS, et al: Prognosis of asthma from childhood to adulthood. Am Rev Respir Dis 140:1325–1330, 1989.
52. Girsh LS, Yu M, Jones J, et al: A study of the risk of mortality of varicella in patients with bronchial asthma or other allergic disease receiving corticosteroid therapy. Ann Allergy 24:690–693, 1966.
53. Goldman J, Muers M: Vocal cord dysfunction and wheezing. Thorax 46:401–404, 1991.
54. Goldman JM, Bennett JR: Gastro-oesophageal reflux and asthma; a common association, but of what clinical importance. Gut 31:1–3, 1990.
55. Gortmaker SL, Walker DK, Jacobs FH, et al: Parental smoking and the risk of childhood asthma. Am J Public Health 72:574–579, 1982.
56. Green CP, Price JF: Prevention of exercise induced asthma by inhaled salmeterol xinafoate. Arch Dis Child 67:1014–1017, 1992.
57. Gustafsson PM, Kjellman NM, Tibbling L: Bronchial asthma and acid reflux into the distal and proximal oesophagus. Arch Dis Child 65:1255–1258, 1990.
58. Gustafsson PM, Kjellman NI, Tibbling L: A trial of ranitidine in asthmatic children and adolescents with or without pathological gastro-oesophageal reflux. Eur Respir J 5:201–206, 1992.
59. Haas F, Pineda H, Axen K, et al: Effects of physical fitness on expiratory airflow in exercising asthmatic people. Med Sci Sports Exerc 17:585–592, 1985.
60. Halfon N, Newacheck PW: Trends in the hospitalization for acute childhood asthma, 1970–84. Am J Public Health 76:1308–1311, 1986.
61. Halfon N, Newacheck PW: Childhood asthma and poverty: differential impacts and utilization of health services. Pediatrics 91:56–61, 1993.
62. Hendeles L, Weinberger M, Szefler S: Safety and efficacy of theophylline in children with asthma. J Pediatr 177–183, 1992.

63. Henderson FW, Clyde WA, Collier AM, et al: The etiologic and epidemiologic spectrum of bronchiolitis in pediatric practice. J Pediatr 95:183–190, 1979.
64. Herve P, Denjean A, Jian R, et al: Intraesophageal perfusion of acid increases the bronchomaoter response to methacholine and to isocapnic hyperventilation in asthmatic subjects. Am Rev Respir Dis 134:986–989, 1986.
65. Hiller EJ, Milner AD, Lenney W: Nebulized sodium cromoglycate in young asthmatic children. Arch Dis Child 875–876, 1977.
66. Howarth PH, Durham SR, Lee TH, et al: Influence of albuterol, cromolyn sodium, and ipratropium bromide on the airway and circulating mediator responses to allergen bronchial provocation in asthma. Am Rev Respir Dis 132:986–992, 1985.
67. Hunt LW, Rosenow EC: Drug-induced asthma. In Weiss EB, Stein M (eds): Bronchial Asthma: Mechanisms and Therapeutics, 3rd edition. Little, Brown and Company, Boston, 1993, pp 621–631.
68. James AL, Pare PD, Hogg JC: The mechanics of airway narrowing in asthma. Am Rev Respir Dis 139:242–246, 1989.
69. James JM, Bernhisel-Broadbent J, Sampson HA: Respiratory reactions provoked by double-blind food challenges in children. Am J Respir Crit Care Med 149:59–64, 1994.
70. Johnston SL, Pattemore PK, Sanderson G, et al: Role of virus infections in children with recurrent wheeze or cough. Thorax 48:1055, 1993. Abstract.
71. Jusko WJ, Gardner MJ, Mangione A, et al: Factors affecting theophylline clearances: age, tobacco, marijuana, cirrhosis, congestive heart failure, obesity, oral contraceptives, benzodiazepines, barbiturates, and ethanol. J Pharm Sci 1358–1366, 1979.
72. Kaplan BA, Mascie-Taylor CGN: Predicting the duration of childhood asthma. J Asthma 29:39–48, 1992.
73. Kasper WJ, Howe PM: Fatal varicella after a single course of corticosteroids. Pediatr Infect Dis J 9:729–732, 1990.
74. Kerem E, Levison H, Schuh S, et al: Efficacy of albuterol administered by nebulizer versus spacer device in children with acute asthma. J Pediatr 123:313–317, 1993.
75. Kondo S, Ito M, Saito M, et al: Progressive bronchial obstruction during the acute stage of respiratory tract infection in asthmatic children. Chest 106:100–104, 1994.
76. Konig P: The risks and benefits of inhaled corticosteroids. Eur J Respir Dis 15:501–510, 1993.
77. Kowabori I, Pierson WE, Loveday LC, et al: Incidence of exercise-induced asthma in children. J Allergy Clin Immunol 58:447–455, 1976.
78. Lacoste J-Y, Bousquet J, Chanez P, et al: Eosinophilic and neutrophilic inflammation in asthma, chronic bronchitis, and chronic obstructive pulmonary disease. J Allergy Clin Immunol 92:537–548, 1993.
79. Lal S, Dorow PD, Venho KK, et al: Nedocromil sodium is more effective than cromolyn sodium for the treatment of chronic reversible obstructive airway disease. Chest 104:438–447, 1993.
80. Lazaar AL, Albelda SM, Pilewski JM, et al: T lymphocytes adhere to airway smooth muscle cells via integrins and CD44 and induce smooth muscle cell DNA synthesis. J Exp Med 180:807–816, 1994.
81. Leaver R, Weinberg EG: Is Mycoplasma pneumoniae a precipitating factor in acute severe asthma in children? S Afr Med J 68:78–79, 1985.
82. Leff AR, Hamann KJ, Wegner CD: Inflammation and cell-cell interactions in airway hyperresponsiveness. Am J Physiol 260:L189–L206, 1991.
83. Lemanske RF Jr: Patterns of airway responsiveness. J Allergy Clin Immunol 86:653–656, 1990.
84. Lemanske RF Jr: Mechanisms of airway inflammation. Chest 101:372S–377S, 1992.
85. Lemanske RF Jr, Kaliner MA: Late phase allergic reactions. In Middleton E Jr, Reed CE, Ellis EF, et al (eds): Allergy: Principles and Practice, 4th edition. Mosby-Year Book, Inc, St Louis, 1993, pp 320–361.
86. Lindgren SD, Lokshin B, Stromquist A, et al: Does asthma or treatment with theophylline limit children's academic performance? N Engl J Med 926–930, 1992.
87. Lundgren JD, Shelhamer JH: Pathogenesis of airway mucus hypersecretion. J Allergy Clin Immunol 85:399–417, 1990.
88. Macek V, Sorli J, Kopriva S, et al: Persistent adenoviral infection and chronic airway obstruction in children. Am J Respir Crit Care Med 150:7–10, 1994.
89. Martinez F, Cline M, Burrows B: Increased incidence of asthma in children of smoking mothers. Pediatrics 89:21–26, 1992.
90. Martinez FD, Morgan WJ, Wright AL, et al: Initial airway function is a risk factor for recurrent wheezing respiratory illnesses during the first three years of life. Am Rev Respir Dis 143:312–316, 1991. Abstract.
91. Martinez FD, Wright AL, Taussig LM, et al: Asthma and wheezing in the first six years of life. N Engl J Med 332:133–138, 1995.
92. Mazon A, Nieto A, Nieto FJ, et al: Prognostic factors in childhood asthma: a logistic regression analysis. Ann Allergy 72:455–461, 1994.
93. McFadden ER Jr: Perspectives in beta-2-agonist therapy: vox clamantis in deserto vel lux in tenebris? J Allergy Clin Immunol 95:641–651, 1995.
94. McFadden ER Jr, Gilbert IA: Asthma. N Engl J Med 327:1928–1937, 1992.
95. McIntosh K, Ellis EF, Hoffman LS, et al: The association of viral and bacterial respiratory infections with exacerbations of wheezing in young asthmatic children. J Pediatr 82:578–590, 1973.
96. Meltzer EO, Orgel HA, Kemp JP, et al: Vocal cord dysfunction in a child with asthma. J Asthma 28:141–145, 1991.
97. Metzger WJ, Zavala D, Richerson HB, et al: Local allergen challenge and bronchoalveolar lavage of allergic asthmatic lungs. Description of the model and local airway inflammation. Am Rev Respir Dis 135:433–440, 1987.
98. Minor TE, Dick EC, DeMeo AN, et al: Viruses as precipitants of asthmatic attacks in children. JAMA 227:292–298, 1974.
99. Miraglia del Giudice M, Capristo A, Maiello N, et al: Nebulized sodium cromoglycate for the treatment of asthma in children under five years of age. Mod Probl Pediatr 21:122–127, 1982.
100. Morgan WJ, Martinez FD: Risk factors for developing wheezing and asthma in childhood. Pediatr Clin North Am 39:1185–1203, 1992.
101. Morrow PE: Aerosol characterization and deposition. Am Rev Respir Dis 110:88–99, 1974.
102. Murray AB, Morrison BJ: The effect of cigarette smoke from the mother on bronchial responsiveness and severity of symptoms in children with asthma. J Allergy Clin Immunol 77:575–581, 1986.
103. Murray AB, Morrison BJ: Passive smoking and the seasonal difference of severity of asthma in children. Chest 94:701–708, 1988.
104. Murray AB, Morrison BJ: Passive smoking by asthmatics: its greater effect on boys than on girls and on older than on younger children. Pediatrics 84:451–459, 1989.
105. National Asthma Education Program, National Heart, Lung, and Blood Institute, National Institutes of Health: Guidelines for the Diagnosis and Management of Asthma. NIH Publication No 91-3042. US Department of Health and Human Services, Bethesda, MD, 1991.
106. National Asthma Education Program, National Heart, Lung, and Blood Institute, National Institutes of Health: Teach Your Patients About Asthma: A Clinician's Guide #92–2737. US Department of Health and Human Services, Bethesda, MD, 1992.
107. Neddenriep D, Schumacher MJ, Lemen RJ: Asthma in childhood. Curr Probl Pediatr 19:325–388, 1989.
108. Nelson HS: Gastroesophageal reflux and pulmonary disease. J Allergy Clin Immunol 73:547–556, 1984.
109. Newhouse MT: Pulmonary drug targeting with aerosols: principles and clinical applications in adults and children. Am J Asthma Allergy Ped 7:23–35, 1993.
110. Newhouse MT: Emergency department management of life-threatening asthma: are nebulizers obsolete? Chest 103:661–662, 1993.
111. Newhouse MT, Dolovich MB: Control of asthma by aerosols. N Engl J Med 315:870–874, 1986.
112. Nicholson KG, Kent J, Ireland DC: Respiratory viruses and exacerbations of asthma in adults. Br Med J 307:982–986, 1993.
113. Nickerson BG, Bautista DB, Namey MA, et al: Distance running improves fitness in asthmatic children without pulmonary complications or changes in exercise-induced bronchospasm. Pediatrics 71:147–152, 1983.
114. Niemeijer NR, de Monchy JGR: Age-dependency of sensitization to aero-allergens in asthmatics. Allergy 47:431–435, 1992.
115. Nudel DB, Diamant S, Brady T, et al: Chest pain, dyspnea on exertion, and exercise-induced asthma in children and adolescents. Clin Pediatr (Phila) 26:388–392, 1987.
116. O'Connell EJ, Logan GB: Parental smoking in childhood asthma. Ann Allergy 32:142–145, 1974.
117. O'Hollaren MT, Yunginger JW, Offard KP, et al: Exposure to an aeroallergen as a possible precipitating factor in respiratory arrest in young patients with asthma. N Engl J Med 324:359–363, 1991.
118. Orenstein SR, Orenstein DM: Gastroesophageal reflux and respiratory disease in children. J Pediatr 112:847–858, 1988.
119. Pattemore PK, Johnston SL, Bardin PG: Viruses as precipitants of

asthma symptoms. I. Epidemiology. Clin Exp Allergy 22:325–336, 1992.

120. Pearlman DS, Chervinsky P, LaForce C, et al: A comparison of salmeterol with albuterol in the treatment of mild-to-moderate asthma. N Engl J Med 327:1420–1425, 1992.
121. Platts-Mills TAE, Tovey ER, Mitchell EB, et al: Reduction of bronchial reactivity during prolonged allergen avoidance. Lancet 1:675–678, 1982.
122. Quinn JM: The side effects of inhaled corticosteroids. Insights Allergy 9:1–8, 1994.
123. Rachelefsky GS, Coulson A, Siegel SC, et al: Aspirin intolerance in chronic childhood asthma: detected by oral challenge. Pediatrics 56:443–448, 1975.
124. Rachelefsky GS, Katz RM, Siegel SC: Chronic sinus disease with associated reactive airway disease in children. Pediatrics 73:526–529, 1984.
125. Rachelefsky GS, Wo J, Adelson J, et al: Behavior abnormalities and poor school performance due to oral theophylline use. Pediatrics 78:1133–1138, 1986.
126. Rackemann FM: A working classification of asthma. Am J Med 601–606, 1995.
127. Redline S, Gold D: Challenges in interpreting gender differences in asthma. Am J Respir Crit Care Med 150:1219–1221, 1994.
128. Reid MJ, Moss RB, Hsu YP, et al: Seasonal asthma in northern California: allergic causes and efficacy of immunotherapy. J Allergy Clin Immunol 78:590–600, 1986.
129. Robertson CF, Rubinfeld AR, Bowes G: Pediatric asthma deaths in Victoria: the mild are at risk. Pediatr Pulmonol 13:95–100, 1992.
130. Rubin BK, Marcushamer S, Priel I, et al: Emergency management of the child with asthma. Pediatr Pulmonol 8:45–57, 1990.
131. Sabato AR, Martin AJ, Marmion BP, et al: Mycoplasma pneumoniae: acute illness, antibiotics, and subsequent pulmonary function. Arch Dis Child 59:1034–1037, 1984.
132. Salvato G: Some histologic changes in chronic bronchitis and asthma. Thorax 23:168–172, 1968.
133. Salzman GA, Pyszczynski DR: Oropharyngeal candidiasis in patients treated with beclomethasone dipropionate delivered by metered-dose inhaler alone and with Aerochamber. J Allergy Clin Immunol 81:424–428, 1988.
134. Scarfone RJ, Fuchs SM, Nager AL, et al: Controlled trial of oral prednisone in the emergency department treatment of children with acute asthma. Pediatrics 92:513–518, 1993.
135. Schauer U, Alefsen S, Jager R, et al: Blood eosinophils, leukotriene C_4 generation, and bronchial hyperreactivity in formerly preterm infants. Arch Dis Child 71:506–510, 1994.
136. Schauer U, Eckhart A, Muller R, et al: Enhanced leukotriene C_4 production by peripheral eosinophilic granulocytes from children with asthma. Int Arch Allergy Appl Immunol 90:201–206, 1989.
137. Schleimer RP: Glucocorticosteroids. Their mechanisms of action and use in allergic diseases. In Middleton E Jr, Reed CE, Ellis EF, et al (eds): Allergy: Principles and Practice, 4th edition. Mosby-Year Book, Inc, St Louis, 1993, pp 893–925.
138. Sears MR: The definition and diagnosis of asthma. Allergy 48:12–16, 1993.
139. Sears MR, Taylor DR, Print CG, et al: Regular inhaled beta-agonist treatment in bronchial asthma. Lancet 336:1391–1396, 1990.
140. Selner JC, Staudenmayer H, Koepke JW, et al: Vocal cord dysfunction: the importance of psychologic factors and provocation challenge testing. J Allergy Clin Immunol 79:726–733, 1987.
141. Settipane GA, Klein DE, Boyd GK, et al: Adverse reactions to cromolyn. JAMA 811–813, 1979.
142. Shapiro GG, Christie DL: Gastroesophageal reflux in steroid-dependent asthmatic youths. Pediatrics 63:207–212, 1979.
143. Shapiro GG, Sharpe M, DeRouen TA, et al: Cromolyn versus triamcinolone acetonide for youngsters with moderate asthma. J Allergy Clin Immunol 88:742–748, 1991.
144. Sheffer AL: Guidelines for the diagnosis and management of asthma. National Heart, Lung, and Blood Institute National Asthma Education Program Expert Panel Report. J Allergy Clin Immunol 88:425–534, 1991. Abstract.
145. Silk HJ, Guay-Woodford L, Perez-Atayde AR, et al: Fatal varicella in steroid-dependent asthma. J Allergy Clin Immunol 81:47–51, 1988.
146. Simons FER, Soni NR, Watson WTA, et al: Bronchodilator and bronchoprotective effects of salmeterol in young patients with asthma. J Allergy Clin Immunol 90:840–846, 1992.
147. Skobeloff EM, Spivey WH, St Clair SS, et al: The influence of age and sex on asthma admissions. JAMA 268:3437–3440, 1992.
148. Sly PD, Landau LI, Weymouth R: Home recording of peak expiratory flow rates and asthma. Am J Dis Child 139:479–482, 1985.
149. Sly RM, Heimlich EM, Busser RJ, et al: Exercise-induced bronchospasm: evaluation of isoproterenol, phenylephrine and the combination. Ann Allergy 25:324–330, 1967.
150. Sly RM, O'Donnell R: Regional distribution of deaths from asthma. Ann Allergy 62:347–354, 1989.
151. Sontag SJ, O'Connell S, Khandelwal S, et al: Most asthmatics have gastroesophageal reflux with or without bronchodilator therapy. Gastroenterology 99:613–620, 1990.
152. Spitzer WO, Suissa S, Ernst P, et al: The use of beta-agonists and the risk of death and near death from asthma. N Engl J Med 326:501–506, 1992.
153. Sporik R, Chapman MD, Platts-Mills TAE: House dust mite exposure as a cause of asthma. Clin Exp Allergy 22:897–906, 1992.
154. Strunk RC, Mrazek DA, Fukuhara JT, et al: Cardiovascular fitness in children with asthma correlates with psychological functioning of the child. Pediatrics 84:460–464, 1989.
155. Strunk RC, Rubin D, Kelly L, et al: Determination of fitness in children with asthma: use of standardized tests for functional endurance, body fat composition, flexibility, and abdominal strength. Am J Dis Child 142:940–944, 1988.
156. Summer W, Elston R, Tharpe L, et al: Aerosol bronchodilator delivery methods: relative impact on pulmonary function and cost of respiratory care. Arch Intern Med 149:618–623, 1989.
157. Sur S, Crotty TB, Kephart GM, et al: Sudden-onset fatal asthma. A distinct entity with few eosinophils and relatively more neutrophils in the airway submucosa? Am Rev Respir Dis 148:713–718, 1993.
158. Szczklik A, Gryglewski RJ, Czermawska-Hysik G: Relationship of inhibition of prostaglandin biosymthesis by analgesics to asthma attacks in aspirin-sensitive patients. Br Med J 1:67–69, 1975.
159. Szentagothai K, Gyene I, Szocska M, et al: Physical exercise programs in children with bronchial asthma. Pediatr Pulmonol 3:166–172, 1987.
160. Tal A, Levy N, Bearman JE: Methylprednisolone therapy for acute asthma in infants and toddlers: a controlled clinical trial. Pediatrics 86:350–356, 1990.
161. Tan WC, Martin RJ, Pandey R, et al: Effects of spontaneous and simulated gastroesophageal reflux on sleeping asthmatics [see comments]. Am Rev Respir Dis 141:1394–1399, 1990.
162. Taylor WR, Newacheck PW: Impact of childhood asthma on health. Pediatrics 90:657–662, 1992.
163. Tinkelman DG, Reed CE, Nelson HS, et al: Aerosol beclomethasone dipropionate compared with theophylline as primary treatment of chronic, mild to moderately severe asthma in children [see comments]. Pediatrics 92:64–77, 1993.
164. Toogood JH: Helping your patients make better use of MDIs and spacers. J Resp Dis 15:151–165, 1994.
165. Towns SJ, Mellis CM: Role of acetyl salicylic acid and sodium metabisulfite in chronic childhood asthma. Pediatrics 73:631–637, 1984.
166. Twentyman OP, Finnerty JP, Harris A, et al: Protection against allergen-induced asthma by salmeterol [see comments]. Lancet 336:1338–1342, 1990.
167. Van Asperen PP, Mukhi A: Role of atopy in the natural history of wheeze and bronchial hyper-responsiveness in childhood. Pediatr Allergy Immunol 5:178–183, 1994.
168. Van Essen-Zandvliet EE, Hughes MD, Waalkens HJ, et al: Effects of 22 months of treatment with inhaled corticosteroids and/or beta-2-agonists on lung function, airway responsiveness, and symptoms in children with asthma. Am Rev Respir Dis 146:547–554, 1992.
169. Virant FS, Shapiro GG: Evaluation of the child with chronic cough and/or wheezing. In Tinkelman DG, Naspitz CK (eds): Childhood Asthma: Pathophysiology and Treatment, 2nd edition. Marcel Dekker, Inc, New York, 1993, pp 303–327.
170. Vittori E, Marini M, Fasoli A, et al: Increased expression of endothelin in bronchial epithelial cells of asthmatic patients and effect of corticosteroids. Am Rev Respir Dis 146:1320–1325, 1992.
171. Weeke ER: Epidemiology of allergic diseases in children. Rhinol Suppl 13:5–12, 1992. Abstract.
172. Weinberg EG, Tuchinda M: Varicella in asthma children receiving alternate-day corticosteroid therapy. J Med Assoc Thail 56:140–143, 1973.
173. Weinberger M: Analgesic sensitivity in children with asthma. Pediatrics 62:910–915, 1977.

174. Weinberger M, Hendeles L: Theophylline. In Middleton E Jr, Reed CE, Ellis EF, et al (eds): Allergy: Principles and Practice, 4th edition. Mosby-Year Book, Inc, St Louis, 1993, pp 816–855.
175. Weiss KB, Wagener DK: Changing patterns of asthma mortality. JAMA 264:1683–1687, 1990.
176. Weiss ST, Speizer FE: Epidemiology and natural history. In Weiss EB, Stein M (eds): Bronchial Asthma: Mechanisms and Therapeutics, 3rd edition. Little, Brown and Company, Boston, 1993, pp 15–25.
177. Weitzman M, Gortmaker S, Walker DK, et al: Maternal smoking and childhood asthma. Pediatrics 85:505–511, 1990.
178. Weitzman M, Gortmaker SL, Sobol AM, et al: Recent trends in the prevalence and severity of childhood asthma. JAMA 268:2673–2677, 1992.
179. Wiggs BR, Bosken C, Pare PD, et al: A model of airway narrowing in asthma and in chronic obstructive pulmonary disease. Am Rev Respir Dis 145:1251–1258, 1992.
180. Williams MC: Maximizing morphologic data from lung biopsies from normal and asthmatic humans. Am J Respir Crit Care Med 150:S2–S5, 1994.
181. Wilson NM, Charette L, Thomson AH, et al: Gastro-oesophageal reflux and childhood asthma: the acid test. Thorax 40:592–597, 1985.
182. Wolthers OD, Pedersen S: Short term growth during treatment with inhaled fluticasone propionate and beclomethasone dipropionate. Arch Dis Child 68:673–676, 1995.
183. Woodfolk JA, Luczynska CM, de Blay F, et al: The effect of vacuum cleaners on the concentration and particle size distribution of airborn cat allergen. J Allergy Clin Immunol 91:829–837, 1993.
184. Young S, LeSouef PN, Geelhoed GC, et al: The influence of a family history of asthma and parental smoking on airway responsiveness in early infancy. N Engl J Med 324:1168–1173, 1991.
185. Yunginger JW, O'Connell EJ, Logan GB: Aspirin-induced asthma in children. J Pediatr 82:218–221, 1973.
186. Zimmerman B, Lanner A, Enander I, et al: Total blood eosinophils, serum eosinophil cationic protein and eosinophil protein X in childhood asthma: relation to disease status and therapy. Clin Exp Allergy 23:564–570, 1993.

28 Asthma: Pathogenesis and Treatment

DEBORAH ORTEGA WILLIAM W. BUSSE

Asthma is a common disease, affecting about 10% of the population. Although the incidence and morbidity of asthma have increased over the past two decades, the reasons for this are unclear. Moreover, the mechanisms by which asthma develops continue to elude researchers, although great progress is being made in this area.

An interdisciplinary panel, the National Asthma Education Program (NAEP), has defined asthma as a chronic airway disease characterized by recurrent and usually reversible air flow obstruction, inflammation, and hyperresponsiveness, producing symptoms of wheezing and breathlessness.

There is evidence that airway inflammation is associated with airway hyperresponsiveness even when the disease is mild and otherwise well controlled. Earlier studies suggested that the mast cell or eosinophil may be the end effector cell in asthma pathogenesis, producing the asthmatic changes in the airway. More recent observations, however, indicate that airway inflammation in asthma is a multicellular process with cell–cell interactions that produce inflammation and, in turn, chronic changes in the airway. Moreover, various models of this complex process suggest roles for T lymphocytes, eosinophils, basophils, mast cells, neutrophils, platelets, and macrophages, as well as cells of the airway itself, epithelium, neurons, and smooth muscle. The importance of cytokines has also become apparent. Recognition of these factors has stimulated new investigations into the mechanisms involved in the pathogenesis of asthma, with an emphasis on the factors involved in the development and regulation of airway inflammation.

In addition to the advances that have been made in asthma pathogenesis, great strides in asthma management have also helped to better characterize the disease, as well as to improve treatment. A management plan in which the patient takes an active role in its design is now thought to be essential for long-term control. Management plans may prove to be helpful in diagnosis as well as treatment.

PATHOGENESIS OF AIRWAY INFLAMMATION

Several observations support the concept that chronic bronchial inflammation is an essential component of asthma. Postmortem studies have shown an inflammatory process in asthmatic airways: occlusion with mucus, serum proteins, and cellular debris; epithelial sloughing; edema and leukocyte infiltration, with eosinophils predominating; thickening of the epithelial subbasement membrane; hypertrophy of bronchial smooth muscle; and hyperplasia of the mucous glands.[61, 67]

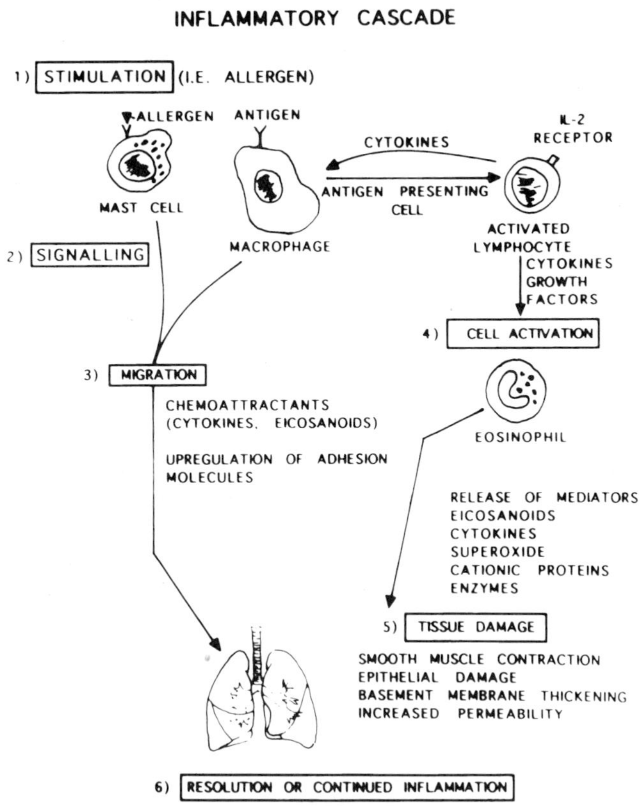

FIGURE 28-1. Inflammation involves various cell types that may themselves act in the inflammatory cascade, producing tissue damage, or release cytokines that recruit additional cells into the inflammatory reaction.

Laitinen and colleagues[156] quantitated bronchial responsiveness to inhaled histamine and then performed bronchial biopsies through a rigid bronchoscope. The bronchial biopsies showed consistent findings of epithelial damage at all levels, with ciliated epithelial cells most likely to be destroyed. The investigators also found that intraepithelial nerves and mast cells were exposed. They concluded that these changes, especially the exposure of sensory nerve endings, could contribute to bronchial hyperresponsiveness and appeared to be related to asthma rather than other causes of airway disease.

Jeffrey and colleagues[130] obtained bronchial biopsy specimens from normal, allergic rhinitis and asthmatic patients. Complete absence of surface epithelium was noted in three of the four asthmatic subjects. There was a tendency for high numbers of inflammatory cells to be present in the lamina propria of the asthmatic patients, although the difference between groups did not achieve significance. The authors concluded that epithelial fragility is closely linked to airway reactivity in asthma and that these changes begin early in the illness.

Beasley and coworkers[12] have found that airway inflammation is an existing component of asthma even in mild disease. In bronchial lavage samples, these investigators found a correlation between epithelial cell numbers and bronchial reactivity. Bronchial biopsy specimens showed extensive deposition of collagen beneath the epithelial basement membrane, mast cell degranulation, and mucosal infiltration by eosinophils. These changes were present even in patients with mild or subclinical disease.

Collectively, these and other studies indicate that inflammation is an important feature of asthma and may also be a driving force in the development of bronchial hyperresponsiveness.[50, 115, 183] Various studies using the airway response to allergen have demonstrated inflammation as an important component of the allergic reaction. Allergic mechanisms appear relevant to over 90% of children with asthma and about 50 to 60% of adults. The next sections will discuss the various cell types that have been identified in the allergic airway reaction and how their participation in an inflammatory cascade may contribute to clinical features of asthma (Fig. 28–1).

MAST CELLS (Fig. 28–2)

Mast cells contain preformed mediators, such as histamine and tryptase, and can generate sulfidopeptide leukotrienes and a variety of other mediators when activated. Both histamine and the mast cell–derived leukotrienes (LTC_4, LTD_4, LTE_4) cause immediate airway smooth muscle contraction and edema. Tryptase is unique to the mast cell, and its release provides a specific marker of mast cell activation.[36, 37] In addition, mast cells have been shown to generate an increasingly comprehensive number of cytokines (see Chapter 10).[27, 217, 285] Mast cell–derived cytokines may have profound effects on recruitment, priming, and activation of various leukocytes and may be linked to the generation of inflammatory infiltrates. Thus the mast cell's influence is important not only in acute airway changes but also in the late inflammatory reaction.

The role of mast cells in asthma and in chronic airway inflammation is undergoing reevaluation and expansion. Mast cells are present at environmental interfaces, such as the skin, gastrointestinal tract, and the respiratory tract. In the lung, they are found at several levels, including the airway lumen, epithelium, submucosa, and lung parenchyma. Evidence shows that mast cells are activated in

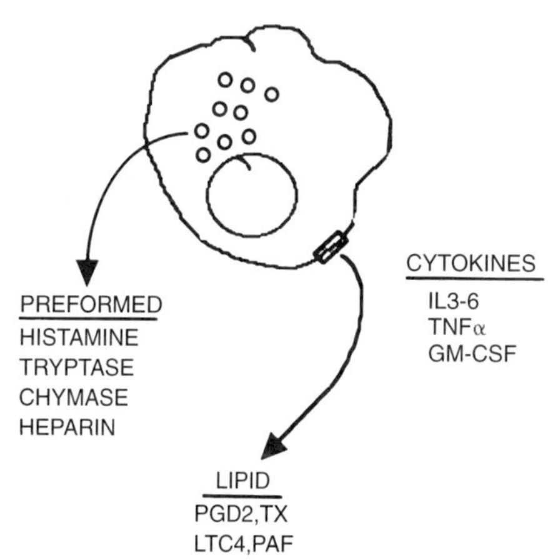

FIGURE 28-2. Mast cells contain preformed mediators, such as histamine, tryptase, and ECF, that are released quickly during mast cell activation. Mast cells also generate lipid mediators (from cell membrane) that can produce airway smooth muscle contraction. Cytokines are polypeptides synthesized from mRNA and can recruit additional cells to the area.

asthma, with several metabolic pathways assuming functional significance in this process. For example, antigen bronchoprovocation causes the acute release of histamine that can be detected in both the circulation[30] and BAL fluid.[35] In addition, the baseline concentrations of histamine in BAL fluid correlate with bronchial responsiveness[35] and the degree of air flow obstruction.[129] Tryptase, a specific marker for mast cell activation, has also been identified in the BAL fluid of patients with stable allergic asthma.[281] Furthermore, although tryptase itself has no effect on airway smooth muscle, there is evidence that it enhances bronchial smooth muscle responsiveness,[245] suggesting another mechanism for its role in the pathogenesis of asthma. These observations indicate that airway mast cells are activated with antigen, leading to an airway environment of mast cell mediators in asthma. Such effects can contribute to enhanced airway tone.

The role of leukotrienes in asthma, especially in specific subgroups of asthmatic patients, has become more apparent. LTD_4 antagonists prevent exercise-induced asthma.[173] Moreover, inhibitors of the 5-lipoxygenase pathway modify nasal allergic reactions and diminish bronchoconstriction induced by isocapnic hyperventilation.[127, 143] Finally, antagonists of LTD_4 cause immediate bronchodilation and diminish airway obstruction that is not fully responsive to beta-agonists.[87, 124]

The importance of pulmonary mast cells in the late inflammatory asthmatic reaction may be further suggested by the fact that mast cell–derived chemotactic factors (for eosinophils and neutrophils) influence recruitment of inflammatory cells to the airway. In addition, mast cells produce several proinflammatory cytokines, including IL-4, IL-5, and IL-6,[285] and express mRNA for other cytokines, such as IL-3 and interferon-γ (IFN-γ). Following FcϵRI activation,[27] these molecules can influence function of airway inflammatory cells, as well as the recruitment of other cells. This evidence supports a role for mast cells in the development of late-phase inflammatory responses. Activation of endothelial cells by mast cell products may also contribute to cell migration via induction of adhesion molecules and endothelial cell secretion of cytokines/chemokines. In addition, observations from cutaneous late-phase reactions (LPRs) indicate that mast cells participate in the initiation of these inflammatory responses, whereas cytokine interactions can lead to cell activation in the absence of IgE or antigen.[63] However, macrophages and lymphocytes also express FcϵRII on their surface membranes and can likewise be activated by allergen[134, 179, 180] to initiate or perpetuate the process. Until the identity of all the activated cells involved in cytokine production are confirmed, the role of the mast cell in the pulmonary LPRs will remain incompletely understood and appreciated.

EOSINOPHILS

Eosinophils mature in the bone marrow under the influence of a number of cytokines, including IL-2, IL-3, IL-5, and granulocyte-macrophage colony-stimulating factor (GM-CSF).[179, 180] The cytoplasmic granules of the eosinophil contain preformed mediators that are released upon stimulation. In addition, the eosinophil has the capacity to synthesize a variety of mediators, including cytokines, leukotrienes, prostaglandins, and platelet activating factor (PAF). There is evidence that eosinophils release various mediators in response to cell activation and that many of these metabolic products play a significant role in the pathogenesis of asthma. Activation of arachidonic acid metabolism leads to the generation of prostaglandin E_2 (PGE_2) and prostacyclin (PGI_2). Eosinophils also produce LTC_4 via the 5-lipoxygenase pathway.[208] LTC_4 and its derivatives LTD_4 and LTE_4 are potent stimulators of smooth muscle constriction and mucous secretion. Furthermore, eosinophil secretion of LTC_4 is enhanced by exposure of the eosinophil to LTB_4 PAF, IL-3, IL-5, and GM-CSF.[280] There is also evidence that eosinophils generate PAF.[160] However, whether PAF is released following cell activation and contributes to altered airway function has yet to be established.

Eosinophils in Asthma (Fig. 28–3)

The eosinophil is believed to be a critical effector cell in the pathogenesis of asthma. In fact, some describe the pathology of asthma as chronic eosinophilic desquamative bronchitis. Evidence that the eosinophil is important in asthma is noted in a number of observations. First, the degree of peripheral blood eosinophilia correlates with asthma severity. Serum eosinophil cationic protein (ECP), suggesting eosinophil activation, has also been found as a marker for asthma severity.[288] Eosinophilia has likewise been identified in the BAL fluid[274] and bronchial mucosal biopsies[12] of subjects with asthma and correlates with disease severity. Several eosinophil products, major basic protein (MBP)[274] and LTC_4,[275] have been identified in the BAL fluid of patients with asthma. Similarly, other markers of degranulation, MBP[78] and ECP,[6, 23] have been found in the bronchial biopsies as well. These data suggest that eosinophils are present, are activated, and release their mediators, which then can play a role in the development of airway inflammation, hyperresponsiveness, and air flow obstruction.

de Monchy and colleagues[58] found striking eosinophilia in the BAL fluid of patients with late allergic responses (LAR) to inhaled antigen. Their finding has been confirmed by

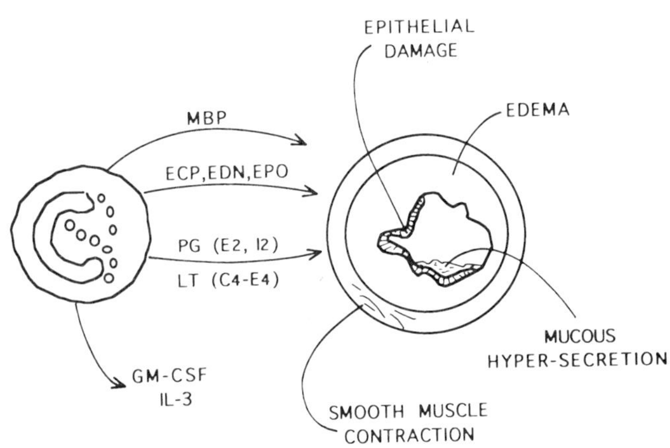

FIGURE 28-3. The eosinophil is potentially one of the most potent effector cells in the pathogenesis of asthma and produces a variety of proteins, enzymes, and lipid mediators (MBP, ECP, EDN, EPO) that may lead to epithelial damage and mucous hypersecretion. Eosinophils also generate prostaglandins (PG) and leukotrienes (LT), which may play a role in bronchoconstriction and airway edema. The release of cytokines (GM-CSF) may prolong the response and recruit additional cells to the area.

other investigators.[60, 183, 244] Frick and coworkers[84] demonstrated a rise in peripheral blood low-density eosinophils in patients experiencing an LAR following inhaled antigen; the low-density cells were felt to represent an increase in activated eosinophils. To more specifically characterize the allergic response in the airway and the role of eosinophils in this process, Sedgwick and colleagues[244] studied BAL fluid obtained following segmental antigen bronchoprovocation in allergic subjects. Lavage samples obtained immediately following antigen challenge had elevated concentrations of histamine and tryptase but no significant changes in cellularity. In BAL samples obtained 48 hours after antigen challenge, tryptase concentrations had returned to baseline; histamine levels, however, remained slightly elevated, which may indicate basophil activation. In contrast, late lavage samples demonstrated a marked increase in cellularity, with eosinophils predominating. Furthermore, the 48-hour lavage samples had dramatic increases in LTC_4, eosinophilic granular proteins (MBP, ECP, EPO, EDN), and IL-5, suggesting that the cells recruited to the airway were activated. These data support the possibility that eosinophils contribute to the bronchial inflammation and hyperresponsiveness associated with the late reaction to an antigen challenge.

Several studies provide evidence that the degree of eosinophilia in blood,[69] BAL,[270, 157, 274] and bronchial mucosal biopsies[6, 23] correlates with the magnitude of airway hyperresponsiveness in subjects with asthma. Gundel and coworkers[108] have further shown that the instillation of purified MBP into the airway of primates induces bronchial hyperresponsiveness. The precise mechanism of this effect is not entirely clear but likely results from injury to the airway epithelium and subsequent development of bronchial hyperresponsiveness.[44]

The mechanisms that control selective eosinophil recruitment to the lung and eosinophil activation have not been fully established. However, one factor in the influx of eosinophils is activation of lymphocytes, possibly the Th2 subclass, with the subsequent release of several proinflammatory cytokines (IL-2–IL-5, GM-CSF). Eosinophil activation may also occur by stimulation of FcϵRII by specific antigen,[85] binding of leukocyte adhesion molecules to their ligands on vascular endothelium and/or airway epithelium,[278] and stimulation of degranulation by IgA complexes,[2] PAF,[152] IL-5, or chemokines, such as RANTES and MCP-3.[85] The precise mechanism of eosinophil activation in the lung is not identified.

An important step in the participation of eosinophils in asthma is cell adhesion. Wegner and Gundel[278] have shown that pretreatment of sensitized monkeys with monoclonal antibody to intercellular adhesion molecule-1 (ICAM-1) blocks both the airway eosinophilia and bronchial hyperresponsiveness, which otherwise follows repetitive antigen challenge. This suggests that eosinophils are important in the generation of airway hyperresponsiveness and that vascular adhesion and transendothelial migration are a necessary step in this response. Antibodies to adhesion molecules may represent a novel form of treatment for disorders characterized by eosinophilia.

It is apparent that the participation of the eosinophil in the generation of airway inflammation and hyperresponsiveness is complex and involves an intricate relationship between cell adhesion, migration, and activation. Selected cytokines produced by inflammatory cells, including the eosinophil itself, can increase the survival, maturation, and activation of the eosinophil to enhance its inflammatory activity.

T LYMPHOCYTES

T lymphocytes possess several functional pathways that play a central role in the inflammatory process of asthma. T cells recognize and respond directly to processed antigen. They synthesize and release various regulatory cytokines, orchestrate the recruitment and activation of eosinophils, neutrophils, and basophils; and promote the development of the inflammatory reaction in asthma.[88] In addition, T cells have an important role in IgE-mediated hypersensitivity, as they initiate and regulate the production of IgE by B lymphocytes[257] and cytokines, such as IL-4.

Two types of T lymphocytes have been described in a murine model, Th1 and Th2,[191] which are differentiated by their respective cytokine profile. Th1 cells produce IL-2 and IFN-γ but little IL-4 and IL-5. In contrast, Th2 clones produce IL-4 and IL-5 but little IL-2 and IFNγ. IL-3 and GM-CSF are produced by both sets of clones. Th1 lymphocytes mediate classic delayed-type hypersensitivity reactions and immunity against intracellular organisms, like viruses or fungi; Th2 lymphocytes promote B-cell production of IgE and allergic inflammation.[39, 82, 192, 254] Wierenga and colleagues[279] have identified a Th2-like pattern of cytokine secretion following stimulation with specific antigen from lymphocyte clones derived from atopic dermatitis patients. Robinson and colleagues[231] used in situ hybridization to show that airway cells from patients with atopic asthma had a cell mRNA for cytokines compatible with a Th2-like profile: IL-4 and IL-5 but little INF-γ.

Role of T Lymphocytes in Asthma (Fig. 28–4)

Several investigators have used the late response to antigen (LPR) in sensitized individuals to define a role for T lymphocytes and other cells in the pathogenesis of airway inflammation and asthma. Antigen challenge of allergic asthmatic patients provokes acute airway obstruction, the immediate response. This reaction peaks within 10 to 30 minutes of antigen challenge and resolves within 1 to 2 hours. The second phase, or the late asthmatic response (LAR), appears 3 to 8 hours after antigen challenge in approximately 50% of asthmatic subjects challenged. Compared with the bronchoconstriction in the immediate reaction, airway obstruction in the LAR is often more prolonged and less responsive to bronchodilator therapy. Pathologic findings of the airway in the LAR show cellular infiltration of the airway mucosa and lumen, plasma exudation, and edema. In addition, there is an increase in bronchial responsiveness in those subjects with an LAR. All of these changes are characteristic of airway inflammation, as well as features of chronic asthma making the LAR a useful model to study the mechanisms of inflammation in asthma.

Metzger and colleagues[183] found that segmental airway allergen challenge in patients with allergic asthma increased the number of T lymphocytes in the BAL fluid 48 and 96 hours following challenge; the majority of these were of

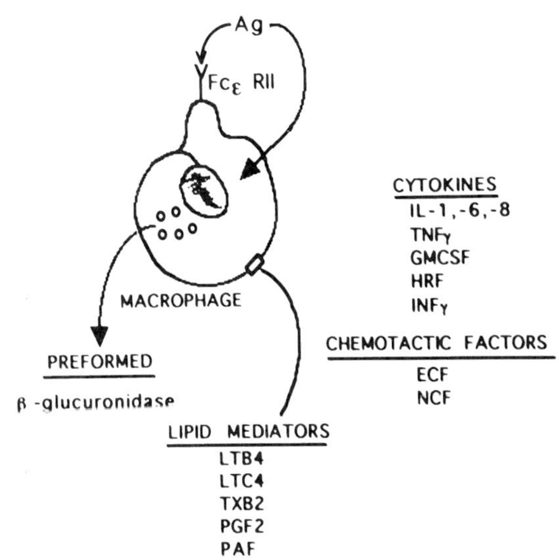

FIGURE 28-4. Activation by antigen (Ag) leads to the production and release of several mediators with multiple proinflammatory effects. These mediators include lysosomal enzymes, toxic oxygen metabolites via the respiratory burst, membrane-derived lipids, cytokines, and chemotactic factors.

the T-helper subtype. Frew and Kay[83] likewise found T-lymphocyte infiltration in cutaneous LPRs of atopic subjects challenged with allergen; the majority of these infiltrating cells were of the Th2 subtype. Furthermore, eosinophilic infiltration was identified, and both eosinophils and T cells expressed markers of activation: increased IL-2 receptor expression in T cells (CD25) and an increased presence of EG-2 staining (a marker of eosinophil degranulation) in eosinophils. There was also a strong correlation between the number of eosinophils and activated T helper cells at 24 hours, suggesting that the recruitment and activation of eosinophils may be the result of activation of T lymphocytes.

Several other studies have identified markers of T-lymphocyte activation in subjects with asthma. Timonen and colleagues[259] found enhanced natural killer activity in the peripheral blood of asthmatics. In addition, Corrigan and colleagues[44, 45] and Walker and colleagues[270] found the increased expression of IL-2 receptors, class II histocompatibility antigens (HLA-DR), and very late activation antigen (VLA-1) on peripheral blood T lymphocytes isolated from patients with acute severe asthma. Furthermore, IL-2 receptor and HLA-DR expression decreased with appropriate treatment of asthma and clinical improvement in markers of disease severity.

Similar findings have been identified in both the BAL fluid and bronchial mucosal biopsies of individuals with asthma. Jeffery and colleagues[130] found that symptomatic asthmatic patients have increased populations of irregularly shaped atypical lymphocytes in the lamina propria and submucosa of bronchial biopsies compared with healthy controls. Increased T-lymphocyte IL-2 receptor expression was also identified in bronchial biopsies[6, 23] and the BAL fluid[270] in asthma, although there was no difference in lymphocyte number compared with atopic nonasthmatics and normal controls. Increased T-lymphocyte IL-2 receptor expression correlated with both eosinophilia and airway hyperresponsiveness. Robinson and colleagues[231] demonstrated an increased frequency of mRNA for IL-2 through IL-5 and GM-CSF by in situ hybridization of airway cells in individuals with atopic asthma. Greater than 90% of the mRNA for IL-4 and IL-5 was T-lymphocyte associated, raising the possibility that atopic asthma has a predominant Th2-like collection of lymphocytes in the airways.

Collectively, these data support a role for T cells in the pathogenesis of asthma, with the Th2-like subtype of greatest interest. Studies in animals also suggest that the components of the late airway response to allergen can be reproduced with the transfer of sensitized T helper cells.[109] However, further studies are necessary to fully establish the role of the T cell in asthma. These investigations should be designed to supply more information on the temporal course of asthmatic inflammation, the relationship with subsequent bronchial hyperresponsiveness, the cytokine pattern of airway mucosal T cells, and the nature of T-cell sensitization and regulation of altered airway function antigen.

MONONUCLEAR PHAGOCYTES (Fig. 28–5)

Macrophages develop from promonoblasts in the bone marrow, are released into the circulation as monocytes, and continue to differentiate morphologically and functionally into macrophages in select tissues (lung, peritoneal cavity, liver). The macrophage has a unique role in the induction

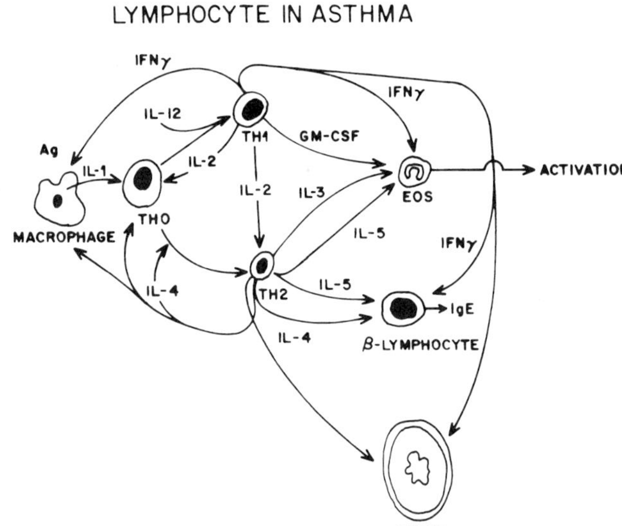

FIGURE 28-5. Macrophage processing of antigen results in the release of IL-1, which induces CD4+ T lymphocytes to proliferate and differentiate in two distinct subsets, Th1 and Th2. Th1 lymphocytes produce several cytokines whose cumulative effects are more involved in the mediation of delayed-type hypersensitivity responses than IgE-mediated allergic inflammatory responses. IFN-γ is a potent macrophage activator that also promotes eosinophil survival but inhibits the production of IgE by B lymphocytes. IL-2 stimulates the proliferation of T lymphocytes. IL-3 and GM-CSF have multiple proinflammatory effects on the eosinophil, including enhanced maturation, chemotaxis adhesion, activation, and survival. Th2 cells also produce IL-4, whose primary effect is the stimulation of IgE synthesis by B lymphocytes. IL-5 promotes eosinophil functions and the proliferation and differentiation of B lymphocytes. Supportive evidence for the importance of lymphocytes in asthma is suggested by the effects of corticosteroid therapy, which show decreases in BAL IL-4 and increases in IFN-γ that go along with decreases in airway hyperresponsiveness.

and proliferation of the host inflammatory responses in that it is a cell capable of processing native antigen into a form recognized by other cells. During antigen processing, mononuclear cells produce IL-1; this cytokine can induce T-lymphocyte IL-2 receptor expression, as well as IL-2 and IL-4 secretion. In addition, IL-1 promotes B-cell antibody production and proliferation. As an initiator of lymphocyte activation, the macrophage may be considered one gatekeeper of the immune response.

In addition to its afferent role, the macrophages can bind, phagocytose, and enzymatically degrade numerous biologic substrates. These properties confer multiple diverse functions, including tissue and bone remodeling, tumor cell destruction, inactivation of exotoxins and endotoxins, iron storage and recycling, and wound healing. These functions involve the release of lysosomal enzymes and the generation of free oxygen radicals. Mononuclear phagocytes are also capable of releasing several proinflammatory cytokines, lipid mediators, and chemotactic factors to recruit and activate various leukocytes that are involved in the inflammatory airway response.

Although mast cell activation is responsible for the initiation of immediate reaction to antigen, additional cells are likely necessary in the pathogenesis of allergic inflammation and asthma. Less than 1% of cells recovered in BAL fluid in asthma are mast cells, whereas more than 90% are macrophages.[224] Metzger and colleagues[183] demonstrated an increase in the total number of mononuclear phagocytes in the BAL fluid of atopic asthmatics 48 to 96 hours following antigen challenge, suggesting active involvement of this cell in late-phase inflammatory responses. The finding of FcεRII on the surfaces of macrophages[134, 179, 180] provides additional mechanisms by which macrophages contribute to allergic asthma.

FcεRII differs both in structure and function from FcεRI expressed on mast cells and basophils. The most important functional difference between the two types of IgE receptors is the binding affinity for the Fc portion of the IgE molecule. FcεRII is a relatively low-affinity receptor, whereas FcεRI forms a very high affinity bond to IgE antibody. Melewicz and colleagues[181] have demonstrated that whereas only 5% to 10% of peripheral blood monocytes (PBM) and lung macrophages from nonatopic individuals express FcεRII, approximately 20% of mononuclear phagocytes from atopic asthmatics have this receptor. Activation of mononuclear FcεRII leads to a variety of effects, including lysosomal enzyme release, stimulation of the respiratory burst, generation of lipid mediators, and production of proinflammatory cytokines.

Joseph and colleagues[134] incubated human alveolar macrophages (AMs) with serum from allergic subjects, added anti-IgE antibody, and found augmented β-glucuronidase and neutral protease release, as well as enhanced O_2^- production. Removal of IgE antibody from the sensitizing serum attenuated this response, suggesting an involvement of FcεRII. In a variation of this method, AMs from atopic subjects were challenged with specific antigen and demonstrated similar results.[134] Cluzel and colleagues[41] showed that AMs from asthmatic individuals have an augmented respiratory burst. Joseph and colleagues[134] have provided evidence that at least part of this mechanism occurs through stimulation of FcεRII. Rankin and coworkers demonstrated that AMs could be activated to release LTB_4[222] and LTC_4[223] by monoclonal anti-IgE antibody or specific antigen. Fuller et al[86] likewise found rapid secretion of various lipid mediators (thromboxane B2, PGF_2, LTB_4) following stimulation of isolated human AMs with anti-IgE. These data suggest that the *in vivo* release of leukotrienes from AMs might contribute to the bronchospasm associated with antigen challenge.

In subsequent studies, Rankin and colleagues[225] showed that IFN-γ, itself a macrophage product, primes cultured AM for the subsequent IgE-dependent release of LTB_4. There is now a substantial amount of evidence that stimulation of AM FcεRII leads to the release of several proinflammatory cytokines and chemotactic factors. Gosset and coworkers[99] detected a low molecular weight chemotactic factor for neutrophils and eosinophils from sensitized AMs following stimulation with either specific antigen or anti-IgE. IL-8 or RANTES may be among the responsible factors. Secretion of tumor necrosis factor-alpha (TNF-α) was identified from AMs isolated during the LAR from atopic asthmatics challenged with specific antigen.[100]

AMs can influence granulocyte function. Howell and colleagues[122] have shown that AMs from asthmatic subjects release a product capable of enhancing the eosinophil generation of LTC_4 and PAF. Using neutralizing antibodies, this substance was identified as GM-CSF. Wilkinson and coworkers[284] also identified a smaller peptide (approximately 3 kD) from peripheral blood monocytes (PBMs) of asthmatics that is capable of increasing neutrophil LTB_4 production and eosinophil LTC_4 generation. Finally, mononuclear phagocytes produce histamine-releasing factors, which can cause histamine release from basophils and mast cells via either an IgE-dependent[164] or a non–IgE-dependent means.

In summary, mononuclear phagocytes play a central role in the initiation and propagation of the airway inflammatory response by virtue of their antigen processing and presenting function, phagocytic and cytolytic activities, capacity to be activated via FcεRII, and ability to generate proinflammatory cytokines and lipid mediators. Further investigation into the subpopulations of macrophages involved in these processes, as well as the relationship between AMs and other effector cells in asthma, is necessary to better establish the role of AMs in asthma.

NEUTROPHILS

Neutrophils are important host defense cells against bacterial and fungal infections. The destruction of fungal and bacterial elements is mediated by the generation and release of oxidative metabolites and lysosomal enzymes. In addition, activated neutrophils can recruit other inflammatory cells to further perpetuate the inflammatory cascade. The same oxidative and nonoxidative mechanisms that are beneficial in host defense can also cause tissue damage, including the lung. Neutrophil-induced tissue damage has been implicated in several respiratory disease states, including adult respiratory distress syndrome, emphysema, and asthma.[172]

Following activation, neutrophils, eosinophils, and monocytes increase oxygen uptake and produce oxygen radicals, including large amounts of superoxide and H_2O_2. Due to the marked increase in oxygen uptake (up to 50-fold), this process has been termed the respiratory burst. In the presence of superoxide dismutase, the majority of O_2^- anion is rapidly metabolized to H_2O_2 and oxygen. Both O_2^- anion and H_2O_2 have minimal microbicidal activity; however, they produce active oxidants, including hypohalous acids and oxidizing radicals (OH•), which damage host tissue.

The evidence that neutrophils play a significant role in the pathogenesis of asthma remains controversial. Similar numbers of neutrophils can be found in the bronchial wash[274] and mucosal biopsies[6, 23] of patients with asthma compared with atopic nonasthmatics and normal controls. Diaz and colleagues[60] identified an increased number of neutrophils in the BAL fluid of subjects experiencing an LPR following bronchial challenge. Despite a lack of neutrophil accumulation in the airway, a few studies provide direct evidence that neutrophils are activated in asthma. Papageorgiou and colleagues[213] and Moqbel and colleagues[188] found increased complement receptor expression and enhanced cytotoxicity, respectively, in peripheral blood neutrophils obtained from subjects with asthma following exercise bronchoprovocation. Kelly and colleagues[138] likewise found a twofold increase in chemiluminescence in airway neutrophils from asthmatics compared with normal controls.

Other studies demonstrate an association between the development of airway hyperresponsiveness and neutrophil influx and activation. In animals, neutrophil infiltration of the airway after exposure to ozone correlated with the development of bronchial hyperresponsiveness,[117] which may be prevented by neutrophil depletion[200] and restored by repletion with highly purified populations of neutrophils.[194] Kelly and colleagues[138] found that airway responsiveness (PD_{20} FEV_1) correlated with the percentage of neutrophils in the BAL fluid of asthmatic humans. Other studies have demonstrated a correlation between airway responsiveness and reactive oxygen species following exposure to ozone.[253] Despite the potential of neutrophils to cause tissue damage, their role in the pathologic and physiologic features of asthma remains to be established.

BASOPHILS

The role of basophils in allergic inflammation is not fully established. There is evidence that basophils may be a component of the late asthmatic reaction to antigen.[244] The contribution that basophils can make to the inflammatory response includes release of inflammatory mediators and cytokines. However, because so few basophils appear in response to allergen when compared with other cells, such as the eosinophil, it is difficult to precisely define their importance. The protracted histamine release seen in cutaneous late-phase reactions is, however, attributable to basophil degranulation.

PLATELETS

Platelets represent the fragmented cytoplasm of bone marrow megakayocytes. Ultrastucturally, three types of secretory granules are present in platelets: alpha granules, lysosomes, and dense granules. Alpha granules are by far the most numerous and contain a large variety of secretory proteins, including fibronectin, fibrinogen, platelet factor 4 (PF4), and β-thromboglobulin. Lysosomes are morphologically indistinguishable from alpha granules. The functions of their constitutive acid hydrolase enzymes are unknown but probably involve the clearance of cellular debris following hemostasis. Dense granules contain high concentrations of calcium, pyrophosphate, serotonin, and adenine nucleotides.

Although once thought to represent an innocent bystander, several studies suggest that the platelet plays an active role in the generation of bronchial smooth muscle constriction and airway inflammation. In both animals and humans, allergen challenge induces the release of platelet-specific proteins, such as PF4[144] and β-thromboglobulin,[106] into the circulation. Metzger and colleagues[182] found elevated levels of β-thromboglobulin in the BAL fluid of asthmatic subjects during early- and late-phase responses following allergen challenge. Although other investigators have found conflicting data,[68, 105] these observations suggest that such products may mark platelet activation and contribute to altered lung function.

Human platelets have the capacity to bind IgE in vitro. Stimulation by specific antigen or anti-IgE antibody induces platelet activation and secretion. Joseph and colleagues demonstrated that activation of platelets isolated from patients with atopic asthma or Hymenoptera venom hypersensitivity with either specific allergen or anti-IgE caused *Schistosoma mansoni* larvae[132] death or the generation of free oxygen radicals.[133] Similar results were obtained when normal platelets were passively sensitized with serum from allergic individuals. The IgE-dependent nature of this response was confirmed by inhibition with antibody to FcεRII.[34, 251]

Platelets may be activated by non–IgE-dependent mechanisms. Pancre and coworkers[212] incubated normal platelets with culture supernatants from mitogen or antigen-stimulated $CD4^+$ T cells; platelet-dependent helminth cytotoxicity was observed even in the absence of IgE (possibly due to the secretion of a lymphokine that acts independent of FcεRII). INF-γ was implicated in this process, since the investigators found this cytokine in the T-cell supernatant; recombinant INF-γ had a direct cytotoxic effect, and this reaction was attenuated with antibody to IFN-γ. Molinas and colleagues[186] then identified a human platelet receptor for INF-γ. Pancre and coworkers[212] extended their observations in vivo by demonstrating that normal rat platelets treated with recombinant IFN-γ, passively transferred to syngeneic recipients, and subsequently challenged with parasitic infection conferred protection to the animal. Similar results were obtained with $CD4^+$-derived recombinant TNF,[64] although a specific platelet receptor for TNF has yet to be identified. These data suggest that platelets can be activated via IgE-independent mechanisms. Moreover, IFN-γ has been shown to up-regulate platelet FcεRII expression,[211] suggesting that this cytokine may affect IgE-dependent mechanisms.

In contrast to $CD4^+$ T lymphocytes, antigen-stimulated $CD8^+$ T cells release a factor that inhibits IFN-γ and TNF-dependent platelet cytotoxicity toward parasitic larvae.[209] IgE-dependent production of free oxygen radicals was likewise inhibited with this lymphokine, termed platelet activity suppressive lymphokine (PASL). Recipient rats challenged with parasitic infection were more susceptible when they received syngeneic platelets treated with PASL.[210] Platelets isolated from patients with Hymenoptera venom hypersensitivity and undergoing rush immunotherapy lost their specific reactivity to allergen in vitro.[263] It was further demonstrated that lymphocyte supernatants from these patients were able to suppress the reactivity of platelets from normal individuals. One proposed mechanism of immunotherapy is the induction of allergen-specific suppressor T cells; it is therefore hypothesized that PASL or other unidentified cytokines down-regulate platelet reactivity to allergen. Thus a complex relationship exists between $CD4^+$ and $CD8^+$ T-lymphocyte–derived mediators and their effect on platelet surface receptors to ultimately determine platelet activation.

PAF was initially identified as a substance that caused platelet aggregation and was released by rabbit basophils following IgE-dependent stimulation.[15] PAF is a potent inflammatory mediator that causes airway edema, hyperresponsiveness, and eosinophil recruitment and activation.[8] In some species, the PAF-induced bronchoconstriction is dependent on the presence of platelets.[240] In canine airways, Popovich and colleagues[219] demonstrated serotonin release from PAF-activated platelet, suggesting that serotonin is the mediator of altered airway function. However, secondary mediators involved in PAF-induced bronchoconstriction are not fully established and likely depend on the route of PAF administration and species studied. There are also data that PAF-activated platelets release an eosinophil chemotactic factor, as platelet depletion decreases PAF and allergic-mediated eosinophil infiltration into the lungs of normal and sensitized animals, respectively.[161] RANTES, a product of platelets as well as T lymphocytes, may represent this factor. Finally, PAF has a number of platelet-independent effects, and its effects on the platelet, per se, may be minor in comparison to actions on other cells in the development of airway inflammation.

CYTOKINES

Evidence suggests that cytokines, a diverse family of oligopeptides, play an integral role in the development of airway inflammation and the pathogenesis of asthma.

Interleukin-1 (IL-1)

IL-1 is produced primarily by mononuclear phagocytes; additional sources include endothelial cells, synovium, astrocytes, and osteoclasts. The effects of IL-1 (endogenous pyrogen) are diverse and include many of the signs and symptoms associated with acute illness, such as fever and fatigue. The principal effect of IL-1 on the immune response is an activation of T lymphocytes. In the absence of IL-1, either no immune response occurs or a state of tolerance develops. Finally, IL-1 is a potent endothelial activator of adhesion molecule expression and may function in immune responses by modulating leukocyte regression.[218]

Three lines of evidence exist for the participation of IL-1 in IgE-mediated allergic responses. First, Mazingue and colleagues[178] found increased IL-1 production in purified rat peritoneal macrophages stimulated with splenocyte-bound IgE or antibody to FcεRII. Second, Bochner and colleagues[19] found IL-1 in skin biopsies from atopic subjects following cutaneous allergen challenge, but not in normal controls. Finally, Gosset and coworkers[98] compared IL-1 release by human AM and PBMs from patients with allergic asthma and normal controls to both nonspecific polysaccharide antigen and specific antigen or anti-IgE. When stimulated with polysaccharide antigen, both AMs and PBMs released similar amounts of IL-1. In contrast, when stimulated with allergen or anti-IgE, only PBMs released IL-1; there was no detectable IL-1 activity in AM supernatants, an effect that may relate to the existence of an IL-1 inhibitory factor. Thus in contrast to blood and skin, where IL-1 production by macrophages is accentuated following allergen challenge, IgE-dependent activation of AMs may suppress lymphocyte proliferation via the production of IL-1 inhibitory factor, which may modulate the lower respiratory response to inhaled antigen.

Interleukin-3 (IL-3)

IL-3 has been identified as a myelopoietic cytokine, but its effects on the bone marrow are not limited to granulocyte precursors alone. Its predominant effects are on eosinophils and mast cells. IL-3 possesses a number of proinflammatory effects on the eosinophil and prolongs survival in vitro.[204] In the presence of IL-3, eosinophils have increased antibody-dependent killing of *Schistosoma* larvae, LTC_4 generation to calcium ionophore stimulation, production of free oxygen radicals, and numbers of low-density cells.[177, 234]

IL-3 also promotes the proliferation and differentiation of mast cells. Human bone marrow cells cultured on fibroblast monolayers, in the presence of IL-3 for up to 3 weeks, leads to the selective predominance of mast cells.[140]

IL-3 is secreted not only by Th1 and Th2 lymphocytes[192] but also by eosinophils and mast cells.[142, 217] IL-3 from eosinophils appears in supernatants as early as 3 hours after activation with calcium ionophore. The survival-enhancing activity of these supernatants is completely attenuated by the addition of monoclonal antibody to IL-3.[142] These data provide evidence for a positive feedback loop whereby IL-3 causes production of eosinophils and mast cells, which in conjunction with T lymphocytes, can cause a continued production of IL-3.

The role of IL-3 in allergic reactions is derived from analyses of BAL fluid and cutaneous late-phase reactions (LPRs). Robinson and colleagues[231] demonstrated elevated levels of mRNA for IL-3 in BAL cells obtained from atopic asthmatics. Massey and colleagues[234] likewise found increased levels of IL-3 in both pulmonary and cutaneous LPRs of atopic subjects following antigen challenge. Kay and coworkers[137] demonstrated increased expression of mRNA for IL-3 in cutaneous LPR of allergic subjects. As eosinophils and mast cells are important effector cells in the pathogenesis of allergic reactions, these data suggest that IL-3 (as both a product and stimulator of mast cells and eosinophils) may represent an important contributor to amplification of allergic inflammatory reactions.

Interleukin-4 (IL-4)

IL-4 is one of the major cytokines involved in T-B cell in teractions and is important for the synthesis of IgE by B lymphocytes, as it causes an isotype switch from IgM to

IgE[57, 171] and up-regulates both class II MHC[221, 233] and FcεRII[55] expression. Under normal circumstances, T lymphocytes are necessary for the production of IgE. Del Prete and colleagues[57] found that the addition of either PHA-stimulated IL-4 containing supernatants or recombinant IL-4 to B-cell suspensions causes IgE synthesis. The capacity of human T-cell clones to support IgE synthesis in vitro is directly proportional to their capacity to produce IL-4.[57] The addition of antibody to IL-4 abrogates the capacity of these clones to support IgE synthesis.[79] In addition to its effect on B-cell IgE synthesis, IL-4 up-regulates the expression of FcεRII on monocytes[269] and B cells[55] and functions as a T-cell growth factor.[77]

Robinson and colleagues[231] concluded that 92% of the mRNA encoding IL-4 in the BAL fluid of atopic asthmatics is T-cell derived. Although the primary source of IL-4 is believed to be the Th2-like lymphocyte, IL-4 has also been identified from stimulated mast cells by Northern blot analysis.[217] It is also prominently produced by human eosinophils.

A logical role of IL-4 in the induction of IgE-mediated allergic reactions is further supported by three studies. First, Wierenga and colleagues[279] demonstrated that *Dermatophagoides pteronyssinus*–specific T-lymphocyte clones from atopic subjects secrete large amounts of IL-4 on exposure to allergen. Second, Kay et al[137] found increased expression of mRNA for IL-4 in cutaneous tissue following an LPR in atopic individuals. Finally, Robinson and colleagues found increased expression of mRNA for IL-4 in the BAL fluid of atopic asthmatics.[231] These data suggest that IL-4 may play a vital role in the induction of allergic inflammatory responses in atopic individuals.

Interleukin-5 (IL-5)

IL-5 augments eosinophil maturation, chemotaxis, adhesion, activation, and in vitro survival.[47, 204] In the presence of IL-5, eosinophils demonstrate increased antibody-dependent cellular cytotoxicity, phagocytosis of serum-opsonized zymosan, and generation of toxic oxygen metabolites.[168] In addition, IL-5 stimulates bone marrow production of eosinophils.[33] Increased levels of IL-5 have been associated with several disease states marked by hypereosinophilia, including episodic angioedema and eosinophilia,[31] the eosinophilia-myalgia syndrome,[205] idiopathic hypereosinophilia,[206] and helminth infections.[165] Coffman and colleagues[43] have demonstrated a functional in vivo role for IL-5 by showing that pretreatment anti–IL-5 antibody attenuated the subsequent development of eosinophilia in parasite-infected mice. In addition to its effect on eosinophils, IL-5 induces the proliferation and differentiation of B lymphocytes.[47, 256]

Like IL-4, IL-5 is proposed to be derived, in large part, from Th2-like lymphocytes.[192] Athymic or T-cell–depleted animals are unable to mount an eosinophilic response, presumably due to a deficiency of IL-5.

Several studies have investigated the role of IL-5 in mediating allergic responses. Hamid and coworkers[110] found mRNA for IL-5 in bronchial biopsies of asthmatics but not normals. Robinson and colleagues[231] demonstrated increased levels of mRNA for IL-5 in the BAL fluid of atopic asthmatics. Furthermore, Sedgwick and colleagues[244] detected elevated levels of IL-5 in the BAL fluid of atopic subjects 48 hours following antigen segmental bronchoprovocation, and the concentration of IL-5 correlated with BAL eosinophilia. Finally, Kay and coworkers[137] showed increased expression of mRNA of IL-5 in biopsies of cutaneous LPRs of atopic individuals. Collectively, these data suggest that IL-5 is likely instrumental in the development of local eosinophilia in allergic inflammation.

GM-CSF

GM-CSF stimulates myelocyte production and other bone marrow cells, including megakaryocyte and erythrocyte progenitors. The effect of GM-CSF on the eosinophil is particularly relevant to the development of inflammation. GM-CSF enhances eosinophil maturation; promotes chemotaxis, adhesion, and activation; and prolongs survival in vitro.[169, 204] Therapeutic trials with GM-CSF induce peripheral eosinophilia.[65] Several functional properties of eosinophils are augmented with GM-CSF treatment, including antibody-dependent killing of *Schistosoma* larvae, the generation of free oxygen radicals, change to a lower-density phenotype,[207] and phagocytosis of serum-opsonized zymosan.[169]

GM-CSF, like IL-3, is produced by both Th1- and Th2-like lymphocytes, as well as eosinophils.[142] Evidence for the role of GM-CSF in allergic inflammatory reactions is derived from mediator analyses following antigen challenge of atopic individuals. As is true of IL-2 through IL-5, Robinson and colleagues[231] found increased mRNA for GM-CSF in the BAL cells of atopic asthmatics. In addition, Kay and colleagues[137] demonstrated mRNA for GM-CSF in cutaneous LPRs.

INTERFERON-γ

IFN-γ can inhibit components of allergic inflammation. For example, IFN-γ inhibits IL-4–mediated effects on B-cell function to decrease IgE synthesis (via inhibition of the isotype switch from IgM to IgE[42, 171, 227]) and the expression of FcεRII[55] and class II MHC antigens.[187] Del Prete and colleagues[57] found that the capacity of T-lymphocyte clones to support IgE synthesis was inversely proportional to IFN-γ production. IFN-γ has a variety of effects on other cells involved in the inflammatory response. It is an important macrophage-activating factor, stimulating not only antigen presentation but also a variety of effector functions, including adherence phagocytosis, secretion, cytokine generation, the respiratory burst, and microcidal and tumoricidal activities. IFN-γ up-regulates the expression of ICAM-1 on endothelial cells and can thus promote leukocyte adherence.[70]

IFN-γ prolongs in vitro eosinophil survival. Dexamethasone (1×10^{-6} M) inhibits the survival of eosinophils mediated by several cytokines.[281] High concentrations of IL-3, IL-5, and GM-CSF can overcome the dexamethasone effect, but increased concentrations of IFN-γ (up to 100 units/ml) do not modify the dexamethasone effect.[271] These observations indicate a difference between the mechanisms of action of INF-γ on eosinophil survival versus other cytokines. These results also support the proposal that high concentrations of cytokines may contribute to corticosteroid resistance.

IFN-γ is derived primarily from Th1-like rather than Th2 lymphocytes.[192] Wierenga and colleagues[279] have demonstrated that stimulation of allergen-specific T-lymphocyte clones from atopic humans generated IL-4; stimulation of allergen-specific clones generated from nonatopic humans results in IFN-γ secretion. Interestingly, stimulation of T-lymphocyte clones from atopic humans with nonallergenic antigens (tetanus toxoid, corpus albicans) also causes IFN-γ secretion. These observations suggest that the atopic status is characterized by the preferential stimulation of a Th2-like profile of cytokines with IL-4 and IL-5 but little IL-2 and IFN-γ. IL-4 itself acts as a stimulant for Th2 differentiation, leading to further IL-4 and IL-5 production, whereas IL-2 stimulates the Th1 response and secretion of IFN-γ and IL-2.

ADHESION MOLECULES

For inflammatory cells to accumulate at sites of inflammation, they are recruited from circulating pools, migrate across vascular endothelium and tissue interstitial spaces, and become activated. The initial steps in this process, endothelial attachment and transendothelial migration, are mediated by receptor molecules on the leukocytes and their counterligands on vascular endothelium. These receptors are known as adhesion molecules and can be broadly divided into those expressed on the surface of leukocytes and other cell surfaces, such as endothelial or epithelial cells. The major leukocyte adhesion molecules include lymphocyte function or associated antigen-1 (LFA-1), which is present on all leukocytes and is responsible for T–B-cell collaboration, and $CD8^+$ or NK cytotoxic activities.[52] Mac-1 is expressed on myeloid cells and is responsible for C3 bi-dependent adherence.[5] VLA-4 is present on eosinophils, basophils, monocytes, and lymphocytes and is utilized in cell matrix and cell-cell adhesions.[111] The major endothelial adhesion molecules include ICAM-1, ICAM-2, endothelial leukocyte adhesion molecule (ELAM-1), and vascular cell adhesion molecule (VCAM-1). ICAM-1 and ICAM-2 are ligands for LFA-1,[4, 141] ICAM-1 is a ligand for Mac-1,[4, 141] and VCAM-1 binds only to VLA-4.[111]

There is evidence that the heterogeneity of inflammatory infiltrates is dependent not only on the capacity of leukocytes to express different adhesion molecules but also on the variability of endothelial cell expression of counterligands. The expression of adhesion molecules is regulated by cytokines. Cotran,[46] Lewis,[163] and Rice and colleagues[228] have demonstrated that ELAM-1, ICAM-1, and VCAM-1 are up-regulated on endothelium during delayed hypersensitivity responses. In contrast, ICAM-1 and ICAM-2 are expressed constitutively on endothelial cells; ELAM-1 and VCAM-1 (as well as ICAM-1) are induced by endothelial cell exposure to the cytokines IL-1 and TNF-α and bacterial lipopolysaccharide.[54, 70, 193, 218, 228, 276, 278] Since macrophages are rich sources of IL-1 and TNF-α, activated macrophages are proposed to be the cell source of these cytokines.

Similar types of responses occur in IgE-mediated allergic reactions. Using an in vivo model, ICAM-1 and ELAM-1 expression are increased in skin biopsies during late-phase responses to antigen.[14, 21, 32, 62, 66, 71, 74, 154, 162, 176, 241, 258, 272] Monoclonal antibodies to ICAM-1 and ELAM-1 inhibit adherence of eosinophils, basophils, and neutrophils to endothelium.

Allergic inflammation is characterized by the selective accumulation of eosinophils. Eosinophils and basophils, but not neutrophils, possess the adhesion molecule VLA-4, which binds to endothelial VCAM-1.[21, 62, 241, 272] Bochner and colleagues[21] have shown that monoclonal antibody to VCAM-1 decreases eosinophil and basophil, but not neutrophil, adherence to IL-1–activated endothelium. Walsh[272] and Dobrina and colleagues[62] similarly showed that anti–VLA-4 antibody inhibits eosinophil adherence to IL-1–activated endothelium. These data suggest that the expression of endothelial VCAM-1 leads to a selective recruitment of eosinophils and basophils. IL-4 will up-regulate VCAM-1 expression.[241] Finally, a synergistic effect between IL-4, IL-1, and TNF-α has been identified in inducing both the endothelial expression of VCAM-1 and eosinophil adherence.[74, 176, 258] These data suggest that the selective induction of VCAM-1 by IL-4 causes eosinophil and basophil recruitment.

Although it has been demonstrated that adhesion molecule expression is up-regulated during inflammatory reactions, the functional effects of this response are not fully established. Wegner and colleagues[278] induced airway eosinophilia and hyperresponsiveness in cynomolgous monkeys by repeated inhalation of *Ascaris suis* antigen. ICAM-1 was demonstrated on both the vascular endothelium and airway epithelium by immunohistochemical staining in the sensitized animals. Administration of anti–ICAM-1 antibodies prevented eosinophilic infiltration and airway responsiveness. As airway hyperresponsiveness is an important feature of asthma, prevention of eosinophilic infiltration represents an exciting strategy for future immunomodulatory therapy.

The heterogeneity of inflammatory infiltrates is dependent on a variable expression of endothelial adhesion molecules and also on a variability in the expression of leukocyte adhesion molecules. This variability involves not only the effects of various cytokines on adhesion molecule expression but also alterations of adhesion molecule avidity for ligands via conformational changes in either the α or β chains of the CD11/CD18 molecule[66, 71] or phosphorylation of the intracytoplasmic tail of CD18.[32] Tomioka and colleagues[260] noted very little Mac-1 expression on unprimed eosinophils when exposed to PAF. Eosinophils treated with GM-CSF had increased Mac-1 expression and adherence to endothelium. These observations suggest that GM-CSF is an important mediator of eosinophil Mac-1 expression and subsequent cell adherence. Bochner and coworkers[22] have demonstrated similar effects in vitro with human basophils primed with IL-3. Extending this observation, Bochner and colleagues[20] monitored Mac-1 expression in vivo in a patient with episodic hypereosinophilia and myalgia. During disease exacerbations, eosinophils became less dense and expressed more Mac-1 when activated by PAF. These changes were temporarily correlated with increased serum levels of GM-CSF. Corticosteroid treatment decreased serum levels of GM-CSF and the number and up-regulated features of eosinophils. These data suggest that GM-CSF is an important contributor to eosinophil-associated disease.

EPITHELIAL CELLS

Airway epithelium is a target of inflammation. Epithelial damage occurs with viral infections,[13, 75] following allergen exposure,[93] and as a consequence of contact with ozone,[93] toluene dissocyanate,[97] and cigarette smoke.[90] Airway epithelium protects airway cells and structures from external stimuli, regulates fluid and ion transport across the airway and into the airway lumen, modulates airway caliber and airway smooth muscle tone, and influences inflammatory cell function. Disruption of these functions has been shown to promote airway obstruction and hyperresponsiveness.

Epithelial cells secrete a complex fluid that covers the airway surface and is important in mucociliary clearance and the active transepithelial transport of solutes.[59] In asthma, it has been suggested that elevated submucosal hydrostatic pressure may drive fluid into the airway lumen.[119, 145] Technical difficulties, however, have created uncertainties about the osmolarity of airway lining fluid and the rate of flows that these physiologic states produce.

Epithelium, in addition to its barrier and fluid transport functions, releases a variety of mediators. Prostaglandins are products of the airway epithelium.[203] PGE_2 can inhibit mast cell mediator release,[123] decrease cholinergic neurotransmission, and diminish airway smooth muscle tone.[249, 273] In addition, Barnett and colleagues[10] collected supernatants from cultured dog airway epithelial cells that had been stimulated with bradykinin; these supernatants inhibited cholinergic neurotransmission in the dog trachealis, presumably via PG synthesis. PGE_2 regulates transport of water and electrolytes by the airway epithelium.[3]

Human airway epithelial lipoxygenase metabolism of arachidonic acid produces 15-hydroxyeicosatetranenoic acid (15-HETE), 14,15-diHETE, and 8,15 diHETE.[125] These products are chemotactic for neutrophils[247] and may also contract airway smooth muscle.[246] Epithelium from other species produces additional chemotactic properties in vitro.[151, 229] Lipid mediators, such as LTB_4, and peptide mediators, such as fibronectin, TNF-α, IL-6, IL-8, and GM-CSF, have also been identified as epithelial products.[40, 116, 150, 195, 198, 248] The possibility of an epithelium-derived relaxing factor has also been suggested[9, 80, 94] but remains a matter of controversy.

The epithelium regulates mucous secretion. Tobacco smoke, sulfur dioxide, ozone, and bacterial products can directly affect goblet cells and stimulate C fibers to cause an antidromic release of secretory cell products.

Accessory cells that express the major histocompatibility complex (MHC) can be involved in antigen presentation.[267] Bronchial epithelial cells possess both MHC class I and class II molecules.[101] Therefore, bronchial epithelial cells, in addition to other airway cells, such as macrophages, may serve as accessory cells and present antigens to T cells.[135]

The epithelium plays a significant role in the endogenous regulation of airway tone. Damaged epithelium, as occurs in asthma, may narrow airway caliber by impairing secretion of relaxing factors or promoting secretion of constricting factors. Damage to the epithelium may also disrupt fluid balance and plasma exudation in the airway; this will cause rheologic changes in mucus, impairment of mucociliary transport, and edema. Activation of epithelium can also generate cytokines. Damaged epithelium may not respond appropriately to signals for normal repair.[282] Finally, alteration in the antigen-presenting capacity of this response or environment-induced perturbations could affect host defense responses.

AIRWAY SMOOTH MUSCLE

The production of asthmatic symptoms involves airway smooth muscle contraction. The patient with asthma has a lower threshold to inhaled bronchospastic agonists and often an exaggerated maximal contractile response.

Woolcock and colleagues[287] have shown that asthmatics not only have a leftward shift in the dose-response curve to methacholine but also have increased maximal responses. One explanation for the altered airway behavior in asthma may relate to increased airway smooth muscle shortening for a given degree of stimulation.[189] The increased maximal contractile response in asthma may be due to a loss of interdependence between lung parenchyma and the airway wall itself. Thus the absence of normal tethering can contribute to an unopposed maximal contraction.[170]

Although the causes of increased airway smooth muscle response in asthma are not established, a number of explanations have been proposed. First, increased airway smooth muscle mass may exist in the airways of asthmatics.[128] Second, epithelial desquamation may remove factors that directly or indirectly regulate smooth muscle function. Third, the subepithelial collagen deposition in asthmatic airways may affect smooth muscle shortening.[232] Fourth, infiltration of inflammatory cells with released mediators excessively shortens smooth muscle, and these cells may act as growth factors. Finally, deposition of connective tissue matrix during the inflammatory process may also contribute to altered smooth muscle function and enhanced contractile activity.

Function of Isolated Smooth Muscle in Asthma

Some investigators have obtained isolated airway smooth muscle from patients with asthma or related disorders. de-Jongste and colleagues[56] evaluated surgery specimens of smooth muscle from patients with chronic obstructive lung disease. All patients had a cough of at least 3 years' duration and an FEV_1 less than 70% of predicted. In comparison with pulmonary tissue from control subjects, the isometric contraction to histamine was significantly greater in airways from subjects with chronic obstructive lung disease. However, when lung responses to methacholine and leukotriene C_4 were evaluated, no differences were noted between these two groups. These observations suggest the possibility of a selective defect in the contractile response and imply that differences between normal and chronic obstructive lung disease tissue are found not only in the isometric response measured but also in the agonist tested.

The next logical step in the investigation of airway smooth muscle responses would be to study tissue from patients with asthma. As previously indicated, one possible mechanism for increased bronchial responsiveness in asthma is an intrinsic alteration in airway smooth muscle properties. Preliminary studies assessing pharmacologic and physical properties of airway smooth muscle have been undertaken but have yet to come to a consensus regarding the features of airway smooth muscle.

Bronchial smooth muscle from asthmatics was obtained at thoracotomy and found to have an enhanced contractile response to histamine, cholinergic agonists, and leukotrienes.[56, 239] In contrast, asthmatic bronchial tissue has been shown to respond normally to histamine and carbachol.[95, 283] Similar inconsistencies have been noted when beta-agonist regulation of airway smooth muscle relaxation is evaluated with asthma tissue.[56, 95, 239, 255, 283] Bai[7] evaluated tracheal smooth muscle from patients with fatal asthma compared with control subjects who died from nonrespiratory causes with normal lungs. The airway smooth muscle was isolated, and its response to acetylcholine, histamine, isoproterenol, and theophylline was evaluated. The maximal response to histamine was significantly increased in tissue from asthmatic subjects even though the EC_{50} value of both groups was similar. In addition, Bai evaluated the isolated airway relaxation response to isoproterenol. The concentration of isoproterenol to achieve IC_{50} (nM) values was significantly greater in asthma (60.3 vs 12.6, $p = 0.01$). These observations led the investigator to conclude that after a fatal attack of asthma, isolated airway smooth muscle had a greater maximal response to contractile agonists and impaired relaxation. The nature of this defect, inherent or acquired, was not established, nor was the influence of persistent and severe asthma determined.

Cerrina and colleagues[38] evaluated patients who were to undergo thoracotomy. Prior to surgery, in vivo bronchial challenges were performed with histamine. Isolated lung tissue was then obtained at surgery, and the in vitro response to histamine was determined. There was no correlation between the in vivo and in vitro response to histamine. However, there was an inverse correlation between the in vivo contractile response to histamine and in vitro relaxation following isoproterenol. These observations again raise the possibility of an association between bronchial responsiveness and altered airway relaxation. These subjects, however, did not have asthma.

Bramley and colleagues[24] evaluated asthma airway tissue and showed enhanced isometric force to electrical field stimulation when compared with responses of eight nonasthmatic tissues. It is not possible to resolve the conflicting data and precisely characterize airway smooth muscle response in asthma. It should be noted that results may simply reflect the spectrum of severity of bronchial asthma and a lack of sufficient studies in which the diagnosis of asthma was well established.[238]

SUMMARY

Our understanding of mechanisms in asthma has advanced but is incomplete.[18, 149] Airway inflammation is recognized as a major factor in asthma pathogenesis. The cells, tissues, and mediator involved in this process act in a complex fashion to orchestrate the clinical disease of asthma. The current focus on inflammation is an important direction for future research and should lead to the development of new therapeutic agents.

ASTHMA DIAGNOSIS

A patient's history is of utmost importance in diagnosing asthma.[136] A patient may describe a history of episodic or fluctuating respiratory distress and may also have experienced specific features of exertional dyspnea or cough; nocturnal awakenings with cough, dyspnea, and wheezing; or possibly a chronic persistent cough. Asthma may begin at any age. Potential risk factors for asthma include a family history of asthma or allergy, IgE production, significant aeroallergen exposure, viral respiratory illness, or low socioeconomic status. Certain specific aeroallergen sensitivities, such as house dust mite, have been associated with the diagnosis of asthma[215, 242]; others may be related to specific subsets of asthmatic patients, such as those with risk factors for sudden death.[1, 126, 201]

Since asthma is often episodic in nature, an important feature for diagnosis and management is an identification of factors that elicit or trigger symptoms. These triggers may be obvious or only determined after extensive investigation (Table 28–1). Several of these triggers, such as aeroallergen from house dust mites, cockroaches, cats, other animal proteins, and molds, cause asthma exacerbations. Viral infections and cigarette smoke exposure are also important triggers for a large numbers of patients. Identification of these factors will help in the care of patients with asthma and improve management.

DIFFERENTIAL DIAGNOSIS

The clinician needs to consider nonasthmatic causes of wheezing. Pulmonary function tests (spirometry with flow volume loops) are helpful and provide objective measures of air flow obstruction.

Mechanical obstruction of the airways, such as vocal cord paralysis, glottic webs, subglottic stenosis secondary to

TABLE 28–1
ASTHMA TRIGGERS

Trigger	Mechanism	Special Features
Aeroallergen (dust mite, mold, pet dander)	IgE-mediated immune response	Can be associated with allergic rhinitis and conjunctivitis
Viral infection	Potentiates IgE-mediated and non–IgE-mediated immune responses	Winter predominates
Aeroirritant (cigarette smoke, ? ozone, other pollutants)	Nonspecific initiation, ? possible airway inflammation	May produce airway hyperreactivity to other agents
Exercise	Nonspecific/cooling and drying of airway → physiologic changes	Running commonly causes symptoms
Aspirin sensitivity	Idiosyncratic/non–IgE-mediated	May be associated with sinusitis/nasal polyps
Occupation	IgE- and/or non–IGE-mediated immunologic response	
Emotion	Unknown	
Meteorologic	Unknown	

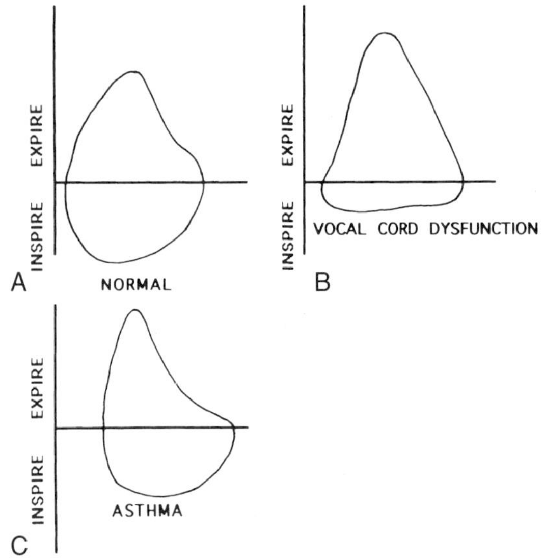

FIGURE 28-6. Flow volume loops. **(A)** Normal airway function. **(B)** Vocal cord dysfunction with inspiratory cutoff. **(C)** Asthma with small airway obstruction.

trauma, tracheomalacia, neoplasm, or extrinsic compression, can produce symptoms of wheezing and breathlessness. There is also a functional disorder of the larynx, vocal cord dysfunction (VCD) that has been identified as somatoform-conversion disorder. Patients with VCD have paroxysmal wheezing and a poor response to standard asthma therapy. VCD has been described as an inappropriate adduction of the vocal cords during inspiration and may also be associated with gastroesophageal reflux. During an acute attack of wheezing from VCD, a flow volume loop can show an abrupt inspiratory cutoff; the pattern is very characteristic (Fig. 28–6).

Other conditions to be considered in the differential diagnosis of asthma include chronic obstructive pulmonary disease, cardiac asthma with congestive heart failure, and rarer conditions, such as Churg-Strauss syndrome, carcinoid tumor, or systemic mastocytosis. Allergic bronchopulmonary aspergillosis, a colonization of the lung by *Aspergillus* with subsequent allergic inflammation and lung infiltrates, may contribute to worsening of symptoms in an asthmatic patient. Constant reassessment of asthmatic patients and their level of control is required to identify nonasthmatic causes of wheezing, especially if they complicate existing asthma.

ASTHMA THERAPY

GOALS OF THERAPY

Optimal asthma management, as delineated in the National Asthma Educational Program (NAEP) expert panel guidelines, includes patient education on the basic principles of asthma and how to effectively monitor and manage this condition. NAEP recommendations also underscore the need to reduce or avoid triggers of asthma, particularly environmental allergens. Furthermore, pharmacologic intervention must include medications to control airway obstruction and inflammation. A successful outcome will be reflected in the patient who has few or no symptoms, normal to near normal spirometry, and little to no limitation in lifestyle. The health care provider must attempt to attain these goals with minimum side effects or disruption to the patient's lifestyle.

PATIENT EDUCATION/OBJECTIVE ASSESSMENT

Patient education is of utmost importance to achieve optimal control of asthma. Patients should understand the goals of treatment and the concept that asthma is a chronic airway disease caused by inflammation. The latter feature must also be appreciated by the physician. To ensure adherence to treatment, patients need to understand why certain medications are used and what their effects are, both therapeutic and nontherapeutic. Patients also must follow a plan that includes the recognition and avoidance of possible triggers and allergens in addition to appropriate medications. The ultimate aim of asthma management, although perhaps not presently achievable, must be to change the natural history of the disease by preventing the long-term asthma risks and pulmonary pathologic sequelae.

Patient Management

A necessary step in the objective assessment of asthma symptoms and therapeutic control depends on a measurement of lung function. This approach is akin to the management of diabetes with blood sugar monitoring or blood pressure measurement in hypertension treatment. Providing the patient with a diary to record peak expiratory flows and a concise plan of action for increased asthma will help improve patient understanding and adherence to medications and increase patient motivation to prevent the progression of asthma attacks. Review of the treatment plan and medication administration, especially inhaler technique, should also be included in subsequent visits.

The importance of objective measurements of air flow obstruction by spirometry or peak flow meters cannot be overemphasized when assessing disease severity in a more precise manner. Peak expiratory flow rate (PEFR) correlates well with FEV_1 measures by spirometry.[199] When PEFR measurements are used as a marker for disease activity, they should be performed twice daily and more frequently during symptomatic periods. During a trial period of 2 weeks, patients can determine their degree of lung function variability and their usual or personal best measure of lung function. The personal best peak flow recording is used as a baseline reference point from which changes in symptoms or treatment can be based. The NAEP has suggested a zone system adapted from traffic lights in the use of PEFR.[76] Using this system, patients can be alerted to early worsening of asthma and the need for an intervention (Fig. 28–7).

GREEN ZONE

At 80% to 100% of personal best PEFR, no change in medication is needed. In patients on chronic treatment who remain in this zone, reductions in medication can be considered.

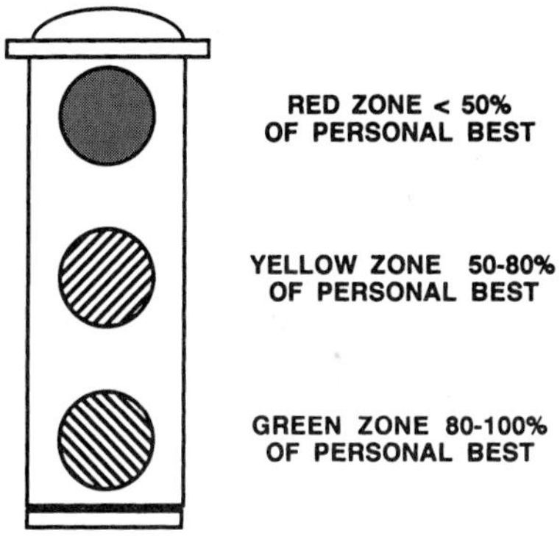

FIGURE 28-7. The use of peak flow measurements to maintain control of asthma.

YELLOW ZONE

At 50% to 80% of personal best PEFR, a patient's asthma is not under optimal control. Alternatively, the patient may be developing an acute exacerbation, and maintenance therapy should be adjusted. If readings do not improve within 24 hours, further evaluation by a medical professional is necessary. These patients are often managed by brief outpatient courses of systemic steroids (oral prednisone at 0.5 to 1 mg/kg/day).

RED ZONE

Less than 50% of personal best PEFR should signal an impending medical emergency. Patients should initiate bronchodilator therapy immediately and notify their physician or appropriate health care provider.

PHARMACOLOGIC THERAPY

Pharmacologic therapy of asthma must address the mechanisms contributing to air flow obstruction: bronchial smooth muscle contraction, edema, mucous secretion, and inflammation. Thus therapy for asthma must be directed toward reducing airway inflammation and, consequently, bronchial hyperresponsiveness. Immediate relief of air flow obstruction from bronchospasm is obtained with bronchodilators, of which inhaled β_2-agonists are most effective. Methylxanthines, such as theophylline, can modify the degree of bronchospasm on a more chronic basis. In addition, the inclusion of chronic anti-inflammatory medications (inhaled corticosteroids, cromolyn sodium, nedocromil sodium) should be indicated for patients with moderate or more severe asthma.

β-Adrenergic Agonists

SPECIFIC ADRENERGIC BRONCHODILATORS

Epinephrine (adrenaline) is a catecholamine and has potent, rapidly acting parenteral and aerosol bronchodilator effects. Its therapeutic use is limited by its short duration of action and a possession of both α-adrenergic and nonspecific β-adrenergic agonist properties. Subcutaneous doses of epinephrine (0.01 mg/kg, maximum 0.3 to 0.5 mg) produce acute bronchodilation, but the coexistence of potent α-adrenergic activity may limit its use in adults, particularly those with underlying cardiac disease or hypertension.[250] Inhaled epinephrine has also been used for acute relief of bronchospasm; its brief duration of action is a significant limitation. Ephedrine, a weak oral bronchodilator, is structurally similar to the catecholamines and has been used in combination oral bronchodilators (Tedral, Marax). Ephedrine has limited use and is not recommended for chronic asthma therapy.

Isoproterenol is a rapidly acting catecholamine-inhaled bronchodilator with β_1 and β_2 activity and a peak response that occurs within 5 minutes of inhalation. Although isoproterenol is β-adrenergic selective, its duration of action is less than 2 hours. Isoproterenol is used in a diagnostic evaluation of reversible air flow obstruction.

Metaproterenol (Alupent), a noncatechol adrenergic bronchodilator, is relatively β_2 selective when used by inhalation; however, it is less β_2 selective than other noncatechol bronchodilators and may have more systemic effects.

NONCATECHOL β_2-ADRENERGIC SELECTIVE BRONCHODILATORS

β_2-selective bronchodilators offer adrenergic selectivity for the airway β-adrenoreceptor and a longer duration of bronchodilation. Structural modifications of catechol compounds increase their selectivity for the β_2-receptor by either increasing the bulk of side chains or placing substituents on the terminal amine group (see Chapter 41). Such compounds have unique structure but give equivalent bronchodilation over 4 hours. Those currently available include albuterol (Proventil, Ventolin), pirbuterol (Maxair), bitolterol (Tornalate), and terbutaline (Brethaire). These compounds are used principally as inhaled β-agonists, but oral preparations are also available. They are effective in the control of acute asthma and offer protection against exercise-induced asthma[91, 92] or the acute response to inhaled allergen.[121]

A new long-acting β_2-selective agonist, salmeterol (Serevent) is now available; another, formoterol, is under investigation. These agents possess bulky lipophilic side chains, which provide for bronchodilation up to 12 hours.[167] In a comparative trial, Pearlman and colleagues[214] showed improved peak flow rates and symptom scores in patients who used salmeterol compared with patients receiving albuterol either four times daily or as needed. Salmeterol may be particularly useful to control nocturnal awakenings due to asthma. These long-acting agents can prevent exercise- and antigen-induced bronchospasm for up to 12 hours.[113, 265]

Reports of possible morbidity associated with salmeterol in certain settings have prompted the American Academy of Allergy and Immunology to recommend its use only with anti-inflammatory therapy. Furthermore, salmeterol's onset of action is delayed compared with shorter-acting β_2-agonists (albuterol, terbutaline), and salmeterol may take up to 30 minutes to achieve maximal bronchodilation. Therefore, salmeterol must not be considered a rescue drug but rather used only as a long-acting bronchodilator.

USE OF β-ADRENERGIC DRUGS IN ADULT ASTHMA THERAPY

B-agonists act on β_2-adrenergic receptors to activate adenylyl cyclase, increase intracellular cyclic adenosine monophosphate (cAMP), and reduce intracellular calcium; the end result is airway smooth muscle relaxation. The rise in cAMP may be linked to the opening of Ca^{2+}-activated K^+ channels (maxi-K channels) in airway smooth muscle.[185] β_2-agonists have also been shown to modulate mediator release from mast cells and basophils; whether this occurs in vivo has not been established, but no clinical anti-inflammatory effect has been documented with β_2-agonists, even those of long duration.[120, 196, 277] Side effects from β_2-agonists include hypokalemia, skeletal muscle tremor, anxiety, and cardiovascular stimulation.

DOSAGE AND ROUTES OF ADMINISTRATION

Episodic administration of selective β_2-agonists is most useful for acute asthma and to prevent exercise-induced asthma. Aerosol or inhaled β_2-agonists are equivalent or superior to oral therapy and have fewer systemic effects such as tachycardia, palpitations, tremor, and anxiety.[159] Furthermore, compared with oral preparations, inhaled β_2-agonists are more rapid in onset of action.[96] For acute asthma, two puffs of an inhaled β_2-agonist at repeated intervals (every 20–30 minutes initially for 1 hour, and then every 3–4 hours) is recommended for rapid symptomatic relief of bronchospasm. Robertson and colleagues[230] have shown that albuterol is more effective when the total dose is divided into three administrations and given at 20-minute intervals than when given as a single dose. Although tachyphylaxis can occur with adrenergic compounds, this phenomenon has not consistently been seen with long-term use of inhaled β_2-agonists.[166, 266] Long-acting β_2-agonists have not shown tachyphylaxis to bronchodilation with long-term scheduled use.[184, 266] Long-acting β_2-bronchodilator should be considered in patients who require (and benefit from) frequent short-acting β_2 use.

The regular use of β-agonists has been linked to a deterioration in asthma control in some situations.[114, 243] Moreover, greater β-agonist use has been associated with increased morbidity and mortality.[252] Although the mechanisms for this increase in morbidity have not been established, nor have investigations identified cause and effect with relationship to β-agonists, underlying poorly controlled asthma may play a role. Increased β-agonist use should be considered a marker for more severe and poorly controlled asthma.

Ideally, short-acting β_2 agonists should be used infrequently or as needed once chronic anti-inflammatory treatment has been established, with symptoms and lung function under good control. Symptom and lung function control may require long-acting bronchodilators in some patients. The mechanisms underlying the deleterious effects proposed to occur with chronic administration of short-acting β_2-agonists have not been established. Nonetheless, frequency of short-acting β-agonist administration should be reviewed periodically, whether used as a rescue agent or as needed.

Theophylline

Although theophylline has been used for years, its mechanisms of action are not fully understood (see Chapter 44). One advantage of theophylline is its many formulations. Sustained-release products are frequently chosen for chronic use, particularly to control nocturnal symptoms of asthma. These preparations provide a slow onset but prolonged duration of action (up to 24 hours) and reduce air flow obstruction. Dosing once a day, especially in the evening, provides good control of asthma symptoms with few side effects in many individuals.[29] For adults, initial therapy with 400 mg/day of a long-acting preparation is given as a single evening dose. If this initial dose is tolerated and serum theophylline levels are not excessive (approaching 10–15 μg/ml), a 25% increase in dose may be attempted at 3-day intervals until either a therapeutic concentration or control of symptoms is achieved. Serum theophylline levels should be used to monitor the dose given.

Although optimal therapeutic concentrations of plasma theophylline are reported to be 10 to 20 μg/ml, the window of efficacy has been changed to 5 to 15 μg/ml, as some patients achieve symptom and pulmonary function control at lower plasma levels. This approach reduces side effects.

The clinical response to theophylline always must be considered along with the plasma theophylline concentration. Some patients experience gastrointestinal side effects, headaches, and irritability at levels in therapeutic ranges. Elderly patients metabolize theophylline slower than do children and young adults, and underlying illnesses, such as congestive heart failure, liver disease, or viral respiratory infections, may prolong the methylxanthine half-life. Special recommendations are available for appropriate reductions in dose in these situations.[230]

Theophylline freely crosses the placenta.[155] Although theophylline therapy in pregnant women has not been associated with any significant birth defects, it may lead to transient toxic effects in the newborn.

Anticholinergics

Atropine, the anticholinergic prototype, has limited use in asthma treatment due to systemic side effects following mucosal absorption.[107] Modification of atropine into quaternary ammonium congeners (ipratropium bromide) decreases systemic absorption but maintains local anticholinergic activity. Ipratropium bromide (Atrovent) and glycopyrrolate (Robinul) are nearly twice as effective as atropine in producing bronchodilation and have greater duration of action. However, the benefits of chronic anticholinergic use in asthma are not established. The availability of ipratropium solution for nebulizer use has increased the utilization of inhaled ipratropium in combination with a β_2-agonist for acute bronchospasm. Anticholinergic use has been most effective in chronic obstructive disease that has a component of reversibility to air flow obstruction and is a first-line agent for chronic bronchitis.

Corticosteroids

Inflammation appears to be an essential component in the development and persistence of asthma. Treatment to interrupt this inflammatory process or limit its progression is now considered a fundamental basis of therapy. Furthermore, anti-inflammatory therapy may prevent the development of irreversible airway epithelial changes that occur in some patients with severe chronic asthma. Although this premise is unproven, current philosophy suggests this approach.

Corticosteroids have multiple effects in the regulation of allergic inflammation, which is discussed in greater depth in Chapter 45. Corticosteroids decrease the production and release of many cytokines and inhibit inflammatory cell recruitment.[17] Studies in adults have shown that pretreatment with oral or inhaled corticosteroids inhibits the late allergic response to antigen challenge. In contrast, the corticosteroid effect on the immediate reaction depends on the dose, duration of treatment, and organ studied, but in general, there is little effect.[49] Finally, dexamethasone and methylprednisolone inhibit mucous secretion in human airways.[175]

Inhaled corticosteroids also reduce bronchial hyperresponsiveness. In children, a progressive reduction in bronchial hyperresponsiveness occurred with a small dose of inhaled budesonide (200 μg daily); the onset of this effect became maximal after 3 months of treatment and was maintained at 6 months.[139] In adults with more severe asthma, inhaled beclomethasone (800 μg daily) decreased bronchial hyperresponsiveness after 10 weeks of treatment.[72] In addition, corticosteroids potentiate the relaxing effects of β_2-agonists.[73] This effect may involve an improvement in β_2-receptor function.[247]

DOSAGE AND ROUTES OF ADMINISTRATION

Oral, parenteral, or inhaled corticosteroids have been used in asthma for many years. Investigators were able to formulate beclomethasone dipropionate (BDP) for metered-dose inhaler administration. This approach allowed oral glucocorticoid doses to be reduced in patients with moderately severe chronic asthma.[190] With the emphasis on the inflammatory component of asthma, inhaled corticosteroids have become the principal anti-inflammatory medication for chronic asthma in order to avoid adrenal suppression and other complications associated with systemically given corticosteroids. Compliance is a major problem in the long-term use of inhaled corticosteroids. Since inhaled corticosteroids do not cause bronchodilation, some patients are less inclined to take them regularly. There is no immediate reinforcement. Local side effects, as well as extra time and difficulty in administration, can also reduce individual patient compliance. This factor reinforces the need to review the technique of inhaler use and to ensure that the regimen is simplified as much as possible.

Inhaled corticosteroids should be considered in asthmatic patients who have moderate disease. This approach has been a change in direction from previous therapeutic programs. Inhaled preparations currently available are listed in Table 28–2. The dose of inhaled corticosteroids is titrated to the severity of asthma and may be given, with equal efficacy, either twice or four times daily. There is some evidence that more frequent dosing offers better control in the more severe asthmatic patient, but this may be associated with diminished compliance.[262] Patients often require a minimum of 2 to 4 weeks of use before symptomatic control becomes evident. High-potency inhaled corticosteroids, such as budesonide, fluticasone, and beclomethasone-forte, are available in Canada and Europe and will probably be the principal agents used in the future.

TABLE 28–2
CURRENT DRUGS FOR MANAGEMENT OF ASTHMA IN THE UNITED STATES

Name	Notes
β-Agonist Bronchodilating Drugs	
Metaproterenol	2–3 hours' duration
Albuterol	4–6 hours' duration
Pirbuterol	4–6 hours' duration
Terbutaline	4–6 hours' duration
Tornolate	4–6 hours' duration
Salmeterol	12 hours' duration
Nonsteroidal Anti-Inflammatory Agents	
Cromolyn sodium (ampules and MDI)	Begin q.i.d., may reduce gradually to b.i.d. if possible
Nedocromil MDI	Begin q.i.d., may reduce gradually to b.i.d. if possible
Oral Corticosteroids	
Prednisone (tablets/liquid)	May be given as single dose or divided doses
Prednisolone (tablets/liquid)	May be given as single dose or divided doses
Methylprednisolone	May be given as single dose or divided doses
Aerosolized Steroids	
Beclomethasone	Administer every 6–12 hours
Triamcinolone	Administer every 6–12 hours
Flunisolide	Administer every 6–12 hours
Theophylline	
Various sustained-release products available	Administer every 8–24 hours
Other Agents	
Anticholinergic (ipratropium bromide)	May increase albuterol bronchodilation

At recommended doses, systemic side effects of inhaled corticosteroids are rare. Local effects, however, including dysphonia, oral candidiasis, and nonspecific cough, occur in about 30% of patients; such effects can be prevented or alleviated with the use of a spacer. Rinsing the mouth immediately after administration may also be helpful in preventing oral candidiasis.

Oral corticosteroids were used before inhaled preparations became available and remain an essential part of the management of acute exacerbations of asthma and in patients with severe disease. Early treatment of acute exacerbations with prednisone prevents progression of asthma symptoms and reduces morbidity.[28] Exacerbations of airway obstruction can usually be managed by prednisone doses of 0.5 to 1 mg/kg daily in divided doses. The higher dosage is used for 1 week and then stepped down or reduced to 10 mg/day for an additional 7 days before stopping. Long tapers of systemic corticosteroids are not required when short courses are given. This is a suggested regimen. Data are unavailable showing optimal or required dosages in both oral and inhaled corticosteroid therapy for the individual patient. A study by Beam and colleagues[11] suggests that dosing between 3 and 5 p.m. may be more effective in controlling asthma symptoms.

It is not possible to control asthma with inhaled corticosteroids alone in all patients. Some patients have poorly controlled symptoms, even with maximal doses of bronchodilators and inhaled steroids, and require frequent bursts or continued daily use of oral corticosteroids. All attempts should be made to lower the daily steroid dose to the minimum possible dose required to control symptoms. Alternate day dosing should be considered if good control is obtained with low daily dose treatment.

The complications of long-term oral corticosteroid administration are well appreciated. Nonetheless, systemic corticosteroids should be used in the treatment of asthma when necessary. Most short-term complications of corticosteroids, such as nervousness, dyspepsia, disturbances in fluid and electrolyte balance, hypokalemia, and hyperglycemia, are present only during treatment. Patients should be advised of these effects. The complications of long-term systemic use, such as subcapsular cataracts, osteoporosis, aseptic necrosis of bone, hyperglycemia, and hypertension, are less frequent with low or intermittent dosing. Osteoporosis, cataracts, stunting of growth, and insulin resistance have been reported with systemic and very high doses of inhaled corticosteroids; however, such side effects with inhaled corticosteroids are very rare.[131, 146, 153, 262] Calcium replacement, vitamin D, and estrogen should be administered to postmenopausal women on long-term corticosteroids.

Sodium Cromoglycate and Nedocromil Sodium

Cromolyn sodium (Intal) prevents both the immediate and late pulmonary response to antigen. Its mechanism of action is not fully established and will be discussed separately (Chapter 43) in greater depth.[25] Cromolyn sodium prevents mast cell mediator release and inhibits cell recruitment and activation in the lung. Cromolyn sodium is an exceptionally safe drug, but its efficiency and anti-inflammatory effects in adults are less predictable than those of inhaled corticosteroids. Consequently, cromolyn sodium is used more frequently in younger patients and those with asthma secondary to allergic disease.

Although nedocromil sodium has many similarities to cromolyn sodium, it has distinct anti-inflammatory effects and may be more potent.[50] Based on these data, nedocromil sodium (Tilade) has been proposed for mild to moderate asthma and possibly as a step prior to topical corticosteroid therapy. Finally, nedocromil sodium may have particular benefits for patients with chronic cough as a component of their asthma.

Cromolyn sodium is available in a metered-dose inhaler preparation as well as a solution for nebulization. For use prior to exercise or allergen exposure, two to four puffs of cromolyn sodium or nedocromil sodium should be taken immediately prior to challenge. This may be accompanied by an inhaled β-agonist. The recommended dosage of nedocromil sodium for chronic use is two puffs four times a day, although simplified regimens are being attempted. Intal has been used in more convenient dosages, such as two to three puffs three times a day, which can be tapered to twice a day in certain patients.

Leukotriene Antagonists

Leukotriene receptor antagonists and 5-lipoxygenase inhibitors may soon be available as oral agents for the treatment of asthma. These compounds have shown beneficial effects in exercise-induced asthma, with improvement in lung function and efficacy for aspirin-induced asthma.

Other Anti-Inflammatory Drugs

Several corticosteroid-sparing medications have been used in the treatment of severe corticosteroid-dependent asthma. Methotrexate, gold, troleandomycin, hydroxychloroquine sulfate, and intravenous immunoglobulin have shown benefit in selected cases. Several trials with methotrexate have shown corticosteroid-sparing effects in severe asthma patients; however, this has not been a consistent finding. Oral gold (auranofin) was used in one open labeled study and reduced the oral corticosteroid dosage and controlled symptoms.[16] Troleandomycin, which reduces the clearance of methylprednisolone, has offered benefit for some patients on chronic steroid dose. The effectiveness of steroid-sparing agents in the overall management of asthma has been inconsistent, and these agents should be used only by physicians experienced in this area.

ENVIRONMENTAL CONTROL

Aeroallergens play a significant role for many patients. Up to 85% of asthmatic patients have positive skin test reactions to common aeroallergens,[197] and environmental control can improve asthma control in many of these individuals.[102] The effectiveness of this approach is most noticeable with indoor allergens, such as house dust mite, insects, and animal dander.

House dust mite exposure is important in the development of allergic asthma.[216] A major source of house dust mite antigen is mattresses, carpets, and area rugs; these should be removed from the sleeping area. Encasing mattresses in airtight covers, washing pillows and bedding weekly in hot water, and removing carpets, particularly if laid on concrete slab floors, will reduce house dust mite levels in the home.[148] Reducing the indoor humidity to less than 50% also diminishes concentrations of house dust mite.[147] Acaricides and denaturing agents, such as tannic acid, may reduce house dust mite levels, but their efficacy has been questioned.[126]

Animal allergens, particularly those due to cats, are potent indoor allergens.[174] It is best to remove the animal from the home. If the pet is not removed, it should at least be excluded from the bedroom. Weekly washing of the cat may reduce the amount of allergen deposited on carpets and furnishings.[53] Although removal of the pet is the most effective form of antigen control, immediate relief of asthma may not occur since cat allergen can persist in the home for many months.[286]

Cockroach allergen is also important in the development of asthma, particularly in warmer climates and inner-city neighborhoods.[158] Appropriate roach control should benefit the patient, although conclusive studies to evaluate this form of management are not available.

IMMUNOTHERAPY

Immunotherapy may be used as adjunctive therapy in patients who have an allergic component to their asthma.

Allergen immunotherapy reduces symptoms of asthma in double-blind studies with a variety of allergens, including house dust mite,[1] cat dander,[202] grass pollen,[226] and *Alternaria*.[118] Studies have also shown that allergen immunotherapy decreases the late pulmonary reaction to allergen.[268] Although maintenance immunotherapy appears safe in pregnancy,[264] initiation of immunotherapy should wait until the pregnancy is completed. Since immunotherapy modifies the allergic reaction to antigen, and may be anti-inflammatory, its use might be most effective early in the course of asthma; such an approach needs to be thoroughly evaluated (considered in detail in Chapter 46).

TREATMENT OF ACUTE ASTHMA

An acute exacerbation of asthma poses an urgent medical problem. The best strategy for management is early recognition, evaluation, and aggressive treatment to prevent deterioration and the development of respiratory compromise. Early recognition by the patient with the use of peak flow measurement and prompt communication between the patient and the health care provider are an essential component of the process. This approach allows the physician to intervene more rapidly and appropriately.

The intensity and outcome of the acute attack are influenced by several factors, including the patient's age (elderly patients have greatest risk), the duration of the current episode, a history of previous life-threatening asthma, a frequent need for acute care, and either current systemic corticosteroid usage or recent withdrawal. Each patient should have and be familiar with an action plan for an acute asthma exacerbation. Peak flow measurements are important and provide a more precise quantitation of air flow obstruction. The basic goal of treatment is a rapid reversal of air flow obstruction. First-line therapy is the use of inhaled β-agonists. Poor or minimal response to β-adrenergic agonists is an indication for an emergent evaluation by medical personnel.

Physical examination often reveals wheezing, accessory muscle use, and tachycardia. These findings may confirm the diagnosis of acute asthma but do not reliably indicate the severity of the asthma episode. Signs of increasing respiratory distress include a widening of the pulsus paradoxus and cyanosis. Objective measurements of pulmonary function and oxygen saturation by either oximetry or arterial blood gas measurements are essential in severe asthma. Early administration of systemic steroids may lead to more rapid improvement of pulmonary function. Close monitoring of the patient with repeated assessment of lung function is used as a guide to management and the need for changes in therapy. Table 28–3 suggests an initial treatment approach for the adult patient with acute asthma.

TREATMENT OF THE HOSPITALIZED ASTHMATIC PATIENT

The decision to hospitalize a patient suffering with acute asthma is made after considering several variables but should not be delayed. Emergency ward treatment for more than 4 hours is unlikely to alter the need for hospitalization. If a patient's asthma is severe and does not improve substantially after a few hours of treatment, intensive monitoring and therapy as an inpatient must be considered. This is particularly relevant for patients with a poor response to β_2-agonists, hypoxia, hypercarbia, a history of respiratory failure, or multiple medical problems or for older patients.

Hospital management of asthma should continue to address the same goals initiated with emergency management, that is, reduce air flow obstruction with intensive bronchodilator therapy and systemic corticosteroids. Initial assessment of lung function with spirometry or peak flow is essential. Arterial blood gases or pulse oximetry is often required to monitor the consequence of air flow obstruction on pulmonary gas exchange. If respiratory failure occurs, the patient will require endotracheal intubation and assisted ventilation; this is often difficult in the severe asthmatic. Early, aggressive, and well-monitored therapy can usually prevent the progression into respiratory failure.

Nebulized β_2-agonist therapy should be continued (or instituted) in the hospitalized patient. Initially, inhaled β-agonists are administered hourly, with a gradual reduction to every 3 to 4 hours as air flow obstruction improves. Subcutaneous administration of β_2-agonists may supplement inhaled therapy. Intravenous administration of β_2-agonists should be avoided in adults because of the risk of myocardial injury.

Therapy with corticosteroids should be initiated if not already begun in the emergency room. An initial dose of methylprednisolone, 1 mg/kg every 6 hours, or hydrocortisone, 2 mg/kg bolus every 4 hours, is recommended.[76] Intravenous dosing is continued until the patient shows improvement in pulmonary function; this usually requires 24 to 48 hours. At that point, oral prednisone, or its equivalent, may be substituted (10–15 mg 3–4 times a day). Oral corticosteroids are usually given at high doses for 7 days and then tapered, and inhaled corticosteroids added to the therapeutic regimen.

Methylxanthines may be considered in hospitalized patients with asthma, especially in those who have received benefit from theophylline therapy in the past. Patients should have plasma theophylline levels monitored, with subsequent adjustment of dosages to achieve levels of 5 to 15 μg/ml. Patients who use theophylline regularly should have plasma theophylline levels determined. If there are no signs of clinical toxicity, patients can be given 2.5 mg/kg loading doses over 30 minutes, followed by constant intravenous infusion. A plasma theophylline level should be obtained 30 to 60 minutes after the loading dose to ascertain if additional theophylline is required. Intravenous theophylline is continued until intravenous corticosteroids are discontinued. The patient then may be placed on an oral sustained-release theophylline preparation, if theophylline is to be continued.

Supplemental oxygen is an integral part of therapy. Although it is commonly recommended that hydration is essential, there is little evidence to support this recommendation. Unless an infectious complication exists, such as sinusitis, pneumonia, or bronchitis, antibiotics are usually not needed. Sinusitis should be strongly considered in a patient with an asthma exacerbation, especially in the patient with a recent respiratory infection.

Morbidity in asthma is increased in the elderly and those with previous episodes of respiratory failure. The use of

TABLE 28–3
TREATMENT OF ACUTE ASTHMA

Step	Treatment	Assessment
1. (After initial assessment) 0–30 minutes	Inhaled (nebulized) β_2-agonist × 2, then β_2-agonist every 20 minutes × 1 hour; systemic corticosteroids if no immediate response or if patient is currently on or recently has been on oral taper; oxygen 2–6 L/min; consider subcutaneous epinephrine 0.3 cc (1:1000)	Peak flow, FEV_1, FVC, physical exam, O_2 saturation if warranted
2. (FEV_1 > 50–70% predicted) 40–120 minutes	If not already initiated, administer systemic corticosteroids; continue treatment with topical or injected β_2-agonists for 1–3 hours if patient is improving (inhaled β_2-agonist, subcutaneous epinephrine, or 0.3 cc 1:1000)	Peak flow, FEV_1, FVC, physical exam
(FEV_1 <50% predicted) 40–120 minutes	Inhaled β_2-agonist hourly or continuous; begin IV corticosteroids (methylprednisolone 60–120 mg IV); oxygen at 6 L/minute or as required	Peak flow, FEV_1, continuous O_2 saturation or arterial blood gases, physical exam (check for cyanosis, fatigue, decreased consciousness, and silent chest)
3. (FEV_1 >70%) 120–180 minutes	Consider disposition: *for discharge home* Patient to continue frequent inhaled β_2-agonist every 3–4 hours as needed, and a short course of oral corticosteroids 40 mg PO × 3–7 days, then either taper by 5 mg/day or give 10–20 mg PO OD × 3–7 days; also include patient education on treatment plan and schedule medical follow-up	Home peak flow monitoring
(FEV_1 <70%) 120–180 minutes	For poor or incomplete response: *hospital admission* Consider intravenous aminophylline, respiratory support with O_2, continue inhaled β_2-agonist hourly (every 3 hours) or continuously, and continue with intravenous corticosteroids Disposition and appropriate follow-up must be determined on an individual basis. A patient with a pertinent medical history such as prolonged symptoms prior to visit, previous severe exacerbations, or pertinent psychosocial history may require closer observation. In addition, any suggestion of deterioration throughout the course of treatment with increasing PCO_2 merits intensive care monitoring	FEV_1, FVC, continuous O_2 saturation or arterial blood gases

From Expert Panel on the Management of Asthma: Guidelines for the diagnosis and management of asthma. J Allergy Clin Immunol 88:425, 1991.

sedatives or withholding corticosteroid therapy increases morbidity. Status asthmaticus is a medical emergency that should have a favorable outcome with proper treatment. To accomplish this goal, the physician and patient must recognize and heed the warnings of severe disease, intervene with bronchodilators and corticosteroids appropriately but aggressively, and monitor pulmonary functions and levels of oxygenation carefully.

SPECIAL SITUATIONS

Pregnancy

Retrospective analyses suggest that approximately one third of asthmatic women will have more severe asthma during pregnancy, another third will improve, and the other third will remain unchanged. Peak severity of asthma usually occurs at 29 to 36 weeks of gestation. Asthma becomes less severe during the last 4 weeks of pregnancy and usually returns to prepregnancy levels 4 weeks postpartum.[235] Poorly controlled asthma has an adverse effect on the fetus, resulting in increased perinatal mortality, increased prematurity, and low birth weight.[236] Optimal perinatal asthma control is essential.

During pregnancy, inhaled medications are preferred. Terbutaline (Brethaire) is the preferred β_2-agonist because there is no evidence from animal studies that teratogenicity occurs. Guidelines of the National Heart, Lung, and Blood Institute also suggest albuterol as a good alternative β-agonist. For most drugs used to treat asthma and rhinitis, with the exception of brompheniramine, hydroxyzine, and epinephrine, there is little evidence to suggest increased risk to the fetus.[104, 237] Because beclomethasone is the only inhaled steroid that has been used in well-controlled studies during pregnancy, it is generally prescribed when such treatment is indicated. Oral β-agonists should be stopped near term since they inhibit uterine contraction.

Acute exacerbations of asthma should be treated aggressively in order to avoid fetal hypoxia. The use of epinephrine has been a subject of controversy. Schatz and associates[236] indicate that epinephrine decreases uteroplacental blood flow and is associated with congenital malformations. Others have not confirmed the findings of epinephrine's teratogenicity.[103] In general, acute asthma treatment should include the nebulized β-agonist, usually terbutaline, oxygen, and systemic corticosteroids when necessary.

Surgery

Primary care physicians and asthma specialists are often asked to participate in the preoperative evaluation of their asthmatic patients. This involves assessing the risk of anesthesia and the surgical procedure itself, as well as taking measures to minimize risk. Preoperative assessment includes careful evaluation of the patient's current respiratory status. Integral to this evaluation is measurement of pulmonary function and its comparison with the patient's recent best values. This comparison allows the physician to determine the degree of improvement that may be required to optimize the patient's lung function. Should the patient have increased asthma or worsening of airway obstruction on spirometry, attempts should be made to improve lung function prior to surgery. This may require a short burst of corticosteroids. The possible adverse effects of systemic corticosteroids on wound healing and suppressive effects on the adrenal-pituitary axis are not a contraindication to their preoperative use.

Immediately prior to surgery, inhaled β-agonists are recommended; this will minimize the risk of bronchoconstriction during endotracheal intubation. Inhaled bronchodilators may be maintained intraoperatively. In mechanically ventilated patients, parameters such as peak inspiratory airway pressures may signal changes in airway resistance requiring modifications in ventilatory management, as well as administration of inhaled bronchodilators. For patients who regularly take theophylline, intraoperative aminophylline may be used to maintain its therapeutic effects. A usual maintenance dosage is 0.5 mg/kg per hour by continuous infusion; rates are modified depending on the metabolism of the patient. For patients with a therapeutic blood level on their oral regimen, aminophylline infusion may be calculated at 1.25 times the total daily theophylline dose over 24 hours.

Patients with moderately severe or severe asthma may be on chronic corticosteroid administration at the time of surgery. These patients should be considered to have a decreased adrenal-pituitary response to stress. To prevent the complications of adrenal insufficiency with surgery, patients should be supplemented intraoperatively and perioperatively with corticosteroids. Stress dose corticosteroid administration should be given to any patient who has received systemic corticosteroids for more than 2 weeks within 6 months of the scheduled surgical procedure. In addition, patients who take high doses of inhaled corticosteroids (more than the conventional recommended doses) should also be considered at risk for adrenal-pituitary suppression with surgery.

The routine dose of corticosteroids for replacement during stress is 300 mg of hydrocortisone per day, or its equivalent,[76] given as 100 mg intravenously preoperatively, 100 mg intraoperatively, and 100 mg by intravenous bolus postoperatively. Systemic corticosteroids may then be tapered over the next few days, depending on the patient's postoperative course.

In patients with compromised lung function, anesthesia may often be modified to decrease perioperative risk. For instance, spinal or local anesthesia may be used rather than general anesthesia for selected procedures. Epidermal postoperative anesthesia can be substituted for parenteral narcotics, which could induce respiratory depression. Good respiratory supportive care following surgery, important in all patients, is essential in the asthmatic patient, who likely has a greater tendency to develop mucous plugging and atelectasis. Inhaled β-agonist therapy and frequent spirometry are important in postoperative care; continual reassessment is the key to optimal asthma management during and after surgery.

Elderly

The elderly patient with asthma poses a problem in recognition, as well as management. Elderly patients with chronic airway obstruction are often considered to have chronic obstructive pulmonary disease, and the diagnosis of asthma is not considered. Chronic sinusitis complicating asthma in elderly patients may occur without being suspected. Some asthma and allergy medications are metabolized slowly in the elderly patient. These patients also may have a lower threshold for toxic effects. These factors must be considered in asthma management.

SUMMARY

Asthma is a complex and often frustrating disease for both the patient and the clinician. Our understanding of its pathogenesis must guide therapeutic principles. Clinicians, however, must keep each patient's individual goals in mind. These goals should include allowing patients to function well without limitation, preventing chronic symptoms, as well as acute exacerbations, and enabling patients to normalize their pulmonary function. These goals are challenging but achievable. Improved knowledge on the pathogenesis of asthma has directed us to establish asthma therapy that is focused at two specific features of the disease: bronchospasm and inflammation. A partnership should be forged between the patient, physician, and additional health care professionals involved in management. This partnership will enable the patient to gain a sense of control of a chronic, often life-disrupting disease. The patient and the clinician together form a therapeutic plan that encompasses medications, environmental control, and continued reassessment. The resulting educated and responsible patient can then assist the clinician in disease management and often bring additional legitimate concerns regarding cost and simplicity of care into the therapeutic process. Such an approach will be most likely to lead to an optimal outcome.

REFERENCES

1. Aas K: Controlled trial of hyposensitization to house dust. Acta Paediatr Scand 60:264, 1971.
2. Abu-Ghazaleh RI, Fujisawa T, Mestecky J, et al: IgA-induced eosinophil degranulation. J Immunol 142:2393, 1989.
3. Al-Bazzaz FG, Yadava VP, Westenfelder C: Modification of Na and Cl transport in canine tracheal mucosa by prostaglandins. Am J Physiol 241:F101, 1981.

4. Albelda SM: Endothelial and epithelial cell adhesion molecules. Am J Respir Cell Mol Biol 4:195, 1991.
5. Anderson CD, Miller LJ, Schmalstieg FC, et al: Contributions of the Mac-1 glycoprotein family to adherence-dependent granulocyte functions: structure-function assessments employing subunit-specific monoclonal antibodies. J Immunol 137:15, 1986.
6. Azzawi M, Bradley B, Jeffery PK, et al: Identification of activated T-lymphocytes and eosinophils in bronchial biopsies in stable atopic asthma. Am Rev Respir Dis 142:1407, 1990.
7. Bai TR: Abnormalities in airway smooth muscle in fatal asthma. Am Rev Respir Dis 141:552, 1990.
8. Barnes PJ, Chung, KF, Page CP: Platelet-activating factor as a mediator of allergic disease. J Allergy Clin Immunol 81:919, 1988.
9. Barnes PJ, Cuss FM, Palmer JB: The effect of airway epithelium on smooth muscle contractility in bovine trachea. Br J Pharmacol 86:685, 1985.
10. Barnett K, Jacoby DB, Nadel JA, Lazarus SC: The effects of epithelial cell supernatant on contractions of isolated canine tracheal smooth muscle. Am Rev Respir Dis 138:780, 1988.
11. Beam WR, Weiner DE, Martin RJ: Timing of prednisone and alterations of airways inflammation in nocturnal asthma. Am Rev Respir Dis 146:1524, 1992.
12. Beasley R, Roche WR, Roberts JA, et al: Cellular events in the bronchi in mild asthma and after bronchial provocation. Am Rev Respir Dis 139:806, 1989.
13. Behrens BL, Clark RA: Comparison of the evolving histopathology of early and late cutaneous and asthmatic response in rabbits after a single antigen challenge. Lab Invest 56:101, 1987.
14. Benenati S, Bochner B, Horn T, et al: Endothelial-leukocyte adhesion to molecule-1 (ELAM-1) expression following cutaneous allergen challenge. J Allergy Clin Immunol 87:304 1991. Abstract.
15. Benveniste J, Henson PM, Cochrane CG: Leucocyte dependent histamine release from rabbit platelets: the role of IgE, basophils and a platelet activating factor. J Exp Med 136:1356, 1972.
16. Bernstein DI, Bernstein IL, Bodenheimer SS, et al: An open study of auranofin in the treatment of steroid-dependent asthma. J Allergy Clin Immunol 81:6, 1988.
17. Blackwell GJ, Carnuccio R, Di Rosa M, et al: Glucocorticoids induce the formation of and release of antiinflammatory proteins into the peritoneal cavity of the rat. Br J Pharmacol 76:185, 1982.
18. Bleecker ER: Cholinergic and neurogenic mechanisms in obstructive airways disease. Am J Med 81:93, 1986.
19. Bochner BS, Charlesworth EN, Lichtenstein LM, et al: Interleukin-1 is released at sites of human cutaneous allergic reactions. J Allergy Clin Immunol 86:830, 1990.
20. Bochner BS, Friedman B, Krishnaswami G, et al: Episodic eosinophilia-myalgia-like syndrome in a patient without L-tryptophan use: association with eosinophil activation and increase serum levels of granulocyte-macrophage colony-stimulating factor. J Allergy Clin Immunol 88:629, 1991.
21. Bochner BS, Luscinskas FW, Gimbrone MA, et al: Adhesion of human basophils, eosinophils, and neutrophils to IL-1-activated human vascular endothelial cells: contributions of endothelial cell adhesion molecules. J Exp Med 173:1553, 1991.
22. Bochner BS, McKelvey AA, Sterbinsky SA, et al: Interleukin-3 augments adhesiveness for endothelial and CD11b expression in human basophils but not neutrophils. J Immunol 145:1832, 1990.
23. Bradley BL, Azzawi M, Jacobson M, et al: Eosinophils, T-lymphocytes, mast cells, neutrophils and macrophages in bronchial biopsy specimens from atopic subjects without asthma: comparison with biopsy specimens from atopic subjects without asthma and normal control subjects and relationship to bronchial hyperresponsiveness. J Allergy Clin Immunol 88:661, 1991.
24. Bramley AM, Thomson RJ, Roberts CR, et al: Hypothesis: excessive bronchoconstriction in asthma is due to decreased airway elastance. Eur Respir J 7:337, 1994.
25. Breslin FJ, McFadden ER, Ingram RJ: The effects of cromolyn sodium on the airway response to hyperpnea and cold air in asthma. Am Rev Respir Dis 122:11, 1980.
26. Bukowskyj M, Nakatsu K, Munt PW: Theophylline reassessed. Ann Intern Med 101:63, 1984.
27. Burd PR, Rogers HW, Gordon JR, et al: Interleukin 3-dependent and independent mast cells stimulated with IgE and antigen express multiple cytokines. J Exp Med 170:245, 1989.
28. Burnette MG, Landis S, Thibodeau LP: Childhood asthma: prevention of attacks with short term corticosteroid treatment of upper respiratory tract infection. Pediatrics 81(5):624, 1988.
29. Busse WW, Bush RK: A comparison of AM and PM dosing with a 24 hour sustained release theophylline, Uniphyl, for nocturnal asthma. Am J Med 79(6A):62, 1985.
30. Busse WW, Swenson CA: The relationship between plasma histamine concentrations and bronchial obstruction to antigen challenge in allergic rhinitis. J Allergy Clin Immunol 84:658, 1989.
31. Butterfield JH, Leiferman KM, Abrams J, et al: Elevated serum levels of interleukin-5 in patients with the syndrome of episodic angioedema and eosinophilia. Blood 79:688, 1992.
32. Buyon JP, Slade SG, Reibman J, et al: Constitutive and induced phosphorylation of the α and β chains of the CD11/CD18 leukocyte integrin family. J Immunol 140:191, 1990.
33. Campbell HD, Tucker WQJ, Hort Y, et al: Molecular cloning, nucleotide sequence and expression of the gene encoding human eosinophil differentiation factor (interleukin-5). Proc Natl Acad Sci USA 84:6629, 1987.
34. Capron M, Jouault T, Prin L, et al: Functional study of a monoclonal antibody to IgE Fc receptor (Fc RII) of eosinophils, platelets, and macrophages. J Exp Med 164:72, 1986.
35. Casale TB, Wood D, Richerson HB, et al: Direct evidence of a role for mast cells in the pathogenesis of antigen-induced bronchoconstriction. J Clin Invest 80:1507, 1987.
36. Caughey GH: Roles of mast cell tryptase and chymase in airway function. Am J Physiol 257:L39, 1989.
37. Caughey GH, Lazarus SC, Viro NF, et al: Tryptase and chymase: comparison of extraction and release in two dog mastocytoma lines. Immunology 63:339, 1988.
38. Cerrina J, Le Roy LM, Labat C, et al: Comparison of human bronchial smooth muscle responses to histamine in vivo with histamine and isoproterenol agonists in vitro. Am Rev Respir Dis 134(1):57, 1986.
39. Cher DJ, Mosmann TR: Two types of murine helper T-cell clone. II. Delayed-type hypersensitivity is mediated by TH1 clones. J Immunol 138:3688, 1987.
40. Churchill L, Freidman B, Schleimer RP, et al: Production of granulocyte-macrophage colony stimulating factor by cultured human tracheal epithelial cells. Immunology 75:189, 1992.
41. Cluzel M, Damon M, Chanez P, et al: Enhanced alveolar cell lumonil-dependent chemiluminescence in asthma. J Allergy Clin Immunol 80:195, 1987.
42. Coffman RL, Carty J: A T-cell activity that enhances polyclonal IgE production and its inhibition by interferon-γ. J Immunol 136:949, 1986.
43. Coffman RL, Seymour BWP, Hudak S, et al: Antibody to interleukin 5 inhibits helminth-induced eosinophilia in mice. Science 245:308, 1989.
44. Corrigan CJ, Hartnell A, Kay AB: T-lymphocyte activation in acute severe asthma. Lancet I:1129, 1988.
45. Corrigan CJ, Kay AB: CD4 T-lymphocyte activation in acute severe asthma. Relationship to disease severity and atopic status. Am Rev Respir Dis 141:970, 1990.
46. Cotran RS, Gimbrone MA, Bevilacqua MP, et al: Induction and detection of a human endothelial activation antigen in vivo. J Exp Med 164:661, 1986.
47. Crawford RM, Finbloom DS, Ohara J, et al: B cell stimulatory factor-1 (interleukin 4) activates macrophages for increased tumoricidal activity and expression of Ia antigens. J Immunol 139:135, 1987.
48. Cushley MJ, Tattersfield AE, Holgate ST: Adenosine-induced bronchoconstriction in asthma. Antagonism by inhaled theophylline. Am Rev Respir Dis 129:380, 1984.
49. Dahl R, Johansson SA: Importance of duration of treatment with inhaled budesonide on the immediate and late bronchial reaction. Eur J Respir Dis Suppl 63 (122):167, 1982.
50. Dahl R, Pedersen B: Influence of nedocromil sodium on the dual asthmatic reaction after challenge: a double placebo controlled study. Eur J Respir Dis Suppl 69(147):263, 1986.
51. Dahl R, Pedersen B, Venge P: Bronchoalveolar lavage studies. Eur Respir Rev 4:272, 1991.
52. Davignon D, Martz E, Reynolds T, et al: Lymphocyte function associated antigen 1 (LFA-1): a surface antigen distinct from Lyt-2.3 that participates in T lymphocyte-mediated killing. Proc Natl Acad Sci USA 78:4535, 1981.
53. DeBlay F, Chapman MD, Platts-Mills TAE: Airborne cat allergen (Fel d I) environmental control with the in situ. Am Rev Respir Dis 143:1334, 1991.

54. deFougerolles AR, Stacker SA, Schwarting R, et al: Characterization of ICAM-2 and evidence for a third counter-receptor for LFA-1. J Exp Med 174:253, 1991.
55. Defrance T, Aubry JP, Rousset F, et al: Human recombinant IL-4 induces Fce receptors (cd23) on normal human B lymphocytes. J Exp Med 165:1459, 1987.
56. deJongste JC, Mons H, Bonta IL, et al: In vitro responses of airways from an asthmatic patient. Eur J Respir Dis 71:23, 1987.
57. Del Prete GF, Maggi E, Parronchi P: IL-4 is an essential factor for the IgE synthesis induced in vitro by human T-cell clones and their supernatants. J Immunol 140:4193, 1988.
58. deMonchy JGR, Kauffman HF, Venge P: Bronchoalveolar eosinophilia during allergen-induced late asthmatic reactions. Am Rev Respir Dis 181:373, 1985.
59. Diamond JM: Osmotic water flow in leaky epithelia. J Membr Biol 51:195, 1979.
60. Diaz P, Gonzalez MC, Galleguillos FR, et al: Leucocytes and mediators in bronchoalveolar lavage during allergen-induced late-phase asthmatic reactions. Am Rev Respir Dis 144:1274, 1991.
61. Djukanovic R, Roche WR, Wilson JW, et al: Mucosal inflammation in asthma. Am Rev Respir Dis 142:434, 1990.
62. Dobrina A. Menegazzi R, Carlos TM, et al: Mechanisms of eosinophil adherence to cultured vascular endothelial cells: eosinophils bind to the cytokine-induced endothelial ligand vascular cell adhesion molecule-1 via the very late activation antigen-4 integrin receptor. J Clin Invest 88:20, 1991.
63. Dolovich J: Late cutaneous allergic responses in isolated IgE-dependent reactions. J Allergy Clin Immunol 52:38, 1973.
64. Domonneville M, Wietzerbin J, Pancre V, et al: Recombinant tumor necrosis factors mediate platelet cytotoxicity to *Schistosoma mansoni* larvae. J Immunol 140:3962, 1988.
65. Donahue RE, Wang EA, Stone DK, et al: Stimulation of hematopoiesis in primates by continuous infusion recombinant human GM-CSF. Nature 321:872, 1986.
66. Dransfield I, Buckle AM, Hogg N: Early events of the immune response mediated by leukocyte integrins. Immunol Rev 114:29, 1990.
67. Dunnill MS: The pathology of asthma with special reference to changes in the bronchial mucosa. J Clin Pathol 13:27, 1960.
68. Durham SR, Dawes J, Kay AB: Platelets in asthma. Lancet 2:36, 1985.
69. Durham SR, Kay AB: Eosinophils, bronchial hyperreactivity and late-phase asthmatic reactions. Clin Allergy 15:411, 1985.
70. Dustin ML, Rothlein R, Bhan AK, et al: Induction by IL-1 and interferon, tissue distribution, biochemistry, and function of a natural adherence molecule (ICAM-1). J Immunol 137:245, 1988.
71. Dustin ML, Springer TA: T-cell receptor cross-linking transiently stimulates adhesiveness through LFA-1. Nature 341:619, 1989.
72. Dutoit JI, Solome CM, Woolcock AJ: Inhaled corticosteroids reduce the severity of bronchial hyperresponsiveness in asthma, but oral theophylline does not. Am Rev Respir Dis 136:1174, 1987.
73. Dvorsky-Gebauer RJ: Potentiation of bronchodilators by glucocorticoids. Lancet 2:306, 1976.
74. Ebisawa M, Bochner BS, Lichtenstein LM, et al: Effect of cytokines on eosinophil transendothelial migration. J Allergy Clin Immunol 89:296, 1992. Abstract.
75. Empey DW, Laitinen LA, Jacobs L, et al: Mechanism of bronchial hyperreactivity in normal and asthmatic subjects after upper respiratory tract infection. Am Rev Respir Dis 113(2):131–139, 1976.
76. Expert Panel on the Management of Asthma: Guidelines for the diagnosis and management of asthma. J Allergy Clin Immunol 88:425, 1991.
77. Fernandez-Botran R, Kramer PH, Diamenstein T, et al: B-cell stimulatory factor 1 (BSF-1) promotes growth of helper T cell lines. J Exp Med 164:580, 1986.
78. Filley WV, Holley KE, Kephart GM, Gleich GJ: Identification by immunofluorescence of eosinophil granule major basic protein in lung tissues of patients with bronchial asthma. Lancet 2:11, 1982.
79. Finkelman FD, Katona IM, Urban JF Jr, et al: Suppression of in vivo polyclonal IgE responses by monoclonal antibody to the lymphokine BSF-1. Proc Natl Acad Sci USA 83:9675, 1986.
80. Flavahan NA, Aarhus LL, Rimele TJ, Vanhoutte PM: Respiratory epithelium inhibits bronchial smooth muscle tone. J Appl Physiol 58:834, 1985.
81. Flavahan NA, Slifman NR, Gleich GJ, et al: Human eosinophil major basic protein causes hyperreactivity of respiratory smooth muscle. Am Rev Respir Dis 138:685, 1988.
82. Fong TA, Mosmann TR: The role of INF-γ in delayed type hypersensitivity mediated by TH1 clones. J Immunol 143:2887, 1989.
83. Frew AJ, Kay AB: The relationship between infiltrating CD4 lymphocytes, activated eosinophils, and the magnitude of the allergen-induced late phase cutaneous reaction in man. J Immunol 141:4158, 1988.
84. Frick WE, Sedgwick JB, Busse WW: The appearance of hypodense eosinophils in antigen-dependent late phase asthma. Am Rev Respir Dis 139:1401, 1989.
85. Fujisawa T, Abu-Ghazaleh R, Kita H, et al: Regulatory effect of cytokines on eosinophil degranulation. J Immunol 144:642, 1990.
86. Fuller RW, Morris PK, Richmond R, et al: IgE-dependent stimulation of human alveolar macrophages: significance in type I hypersensitivity. Clin Exp Immunol 65:416, 1986.
87. Gaddy JN, Bush RK, Margolskee D, et al: The effects of a leukotriene D4 (LTD4) antagonist (MK-571) in mild to moderate asthma. J Allergy Clin Immunol 85:197(A), 1990.
88. Garssen J, Nijamp FP, Vandervliet H, et al: T-cell-medicated induction of airway hyperreactivity in mice. Am Rev Respir Dis 144:931, 1991.
89. Gelber LE, Seltzer LH, Bouzoukis JK, et al: Sensitization and exposure to indoor allergens as risk factors for asthma among patients presenting to hospital. Am Rev Respir Dis 147:573, 1993.
90. Gerrard JW, Cockroft DW, Mink JT, et al: Increased nonspecific bronchial reactivity in cigarette smokers with normal lung function. Am Rev Respir Dis 122:577, 1980.
91. Godfrey S: Controversies in pathogenesis of EIA. Eur J Respir Dis 68:81, 1986.
92. Godfrey S, Konig P: Inhibition of exercise induced asthma by different pharmacological pathways. Thorax 31(2):137–143, 1976.
93. Golden JA, Nadel JA, Boushey HA: Bronchial hyperresponsiveness in healthy subjects after exposure to ozone. Am Rev Respir Dis 118:287, 1978.
94. Goldie RG, Papadimitriou JM, Paterson JW, et al: Influence of the epithelium on responsiveness of guinea pig isolated trachea to contractile and relaxant agonists. Br J Pharmacol 87:5, 1986.
95. Goldie RG, Spina D, Henry PJ, et al: In vitro responsiveness of human asthmatic bronchus to carbachol, histamine, B-adrenoceptor agonists and theophylline. Br J Clin Pharmacol 22:669, 1986.
96. Gongora HC, Wisniewski AFZ, Tattersfield AE: A single dose comparison of inhaled salbutamol and 2 formulations of salmeterol on airway reactivity in asthmatic subjects. Am Rev Respir Dis 144:626, 1991.
97. Gordon T, Sheppard D, McDonald DM, et al: Airway hyperresponsiveness and inflammation induced by toluene diisocyanate in guinea pigs. Am Rev Respir Dis 132:1106, 1985.
98. Gosset P, Cassalle P, Tonnel AB, et al: Production of an interleukin 1 inhibitory factor by human alveolar macrophages from normal and allergic patients. Am Rev Respir Dis 138:40, 1988.
99. Gosset P, Tonnel AB, Joseph M, et al: Secretion of a chemotactic factor for neutrophils and eosinophils by alveolar macrophages from asthmatic patients. J Allergy Clin Immunol 74:827, 1984.
100. Gosset P, Tsicopoulos A, Wallaert B, et al: Increased secretion of tumor necrosis factor alpha and interleukin-6 by alveolar macrophages consecutive to the development of the late asthmatic reaction. J Allergy Clin Immunol 88:561, 1991.
101. Granville AR, Tazalaar HD, Theodore J, et al: The distribution of MHC class I and class II antigens on bronchial epithelium. Am Rev Respir Dis 139:330, 1989.
102. Green WF, Nicholas NR, Salome CM, et al: Reduction of house dust mites and mite allergens: effects of spraying carpets and blankets with Allersearch DMS, an acaricide combined with an allergen reducing agent. Clin Exp Allergy 19:203, 1989.
103. Greenberger PA, Patterson R: Management of asthma during pregnancy. N Engl J Med 3:897, 1985.
104. Greenberger PA, Patterson R: The management of asthma during pregnancy and lactation. Clin Rev Allergy 5(4):317, 1987.
105. Greer IA, Winter JH, Gaffney D, et al: Platelets in asthma. Lancet 2:1479, 1984.
106. Gresele P, Todisco T, Merarte F, et al: Platelet activation and allergic asthma. N Engl J Med 306:549, 1982.
107. Gross NJ, Skorodin MS: Anticholinergic, antimuscarinic bronchodilators. Am Rev Respir Dis 129:856, 1984.
108. Gundel RM, Letts LG, Gleich GJ: Human eosinophil major basic protein induces airway constriction and airway hyperresponsiveness in primates. J Clin Invest 87:1470, 1991.
109. Haczku A, Chung KF, Tsukagoshi H, et al: Adoptive transfer of T cells induces airway hyperresponsiveness (AHR) related to tissue eosino-

philia in brown Norway rats. J Allergy Clin Immunol 1(2):221, 1995. Abstract.
110. Hamid Q, Azzawi MA, Ying S, et al: Expression of mRNA for interleukin-5 in mucosal bronchial biopsies from asthma. J Clin Invest 87:1541, 1991.
111. Hemler HE: VLA proteins in the integrin family: structures, functions and their roles on leukocytes. Ann Rev Immunol 8:365, 1990.
112. Hendeles L, Weinerger M: Theophylline: a state of the art review. Pharmacotherapy 3:2, 1983.
113. Henriksen JM, Agertoft L, Pederson S: Protective effect and duration of action of inhaled formoterol and salbutamol on exercise induced asthma in children. J Allergy Clin Immunol 89:1176, 1992.
114. Holgate ST, Baldwin CJ, Tattersfield AE: Beta-adrenergic agonist resistance in normal human airways. Lancet 2:375, 1977.
115. Holgate ST, Beasley R, Twentyman OP: The pathogenesis and significance of bronchial hyperresponsiveness in airways disease. Clin Sci (Colch) 73:561, 1987.
116. Holtzman MJ, Aizawa H, Nadel JA, et al: Selective generation of leukotriene B4 by tracheal epithelial cells from dogs. Biochem Biophys Res Commun 114:1071, 1983.
117. Holtzman MJ, Fabbri LM, O'Byrne PM, et al: Importance of airway inflammation for hyperresponsiveness induced by ozone. Am Rev Respir Dis 127:686, 1983.
118. Horst M, Hejjaoui A, Horst V, et al: Double-blind, placebo controlled rush immunotherapy with a standardized *Alternaria* extract. J Allergy Clin Immunol 85:460, 1990.
119. House CR: Water transport in cells and tissues. Edward Arnold, London; Williams & Wilkins Co, Baltimore, 1974.
120. Howarth PH: The investigation of the nonbronchodilator properties of asthma therapies in vivo. Eur Respir J 4:399, 1991.
121. Howarth PH, Durham SR, Lee TH, et al: Influence of albuterol, cromolyn sodium and ipratropium bromide on the airway and circulating mediator responses to allergen bronchial provocation in asthma. Am Rev Respir Dis 132:986, 1985.
122. Howell CS, Pujol JL, Crea AEG, et al: Identification of an alveolar macrophage-derived activity in bronchial asthma that enhances LTD4 generation by human eosinophils stimulated by ionophore (A23187) as granulocyte-macrophage-colony stimulating factor (GM-CSF). Am Rev Respir Dis 140:1340, 1989.
123. Hubscher T: Role of eosinophil in the allergic reactions. I. EDI-an eosinophil derived inhibitor of histamine release. J Immunol 114:1379, 1975.
124. Hui KP, Barnes NC: Lung function improvement in asthma with a cysteinyl-leukotriene receptor antagonist. Lancet 337:1062, 1991.
125. Hunter JA, Finkbeiner WE, Nadel JA, et al: Predominant generations of 15-lipoxygenase metabolites of arachidonic acid by epithelial cells from human trachea. Proc Natl Acad Sci USA 82:4633, 1985.
126. Huss R, Huss K, Squire EN, et al: Mite allergen control with acaricide fails. J Allergy Clin Immunol 94:27, 1994.
127. Isreal E, Dermarkarian R, Rosenberg M, et al: The effects of a 5 lipoxygenase inhibitor on asthma induced by cold, dry air. N Engl J Med 323:1740, 1990.
128. James AL, Pare PD, Hogg JC: The mechanism of airway narrowing in asthma. Am Rev Respir Dis 139:242, 1989.
129. Jarjour NN, Calhoun WJ, Schwartz LB, et al: Elevated bronchoalveolar lavage fluid histamine levels in allergic asthmatics are associated with increased airway obstruction. Am Rev Respir Dis 144:83, 1991.
130. Jeffery PK, Wardlaw AJ, Nelson FC, et al: Bronchial biopsies in asthma. An ultrastructural, quantitative study and correlation with hyperreactivity. Am Rev Respir Dis 140(6): 1745, 1989.
131. Jennings BH, Andersson KE, Johansson SA: The assessment of systemic effects of inhaled glucocorticoids: a comparison of the effects of inhaled budesonide and oral prednisolone on adrenal function and markers of bone turnover. Eur J Clin Pharmacol 41 (1):11, 1991.
132. Joseph M, Auriault C, Capron A, et al: A new function for platelets: IgE-dependent killing of schistosomes. Nature 303:810, 1983.
133. Joseph M, Capron A, Ameisen JC, et al: The receptor for IgE on blood platelets. Eur J Immunol 16:306, 1986.
134. Joseph M, Tonnel AB, Topier G, et al: Involvement of immunoglobulin E in the secretory process of alveolar macrophages from asthmatic patients. J Clin Invest 71:221, 1983.
135. Kalb TH, Kuang MT, Marom Z, Mayer L: Evidence for the accessory cell function by class MHC antigen expressing airway epithelial cells. Am J Respir Cell Mol Biol 4:320, 1991.
136. Kaliner MA, Lemanske RL: Rhinitis and asthma. JAMA 268:2807, 1992.
137. Kay AB, Ying S, Varney V, et al: Messenger RNA expression of the cytokine gene cluster IL-3, IL-4, IL-5 and GM-CSF in allergen-induced late phase cutaneous reactions in atopic subjects. J Exp Med 173:775, 1991.
138. Kelly C, Ward C, Stenton CS, et al: Number and activity of inflammatory cells in bronchoalveolar lavage fluid in asthma and their relation to airway responsiveness. Thorax 43:684, 1988.
139. Kerrebijn KF, Von Essen-Zandvliet EEM, Neijens HJ: Effect of long term treatment with inhaled corticosteroids and beta-agonists on bronchial responsiveness in asthmatic children. J Allergy Clin Immunol 79:653, 1987.
140. Kirshenbaum AS, Goff JP, Dreskin SC, et al: IL-3-dependent growth of basophil-like cells and mast-like cells from human bone marrow. J Immunol 142:2427, 1989.
141. Kishimoto TK, Larsen RS, Corbi AL, et al: The leukocyte integrins. Adv Immunol 46:149, 1989.
142. Kita H, Ohnishi T, Okubo Y, et al: Granulocyte/macrophage colony-stimulating factor and interleukin 3 release from human peripheral blood eosinophils and neutrophils. J Exp Med 174:745, 1991.
143. Knapp HR: Reduced allergen-induced nasal congestion and leukotriene synthesis with an orally active 5 lipoxygenase inhibitor. N Engl J Med 323:1745, 1990.
144. Knauer KA, Lichtenstein LM, Adkinson NF, et al: Platelet activation during antigen-induced airway reactions in asthmatic subjects. N Engl J Med 304:1404, 1981.
145. Kondo M, Finkbeiner WE, Widdicombe JH: Changes in permeability of dog tracheal epithelium in response to hydrostatic pressure. Am J Physiol 262:L176, 1992.
146. Konig P: Inhaled corticosteroids—their present and future role in the management of asthma. J Allergy Clin Immunol 82:297, 1988.
147. Korsgaard J: House dust mites and absolute indoor humidity. Allergy 38:88, 1983.
148. Korsgaard J: Preventative measures in house dust allergy. Am Rev Respir Dis 125:80, 1982.
149. Kowalski ML, Diddier A, Kaliner MA: Neurogenic inflammation in the airways. Am Rev Respir Dis 140:101, 1989.
150. Koyama S, Rennard SI, Leikauf GD, et al: Endotoxin stimulates bronchial epithelial cells to release chemotactic factor for neutrophils. J Immunol 147:4293, 1991.
151. Koyama S, Rennard SI, Leikauf GD, et al: Bronchial epithelial cells release monocyte chemotactic activity for monocytes. Am J Physiol 257:L130, 1989.
152. Kroegel C, Yukawa T, Dent G, et al: Stimulation of degranulation from human eosinophils by platelet-activating factor. J Immunol 142:3518, 1989.
153. Kruszynska YT, Greenstone M, Home PD, et al: Effect of high dose inhaled beclomethasone dipropionate on carbohydrate and lipid metabolism in normal subjects. Thorax 42:881, 1987.
154. Kyan-Aung U, Haskard DO, Poston RN, et al: Endothelial leukocyte adhesion molecule-1 and intercellular adhesion molecule-1 mediate the adhesion of eosinophils to endothelial cells in vitro and are expressed by endothelium in allergic cutaneous inflammation in vivo. J Immunol 146:521, 1991.
155. Labovitz E, Spector S: Placental theophylline transfer in pregnant asthmatics. JAMA 247:786, 1982.
156. Laitinen LA, Heino M, Laitinen A, et al: Damage of the airway epithelium and bronchial reactivity in patients with asthma. Am Rev Respir Dis 131:599, 1985.
157. Lam S, LeRiche J, Phillips D, et al: Cellular and protein changes in bronchial lavage fluid after late asthmatic reactions in patients with red cedar asthma. J Allergy Clin Immunol 80:44, 1987.
158. Lan J-L, Lee D-T, Wu C-H, et al: Cockroach hypersensitivity: preliminary study of allergic cockroach asthma in Taiwan. J Allergy Clin Immunol 82:736, 1988.
159. Larsson S, Svedmyr N: A comparison of 2 modes of administering beta-2 adrenoreceptor stimulants in asthmatics: tablets and metered aerosol. Scand J Respir Dis 101:79, 1977.
160. Lee T, Lenihan DJ, Malone B, et al: Increased biosynthesis of platelet activating factor in activated human eosinophils. J Biol Chem 259:5526, 1984.
161. Lellouch-Tubiana A, Lefort J, Simon MT, et al: Eosinophil recruitment into guinea pig lungs after PAF-acether and allergen administration, modulation by prostacyclin, platelet depletion, and selective antagonists. Am Rev Respir Dis 137:948, 1988.
162. Leung DYM, Pober JS, Cotran RS: Expression of endothelial-leukocyte

adhesion molecule-1 in elicited late phase allergic reactions. J Clin Invest 87:1805, 1991.
163. Lewis RE, Buchsbaum T, Whitaker D, et al: Intercellular adhesion molecule in the evolving human cutaneous delayed hypersensitivity reaction. J Invest Dermatol 93:672, 1989.
164. Lichtenstein LM: Histamine-releasing factors and IgE heterogeneity. J Allergy Clin Immunol 81:814, 1988.
165. Limaye AP, Abrams JS, Silver JE, et al: Regulation of parasite-induced eosinophilia: selectively increased interleukin-5 production in helminth-infected patients. J Exp Med 172:399, 1990.
166. Lipworth BJ, Struthers AD, McDevitt DG: Tachyphylaxis to systemic but not airway responses during prolonged therapy with high dose inhaled salbutamol in asthmatics. Am Rev Respir Dis 140:586, 1989.
167. Lofdahl CG, Chung KF: Long acting beta-2 adrenoreceptor agonists: a new perspective in the treatment of asthma. Eur J Respir Dis 4:218, 1991.
168. Lopez AF, Sanderson CJ, Gamble JR, et al: Recombinant human interleukin-5 is a selective activator of eosinophil function. J Exp Med 167:219, 1988.
169. Lopez AF, Williamson DJ, Gamble JR, et al: Recombinant human granulocyte-macrophage colony-stimulating factor stimulates in vitro mature human neutrophil and eosinophil function, surface receptor expression, and survival. J Clin Invest 78:1220, 1986.
170. Macklem PT: Bronchial hyporesponsiveness. Chest 87 (suppl): 158S, 1985.
171. Maggi E, Del Prete GF, Macchia D, et al: Profile of lymphokine activities and helper function for IgE in human T-cell clones. Eur J Immunol 18:1045, 1988.
172. Malech HL, Gallin JI: Neutrophils in human disease. N Engl J Med 317:687, 1987.
173. Manning PJ, Watson RM, Margolskee DJ, et al: Inhibition of exercise-induced bronchoconstriction by MK-571, a potent leukotriene D4-receptor antagonist. N Engl J Med 323:1736, 1990.
174. Mansfield LE, Nelson HS: Allergens of commercially available house dust. Ann Allergy 48:205, 1982.
175. Marom Z, Shelhamer J, Alleny D, et al: The effect of corticosteroids on mucous glycoprotein secretion from human airways in vitro. Am Rev Respir Dis 129:62, 1984.
176. Masinovsky B, Urdal D, Gallatin WM: IL-4 acts synergistically with IL-1N to promote lymphocyte adhesion microvascular endothelium by induction of vascular cell adhesion molecule-1. J Immunol 145:2886, 1990.
177. Massey W, Friedman B, Kato M, et al: Allergen-induced late-phase reaction sites contain IL-3 and GM-CSF activity. J Allergy Clin Immunol 87:207, 1991. Abstract.
178. Mazingue C, Carriere V, Dessaint J-P, et al: Regulation of IgE synthesis by macrophages expressing FcE receptors: role of interleukin 1. Clin Exp Immunol 67:587, 1987.
179. Melewicz FM, Kline NE, Cohen AB, et al: Characterization of Fc receptor for IgE on human alveolar macrophages. Clin Exp Immunol 49:364, 1982.
180. Melewicz FM, Spiegelberg HL: Fc receptors for IgE on a subpopulation of human peripheral blood monocytes. J Immunol 125:1026, 1980.
181. Melewicz FM, Zeiger RS, Mellon MH, et al: Increased peripheral blood monocytes with Fc receptors for IgE in patients with severe allergic disorders. J Immunol 126:1592, 1981.
182. Metzger WJ, Hunninghake GW, Richerson HB: Late asthmatic response: inquiry into mechanisms and significance. Clin Rev Allergy 3:145, 1985.
183. Metzger WJ, Zavala D, Richerson HB, et al: Local allergen challenge and bronchoalveolar lavage of allergic asthmatic lungs. Am Rev Respir Dis 135:433, 1987.
184. Minton NE, Kensington JE, Maconachie JG, et al: Does tachyphylaxis occur to the non-pulmonary effects of salmeterol? Br J Clin Pharmacol 31:241, 1991.
185. Miura M, Belvisi MG, Stretton CP, et al: Role of potassium channels in bronchodilator responses in human airways. Am Rev Respir Dis 146:132, 1992.
186. Molinas FC, Wietzerbin J, Fallcoff E: Human platelets possess receptors for a lymphokine: demonstration of high specific receptors for Hu IFN. J Immunol 138:802, 1987.
187. Mond JJ, Carman J, Sarma C, et al: Interferon-γ suppresses B-cell stimulation factor (BSF-1) induction of class II MHC determinants on B cells. J Immunol 137:3534, 1986.
188. Moqbel R, Durham SR, Shaw RJ, et al: Enhancement of leukocyte cytotoxicity after exercise-induced asthma. Am Rev Respir Dis 133:609, 1986.
189. Moreno RH, Hogg JC, Pare PD: Mechanisms of airway narrowing. Am Rev Respir Dis 133:1171, 1986.
190. Morrow-Brown H, Storey G, George WHS: Beclomethasone dipropionate: a new steroid aerosol for the treatment of allergic asthma. Br J Med 1:585, 1972.
191. Mosmann TR, Cherwinski H, Bond MW, et al: Two types of murine helper T cell clone. I. Definition according to profiles of lymphokine activities and secreted proteins. J Immunol 136:2348, 1986.
192. Mosmann TR, Coffman RL: TH1 and TH2 cells: different patterns of lymphokine secretion lead to different functional properties. Annu Rev Immunol 7:145, 1989.
193. Munro JM, Pober JS, Cotran RS: TNF and INF gamma induce distinct patterns of endothelial cell activation and associated leukocyte accumulation in skin of *Papio anubis*. Am J Pathol 135:121, 1989.
194. Murphy KR, Wilson MC, Irvin CG, et al: The requirement for polymorphonuclear leukocytes on the late asthmatic response and heightened airways reactivity in an animal model. Am Rev Respir Dis 134:62, 1986.
195. Nakamura H, Yoshimura A, Jaffe HA, Crystal RG: Interleukin 8 gene expression in bronchial epithelial cells. J Biol Chem 29:19611, 1991.
196. Nelson HS: Adrenergic therapy of bronchial asthma. J Allergy Clin Immunol 77:771, 1986.
197. Nelson HS: The atopic diseases. Ann Allergy 55:441, 1985.
198. Noah TL, Paradiso AM, Madden MC, et al: The response of human bronchial epithelial cell line to histamine: intracellular calcium changes and extracellular release of inflammatory mediators. Am J Respir Cell Mol Biol 5:484, 1991.
199. Nowak RM, Pensler MI, Parker DD: Comparison of peak expiratory flow and FEV1: admission criteria for acute bronchial asthma. Ann Emerg Med 11:64, 1982.
200. O'Byrne PM, Walters EH, Gold BP, et al: Neutrophil depletion inhibits airway hyperresponsiveness induced by ozone exposure. Am Rev Respir Dis 130:214, 1984.
201. O'Hollaren MT, Yunginger J, Offord KP, et al: Exposure to an aeroallergen as a possible precipitating factor in respiratory arrest in young patients with asthma. N Engl J Med 324:359, 1991.
202. Ohman JL Jr, Findlay SR, Leiterman KM: Immunotherapy in cat induced asthma: double blind trial with evaluation of in vivo and in vitro responses. J Allergy Clin Immunol 74:230, 1984.
203. Orochek J, Doudlas JS, Bouhuys A: Contractile responses to guinea-pig trachea in vitro: modification by prostaglandin synthesis-inhibiting drugs. J Pharmacol Exp Ther 194:554, 1975.
204. Owen WF: Cytokine regulation of eosinophil inflammatory disease. Allergy Clin Immunol News 3:47, 1991.
205. Owen WF, Petersen J, SheffD, et al: Hypodense eosinophils and interleukin-5 activity in the blood of patients with the eosinophiliamyalgia syndrome. Proc Natl Acad Sci USA 87:8647, 1990.
206. Owen WF, Rothenberg ME, Petersen J, et al: Interleukin-5 and phenotypically altered eosinophils in the blood of patients with the idiopathic hypereosinophilic syndrome. J Exp Med 170:343, 1989.
207. Owen WF Jr, Rothenberg ME, Silberstein DS, et al: Regulation of human eosinophil viability, density, and function by granulocyte/macrophage colony-stimulating factor in the presence of 3T3 fibroblasts. J Exp Med 166:129, 1987.
208. Owen WF Jr, Soberman RJ, Yoshimoto T, et al: Synthesis and release of leukotriene C4 by human eosinophils. J Immunol 138:532, 1987.
209. Pancre V, Auriault C, Joseph M, et al: A suppressive lymphokine of platelet cytotoxic functions. J Immunol 137:585, 1986.
210. Pancre V, Joseph M, Capron A, et al: Characterization of a suppressive factor of platelet cytotoxic functions in human and rat schistosomiasis mansoni. Clin Exp Immunol 76:417, 1989.
211. Pancre V, Joseph M, Capron A, et al: Recombinant human interferon induces increased IgE receptor expression on human platelets. Eur J Immunol 18:829, 1988.
212. Pancre V, Joseph M, Mazingue C, et al: Induction of platelet cytoxic functions by lymphokine: role of γ-IFN. J Immunol 138:4490, 1987.
213. Papageorgiou N, Carroll M, Durham SR, et al: Complement receptor enhancement as evidence of neutrophil activation after exercise-induced asthma. Lancet 2:1220, 1983.
214. Pearlman DS, Chervinsky P, LaForce C, et al: A comparison of salmeterol with albuterol in the treatment of mild-to-moderate asthma. N Engl J Med 327:1420, 1992.
215. Platts-Mills TAE: Dust mite cockroach and other arthropods. In Pope

AM, Patterson R, Burge H (eds): Indoor Allergens: Assessing and Controlling Adverse Health Effects. Public Institute of Medicine, Washington, DC, 1993.
216. Platts-Mills TAE, deWeck AL, et al: Dust mite allergens and asthma—world wide problem. J Allergy Clin Immunol 83:416, 1989.
217. Plaut M, Pierce JH, Watson CJ, et al: Mast cell lines produce lymphokines in response to crosslinkage of Fc RI or to calcium ionophores. Nature 339:64, 1989.
218. Pober JS, Gimbrone MA Jr, Lapierre LA, et al: Overlapping patterns of activation of human endothelial cells by IL-1, TNF and INF gamma. J Immunol 137:1893, 1986.
219. Popovich KJ, Sheldon G, Mack M, et al: Role of platelets in contraction of canine tracheal muscle elicited by PAF in vitro. J Appl Physiol 65:914, 1988.
220. Powell JR, Rogers JF, Wargin WA, et al: Inhibition of theophylline clearance by cimetidine but not ranitidine. Arch Intern Med 144:484, 1984.
221. Randolph N, Krammer PH, Ohara J, et al: Increased expression of Ia antigens on resting B cells: an additional role for B-cell growth factor. Proc Natl Acad Sci USA 81:6149, 1984.
222. Rankin JA: IgE immune complexes induce LTB4 release from rat alveolar macrophages. Ann Inst Pasteur Immunol 137:364, 1986.
223. Rankin JA, Hitchcock M, Merrill WW, et al: IgE-dependent release of leukotriene C4 from alveolar macrophages. Nature 297:329, 1982.
224. Rankin JA, Kaliner M, Reynolds HY: Histamine levels in bronchoalveolar lavage from patients with asthma, sarcoidosis and idiopathic pulmonary fibrosis. J Allergy Clin Immunol 79:371, 1987.
225. Rankin JA, Schrader CE, Smith SM, et al: Recombinant IFN-γ primes alveolar macrophages culture in vitro for the release of leukotriene B4 in response to IgE stimulation. J Clin Invest 83:1691, 1989.
226. Reid MJ, Moss RB, Hsu YP: Seasonal asthma in northern California: allergy causes and efficacy of immunotherapy. J Allergy Clin Immunol 78:590, 1986.
227. Reynolds DS, Boom WH, Abbas AK: Inhibition of B-lymphocyte activation by interferon-γ. J Immunol 139:767, 1987.
228. Rice GE, Munro JM, Bevilacqua MP: Inducible cell adhesion molecule 110 is an inducible endothelial cell receptor for lymphocytes. J Exp Med 171(4):1369, 1990.
229. Robbins RA, Shoji S, Linder J, et al: Bronchial epithelial cells release chemotactic activity for lymphocytes. Am J Physiol 257:L109, 1989.
230. Robertson CF, Smith F, Beck R, et al: Response to frequent low doses of nebulized salbutamol in acute asthma. J Pediatr 106:672, 1985.
231. Robinson DS, Hamid Q, Ying S, et al: Predominant TH2-like bronchoalveolar T-lymphocyte population in atopic asthma. N Engl J Med 326:298, 1992.
232. Roche WR, Beasley R, Williams JH, Holgate ST: Subepithelial fibrosis in the bronchi of asthmatics. Lancet i:520, 1989.
233. Roehm N, Herron L, Cambier J, et al: The major histocompatibility complex-restricted antigen receptor on T cells: distribution on thymus and peripheral T cells. Cell 38:577, 1984.
234. Rothenberg ME, Owen WF Jr, Silberstein DS, et al: Human eosinophils have prolonged survival, enhanced functional properties, and become hypodense when exposed to human interleukin 3. J Clin Invest 81:1986, 1988.
235. Schatz M, Harden KM, Forsythe A, et al: The course of asthma during pregnancy, post-partum, and with successive pregnancies: a prospective analysis. J Allergy Clin Immunol 81:509, 1988.
236. Schatz M, Hoffman CP, Zeiger RS, et al: In Middleton E, Reed CE, Ellis EF, et al (eds): Allergy: Principles and Practice, 4th edition. Mosby Yearbook Co, St Louis, MO, 1992, pp1301–1342.
237. Schatz M, Zeiger RS, Harden KM, et al: The safety of inhaled beta-agonist bronchodilators during pregnancy. J Allergy Clin Immunol 82:686, 1988.
238. Schellenberg RR: Evidence for smooth muscle dysfunction in asthma. In Busse WW, Holgate ST (eds): Asthma and Rhinitis. Blackwell Scientific Publications, Cambridge, 1995, p1153.
239. Schellenberg RR, Duff MJ, Foster A, et al: Asthmatic bronchial reactivity in vitro. Proc Can Soc Clin Invest. Abstract 1985;8:A202.
240. Schellenberg RR, Walker B, Snyder F: Platelet-dependent contraction of human bronchi by platelet-activating factor. J Allergy Clin Immunol 71:145, 1983.
241. Schleimer RP, Sterbinsky SA, Kaiser J, et al: Interleukin-4 induces adherence of human eosinophils and basophils but not neutrophils to endothelium: association with expression of VCAM-1. J Immunol 148:1086, 1992.
242. Sears MR, Hervison GP, Holdaway MD, et al: The relative risks of sensitivity to grass pollen, house dust mite and cat dander in the development of childhood asthma. Clin Exp Allergy 19:419, 1989.
243. Sears MR, Taylor DR, Print CG, et al: Regular inhaled beta-agonist treatment in bronchial asthma. Lancet 336:1391, 1990.
244. Sedgwick JB, Calhoun WJ, Gleich GJ, et al: Immediate and late airway response of allergic rhinitis patients to segmental antigen challenge: characterization of eosinophil and mast cell mediators. Am Rev Respir Dis 144:1274, 1991.
245. Sekizawa K, Caughey GH, Lazarus SC, et al: Mast cells by bronchoalveolar allergen challenge. Am Rev Respir Dis 137:1002, 1988.
246. Serhan CN, Nicolaou KC, Webber SE, et al: Lipoxin A. Stereochemistry and biosynthesis. J Biol Chem 261:16340, 1986.
247. Shak S, Perez HD, Goldstein IM: A novel deoxygenation product of arachidonic acid possesses potent chemotactic activity for human polymorphonuclear leukocytes. J Biol Chem 258:14948, 1983.
248. Shoji S, Rickard KA, Ertl RF, et al: Bronchial epithelial cells produce lung fibroblast chemotactic factor: fibronectin. Am J Respir Cell Mol Biol I:13, 1989.
249. Shore S, Collier B, Martin JG: Effect of endogenous prostaglandins on acetylcholine release from dog trachealis muscle. J Appl Physiol 62:1837, 1987.
250. Sly RM, Anderson JA, Bresman CW, et al: Adverse effects and complications of treatment with beta-adrenergic agonist drugs. J Allergy Clin Immunol 75:433, 1985.
251. Spielgelberg HL: Structure and function of Fc receptors for IgE on lymphocytes, monocytes and macrophages. Adv Immunol 35:61, 1981.
252. Spitzer WO, Suissa S, Ernst P, et al: The use of beta-agonists and the risk of death and near death from asthma. N Engl J Med 326(8):501, 1992.
253. Stelzer J, Bigby BG, Stulbarg M, et al: O3-induced change in bronchial reactivity to methacholine and airway inflammation in humans. J Appl Physiol 60:1321, 1986.
254. Stevens TL, Bossie A, Sanders VM, et al: Subsets of antigen-specific helper T-cells regulate isotype secretion by antigen-specific B-cells. Nature 334:255, 1988.
255. Svedmyr NL, Larsson SA, Thiringer GK: Development of resistance in beta-adrenergic receptors of asthmatic patients. Chest 69:479, 1976.
256. Takatsu K, Tominaga A, Hamaoka T: Antigen-induced T cell-replacing factor (TRF). J Immunol 124:2414, 1980.
257. Teale JM, Abraham KM: The regulation of antibody class expression. Immunol Today 8:122, 1987.
258. Thornhill MH, Haskard DO: IL-4 regulates endothelial cell activation by IL-1, tumor necrosis factor, or IFN-γ. J Immunol 145:865, 1990.
259. Timonen T, Stenius-Aarnala B: Natural killer cell activity in asthma. Clin Exp Immunol 59:85, 1985.
260. Tomioka K, Bochner BS, Derse-Anthony C, et al: GM-CSF enhances PAF- and FMLP-induced adherence to endothelial cells. J Allergy Clin Immunol 87:303, 1991. Abstract.
261. Toogood JH: Complications of topical steroid therapy for asthma. Am Rev Respir Dis 141:S89, 1990.
262. Toogood JH, Baskerville JC, Jennings B, et al: Influence of frequent dosing schedule on the response of chronic asthmatics to the aerosol steroid, budesonide. J Allergy Clin Immunol 122:288, 1982.
263. Tsicopoulos A, Tonnel AB, Wallaert B, et al: Decrease of IgE-dependent platelet activation in Hymenoptera hypersensitivity after specific rush desensitization. Clin Exp Immunol 71:433, 1988.
264. Turner ES, Greenberger PA, Patterson R: Management of the pregnant asthmatic patient. Ann Intern Meal 93:905, 1980.
265. Twentyman OP, Finnerty JP, Harris A, et al: Protection against allergen induced asthma by salmeterol. Lancet 336:1338, 1990.
266. Ullman A, Hedner J, Svedmyr N: Inhaled salmeterol and salbutamol in asthmatic patients. An evaluation of asthma symptoms and the possible development of tachyphylaxis. Am Rev Respir Dis 142:571, 1990.
267. Unanue ER, Beller DI, Lu CY, et al: Antigen presentation: comments on its regulation and mechanism. J Immunol 132:1, 1984.
268. Van Bever HP, Stevens WJ: Suppression of the late asthmatic reaction by hyposensitization in asthmatic children allergic to house dust mites (Dermatophagoides pteronyssinus). Clin Exp Allergy 19:399, 1989.
269. Vercelli D, Jabara HH, Lee B-W, et al: Human recombinant interleukin 4 induced Fc RII/CD23 on normal human monocytes. J Exp Med 167:1406, 1988.
270. Walker C, Kaegi MK, Braun P, et al: Activated T-cells and eosinophilia

in bronchoalveolar lavages from subjects with asthma correlated with disease severity. J Allergy Clin Immunol 88:935, 1991.
271. Wallen N, Kita H, Weiler D, et al: Glucocorticoids inhibit cytokine-mediated eosinophil survival. J Immunol 147:3490, 1991.
272. Walsh GM, Mermod J, Hartnell A, et al: Human eosinophil, but not neutrophil, adherence to IL-1–stimulated human umbilical vascular endothelial cells is a4B1 (very late antigen-4) dependent. J Immunol 146:3419, 1991.
273. Walters EH, O'Byrne PM, Fabbri LM, et al: Control of neurotransmission by prostaglandins in canine trachealis smooth muscle. J Appl Physiol 57:129, 1984.
274. Wardlaw AJ, Dunnette S, Gleich GJ, et al: Eosinophils and mast cells in bronchoalveolar lavage in mild asthma, relationship to bronchial hyperreactivity. Am Rev Respir Dis 137:62, 1988.
275. Wardlaw AJ, Hay H, Cromwell O, et al: Leukotrienes, LTC4 and LTB4, in bronchoalveolar lavage fluid in bronchial asthma and other respiratory diseases. J Allergy Clin Immunol 84:19, 1989.
276. Watson ML, Kingsmore SF, Johnston GI, et al: Genomic organization of the selection family of leukocyte adhesion molecules on human and mouse chromosome I. J Exp Med 172:263, 1990.
277. Webb-Johnson DC, Andrews JL: Bronchodilator therapy. N Engl J Med 297(9):476, 1977.
278. Wegner CD, Gundel RH, Reilly P, et al: Intercellular adhesion molecule-1 (ICAM-1) in the pathogenesis of asthma. Science 247:456, 1990.
279. Weirenga EA, Snoek M, DeGroot C, et al: Evidence for compartmentalization of functional subsets of CD4+ T-lymphocytes in atopic patients. J Immunol 144:4651, 1990.
280. Weller PF, Lee CW, Foster DW, et al: Generation and metabolism of 5-lipoxygenase pathway leukotrienes by human eosinophils: predominant production of leukotriene C4. Proc Natl Acad Sci USA 80:7626, 1983.
281. Wenzel SE, Fowler AA III, Schwartz LB: Activation of pulmonary mast cells by bronchoalveolar allergen challenge. Am Rev Respir Dis 137:1002, 1988.
282. White SR, Left A: Epithelial damage in asthma. In Busse WW, Holgate ST (eds): Asthma and Rhinitis. Blackwell Scientific Publications, Cambridge, 1995, pp 599–611.
283. Wicker S, Armour C, Black J: Responsiveness of bronchial smooth muscle from asthmatic subjects to contractile and relaxant agonists. Pulm Pharmacol 1:25, 1988.
284. Wilkinson JRW, Crea AEG, Clark TJH, et al: Identification and characterization of a monocyte-derived neutrophil activating peptide in corticosteroid resistant bronchial asthma. J Clin Invest 84:1930, 1989.
285. Wodnar-Filipowicz A, Heusser CH, Moroni C: Production of haemopoietic growth factors GM-CSF and interleukin-3 by mast cells in response to IgE receptor-mediated activation. Nature 339:150, 1989.
286. Wood RA, Chapman MD, Adkinson NF Jr, et al: The effect of cat removal on allergen content in household dust samples. J Allergy Clin Immunol 83:730, 1989.
287. Woolcock AJ, Salome CM, Yan K: The shape of the dose response curve to histamine in asthmatic and normal subjects. Am Rev Respir Dis 130:72, 1984.
288. Zimmerman B, Lanner A, Enander I, et al: Total blood eosinophils, serum ECP and eosinophil protein X in childhood asthma, relationship to disease status and therapy. Clin Exp Allergy 23:564, 1993.

29 Exercise and Asthma

E. R. McFADDEN, JR.

Bronchial asthma is a common disorder. Perhaps as many as 10 to 12 million Americans are affected by this illness, and of all the stimuli that induce acute episodes, one of the most commonly encountered in practice is physical exertion. In a survey of more than 400 consecutive patients with asthma who were referred to my institution for evaluation, 94% indicated that physical exertion was a major cause of their air flow limitation. Because of its high prevalence and the fact that exercise is a real world stimulus that is potentially operational in the everyday lives of asthmatics, exercise-induced asthma can greatly contribute to the overall morbidity of this condition.

Supported in part by Grant HL3/3791 and Specialized Center of Research Grant (SCOR) HL 37117 from the National Heart Lung and Blood Institute and General Clinical Research Center Grant MO1 RR0080 from the National Center for Research Resources

DEFINITION AND PREVALENCE

Exercise-induced asthma (EIA) is a condition in which vigorous physical activity triggers acute airway narrowing in persons with heightened airway reactivity. Exercise-induced asthma is not a specific disease but, rather, part of the overall asthmatic diathesis in which exercise is but one of many stimuli that induce air flow limitation. Frequently, physical exertion is the first precipitant of asthma to appear; with time, however, others also emerge.

The prevalence of exercise-induced symptoms in asthmatics has been reported to range from 40% to 90%.[44, 68] The reasons for this variability are related to such factors as the severity of the exercise stress employed, the means used to measure the response, and failure to standardize the environmental variables that control the magnitude of the obstruction, such as the temperature and water content of the air breathed when the challenge was performed. In many studies in the past, purely arbitrary criteria have been used to define whether a subject developed EIA. These have varied from the detection of wheezing on auscultation to the recording of falls of various magnitudes in airway conductance or forced expiratory volumes or flow rates. At present, most authorities would agree that EIA is present when a 15% or greater decrease in 1-second forced expiratory volume (FEV_1) or peak expiratory flow rate (PEFR) develops in response to a challenge.

In experienced laboratories, virtually all asthmatics demonstrate a reduction in pulmonary mechanics to thermal provocations (i.e., exercise and hyperventilation) if the stimulus is intense enough. Airway obstruction with exertion is never seen in normals, but it can occur in first-degree relatives of asthmatics, atopic nonasthmatics, and patients with cystic fibrosis.[19, 34] It is important to make some objective measurement of lung function, and not merely to rely on the patient's subjective responses or physical findings to make a diagnosis. As many as 30 to 50% of people with exercise-induced asthma may be unaware that their resistance to airflow has increased. Occasionally, this increase can happen in the most unlikely individuals. For example, testing of members of the 1984 U. S. Olympic Team showed that 11% had asthma or experienced EIA.[66]

PATHOGENESIS

RESPIRATORY HEAT EXCHANGE

The mechanism for EIA has not fully been elucidated. It is known, however, that the pathogenesis of this condition is related to the transfer of thermal energy from the airway mucosa to the air stream and back during periods of hyperpnea.[6, 15, 16, 21, 22, 78, 79, 81] Whenever minute ventilation rises, the intrathoracic airways are forced to participate in the warming and humidification of the incoming air. Large minute ventilations and/or low temperatures (and so, low water contents) of the inspirate increase the thermal load on the airways and necessitate greater movement of heat and water from the mucosal surface to bring the air to body conditions of temperature and humidity. The greater the quantities of heat and water that have to be transferred, the larger the subsequent obstructive response. Conversely, low ventilations and high inspired air temperatures and humidity minimize the transfers, and so decrease the magnitude of the response. When there is no movement of heat and water from the respiratory tract during hyperpnea, airway obstruction does not develop at all. Quantitating this phenomenon in terms of respiratory heat exchange (RHE) has shown a direct relationship with the severity of EIA in any given patient.[21] Because airway cooling was an essential part of RHE, it was postulated that this event was somehow related to the development of airway narrowing.

The existence of cooling of the intrathoracic airways in humans was first inferred from measurement of temperature changes in the retrotracheal esophagus during hyperpnea.[18] Subsequently, techniques for directly measuring thermal fluxes within the tracheobronchial tree in exercising humans were developed, and they have confirmed this phenomenon.[31, 33, 52, 54] Construction of thermal maps from the mouth to the subsegmental bronchi of normal and asthmatic subjects under a variety of ventilatory circumstances, ranging from sedentary activity to strenuous exertion in ambient and frigid environments,[31, 33, 52] demonstrates that cooling of the intrathoracic airway is a normal physiologic event that occurs whenever ventilation rises and heat and water move from the mucosa to the air. Conditioning of inspired air is not confined to a single region of the respiratory tract, as formerly thought. Rather, it is a continuum that begins at the portal of entry and involves as much of the airways as is necessary to complete the task. As the air flows from the mouth toward the periphery of the lung, heat and water are added continuously to it as a function of the gradients that exist between the air stream and the mucosa. The higher the ventilation and the colder the air, the more the transfers, the lower the temperature at any point in the airways, and the farther out into the lung the air flows before it becomes fully saturated at body temperature. At levels of hyperpnea associated with heavy exercise, the inhalation of subfreezing air does not reach body conditions until well beyond the 8th- to 10th-generation airways.[31, 33, 52] It is likely that the heat required to bring the air to body conditions comes from the bronchial circulation, and as will be developed, this vascular bed is believed to play a prominent part in the pathogenesis of EIA.

The net effect of the thermal exchanges that occur during inspiration is to cool the airways so that, on expiration, recovery of heat and water can occur. The temperature of the airway surface is lowered both by the direct loss of heat energy to the air and by the evaporation of water. Of the two, the vast majority of energy is spent in vaporization. The two processes are linked, however, and one can not occur without the other. During expiration, the air exiting the alveoli is now warmer than the airway mucosa, so heat and water are returned from the air to the airway surface. As air stream temperature falls, its ability to hold water decreases, and water condenses back onto the mucosa. If the airways were perfect heat exchangers, input would equal recovery, and no net losses would occur. This is not the case, and environmental losses of heat and water are a normal part of respiration. The majority of them, however, come from the extrathoracic airways, with the mouth and pharynx accounting for approximately 50% of the total heat and water exchange that takes place during hyperpnea.[31, 33] Of the remainder, the central airways (glottis to segmental bronchi) account for only 15%, whereas the rest of the tracheobronchial tree accounts for 35%. Thus, the loss per unit surface is quite small.

The type of longitudinal distribution of heat exchange just described allows the upper airways to act as a thermal reservoir enabling large volumes of frigid or dry air to be inhaled for prolonged periods without materially affecting the status of the mucosal surface fluid of the lower airways. A further safeguard is also in place. The mouth and pharynx are continuously bathed by a hypotonic solution whose main constituent is water;[73] thus, water can be put into the inspirate without depleting the surface fluid of this region or increasing its tonicity. In this fashion, the thermal demands on the lower airways are kept to a minimum.

AIRWAY COOLING VERSUS MUCOSAL DRYING

A series of experiments from a number of laboratories have demonstrated that the severity of the bronchoconstriction following exercise can be manipulated by changing the thermal characteristics of the inspired air. For a fixed ventilation, humidification of the inspirate reduces the severity of the response,[6, 16, 21, 22, 78] whereas drying and cooling the air increase the bronchial narrowing.[19, 21, 22, 79] Inhaling air conditioned to body temperature and humidity during exercise prevents the obstruction from developing.[21, 22, 78, 81] For a given set of inspired conditions, high levels of ventilation result in greater responses than do low levels.[21] Thus, the greater the heat flux (i.e., the product of the evaporative losses from water flux and convective losses from heat movement), the greater the cooling of the airways, and the more marked the subsequent obstruction to air flow.

If a cause-and-effect relationship between heat flux and postexertional obstruction exists, then equivalent thermal burdens should result in equivalent obstruction even without exercise. This postulate was tested by having asymptomatic asthmatic subjects simulate the hyperpnea of moderate and severe workloads by performing eucapnic hyperventilation while breathing air mixtures at several different temperatures and humidities.[21] The airway consequences of voluntary hyperventilation exactly mirrored those seen with exercise when ventilation and inspired air conditions were matched. The severity of the obstruction was the same, as were the extent of airway cooling and the response to various drugs.[12, 13, 19, 20] When it became possible to directly record thermal events in the airways of humans during hyperpnea, Gilbert and colleagues[31] established that both exercise and hyperventilation produce identical triggering events.

It has been postulated that hyperpnea causes an evaporation of mucosal periciliary fluid and an increase in local osmolarity, which then result in mast cell degranulation and constriction of airway smooth muscle.[1, 2, 27, 75] At present, this is a purely theoretic construct without supporting data, and there is no evidence that drying of the intrathoracic airways occurs when ventilation is elevated. In fact, the opposite seems to be the case. Direct assessments of intrathoracic thermal fluxes during hyperpnea indicate that large changes in surface osmolarity do not occur, because the distributed nature of the conditioning process described previously prevents drying.[31, 33] Moreover, if the osmolarity theory were correct, the more time spent breathing desiccated air, the more drying there would be, and the worse the expected obstruction. Further, drugs such as atropine, which alter the availability of airway water, would worsen the effects of exercise; yet none of these events occurs.[12, 20, 36, 51, 74]

Those who favor the hyperosmolar postulate point to the fact that nonisotonic aerosols produce airway obstruction in asthma[77] and that this response correlates with that seen with exercise.[2, 5] Unfortunately, these associations cannot be construed as cause and effect. Nonisotonic aerosols produce disruption of airway mucosal integrity; exercise and hyperventilation do not.[37] Thus, osmotic and thermal stimuli do not appear to have the same pathogenesis. Equally important, association does not equal causality. The response to histamine and methacholine challenges correlate with each other and with exercise,[4, 5, 45, 62] yet no one assumes that they all have the same mechanism of action.

EIA AS A VASCULAR PHENOMENON

It has become apparent that airway cooling alone is only part of the story and that it must be followed by rapid rewarming for obstruction to develop.[32, 51, 57, 72, 81] The lower the fall in air stream temperatures during hyperpnea, the greater will be the initial rewarming and the ensuing air flow limitation. Hence, the size of the temperature differences between cooling and rewarming in the immediate posthyperpnea period directly determines the severity of the subsequent obstruction.[32] Small temperature changes are associated with minimal airway narrowing, whereas large changes produce symptomatic episodes of asthma. If either cooling or rewarming is altered by pharmacologic[32] or physical[29, 51] means, the magnitude of the obstruction follows suit.

For a fixed level of ventilation that produces a constant amount of airway cooling, altering the heat content of the inspired air after the exercise challenge is completed changes the size of obstruction in a very predictable fashion.[51] Inspiring hot humid air augments the response, whereas inspiring cold air attenuates it.[51] This is the exact opposite of what happens when air at these thermal conditions is inspired during exercise.[15, 21, 22, 78, 79] If the size of the temperature gradient is important, so also should be the rate at which the gradient develops. Slow rewarming has been found to abolish the effects of hyperventilation, whereas rapid rewarming increases obstruction.[51] Because the bronchial circulation is the primary blood supply and heat source for the tracheobronchial tree, it has been suggested that the findings just described could derive from a sudden increase in local blood flow and/or a change in vascular permeability.[29, 31–33, 51, 55, 70] The bronchial circulation is a systemic vascular bed and, like the capillaries in the skin, is exposed to fluctuations in local temperature.[52, 54] If it were thermally reactive, so that cooling induced a reactive hyperemia and edema of the walls, all of the preceding observations could be explained. In support of this theory, asthmatic airways have a hyperplastic capillary bed[25] that appears to be more permeable than normal.[74, 75] Constriction or dilatation of these vessels through the use of α or β agonists, fluid administration, or volume shifts with shock trousers during and/or after hyperpnea influences cooling and reheating as well as the associated changes in pulmonary mechanics.[29, 32]

MEDIATORS OF IMMEDIATE HYPERSENSITIVITY

Many argue that mediators of immediate hypersensitivity may play an important part in EIA. Unfortunately, experiments designed to document this association have been extremely inconsistent, and this issue remains controversial.[7, 11, 14, 23, 24, 38, 43, 48, 58, 60, 67, 76] Searches for various inflammatory compounds in blood, urine, and bronchial lavage fluid before and after exercise have produced conflicting results. Indirect assessments with the use of pharmacologic probes have also been problematic. Some drugs with activity against inflammatory cells or their products, such as cromolyn and nedocromil, are purported to be important in treating asthma and also influence exercise-induced asthma.[42, 69, 76] The specificity and selectivity of the available and experimental agents used thus far, however, are not sufficiently narrow to permit unequivocal conclusions to be reached.

CLINICAL FEATURES

Exercise-induced asthma is most commonly seen in children and young adults because of their high levels of physical activity, although patients of all ages can be affected. The intensity of expression rises and falls with the state of the underlying airway reactivity. In unusual circumstances, exposure to antigens or respiratory viruses may so increase bronchial lability that disabling episodes of obstruction can follow even minimal exertion.

During exercise, the airways dilate.[3] When the workload period is over, airway obstruction begins almost immediately, peaks in about 5 to 10 minutes, and then spontaneously resolves over the next 30 minutes.[3] For symptoms to occur, exertion needs to be sustained.[3] Short intense bouts of work lasting less than 2 minutes produce fewer problems than do longer periods of effort. Other than these caveats, there is little that is important about the duration of work. It was originally thought that a patient had to exercise for 6 to 8 minutes to produce a maximum response. This is now known not to be the case, and significant obstruction can be induced in the laboratory with 4 minutes of maximum effort.

Because of the effects of ventilation and heat content of the inspired air on determining the airway response, the severity of obstruction varies with both the exercise task and the environment in which it is undertaken. The more strenuous the work, the greater the ventilation required to meet metabolic demands, and the more intense the asthma attack. Thus, running produces more severe air flow limitation than jogging, which, in turn produces a more severe limitation than walking.[6, 15, 16, 21, 22, 78] It is important to appreciate that there is nothing inherently unique about the exercise task. Exercise serves only to increase ventilation, so there are no specific activities that an asthmatic should or should not undertake. This basic pattern is modified by the temperature profile of the air inhaled during each form of work. As described, when the inspirate is cold (which by definition is dry), or dry at any other temperature, obstruction maximizes, and when the air is warm and humid, it minimizes.[6, 15, 16, 21, 22, 78, 79] Clinically, these interactions cause identical types of exertion to have different consequences as the seasons change or as the activities move in and out of doors.

PHYSIOLOGIC FEATURES

The attacks of asthma precipitated by exertion are indistinguishable from those that follow other stimuli. Wheezing, dyspnea, cough, and chest tightness in association with hyperinflation, air flow limitation, and hypoxemia are the usual symptomatic and physiologic manifestations.[3] In atypical circumstances, cough may be the sole complaint. The chief difficulty with exercise is not so much the severity of the attacks, but the propensity for it to interfere daily in the lives of affected individuals by forcing them to limit their activities. In contrast to antigen, aspirin, β blockers, and viral infection, exercise does not cause prolonged and/or intense obstruction that threatens the patient's safety or requires hospitalization for resolution.

Exercise is the only natural precipitant of asthma that induces tachyphylaxis.[26, 56] When bouts of work are repetitively performed within 40 minutes or less of each other, the bronchial narrowing progressively decreases. Clinically, this means that a patient can limit the obstructive consequences of vigorous activity by first undertaking a short warm-up period. Experience indicates, however, that there is little or no protection unless the warm-up is fairly strenuous and task specific. The loss of response to repetitive exercise has been called the "refractory period," but the term is misleading. The airways are only "refractory" to exercise and will readily constrict with other stimuli.[84] The latest evidence suggests that a loss of vascular responsiveness with a consequent disruption of the cooling-rewarming gradient may be important.[30]

LATE REACTIONS

The tendency toward spontaneous remission is a hallmark of EIA. In fact, it is a therapeutic maxim that one needs only to reverse the acute event and the patient will continue to be free of symptoms. Recurrent episodes of asthma such as those that follow antigen or viral exposure have never been reported in the days following single or multiple bouts of exercise. Despite these clinical data, some have suggested that exercise produces a dual obstructive pattern[9–11, 28, 39, 40] associated with the elaboration of mediators of immediate hypersensitivity.[50] However, not all investigators have found a late reaction with exercise,[17, 72, 86] and some positive studies have not used appropriate analysis or controls.[10, 11, 40, 41] Consequently, the issue remains contentious.

Well-controlled studies involving more than 100 patients have demonstrated that exercise produces self-limited, spontaneously remitting, nonrecurrent airway narrowing in the majority.[72, 86] A small number of patients can have a second wave of bronchoconstriction, but it appears to be a nonspecific phenomenon related to the withdrawal of medication.[72, 86] For example, the patients with cyclic changes in lung function due to EIA develop the same phenomenon even when the initial phase of obstruction is eliminated by the inhalation of hot humid air (thermal manipulation known to prevent the release of mediators[49]) and when they are given methacholine to inhale. More importantly, even if late reactions do occur, they do not have any secondary sequelae. There is no increase in airway reactivity following an exercise challenge, nor do late reactions induce nocturnal asthma.[85] Late reactions have not been repeated with isocapnic hyperventilation[82] even though this stimulus produces the same thermal and physiologic events as exercise.

DIAGNOSIS

The diagnosis of exercise-induced asthma is readily made. Salient historical points are the types and levels of exercise that produce the problem, the conditions that modify it, the timing of the onset of the obstruction, and symptoms that develop. It is also important to determine medication use, because drugs such as calcium channel blockers, H_1 antihistamines, and α agonists and antagonists, if taken before a challenge, can produce false-negative results. Many in clinical practice make the diagnosis of exercise-induced asthma solely on the basis of historical criteria. As previously indicated, however, such information can be misleading. For example, glottic dysfunction and tracheal narrowing produce obstructive symptoms whenever ventilation rises. The correct diagnosis can be established only by a detailed assessment of pulmonary mechanics following an appropriate challenge.

The presence of EIA is confirmed by recording a fall in peak expiratory flow rates or 1-second forced expiratory volume of 15% or greater after a thermal challenge. This is an arbitrarily defined end point, but one that has long been in use. Exercise protocols based upon duration of work or achieving a fixed heart rate have been proposed as standards; however, they are complex and unfortunately do not monitor the relevant variables. Again, the key elements in a challenge are the level of ventilation, the heat content of the inspired air, and the presence or absence of a warm-up or its thermal equivalent. To produce a maximum response, taking large ventilations while inhaling frigid air followed by abrupt recovery on room air are required. This translates into maximum workloads. It is immaterial physiologically whether the increase in ventilation is arrived at on a treadmill or bicycle or by voluntary hyperventilation.[31] Typically, if the FEV_1 is 65% of predicted or greater, an exercise challenge can be safely undertaken.

Exercise testing in clinical practice has both diagnostic and therapeutic indications. This form of challenge has the advantage that it is a naturally occurring stimulus that is technically simple to perform and is maximally selective for asthmatics. Thus, it is indicated in any patient who gives a history of exertionally induced airway symptoms such as cough, dyspnea, and/or wheezing. Exercise challenges are also quite useful in individuals who give a history compatible with EIA but do not respond to the usual therapeutic approaches. In these patients, the effects of various bronchodilator agents or other medications on the subjects' exercise response can be directly evaluated in the laboratory. The only absolute contraindication to the performance of exercise is concomitant cardiac disease that produces arrhythmias or coronary ischemia or otherwise limits exercise performance.

My colleagues and I find it easier to use cycle ergometers than treadmills, because the workload in the latter involves controlling speed, inclination, and patient interactions with the device. With a cycle, obstruction can readily be induced with 4 minutes of work at 50% to 60% of the subject's predicted maximum oxygen consumption ($\dot{V}O_2max$). With this load, ventilation reaches significantly high levels to cause a response in all but the most fit subjects; in which case, 90% $\dot{V}O_2max$ may be required. In some elite athletes, it may be difficult to provide a challenge in the laboratory sufficient to evoke symptoms because of the combination of activities and muscle groups used. This is particularly true for sports requiring high-intensity effort of variable duration (e.g., boxing, hockey, figure skating, track sprints, basketball). When we encounter this situation, we test the subjects in their local environment while they perform the activities that induce their problems.

The disadvantages of exercise provocations are that they represent only a single point on a stimulus-response curve and that their applicability is confined to individuals capable of performing and sustaining vigorous exertion. To extend the utility of thermal provocations, isocapnic hyperventilation with dry air at frigid or ambient temperatures has been employed.[21, 76] Despite notions to the contrary, there are no inherent differences between these techniques save for the temperature of the air. As pointed out earlier, frigid air by definition is dry. Its low heat content simply adds an additional thermal burden to that of dry air at room temperature. Because voluntary hyperpnea does not require the subjects to physically work, it is free of any cardiac or systemic stresses and can be safely used in anyone. Stimulus-response curves can also be easily generated to examine overall airway reactivity.

THERAPY

Exercise-induced asthma can occur as an isolated event episodically in the life of an asthmatic or as part of the overall symptom complex. When EIA is one of many stimuli that induce problems for the patient, treatment aimed at lowering airway reactivity is essential. As the underlying bronchial hyperresponsiveness improves with inhaled anti-inflammatory agents, the obstructive consequences of hyperpnea diminish. Ultimate control of the patient's acute problems depends, however, upon pretreating, before exertional activities are undertaken.

If the patient has only EIA, regularly scheduled medications are not necessary, and therapy consists of aerosols of β_2 agonists, cromolyn, or nedocromil given 10 to 15 minutes before exertion on an as-needed basis.[35, 47, 71, 80] The adrenergic aerosols are the treatment of choice, and they typically protect patients from all but the most severe exertional activities. They can also be used to reverse obstruction once it develops. The chief difficulty with the current short-acting β_2 agonists is that the protective effects only last a few hours. Thus, if exercise is to be repeated over the course of the day, repetitive doses of medication are required. Cromolyn and nedocromil only attenuate the response to exercise and do not abolish it totally. They, too, have a relatively short duration of protection that rarely exceeds several hours. The advent of long-acting β_2 agonists, such as salmeterol and formoterol, have solved these problems. These drugs prevent thermally induced obstruction from developing over the course of 10 to 12 hours, but it takes 20 to 30 minutes for selmeterol to have an effect. For breakthrough wheezing, a short-acting β_2 agonist, and not more salmeterol, is required.[35]

Oral sympathomimetics and methylxanthines are not very effective agents for treating this condition because of the difficulty of coordinating physical activity with the development of therapeutic blood levels. Similarly, anticholinergics do not work well because of their slow onset of action and inconsistent effects on the bronchoconstriction. The use of glucorticoids before exercise is ineffective; however, lowering airway reactivity with these compounds may provide some benefit. Antihistamines, α_1-adrenergic antagonists, calcium channel blockers, and inhaled diuretics offer little, and their use should be considered experimental.

REFERENCES

1. Aitken ML, Marini JJ: Effect of heat delivery and extraction on airway conductance in normal and asthmatic subjects. Am Rev Respir Dis 131:357–361, 1985.

2. Anderson SD: Is there a unifying hypothesis for exercise induced asthma? J Allergy Clin Immunol 73:660–665, 1984.
3. Anderson SD, Silverman M, Konig P, Godfrey J: Exercise-induced asthma. Br J Dis Chest 69:1–39, 1975.
4. Anderton RC, Cuff MT, Frith PA, et al: Bronchial responsiveness to inhaled histamine and exercise. J Allergy Clin Immunol 63:315–320, 1979.
5. Aquilina AT: Comparison of airway reactivity induced by histamine, methacholine, and isocapnic hyperventilation in normal and asthmatic subjects. Thorax 38:766–770, 1983.
6. Bar-Or O, Neuman I, Dotan R: Effects of dry and humid climates on exercise-induced asthma in children and preadolescents. J Allergy Clin Immunol 60:163–168, 1977.
7. Barnes PJ, Brown MJ: Venous plasma histamine in exercise and hyperventilation induced asthma in man. Clin Sci 61:159, 1962.
8. Belcher NG, Murdoch R, Dalton N, et al: Circulating concentrations of histamine, neutrophile chemotactic activity and catecholamines during the refractory period in exercise induced asthma. J Allergy Clin Immunol 81:100–115, 1988.
9. Bierman CW, Spiro SG, Petheram I: Characterization of the late response in exercise-induced asthma. J Allergy Clin Immunol 74:701, 1984.
10. Boner A, Niero E, Antolini I, et al: Biphasic (early and late) asthmatic responses to exercise in children with severe asthma, resident at high altitude. Eur J Pediatr 144:164, 1985.
11. Boulet LP, Legris C, Turcotte H, et al: Prevalence and characteristics of late asthmatic response to exercise. J Allergy Clin Immunol 80:655, 1987.
12. Breslin FJ, McFadden ER Jr, Ingram RH Jr, et al: Effects of atropine on respiratory heat loss in asthma. J Appl Physiol Respir Envir Exerc Physiol 48:619–623, 1980.
13. Breslin FJ, McFadden ER Jr, Ingram RH Jr: The effect of cromolyn sodium on the airway response to hyperpnea and cold air in asthma. Am Rev Respir Dis 122:11–16, 1980.
14. Brode DH, Eisman S, Ramsdell JW, et al: Airway levels of mast cell–derived mediators in exercise-induced asthma. Am Rev Respir Dis 141:503–508, 1990.
15. Bundgaard A, Ingemann-Hansen J, Schmidt A, et al: Influence of temperature and relative humidity of inhaled gas on exercise-induced asthma. Eur J Respir Dis 63:239–244, 1982.
16. Chen WY, Horton DJ: Heat and water loss from the airways and exercise-induced asthma. Respiration 34:305–313, 1977.
17. Dahl R, Henriksen JM: Development of late asthmatic reactions after allergen or exercise challenge tests. Eur J Respir Dis 61:320–324, 1980.
18. Deal EC Jr, McFadden ER Jr, Ingram RH Jr, et al: Esophageal temperature during exercise in asthmatic and unasthmatic subjects. J Appl Physiol 46:484–490, 1979.
19. Deal EC Jr, McFadden ER Jr, Ingram RH Jr, et al: Airway responsiveness to cold air and hyperpnea in normal subjects and in those with hay fever and asthma. Am Rev Respir Dis 121:621–628, 1980.
20. Deal EC Jr, McFadden ER Jr, Ingram RH Jr, et al: Effects of atropine on potentiation of exercise-induced bronchospasm by cold air. J Appl Physiol Respir Envir Exerc Physiol 45:238–243, 1978.
21. Deal EC Jr, McFadden ER Jr, Ingram RH Jr, et al: The role of respiratory heat exchange in the production of exercise-induced asthma. J Appl Physiol 46:467–475, 1979.
22. Deal EC Jr, McFadden ER Jr, Ingram RH Jr, et al: Hyperpnea and heat flux: Initial reaction sequence in exercise-induced asthma. J Appl Physiol 46:467–483, 1979.
23. Deal EC Jr, Wasserman SI, Soter NA, et al: Evaluation of role played by mediators of immediate hypersensitivity in exercise induced asthma. J Clin Invest 65:659–665, 1980.
24. Del Bono N, Petrini M, Dente F, et al: L'Attivita' chemotattica per I neutrofili (NCA) dopo bronchospasms indotto da esercizio fisico (EIB) in asmatici atropici. Folia Allergol Immunol Clin 31:111, 1984.
25. Dunill MD: The pathology of asthma with special reference to changes in the bronchial mucosa. J Clin Pathol 13:27–33, 1960.
26. Edmunds AT, Tooley M, Godfrey S: The refractory period after exercise-induced asthma: its duration and relationship to the severity of exercise. Am Rev Respir Dis 117:247–254, 1978.
27. Eschenbacher WL, Sheppard D: Respiratory heat loss is not the sole stimulus for bronchoconstriction induced by isocapnic hyperpnea with dry air. Am Rev Respir Dis 131:894–901, 1985.
28. Foresi A, Mattoli S, Corbo GM, et al: Late bronchial response and increase in methacholine hyperresponsiveness after exercise and distilled water challenge in atopic subjects with asthma with dual asthmatic response to allergen inhalation. J Allergy Clin Immunol 78:1130–1139, 1986.
29. Gilbert IA, Regnard J, Lenner KA, et al: Intrathoracic airstream temperatures during acute expansions of thoracic blood volume. Clin Sci 81:655–666, 1991.
30. Gilbert IA, Fouke JM, McFadden ER Jr: The effect of repetitive exercise on airway temperature. Am Rev Respir Dis 142:826–831, 1990.
31. Gilbert IA, Fouke J, McFadden ER Jr: Intra-airway thermodynamics during exercise and hyperventilation in asthmatics. J Appl Physiol 64:2167–2174, 1988.
32. Gilbert IA, McFadden ER Jr: Airway cooling and rewarming: the second reaction sequence in exercise induced asthma. J Clin Invest 90:699–704, 1991.
33. Gilbert IA, Fouke JM, McFadden ER Jr: Heat and water flux in the intrathoracic airways and exercise induced asthma. J Appl Physiol 63:1681–1691, 1987.
34. Godfrey S, Konig P: Exercise induced bronchial lability in wheezing children and their families. Pediatrics 56:851–854, 1975.
35. Green CP, Price JF: Prevention of exercise-induced asthma by inhaled salmeterol xinafoate. Arch Dis Child 67:1014–1017, 1992.
36. Griffin MP, Fung KJ, Ingram RH Jr, et al: Dose-response effects of atropine on thermal stimulus-response relationships in asthma. J Appl Physiol 53:1576–1582, 1982.
37. Higenbottam T, Stokes T, Jamieson S, et al: A comparison of exercise, hyperventilation with cold air and warm air and the inhalation of "fog" in the provocation of asthma. Eur J Respir Dis 64(suppl 128):421, 1983.
38. Holgate ST, Church MK, Cushley MJ, et al: Pharmacologic modulation of airway caliber and mediator release in human models of bronchial asthma. In Kay B, Austen KF, Lichtenstein L (eds): Asthma: Physiology, Immunopharmacology and Treatment. Third International Symposium. Academic Press, London, 1984, p 391.
39. Horn CR, Jones RM, Lee D, et al: Late response in exercise-induced asthma. Clin Allergy 14:307–309, 1984.
40. Iikura Y, Nagakura T, Lee TH: Factors predisposing to exercise-induced late asthmatic responses. J Allergy Clin Immunol 75:285, 1985.
41. Inman MD, Watson RM, Killian KJ, et al: Methacholine airway responsiveness decreases during exercise in asthmatic subjects. Am Rev Respir Dis 141:1414–1417, 1990.
42. Israel E, Demarkarin R, Rosenberg M, et al: The effects of a 5-lipoxygenase inhibition on asthma induced by cold dry air. N Engl J Med 323:1740–1744, 1990.
43. Jarjour NN, Calhoun WJ: Exercise-induced asthma is not associated with mast cell activation or airway inflammation. J Allergy Clin Immunol 89:60–68, 1992.
44. Jones RS, Buston MH, Wharton MJ: The effect of exercise on ventilatory function in children with asthma. Br J Dis Chest; 56:78–86, 1962.
45. Juniper EF, Frith PA, Dunnett E, et al: Reproducibility and comparison of responses to inhaled histamine and methacholine. Thorax 33:705–710, 1978.
46. Laitinen LA, Laitinen A, Widdicombe J: Effects of inflammatory and other mediators on airway vascular beds. Am Rev Respir Dis 135:S67–S70, 1987.
47. Latimer KM, O'Byrne PM, Morris MM, et al: Bronchoconstriction stimulated by airway cooling: better protection with combined inhalation of terbutaline sulfate and cromolyn sodium than either alone. Am Rev Respir Dis 128:440–443, 1983.
48. Lee TH, Brown MJ, Nagy L, et al: Exercise-induced release of histamine and neutrophil chemotactic factor in atopic asthmatics. J Allergy Clin Immunol 70:73, 1982.
49. Lee TH, Assoufi BK, Kay AB: The link between exercise, respiratory heat exchange, and the mast cell in bronchial asthma. Lancet 1:520–552, 1983.
50. Lee TH, Nagakura T, Papageorgiou N, et al: Exercise-induced late asthmatic reactions with neutrophil chemotactic activity. N Engl J Med 308:1502–1505, 1983.
51. McFadden ER Jr, Lenner KA, Strohl KP: Post-exertional airway rewarming and thermally-induced asthma. J Clin Invest 78:18–25, 1986.
52. McFadden ER Jr, Pichurko B, Bowman F, et al: Thermal mapping of the airways in man. J Appl Physiol 58:564–570, 1985.
53. McFadden ER Jr, Gilbert IA: Asthma. N Engl J Med 327:1928–1937, 1992.
54. McFadden ER Jr: Respiratory heat and water exchange: physiological and clinical implications. J Appl Physiol 54:331–335, 1983.
55. McFadden ER Jr: Exercise-induced asthma as a vascular phenomenon. Lancet 335:880–883, 1990.

56. McNeill RS, Nairn JR, Millar J, et al: Exercise-induced asthma. Q J Med 35:55–67, 1966.
57. Mihalyka M, Wong J, James AL, et al: The effect on airway function of inspired air conditions following isocapnic hyperventilation with dry air. J Allergy Clin Immunol 82:842–848, 1988.
58. Morgan DJR, Phillips MJ, Moodley I, et al: Histamine, neutrophil chemotactic factor and circulating basophil levels following exercise in asthmatic and control subjects. Clin Allergy 12:29, 1982.
59. Mussaffi H, Springer C, Godfrey S: Increased bronchial responsiveness to exercise and histamine after allergen challenge in children with asthma. J Allergy Clin Immunol 77:48–52, 1986.
60. Nagakura T, Lee TH, Assoufi BK, et al: Neutrophil chemotactic factor in exercise and hyperventilation induced asthma. Am Rev Respir Dis 128:294, 1983.
61. National Asthma Education Program Expert Panel Report: Guidelines for the diagnosis and management of asthma. US Department of Health and Human Services Publication No. 01:3042, 1991, pp 119–125.
62. O'Byrne PM, Ryan G, Morris M, et al: Asthma induced by cold air and its relation to nonspecific bronchial responsiveness to methacholine. Am Rev Respir Dis 125:281–285, 1982.
63. Persson CGA: Leakage of macromolecules from the tracheobronchial microcirculation. Am Rev Respir Dis 135(suppl):71–75, 1987.
64. Persson CGA: Role of plasma exudation in asthmatic airways. Lancet 2:1126–1129, 1968.
65. Philips YY, Jaeger JJ, Laube BL, et al: Eucapnic voluntary hyperventilation of compressed gas mixture: a simple system for bronchial challenge by respiratory heat loss. Am Rev Respir Dis 131:31–35, 1985.
66. Pierson WE, Voy RO: Exercise-induced bronchospasm in the XXIII summer Olympic games. N Engl Reg Allergy Proceed 9:209–213, 1988.
67. Pliss LB, Ingenito EP, Ingram RK Jr, et al: Assessment of bronchoalveolar cell and mediator response to isocapnic hyperpnea in asthma. Am Rev Respir Dis 142:73–78, 1990.
68. Poppins H, Morttari A, Krens KE, et al: Exercise asthma and disodium cromoglycate. Br Med J 4:337–339, 1970.
69. Roberts JA, Thomson NC: Attenuation of exercise-induced asthma by pretreatment with nodocromil sodium and minocromil. Clin Allergy 15:377–381, 1985.
70. Robinson PJ, Hillian CH, Blackie SW, et al: Airway rewarming and rehydration elicits bronchoconstriction despite continued hyperventilation is asthmatic subjects (abstract). Am Rev Respir Dis 141:A476, 1990.
71. Rossing TH, Weiss JW, Breslin FJ, et al: Effects of inhaled sympathomimetics on obstructive response to respiratory heat loss. J Appl Physiol 52:1119–1123, 1982.
72. Rubinstein I, Hak H, Wells J, et al: Immediate and delayed bronchoconstriction after exercise in patients with asthma. N Engl J Med 317:482, 1987.
73. Schneyer LH, Schneyer CA: Inorganic composition of saliva. In Code CF (ed): Handbook of physiology, vol 2: Alimentary Canal: Secretion. American Physiological Society, Washington DC, 1968, pp 497–530.
74. Sheppard E, Epstein J, Holtzman MJ, et al: Dose-dependent inhibition of cold-air-induced bronchoconstriction by atropine. J Appl Physiol 53:169–174, 1982.
75. Sheppard D, Eschenbacher WL: Respiratory water loss as a stimulus to exercise-induced bronchoconstriction asthma. J Allergy Clin Immunol 73:640–642, 1984.
76. Smith CM, Christie PE, Hawksworth RJ, et al: Urinary leukotriene E_4 levels after allergen and exercise challenge in bronchial asthma. Am Rev Respir Dis 144:1411–1413, 1991.
77. Smith CM, Anderson SD: Inhalation provocation tests using nonisotonic aerosols. J Allergy Clin Immunol 84:781–790, 1989.
78. Strauss RH, McFadden ER Jr, Ingram RH Jr, et al: Influence of heat and humidity on the airway obstruction induced by exercise in asthma. J Clin Invest 61:433–440, 1978.
79. Strauss RH, McFadden ER Jr, Ingram RH Jr, et al: Enhancement of exercise-induced asthma by cold air breathing. N Engl J Med 297:743–747, 1977.
80. Tullett WM, Tan KM, Wall RJ, et al: Dose-response effect of sodium cromoglycate pressurized aerosol in exercise induced asthma. Thorax 45:41–44, 1985.
81. Turcotte H, Boulet LP: Effects of inspired air and water content on exercise-induced bronchospasm in asthma. Eur Respir J 4:979–984, 1991.
82. Varga EM, Eger E, Zach MS: Cold air challenge for measuring airway reactivity in children: Lack of a late reaction. Lung 108:267–272, 1990.
83. Venge P, Herikson J, Pahl R, et al: Exercise-induced asthma and the generation of neutrophil chemotactic activity. J Allergy Clin Immunol 84:293–295, 1990.
84. Weiler-Ravell D, Godfrey S: Do exercise and antigen-induced asthma utilize the same pathways? J Allergy Clin Immunol 67:391–399, 1981.
85. Zawadski DK, Lenner KA, McFadden ER Jr: Effect of exercise on nonspecific airway reactivity in asthmatics. J Appl Physiol 64:812–816, 1988.
86. Zawadski DK, Lenner KA, McFadden ER Jr: Re-examination of the late asthmatic response to exercise. Am Rev Respir Dis 137:837–841, 1988.

30 Occupationally Induced Asthma

JONATHAN A. BERNSTEIN I. LEONARD BERNSTEIN

Occupational asthma (OA) can be defined as "a disease characterized by variable airflow limitation and/or airway hyperresponsiveness due to causes and conditions attributable to a particular occupational environment and not to stimuli encountered outside the workplace."[1] A more complete definition of OA should always consider the onset of disease in the presence or absence of an initial latency period of exposure. If a defined latency period exists, the underlying mechanism of OA is more apt to be immunologically mediated, although in many instances, specific immunologic mechanisms have not been confirmed or identified. OA in the absence of a latency period is referred to as *irritant-induced asthma* or the *reactive airways dysfunction syndrome* (RADS), which is characterized by the sudden onset of asthma (12 to 24 hours) after a single exposure to irritant concentrations of a chemical or solvent. RADS is discussed in more detail later in this chapter.[21]

Certain asthma-like disorders have not been included as part of the definition of OA because bronchial hyperresponsiveness (BHR) or eosinophilia is not an associated feature. Asthma-like disorders include byssinosis, which occurs in textile workers exposed to a variety of dusts from cotton, flax, hemp, or jute.[21]

INCIDENCE

Occupational asthma is estimated to account for 2% to 15% of all new cases of asthma worldwide each year.[19] However, the actual prevalence or incidence of OA has been difficult to establish because of international differences in reporting systems designed to document new cases of OA. Another reason for this information gap is physician apathy in reporting new cases of OA. More than 200 agents have been recognized to cause OA, and the list is expanding as industrial technology becomes more sophisticated.[22]

Because of the general consensus that the diagnosis of OA should be established as soon as possible in order to minimize long-term morbidity, some countries have established government-supported programs to compile information about the prevalence, causes, and natural course of OA.[18, 76] These programs have been helpful in the evaluation and monitoring of large populations of workers in a variety of industries.[10] The Surveillance of Work Related and Occupational Respiratory Disease (SWORD) has been established in the United Kingdom to facilitate the voluntary reporting of occupational respiratory illnesses by pulmonologists and occupational health physicians.[76] After 1 year of operation, SWORD reported that 26.4% of all work-related respiratory diseases were secondary to OA and that the most common cause (22%) was diisocyanates. One criticism of SWORD is that it uses only case definitions to establish a diagnosis of OA and does not require objective tests to confirm reported cases.[76]

A comparable program established in the United States is the Sentinel Health Notification System for Occupational Risks (SENSOR).[8] This system, currently operational in 10 states, was originally established in Michigan, which by law requires that all physicians report all cases of occupational disease. However, preliminary results have revealed that new cases of occupational lung disease were reported by only 0.7% of the physicians targeted to participate in SENSOR, in contrast to 83% participation by physicians in SWORD.[8] This discrepancy has been accounted for by the lack of a focused group of reporting physicians as well as of a standardized approach to collecting information for the SENSOR database.

Finland has a well-established and effective national registry for identification of all new cases of occupational respiratory diseases and their specific causes.[8] This registry has succeeded in compiling sufficiently accurate data to enable yearly estimates of the incidence of both OA and hypersensitivity pneumonitis. These national registries are also intended to shed light on relevant risk factors for developing OA in specific industries, thereby improving the current approaches of surveillance and prevention of OA.[8]

PATHOGENESIS

Knowledge of the pathogenesis of OA has been significantly enhanced by the use of bronchoalveolar lavage (BAL) and transbronchial biopsy techniques in the evaluation of workers with OA.[42, 47] Compared with patients with nonoccupational asthma, workers with OA exhibit very similar patterns of airway inflammation. The characteristic pathologic findings in OA are bronchial mucosal edema, smooth muscle hypertrophy, and basement membrane thickening characterized by subepithelial deposition of collagen beneath the lamina reticularis.[7, 50, 88] Bronchoalveolar lavage analysis of asymptomatic subjects with nonoccupational asthma and subjects with inactive OA shows similar distributions of inflammatory cells, consisting of 90% to 95% alveolar macrophages, 5% to 10% lymphocytes, and <1% leukocytes and epithelial cells.[50] However, the BAL inflammatory cell profile from workers with active OA differs, in that eosinophils and neutrophils are more prominent.[50]

Serial bronchial biopsies of workers with toluene diisocyanate (TDI) induced OA have also found increased numbers of eosinophils, mast cells, and activated lymphocytes with a thickened reticular basement membrane secondary to collagen deposition (types I, III, and V) compared with normal nonasthmatic subjects.[89, 90] The eosinophilia in these workers directly correlated with mRNA expression of interleukin-5 (IL-5), the interleukin responsible for growth, differentiation, and activation of eosinophils.[89] Electron microscopic evaluation of these biopsy specimens has also revealed widening of interepithelial cell spaces. This finding has led to speculation that a loss of tight junctions and intercellular adhesion molecules could potentiate the influx of inflammatory cells into the airways.[104]

Increased levels of the bioactive mediators histamine and leukotriene E_4 (LTE_4) have been demonstrated in workers with western red cedar OA immediately after plicatic acid bronchoprovocation. Similarly, increased concentrations of LTB_4 and LTE_4 were detected in the BAL fluid and urine, respectively, after TDI bronchoprovocation.[39, 107]

PHYSIOLOGY

Bronchoprovocation using specific agents corresponds very well with the worker's occupational history and the histopathologic changes demonstrated by BAL and transbronchial biopsy.[42, 47] Workers sensitized to high molecular weight (HMW) substances primarily exhibit either isolated immediate or dual airway responses, whereas workers sensitized to low molecular weight (LMW) chemical xenobiotics manifest more diverse patterns of bronchospastic reactions. For example, 10% to 20% of workers with diisocyanate or red cedar OA responded with isolated early asthmatic reactions (EARs), 30% to 50% of workers exhibited isolated late asthmatic reactions (LARs), and 30% to 60% of workers experienced dual asthmatic reactions (DARs).[50]

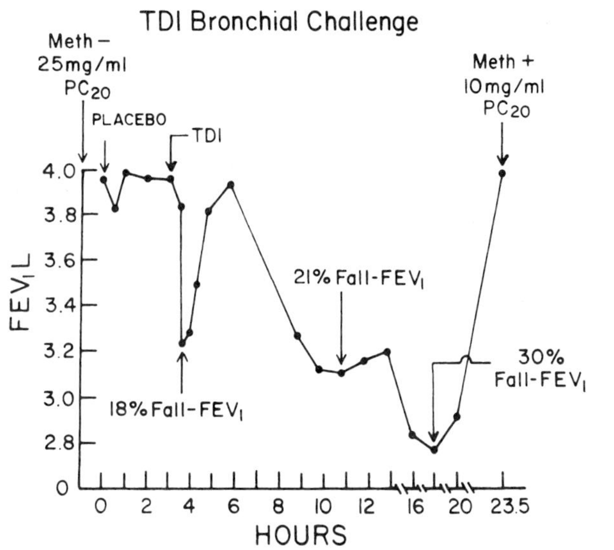

FIGURE 30–1. A dual-phase response in a polyurethane foam worker after bronchial provocation with toluene diisocyanate (TDI). Early-phase bronchospasm is followed by spontaneous recovery, which in turn is followed by late-phase bronchospasm. The concentration of methacholine required to reduce the forced expiratory volume in 1 second (FEV_1) by 20% (PC_{20}) fell from a baseline normal of 25 mg/mL to 10 mg/mL the day after TDI challenge. (From Bernstein DI: Occupational asthma. Med Clin North Am 76:917, 1992.)

The EAR correlates with the release of preformed and newly formed bioactive mediators, whereas the LAR, which occurs 4 to 12 hours after exposure to a specific antigen, correlates with the influx of inflammatory cells into the airways.[50] Resolution of the LAR is typically associated with a measurable increase in nonspecific bronchial hyperresponsiveness (NSBH). However, studies in our laboratory, which were subsequently confirmed in another research center, demonstrated that increased NSBH may actually precede the LAR as early as 2 hours. A dual asthmatic reaction after TDI bronchoprovocation in a worker suspected of having occupational asthma is illustrated in Figure 30–1.[9] It should be noted that 24 hours after the specific challenge, nonspecific bronchial hyperresponsiveness as measured by methacholine challenge increased over the prechallenge, baseline level.[9]

ANIMAL MODELS FOR OCCUPATIONAL ASTHMA

A number of animal models have been used to investigate potential immunologic and nonimmunologic mechanisms of OA. Guinea pigs sensitized to diisocyanates were initially used to detect haptenic determinant specific immunoglobulin IgE and IgG antibodies. Guinea pigs have also been used to study the direct effect of diisocyanates on lung immunopathology and to evaluate the role of neurogenic inflammation induced by neuropeptides after TDI exposure. Guinea pig afferent nerve endings exposed to toluene diisocyanate have been demonstrated to release the tachykinins substance P and neurokinin A, resulting in increased airway responsiveness.[50, 93] Bronchial hyperresponsiveness was reversed by depleting these nerve endings of tachykinins by pretreatment with capsaicin and was potentiated by TDI's direct inhibition of neutral endopeptidase, the enzyme responsible for tachykinin degradation.[93] Rhesus monkeys and Sprague-Dawley rats have also been used to study the various immune mechanisms associated with platinum salt and acid anhydride sensitization.[11]

One of the most intriguing uses of animal models thus far has been that of BALB/c mice to study the role of T lymphocytes in the pathogenesis of OA induced by LMW chemical xenobiotics. This model has been used to study the differential production of cytokines by helper T-cell subsets (Th1 and Th2) after sensitization and reexposure to a variety of reactive chemicals.[45, 46] Normally, helper T-cell mediated immune responses in BALB/c mice may be directed to two pathways: (1) Th1 lymphocytes, which primarily secrete IL-2, gamma interferon (γ-IFN), and tumor necrosis factor–β (TNF-β); and (2) Th2 lymphocytes, which secrete IL-4, IL-5, IL-6, IL-10, and IL-13.[79, 80] A predominance of Th2 cells is associated with IgE immune responses, whereas a predominance of Th1 cells heralds the development of IgG and cell-mediated immune responses.[79, 80] Dearman and colleagues[45, 46] demonstrated preferential activation of T lymphocytes with a Th2 cytokine profile when mice were immunized with phthalic anhydride (PA), trimellitic anhydride (TMA), or methylenediphenyldiisocyanate (MDI); in contrast, Th1 immune profiles were induced after immunization with dinitrochlorobenzene (DNCB), a common contact-sensitizing agent. These experiments suggested that the chemical structure of occupational allergens may be an important determinant in the induction of IgE immune responses.[45, 46]

COGNATE AND NONCOGNATE MECHANISMS

Occupational asthma occurs in a spectrum of work environments, including pharmaceutical, textile, and automobile manufacturing, food processing, hair care, printing, farming, smelting, soldering, metal plating, tanning, and brewing.[22] The classification of occupational asthma mechanisms is summarized in Table 30–1.[22] Specific etiologic agents of OA may exert their effects through either cognate (immune) or noncognate pathways. Traditionally, these agents have been

TABLE 30–1
CLASSIFICATION OF OCCUPATIONAL ASTHMA MECHANISMS

Nonimmunologic mechanisms	Reflex bronchoconstriction
	Irritant bronchoconstriction (i.e., reactive airways dysfunction syndrome)
	Pharmacologically induced bronchoconstriction
Immunologic mechanisms	Immediate hypersensitivity response (IgE mediated)
	High molecular weight allergens
	Low molecular weight allergens (e.g., haptens)
	Mixed (immunologic and nonimmunologic) allergens
	IgG antibody and/or immune (antigen-antibody) complex response
	Complement pathway activation
	Cell-mediated

From Bernstein JA: Occupational asthma. Postgrad Med 92:109, 1992.

classified according to their respective molecular weights and biologic sources. Separating etiologic agents of OA into high and low molecular weight categories permits a clearer distinction between the underlying mechanisms of these disorders (Tables 30–2 and 30–3).[43]

HIGH MOLECULAR WEIGHT AGENTS

High molecular weight agents (>1,000 kD) induce OA primarily through IgE-mediated mechanisms.[9] Atopic individuals in occupations that require persistent contact with HMW proteins (e.g., laboratory technicians, food processors, veterinarians, enzyme workers, farmers) are at greater risk of being sensitized and developing OA.[16] Cutaneous testing to many HMW protein allergens is useful for confirming the specific agent responsible for inducing OA.[9]

LOW MOLECULAR WEIGHT AGENTS

Low molecular weight substances (<1,000 kD) induce OA by both immunologic and nonimmunologic mechanisms (see Table 30–1).[22] LMW agents must be linked with an endogenous protein carrier such as albumin prior to acquisition of immunogenic potential.[18] This reaction, referred to as *haptenation*, results in the formation of a new antigenic determinant (NAD).[18] Acid anhydrides and polyisocyanates are good examples of chemical compounds capable of inducing specific IgE antibody responses after haptenation.[13, 54, 68]

Other immunologic mechanisms through which LMW agents exert their effects are as follows:

1. A type II, cytotoxic reaction, as exemplified by the hemolytic anemia and pulmonary hemorrhage syndrome observed in workers exposed to high concentrations of trimellitic anhydride (TMA) fumes.[106]
2. A type III, immune complex–mediated reaction that has been postulated to account for the late respiratory systemic syndrome (LRSS) (see later) in TMA workers who develop cough, wheezing, shortness of breath, and the systemic symptoms chills, myalgias, and arthralgias.[106]
3. Type IV, cell-mediated hypersensitivity responses that can be demonstrated after exposure to many LMW chemicals.

There is an impressive body of evidence supporting a central role for T lymphocytes in the pathogenesis of diisocyanate-induced OA.[19] Avery and coworkers[2] first demonstrated lymphocyte blast transformation in symptomatic diisocyanate workers, and Gallagher and colleagues[54] later confirmed this finding by demonstrating the presence of in vitro leukocyte inhibitory factor produced by peripheral blood leukocytes from symptomatic workers stimulated with TDI-HSA (human serum albumin). Increased numbers of CD8+ cells have been found in the peripheral blood of workers with TDI-induced OA after TDI challenge, and increased numbers of CD8+ cells and eosinophils have been found in BAL fluids from workers with confirmed TDI asthma.[50, 51] Furthermore, peripheral blood mononuclear cells from workers with nickel- and cobalt-induced OA have been found to proliferate when co-incubated with nickel and cobalt metallic salts, respectively.[59, 61]

Preliminary data also suggest that workers susceptible to developing nickel-induced OA may have preferential expression of the T-cell receptor (TCR) Vβ 14 gene segment.[59] Similar observations of selective TCR Vβ gene segment (1 and 5) expansion in response to diisocyanate exposure in workers with diisocyanate-induced OA have been noted.[24b] Secretion of an antigen-dependent histamine-releasing factor has been demonstrated in association with diisocyanate-induced OA.[58] Peripheral blood basophil cells from some workers with western red cedar asthma have been shown to release histamine when incubated with low concentrations of plicatic acid, but it is still unclear whether complement fragments (i.e., C3a and C5a) or plicatic acid itself is responsible for this response.[37]

IRRITANT-INDUCED ASTHMA

Irritant-induced asthma or RADS was initially described as occurring after a single exposure to high concentrations of fumes, gases, acids, anhydrous ammonium, or other toxic chemicals, resulting in acute-onset bronchial hyperresponsiveness (BHR) and asthma symptoms.[27, 29] As more cases are recognized, it has become apparent that repetitive exposures to smaller concentrations of these substances may also evoke a slower-onset form of RADS. The classic form of RADS is characterized by absence of a latency period, but this may not be as clear-cut in slower-onset RADS.

The RADS syndrome is histopathologically very similar to asthma. Nonspecific bronchial hyperresponsiveness (NSBH) and asthma symptoms may persist in affected individuals for months or years after exposure.[27, 29] Nonimmunologic (noncognate) or neurogenic mechanisms are thought to account for this syndrome. Damage to bronchial epithelial cells by these air toxics could permit their easier access into the lamina propria and subepithelial tissues, accounting for the persistent NSBH that these patients experience.

RADS-inciting substances could also exert direct effects on inflammatory cells and the bronchial microvasculature.[92] For instance, phthalic anhydride has been shown to exhibit a neurogenic effect by stimulating local release of substance P and calcitonin gene related peptide (CGRP) from afferent nerve endings, independent of the central nervous system.[99] Substance P has been demonstrated to activate mast cells in the skin but not in the respiratory tract. However, it and other tachykinins may cause degranulation of airway eosinophils and monocytes, causing the release of mediators and cytokines that are capable of inducing and perpetuating airway inflammation.[3, 4] Diisocyanates have been reported to cause RADS in several instances, leading one to consider whether noncognate mechanisms may play a significant role in the underlying pathogenesis of diisocyanate-induced OA.[66]

PHARMACOLOGICALLY INDUCED ASTHMA

The pharmacologically induced form of OA includes bronchospasm induced by organophosphate insecticides and cholinesterase inhibitors. These substances exert their effect by inhibiting the degradation of acetylcholine with subsequent accumulation of this transmitter in the neuronal synaptic clefts.[19] Pharmacologic mechanisms have also been proposed

TABLE 30–2
CAUSES OF OCCUPATIONAL ASTHMA: ALLERGIC MECHANISM IN HIGH MOLECULAR WEIGHT COMPOUNDS*

Agents	Occupations	No. of Subjects	Prevalence	Skin Test	Specific IgE	Precipitin Test	Bronchoprovocation
Animal products,	Laboratory workers						
insects, others	Veterinarians	1,487	3.1%				
Laboratory animals	Animal handlers	399	7.5%	+			+ (12/12)
rats, mice,		179	11.7%	+		−	
rabbits, guinea		130	30.4%	+			
pigs		146	10.3%	+			
		5		+	+	−	+ (5/5)
		11					
Birds							
Pigeon, budgerigar	Pigeon breeders						+ (9/10)
Chicken	Poultry workers	10		+			+ (1/1)
	Bird fanciers	14		+	+		
Insects							
Grain mite	Grain workers	1		+		+	+
Locust	Research laboratory	119	26%	+	+		
River fly	Workers in power plants along rivers	1,284	3.1%	+			
Screw worm fly	Flight crews	182	70%	+			
Cockroach	Laboratory workers	10		+			+ (4/10)
Cricket	Field contact	1		+	−	−	+
Bee moth	Fish bait breeders	18	5.5%	+		−	+
Moth and butterfly	Entomologists	2		+			
Plants							
Grain dust	Grain handlers	17		+		+	+ (8/15)
		22		−	−	−	+ (6/22)
		11		+		+	+ (5/11)
Wheat/rye flour	Bakers, millers	1		+	+	−	
		2		+		+	+ (2/2)
		4		+	+		+ (1/2)
		7		+	+		+ (4/7)
		31		+	+		+ (22/31)
Buckwheat	Bakers	3		+			+ (2/3)
Coffee beans	Food processors	6		+	+		+
Castor bean	Oil industry	5			+		
Tea	Teaworker	1		+			
Tobacco leaf	Tobacco manufacturing	1		+			
Hops *(Humulus lupulus)*	Brewery chemist	1		+			
Biologic enzymes							
Bacillus subtilis	Detergent industry	3		+	+		+ (3/3)
		98	50%	+			
		38	66%	+	+	+	+ (9/10)
Trypsin	Plastic, pharmaceutical	14	29%	+	+	−	+ (3/4)
Pancreatin	Pharmaceutical	5					
Papain	Laboratory packaging	1		+	+	+	+ (8/9)
		33	46%	+	+	−	+
Pepsin	Pharmaceutical	1		+	+		
Flaviastase	Pharmaceutical	3		+	+	+	+ (2/2)
Bromelin	Pharmaceutical	2		+			
Fungal amylase	Manufacturing, bakers	5		+			
Vegetable Gums							
Gum acacia	Printers	2		+			+ (1/1)
		63					
Gum tragacanth	Gum manufacturing	1	51%	+			
Others							
Crab	Crab processing	303	16%	+	+		+ (33/57)
Prawns	Prawn processing	50	36%	+	+		+ (2/2)
Hoya	Oyster farm	1,413	29%	+	+		
Larva of silkworm	Sericulature	5,519	0.2%	+	+		+ (9/9)

From Chan-Yeung M: Occupational asthma—state of the art. Am Rev Respir Dis 133:686, 1986.
*A blank indicates test not performed. The parentheses under bronchoprovocation indicate number positive of those tested.

TABLE 30–3
CAUSES OF OCCUPATIONAL ASTHMA: ALLERGIC OR POSSIBLY ALLERGIC MECHANISM IN LOW MOLECULAR WEIGHT*

Agents	Occupations	No. of Subjects	Prevalence	Skin Test	Specific IgE	Precipitin Test	Bronchoprovocation	
Diisocyanates								
Toluene diisocyanate	Polyurethane industries, plastics, varnish	4					+	(4/4)
		21	38%	−		−		
		112	12.5%	+	−	−	+	(5/11)
		23	17.4%		+			
		15		+	−			
		26			+		+	(26/26)
		17			−		+	(14/17)
		195						
			28%		+		+	(12/17)
Diphenylmethane diisocyanate	Foundries	57	5%	−				
		1		−	+			
		11			+		+	(6/11)
		1			−	+	+	
Hexamethylene diisocyanate	Automobile spray painting							
Anhydrides								
Phthalic anhydride	Epoxy resins, plastics	4					+	(3/3)
		1		+	+		+	
Trimellitic anhydride	Epoxy resins, plastics	14	29%	+	+		+	(1/1)
Tetrachlorophthalic anhydride	Epoxy resins, plastics	14	36%		+			
		5			−	−	+	(3/3)
Wood dust								
Western red cedar *(Thuja plicata)*	Carpenter, construction, cabinetmaker, sawmill worker	6						
		1,320	3.4%	+				
		22		+		−	+	(18/22)
		185			+		+	(185/185)
California redwood *(Sequoia sempervirens)*		2		−		−	+	(2/2)
Cedar of Lebanon *(Cedra libani)*		6		−		−		
Cocabolla *(Dalbergia resusa)*		2		−				
Iroko *(Chlorophora excelsa)*		1		+		+	+	
Oak *(Quercus robur)*		1		−		+	+	
Mahogany (*Shorreal* sp)		1		−		+	+	
Abiruana *(Pouteria)*		2		+		−	+	(2/2)
African maple *(Triplochiton scleroxylon)*		2		+	+		+	(2/2)
						−		
Tanganyika *Aningre*		3		+	−		+	(3/3)
Central American walnut *(Juglans olanchana)*		1		−	−	−	+	
Kejaat *(Pterocarpus angolensis)*		1		+		−		
African zebra wood *(Microberlinia)*		1		+	+		+	
Metals								
Platinum	Platinum refinery	91	57%	+				
		16		+			+	(10/16)
Nickel	Metal plating	1		+		−	+	
		1		+	−	−	+	
		1		+	+	+	+	
Chromium	Tanning	1	−	+		+		
		1	+					
		1	+					
Cobalt	Hard metal industry	4		+		+	+	(2/4)
Vanadium	Hard metal industry	12	33%					
Tungsten carbide	Hard metal industry	1						

TABLE 30–3
CAUSES OF OCCUPATIONAL ASTHMA: ALLERGIC OR POSSIBLY ALLERGIC MECHANISM IN LOW MOLECULAR WEIGHT* *(Continued)*

Agents	Occupations	No. of Subjects	Prevalence	Skin Test	Specific IgE	Precipitin Test	Bronchoprovocation
Fluxes							
Aminoethyl ethanolamine	Aluminum soldering	3					+ (3/3)
		2		–			+ (2/2)
Colophony	Electronic	51					+ (34/51)
Drugs							
Penicillins	Pharmaceutical	4		–			+ (3/4)
Cephalosporins	Pharmaceutical	2		+			+ (2/2)
Phenylglycine acid chloride	Pharmaceutical	24	29%	+	+		+ (2/2)
				+	+		
Piperazine hydrochloride	Chemist	2		+			+ (2/2)
Psyllium	Laxative manufacturer	3		+			+ (2/3)
Methyldopa	Pharmaceutical	1		–			+
Spiramycin	Pharmaceutical	1		+			+
Salbutamol intermediate	Pharmaceutical	1					+
Amprolium hydrochloride	Poultry feed mixer	1					+
Tetracycline	Pharmaceutical	1					+
Sulphone chloramides	Manufacturers, brewery	12		+			
Other chemicals							
Dimethyl ethanolamine	Spray painting	1		–			+
Persulfate salts and henna	Hairdressing	2		+			+ (2/2)
				–			+
Ethylenediamine	Photography	1	18.5%	–			
Azodicarbonamide	Plastics and rubber	151					
Diazonium salt	Photocopying and dye	1					+
Hexachlorophene (sterilizing agent)	Hospital staff	1	29%				+
Formalin	Hospital staff	28		–			+ (2/4)
Urea formaldehyde	Insulation, resin	2					+ (2/2)
	Refrigeration	1					+
Freon		1	37.5%	+			
Paraphenylene diamine	Fur dyers	80					+
Furfuryl alcohol (furan-based resin)	Foundry mold makers	1					+

From Chan-Yeung M: Occupational asthma—state of the art. Am Rev Respir Dis 133:686, 1986.
*A blank indicates test not performed. The parentheses under bronchoprovocation indicate number positive of those tested.

to explain bronchoconstrictive responses observed after inhalation of endotoxin by workers exposed to cotton dust and swine excreta.[75] The cross-shift decrements in lung function observed in pharmaceutical workers continuously exposed to opiate byproducts are presumably secondary to the direct pharmacologic release of histamine from mast cells.[26] Pharmacologic mechanisms have also been postulated to be involved in meat wrapper's asthma and wood dust asthma.[37, 100]

CAUSES

HMW AGENTS

High molecular weight agents account for most of the known causes of OA in industry and are primarily derived from animal sources (i.e., saliva, urine, skin, and dander) and plant byproducts (see Table 30–2).[16]

Occupational asthma has been associated with exposure to insects and their byproducts in grain workers, insect breeders, entomologists, and fishbait (e.g., mealworm larvae) handlers.[12, 74] The storage mites *Glycyphagus destructor, Acarus siro,* and *Tyrophagus putrescentiae,* which are known contaminants of grain and flour, have been well documented to cause OA.[16] Grain dust asthma has been described in farmers sensitized to different byproducts of grain dust, including these storage mites.[40] Specific bronchoprovocation studies using crude grain dust or grain dust mite extracts have been useful for confirming this diagnosis.[40] However, it should be noted that granary workers are more likely to develop chronic bronchitis.[40]

Flour dust is a plant byproduct containing a number of potentially sensitizing allergens, including cereal proteins, mold spores, grain mites, and microbial enzymes. Workers with baker's asthma become sensitized to soluble and insoluble wheat fractions. Albumin derived from wheat allergen has been found to be the most common sensitizing allergen in bakers, but barley, rye, oat, and triticale cereal proteins and, less frequently, buckwheat and soy flour proteins have also been found to be sensitizing.[16] Baker's asthma can also result from sensitization to the enzymes α-amylase and hemicellulase, which are commonly used as dough conditioners.[6]

Latex has also been recognized as an important occupational allergen in health care professionals. The rubber antigen in latex gloves derived from the rubber plant, *Hevea brasiliensis*, may induce OA in approximately 6% of exposed health care professionals.[98] Latex may also cause systemic anaphylaxis, urticaria, or angioedema with or without respiratory symptoms.

Food-processing workers who are exposed to egg white proteins (conalbumin, ovalbumin, ovomucoid, and lysozyme), coffee beans, spices, and soy proteins are at risk for OA.[15, 95] Other food-derived agents associated with OA are tea and garlic dusts, pectin, mushroom powder, green coffee beans, and seeds (flaxseed and linseed).[16]

Enzymes derived from animals or plants are also well-known causes of OA. Occupational asthma secondary to microbial detergent enzymes at one time occurred in up to 30% of exposed workers and was more prevalent among those with an atopic history.[53, 84, 85] These enzymes are derived primarily from *Bacillus subtilis* and *Aspergillus* species. Egg lysozyme, used in the food and pharmaceutical industries, has been shown to be a specific inducer of OA by inhalational exposure.[23] Skin prick testing is a more sensitive method for longitudinal monitoring and detection of workers at risk for sensitization to enzymes than in vitro tests such as enzyme-linked immunosorbent assay (ELISA) and radioallergosorbent test (RAST).[17]

Vegetable gums are HMW carbohydrate products used as thickening agents in foods, as emulsifying agents in lotions and creams, as substrates in pills, and as sizing material for paper and textiles.[33] Printer's asthma was once the most common cause of OA induced by vegetable gums.[52] The causative agent, gum acacia, has been subsequently replaced by other materials in the printing industry because of the increased frequency with which workers experienced symptoms.[33, 52] Sensitization to the vegetable gum guar gum, detected by skin prick testing, has been found in 5% of exposed carpet factory workers, 2% of whom were confirmed to have OA by specific bronchial challenge.[70]

LOW MOLECULAR WEIGHT AGENTS

A variety of LMW substances are known to induce OA (see Table 30–3).[43]

Diisocyanates

Diisocyanates are the most common cause of OA among LMW chemicals, as 5% to 10% of diisocyanate-exposed workers develop OA.[18] Diisocyanates have reactive N=C=O side groups, making this chemical class useful in the production of polyurethane foams, plastimers, adhesives, varnishes, coatings, and paint hardeners.[18] It has been estimated that more than 100,000 workers in the United States are exposed to diisocyanates in their work environment each year. The three most commonly used diisocyanate compounds in industry are hexamethylene diisocyanate (HDI), methylenediphenyldiisocyanate (MDI), and toluene diisocyanate (TDI).[60] Although the chemical properties of diisocyanate compounds vary, workers sensitized to one compound may exhibit significant bronchial cross-reactivity to other diisocyanate chemicals.[5, 60]

The natural history of diisocyanate-induced OA is variable, in that some workers may have complete remission following cessation of exposure, whereas others may experience NSBH for years after removal of workplace exposure.[78] Risk factors for development of diisocyanate-induced OA have not been thoroughly identified, but repetitive exposure to accidental spills is a recurrent theme in the history of many workers with OA.[73]

As mentioned earlier, workers with diisocyanate-induced OA demonstrate a variable spectrum of serum-specific antibody responses to diisocyanate antigens.[5, 60] Specific IgG antibodies to diisocyanate conjugates are observed in as many as 70% of HDI- and MDI-exposed workers with OA, whereas TDI-exposed workers commonly fail to demonstrate specific antibody responses.[57, 64, 67] Serum-specific antibody assays with diisocyanate-HSA conjugates are of limited value in the diagnosis of diisocyanate OA, because increased antibody levels can be detected in workers with either positive or negative responses to inhalational diisocyanate challenge.[34] Skin testing with diisocyanate conjugates is less sensitive than assays for serum-specific IgE.[34, 54] Diisocyanates have also been demonstrated to cause RADS and hypersensitivity pneumonitis syndromes.[54, 66]

Acid Anhydrides

Acid anhydrides are reactive organic compounds that are constituents of alkyd and epoxy resins found in paints, varnishes, and plastics.[101] TMA is a useful plasticizing agent for the production of wire and cable coatings and in the manufacturing of paints, textiles, and paper goods.[101]

Exposure to acid anhydride chemicals has the broadest spectrum of clinical presentation among LMW agent exposures. Several immunologic mechanisms have been implicated, as described earlier.[101] Workers with anhydride exposure can present with rhinitis and asthma symptoms that begin after a latency period of exposure and recur after reexposure. This presentation has been confirmed to be a type I IgE-mediated mechanisms for phthalic (PA), trimellitic (TMA), hexahydrophthalic (HHPA), himic (HA), and tetrachlorophthalic (TCPA) anhydrides.[101] ELISA, in conjunction with skin testing to acid anhydride conjugates, have acted as sensitive markers of exposure and subsequent development of OA.[105] However, some exposed workers may present with cough, wheezing, malaise, chills, myalgias, and arthralgias 4 to 12 hours after anhydride exposure, a presentation that may resemble hypersensitivity pneumonitis. This has been termed the *late respiratory systemic syndrome*.[101] Anhydride workers have experienced hemoptysis, pulmonary infiltrates on chest radiographs, anemia, and restrictive lung disease after a high-dose, long-term exposure to TMA fumes, whereas RADS has been reported in workers after their first exposure to TMA fumes.[101]

Wood Dusts

Wood dusts cause a variety of occupationally related lung disorders, including hypersensitivity pneumonitis, organic dust syndrome, asthma, chronic bronchitis, and a mucous membrane irritation syndrome.[38, 49]

Longitudinal studies of workers exposed to western red cedar dust have found that approximately 5% develop OA.[40] Western red cedar wood dust contains a variety of chemicals, including tannin, dyes, pitch, resins, and gums.[38] These chemicals are extracted by steam distillation from the cedar wood to form volatile and nonvolatile components.[38] The volatile components contain primarily tropolones and natural fungicides, which protect the wood from decay, whereas nonvolatile residues include plicatic acid, the organic component responsible for red cedar OA.[38] Atopy and nonspecific bronchial hyperresponsiveness are not risk factors for developing red cedar OA. In fact, nonsmokers and ex-smokers have been found to have a greater likelihood for developing red cedar OA compared with active smokers.[40] Specific inhalation tests to plicatic acid are characterized by either DARs or isolated LARs.[40] Because immediate skin testing and serum IgE antibodies are not diagnostically useful, specific bronchial challenge to plicatic acid is often necessary to confirm a diagnosis of OA.[82]

Several other wood dusts that have been recognized as causes of OA are African maplewood and zebrawood, mahogany, and Quillaja bark.[40] Microbial contaminants of wood dusts have been identified as causes of hypersensitivity pneumonitis disorders in maple bark disease, sequoiosis, suberosis, and wood pulp worker's disease. These diseases are caused by immunologic responses to a variety of fungi, such as *Cryptostroma corticale* (maple bark disease), *Alternaria* species (wood pulp worker's disease), *Aspergillus* species, and *Thermoactinomyces vulgaris* (sawmill worker's disease) that contaminate the wood dust or bark of the tree.[40] Wood dusts have also been implicated in other nonrespiratory symptoms, including allergic conjunctivitis, rhinitis, dermatitis, and adenocarcinoma of the nasal pharynx.[40]

Metallic Salts

Metallic salts have been documented to cause OA in addition to chemical pneumonitis, bronchitis, pulmonary emphysema, and adult respiratory distress syndrome (ARDS).[81] Metallic salts cause respiratory diseases through both immunologic and nonimmunologic mechanisms.[20] The most extensively studied metallic salts are platinum, nickel, chromium, and cobalt salts.[20]

Platinum salts are highly allergenic and have a high prevalence of skin sensitization compared with other metallic salts.[20, 28] Atopy and cigarette smoking constitute known risk factors for cutaneous and bronchial sensitizations to halide platinum salts.[25] The immunopathogenesis of platinum salt induced OA has been demonstrated to be primarily IgE-mediated, although the presence of platinum-HSA specific reaginic IgG_4 antibody has also been reported.[25]

Nickel is widely used in mining, milling, smelting, and refinishing processes and can be extremely toxic to the central nervous system. Nickel-induced OA is very rare, and nickel-specific IgE antibodies have been found in only a few, individual cases.[20, 71] Chromium is used in electroplating processes, leather tanning, and the production of cement. Exposure to the hexavalent chromium salt has been associated with OA.[32, 77] IgE- and cell-mediated immune responses may be involved in chromium metallic salt induced asthma.[32, 77] Cobalt salts induce OA in approximately 5% of exposed workers, and this condition should be distinguished from hard metal diseases, which can result in interstitial pneumonia and pulmonary fibrosis.[56, 94] Some workers with cobalt-induced OA have been found to produce specific IgE antibodies.[94]

The metallic salts vanadium pentoxide, zinc oxide, cadmium, and aluminum (potroom asthma) have also been associated with respiratory diseases.[20] For instance, patients with metal fume fever and potroom asthma present with shortness of breath, wheezing, chest tightness, and coughing that begin hours after exposure.[20] These two disorders can be differentiated, because symptoms of metal fume fever usually subside 1 to 2 days after the patient's removal from the workplace, whereas symptoms of potroom asthma may persist.[20]

Colophony

Colophony fumes may cause OA in susceptible electronic soldering workers.[30] Colophony is derived from pine tree resin containing abietic, pumaric, and dihydroabietic acids, the putative causative compounds in OA.[30, 31] Atopic workers with preexisting asthma are at greatest risk for developing OA due to colophony fumes.[31] Immune mechanisms have not been demonstrated for colophony-induced OA, and therefore, confirmation often depends on specific inhalational challenges or serial peak expiratory flow rate (PEFR) studies performed at work. Persistence of BHR and asthma symptoms is common among affected workers even after they have been removed from the workplace.[30, 31]

Other Chemicals

Other LMW chemicals identified or suspected of causing OA are primary, secondary, tertiary, and quaternary amines; formaldehyde; sulfonechloramide (chloramine T); azo-reactive dyes; persulfates; diazonium salts; and a variety of pharmaceutical agents (i.e., β-lactam, macrolide, and tetracycline antibiotics, hydralazine, isoniazid, penicillamine, and methyldopa).[24a, 69] Pyrolysis fumes emitted from polyvinyl chloride (PVC) have been associated with meat wrapper's asthma.[83, 100] Other chemicals associated with OA but for which immune mechanisms have not been defined are methyl methacrylates, freon, hexachlorophene, furan, styrene, machining fluid, and noxious fumes from concentrated acids.[69] Many of these chemical agents could be inducing OA through noncognate mechanisms such as those described for irritant-induced asthma or RADS.

EPIDEMIOLOGY

Well-designed epidemiologic studies can yield important information regarding prevalence, exposure-response relationships, and risk factors associated with specific causes of OA. Most of the OA epidemiologic studies thus far have been "cross-sectional" surveys that can only estimate the prevalence data within specific industries.[18] One major criticism of cross-sectional surveys therefore has been the great potential for underestimation of the true incidence of OA, because many symptomatic workers quit their jobs prior to a medical diagnosis, the so-called healthy worker effect.[8] Few well-designed, prospective, longitudinal studies have been performed to study OA because of cost factors and insufficient access to exposed worker populations.[14, 55, 76]

A properly designed epidemiologic study should evaluate the temporal association between a worker's environmental exposure and clinical symptoms.[96] Occupational questionnaires have been used to identify symptomatic individuals, but these often lack adequate specificity for OA and alone are not reliable for diagnosing OA.[8, 72] A well-designed questionnaire should elicit detailed information about previous work history, current job description, previous or current exposures at home or work, asthma and rhinitis symptoms, and smoking history as well as the personal and familial atopic histories.[96]

Workers who satisfy a case definition on the basis of questionnaire responses should be further evaluated using physiologic lung function tests at work and any appropriate immunologic methods to confirm or refute the diagnosis of OA. Such data could also be used to estimate disease prevalence and host risk factors.

RISK FACTORS FOR OCCUPATIONAL ASTHMA

The relationship between exposure and OA has been well demonstrated for laboratory animal handlers, locust research workers, snowcrab and prawn processors, bakers, papain workers, enzyme detergent processors, sawmill and furniture factory workers, electronic and steel coating workers, and TDI production workers.[16, 34] *Atopy,* defined as cutaneous reactivity to environmental aeroallergens, has been implicated as an important risk factor for OA in workers exposed to certain HMW (>1,000 kD) compounds, such as detergent enzymes and laboratory animal proteins. A similar relationship between atopy and OA has not been established for most LMW (< 1,000 kD) compounds.[8, 16]

Cigarette smoking is a risk factor among platinum workers and snowcrab processors.[8] Venables and associates[103] reported that cigarette smoking and atopy were coassociation risk factors for IgE-mediated sensitization to tetrachlorophthalic anhydride (TCPA). However, Liss and coworkers[63] found contradictory results, in that nonsmokers were more likely to become sensitized to TCPA than smokers.[63] Chan-Yeung and colleagues[41] found a similar increased association between red cedar induced OA and absence of cigarette smoking. NSBH has not been established to be a risk factor for OA at present.[33]

DIAGNOSIS

HISTORY

An algorithmic approach for establishing a diagnosis of OA is strongly recommended.[9] It begins with obtaining an accurate occupational history to establish a relationship between respiratory symptoms and work environment. Workers may present with a spectrum of lower respiratory symptoms, including dyspnea, chest tightness, wheezing, and cough, in addition to concomitant upper airway symptoms, such as rhinorrhea, nasal congestion, and ocular pruritus. The onset of symptoms is variable, as they can begin minutes, hours, or days after the worker comes to work. Symptoms typically improve when the worker is away from work and recur with reexposure but also may appear to be worse when away from work in those workers who exhibit an isolated LAR.[9, 10] Furthermore, it may not be possible to readily observe improvement of symptoms if a worker's OA has been chronic and severe. Individuals with preexisting asthma can sometimes be mistakenly diagnosed with OA if they work in places where irritants, cold temperatures, or exercise can aggravate their symptoms.[9] However, a preexisting history of asthma does not exclude a diagnosis of OA, particularly if there is a long hiatus between the last appearance of natural asthma and current work-related symptoms.[9]

A detailed environmental employment history should also be obtained to identify direct and indirect exposures to suspected agents. It includes an accurate description of the work environment and specific duties, which should contain information about the physical form of exposure, such as fumes, dusts, or aerosols. Information should be obtained on accidental spills, which often are associated with high-dose toxic exposures to fumes, smoke, or chemicals and may predispose the worker to develop OA.[9, 10] Material safety data sheets (MSDSs), should be obtained for review of all potential agent(s) that could be responsible for inducing OA. Industrial hygienists may be able to assist in providing information about the worksite's exposure levels if these are available.[9, 10]

DIFFERENTIAL DIAGNOSIS

The differential diagnosis of OA includes chronic obstructive pulmonary disease (COPD), hypersensitivity pneumonitis, bronchiolitis obliterans, grain fever, metal fume fever, mill fever, and byssinosis. The history and objective testing can be helpful in differentiating OA from these diseases. Workers with COPD usually have a history of significant tobacco abuse, and their respiratory symptoms do not correlate with workplace exposure. Bronchiolitis obliterans can be very difficult to differentiate definitively from asthma, especially when it is associated with asthma. In certain cases, bronchiolitis obliterans has been noted to occur within weeks after exposure to irritant gas inhalation, which may be confused with RADS as discussed earlier.[29] Allergic bronchopulmonary aspergillosis can be a cause of bronchiolitis obliterans (see Chapter 31).

Workers with byssinosis usually present with chest tightness 2 to 3 hours after exposure that persists and may get worse away from exposure, indicating that there is a loss of exposure tolerance.[40] This symptom may occur with new exposure after a vacation or at the start of the work week, since many experience tolerance of some sort later in the week with repeated exposure. Workers with mill fever or grain fever experience chills, headache, nausea or vomiting, fever, and fatigue 8 to 12 hours after exposure to cotton dust or grain dust, respectively, that subside over a few days after their removal from exposure.[40] Metal fume fever has been described as a nonasthmatic syndrome in welders consisting of fever, myalgias, cough, and shortness of breath lasting 1 to 2 days after welding fume inhalation.[20] This syndrome may also have a tolerance phenomenon with repeated exposure. A diagnosis of hypersensitivity pneumonitis requires a consistent clinical history and environmental and serologic evidence of exposure to known causative agents, such as mold spores or bacteria (see Chapter 32). Abnormal chest radiograph findings, a reduction in diffusing capacity (DLCO), and hypoxia are usually present. In some instances, histologic confirmation or a specific bronchoprovocation test for the suspected agent is required to make a definitive diagnosis.[40]

RADIOGRAPHY AND LABORATORY TESTING

Chest radiographs should be performed in all workers being evaluated for OA. Measurement of DLCO, although typically normal in asthma patients, can be helpful in distinguishing restrictive disorders from OA.[9, 10] Methacholine or histamine inhalation tests, when negative, are helpful in excluding a diagnosis of OA because of their high negative predictive value. A positive methacholine test for NSBH still requires demonstration that symptoms and lung function improve when the worker is away from work and recur after the worker returns to work. Serial PD_{20} measurements—provocative dose of methacholine or histamine required to cause a 20% decrease in FEV_1 (1-second forced expiratory volume)—made with the worker at and away from work are useful for demonstrating changes in NSBH. They are considered to be useful adjunctive objective tests for establishing a diagnosis of OA.[9, 44]

Serial PEFRs are the simplest screening tests available for measuring lung function at and away from the workplace. PEFRs should be recorded for at least 2 weeks, every 2 to 3 hours, with the worker at and away from work while work exposure and asthma medication usage are documented. A 24-hour PEFR showing variability of at-work values of more than 15% to 20% from at-home values is considered an abnormal response compatible with OA. However, it should be noted that PEFR variability measurements can be problematic, inasmuch as recordings can be falsified and do not identify specific causative agents responsible for OA. The availability of computerized PEFR devices that prohibit a worker from tampering with readings circumvents the malingering factor to some extent, but close supervision is still required to ensure compliance.[9, 10]

The specific inhalation challenge test is considered the standard test for diagnosing OA if a suspect substance in the workplace can be identified and if the test is performed within a reasonable period after OA is diagnosed.[36] Because the technology and personnel required for specific inhalation challenge tests increase the diagnostic costs, the use of these tests is reserved to document new causative substances for OA, for medical/legal purposes such as proving a worker's eligibility under workers' compensation or disability benefits regulations, and when there is uncertainty about the diagnosis of OA.[36] A positive specific challenge test provides a definitive diagnosis of OA, but a negative challenge study does not always exclude the diagnosis, because sensitivity to a suspected agent may decrease in workers removed from the workplace after varied periods.[36] Therefore, specific challenge tests should be performed before or soon after a worker is removed from the workplace.[36] Because of the risks and technical problems inherent in challenge testing, only experienced individuals at specialized medical centers should perform these tests.[36]

Immunologic studies may be helpful in establishing a diagnosis of OA. Workers should always be assessed for atopy by skin testing to common seasonal and perennial aeroallergens, because atopy represents a potential risk factor for HMW agent induced OA.[9, 16] Skin prick tests to such substances as cereal proteins in flour, coffee beans, castor beans, *B. subtilis* derived enzymes, and egg white proteins are often diagnostic in the detection of allergic sensitization.[9, 16] In vitro assays to measure specific IgE to these proteins have been found to be less sensitive than in vivo skin testing.[16]

The presence of cutaneous reactivity or elevated serum-specific IgE to one of these agents only indicates that sensitization has occurred but does not necessarily confirm a diagnosis of OA.[10, 16] Serum-specific IgE assays by RAST or ELISA methods have been more useful as screening tests in identifying workers sensitized to acid anhydrides.[9, 91] Elevated serum-specific IgE antibodies are detectable in only a minority (5% to 15%) of workers diagnosed with diisocyanate OA as confirmed by inhalational challenge.[35] The significance of specific IgG antibodies is unclear but has been proposed to represent a marker of exposure to the causative agent. In vitro techniques, such as leukocyte histamine release, peripheral blood mononuclear cell proliferation, and leukocyte inhibitory factor, are reserved primarily for research purposes.[9, 10]

TREATMENT

Treatment of OA requires that the worker be removed from further potentially harmful exposure as soon as possible. The persistence of asthma after leaving the worksite is directly related to the duration of symptoms prior to diagnosis.[9] Workers diagnosed early in the course of their disease, who have well-preserved lung function and minimal airway hyperresponsiveness, are more likely to improve after removal from the workplace.[86] This feature is exemplified by red cedar OA workers, 50% of whom experienced deterioration of their lung function and an increase in symptoms and medication requirements after remaining in their workplace where they were continuously exposed to the causative agent.[10]

Treatment of acute or chronic occupational asthma parallels the treatment of nonoccupational asthma and should include a combination of bronchodilator medication (β_2 selective agonists, theophylline) and anti-inflammatory agents (cromolyn sodium, inhaled and systemic corticosteroids) in various combinations chosen according to the severity and persistence of the worker's symptoms when away from the workplace.[9, 10] Pharmacotherapy is not considered an alternative to avoidance measures. Immunotherapy using specific animal extracts (i.e., rat, dog, cat) has been successful in treating laboratory animal workers and in shellfish handlers with sea squirt asthma but is not useful in treatment of OA induced by LMW haptens.[1, 9]

PREVENTION

The prevention of OA requires cooperation between management and labor in organizing comprehensive immunosurveillance programs for detecting and monitoring all workers who are at increased risk for exposure to known inducers of OA.[102] Implementation of comprehensive immunosurveillance programs in the workplace can significantly reduce the incidence of OA.[14] Newly hired employees should be screened for risk factors that may place them at greater risk if they work in certain jobs (i.e., atopic persons in enzyme or pharmaceutical companies).

The level of exposure necessary to initiate or perpetuate sensitization in susceptible workers is not available for most causative agents.[87] For chemical xenobiotics, such as diisocyanates and most other protein agents, the levels eliciting sensitization have ranged from 1 to 30 ng/m^3.[87] Therefore, good industrial hygiene is essential to minimize a worker's exposure to potentially causative agent(s) and should include careful handling procedures for toxic chemicals, avoidance of accidental spills, and upgrading of ventilation and filtration systems in the workplace.[102] In certain situations, special air-fed body suits have been demonstrated to reduce a worker's exposure to potentially sensitizing agents. Use of respirators in the work environment does not reduce exposure or prevent clinical deterioration in workers, although special fitting air stream helmets can be tried to offer better protection against an offending agent than other devices.[10] Encapsulation of enzymes, along with improved dust control measures, is one example whereby modification of a product has reduced the worker's risk of sensitization.[65]

SUMMARY

Occupational asthma is projected to increase worldwide as industrial technology becomes more sophisticated and additional chemicals are introduced into the workplace. To make the workplace safer, it is essential to identify susceptibility risk factors, which can be used to screen employees at greater risk for developing OA if exposed to specific causative agents. Until the necessary longitudinal prospective studies fully identify inherent risk factors, the diagnosis of OA depends on obtaining a careful occupational history and performing physical examination, objective assessment of lung function in and out of the workplace, and immunologic testing if appropriate. Once a diagnosis of OA is established, removal of the employee from further exposure is imperative to reduce the long-term morbidity often associated with occupational asthma.

REFERENCES

1. Armentia A, Arranz M, Martin JM, et al: Evaluation of immune complexes after immunotherapy with wheat flour in bakers' asthma. Ann Allergy 69:441, 1992.
2. Avery SB, Stetson DM, Pan PM, Mathews KP: Immunological investigation of individuals with toluene diisocyanate asthma. Clin Exp Immunol 4:585, 1969.
3. Barnes PJ, Baraniuk JN, Belvisi MG: Neuropeptides in the respiratory tract: Part I. Am Rev Respir Dis 144:1187, 1991.
4. Barnes PJ, Baraniuk JN, Belvisi MG: Neuropeptides in the respiratory tract: Part II. Am Rev Respir Dis 144:1391, 1991.
5. Baur X: Immunologic cross-reactivity between different albumin-bound isocyanates. J Allergy Clin Immunol 71:197, 1983.
6. Baur X, Fruhmann G, Haug B, et al: Role of *Aspergillus amylase* in baker's asthma. Lancet 1:43, 1986.
7. Beasley R, Roce WR, Roberts JA, et al: Cellular events in the bronchi in mild asthma and after bronchial provocation. Am Rev Respir Dis 139:806, 1989.
8. Becklake MR: Epidemiology: Prevalence and determinants. In Bernstein IL, Chan-Yeung M, Malo JL (eds): Asthma in the Workplace. Marcel Dekker, New York, 1992, p 29.
9. Bernstein DI: Occupational asthma. Clin Allergy 76:917, 1992.
10. Bernstein DI: Clinical assessment and management of occupational asthma. In Bernstein IL, Chan-Yeung M, Malo JL (eds): Asthma in the Workplace. Marcel Dekker, New York, 1993, 103.
11. Bernstein DI: Animal models of occupational asthma. In Bernstein IL, Chan-Yeung M, Malo JL (eds): Asthma in the Workplace. Marcel Dekker, New York, 1993, p 93.
12. Bernstein DI, Gallagher JS, Bernstein IL: Meal worm asthma: Clinical and immunologic studies. A new occupational disease. J Allergy Clin Immunol 72:475, 1983.
13. Bernstein DI, Gallagher JS, D'Souza L, et al: Heterogeneity of specific-IgE responses in workers sensitized to acid anhydride compounds. J Allergy Clin Immunol 74:794, 1984.
14. Bernstein DI, Korbee L, Stauder T, et al: The low prevalence of occupational asthma and IgE mediated sensitization to diphenylmethane diisocyanate (MDI) in a plant engineered for minimal exposure to diisocyanates. J Allergy Clin Immunol 92:387, 1993.
15. Bernstein DI, Smith AB, Moller DR, et al: Clinical and immunologic studies among egg-processing workers with occupational asthma. J Allergy Clin Immunol 80:791, 1987.
16. Bernstein DI, Malo JL: High molecular weight agents. In Bernstein IL, Chan-Yeung M, Malo JL (eds): Asthma in the Workplace. *lst edition,* Marcel Dekker, New York, 1993, p 373.
17. Bernstein DI, Bernstein IL, Gaines WG, et al: Characterization of skin prick testing responses for detecting sensitization to detergent enzymes at extreme dilutions: Inability of the RAST to detect lightly sensitized individuals. J Allergy Clin Immunol 94:498, 1994.
18. Bernstein IL: Isocyanate-induced pulmonary diseases: a current perspective. J Allergy Clin Immunol 70:24, 1982.
19. Bernstein IL: Pulmonary hypersensitivity disorders. In Newcombe DS, Rose NR, Blood JC (eds): Pulmonary Hypersensitivity Disorders. Raven Press, New York, 1992, p 191.
20. Bernstein IL, Brooks SM: Metals. In Bernstein IL, Chan-Yeung M, Malo JL (eds): Asthma in the Workplace. Marcel Dekker, New York, 1993, p 459.
21. Bernstein IL, Chan-Yeung M, Bernstein DI: Definition and classification of asthma. In Bernstein IL, Chan-Yeung M, Malo JL (eds): Asthma in the Workplace. Marcel Dekker, New York, 1993, p 1.
22. Bernstein JA: Occupational asthma: "My job is making me sick." Postgrad Med 92:109, 1992.
23. Bernstein JA, Kraut A, Bernstein DI, et al: Occupational asthma induced by inhaled egg lysozyme. Chest 103:532, 1993.
24a. Bernstein JA, Stauder T, Bernstein DI, et al: A combined respiratory and cutaneous hypersensitivity syndrome induced by work exposure to quaternary amines. J Allergy Clin Immunol 94:257, 1994.
24b. Bernstein JA, Munson J, Herd ZL, et al: T-cell receptor V-beta gene segment expression in diisocyanate occupational asthma. J Allergy Clin Immunol (In press).
25. Biagini RE, Bernstein IL, Gallagher JS, et al: The diversity of reaginic immune responses to platinum and palladium metallic salts. J Allergy Clin Immunol 76:794, 1985.
26. Biagini RE, Klincewicz SL, Henningsen GM, et al: Antibodies to morphine in workers exposed to opiates at a narcotics manufacturing facility and evidence for similar antibodies in heroin abusers. Life Sci 47:897, 1990.
27. Boulet LP: Increases in airway hyperresponsiveness following acute exposure to respiratory irritants: reactive airways dysfunction syndrome or occupational asthma. Chest 94:47, 1988.
28. Brooks SM, Baker DB, Gann PH, et al: Cold air challenge and platinum skin reactivity in platinum refinery workers. Chest 97:1401, 1990.

29. Brooks SM, Bernstein IL: Reactive airways dysfunction syndrome or irritant-induced asthma. In Bernstein IL, Chan-Yeung M, Malo JL (eds): Asthma in the Workplace. Marcel Dekker, New York, p 533, 1993.
30. Burge PS: Occupational asthma due to soft soldering fluxes containing colophony (rosin, pine, resin). Eur J Respir Dis 63:65, 1982.
31. Burge PS: Occupational asthma in electronics workers caused by colophony fumes: followup of affected workers. Thorax 37:348, 1982.
32. Burrows D: The dichromate problem. Int J Dermatol 23:215, 1984.
33. Bush RK: Occupational asthma from vegetable gums. J Allergy Clin Immunol 86:443, 1990.
34. Butcher BT, Mapp CE, Fabbri LM: Polyisocyanates and their prepolymers. In Bernstein IL, Chan-Yeung M, Malo JL (eds): Asthma in the Workplace. Marcel Dekker, New York, 1993, p 415.
35. Cartier A, Grammer L, Malo JL, et al: Specific serum antibodies against isocyanates. J Allergy Clin Immunol 84:507, 1989.
36. Cartier A, Malo JL: Occupational challenge tests. In Bernstein IL, Chan-Yeung M, Malo JL (eds): Asthma in the Workplace. Marcel Dekker, New York, 1993, p 215.
37. Chan-Yeung M: Immunologic and nonimmunologic mechanisms in asthma due to western red cedar (*Thuja plicata*). J Allergy Clin Immunol 70:32, 1982.
38. Chan-Yeung M, Barton G, MacLean L, et al: Occupational asthma and rhinitis due to western red cedar (*Thuja plicata*). Am Rev Respir Dis 108:1094, 1973.
39. Chan-Yeung M, Chan H, Tse KS, et al: Histamine and leukotriene release in bronchoalveolar lavage fluid during plicatic acid induced bronchoconstriction. J Allergy Clin Immunol 84:762, 1989.
40. Chan-Yeung M, Kennedy S, Enarson D: Grain dust-induced lung diseases. In Bernstein IL, Chan-Yeung M, Malo JL (eds): Asthma in the Workplace. Marcel Dekker, New York, 1993, p 577.
41. Chan-Yeung M, Lam S, Koerner S: Clinical features and natural history of occupational asthma due to western red cedar, *Thuja plicata*. Am Rev Respir Dis 72:411, 1982.
42. Chan-Yeung M, Leriche J, MacLean L, et al: Comparison of cellular and protein changes in bronchial lavage fluid of symptomatic and asymptomatic patients with red cedar asthma on follow-up examination. Clin Allergy 18:359, 1988.
43. Chan-Yeung M: Occupational asthma—state of the art. Am Rev Respir Dis 137:686, 1986.
44. Cote J, Kennedy S, Chan-Yeung M: Sensitivity and specificity of PC_{20} and peak expiratory flow rate in cedar asthma. J Allergy Clin Immunol 14:592, 1990.
45. Dearman RJ, Kimber I: Differential stimulation of immune function by respiratory and contact chemical allergens. Immunology 72:563, 1991.
46. Dearman RJ, Kimber I: Divergent immune responses to respiratory and contact chemical allergens: antibody elicited by phthalic anhydride and oxazolone. Clin Exp Allergy 22:241, 1992.
47. De Monchy GR, Kauffman HF, Venge P, et al: Bronchoalveolar eosinophils following allergen-induced late-phase asthmatic reactions. Am Rev Respir Dis 131:373, 1985.
48. Durham SR, Graneck BJ, Hawkins R, et al: The temporal relationship between increases in airway responsiveness to histamine and late asthmatic responses induced by occupational agents. J Allergy Clin Immunol 79:398, 1987.
49. Enarson DA, Chan-Yeung M: Characterization of health effects of wood dust exposures. Am J Ind Med 17:33, 1990.
50. Fabbri LM, Ciaccia A: Pathophysiology of occupational asthma. In Bernstein IL, Chan-Yeung M, Malo JL (eds): Asthma in the Workplace. Marcel Dekker, New York, 1993, p 61.
51. Finotto S, Fabbri LM, Rado V, et al: Increase in numbers of CD8+ lymphocytes and eosinophils in peripheral blood of subjects with late asthmatic reactions induced by toluene diisocyanate. Br J Ind Med 48:116, 1991.
52. Fowler PBS: Printers' asthma. Lancet 2:755, 1952.
53. Franz T, McMurrain KD, Brooks S, et al: Clinical, immunologic and physiologic observations in factory workers exposed to *B. subtilis* enzyme dust. J Allergy 47:170, 1971.
54. Gallagher JS, Tse CST, Brooks SM, et al: Diverse profiles of immunoreactivity in toluene diisocyanate (TDI) asthma. J Occup Med 23:610, 1981.
55. Gannon PFG, Burge PS: A preliminary report of a surveillance scheme of occupational asthma in the West Midlands. Br J Ind Med 48:579, 1991.
56. Gheysens B, Auwerx J, Van den Eeckkhout A, et al: Cobalt-induced bronchial asthma in diamond polishers. Chest 88:740, 1985.
57. Grammer LC, Eggum P, Silverstein M, et al: Prospective immunologic and clinical study of a population exposed to hexamethylene diisocyanate. J Allergy Clin Immunol 82:627, 1988.
58. Herd ZL, Bernstein DI: Antigen-specific stimulation of histamine releasing factors in diisocyanate-induced occupational asthma. Am J Respir Crit Care Med 150:988, 1994.
59. Herzog CH, Villiger B, Braun P: Nickel-specific T cell clones in asthma—preferential use of V-beta 14 in T cell receptor beta chain. Third International Conference on Bronchoalveloar Lavage. Vienna, June 20–22. Eur Respir Rev 33S, 1991.
60. Kennedy AL, Brown WE: Isocyanates and lung disease: experimental approaches to molecular mechanisms. Occup Med 7:301, 1992.
61. Kusaka Y, Nakona Y, Shirakawa T, et al: Lymphocyte transformation with cobalt in hard metal asthma. Ind Health 27:155, 1989.
62. Lam S, Wong R, Chan-Yeung M: Nonspecific bronchial reactivity in occupational asthma. J Allergy Clin Immunol 63:28, 1979.
63. Liss GM, Bernstein DI, Genesove L, et al: Assessment of risk factors for IgE mediated sensitization to tetrachlorophthalic anhydride. J Allergy Clin Immunol 92:237–247, 1993.
64. Liss GM, Bernstein DI, Moller DR, et al: Pulmonary and immunologic evaluation of foundry workers exposed to methylene diphenyldiisocyanate (MDI). J Allergy Clin Immunol 85:1076, 1990.
65. Liss GM, Kominsky JR, Gallagher JS, et al: Failure of enzyme encapsulation to prevent sensitization of workers in the dry bleach industry. J Allergy Clin Immunol 73:348, 1984.
66. Luo JD, Nelsen KG, Fischbein A: Persistent reactive airway dysfunction syndrome after exposure to toluene diisocyanate. Br J Ind Med 47:239, 1990.
67. Lushniak BD, Reh CM, Gallagher JS, et al: Indirect assessment of exposure to MDI by evaluation of specific immune responses to MDI-HSA in foam workers. J Allergy Clin Immunol 85:251, 1990.
68. Maccia CA, Bernstein IL, Emmett EA, et al: In vitro demonstration of specific IgE in phthalic anhydride hypersensitivity. Am Rev Respir Dis 113:701, 1976.
69. Malo JL, Bernstein IL: Other chemical substances causing occupational asthma. In Bernstein IL, Chan-Yeung M, Malo JL (eds): Asthma in the Workplace. Marcel Dekker, New York, 1993, p 481.
70. Malo JL, Cartier A, L'Archeveque J, et al: Prevalence of occupational asthma and immunological sensitization to guar gum among employees at a carpet-manufacturing plant. J Allergy Clin Immunol 86:562, 1990.
71. Malo JL, Cartier A, Doepner M, et al: Occupational asthma caused by nickel sulfate. J Allergy Clin Immunol 69:55, 1982.
72. Malo JL, Ghezzo H, L'Archeveque J, et al: Is the clinical history a satisfactory means for diagnosing occupational asthma? Am Rev Respir Dis 143:528, 1991.
73. Mapp CE, Boschetto P, Dal Vecchio, et al: Occupational asthma due to isocyanate. Eur Respir J 1:273, 1988.
74. Matthews KP: Inhalant insect-derived allergens. Immunol Allergy Clin North Am 2:2, 1989.
75. Merchant JA, Bernstein IL: Cotton and other textile dusts. In Bernstein IL, Chan-Yeung M, Malo JL (eds): Asthma in the Workplace. Marcel Dekker, New York, 1992, p 551.
76. Meredith SK, Taylor VM, McDonald JC: Occupational respiratory disease in the United Kingdom 1989: a report to the British Thoracic Society and the Society of Occupational Medicine by the SWORD project group. Br J Ind Med 48:292, 1991.
77. Moller DR, Brooks SM, Bernstein DI, et al: Delayed anaphylactoid reaction in a worker exposed to chromium. J Allergy Clin Immunol 77:451, 1986.
78. Moller DR, McKay RT, Bernstein IL, et al: Persistent airways disease caused by toluene diisocyanate. Am Rev Respir Dis 134:175, 1986.
79. Mosmann TR, Coffman RL: Heterogeneity of cytokine secretion patterns and functions of helper T cells. Adv Immunol 46:111, 1989.
80. Mosmann TR, Schumacher JH, Street NF, et al: Diversity of cytokine synthesis and function of mouse CD4+ T cells. Immunol Rev 123:209, 1991.
81. Nemery B: Metal toxicity and the respiratory tract. Eur Respir J 3:202, 1990.
82. Paggiaro PL, Chan-Yeung M: Pattern of specific airway response in asthma due to western red cedar (*Thuja plicata*): relationship with length of exposure and lung function measurements. Clin Allergy 17:333, 1987.
83. Pauli G, Bessot JC, Kopferschitt MC, et al: Meat wrapper's asthma: identification of the causal agent. Clin Allergy 10:263, 1980.

84. Pepys J, Longbottom JL, Hargreave FE, et al: Allergic reactions of the lungs to enzymes of *Bacillus subtilis*. Lancet 1:1811, 1969.
85. Quirce S, Cuevas M, Diez-Gomz M, et al: Respiratory allergy to Aspergillus-derived enzymes in bakers' asthma. J Allergy Clin Immunol 90:970, 1992.
86. Reports of the Working Groups, Workshop on Environmental and Occupational Asthma. Chest 96:240S, 1990.
87. Reed CE, Swanson MC, Li JTC: Environmental monitoring of protein aeroallergens. In Bernstein IL, Chan-Yeung M, Malo JL (eds): Asthma in the Workplace. Marcel Dekker, New York, 1992, p 249.
88. Roche WR, Beasley R, Williams JH, et al: Subepithelial fibrosis in the bronchi of asthmatics. Lancet 1:520, 1989.
89. Saetta M, Di Stefano A, Maestrelli P, et al: Airway mucosal inflammation in occupational asthma induced by toluene diisocyanate. Am Rev Respir Dis 145:160, 1992.
90. Saetta M, Maestrelli P, De Stefano A, et al: Effect of cessation of exposure to toluene diisocyanate (TDI) on bronchial mucosa of subjects with TDI-induced asthma. Am Rev Respir Dis 145:169, 1992.
91. Sarlo K, Clark ED, Ryan CA, et al: ELISA for human IgE antibody to subtilisin. A (Alcalase): Correlation with RAST and skin test results with occupationally exposed individuals. J Allergy Clin Immunol 83:393, 1990.
92. Sheppard D: Airway hyperresponsiveness mechanisms in experimental models. Chest 96:2265, 1989.
93. Sheppard D, Thompson JE, Scypinski L, et al: Toluene diisocyanate increases airway responsiveness to substance P and decreases airway neutral endopeptidase. J Clin Invest 81:1111, 1988.
94. Shirakawa T, Kusaka Y, Fujimura N, et al: The existence of specific antibodies to cobalt in hard metal asthma. Clin Allergy 18:451, 1988.
95. Smith AB, Bernstein DI, Tar-Ching AW, et al: Occupational asthma from inhaled egg protein. Am J Ind Med 12:205, 1987.
96. Smith AB, Castellan RM, Lewis D, et al: Guidelines for the epidemiologic assessment of occupational asthma. J Allergy Clin Immunol 94:794, 1989.
97. Steinberg DR, Bernstein DI, Bernstein IL, et al: Bronchial reactivity increases early in both immediate and dual phase responders to allergen. J Allergy Clin Immunol 79:249, 1987.
98. Tarlo SM, Wong L, Roos J, et al: Occupational asthma caused by latex in a surgical glove manufacturing plant. J Allergy Clin Immunol 85:626, 1990.
99. Thompson JE, Scypinsky LA, Gorton T, et al: Tachykinins mediate the acute increase in airway responsiveness caused by toluene diisocyanate in guinea pigs. Am Rev Respir Dis 136:43, 1987.
100. Vandervort R, Brooks SM: Polyvinyl chloride film thermal decomposition products as an occupational illness. 1: Environmental exposures and toxicology. J Occup Med 19:188, 1977.
101. Venables K: Low molecular weight chemicals, hypersensitivity and direct toxicity: the acid anhydrides. Br J Ind Med 46:222, 1989.
102. Venables KM: Preventing occupational asthma. Br J Ind Med 49:817, 1992.
103. Venables KM, Topping MD, Howe W, et al: Interaction of smoking and atopy in producing specific IgE antibody against a hapten protein cojugate. Br Med J 290:201, 1985.
104. Wagner CD, Gundel RH, Reilly P, et al: Intercellular adhesion molecule-1 (ICAM-1) in the pathogenesis of asthma. Science 247:456, 1990.
105. Zeiss CR, Mitchell JH, Van Peenen PFD, et al: A twelve year clinical and immunologic evaluation of workers involved in the manufacture of trimellitic anhydride (TMA). Allergy Proc 11:71, 1990.
106. Zeiss CR, Wolkonsky P, Pruzansky JJ, et al: Clinical and immunologic evaluation of trimellitic anhydride workers in multiple industrial settings. J Allergy Clin Immunol 70:15, 1982.
107. Zocca E, Fabbri LM, Boschetto P, et al: Leukotriene B4 and late asthmatic reactions induced by toluene diisocyanate. J Appl Physiol 68:1576, 1990.

31 Allergic Bronchopulmonary Aspergillosis

MANUEL LOPEZ JOHN E. SALVAGGIO

Allergic bronchopulmonary aspergillosis (ABPA) is a hypersensitivity disease of the lungs caused by *Aspergillus fumigatus* and characterized by asthma, productive cough with mucus plugs, low-grade fever, pulmonary infiltrates, and central bronchiectasis. In 1952, Hinson and coworkers[24] reported three patients with episodes of reversible bronchospasm, recurrent lung infiltrates with fever occurring over months or years, sputum and blood eosinophilia, mucus plugs obstructing airways, *Aspergillus* hyphae in sputum, and central saccular bronchiectasis. Most of the initial studies were performed in Europe,[57] and it was believed that the condition was rare in the United States. Since then, however, many cases has been reported from this country.[4, 17, 25] ABPA has been reported to occur with a frequency as high as 22% in patients with asthma seen in chest clinics in Great Britain[21] and 9% in corticosteroid-dependent asthmatics in the United States.[3] Patients with cystic fibrosis (CF) have a particularly high incidence of the disease, ranging between 8% and 11%.[51, 82]

Some of the discrepancies between estimates of the incidence of ABPA in Great Britain and the United States may be due to antigen selection.[34] Hoehne and collaborators[25] demonstrated that commercially prepared antigens did not induce positive skin tests or serum precipitins in patients with ABPA. Furthermore, Malo and associates[39] found that the prevalence of serum antibodies to *Aspergillus* was related to the number of antigen preparations tested.[39] Another possible reason for the apparently higher incidence of ABPA in Great Britain is the high level of exposure to *Aspergillus* spores. However, Schwartz and colleagues[73] found similar incidences of positive immediate skin tests to *Aspergillus* in atopic asthmatics in London and in Cleveland, Ohio, indicating that sufficient *Aspergillus* was present on both sides of the Atlantic to sensitize susceptible individuals. In the study by Malo and associates,[39] the incidence of immediate sensitivity to *A. fumigatus* in asthmatic patients in North America was at least equal to that found in Great Britain. In a later study of 531 patients with asthma and positive immediate skin tests to *Aspergillus*, Greenberger and Patterson[17] reported 19 patients (3.6%) with ABPA who had central bronchiectasis and 13 patients (2.4%) without bronchiectasis.

ABPA should be considered a complication of asthma, because virtually all cases have been reported in asthmatics, most of whom are allergic. The clinical spectrum of ABPA overlaps those of other pulmonary disorders. Eosinophilic pneumonia, bronchocentric granulomatosis, and mucoid impaction are other clinical, radiologic and pathologic diagnoses that are readily confused with ABPAQ. If *Aspergillus* is present, it may be the same entity. However, these conditions are not necessarily associated with *Aspergillus*. *Aspergillus fumigatus* is the most common cause of ABPA, but other species of *Aspergillus* (*flavus*, *niger*, and *terreus*), as well as *Ghialisegtus*,[36] *Helminthosporium* and *Penicillium* species,[41] the dematiaceous hypomycetes *Curvularia* and *Drechslera*,[42] and *Candida* species[81] can also cause ABPA (prompting some to suggest that the term allergic bronchopulmonary mycosis might be better suited to describe this condition).

THE FUNGUS

Aspergillus is a ubiquitous environmental fungus belonging to the Fungi Imperfecti classification. It is commonly found in decaying organic matter, and its spores are frequently isolated in the air. *Aspergillus* species are associated with a wide spectrum of illness; they may colonize paranasal sinuses, causing chronic sinusitis.[30] They may also cause asthma in sensitized individuals, proliferate in the bronchi, leading to causing ABPA; induce hypersensitivity pneumonitis; grow in perforated lung cavities, producing aspergilloma[68]; colonize the pleural cavity; and, in immunocompromised patients, produce severe systemic infection.[12, 74] *Aspergillus* frequently colonizes the lung for reasons not clearly understood. The spores are small, facilitating their penetration to the smaller bronchi. The organisms grow best at body temperature (37°C), making them ideal for growth in bronchi and pulmonary tissues with subsequent release of a variety of antigens into tissues and generation of strong immune responsiveness. *Aspergillus* growth may be enhanced by cytotoxic metabolites, mainly gliotoxin and fumagillin, which are thought to facilitate growth by inhibiting macrophage function and causing immunosuppression. The fungus also produces important hydrolytic enzymes[20] and toxins. On the other hand, *Aspergillus* seldom invades tissues in healthy individuals and becomes invasive only in immunocompromised patients.

PATHOLOGY

The diagnosis of ABPA is usually based on clinical and laboratory changes. For this reason, there is a paucity of information regarding pathologic changes in the lung.

Postmortem or lobectomy specimens from patients with ABPA have the histologic features of asthma, i.e., hypertrophy of bronchial muscle, thickening of the basement membrane, goblet cell hyperplasia, oversecretion of mucus, and infiltration with inflammatory cells, especially eosinophils. In addition, central bronchiectasis, at times with mucus plugs in place, abscesses, bronchiolar destruction, bronchocentric granulomatosis, pleuritis, and eosinophilic pneumonia are often present.[8, 22, 31, 65, 85]

In a lung biopsy study of 18 patients reported by Bosken and collaborators,[5] the more common features were: (1) bronchocentric granulomatosis with replacement of the bronchial wall by granulomatous inflammation consisting mainly of histiocytes, lymphocytes, plasma cells, and eosinophils; (2) mucoid impactation of bronchi, with the mucin containing a large number of eosinophils and Charcot-Leyden crystals; (3) exudative bronchiolitis with dense peribronchial infiltrates of lymphocytes and eosinophils; (4) tissue eosinophilia; and (5) frequent fungal hyphae without invasion of the bronchial wall or lung parenchyma. Although bronchocentric granulomatosis can have causes other than ABPA, 9 of the 23 cases described by Katzenstein and associates[31] had demonstrable hyphal remnants compatible with *Aspergillus* on histologic examination.

Slavin and collaborators[71] demonstrated the presence of major basic protein freely deposited outside eosinophils, especially in the interlobular septum, on biopsy and immunofluorescence studies of a patient with ABPA.[77] A significant increase in interleukin-2 positive staining T cells was also observed.

IMMUNOPATHOGENESIS

The mechanism of tissue damage in ABPA is not clearly understood. *Aspergillus* organisms likely live and grow in viscid bronchial secretions in affected patients, constantly liberating antigens onto bronchial mucosal surfaces. It is thought that specific immunoglobulin E (lgE) on mast cells present in the bronchial tissue combines with *Aspergillus* antigens to cause mast cell degranulation with mediator release, and consequent vasodilation and vascular leakage, so that serum components (including anti-*Aspergillus* IgG and IgA) enter the bronchi and combine with *Aspergillus* antigen to form immune complexes containing IgG and IgA. Subsequent activation of the complement cascade, with attraction of acute inflammatory cells and enzyme release, causes immune-complex or Arthus-type inflammation and pulmonary damage in the bronchial wall.

The following findings are supportive of this hypothesis: the elevated levels of specific serum IgE, IgG, and IgA directed against *Aspergillus*[84]; B cells with significantly increased preformed IgE and increased spontaneous de novo IgE synthesis[35]; prolonged presence of antigen in the damaged bronchi; the presence of circulating immune complexes and complement activation[14]; and primate animal models in which anti-*Aspergillus* IgE and IgG are both required to cause susceptibility to lung damage following inhalation of *Aspergillus* antigen.[76]

It is possible that the pathogenesis of ABPA also involves the pulmonary equivalent of "late-phase," eosinophil-mediated, IgE-dependent reactions. In such reactions, mediators released from basophils, mononuclear cells, and endothelial cells (e.g., leukotriene B_4, histamine, and eosinophilic chemotactic factors) are thought to result in attraction of eosinophils and other cells, plus the deposition of fibrin in tissue sites of prior IgE-mediated immediate reactions. The presence of major basic protein in the interstitium[28] suggests that eosinophils play an important role in the inflammatory process. These inflammatory reactions have been studied in the skin as well as the bronchi. Unlike the early response, these late-phase reactions can be inhibited by corticosteroids. However, the pathology of ABPA is puzzling; some of the more important histologic features, such as infiltrates with lymphocytes and other chronic inflammatory cells, granuloma formation, and the presence of activated T lymphocytes, are features suggestive of delayed hypersensitivity. In vitro lymphoproliferative responses to *Aspergillus* antigens have also been demonstrated in patients with ABPA, although the findings do not correlate with disease activity and are not different from the responses of patients who demonstrate only positive skin test reactivity to *Aspergillus*.[78] Delayed skin test reactivity to *Aspergillus* antigen is usually not demonstrable. It has also been shown that increased T-cell suppressor activity occurs in patients with CF and ABPA.[35] These facts notwithstanding, the importance of delayed hypersensitivity in the immunopathogenesis of ABPA remains to be determined.

CLINICAL PRESENTATION

Patients with ABPA may progress through various stages (Table 31–1).[54] These range from the acute form to a stage of recurrent exacerbations and remissions, and finally to corticosteroid-dependent and fibrotic stages. Treatment with corticosteroids at earlier stages can prevent advancement to the final fibrotic stage. In the initial acute stage, when most cases are diagnosed, patients usually present with findings of cough and wheezing identical with those seen in bronchial asthma together with systemic symptoms of malaise and fever. Small brownish or golden sputum plugs may be present in sputum samples, and there may be temporary or migratory lesions on chest radiograph, usually with intense peripheral eosinophilia. Occasionally, eosinophilia is only minimal, and the patient may present with fleeting radiologic abnormalities in the absence of wheezing. At this stage, regardless of the presentation, there is usually excellent response to prednisone.

TABLE 31–1
CLINICAL STAGES OF ALLERGIC BRONCHOPULMONARY ASPERGILLOSIS

Stage	
I:	Acute Asthma, pulmonary infiltrates, eosinophilia, productive cough, and serologic changes
II:	Remission After treatment with corticosteroids: symptoms improve, chest radiograph normal, eosinophilia decreases, serologic changes decrease
III:	Recurrent exacerbation Recurrence of symptoms and laboratory changes
IV:	Corticosteroid-dependent asthma
V:	Fibrotic end stage

From Patterson R, Greenberger PA, Lee TM, et al: Prolonged evaluation of patients with corticosteroid-dependent asthma stage of allergic bronchopulmonary aspergillosis. J Allergy Clin Immnol 80:663–668, 1987.

Following therapy, the patient may remain in a remission stage with either very mild asthma or no respiratory symptoms at all. During this stage, radiologic findings disappear, as do systemic symptoms, whereas many of the serologic abnormalities, such as elevated serum IgE and precipitating antibody, may remain. Following this stage, the patient may again slowly progress to the stage of recurrent exacerbations responsive to prednisone therapy. Gradually, these exacerbations may progress to a more permanent, corticosteroid-dependent type of wheezing, cough, and dyspnea, usually associated with elevated total serum IgE, serum precipitins, and eosinophilia. In all of these stages, central bronchiectasis may or may not be present. The reasons for the progression of asthma through these various stages in some ABPA patients is unknown. Some individuals may illustrate a coincidental progression in severity of symptoms, and most develop increasing degrees of airways hyperreactivity during this process.

In the fibrotic end stage of the disease, severe corticosteroid-dependent asthma remains, and the patient usually manifests severe cough, dyspnea on exertion, and production of profuse amounts of sputum associated with increasing bronchiectasis. Honeycombing and other fibrotic changes are evident on chest radiographs, and the disease is poorly controlled even with high doses of prednisone. Fatalities may occur from such conditions as respiratory failure, septicemia, severe bronchospasm, and terminal fibrotic lung disease. These fatalities often occur in the fourth decade of life and usually reflect damage that has occurred in the very early stages of the disease process.

APBA AND CYSTIC FIBROSIS

ABPA was first demonstrated to be associated with cystic fibrosis by Mearns and collaborators.[45] This association was subsequently confirmed by other studies.[37, 38, 51] In the United States, ABPA has been reported in approximately 11% of patients with cystic fibrosis. Schonheyder and associates,[71] reported from Denmark that during 5 years of observation of a group of CF patients, 0.9/100 patients/year developed ABPA. Similar results have been reported by Henry and collaborators[23] in Australia. Colonization with *A. fumigatus* is common in CF, and for this reason, immune responses, particularly development of IgE and IgG antibodies against *Aspergillus*, are commonly seen. According to Nelson and collaborators,[51] up to 57% of CF patients are colonized by *A. fumigatus*. In a retrospective autopsy study of 63 patients with CF, Bhargava and colleagues[4] reported the presence of fungi in the tissues of 21% of the patients, in most cases representing colonization.

ABPA is difficult to diagnose in CF, because patients with CF and those with ABPA often have frequent bronchial bacterial infections (mainly *Pseudomonas aeruginosa*) that may result in complications such as pulmonary infiltrates, bronchiolitis obliterans, bronchiectasis, and interstitial fibrosis. Patients with CF also commonly demonstrate IgE and IgG anti-*Aspergillus* antibodies and elevated IgE levels.[59] In a study by Zeaske and coworkers[86] of a group of 75 cystic fibrosis patients, 77% of the patients had at least one immunologic response to *A. fumigatus,* 58% had a positive immediate skin test, 42% demonstrated precipitins, 16% demonstrated elevated total IgE levels, and 10.7% met the criteria for diagnosis of ABPA. According to Slavin and associates,[76] the diagnosis of ABPA in CF should not be based soley on serology and skin test results, because patients with CF may demonstrate multiple responses to *A. fumigatus* without sustained pulmonary deterioration as well as spontaneous reversal of the serologic changes.[26]

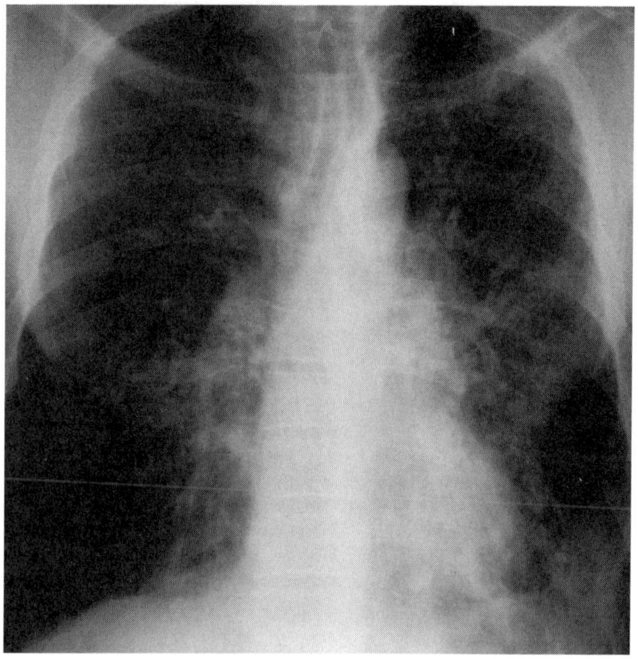

FIGURE 31–1. Chest x-ray of a patient with ABPA showing patchy linear, nodular, and larger areas of consolidation, most prominent in the left middle zone. (Courtesy of Lawrence Goodman, Medical College of Wisconsin, Milwaukee, WI.)

RADIOLOGIC FEATURES

The major radiographic changes in ABPA are lung infiltrates, mucous plugging, and central bronchiectasis. In general, radiographic reactions can be classified as acute or transient and chronic or permanent. Table 31–2 lists the more important radiologic features.

ACUTE CHANGES

The most common finding is ill-defined homogeneous shadows, which may be small (5 to 15 mm) or massive (lobar).[40, 43, 49] These shadows can appear in any part of the lung but predominate in the upper lobes and are presumably caused by bronchial obstruction with plugs, localized eosinophilic pneumonia, or both. They resolve often after expectoration of a bronchial plug, and corticosteroid therapy hastens resolution. Half of the shadows leave permanent changes, mainly ring shadows.[40] Bronchial abnormalities, occurring in 50% to 70% of episodes of acute ABPA, consist of tramline, ring shadows, and glove finger shadows. (Glove finger shadows are branched tubular radiodensities 2 to 3 cm long that branch distally from the hilus and represent dilated branching bronchi filled with inflammatory exudates.[43])

Atelectasis of a lobe of a lung with evidence of shrinkage due to occlusion of a bronchus with a plug is present in 10% to 20% of patients with acute ABPA. Mintzer and associates[46] emphasized the occurrence of perihilar infiltrates simulating hilar adenopathy in 40% of episodes of ABPA (Fig. 31–1). This is secondary to central dilated bronchi filled with fluid and debris associated with perihilar parenchymal infiltrates.[46] Other acute changes are abscesses with air-fluid levels, diffuse nodulation, avascular areas, and signs of hyperinflation (10% to 30%). Pleural effusion occurs infrequently, in less than 5% of episodes.[40, 49]

TABLE 31–2
RADIOLOGIC FEATURES OF ALLERGIC BRONCHOPULMONARY ASPERGILLOSIS

Abnormality	Approximate Frequency (%)
Homogeneous shadows (fleeting infiltrates)	80–90
Parallel line shadows	70
Ring shadows	45
Lobar shrinkage	35
Toothpaste shadows	35
Honeycomb shadows (pulmonary fibrosis)	25
Tramline shadows	20
Atelectasis	20
Cavitation	15
Gloved finger shadows	10
Central bronchiectasis	100

CHRONIC CHANGES

Chronic permanent radiographic findings result from irreversible damage and include central bronchiectasis, and interstitial fibrosis. Radiographic changes of central bronchiectasis include parallel line shadows and ring shadows that are often bilateral and occur more commonly in the upper lobes.[43] In addition, pulmonary fibrosis, usually of the upper lobes, may be present. The association between ABPA and interstitial fibrosis with upper lobe predominance is so strong in Great Britain that a patient with this radiologic finding, a negative tuberculin skin test, and positive immediate *Aspergillus* skin test reaction is assumed to have ABPA.[81]

Late sequelae include radiologic evidence of cavitation, contracted upper lobes, local emphysema, and honeycomb fibrosis.[43] In patients with ABPA, radiographs obtained every 3 to 6 months for the first year after diagnosis and yearly thereafter are recommended to avoid missing symptomatic relapses.[62]

Central bronchiectasis is a unique feature of ABPA. It is associated with normal small bronchi and bronchioles,[69] in contrast to saccular bronchiectasis, in which small bronchi and bronchioles are occluded so that dilated bronchi end

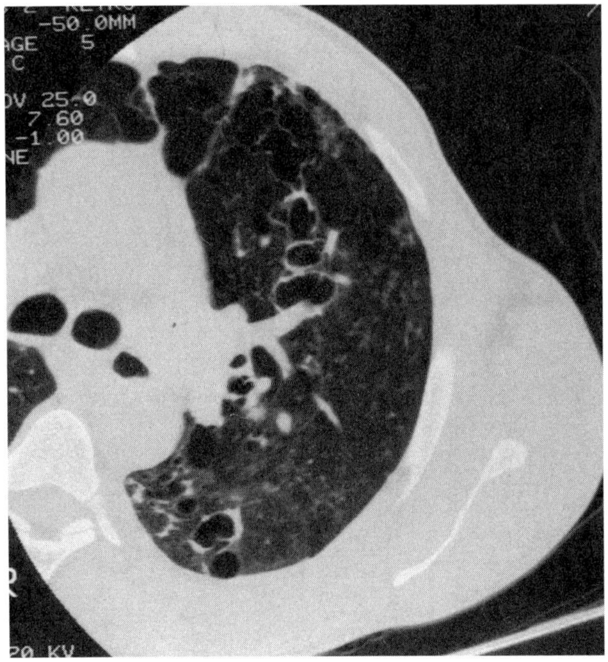

FIGURE 31–2. CT showing mainly central bronchiectasis, with some emphysema and scattered areas of consolidation. (Courtesy of Lawrence Goodman, Medical College of Wisconsin, Milwaukee, WI.)

blindly when examined with bronchographic dye. Bronchography is considered the definitive test for the detection of bronchiectasis. However, bronchography is invasive, and minor complications are common.[52] Filling of the bronchial tree may be incomplete owing to bronchospasm or mucus plugs. Computerized tomography (CT) has become a very useful technique in the detection and localization of bronchiectasis.[18, 29, 47, 48, 58] High-resolution CT scans utilizing thin (1.5-mm) sections has been shown to be reliable for the assessment of bronchiectasis, with a sensitivity and specificity similar to those of bronchography.[29] In a study of high-resolution CT in patients with ABPA, Neeld and coworkers[50] concluded that this method is useful in the detection of bronchiectasis in patients with asthma who are suspected of having ABPA and may provide information about the severity of the inflammatory process. Compared with chest radiography, CT scanning demonstrates up to twice as many radiographic abnormalities in ABPA (Fig. 31–2).[11]

DIAGNOSIS

The diagnosis of ABPA is based on clinical, radiologic, and immunological criteria (Table 31–3). However, many of the diagnostic criteria are not specific for ABPA, and there is no individual test to establish the diagnosis. It is very important to make an early diagnosis in an effort to prevent progression of the disease to severe irreversible lung damage.[55] Currently, the most important diagnostic criteria for ABPA are: (1) history of asthma; (2) peripheral blood eosinophilia; (3) immediate skin test reactivity to *A. fumigatus* allergens; (4) precipitating antibodies to *Aspergillus* antigens; (5) markedly elevated total serum IgE levels; (6) history of transient or fixed pulmonary infiltrates; and (7) central bronchiectasis. Ancillary findings are: *Aspergillus* observed or grown from sputum; a history of expectoration of brown plugs; sputum eosinophilia; and late (4 to 6 hours) Arthus-type skin reactivity to *Aspergillus* antigens.

A stepwise method for the diagnosis or exclusion of ABPA has been proposed by Patterson and collaborators.[56] With this method, one initially performs a skin prick test with *Aspergillus* mixed extract, 1:20 w/v in 50% glycerine; if negative, an intradermal test with 1:1000 w/v is performed. If the skin test is negative, ABPA is excluded. If the *Aspergillus* skin prick or intradermal test is positive, one assesses total serum IgE levels and tests for precipitins against *Aspergillus* antigens. If total IgE levels are greater than 500 U/mL and the precipitin tests (see later) are positive, measurements of IgE and IgG antibodies against *A. fumigatus* by ELISA are obtained and compared with levels in asthmatic controls. If levels are greater than 2 times those of controls, one can diagnose ABPA. Hilar pulmonary tomography or CT scan should be performed to assess the presence of bronchiectasis.[50]

The measurement of specific anti-*Aspergillus* IgG antibodies is very important in the evaluation of patients in whom ABPA is suspected. The most common methods for the detection of IgG anti-*Aspergillus* antibodies are the precipitin test by double diffusion and the ELISA method. The precipitin test is a qualitative method of low sensitivity. The ELISA method has greater sensitivity, but with low titers, one may experience difficulty in discriminating between those with ABPA and normals.[61] There is good correlation between double diffusion and ELISA values among sera with high levels of anti-*Aspergillus* antibodies[19, 32, 33, 75]; however, weakly positive reactions by double diffusion in most instances correspond to ELISA titers within the normal range.[7] False-negative results with ELISA may be due to failure in binding of *Aspergillus* antigens to microtiter plates or to the presence of IgM rather than IgG antibodies.[15] Increased ELISA titers may be due in some cases to cross-reacting antibodies.[3] Immunoblotting analysis may be used as a confirmatory test to identify relevant antigens, i.e., *A. fumigatus* for those sera with negative precipitin and positive ELISA.[7] By this technique, sera from patients with ABPA demonstrate characteristic combinations of intensive reactivity with all IgG subclasses, particularly IgG4.[80] An index for serum IgG anti-*Aspergillus* in patients with ABPA compared with a serum pool from *Aspergillus* skin test positive asthmatic controls has been established by Patterson and colleagues.[53]

TABLE 31–3
ALLERGIC BRONCHOPULMONARY ASPERGILLOSIS: CRITERIA FOR DIAGNOSIS*

Major	Asthma
	Blood eosinophilia
	Immediate skin reactivity to *Aspergillus* allergens
	Precipitating antibodies to *Aspergillus* antigens
	Elevated total IgE levels
	History of pulmonary infiltrates
	Central bronchiectasis
Minor	*Aspergillus fumigatus* in sputum
	History of expectoration of brown plugs
	Arthus-type skin reactivity to *Aspergillus* antigens

From Rosenberg M, Patterson R, Mintzer R, et al: Clinical and immunologic criteria for the diagnosis of ABPA. Ann Intern Med 86:405, 1977.

*Presence of six of the seven major criteria indicates that the diagnosis is very likely. Diagnosis is certain if all seven are present.

TREATMENT

Treatment is directed toward two goals: resolution of the acute symptoms and prevention of bronchiectasis and pulmonary fibrosis. McCarthy and Pepys[44] demonstrated that treatment with prednisone, 20 to 40 mg/day, significantly hastens clearing of pulmonary infiltrates and reverts sputum cultures for *A. fumigatus* to negative. Safirstein and associates,[69] in a retrospective review of patients followed for 5 years, found that therapy with 7.5 mg of prednisone or more daily prevented the appearance of new radiologic shadows, whereas new persistent shadows appeared in 7 of 19 patients who were not treated with steroids. Thirty-five percent of flares were asymptomatic and could be detected only radiologically.[40, 69]

The striking increase in serum total IgE levels in patients with ABPA has been used to monitor patients.[27, 28] Rosenberg and colleagues[66, 67] found that IgE increases during and prior to the flares of ABPA. In serial measurements of total IgE levels in patients with ABPA, Wang and collaborators[83] demonstrated a significant increase in total IgE before the development of pulmonary infiltrates. In Chicago, most ABPA exacerbations occur between June and November, and an increase of 100% in total IgE levels over baseline signifies an exacerbation of the disease.[60] Patterson and coworkers[55] reported that when total IgE level doubles or triples over a stable baseline level, an active infiltrate caused by ABPA should be suspected, and a chest radiograph should be obtained. Total IgE levels may remain elevated following corticosteroid treatment. Thus, therapy should not be directed to bring total IgE levels to normal but can be used as index of activity.

The treatment of acute ABPA includes prednisone, 40 to 60 mg (0.5 to 0.8 mg/k), with gradual decrease of the dose based on clinical response and reduction in total IgE levels. Serial measurement of total IgE levels is important in determining the evolution of treatment; a 100% or more increase over the baseline is associated with new infiltrates, whereas a decrease in levels of at least 35% following prednisone correlates with resolution of infiltrates. Follow-up consists of monthly serum IgE measurements for 1 year, followed by bimonthly measurements for 1 to 2 years if there are no flares; IgE monitoring can then be performed at semiannual intervals. Chest radiographs rays should be obtained every 3 to 6 months during the first year, and yearly there after to avoid missing intercurrent pulmonary damage.[62]

Exacerbations should be treated with prednisone, 20 to 40 mg/day for 2 weeks, followed by changing to every-other-day therapy for 3 months with gradual decrease of the dose. Inhaled corticosteroids are ineffective in the treatment of ABPA,[63, 66, 83] but are used for the treatment of the underlying asthma. Immunotherapy with *Aspergillus* is not effective, and may cause anaphylaxis because of the high degree of sensitivity to *Aspergillus* in these patients. It would also increase specific anti-*Aspergillus* IgG and could theoretically worsen the disorder. Management of ABPA also includes environmental control to decrease exposure to molds and other aeroallergens, and optimal pharmacologic treatment of the coexisting asthma.

Antifungal agents have been used in ABPA with some degree of success.[9, 10, 79] Denning and coworkers[13] treated six ABPA patients with itraconazole, an orally administered antifungal agent. Most of the patients had marked improvement in subjective exercise tolerance and decreased serum IgE levels. Corticosteroid dosage was reduced in five of the six patients. Although these observations are interesting, the administration of antifungal agents for the treatment of ABPA is considered experimental at present.

REFERENCES

1. Ansell G: Complications in Diagnostic Radiology. Blackwell Scientific, Oxford, 1976, 286–290.
2. Bardana EJ Jr., McClatchy JK, Farr RS, Minden P: The primary interaction of antibody to components of aspergilli. J Allergy Clin Immunol 50:222–234, 1972.
3. Basisch JE, Graves TS, Nasir Baz M, et al: Allergic bronchopulmonary aspergillosis in corticosteroid-dependent asthmatics. J Allergy Clin Immunol 68:98–102, 1981.
4. Bhargava V, Tomashefski JF Jr, Stern RC, Abramowsky CR: The pathology of fungal infection and colonization in patients with cystic fibrosis. Hum Pathol 20:977–986, 1989.
5. Bosken CH, Myers JL, Greenberger PA, Katzenstein AL: Pathologic features of allergic bronchopulmonary aspergillosis. Am J Surg Pathol 12:216–222, 1988.
6. Brouwer J: Detection of antibodies against *Aspergillus fumigatus*: comparison between double immunodiffusion, ELISA and immunoblot analysis. Int Arch Allergy Appl Immunol 85:244–249, 1988.
7. Brummund W, Resnick A, Fink JN, Kurup VP: *Aspergillus fumigatus*–specific antibodies in allergic bronchopulmonary aspergillosis and aspergilloma: evidence for a polyclonal antibody response. J Clin Micro Biol 25:5–9, 1987.
8. Chan-Yeung M, Chase WH, Trapp W, Gryzbowski S: Allergic bronchopulmonary aspergillosis. Chest 59:33–39, 1971.
9. Crompton GK, Milne LJ: Treatment of bronchopulmonary aspergillosis with clotrimazole. Br J Dis Chest 67:301–307, 1973.
10. Currie DC, Lueck C, Milburn HJ, et al: Controlled trial of natamycin in the treatment of allergic bronchopulmonary aspergillosis. Thorax 45:447–450, 1990.
11. Currie DC, Goldman JM, Cole PJ, Strickland B: Comparison of narrow section computed tomography and plain chest radiography in chronic allergic bronchopulmonary aspergillosis. Clin Radiol 38:593–596, 1987.
12. Denning DW, Follansbee SE, Scolaro M, et al: Pulmonary aspergillosis in the acquired immunodeficiency syndrome. N Engl J Med 324:654–662, 1991.
13. Denning DW, Van Wye JE, Lewiston NJ, Stevens DA: Adjunctive therapy of allergic bronchopulmonary aspergillosis with itraconazole. Chest 100:813–820, 1991.
14. Geha RS: Circulating immune complexes and activation of the complement sequence in acute allergic bronchopulmonary aspergillosis. J Allergy Clin Immunol 60:357–359, 1977.
15. Golbert TM, Patterson R: Pulmonary allergic aspergillosis. Ann Intern Med 72:395–403, 1970.
16. Greenberger PA, Miller TP, Roberts M, Smith LL: Late sequelae of allergic bronchopulmonary aspergillosis. J Allergy Clin Immunol 66:327–335, 1980.
17. Greenberger PA, Patterson R: Allergic bronchopulmonary aspergillosis and the evaluation of the patient with asthma. J Allergy Clin Immunol 81:646–650, 1988.
18. Grenier P, Frantz M, Musset D, et al: Bronchiectasis: assessment by thin section CT. Radiology 161:95–99, 1986.
19. Hearn VM, Donaldson GC, Healy MJ, Trotman DM: A method to determine significant levels of immunoglobulin G to *Aspergillus fumigatus* antigens in an ELISA system and a comparison with counter immunoelectrophoresis and double diffusion techniques. J Immunoassay 6:137–158, 1985.
20. Hearn VM: Antigenicity of Aspergillus species. J Med Vet Mycol 30:11–25, 1992.
21. Henderson AH, English MP, Vecht RJ: Pulmonary aspergillosis: a survey of its occurrence in patients with chronic lung disease and a discussion of the significance of diagnostic tests. Thorax 23:513–518, 1968.

22. Henderson AH: Allergic aspergillosis: review of 32 cases. Thorax 23:501–512, 1968.
23. Henry RL, Mellis CM, Simpson SJ, South RT: Allergic bronchopulmonary aspergillosis in cystic fibrosis. Aust Paediatr 18:110–113, 1982.
24. Hinson KF, Moon AJ, Plummer NS: Bronchopulmonary aspergillosis. Thorax 7:317–333, 1952.
25. Hoehne JH, Reed CE, Dickie HA: Allergic bronchopulmonary aspergillosis is not rare. Chest 63:177–181, 1973.
26. Hutcheson PS, Rejent AJ, Slavin RG: Variability in parameters of allergic bronchopulmonary aspergillosis in patients with cystic fibrosis. J Allergy Clin Immunol 88:390–394, 1991.
27. Imbeau SA, Nichols D, Flaherty D, et al: Relationships between prednisone therapy, disease activity, and the total serum IgE level in allergic bronchopulmonary aspergillosis. J Allergy Clin Immunol 62:91–95, 1978.
28. Jarmoc LM, Maton MC, Hutcheson PS, et al: The immunopathology of cystic fibrosis with and without allergic bronchopulmonary aspergillosis. J Allergy Clin Immunol 81:185, 1988.
29. Joharjy IA, Bashi SA, Abdullah AK: Value of medium thickness CT in the diagnosis of bronchiectasis. Am J Roentgenol 149:1133–1137, 1987.
30. Katzenstein AL, Sale SR, Greenberger PA: Allergic *Aspergillus* sinusitis: a newly recognized form of sinusitis. J Allergy Clin Immunol 72:89–93, 1983.
31. Katzenstein AL, Liebow AA, Friedman PJ: Bronchocentric granulomatosis, mucoid impaction and hypersensitivity reactions to fungi. Am Rev Respir Dis 111:497–537, 1975.
32. Kauffman HF, Beaumont F, Meurs H, et al: Comparison of antibody measurements against *Aspergillus fumigatus* by means of double-diffusion and enzyme-linked immunosorbent assay (ELISA). J Allergy Clin Immunol 72:255–261, 1983.
33. Khan ZU, Richardson MD, Warnock DW: Evaluation of a rapid enzyme-linked immunosorbent assay for IgG antibodies to *Aspergillus fumigatus* in the serological diagnosis of allergic aspergillosis. Int Arch Allergy Appl Immunol 73:205–211, 1984.
34. Kim SJ, Chaparas SD: Characterization of antigens from *Aspergillosis fumigatus* III: comparison of antigenic relationships of clinically important aspergilli. Am Rev Respir Dis 120:1297–1303, 1979.
35. Knutsen AP, Slavin RG: In vitro T cell responses in patients with cystic fibrosis and allergic bronchopulmonary aspergillosis. J Lab Clin Med 113:428–435, 1989.
36. Laham MN, Allen RC, Greene JC: Allergic bronchopulmonary aspergillosis (ABPA) caused by *Aspergillus terreus*: specific lymphocyte sensitization and antigen-directed serum opsonic activity. Ann Allergy 46:74–80, 1981.
37. Laufer P, Fink JN, Bruns WT, et al: Allergic bronchopulmonary aspergillosis in cystic fibrosis. J Allergy Clin Immunol 73:44–48, 1984.
38. Laufer P, Fink JN, Bruns WT, et al: Allergic bronchopulmonary aspergillosis in cystic fibrosis. J Allergy Clin Immunol 73:44–48, 1984.
39. Malo JL, Paguin R, Longbottom JL: Prevalance of precipitating antibodies to different extracts of *Aspergillus fumigatus* in a North American asthmatic population. Clin Allergy 11:333–341, 1981.
40. Malo JL, Pepys J, Simon G: Studies in chronic allergic bronchopulmonary aspergillosis 2: radiological findings. Thorax 32:262–268, 1977.
41. Matthiesson AM: Allergic bronchopulmonary disease caused by fungi other than *Aspergillus*. Thorax 36:719, 1981.
42. McAleer R, Kroenert DB, Elder JL, Froudist JH: Allergic bronchopulmonary disease caused by *Curvularia lunata* and *Drechslera hawaiiensis*. Thorax 36:338–344, 1981.
43. McCarthy DS, Simon G, Hargreave FE: The radiological appearances in allergic bronchopulmonary aspergillosis. Clin Radiol 21:366–375, 1970.
44. McCarthy DS, Pepys J: Allergic bronchopulmonary aspergillosis: clinical immunology: (1) clinical features. Clin Allergy 1:261–286, 1971.
45. Mearns M, Young W, Batten J: Transient pulmonary infiltrations in cystic fibrosis due to allergic aspergillosis. Thorax 20:385–392, 1965.
46. Mintzer RA, Rogers LF, Kruglik GD, et al: The spectrum of radiologic findings in allergic bronchopulmonary aspergillosis. Radiology 127:301–307, 1978.
47. Mootoosamy IM, Reznek RH, Osman J, et al: Assessment of bronchiectasis by computed tomography. Thorax 40:920–924, 1985.
48. Muller NL, Bergin CJ, Ostrow DN, Nichols DM: Role of computed tomography in the recognition of bronchiectasis. Am J Roentgenol 143:971–976, 1984.
49. Murphy D, Lane DJ: Pleural effusion in allergic bronchopulmonary aspergillosis: two case reports. Br J Dis Chest 75:91–95, 1981.
50. Neeld DA, Goodman LR, Gurney JW, et al: Computerized tomography in the evaluation of allergic bronchopulmonary aspergillosis. Am Rev Respir Dis 142:1200–1205, 1990.
51. Nelson LA, Callerame ML, Schwartz RH: Aspergillosis and atopy in cystic fibrosis. Am Rev Respir Disease 120:863–873, 1979.
52. O'Neill JJ: Bronchography: a report of the Committee on Bronchoesophagology, American College of Chest Physicians. Dis Chest 51:663–668, 1967.
53. Patterson R, Greenberger PA, Ricketti AJ, Roberts M: A radioimmunoassay index for allergic bronchopulmonary aspergillosis. Ann Intern Med 99:18–22, 1983.
54. Patterson R, Greenberger PA, Radin RC, Roberts M: Allergic bronchopulmonary aspergillosis: staging as an aid to management. Ann Intern Med 96:256–291, 1982.
55. Patterson R, Greenberger PA, Lee TM, et al: Prolonged evaluation of patients with corticosteroid-dependent asthma stage of allergic bronchopulmonary aspergillosis. J Allergy Clin Immunol 80:663–668, 1987.
56. Patterson R, Greenberger PA, Halwig JM, et al: Allergic bronchopulmonary aspergillosis: natural history and classification of early disease by serologic and roentgenographic studies. Arch Intern Med 146:916–918, 1986.
57. Pepys J: Hypersensitivity diseases of the lungs due to fungi and organic dusts. Monographs in Allergy 4:1–147, 1969.
58. Phillips MS, Williams MP, Flower CD: How useful is computed tomography in the diagnosis and assessment of bronchiectasis? Clin Radiol 37:321–325, 1986.
59. Rachelefsky GS, Osher A, Dooly RE, et al: Coexistent respiratory allergy and cystic fibrosis. Am J Dis Child 128:355–359, 1974.
60. Radin RC, Greenberger PA, Patterson R, Ghory A: Mold counts and exacerbations of allergic bronchopulmonary aspergillosis. Clin Allergy 13:271–275, 1983.
61. Richardson MD, Warnock DW: Antigen and antibody attachment in ELISA for *Aspergillus fumigatus* IgG antibodies. J Immunol Methods 66:119–132, 1984.
62. Ricketti AJ, Greenberger PA, Mintzer RA, Patterson R: Allergic bronchopulmonary aspergillosis. Chest 86:773–778, 1984.
63. Ricketti AJ, Greenberger PA, Patterson R: Serum IgE as an important aid in management of allergic bronchopulmonary aspergillosis. J Allergy Clin Immunol 74:68, 1984.
64. Riddle HF, Channell S, Blyth W, et al: Allergic alveolitis in a maltworker. Thorax 23:271–280, 1968.
65. Riley DJ, Mackenzie JW, Uhlman WE, Edelman NH: Allergic bronchopulmonary aspergillosis: evidence of limited tissue invasion. Am Rev Respir Dis 111:232–236, 1975.
66. Rosenberg M, Patterson R, Roberts M, Wang J: The assessment of immunologic and clinical changes occurring during corticosteroid therapy for allergic bronchopulmonary aspergillosis. Am J Med 64:599–606, 1978.
67. Rosenberg M, Patterson R, Roberts M: Immunologic responses to therapy in allergic bronchopulmonary aspergillosis: serum IgE value as an indicator and predictor of disease activity. J Pediatr 91:914–917, 1977.
68. Rosenberg IL, Greenberger PA: Allergic bronchopulmonary aspergillosis and aspergilloma: long-term follow-up without enlargement of a large multiloculated cavity. Chest 85:123–125, 1984.
69. Safirstein BH, D'Souza MF, Simon G, et al: Five-year follow-up of allergic bronchopulmonary aspergillosis. Am Rev Respir Dis 108:450–459, 1973.
70. Scadding JG: The bronchi in allergic aspergillosis. Scand J Respir Dis 48:372–377, 1967.
71. Schonheyder H, Jensen T, Hoiby N, Koch C: Clinical and serological survey of pulmonary aspergillosis in patients with cystic fibrosis. Int Arch Allergy Appl Immunol 85:472–477, 1988.
72. Schwartz RH, Hollick GE: Allergic bronchopulmonary aspergillosis with low serum immunoglobulin E. J Allergy Clin Immunol 68:290–294, 1981.
73. Schwartz HJ, Citron KM, Chester EH, et al: A comparison of the prevalence of sensitization to Aspergillus antigens among asthmatics in Cleveland and London. J Allergy Clin Immunol 62:9–14, 1978.
74. Schwartz RS, Mackintosh FR, Schrier SL, Greenberg PL: Multivariate analysis of factors associated with invasive fungal disease during remission induction therapy for acute myelogenous leukemia. Cancer 53:411–419, 1984.
75. Sepulveda R, Longbottom JL, Pepys J: Enzyme linked immunosorbent assay (ELISA) for IgG and IgE antibodies to protein and polysaccharide antigens of *Aspergillus fumigatus*. Clin Allergy 9:359–371, 1979.

76. Slavin RG, Fischer VW, Levine EA, et al: A primate model of allergic bronchopulmonary aspergillosis. Int Arch Allergy Appl Immunol 56:325–333, 1978.
77. Slavin RG, Bedrossian CW, Hutcheson PS, et al: A pathologic study of allergic bronchopulmonary aspergillosis. J Allergy Clin Immunol 81:718–725, 1988.
78. Slavin RG, Hutcheson PS, Knutsen AP: Participation of cell-mediated immunity in allergic bronchopulmonary aspergillosis. Int Arch Allergy Appl Immunol 83:337–340, 1987.
79. Stark JE: Allergic pulmonary aspergillosis successfully treated with inhalations of nystatin. Dis Chest 51:96–99, 1967.
80. Trompelt J, Becker WM, Schlaak M: Analysis of IgG subclass and IgE response in allergic disease caused by Aspergillus fumigatus by immunoblotting techniques. Int Arch Allergy Immunol 104:390–398, 1994.
81. Turner-Warwick M: Immunologic lung disease due to *Aspergillus*. Chest 68:346–355, 1975.
82. Voss MJ, Bush RK, Mischler EH, Peters ME: Association of allergic bronchopulmonary aspergillosis and cystic fibrosis. J Allergy Clin Immunol 69:539–546, 1982.
83. Wang JL, Patterson R, Roberts M, Ghory AC: The management of allergic bronchopulmonary aspergillosis. Am Rev Respir Dis 120:87–92, 1979.
84. Wang JL, Patterson R, Rosenberg M, et al: Serum IgE and IgG antibody activity against *Aspergillus fumigatus* as a diagnostic aid in allergic bronchopulmonary aspergillosis. Am Rev Respir Dis 117:917–927, 1978.
85. Warnock ML, Fennessy J, Ripon J: Chronic eosinophilic pneumonia, a manifestation of allergic aspergillosis. Am J Clin Pathol 62:73–81, 1974.
86. Zeaske R, Bruns WT, Fink JN, et al: Immune responses to *Aspergillus* in cystic fibrosis. J Allergy Clin Immunol 82:73–77, 1988.

32 Hypersensitivity Pneumonitis

JORDAN N. FINK

Hypersensitivity pneumonitis comprises a group of immunologic lung disorders occurring as a result of sensitization and repeated exposure to any of a wide variety of inhaled organic dusts. The disease is a diffuse, predominantly mononuclear inflammation of the lung parenchyma, particularly of the terminal bronchioles and alveoli. The inflammation often organizes into granulomas and may progress to fibrosis. A wide variety of dusts can cause the disease, including moldy fodder in farmer's lung, moldy sugar cane in bagassosis, bird droppings or other avian proteins in bird handler's lung, and mold spores in cheese washer's lung. Most individuals who develop hypersensitivity pneumonitis are exposed through their occupation; however, organisms can also contaminate and be dispersed through forced air heating, humidification, or air conditioning systems, causing pulmonary disease in home and office occupants.

No single clinical feature or laboratory test is diagnostic of the disease. Rather, the diagnosis can be made from a combination of characteristic symptoms, physical findings, radiologic abnormalities, and pulmonary function and immunologic tests. The demonstration of serum-precipitating antibodies to a suspected inhaled antigen is particularly helpful. Inhalation challenge with the suspected offending agent, evaluation of bronchalveolar lavage cells, or lung biopsy may be useful in clarifying the diagnosis.

Hypersensitivity pneumonitis should be suspected in patients with a history of exposure to one of the offending antigens and who have either repeated bouts of influenza-like pneumonitis or active interstitial lung disease. A number of the other interstitial lung diseases bear clinical and pathologic similarities to hypersensitivity pneumonitis and should be considered in the differential diagnosis. Although the clinical and laboratory abnormalities tend to disappear when the offending antigen is avoided, continued exposure has been shown to result in irreversible pulmonary damage. The immune mechanisms and pathogenesis responsible for the development of hypersensitivity pneumonitis are incompletely understood. Most individuals exposed to an offending antigen fail to develop disease.

Certain types of hypersensitivity pneumonitis are of particular importance. Maple bark stripper's disease, for example, is a hypersensitivity pneumonitis essentially eliminated by recognizing the conditions necessary for its development. Maple logs are no longer stored in the open, where they may get wet and foster the growth of the offending organism under the wet bark. Hypersensitivity pneumonitis secondary to contaminated forced air heating, cooling, and humidification systems is potentially of great practical importance, considering the widespread use of such systems.

ETIOLOGY

Hypersensitivity pneumonitis may occur following the inhalation of and subsequent sensitization to any of a wide variety of antigens in the environment. Offending agents may be bacterial (thermophilic actinomycetes), fungal (*Alternaria, Aspergillus*), serum proteins (avian proteins), chemical (anhydrides), or yet undefined (coffee dust) (Table 32–1).

The major occupations and industries associated with hypersensitivity pneumonitis are those in which moldy vegetable compost is handled, which by its very wet nature is contaminated with the thermophilic actinomycetes. Thus, dairy farmers,[14, 18] sugar cane workers,[12] and mushroom compost handlers[11] may be exposed, as are individuals living or working in environments with ventilation systems contaminated with these same organisms.[5, 29, 30, 43, 52]

Industries in which raw wood products are processed have also been shown to be prone to the development of hypersensitivity pneumonitis. Suberosis (cork),[4] sequoiosis (redwood),[16] maple bark,[24] and wood pulp industries[9, 67] have reported cases. Individuals involved in bird handling (pigeon racers, pigeon fanciers, budgerigar breeders) develop disease as a result of the inhalation of proteins from droppings, dander, saliva, or urine.[2, 26, 34, 58, 61]

The disease had also been described in chemical manufacturing and processing, especially when isocyanates and anhydrides are used.[32, 66] Such areas include paint spray, epoxy, and other plastics manufacturing. As additional areas of exposure and subsequent diseases have been detected, it has become apparent that a broad variety of inhalant organic dusts are capable of inducing the syndrome hypersensitivity pneumonitis.

Statistical reports of respiratory disease incidence do not commonly categorize "hypersensitivity pneumonitis," because the disorder has not become widely recognized. Cases of this disease may therefore be categorized as inhalation diseases, interstitial diseases, or occupational airway diseases.[57]

Little information is available regarding a relationship between antigens, exposure, and disease. In a particular population similarly exposed to a sensitizing inhalational antigen, the number of individuals with detectable pulmonary disease has ranged from 3% to 15%.[15, 54] Yet, up to 50% of exposed but asymptomatic individuals in similar environments have detectable humoral or cellular immune responses to the antigen without clinical evidence of disease. Thus, some other unknown factor is important in the genesis of hypersensitivity pneumonitis. The possibilities are as follows:

Genetic Factors. Farmer's lung or pigeon breeder's disease may be under genetic control, because increased frequencies of specific HLA haplotype have been demonstrated in ill individuals.[1, 35] Other evidence has suggested that pigeon breeder's disease is not associated with immunologic responsiveness as determined by HLA typing of ill and well pigeon breeders.[64]

Infection. Animal models of hypersensitivity pneumonitis have suggested that some inflammatory event must occur in the lung in addition to recurrent antigen inhalation exposure for disease to develop. Animals subjected to long-term exposed to pigeon antigens develop an immune response but

TABLE 32–1
ANTIGENS OF HYPERSENSITIVITY PNEUMONITIS

Agent	Disease	Exposure
Thermophilic actinomycetes		
Micropolyspora faeni	Farmer's lung	Moldy compost
Thermoactinomyces vulgaris	Farmer's lung and mushroom worker's lung	
Thermoactinomyces sacchari	Bagassosis	Moldy sugar cane
Thermoactinomyces candidus, Thermoactinomyces viridis, Naegleria gruberii (an amoeba), and unidentified fungi and slime molds	Ventilation pneumonitis	Contaminated forced-air system
Fungi		
Aspergillus clavatus	Malt worker's lung	Moldy malt
Penicillium frequentans	Suberosis	Moldy work dust
Penicillium caseii, Penicillium roquefortii	Cheese worker's lung	Cheese mold
Alternaria species	Wood worker's lung	Moldy wood chips and sawdust
Rhizopus species		
Pullularia species	Sequoiosis	Moldy redwood dust
Cryptostroma corticale	Maple bark stripper's disease	Moldy maple bark
Trichosporon cutaneum	Summer hypersensitivity pneumonitis in Japan	Contaminated house dust
Arthropods		
Sitophilus granarius	Wheat weevil disease	infested wheat
Animal proteins		
Avian proteins	Bird breeder's lung	Avian droppings
Bovine and porcine proteins	Pituitary snuff user's lung	Pituitary snuff
Phthalic anhydride	Epoxy resin worker's lung	Epoxy resin
Toluene diisocyanate	Porcelain refinisher's lung	Paint catalyst
Trimellitic anhydride (TMA)	TMA disease	Trimellitic anhydride
Other		
Amebae, various fungi	Ventilation pneumonitis	Contaminated systems
Bacillus subtilis	Enzyme worker's lung	Detergent enzymes
Hair dust	Furrier's lung	Animal proteins
Coffee dust	Coffee worker's lung	?

no pulmonary inflammation until an agent such as BCG or carageenen is given.[55] Such agents may stimulate the immune response by adjuvant action or by enhancement of antigen absorption and subsequent availability to immunologically active cells through inflamed mucosa.

Toxic Factors. The induction, progression, and severity of hypersensitivity pneumonitis may be related to a variety of toxic exposures. Possible toxicants include tobacco smoke, air pollution, and industrial exposures. One study has linked the occurrence of pigeon breeder's disease with the use of hexachlorobenzene as a disinfectant in pigeon lofts.[1] These factors may enhance absorption of antigens as a result of pulmonary inflammation. They may also increase local immune responses or may act systemically as adjuvants.

Altered Immunoregulation. Suppressor cell activity utilizing peripheral blood cells and lymphocytes obtained by bronchoalveolar lavage from symptomatic and asymptomatic but similarly exposed individuals has been evaluated in in vitro culture systems. Such studies have demonstrated that suppressor cell activity, present in the asymptomatic group, cannot be detected in the symptomatic group.[46] These findings suggest that abnormalities in immunoregulation may be basic to the development of hypersensitivity pneumonitis.

EPIDEMIOLOGY

Hypersensitivity pneumonitis is not categorized in statistical reports of respiratory disease incidence. Because of its clinical presentation and pathophysiology, the disease may be classified with inhalation diseases, interstitial diseases, occupational diseases, or even diseases of the airways. However, some data are available on a few specific forms, especially farmer's lung, which has been studied in England and the United States. Information available is sketchy, because closed populations of farmers have seldom been studied; and although some prevalence data are available, few or no incidence data have been published. There is little doubt that farmer's lung is an important occupational illness in farmers in the United States, but the diagnosis may be commonly overlooked because of a lack of patient and/or physician awareness.

Grant and associates,[38] in a study of 655 farm workers in Scotland, found the prevalence of farmer's lung to range from 2.3% to 8.6% in three counties. Staines and Froman[71] estimated the prevalence of farmer's lung in British farm communities to range from 0.5% to 1% of the population.[71] A study of 93 farmers by Morgan and coworkers,[56] in an area endemic for farmer's lung, showed that 9 (9.6%) had clinical histories compatible with farmer's lung. Smyth and associates[70] found that fewer than 45% of patients with farmer's lung were diagnosed during the first year of their illness.

A U.S. study surveyed 471 people associated with farming or dairy production.[50] A history typical of farmer's lung syndrome was given by 14 (3.9%) people. The prevalence of farmer's lung in this western Wyoming community was comparable to those in the British and Scottish studies.

More than 1,000 dairy farmers in central Wisconsin were surveyed for the presence of serum precipitins to a panel of antigens including thermophilic actinomycetes, *Aspergillus*, and pigeon serum[51]; 8.5% of the group had precipitating antibodies to one or more of the thermophilic actinomyces, whereas 0.4% had precipitins to *Aspergillus*. All of the individuals with precipitins were further evaluated. Thirty-six percent had a positive history and 10% had a questionable history of farmer's lung.

On the basis of these findings, there is a potential development of approximately 32 cases of farmer's lung per 1,000 in the dairy farming population of Wisconsin. This would result in 4,800 farmers at risk, a figure exceeding the frequency of many other pulmonary diseases. Such a high estimated prevalence is alarming, because these individuals are at risk of developing the chronic irreversible lung damage associated with hypersensitivity pneumonitis.

Estimates of the socioeconomic impact of farmer's lung are difficult to obtain. If the definitive treatment is to remove the farmer from the offending environment, the consequences of such changes are far-reaching. The average dairy farmer, a 45-year-old man, knows no other occupation. His farm, which is his home as well as his place of business, often represents a considerable investment that may not be easily liquidated. Furthermore, farm spouses seldom have outside employment and are usually not prepared to become part of an outside work force. Thus the impact of such a situation on the family is considerable.

Changing farm practices and purchasing additional equipment could produce an environment relatively free of exposure to the thermophilic actinomycetes. However, sufficient information is not available to determine the cost and effectiveness of such changes. There have been instances in which the farm environment and practices have been altered, but at a cost of $50,000 to $100,000 (F. Wenzel, personal communication, 1985).

Of the more than 600 cases of bagassosis in the literature, approximately 500 have been detected in Louisiana. However, the disease is of worldwide distribution and occurs wherever sugar cane is processed. Cases have been reported from Louisiana, Texas, Missouri, Illinois, Puerto Rico, India, Cuba, Italy, England, and Peru.[58] A number of cases have been seen in nonoccupationally exposed individuals, such as persons using the material as a garden mulch, homemakers residing in homes several miles downwind from sugar cane processing areas, and employees working in air conditioned offices at or near the processing site.

Pigeon breeder's disease has been estimated to occur in 6% to 15% of individuals who raise pigeons as a hobby.[15, 33] There are approximately 75,000 breeders in the United States; therefore if the estimated prevalence is correct, up to 10,000 of these individuals could develop irreversible lung damage.

Studies of several office worker populations exposed to contaminated air cooling systems have demonstrated a prevalence of hypersensitivity pneumonitis ranging from 15% in one such outbreak[5] to less than 1% in another.[3]

Thus although no specific prevalence and incidence data are available for each type of hypersensitivity pneumonitis, it is known that the disease represents a serious health problem in many occupations. It is also believed to occur more commonly in home and office environments than has been recognized.[28, 37]

CLINICAL FEATURES

The onset of hypersensitivity pneumonitis may be acute or insidious.[27, 58] When exposure is intermittent, as in the hobby of pigeon breeding, symptoms begin abruptly 4 to 6 hours later. Chills, fever of 101 to 104°F, malaise, dry cough, dyspnea, and easy fatigue may persist for up to 18 hours. With frequent and repeated exposure, anorexia and weight loss of 10 to 20 lb is usual. Bronchospastic involvement of the airways is exceptional, and most patients do not develop both asthma and hypersensitivity pneumonitis. Fatalities have been reported.[8, 39]

When exposure is less intense but more continuous, chills and fever may not occur. Exertional dyspnea, cough with scanty mucopurulent sputum, easy fatigue, anorexia, and weight loss are usual symptoms. In an affected individual, an acute episode is rare unless exposure is exceptionally intense.

In the chronic form of the disease, the symptoms are mainly respiratory and consist of progressive shortness of breath leading to pulmonary disability. There may be associated anorexia and weight loss with mucopurulent sputum, but acute episodes do not usually occur.[33]

The physical examination reveals characteristic inspiratory rales resembling crackling cellophane; these can be heard throughout the lungs but are loudest at the bases. The rales may be heard only at the peak of an acute illness or may persist for weeks or months. Wheezing or prolonged expiration occur occasionally in patients also allergic (immunoglobulin E–mediated) to birds but does not usually occur with exposure to thermophilic actinomycetes. Ankle edema and enlargement of the liver are rare and indicate complicating right-sided heart failure.

Other aspects of the physical examination serve mainly to exclude other diagnoses. Peripheral lymphadenopathy or splenomegaly does not occur, and hilar adenopathy is unusual. Complicating arthritis or skin rashes are not observed.

LABORATORY FINDINGS

BLOOD STUDIES

A polymorphonuclear leukocytosis of up to 25,000 cells/mm^3 with a shift to young forms is the usual finding in the acute episode. The leukocytosis resolves with recovery and is not seen between attacks. Eosinophilia of up to 10% may be found. The erythrocyte sedimentation rate is within normal limits.

There is broad elevation of all immunoglobulins (Igs), except for IgE. Rheumatoid factor levels are often elevated but are not evident after prolonged avoidance.

PULMONARY FUNCTION STUDIES

A number of pulmonary function abnormalities can occur, depending on the clinical form and stage of the hypersensitivity pneumonitis.[58, 65]

During acute episodes, the most common response occurs within 4 to 6 hours after exposure to the offending antigen. There is a decrease in forced vital capacity (FVC) and 1-second forced expiratory volume (FEV_1), with a constant ratio between these two parameters, indicating restriction. There is little change in expiratory flow rates. A fall in the diffusion capacity and a decrease in compliance indicating increased lung stiffness also occur during acute episodes. As the attack subsides over the next 12 to 24 hours, these abnormalities resolve; if the attack is severe, the abnormalities may persist for several days. With parenchymal damage, volume and flow abnormalities as well as hypercapnia may be detected during asymptomatic phases.

Some individuals with hypersensitivity pneumonitis exhibit a two-stage pulmonary reaction. Immediately after exposure, an asthmatic response occurs with a decrease in forced vital capacity, forced expiratory flow volume, and expiratory flow rates indicative of medium and small airway obstruction. This response is followed by the late 4- to 6-hour response described previously. Controlled laboratory challenge studies have demonstrated that the immediate pulmonary function response can be reversed with bronchodilators; the late response is resistant to these drugs. Pretreatment with corticosteroids blocks the late response, and cromolyn may block both responses. These findings suggest that different pathophysiologic mechanisms may be involved in the two distinct types of response.

In the subacute form of hypersensitivity pneumonitis, a more persistent restrictive impairment and diffusion defect may be demonstrated during exposure and even for some time after cessation of contact with the antigen.[68] In patients with the chronic form of hypersensitivity pneumonitis, irreversible pulmonary function abnormalities may be demonstrated. In fact, the most marked physiologic alterations have been found in patients with the chronic form of hypersensitivity pneumonitis, such as individuals with pigeon breeder's disease[34] or farmer's lung.[6] A severe restrictive impairment with a moderate to marked diffusion defect has been shown to persist in some of these patients; the defect may be physiologically correlated with the pulmonary fibrosis demonstrable on chest radiography and lung biopsy.

Other individuals with chronic hypersensitivity pneumonitis may demonstrate poorly reversible and progressive obstructive disease with hyperinflation and elevation of residual volume. A loss of pulmonary elasticity with increased static compliance can also be demonstrated in these individuals.[68] Some of the latter group may also have decreased diffusion capacity. These findings may correlate with biopsy evidence of obliterative bronchiolitis and destructive emphysema.[34]

RADIOLOGIC STUDIES

Chest radiography of patients with hypersensitivity pneumonitis can be normal if recurrent episodes are infrequent. In active cases one may see fine, sharp nodulations (Fig. 32–1) and reticulations with general coarsening of bronchovascular markings. During an acute attack, soft, patchy, ill-defined diffuse parenchymal densities that tend to coalesce may be seen in both lung fields. Chronic or end-stage disease may present as diffuse fibrosis with parenchymal contraction or even honeycombing.[71, 75]

IMMUNOLOGIC STUDIES

The characteristic immunologic feature of hypersensitivity pneumonitis is the demonstration of serum-precipitating an-

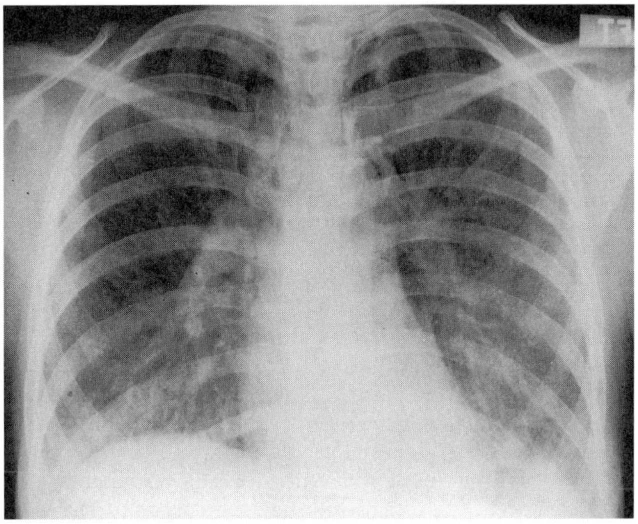

FIGURE 32–1. Chest x-ray of patient with hypersensitivity pneumonitis due to contamination of a home humidifier. Fine reticulations are evident in the bases.

tibodies against the offending organic dust antigen. Agar gel diffusion techniques using the suspect antigen and patient serum can detect antibodies in almost all ill individuals[7] (Fig. 32–2). However, these tests must be evaluated in light of the other clinical findings, because up to 50% of similarly exposed but asymptomatic individuals may also have moderate to high titers of serum-precipitating antibodies to the same antigen.[34] The antibodies in symptomatic and asymptomatic individuals belong largely to the IgG class of immunoglobulins, but IgA and IgM antibodies have also been detected in serum and bronchoalveolar lavage fluids of ill pigeon breeders.[13]

Skin tests with bird sera and some of the mold antigens may evoke a dual-phase skin reaction. A positive response consists of an immediate wheal-and-erythema reaction followed 3 to 8 hours later by an area of dermal and subcutaneous swelling several centimeters in diameter. Biopsy of such sites may demonstrate a mild vasculitis with immunofluorescent detection of immunoglobulin and complement.

Cell-mediated immunity to organic dust antigens has been detected with the peripheral lymphocytes of patients with hypersensitivity pneumonitis.[31–36] Studies of bronchoalveolar lavage cell populations from symptomatic individuals have detected marked increases in T cells with a predominance of the CD8 or suppressor cell phenotype.[46] Such cells are activated and have heightened responses to the specific environmental substances as well as nonspecific mitogens.[72] Activated macrophages, natural killer (NK) cells, and cells with activated adhesion molecules are also present.[72]

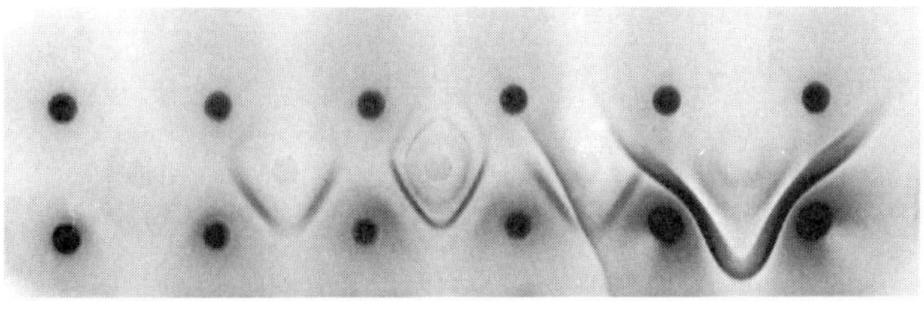

FIGURE 32–2. Gel immunodiffusion of sera from patients with pigeon breeder's disease (center wells) against pigeon antigens (peripheral wells). Serum on far left is control.

Asymptomatic but similarly exposed individuals also have increases in alveolar T cells but no evidence of active alveolitis.[46] These tests may thus be useful and specific for hypersensitivity pneumonitis and may more readily discriminate than do antibody tests between exposed individuals who are ill compared with those who are asymptomatic.

DIAGNOSTIC CHALLENGE

Purposeful inhalation challenge may be carried out by cautiously exposing the patient to the suspect environment or by utilizing the suspect antigen in the laboratory. The technique may reproduce the typical acute episode, with fever, chills, cough, rales, leukocytosis, and pulmonary function abnormalities occurring 4 to 6 hours after the exposure. Once an episode has begun, it should be aborted with corticosteroids to prevent further pulmonary changes.

PATHOLOGY

The lung is a unique organ, in that it is presented with an extremely large number and variety of potential antigens. Important antigenic agents present in the inhaled organic dusts are derived from fungal, bacterial, or serum protein sources. Because of the small particle size of these dusts (usually less than 5 μm), large quantities of antigenic material can be deposited at the alveolar level as well as in the airways. Under certain circumstances, this antigenic challenge can result in an immunologic response producing reactions in the airways and lung parenchyma. The clinical response to this challenge depends on the person's immunologic reactivity, the nature of the dust, the size of the particles, and the intensity of the exposure.[58]

The pathologic variation of the response depends more on the timing of the antigen exposure than on the character of the offending antigen, because pathologic events are similar during the disease course for the various clinical entities. The intensity of any acute inflammatory events appears to vary with the dose of the specific antigen delivered to the lung and with the interval between the acute and past episodes.

The lung morphology during the acute clinical episodes is that of acute interstitial pneumonitis. The alveolar spaces contain numerous macrophages and foreign body giant cells, as well as neutrophils and a modest number of eosinophils. The macrophages commonly contain some stainable neutral fat. The alveolar walls are often thickened, edematous, and infiltrated by neutrophils, a few eosinophils, and macrophages (Fig. 32–3).

As the chronicity of the process develops, the inflammatory exudate within the interstitial tissue has more of a plasmacytic or lymphocytic character. The inflammatory exudate is paucicellular in the earliest stages; some fibrinous exudate may also precede the inflammatory cells. The granulomatous lesions that develop later consist of dense collections of plump epithelioid cells arranged in palisade fashion and often surround zones of liquefaction necrosis in which some necrotic tissue debris and a few inflammatory cells

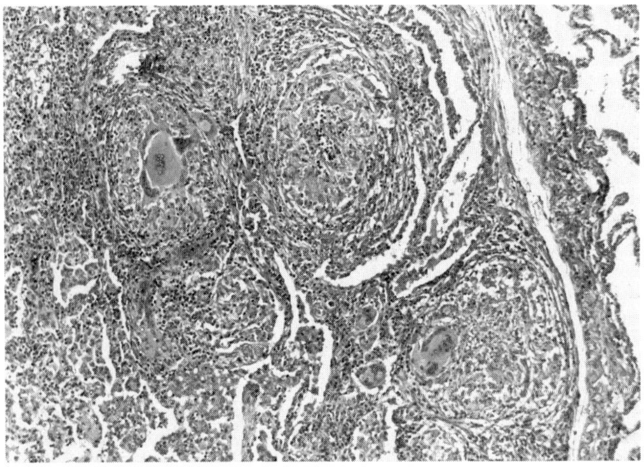

FIGURE 32–3. Lung biopsy of patient with pigeon breeder's disease demonstrating lymphocytic interstitial pneumonitis, foamy macrophages, and granuloma formation.

remain. Bronchioles are often involved in the process and demonstrate necrosis, which destroys portions of their mural structure and occludes the bronchiolar lumen with macrophages, inflammatory cells, and tissue debris. The bronchiolar epithelium may be destroyed and replaced by flat, regenerating epithelium. The involved adjacent alveoli are lined by hypertrophied, cuboidal, epithelial cells.[69]

As the process unfolds, its course may be influenced by several factors: (1) the degree of sensitization to the offending, specific antigenic material, and the subsequent immune response; (2) the amount of antigen presented in the current episode; and (3) the number and timing of any repeat exposures to the same antigen. If the degree of sensitivity is minimal or the antigen dose encountered during the inciting episode small, and the encounter is not repeated, the inflammatory episode may resolve with little or no residual tissue change. If the inflammatory process persists—owing to either persistence of the chronic reaction or the periodic recurrence of acute exacerbations—the lung suffers insidious or episodically overt, continued tissue destruction. Noncaseating granulomas may then be seen with greater frequency. The inflammatory exudate within alveolar spaces and bronchiolar lumens may become invaded with fibroblastic cells and contain distinctive Masson bodies, which are evidence of organization of alveolar exudate. The chronic inflammatory exudate within the interstitial and alveolar septa increase in amount, are characterized by a greater number of plasma cells, and become thickened by fibroblastic invasion and hypertrophied, alveolar epithelial cells.[23]

After a prolonged period of repeated acute insults and persistent chronic inflammation, diffuse interstitial fibrosis or honeycomb lung may develop. Within the fibrosis, inflammation may persist in the interstitial and alveolar septa, which have been thickened by mature collagenous connective tissue and some residual chronic inflammatory cells. Noncaseating granulomas are infrequent or absent and may be replaced by collagen or hyalinized tissue. The alveolar spaces are modestly enlarged and the walls thickened by fibrosis and alveolar cell hyperplasia. Intraalveolar organizing Masson bodies are seen. Small muscular arteries are thickened and sclerotic. In honeycomb lung, a similar residual chronic inflammatory process may be present in the interstitial and intraalveolar spaces, and the air spaces are enlarged and cyst-like, reaching a dimension of 0.5 to 1.0 cm. The walls of these spaces are fibrotic, contain elements of hypertrophied smooth muscle, plasmacytes, and lymphocytes, and are commonly lined by hypertrophied bronchial epithelial cells. The muscular arteries and arterioles are markedly thickened.[69]

The characteristic abnormality in an acute reaction is the response described earlier along with granulomas composed of epitheloid cells plus necrosis and tissue destruction. The presence of large foamy macrophages has been most commonly observed in bird fancier's lung.[42]

Although bronchioles may be involved with a resulting obstructive organizing bronchiolitis, the lesion is clearly alveolar, inflammatory, and capable of tissue destruction. Because the involvement is usually focal and does not involve large amounts of lung tissue, the functional abnormalities observed may reflect alveolar wall involvement and, to a lesser degree, airway disease, producing a decrease in the diffusion capacity of the lung and slight compromise in tests of ventilation. In later stages, the lesions show evidence of tissue loss with fibrosis or scarring.

NATURAL HISTORY AND PROGNOSIS

With the exception of farmer's lung and pigeon breeder's disease, the number of patients with hypersensitivity pneumonitis seen by one group of investigators is small. This has made large-scale longitudinal studies difficult. In addition, only a few individuals develop disease after antigen exposure. As a result, the problem may not be recognized in a particular case. Often there is voluntary avoidance of exposure by the affected person, even though the exact cause-and-effect relationship is not understood.

The clinical course of the disease depends to a large extent on the intensity and duration of exposure. In general, a brief exposure, even though intense, results in an acute reaction in a sensitive individual followed, within several days to weeks of avoidance, by complete resolution of symptoms and return of pulmonary function to normal or near normal. Recovery can be accelerated by the use of corticosteroids. However, with repeated exposure to the antigen or with chronic low-level exposure, progressive disabling respiratory symptoms and irreversible physiologic changes may result. This type of exposure has been found in patients with farmer's lung.[18] Intense exposure to mold spores, as found when silos are "uncapped," may precede some patients' development of farmer's lung.[25]

Only limited data are available on the long-term prognosis and physiologic abnormalities in the chronic phase of hypersensitivity pneumonitis. A study of 50 patients with farmer's lung over an average of 6 years showed a mortality rate of 10%.[6] In this same group, 30% had persistent respiratory symptoms and physiologic abnormalities, with pulmonary fibrosis being the major problem. In a retrospective study of 24 patients, 4 died during the period of observation after a 2- to 10-year duration of illness.[23] Three of 5 patients who had a lung biopsy in the acute stage and subsequently progressed to the chronic stage have been reported.[69] A study of farmer's lung in Devon, England, included 200 patients diagnosed between 1939 and 1971.[70] There were four deaths from farmer's lung, and severe disability was present in approximately one third of patients. Disability was commonly associated with restriction and reduced diffusing capacity and with airways obstruction in severe cases. Both face masks and steroids were utilized by many of the farmers included in this study.

A review dealing with bagassosis reported that 4 of 53 patients with the disease had died, representing a mortality rate of 7.5%.[12] However, the figure was believed to be falsely high, because milder cases likely escaped medical attention. Several other studies of acute bagassosis outbreaks showed that with exposure avoidance, even without corticosteroids, the restrictive impairment and abnormal diffusing capacity returned to normal.[44, 76] In contrast, another study found similar functional changes during the course of the acute illness, and chest radiographs returned to normal; however, the restrictive impairment and reduction in diffusing capacity, although improved, persisted even after 12 months of follow-up.[60]

Ten patients with pigeon breeder's disease followed with serial pulmonary function studies for 20 years have shown a variable pattern. Individuals who had normal function at the time they were first seen have tended to remain within normal limits despite occasional acute episodes. Patients who had either a restrictive impairment or, as in two cases, severe airway obstruction were found to show slight improvement but, in some cases, a more rapid deterioration in function than normally expected, even in the absence of further pigeon exposure (Schlueter and Fink, personal observations, 1995). Another study with a shorter follow-up period reported a similar finding, particularly with regard to the diffusing capacity.[19]

A study of nine afflicted breeders showed complete recovery in four patients 8 to 30 months after they had ceased exposure to the antigen. The other five had evidence of interstitial damage; three had a progressive increase in the degree of airway obstruction, and one had loss of elastic recoil. The patients were nonsmokers, and occult antigen exposure was ruled out because the precipitating antibody studies became negative.[2] Neither the nature or degree of lung function abnormality nor the form of clinical presentation was related to the development of residual damage. The period of continued exposure after symptoms developed and the patient's age seemed to be the most important factors determining recovery of lung function.

Although the spectrum of response to antigen exposure in patients with hypersensitivity pneumonitis is broad, exposure avoidance appears to result in complete resolution of abnormalities in most, but not all, cases. It seems, however, that continued exposure can lead to progressive and irreversible disease. When a substantial volume of lung tissue is involved and alveolar hypoxia is chronic, pulmonary hypertension develops. Chronic and sustained pulmonary hypertension leads to right ventricular enlargement and ultimately to right ventricular failure. Respiratory failure as a result of extensive destruction and fibrosis of lung tissue may be seen in the end stages of chronic, progressive lung disease.

PATHOGENESIS

The potential antigens for hypersensitivity pneumonitis are almost infinite when one considers the varieties of dusts inhaled into the lungs during a lifetime. It is likely that a relationship exists between the character and dose of inhaled antigen, the pulmonary removal mechanisms, and defense systems.

The immunologic hallmark of hypersensitivity pneumonitis is the presence of serum precipitins to the inhaled antigen[58] (see Fig. 32–2). Precipitins are present in more than 90% of patients with clinical disease and are of the IgG class of immunoglobulins. However, as many as 50% of individuals with similar antigen exposure also have precipitins but are asymptomatic.[27] There is considerable overlap in the titers of symptomatic and asymptomatic individuals; therefore, the titer itself is neither diagnostic nor prognostic. Hence, the precipitin reaction must be considered in light of the clinical presentation of the patient.

With the exception of patients who have an asthmatic (IgE) response to an inhaled antigen, the role of serum antibodies is not clear and may represent a natural immune response to an inhaled antigen with the formation of immune complexes as a clearing mechanism. Elevated specific IgE antibody is present only in atopic individuals who have the immediate airways obstructive reaction characteristic of asthma.

The immunologic events responsible for the physiologic and anatomic abnormalities in the acute and chronic forms of hypersensitivity pneumonitis are not understood. There is evidence for and against an immune complex role. The presence of antigen-specific IgG precipitating antibodies in the patients and the temporal relationship between antigenic exposure and the onset of acute illness (4 to 10 hours) are compatible with an immune complex, complement-dependent (Arthus-type) immunologic reaction. In addition, lung biopsies obtained during the acute reaction have demonstrated infiltration of the alveolar walls with lymphocytes and plasma cells, whereas polymorphonuclear leukocytes and eosinophils have been seen in only modest numbers. Within the alveoli are foamy macrophages that contain C3.[78] In contrast to the experimental Arthus-type reaction, there is no direct relationship between the antibody titer and the severity of the acute reaction in patients with hypersensitivity pneumonitis. In some patients, the precipitin titers may fall below the level of detection by immunodiffusion, yet clinical sensitivity persists.[53] Patients with hypersensitivity pneumonitis may have low antibody levels in their sera, although their bronchoalveolar lavage fluids contain increased concentrations of IgG and, in many instances, increased titers of antibody of several immunoglobulin classes against the etiologic agent.[58] Attempts to demonstrate immune complexes within alveolar lesions have been unsuccessful, but complement activation with the release of chemotactic factors has been detected in the lung.[79]

Additional evidence that IgG-mediated reactions are not solely responsible for hypersensitivity pneumonitis comes from animal studies. In guinea pigs immunized to produce an antibody response, hemorrhagic alveolitis not morphologically compatible with farmer's lung was induced after antigen challenge.[63] Moreover, it has not been possible to passively transfer the disease to monkeys with antibody-containing serum followed by antigen challenge.[41] Thus even though skin testing of persons with pigeon breeder's disease with pigeon serum produces Arthus-type responses at 4 to 6 hours, current evidence suggests that this reaction, like the serum precipitins, is a consequence of antigenic exposure. Its relationship to the pathogenesis of the disease is unclear. Additional evidence for the participation of humoral factors in hypersensitivity pneumonitis includes the demonstration that the alternate pathway of complement fixation is activated by spores of thermophilic actinomycetes.[20] This pathway may play a direct role in the genesis of inflammatory mediators within the pulmonary parenchyma or may interact with the circulating immune complexes to induce lesions, or products such as Ba may activate alveolar macrophages.

Bronchoalveolar lavage studies have demonstrated a marked lymphocytic alveolitis in patients with hypersensitivity pneumonitis, with more than 60% of the cells being T cells that are largely of the CD8 or suppressor phenotype.[46, 72] The cells are markedly activated, as shown by the presence of HLA-DR and activated T-cell markers.[72] Such lymphocytes have enhanced reactivity to specific antigen as well as to nonspecific mitogens but have defective suppressor cell activity.[46] An increase in soluble IL-2 receptor and Il-2 receptor expression on macrophages reflects T cell and macrophage activation.[58a] Further, there are increases in NK cell numbers and NK cell activity,[16b] and in adhesion molecule cell markers such as intracellular adhesion molecule 1 (ICA-1) on activated alveolar macrophages.[59] Additional findings indicate that mast cell activities and numbers are increased.[45] This increase results in secretion of proinflammatory cytokines and other immunoregulatory molecules.[45]

These studies explain the finding of enhanced cellular activation along with immunoregulatory imbalance to lead to lymphocytic alveolitis and granuloma formation.

Animal models have supported cellular mechanisms in the pathogenesis of hypersensitivity pneumonitis. Sensitized lymph node and spleen cell transfer followed by antigen challenge has resulted in the development of pulmonary lesions resembling those seen in human hypersensitivity pneumonitis. Such changes are not reproduced with transfer of serum antibodies. Such induced lesions are marked by activated T cells and alveolar macrophages.[10] Soluble proinflammatory factors such as interleukin-1 and tumor necrosis factor–α (TNF-α) can also be detected in the lungs.[16a, 16b, 17, 45] In other animal models, immunoregulatory imbalances induced with cyclosporin, antimacrophage antibody, and neonatal thymectomy inhibit the lesions.[47]

Although these observations suggest a role for cell-mediated immunity in the pathogenesis of hypersensitivity pneumonitis, they do not exclude the likely possibility that a combination of immune complex and complement along with cell-mediated reactions is necessary for production of clinical hypersensitivity pneumonitis in exposed individuals. Because most patients with hypersensitivity pneumonitis have demonstrable precipitating antibodies and cellular immune reactions to an offending antigen, it is likely that a multiplicity of immune reactions are important in the pathogenesis of the disease.

PATHOPHYSIOLOGY

The nature and extent of the physiologic events occurring in hypersensitivity pneumonitis depend primarily on the clinical form of the disease. The acute form of hypersensitivity pneumonitis is characterized clinically by chills, fever, cough, breathlessness without wheezing, and malaise 4 to 8 hours after antigen exposure.[34] There is some correlation between the severity of the acute episode and the magnitude of the antigenic challenge; however, immunologic responsiveness also influences the severity of an attack. In general, an acute attack subsides after 18 to 24 hours.

The classic response to antigen exposure results in maximum changes 8 to 10 hours after exposure.[62] Pulmonary changes are primarily restrictive, with a decrease in FVC, FEV_1, and total lung capacity (TLC). There is little change in flow rates, but small airways obstruction can be demonstrated on flow volume curves. There is a decrease in static compliance, and dynamic compliance becomes frequency dependent. Changes in the small airways result in a nonuniform ventilation distribution and, in turn, disturbance in ventilation-perfusion relationships. Hypoxemia and impaired diffusing capacity result from this mismatching.[68, 76] Hypoxemia may also be caused by redistribution of blood flow with resulting ventilation-perfusion inequality, or it can be secondary to intrapulmonary shunting of blood. The pulmonary circulatory response is unclear in the acute form of hypersensitivity pneumonitis.

Several other patterns of response are seen. The late reaction can be preceded by an immediate asthmatic reaction with a decrease in FEV_1 and expiratory flow rates. The immediate changes resolve within 1 to 2 hours even if untreated.

In atopic subjects, an acute asthmatic response (with wheezing and evidence of air flow obstruction on standard testing) may occur within minutes after antigen inhalation.[35, 65] This attack may subside with or without treatment, but 4 to 10 hours later, the typical late response occurs. In addition, the immediate asthmatic reaction can, in some subjects, persist for 4 to 6 hours.[53]

In the majority of patients with the acute disease form, pulmonary function returns to normal within a few weeks to months, particularly with avoidance of exposure. Even with repeated acute attacks, if the exposure is not intense or frequent, physiologic function may remain normal between exposures.

A small number of patients show a more insidious disease or a subacute form resembling progressive chronic bronchitis with productive cough, dyspnea, easy fatigue, and weight loss.[27, 34, 58] Both restrictive and obstructive defects in pulmonary function can be observed; the former, however, predominate along with a decrease in static lung compliance and diffusing capacity. Hypoxemia, although only mild at rest, may show a substantial worsening with exercise. Long-term avoidance of exposure and administration of corticosteroids usually result in resolution of these functional abnormalities.

Prolonged and intense exposure to a sensitizing organic dust can lead to the gradual development of disabling respiratory symptoms with irreversible physiologic changes.[27, 58] Pulmonary fibrosis is the predominant finding, particularly in farmer's lung or in patients with chronic low-level exposure to antigens.[6] These patients have progressive restrictive impairment, a diffusion defect, hypoxemia, and decreased lung compliance. Pulmonary fibrosis may progress, even without further exposure and despite corticosteroid therapy, eventually resulting in respiratory failure. A few patients with the chronic form of the disease have also shown signs and symptoms of obstructive disease.[68] Physiologic studies show diminished flow rates, hyperinflation with markedly elevated residual volume, decreased diffusing capacity, and a loss of pulmonary elastic recoil pressure suggestive of emphysema. Biopsy specimens in these cases have revealed an obstructive bronchiolitis with distal destruction of alveoli. Avoidance of exposure (even for prolonged periods), corticosteroids, and bronchodilator therapy afford only minimal improvement; the disease tends to be progressive.[34]

DIAGNOSTIC CRITERIA

The diagnosis of hypersensitivity pneumonitis depends upon an association of the pulmonary and/or systemic response of the patient with the inhalation of a specific environmental dust. The disorder should be suspected in individuals with recurrent "flu"-like episodes, chronic unexplained cough, sputum, and dyspnea, or in individuals with chronic progressive pulmonary impairment. The history may be important in differentiating hypersensitivity pneumonitis from other forms of interstitial pneumonitis, in that it may bring out a temporal relationship between exposures (e.g., hobby or occupation) and symptoms. However, if the exposure is constant, the symptoms may be insidious and progressive, and the diagnosis more obscure.

The physical examination is not specific for hypersensitivity pneumonitis. The acute attack is characterized by the presence of diffuse bibasilar rales indicative of an interstitial process. Fever and leukocytosis occur during the acute episode, and these features disappear with recovery. This spontaneous recovery and subsequent recurrence should suggest the diagnosis.

Pulmonary function abnormalities are not specific. An acute episode is associated with transient restriction, diffusion defect, and more persistent functional defects, including high-grade irreversible obstruction or severe restriction and diffusion impairment.

The radiologic features of hypersensitivity pneumonitis are variable with findings ranging from no abnormality to diffuse interstitial fibrosis. The most common feature is diffuse nodular infiltrates and coarse bronchovascular markings that disappear with avoidance. Hilar adenopathy is rare.

The clinical features of hypersensitivity pneumonitis may be present in most other interstitial lung diseases as well, e.g., chronic eosinophilic pneumonia, the collagen-vascular diseases, lymphogenous spread of carcinoma, desquamative pneumonitis, and sarcoidosis. The finding of extrapulmonary involvement such as splenomegaly or lymphadenopathy is rare in hypersensitivity pneumonitis. At times, lung biopsy is necessary to confirm the diagnosis.

The most consistent feature of hypersensitivity pneumonitis is the presence of serum-precipitating antibodies to an offending organic dust in affected individuals. However, these antibodies can also be detected in the serum of up to 50% of exposed but well individuals. Therefore, the finding of these antibodies must be evaluated in light of a patient's clinical features. Evidence has suggested that cellular immune responses to offending antigens may be important in the diagnosis of hypersensitivity pneumonitis. Additional studies are necessary to confirm these observations.

A suspected diagnosis may be confirmed by observation of the patients for clinical and pulmonary function changes following natural exposure to the environmental dust or after provocative challenge by controlled insufflation. Observation following removal of the individual from the suspect environment may also aid in confirming the diagnosis. These measures have been shown to be specific for the etiologic agent in hypersensitivity pneumonitis and are likely the key in diagnostic confirmation.

TREATMENT

The major therapy for hypersensitivity pneumonitis is the same as for all allergic disorders once the offending antigen is known, i.e., avoidance of the sensitizing antigen or environment. Because many of these disorders are occupational and the antigen size is known, the use of masks with filters capable of removing the antigen, appropriate ventilation of working areas, or, as a last resort, changing of occupations may be necessary.[27, 58]

When avoidance cannot be quickly achieved in the acute or subacute forms of hypersensitivity pneumonitis, drug therapy may be utilized. Corticosteroids, the drugs of choice, abort and prevent the episodic acute attack. Antihistamines and bronchodilators have no effect on the disease. If the corticosteroids are administered while avoidance is practiced, reversibility of the clinical and laboratory abnormalities is usually possible. Immunotherapy, as used for treatment of atopic diseases such as asthma and allergic rhinitis, is contraindicated in hypersensitivity pneumonitis because of the possibility of immune complex–induced vascular damage.

PREVENTION

The most effective control measure for abnormalities associated with hypersensitivity pneumonitis is removal of the affected worker from the occupational exposure, a step often quite disruptive to the individual involved. A more satisfactory approach would be prevention of the disease through the lowering of antigen levels in the work environment. In a few instances, e.g., the lumber industry, exposure of workers to potentially problematic dusts has been prevented by operational changes. For example, maple bark stripper's disease has been eliminated by altering handling of the logs. The disease is caused by the inhalation of the spores of *Cryptostroma corticale*, a mold found growing beneath the bark of maple logs. The disease was first described in a group of bark peelers in northern Michigan in 1932.[74] The next report of the illness occurred in a paper mill in northern Wisconsin. Out of 35 men tested at the site, 5 had severe clinical disease, 9 had subclinical disease, and the others appeared normal.[77]

High dust concentrations occurred in the wood room, and it was shown that most of the dust material consisted of spores of *C. corticale*. Clouds of spores could be seen each time an infected maple log entered the saw area. The spore counts were particularly high during the winter because of the poor ventilation of the wood room. To combat these conditions, changes were made, such as eliminating the saw area by installing debarking drums, spraying the drums continuously with water containing a detergent, isolating the chippermen from the wood room with a glass positive-pressure room, and cautioning the work room crew against spending excessive time in areas of high dust concentrations. These changes resulted in a dramatic fall in spore counts during the winter of 1964, and there have been no further cases of maple bark stripper's disease at the plant since that time.

Attempts to prevent bagassosis have included drying the material and treatment with propionic acid to prevent growth of microorganisms.[48] Bagassosis has also been reported to have been eliminated from a Louisiana paper mill by process changes.[49] These changes involved both storage and processing modifications that retarded microbial growth and reduced the generation of organic dust.

Hypersensitivity pneumonitis due to the inhalation of microorganisms present in industrial air handling systems may also be amenable to engineering control. The microorganisms reported to have been associated with this type of pneumonitis have varied, presumably because of differing environmental conditions.[21, 22, 37, 73] In an industrial context, contaminated humidifier water is likely to cause problems. This type of pneumonitis constitutes a serious health problem that probably occurs more commonly than is generally realized.

In situations in which such preventive approaches are not possible or feasible, it would be helpful to be able to screen applicants for sensitivity to antigens and selectively prevent those susceptible from contacting the offending dusts. However, such testing is not currently available, because factors that lead to sensitization other than exposure are not known.

Immediate, practical measures for hypersensitivity pneumonitis prevention and control include the education of individuals and industries at risk. Workers exposed to incriminated organic dusts must be made aware of potential hazards. Pertinent industries must be encouraged to reduce sensitizing and challenging exposures. Industrial physicians, public health officials, primary care physicians, and consultants must be alerted to the importance of prevention as well as diagnosis and treatment of this group of diseases.

The limited current control of hypersensitivity pneumonitis is primarily confined to manipulations of an afflicted individual's environment. Environmental factors have been clarified by studies of potential causative agents and their sources, and individual patients have benefited greatly by these studies. Of greater economic and epidemiologic importance, however, will be predictive and preventive measures affecting whole environments and communities of workers that will result from better understanding of sensitizing events and host factors. Further research is required to establish knowledge necessary for the design of feasible preventive programs and the maintenance of a healthy, stable work force in relevant environments.

REFERENCES

1. Allen DH, Barten A, Woolcock AJ: Familial hypersensitivity pneumonitis. Am J Med 59:505, 1975.
2. Allen DH, Williams GV, Woolcock AJ: Bird breeder's hypersensitivity pneumonitis: progress studies of lung function after cessation of exposure to provoking antigen. Am Rev Respir Dis 114:555, 1976.
3. Arnow PM, Fink JN, Schlueter DP, et al: Early detection of hypersensitivity pneumonitis in office workers. Am J Med 64:236, 1978.
4. Avila R, Villar TG: Suberosis: respiratory disease in cork workers. Lancet 1:620, 1968.
5. Banaszak EF, Thiede WH, Fink JN: Hypersensitivity pneumonitis due to contamination of an air-conditioner. N Engl J Med 283:271, 1965.
6. Barbee RA, Callies O, Dickie HA, et al: The long-term prognosis in farmer's lung. Am Rev Respir Dis 97:223, 1966.
7. Barboriak JJ, Sosman AJ, Reed CE: Serologic studies in pigeon breeders' disease. J Lab Clin Med 65:600, 1965.
8. Barrowcliff DF, Arblaster PG: Farmer's lung: a study of an early acute fatal case. Thorax 23:490, 1968.
9. Belin KWL: Recognition of allergic alveolitis in the trimming department of a Swedish sawmill. Eur J Respir Dis 107(Suppl 61):169, 1980.
10. Bice D, Salvaggio JE, Hoffman E: Passive transfer of experimental hypersensitivity pneumonitis with lymphoid cells in the rabbit. J Allergy Clin Immunol 58:250, 1976.
11. Bringhurst LS, Byrne RN, Gershon-Cohen J: Respiratory disease of mushroom workers. JAMA 171:15, 1959.
12. Buechner HA, Prevatt AL, Thompson J, et al: Bagassosis—a review with further historical data, studies of pulmonary function and results of adrenal steroid therapy. Am J Med 25:234, 1958.
13. Calvanico NJ, Ambegaonkar SP, Schlueter DP, et al: Immunoglobulin levels in bronchoalveolar lavage fluid from pigeon breeders. J Lab Clin Med 96:129, 1980.
14. Campbell JM: Acute symptoms following work with hay. Br Med J 2:1143, 1932.
15. Christensen LT, Schmidt CD, Robbins L: Pigeon breeder's disease: a prevalence study and review. Clin Allergy 5:417, 1975.
16. Cohen HI, Merigan TC, Kosek JC, et al: A granulomatous pneumonitis associated with redwood sawdust inhalation. Am J Med 43:785, 1967.

16a. Denis M: Proinflammatory cytokines in hypersensitivity pneumonitis. Am J Respir Crit Care Med 151:164, 1995.

16b. Denis M, Bedard M, Laviolette M, et al: A study of monokine release and natural killer activity in the bronchoalveolar lavage of subjects with farmer's lung. Am Rev Respir Dis 147:934, 1993.

17. Denis M, Cormier Y, Fournier M, et al: Tumor necrosis factor plays an essential role in determining hypersensitivity pneumonitis in a mouse model. Am J Respir Cell Mol Biol 5:477, 1991.
18. Dickie HA, Rankin J: Farmer's lung: an acute granulomatous interstitial pneumonitis occurring in agricultural workers. JAMA 167:1069, 1958.
19. Dinda P, Chatterjee SS, Reding WD: Pulmonary function in bird breeder's lung. Thorax 24:374, 1969.
20. Edwards JH, Baker JT, Davies BH: Precipitin test negative farmer's lung: activation of the alternative pathway of complement by mouldy hay dusts. Clin Allergy 4:379, 1974.
21. Edwards JH, Griffiths AJ, Mullins J: Protozoa as a source of humidifier fever. Nature 264:438, 1976.
22. Edwards JH, Harbord PP, Skidmore JW, et al: Humidifier fever. Thorax 32:653, 1977.
23. Emanuel DA, Wenzel FJ, Bowerman CI, et al: Farmer's lung: clinical pathologic and immunologic study of twenty-four patients. Am J Med 37:392, 1964.
24. Emanuel DA, Wenzel FJ, Lawton BR: Pneumonitis due to *Cryptostroma corticale* (maple-bark disease). N Engl J Med 274:1413, 1966.
25. Emanuel DA, Wenzel FJ, Lawton BR: Pulmonary mycotoxicosis. Chest 67:293, 1975.
26. Faux JA, Wide L, Hargreave FE, et al: Immunological aspects of respiratory allergy in budgrigar *(Melopsittacus undulatus)* fanciers. Clin Allergy 1:149, 1971.
27. Fink JN: Hypersensitivity pneumonitis. J Allergy Clin Immunol 52:309, 1973.
28. Fink JN: The environment and pulmonary hypersensitivity. Ann Intern Med 74:293, 1971.
29. Fink JN, Banaszak EF, Barboriak JJ, et al: Interstitial lung disease due to contamination of forced air systems. Ann Intern Med 84:406, 1976.
30. Fink JN, Banaszak EF, Thiede WH, et al: Interstitial pneumonitis due to hypersensitivity to an organism contaminating a heating system. Ann Intern Med 74:80, 1971.
31. Fink JN, Moore VL, Barboriak JJ: Cell-mediated hypersensitivity in pigeon breeders. Int Arch Allergy Appl Immunol 49:831, 1975.
32. Fink JN, Schlueter DP: Bathtub refinisher's lung: an unusual response to toluene diisocyanate. Am Rev Respir Dis 118:955, 1978.
33. Fink JN, Schlueter DP, Sosman AJ, et al: Clinical survey of pigeon breeders. Chest 62:277, 1972.
34. Fink JN, Sosman AJ, Barboriak AJ, et al: A clinical survey of a hypersensitivity pneumonitis. Ann Intern Med 68:1205, 1968.
35. Flaherty DK, Iha T, Chemlik F, et al: HLA B-8 and farmer's lung disease. Lancet 2:507, 1975.

36. Flaherty DK, Surfaus JE, Chemlik F, et al: Lymphocyte subpopulation in the peripheral blood of patients with farmer's lung. Am Rev Respir Dis 114:1093, 1976.
37. Friend JAR, Goodie J, Palmer KNV, et al: Extrinsic allergic alveolitis and contaminated cooling-water in a factory machine. Lancet 1:297, 1977.
38. Grant IWB, Blyth W, Gordon RM, et al: Prevalence of farmer's lung in Scotland: a pilot survey. Br Med J 1:530, 1972.
39. Greenberger PA, Pien LC, Patterson R, et al: End stage lung and ultimately fatal disease in a bird fancier. Am J Med 85:119, 1989.
40. Hansen PJ, Penny R: Pigeon breeder's disease: study of cell-mediated immune response to pigeon antigens by the lymphocyte culture technique. Int Arch Allergy Appl Immunol 47:398, 1974.
41. Hensley GT, Fink JN, Barboriak JJ: Hypersensitivity pneumonitis in the monkey. Arch Pathol 97:33, 1974.
42. Hensley GT, Garancis GC, Cherayil GA, et al: Lung biopsies of pigeon breeder's disease. Arch Pathol 87:572, 1969.
43. Hodges GR, Fink JN, Schlueter DP: Hypersensitivity pneumonitis caused by a contaminated coolmist vaporizer. Ann Intern Med 80:501, 1974.
44. Jenkins DE, Malik SK, Figueroa-Casas JC, et al: Sequential observations in pulmonary functional derangements in bagassosis. Arch Intern Med 128:535, 1975.
45. Kaltreider HP: Hypersensitivity pneumonitis. West J Med 159:547, 1993.
46. Keller RH, Swartz S, Schlueter DP, et al: Immunoregulation in hypersensitivity pneumonitis: phenotypic and functional studies of bronchoalveolar lavage lymphocytes. Am Rev Respir Dis 130:766, 1984.
47. Kopp WC, Dierks SE, Butler JE, et al: Cyclosporin immunomodulation in a rabbit model of chronic hypersensitivity pneumonitis. Am Rev Respir Dis 123:1027, 1985.
48. Lacey J: Moulding of sugar cane bagasse and its prevention. Ann Appl Biol 76:63, 1974.
49. Lehrer SB, Turer H, Weill H, et al: Elimination of bagassosis in Louisiana paper manufacturing plant workers. Clin Allergy 8:15, 1978.
50. Madsen D, Klock LE, Wenzel FJ, et al: The prevalence of farmer's lung in an agricultural population. Am Rev Respir Dis 113:171, 1976.
51. Marx JJ, Emanuel DA, Dovenbarger WV, et al: Farmer's lung disease among farmers with precipitating antibodies to the thermophilic actinomycetes: a clinical and immunologic study. J Allergy Clin Immunol 62:185, 1978.
52. Miller M, Patterson R, Fink JN, et al: Chronic lung disease with recurrent episodes of hypersensitivity pneumonitis due to a contaminated central humidifier. Clin Allergy 6:451, 1976.
53. Moore VL, Fink JN: Immunologic studies in hypersensitivity pneumonitis—quantitative precipitins and complement-fixing antibodies in symptomatic and asymptomatic pigeon breeders. J Lab Clin Med 85:504, 1975.
54. Moore VL, Fink JN, Barboriak JJ, et al: Immunologic events in pigeon breeders disease. J Allergy Clin Immunol 53:314, 1974.
55. Moore VL, Hensley GT, Fink JN: An animal model of hypersensitivity pneumonitis. J Clin Invest 56:937, 1975.
56. Morgan DC, Smyth JT, Lester RW, et al: Chest symptoms and farmer's lung: a community survey. Br J Ind Med 30:259, 1973.
57. Mushkin S: Report to NHLBI Task Force on Hypersensitivity Pneumonitis. 1976.
58. Pepys J: Hypersensitivity disease of the lungs due to fungi and other organic dusts. Monogr Allergy 4:1, 1969.
58a. Pforte A, Brunner A, Gais P, et al: Increased levels of soluble serum interleukin-2 receptor in extrinsic allergic alveolitis correlate with interleukin-2 receptor expression on alveolar macrophages. J Allergy Clin Immunol 94:1057, 1994.
59. Pforte A, Schiessler A, Gais P, et al: Expression of the adhesion molecule ICAM-1 on the alveolar macrophages and in serum in extrinsic allergic alveolitis. Respiration 60:221, 1993.
60. Pierce AK, Nicholson DP, Miller JM, et al: Pulmonary function in bagasse worker's lung disease. Am Rev Respir Dis 97:561, 1968.
61. Reed CE, Sosman A, Barbee RA: Pigeon breeder's lung. JAMA 193:261, 1965.
62. Reynolds HY, Fulmer JD, Kazmierowski JA, et al: Analysis of cellular and protein content of bronchoalveolar lavage fluid from patients with idiopathic pulmonary fibrosis and chronic hypersensitivity pneumonitis. J Clin Invest 59:165, 1977.
63. Richerson HB: Acute hypersensitivity pneumonitis in the guinea pig. J Lab Clin Med 70:745, 1972.
64. Rodey G, Fink JN, Koethe S, et al: A study of HLA-A,B,C and DR specificities in pigeon breeder's disease. Am Rev Respir Dis 119:755, 1979.
65. Schlueter DP: Response of the lung to inhaled antigens. Am J Med 57:476, 1974.
66. Schlueter DP, Banaszak EF, Fink JN, et al: Occupational asthma due to tetrachlorophthalic anhydride. J Soc Occup Med 20:183, 1978.
67. Schlueter DP, Fink JN, Hensley GT: Wood pulp worker's disease: a hypersensitivity pneumonitis. Ann Intern Med 77:907, 1972.
68. Schlueter DP, Fink JN, Sosman AJ: Pulmonary function in pigeon breeder's disease: a hypersensitivity pneumonitis. Ann Intern Med 70:457, 1969.
69. Seal RME, Hapke EJ, Thomas GO: The pathology of acute and chronic farmer's lung. Thorax 23:469, 1968.
70. Smyth JT, Adkins GE, Lloyd M, et al: Farmer's lung in Devon. Thorax 30:197, 1975.
71. Staines FH, Froman JAS: A survey of farmer's lung. J R Coll Gen Pract 4:351, 1961.
72. Szemenzato G, Agostini C, Zambello R, et al: Lung T-cells in hypersensitivity pneumonitis: phenotypic and functional analyses. J Immunol 137:1164, 1986.
73. Tourville DR, Weiss W, Wertlake PT, et al: Hypersensitivity pneumonitis due to contamination of home humidifier. J Allergy Clin Immunol 49:245, 1972.
74. Towey JW, Swoany HC, Huron WH: Severe bronchial asthma apparently due to fungus spores found in maple bark. JAMA 99:453, 1932.
75. Unger GF, Scanlon GT, Fink JN, et al: A radiologic approach to hypersensitivity pneumonitis. Radiol Clin North Am 11:339, 1973.
76. Weill H, Buechner HA, Gonzales E: Bagassosis: a study of pulmonary function in 20 cases. Ann Intern Med 64:737, 1966.
77. Wenzel FJ, Emanuel DA: The epidemiology of maple bark disease. Arch Environ Health 14:385, 1967.
78. Wenzel FJ, Emanuel DA, Gray RL: Immunofluorescent studies in patients with farmer's lung. J Allergy Clin Immunol 48:224, 1971.
79. Yoshizawa Y, Nomura A, Ohdama S, et al: The significance of complement activation in the pathogenesis of hypersensitivity pneumonitis: sequential changes of complement components and chemotactic activities in bronchoalveolar lavage fluids. Int Arch Allergy Appl Immunol 87:417, 1988.

33 Adverse Reactions to Foods

PHILIPPE A. EIGENMANN HUGH A. SAMPSON

What is food to one, is to others bitter poison.
De Rerum Natura, Lucretius (95–51 BC)

Foods have always played a major role in the cultural identity of humanity. It is not surprising, then, that foods have very often been implicated as the pathogenic factor in a broad variety of diseases. As a result, many "reactions" to foods have been designated "allergies," mainly because of the absence of a well-known pathogenic mechanism. Food allergy has become part of modern immunology, and a clear nomenclature of adverse reactions to foods has been established according to their pathogenic mechanisms.[1]

Adverse reaction to food is a global term that embodies any syndrome directly resulting from the ingestion of an identified food with which there is a clear causal and temporal relationship. Adverse reactions to food can be further subdivided into food hypersensitivity and food intolerance. *Food hypersensitivities* are the result of abnormal responses of the immune system to ingested nutrients. They include the classical immunoglobulin E (IgE) mediated reactions with immediate symptoms provoked by degranulation of mast cells after contact with specific food antigen, as well as immune mechanisms primarily involving lymphocyte and/or cytokine mediation or other effector cells of the immune system. *Food intolerances* are the result of nonimmunologic mechanisms and can be due to toxic contaminants in the ingested foods (e.g., *Escherichia coli* toxins), to pharmacologic properties of food ingredients (e.g., caffeine), to enzymatic deficiencies of the patient (e.g., lactase deficiency), to idiosyncratic reactions (e.g., individual sensitivity to tyramine in aged cheese), or to psychogenic reactions. The appropriate use of these terms aids in the diagnostic approach and appropriate therapeutic counseling of patients experiencing adverse food reactions.

HISTORICAL ASPECTS

For centuries, foods have been known to possess the potential to induce adverse reactions. Possibly the oldest report of a reaction related to foods comes from China, where around 2500 BC, emperor Shen-Nung advised pregnant women not to eat meat, chicken, or shrimp, foods likely to provoke ulcerations of the skin.[42] Two thousand years later, Hippocrates (460–370 BC) reported development of headache, fever, abdominal distention, thirst, and bilious and bloody stools in a patient after ingestion of cow's milk. Several centuries later, Discorides (around 50 AD) and Galen (130–200 AD) described other cases of reactions to cow's milk.[43] The potentially harmful effect of cow's milk was therefore well-known by the Greeks and possibly prompted them to avoid cow's milk and to drink mostly goat's and ewe's milk. Contemporary observations of repeated adverse reactions to foods in specific subjects probably inspired the Roman philosopher Lucretius (95–51 BC), when he wrote in *De Rerum Natura*, "What is food to one, is to others bitter poison."

In the early twentieth century, the specific role of the immune system in adverse reactions became recognized. In 1906, high levels of precipitating antibodies to cow's milk in the serum of a marasmic infant were noted by Moro.[137] Prausnitz and Küstner[170] demonstrated in 1921 that sensitivity to fish could be passively transferred by injecting the serum of an allergic individual into the skin of a nonallergic individual; when the passively sensitized subject ingested fish, local swelling developed at the injection site. This observation was the first evidence of a serologic factor involved in the pathogenesis of food hypersensitivity. In a review article, Piness and Miller[165] reported that protein sensitization could affect patients differently and result in allergic reactions in variable organ systems. They also described hypersensitivity to egg proteins, also called "egg-poisoning," as an immediate reaction following ingestion of minute quantities of egg, which leads to a burning sensation of the upper gastrointestinal tract, swelling of the mucous membranes, breathing difficulties, vomiting and diarrhea, convulsions, and a state of collapse. They noted that patients "usually experienced gradual recovery."[165]

However, it was not until the second half of the twentieth century that controlled studies and accurate diagnostic methods were first reported. Standardized diagnosis of cow's milk allergy by food provocation challenges was first proposed by Goldman and colleagues.[72] In their protocol, children suspected of having milk allergy were diagnosed as being "milk allergic" if they experienced three positive open challenges to 100 ml of skim milk. This method was not generally accepted because of the risk of carrying out three challenges in highly sensitized patients, and because nonallergic etiologies could fulfill the diagnostic criteria, e.g., lactase deficiency. The double-blind placebo-controlled food challenge (DBPCFC) was first proposed by May[132] in 1975. This protocol was initially set up to study severe asthmatic children suspected of being allergic to different foods. Besides asthma, the investigators also documented gastrointestinal and skin symptoms, and all symptoms occurred with 8 gm or less of dehydrated food product. Variations of this procedure have now become the standard for establishing the diagnosis of food hypersensitivity.

PREVALENCE OF FOOD HYPERSENSITIVITY

Food hypersensitivity is a commonly encountered complaint seen by allergists because many people of all ages believe that they have, or have had food "allergy." It is therefore important to review epidemiologic studies that clearly identify common food allergens and related clinical manifestations. Symptoms reported can range from classic manifestations, such as hives or upper airway obstruction occurring within a few minutes, to vague symptoms, such as fatigue without definite temporal link to a particular food ingestion. A survey on popular perceptions of food allergies in the United States showed that one third of the population studied had some concern about a food allergy and that 14% believed that their food allergy was a major health problem.[202] Foods most commonly mentioned were chocolate, milk, eggs, tomatoes, orange, corn, cheese, wheat, cucumbers, and coffee. Chocolate, a food very rarely proven by controlled challenges to cause allergies, was reported three times more often than milk.

Early epidemiologic observations emphasized the importance of food hypersensitivity, mainly cow's milk hypersensitivity in childhood. In 1955, Collins-Williams[44] reported an epidemiologic study on the incidence of cow's milk allergy in his general pediatric practice in which 3,000 patients were screened for a suggestive history. Nine patients (0.3%) with predominantly gastrointestinal symptoms were identified as cow's milk allergic and responded to a milk elimination diet. In another study, 403 healthy newborns from a "well baby clinic" were prospectively studied by Bachman and Dees[8] for possible symptoms of cow's milk allergy. These researchers diagnosed 4 infants (1%) who presented with colic, diarrhea, a skin rash, frequent colds, or wheezing, and who fulfilled their criteria of repeated reactions upon exposure to milk.

Positive scratch and intradermal skin tests were part of the diagnostic criteria for cow's milk allergy in a study published by Mueller and associates[141] in 1963. Out of a series of 299 healthy infants, these researchers identified 16 children with atopic dermatitis, 6 children with wheezing, and 6 with recurrent rashes. In this series, only 2 of 13 children with atopic dermatitis had significant improvement of their symptoms when switched to a soy formula. Interestingly, most of the children also had positive skin test reactions to other foods, mainly egg and wheat. However, no further work-up was undertaken for these foods.

Similarly, 10 years later Gerrard and coworkers[70] studied the prevalence of cow's milk allergy in healthy infants by identifying children with suggestive symptoms and by confirming the diagnosis with two subsequent open challenges. Fifty-nine of 787 infants (7.5%) were found to be sensitized to milk, with mainly gastrointestinal (diarrhea, vomiting, and colic), cutaneous (eczema), or respiratory manifestations. However, symptoms such as recurrent rhinitis and bronchitis, rarely related to food allergy, were reported frequently in this series, possibly explaining the much higher prevalence of food allergy than observed in other studies. Several children were also found to be sensitive to other foods, mainly soy, orange, egg, and wheat.

Later studies have utilized prospective evaluations and more rigorous diagnostic methods to estimate the prevalence of food allergy. In a large prospective study, Bock[19] recruited 480 children at birth and followed them until their third birthday. Twenty-eight percent of the children were suspected by their parents of having reactions to foods, with 80% of the complaints occurring during the first year of life. When suspected foods were eliminated and then re-introduced by either blinded or open challenges, symptoms were reproduced in only 8% of the children. Most reactions were suspected to be non–immunoglobulin E (IgE) mediated, because skin prick tests were commonly negative. Bock[19] concluded that all reported "food allergies" need to be carefully evaluated before the patient is definitely labeled with this diagnosis.

Jakobsson and Lindberg[100] followed 1,079 Swedish newborns prospectively to determine the prevalence of adverse reactions to cow's milk. They found that 1.9% developed a sensitivity to milk with predominantly cutaneous and gastrointestinal symptoms. A majority of the children also reacted to other foods, mostly soy. Similarly, a 3-year prospective study in Denmark evaluated 1,759 children and found 2.2% to be the overall rate of cow's milk allergy. Almost identical rates were found in a population of Dutch infants who were diagnosed by open challenges (2.8%) as well as by a survey in infants from the Isle of Wight (2.5%).[84] Overall, it appears that about 2.5% of children less than 2 years of age experience cow's milk allergy.

Food additives are commonly incriminated in adverse food reactions. Fuglsang and coworkers[66] studied the prevalence of intolerance to additives in 4,274 Danish school children by questionnaires. Reactions to additives were reported in 281 children (6.6%), of whom 271 were challenged. Open challenges reproduced symptoms in 17 children (6.2%), and DBPCFC reproduced symptoms in 6 (2.2%). Synthetic dyes were most often incriminated, and all children reacted with skin symptoms (5 eczema, 1 urticaria). This study suggests that although commonly incriminated, food additives are seldom real triggers of adverse reactions to foods. The pathophysiologic mechanisms of these reactions remain unknown.

Besides prospective studies in infants and children, which have dealt mainly with the prevalence of cow's milk hypersensitivity, only a few studies have evaluated the prevalence of food hypersensitivity in the adult population. In the Netherlands, a 1994 survey indicated that more than 10% of a random sample of 1,483 adults reported adverse food reactions.[144] After DBPCFC, however, about 2.2% had confirmed reactions, with only 1 subject having a proven IgE-mediated reaction to kiwi fruit, and 11 others having manifestations of food intolerance. A further survey from the

United Kingdom reported that 20% of a random adult and child population complained about adverse reactions to food, with women between the ages of 21 and 50 years reporting the highest frequency of reactions.[226] Double-blind placebo-controlled challenges using common foods substantiated a reaction in less than 2% of the study population. The most common symptoms were arthralgias, gastrointestinal tract complaints, headaches, and multiple subjective symptoms. Classic IgE-mediated reactions were rare (asthma in 1 and urticaria in 2). Children had the highest rate of positive reactions (3 of 5 challenges).

It is generally accepted that open challenges are not diagnostic of adverse food reactions, and that accurate diagnosis requires DBPCFCs. Consequently, appropriate epidemiologic studies on food hypersensitivity are very difficult, time-consuming, and costly. Considering the few available studies, it is probable that 1% to 2% of a general population have proven food hypersensitivity, with a slightly higher prevalence in young children. It is also possible that although the prevalence does not change from one geographical area to another, the types of foods implicated vary in relation to cultural eating habits.

PATHOPHYSIOLOGY

Food hypersensitivity may manifest either as diverse clinical symptoms (e.g., gastrointestinal, respiratory, cutaneous, and/or cardiovascular symptoms) or as definite clinical entities (e.g., celiac disease, Heiner's syndrome). However, food hypersensitivity is mediated by a homogeneous cellular population of the gut, with different immunologic reaction pathways. Conventionally, food hypersensitivity is classified as IgE-mediated or non–IgE-mediated, according to clinical expression and laboratory findings. However, in reality, there often is no clear distinction between these two types of immunologic mechanisms. Furthermore, the same patients can have a combination of symptoms classically attributed to both types (e.g., eosinophilic gastroenteritis and anaphylactic reactions), and cells from the immune system involved in adverse reactions to foods can mediate both classic "cellular" and "humoral" reactions, although one pathway is usually dominant. In this section, the pathogenic mechanisms of food hypersensitivity are discussed as a coherent entity, but mention of the different patterns of cell expression is made when clinically relevant.

THE GUT AS A BARRIER TO FOOD ALLERGENS

In addition to processing and absorbing food nutrients, the gastrointestinal tract functions as a barrier to potentially harmful antigens. The human gut is colonized by microorganisms that may be involved in the digestive process (e.g., lactose digestion),[130, 192] and the mucosa must provide them with a viable environment but also prevent them from invading the blood stream. Foods are broken down into elements of absorbable size (e.g., short sugars or small proteins) that potentially can be antigenic substances. Therefore, the gastrointestinal mucosa must function as a barrier that selectively absorbs nutrients. A wide variety of immunologic and nonimmunologic mechanisms are involved in this process (Fig. 33–1). First, the digestion of food proteins is initiated by gastric and pancreatic enzymes. Then, physical barriers composed of intestinal peristalsis, the intestinal mucous coat, and the microvilli and cell barrier intercede. Secretory IgA (s-IgA) coating the mucosa and various cells in the reticuloendothelial system are the main effectors of the immunologic barrier. Finally, the mucosa contains cells belonging to the immune system and capable of clearing away foreign antigens. The combined action of all these effector barriers largely contains foreign allergen in the gut and prevents them from invading the blood stream or inducing a local reaction.

Chemical digestion begins prior to passage of the nutrients through the small intestine, where absorption then occurs. Besides breaking down foods into substances of absorbable size, proteolysis reduces the size of potentially antigenic proteins and denatures major antigenic epitopes. However, this protective mechanism is immature in newborns, because basal acid secretion attains adult levels only after 1 month of age.[96] Furthermore, protease secretion by the pancreas and the gut fully matures during infancy.[123] Suboptimal digestion results in potential exposure to larger amounts of major antigens in young infants.

Nutrients that escape optimal digestion are generally pre-

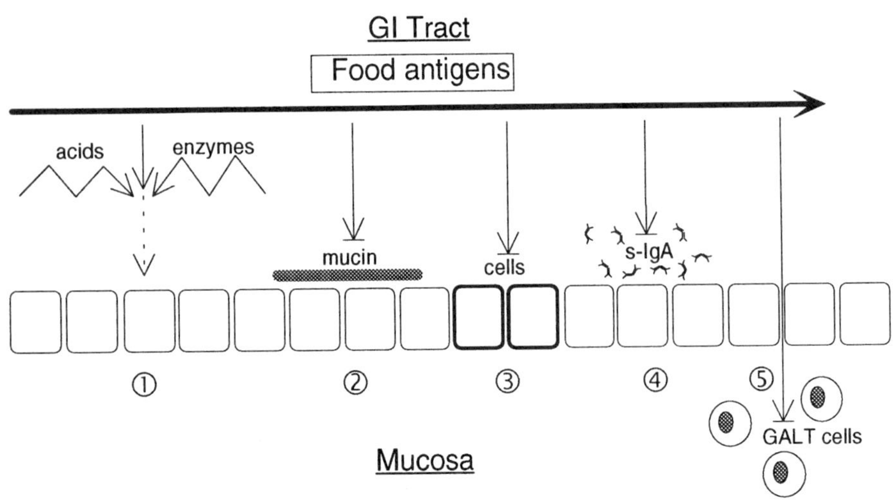

FIGURE 33–1. Barriers to antigen penetration through the gut. (1) Gastric and enzymatic digestion. (2) Mucin layer preventing antigen absorption. (3) Cell barrier to antigen absorption. (4) Antigen binding to s-IgA. (5) Clearing of antigen from the submucosa by cells from the gut-associated immune system (GALT).

vented from invading the blood stream by physical barriers. First, mucin forms a protective layer on the mucosal surface. However, animal studies suggest that this protection may be only partially effective in the first weeks of life, because mucin is present in reduced amounts in newborn rats.[200] Furthermore, in an immature gut rabbit model, increased glycosylation of the mucous layer led to enhanced binding of macromolecules.[25] This resulted in increased binding of cholera enterotoxin on the microvillous membranes and was postulated to be associated with increased crossing of foreign antigens through the mucosa. Similarly, increased binding of food antigen on gastrointestinal mucosa in immature rats was also observed.[205] Altogether, the maturational pattern of protective mechanisms is responsible for increased penetration of intestinal antigens through the gut mucosa in newborn animals.[212]

Reduction of both proteolytic digestion and physical barriers may leave the young infant particularly prone to sensitization to food antigens. Mucosal plasma cells synthesize large quantities of antigen-specific antibodies, with a large majority (80% to 90%) being IgA. These antibodies are transported as dimeric s-IgA through the gut mucosa, where they play a protective role.[197] Foreign antigens then bind to s-IgA and are cleared away in the gut. Secretory IgA is found mainly on the lumen of the mucosal surface, but IgA can also bind antigens on the basolateral side of the epithelial cells, and by epithelial transcytosis eliminate foreign antigen.[108] It has been suggested that transient maturational IgA deficiency in young infants and the paucity of IgA-producing plasma cells in the lamina propria of the newborn could account for the higher prevalence of food hypersensitivity in this age group,[219] but conformational data are lacking.

ORAL TOLERANCE

In conjunction with the age-related immaturity of the gut barrier in the newborn, a tolerizing phenomenon called oral tolerance takes place that subsequently plays an important role in normal processing of food antigens in childhood and adult life. Although not completely understood, *oral tolerance* can be defined as the state of specific immunologic unresponsiveness induced by prior oral administration of antigens.[140] Oral tolerance applies only to thymus-dependent soluble antigens, and the potential immune responses they can induce are therefore mediated by thymus-dependent lymphocytes (T cells).

Like autoantigens recognized as self, food allergens can act as tolerizing antigens. Murine models demonstrated that newborn mice primed with ovalbumin developed a hypersensitivity reaction, whereas ovalbumin exposure after 2 to 3 days of life induced a state of immune tolerance.[80, 207] It is not clear how long the immune system has the ability to recognize a foreign antigen as a tolerogen, because several observations emphasize that the ability to induce tolerance is lost in older animals. Furthermore, oral tolerance appears to occur primarily before or during the period of weaning.[80, 207]

Besides the age of the animal at the time of exposure to antigens, tolerance is dose dependent. Mice exposed to low doses of ovalbumin (< 1 mg) developed a hypersensitivity response, whereas higher doses induced tolerance.[140] Lymphocyte proliferation assays suggest that the response of $CD4^+$ (helper) lymphocytes to clinically tolerated food antigens was markedly reduced.[39] However, suppressor T cells also are implicated in this phenomenon, because oral tolerance could be transferred between animals by adoptive transfer of $CD8^+$ suppressor cells.[209] Furthermore, oral tolerance was lost when the $CD8^+$ cells were depleted by cyclophosphamide or 2′-deoxyguanosine, confirming a predominant role of suppressor T cells in development and maintenance of oral tolerance.[138, 139] Finally, γ/δ–T-cell receptor (TCR) bearing $CD3^+$, $CD4^-$, and $CD8^-$ T cells have been shown to reverse oral tolerance when adoptively transferred.[63] The exact immunologic mechanism responsible for oral tolerance remains unclear. However, clonal anergy seems to be one of the principal phenomena.[135, 171]

Clinical implications of oral tolerance are evident. The aforementioned animal studies suggest that early feedings of small amounts of foreign food antigens can sensitize the newborn or small infant. Therefore, the benefit of breast-feeding and delayed antigen exposure may be lost by starting with supplemental feeds of formula in the nursery. However, one clinical study contradicts these findings. Lindfors and Enocksson[127] demonstrated that newborn infants, initially bottle-fed until their mother's lactation started, had significantly fewer symptoms of atopic diseases than exclusively breast-fed infants at the end of the 18-month follow-up period.[127] Exclusively breast-fed infants are exposed to small amounts of food antigens passed into breast milk. Unlike nonatopics, infants predisposed to develop sensitivity to foods (already allergic to other foods, or by heredity) can be primed by small amounts of food antigen in breast milk, because positive skin tests can be seen in infants who never overtly ingested the incriminated food. In practice, early feeding with major food allergens (peanut, egg, milk) should be avoided in infants at high risk for atopy, and young infants should be fed consistently with the same formula. Supplements of formula and formula switching should be avoided, as they may lead to antigen priming and eventually to food hypersensitivity.

ABSORPTION OF FOOD ANTIGEN

In 1921, Prausnitz and Küstner[170] first showed that food proteins frequently elude the protective barriers already described and invade the blood stream. In their classic experiment, the serum of Küstner, who was allergic to fish, was injected into the skin of Prausnitz. Shortly after eating fish, Prausnitz experienced a local urticarial reaction at the passively sensitized site, but not at the control site, proving that fish protein had passed through the gut and traveled via the blood stream to the site of injection.

Antigen absorption was later studied by Walzer[220] in a series of elegant experiments. Sera from egg- or fish-allergic children were injected into their mothers' arms, who then experienced immediate local reactions after ingesting the implicated foods.[220] Removing the offending foods from the childrens' diets resulted in a significant improvement of their symptoms (e.g., eczema, asthma, urticaria). In a second set of experiments, Gray and Walzer[74] administered peanut protein to passively sensitized subjects either by mouth or by placement into the duodenum or the rectum. Absorption time was found to be between 18 and 25 minutes, the absorption being most rapid from the duodenum and rectum, or by mouth in patients with decreased gastric acidity. In addition, two patients who had undergone colostomy previously for other reasons were locally sensitized by intramucosal injection of a "peanut-reagin bearing" serum and were subsequently challenged orally and locally with peanut proteins.[73] The research group observed similar reactions, consisting of edema, hyperemia, and excessive mucus secretion, regardless of the route of administration. The group unequivocally demonstrated that potentially allergenic food proteins are absorbed immunologically intact and that they can elicit typical allergic reactions either locally or at distant organ sites following transport through the blood stream.

These experiments have been confirmed by later investigators utilizing intragastric challenges under endoscopy. Hypersensitivity responses to foods generally resulted in edema within a few minutes, increased permeability, as well as bleeding of the gut mucosa.[83, 172, 221] The gastrointestinal barrier function is generally altered after allergen challenges; for example, increased serum levels of milk antigen have been demonstrated in celiac patients after gluten challenge.[95] Increased mucosal permeability can also be observed under baseline conditions in patients with underlying atopic diseases,[99, 164] but has not been consistently seen by all investigators.[16, 51] It has been suggested that "intestinal closure" occurs soon before birth in humans, defining the first few days of life in premature babies as a high-risk period for food protein absorption and sensitization.[173] By measuring serum ovalbumin levels before and after food challenges at different ages (3 to 11 months) in infants with food-induced colitis, Powell and associates[169] could not demonstrate any difference in ovalbumin levels related to the results of the challenge. The normal protective mucous layer can be affected in allergic enteropathy; the glycocalyx has been shown to be absent in children with this condition.[166] Mucin is secreted as a protective mechanism by goblet cells during intestinal anaphylaxis, with copious amounts produced during hypersensitivity reactions.[121]

Radiologic studies in the 1930s focused on intestinal motility after allergen challenge. Rowe[176] and later Fries and Zizmor[64] performed blinded crossover allergen challenges in food-allergic children. Patients received a barium meal both with and without the offending food. During positive challenges, most patients were observed to experience gastric retention, increased or decreased motility of the gastrointestinal tract, and spasms or dilatation of the stomach or intestines. Rapid transit in the proximal small bowel has been confirmed in patients with milk hypersensitivity and gastrointestinal symptoms.[128]

ORGANIZATION OF THE IMMUNE SYSTEM IN THE GASTROINTESTINAL TRACT

After antigen penetration through the mucosal layer, an effective and rapid response is generated by the gut-associated lymphoid tissue (GALT). This immunologic barrier is composed of organized lymphoid tissue mainly in the ileum (Peyer's patches) as well as a large variety of isolated cells (B and T lymphocytes, plasma cells, macrophages, mast cells, eosinophils, and basophils) infiltrating the gastrointestinal mucosa.[206] Specialized epithelial cells (also called M cells) have been found overlying Peyer's patches, that act as antigen-presenting cells (APCs).[24] These cells are thought to be the major site of particulate antigen entry into mucosal lymphoid follicles.[109] Dendritic cells and macrophages located in Peyer's patches also transport antigens and are the predominant APCs to local T and B lymphocytes.

Intraepithelial lymphocytes (IELs) are mainly T cells. A majority (75%) have a $CD8^+$ phenotype and express a γ/δ TCR. Murine $CD8^+$ and γ/δ TCR^+ IELs were shown to be involved in regulation of the immune response, because adoptive transfer could abrogate a state of tolerance to an antigen and elicit an immune response.[68] Furthermore, α/β TCR+ IELs produce interleukin-5 (IL-5) and function as helper cells.[67] It is therefore suspected that IELs play a major role in host mucosal cell mediated immunity. In contrast, the majority of T cells in the lamina propria express CD4 and are involved in antibody and T-cell mediated immune responses.[109] Seventy to 80% of gut-infiltrating lymphocytes were shown to be $CD45RO^+$ memory cells.[79]

B lymphocytes are predominantly IgA-specific precursors.[69] It is still unclear at what site IgE-specific B-cell stimulation occurs, because IgE-specific B cells constitute less than 2% of the intestinal plasmocyte population.[27] However, large numbers of plasma cells secrete s-IgA, which functions in conjunction with the mucosal barrier, as explained earlier. Furthermore, unlike IgG or IgM, s-IgA does not activate the classical complement pathway. Dysregulation of IgA function has been incriminated in the pathogenesis of gastrointestinal inflammatory conditions such as celiac disease and inflammatory bowel disease.[109]

Several cytokines are involved either to promote interleukins (IL-1, IL-4, IL-5) or to downregulate the interferon-γ (IFN-γ) immune response. Eckmann and associates[52] found that IL-8 is secreted by intestinal epithelial cells, suggesting that it may act as an activator of the inflammatory response by promoting chemotaxis.

MECHANISMS OF FOOD HYPERSENSITIVITY

At the cellular level, priming occurs with the first exposure of an antigen to the GALT.[206] If the food antigen escapes the mucosal barrier defense mechanisms, it migrates through the mucosa and will be endocytosed by an APC (e.g., macrophage, dendritic cell, M cell) and presented to $CD4^+$ T cells. The contact with an antigen-specific T cell finally leads to an immune response. Various cytokines promote cell maturation and differentiation, and initiate an immune response. IL-2 acts as an autocrine growth factor for T cells, whereas IL-4 secretion and T-cell–B-cell interaction promote specific IgE production, which may result in generation of specific IgE antibodies. IL-5 secreted by T cells activates eosinophil maturation. Eosinophils are involved in IgE-mediated late-phase responses but also in syndromes without well-defined mechanisms (e.g., allergic eosinophilic gastroenteritis). Several populations of lymphocytes, in conjunction with cytokines, are probably responsible for the "cellular type"—or delayed—symptoms. Furthermore, a subset of activated $CD4^+$ T cells then differentiates into memory T cells ($CD45RO^+$) and provides immunologic memory until a later exposure to the antigen (Fig. 33–2).

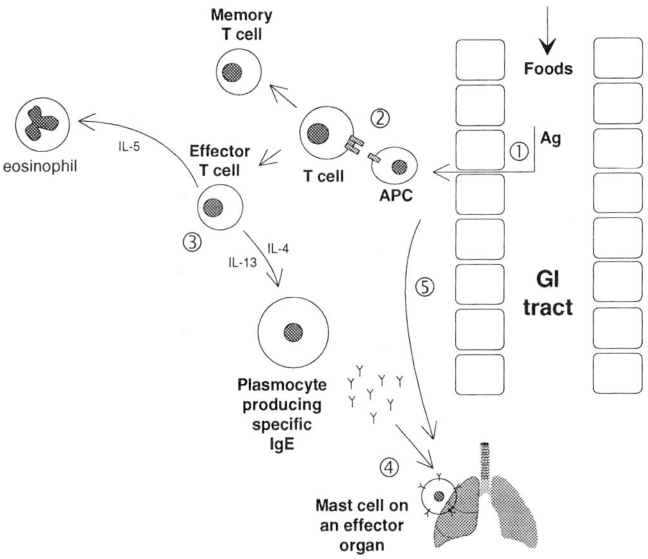

FIGURE 33–2. Schematic representation of mechanisms of food allergy. (1) Antigen (Ag) passage is facilitated by lack of integrity of the physical barrier. (2) Coupling of the Ag on an antigen-presenting cell (APC) induces Ag-specific T-cell differentiation in either memory T cells or effector T cells. (3) Cytokines stimulate plasmocytes to secrete Ag-specific antibodies (Ab) and recruit other inflammatory cells such as eosinophils. (4) Mast cells in target organs are coated with specific Ab. (5) Subsequent exposure to the antigen provokes allergy mediator release by mast cells in target organs.

After initial priming and mast cell coating with antigen-specific IgE, subsequent exposures to antigens provoke mediator release when antigen bridges specific IgE bound to high-affinity Fcε1 receptors on mast cells, basophils, and macrophages in target organs. Immediate symptoms result after release of histamine, prostaglandins, leukotrienes, and cytokines by activated mast cells or basophils.[178] Evidence of IgE involvement in gastrointestinal food hypersensitivity was demonstrated by the finding of IgE both in secretions collected from the proximal gut[12] and in the feces of allergic children.[118] However, contradictory results were reported on the number of IgE-specific plasma cells in the gastrointestinal mucosa of food-allergic patients.[162, 175, 215] McDonald and colleagues[134] investigated the roles of food-specific IgA, IgM, and IgG in food protein-induced enterocolitis by measuring circulating levels before and after food challenge.[134] Food-specific IgG and IgA antibody titers rose after positive challenges to soy and egg; and soy-specific IgM decreased with a positive challenge. In this disease of "nonreaginic food hypersensitivity," the investigators suggest an involvement of food-sensitized helper T lymphocytes, which would promote a switch to IgA and IgG isotypes and reduce IgM antibody production.

Furthermore, repeated ingestions of antigen may trigger mononuclear cells to secrete cytokines, chemokines, and IgE-dependent histamine-releasing factor (HRF). This form of HRF interacts with basophil membrane bound IgE and increases the susceptibility of the cell to release histamine. The greater susceptibility may lead to increased bronchial hyperactivity in asthmatic patients or skin irritability in patients with atopic dermatitis.[187] Mast cell involvement has been extensively studied in rat models, because intestinal mucosal mast cells secrete rat mast cell protease type II (RMCP II), a specific marker reflecting mast cell activation.[136] Mast cell involvement could be demonstrated in ovalbumin-sensitized Sprague-Dawley rats, in which increased RMCP II secretion and greater permeability could be documented after jejunal challenge with the antigen.[45] Similarly, other investigators observed increased RMCP II secretion after antigen challenge.[211] RMCP II release was found to be modulated by the duration of antigen avoidance; repeated challenges after short periods could elicit smaller amounts of RMCP II release. Several other investigators have demonstrated mast cell involvement in humans either by a decrease in the number of staining mast cells in the jejunum, reflecting degranulation after in vitro food challenge,[198] or by mediator (e.g., histamine) release from intestinal mucosa after challenge.[9, 10]

Animal models of food hypersensitivity have shown that antigen challenge produces rapid elevation of cyclic adenosine monophosphate (cAMP) in the gut mucosa, together with a subsequent increase in secretion of chloride ions.[161] Specific mast cell mediators are involved in intestinal anaphylaxis, independent of histamine, because histamine receptor antagonists (diphenhydramine or cimetidine) have no effect on ion transport abnormalities.[160] Furthermore, release of RMCP II after jejunal antigen challenge was accompanied by increased intestinal absorption of antigen as well as ethylenediaminetetra-acetic acid labeled with a chromium radioisotope (^{51}Cr-EDTA).[45] Together, these observations suggest that mast cell mediators change mucosal permeability. Clinically, release of histamine in the serum could be observed in patients with food hypersensitivity and atopic dermatitis following food challenges.[189]

The preferential involvement of specific organs in a hypersensitivity response may be explained by the presence of homing receptors on circulating T cells. Lymphocytes expressing these cell surface receptors "home," or are directed, to specific organs. Antigen-specific T cells in the skin express cutaneous lymphocyte antigen (CLA) and are found in the skin of patients with atopic dermatitis.[163] Similarly, T cells derived from pulmonary lavage fluid did not express CLA but did express the specific homing receptor αEβ7, suggesting a preferential distribution of a subpopulation of lymphocytes to the lung. Antigen-specific lymphocytes in target organs therefore express a peculiar affinity for their designated tissues, although it is not known to what extent they preferentially mediate certain types of allergic responses. Several investigators have studied cell-mediated mechanisms utilizing lymphocyte proliferation assays. Van Sickle and associates[214] stimulated in vitro peripheral blood mononuclear cells from children with milk- or soy protein–induced enterocolitis. The respective antigens reportedly demonstrated a direct correlation between symptoms and lymphocyte response. The investigators concluded that T cells are probably involved in the pathogenesis of this form of food allergy.[214] Other studies have made similar observations.[98, 119, 120] Very little information exists on the role of T-cell secreted cytokines in food allergy. In a preliminary report, one antigen-specific T-cell line isolated from an egg-allergic individual was found by enzyme-linked immunosorbent assay (ELISA) to secrete IL-5, but not IL-2, IL-4 or IFN-γ, into the culture supernatant.[199] Ovomucoid cell lines and clones specific to ovomucoid have been generated from several egg-allergic individuals.[54] Amplification of messenger RNA (mRNA) by reverse-transcriptase polymerase-chain reaction (PCR) disclosed a constant expression pattern of IL-5, sometimes associated with IL-4, IL-13, and/or IFN-γ. These results may suggest that IL-5 plays an important role in the mediation of the food hypersensitivity, possibly by eosinophil recruitment and activation.

Reactions secondary to other hypersensitivity mechanisms are very uncommon. A cytotoxic reaction was thought to be responsible for thrombocytopenia secondary to milk in one report.[38] The mechanism postulated involved complement activation by a specific antibody bound to a surface tissue antigen, resulting in cell damage.[185] Antigen-antibody mediated disease has also been implicated as a pathogenic mechanism in food hypersensitivity. Food-specific antigen-antibody complexes have been reported in the serum of food-sensitive patients.[156] However, antigen-antibody complexes can also be found in milk-tolerant children and adults after meals.[155]

FOOD ALLERGENS

SPECIFIC FOOD ALLERGENS IN ADVERSE REACTIONS

Prevalence of food hypersensitivity to specific food allergens is related to the dietary habits in a population. Furthermore, eating patterns have been changing over the centuries. For example, peanuts originated in Peru but are now one of the most prevalent food antigens in North America.

In an attempt to define the prevalence of food allergic reactions, it is often difficult to compare published studies because of variations in patient ages, diagnostic criteria utilized, and/or recruitment bias (Table 33–1). In our studies on the prevalence of food hypersensitivity in children with atopic dermatitis, egg, milk, peanut, soy, and wheat were found to be the most common causes of allergic reactions. In another study from the United States, food-allergic children more than 3 years of age were found to be predominantly allergic to peanut, egg, and milk.[18]

A retrospective study from Switzerland with predominantly adult subjects disclosed that 45% of the patients had a reaction to celery and the second most common food sensitivity was to carrots.[142] More common food allergens, such as milk, egg, and seafood, were also seen, but peanut sensitivity was rarely observed. A Swedish study on food hypersensitivity in patients with respiratory allergies found that nuts, apple, and shellfish were most commonly reported.[57] A study from Israel evaluated 112 food allergic patients whose symptoms developed after the age of 10 years.[117] Most of the patients had positive skin tests to peach, sunflower, soy, and peanuts. A minority of the patients were found to be sensitive to egg or milk. Reactions to peaches could be reproduced by blinded challenges in close to 75% of the patients, whereas other foods induced a reaction in less than one third of the patients. Furthermore, it was observed that reactions to foods were commonly associated with exercise.

Atkins and colleagues[7] studied an exclusively adult referral population by blinded food challenges. Foods found to provoke symptoms included shrimp (4 patients), peanut (2 patients), and crab, eggs, beer, and carrots (each in 1 patient). The patients had a history of reactions persisting over an average of 17 years.

CHARACTERISTICS OF FOOD ALLERGENS

Cow's Milk Proteins

In young infants, cow's milk protein generally represents the largest portion of ingested antigens. Cow's milk proteins (as well as peanut, egg, and other proteins) can be found in breast milk, and therefore, exclusively breast-fed infants may be exposed and sensitized to cow's milk before ever ingesting plain cow's milk.[116] β-Lactoglobulin was found in samples of breast milk from nursing mothers, 50% of whom had increased levels after drinking milk.[203] Casein and the whey proteins (β-lactoglobulin and α-lactalbumin) appear to be the major allergens among about 20 different cow's milk proteins.[17]

Casein is composed of five basic fractions and constitutes approximately 80% of the proteins in cow's milk. The most prevalent subfractions are α-casein and α_s-casein with molecular weights of 27 and 23 kD, respectively. The three other fractions, β-, κ-, and γ-casein, have molecular weights of 24, 19, and 21 kD, respectively. The second major group is composed of the whey proteins. β-Lactoglobulin (molecular weight 36 kD) constitutes 10% of the milk proteins, and α-lactalbumin (14.4 kD) less than 5%. Other cow's milk protein fractions (e.g., bovine serum albumin, bovine immunoglobulin, lactoferrin) are present in only minute quantities.

The clinical significance of the different cow's milk protein fractions is not yet well defined. In a report on T-lymphocyte specific responses to casein, α-lactalbumin and β-lactoglobulin in cow's milk allergic patients failed to demonstrate clear dominance of any protein.[53] The reactive T-cell repertoire in cow's milk allergic patients probably comprises several different clones specific to a number of casein and whey protein epitopes. Future studies of T-cell epitopes should allow a more definitive understanding of cow's milk antigen processing by APCs and T cells. The prevalence of IgE specificity to milk proteins was studied in milk-allergic patients by skin testing.[72] Skin tests were positive for casein in 40%, α-lactalbumin in 26%, bovine serum albumin in 25%, and β-lactoglobulin in 24% of 85 cow's milk allergic patients diagnosed by positive challenges.

Milk ingestion can produce either immediate or delayed-type symptoms. IgE-mediated reactions, which occur in about half of the patients, consist of eczema, urticaria, vomiting, diarrhea, rhinitis, and wheezing. Non–IgE-mediated reactions occur in approximately one half of the patients and consist mainly of gastrointestinal symptoms.[47, 97, 100] Cow's milk protein-induced enterocolitis syndrome is one of the more common disorders in infants. It usually manifests as recurrent vomiting and diarrhea during the first several months of life. Other clinical entities, such as cow's milk induced colitis and pulmonary hemosiderosis, can be milk protein mediated and are discussed later.

Egg Protein

The major allergens of hen's egg are found in egg white. Ovalbumin (*Gal d* II), the most abundant egg white protein

TABLE 33–1
PERCENTAGES OF PATIENTS REACTING TO FOODS IN RESPECTIVE STUDY GROUPS

	Bock[18]	Sampson*	Mühlemann and Wüthrich[142]	Eriksson[57]	Kivity et al[117]
Country	U.S.	U.S.	Switzerland	Sweden	Israel
Parameters	Double-blind placebo-controlled food challenge in a population of pediatric patients with food hypersensitivity	Double-blind placebo-controlled food challenge in a population of pediatric patients with atopic dermatitis	Skin tests and history in a population of predominantly adult patients with a history of food hypersensitivity	History in a population of adult patients with respiratory symptoms	Blinded food challenges in patients >10 years of age with a history of food hypersensitivity
Foods					
Egg	21%	54%	5%	3%	—
Milk	13%	28%	10%	<1%	—
Nuts					
Peanut	39%	22%	—	—	31%
Walnut	8%	—	—	5%	—
Cashew	6%	—	—	—	—
Hazelnut	—	—	—	10%	—
Almond	—	—	—	—	39%
Soy	—	12%	—	—	—
Fish/shellfish					
Fish	5%	9%	—	—	—
Shellfish	—	—	6%	6%	—
Fruits/vegetables					
Apple	—	—	—	8%	—
Peach	—	—	—	—	75%
Orange	—	—	—	—	9%
Celery	—	—	45%	—	—
Carrot	—	—	14%	—	6%
Cereals					
Wheat	—	10%	—	—	—
Others			6%		
Curry	—	—	—	—	—
Sunflower	—	—		—	35%

*Unpublished.

(54%), has a molecular weight (MW) of 45 kD. Ovotransferrin (*Gal d* I; MW 77 kD) and ovomucoid (*Gal d* III; MW 28 kD) are the second most prevalent protein components. In a study of 18 egg-allergic patients, the allergenicity of ovomucoid was compared with that of ovalbumin.[13] The major response previously attributed to ovalbumin in various diagnostic tests was found to be due to contamination of commercial ovalbumin by trace amounts of ovomucoid. Results of skin tests and quantification of serum antigen-specific IgE antibodies indicated that ovomucoid is the predominant egg white allergen.

Ovomucoid is composed of three major domains of equal length (approximately 60 residues).[110] T cells from egg-allergic individuals have been found to recognize different domains.[54] These results indicate that T cells from different patients are likely to recognize different ovomucoid epitopes.

The majority of symptoms provoked in egg hypersensitivity are of the immediate type. They involve the skin (eczema, facial angioedema), the respiratory tract (asthma and rhinitis), and the gastrointestinal tract (vomiting, abdominal pain, diarrhea).[59]

Allergic reactions to the mumps-measles-rubella (MMR) vaccine, which is grown on chicken embryo fibroblasts, is a feared complication in children with egg allergy. Current recommendations by the American Academy of Pediatrics (AAP) are to first skin-test egg-allergic patients with the MMR vaccine and subsequently to desensitize patients who have a positive skin test. However, James and coworkers[102] reported that more than 1,200 egg-allergic patients have been safely immunized in the routine manner, regardless of vaccine skin test results or severity of reactions to egg. Similarly, an Australian series reported that egg-sensitive children could be routinely vaccinated without any adverse reaction.[114] A large series evaluated 500 children with histories of reactions to egg.[62] One hundred twenty patients initially enrolled were skin tested and then immunized. However, there was little correlation between the result of the skin tests and suspicion of a reaction to the vaccine. Consequently, subsequent patients were immunized without skin testing. A total of 5 patients had minor reactions to the vaccine, mostly localized rashes. Adverse reactions to MMR are most commonly reported in non–egg allergic children. From all reviewed studies, it seems that the current (AAP) recommendations are overcautious and should be revised.

Peanut Proteins

Peanut, a legume, is one of the most prevalent food allergens in North America. Peanut is composed of 16 protein fractions, as determined by sodium dodecyl sulfate–polyacrylamide gel electrophoresis (SDS-PAGE) (see Fig. 33–

3). Two of these proteins, *Ara h I* (MW 63.5 kD) and *Ara h II* (MW 17 kD), have been isolated and characterized as major peanut allergens.[32, 33] Serum from more than 90% of peanut-allergic patients have been found to have specific IgE to these two fractions.[32] The proteins are heat stable, and in vitro chemical denaturation mimicking digestion was found to only partially denature the proteins.[34] Although distilled peanut oil is free of antigen, several brands of cold-pressed or "extruded" oil have been found to contain significant amounts of peanut proteins.[91]

Peanut allergy is a major health problem in the United States with many social implications. Peanut proteins are ubiquitous in the contemporary diet of children and teenagers and furthermore are used as a cheap source of protein in many processed foods. This situation can lead to early sensitization, often resulting in life-long sensitivity.[181] Peanuts are also responsible for numerous, often life-threatening reactions and are among the most common causes of severe reactions to foods in the United States. Two reviews of fatal or near-fatal anaphylaxis to foods implicated peanuts in a majority of the cases.[190, 227]

Soybean Proteins

Soybeans are also members of the legume family and account for numerous hypersensitivity reactions, predominantly in children. There are 21 soy protein fractions (Fig. 33–3). Although the major allergens have not been completely characterized, four major fractions have been isolated by ultracentrifugation from crude soy proteins. Two soy protein fractions, 7S and 11S, have been isolated from the whey fraction. These proteins are heat stable but are partially denatured by chemical digestion, with IgE binding reduced by tenfold.[34] In one study, serum IgE antibody from soy-allergic children showed no difference in binding to either fraction,[35] whereas in another study, IgE antibodies bound strongly to a unique protein (MW 30 kD) from the 7S-globulin fraction.[150] This protein appears to be a major allergen and was named *Gly m* Bd 30K by the investigators.

Immunoblots of IgE binding to proteins of various commercial and crude soybean extracts were compared using sera from patients allergic to soy, peanut, and other beans.[82] Serum IgE from individuals allergic to both peanuts and soy bound to different protein fractions in the various extracts, explaining the low accuracy rate for skin tests and insufficient stability of commercial extracts.

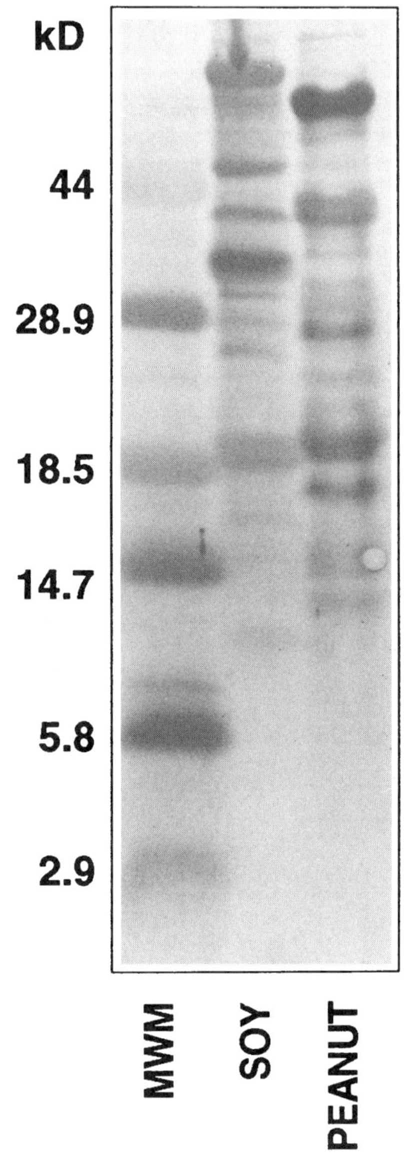

FIGURE 33–3. Low molecular weight SDS-PAGE of soy and peanut protein extracts.

Cereal Proteins

Hypersensitivity to cereals is not uncommonly seen in children. Wheat is most commonly implicated, but reactivity to barley, oat, and rye is also seen. Rice hypersensitivity is very rare in the western hemisphere, but fairly common in Asian countries. Corn hypersensitivity is very rare and seldom proven by DBPCFC. The gliadin found in wheat, oat, barley, and rye is responsible for celiac disease, which is discussed briefly later. Twenty-seven to 31 protein bands with molecular weight between 7.8 kD and 66.5 kD were identified in various cereal grains by SDS-PAGE and immunoblot analysis utilizing sera from patients sensitized to cereals.[106] Extensive immunologic cross-reactivity was noted on skin testing. This extensive cross-reactivity was confirmed by other investigators who found extensive cross-reactivity between wheat, barley, and rye on immunoblots developed for IgE antigen specific antibodies from cereal-sensitive patients.[216] Further evidence for cross-reactivity among grains and airborne pollens was found by other investigators utilizing radioallergosorbent test (RAST) inhibition assays.[50]

Nut Proteins

Tree nut hypersensitivity is most prominent in adults, probably because of the later introduction of nuts into the human diet and the life-long sensitivity to these antigens. Nuts frequently implicated in allergic reaction are almonds, Brazil nuts, cashews, filberts, hazelnuts, pecans, walnuts, and pistachios. It has also been shown that IgE-containing sera from walnut-allergic patients predominantly bound a 65 kD protein that was found to have significant homology to the vicilin, storage proteins found in a large number of legumes, including peanuts.[208] Patients often show cross-reactivity between different nuts on skin testing, leading to the recommendation that a patient allergic to one tree nut should avoid all tree nuts (but not peanuts). Cross-reactivity with nonfood allergens can also occur. Particularly prevalent in Scandinavian countries is the clinical cross-reactivity between hazelnuts and birch pollen.[58] Interestingly, the birch sensitivity was reported to be more severe in patients who also had hazelnut sensitivity. An isolated case of clinical sensitivity to chestnut and latex, confirmed by serum IgE binding to both proteins on SDS-PAGE immunoblots, has been reported.[6] Nut-allergic patients should be cautious when eating commercially roasted peanuts or other nuts, because contamination may occur in the processing and packaging lines.

Fish and Seafood Proteins

Fish and seafood sensitivities are commonly seen in food-allergic adults. Immunoblot analysis of fish extracts showed that most fish species have a prominent band at 12.25 kD, corresponding to *Gad C 1*, the major allergen of codfish. This protein has been isolated from the myogen of the white meat, is heat stable, and resists proteolytic digestion.[56] To study possible cross-reactivity, 11 fish allergic patients were skin tested and challenged to several fish species.[14] All patients had positive skin reactions to most of the species, but only 3 patients had a positive reaction by challenge to more than one of the species ingested.

A major allergen of the major brown shrimp, *Pen a* I was found to be the muscle protein tropomyosin.[48] Similarly, *Par f* I, a 39 kD protein, has been isolated from another shrimp species and was found to have allergenic activity.[126] In this study, a protein from crab with a similar weight had 62% to 83% sequence homology to *Par f* I. Furthermore, cross-reactivity by skin prick testing and RAST analysis has been shown between different crustaceans.[222] Shrimp and fish sensitivities frequently produce anaphylactic reactions of diverse severity. Of 14 patients with a history of shrimp sensitivity, more than half experienced a potentially life-threatening reaction.[222]

Fruit Protein

Allergies to fruits and vegetables are seen more often in adults than in children. Celery and carrot sensitivities are frequently reported to develop later in life.[142] In one study, peach was the most prevalent food allergen in patients more than 10 years of age.[117] In an attempt to characterize fruit allergens in patients sensitive to peaches and several other fruits, Wadee and associates[218] isolated a 30 kD protein by SDS-PAGE and immunoblotting using sera from fruit-allergic patients.[218] This protein was present in extracts from peaches, strawberries, and mandarins. In another series of experiments, pooled sera from six individuals was used to investigate cross-reactivity among extracts of celery, cucumber, carrot, and watermelon.[107] Each patient demonstrated clinical allergy to one or more study foods, and most of them were found to have specific IgE for all four extracts by skin test or ELISA. Furthermore, immunoblots showed a 15 kD protein band common to all four foods.

Efforts to characterize apple allergens have shown that sera from apple-allergic patients are bound predominantly to two proteins, an 18 kD fraction and a 31 kD fraction.[94] The *N*-terminal amino acid sequence of both proteins showed a 60% to 70% homology with birch pollen.

Another common cross-reactivity has been reported between latex and banana.[129] Common clinical cross-reactivities between different foods are listed in Table 33–2. Raw fruits and vegetables are commonly implicated in oral allergy syndrome, which is discussed later.

Other Food Proteins

Other foods are less common causes of food hypersensitivity reactions. Beef, especially rare, can provoke reactions in some milk-sensitized individuals. Positive skin tests to chicken, with or without clinical reactivity, are seen frequently in highly egg-allergic individuals. Among commonly ingested meats, turkey and lamb sensitivities are rarely diagnosed.

Anaphylactic reactions to psyllium, a water-soluble mucilloid contained in bulk laxatives and some breakfast cereals, have been reported.[103] Interestingly, the patients (predominantly nurses) had been previously sensitized by inhaling aerosolized particles when dispensing laxatives to patients.

Food dyes are commonly implicated in adverse reactions, but true sensitivity is rarely proven. In one study, 335 children were evaluated for adverse reactions to food additives by means of an initial washout period followed by open challenges.[65] Six percent of the children had a reaction following an open challenge, but only 2% of the reactions were confirmed by double-blind challenge. Symptoms were

TABLE 33–2
CROSS-REACTIVITY AMONG DIFFERENT FOODS

Allergen	Cross-Reactivities						
Tree nuts	Hazelnuts	Walnuts	Pecan	Brazil nut	Pistachio	Cashews	
Apple family	Apple	Pear					
Plum family	Plum	Cherry	Peach	Apricot	Almond		
Grains	Wheat	Rye	Barley	Oats			
Fish	Salmon	Flounder	Trout	Bass	Perch	Mackerel	Codfish
Shellfish	Crab	Crayfish	Shrimp	Lobster			
Diverse	Milk	Rare beef					
	Soybean	Peanut					
	Egg	Chicken meat					

related predominantly to the skin (atopic dermatitis or urticaria) or to the respiratory tract (asthma or rhinitis).

CLINICAL MANIFESTATIONS OF FOOD HYPERSENSITIVITY

Food hypersensitivity may manifest clinically as a variety of different syndromes and symptoms involving various target organs. This variability of symptoms often generates confusion and frequently leads to erroneous diagnosis of "food allergy." In this section, clinical manifestations of food allergies reported by target organ are reviewed with reference to the immune mechanism involved; and a later section deals with specific syndromes classified as clinical entities (Table 33–3).

RESPIRATORY TRACT

Symptoms of food hypersensitivity in the respiratory tract are common, with some form of airway reaction occurring in up to 60% of patients in one series of more than 200 food-allergic patients diagnosed by blinded food challenges.[188] Sixty-six percent of patients had nasal symptoms, 43% had laryngeal symptoms, and 24% developed lower respiratory tract symptoms. Nasal symptoms rarely occur in isolation and may consist of watery rhinorrhea, nasal pruritus, and sneezing.

Laryngeal symptoms may range from dysphonia or hoarseness of the voice and a sensation of tickling in the throat, to acute laryngeal edema causing life-threatening upper airway obstruction. Laryngeal involvement can occur either as a symptom of an anaphylactic reaction or sometimes as an isolated manifestation of hypersensitivity. In any case, involvement of the larynx may portend a potentially life-threatening reaction, so aggressive therapy, including subcutaneous injections of epinephrine, must be initiated rapidly.

Wheezing due to bronchoconstriction is rarely seen as an isolated symptom. In asthmatic patients, it is often an indicator of the severity of the reaction. In a series of patients referred for evaluation of respiratory symptoms over an 18-year period, Bock found that 24% of patients with asthma and a history of food hypersensitivity had a positive food challenge with wheezing.[20] Most of these patients also had upper respiratory symptoms. Furthermore, in 5% of children without asthma who had a positive food challenge, wheezing was one of the symptoms provoked. In a series of 320 patients referred for evaluation of atopic dermatitis and food hypersensitivity by DBPCFC, 59% of the patients experiencing a positive challenge had some respiratory reaction, with only 17% having wheeze or cough.[101] Only 6 of 13 of this latter group had a decrease of 1-second forced expiratory volume (FEV_1) greater than 20%. These results suggest that chest symptoms are not generally severe in food challenge positive subjects with atopic dermatitis. Furthermore, it has been noted that in some patients with asthma and positive food challenges that provoked no significant respiratory symptoms, institution of an appropriate food elimination diet frequently led to improvement in the asthma.

Several investigators have hypothesized that bronchial hyperactivity not recognized with standard spirometry could be attributed to food hypersensitivity.[188, 230] Utilizing methacholine inhalation challenges before and after double-blind placebo-controlled challenges, James and colleagues[104] studied food-allergic patients with asthma. They observed that 7 of 12 patients with chest symptoms (cough or mild wheezing) provoked during DBPCFC experienced increased responsiveness to methacholine after the food challenge, generally without significant changes in routine spirometry. Negative challenges were not associated with a change in bronchial hyperreactivity. This study confirmed that food-allergic patients with asthma can have significant bronchial hyperresponsiveness after oral food challenges, even without having obvious wheezing. It also suggests that lower respiratory symptoms in food allergy may be more common than the 2% to 8% rate previously reported.[147, 149, 151] It should be noted that most patients with food-induced wheezing have atopic dermatitis or a history of eczema.

Heiner's Syndrome

Heiner's syndrome is a well-defined clinical entity predominantly involving the lungs. It was first described in the 1960s as a rare form of pulmonary hemosiderosis in children linked to cow's milk ingestion. Seven infants or children with chronic cough, wheezing, recurrent lung infiltrates on chest films, hemosiderosis, persistent rhinitis, gastrointestinal symptoms, and anemia were initially described.[81] The pathogenesis of this syndrome involves immunoglobulin deposi-

TABLE 33–3
SIGNS, SYMPTOMS, AND SYNDROMES OF FOOD HYPERSENSITIVITY REPORTED BY TARGET ORGAN

Target Organ	IgE-mediated	Non–IgE-mediated
Airways	Asthma	Heiner's syndrome
	Upper airway constriction	
	Bronchial hyperactivity	
	Rhinitis	
Skin	Urticaria/angioedema	Papulovesicular rash of dermatitis herpetiformis
	Atopic dermatitis	
Gastrointestinal	Diarrhea	Colitis
	Vomiting	Enterocolitis
	Oral pruritus (oral allergy syndrome)	Celiac disease
	Allergic eosinophilic gastroenteritis	Allergic eosinophilic gastroenteritis
Cardiovascular	Collapse (systemic anaphylaxis)	
Other		Migraines

tion in the lung tissue. The classical in vitro test relies on positive serum precipitins to several constituents of cow's milk.[124] A later study established no definitive diagnostic laboratory parameters in Heiner's syndrome, because milk-specific immunoglobulins of diverse isotypes and lymphocyte proliferation assays were not discriminatory between patients with milk-induced pulmonary hemosiderosis and those with other milk hypersensitivity syndromes.[204]

SKIN

Acute urticaria/angioedema, which may be an early sign of a systemic anaphylactic reaction, is commonly related to food ingestion. It is believed to be the most common clinical manifestation of immediate-onset food hypersensitivity, and its cause-and-effect relationship with the incriminated food is often obvious because symptoms appear within minutes. Food hypersensitivity is also frequently suspected as a possible cause of chronic urticaria. In a study on 226 children with chronic urticaria, positive skin prick tests to food were found in 31% of the patients. However, food hypersensitivity could be confirmed by DBPCFC in only 4% of the children.[217] Adverse reactions to food additives (tartrazine and salicylates) were found in 2.6% of the study population. Similarly, chronic urticaria in adults is rarely secondary to food allergy which probably accounts for less than 2% of cases.[40]

Food allergy is clearly a trigger of skin symptoms in some patients with atopic dermatitis. The earliest report linking the two diseases came 10 centuries ago from the Central Asian physician Avicenna, who reported that milk and fish could cause a chronic scabrous skin disease. More than 50 years ago, Grulee and Sanford[75] published their observation of an increased prevalence of atopic dermatitis in infants fed artificial formulas. In 1992, Guillet and Guillet[77] reported that 50% of 169 patients with moderate or severe atopic dermatitis and 96% of patients with severe atopic dermatitis were sensitized to foods. The pathogenic role of foods was confirmed by double-stage open and single-blinded challenges. Foods incriminated were, in decreasing frequency: eggs, milk, shellfish, peanuts, fish, and soy. In our series, 364 patients with atopic dermatitis have undergone a total of 1,613 DBPCFCs. Six hundred eight challenges were positive, with skin symptoms in 76%, gastrointestinal symptoms in 50%, and respiratory symptoms in 44%. Fifty-four percent of the patients reacted to egg, 28% to milk, 22% to peanut, 12% to soy, 10% to wheat, and 9% to fish. The role of food hypersensitivity in atopic dermatitis has been confirmed by other researchers[29, 37] and is believed to be pathogenic in 20% to 40% of children with eczema. Food-specific IgE-mediated and cellular responses are believed to be pathogenic in this disorder.[2, 178]

GASTROINTESTINAL TRACT

Diarrhea and vomiting as immediate symptoms following food ingestion are often part of a generalized anaphylactic reaction. Such a relationship is obvious when the symptoms closely follow the ingestion of the offending food and accompanies other anaphylactic symptoms but can be rather difficult to implicate, especially in infants, when diarrhea or vomiting occurs as an isolated late symptom. A positive skin test or the presence of specific IgE antibodies in the serum can help to determine sensitivity to a specific food.

Gastrointestinal symptoms are seen most commonly in young children with food-induced *colitis* and *enterocolitis*. These syndromes are most commonly reported to be related to milk or soy. Burks and associates[35] challenged 43 patients younger than 27 months of age who were suspected of having food-induced enterocolitis using milk and soy.[28] More than half of the patients had positive challenges to soy or milk—55% to soy, and 18% to milk. Twenty-seven percent had a positive challenge to both milk and soy. Furthermore, patients with soy sensitivity almost always reacted to the partially hydrolyzed soy formula, suggesting that protein epitopes were still intact and recognized by the cells involved in the pathogenesis of enterocolitis. An isolated case of enterocolitis due to an extensively hyrolyzed casein formula has also been reported.[113]

In their prospective study on milk sensitivity in young children, Host and Halken[92] found that 59% of the patients sensitive to milk had non–IgE-mediated gastrointestinal symptoms, mostly vomiting and/or diarrhea.[92] In some cases of enterocolitis, the diarrhea can be protracted and may lead to dehydration, so may be misdiagnosed as a mucosal enzyme deficiency.[168] The symptoms are generally delayed up to 2 to 4 hours following a food challenge.[89, 97] In a clinical trial with young infants having protracted diarrhea, loose stools with blood and leukocytes were observed within 24 hours of initiation of the challenge with soy and/or milk.[168] Similarly, acute colitis with crypt abscesses and polymorphonuclear cells in the lamina propria could be demonstrated by rectal biopsy after soy-induced colitis.[78]

The following diagnostic features have been established for food-induced enterocolitis: vomiting and/or diarrhea occurring within 24 hours of the challenge; stool containing blood and leukocytes; and a rise in peripheral blood polymorphonuclear cells of greater than 3,500/mm^3 6 to 8 hours after the challenge.[168]

Although enterocolitis is predominantly a disease of the infant and young toddler, Powell described two cases of low-birth-weight newborns who presented with classic symptoms of necrotizing enterocolitis and improved only on an extensively hydrolyzed formula diet.[167] In both patients, elevated peripheral blood leukocyte counts were a constant feature until an appropriate diet was initiated. Subsequent food challenges confirmed the diagnosis of milk hypersensitivity for one patient and of milk and soy hypersensitivities for the second patient. Infants with food-induced enterocolitis generally "outgrow" their sensitivity in 1 to 2 years, but some cases persist through the first decade.

Isolated colitis is a slightly less common manifestation of food hypersensitivity. It can manifest as gross or microscopic blood in the stool. It is almost exclusively a problem of the young infant and is generally limited in time, as shown by Hill and Milla.[90] Lake and associates[122] reported six exclusively breast-fed infants who presented with blood-streaked diarrhea. Rectal biopsies showed chronic inflammation with eosinophilic infiltration in two patients. Restriction from cow's milk in the maternal diets led to resolution of the symptoms. The investigators concluded that the colitis was induced by cow's milk protein secreted in the breast milk.[122]

Gastrointestinal Syndromes

Certain types of gastrointestinal symptoms are typical features of well-characterized clinical entities. *Oral allergy syndrome* is a symptom complex almost exclusively localized to the oropharynx and is a "mucosal equivalent" of urticaria. It is usually associated with the ingestion of fresh fruits and vegetables, which provoke pruritus and swelling of the lips, the oropharynx, and/or the laryngeal pharynx. In an initial report, Amlot and colleagues[5] reported about 80 adult food-allergic patients who were experiencing frequent symptoms of oral irritation and throat tightness.[5] One fifth of the patients experienced other symptoms of food allergy (gastrointestinal, respiratory, or cutaneous) immediately following the initial oral symptoms on at least one occasion. Subsequently, Ortolani and associates[153] described 262 adult patients with oral allergy syndrome, most of whom had allergic rhinitis. Foods most commonly implicated were fruits, nuts, and vegetables (i.e., apple 53%, peach 40%, hazelnut 37%), and symptoms were only rarely systemic (anaphylactic reaction in less than 1%). Frequent cross-reactivity was observed within botanical families (e.g., apple and pear; melon, apricot, peach and plum), and with certain aeroallergens, especially birch and grass pollens. The diagnosis of oral allergy syndrome relies on clinical history and the demonstration of specific IgE antibody by positive RAST or skin tests. Skin testing with commercial extracts of fruits and vegetables has been found to be unreliable because many of the allergenic fractions are very labile. However, use of the fresh material has been demonstrated to have acceptable predictive accuracy.[154]

Clinically, *allergic eosinophilic gastroenteritis* may cause symptoms similar to those of non–IgE-mediated enterocolitis. The main clinical features are postprandial abdominal pain, nausea, vomiting, early satiety, anorexia, and diarrhea. Weight loss in adults and older children, or failure to thrive in toddlers, also occurs. In a series reported by Naylor,[143] 220 adult patients were evaluated; predominant symptoms were abdominal pain (77%), anorexia, nausea and vomiting (48%), and diarrhea (42%). Food hypersensitivity was suspected in 8% of the patients, and most patients responded favorably to oral steroids. However, significant eosinophil infiltration can be seen in the gastrointestinal tracts of both patients with allergic eosinophilic gastroenteritis and those with gastrointestinal cow's milk sensitivity.[111] Kelly and coworkers[112] studied 10 children with symptoms consistent with allergic eosinophilic gastroenteritis and gastroesophageal reflux (GER); for all 10, medical management failed and for 6 of 10, surgical management of GER also failed. After 6 weeks on an elemental amino-acid based formula symptoms completely resolved in 8 of 10 patients and substantially improved in the remaining 2 patients. Furthermore, biopsies performed before and after the dietary change, showed a significant, marked decrease in intraepithelial eosinophils in the lower esophagus and resolution of inflammation.

Inflammatory bowel diseases (IBDs) have been linked to food hypersensitivity in several reports. In one series of 78 patients with IBDs, 8.5% of patients with Crohn's disease and 21% of patients with ulcerative colitis had a history of cow's milk allergy during infancy.[71] Patients with a history of cow's milk allergy also developed the first symptoms of IBD earlier in life. In another study, food-specific in vitro tests were positive more commonly in patients with IBDs than in healthy controls.[26] Finally, almost 50% of patients with Crohn's disease on an exclusion diet were found to experience a relapse after food was re-introduced into their diet.[158] It is not clear to what extent there is a direct relationship between IBDs and food hypersensitivity or whether increased mucosal permeability due to inflammation accounts for food-specific IgE in the serum and for food-related symptoms.

Celiac disease is a well-described food hypersensitivity to gluten (a protein contained in wheat, barley, oat, and rye). The classic clinical presentation consists of steatorrhea, flatulence, weight loss, and fatigue, with a flattening of villi in the small bowel noted on biopsy. However, symptoms can vary tremendously from patient to patient.[210] Detection of serum IgA specific to gliadin suggests the diagnosis.[196] Besides plasma cells, lymphocytes can also be observed in the intestinal mucosa.[61] These cells are thought to contribute to the pathogenesis of the disease. In affected individuals, peripheral blood lymphocytes are reactive to gluten in vitro.[201] In patients with untreated celiac disease, an increased number of $CD45RO^+$ lymphocytes were found in the gut epithelium, suggesting an influx of primed memory T cells.[79] Celiac disease is reported to occur in association with a number of other immunologic disorders, including dermatitis herpetiformis, insulin-dependent diabetes, and selective IgA deficiency. The prevalence of HLA-DR3 and DQw2 is also reported to be increased in celiac disease.[210]

Although commonly incriminated, a definite pathogenic link between the syndrome *infantile colic* and food hypersensitivity is rarely established. The syndrome is vaguely defined as paroxysms of intense and inconsolable crying in very young infants, commonly assumed to originate from abdominal pain. Several reports suggest an association with milk allergy. A well-designed crossover study alternating milk and hydrolyzed casein formulas showed significant improvement in a very low percentage of infants.[60] Demonstrating an association between infantile colic and IgE antibodies to food proteins is difficult owing to the low specific IgE antibody concentrations in the serum of young infants and to the low skin reactivity seen at this young age. Furthermore, studies requiring multiple crossover trials can make interpretation of late-phase reactions difficult.[180]

SYSTEMIC ANAPHYLAXIS

Although most immediate reactions to foods involve more than one organ, they are generally mild to moderate and are often self-limited or easily controlled with over-the-counter medication. However, foods may represent the most common trigger of severe anaphylactic reactions developing outside the hospital setting.[225] Two reviews of cases of fatal or near-fatal anaphylactic reactions to foods are summarized in Table 33–4. In one study, 13 food-induced anaphylactic reactions—6 fatal and 7 near-fatal—in children or adolescents were recorded from three cities over 14 months.[190] Peanut was the most frequently implicated allergen in the fatal cases (3/6), and nuts were most common in the near-fatal reactions (4/7). All 13 patients had had a known history of previous "allergic" reactions "to the food." Of major concern was the fact that none of the patients who died had received epinephrine before severe respiratory symptoms de-

TABLE 33–4
CHARACTERISTICS OF FATAL OR SEVERE ANAPHYLAXIS DUE TO FOODS AS REPORTED IN TWO STUDIES

	Sampson *et al*[190]	Yunginger *et al*[227]
Number of patients	6 (fatal); 7 (nonfatal)	7 (all fatal)
Median age (range)	13 years (2–17 years)	19 years (11–43 years)
Number of asthmatics	13/13	5/7†
Previous reaction	12/13	7/7
Food	nuts 6; peanut 4; milk 2; egg 1	peanut 4; pecan 1; shrimp 1; fish 1
Location	Friend's or relative's house 4; school 4*; home 3; carnival 1	Restaurant 4; college or school 2; home 1

*All children in this group had fatal anaphylaxis.
†Two patients with unknown previous medical history.

veloped. Furthermore, none of these patients had self-injectable epinephrine available at the time of the reaction, either because they had left it at home, or because it had never been prescribed. The second report on teenagers and adults reported similar events prior to the fatal outcome.[227] All incriminated foods contained either peanuts, nuts, fish, or shellfish and were ingested, in all but one case, outside the home. Again, proper medical management was delayed by the nonavailability of appropriate emergency medication. In both series, risk factors were identified: most of the patients had asthma, and respiratory distress generally occurred *without* commonly expected reactions such as hives. The severity of the situation was often not appreciated, thereby delaying appropriate medical management. This factor was often due to a lack of education on the part of people dealing with the patient. Another major problem was the lack of knowledge about the potential contaminants in processed foods, on the part of both of the patients and the individuals who dispensed the foods in restaurants or schools. A better understanding of allergic reactions to foods by health professionals might also have reduced the number of fatalities in both series.

Food-dependent exercise-induced anaphylaxis is another form of systemic anaphylaxis. An initial report by Maulitz and associates[131] in 1979 described the case of a long-distance runner who suffered recurrent episodes of systemic allergic reactions following exercise each time he ingested shrimp 5 to 24 hours prior to exercise. Skin tests were positive for shrimp. The patient did not experience any more symptoms once he strictly avoided eating shrimp. In addition to several case reports, two small series of patients with food-dependent exercise-induced anaphylaxis have been published. In the first series, three adults reacted about 2 hours after ingesting celery and were found by skin test to be reactive to this food.[115] The investigators failed in this report to identify any food sensitivity in the fourth patient; however, avoiding the ingestion of a specific food 2 hours prior to exercise resulted in a complete resolution of the symptoms. The second study reported 11 patients between the ages of 18 and 43 years.[49] The offending food could be identified in 7 patients: 3 patients reacted to wheat, 3 to seafood, and 1 to grapes. Our current knowledge about this unusual manifestation of food hypersensitivity suggests that it occurs mainly in young adults (20–40 years) and that an additional trigger related to exercise acts as a cofactor in the pathogenesis of this syndrome. An increase of plasma histamine has been found in several patients experiencing symptoms[49] suggesting an increased releasability of mast cells during exercise.

Other Symptoms

A variety of other symptoms have been associated with adverse reactions to foods. Sixteen patients who reported *arthritis* after food ingestion underwent a double-blind challenge in a study reported by Panush,[157] but only three had reproducible symptoms, one each to milk, shrimp, and nitrates. However, no clear mechanism could be delineated.

In one study, a third of patients suffering from *migraine* associated their symptoms with food ingestion, mainly chocolate, cheese, or citrus fruits.[159] In a study of patients with three or more migraine headaches per week, symptoms were reproduced by placebo-controlled food challenges in about 15% of patients. Foods implicated included wheat, egg, corn, cheese, coffee, milk, and beans. Some patients reportedly had positive skin prick tests to food, suggesting an IgE-mediated reaction, but a review of several studies failed to identify a definite immunologic mechanism.[224]

Controversy regularly resurfaces regarding the possible role of adverse reactions to food in the etiology of *attention deficit disorder and hyperkinetic syndrome*. A 1993 review by Warner[223] emphasizes that association of food ingestion and behavioral changes can occur in a number of circumstances. However, true hyperactivity (a neurologic problem) is very rare and should not be mistaken for a nonspecific behavioral problem (a psychosocial problem). Overall, a clear association between adverse reactions to foods and behavioral disorders can only rarely be demonstrated, and Warner concluded that "obsession with diet only detracts from the real cause of the problem and its solution."[223] Only carefully designed, double-blind, placebo-controlled scientific studies, especially in dealing with polymorphic symptoms, can address a possible link between hyperkinetic syndrome and food hypersensitivity. Other common complaints not proven to be provoked by food hypersensitivity are listed in Table 33–5.

DIAGNOSTIC APPROACH TO FOOD HYPERSENSITIVITIES

An appropriate and cost-effective work-up of possible adverse food reactions requires a well-structured history. The following issues must be addressed: (1) type of symptoms,

TABLE 33–5
SOME SYMPTOMS NOT SUBSTANTIATED TO BE RELATED TO FOOD HYPERSENSITIVITY

Hyperkinetic syndrome/attention deficit disorder/aggressive disorders
Chronic fatigue
Tics
Seizures
Chronic upper airway infections
Bed wetting

TABLE 33–6
VALUE OF DIAGNOSTIC TESTS ACCORDING TO SYMPTOMS OR SYNDROMES*

Test	Immediate Symptoms	Enterocolitis	Eosinophilic Gastroenteritis	Celiac Disease	Heiner's Syndrome
Food challenge	+ + +	+ + +	+ + +	+ +	?
Skin test	+ + +	–	+	–	–
Specific IgE (CAP-RAST)	+ +	–	+	–	–
Precipitins	–	–	–	–	+ + +
Lymphocyte proliferation	(+)	(+)	(+)	(+)	?
Endoscopy	–	+	+ + +	+ + +	+ +

*– = nonrelevant or not studied; (+) = experimental or unproved; + = low value; + + = definite value; + + + = standard procedure.

(2) temporal relationship between the ingestion of a food and the symptoms, (3) reproducibility and frequency of the symptoms, (4) when the last reaction occurred, (5) amount of food necessary to trigger the symptoms, and (6) other concomitant factors (e.g., exercise).

Appropriate and systematic history of food-related adverse events will direct further in vitro and/or in vivo testing in the majority of the cases (Table 33–6). Appropriate testing must be for specific foods, directed either by patient history or the likelihood that a specific food would provoke the clinical picture. A large variety of in vitro tests are available to physicians for diagnosing food hypersensitivity. However, it is in the patient's best interest to use diagnostic testing as specifically as possible, because the lack of specificity of these tests can lead to inappropriate, and sometimes harmful, exclusion diets. In some cases, if the history is unclear or confusing, a dietary record may be helpful in the primary assessment to identify foods implicated in the pathogenesis of the symptoms.[31]

SKIN PRICK TEST

Skin prick tests are easy to perform and inexpensive, and the results are available in about 15 minutes. Glycerinated food extracts are available from a number of commercial laboratories. However, the absence of standardized extracts results in considerable variability of results between one company's extract and another's. The accuracy of skin tests for six common food allergens was compared with the outcome of food challenges in children with atopic dermatitis.[186] The sensitivity was good overall, ranging from 73% (egg) to 100% (peanut, soy, fish). The specificity was significantly lower for all extracts tested. Overall, the positive predictive accuracies of these tests were poor, whereas the negative predictive accuracies were excellent. Skin prick tests are useful only in the diagnosis of IgE-mediated food hypersensitivity and are of no diagnostic value in non–IgE-mediated disorders, such as milk-induced enterocolitis.[86, 97, 133]

In some circumstances, the reliability of skin tests must be questioned. For example false-negative skin prick test results are seen frequently in very young infants because of the low reactivity of their skin, and in patients maintained on immunosuppressive medications or prolonged courses of high-dose systemic steroids. As a general rule, antihistamines should be discontinued for at least 4 to 5 days (up to 6 weeks for astemizole) prior to skin testing in order to avoid false-negative results. Furthermore, commercially available extracts of many fruits and vegetables are unreliable because of the lability of relevant allergens. In cases in which history is highly suggestive but the skin tests are negative or equivocal, the tests should be repeated with fresh products.[154] Intradermal skin tests do not provide clinically relevant improvement in sensitivity over skin prick tests, but carry an increased risk of adverse systemic reactions. Therefore, intradermal tests should not be considered routine diagnostic procedures. Scratch tests have no advantage over skin prick tests and are less quantitative.

SPECIFIC IgE TESTS

Specific in vitro IgE tests consist of isotope or enzyme-linked immunosorbent tests—RAST, CAP-RAST or ELISA—for detecting food-specific IgE antibodies circulating in a patient's serum. They are commonly used by nonallergists as screening tests in patients suspected of food hypersensitivity, and their diagnostic accuracy is comparable or slightly inferior to that of skin tests.[89, 186] However, there is generally no advantage in combining skin tests with specific IgE antibody determination.[186] Skin prick tests are generally preferred over in vitro IgE tests in the initial work-up, mainly because of their sensitivity and the immediate availability of results. In vitro tests are used routinely in selected cases in which skin tests cannot be performed (e.g., severe eczema, exquisite sensitivity, marked dermographism, antihistamine therapy).

There is no established diagnostic value for the determination of antigen-specific IgG, IgG_4, IgA, or IgM antibodies, because they are frequently found in sera of food-tolerant subjects.[46]

LYMPHOCYTE PROLIFERATION ASSAYS

The diagnostic value of in vitro peripheral blood antigen-specific lymphocyte proliferation assays has now been reassessed. Although earlier studies showed limited diagnostic value,[194, 214] partially because of significant lymphocyte proliferation in controls, some later studies have regenerated interest in this diagnostic procedure. Some studies are highly enthusiastic with claims of specific results,[4] whereas others report a limited diagnostic value for this test in disorders with delayed-type symptoms.[214] Overall, the broad interindividual variability of antigen-induced cell proliferation as well as nonstandardized methods used by investigators makes it highly unlikely that lymphocyte proliferation tests will be of significant value in the diagnosis of food hypersensitivity.[183] These procedures should be restricted to research studies, mainly for the evaluation of T-cell modulation of the food antigen response. Furthermore, the cost and time required for such tests make their widespread use impractical.

BASOPHIL HISTAMINE RELEASE TESTS

Basophil histamine release testing has become increasingly popular, and semiautomated methods have been introduced in some commercial laboratories. The predictive values of antigen-induced basophil histamine release and skin prick tests were compared in a study of 57 children admitted for DBPCFC. The positive predictive accuracy was found to be much lower for basophil histamine release (16% to 30%) than for skin prick tests (25% to 69%) for milk, egg, and peanut.[184] It has been determined that food-allergic children with atopic dermatitis have higher rates of spontaneous basophil histamine release than normal controls and children with atopic dermatitis who do not have food allergies.[187] Furthermore, in food-allergic patients, basophil histamine release from intestinal mast cells could be correlated with RASTs, skin prick tests, and food challenges.[145] The basophil histamine release assay cannot be recommended for routine diagnostic testing, but it may have a limited clinical value in the follow-up of food-allergic children with severe symptoms, because spontaneous basophil releasability is lost after 4 to 6 months of an appropriate allergen elimination diet.

ELIMINATION DIETS

Special care must be taken in ordering a diagnostic elimination diet. When a causal relationship is seen between a food and a reaction, such as repeated immediate hives after a single food, the food should be removed from the diet as soon as the food is identified. The remission of symptoms in the presence of a positive skin reaction strongly implicates the pathogenic role of the food. However, more caution must be exercised when the relationship is less clear, and further work-up must proceed in a stepwise fashion. First, skin tests, in vitro testing, and/or challenges directed to test foods suspected on the basis of their prevalence in the pathogenesis of a given clinical picture may help to detect the food(s). Second, if the initial work-up is negative, careful removal of highly allergenic foods under dietary supervision may be helpful. In some patients with severe symptoms, only the utilization of an amino acid based formula (elemental formula), with one or two low-allergenic foods, such as corn or rice, is effective in eliminating symptoms. Third, after stabilization of the clinical condition, physician-supervised food challenges help to delineate specific food sensitivities.

DOUBLE-BLIND PLACEBO-CONTROLLED FOOD CHALLENGE (DBPCFC)

A large number of factors may induce symptoms that mimic adverse reactions to foods, making the interpretation of equivocal and subjective symptoms difficult during an open challenge. At present, the standard for the diagnosis of food hypersensitivity remains a standardized double-blind placebo-controlled food challenge, which has been extensively and successfully utilized in children and adults by many investigators.[22, 151, 177] The "blinding" of both the physician and the patient and family eliminates any possibility of an interpretational bias.[179] This procedure has been published in detail[23] and is summarized in Table 33–7.

Briefly, the suspected food should be eliminated from the patient's diet for 2 weeks prior to the DBPCFC. If the patient has atopic dermatitis or urticaria, the skin should be cleared before challenges are initiated. Asthmatic patients should have their symptoms stabilized, and ideally, β_2-agonist medication should be discontinued at least 4 to 8 hours prior to the challenges. An intravenous line should be available during challenges if major allergic reactions are suspected. The timing of the challenge is dictated by the history of the reactions. If immediate reactions are suspected, two challenges, one with a placebo and one with the suspected food, may be administered each day. If the patient presents with a history of delayed reactions, the individual challenges must be spaced accordingly in order to detect late reactions.

The food is hidden in a vehicle, often a liquid (fruit juice, formula), in a low-allergenic solid food (applesauce, oatmeal), or in opaque capsules. A low dose (less than that thought to have provoked a reaction) is administered first, and then gradually the dose is increased every 15 minutes. However, the timing between doses must be determined initially according to the time between the ingestion of the food and expected reactions. The initial dose is increased up to a total of 8 to 10 gm of dehydrated food, generally between 60 and 90 minutes for immediate reactions. During the challenge, symptoms are recorded by an observer who is unaware of the content of the challenge.

Patients with suspected immediate reactions should be monitored for at least 2 hours after completion of the challenge, because most immediate reactions occur within this

TABLE 33–7
PROCEDURE FOR DOUBLE-BLIND PLACEBO-CONTROLLED FOOD CHALLENGES (DBPCFCs)

1. Restriction of the tested food(s) from diet 2 weeks prior to challenge.
2. Admission to clinic, ± insertion of IV line for following emergency medications:
   a. Epinephrine 0.01 mg/kg/dose SC (max 0.3 mg).
   b. Diphenhydramine, 1 mg/kg/dose PO or IV (max 75 mg).
   c. Solu-Medrol, 1–2 mg/kg/dose IV (max. 150 mg).
   d. Albuterol nebulizations, 2.5 mg in 0.9% NaCl.
   e. Cimetidine, 5–10 mg/kg/dose (max. 400 mg).
3. Prepare test substance: Hide 8 to 10 gm of dehydrated food in a liquid vehicle (e.g., total of 100 ml of formula or juice) or an opaque capsule.
4. Randomize the following AM/PM challenges as either test food or placebo:
   a. 5% of test substance; wait 15 minutes.
   b. 10% of test substance; wait 10 minutes.
   c. 20% of test substance; wait 10 minutes.
   d. 20% of test substance; wait 10 minutes.
   e. 20% of test substance; wait 10 minutes.
   f. 25% of test substance; end of the test.
5. Have symptoms recorded by a blinded investigator.
6. Discharge patient or give further DBPCFC on next day.
7. After last DBPCFC of the series, "break the code" and give the foods with negative DBPCFC openly in usual quantities.

time. Special caution must be exercised in young patients with soy or cow's milk enterocolitis, because vomiting and/or diarrhea may occur for several hours after the challenge and may lead to severe dehydration and hypotension. The challenge should be discontinued if a reaction occurs, and on-site available emergency medication—diphenhydramine, 1–1.5 mg/kg PO or IV (up to 75 mg); epinephrine, 0.01 mg/kg SC (up to 0.3 mg); β_2-agonist nebulization; cimetidine, 5–10 mg/kg IV (up to 400 mg)—is administered according to the severity of the symptoms.[23]

As a general rule, the diagnostic approach to suspected adverse reactions to food proceeds in the following steps (Fig. 33–4): (1) a careful medical history; (2) a physical examination to assess atopic features and the nutritional status of the patient; and (3) if an IgE-mediated disorder is suspected, skin tests to foods selected on the basis of history and the likelihood of their inducing certain symptoms. In patients with non–life-threatening reactions, a definite diagnosis can be obtained only by allergen elimination followed by DBPCFC or, in selected cases, by single blind challenge or occasionally by open challenges.

THERAPEUTIC OPTIONS IN FOOD HYPERSENSITIVITY

Once the diagnosis of food hypersensitivity is established and the causal food(s) identified, the symptoms should resolve if the incriminated food(s) are strictly eliminated from the diet. However, only foods proven to elicit symptoms should be removed from the patient's diet. Overzealous diets can be detrimental, especially in children, in whom they can result in failure to thrive.[174] Elimination diets are complicated by the extensive utilization of food proteins such as soy, egg, peanut, and milk in many manufactured food products. Patients and/or their parents must be carefully instructed to read product ingredient labels, because relevant antigens can be "hidden" under various designations[11] (Table 33–8). The assistance of a dietitian well trained in the management of food elimination diets is invaluable in the proper care of food-allergic patients. The dietitian can also give the patient valuable advice for a balanced diet comprising all required nutrients, especially for younger patients, who may need to eliminate several foods from their diet. Parent support groups are of great help in providing information about substitute foods, i.e., for baking or cooking, and updates on the composition of manufactured foods (in the United States, such updates are available from The Food Allergy Network, Fairfax VA 22030; phone 800-929-4040).

In cow's milk–allergic children who are not being breastfed, extensively hydrolyzed formulas represent the best substitution for cow's milk formula. The protein sources of these formulas are extensively hydrolyzed casein and/or whey proteins with residual peptides of very low molecular weight (<1.5 kD). However, even though hydrolysates are safe in most milk-allergic patients, reactions have rarely been re-

TABLE 33–8
INGREDIENTS THAT MAY INDICATE EGG PROTEIN IN PROCESSED FOODS

Albumin	Mayonnaise
Egg (white, yolk, dried, powdered, solids)	Meringue
Egg substitutes	Ovalbumin
Eggnog	Ovomucin
Globulin	Ovomucoid
Livetin	Ovovitellin
Lysozyme	Simplesse

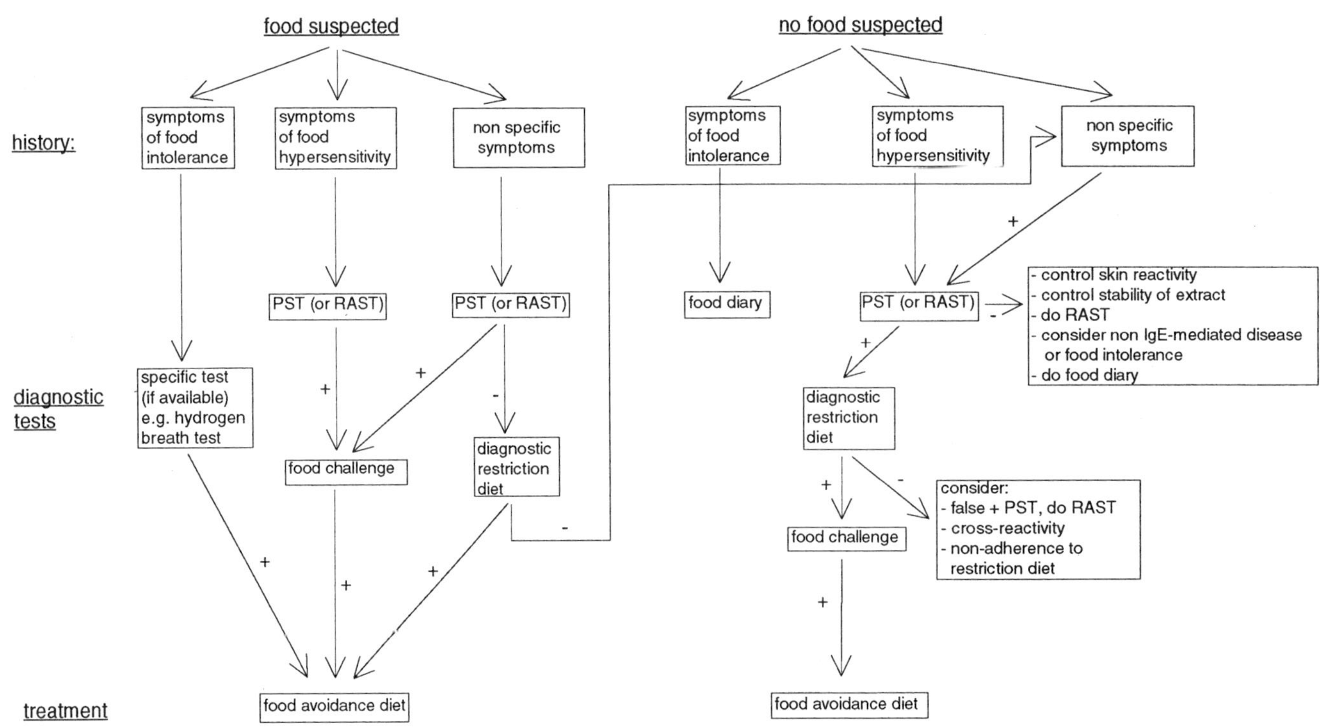

FIGURE 33–4. Diagnostic protocol for adverse reactions to foods.

ported in milk-sensitive children.[55, 113, 193] In older patients with severe symptoms and reactions to several foods, a balanced diet with sufficient caloric intake may require the use of an elemental formula composed of amino acids. Such a diet should be instituted only under supervision of a dietitian.

At present, there is no proactive treatment for food hypersensitivity. As opposed to immunotherapy for Hymenoptera venom or certain aeroallergen sensitivities, only a few studies on immunotherapy to food have been published. Peanut would be an ideal candidate for immunotherapy, because peanut sensitivity is only rarely "outgrown." However, peanut is an allergen that commonly provokes life-threatening reactions and has been found to induce significant adverse side effects with immunotherapy.[152, 182]

Sodium cromoglycate has been investigated in various clinical trials for its efficacy in preventing adverse reactions to foods. Burks and associates[30] reported a study of 10 egg-sensitive children with atopic dermatitis enrolled in a double-blind crossover trial receiving either placebo or cromolyn (40 mg/kg/day of challenge). There was no difference in symptoms, or in the responses to food challenges between the groups.[30] Some studies have reported benefits from treatment with cromolyn. However, a large variety of doses have been tested, and most studies have not validated the food sensitivity of their patients with blinded challenges.[36, 155] Thus, there is no conclusive evidence to support the use of oral cromolyn in food-allergic patients. Animal studies support these findings since sodium cromoglycate failed to prevent mast cell histamine release.[160] In an isolated study with a double-blind design, antihistamine therapy (astemizole) was reported to decrease the severity of oral pruritus in patients with oral allergy syndrome to hazelnut.[15] It should be emphasized, however, that antihistamines may mask early symptoms of anaphylaxis, potentially delaying the initiation of treatment of a life-threatening reaction.

In the last few years, the role of antigen-specific T cells in the modulation of allergic responses has been studied extensively.[93, 148] In the future, synthesis of peptides acting as tolerogens could provide an important agent in the treatment of allergic disease. Clinical immunotherapy trials have been performed with peptides to several aeroallergens.[125, 146] Promising preliminary results show limited adverse side effects, suggesting that this form of immunotherapy may someday be applied safely in food-allergic patients with potentially severe reactions.

Currently, measures to prevent accidental ingestions of foods should be emphasized by health care professionals, and proper food avoidance diets must be thoroughly explained. Patients at high risk must be identified, and the patients or their parents, spouses, teachers, and so on, should be educated to recognize the onset of a reaction. The high-risk group comprises any patient with asthma, a history of a previous severe reaction, or hypersensitivity to life-threatening allergens such as peanut, nuts, or shellfish.

If such a patient experiences any severe symptom, but also any respiratory symptom (laryngeal, lung tightness), epinephrine (0.01 mg/kg, up to 0.3 mg) should be injected subcutaneously or intramuscularly. After on-site injection of epinephrine, the patient should be transported as rapidly as possible to a medical facility, where blood pressure and other vital signs can be monitored, and intubation can be performed if necessary. Epinephrine, in a ready-to-use, self-injectable form (Epi-Pen, Anaguard, Anakit) must be available to all patients with a history of a previous severe allergic reaction to food or a history of food allergy and asthma.

Less severe reactions (usually localized skin or gastrointestinal symptoms) can often be treated with oral antihistamines (e.g., diphenhydramine, 1 to 1.5 mg/kg/dose up to 75 mg, or hydroxyzine 1 to 2 mg/kg/dose up to 75 mg).

Patients (and/or their parents), daycare providers, school teachers, and so on, must be trained in the proper evaluation and initial management of anaphylaxis in case of an accidental ingestion of a food allergen. In some severe cases, proper initial care can be life-saving.[190, 227] Rapid access to adequate medical treatment is one of the most favorable predictive factors of outcome in food-related anaphylaxis.[190]

PROPHYLAXIS OF FOOD HYPERSENSITIVITY

The increasing prevalence of atopic disorders and an awareness of the potential role that early feeding may play in the development of atopy have generated speculation about the pathogenicity of foods (e.g., cow's milk, egg, and peanut) in the diet of infants and young children. Since the studies by Grulee and Sanford,[75] conflicting reports on the benefits of exclusive breast-feeding for prevention of atopy and food allergy have been published.

In a carefully designed study, Zeiger and colleagues,[229] randomized pregnant women in atopic families into a prophylactically treated group (maternal avoidance of egg, milk, and peanut during the third trimester of pregnancy as well as during lactation and breast-feeding, supplementation with hydrolyzed formula until 12 months of age, and delayed introduction of solid foods) and a control group (unrestricted maternal diet and infant feeding following guidelines of the AAP).[229] The prevalence of atopic diseases (food-induced atopic dermatitis, urticaria, and/or gastrointestinal diseases) was lower at 12 months in the prophylactic group, as was the prevalence of positive skin reactions to foods by 24 months. However, no difference was seen in the prevalence of respiratory allergies. In a 7-year follow-up of the same groups of patients, Zeiger and Heller[226] found no overall difference in the prevalence of atopic disease. Interestingly, the prevalence of asthma and allergic rhinitis in children who were diagnosed with food allergy at 4 years of age was almost two times greater when they were 7 years old than in children who did not have food allergies. Comparable results were noted by some investigators in preventive food allergen avoidance studies with similar designs,[41, 76] but other studies have not supported the preventive effect of breast-feeding.[85, 213]

As a general rule, a maternal diet restricting highly allergenic foods (peanuts and nuts) combined with delayed introduction of solid foods until after 6 months (milk after 12 months, eggs after 24 months, fish and peanuts after 36 months) is indicated in high-risk patients (both parents with atopic disease and/or siblings with food allergy). However, such dietary measures are very restrictive and need to be carefully discussed with the mothers, because the dropout rate may be high. Avoidance diets during the third trimester of pregnancy are probably without benefit and add unnecessary constraints to already severe restrictions.[229]

NATURAL HISTORY

It is commonly observed that clinical tolerance to foods eventually develops in most children. The phenomenon is often referred to as "outgrowing" food allergy. This favorable outcome was observed in 87% of cow's milk–allergic infants in a prospective study over 3 years.[92] However, several factors appear to influence the development of tolerance. The age at diagnosis is important, because it was observed that children younger than 3 years of age appeared to outgrow their food allergy more often than older children.[18] Furthermore, sensitivity to certain foods may be lifelong.[18, 191] As outlined previously, peanut sensitivity is only rarely outgrown. Bock and Atkins[21] evaluated 32 peanut-allergic patients 2 to 14 years after their initial positive double-blind challenge. None of the patients had outgrown the peanut sensitivity or lost positive skin test reactions. Also, children with one food hypersensitivity are more likely to develop sensitivity to other foods. Hill and associates[87] showed that children with persistent IgE-mediated cow's milk allergy were more prone to be sensitized to egg and peanut than those who had lost their sensitivity during the 2 years of prospective follow-up. However, the same study showed no increase in asthma or atopic dermatitis in children who remained milk sensitive.

It also has been observed that children who develop tolerance to a food frequently maintain positive skin reactions for several years. Therefore skin tests are not predictive of outgrowing a food sensitivity.[18, 191] Two studies on serum specific IgE and IgG showed a certain predictive value regarding the outcome of future food challenges. A low ratio of IgE/IgG early in the follow-up of 82 egg-, milk-, and fish-allergic children studied by Dannaeus and colleagues[47] suggested a rapid outgrowing of the sensitivity. A rise in casein and β-lactoglobulin specific IgG_4 concomitant with a decrease in specific IgE was observed by James and Sampson[105] in children with cow's milk allergy who developed tolerance. However, quantification of specific antibodies alone is reported not to be predictive of outcome in cow's milk–allergic patients.[88] In a study reported by Isolauri and associates,[97] the number of IgA-secreting cells as determined by a solid-phase enzyme-linked immunoassay was found to be higher in children with cow's milk allergy and positive follow-up challenges. These investigators speculate that the ability to mount a local IgA response is related to the subsequent loss of the sensitivity.

In a study on modulation of cellular mechanisms in children with eczema and food hypersensitivity, lymphocyte responses to antigen were found to be partially suppressed during an elimination diet; however, definite conclusions regarding the predictive value of this test cannot be drawn.[3] Repeated challenges will be necessary until a reliable test to predict loss of the sensitivity is available.

Individual schedules for repeated challenges must be established. As a rule, a patient with a recent significant reaction to a food should not be rechallenged within the following year. Patients with peanut, nuts, fish, and shellfish allergy usually need not be rechallenged for at least several years after a reaction. Accidental ingestions often occur even in carefully managed diets and thereby reveal the status of the sensitivity. Sensitivity to milk is often lost early in childhood,[92] so yearly challenges may be indicated for this food. In our experience, the egg-allergic patient should be rechallenged only every 2 to 3 years, especially the patient who reacts to low doses with immediate symptoms. Patients allergic to soy and wheat should be rechallenged every 1 or 2 years. Otherwise, the decision to rechallenge a patient with a specific food is dictated by nutritional requirements and the time elapsed since the last reaction to the food.

SUMMARY

Food hypersensitivity can be identified in about 2% of a general population, with a peak occurrence in infancy and early childhood. The pathogenesis of the symptoms can be attributed to immunologic reactions in the intestinal mucosa and other target organs with subsequent liberation of mediators and cytokines responsible for clinical symptoms and further reactions to the food. Target organs may vary according to the mechanism involved. Immediate clinical response such as systemic anaphylaxis may involve the gastrointestinal tract, the lungs, the skin, and the cardiovascular system with possible life-threatening reactions. Delayed reactions such as enterocolitis due to milk or soy sensitivity may be difficult to link to a specific food, because the symptoms may be nonspecific and may mimic other diseases. In any case, an appropriate history and diagnostic testing should lead to early recognition of the offending food(s), and the symptoms will resolve after a careful elimination diet. Special care must be applied in the management of patients at high risk for a fatal reaction, for example, asthmatics and patients sensitive to a very potent allergen (nuts, peanuts, shellfish). Prophylactic measures (self-injectable epinephrine available at all times, proper education of potential care providers) must be emphasized for all patients. Only a risk-conscious management program conducted by health care providers will keep the morbidity and mortality of food allergy as low as possible until a proactive treatment becomes available.

REFERENCES

1. American Academy of Allergy and Immunology/NIAID: Adverse reactions to foods. Anderson JA, Sogn DD (eds). NIH Publication 84–2442, 1984, p 1.
2. Abernathy-Carver KJ, Sampson HA, Picker LJ, et al: Milk-induced eczema is associated with the expansion of T cells expressing cutaneous lymphocyte antigen. J Clin Invest 95:913–918, 1995.
3. Agata H, Kondo N, Fukutomi O, et al: Effect of elimination diets on food-specific IgE antibodies and lymphocyte proliferative response to food antigens in atopic dermatitis patients exhibiting sensitivity to food allergens. J Allergy Clin Immunol 91:668–679, 1993.
4. Albani S, Avanzini MA, Plebani A, et al: Diagnostic value of a lymphocyte stimulation test in cow milk protein intolerance. Ann Allergy 63:489–492, 1989.
5. Amlot PL, Kemeny DM, Zachary C, et al: Oral allergy syndrome (OAS): symptoms of IgE mediated hypersensitivity to foods. Clin Allergy 17:33–42, 1987.
6. Anibarro B, Garcia-Ara MC, Pascual C: Associated sensitization to latex and chestnut. Allergy 48:130–131, 1993.
7. Atkins FM, Steinberg SS, Metcalfe DD: Evaluation of immediate adverse reactions to foods in adult patients. I: Correlation of demographic, laboratory, and prick skin test data with response to con-

trolled oral food challenges. J Allergy Clin Immunol 75:348–355, 1985.

8. Bachman KD, Dees SC: Milk allergy. I: Observations on incidence and symptoms in well babies. Pediatrics 20:393–399, 1957.
9. Baenkler HW, Lux G: Antigen-induced histamine-release from duodenal biopsy in gastrointestinal food allergy. Ann Allergy 62:449–452, 1989.
10. Baenkler HW, Lux G, Oltsch H: Food-induced histamine release from gastric and duodenal mucosa. Hepatogastroenterology 31:233–235, 1984.
11. Barnes Koerner C, Sampson HA: Diets and nutrition. In Metcalfe DD, Sampson HA, Simon RA (eds): Food allergy: Adverse reactions to Foods and Food Additives. Blackwell Scientific Publications, Boston, 1991, p 332.
12. Belut D, Moneret-Vautrin DA, Nicolas JP, et al: IgE levels in intestinal juice. Dig Dis Sci 25:323–332, 1980.
13. Bernhisel-Broadbent J, Dintzis HM, Dintzis RZ, et al: Allergenicity and antigenicity of chicken egg ovomucoid (*Gal d* III) compared with ovalbumin (*Gal d* I) in children with egg allergy and in mice. J Allergy Clin Immunol 93:1047–1059, 1994.
14. Bernhisel-Broadbent J, Scanlon SM, Sampson HA: Fish hypersensitivity. I: In vitro and oral challenge results in fish-allergic patients. J Allergy Clin Immunol 89:730–737, 1992.
15. Bindslev-Jensen C, Vibits A, Stahl Skov P, et al: Oral allergy syndrome; the effect of astemizole. Allergy 46:610–613, 1991.
16. Bjarnason I, Goolamali SK, Levi AJ, et al: Intestinal permeability in patients with atopic eczema. Br J Dermatol 112:291–297, 1985.
17. Bleumink E, Young E: Identification of the atopic allergen in cow's milk. Int Arch Allergy Appl Immunol 34:521–543, 1968.
18. Bock SA: The natural history of food sensitivity. J Allergy Clin Immunol 69:173–177, 1982.
19. Bock SA: Prospective appraisal of complaints of adverse reactions to foods in children during the first 3 years of life. Pediatrics 79:683–688, 1987.
20. Bock SA: Respiratory reactions induced by food challenges in children with pulmonary disease. Pediatr Allergy Immunol 3:188–194, 1992.
21. Bock SA, Atkins FM: The natural history of peanut allergy. J Allergy Clin Immunol 83:900–904, 1989.
22. Bock SA, Atkins FM: Patterns of food hypersensitivity during sixteen years of double-blind, placebo-controlled food challenges. J Pediatr 117:561–567, 1990.
23. Bock SA, Sampson HA, Atkins FM, et al: Double-blind, placebo-controlled food challenge (DBPCFC) as an office procedure: A manual. J Allergy Clin Immunol 82:986–997, 1988.
24. Bockman DE, Cooper MD: Pinocytosis by epithelium associated with lymphoid follicles in the bursa of Fabricius, appendix, and Peyer's patches: an electron microscopic study. Am J Anat 136:455–478, 1973.
25. Bresson JL, Pang KY, Walker WA: Microvillus membrane differentiation: quantitative difference in cholera toxin binding to the intestinal surface of newborn and adult rabbits. Pediatr Res 18:984–987, 1984.
26. Brignola C, Miniero R, Campieri M, et al: Dietary allergy evaluated by PRIST and RAST in inflammatory bowel disease. Hepatogastroenterology 33:128–130, 1986.
27. Brown WR, Borthistle BK, Chen ST: Immunoglobulin E (IgE) and IgE-containing cells in human gastrointestinal fluids and tissues. Clin Exp Immunol 20:227–237, 1975.
28. Burks AW, Casteel HB, Fiedorek SC, et al: Prospective oral food challenge study of two soybean protein isolates in patients with possible milk or soy protein enterocolitis. Pediatr Allergy Immunol 5:40–45, 1994.
29. Burks AW, Mallory SB, Williams LW, et al: Atopic dermatitis: clinical relevance of food hypersensitivity reactions. J Pediatr 113:447–451, 1988.
30. Burks AW, Sampson HA: Double-blind placebo-controlled trial of oral cromolyn in children with atopic dermatitis and documented food hypersensitivity. J Allergy Clin Immunol 81:417–423, 1988.
31. Burks AW, Sampson HA: Diagnostic approaches to the patient with suspected food allergies. J Pediatr 121:S64–S71, 1992.
32. Burks AW, Williams LW, Connaughton C, et al: Identification and characterization of a second major peanut allergen, Ara h II, with use of the sera of patients with atopic dermatitis and positive peanut challenge. J Allergy Clin Immunol 90:962–969, 1992.
33. Burks AW, Williams LW, Helm RM, et al: Identification of a major peanut allergen, Ara h I, in patients with atopic dermatitis and positive peanut challenges. J Allergy Clin Immunol 88:172–179, 1991.
34. Burks AW, Williams LW, Thresher W, et al: Allergenicity of peanut and soybean extracts altered by chemical or thermal denaturation in patients with atopic dermatitis and positive food challenges. J Allergy Clin Immunol 90:889–897, 1992.
35. Burks AW, Jr, Brooks JR, Sampson HA: Allergenicity of major component proteins of soybean determined by enzyme-linked immunosorbent assay (ELISA) and immunoblotting in children with atopic dermatitis and positive soy challenges. J Allergy Clin Immunol 81:1135–1142, 1988.
36. Businco L, Cantani A, Meglio P, et al: Sodium cromoglycate in the management of food allergy in children. In Harms HK, Wahn U (eds): Food Allergy in Infancy and Childhood. Springer, Berlin, 1989, p 189.
37. Businco L, Meglio P, Ferrara M: The role of food allergy and eosinophils in atopic dermatitis. Pediatr Allergy Immunol 4(suppl 4):33–37, 1993.
38. Caffrey EA, Sladen GE, Isaacs PET, et al: Thrombocytopenia caused by cow's milk. Lancet 2:316, 1981.
39. Challacombe SJ, Tomasi TB: Systemic tolerance and secretory immunity after oral immunization. J Exp Med 152:1459–1472, 1980.
40. Champion RH, Roberts SOB, Carpenter RG, et al: Urticaria and angiooedema: a review of 554 patients. Br J Dermatol 81:588–597, 1969.
41. Chandra RK, Puri S, Cheema PS: Predictive value of cord blood IgE in the development of atopic disease and role of breast feeding in its prevention. Clin Allergy 15:517–522, 1985.
42. Cohen SG, Saavedra-Delgado AM: Through the centuries with food and drink, for better or worse. Allergy Proc 10:281–290, 1989.
43. Cohen SG, Saavedra-Delgado AM: Through the centuries with food and drink, for better or worse II. Allergy Proc 10:363–373, 1989.
44. Collins-Williams C: The incidence of milk allergy in pediatric practice. J Pediatr 48:39–47, 1956.
45. Crowe SE, Soda K, Stanisz AM, et al: Intestinal permeability in allergic rats: nerve involvement in antigen-induced changes. Am J Physiol 264:G617–G623, 1993.
46. Dannaeus A: Age-related antibody response to food antigens. Pediatr Allergy Immunol 4(suppl 3):21–24, 1993.
47. Dannaeus A, Inganäs M: A follow-up study of children with food allergy: clinical course in relation to serum IgE- and IgG-antibody level to milk, egg and fish. Clin Allergy 11:533–539, 1981.
48. Daul CB, Slattery M, Reese G, et al: Identification of the major brown shrimp *(Penaeus aztecus)* allergen as the muscle protein tropomyosin. Int Arch Allergy Immunol 105:49–55, 1994.
49. Dohi M, Suko M, Sugiyama H, et al: Food-dependent, exercise-induced anaphylaxis: a study on 11 Japanese cases. J Allergy Clin Immunol 87:34–40, 1991.
50. Donovan GR, Baldo BA: Crossreactivity of IgE antibodies from sera of subjects allergic to both ryegrass pollen and wheat endosperm proteins: evidence for common allergenic determinants. Clin Exp Allergy 20:501–509, 1990.
51. DuMont GCL, Beach RC, Menzies IS: Gastrointestinal permeability in food-allergic eczematous children. Clin Allergy 14:55–59, 1984.
52. Eckmann L, Jung HC, Schurer-Maly C, et al: Differential cytokine expression by human intestinal epithelial cell lines: regulated expression of interleukin 8. Gastroenterology 105:1689–1697, 1993.
53. Eigenmann PA, Belli DC, Ludi F, et al: In-vitro lymphocyte proliferation with milk and a casein/whey protein hydrolyzed formula in cow's milk allergic children. J Allergy Clin Immunol 96:549–557, 1995.
54. Eigenmann PA, Huang SK, Ho DG, Sampson HA: Characterization of ovomucoid specific T-cell lines and clones from egg allergic individuals. Pediatr Allergy Immunol 7:12–21, 1996.
55. Ellis MH, Short JA, Heiner DC: Anaphylaxis after ingestion of a recently introduced hydrolyzed whey protein formula. J Pediatr 118:74–77, 1991.
56. Elsayed S, Bennich H: The primary structure of allergen M from cod. Scand J Immunol 4:203–208, 1975.
57. Eriksson NE: Food sensitivity reported by patients with asthma and hay fever. Allergy 33:189–196, 1978.
58. Agglé-Hansson M, Bende M: The significance of hypersensitivity to nuts in patients with birch pollen allergy. Allergy 48:282–284, 1993.
59. Ford RPK, Taylor B: Natural history of egg hypersensitivity. Arch Dis Child 57:649–652, 1982.
60. Forsyth BWC: Colic and the effect of changing formulas: a double-blind, multiple-crossover study. J Pediatr 115:521–526, 1989.
61. Freedman AR, Macartney JC, Nelufer JM, et al: Timing of infiltration of T lymphocytes induced by gluten into the small intestine in coeliac disease. J Clin Pathol 40:741–745, 1987.

62. Freigang B, Jadavji TP, Freigang DW: Lack of adverse reactions to measles, mumps, and rubella vaccine in egg-allergic children. Ann Allergy 73:486–488, 1994.
63. Friedman A, al-Sabbagh A, Santos LM, et al: Oral tolerance: a biologically relevant pathway to generate peripheral tolerance against external and self antigens [review]. Chem Immunol 58:259–290, 1994.
64. Fries JH, Zizmor J: Roentgen studies of children with alimentary disturbances due to food allergy. Am J Dis Child 54:1239–1251, 1937.
65. Fuglsang G, Madsen C, Halken S, et al: Adverse reactions to food additives in children with atopic symptoms. Allergy 49:31–37, 1994.
66. Fuglsang G, Madsen C, Saval P, et al: Prevalence of intolerance to food additives among Danish school children. Pediatr Allergy Immunol 4:123–129, 1993.
67. Fujihashi K, Taguchi T, Aicher WK, et al: Immunoregulatory functions for murine intraepithelial lymphocytes: gamma/delta T cell receptor-positive (TCR+) T cells abrogate oral tolerance, while alpha/beta TCR+ T cells provide B cell help. J Exp Med 175:695–707, 1992.
68. Fujihashi K, Taguchi T, McGhee JR, et al: Regulatory function for murine intraepithelial lymphocytes. Two subsets of CD3+, T cell receptor-1+ intraepithelial lymphocyte T cells abrogate oral tolerance. J Immunol 145:2010–2019, 1990.
69. Gearhart PJ, Cebra JJ: Differentiated B lymphocytes: potential to express particular antibody variable and constant regions depends on site of lymphoid tissue and antigen load. J Exp Med 149:216–227, 1979.
70. Gerrard JW, MacKenzie JWA, Goluboff N, et al: Cow's milk allergy: prevalence and manifestations in an unselected series of newborns. Acta Paediatr Scand Suppl 234:1–21, 1973.
71. Glassman MS, Newman LJ, Berezin S, et al: Cow's milk protein sensitivity during infancy in patients with inflammatory bowel disease. Am J Gastroenterol 85:838–840, 1990.
72. Goldman AS, Anderson DW, Sellers WA, et al: Milk allergy I: oral challenge with milk and isolated milk proteins in allergic children. Pediatrics 32:425–443, 1963.
73. Gray I, Harten M, Walzer M: Studies in mucous membrane hypersensitiveness. IV: the allergic reaction in the passively sensitized mucous membranes of the ileum and colon in humans. Ann Intern Med 13:2050–2056, 1940.
74. Gray I, Walzer M: Studies in absorption of undigested protein in human beings. VIII: absorption from the rectum and a comparative study of absorption following oral, duodenal, and rectal administrations. J Allergy 11:245–250, 1940.
75. Grulee CG, Sanford HN: The influence of breast feeding and artificial feeding in infantile eczema. J Pediatr 9:223–225, 1936.
76. Gruskay FL: Comparison of breast, cow and soy feedings in the prevention of onset of allergic disease. Clin Pediatr 21:486–491, 1982.
77. Guillet G, Guillet MH: Natural history of sensitizations in atopic dermatitis. Arch Dermatol 128:187–192, 1992.
78. Halpin TC, Byrne WJ, Ament ME: Colitis, persistent diarrhea, and soy protein intolerance. J Pediatr 91:404–407, 1977.
79. Halstensen TS, Scott H, Brandtzaeg P: Human intraepithelial T lymphocytes are mainly CD45Ra-RB+ and show increased co-expression of CD45RO in coeliac disease. Eur J Immunol 20:1825–1830, 1990.
80. Hanson DG: Ontogeny of orally induced tolerance to soluble proteins in mice; priming and tolerance in newborn. J Immunol 127:1518–1524, 1981.
81. Heiner DC, Sears JW, Knicker WT: Multiple precipitins to cow's milk in chronic respiratory disease. Am J Dis Child 103:634–654, 1962.
82. Herian AM, Bush RK, Taylor SL: Protein and allergen content of commercial skin test extracts for soybeans. Clin Exp Allergy 22:461–468, 1992.
83. Heyman M, Grasset E, Ducroc R, et al: Antigen absorption by the jejunal epithelium of children with cow's milk allergy. Pediatr Res 24:197–202, 1988.
84. Hide DW, Guyer BM: Cow milk intolerance in Isle of Wright infants. Br J Clin Pract 37:285–287, 1983.
85. Hide DW, Guyer BM: Clinical manifestations of allergy related to breast- and cow's milk–feeding. Pediatrics 76:973–975, 1985.
86. Hill DJ, Ball G, Hosking CS: Clinical manifestations of cow's milk allergy in childhood I: Associations with in-vitro cellular immune responses. Clin Allergy 18:469–479, 1988.
87. Hill DJ, Bannister DG, Hosking CS, et al: Cow milk allergy within the spectrum of atopic disorders. Clin Exp Allergy 24:1137–1143, 1994.
88. Hill DJ, Firer MA, Ball G, et al: Recovery from milk allergy in early childhood: antibody study. J Pediatr 114:761–766, 1989.
89. Hill DJ, Firer MA, Shelton MJ, et al: Manifestations of milk allergy in infancy: clinical and immunological findings. J Pediatr 109:270–276, 1986.
90. Hill SM, Milla PJ: Colitis caused by food allergy in infants. Arch Dis Child 65:132–133, 1990.
91. Hoffman DR, Collins-Williams C: Cold-pressed peanut oils may contain peanut allergen. J Allergy Clin Immunol 93:801–802, 1994.
92. Host A, Halken S: A prospective study of cow milk allergy in Danish infants during the first 3 years of life. Allergy 45:587–596, 1990.
93. Hoyne GF, O'Hehir RE, Wraith DC, et al: Inhibition of T cell and antibody response to house dust mite allergen by inhalation of the dominant T cell epitope in naive and sensitized mice. J Exp Med 178:1783–1788, 1993.
94. Hsieh LS, Moos M, Lin Y: The study of apple allergens [abstract]. J Allergy Clin Immunol 95:328, 1995.
95. Husby S, Foged N, Host A, et al: Passage of dietary antigens into the blood of children with coeliac disease: quantification and size distribution of absorbed antigens. Gut 28:1062–1072, 1987.
96. Hyman PE, Clarke DD, Everett SL, et al: Gastric acid secretory function in pre-term infants. J Pediatr 106:467–471, 1985.
97. Isolauri E, Suomalainen H, Kaila M, et al: Local immune response in patients with cow milk allergy: follow-up of patients retaining allergy or becoming tolerant. J Pediatr 120:9–15, 1992.
98. Isolauri E, Virtanen E, Jalonen T, et al: Local immune response measured in blood lymphocytes reflects the clinical reactivity of children with cow's milk allergy. Pediatr Res 28:582–586, 1990.
99. Jackson PG, Lessof MH, Baker RWR, et al: Intestinal permeability in patients with eczema and food allergy. Lancet 1:1285–1286, 1981.
100. Jakobsson I, Lindberg T: A prospective study of cow's milk protein intolerance in Swedish infants. Acta Pediatr Scand 68:853–859, 1979.
101. James JM, Bernhisel-Broadbent J, Sampson HA: Respiratory reactions provoked by double-blind food challenges in children. Am J Respir Crit Care Med 149:59–64, 1994.
102. James JM, Burks AW, Roberson PK, et al: Safe administration of measles vaccines to egg-allergic patients. N Engl J Med 332:1262–1266, 1995.
103. James JM, Cooke SK, Barnett A, et al: Anaphylactic reactions to a psyllium-containing cereal. J Allergy Clin Immunol 88:402–408, 1991.
104. James JM, Eigenmann PA, Eggleston PA, et al: Airway reactivity changes in food-allergic, asthmatic children undergoing double-blind placebo-controlled food challenges. Am J Respir Crit Care Med 153:597–603, 1996.
105. James JM, Sampson HA: Immunologic changes associated with the development of tolerance in children with cow milk allergy. J Pediatr 121:371–377, 1992.
106. Jones SM, Magnolfi CF, Cooke SK, Sampson HA: Immunologic cross-reactivity among cereal grains and grasses in children with food hypersensitivity. J Allergy Clin Immunol 96:341–351, 1995.
107. Jordan-Wagner DL, Whisman BA, Goetz DW: Cross-allerginicity among celery, cucumber, carrot, and watermelon. Ann Allergy 71:70–79, 1993.
108. Kaetzel CS, Robinson JK, Lamm ME: Epithelial transcytosis of monomeric IgE and IgG cross-linked through antigen to polymeric IgA: a role for monomeric antibodies in the mucosal immune system. J Immunol 152:72–76, 1994.
109. Kagnoff MF: Immunology of the intestinal tract [review]. Gastroenterology 105:1275–1280, 1993.
110. Kato I, Schrode J, Kohr WJ, et al: Chicken ovomucoid: determination of its amino acid sequence, determination of the trypsin reactive site, and preparation of all three of its domains. Biochemistry 26:193–201, 1987.
111. Katz AJ, Twarog FJ, Zeiger RS, et al: Milk-sensitive and eosinophilic gastroenteropathy: similar clinical features with contrasting mechanisms and clinical course. J Allergy Clin Immunol 74:72–78, 1984.
112. Kelly KJ, Lazenby AJ, Rowe PC, et al: Eosinophilic esophagitis attributed to gastroesophageal reflux: improvement with an amino-acid based formula. Gastroenterology 109:1503–1512, 1995.
113. Kelso JM, Sampson HA: Food protein-induced enterocolitis to casein hydrolysate formulas. J Allergy Clin Immunol 92:909–910, 1993.
114. Kemp A, Van Asperen P, Mukhi A. Measles immunization in children with clinical reactions to egg protein. Am J Dis Child 144:33–35, 1990.
115. Kidd JM III, Cohen SH, Sosman AJ, et al: Food-dependent exercise-induced anaphylaxis. J Allergy Clin Immunol 71:407–411, 1983.
116. Kilshaw PJ, Cant AJ: The passage of maternal dietary proteins into human breast milk. Int Arch Allergy Appl Immunol 75:8–15, 1984.

117. Kivity S, Dunner K, Marian Y: The pattern of food hypersensitivity in patients with onset after 10 years of age. Clin Exp Allergy 24:19–22, 1994.
118. Klomannskog S, Haneberg B: Immunoglobulin E in feces from children with allergy: evidence of local production of IgE in the gut. Int Arch Allergy Appl Immunol 76:133–137, 1985.
119. Kondo N, Agata H, Fukutomi O, et al: Lymphocyte response to food antigens in patients with atopic dermatitis who are sensitive to food. J Allergy Clin Immunol 86:253–260, 1990.
120. Kondo N, Fukutomi O, Agata H, et al: The role of T lymphocytes in patients with food-sensitive atopic dermatitis. J Allergy Clin Immunol 91:658–668, 1993.
121. Lake AM, Bloch KJ, Sinclair KJ, et al: Anaphylactic release of intestinal goblet cell mucus. Immunology 39:173–178, 1980.
122. Lake AM, Whitington PF, Hamilton SR: Dietary protein-induced colitis in breast-fed infants. J Pediatr 101:906–910, 1982.
123. Lebenthal E, Lee PC: Development of functional responses in human exocrine pancreas. Pediatrics 66:556–560, 1980.
124. Lee SK, Kniker WT, Cook CD, et al: Cow's milk–induced pulmonary disease in children. Adv Pediatr 25:39–57, 1978.
125. Lichtenstein LM, Creticos PS, Norman PS, et al: Initial clinical experience with T cell epitope defined peptides from ragweed allergen *Amb a* 1 [abstract]. J Allergy Clin Immunol 95:390, 1995.
126. Lin RY, Shen HD, Han SH: Identification and characterization of a 30 kd major allergen from *Parapenaeus fissurus*. J Allergy Clin Immunol 92:837–845, 1993.
127. Lindfors A, Enocksson E: Development of atopic disease after early administration of cow milk formula. Allergy 43:11–16, 1988.
128. Liu HY, Whitehouse WM, Giday Z: Proximal small bowel transit pattern in patients with malabsorption induced by bovine milk protein ingestion. Radiology 115:415–420, 1975.
129. M'Raihi L, Charpin D, Pons A, et al: Cross-reactivity between latex and banana. J Allergy Clin Immunol 87:129–130, 1991.
130. Martini MC, Lerebours EC, Lin WJ, et al: Strains and species of lactic acid bacteria in fermented milks (yogurts): effect on in vivo lactose digestion. Am J Clin Nutr 54:1041–1046, 1991.
131. Maulitz RM, Pratt DS, Schocket AL: Exercise-induced anaphylactic reaction to shellfish. J Allergy Clin Immunol 63:433–434, 1979.
132. May CD: Objective clinical and laboratory studies of immediate hypersensitivity reactions to food in asthmatic children. J Allergy Clin Immunol 58:500–515, 1976.
133. May CD, Alberto R: In-vitro response of leucocytes to food proteins in allergic and normal children: lymphocyte stimulation and histamine release. Clin Allergy 2:335–344, 1972.
134. McDonald PJ, Goldblum RM, Van Sickle GJ, et al: Food protein-induced enterocolitis: altered antibody response to ingested antigen. Pediatr Res 18:751–755, 1984.
135. Melamed D, Friedman A: Direct evidence for anergy in T lymphocytes tolerized by oral administration of ovalbumin. Eur J Immunol 23:935–942, 1993.
136. Miller HR, Woodbury RG, Huntley JF, et al: Systemic release of mucosal mast-cell protease in primed rats challenged with *Nippostrongylus brasiliensis*. Immunology 49:471–479, 1983.
137. Moro E: Kuhmilchpräzipitine im Serum eines 4 1/2 Monate alten Atrophikern. Muench Med Wochenschr 53:214, 1906.
138. Mowat AM: Depletion of suppressor T cells by 2′-deoxyguanosine abrogates tolerance in mice fed ovalbumin and permits the induction of intestinal delayed-type hypersensitivity. Immunology 58:179–184, 1986.
139. Mowat AM, Strobel S, Drummond HE, et al: Immunological responses to fed protein antigens in mice I: reversal of oral tolerance to ovalbumin by cyclophosphamide. Immunology 45:105–113, 1982.
140. Mowat AM: The regulation of immune responses to dietary protein antigens. Immunol Today 8:93–98, 1987.
141. Mueller HL, Weiss RJ, O'Leary D, et al: The incidence of milk sensitivity and the development of allergy in infants. N Engl J Med 268:1220–1224, 1963.
142. Mühlemann RJ, Wüthrich B: Nahrungsmittelallergien 1983–1987. Schweiz Med Wochenschr 121:1696–1700, 1991.
143. Naylor AR: Eosinophilic gastroenteritis. Scott Med J 35:163–165, 1990.
144. Niestijl Jansen JJ, Kardinaal AFM, Huijbers GH, et al: Prevalence of food allergy and intolerance in the adult Dutch population. J Allergy Clin Immunol 93:446–456, 1994.
145. Nolte H, Schiotz PO, Kruse A, et al: Comparison of intestinal mast cell and basophil histamine release in children with food allergic reactions. Allergy 44:554–565, 1989.
146. Norman PS, Ohman JL, Long AA, et al: Follow on study of the first clinical trial with T cell defined peptides from cat allergen *Fel d* 1 [abstract]. J Allergy Clin Immunol 95:259, 1995.
147. Novembre E, de Martino M, Vierucci A: Foods and respiratory allergy. J Allergy Clin Immunol 81:1059–1065, 1988.
148. O'Hehir RE, Busch R, Rothbard JB, et al: An in vitro model of peptide-mediated immunomodulation of the human T cell response to *Dermatophagoides* spp (house dust mite). J Allergy Clin Immunol 87:1120–1127, 1991.
149. Oehling A, Cagnani CEB: Food allergy and child asthma. Allergol Immunopathol 8:7–14, 1980.
150. Ogawa T, Bando N, Tsuji H, et al: Investigation of the IgE-binding proteins in soybeans by immunoblotting with the sera of the soybean-sensitive patients with atopic dermatitis. J Nutr Sci Vitaminol (Tokyo) 37:555–565, 1991.
151. Onorato J, Merland N, Terral C, et al: Placebo-controlled double-blind food challenge in asthma. J Allergy Clin Immunol 78:1139–1146, 1986.
152. Oppenheimer JJ, Nelson HS, Bock SA, et al: Treatment of peanut allergy with rush immunotherapy. J Allergy Clin Immunol 90:256–262, 1992.
153. Ortolani C, Ispano M, Pastorello E, et al: The oral allergy syndrome. Ann Allergy 61:47–52, 1988.
154. Ortolani C, Ispano M, Pastorello EA, et al: Comparison of results of skin prick tests (with fresh foods and commercial food extracts) and RAST in 100 patients with oral allergy syndrome. J Allergy Clin Immunol 83:683–690, 1989.
155. Paganelli R, Levinsky RJ, Brostoff J, et al: Immune complexes containing food proteins in normal and atopic subjects after oral challenge and effect of sodium cromoglycate on antigen absorption. Lancet 1:1270–1272, 1979.
156. Paganelli R, Matricardi PM, Aiuti F: Interactions of food antigens, antibodies, and antigen-antibody complexes in health and disease. Clin Rev Allergy 2:69–74, 1984.
157. Panush RS: Food induced ("allergic") arthritis: clinical and serologic studies. J Rheumatol 17:291–294, 1990.
158. Pearson M, Teahon K, Levi AJ, et al: Food intolerance and Crohn's disease. Gut 34:783–787, 1993.
159. Peatfield RC, Glover V, Littlewood JT, et al: The prevalence of diet-induced migraine. Cephalalgia 4:179–183, 1984.
160. Perdue MH, Gall DG: Transport abnormalities during intestinal anaphylaxis in the rat: effect of antiallergic agents. J Allergy Clin Immunol 76:498–503, 1985.
161. Perdue MH, Gall DG: Intestinal anaphylaxis in the rat: jejunal response to in vitro antigen exposure. Am J Physiol 250:G427–G431, 1986.
162. Perkkiö M: Immunohistochemical study of intestinal biopsies from children with atopic eczema due to food allergy. Allergy 35:573–580, 1980.
163. Picker LJ, Martin RJ, Trumble A, et al: Differential expression of lymphocyte homing receptors by human memory/effector T cells in pulmonary versus cutaneous immune effector sites. Eur J Immunol 24:1269–1277, 1994.
164. Pike MG, Heddle RJ, Boulton P, et al: Increased intestinal permeability in atopic eczema. J Invest Dermatol 86:101–104, 1986.
165. Piness G, Miller H: Allergic manifestations in infancy and childhood. Arch Pediatr 42:557–562, 1925.
166. Poley JR: Loss of the glycocalyx of enterocytes in small intestine: a feature detected by scanning electron microscopy in children with gastrointestinal intolerance to dietary protein. J Pediatr Gastroenterol Nutr 7:386–394, 1988.
167. Powell GK: Enterocolitis in low-birth-weight infants associated with milk and soy protein intolerance. J Pediatr 88:840–844, 1976.
168. Powell GK: Milk- and soy-induced enterocolitis of infancy. J Pediatr 93:553–560, 1978.
169. Powell GK, McDonald PJ, Van Sickle GJ, et al: Absorption of food protein antigen in infants with food protein-induced enterocolitis. Dig Dis Sci 34:781–788, 1989.
170. Prausnitz C, Küstner H: Studies on supersensitivity. Centrabl Bakteriol 86:160–169, 1921.
171. Ramsdel F, Fowlkes BJ: Clonal deletion versus clonal anergy: the role of the thymus in inducing self tolerance. Science 248:1342–1348, 1990.
172. Reimann HJ, Lewin J: Gastric mucosal reactions in patients with food allergy. Am J Gastroenterol 83:1212–1219, 1988.

173. Robertson DM, Paganelli R, Dinwiddie R, et al: Milk antigen absorption on the preterm and term neonate. Arch Dis Child 57:369–372, 1982.
174. Roesler TA, Barry PC, Bock SA: Factious food allergy and failure to thrive. Arch Pediatr Adolesc Med 148:1150–1155, 1994.
175. Rosekrans PCM, Meijer CJLM, Cornelisse CJ, et al: Use of morphometry and immunohistochemistry of small intestinal biopsy specimens in the diagnosis of food allergy. J Clin Pathol 33:125–130, 1980.
176. Rowe AH: Roentgen studies of patients with gastro-intestinal food allergy. JAMA 100:394–400, 1933.
177. Sampson HA: Immediate hypersensitivity reactions to foods: blinded food challenges in children with atopic dermatitis. Ann Allergy 57:209–212, 1986.
178. Sampson HA: The role of food allergy and mediator release in atopic dermatitis. J Allergy Clin Immunol 81:635–645, 1988.
179. Sampson HA: Immunologically mediated food allergy: the importance of food challenge procedures. Ann Allergy 60:262–269, 1988.
180. Sampson HA: Infantile colic and food allergy: fact or fiction? J Pediatr 115:583–584, 1989.
181. Sampson HA: Peanut anaphylaxis. J Allergy Clin Immunol 86:1–3, 1990.
182. Sampson HA: Food allergy and the role of immunotherapy. J Allergy Clin Immunol 90:151–152, 1992.
183. Sampson HA: Food antigen-induced lymphocyte proliferation in children with atopic dermatitis and food hypersensitivity [editorial]. J Allergy Clin Immunol 91:549–550, 1993.
184. Sampson HA: *In vitro* diagnosis and mediator assays for food allergies. Allergy Proc 14:259–261, 1993.
185. Sampson HA: Adverse reactions to foods. In Middleton EJ, Reed CE, Ellis EF, et al (eds): Allergy: Principles and Practice, 4th edition. CV Mosby, St Louis, 1993, p 1661.
186. Sampson HA, Albergo R: Comparison of results of skin tests, RAST, and double-blind, placebo-controlled food challenges in children with atopic dermatitis. J Allergy Clin Immunol 74:26–33, 1984.
187. Sampson HA, Broadbent KR, Bernhisel-Broadbent J: Spontaneous release of histamine from basophils and histamine-releasing factor in patients with atopic dermatitis and food hypersensitivity. N Engl J Med 321:228–232, 1989.
188. Sampson HA, James JM: Respiratory reactions induced by food challenges in children with atopic dermatitis. Pediatr Allergy Immunol 3:195–200, 1992.
189. Sampson HA, Jolie PL: Increased plasma histamine concentrations after food challenges in children with atopic dermatitis. N Engl J Med 311:372–376, 1984.
190. Sampson HA, Mendelson LM, Rosen JP: Fatal and near-fatal anaphylactic reactions to food in children and adolescents. N Engl J Med 327:380–384, 1992.
191. Sampson HA, Scanlon SM: Natural history of food hypersensitivity in children with atopic dermatitis. J Pediatr 115:23–27, 1989.
192. Sanders ME: Summary of conclusions from a consensus panel of experts on health attributes of lactic cultures: significance to fluid milk products containing cultures. J Dairy Sci 76:1819–1828, 1993.
193. Saylor JD, Bahna SL: Anaphylaxis to casein hydrolysate formula. J Pediatr 118:71–74, 1991.
194. Scheinmann P, Gendrel D, Charlas J, et al: Value of lymphoblast transformation test in cow's milk protein intestinal intolerance. Clin Allergy 6:515–521, 1976.
195. Schrander JJP, van den Bogart JPH, Forget PP, et al: Cow's milk protein intolerance in infants under 1 year of age: a prospective epidemiological study. Eur J Pediatr 152:640–644, 1993.
196. Scott H, Ek J, Havnen J, et al: Serum antibodies to dietary antigens: a prospective study of the diagnostic usefulness in celiac disease of children. J Pediatr Gastroenterol Nutr 11:215–220, 1990.
197. Scott H, Halstensen TS, Brandtzaeg P: The immune system of the gastrointestinal tract. Pediatr Allergy Immunol 4(suppl 3):7–15, 1993.
198. Selbekk BH, Aas K, Myren J: In vitro sensitization and mast cell degranulation in human jejunal mucosa. Scand J Gastroenterol 13:87–92, 1978.
199. Shimojo N, Katsuki T, Coligan JE, et al: Identification of the disease-related T cell epitope of ovalbumin and epitope-targeted T cell inactivation in egg allergy. Int Arch Allergy Appl Immunol 105:155–161, 1994.
200. Shub MD, Pang KY, Swann DA, et al: Age-related changes in chemical composition and physical properties of mucus glycoproteins from rat small intestine. Biochem J 215:405–411, 1983.
201. Sikora K, Anand BS, Truelove SC, et al: Stimulation of lymphocytes from patients with coeliac disease by a subfraction of gluten. Lancet 2:389–391, 1976.
202. Sloan AE, Powers ME: A perspective on popular perceptions of adverse reactions to foods. J Allergy Clin Immunol 78:127–133, 1986.
203. Sorva R, Mäkinen-Kiljunen S, Juntunen-Backman K: Beta-lactoglobulin secretion in human milk varies widely after cow's milk ingestion in mothers of infants with cow's milk allergy. J Allergy Clin Immunol 93:787–792, 1994.
204. Stafford HA, Polmar SH, Boat TF: Immunologic studies in cow's milk–induced pulmonary hemosiderosis. Pediatr Res 11:898–903, 1977.
205. Stern MS, Pang KY, Walker WA: Food proteins and gut mucosal barrier II: Differential interaction of cow's milk protein with the mucous coat and the surface membrane of adult and immature rat jejunum. Pediatr Res 18:1252–1257, 1984.
206. Strobel S: Mechanisms of mucosal immunology and gastrointestinal damage. Pediatr Allergy Immunol 4(suppl 3):25–32, 1993.
207. Strobel S, Ferguson A: Immune response to fed protein antigens in mice 3: systemic tolerance or priming is related to age at which antigen is first encountered. Pediatr Res 18:588–594, 1984.
208. Teuber SS, Dandekar AM, Uratsu SL, et al: Cloning and sequencing of one of the walnut (*Juglans regia*) food allergens [abstract]. J Allergy Clin Immunol 95:332, 1995.
209. Thomas HC, Ryan CJ, Benjamin IS, et al: The immune response in cirrhotic rats: the induction of tolerance to orally administered protein antigens. Gastroenterology 71:114–117, 1976.
210. Trier JS: Celiac sprue. N Engl J Med 325:1709–1719, 1991.
211. Turner MW, Barnett GE, Strobel S: Mucosal mast cell activation patterns in the rat following repeated feeding of antigen. Clin Exp Allergy 2090:421–427, 1990.
212. Udall JN, Pang K, Fritze L, et al: Development of gastrointestinal mucosal barrier I: the effect of age on intestinal permeability to macromolecules. Pediatr Res 15:241–244, 1981.
213. Van Asperen PP, Kemp AS, Mellis CM: Relationship of diet in the development of atopy in infancy. Clin Allergy 14:525–532, 1984.
214. Van Sickle GJ, Powell GK, McDonald PJ, et al: Milk- and soy protein–induced enterocolitis: evidence for lymphocyte sensitization to specific food proteins. Gastroenterology 88:1915–1921, 1985.
215. Van Spreeuwel JP, Lindeman J, Van Maanen J, et al: Increased numbers of IgE containing cells in gastric and duodenal biopsies: an expression of food allergy secondary to chronic inflammation. J Clin Pathol 37:601–606, 1984.
216. Varjonen E, Savolainen J, Mattila L, et al: IgE-binding components of wheat, rye, barley and oats recognized by immunoblotting analysis with sera from adult atopic dermatitis patients. Clin Exp Allergy 22:481–489, 1994.
217. Volonakis M, Katsarou-Katsari A, Stratigos J: Etiologic factors in childhood chronic urticaria. Ann Allergy 69:61–65, 1992.
218. Wadee AA, Boting LA, Rabson AR: Fruit allergy: demonstration of IgE to a 30 kd protein present in several fruits. J Allergy Clin Immunol 85:801–807, 1990.
219. Walker WA: Pathophysiology of intestinal uptake and absorption of antigens in food allergy. Ann Allergy 59:7–16, 1987.
220. Walzer M: Studies in absorption of undigested proteins in human beings I: a simple direct method of studying the absorption of undigested protein. J Immunol 14:143–174, 1927.
221. Walzer M: Allergy of the abdominal organs. J Lab Clin Med 26:1867–1877, 1941.
222. Waring NP, Daul CB, deShazo RD, et al: Hypersensitivity reactions to ingested crustacea: clinical evaluation and diagnostic studies in shrimp-sensitive individuals. J Allergy Clin Immunol 76:440–445, 1985.
223. Warner JO: Food and behavior: allergy, intolerance or aversion. Pediatr Allergy Immunol 4:112–116, 1993.
224. Weber RW, Vaughan TR: Food and migraine headache. Immunol Allergy Clin North Am 11:831–841, 1991.
225. Yocum MW, Khan DA: Assessment of patients who have experienced anaphylaxis: a 3-year survey. Mayo Clin Proc 69:16–23, 1994.
226. Young E, Stoneham MD, Petruckevitch A, et al: A population study of food intolerance. Lancet 343:1127–1130, 1994.
227. Yunginger JW, Sweeney KG, Sturner WQ, et al: Fatal food-induced anaphylaxis. JAMA 260:1450–1452, 1988.
228. Zeiger RS, Heller S: The development and prediction of atopy in high-

risk children: follow-up at age seven years in a prospective randomized study of combined maternal and infant food allergen avoidance. J Allergy Clin Immunol 95:1179–1190, 1995.
229. Zeiger RS, Heller S, Mellon MH, et al: Effect of combined maternal and infant food-allergen avoidance on development of atopy in early infancy: a randomized study. J Allergy Clin Immunol 84:72–89, 1989.
230. Zwetchkenbaum JF, Skufca R, Nelson HS: An examination of food hypersensitivity as a cause of increased bronchial responsiveness to inhaled methacholine. J Allergy Clin Immunol 88:360–364, 1991.

34 *Anaphylaxis*

STEPHEN I. WASSERMAN

Anaphylaxis has been a clinically recognized entity for millennia. However, it has only been within the past 100 years that a more complete understanding of this disorder has developed. Initial observations by Portier and Richet[26] early in this century led to coining of the term *anaphylaxis,* meant to distinguish an adverse event after experience with a particular material in contrast to prophylaxis. Early in this century, anaphylaxis was increasingly recognized after the use of therapeutic heterologous serum, primarily horse serum, for the treatment of diphtheria. With the advent of penicillin and the antibiotic era, a number of new causes of anaphylaxis were identified. The continued development of new therapeutic and diagnostic materials, environmental agents, foods, and food additives have continued to add to a long list of agents demonstrated to be responsible for the induction of anaphylaxis in humans. Although an exact enumeration is not possible, hundreds of deaths annually and numerous hospitalizations and emergency room visits can be directly attributed to anaphylactic reactions in the United States.

EPIDEMIOLOGY

No specific role for age, race, sex, or occupation has been demonstrated in susceptibility to anaphylaxis except insofar as particular exposure patterns may be due to these variables (e.g., exposure to latex antigen is more likely in medical personnel). General and specific rates of anaphylaxis are difficult to state with certainty. It has been estimated that approximately 1 out of every 2,700 hospitalized patients has suffered from an anaphylactic reaction.[21] This total represents (approximately) 0.5% of Hymenoptera sting episodes, 1 in 10,000 radiographic contrast dye exposures, 1% of exposures to penicillin, 1 in every 5,000 to 25,000 exposures to general anesthetic agents, 1 in every 3,000 to 5,000 hemodialyses, and 1 in every 10,000,000 allergy injections.[21] The case rate for fatal anaphylaxis is even more difficult to discern and has been estimated to be 0.002% for penicillin and 0.001% for Hymenoptera.[20] It is believed that repeated interrupted exposures to antigens enhance the likelihood of an anaphylactic response. Debate continues as to whether atopic individuals are at higher risk of anaphylactic reactions, but once sensitized, atopic individuals (particularly those with asthma) may be more at risk for severe or fatal anaphylaxis.

CLINICAL MANIFESTATIONS AND ETIOLOGY

Anaphylaxis, by definition, is a critically important allergic emergency. It is very often abrupt and potentially fatal. It results from the activation of a variety of potent mediator-generating systems through several different activating cascades. Although many writers use the terms *anaphylactoid* and *anaphylaxis* to differentiate immunochemical mechanisms,[22] these semantic differences are not of relevance to the clinician faced with a patient experiencing anaphylaxis. For this reason, *anaphylaxis* is used in this chapter to reflect the pathophysiologic and clinical manifestations that characterize anaphylaxis, and the mechanisms by which anaphylaxis may be engendered are then discussed.

As a clinical diagnosis, anaphylaxis is manifested as a number of nonspecific findings as well as specific organ changes. Nonspecific events include patient historical information of a "funny" or metallic taste in the mouth as well as a sense of warmth, flushing, and pruritus, particularly in intertriginal areas. Some patients even describe a feeling of impending doom.

More organ-specific changes can be seen in the respiratory, cutaneous, cardiovascular, gastrointestinal, or reproductive tracts. Cutaneous findings range from flushing, particularly of the face and upper chest and accompanied by pruritus, to urticaria and angioedema, especially of the face, mouth parts, and upper airway, which may contribute to respiratory dysfunction. Cutaneous findings in and of themselves are generally not life-threatening, are usually transient, and almost always clear within 24 to 48 hours.

Respiratory effects include obstruction of the upper airway due to laryngeal edema or of the lower airway mimicking asthma. Fatal anaphylaxis is more likely in patients who have underlying asthma, and in a series of fatal anaphylaxis events, more than two thirds of the patients died of respiratory complications.[18] Respiratory manifestations may induce asphyxia, and thus, the early recognition of these changes is essential. Early manifestations may be as mild as a lump in the throat or hoarseness but may quickly progress to the inability to swallow or to handle oral secretions. Tightness in the chest and wheezing are clear manifestations of lower respiratory involvement.

Cardiovascular effects include tachycardia, atrial and ventricular dysrhythmias, and cardiovascular collapse.[10] In many instances, it is difficult to differentiate cardiovascular collapse as a primary cardiac event from secondary manifestations due to hypotension or hypoxia. Hypotensive manifestations may occur because of primary cardiac pump failure[27] or, more frequently, from profound third space fluid losses associated with hemoconcentration and intravascular volume depletion.[4] Myocardial infarction may occur as a manifestation of anaphylaxis or as a consequence of its treatment, and approximately a quarter of patients dying of anaphylaxis do so because of cardiovascular manifestations.[7]

Gastrointestinal manifestations of anaphylaxis include cramping, nausea, vomiting, and diarrhea, which may be bloody. It has been stated that food-induced anaphylaxis is more likely to include these gastrointestinal manifestations, but proof of this opinion is lacking. Cramping of other hollow organs, such as the uterus, may also complicate anaphylactic reactions.

Additional manifestations of anaphylaxis are rhinorrhea, nasal and palatal pruritus, conjunctival injection, and diaphoresis. Hypotension may lead to cardiac dysrhythmia and/or hypoxia, disorientation, incontinence, and loss of consciousness. Death has been documented to occur within a few minutes[13] but may be delayed and occur days to weeks later as a consequence of cardiovascular or central nervous system (CNS) insults incurred at the time of initial hypotension and/or hypoxia. The more severe the reaction, the earlier its manifestations are likely to be apparent, although slowly developing anaphylaxis should not be ignored. A biphasic expression of anaphylaxis, similar to the biphasic response in the airway due to inhaled antigen, has been reported, although its frequency is debated.[8, 33] These manifestations may represent a true biphasic event or may be due to delayed absorption of antigen or to treatment whose effect is transient, permitting recrudescence of symptoms.

MECHANISMS OF ANAPHYLAXIS

The mechanisms of anaphylaxis are listed in Table 34–1.

TABLE 34–1
MECHANISMS OF ANAPHYLAXIS

I	IgE mediated
II	Immune complex mediated
III	Abnormalities of arachidonic acid metabolism
IV	Direct degranulation of mast cells and basophils
V	Idiopathic

IMMUNOGLOBULIN E–MEDIATED ANAPHYLAXIS

The classic descriptions of anaphylaxis and most of the research in this area have focused on immunoglobulin IgE-mediated mechanisms of its induction. IgE-mediated anaphylaxis may occur in patients known to have an atopic diathesis or in isolation in otherwise nonatopic individuals. Such processes are thought to be central to the expression of anaphylaxis to foods, many drugs and antibiotics, preservatives, proteins, and foreign sera, Hymenoptera venoms, and allergen immunotherapy. The list of materials that have been demonstrated to cause IgE-mediated anaphylaxis is virtually endless.

Because of their frequent use and intense study, penicillin and its congeners as well as the cephalosporins have been best studied and most commonly implicated as causes of anaphylaxis. Cross-reactivity between penicillin and first-generation cephalosporins is a matter of some debate, and its rate has been reported to range as high as 30%, although most workers believe that less than 10% true cross-reactivity exists[1] and that it is even lower with second- and third-generation cephalosporins.[23] Antibodies to both the major and minor determinants of penicillin exist, although antibodies to the minor determinant mixture seem most predictive of severe anaphylactic sensitivity to penicillin.[16] Antibiotic allergy outside the penicillin/cephalosporin family has been less well studied and is much more difficult both to diagnose and to understand. Anaphylactic reactions to antibiotics are said to be less common and less severe when the materials are administered by the oral route; however, every route imaginable has been implicated in anaphylactic episodes.

Foreign proteins, initially horse serum and later many other therapeutic proteins, have been demonstrated to cause IgE-mediated anaphylaxis. Venom of hymenopterans, including fire ants, enzymes such as chymopapain, and free latex as a contaminant of gloves and appliances used in medical devices have also been demonstrated to be important inducers of IgE-mediated anaphylaxis.

Many foods have been demonstrated to be responsible for causing IgE-mediated anaphylaxis. Most important are peanuts, followed by eggs, milk, tree nuts, and shellfish.[29] However, nearly every food has been demonstrated to induce anaphylaxis on occasion. Foods that cross-react with latex, such as chestnut, avocado, kiwi, and banana, have also been demonstrated to be important inducers of anaphylaxis in latex-sensitive individuals.[2, 19] Various other drugs, both therapeutic and diagnostic agents, have also been shown to induce IgE-mediated anaphylaxis. They include anesthetic agents, muscle relaxants, some synthetic hormones, medicinal fillers, and sterilizing agents. For example, ethylene oxide, which is used to sterilize dialysis membranes, has been shown to induce anaphylaxis in patients undergoing dialysis. Another important cause of IgE-mediated anaphylaxis is therapeutic immunotherapy injections. Anaphylactic reactions to injections are thought to occur as a serious problem in relatively few patients. However, a substantial number of patients undergoing hymenopteran immunotherapy have been reported to suffer anaphylactic reactions during the buildup period of their treatment.

An interesting group of patients with exercise-induced anaphylaxis has been identified.[12] Many of these individuals experience their anaphylactic episodes upon exercise only after eating, and some, only after eating a specific food. In those individuals who experience anaphylaxis after exercise and eating a specific food, an IgE-mediated food sensitivity (e.g., to shellfish, celery) has been identified.[13]

IMMUNE COMPLEX–MEDIATED ANAPHYLAXIS

Reactions to blood and blood products, such as immunoglobulins, plasma, and other fractionated serum constituents that contain IgA, have been demonstrated to be due to antibody to IgA. On rare occasions, reactions to blood products may be due to IgE antibody to IgA,[3] but the currently accepted explanation for most such reactions is host IgG directed against IgA antibody.[38] Immunoglobulin G binds to the transfused IgA and activates complement, thereby inducing generation and release of mediators. In the past, aggregated IgG in various immunoglobulin preparations was also implicated in such complement activation. Complement activation has also been demonstrated to occur in serum upon the addition of a radiocontrast medium, although the participation of this process in the adverse reactions to contrast media is uncertain. Finally, first use syndrome in patients undergoing dialysis may in some instances be due to contact activation of the complement system.[37]

ALTERED ARACHIDONIC ACID METABOLISM

Sensitivity to aspirin and other nonsteroidal anti-inflammatory drugs (NSAIDs) is generally separable from anaphylaxis, but those episodes that are severe or include urticaria may be difficult to distinguish from it. In general, reactions to NSAIDs occur and progress more slowly than classic anaphylaxis. In addition, reactions tend to be restricted to the respiratory tract, to manifest primarily as profuse rhinorrhea, nasal obstruction, and asthma, and to occur most commonly in patients with pre-existing rhinitis and asthma.[5] In some patients, however, rapidly progressive and severe reactions, including collapse, may occur upon the ingestion of NSAIDs. The common theme shared by these drugs is the ability to inhibit the cyclooxygenase enzymes COX 1 and COX 2, and these drugs' relative potency in inducing the syndrome appears related to their potency in inhibiting prostaglandin synthesis. Individuals with this syndrome produce excessive amounts of sulfidopeptide leukotrienes and do so especially in the presence of NSAIDs.[14] It is unclear whether these potent leukotriene mediators are responsible for the syndrome or are merely markers. In NSAID-induced asthma, however, leukotriene inhibitors have proved beneficial, suggesting the direct participation of these mediators in the clinical syndrome.[6]

DIRECT MAST CELL DEGRANULATION

In the absence of identifiable antibodies, opiates, highly cationic antibiotics, some muscle relaxants, some agents used as plasma volume expanders, and radiocontrast media have all been demonstrated to release histamine into the plasma and/or urine, suggesting their ability to directly degranulate mast cells. This ability has been demonstrated for opiates and radiocontrast media in a variety of model systems. Because these agents directly degranulate mast cells, prior sensitization is not required. For example, reactions to radiocontrast media may occur in up to 10% of persons on first exposure (although the majority of these reactions are very difficult to classify). Those patients who have had clear-cut anaphylactic reactions to radiocontrast media have a 20% to 40% risk of subsequent anaphylaxis upon reexposure.[17] Reactions to contrast media are more common when they are given intravenously and when high osmotic strength agents are employed. Allergy to shellfish or iodine does not play a role in these reactions. As previously noted, complement activation as well as histamine release occurs in all individuals receiving contrast media, and the responsible pathogenetic events are uncertain.

IDIOPATHIC ANAPHYLAXIS

A syndrome of recurrent anaphylactic episodes in the absence of identifiable factors is a well-known clinical challenge. In individuals presenting with anaphylaxis, intense evaluation often elucidates a responsible agent and mechanism. However, in a small group of patients, no clear-cut precipitin can be identified, and the term *idiopathic anaphylaxis* is justified. Of patients in this category, approximately half are atopic, and many have recurrent severe episodes of anaphylaxis that may be refractory to commonly used therapy.[24]

PATHOLOGIC CHANGES IN ANAPHYLAXIS

There are no pathognomonic changes that can unequivocally identify anaphylaxis. In many fatal cases of anaphylaxis, however, laryngeal edema, visceral congestion, pulmonary edema, hyperinflation, and intraalveolar hemorrhage as well as the cutaneous findings of urticaria and angioedema are identified. Occasionally, infiltration of the airway and spleen with eosinophils is noted.[13] Pulmonary hyperinflation, accompanied by atelectasis, hemorrhage, and edema, has been found in a significant minority of fatal cases of anaphylaxis. Increased bronchial secretions and vascular congestion with eosinophil infiltration have been reported. Upper airway obstruction due to laryngeal edema is seen in a majority of fatalities, although vascular collapse leaves no footprints. Occasionally, myocardial infarction may be seen, either as a direct effect of anaphylaxis or as a secondary manifestation of hypotension.

In contrast to the anatomic pathology laboratory, the clinical laboratory can be helpful in the evaluation of patients with anaphylaxis. Obviously, airway obstruction can be identified through a variety of pulmonary functional maneuvers, and chest radiographs may demonstrate areas of hyperinflation. In patients manifesting shock, hemoconcentration and elevated hematocrit occur. Defects in coagulation have been reported and are believed to be due to mast cell heparin release or to degradation of coagulation proteins by proteases. Serum enzymes reflective of myocardial injury may be evident in patients suffering this consequence of anaphylaxis. In such cases, electrocardiographic manifestations of infarction are not uncommon. More commonly, however, electrocardiographic manifestations of anaphylaxis include tachyarrhythmias, usually supraventricular, T-wave abnormalities and bundle branch block or other intraventricular conduction delays.[39] Elevations in plasma and urinary histamine and in serum or plasma tryptase have been reported.[30, 32] The latter, because of its exclusive mast cell origin and its half-life of 1 to 2 hours, is a particularly useful marker of anaphylaxis. A variety of complement abnormalities whose significance is uncertain have also been reported.

THE DIAGNOSIS AND DIFFERENTIAL DIAGNOSIS OF ANAPHYLAXIS

The diagnosis of anaphylaxis is usually apparent, because its rapid onset and severe manifestations are rarely overlooked. The presence of flushing, premonitory signs and symptoms of pruritus, and sense of oppression and fear on the part of the patient as well as an associated event such as an ingestion or injection make the diagnosis that much more obvious. The presence of tachycardia, hypotension, upper or lower respiratory obstruction, and other accompanying symptoms, such as abdominal discomfort, vomiting, cramping, urticaria, and angioedema, are all helpful to the astute clinician. Obviously, the setting in which anaphylaxis occurs is often associated with a number of other potential adverse patient outcomes, and the differential diagnosis of syncope, collapse, hypotension, flushing, and other overlapping syndromes is important.

The most common occurrence that mimics anaphylaxis is vasovagal syncope. This syndrome occurs after a stressful, painful event such as an injection, and collapse under these circumstances may be confused with anaphylaxis. In general, the patient suffering vasovagal collapse is pale and cool, notes nausea before fainting, and generally faints in a slow and controlled fashion. Rarely does injury occur during a vasovagal collapse. Patients do not flush or itch and usually do not have respiratory difficulty during a vasovagal episode. Symptoms are rapidly reversed by recumbency. Associated events, including diaphoresis, bradycardia, slow pulse, and generally normal blood pressure, differentiate vasovagal syncope from anaphylaxis. In some patients, hyperventilation after a stressful or painful event may cause breathlessness and fainting. Premonitory signs and symptoms of perioral numbness and tingling may be mentioned. Blood pressure and pulse are generally unaffected.

The cutaneous manifestations of anaphylaxis, urticaria and angioedema, may occur through all of the mechanisms known to induce anaphylaxis, and in fact, anaphylaxis limited to urticaria/angioedema may merely be a semantic differentiation. Flushing disorders, including those due to alcohol ingestion, particularly in persons of Asian background, post/perimenopausal flushing, and the flushing syndromes associated with mastocytosis and carcinoid syndrome, may be confused with anaphylaxis. Angioedema due to hereditary angioedema (see Chapter 35), particularly when it manifests as laryngeal edema, may in rare instances be confused with anaphylaxis. However, the slow onset of this disorder, its hereditary nature, and its lack of urticaria or hypotension should make it clearly separable. In addition, the lack of response of hereditary angioedema to the usual therapeutic interventions is helpful in differentiating it from anaphylactic laryngeal edema. Patients with globus hystericus (lump in the throat) have chronic, persistent, nonprogressive symptoms associated with no anatomic abnormalities in the pharynx or hypopharynx. Serum sickness should in no way be confused with anaphylaxis, because of its delay in onset and its manifestations, primarily of fever, lymphadenopathy, arthralgia, urticaria, and, occasionally, nephritis. Physical urticarias, particularly, severe episodes of cholinergic or cold urticaria, can be mistaken for anaphylaxis. Severe cholinergic urticaria can mimic exercise-induced anaphylaxis, whereas in cold urticaria, collapse following immersion in cold water could also be confusing. These entities may be diagnosed through physical challenges once the patient has recovered. Other causes of acute collapse, including pulmonary embolism, cardiac dysrhythmia, myocardial infarction, cerebral vascular accident, and even unsuspected trauma, must be recognized and differentiated from anaphylactic collapse. Epidemiologic evidence suggests that fatal asthma may occur abruptly upon interaction with antigens and could be considered by some to be anaphylaxis.

The diagnosis and differential diagnosis of anaphylaxis may be supported by in vivo and in vitro tests, including assessment of antigen-specific IgE as well as physical and other environmental challenges. Such challenges include the application of an ice cube to the forearm to identify cold urticaria and having individuals exercise in a warm environment to investigate cholinergic urticaria. Systemic mastocytosis may be identified by a thorough skin examination, skin biopsy, 24-hour urine histamine level, or by other tests such as technetium 99m bone scans (see Chapter 53). The finding of metabolites of serotonin in the urine of patients with carcinoid syndrome may identify this disorder. Obviously, patients who are suspected of suffering from pulmonary embolism, cerebrovascular accident, myocardial infarction, or cardiac dysrhythmia should be investigated by tests appropriate to those entities, including computed tomography, electrocardiography, echocardiography, ventilation/perfusion scanning, and/or pulmonary angiography.

The presence of IgE antibody to specific agents may be identified in allergic patients by in vivo (skin) testing, or by in vitro tests capable of measuring antigen-specific IgE (see Chapter 19). Research technologies have also employed direct antigen induced peripheral blood leukocyte histamine release or have used patient serum to sensitize donor leukocytes to release histamine in the presence of specific antigens. These latter procedures are insensitive, are poorly standardized, and are not recommended for routine evaluation of anaphylaxis. Laboratory identification of mast cell participation in allergic disease (as noted previously) includes the measurement of histamine in plasma or urine and the identification of tryptase in serum following anaphylactic episodes.

Histamine is rapidly metabolized, and its presence in plasma would not be expected long after an anaphylactic episode, whereas tryptase elevations may persist for several hours. Neither measurement is of much use in the diagnosis of an anaphylactic episode 6 or more hours after the event. The laboratory diagnosis of non–IgE-mediated anaphylactic reactions is less clear. The presence of host antibodies to IgA has been demonstrated in some research laboratories investigating patients with blood product associated anaphylactic episodes. Measurements of complement during an acute anaphylactic episode are not readily available, are unlikely to be helpful, and may reflect secondary alterations. The ability of NSAIDs to cause anaphylaxis has generally been investigated through controlled challenge tests that have been reproducible in patients sensitive to these agents. Obviously, patients undergoing such challenges must be closely monitored in controlled settings to preserve pulmonary and cardiovascular function. Direct release of histamine from peripheral blood basophils or cutaneous mast cells has been used to identify some agents capable of inducing anaphylaxis. Opioids cause positive skin test responses in all individuals (as do other agents implicated in direct degranulation). Unfortunately, many of these agents are ineffective in causing leukocyte histamine release, and therefore, only direct skin testing may permit their identification. The tip-off to their ability to cause degranulation in the absence of antibody may come from the response of normal individuals, who do not experience adverse reactions to these agents but do demonstrate positive wheal and flare responses upon their intracutaneous injection.

PATHOGENIC MECHANISMS IN ANAPHYLAXIS

Although the immunopharmacologic pathways responsible for the manifestations of anaphylaxis to some degree depend on the particular cascade initiated by the inciting agent, it appears that the mast cell and its constituent mediators are critically important. Best studied are IgE-mediated processes where IgE bound to high-affinity Fc receptors on mast cells and basophils cross-link on the cell membrane upon interaction with antigen. Cross-linking then transmits signals that eventuate generation and release of mediators (see Chapters 8 and 9). Although many of the antigens capable of activating IgE-mediated processes are peptides, a whole host of other haptens and nonpeptide materials have been implicated, and no common features can be discerned to predict the likelihood of IgE reactivity to any particular agent. Mast cells and basophils are capable of generating mediators that can cause the manifestations of anaphylaxis, including vasoactive-spasmogenic mediators, active enzymes, proteoglycans, and chemoattractant factors. Although some of these mediators may have more relevance to chronic allergic inflammatory states, such as asthma and rhinitis, vasoactive and spasmogenic mediators also appear to be critical to the expression of anaphylaxis.

The presence of histamine in human anaphylactic episodes has been documented (see earlier), and it is clear that injection of histamine into humans can cause a wheal and flare urticarial response, angioedema, flushing, and, at sufficient dose, hypotension and vomiting. This substance can also cause endothelial cell gaps, thereby augmenting permeability, and may be responsible for third space fluid accumulation and airway edema in anaphylactic episodes. Histamine can diminish coronary blood flow and thus could be important in the expression of hypotension and cardiac dysrhythmias. The metallic taste described by some patients experiencing anaphylaxis has been reproduced by the intravenous and intra-arterial injection of histamine in human volunteers. The sulfidopeptide leukotrienes, platelet-activating factor, and adenosine are also capable of causing many of the same manifestations, particularly third space fluid loss, hypotension, and diminished cardiac output, but their direct role in anaphylaxis is less certain.

The coming availability of leukotriene synthesis antagonists and receptor blockers may elucidate the role of arachidonate metabolites in anaphylaxis. Leukotrienes may be generated by a variety of inflammatory cells (i.e., eosinophils, macrophages) in addition to the mast cell and could be secondary sources of such mediators. No direct role for chemoattractant molecules has been postulated in anaphylaxis. Similarly, although the neutral protease tryptase has been a useful marker for identifying anaphylaxis, no credible role for this enzyme or for other mast cell neutral proteases (e.g., chymase) has been identified in anaphylaxis. Similarly, although in the human mast cell, heparin has been implicated in some of the hemostatic defects seen in the patients suffering anaphylaxis, the role of hypotension and important fluid and electrolyte shifts may confound these interpretations. In contrast to the evolving understanding of IgE-mediated anaphylaxis, the ability to elucidate the pathways by which non–IgE-mediated anaphylaxis occurs is virtually nil.

The generation of complement protein fragments C3a and C5a by immune complexes is believed responsible for directly affecting vascular and respiratory smooth muscle and activating mast cells to release histamine, and is assumed to be the mechanism whereby anaphylaxis is engendered during reactions to immune complexes.

MANAGEMENT OF THE PATIENT WITH ANAPHYLAXIS

The clinician's approach to the problem of anaphylaxis is multifaceted. Obviously, treatment of the acute episode requires knowledge of its pathophysiology and the appropriate therapeutic options available. After the acute situation has been controlled, the prevention of future anaphylactic episodes requires understanding of the principles of prevention, identifying causative agents, counseling patients, and educating the community in which they live or work. Finally, the clinician needs to understand strategies useful to prevent anaphylaxis in high-risk patients if encounters with eliciting agents are unavoidable.

TREATMENT OF ACUTE ANAPHYLAXIS

Acute anaphylaxis is the sine qua non of the allergic emergency. Although fatalities may occur within minutes despite the availability of medical therapy, it is clear that the earlier the treatment, the more likely the patient is to survive.[28]

Initial measures require identification of the patency of both the upper and lower airways and assessment of the cardiovascular status, including blood pressure, central and peripheral perfusion, and volume status. Simple measures, such as placing the patient in a recumbent position with the legs elevated, may be all that is needed in mild episodes. Obviously, upper airway obstruction needs to be rapidly assessed and may require early nasotracheal intubation, or, in cases of advanced upper airway edema, tracheostomy. If possible, a patient with upper airway edema seen in an emergent setting should be evaluated by surgeons competent in the performance of tracheostomy well in advance of its potential need. Because of third space losses, fluid resuscitation is generally required for patients with marked hypotension.

In addition to initiation of these nonspecific treatments, the primary drug of choice for treatment of anaphylaxis is epinephrine. For most patients, 0.1 to 0.5 mL of a 1:1,000 solution of epinephrine should be given subcutaneously. For most adults, 0.3 mL is sufficient, and for small children, 0.1 to 0.15 mL may be all that is required. Obviously, in the elderly and in patients with preexisting hypertension or cardiac disease, consideration must be given to using smaller doses in a sequential manner. As tolerated and needed, doses can be repeated at 15- to 30-minute intervals. Intravenous epinephrine should be reserved for patients with failure of response to subcutaneous administration. If intravenous epinephrine is to be used intravenously, it should be diluted 1:10,000 prior to administration. Intravenous epinephrine may increase cardiac oxygen demands, precipitate myocardial infarction, and, particularly in the setting of hypoxia, induce arrhythmias. In addition to epinephrine, antihistaminics have been proven beneficial. They are particularly useful for the less severe symptoms, such as pruritus, flushing, and urticaria. However, some evidence suggests that these agents may also be beneficial in ameliorating refractory hypotension. Intravenous use of a traditional H_1 antihistamine may be supplemented with the use of a H_2 receptor antagonist as well.[40]

The role of glucocorticosteroids in the treatment of acute anaphylaxis remains unclear. Because steroid action is delayed, many authorities advocate using these agents early, so that any beneficial effect would occur as soon as possible. Those who believe that delayed or biphasic anaphylaxis is a major clinical problem advocate steroid use as well. Glucocorticoids may be particularly useful in the patient with severe asthma either as a manifestation of or as a complicating factor in anaphylaxis.

Treatment of asthmatic symptoms with $beta_2$ selective agonists or methylxanthines should be considered as well. For patients continuing to suffer from hypotension, the use of intravenous epinephrine or other presser agents must be considered. Although dopamine has been advocated, norepinephrine is sometimes effective in patients in whom dopamine is ineffective. Treatment of complicating factors such as myocardial infarction, ventricular dysrhythmia, and other organ failure would be directed by the particular manifestation.

A special problem in the treatment of anaphylaxis occurs in patients who are taking beta-blocking agents. In the presence of a beta blocker, epinephrine should still be used, with the recognition that only its alpha action is likely to be effective. For patients taking beta blockers who are suffering severe anaphylaxis despite the use of H_1 and H_2 antagonists and epinephrine, two schools of thought exist as to how to proceed. First, case reports suggest that the use of glucagon, 1 mg intravenously, may overcome beta blockade,[41] although no large studies of this maneuver in anaphylaxis exist. This drug is a positive inotropic agent acting by non–beta receptor means. Second, others suggest the careful intravenous use of combined $beta_1$ and $beta_2$ agonist agents titrated against heart rate and the clinical response. This, too, is an unproven and potentially risky maneuver. Most patients who are treated briskly and thoroughly survive their anaphylactic episode, but there are reports of properly treated individuals who died within hours or even minutes.

Angiotensin-converting enzyme inhibitor drugs, increasingly popular in the treatment of congestive heart failure and hypertension, have also been implicated in the direct induction of cough and angioedema and, in some instances, in exacerbation of anaphylaxis.[37] No modifications in the treatment protocols for anaphylaxis have been suggested for patients taking such agents.

PREVENTION OF ANAPHYLAXIS

Any physician who has had the opportunity to care for a patient experiencing anaphylaxis will appreciate the need for prevention of this emergency. Although nothing can completely eliminate the risk, a number of general principles combined with specific information can be utilized to help patients and their families prevent episodes of anaphylaxis. It is essential for the physician to obtain a complete allergic history and to identify the agents that may have previously caused anaphylaxis in the patient. The physician should be aware of cross-reacting agents and should educate the patient about the sources of cross-reacting materials or hidden sources of the known anaphylactic agent. If possible, the patient should be tested for sensitivity, either in vitro or in vivo, to solidify clinical impressions. Clearly, patients should be asked to eliminate causative antigens from their environment—at home, work, and school, including hobby and play activities. To prevent sensitization, no drugs should be used without clear cause. If feasible, drugs should be administered by the oral route, and patients should be observed for at least half an hour after the administration of medications. These simple procedures, used on a regular basis, should give the greatest degree of protection to patients at risk of anaphylaxis. It is clear that patients may suffer life-threatening or even fatal anaphylaxis as the first manifestation of allergy to a compound, but in many patients, premonitory symptoms indicate sensitization. Eliciting the history of such symptoms may be life-saving.

Three maneuvers are available to the physician in situations in which a sensitized patient must receive an allergen for important diagnostic or therapeutic reasons: desensitization, immunotherapy, and premedication. Desensitization, or the incremental administration of a drug or agent to which the patient is known to be sensitive, has been demonstrated to permit patients to receive life-saving therapeutic agents in the presence of anaphylactic reactivity. The technique requires a clear-cut diagnosis of allergic sensitization, by either skin test or in vitro test, combined with a previous positive history of anaphylactic reaction to the agent. Both skin testing and the administration of allergen through desensitization have risks, and systemic or even fatal reactions may occur. Desensitization has been best demonstrated to be effective with penicillin and other beta-lactam antibiotics[35] but has also been used for NSAIDs.[34] Its mechanism of action is unclear but may be due to a short-term inability of mediator-releasing cells to respond to the antigen. Studies have suggested that oral desensitization, if feasible, is the best and safest route. Unfortunately, desensitization provides protection only for the episode in question, and if repeated courses of an antibiotic or an agent are necessary, repeated desensitization maneuvers are required. Because of its attendant risks, desensitization should be performed in an environment in which emergency medical treatment can be immediately available. It should also be reserved only for the administration of life-saving treatments (e.g., the use of penicillin in a pregnant woman with syphilis or in a patient with acute bacterial endocarditis due to an organism exquisitely sensitive to penicillin). Numerous published protocols exist for desensitization, most achieving desired results over 4 to 8 hours. Aspirin desensitization may prove useful in patients with recurrent severe reactions to this compound and have in some instances proven beneficial in the control of rhinitis and asthma in sensitive patients.[36]

In contrast to the acute, but transient effects of desensitization, immunotherapy has proved useful in providing long-term protection against anaphylactic reactivity, especially in patients sensitive to hymenopterans. In this technique, increasing amounts of antigen are administered over a period of several years, and protection is conferred not acutely, but over a period of months to years. Protection is thought to be due to altered T-cell reactivity, diminished IgE production, and increased production of antigen specific IgG "blocking" antibody. Unfortunately, this technique does not appear to be helpful in control of antibiotic sensitivity, and although it has shown promise in experimental treatment of food allergy, its attendant risks are such that it has not been made available for routine clinical use.

A final option available to the physician for preventing anaphylactic manifestations is to premedicate patients who are known to require exposure to an agent to which they are sensitive. This technique has proved useful in permitting the use of radiocontrast media in patients who have previously experienced reactions to these compounds. When combined with a change to low ionic strength contrast media in such patients, the administration of an H_1 antagonist (50 mg diphenhydramine), a glucocorticoid (50 mg prednisone), and a beta agonist (25 to 50 mg ephedrine) 12 hours, 6 hours, and 1 hour prior to the contrast study, has been demonstrated to markedly diminish the incidence of anaphylaxis.[11] The addition of an H_2 antagonist does not appear to be beneficial in this setting. The use of such a premedication regimen for other agents has not been as well studied and cannot routinely be recommended.

Patients with chronic, recurrent idiopathic anaphylaxis are best managed with a regimen of a regular antihistamine (e.g., hydroxyzine, 50 mg. t.i.d.), an oral sympathomimetic agent (e.g., albuterol, 2 mg t.i.d.), and prednisone. The dosage of prednisone should be 60 to 100 mg per day for 1 week or until control is achieved, then converted to an alternate-day schedule. The prednisone dosage may then be decreased by no more than 5 to 10 mg each month, as tolerated. If symptoms persist, requiring 60 mg prednisone on alternate days or 20 mg per day, cromolyn sodium (Gastrocrom) or ketotifen (not available in the United States) may be tried.[25]

Obviously, for all patients known to be anaphylactically sensitive, strict instructions as to how best avoid the allergen(s) to which they are sensitive must be given. They include education about the various forms that these antigens and cross-reacting compounds may take, about the lifestyles of the insects to which they may be sensitive, and to the various unsuspected sources of food antigens likely to be encountered. Anaphylactically sensitive persons should carry medical information at all times, such as in a bracelet or in a laminated card in a wallet or purse. Various immunizations should be kept up to date, so that use of heterologous antiserum is not necessary, and such patients should avoid treatment with beta-adrenergic blocking drugs, if at all possible. Some authorities advocate avoiding angiotensin-converting enzyme inhibitors and calcium channel-blocking agents as well. Finally, anaphylactically sensitive patients should carry, at all times, a preloaded syringe of epinephrine.

OUTLOOK FOR PATIENTS WITH ANAPHYLAXIS

Nearly all patients suffering acute anaphylaxis will survive if appropriate medical therapy is instituted promptly. Recovery is usually quick and complete unless secondary organ damage occurs as a result of hypoxia, hypovolemia, or hypotension. Long-term prognosis in such patients is affected by (1) education to avoid the same or cross-reacting agent(s); (2) the provision of readily usable epinephrine and appropriate instructions; (3) accurate diagnosis of the cause and (when feasible) use of desensitization, immunotherapy or prophylactic therapy.

ANAPHYLAXIS IN SPECIAL CIRCUMSTANCES

Two unique circumstances in which anaphylaxis may occur require special attention of the clinician. Anaphylaxis in the pregnant patient is of particular importance, because two individuals are at risk. A unique clinical event in anaphylaxis of importance in the pregnant patient is uterine cramping, which may mimic impending delivery; however, miscarriage is not a common complication of anaphylaxis. The fall in uterine blood flow that may occur during cardiovascular collapse may be of particular importance to fetal well-being. Other important clinical points in anaphylaxis in the pregnant patient surround the unique medications to which such patients are exposed. Obviously, in most pregnancies, drugs are avoided. However, oxytocin, which may be used to induce labor, has been associated with mast cell degranulation.[15] In addition, many of the drugs and exposures associated with the operating theater (see later) may be used in pregnant patients undergoing surgical procedures such as episiotomy and cesarean section. For the pregnant patient experiencing anaphylaxis, epinephrine remains the treatment of choice, although some obstetricians are concerned about its alpha-adrenergic mediated decrease in uterine blood flow. Therefore, some advocate the use of ephedrine as a first-line treatment, although this is less effective in anaphylaxis than epinephrine.[9] The other agents useful in the treatment of anaphylaxis are also useful in the pregnant patient.

A second unique setting in which anaphylaxis may require special attention of the clinician is the operating room. This is a particularly difficult setting in which to evaluate anaphylaxis, first because patients are often intubated and sedated, and a clear history may be difficult to obtain. Second, patients in this setting are often exposed to a wide variety of agents, including antibiotics, muscle relaxants, opiates, neuromuscular blocking drugs, and latex. In addition, plasma expanders and protamine may be administered in special circumstances. Many of the clinical clues to impending anaphylaxis are not available in the operating room, so the first sign may be hypotension or difficulty in ventilating an unconscious patient. Obviously, in the operating room, management of the airway and blood pressure may be facilitated, because the patient generally has already been intubated and is receiving intravenous fluids. Postoperative analysis of the causative agents may require not only a very careful sifting through the medical records but also evaluation of prior interactions with similar compounds, supplemented by skin testing when available. Highest on the list of suspected agents in this setting would be latex, neuromuscular blocking agents, and antibiotics. Clearly, the history of anaphylaxis during an operative procedure requires full investigation, and if an etiology cannot be identified, it is essential that on subsequent operative interventions, different classes of drugs be chosen to reduce the risk of repeated anaphylaxis. In addition, all medical personnel, particularly the anesthesiologist, must be prepared to intervene should anaphylaxis ensue.

REFERENCES

1. Anderson J: Cross reactivity to cephalosporins in patients allergic to penicillin. Pediatr Infect Dis 5:557, 1986.
2. Blanco C, Carillo T, Castillo R, et al: Avocado hypersensitivity. Allergy 49:454, 1994.
3. Burks AW, Sampson HA, Buckley RH: Anaphylactic reactions after gamma globulin administration in patients with hypogammaglobulinemia: detection of IgE antibodies to IgA. N Engl J Med 314:560, 1986.
4. Carlson RW, Schaeffer RC, Puri VK, et al: Hypovolemia and permeability pulmonary edema associated with anaphylaxis. Crit Care Med 9:883–885, 1981.
5. Chafee FH, Sottipane GA: Aspirin intolerance I: frequency in an allergic population. J Allergy Clin Immunol 53:193, 1974.
6. Christie PE, Smith CM, Lee TH: The potent and selective sulphidopeptide leukotriene antagonist SK&F 104353 inhibits aspirin-induced asthma. Am Rev Respir Dis 144:957, 1991.
7. Delage C, Irey NS: Anaphylactic deaths: a clinicopathologic study of 43 cases. J Forensic Sci 17:525–540, 1972.
8. Douglas DM, Sukenick E, Andrade P, Brown JS: Biphasic systemic anaphylaxis: an inpatient and outpatient study. J Allergy Clin Immunol 93:977–985, 1994.
9. Entman SS, Marse KJ: Anaphylaxis in pregnancy. South Med J 77:402, 1984.
10. Fisher MM: Clinical observation on the pathophysiology and treatment of cardiovascular collapse. Anaesth Intens Care 14:17–21, 1986.
11. Greenberger PA, Patterson R, Rodin RC: Two pretreatment regimens for high-risk patients receiving radiographic contrast media. J Allergy Clin Immunol 74:540, 1984.
12. Horan RF, Sheffer AL: Exercise-induced anaphylaxis. Immunol Allergy Clin North Am 12:559, 1992.
13. James LP, Austen KF: Fatal systemic anaphylaxis in man. N Engl J Med 270:597–603, 1964.
14. Jurgens U, Christiansen SC, Stevenson DD, Zurow BL: Arachidonic acid metabolism in monocytes of aspirin-sensitive asthmatic patients before and after oral aspirin challenge. J Allergy Clin Immunol 90:636, 1992.
15. Kawarabyashi T, Narisawa Y, Nakimura K, et al: Anaphylactoid reactions to oxytocin during caesarian section. Gynecol Obstet Invest 25:277, 1988.
16. Levine BB, Redmond AP: Minor haptenic determinate-specific reagins of penicillin hypersensitivity in man. Int Arch Allergy Appl Immunol 35:445, 1969.
17. Lieberman P: Anaphylactoid reactions to radiocontrast material. Immunol Allergy Clin North Am 12:649, 1992.
18. Lockey RF, Benedict LM, Turkeltaub PC, et al: Fatalities from immunotherapy and skin testing. J Allergy Clin Immunol 79:660, 1987.
19. Makinen-Kiljunen S: Banana allergy in patients with immediate-type hypersensitivity to natural rubber latex. J Allergy Clin Immunol 93:990, 1994.
20. Marquardt DL, Wasserman SI: Anaphylaxis. In Middleton EE, Reed CE, Ellis E, et al (eds): Allergy Principles and Practice, 4th edition. CV Mosby, St Louis, 1993, pp 1525–1536.
21. Metcalfe DD: Acute anaphylaxis and urticaria in children and adults. In Schochet AL (ed): Clinical Management of Urticaria and Anaphylaxis. Marcel Dekker, New York, 1992, pp 70–96.
22. Moneret-Vautrin D-A, Laxenaire M-C: Anaphylactic and anaphylactoid reactions. Clin Rev Allergy 9:249–258, 1991.
23. Neu HD: The new beta-lactamase-stable cephalosporins. Am Intern Med 97:408, 1982.
24. Patterson R, Hogan MB, Yarnold PR, Harris KE: Idiopathic anaphylaxis. Arch Intern Med 155:869, 1995.
25. Patterson R, Stoloff RS, Greenberger PA, et al: Algorithms for the diagnosis and management of idiopathic anaphylaxis. Ann Allergy 71:40, 1993.
26. Portier P, Richet C: De l'action anaphylactique de certains venins. CR Soc Biol (Paris) 54:170, 1902.
27. Raper RF, Fisher MM: Profound reversible myocardial depression after anaphylaxis. Lancet 1:386–388, 1988.
28. Sampson HA, Mendelson L, Rosen JP: Fatal and near fatal anaphylactic reactions to food in children and adolescents. N Engl J Med 327:380, 1992.
29. Sampson HA, Scanlon SM: Natural history of food hypersensitivity in children with atopic dermatitis. J Pediatr 115:23, 1989.
30. Schwartz LB, Yuninger JW, Miller J, et al: Time course of appearance and disappearance of human mast cell tryptase in the circulation after anaphylaxis. J Clin Invest 83:1551, 1989.
31. Silverstein SR, Frommer DA, Dobozin B, et al: Celery-dependent exercise-induced anaphylaxis. J Emerg Med 4:195, 1986.
32. Smith PL, Kagey-Sobotka A, Bleeker ER, et al: Physiologic manifestations of human anaphylaxis. J Clin Invest 66:1072, 1980.
33. Stark BJ, Sullivan TJ: Biphasic and prolonged anaphylaxis. J Allergy Clin Immunol 78:76–83, 1986.
34. Stevenson DD, Pleskow WW, Simon RA, et al: Aspirin-sensitive rhinosinusitis-asthma: a double blind crossover study of treatment with aspirin. J Allergy Clin Immunol 73:500, 1984.
35. Sullivan TJ, Yecies LD, Shatz GS, et al: Desensitization of patients allergic to penicillin using orally administered beta-lactam antibiotics. J Allergy Clin Immunol 69:275, 1982.
36. Sweet JM, Stevenson DD, Simon RA, Mathison DA: Long-term effects of aspirin desensitization: treatment for aspirin-sensitive rhinosinusitis-asthma. J Allergy Clin Immunol 85:59, 1990.
37. Verresen L, Waer M, Vanrenterghem Y, et al: Angiotensin-converting enzyme inhibitors and anaphylactic reactions to high-flux membrane dialysis. Lancet 336:1360, 1990.
38. Vyas GN, Perkins HA, Fudenberg HH: Anaphylactoid transfusion reactions associated with anti-IgA. Lancet 2:312, 1968.
39. Wasserman SI: The heart in anaphylaxis. J Allergy Clin Immunol 87:663, 1986.
40. Yarbrough JA, Moffitt JE, Brown DA, Stafford CT: Cimetidine in the treatment of refractory anaphylaxis. Ann Allergy 63:235, 1989.
41. Zaloga GP, Delacey W, Holmboe E, et al: Glucagon reversal of hypotension in a case of anaphylactic shock. Ann Intern Med 105:65, 1986.

35 Urticaria and Angioedema

ALLEN P. KAPLAN

DEFINITIONS

Urticaria is characterized by the appearance of pruritic, erythematous, cutaneous elevations that blanch with pressure, indicating the presence of dilated blood vessels and edema. In its simplest form, urticaria is envisioned to represent the same sort of wheal-and-flare reaction observed when histamine is injected into the skin. Biopsy of acute urticarial lesions reveals dilation of small venules and capillaries located in the superficial dermis with widening of the dermal papillae, flattening of the rete pegs, and swelling of collagen fibers. *Angioedema* is caused by the same (or similar) pathologic alterations that occur in the deep dermis and subcutaneous tissue. Thus, an area involved with angioedema has swelling as the prominent manifestation, and the appearance of the skin itself may be normal.

Because angioedema occurs in deeper skin layers, where there are fewer mast cells and sensory nerve endings, the lesions have little or no associated pruritus, and the swelling may be described as painful or burning in nature. Urticaria may occur on virtually any part of the body, whereas angioedema (in the absence of hives) often involves the face, tongue, extremities, or genitalia. Unlike other forms of edema, angioedematous swellings do not characteristically occur in dependent areas, are asymmetrically distributed, and are transient.

Of course, urticaria and angioedema can occur together, and often do so; in one series, approximately half the referred patients had both urticaria and angioedema. The incidence of the various types of urticaria and angioedema is unknown and the frequencies seen in clinical practice can vary greatly. Chronic idiopathic urticaria is commonly seen in clinical practice and may account for 75% to 80% of patients seen; the physical urticarias, taken together, compose another 15%, and all the others about 5%.

ACUTE URTICARIA OR ANGIOEDEMA

Acute urticaria or angioedema is a self-limited disorder typically caused by an allergic reaction to a food or drug that lasts from a few days to as long as 6 weeks. Thereafter, the disorder is arbitrarily designated "chronic."

When such a reaction is suspected, food skin testing can be helpful to identify or confirm an immunoglobulin IgE-dependent reaction. Oral provocation testing at this stage is risky, and is best avoided. An IgE-dependent reaction directed against a particular antigen does not, however, prove a pathogenic role, and the observation must be correlated with the history and the patient's experience. Common foods causing acute urticaria (and/or angioedema) are shellfish, nuts (particularly peanuts), eggs, and soft fruits. Patients with food allergies are typically sensitive to one or two foods; thus, the reaction should be relatively obvious and reproducible.

Penicillin allergy is among the most common of the *drug allergies* as well as the best studied. Urticaria may commence any time from minutes after its administration to 10 days later. The reaction is IgE mediated and can be associated with other systemic symptoms, such as wheezing, laryngeal edema, and hypotension (anaphylaxis).

Urticaria or angioedema occurring 10 days to 2 weeks after antibiotic administration may also represent a serum sickness reaction, in which there are circulating immune complexes (usually antigen-IgG), complement fixation, and a small vessel vasculitis with predominantly neutrophilic infiltration. Histamine release can be due to anaphylatoxins (primarily C3a and C5a)[19, 199] and, to a lesser extent, C4a, as well as any IgE antibody present. Serum sickness may be associated with fever, lymphadenopathy, or proteinuria (glomerulonephritis) in addition to urticaria and/or angioedema. Urticaria due to penicillin can result from the penicilloyl major determinant[97] or one of the minor determinants. One must watch out for traces of penicillin contaminating food, drink, or vaccines, although the practice of prophylactically injecting cattle with penicillin and thereby contaminating milk products was abandoned in the United States many years ago.

Penicillins, in general, share the 6-amino penicillinic acid nucleus and cross-react. Cephalosporins, which are derivatives of 6-amino cephalosporanic acids, exhibit cross-reactivity to penicillin of a high degree in vitro, but in practice, cephalosporins cause reactions in about 15% to 20%.[181] The figure is high enough, however, to warrant caution. Aztreonam, a broad-spectrum semisynthetic penicillin derivative, is not cross-reactive,[121] nor is penicillamine, which is used to treat chronic arthritis or cystinuria. Other classes of drugs that commonly cause urticaria or angioedema are sulfonamides, analgesics, sedatives, tranquilizers, diuretics, antiseizure medications, and radiocontrast agents. One should be aware of structural similarities of certain drugs; for example, sulfonylurea-type oral hypoglycemic agents, thiazide diuretics or furosemide, carbonic anhydrase inhibitors, and procaine-type local anesthetics are structurally related to sulfonamides.

Except for penicillin, no routine tests are available that can confirm or refute the diagnosis of drug-induced urticaria (or angioedema), and an empiric approach is indicated. Some progress has been made in defining the allergenicity and immune response in sulfonamide allergy.[140]

Urticaria and angioedema may result from *cytotoxic reactions*, for example, after a blood transfusion. In such a case, the cause is obvious, and the symptoms are self-limited. Occasionally, a patient may have symptoms that recur with a seasonal pattern. One then must regard urticaria or angioedema as a manifestation of some allergen with a seasonal pattern that is either inhaled, ingested, or contacted. There may be associated symptoms of allergic rhinitis or asthma to the same allergen, but it is not known why, in some cases, skin manifestations of these presumably IgE-mediated reactions are evident.[188] In general, inhaled allergens cause respiratory symptoms, whereas ingested allergens cause urticaria, angioedema, or gastrointestinal symptoms. Volatilization of foods, during cooking for example, is a way that foods can produce respiratory symptoms.

Contact urticaria follows contact of an antigen with intact skin. For example, patients extremely sensitive to dogs or cats may have urticaria where they have been licked, or a subject highly sensitive to a food may develop hives on skin contact. Mucosal surfaces may be particularly susceptible to this kind of reaction. Physical urticarias, such as cold urticaria, local heat urticaria, and aquagenic urticaria, are excluded from the usual definition but are a form of contact-induced hives.

Contact urticarial reactions are IgE mediated and therefore depend on mast cell degranulation. Skin tests or radioallergosorbent tests (RASTs) for the offending substance will be positive. The most common history is acute lip swelling after ingestion of fish, eggs, or nuts by atopic subjects. Also, reactions to latex materials (surgical gloves, condoms) have been recognized as a form of contact urticaria,[79] and cross-reactivity of the antigen with certain foods has been noted. These can include bananas, kiwis, and avocados. Nonimmunologic contact urticaria can be caused by agents that penetrate skin and cause pharmacologic mast cell degranulation, such as ammonium persulfate,[106] dimethylsulfoxide,[125] and cinnemaldehyde.[93]

Virtually all of the aforementioned types of urticaria are initiated by an IgE-mediated reaction caused by combination with antigen at the cell membrane surface of the mast cell. The wheal-and-flare reaction seen is due to a combination of vasodilatation and increased vascular permeability caused by secretion of histamine, prostaglandin (PG) D_2, leukotriene C_4, and platelet-activating factor (PAF). Each of these causes a hive-like lesion when injected intradermally, and PAF is the most potent on a molar basis. However, histamine is predominant because the quantities are 100 to 1,000 times more than the other constituents. Histamine also causes the axon reflex by stimulation of sensory unmyelinated type C fibers in the skin, which, en route to the spinal cord, intersect other fibers and by retrograde (antidromic) conduction release substance P from adjacent nerve endings. This vasodilatory flare markedly enlarges the diameter of the erythema far beyond that due to diffusion of histamine.

Substance P can also directly degranulate cutaneous mast cells and further augment the reaction seen. However, it has been observed that during skin testing, the immediate wheal-and-flare reaction may disappear (10 to 15 minutes), to be followed by a local swelling 4 to 6 hours later, known as the late-phase reaction.[33] A mixed cellular infiltrate is seen, consisting of neutrophils, eosinophils, basophils, and mononuclear cells[41, 168] with evidence of protracted release of histamine and other vasoactive substances[139, 154] that is no longer strictly IgE dependent. It may be that mast cell degranulation that persists over time and/or persistence of antigenic stimulation is required to induce this late phase. Persistence of hives in food or drug reactions over days to weeks may be related to this phenomenon. Although antihistamine therapy in high dosage is used to treat acute urticaria or angioedema, the response of severe and/or protracted urticaria/angioedema to corticosteroid therapy may be related to the effects of steroids upon this late-phase response.

Urticaria and angioedema can result from foods or drugs by mechanisms that are not mediated by IgE antibody and may, in fact, not be immunologic. Thus, although allergy to strawberries may be IgE mediated, strawberries contain histamine-releasing substances that can directly cause mast cell degranulation. A small percentage of patients may have urticaria due to aspirin or other nonsteroidal anti-inflammatory drugs (NSAIDs). These reactions are not immunologic,[148] and such patients may also be sensitive to coal tar dye derivatives, such as tartrazine (yellow No. 5), used to color foods and medications. Certainly, when confronted with a patient with a history that suggests sensitivity to a long listing of medications or foods, the clinician should consider the possibility that urticaria is due to sensitivity to an ingredient common to them such as tartrazine. We have found, however, that the longer the list, the less likely any will prove to be correct, particularly when the hives are chronic. Most NSAIDs share the property of being inhibitors of prostaglandin synthetase,[187] and aspirin may directly acetylate and inactivate the enzyme.[144] Other salicylates, such as choline salicylate, sodium salicylate, and diacetylates, are much weaker inhibitors of prostaglandin synthetase and are usually tolerated. The same is true of acetaminophen (Tylenol). Sulfites have been considered a possible cause of urticaria due to food additives but such reactions are not well documented; an asthmatic reaction is far more common.

Papular urticaria is a rash typically seen in childhood that is caused by bites of insects, including mosquitoes, bedbugs, fleas, lice, and mites. There may be hypersensitivity to the saliva, mouth parts, or excreta of the causative insect. The bite reaction is typically biphasic, with an acute wheal-and-flare reaction that is possibly IgE mediated (not proven), followed by the appearance of indurated papules with lymphocytic infiltrates that resemble those in a late-phase reaction or a bona fide delayed hypersensitivity reaction.[153] Groups of delayed linear papules are seen that are extremely pruritic and can become secondarily infected (impetiginous) by scratching. Papular urticaria is most commonly seen in the summer, and application of calamine lotion usually suffices. In the case of flea bites, all clothing, bed linen, and soft furnishings need to be cleaned thoroughly, and pets treated for fleas.

Infection is rarely a cause of urticaria. Children may have transient urticaria (a few days to 6 weeks) with a viral illness with gradual improvement within that period. Adults may have transient urticuria as a prodrome to hepatitis B (serum sickness–like reaction) or with EBV infection (infectious mononucleosis). Urticaria is not due to bacterial or fungal infections. It may be seen with parasitic infections associated with eosinophilia.

PHYSICAL URTICARIAS AND ANGIOEDEMA

The group of disorders known as physical urticarias and angioedema share the common property of being reproducibly induced by environmental factors, such as a change in temperature, or by direct stimulation of the skin by pressure, stroking, vibration, or light.[60] A classification of this group of disorders in given in Table 35–1.

COLD URTICARIA AND RELATED DISORDERS

Cold urticaria is a disorder characterized by the rapid onset of pruritus, erythema, and swelling after exposure to a

TABLE 35–1
CLASSIFICATION OF PHYSICALLY INDUCED URTICARIA AND ANGIOEDEMA

Cold-dependent disorders
- Idiopathic cold urticaria
- Cold urticaria associated with abnormal serum proteins: cold agglutinins, cryoglobulin, cryofibrinogen, Donath-Landsteiner antibody
- Systemic cold urticaria
  - Cold-induced cholinergic urticaria
  - Cold-dependent dermographism
- Delayed cold urticaria
- Localized cold urticaria
- Localized cold reflex urticaria

Exercise-induced disorders
- Exercise-induced anaphylaxis (idiopathic or food-dependent)
  - Cholinergic urticaria (cold-dependent variant: cold-induced cholinergic urticaria)
- Exercise-induced angioedema

Local heat urticaria
- Familial variant

Dermographism
- Urticaria pigmentosa–systemic mastocytosis
- Cold-dependent variant (cold-dependent dermographism)
- Delayed dermographism

Pressure-induced urticaria-angioedema (delayed)
- Immediate pressure urticaria

Solar urticaria
- Types I–VI

Aquagenic urticaria

Vibratory angioedema
- Familial
- Sporadic

From Kaplan AP: Urticaria and angioedema. In Samter's Immunologic Diseases, 5th edition. Vol II. Frank MM, Ansten KF, Claman HN, Unanue ER (eds): Little Brown and Co, Boston, 1995.

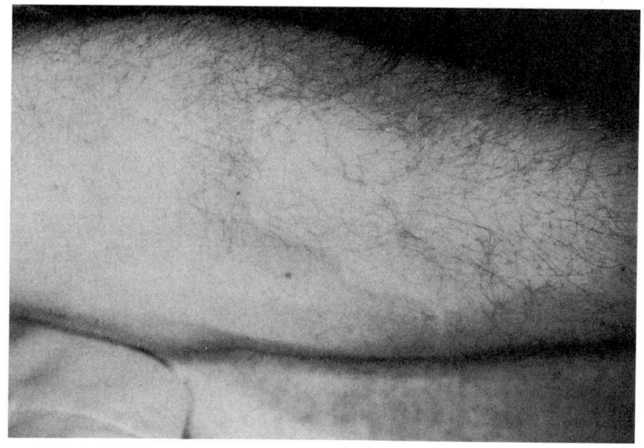

FIGURE 35–1. Positive ice cube test in a patient with cold urticaria demonstrating a wheal the shape of the cube and a track where ice water had dripped along the arm.

cold stimulus. The location of the swelling is confined to those portions of the body that have contacted the cold, although the symptoms are often maximal after the exposed area is warmed. Patients typically experience symptoms while outside on cold, windy days, but holding cold objects can cause hand swelling, and eating cold foods may cause lip swelling. Swelling of the tongue and pharynx is less common, and laryngeal edema or abdominal complaints are rarely, if ever, seen. Total body exposure, such as occurs while swimming, can cause massive mediator release, resulting in hypotension. Because fatalities by drowning have been reported secondary to cold-induced hypotension,[77] patients should be warned that swimming is dangerous.

This disease can begin in any age group and has no obvious sex predilection. When the diagnosis is suspected, a simple test that can confirm the initial impression is to place an ice cube on the patient's forearm for 4 minutes and to observe the area for 10 minutes afterward. If the patient has cold urticaria, the area becomes pruritic about 2 minutes after removal of the ice cube, and by 10 minutes, a large hive the shape of the ice cube will form, as shown in Figure 35–1. Cold urticaria has been reported in association with a variety of diseases characterized by abnormal immunoglobulins that have some cold-dependent property. Thus, it may be seen in cryoglobulinemia, cold agglutinin disease, cryofibrinogenemia, and paroxysmal cold hemoglobinuria (the Donath-Landsteiner antibody associated with secondary syphilis[119]). The mechanism of production of urticaria in these diseases in unknown; however, in some studies, isolated cryoglobulins have been shown to be capable of transferring the sensitivity.[23, 24] These proteins can fix complement when aggregated by cryoprecipitation; thus, it is possible that histamine release may occur through the release of anaphylatoxins.

Therapy consists of measures directed toward the underlying disease plus antihistamines. It is clear that a disorder such as cryoglobulinemia can be associated with cutaneous vasculitis as well as cold urticaria; in addition, other associations between these two entities have been reported. Eady and Greaves[42] reported that frequent and repeated cooling of the skin in patients with idiopathic cold urticaria can cause vasculitic lesions. In one case, immune reactants (IgM and

C3) were deposited in the vessels of such lesions.[43] In two other patients, leukocytoclastic vasculitis was seen in association with cold urticaria, and circulating immune complexes were clearly evident.[171, 191] It appears that the mediator release caused by cold challenge could localize immune complexes to cutaneous sites, where they then caused a vasculitis.[171] Sites of typical urticarial vasculitis independent of temperature change were also evident.[191]

In most patients, however, an abnormal circulating protein is not evident, and the disorder is termed "idiopathic." My colleagues and I[86] have studied mediator release in more than 40 such patients with a simple procedure, placing one of the patient's hands in ice water for 4 minutes and serially determining the plasma histamine level in the brachial vein draining that hand (Fig 35–2). In all patients, a peak of histamine release was observed between 4 and 8 minutes after the hand was removed from the ice water. Figure 35–3 shows the histamine release curve in a single patient with a history of repeated episodes of hypotension while wading in the ocean. A 50-mm Hg drop in diastolic blood pressure was observed coincident with the peak histamine level. Thus, histamine likely contributes to both the urticaria and the hypotension characteristic of this disorder. In 2 of 12 such patients, the cold urticaria could be passively transferred to normal individuals and was shown to be mediated by IgE; however, the mechanism by which temperature changes lead to IgE-dependent histamine release is unknown.

IgE-mediated cold urticaria has also been reported in another series of such patients and at a somewhat higher incidence.[73] However, the true incidence of IgE-dependent cold urticaria may be underestimated in general, because the passive transfer test is far less sensitive than an ice cube test in the propositus. Furthermore, only those patients with sufficient pathogenic antibody in the circulation (beyond that bound to cutaneous mast cells) are detected. In two cases, an IgM antibody was shown to mediate cold urticaria[190]; passive transfer was positive after a short interval (3 to 6 hours) but was negative at 48 hours, whereas IgE-mediated reactions remained positive at 48 hours. We have reported a similar patient with short-term passive sensitization that seemed to be caused by an IgG antibody.[67]

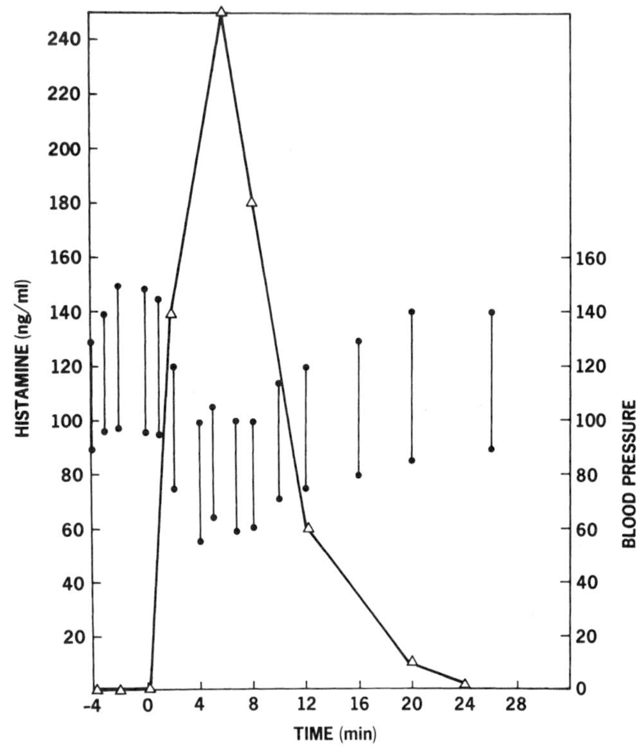

FIGURE 35–3. Plasma histamine levels in the patient shown in Figure 35-2. The hand is placed in ice water at 4 minutes and removed at 0 time. Serial histamine determinations are made at 4-minute intervals. The vertical lines indicate systolic and diastolic blood pressure.

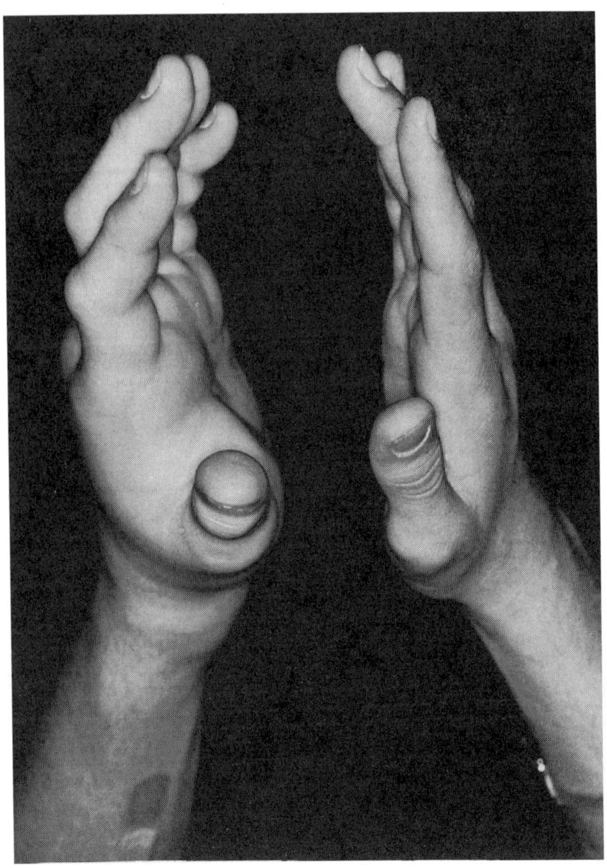

FIGURE 35–2. Hand swelling observed after submersion of one hand in ice water for 4 minutes in a patient with cold urticaria. Maximal swelling is observed 4 to 8 minutes thereafter.

Challenge studies have documented release of other mast cell constituents in addition to histamine, including eosinophilotactic peptides,[174, 194] neutrophil chemotactic factor (NCF),[195] PAF,[65] and PGD_2.[126]

Although this disease generally responds to antihistamines, cyproheptadine (Periactin) appears to be particularly effective.[189, 192] I have found that 16 to 32 mg of cyproheptadine daily in divided doses renders the ice cube test negative in most patients and affords considerable objective relief of their symptoms when exposed to cold. Cyproheptadine does not inhibit histamine release and appears to act as a classic H_1 receptor antagonist.[163] Thus, any antihistamine given in sufficient dosage may be effective. Nevertheless, cyproheptadine remains the drug of choice. It is possible that vasoactive factors other than histamine have a significant contribution to the urticarial reaction of those patients who do not show good response to cyproheptadine or other antihistamines or whose symptoms are less well correlated with histamine release.[65, 89] Attempts to desensitize patients with cold urticaria using ice baths[8] have been reported, but caution must be exercised, because highly sensitive patients could have anaphylactoid symptoms. Because this approach is effective, it can be considered for patients unresponsive to alternative therapeutic modalities.

Studies of the mechanism by which a temperature change can lead to mediator release have failed to demonstrate the presence of an IgE cryoglobulin but have succeeded in obtaining cold-dependent release of histamine from skin biopsy specimens that have been chilled and then warmed.[85] However, chilling and warming the basophils of patients did not result in histamine release, including patients in whom IgE-mediated disease was demonstrable. Thus, cutaneous mast cells seem to be essential. Although cryoaggregation of an abnormal protein might explain the cold dependence of the reaction, it is also possible that patients have an IgE antibody to a cold-induced skin antigen. Which of these possibilities, if any, is operative is not yet clear.

The prognosis and severity of cold urticaria vary considerably. Occasionally, the problem may resolve spontaneously in a few months. However, it can last for many years, and the course is not predictable.

Other cold-dependent syndromes have been reported, although the incidence of such cases in unknown. A delayed form of cold urticaria was described in which swelling appeared 9 to 18 hours after cold exposure.[177] Studies of mediator release were unrevealing; the cold sensitivity could not be passively transferred, and biopsy of a lesion revealed edema and a mononuclear cell infiltrate. Family studies suggested a dominant mode of inheritance.

A series of four patients have been described in whom exercise in a cold environment induced hives similar to those seen with cholinergic urticaria; however, hive formation did not occur if exercise was performed in a heated environment. In this disorder, the cold exposure is systemic rather than local, and it should be suspected for any patient with symptoms suggestive of either cold urticaria or cholinergic urticaria in whom standard tests for each disorder are negative.[84] Exercise in a cold room or running on a winter's day will lead to generalized urticaria and confirm the diagnosis. Because of the visual resemblance of the lesions seen to those typical of cholinergic urticaria, the disorder has been called *cold-induced cholinergic urticaria.* Cholinergic urticaria observed only in winter[186] may represent this disorder. A study of thirteen patients with symptoms suggestive of cold urticaria and cholinergic urticaria revealed two who did not have both disorders but had the cold-induced cholinergic type.[127]

Another related disorder, called *systemic cold urticaria,* yields severe generalized hive formation upon systemic cold challenge occurring over covered or uncovered parts of the body. Symptoms are unrelated to exercise or other activities,[82] and the ice cube test is negative. Histamine release upon cold challenge (with or without exercise as appropriate) has been seen in cold-induced cholinergic urticaria as well as in systemic cold urticaria. A treatment regimen of hydroxyzine (Atarax) plus cyproheptadine in high dosage has been utilized successfully.

In addition, a disorder called *cold-dependent dermographism* has been reported in which prominent hive formation is seen if the skin is scratched and then chilled.[82] In this disorder, the ice cube test and systemic cold challenge yield no hives. Simply scratching the skin yields a weakly positive dermographic response, but dramatic accentuation is seen when the scratched area is chilled. Treatment once again is high-dose antihistamines, for example diphenhydramine, 200 mg/day, or a combination of hydroxyzine, 100 to 200 mg/day, and cyproheptadine, 8 to 16 mg/day. Experimental cromolyn-like drugs, which inhibit mast cell degranulation, are effective in controlling symptoms and suppressing the ice cube test in patients with poor response to cyproheptadine.[133] Ketotifen, in particular, has been shown to inhibit histamine release and is effective in a variety of physically induced urticarias.[78]

Localized cold urticaria in which only certain areas of the body urticate with cold contact has been reported after predisposing conditions, such as cold injury, or at sites of intracutaneous allergen injections, ragweed immunotherapy, or insect bites. Kurtz and Kaplan[96] have described a patient with cold urticaria confined to the head and face in which there was no identifiable antecedent or associated event. Such cases argue against the presence of a circulating pathogenic factor and speak in favor of a local abnormality of mast cells.

Finally, a disorder called *localized cold reflex urticaria* has been reported in which the ice cube test is positive but hives form in the vicinity of the contact site, but not where the ice cube is applied.[183] In appearance, the hives resemble the punctate lesions of cholinergic urticaria, and there is no confluent hive where the ice cube is applied. A methacholine or acetylcholine skin test for cholinergic urticaria is negative, although the symptoms in one such patient resembled cold-induced cholinergic urticaria, because exercise-induced hives were seen in a cold environment.[29]

CHOLINERGIC URTICARIA AND LOCAL HEAT URTICARIA

Heat urticaria can occur in a local or generalized form. The local form is observed when a warm stimulus is in contact with the skin and, when suspected, can be tested for by applying a test tube of warm water[69] at 44°C to the arm for 4 to 5 minutes. In a positive reaction, a hive is seen a few minutes after the test tube is removed. Local heat urticaria is an extremely rare disorder, and studies have demonstrated histamine and NCF release on warming of the skin,[61] although some heterogeneity in disease pathogenesis may exist.[30] Mast cell degranulation seems likely even though passive transfer studies have been negative.

Association with other forms of physical allergy is also sometimes seen, for example, combined cold urticaria and local heat urticaria.[180] Therapy has been problematic, because antihistamines such as hydroxyzine and cyproheptadine as well as oral cromolyn have been ineffective. One patient was successfully desensitized by repeated daily immersion in hot baths, but caution is in order with such measures because systemic reactions are possible.[30] A variant of local heat urticaria has been described that was familial; urticaria occurred 1.5 to 2 hours after application of a warm stimulus[115] and persisted for 6 to 10 hours. Sunbathing with pronounced heating of skin could produce wheals from the temperature effect, whereas sunlight itself could be tolerated. Desensitization of an area would be achieved with repeated

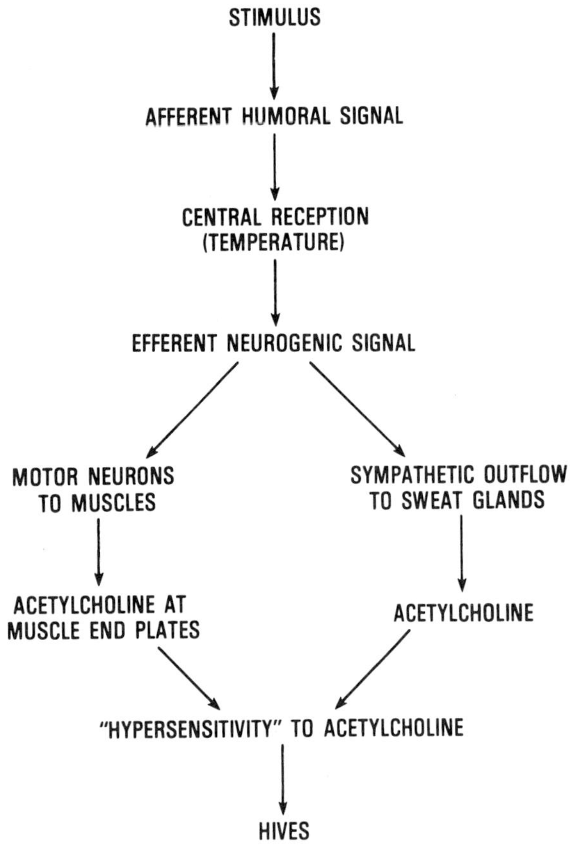

FIGURE 35–4. Diagrammatic representation of the pathogenic sequence that underlies urticaria development in patients with cholinergic (generalized heat) urticaria.

challenge every few days. Skin biopsy demonstrated a pronounced inflammatory cell infiltrate in the upper dermis and around hair follicles. The pathogenesis of this form of local heat urticaria is unknown; however, partial control could be achieved with oral antihistamines.

Generalized heat (cholinergic) urticaria is characterized by the onset of small punctate wheals surrounded by a prominent erythematous flare associated with exercise, hot showers, sweating, and anxiety.[62] It tends to appear first over the upper thorax and neck but can spread distally to involve virtually the entire body. In some patients, these hives can become confluent and resemble angioedema, whereas other patients may have symptoms characteristic of cholinergic stimulation, such as lacrimation, salivation, and diarrhea. These various stimuli have the common feature of being mediated by cholinergic nerve fibers, which innervate the musculature by way of parasympathetic neurons and innervate the sweat glands by cholinergic fibers that travel with the sympathetic nerves[75] (Fig. 35–4).

The characteristic lesion of cholinergic urticaria can be reproduced by an intradermal injection of 0.1 mg methacholine (Mecholyl) in 0.1 ml saline; a localized hive surrounded by smaller satellite lesions is diagnostic.[69] Affected patients therefore demonstrate a hypersensitivity to cholinergic mediators, but they have no evidence of an immunoglobulin-mediated allergy. However, we have found that only about one third of patients give a clearly positive skin test; these generally are the most severe cases. Challenge by exercise (e.g., running in an 85°F warmed room or using a bicycle ergometer for 10 to 15 minutes) is a far more sensitive test. Thus, the skin test can be used to confirm the diagnosis but cannot be used as a diagnostic test.[21, 86]

Cholinergic urticaria may be due to an intrinsic cellular abnormality that leads to mediator release in the presence of cholinergic agents. One study addressing this issue demonstrated an increased number of muscarinic receptors in urticarial sites. These receptors were further augmented when exercise followed patch testing to copper-containing materials.[162] The higher number of acetylcholine binding sites may be an important key to understanding the pathogenesis of cholinergic urticaria. The importance of copper is unclear, but it may affect ligand receptor affinity. Evidence that a neurogenic reflex is involved is provided by the observation that placing a patient's hand in warm water with a tourniquet tied proximally does not cause localized hives, whereas removal of the tourniquet can lead to a generalized eruption. Thus, a central perception of the temperature change appears to be followed by an efferent reflex, leading to the urticaria. Such a reflex could also account for the association of hives with anxiety, although it should be emphasized that in these instances, the emotional reaction itself may be normal.

A photograph of typical cholinergic urticaria is shown in Figure 35–5, in which lesions were induced by having the patient run in place for 10 minutes. Studies of mediator release during attacks of cholinergic urticaria have demonstrated that in most cases, elevated plasma histamine levels parallel the onset of pruritus and urticaria[86] (Fig. 35–6). Subsequent studies confirmed the presence of histaminemia in association with cholinergic urticaria[88, 164, 175] and have also observed release of eosinophilotactic peptides and NCF.[175]

When patients were challenged while wearing a plastic occlusive suit to produce maximal changes in cutaneous and core body temperature, significant falls in 1-second forced expiratory volumes (FEV_1), maximal midexpiratory flow rate, and specific conductance were seen in association with a rise in residual volume. Four of seven patients also had wheezing detected by auscultation. Thus, under such conditions, an abnormality in pulmonary function can be detected, reflecting either primary pulmonary involvement or altered pulmonary mechanics secondary to circulating mediators. A

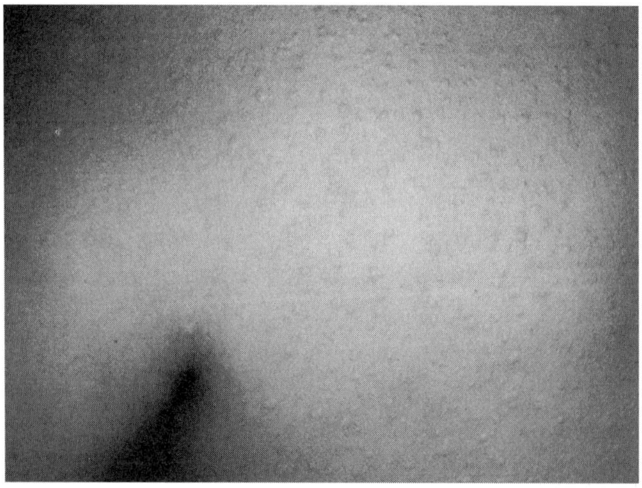

FIGURE 35–5. Urticarial lesions induced in a patient with cholinergic urticaria by running in place for 10 minutes.

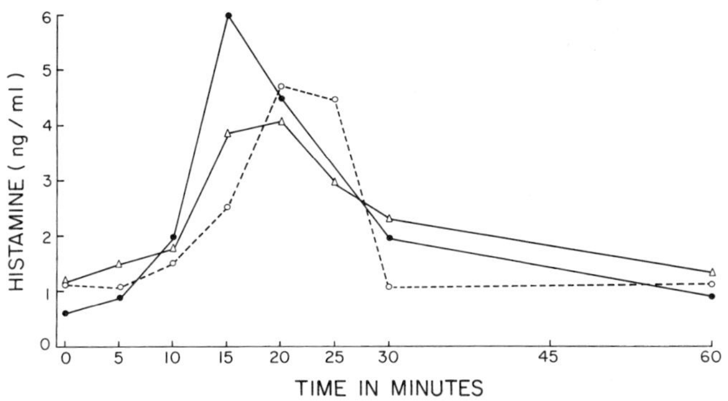

FIGURE 35–6. Histamine release in three patients with cholinergic urticaria after running for 10 minutes.

clinically significant alteration in pulmonary function is unusual in cholinergic urticaria, and it has no known association with exercise-induced asthma.

The drug of choice for the management of cholinergic urticaria is hydroxyzine, and most patients respond to a dose between 100 and 200 mg every 24 hours.[117] Hydroxyzine is considerably more effective than conventional antihistamines, suggesting that it has some additional action; it might, for example, interrupt the neurogenic reflex that leads to the urticaria. Anticholinergic agents given orally are generally ineffective, perhaps because of an inability to attain a sufficient systemic level. However, injected atropine can reverse the methacholine skin test.[164]

Patients with combined cold and cholinergic urticaria have been reported, and the time course of histamine release seen is characteristic of each disorder.[127, 164] Such patients respond well to therapy with hydroxyzine plus cyproheptadine but are to be distinguished from patients with cold-induced cholinergic urticaria.[84]

EXERCISE-INDUCED ANAPHYLAXIS

The syndrome of exercise-induced anaphylaxis was first described in a series of patients in whom combinations of pruritus, urticaria, angioedema, wheezing, and hypotension occurred as a result of exercise. Symptoms did not occur with each exercise experience, and most described patients were accomplished athletes.[155] The disorder is distinguished from cholinergic urticaria by the following criteria: First, although exercise is the precipitating stimulus of each disorder, hot showers, sweating in the absence of exercise, and anxiety do not trigger attacks in exercise-induced anaphylaxis as they do in cholinergic urticaria.[62] Second, the hives seen with exercise-induced anaphylaxis are large (10 to 15 mm) rather than the small punctate lesions characteristic of cholinergic urticaria. Finally, when patients with exercise-induced anaphylaxis were challenged in an occlusive body suit, no change in pulmonary function was seen, although histamine release was documented.[161]

Kaplan and associates[88] have described two cases of typical cholinergic urticaria in which lesions became confluent, were associated with prominent elevation of plasma histamine, and were associated with recurrent episodes of hypotension. Thus, it is clear that some extreme cases of cholinergic urticaria can resemble the exercise-induced anaphylactic syndrome. An important distinguishing feature is that an increase in core body temperature of greater than 0.7°C using hyperthermic blankets or submersion in warmed water causes hives, histamine release, and anaphylactic symptoms in cholinergic urticaria patients with anaphylactic-like symptoms but not in the exercise-induced anaphylactic syndrome.[15]

Lewis and associates[98] reported on an additional six patients with exercise-induced symptoms. Upon exercise challenge, three patients developed cholinergic urticaria; two had associated angioedema, and one became hypotensive. Challenge of one patient caused giant hives and hypotension (clearly, exercise-induced anaphylaxis), whereas challenge of another patient caused periorbital angioedema without hive formation. Thus, various combinations of exercise-induced hives, angioedema, and hypotension are possible. Other studies have demonstrated histologic changes consistent with mast cell degranulation upon exercise challenge of such patients.[160] Elevated levels of plasma histamine were also documented but did not necessarily correlate with induction of any particular symptom. There is no generally agreed-upon therapy for the exercise-induced anaphylactic syndrome, and attempts at prophylaxis utilizing H_1 and H_2 antagonists have not generally been effective.[98] In contrast, classic cholinergic urticaria is usually responsive to prophylactic use of hydroxyzine.

Patients with the exercise-induced anaphylactic syndrome, in contrast to those with most other "physical urticarias," have high incidences of atopy (half to two thirds)[161] and also of other types of physically induced hives, particularly cold urticaria.[98] Subtypes of exercise-induced anaphylaxis have also been described that are food related. In one patient, exercise-induced anaphylaxis occurred if the patient exercised between 5 and 24 hours after eating shellfish, whereas taking exercise alone or eating shellfish alone did not cause any symptoms.[111] In five other reported cases, two patients had symptoms only if exercise followed the ingestion of any food within 2 hours,[92, 124] whereas in three other patients, symptoms were precipitated by the specific ingestion of celery within 2 hours of exercise.[92] These latter patients also had positive skin tests to celery.

Various forms of food-dependent exercise-induced anaphylaxis are therefore possible, and treatment requires avoiding specific foodstuffs prior to exercising or avoiding exercise within certain time intervals after eating. Patients usually continue to exercise but carry an epinephrine kit and diphenhydramine (Benadryl) with them. There have been no reported fatalities. Kivity and associates[94] performed skin tests using compound 48/80 in subjects with food-related (skin test positive) exercise-induced anaphylaxis. Food or exercise alone did not affect the 48/80 response; however, an augmented wheal-and-flare response was observed with food intake plus exercise. The data suggest increased mast cell releasability caused by the combination of food plus exercise. Also of interest is that one patient with cholinergic urticaria and associated anaphylaxis was successfully treated by vigorous daily exercise such that desensitization occurred within a week.[88] The number of patients with cholinergic urticaria or the exercise-induced anaphylactic syndrome that might respond to such treatment is unknown, although it is more likely to be effective in cholinergic urticaria with or without hypotension, because symptoms occur reproducibly each time an exercise challenge is performed.

PRESSURE URTICARIA (ANGIOEDEMA)

Pressure-induced urticaria differs from most of the aforementioned types of hives or angioedema in that symptoms typically occur 4 to 6 hours after pressure has been applied. The disorder is clinically heterogeneous, as some patients may complain of swelling secondary to pressure with normal-appearing skin (i.e., no erythema or superficial infiltrating hive); therefore, the term *angioedema* is more appropriate. Other patients have predominantly urticaria that may or may not be associated with significant swelling. When urticaria is present, an infiltrative lesion is seen consistent with biopsy studies characterized by a perivascular mononuclear cell infiltrate and dermal edema similar to that seen with chronic urticaria.[47] Immediate dermographism is not present, but delayed dermographism is seen and may represent the same disorder.[47, 81, 146]

Symptoms occur around tight clothing, the hands may swell with activity such as hammering, foot swelling is common after walking, and buttock swelling may be prominent after sitting for a few hours. Testing can be done by placing a sling with a 5- to 15-lb weight attached over the forearm or shoulder for 10 to 20 minutes. Gradual pressure-applying devices measuring in grams per square millimeter can also be used.[47]

There are few available studies regarding the pathogenesis of pressure urticaria; however, mediators that cause pain rather than pruritus (e.g., kinins) have been considered, because the lesions are typically described as burning or painful. Nevertheless, induced blisters over lesions revealed histamine release following the time course of hive formation.[87] Antihistamines, however, have little effect upon the disorder, and patients with severe disease often have to be treated with corticosteroids. For long-term treatment, we utilize the lowest dose given on alternate days that allows a significant diminution of symptoms. The usual range required is 15 to 30 mg of prednisone every other day. Although pressure urticaria (angioedema) can occur as an isolated disorder, it is most often seen in association with chronic urticaria, in which case therapy is usually directed toward the chronic urticaria.

Immediate pressure urticaria has been described in patients with the hypereosinophilic syndrome. It is characterized by an acute wheal-and-flare reaction within 1 to 2 minutes of applied pressure, for example, pressing on the patient's back with a thumb. Those patients also were dermographic; however, dermographic patients typically do not have immediate pressure urticaria and require a stroking motion to produce a hive.[128]

DERMOGRAPHISM

The ability to "write on skin," termed *dermographism,* can occur as an isolated disorder that often presents as traumatically induced urticaria. It can be diagnosed by observing the skin after stroking it with a tongue blade or fingernail. In these patients, the white line secondary to reflex vasoconstriction is followed by pruritus, erythema, and linear swelling as in a classic wheal-and-flare reaction (Fig. 35–7). It is said to be present in 2% to 5% of the population,[109, 173] although only a small fraction of such patients are sufficiently severe to warrant treatment.

In approximately 50% of the patients, passive transfer studies have suggested an IgE-mediated reaction,[123] but an antigen has not been identified. Thus, many patients have an abnormal circulating IgE that confers a particular form of pressure sensitivity to dermal mast cells. Such observations further suggest that histamine is one of the mediators of dermatographism, although demonstration of such release has been difficult because of the localized and fleeting nature of the reaction. Early studies, however, did suggest that (1) histamine is released into whole blood,[142] (2) induced blisters over lesions contain elevated histamine levels,[87] (3) 24-hour urine histamine levels are elevated,[63] and (4) histamine is increased in the perfusate obtained during in vivo subcutaneous perfusion studies.[64] In a single unusually severe case of IgE-mediated dermographism, elevation of plasma histamine levels was documented within 1 minute of stroking of the skin and the baseline histamine level was abnormal in multiple determinations, suggesting that "leakage" of histamine is ongoing at all times.[53]

Although anecdotal, because a formal study has not yet been performed, dermographism has been observed as a consequence of drug reactions.[109] In one case, dermographism could be observed only upon challenge with the offending agent, in this instance penicillin.[167]

The drug of choice for this disease is diphenhydramine (Benadryl), although different patients may prefer different antihistamines, depending on their relative efficacy rather than adverse side effects. The initial objective of therapy is to decrease pruritus so that the stimulation for scratching is diminished. Many patients complain of a sensation of itching or "skin crawling" that is readily relieved by antihistamines. At higher antihistamine doses, one can show that the wheal-and-flare reaction to stroking is also markedly diminished.

Dermatographism may also be seen in patients with chronic urticaria from a variety of different causes, as is discussed subsequently. Severe dermographism is seen in association with urticaria pigmentosa and systemic mastocytosis, and in the systemic disease, the wheals may last for many hours. Large doses of antihistamines are required to relieve the symptoms, and evidence of histamine release in

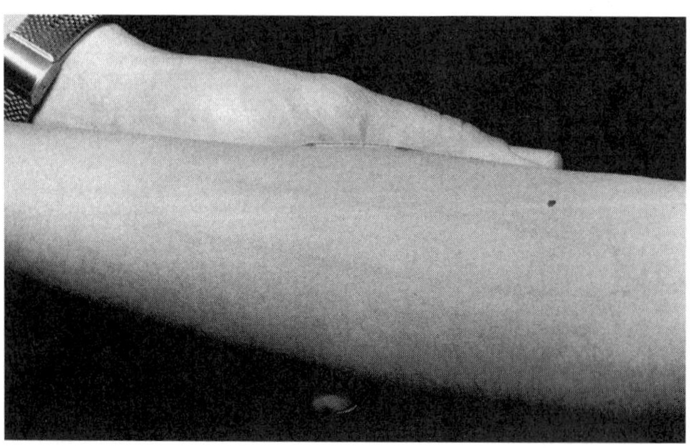

FIGURE 35–7. Severe dermographism induced by stroking the forearm.

urticaria pigmentosa as well as in idiopathic dermographism has been reported.[53, 64]

It is also possible that other vasoactive agents released from cutaneous mast cells can be implicated in dermographism and, in fact, in all forms of physically induced urticaria. An example is the elevation of prostaglandin D_2 metabolites seen in the urine of patients with systemic mastocytosis, which may relate to the hypotension associated with this disorder.[141]

SOLAR URTICARIA

Solar urticaria is a rare disorder in which brief exposure to light causes the development of urticaria within 1 to 3 minutes. Typically, pruritus occurs first, at about 30 seconds, followed by erythema and edema confined to the light-exposed area and surrounded by a prominent erythematous zone caused by an axon reflex. The lesions then usually disappear within 1 to 3 hours. When large areas of the body are exposed, systemic symptoms may occur, including hypotension and asthma. Although most patients reported have been in the third and fourth decades, this disorder can occur in any age group and has no association with other allergic disorders.

Solar urticaria has been classified into six types according to the wavelength of light that induces lesions and the ability or inability to passively transfer the disorder with serum.[69, 70, 147] Types I and IV can be passively transferred and may therefore be antibody (IgE?) mediated and are associated with wavelengths of 2800 to 3200 angstroms (Å) and 4000 to 5000 Å, respectively. The antigen has not been identified. Release of histamine[74] and chemotactic factors for neutrophils and eosinophils[176] after experimental challenge of solar urticaria patients has been reported, suggesting degranulation of mast cells. Type VI solar urticaria, activated at 4000 Å, is clearly a metabolic disorder, in which protoporphyrin IX acts as a photosensitizer, and is synonymous with erythropoietic protoporphyria; it is caused by ferrochelatase deficiency.[11] Unlike other forms of porphyria, urinary porphyrin excretion is normal; however, red cell protoporphyrin levels and fecal protoporphyrin and coproporphyrin levels are elevated.

Evidence for complement activation when plasma of patients with protoporphyria is exposed to light of appropriate wavelengths has been presented.[101] There is generation of C5a chemotactic activity, which is proportional to the serum level of protoporphyrin.[59] Irradiation of the forearms of two such patients also resulted in in vivo complement activation as assessed by a diminution of titers of C3 and C5 and generation of C5a.[102] Consistent with these observations is that (1) deposition of C3 and accumulation of neutrophils are seen in the dermis of patients[7, 46] and (2) complement fragments can be detected in the serum and suction blister fluid of irradiated skin.[7] Hereditary protoporphyria responds to oral beta-carotene, which absorbs light at the same wavelengths as protoporphyrin IX.[120]

The mechanism producing solar urticaria in types II, III, and V is unknown, but these types are induced by inciting wavelengths of 3200 to 4000 Å, 4000 to 5000 Å, and 2800 to 5000 Å, respectively, and cannot be passively transferred with serum. As a simple screen, fluorescent tubes that emit a broad, continuous spectrum can be used to test the patient, and filters can then be used to define the spectrum that causes urticaria.

Ordinary window glass 3 mm thick absorbs most ultraviolet radiation below 3200 Å and thereby protects patients with type I solar urticaria. Therapy of this disease requires avoidance of sunlight, protective garments to cover the skin, and use of topical preparations to absorb or reflect light. A 5% solution of para-aminobenzoic acid in ethanol, as in sunscreen lotions, can be helpful to screen out light in the 2800 to 3200 Å range; however, it is more difficult to screen out the visible spectrum. The most effective agents for this purpose contain titanium oxide or zinc oxide, or both. The efficacy of antihistamines, antimalarials, and corticosteroids in these disorders is not clear and must be evaluated for each type.

AQUAGENIC URTICARIA

Thirteen cases have been reported of patients who developed small wheals after contact with water, regardless of its temperature, that were distinguishable from those of cold urticaria or cholinergic urticaria. This entity, termed *aquagenic urticaria,*[16, 185] can be tested for by direct application of a compress of tap water or distilled water to the skin. The diagnosis should be reserved for those rare individuals who show a positive reaction to water and in whom tests for all other forms of physical urticaria are negative. Combined cholinergic urticaria and aquagenic urticaria has been reported, and histamine release into the circulation was documented upon challenge with water.[32]

HEREDITARY FORMS OF URTICARIA AND ANGIOEDEMA

FAMILIAL COLD URTICARIA

Familial cold urticaria is a rare form of cold intolerance that is inherited as an autosomal dominant trait and histologically is not truly urticaria. Approximately 30 minutes after exposure to cold, a systemic reaction occurs consisting of burning papular skin lesions accompanied by fever, chills, arthralgias, myalgias, headache, and leukocytosis. Biopsy of the skin lesions reveals edema and an intense inflammatory infiltrate consisting almost entirely of polymorphonuclear leukocytes with eosinophils prominent about dilated capillaries.[40, 182]

HEREDITARY VIBRATORY ANGIOEDEMA

Hereditary vibratory angioedema has been described in a single family in whom it was inherited in an autosomal dominant pattern. It is properly viewed as a physically induced angioedema, because patients complain of intense pruritus and swelling within minutes after vibratory stimuli.[129] The patients are not dermographic and do not have pressure urticaria. Lesions can be reproduced by gently stimulating a patient's forearm with a laboratory vortex for 4 minutes. Rapid swelling of the entire forearm and a portion of the upper arm ensues, and histamine has been shown to be released secondary to such a vibratory stimulus.[114] With care, patients can avoid vibratory stimuli, and their symptoms can otherwise be partially relieved with diphenhydramine (Benadryl). Nonfamilial sporadic cases have also recently been described.[184, 197]

C3b INACTIVATOR DEFICIENCY

Three patients have been reported who are deficient in the C3b inactivator. The complement profile in such patients suggests spontaneous activation of the alternative complement pathway, consisting of depletion of factor B, markedly depressed C3 levels, and a circulating inactive C3 byproduct without evidence of further degradation to C3c or C3d.[2] However, intravenous replacement with C3b inactivator leads to elevation of the patient's C3. Of particular interest is that some patients have histaminuria, and one of the presenting symptoms can be urticaria. Urticaria may reflect rapid degradation of C3 with liberation of C3a anaphylatoxin. Family members can have half-normal levels of the C3b inactivator, suggesting an autosomal recessive inheritance.

URTICARIA AND AMYLOIDOSIS

Familial urticaria has also been seen in conjunction with the combination of amyloidosis, nerve deafness, and limb pain.[90, 105] It appears to be inherited as an autosomal dominant condition[4, 10] in which the urticaria has been described as having features of cholinergic urticaria, angioedema, or classic hives. The rash is associated with limb pain and seems to be intensified by cold weather.

SCHNITZLER'S SYNDROME

Schnitzler's syndrome consists of chronic urticaria in the setting of an IgM monoclonal plasma component with associated fever, bone pain, and lymphadenopathy.[9] In addition, there may be an elevated erythrocyte sedimentation rate (ESR) and a leukocytosis. The patients do not, however, have overt multiple myeloma. There is hyperostosis involving the tibia and pelvic bones. There is no vasculitis or cryoprotein, and the antinuclear antibody (ANA) and rheumatoid factor tests are negative. Some patients have been found to have an IgG autoantibody to interleukin-1α.[149]

HEREDITARY ANGIOEDEMA AND ACQUIRED C1 INH DEFICIENCY

Hereditary angioedema is an autosomal dominant disorder caused by absence of the C$\bar{1}$ inhibitor (C$\bar{1}$ INH)[35] in which patients may have attacks of swelling involving almost any portion of the body. A traumatic episode or infection may initiate an attack. However, such a triggering event may not be evident, and the swelling appears to occur spontaneously. This disorder is *not* associated with urticaria, and patients with both urticaria and angioedema without a family history invariably have a normal C$\bar{1}$ INH level.

In addition to the family history, the presence of visceral involvement suggests the hereditary disorder. The most severe complication is laryngeal edema, which has been a major cause of mortality in this disease. Patients can also have abdominal attacks[38] lasting 1 to 2 days and consisting of vomiting, severe abdominal pain, and guarding in the absence of fever, leukocytosis, or abdominal rigidity. This presentation can occasionally be difficult to distinguish from that of an acute abdominal condition; however, the attacks are self-limited and have been shown to be caused by edema of the bowel wall.[131] The ultrastructural lesion seen in tissues of patients with hereditary angioedema consists of gaps in the postcapillary venule endothelial cells, edema, and virtually no cellular infiltrate,[157] consistent with release of a vasoactive factor such as a kinin.

Patients with hereditary angioedema have measurable levels of the activated first component of complement (C$\bar{1}$), although this protein generally circulates as an unactivated enzyme. The serum level of C4 is diminished even when the patient is free of symptoms and is usually undetectable during an attack.[145] A C4 determination is therefore the simplest test utilized to diagnose hereditary angioedema. Rocket immunoelectrophoresis for C4d is a very sensitive assay, indicating that C4 has been cleaved, which is more sensitive than C4 quantitation.[202] C2, the other substrate of C$\bar{1}$, is usually within normal limits when the patient is asymptomatic, but it also is diminished during at attack.[6]

When a diminished C4 level is obtained, a direct assay of protein C$\bar{1}$ INH level should be performed. A diminished level or absence of C$\bar{1}$ INH confirms the diagnosis. However, approximately 15 to 20% of patients have a normal or elevated C$\bar{1}$ INH protein.[143] In these cases, the protein is not functional and often has an abnormal electrophoretic mobility. Thus, a functional C$\bar{1}$ INH assay is then necessary to determine whether the diagnosis is really hereditary angioedema.

The pathogenesis of the swelling appears to involve both the complement pathway and the plasma kinin-forming pathway. Intracutaneous injection of C$\bar{1}$ into normal individuals causes the formation of a small wheal, whereas injection into a patient with hereditary angioedema yields localized angioedema.[95] A kinin-like peptide has been isolated from these patients, and its formation appears to be inhibited in C2-deficient plasma.[37] However, direct demonstration of such a kinin-like peptide on interaction of C$\bar{1}$ with C4 and C2 or with C2 alone is lacking. Most evidence regarding this peptide suggests that cleavage of C2b by plasmin generates a kinin[39]; however, attempts to confirm this experiment have failed.[28, 49] The only identifiable kinin seen in these latter studies was bradykinin.

On the other hand, the amino acid sequence of C2b is known, and Strang and colleagues[178] have synthesized peptides of various lengths and tested each for kinin-like activity. A peptide of 25 amino acids was shown to cause edema when injected intracutaneously, reminiscent of the "C2-kinin" originally described. However, this peptide has not yet been shown to be a cleavage product of C2b, nor to be present during attacks of swelling in patients with hereditary angioedema. Thus, at this point, the data suggest but do not prove that a kinin-like molecule is derived from C2b. The presence of bradykinin has been documented, however, and it is a likely contributor to the swelling that is seen. Perhaps more than one kinin-like moiety will ultimately be shown to be the cause of the angioedema.

Twenty-four hour urine histamine excretion is also increased during attacks of angioedema, suggesting that C3a, C4a, or C5a is being generated. Although the plasma levels of C3 and C5 are normal in this disorder, C3 turnover is enhanced.[14] The lesions, however, are not pruritic, and antihistamines have no effect on the clinical course of the disease.

C$\bar{1}$ INH also inhibits activated Hageman factor,[151] kallikrein,[58] and plasmin.[151] Thus, it is also an important modulator of bradykinin generation. Patients appear to be hyperresponsive to injections of kallikrein,[80] as they are to C$\bar{1}$, and elevated levels of plasma bradykinin have been observed during attacks.[179] There is also evidence that the C1 activation observed in hereditary angioedema may be Hageman factor dependent.[34, 44] Thus, some Hageman factor–dependent enzyme may be initiating the classic complement cascade. Plasmin has been shown to be capable of activating C1s[138] and may represent one such enzyme. Ghebrehiwet and colleagues[57] have demonstrated that HFf (Hageman factor fragment) can directly initiate the classic complement cascade by activation of C1,[56] and Kaplan and Austen[83] have shown that plasmin can cleave HF to form HFf. Plasmin-α_2 antiplasmin levels increase during attacks of swelling, indicating conversion of plasminogen to plasmin. This may represent a critical link between the intrinsic coagulation-kinin cascade, fibrinolysis, and complement activation. The presence of kallikrein-like activity in induced blisters of patients with hereditary angioedema supports this notion,[27] as do the progressive generation of kinin upon incubation of hereditary angioedema plasma in plastic (non–contact-activated tubes)[49] and the low prekallikrein and high molecular weight kininogen levels seen during attacks.[150]

The treatment for attacks of hereditary angioedema generally involves intermittent administration of subcutaneous epinephrine. However, there are no studies to support its efficacy, because attacks usually abate in 3 to 4 days even if no medication is given. A tracheostomy is indicated if laryngeal edema occurs, and mild analgesics may be used to relieve the discomfort of severe swelling and/or abdominal pain. Intravenous fluids may be necessary if the patient is unable to eat or drink.

Successful prevention of attacks has been reported with androgens[31] and with large doses of antifibrinolytic agents such as ϵ-aminocaproic acid[50, 104] or tranexamic acid.[156] The precise mechanism of action of these latter agents is unknown. Their primary effect is to inhibit conversion of plasminogen to plasmin; in higher concentration, they also inhibit plasmin, which may activate C1 as well as Hageman factor[83] and, perhaps, cleave C2b further. These agents also inhibit the activation of C1 by immune complexes, suggesting a direct effect on the C1 molecule.[169] At present, the drugs of choice are androgen derivatives such as danazol or stanozolol, which not only prevent attacks of swelling in patients with hereditary angioedema but also induce synthesis of normal C$\bar{1}$ INH and cause the C4 level to return toward normal.[55]

These drugs may also have other as yet unknown effects, because many patients respond to low doses that are insufficient to raise C4 and C$\bar{1}$ INH.[158, 159, 193] Alternatively, tissue levels may be more important than plasma levels and may be affected first. Patients with hereditary angioedema are heterozygotes and therefore possess one normal gene. However, levels may be less than 25% of normal rather than the expected 50%, owing to depletion by binding to activated enzymes. Patients with functionally abnormal C$\bar{1}$ INH also respond to androgen therapy.[51] Such patients possess single amino acid substitutions at the active site of the inhibitor.[166] With treatment, normal C$\bar{1}$ INH is synthesized along with the abnormal protein, suggesting that such patients possess one gene that manufactures an abnormal protein (structural gene defect) and a second gene that codes for a normal product but is inhibited, or that the product is catabolized excessively.[137] A proposed model for the pathogenesis of hereditary angioedema is shown in Figure 35–8, indicating the reactions inhibited by C$\bar{1}$ INH.

An acquired form of this disease has been described in patients with lymphoma who have circulating low molecular weight IgM and depressed C$\bar{1}$ INH levels. This entity has an unusual complement utilization profile, in that C1 levels are low in addition to depletion of C4, C2, and C3. Usually, it is the C1q subcomponent that is quantitated. The low C1 distinguishes this acquired disorder from the hereditary form.[13, 72, 152] The depressed C$\bar{1}$ INH level may be caused by depletion secondary to C1 activation by immune complexes or C1 interaction with the tumor cell.[152] In the latter instance, C1 fixation and C$\bar{1}$ INH depletion have been shown to be caused by an anti-idiotypic antibody bound to immunoglobulin on the surface of a B-cell lymphoma.[54] Other patients with connective tissue disorders, primarily systemic lupus erythematosus[36] and carcinoma,[20] have acquired C$\bar{1}$ INH deficiency and respond to androgen therapy, which is helpful in these disorders because it enhances C$\bar{1}$ INH synthesis.

A second form of acquired C$\bar{1}$ INH deficiency has been described that is due to synthesis of an autoantibody (IgG) directed to C$\bar{1}$ INH.[3] Like the aforementioned acquired forms of C$\bar{1}$ INH deficiency, C4 and C$\bar{1}$ INH levels are low in the absence of a family history, but C1 levels are usually within normal limits. Under normal circumstances, C$\bar{1}$ INH is a substrate for the enzymes it inactivates; that is, the enzyme cleaves C$\bar{1}$ INH, which exposes the active site in the inhibitor. The cleaved C$\bar{1}$ INH then binds stoichiometrically to the enzyme and inactivates it. When antibody to C$\bar{1}$ INH is present, C$\bar{1}$ INH is cleaved, but the antibody inhibits its ability to inactivate the enzyme. Cleaved, functionless C$\bar{1}$ INH then circulates,[201] and unopposed activation of the complement and kinin-forming cascades takes place.[107] Fibrinolysis is also activated as indicated by increased levels of plasmin-antiplasmin complexes, and this abnormality appears particularly prominent in this autoimmune form of C$\bar{1}$ INH deficiency.[25]

Therapeutic modalities other than androgen therapy are required for this disorder, including the use of fibrinolytic inhibitors,[25] plasmapheresis, and immunosuppressive agents. The complement profile in this autoimmune disorder more closely resembles that of the occasional hereditary angioedema patient, who has no relevant family history (e.g., patient with a new mutation) and because C1 or C1q levels are normal. The diagnosis, if suspected, can be corroborated by performing an immunoblot analysis of C$\bar{1}$ INH and noting

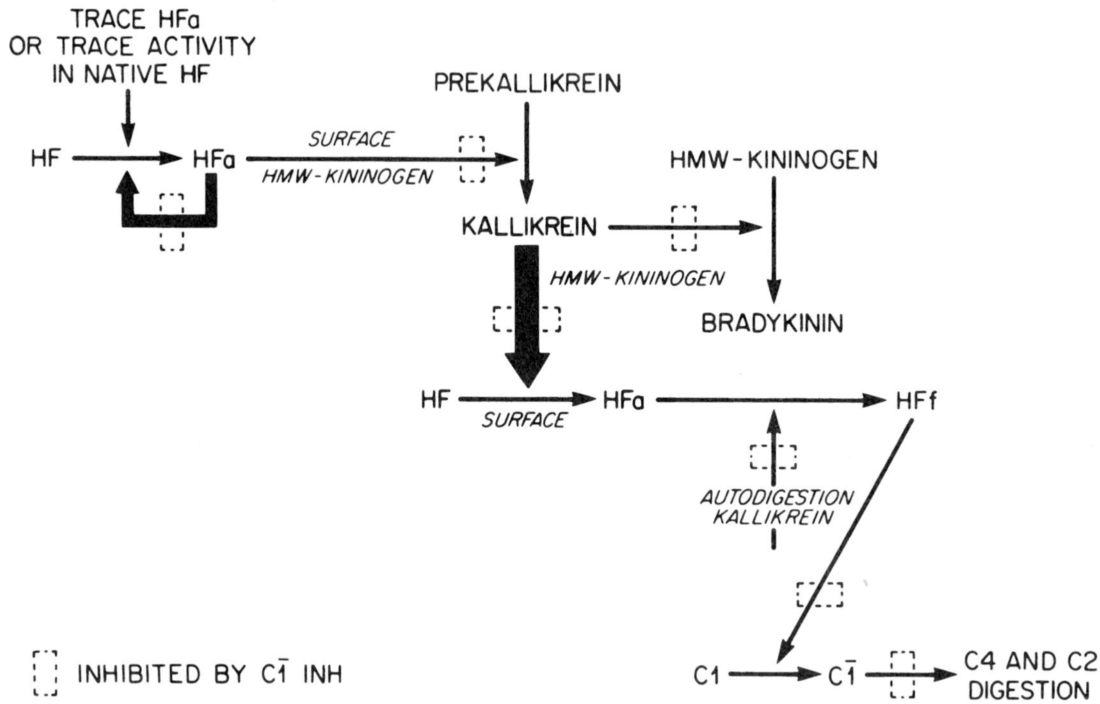

FIGURE 35–8. Pathway for bradykinin formation and linkage to the complement cascade indicating all steps that are inhibitable by C1̄ INH.

increased levels of a 95 Kd cleaved form that increases noticeably during attacks of swelling.[25, 201]

CHRONIC URTICARIA AND IDIOPATHIC ANGIOEDEMA

Reports of the rate of identification of the etiologic agent in chronic urticaria and angioedema vary from 10% to as high as 80%. However, the rate of successful diagnosis in most studies is probably not greater than 20% and is likely much less. Of course, different physicians, clinics, or allergy centers see different populations of patients, perhaps in part accounting for the wide variance reported. One may also confuse chronic urticaria with recurrent urticaria due to a repeatedly encountered allergen.

We have studied more than 700 patients with chronic urticaria for whom no etiologic agent could be identified after evaluation by physicians in the community, many of whom are allergists or dermatologists. Our rate of successful subsequent identification of a causal factor is less than 2%. As a group, these patients are not atopic individuals; that is, they do not have higher incidence of eczema, allergic rhinitis, or asthma compared with the incidence of these disorders in the absence of chronic urticaria. Their IgE levels as a group are within normal limits. Some patients are dermographic, although the disorder is usually of milder degree than is seen with the IgE-dependent dermographism described earlier, and curiously, the dermographism may wax and wane just as the urticaria may vary from severe to mild or may intermittently subside. Some patients have symptoms consistent with pressure urticaria, i.e., areas subject to pressure are particularly likely to erupt with hives, but most hives are unassociated with pressure. These patients have normal white blood counts and ESRs and no evidence of systemic disease.

PATHOGENESIS

The lesion seen in chronic urticaria is different from that seen in most of the physically induced urticarial disorders. Biopsy of lesions of patients with cold urticaria or dermatographism reveals evidence of increased vascular permeability and edematous tissue, but there is no cellular infiltrate. The lesions appear quickly, usually disappear in less than 2 hours, and do *not* have a late-phase component. Thus, a single burst of mast cell degranulation may be insufficient to cause a late-phase reaction.[5] Reactions to foods or drugs may be similar; however, there can be a late-phase component with a cellular infiltrate, so such lesions may resemble those seen in chronic urticaria. Of the physically induced disorders discussed herein, only skin biopsy specimens of patients with delayed pressure urticaria reveal pathology that is virtually indistinguishable from that seen in chronic urticaria.

External examination of patients with chronic urticaria reveals infiltrative hives with palpably elevated borders, sometimes varying greatly in size and/or shape but generally being rounded (Fig. 35–9). The typical lesion consists of a nonnecrotizing perivascular mononuclear cell infiltrate (Fig. 35–10). However, many types of histopathologic processes can occur in the skin and manifest as hives. For example, patients with hypocomplementemia and cutaneous vasculitis can have urticaria (angioedema), and biopsies of patients with urticaria, arthralgias, myalgias, and elevated ESR as a manifestation of necrotizing venulitis revealed fibroid necrosis with a predominant neutrophilic infiltrate.[170, 172] Yet the urticarial lesions were indistinguishable from those seen in the more typical, nonvasculitic cases.

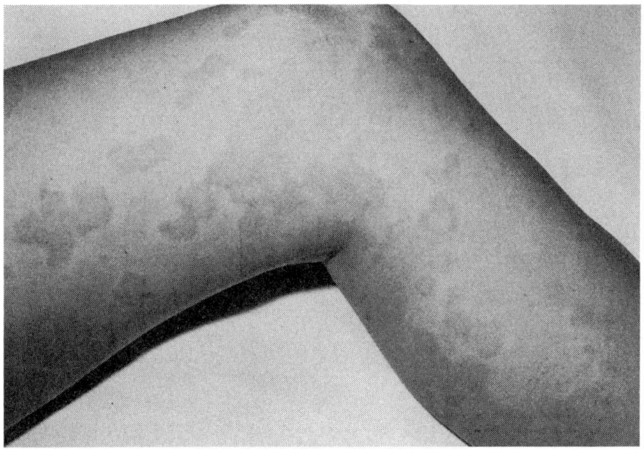

FIGURE 35–9. Typical rounded, slightly indurated lesions of chronic urticaria demonstrating variability in size and shape.

Other studies have examined the incidence of vasculitis in patients with urticaria, with a wide variety of results.[110, 116, 122, 134] Mathison and colleagues[110] found that 10 of 78 patients had hypocomplementemia, many with evidence of activation of the classic complement pathway; 6 of the 10 had elevated levels of circulating immune complexes. If hypocomplementemia and vasculitis are equated, the incidence of presumed vasculitis was 14%. Monroe and coworkers[116] found neutrophilic leukocytoclastic angiitis in 20% of patients; the other 80% had a perivascular infiltrate (not true vasculitis) of mononuclear cells that was classed as dense or sparse. Interestingly, the "vasculitis," "dense," and "sparse" groups had circulating immune complex levels of 33%, 29%, and 13%, respectively, as measured by multiple assays. Phanuphak and associates[134] used the criterion of significant cellular infiltrate within vessel walls to define vasculitis rather than endothelial damage, nuclear dust, fibrin deposition, or red cell extravasation. They found a 52% incidence of vasculitis with various types of predominant cells and a 48% incidence of perivascular mononuclear cell infiltrate. Deposition of immune complexes in the skin was seen in 18% of the vasculitis patients—almost exclusively in those with an abundance of neutrophils.

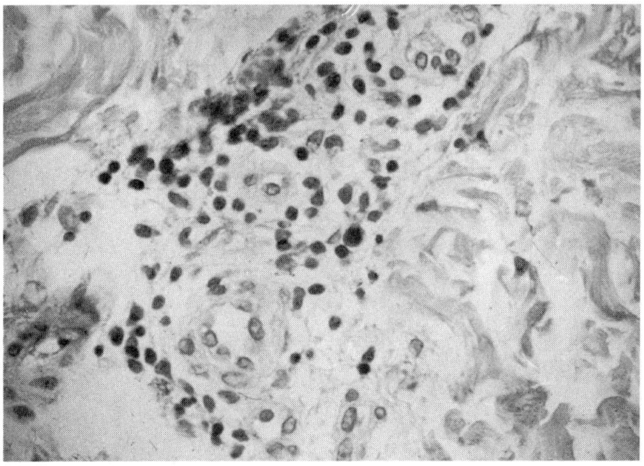

FIGURE 35–10. Skin biopsy of patient with chronic urticaria demonstrating a nonnecrotizing, predominantly mononuclear cell infiltrate surrounding small superficial venules of the skin.

My colleagues and I[122] have reported results of a histopathologic study of chronic idiopathic urticaria in 43 consecutive patients. All but 1 patient had a nonnecrotizing perivascular infiltrate consisting primarily of lymphocytes. We therefore found vasculitis to be a rare cause of urticaria, and we believe that our group is comparable to (1) the group without vasculitis in the study by Mathison and colleagues,[110] (2) the "sparse" and/or "dense" infiltrate groups of Monroe and coworkers,[116] and (3) the perivasculitis group of Phanuphak and associates.[134] We also noted a tenfold increase in number of mast cells and a fourfold increase in number of mononuclear cells in skin biopsy specimens from the patients with chronic urticaria compared with those from normal controls. No increase in basophil number was seen, although basophils of patients with chronic urticaria are reported to be less responsive to anti-IgE than cells of normal control subjects, suggesting in vivo desensitization.[91] Thus, the increase in mast cells observed may relate to the higher amount of histamine found in blister fluid sunctioned from patients with chronic urticaria compared with that from normal control subjects[87] and to the elevation in total skin histamine content reportedly present in such patients.[135]

Later studies have attempted to subtype the mononuclear cell infiltrate using monoclonal antibodies. A predominance of helper T lymphocytes has been reported.[113] We have found 50% T lymphocytes, no B cells, 20% monocytes, and 10% mast cells[45]; however, we found T-cell subtyping to reveal no predominant pattern, as the subtype (CD4 versus CD8) varied greatly among patients. Eosinophils were not often seen in the skin specimens from our series of patients; when they were considered as a group, an occasional patient had a prominent eosinophil accumulation. Deposition of eosinophil major basic protein in skin specimens of 40% of patients with chronic urticaria has also been demonstrated, although only a fraction of the patients had obvious eosinophil infiltration.[132] Thus, degranulated eosinophils may be present.

The 20% unidentified mononuclear cells may represent γ/δ T lymphocytes, and this matter will require reassessment with additional antisera. Because lymphocytes, monocytes, and mast cells accumulate, we propose that a lymphokine or monokine may be released that causes mast cell proliferation (or accumulation) and degranulation. Histamine-releasing factors (HRFs) that can cause cutaneous mast cell degranulation are being sought as a potential cause of histamine release in this disorder. Evidence for HRF release in patients with chronic urticaria has, in fact, been reported[18]; however, identification of the specific factor (? chemokine) was not pursued.

We have concluded that chronic urticaria is characterized by a nonnecrotizing perivascular lymphocyte infiltrate with an accumulation of mast cells. The cause is unknown, and we cannot as yet even state whether the process is or is not immunologically mediated. We consider patients with vasculitis and urticaria a separate subpopulation in whom the cause and pathogenesis of hive formation probably involve immune complexes, complement activation, anaphylatoxin formation, histamine release, and neutrophil accumulation, activation, and degranulation.

There has been considerable renewed interest in the possibility that chronic urticaria may be an autoimmune disorder. Perhaps the first suggestion was engendered by data that demonstrated an association of chronic urticaria with autoimmune hypothyroidism (Hashimoto's thyroiditis) and, more specifically, with the presence of antibodies to peroxidase or thyroglobulin. The incidence was 12% to 14% in two studies of patients with chronic urticaria.[99, 100] However, it was noted that a person's thyroid status did not relate to the occurrence of urticaria and that, typically, hives did not remit when a euthyroid status was achieved. On the other hand, the autoantibodies typically persist.

A more direct approach was taken by Gruber and associates,[66] who reported the incidence of circulating IgG or IgM anti-IgE antibodies in subjects with chronic urticaria to be 10%. The antibodies were not seen in normal controls or in patients with other types of urticaria except cold urticaria, in which such antibodies were also detected. The underlying hypothesis was that such an antibody could degranulate cutaneous mast cells in vivo and lead to acute hives or even a late-phase reaction and its concomitant cellular infiltrate.

Hide and coworkers[76] reported the presence of anti-IgE receptor antibodies in 30% to 40% of patients with chronic urticaria and of anti-IgE antibodies in an additional 10%. These studies demonstrated autoreactivity to autologous serum in such subjects, i.e., injections of serum into the patient induced a wheal-and-flare reaction.[76] The sera could degranulate basophils to release histamine, and those sera reactive with cells stripped of their IgE were presumed reactive with the IgE receptor. The sera were inhibitable with either the α subunit of their IgE receptor or with IgE itself, confirming the functional reactivity. Our preliminary data confirm the presence of reactivity with the α subunit of the IgE receptor in about one third of patients, using activated rat basophil leukemia cells transfected with the α subunit of the IgE receptor. Thus, if this finding turns out to be pathogenic in the disease and not an epiphenomenon, an autoimmune etiology can be inferred in 40% to 50% of patients with chronic urticaria. The cause in the others remains uncertain.

The preceding data suggest that the perivascular infiltrate seen in patients with chronic urticaria is a late-phase reaction or at least a variant thereof. However, there are some discrepancies between the histologic description of late-phase reactions and the lesions described in chronic urticaria. For example, basophils are prominent in the late-phase reaction in the nose, lung, or skin,[17, 68] but no increase in basophils was seen in chronic urticaria.[45] Eosinophils are very prominent in asthma or nasal polyps, and in induced or naturally occurring late-phase reactions in the lung and nose. They are somewhat less prominent in the skin; however, the lesions of chronic urticaria vary from having very prominent eosinophils to having none at all; the latter is the more common scenario. Hence, the presence of major basic protein in many biopsy specimens from chronic urticaria subjects suggests that eosinophils are present transiently or are missed for unknown technical reasons. Monocytes are minimally elevated in late-phase reactions of the lung, nose, and skin, but constitute 20% of the cells in chronic urticaria. This is a significant difference. Lymphocytes are also more prominent in chronic urticaria. Thus, much more information is needed to relate the lesions we see to the consequences of an autoimmune reaction involving cutaneous mast cells. Further, some explanation is needed that localizes such reactions to the skin, because mast cells in the nose or lung should be responsive to the same autoantibody. A theoretic diagram depicting this mechanism for hive induction in chronic urticaria is shown in Figure 35–11.

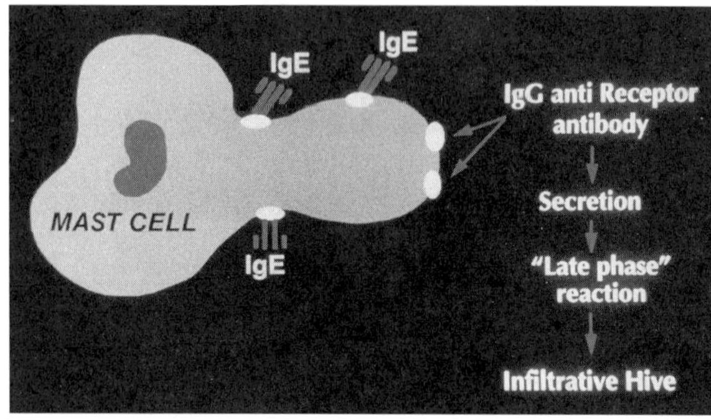

FIGURE 35–11. A possible mechanism of hive formation in a third of patients with chronic urticaria who also have circulating IgG antibody to the α subunit of the IgE receptor ($Fc_{\epsilon}RI\alpha$).

URTICARIA AND VASCULITIS

It is clear that patients with an immune complex disease such as serum sickness[1] or systemic lupus erythematosus (SLE)[130, 136] can have urticaria as a manifestation of their underlying disease. Biopsy of such lesions shows evidence of a necrotizing vasculitis involving small venules (hypersensitivity angiitis)[12, 22] (Fig. 35–12), and immunofluorescent studies demonstrate deposition of immunoglobulins and complement. In patients with serum sickness, IgE-dependent histamine release as well as histamine release secondary to complement activation may contribute to the urticaria seen.

Patients with urticaria secondary to cutaneous vasculitis have been described who could not be readily classified as having an underlying collagen vascular disease.[170] An elevated ESR, arthralgias, and myalgias as well as fever and leukocytosis were the main associated abnormalities. Like patients with palpable purpura associated with a variety of diseases, these patients could be divided into a group with

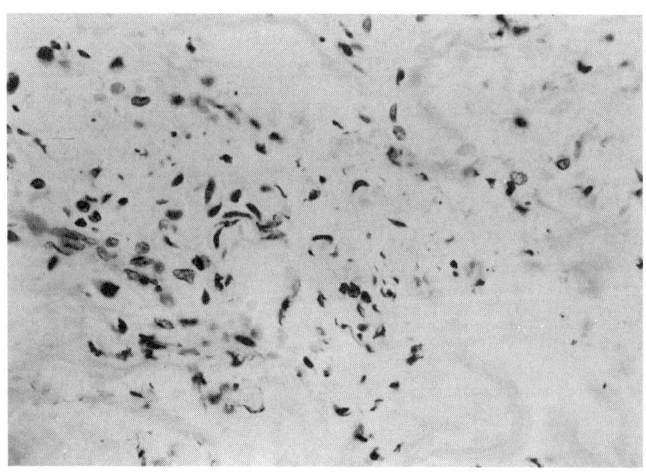

FIGURE 35–12. Skin biopsy of a patient with leucocytoclastic angiitis demonstrating necrosis of the vessel, neutrophilic infiltration, karyolysis, and nuclear debris.

serum hypercomplementemia and a group in whom the serum complement level was normal.[110] The group with hypocomplementemia had lesions characterized by infiltration with neutrophils, fibrin deposition, and prominent nuclear debris. The normocomplementemic group had lesions in which lymphocytes predominated, and there was prominent perivenular fibrin deposition. In each group, there was evidence of mast cell degranulation and true vessel wall necrosis.

Other isolated cases of chronic urticaria have also been reported to involve cutaneous vasculitis and hypocomplementemia in whom the ANA test is negative.[52, 108, 112] This syndrome is reminiscent of connective tissue diseases, but it does not fall into one of the standard diagnostic categories and is termed the *hypocomplementemic urticarial vasculitic syndrome*.

It is now appreciated that other organ involvement can occur in this syndrome, for example, uveitis, glomerulonephritis,[103, 118] pseudotumor cerebri,[48, 103] angioedema, arthralgias, or myalgias. Low molecular weight precipitins that interact with C1q and thereby lower C1q levels appear to be characteristic.[1, 26, 108, 200] Some studies indicate that the binding protein is IgG and may therefore be an autoantibody directed to C1q.[198] Thus, the hypocomplementemic urticarial vasculitic syndrome is an immune complex–mediated disorder in which activation of the classic complement pathway is seen with tissue deposition of immune complexes and inflammation. The urticaria in particular may therefore be a result of anaphylatoxin generation and cutaneous mast cell degranulation. In one report, potassium iodide sensitivity was suspected as a precipitating factor.[26] This disorder is unique because the hives are often responsive to hydroxychloroquine (Plaquanil), at 200 to 400 mg/day.

DIAGNOSTIC TESTS

The recommended work-up for patients with the various types of urticaria is evolving, but in general, few tests are required if the history and physical examination do not reveal evidence of some underlying systemic disease. For patients with acute urticaria, the history is critical in terms of possible exposure to foods, drugs, contact allergens, viral illness in children, and so on. Those with a serum sickness–like presentation, with fever and lymphadenopathy, should have a complete blood count (CBC) with differential, ESR, blood urea nitrogen (BUN), and creatinine measurements, urinalysis, and perhaps an ANA titer. A CBC looking for eosinophilia and/or a stool analysis for ova and parasites may be indicated in selected cases.

Patients with suspected physically induced urticaria or angioedema can be challenged in order to document the reaction. The specific tests are described earlier for each disorder. Blood tests are not revealing in general; however, patients with cold urticaria should be tested for cryoglobulinemia, cold agglutinins, and, if syphilis is a realistic possibility, the Donath-Landsteiner antibody. It is uncertain whether cryofibrinogenemia has any specificity or whether its presence can lead to symptoms.

Criteria for optimal evaluation of a patient with chronic urticaria are in flux, but very few tests are truly indicated. Certainly, anyone with symptoms or signs of illness requires further evaluation; however, the findings may not be related to the urticaria. For example, a patient with chronic urticaria who has symptoms of chronic sinusitis may need sinus films or a limited computed tomography (CT) scan or a nasal culture, but such tests are not done because the sinusitis is related to the urticaria. The same is true for evaluation of other organ system abnormalities.

Only an occasional patient has an abnormal CBC, differential blood count, or ESR, so even these measurements are not recommended as routine. Although an occasional patient with SLE may present with urticaria, whose underlying disease would be missed were ANA and ESR measurements not done, the incidence is so low such tests are not really cost effective as *screening* tools. If SLE is missed, other symptoms will soon reveal themselves and mandate further evaluation. Sometimes, periarticular hives can cause "joint" pain. Such symptoms or associated myalgias would probably lead one to order these tests. Even though antimicrosomal antibodies are associated with chronic urticaria, these tests are once again not indicated as screening tools in an otherwise euthyroid subject. Nonetheless, many such patients have a history of hypothyroidism and may be receiving replacement therapy; thus, a positive test provides some insight, by association. Therapy is unaffected, however. Likewise, skin biopsy is really a research tool rather than part of a clinical assessment, unless other information is suggestive of a cutaneous or systemic vasculitis.

Autologous skin testing in search of an autoantibody is safe, costs nothing, and can easily be done, but requires some experience and a series of negative control subjects to allow interpretation. This area is still evolving and, as of this writing, is not yet adequately confirmed or accepted as part of the routine evaluation of chronic urticaria.

TREATMENT

Therapy for chronic urticaria is aimed at providing symptomatic relief rather than suppressing the urticaria. It consists of the use of antihistamines and, at times, of corticosteroids. Although antihistamines do not always decrease the number of urticarial lesions or the frequency of eruptions, they significantly diminish pruritus.

One often begins with hydroxyzine (Atarax, Vistaril), a histamine H_1-receptor blocker, at 75 to 200 mg/day (25- or 50-mg tablets) divided into three or four doses. The dose is based on the severity of the urticaria and the patient's tolerance of the somnolent effect of the drug. Most patients adapt to these effects within a week. When prescribing the drug, one should stress that it must be taken as prescribed and not just as needed. Daily administration has the object of minimizing or preventing what may be intermittent outbreaks; use of antihistamines after the onset of lesions is too late.

A combination of cyproheptadine (Periactin) and hydroxyzine often gives greater relief than hydroxyzine alone.[95] A typical regimen might be 25 mg of hydroxyzine and 4 mg of cyproheptadine taken together four times a day for a total daily dose of 100 mg of the former and 16 mg of the latter. Maximal daily doses of 200 mg of hydroxyzine and 32 mg of cyproheptadine can be given on the basis of the frequency and severity of outbreaks.

Patients can sometimes tolerate the side effects of one antihistamine better than those of another, even though the doses used are comparable. Diphenhydramine (Benadryl) or tripelennamine (PBZ), both in 25- or 50-mg tablets, can be substituted for hydroxyzine in the same dosage; azatidine (Optimine) in 1-mg tablets can be substituted for cyproheptadine in the same dosage. Histamine H_1-receptor blockers can usually ameliorate the symptoms of chronic urticaria, that is, relieve the pruritus and minimize lesions. They allow most patients to be reasonably comfortable and to function normally. No further intervention is required.

The newer, nonsedating antihistamines such as terfenadine (Seldane), loratidine (Claritin) or astemizole (Hismanal), cetirizine (Zirtec), can be used in place of the aforementioned antihistamines at the recommended dosage; however, their potency at this dose range is less than for the aforementioned regimens. Nevertheless, many milder cases of urticaria may be treated with them, and each may be added to traditional antihistamines such as hydroxyzine or diphenhydramine to try to achieve additional H_1-receptor blockade without additional sedation.

Patients with severe chronic urticaria, however, may not respond satisfactorily to any of the regimens discussed. When urticaria involves the face (particularly with facial angioedema) or when hives are florid and pruritus is severe, additional therapy is required. A small number of patients obtain relief when an antihistamine that blocks histamine H_2 receptors is added to one of the regimens given. Cimetidine (Tagamet), 300 mg four times a day, or ranitidine (Zantac), 150 mg twice a day, as is used in the treatment of ulcer disease, may therefore be added.[71] The rationale is that the cutaneous vasculature possesses not only a large number of H_1 receptors that have been blocked but also H_2 receptors; the addition of an antihistamine that binds to H_2 receptors augments the antihistaminic effect. Use of an H_2-receptor antagonist alone has no effect on urticaria; only with significant H_1-receptor blockade is any effect observable. I discontinue H_2 blockers in 3 weeks unless their use has clearly improved a patient's urticaria.

If antihistamines alone are insufficient to control chronic urticaria, addition of a corticosteroid is indicated. It is necessary to determine the lowest possible effective dose. I usually start with prednisone, giving 40 mg in one morning dose for the first 3 days and then decreasing the dose by 5 mg/day. When the dose is down to 25 mg/day, I begin to decrease it by 5 mg on alternate days. Thus, the daily dose becomes 25 mg, 20 mg, 25 mg, 15 mg, 25 mg, 10 mg, and so on until a dose of 25 mg every second day is achieved. This alternate-day regimen is effective in the vast majority of patients. The steroid should then be slowly withdrawn by decreasing the dose 5 mg every 2 weeks.

The decision to keep decreasing the steroid dose depends on achievement of considerable improvement with the 25-mg alternate-day dose and no obvious worsening of symptoms as the dose is decreased. Optimally, close to 3 months would be needed to discontinue the steroid. Antihistamines are continued with the corticosteroid and should probably not be tapered until the patient no longer requires the steroid. Sometimes, the duration of steroid therapy must be extended because the drug cannot be tapered below a certain dose. This is maintained for a while (usually 1 to 2 months), and then the physician should try again to taper the patient's dose.

Occasionally, urticaria is so severe that it does not respond to the described steroid regimen. In this case, I increase the alternate-day dose to 40 mg and slowly taper from that point. Daily corticosteroids should not be used except for the first week or 10 days of therapy, regardless of the severity of the urticaria. A not uncommon difficulty is achievement of good control of hives during the steroid "on" day with prominent exacerbation during the "off" day. I approach this situation by giving the prednisone in two doses, that is, 30 mg in the morning and 10 mg in the evening every second day. Once the urticaria is under reasonable control, the evening dose is gradually decreased and the decrement added to the morning dose until the evening dose has been discontinued. At this point, the steroid doses are tapered as previously described.

Sometimes, there is no response to prednisone regardless of the dose used. In this case an equivalent dose of methylprednisolone (Medrol) can be tried. Occasionally a patient may be unable to metabolize prednisone to prednisolone; in such a patient, a low dose of methylprednisolone is often effective whereas a high dose of prednisone is not. As of this writing, drugs with cromolyn-like properties are not available for oral use in the United States except by research protocol. They may prove to be a useful adjunct for the therapy of urticaria or angioedema in the future.

A small number of patients have severe urticaria that does not respond to corticosteroids. There is no therapy available as yet for such patients, and it is probably best to use only antihistamines to relieve the pruritus. There are few data regarding the use of immunosuppressive agents in patients with chronic urticaria that is either unresponsive to steroids or requires inordinate dosage. Thus, this approach is not recommended but is an area for future investigation. Some of these patients have cutaneous vasculitis with urticarial lesions, but this is not true of all. At present, the histologic pattern seen on skin biopsy does not correlate with severity of urticaria, nor can it be used as a guide to therapy. In view of data indicating that chronic urticaria may be due to a circulating autoantibody, trials of plasmapheresis, or intravenous γ-globulin, or specific immunosuppressive regimens, such as methotrexate or cyclosporine, can be considered, but should be limited to properly controlled therapeutic trials.

Biopsy of patients with chronic idiopathic angioedema reveals pathologic findings similar to those shown in Figure 35–10 but involving deeper vessels. These patients typically have swelling of the face, extremities, and genitalia as well as of the lips, tongue, and pharynx. However, laryngeal edema rarely if ever occurs. Some patients may be pressure sensitive, so that tight garments or certain types of work or physical exercise can induce localized swelling in addition to episodes that appear to arise spontaneously. Typically, they have no systemic symptoms, are not an atopic group of people, and have no serologic abnormalities. Therapy is usually attempted with high doses of antihistamines such as diphenhydramine and corticosteroids, as outlined for chronic urticaria, if the frequency and severity of attacks warrant it. A small number of patients have been described with complement abnormalities,[165, 196] suggesting that chronic angioedema also probably represents a heterogeneous group of diseases.

Much has been written describing the clinical presentation of therapy of chronic urticaria and angioedema. However, it is clear that in most cases, the cause and pathogenesis are unknown. It is hoped that future studies will provide further insight into the nature of these diseases and lead to improved methods of therapy.

REFERENCES

1. Agnello V, Koffler D, Eisenberg JW: C1q precipitation in the sera of patients with systemic lupus erythematosus and other hypocomplementemia states: characterization of high and low molecular weight types. *J Exp Med* 134:228, 1971.
2. Alper CA, Rosen FS, Lachmann PJ: Inactivator of the third component of complement as an inhibitor of the properdin pathway. *Proc Natl Acad Sci USA* 69:2910, 1972.
3. Alsenz J, Bork K, Loos M: Autoantibody-mediated acquired deficiency of C1 inhibitor. *N Engl J Med* 316:1360, 1987.
4. Anderson V, Buch NH, Jensen MK, et al: Deafness, urticaria, and amyloidosis: a sporadic case with chromosomal aberration. *Am J Med* 42:449, 1967.
5. Atkins PC, Schwartz LB, Adkinson NF, et al: In vivo antigen-induced cutaneous mediator release: simultaneous comparisons of histamine, tryptase, and prostaglandin D_2 release and the effect of oral corticosteroid administration. *J Allergy Clin Immunol* 86:360, 1990.
6. Austen KF, Sheffer AL: Detection of hereditary angioneurotic edema by demonstration of a reduction in the second component of human complement. *N Engl J Med* 272:649, 1965.
7. Baart DLFH, Beerens EGJ, Van Weelden H, et al: Complement components in blood serum and suction blister fluid in erythropoietic protoporphyria. *Br J Dermatol* 99:401, 1978.
8. Bently-Phillips DB, Black AK, Greaves MW: Induced tolerance in cold urticaria caused by cold-evoked histamine release. *Lancet* 2:63, 1976.
9. Berdy SS, Block KJ: Schnitzler's syndrome: A broader clinical spectrum. *J Allergy Clin Immunol* 87:849, 1991.
10. Black JT: Amyloidosis, deafness, urticaria, and limb pains: a hereditary syndrome. *Ann Intern Med* 70:989, 1969.
11. Bonkowsky HL, Bloomer JR, Ebert PS, et al: Heme synthetase deficiency in human protoporphyria: demonstration of the defect in liver and cultured skin fibroblasts. *J Clin Invest* 56:1139, 1975.
12. Braveman FM, Yen A: Demonstration of immune complexes in spontaneous and histamine-induced lesions and normal skin of patients with leucocytoclastic angiitis. *J Invest Dermatol* 64:105, 1975.
13. Caldwell JR, Ruddy S, Schur P, et al: Acquired C1 inhibitor deficiency in lymphosarcoma. *Clin Immunol Immunopathol* 1:39, 1972.
14. Carpenter CB, Ruddy S, Shehadeh IH, et al: Complement metabolism in man: hypercatabolism of the fourth (C4) and third (C3) components in patients with renal allograft rejection and hereditary angioedema. *J Clin Invest* 48:1495, 1969.
15. Casale TB, Keahey TM, Kaliner M: Exercise-induced anaphylactic syndromes: insights into diagnostic and pathophysiologic features. *JAMA* 255:2049, 1986.
16. Chalamidas SL, Charles CR: Aquagenic urticaria. *Arch Dermatol* 104:541, 1971.
17. Charlesworth CN, Hood AF, Soter NA, et al: Cutaneous late-phase response to allergen: mediator release and inflammatory cell infiltration. *J Clin Invest* 83:1519, 1989.
18. Claveau J, Lavoie A, Brunet C, et al: Chronic idiopathic urticaria: possible contribution of histamine-releasing factor to pathogenesis. *J Allergy Clin Immunol* 92:132, 1993.
19. Cochrane CG, Muller-Eberhard HJ: The derivation of two distinct anaphylatoxin activities from the third and fifth component of human complement. *J Exp Med* 127:371, 1968.
20. Cohen SH, Koethe SM, Kozin F, et al: Acquired angioedema associated with rectal carcinoma and its response to danazol therapy. *J Allergy Clin Immunol* 62:217, 1978.
21. Commens CA, Greaves CA: Tests to establish the diagnosis in cholinergic urticaria. *Br J Dermatol* 98:47, 1978.
22. Copeman PWM, Ryan JJ: The problems of classification of cutaneous angiitis with reference to histopathology and pathogenesis. *Br J Dermatol* 82:2, 1970.
23. Costanzi JJ, Coltman CA Jr: Kappa chain cold precipitable immunoglobulin (IgG) associated with cold urticaria. I. Clinical observations. *Clin Exp Immunol* 2:167, 1967.
24. Costanzi JJ, Coltman CA Jr, Donaldson VH: Activation of complement by a monoclonal cryoglobulin associated with cold urticaria. *J Lab Clin Med* 74:902, 1969.
25. Cugno M, Cicardi M, Agostini A: Activation of the contact system and fibrinolysis in autoimmune acquired angioedema: a rationale for prophylactic use of tranexamic acid. *J Allergy Clin Immunol* 93:870, 1994.
26. Curd JG, Milgrom H, Stevenson DD, et al: Potassium iodide sensitivity in four patients with hypocomplementemic vasculitis. *Ann Intern Med* 91:853, 1979.
27. Curd JG, Prograis LF Jr, Cochrane CG: Detection of active kallikrein in induced blister fluids of hereditary angioedema patients. *J Exp Med* 152:742, 1980.
28. Curd JG, Yelvington M, Burridge N, et al: Generation of bradykinin during incubation of hereditary angioedema plasma. *Mol Immunol* 19:1365, 1983.
29. Czarnetzki BM, Frosch PJ, Sprekeler R: Localized cold reflex urticaria. *Br J Dermatol* 104:83, 1981.
30. Daman L, Lieberman P, Garner M, et al: Localized heat urticaria. *J Allergy Clin Immunol* 61:273, 1978.
31. Davis PJ, Davis FB, Charache P: Long-term therapy of hereditary angioedema (HAE): preventive management with fluoxymesterone and oxymetholone in severely affected males and females. *Johns Hopkins Med J* 135:391, 1974.
32. Davis RS, Remigio LK, Schocket AL, et al: Evaluation of a patient with both aquagenic and cholinergic urticaria. *J Allergy Clin Immunol* 68:479, 1981.
33. Dolovich J, Little DC: Correlates of skin test reactions to *Bacillus subtilis* enzyme preparations. *J Allergy Clin Immunol* 49:43, 1972.
34. Donaldson VH: Mechanisms of activation of C1 esterase in hereditary angioneurotic edema plasma in vitro: the role of Hageman factor, a clot-promoting agent. *J Exp Med* 127:411, 1968.
35. Donaldson VH, Evans RR: A biochemical abnormality in hereditary angioneurotic edema. *Am J Med* 35:37, 1963.
36. Donaldson VH, Hess EV, McAdams PJ: Lupus-erythematosus-like disease in three unrelated women with hereditary angioneurotic edema. *Ann Intern Med* 86:312, 1977.
37. Donaldson VH, Ratnoff OD, DaSilva WD, et al: Permeability-increasing activity in hereditary angioneurotic edema plasma. II. Mechanism of formation and partial characterization. *J Clin Invest* 48:642, 1969.
38. Donaldson VH, Rosen FS: Hereditary angioneurotic edema: a clinical survey. *Pediatrics* 37:1017, 1966.
39. Donaldson VH, Rosen FS, Bing DH: Role of the second component of complement (C2) and plasmin in kinin release in hereditary angioneurotic edema (H.A.N.E.). *Plasma Trans Assoc Am Physicians* 40:174, 1977.
40. Douglas HMG, Bleumink E: Familial cold urticaria. *Arch Dermatol* 110:382, 1974.
41. Durham SR, Lee TH, Cromwell O, et al: Immunologic studies in allergen-induced late phase asthmatic reactions. *J Allergy Clin Immunol* 74:49, 1984.
42. Eady RA, Greaves MW: Induction of cutaneous vasculitis by repeated cold challenge in cold urticaria. *Lancet* 1:336, 1978.
43. Eady RAJ, Keahey TM, Sibbald RG, et al: Cold urticaria with vasculitis: report of a case with light and electron microscopic, immunofluorescence, and pharmacological studies. *Clin Exp Dermatol* 6:355, 1981.
44. Eisen V, Loveday C: Activation of arginine and tyrosine esterase in serum from patients with hereditary angioedema. *Br J Pharmacol* 46:157, 1972.
45. Elias J, Boss E, Kaplan AP: Studies of the cellular infiltrate of chronic idiopathic urticaria: prominence of T-lymphocytes, monocytes, and mast cells. *J Allergy Clin Immunol* 78:914, 1986.
46. Epstein JH, Tuffanelli DL, Epstein WL: Cutaneous changes in the porphyrias: a microscopic study. *Arch Dermatol* 107:6789, 1979.
47. Estes SA, Yang CW: Delayed pressure urticaria: an investigation of some parameters of lesion induction. *J Am Acad Dermatol* 5:25, 1981.
48. Feig PJ, Soter NA, Yuger HM, et al: Vasculitis with urticaria, hypocomplementemia, and multiple system involvement. *JAMA* 236:2065, 1976.
49. Fields T, Ghebrehiwet B, Kaplan AP: Kinin formation in hereditary angioedema plasma: evidence against kinin derivation from C2 and in support of "spontaneous" formation of bradykinin. *J Allergy Clin Immunol* 72:54, 1983.

50. Frank MM, Sergent JS, Kane MA, et al: Epsilon aminocaproic acid therapy of hereditary angioneurotic edema: a double blind study. *N Engl J Med* 286:808, 1972.
51. Gadek JE, Hosea SW, Gelfand JA, et al: Response of variant hereditary angioedema phenotypes of danazol therapy. *J Clin Invest* 64:280, 1979.
52. Gammon WR, Wheeler CE Jr: Urticarial vasculitis. *Arch Dermatol* 115:76, 1979.
53. Garofalo J, Kaplan AP: Histamine release and therapy of severe dermatographism. *J Allergy Clin Immunol* 68:103, 1981.
54. Geha RS, Quinti I, Austen KF, et al: Acquired C1-inhibitor deficiency associated with antiidiotypic antibody to monoclonal immunoglobulin. *N Engl J Med* 312:534, 1985.
55. Gelfand JA, Sherms RJ, Alling DW, et al: Treatment of hereditary angioedema with danazol; reversal of clinical and biochemical abnormalities. *N Engl J Med* 295:1444, 1976.
56. Ghebrehiwet B, Randazzo BP, Dunn JT, et al: Mechanism of activation of the classical pathway of complement by Hageman factor fragment. *J Clin Invest* 71:1450, 1983.
57. Ghebrehiwet B, Silverberg M, Kaplan AP: Activation of the classical pathway of complement by Hageman factor fragment (HFf). *J Exp Med* 153:665, 1981.
58. Gigli I, Mason JW, Coleman RW, et al: Interaction of plasma kallikrein with the C1 inhibitor. *J Immunol* 104:574, 1970.
59. Gigli I, Schothorst AA, Soter NA, et al: Erythropoietic protoporphyria: photoactivation of the complement system. *J Clin Invest* 66:517, 1980.
60. Gorevic P, Kaplan AP: The physical urticarias. *Int J Dermatol* 19:417, 1980.
61. Grant JA, Findlay JR, Thueson DO: Local heat urticaria/angioedema: evidence for histamine release without complement activation. *J Allergy Clin Immunol* 67:75, 1981.
62. Grant RT, Pearson RSB, Comeau WJ: Observations on urticaria provoked by emotion, by exercise, and by warming the body. *Clin Sci* 2:266, 1935.
63. Greaves MW: Histamine excretion and dermographism in urticaria pigmentosa before and after administration of a specific histidine-decarboxylase inhibitor. *Br J Dermatol* 85:467, 1971.
64. Greaves MW, Sundergoard J: Urticaria pigmentosa and factitious urticaria: direct evidence for release of histamine and other smooth muscle–contracting agents in dermographic skin. *Arch Dermatol* 101:418, 1970.
65. Grendel KE, Farr RS, Wanderer AA, et al: Association of platelet activating factor with primary acquired cold urticaria. *N Engl J Med* 313:405, 1985.
66. Gruber BL, Baeza M, Marchese M, et al: Prevalence and functional role of anti-IgE autoantibodies in urticarial syndromes. *J Invest Dermatol* 90:213, 1988.
67. Gruber BL, Marchese M, Ballan D, et al: Anti IgG autoantibodies: detection in urticarial syndromes and ability to release histamine from basophils. *J Allergy Clin Immunol* 77:187, 1986.
68. Guo C-B, Liu MC, Galli SJ, et al: Identification of IgE-bearing cells in the late-phase response to antigen in the lung as basophils. *Am J Respir Dis* 10:384, 1994.
69. Gorevic P: Cryopathies: Cryoglobulins and cryofibrinogenemia. In Samter's Immunologic Diseases, 5th edition. Vol II. Frank MM, Ansten KF, Claman HN, Unanue ER (eds). Little Brown and Co, Boston, 1995, pp 956–974.
70. Harber LC, Holloway RM, Sheatley VR, et al: Immunologic and biophysical studies in solar urticaria. *J Invest Dermatol* 41:439, 1963.
71. Hathaway WE, Belhausen LP, Hathaway HS: Evidence of a new plasma thromboplastin factor I: case report, coagulation studies and physiocochemical properties. *Br J Haematol* 26:521, 1965.
72. Hauptmann G, Lang JM, North ML, et al: Acquired C1 inhibitor deficiencies in lymphoproliferative diseases with serum immunoglobulin abnormalities. *Blut* 32:155, 1976.
73. Hauser DD, Arbesman CE, Ito K, et al: Cold urticaria: immunologic studies. *Am J Med* 49:23, 1970.
74. Hawk JLM, Eady RAJ, Challiner AVJ: Elevated blood histamine levels and mast cell degranulation in solar urticaria. *Br J Clin Pharmacol* 9:183, 1980.
75. Herxheimer A: The nervous pathway mediating cholinergic urticaria. *Clin Sci* 15:195, 1956.
76. Hide M, Francis DM, Grattan CEH, et al: Autoantibodies against the high-affinity IgE receptor as a cause of histamine release in chronic urticaria. *N Engl J Med* 328:1595, 1993.
77. Horton BT, Brown GE, Roth GM: Hypersensitivities to cold with local and systemic manifestations of a histamine-like character: its amenability to treatment. *JAMA* 107:1263, 1936.
78. Houston DP, Bressler RB, Kaliner M, et al: Prevention of mast-cell degranulation by ketotifen in patients with physical urticaria. *Ann Intern Med* 204:507, 1986.
79. Jaeger D, Kleinhaus D, Czuppon AB, et al: Latex-specific proteins causing immediate-type cutaneous, nasal, bronchial, and systemic reactions. *J Allergy Clin Immunol* 89:759, 1992.
80. Juhlin L, Michaelsson G: Vascular reactions in hereditary angioedema. *Acta Derm Venereol* 49:20, 1969.
81. Kalz F, Bower CM, Prichard H: Delayed and persistent dermographia. *Arch Dermatol* 61:772, 1950.
82. Kaplan AP: Unusual cold-induced disorders: cold dependent dermatographism and systemic cold urticaria. *J Allergy Clin Immunol* 73:453, 1984.
83. Kaplan AP, Austen KF: A prealbumin activator of prekallikrein II: derivation of activators of prekallikrein from active Hageman factor by digestion with plasmin. *J Exp Med* 133:696, 1971.
84. Kaplan AP, Garofalo J: Identification of a new physically induced urticaria: cold induced cholinergic urticaria. *J Allergy Clin Immunol* 68:438, 1981.
85. Kaplan AP, Garofalo J, Sigler R, et al: Idiopathic cold urticaria: in vitro demonstration of histamine release upon challenge of skin biopsies. *N Engl J Med* 305:1074, 1981.
86. Kaplan AP, Gray L, Snadt RE, et al: In vivo studies of mediator release in cold urticaria and cholinergic urticaria. *J Allergy Clin Immunol* 55:394, 1975.
87. Kaplan AP, Horakova Z, Katz SI: Assessment of tissue fluid histamine levels in patients with urticaria. *J Allergy Clin Immunol* 61:350, 1978.
88. Kaplan AP, Natbony SF, Tawil AP: Exercise-induced anaphylaxis as a manifestation of cholinergic urticaria. *J Allergy Clin Immunol* 68:319, 1981.
89. Keahey TM, Greaves MW: Cold urticaria: dissociation of cold-evoked histamine release and urticaria following cold challenge. *Arch Dermatol* 116:174, 1980.
90. Kennedy DD, Rosenthal FD, Sneddon IB: Amyloidosis presenting as urticaria. *Br Med J* 1:31, 1966.
91. Kern F, Lichtenstein LM: Defective histamine release in chronic urticaria. *J Clin Invest* 57:1360, 1977.
92. Kidd JM III, Cohen SH, Sosman AJ, et al: Food dependent exercise-induced anaphylaxis. *J Allergy Clin Immunol* 71:407, 1983.
93. Kirton V: Contact urticaria and cinnamic aldehyde. *Contact Dermatitis* 4:374, 1978.
94. Kivity S, Sneh E, Greif J, et al: The effect of food and exercise on the skin response to compound 48/80 in patients with food-associated exercise-induced urticaria-angioedema. *J Allergy Clin Immunol* 81:1155, 1987.
95. Klemperer MR, Donaldson VH, Rosen FS: The vasopermeability response in man to purified C1 esterase. *J Clin Invest* 47:604, 1968.
96. Kurtz AS, Kaplan AP: Regional expression of cold urticaria. *J Allergy Clin Immunol* 86:272, 1990.
97. Levine BB: Immunochemical mechanisms of penicillin allergy. *N Engl J Med* 275:1115, 1966.
98. Lewis J, Lieberman P, Treadwell G, et al: Exercise-induced urticaria, angioedema, and anaphylactoid episodes. *J Allergy Clin Immunol* 68:432, 1981.
99. Leznoff A, Josse RG, Denberg J, et al: Association of chronic urticaria and angioedema with thyroid autoimmunity. *Arch Dermatol* 119:636, 1983.
100. Leznoff A, Sussman GL: Syndrome of idiopathic chronic urticaria and angioedema with thyroid autoimmunity: a study of 90 patients. *J Allergy Clin Immunol* 84:66, 1989.
101. Lim HW, Perez HD, Poh-Fitzpatrick M: Generation of chemotactic activity in serum from patients with erythropoietic protoporphyria and porphyria cutanea tarda. *N Engl J Med* 304:212, 1981.
102. Lim HW, Poh-Fitzpatrick MB, Gigli I: Activation of the complement system in patients with porphyrias after irradiation in vivo. *J Clin Invest* 74:1961, 1984.
103. Ludivico CL, Myers AR, Maurer K: Hypocomplementemic urticarial vasculitis with glomerulonephritis and pseudotumor cerebri. *Arthritis Rheum* 22:1024, 1979.
104. Lundh B, Laurell A, Wetterqvist H, et al: A case of hereditary angioneurotic edema successfully treated with ε-aminocaproic acid. *Clin Exp Immunol* 3:733, 1968.
105. Mackle TJ, Wells M: Urticaria, deafness, and amyloidosis: a new heredo-familial syndrome. *Q J Med* 31:235, 1962.

106. Mahzoon S, Yamamoto S, Greaves MW: Response of skin to ammonium persulphate. *Acta Derm Venereol* 57:125, 1977.
107. Malbran A, Hammer CH, Frank MM, et al: Acquired angioedema: observations on the mechanism of action of autoantibodies directed against C1 esterase inhibitor. *J Allergy Clin Immunol* 81:1199, 1988.
108. Marder RJ, Rent R, Choi EYC, et al: C1q deficiency associated with urticaria-like lesions and cutaneous vasculitis. *Am J Med* 61:560, 1976.
109. Mathews KP: Urticaria and angioedema. *J Allergy Clin Immunol* 72:11, 1983.
110. Mathison DA, Arroyave CM, Bhat KN, et al: Hypocomplementemia in chronic idiopathic urticaria. *Ann Intern Med* 86:534, 1977.
111. Maulitz RM, Pratt DS, Schocket AL: Exercise-induced anaphylactic reaction to shellfish. *J Allergy Clin Immunol* 63:433, 1979.
112. McDuffie FC, Sams W Jr, Maldonado JE: Hypocomplementemia with cutaneous vasculitis and arthritis: possible immune complex syndrome. *Mayo Clin Proc* 48:340, 1973.
113. Mekori YA, Giorno RC, Anderson P, et al: Lymphocyte subpopulations in the skin of patients with chronic urticaria. *J Allergy Clin Immunol* 72:681, 1983.
114. Metzger WJ, Kaplan AP, Beaven MA: Hereditary vibratory angioedema: confirmation of histamine release in a type of physical hypersensitivity. *J Allergy Clin Immunol* 57:605, 1976.
115. Michaelsson G, Ros A: Familial localized heat urticaria of delayed type. *Acta Derm Venereol* 51:279, 1971.
116. Monroe EW, Schulz CI, Maize JC, et al: Vasculitis in chronic urticaria: an immunopathologic study. *J Invest Dermatol* 76:103, 1981.
117. Moore-Robinson M, Warin KP: Some clinical aspects of cholinergic urticaria. *Br J Dermatol* 80:794, 1968.
118. Moorthy AV, Pringle D: Urticaria, vasculitis, hypocomplementemia, and immune complex glomerulonephritis. *Arch Pathol Lab Med* 106:68, 1982.
119. Gorevic P: Cryopathies: Cryoglobulins and cryofibrinogenemia. In Samter's Immunologic Diseases, 5th edition. Vol II. Frank MM, Ansten KF, Claman HN, Unanue ER (eds). Little Brown and Co, Boston, 1995, pp 956–974.
120. Moshell AN, Bjornson L: Protection in erythropoietic protoporphyria: mechanism of protection by β carotene. *J Invest Dermatol* 68:157, 1977.
121. Moss RB: Sensitization to aztreonam and cross-reactivity with other beta-lactam antibiotics in high-risk patients with cystic fibrosis. *J Allergy Clin Immunol* 87:78, 1990.
122. Natbony SF, Phillips ME, Elias JM, et al: Histologic studies of chronic idiopathic urticaria. *J Allergy Clin Immunol* 71:177, 1983.
123. Newcomb RW, Nelson H: Dermographism mediated by IgE. *Am J Med* 54:174, 1973.
124. Novey HS, Fairshter RD, Salness K, et al: Postprandial exercise-induced anaphylaxis. *J Allergy Clin Immunol* 71:498, 1983.
125. Odom RB, Maibach HI: Contact urticaria: a different contact dermatitis. *Cutis* 18:672, 1976.
126. Ormerod AD, Kobza-Black A, Dawes J, et al: Prostaglandin D_2 and histamine release in cold urticaria unaccompanied by evidence of platelet activation. *J Allergy Clin Immunol* 82:586, 1988.
127. Ormerod AD, Kobza-Black A, Milford-Ward A, et al: Combined cold urticaria and cholinergic urticaria—clinical characterization and laboratory findings. *Br J Dermatol* 118:621, 1988.
128. Parrillo JE, Lawley TJ, Frank MM: Immunologic reactivity in the hypereosinophil syndrome. *J Allergy Clin Immunol* 64:113, 1979.
129. Patterson R, Mellies CJ, Blankenship ML, et al: Vibratory angioedema: a hereditary type of physical hypersensitivity. *J Allergy Clin Immunol* 50:174, 1972.
130. Paver WK: Discoid and subacute systemic lupus erythematosus associated with urticaria. *Aust J Dermatol* 12:113, 1971.
131. Pearson KD, Buchignani JS, Shimkin PM, et al: Hereditary angioneurotic edema of the gastrointestinal tract. *Am J Roentgenol Radium Ther Nucl Med* 116:256, 1972.
132. Peters MS, Schroeter AL, Kephart GM, et al: Localization of eosinophil granule major basic protein in chronic urticaria. *J Invest Dermatol* 81:39, 1983.
133. Petillo JJ, Natbony SK, Zisblatt M, et al: Preliminary report of the effects of tiaramide on the ice cube test in patients with idiopathic cold urticaria. *Ann Allergy* 51:511, 1983.
134. Phanuphak P, Kohler PF, Stanford RE, et al: Vasculitis in chronic urticaria. *J Allergy Clin Immunol* 65:436, 1980.
135. Phanuphak P, Schocket AL, Arroyave CM, et al: Skin histamine in chronic urticaria. *J Allergy Clin Immunol* 65:371, 1980.
136. Provost TT, Zone JJ, Synkowski D, et al: Unusual clinical manifestations of systemic lupus erythematosus. I. Urticaria-like lesions: correlations with clinical and serological abnormalities. *J Invest Dermatol* 75:495, 1980.
137. Quastel M, Harrison R, Cicardi M, et al: Behavior in vivo of normal and dysfunctional C1 inhibitor in normal subjects and patients with hereditary angioedema. *J Clin Invest* 71:1041, 1983.
138. Ratnoff OD, Naff GB: The conversion of C'1S to C'1 esterase by plasmin and trypsin. *J Exp Med* 125:337, 1967.
139. Reshef A, Kagey-Sobotka A, Adkinson NF Jr, et al: The pattern and kinetics in human skin of erythema and mediators during the acute and late-phase response (LPR). *J Allergy Clin Immunol* 84:678, 1989.
140. Rieder MJ, Uetrecht J, Shear NH, et al: Diagnosis of sulfonamide hypersensitivity reactions by in-vitro "rechallenge" with hydroxylamine metabolites. *Ann Intern Med* 110:286, 1989.
141. Roberts LJ II, Sweetman BJ, Lewis RA: Increased production of prostaglandin D_2 in patients with systemic mastocytosis. *N Engl J Med* 303:1400, 1980.
142. Rose B: Studies on blood histamine in cases of allergy. I. Blood histamine during wheal formation. *J Allergy* 12:327, 1941.
143. Rosen FS, Alper CA, Pensky J, et al: Genetic heterogeneity of the C1 esterase inhibitor in patients with hereditary angioneurotic edema. *J Clin Invest* 50:2143, 1971.
144. Roth GJ, Stanford N, Majerus PW: Acetylation of prostaglandin synthase by aspirin. *Proc Natl Acad Sci USA* 72:3073, 1975.
145. Ruddy S, Gigli I, Sheffer AL, et al: The laboratory diagnosis of hereditary angioedema. In Rose B, et al (eds): *Allergology: Proceedings of the Sixth International Congress of Allergology.* Excerpta Medica, Amsterdam, 1968.
146. Ryan TJ, Shim-Young N, Turk JL: Delayed pressure urticaria. *Br J Dermatol* 80:485, 1968.
147. Sams WM Jr, Epstein JH, Winkelmann RK: Solar urticaria: investigation of pathogenic mechanisms. *Arch Dermatol* 99:390, 1969.
148. Samter M, Beers RF Jr: Concerning the nature of intolerance to aspirin. *J Allergy* 40:281, 1967.
149. Saurat J-H, Schifferli J, Steiger G, et al: Anti-interleukin-1α autoantibodies in humans: characterization, isotype distribution, and receptor-binding inhibition—higher frequency in Schnitzler's syndrome (urticaria and macroglobulinemia). *J Allergy Clin Immunol* 88:244, 1991.
150. Schapira M, Silver LD, Scott CF, et al: Prekallikrein activation and high molecular weight kininogen consumption in hereditary angioedema. *N Engl J Med* 308:1050, 1983.
151. Schreiber RD, Kaplan AP, Austen KF: Inhibition by C1 INH of Hageman factor fragment activation of coagulation, fibrinolysis, and kinin generation. *J Clin Invest* 52:1402, 1973.
152. Schreiber RD, Zweiman B, Atkins P, et al: Acquired angioedema with lymphoproliferative disorder: association of C1 inhibitor deficiency with cellular abnormality. *Blood* 48:567, 1976.
153. Shaffer B, Jacobsone Pori PP: Papular urticaria and its relationships to insect allergy. *Ann Allergy* 10:411, 1952.
154. Shalit M, Schwartz LB, vonAllmen C, et al: Release of histamine and tryptase during cutaneous and interrupted cutaneous challenge with allergen in humans. *J Allergy Clin Immunol* 86:117, 1990.
155. Sheffer AL, Austen KF: Exercise-induced anaphylaxis. *J Allergy Clin Immunol* 66:106, 1980.
156. Sheffer AL, Austen KF, Rosen FS: Tranexamic acid therapy in hereditary angioneurotic edema. *N Engl J Med* 287:452, 1972.
157. Sheffer AL, Craig JM, Willms-Kretschmer K: Histopathological and ultrastructural observations on tissues from patients with hereditary angioneurotic edema. *J Allergy* 47:292, 1971.
158. Sheffer AL, Fearon DT, Austen KF: Clinical and biochemical effects of stanozolol therapy for hereditary angioedema. *J Allergy Clin Immunol* 68:181, 1981.
159. Sheffer AL, Fearon DT, Austen KF: Hereditary angioedema: a decade of management with stanozolol. *J Allergy Clin Immunol* 80:855, 1987.
160. Sheffer AL, Fonferko EB, Murphy GF, et al: Ultrastructural changes of cutaneous mast cells (MC) in response to defined stimuli of the physical allergy class. *J Allergy Clin Immunol* 75:114, 1985.
161. Sheffer AL, Soter NA, McFadden ER Jr, et al: Exercise-induced anaphylaxis: a distinct form of physical allergy. *J Allergy Clin Immunol* 71:311, 1983.
162. Shelley WB, Shelley CD, Ho AKS: Cholinergic urticaria: acetylcholine-receptor dependent immediate-type hypersensitivity reaction to copper. *Lancet* 1:843, 1983.
163. Sigler RW, Evans R III, Horakova Z: The role of cyproheptadine in the treatment of cold urticaria. *J Allergy Clin Immunol* 65:309, 1980.

164. Sigler RW, Levinson AI, Evans R III, et al: Evaluation of a patient with cold and cholinergic urticaria. *J Allergy Clin Immunol* 63:35, 1979.
165. Sissons JGF, Williams DG, Peters KK, et al: Skin lesions, angioedema, and hypocomplementemia. *Lancet* 2:1350, 1974.
166. Skriver K, Radziejewska E, Silbermann JA, et al: CpG mutations in the reactive site of human C1 inhibitor. *J Biol Chem* 264:3066, 1989.
167. Smith JA, Mansfield LE, Fokakis A, et al: Dermographism caused by IgE mediated penicillin allergy. *Ann Allergy* 57:30, 1983.
168. Solley GO, Gleich GJ, Jordan RE, et al: The late phase of the immediate wheal and flare skin reaction: its dependence upon IgE antibodies. *J Clin Invest* 58:408, 1976.
169. Soter NA, Austen KF, Gigli I: Inhibition by ε-aminocaproic acid of the activation of the first component of the complement system. *J Immunol* 114:928, 1975.
170. Soter NA, Austen KF, Gigli I: Urticaria and arthralgias as a manifestation of necrotizing angiitis. *J Invest Dermatol* 63:489, 1974.
171. Soter NA, Mihm MC Jr, Dvorak HF, et al: Cutaneous necrotizing venulitis: a sequential analysis of the morphological alterations occurring after mast cell degranulation in a patient with a unique syndrome. *Clin Exp Immunol* 32:46, 1978.
172. Soter NA, Mihm MC Jr, Gigli I, et al: Two distinct cellular patterns in cutaneous necrotizing angiitis. *J Invest Dermatol* 66:334, 1976.
173. Soter NA, Wasserman SI: Physical urticaria/angioedema: an experimental model of mast cell activation in humans. *J Allergy Clin Immunol* 66:358, 1980.
174. Soter NA, Wasserman SI, Austen KF: Cold urticaria: release into the circulation of histamine and eosinophil chemotactic factor of anaphylaxis during cold challenge. *N Engl J Med* 294:687, 1976.
175. Soter NA, Wasserman SI, Austen KF, et al: Release of mast-cell mediators and alterations in lung function in patients with cholinergic urticaria. *N Engl J Med* 302:604, 1980.
176. Soter NA, Wasserman SI, Pathak MA: Solar urticaria: release of mast cell mediators into the circulation after experimental challenge. *J Invest Dermatol* 72:283, 1979.
177. Soter NA, Joski NP, Twarog FJ: Delayed cold-induced urticaria: a dominantly inherited disorder. *J Allergy Clin Immunol* 54:294, 1977.
178. Strang CJ, Cholin S, Spragg J, et al: Angioedema induced by a peptide derived from complement component C2. *J Exp Med* 168:1685, 1988.
179. Talamo RC, Haber E, Austen KF: A radioimmunoassay for bradykinin in plasma and synovial fluid. *J Lab Clin Med* 74:816, 1969.
180. Tennenbaum JT, Lowney E: Localized heat and cold urticaria. *J Allergy Clin Immunol* 51:57, 1973.
181. Thoburin R, Johnson JE III, Cliff LE: Studies on the epidemiology of adverse drug reactions. IV. The relationship of cephalothin and penicillin allergy. *JAMA* 198:315, 1966.
182. Tindall JP, Beeker SK, Rosse NF: Familial cold urticaria: a generalized reaction involving leucocytosis. *Arch Intern Med* 124:129, 1969.
183. Ting S, Mansfield LE: Localized cold reflex urticaria. *J Allergy Clin Immunol* 75:421, 1985.
184. Ting S, Reiman BEF, Rauls DO, et al: On familial vibration-induced angioedema. *J Allergy Clin Immunol* 71:546, 1983.
185. Tromovitch TA: Urticaria from contact with water. *Calif Med* 106:400, 1967.
186. Udassin R, Harari Z, Shoenfeld Y, et al: Cholinergic urticaria—a seasonal disease. *Arch Intern Med* 141:1029, 1981.
187. Vane JR: Inhibition of prostaglandin synthesis as a mechanism of action for aspirin-like drugs. *Nature (New Biol)* 231:232, 1971.
188. Waldbott GL, Merkle K: Urticaria due to pollen. *Ann Allergy* 10:30, 1952.
189. Wanderer AA, Ellis EF: Treatment of cold urticaria with cyproheptadine. *J Allergy Clin Immunol* 48:366, 1971.
190. Wanderer AA, Maselli R, Ellis EF, et al: Immunologic characterization of serum factors responsible for cold urticaria. *J Allergy Clin Immunol* 48:13, 1971.
191. Wanderer AA, Nuss DP, Tormey AD, et al: Urticarial leukocytoclastic vasculitis with cold urticaria: report of a case and review of the literature. *Arch Dermatol* 119:145, 1983.
192. Wanderer AA, St. Pierre JP, Ellis EF: Primary acquired cold urticaria and double blind comparative study of treatment with cyproheptadine, chlorpheniramine, and placebo. *Arch Dermatol* 131:1375, 1977.
193. Warin AP, Greaves MW, Gatecliff M, et al: Treatment of hereditary angioedema by low-dose attenuated androgens: dissociation of clinical response from levels of C1 esterase inhibitor and C4. *Br J Dermatol* 103:405, 1980.
194. Wasserman SI, Austen KF, Soter NA: The functional and physicochemical characterization of three eosinophilotactic activities released into the circulation by cold challenge of patients with cold urticaria. *Clin Exp Immunol* 47:570, 1982.
195. Wasserman SI, Soter NA, Center DM, et al: Cold urticaria: recognition and characterization of a neutrophil chemotactic factor which appears in serum during experimental cold challenge. *J Clin Invest* 60:189, 1977.
196. Webb DR, Pearsall HR, Sumida SE: Depression of third component of complement (C3) in chronic angioedema (abstract). *J Allergy Clin Immunol* 55:106, 1975.
197. Weiner MH, Metzger J, Simon RA: Occupationally acquired vibratory angioedema with secondary carpal tunnel syndrome. *Ann Intern Med* 98:44, 1983.
198. Wisnieski JJ, Naff GB: Serum IgG antibodies to C1q in hypocomplementemic urticarial vasculitis syndrome. *Arthritis Rheum* 32:1119, 1989.
199. Wuepper KD, Bokisch VA, Muller-Eberhard HJ, et al: Cutaneous responses to human C3a anaphylatoxin in man. *Clin Exp Immunol* 11:13, 1972.
200. Zeiss CR, Burch FX, Marder RJ: A hypocomplementemic vasculitis urticarial syndrome: report of four new cases and definition of the disease. *Am J Med* 68:867, 1980.
201. Zuraw BL, Curd JG: Demonstration of modified inactive first component of complement (C1) inhibitor in the plasmas of C1 inhibitor deficient patients. *J Clin Invest* 78:567, 1986.
202. Zuraw BL, Sugimoto S, Curd JG: The value of rocket immunoelectrophoresis for C4 activation in the evaluation of patients with angioedema or C1-inhibitor deficiency. *J Allergy Clin Immunol* 78:1115, 1986.

36 Atopic Dermatitis, Contact Dermatitis, and Photoallergic Reactions

LEONARD KRISTAL RICHARD A. F. CLARK RICHARD KALISH

ATOPIC DERMATITIS

LEONARD KRISTAL RICHARD A. F. CLARK

The term *atopic dermatitis* was coined by Wise and Sulzberger[16] in 1933 to name an eruption, previously described by Besnier,[5] that was associated with a family history of other atopic diseases, namely asthma and allergic rhinitis. Atopic dermatitis is characterized by a pruritic eruption that follows a chronically relapsing course, with a tendency to involve specific body areas according to the age of the patient. There is usually a family history of atopy in patients affected by the condition. The etiology is unknown, although it appears to be influenced by a complex interaction of genetic factors, immune dysregulation, environmental factors, and defects in the skin's permeability barrier.

EPIDEMIOLOGY

The prevalence of atopic dermatitis has been increasing over the last three decades.[73, 142, 157] Whereas studies from the 1930s through the 1950s revealed that 2% to 3% of children had atopic dermatitis,[34, 131, 152] later epidemiologic studies have shown that the incidence of atopic dermatitis is 9% to 12% in childhood,[71, 72] with 80% to 90% of patients developing the disease before the age of 7 years.[108] A 1994 study evaluating the prevalence of atopic dermatitis in the general community found a lifetime prevalence of 20% in children aged 3 to 11 years.[65] In 60% of these children, the condition developed in the first year of life; 75% of these developed it by 6 months of age.[65] Monozygotic twins have a significantly greater pairwise concordance rate of atopic dermatitis than dizygotic twins and nontwin siblings, thereby supporting the involvement of genetic factors in atopic dermatitis.[71] The linkage of genes on chromosome 11q13 to atopic dermatitis is under investigation.[20, 126]

The frequency of atopic diseases in first-degree relatives of patients with atopic dermatitis ranges between 43% and 73%.[30] When both parents suffer from an atopic disease, there is a risk as high as 72% that their child will have an atopic disease as well.[30]

Vickers[152] found that only about 10% of children with atopic dermatitis in childhood develop persistent dermatitis into adulthood. Yet as many as 83% of patients with severe dermatitis in childhood have persistent disease as adults.[11, 113, 117]

CLINICAL MANIFESTATIONS

The diagnosis of atopic dermatitis is based upon a set of diagnostic criteria derived by Hanifin and Rajka (Table 36–1)[52]. Although these criteria have become a diagnostic standard, attempts have been made to modify them by looking at the relevance of the individual criteria (Table 36–2).[29, 139] A study in Britain attempted to validate the criteria and recommended new diagnostic guidelines for the diagnosis of atopic dermatitis on the basis of the original criteria (Table 36–3).[158–160]

Atopic dermatitis can manifest as acute, subacute, or chronic skin changes. Acute lesions are characterized by erythematous papules, papulovesicles, or weeping skin lesions. Subacute lesions are characterized by ill-defined erythematous, scaling papules and plaques. Chronic changes consist of skin thickening manifested by increased skin markings and hyperpigmentation, known as *lichenification.* Excoriations may be present in all three stages. Patients may present with acute, subacute, or chronic skin changes or may have two or three of these changes superimposed upon one another at one time. A patient with lichenified lesions may undergo an exacerbation and develop acute and/or subacute dermatitis as well.

Atopic dermatitis skin lesions vary in location with the age of the patient. In infancy, the rash is concentrated on the scalp, face, and extensor surfaces of the extremities. Changes of acute dermatitis are seen on the face, especially on the cheeks and chin. Localization to these areas in early infancy may result from rubbing of the face into the sheets and in later infancy from irritation by the saliva associated with drooling. Infra-auricular eczematous changes known as "infra-auricular fissures" are also commonly seen at this age. Although they are not listed as a criteria for atopic dermatitis, one study found them to be present in more than 80% of

TABLE 36–1
DIAGNOSTIC FEATURES OF ATOPIC DERMATITIS

Major Features (must have 3 or more)	Minor Features (must also have 3 or more)
Pruritus Typical morphology and distribution Flexural lichenification or hyperlinearity in adults Facial and extensor involvement in infants and children Chronic or chronically relapsing course Personal or family history of atopy (asthma, allergic rhinitis, or atopic dermatitis)	Xerosis Ichthyosis/palmar hyperlinearity/keratosis pilaris Immediate (type I) skin test reactivity Elevated serum IgE Early age of onset Tendency toward cutaneous infections/impaired cell-mediated immunity Tendency toward nonspecific hand or foot dermatitis Nipple eczema Cheilitis Recurrent conjunctivitis Dennie-Morgan infraorbital fold Keratoconus Anterior subcapsular cataracts Orbital darkening Facial pallor/facial erythema Pityriasis alba Itch when sweating Intolerance to wool and lipid solvents Perifollicular accentuation Food hypersensitivity Course influenced by environmental/emotional factors White dermographism/delayed blanch

Adapted from Hanifin JM, Rajka G: Diagnostic features of atopic dermatitis. Acta Derm Venereol Suppl (Stockh) 92:44–47, 1980.

patients with atopic dermatitis and in 98% of patients with severe dermatitis.[140] Truncal involvement is usually present in infancy, although the diaper area is generally spared owing to the occlusive hydrating of wearing diapers. Children of school age tend to develop involvement of the lower buttocks and posterior thighs. Cheilitis is common as well and is exacerbated by recurrent lip licking, especially in the wintertime. In older children and adults, the eruption is concentrated in flexural areas such as the neck, flexural trunk, antecubital and popliteal fossae, wrists, and ankles (Fig. 36–1). Young women may present with nipple dermatitis, an uncommon but specific finding in atopic dermatitis. Older

TABLE 36–2
MODIFIED CRITERIA FOR DIAGNOSIS OF ATOPIC DERMATITIS IN INFANTS

Major features	Family history of atopic disease Typical facial or extensor eczematous or lichenified dermatitis Evidence of pruritus
Minor features	Xerosis, ichthyosis, hyperlinear palms Perifollicular accentuation Postauricular fissures Chronic scalp scaling

Adapted from Seymour JL, Keswick BH, Hanifin JM, et al: Clinical effects of diaper types on the skin of normal infants and infants with atopic dermatitis. J Am Acad Dermatol 17:988–997, 1987.

TABLE 36–3
NEWLY PROPOSED DIAGNOSTIC GUIDELINES OF ATOPIC ECZEMA

Must have	An itchy skin condition (or parental report of scratching or rubbing in a child).
Plus 3 or more of the following	History of involvement of the skin creases such as folds of elbows, behind the knees, fronts of ankles or around the neck (including cheeks in children younger than 10 years). A personal history of asthma or hay fever (or history of atopic disease in a first-degree relative in children younger than 4 years). A history of a general dry skin in the last year. Visible flexural eczema (or eczema involving the cheeks/forehead and outer limbs in children younger than 4 years). Onset before the age of 2 years (not used if child is younger than 4 years).

Adapted from Williams HC, Burney PJG, Pembroke AC, et al: The U.K. Working Party's Diagnostic Criteria for Atopic Dermatitis III: independent hospital validation. Br J Dermatol 131:406–416, 1994.

patients who also have extensor involvement tend to have a poorer prognosis.[152]

The hands and feet are commonly involved in children with atopic dermatitis. Involvement of the hands in childhood is a significant factor for the development of adult hand dermatitis.[116] The nails may be dystrophic, with ridging and coarse pitting. Atopic dermatitis involving the feet tends to be worse in winter, although many patients have flares in the summer in association with swimming in chlorinated pools.

Patients with atopic dermatitis tend to have xerosis, or dry skin. Xerosis is associated with reduced water-binding capacity, increased transepidermal water loss, and decreased water content.[83] Atopic dermatitis is also associated with hyperlinear palms and soles[90, 142] (Fig. 36–2) as well as keratosis pilaris, a condition characterized by hyperkeratotic follicular papules located on the extensor surfaces of the arms, thighs, and buttocks. Hyperlinear palms and soles and keratosis pilaris are also found in patients with ichthyosis vulgaris.

Postinflammatory pigmentary changes consisting of either hypopigmentation or hyperpigmentation commonly develop in patients with atopic dermatitis. These pigmentary changes are usually transient and generally resolve months after the dermatitis is brought under control. Pityriasis alba, a condition characterized by hypopigmented scaly patches located on the cheeks, upper arms, or shoulders, is also commonly seen[162] (Fig. 36–3). The condition is more pronounced in the summer months, when the surrounding areas of skin tan and the involved areas do not. Pityriasis alba is also seen in patients without atopic dermatitis.

Pruritus is a major factor in atopic dermatitis. The pruritus can be present throughout the day but is usually worse in the evening and at night. Whereas older infants and children are able to express their itching verbally or by scratching, the young infant is unable to do so. Coordinated itch-scratch does not appear until the age of about 3 months, although before this age, parents may note irritability in the affected infant. Many authorities believe that the eruption in atopic dermatitis is secondary to scratching and that there is no primary lesion, yet it is noteworthy that the rash occurs in

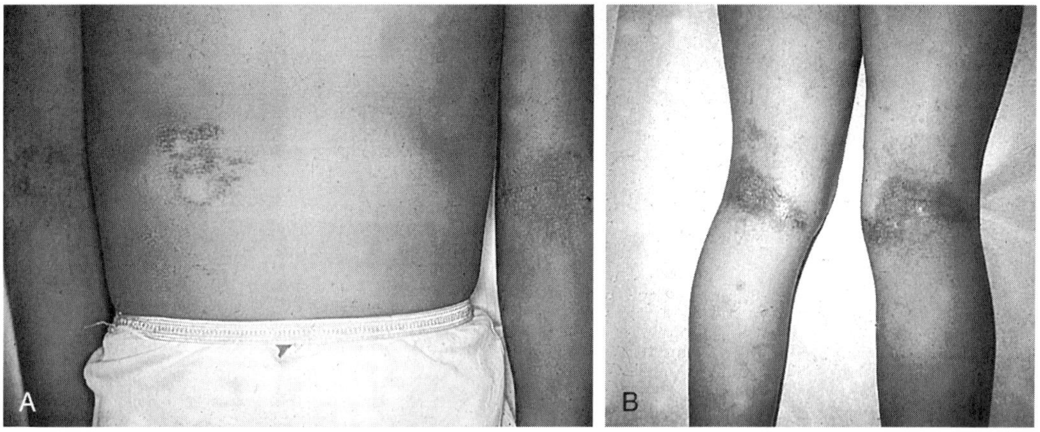

FIGURE 36–1. Distribution of atopic dermatitis lesions in an older child. **(A)** Subacute eczema patches of the antecubital fossa and flexural trunk area. **(B)** Subacute eczema of the popliteal fossae.

very young infants who clearly do not have coordinated itch-scratch mechanisms.

On rare occasions, patients with atopic dermatitis may progress to develop an exfoliative erythroderma. These patients develop generalized erythema and scaling accompanied by fever and lymphadenopathy. Patients with an exfoliative erythroderma are at risk for increased fluid losses, high-output cardiac failure, heat loss secondary to cutaneous vasodilation, and protein depletion.

OCULAR CHANGES

The incidence of ocular complications in atopic dermatitis varies, with estimates as high as 40%.[43, 111] The eyes in patients with atopic dermatitis may present with changes that are more common but not limited to patients with the condition as well as changes that are a direct result of the disease or of complications secondary to treatment. Atopic dermatitis may involve the eyelids, conjunctiva, cornea, or retina. Associated conditions include eyelid dermatitis, keratoconjunctivitis, keratoconus, anterior and posterior subcapsular cataract (Fig. 36–4), retinal detachment, and ocular herpes simplex.

Periorbital darkening, also known as "allergic shiners," is one of the minor criteria for atopic dermatitis that is also seen in patients without the condition. The darkening appears be caused by chronic edema, lichenification, and postinflammatory hyperpigmentation. The Dennie-Morgan fold, clinically seen as a single or double infraorbital fold, has been the subject of many studies to determine its significance as a marker for atopic dermatitis. The studies vary in their results, with some finding an increased incidence[88, 106, 139] and others finding no difference in incidence between patients with atopic dermatitis and controls.[89] Uehara[145] found that the fold can develop when the lower eyelid is subjected to an eczematous dermatitis of many different causes. Loss of the lateral eyebrow, known as Hertoghe's sign, may occur secondary to habitual rubbing.[106]

Keratoconus, or cone-shaped cornea, is another ophthalmologic complication found in 0.5%[9] to 6.7%[39] of patients with atopic dermatitis. Excessive eye rubbing in atopic dermatitis may result in a thinned cornea that then takes on a cone-shaped appearance, which can result in significant visual impairment. Severe cases may require a corneal transplant.[102]

Cataracts can occur in patients with atopic dermatitis and

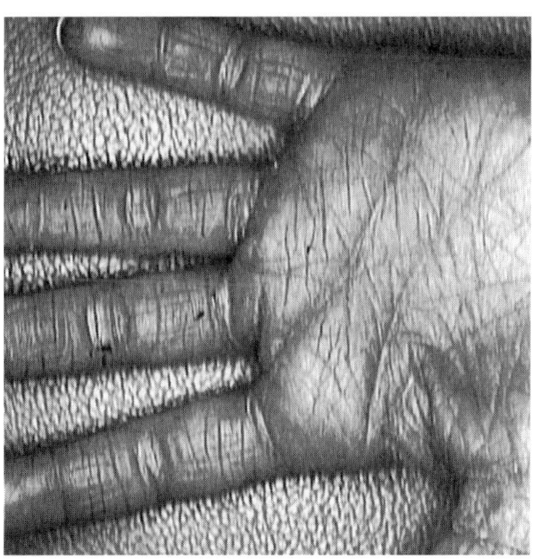

FIGURE 36–2. Hyperlinear palms of a patient with atopic dermatitis.

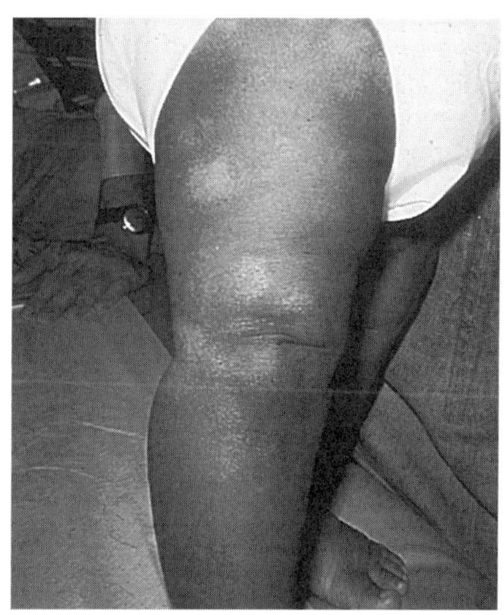

FIGURE 36–3. Pityriasis alba on the anterior thigh of a patient with atopic dermatitis.

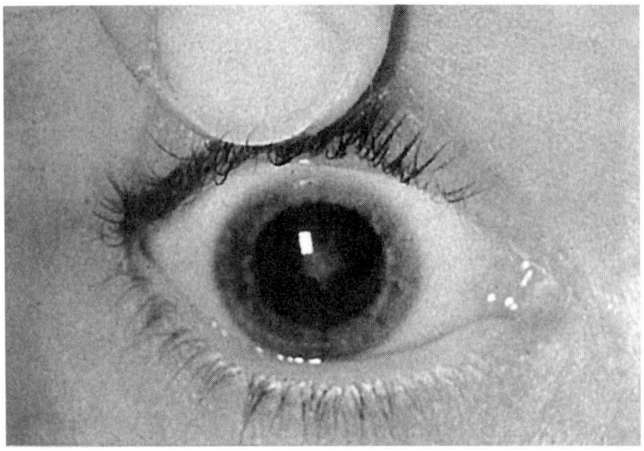

FIGURE 36–4. Anterior cataract of a patient with atopic dermatitis.

are either of the anterior or posterior subcapsular types. Earlier studies revealed a prevalence of cataracts in atopic dermatitis as high as 21%,[63] although later studies have shown the rate to be in 0%[15] to 12%.[146] Anterior subcapsular cataracts tend to occur in younger patients, usually between the ages of 15 and 25 years. Once they develop, they may mature rapidly.[2] Posterior subcapsular cataract formation may result from use of systemic steroids or topical steroids around the eye.[13] Patients with atopic dermatitis are at higher risk of retinal detachment, which may be secondary to self-inflicted ocular contusion by tapping the eyes.[101]

INFECTIONS

BACTERIAL INFECTIONS

Secondary bacterial infection is common in patients with atopic dermatitis. *Staphylococcus aureus* colonizes the skin in more than 95% of patients with atopic dermatitis and is found in higher concentrations in areas of active dermatitis.[82] The patient may present with what appears to be an acute, worsening dermatitis that is not responding to previously successful measures. In addition, small superficial pustules and crusted, weeping skin lesions should be sought (Fig. 36–5). Although these patients are colonized with *S. aureus,* they do not appear to be at increased risk of deeper cutaneous or systemic infection with the organism. There is excellent clinical response to treatment with antistaphylococcal medication, but treatment usually does not eradicate the staphylococcal colonization.

VIRAL INFECTIONS

Patients with atopic dermatitis are at an increased risk of developing viral infections such as herpes simplex, molluscum contagiosum, and, possibly, warts secondary to breaks in their skin.

Herpes simplex infection in these patients may spread locally and possibly become generalized, a condition known as eczema herpeticum or Kaposi's varicelliform eruption. Younger patients may have a toxic appearance and are at risk for systemic involvement. The eruption manifests clinically as vesicopustules that become umbilicated and then at times hemorrhagic. Umbilicated lesions should be sought in patients who have pustules that are not responding to appropriate antibacterial therapy. Lesions occurring on the face can spread to involve an entire side of the face, mimicking herpes zoster. Patients with lesions around the eye should be referred for an ophthalmologic examination to rule out ocular involvement. Herpes simplex infections are generally self-limited, although the patients improve markedly and rapidly from treatment with oral acyclovir.

A 1993 study does not find an increased risk of viral warts in patients with atopic dermatitis.[156] Warts and molluscum contagiosum in patients with atopic dermatitis may be more difficult to treat and more widespread. Patients with molluscum contagiosum may develop an eczematous dermatitis surrounding the molluscum lesions.

FUNGAL INFECTIONS

In atopic dermatitis, there is an increased susceptibility to chronic dermatophyte infections, especially of the hands and feet, caused by *Trichophyton rubrum.*[53, 57] As noted previously for bacterial and viral infections, fungal infections are capable of initiating flares of atopic dermatitis. Patients with persistent areas of dermatitis that is unresponsive to aggressive topical therapy should be evaluated for the presence of a fungal infection. Dermatophytes thrive in a milieu of topical steroids, and fungal infections may present atypically in areas treated with topical steroids, a condition known as *tinea incognito. Pityrosporum ovale* may cause flares of head and neck dermatitis.[138] Treatment with ketoconazole has improved flares of head and neck dermatitis in some patients.[18]

TRIGGERING FACTORS

IRRITANTS

The dry, sensitive skin in patients with atopic dermatitis is easily irritated by exposure to fabrics made of wool and

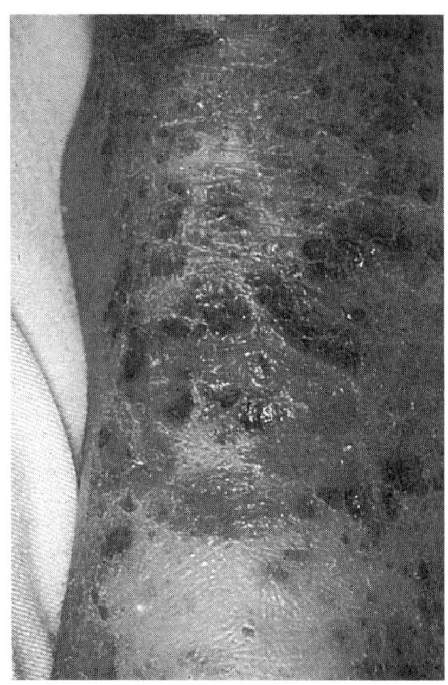

FIGURE 36–5. Impetiginous atopic eczema of the ankle with erosions and dark honey-colored crusts.

nylon as well as to soaps and solvents. Adults with atopic dermatitis are at increased risk of developing hand dermatitis and are more susceptible to occupational irritants.[70] The use of soaps with minimal defatting activity and a neutral pH should be used. Affected patients, especially those with dermatitis of the hands, should avoid jobs that require exposure to irritants and frequent hand washing.

Sweating may cause itching, leading to eczematous skin changes in patients with atopic dermatitis. There may be increased sweat production in these patients,[108] although the mechanism causing the pruritus is unknown. Patients should try to work and live in surroundings that minimize sweating and in which constant temperature and humidity are maintained. There is great variability among patients with regard to the effects of weather on their skin conditions. Some patients experience flares of dermatitis during the cold, dry winter months, whereas others have flares during the spring, autumn, or summer months. Some of this variation may be attributable to aeroallergen sensitivity to pollens[16] (also see later). During the summer months, some patients may experience flares of dermatitis owing to sun exposure, a condition known as *actinic prurigo*.[40]

ALLERGENS

As noted previously, there seems to be a relationship between sensitization to aeroallergens and exacerbation of atopic dermatitis. In cases where aeroallergen sensitivity is suspected, efforts to reduce exposure to the antigen should be instituted. Dust mite control measures include encasement of pillows and mattresses in plastic. Classic hyposensitization is not an established therapeutic intervention to minimize dermatitis in patients with known allergen sensitivity.[44, 65, 99]

When positive results of double-blind food challenges implicate food allergies as causal factors in the exacerbation of atopic dermatitis, the avoidance of those foods can be beneficial to the patients. It is important to avoid restrictive diets that can possibly lead to malnutrition.

A history of pet exposure or recent pet acquisition should be sought from patients with flaring or recalcitrant dermatitis, because pet dander can cause flares of dermatitis.[16, 17] Contact allergic reactions to topical agents should be considered in patients showing no response to appropriate therapy or having flares on therapy.[26]

INFECTION

Infectious agents commonly cause flares of atopic dermatitis. *Staphylococcus aureus* is the most common organism responsible for flares in affected patients. Viral or fungal infections should be ruled out in patients with flares or whose dermatitis is difficult to control. Localized areas of recalcitrant dermatitis may reveal a dermatophyte infection.

STRESS

Psychologic factors, such as stress, frustration, and anxiety, can lead to itching and scratching that exacerbate the dermatitis.[35, 42] The chronicity of the condition as well as poor therapeutic response in a child with atopic dermatitis can cause frustration and anxiety, leading to dysfunctional parent-child relationships.[69] Nighttime pruritus can lead to sleep deprivation in both parent and child, contributing to the psychologic stress.[164] Physicians should be aware of the psychosocial factors that can interfere with the effective therapy of their patients with severe atopic dermatitis and should recommend counseling to families that are having difficulties coping with their affected child. Insight-oriented psychotherapy[68] and group psychotherapy have also been found to be helpful.[19]

PATHOLOGY AND PATHOGENESIS

A healthy immune system is regulated by the complex interactions of the cellular and humoral components of that system. In patients with atopic dermatitis, there is significant evidence of immune system dysregulation. Patients with atopic dermatitis have been found to have abnormalities that include the increased production of immunoglobulin (Ig) E by B cells, abnormal lymphokine secretion profiles, abnormalities of Langerhans cells, and elevated levels of prostaglandin (PG) E_2. The relationships among these abnormalities and how they collectively produce the clinical lesions of atopic dermatitis are just beginning to be understood.

The histopathologic changes in atopic dermatitis vary with the clinical presentation as acute, subacute, or chronic dermatitis. Acute lesions are characterized by epidermal intercellular edema known as spongiosis, papillary dermal edema, and a perivascular and slight interstitial mixed infiltrate with lymphocytes, neutrophils, and few eosinophils. The spongiosis in some acutely inflamed and oozing areas can lead to microvesiculation. The subacute and chronic changes are characterized by varying degrees of spongiosis and epidermal thickening, known as acanthosis. Chronic lesions tend to have less spongiosis, although marked acanthosis, thickened collagen bundles in the papillary dermis, and a perivascular lymphohistiocytic infiltrate are present.[80, 91] Clinically, noninflamed skin in patients with atopic dermatitis reveals epidermal spongiosis and a mild dermal inflammatory infiltrate.[91]

More than 80% of patients with atopic dermatitis have elevated serum IgE levels.[48, 137] The extent of elevation varies such that when patients have associated asthma or allergic rhinitis, the serum IgE levels are at times markedly elevated,[58] whereas those with only skin involvement may have mildly elevated levels.[100]

Immunohistochemical evaluation of the inflammatory infiltrate in atopic dermatitis reveals mainly $CD4^+$ helper T lymphocytes,[77] in a ratio as high as 7:1 compared with $C8^+$ suppressor T lymphocytes.[81] This finding is similar to that in other inflammatory skin conditions such as allergen contact dermatitis.

Helper T ($CD4^+$) cells can be classified into two subsets, designated Th1 and Th2 cells, that are differentiated according to their lymphokine secretion profiles.[94] Although the designations were initially derived from mouse studies, these populations of cells have since been found in the human immune system.[62, 114] Th1 cells produce interferon-γ (IFN-γ) and interleukin-2 (IL-2); Th2 cells secrete interleukins IL-4, IL-5, IL-6, and IL-10. The cytokines IL-4, IL-5, and IL-6 are important for the production of IgE. IL-4 induces IgE synthesis by B cells, IL-5 enhances IL-4–induced IgE synthesis, and IL-6 potentiates plasma cell production of IgE. There is mutual negative feedback between these T cell subsets. IFN-γ produced by the Th1 cells inhibits both IL-4 and IgE production.[104] IL-10 produced by Th2 cells inhibits the production of IL-2 and IFN-γ by the Th1 cells.[95] Patients with atopic dermatitis appear to have a predominant Th2 cell profile,[155] which can help explain the elevation of IgE that occurs in up to 85% of patients with the disease.[48, 58] This Th2 predominance has been found to occur in peripheral blood as well as in lesional skin of patients with atopic dermatitis.[150]

Peripheral blood eosinophilia is often noted as well in patients with atopic dermatitis and may correlate with disease severity. As with IgE levels, patients with a personal or family history of asthma tend to have very high elevations, whereas those without a history of asthma may have normal or mildly elevated levels.[148] Eosinophil cationic protein (ECP), an eosinophil granular protein, has been found to be elevated in the serum of patients with atopic dermatitis; increased ECP levels correlate with disease severity.[27, 61] Although there are only a few eosinophils in the lesional skin in atopic dermatitis, deposition of major basic protein, a remnant of eosinophilic degranulation, is noted.[75]

When T cells are activated, IL-2 is produced, and the cells express their specific cell surface receptors. Besides being expressed on the cell surface, the IL-2 receptor is also released into serum in a soluble form (sIL-2R),[115] which appears to be a good marker for T cell activation. The sIL-2R is elevated in atopic dermatitis and correlates with disease severity.[22]

The primary defect in atopic dermatitis may be a dysregulation of phosphodiesterase. Elevations in cyclic AMP (cAMP) phosphodiesterase levels are noted in monocytes from patients with atopic dermatitis,[55] and appear to be a consistent finding even in patients in clinical remission,[51] as well as in the cord blood of some infants of atopic parents.[54] The elevated phosphodiesterase levels increase cAMP hydrolysis, thereby causing a decrease in intracellular cAMP.[45] Such peripheral blood monocytes produce elevated levels of PGE_2, which inhibit IFN-γ production by Th1 cells.[66] Furthermore, the cAMP dysregulation is also found in T cells and may decrease production of IFN-γ directly. In either case, the decrease in IFN-γ leads to unregulated IgE stimulation by IL-4.[14]

The density of Langerhans cells is increased in lesions of chronic atopic dermatitis.[112, 149, 165] The Langerhans cells in affected patients also have a receptor for the Fc portion of IgE (FcεR1),[6] by which it binds IgE.[154] Cell surface IgE may function as a high-affinity capture mechanism for allergen, enabling the Langerhans cells to present allergens with great efficiency. This possibility was tested in a study evaluating the ability of Langerhans cells from patients with atopic dermatitis to present house dust mite antigen. Langerhans cells with surface IgE evoked a T-cell response to the house dust antigen with greater efficacy.[96] Langerhans cells in patients with atopic dermatitis also have the ability to activate resting $CD4^+$ T cells without any antigenic stimulation, a phenomenon known as autologous T-cell reactivity.[141]

Mast cells are also increased in chronic lesions of atopic dermatitis.[91] Mast cells have the capacity to produce and release IL-4.[8] IL-4 produced by mast cells may help induce a Th2 T-cell response to allergens. Intermittent mast cell degranulation in atopic patients also causes the release of tumor necrosis factor–alpha (TNF-α) which in turn may inhibit the growth of Th1 clones but not Th2 clones.[23]

Staphylococcus aureus

Staphylococcus aureus colonizes the skin of patients with atopic dermatitis and is commonly responsible for flares of the disease. Staphylococcal cell wall products, teichoic acid and peptidoglycan, and enterotoxin B, when combined with IL-4, have been found to lead to increased IgE synthesis and CD23 expression in patients with atopic dermatitis.[97] Staphylococcal exotoxins possess superantigenic properties that can cause T-lymphocyte activation, leading to significant cytokine release and inflammation.[87] IgE antibody directed to staphylococcal antigens may be pathogenic in terms of mast cell activation and a late-phase response.[78]

ALLERGIC ASSOCIATIONS

There were numerous reports of allergen sensitivity as a cause of atopic dermatitis from the 1930s to the 1950s. Then, interest in the subject waned until the 1980s, when Sampson (see Chapter 33) demonstrated the role of food hypersensitivity in the pathogenesis of childhood atopic dermatitis using double-blind food challenges. Since then, there has been renewed interest in food and aeroallergen sensitivity in patients with atopic dermatitis.

Food Allergies

In the mid-1970s, the first controlled studies were done showing an association of food hypersensitivities with flares of atopic dermatitis.[7, 86] Studies using double-blind, placebo controlled food challenges have shown that in some patients, atopic dermatitis is exacerbated by food allergens. Food allergies in patients with atopic dermatitis tend to be limited to infants and children. The prevalence of food allergies in patients with atopic dermatitis has been difficult to ascertain, because many of the studies evaluating this association have been conducted in patients referred to tertiary care centers in university hospitals; these study populations may be skewed to those with more severe skin problems. One study revealed that food hypersensitivity contributed to skin symptoms in approximately one third of children with atopic dermatitis who were tested with double-blind placebo-controlled oral food challenges.[10] Another study revealed that elimination of foods that were associated with positive food challenges in some patients resulted in improvement in the dermatitis, but there was no significant change in patients who did not follow an elimination diet.[124] Several patients in this study also showed improvement in their coexisting asthma. Some patients following an elimination diet eventually lost their food hypersensitivities.[125]

Sampson,[120] studying 320 patients with atopic dermatitis over 10 years using double-blind placebo-controlled oral food challenges, found that cutaneous reactions developed in 75% of positive challenges, with only 30% of the positive responses involving the skin alone.[120] The skin findings usually consisted of a markedly pruritic, erythematous, morbilliform rash that developed at the patient's predilection sites for eczema. More than two thirds of the reactions were caused by egg, peanut, and milk.

A study by Guillet and Guillet[46] evaluating IgE sensitization to food allergens found no evidence of food sensitization in children with mild atopic dermatitis but did find food sensitization in 93% of patients with severe atopic dermatitis. There is evidence for IgE-mediated immediate and late-phase effects associated with positive double-blind placebo-controlled oral food challenges.[121–123] Patients with more severe atopic dermatitis were also found to have activated circulating basophils in vivo and increased basophil releasibility, as opposed to those with mild disease. Food hypersensitivity is not generally seen in an adult population with atopic dermatitis.[122]

Numerous studies have shown that there is no difference in the occurrence of atopic dermatitis between newborns fed cow's milk and those who were fed breast or soy milk,[50] even those with a family history of atopy.[49, 67] Withholding highly allergenic foods from mothers with atopic dermatitis in their last trimester of pregnancy and lactation as well as from their children during the first 2 years of life reduced the prevalence of food allergy or atopic dermatitis in the first year but effected no difference in the prevalence of food allergy or atopic dermatitis by the age of 4 years when compared with a control group.[166]

Aeroallergens

In the 1930s, clinical studies revealed that allergens such as feathers, house dust, and seasonal inhalant allergens, especially ragweed, were associated with the development of atopic dermatitis in some patients.[36, 103, 143, 144] Later studies demonstrated the development of eczematous lesions when aeroallergens are applied epicutaneously to patients with atopic dermatitis.[1, 110] Clark and Adinoff[16, 17] provided evidence that aeroallergen contact can cause flares of atopic dermatitis, especially in adults (Fig. 36–6). Guillet and Guillet[46] showed that children with severe atopic dermatitis are most likely to have an associated food allergy and are at risk for aeroallergen-related respiratory symptoms.

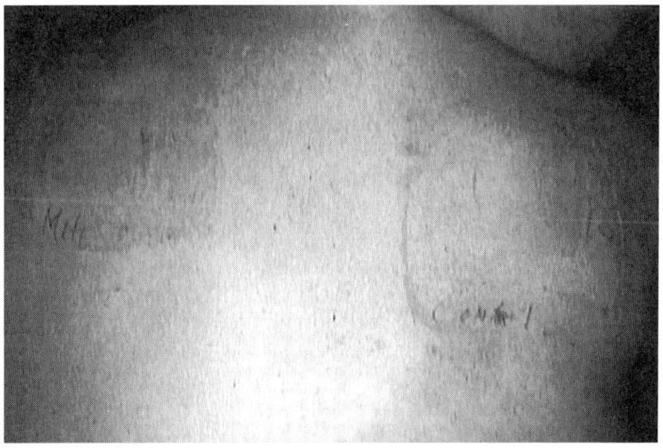

FIGURE 36–6. Positive dust mite patch test at 72 hours of a child with atopic dermatitis.

Eczematous skin changes have been seen in patients with high IgE antibody levels to dust mite.[92] There were higher densities of dust mites in the homes of patients with moderate to severe atopic dermatitis than in those of nonatopic patients,[4] and the magnitude of dust mite exposure correlated positively with the frequency of disease.[21] Sanda and colleagues[127] demonstrated that patients with atopic dermatitis who were sensitized to dust mites showed a long-term remission of their symptoms when hospitalized in a room with low mite counts. Mite-sensitive patients placed in a hospitalized room with no mite precautions showed no improvement in symptoms.

Asthma

The incidence of asthma in patients with atopic dermatitis is higher in those with severe skin disease if (1) there is a family history of asthma and (2) the dermatitis begins early in life.[37, 85, 107, 117] Studies of the prevalence of asthma in children with atopic dermatitis have yielded results that vary widely, ranging from 20% to 76%.[118] The highest incidence was reported by Salob and Atherton[118] from a study of patients referred to a pediatric dermatology clinic, possibly reflecting a population of patients with more severe skin disease.[118] The same researchers found that there was a strong association between atopic dermatitis and bronchial hyperresponsiveness even in the absence of overt symptoms.[119]

Contact Dermatitis

Studies evaluating the incidence of contact dermatitis in patients with atopic dermatitis vary greatly in their results. Some studies reveal an increased incidence,[33, 132] and others report a similar[25] or decreased[28, 59] incidence. What is clear is that patients with atopic dermatitis can and do get contact dermatitis and that refractory dermatitis may in some cases be due to contact sensitization. In addition to the common allergens that have the propensity to sensitize, patients with atopic dermatitis may become sensitive to their medications, particularly because these medications are being applied to skin with damaged barrier function.

DIFFERENTIAL DIAGNOSIS

The differential diagnosis of atopic dermatitis is summarized in Table 36–4.

SEBORRHEIC DERMATITIS

Seborrheic dermatitis can be difficult to differentiate from atopic dermatitis in early infancy. Seborrheic dermatitis generally begins in the first few weeks of life, whereas atopic dermatitis develops in the second to third month of life. At times, the two conditions can occur together. The dermatitis of each condition involves the scalp, postauricular areas and

TABLE 36–4
DIFFERENTIAL DIAGNOSIS OF ATOPIC DERMATITIS

Seborrheic dermatitis
Contact dermatitis
Infections
Dermatophyte
Scabies
Immunologic disorders
Wiskott-Aldrich syndrome
Ataxia telangiectasia
Agammaglobulinemia
Hyper-IgE syndrome
Selective IgA deficiency
Metabolic disorders
Phenylketonuria
Tyrosinemia
Histidinemia
Acrodermatitis enteropathica
Neoplastic disorders
Histiocytosis X
Mycosis fungoides
Genodermatoses
Netherton's syndrome
Erythrokeratoderma variabilis

face as well as the intertriginous areas. The diaper area, which is commonly involved in seborrheic dermatitis, is usually spared in atopic dermatitis. In rare instances, seborrheic dermatitis can generalize to involve most of the body with sparing of the hands and feet. Unlike with atopic dermatitis, pruritus in seborrheic dermatitis is usually absent or mild.

ALLERGIC CONTACT DERMATITIS

Allergic contact dermatitis can become generalized in some affected patients. In addition, localized forms of contact dermatitis, including that of the hands and feet, can mimic atopic dermatitis.

INFECTIONS

The clinical changes of scabies include severe pruritus and erythematous papules and plaques that can appear eczematous and excoriated. Scabies is generally more papular than atopic dermatitis, and burrows that contain the scabies mite should be carefully sought. Dermatophyte infections, especially of the palms and soles, manifest as erythema, scaling, and, at times, vesicles. KOH examination or fungal culture reveals fungal hyphae.

IMMUNOLOGIC DISORDERS

Immunologic disorders, such as Wiskott-Aldrich syndrome, ataxia telangiectasia, agammaglobulinemia, and the hyper-IgE syndrome, all can cause skin changes identical to those of atopic dermatitis. Children with recalcitrant dermatitis and recurrent systemic infections should undergo diagnostic work-up to exclude an immunodeficiency disorder.

METABOLIC DISORDERS

Metabolic disorders that manifest as skin changes resembling atopic dermatitis include phenylketonuria, tyrosinemia, histidinemia, and acrodermatitis enteropathica.

NEOPLASTIC DISEASES

Histiocytosis X may cause eczematous skin changes in children, although there is evidence of purpura in affected skin. Adults with mycosis fungoides and Sèzary's syndrome can present with eczematous skin changes. Furthermore, patients with life-long severe atopic dermatitis may develop mycosis fungoides or Sezary's syndrome.

ICHTHYOTIC GENODERMATOSES

The ichthyotic genodermatoses include Netherton's syndrome and erythrokeratoderma variabilis. Patients with erythrokeratoderma variabilis present with well-demarcated, relatively fixed, erythematous, scaly plaques that tend to occur on extensor surfaces. Patients with Netherton's syndrome develop patches of ichthyosis linearis circumflexa, which are erythematous plaques that have a double-edged scale.

THE TREATMENT OF ATOPIC DERMATITIS

GENERAL MEASURES

In the treatment of patients with atopic dermatitis, it is important to search beyond the skin and attempt to recognize external factors that may cause flare-ups of the dermatitis. The history should include the frequency of bathing, soaps used, and any type of preparations that are applied to the skin. Soaps or cleansers with minimal defatting activity and a neutral pH, such as Dove, Tone, and Cetaphil, should be used. Antibacterial cleansers can be irritating to the skin of these patients and should be avoided. Because the skin in atopic dermatitis tends to be dry and easily irritated, it is important to maintain adequate hydration through bathing and the frequent use of emollients. In the 1960s, the Scholtz regimen[129] prohibited bathing and recommended cleansing with Cetaphil lotion. However, bathing is clearly helpful in atopic dermatitis, although only if emollients or occlusives are applied immediately after skin hydration to prevent evaporation.

Patients with acute dermatitis benefit from the soothing effects of bathing in tepid water. The bath also serves to remove crusts and hydrates the skin prior to the application of topical medication. Upon completion of the bath, an emollient must be applied within 3 to 5 minutes to prevent evaporation that can lead to further dryness. The skin should be patted dry, not rubbed, prior to the application of topical preparations. Hydration of the skin from bathing can increase the penetration of topical medications significantly if they are applied immediately. Bath oils should not be used in place of emollients, because they do not have the same capacity to retain moisture.

Patients with chronic disease as well as those with significant skin dryness may become more dry and pruritic when bathing without subsequent application of emollients, especially in the winter and at other times of low humidity. It is very important that such patients apply emollients frequently, two to three times daily, and immediately after taking baths. In dry climates, occlusive preparations such as petrolatum or Aquaphor may be used. Some patients, especially those living in warmer climates, find that the use of occlusives induces sweating and pruritus. These patients benefit from the use of cream moisturizers. Lactic acid preparations are effective for removing scales in patients with ichthyosis vulgaris but may cause stinging if applied to skin that is fissured or has the changes of acute dermatitis.

Sweating can provoke itching in patients with atopic dermatitis. These patients benefit from wearing protective clothing that is loose fitting and made of cotton as well as from being in indoor environments with a fairly constant temperature of 68° to 75°F and 45% to 55% humidity.

ANTIPRURITICS

Antihistamines have been the predominant oral medications used to control the pruritus of atopic dermatitis. The therapeutic effectiveness of antihistamines is equivocal, with many studies showing little effect in controlling the pruritus or improving the dermatitis.[41, 128] Although the effectiveness of antihistamines remains unproven, they are used quite regularly and may be helpful because of their central sedative effects. In the severely pruritic patient, antihistamines are worth trying in an attempt to lessen the itching. Antihistamines from the hydroxyzine group, e.g., Atarax, are most commonly used, although antihistamines from other groups may be tried. Doxepin, a tricyclic antidepressant with H_1 and H_2 receptor blocking properties, may be tried in patients with severe dermatitis. This medication can cause significant sedation and should be used at lower dosages than those used to treat depression. A new topical preparation of doxepin shows some efficacy in reducing pruritus in patients with atopic dermatitis, although there are risks of sensitization to the medication as well as the absorption of significant amounts of medication when it is used over large surface areas.[32] Although the use of antihistamines is controversial, patients with an allergic component to their condition may benefit from them.[31]

TOPICAL CORTICOSTEROIDS

Topical corticosteroids are important and frequently used agents for the treatment of atopic dermatitis. When topical corticosteroids are used, the lowest-potency agent that is effective should be chosen. Especially with infants and children, weaning to low-potency (1% or 2.5%) hydrocortisone or to a nonhydrocortisone equivalent preparation should be done when the dermatitis is brought under control. Topical corticosteroids are best applied within 3 to 5 minutes of bathing. Ointments are more occlusive and tolerated better on very dry skin and during the winter months. During the summer, especially in humid environments, patients may develop increased pruritus and folliculitis and, therefore, may tolerate a cream better.

Topical corticosteroids should not be applied more than twice daily, as efficacy does not increase with more frequent applications. Mid- to high-potency preparations should be used with great caution on the face and in intertriginous areas such as the neck, axilla, and groin. Topical corticosteroids should be used sparingly in the treatment of patients with chronic atopic dermatitis.

SYSTEMIC CORTICOSTEROIDS

The use of systemic corticosteroids should be avoided in atopic dermatitis. Patients with severe disease experience a flare of their dermatitis when systemic corticosteroids are tapered, which may be even more difficult to control. The side effects of long-term systemic corticosteroid use are dangerous and include osteoporosis, cataract formation, and avascular hip necrosis. Patients with dermatitis severe enough to warrant a brief course of systemic corticosteroids may benefit from a brief hospitalization so that intensive topical therapy can be given in a clean environment. This therapy may enable control of the dermatitis to be obtained with the patient removed from the stresses of daily life, which are compounded by having a chronic disease.

ANTIBIOTICS

Systemic antibiotics are indicated for the treatment of bacterial infections in atopic dermatitis. Treatment should be instituted with systemic antistaphylococcal therapy when staphylococcal impetiginization is clinically suspected or is proven by culture. In many areas of the country, *S. aureus* has shown less susceptibility to erythromycin, which is becoming less a first-line agent than it was in the past. Erythromycin also elevates blood levels of theophylline. Oral dicloxacillin and cephalexin are acceptable alternatives.

Topical antibiotics, with the exception of mupirocin (Bactroban), are not recommended. Mupirocin is best used for localized areas that are impetiginized; it should not be used for prolonged periods or over large surface areas, so as to avoid drug resistance as well as sensitization.

Extensive local or generalized herpes simplex infections respond rapidly to therapy with systemic acyclovir. Infants and immunocompromised patients also benefit from systemic therapy. Mild herpes simplex infections are self-limited and require no topical or systemic antiviral treatment.

Dermatophyte infections respond to topical antifungal preparations, although systemic antifungal therapy may be required for recalcitrant infections. Patients who are proven to have *Pityrosporon*-induced flares may benefit from topical ketoconazole preparations.

TAR

Tar preparations were used extensively in the past, but with the advent of more potent topical corticosteroids, their use has unfortunately diminished. Tars may be used to reduce the use of topical corticosteroids in the maintenance of chronic disease. Tar preparations come in creams, gels, liquor carbonis detergens (LCD) solution, which can be compounded with an emollient to desired strengths, and as shampoos. Tar preparations can be placed in the bath or applied directly to the skin. A mixture of 2.5% to 5% LCD in Aquaphor has acceptable cosmetic properties. Gel preparations, which also tend to be acceptable cosmetically, may prove too irritating because of their alcohol content.

ULTRAVIOLET LIGHT THERAPY

Patients with recalcitrant atopic dermatitis may benefit from treatment with a combination of ultraviolet B (UVB) and ultraviolet A (UVA), or psoralens plus UVA (PUVA) therapy.[93] PUVA therapy on its own may achieve clearing, but UVB therapy requires adjunctive treatment with topical corticosteroids. PUVA therapy has also been shown effective when used in adolescence, with patients achieving significant growth responses as determined on percentile curves.[3] Combination UVA-UVB therapy has been found to be more effective than the use of UVB alone.[56] Medium dose UV-A1 treatment alone has also been found to be effective in treating severe atopic dermatitis but the phototherapy units needed are not readily available. Before phototherapy is begun, it is important to know whether the patient has any photoexacerbated dermatoses, such as lupus erythematosus, polymorphic light eruption, or photoexacerbated atopic dermatitis.

NEWER AGENTS AND MODALITIES

Over the past few years, as the defects in immune dysregulation have been identified in patients with atopic dermatitis, newer drugs with immunomodulatory effects have been tried.

Interferon-γ

Interferon (IFN-γ) is produced by Th1 cells and inhibits the production of IL-4 by Th2 cells. IL-4 has a central role in atopic disease, being necessary for the production of IgE. With the knowledge that IFN-γ levels are decreased and IL-4 levels are increased in patients with atopic dermatitis, therapeutic trials of recombinant IFN-γ were conducted in patients with atopic dermatitis. Initial studies found that patients obtain significant improvement in their dermatitis but experience dermatitis flares once the medication is discontinued. The treatment is associated with a reduction in the eosinophil count but, surprisingly, has no effect on the serum IgE. A later study found that the overall response to treatment with IFN-γ was not significantly better than that to conventional therapy in a control group.[98]

Cyclosporine

Cyclosporine, an immunosuppressive agent, has shown remarkable clinical effects when used in patients with severe atopic dermatitis.[135, 151] Unfortunately, there is a rapid relapse when the drug is discontinued. Patients must also be followed closely for the serious side effects associated with cyclosporine use, such as hypertension and elevations in serum creatinine.

Thymopentin

Thymopentin mimics thymopoietin, a thymic hormone that influences the differentiation of thymocytes and the function of mature T cells. The medication, like IFN-γ, is administered by subcutaneous injection. Studies have obtained efficacious results with the use of thymopentin, although it can require up to 6 weeks to take effect.[60, 79, 136] In addition, patients have had relapses while on the medication.[79]

Oral Lipid Supplementation

Because metabolites of linoleic and γ-linoleic acids have been shown to be deficient in patients with atopic dermatitis,[12, 84] there have been therapeutic trials with dietary supplementation using these lipids. Some of these studies have found no benefit[47, 109] whereas others have found γ-linoleic acid supplementation beneficial.[38, 163]

Allergen Hyposensitization Therapy

Classic hyposensitization therapy has not proved to be effective in the treatment of atopic dermatitis.[44, 64, 99] Later studies, though, have shown that patients with atopic dermatitis who are allergen sensitive do benefit from injections of allergen combined with $F(ab')_2$ fragments of specific antibodies.[76] More studies are needed to assess the efficacy of this treatment.

Chinese Herbal Therapy

There has also been interest in the use of traditional Chinese herbal therapy in the treatment of atopic dermatitis. Studies in both adults and children yielded significant clinical effects in patients with recalcitrant dermatitis, although further studies are warranted.[132–134] An in vitro study found that the Chinese herbal therapy significantly inhibited IL-4–induced CD23 expression on peripheral blood monocytes in nonatopic patients.[74]

Phosphodiesterase Inhibitors

Phosphodiesterase inhibitors have shown in vitro activity,[23] but work is in progress to develop phosphodiesterase inhibitors that have a significant clinical effect.

Extracorporeal Photopheresis

A 1994 study evaluated the use of extracorporeal photopheresis using UVA irradiation of enriched lymphocytes in the presence of 8-methoxypsoralen in three patients with severe atopic dermatitis.[105] The study patients all improved dramatically with the therapy. Extracorporeal photopheresis may be another treatment option for patients with severe, recalcitrant dermatitis.

CONTACT DERMATITIS AND PHOTOALLERGIC REACTIONS

RICHARD S. KALISH

ALLERGIC CONTACT DERMATITIS AND IRRITANT CONTACT DERMATITIS

Contact dermatitis results from exposure to environmental substances. Localization and morphology of lesions are thus a function of exposure. Contact dermatitis is classified as irritant contact or allergic contact dermatitis, and the clinical distinction between them is often difficult.

Dishpan hands is a classic example of irritant contact dermatitis, resulting from prolonged and repeated exposure to water and detergents. Although inflammatory cells have a role in the pathogenesis of irritant contact dermatitis, it is not mediated by immune lymphocytes, and prior sensitization is not required. People vary in their susceptibility to irritants. However, given sufficient exposure, most people would react to an irritant.

In contrast, allergic contact dermatitis is mediated by antigen-specific, sensitized T lymphocytes. Poison ivy dermatitis is an example of allergic contact dermatitis. It is mediated by T cells specific for urushiol, the immunogenic component of poison ivy resin. Following sensitization, a rapid reaction may follow exposure to concentrations of allergen that do not induce inflammation in nonsensitized subjects.

PATHOGENESIS OF ALLERGIC CONTACT DERMATITIS

THE CHEMISTRY OF CONTACT ALLERGENS

Contact allergens are small molecules, and recognition by the immune system requires that they function as haptens and bind macromolecules. Haptens can be classified by their chemical reactivity.[195] Mechanisms used to bind proteins include nucleophilic substitution, electrophilic reactions, free radical reactions, and chelation of metallic salts. Many allergens, such as dinitrochlorobenzene, are chemically reactive and capable of covalently conjugating proteins. Other allergens, such as nickel and chromium,[251] form noncovalent complexes with proteins. A third class of allergens are "prohaptens." These compounds must be activated to a chemically reactive intermediate before they can conjugate proteins. Urushiol, the immunogenic component of poison ivy resin, is a prohapten. Oxidation of the catechol group of urushiol to a quinone makes it a target for nucleophilic substitution by amino acid side chains.

Conjugation of haptens to proteins is also a function of the chemical reactivity of the amino acid side chains.[195] Cysteine, lysine, and histidine (least active) are nucleophiles that will take part in nucleophilic substitutions. Aromatic amino acids such as tyrosine, tryptophan, and phenylalanine can act as electron acceptors and react with free radicals. These last reactions are particularly significant for photoallergic reactions.

INITIATION OF CONTACT DERMATITIS AND THE ROLE OF KERATINOCYTES

Keratinocytes have an active role in the initiation of both allergic contact dermatitis and irritant contact dermatitis. Keratinocytes are capable of producing and secreting many cytokines, including interleukin-1 (IL-1), IL-6, IL-8, tumor necrosis factor–alpha (TNF-α), and granulocyte monocyte colony-stimulating factor (GM-CSF).[210, 224, 225] Many allergens and irritants have been shown to induce keratinocyte activation with synthesis and secretion of these cytokines. It is controversial whether the cytokine profile induced by irritants differs from that induced by allergens. These proinflammatory cytokines have a role in the recruitment of inflammatory cells. Both IL-1 and TNF-α induce expression of the adhesion molecules intercellular adhesion molecule–1 (ICAM-1) and E-selectin on endothelial cells. These molecules are essential for the homing (migration) of inflammatory cells to the involved epidermis.

ANTIGEN PRESENTATION AND THE ROLE OF LANGERHANS CELLS

T-lymphocyte antigen receptors recognize peptides presented in the peptide-binding groove of major histocompatibility complex (MHC) molecules.[179, 180] $CD8^+$ T lymphocytes recognize peptides presented by MHC class I (HLA-A, HLA-B, HLA-C) molecules, and $CD4^+$ T lymphocytes recognize peptides presented by MHC class II (DR, DP, DQ) molecules.[237] Prior to their presentation to T lymphocytes, protein antigens are first cleaved into peptides and then bound to the peptide-binding grooves of MHC molecules. Contact allergens function as haptens and bind proteins either before or after cleavage into peptides.[216] This process of cleaving proteins into peptides and loading the peptides onto MHC molecules is known as *antigen processing*.[214] Antigen processing is a function of antigen-presenting cells (APCs), which have the metabolic functions required for processing along with expression of MHC molecules and costimulatory molecules (e.g., B7).

Langerhans cells are dendritic antigen-presenting cells that serve as the primary APCs of the epidermis.[255, 256, 258, 262] As with other "professional" APCs, Langerhans cells constitutively express cell surface MHC class II molecules (e.g., DR).[257] Unique markers of Langerhans cells include cell surface expression of CD1a[188] and the presence of intracytoplasmic Birbeck granules (shaped like tennis rackets and visible on electron microscopy).[186] Upon interaction with a hapten, Langerhans cells become activated, increase their cell surface expression of MHC class II molecules,[169] and migrate to lymph nodes to present antigen to T cells.[177, 222]

Hapten-conjugated Langerhans cells migrate to the lymph node to present antigen to T cells. On initial sensitization, the number of T cells specific for the hapten is very small, and initial recognition of the hapten is probably within the lymph node. T cells that become activated following recognition of hapten in the lymph node must then home to the inflamed skin.

HOMING OF T LYMPHOCYTES

Homing is the process by which circulating cells recognize and migrate to relevant sites. The proportion of allergen-specific T lymphocytes in a skin lesion of allergic contact dermatitis is less than 1 per thousand.[215] Nevertheless, this proportion represents a several-fold enrichment over the ratio of such T lymphocytes in the peripheral blood and indicates the ability of antigen-specific T lymphocytes to localize at sites of inflammation.

Leukocytes have homing receptors that recognize the endothelium of appropriate tissues. The homing receptor that recognizes the high endothelial venules of lymph nodes is a molecule called L-selectin. This molecule is essential to the homing of lymphocytes to lymph nodes. Addressins are the ligands for homing receptors and signal the lymphocytes as to where to exit the circulation. Addressins expressed on dermal endothelial cells include E-selectin and P-selectin. The ligand for E-selectin (CLA: cutaneous lymphocyte antigen) is believed to be the homing receptor for T lymphocytes that localize in inflamed skin.[181, 246, 247] All three selectins (E-selectin, P-selectin, and L-selectin) belong to a supergene family and have considerable homology.[171] Selectins have an *N*-terminal lectin domain that binds carbohydrate, and there is evidence that the ligands for these selectins are carbohydrates. For example, the ligand for E-selectin is a glycoprotein with a carbohydrate group similar to the Sle^X blood group substance.[174]

Additional adhesion molecule pairs are essential for lymphocyte homing. These include endothelial ICAM-1, which interacts with lymphocyte LFA-1,[196] and endothelial VCAM-1, which interacts with lymphocyte VLA–4.[269] Both LFA-1 and VLA-4 are integrins.

Initial interactions between lymphocytes and endothelial cells are mediated by the selectins (e.g., E-selectin), which induce the lymphocyte to roll along the endothelium.[223] This initial contact permits integrin interactions (e.g., LFA-1), which transmit an activation signal to the cell. The activation signal, mediated by integrins, induces the cell to flatten out and migrate through the vessel wall into the dermis.[213] Activated T lymphocytes express higher levels of cell surface LFA-1 and VLA-4 and probably home nonspecifically to sites of inflammation.

The adhesion molecules ICAM-1, VCAM-1, and E-selectin are expressed on endothelium of inflamed skin in both irritant and allergic contact dermatitis.[192] Allergens and irritants have the ability to induce expression of these molecules either by direct action or through induction of proinflammatory keratinocyte-derived cytokines.[270]

INDUCTION OF INFLAMMATORY CHANGES

Following homing to skin and recognition of hapten, activated T lymphocytes induce disease in the dermis and the epidermis. Because the proportion of T lymphocytes specific for the inciting antigen is less than 1 per thousand, these T lymphocytes must be extremely potent and evoke significant amplification. T lymphocytes have many potential mechanisms for inducing inflammation, including cell-mediated cytotoxicity, recruitment of inflammatory cells, and direct effects of cytokines. It is known that TNF-α has an important role in allergic contact dermatitis, because allergic contact reactions in mice can be blocked by antibody to TNF-α.[248] Which of these potential mechanisms is relevant to the pathogenesis of allergic contact dermatitis is unclear.

DIAGNOSIS OF ALLERGIC CONTACT DERMATITIS

MORPHOLOGY OF CONTACT DERMATITIS

The fundamental characteristic of contact dermatitis is the relationship to environmental exposure. This exposure results in a distribution and morphology which can often be decoded to arrive at a diagnosis and etiology. Linearity and lack of symmetry of lesions are important features that suggest contact dermatitis. Linearity can be evident as a sharp edge to an otherwise amorphous shape or as a sharp cutoff. Plant dermatitis, such as poison ivy, often manifests as linear acute inflammation at sites scratched by branches (Fig. 36–7). These linear lesions may be accompanied by multiple nonlinear eczematous lesions where the resin was transferred from the hands. The presence of a few linear lesions makes the diagnosis.

Many contact allergens seldom produce linear lesions. These include cosmetics, perfume, and topical medications. Localization of the dermatitis may be suggestive of the responsible allergen. Dermatitis localized to sites of application of cosmetics, perfume, or topical medications would suggest the cause (Fig. 36-8). Dermatitis of the waist may result from allergy to rubber components present in the elastic bands of underwear (Fig. 36–9). Rubber allergy can also manifest as linear dermatitis in the distribution of bra straps, as hand

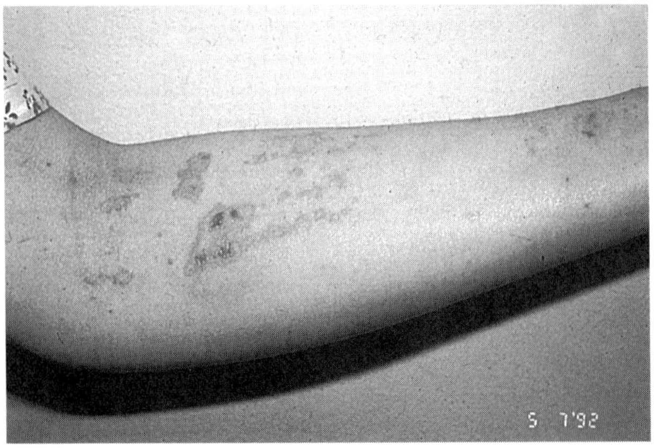

FIGURE 36–7. Allergic contact dermatitis to poison ivy (*Toxicodendron radicans*). Note the linear lesions induced by contact with branches.

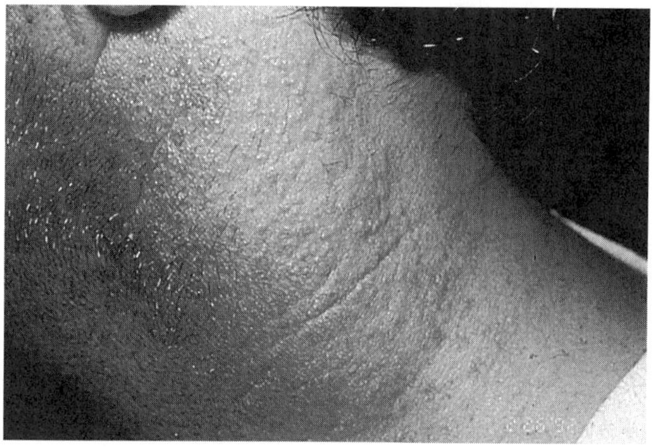

FIGURE 36–8. Allergic contact dermatitis to topically applied cream. Sharp demarcation is obvious.

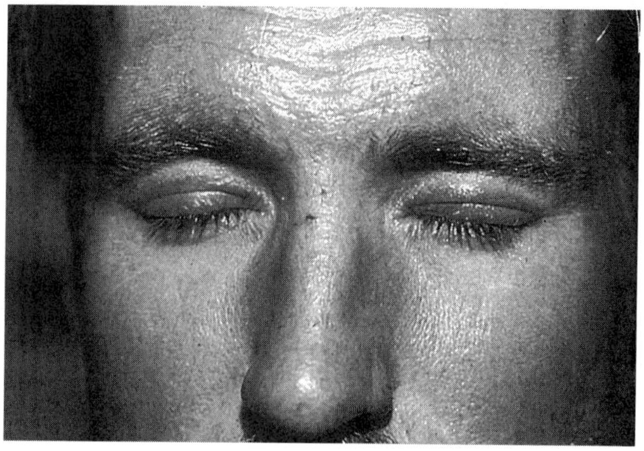

FIGURE 36–10. Allergic contact dermatitis to redwood sawdust in a carpenter. Aeroallergens frequently induce allergic reactions on the face with particular involvement of eyelids.

dermatitis secondary to latex gloves (see later), or as shoe dermatitis. Nickel dermatitis frequently presents at sites of contact with jewelry such as earrings. Aerosol allergens often induce dermatitis of the upper eyelids. This localization is favored by the thin stratum corneum at this site. Upper eyelid dermatitis may also be caused by the toluidine sulfonamide resin in nail polish. However, any aerosol allergen can be implicated, including rosin (colophony) present in spray furniture polish, sawdust (especially cedar and redwood) (Fig. 36–10), spray paints, pollens, and vapors from epoxy or formaldehyde resins.

The principal differential diagnosis of contact dermatitis is between allergic contact dermatitis and irritant contact dermatitis. This distinction is of consequence for treatment. In occupational disability cases, the distinction between allergic contact and irritant contact may determine whether the patient can return to employment and what precautions are

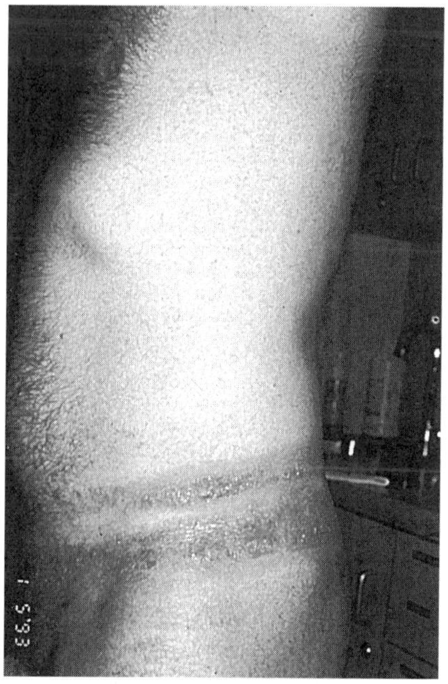

FIGURE 36–9. Elastic in undergarments produced this allergic contact dermatitis. This eruption may be caused by any of the rubber accelerators.

necessary. History, morphology, and location of the eruption are the principal clues to determining etiology. Patch testing is often essential for confirming both the diagnosis and the causative allergen. Identification of the allergen facilitates avoidance and prevention of further dermatitis.

Allergic contact dermatitis and irritant contact dermatitis may be acute, subacute, or chronic. Each phase of dermatitis has a characteristic morphology that is not specific for contact dermatitis. Acute dermatitis is manifested by edema of the epidermis and acute inflammation resulting in vesicle or blister formation and erythema. Subacute dermatitis exhibits erythema, dermal edema, exudate, and crust without vesicle or blister formation. Chronic dermatitis results in a thickening of the epidermis with an increase in skin markings and pigmentation. Erythema and edema are less evident. These chronic changes are described as lichenification. Isolated plaques of lichenified epidermis are described as lichen simplex chronicus. The morphology of a plaque of lichen simplex chronicus is similar whether the cause is contact dermatitis, irritant dermatitis, atopic dermatitis, or neurodermatitis. The diagnosis of contact dermatitis must be made on the basis of location, lack of symmetry, history, and patch test result.

PATIENT HISTORY IN THE DIAGNOSIS OF CONTACT DERMATITIS

History has a major role in the diagnosis of either allergic contact or irritant contact dermatitis and should include both occupational and domestic contactants. Unless the cause is immediately obvious, it is generally necessary to identify all substances the patient applies topically, i.e., moisturizers, cosmetics, soaps, sunscreens, hair dyes, topical medications, shampoos, and miscellaneous toiletry articles. Patients should also be asked about hobbies, sports, gardening, and home improvement projects. Inquiries should be made regarding contact with adhesives, resins, and lubricating oils.

The patient's occupational exposures must be determined. Occupational contactants for construction or industrial workers may include glues and resins, irritant chemicals, solvents, cement, cutting oils, and greases. Hairdressers are exposed to frequent water immersion, hair dyes (paraphenylenediamine), bleaches and boosters (persulfate), and "permanent wave" solutions (thioglycolates). Foresters and horticultural workers are exposed to multiple allergenic plants (see later). Health care workers are exposed to topical medications, gloves, and systemic medications such as penicillin and cancer chemotherapy agents. Improvement of the dermatitis following a vacation may suggest an occupational etiology.

DIFFERENTIAL DIAGNOSIS

The differential diagnosis of contact dermatitis includes most inflammatory skin diseases. Contact dermatitis is usually diagnosed on the basis of location of the lesions. Most skin diseases that are not related to contact have a symmetric distribution. They include atopic dermatitis, drug eruptions, psoriasis, and connective tissue diseases. Atopic dermatitis in older children and adolescents generally involves the popliteal and antecubital fossae. Nummular dermatitis results in round (coin-shaped) eczematous lesions. Seborrheic dermatitis has a typical distribution with a greasy scale.

Photosensitivity diseases may produce lesions with sharp linear cutoffs related to garments. The diagnosis is suggested by the photodistribution of lesions on the sun-exposed skin of the face, upper extensor extremity, and V region of the chest. Skin is relatively spared under the chin and on the volar forearm. The differential diagnosis of photoallergic dermatitis is discussed separately later.

Several conditions may cause diagnostic problems as a result of their morphology. Cutaneous T-cell lymphoma (mycosis fungoides) may have bizarre morphology with lack of symmetry. Fixed drug eruptions are circular and often single. These conditions may be diagnosed by histopathologic examination.

PATHOLOGY

The histologic findings in contact dermatitis are those of inflammation of the epidermis and superficial dermis.[229] Acute contact dermatitis demonstrates edema and a superficial perivascular infiltrate of lymphocytes and monocytes (Fig. 36–11). Small numbers of eosinophils may also be present. Lymphocytes can be observed within the epidermis. The histologic correlate of edema of the epidermis is spongiosis, which is observed as increased intercellular spaces between keratinocytes. These intercellular spaces may fuse, to result in microvesicles, vesicles, and blisters (bullae). Blisters in allergic contact dermatitis are intraepidermal. Irritant dermatitis from caustic materials may result in epidermal necrosis. In the absence of such changes, it is not possible to differentiate irritant from allergic contact dermatitis histologically.

Chronic irritant or allergic contact dermatitis results in a psoriasiform dermatitis with the changes of lichen simplex chronicus (Fig. 36–12). The epidermis is thickened (acanthosis) with irregular elongation of the rete ridges. The collagen of the papillary dermis is thickened with a vertical orientation. There is a perivascular mononuclear cell infiltrate. The same changes are found in chronic dermatitis from many causes. Histologic analysis is usually not useful in the evaluation of contact dermatitis, unless it is needed to rule out other conditions with a specific histologic picture, such as psoriasis, dermatophytosis, herpes virus infection, or cutaneous T-cell lymphoma.

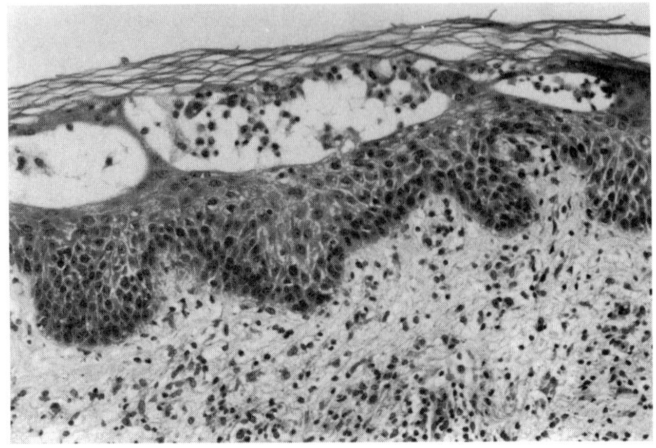

FIGURE 36–11. Acute contact dermatitis demonstrates edema within the epidermis (spongiosis) and an inflammatory infiltrate of lymphocytes and monocytes.

PATCH TESTING IN ALLERGIC CONTACT DERMATITIS

Following a diagnosis of probable allergic contact dermatitis, it is often helpful to identify the allergen. This step has the dual benefit of confirming the diagnosis and providing information required to avoid further contact with the allergen. It may enable a patient with occupational contact dermatitis to return to work with appropriate modifications.[234] It is often possible to find substitutions for contact allergens.[168]

Patients with a history of contact urticaria should never undergo patch testing, because they are at risk for anaphylaxis. Patch testing is designed for the investigation of delayed hypersensitivity reactions only, and not for immunoglobulin E (IgE) mediated disease. Patients with chronic eczematous dermatitis secondary to latex gloves can be tested with rubber accelerators. *Patch testing with latex of a patient with contact urticaria due to latex could be fatal.*

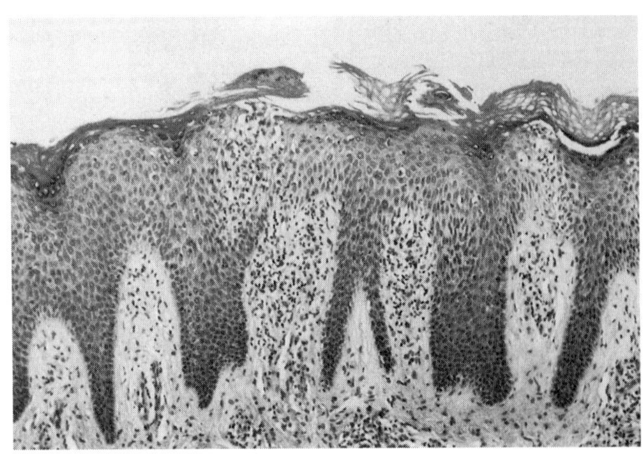

FIGURE 36–12. Chronic contact dermatitis results in a psoriasiform dermatitis with the features of lichen simplex chronicus.

AVAILABILITY OF PATCH TEST ALLERGENS

Currently, patch test allergens are available from only two sources in the United States and are limited to the standard series. Despite a 100-year history of their safe use, the U.S. Food and Drug Administration (FDA) has imposed a substantial regulatory burden on the introduction of each individual allergen. This action has prevented the availability of allergens necessary for appropriate evaluation of many patients.

Within the United States, traditional patch test materials for the standard North American patch test series (Table 36–5) are available from Hermal Pharmaceutical Laboratories (Delmar, NY, 12054; 1-800-HERMAL1). The allergens are supplied in prefilled syringes, and the material is applied to 8-mm cups known as Finn chambers. The Finn chambers are incorporated into strips of Scanpore tape in groups of 10 allergens. Outside the United States, many additional allergens are available in this format from Hermal.

An alternative testing system is marketed in the United States by Glaxo Dermatology (Research Triangle Park, North Carolina 27709) under the name "TRUE Test." This convenient system consists of two strips of tape preloaded with allergens. The backing is removed, and the patches are applied. This convenience comes, however, at significantly greater expense.

PATCH TESTING PROCEDURES

Patch testing requires three visits. The allergens ("patches") are applied to the patient's back on the first visit. Two days (48 hours) later, the patches are removed, and the skin is examined. The patient then returns the following day (72 hours) for a final reading of skin reactivity.

TABLE 36–5
STANDARD PATCH TEST ANTIGEN SERIES

Adhesives	Epoxy resin 1%
	Formaldehyde 1%
	p-Tertiary-butylphenol formaldehyde resin 1%
	Rubber compounds in rubber adhesives (see below)
Antimicrobials	Formaldehyde 1%
	Imidazolidinyl urea 2%
	Neomycin sulfate 20%
	Quaternium-15 2%
Fragrances	Balsam of Peru 25%
	Cinnamic aldehyde 1%
Hair dye	Paraphenylenediamine 1%
Metals	Nickel sulfate 2.5%
Rubber compounds	Black rubber mix 0.6%
	Carbamate mix 3%
	Mercaptobenzothiazole 1%
	Mercapto mix 1%
	Paraphenylenediamine 1%
	Thiuram mix 1%
Topical medicaments	Benzocaine 5%
	Ethylenediamine dihydrochloride 1%
	Lanolin alcohol 30%
	Neomycin sulfate 20%
Other	Colophony 20% (rosin; wax, polish)
	Potassium dichromate 0.25% (cement, leather)

Patch testing is performed on the back. Allergens are standardized for this site and should not be applied elsewhere. It is thus necessary that the skin of the back not be inflamed. Patch testing can induce a flare of contact dermatitis. For this reason, it is preferable that the testing be performed after the dermatitis has resolved. Topical steroids can interfere with patch testing results. Thus, application of topical steroids to the back and use of systemic steroids should be avoided for at least 2 weeks prior to patch testing.

If Finn chambers on Scanpore tape are used, the backing is removed from the chambers, and the tape is laid out on a counter. Chambers are arranged on the Scanpore tape in two rows of five chambers each. Two tapes are required for the standard 20-allergen series. A mark is made in the upper left corner of each tape, and the allergens are placed in the Finn chambers as labeled in a diagram. For allergens in petrolatum, a "ribbon" approximately 4 mm long is added to each chamber. Allergens in solution are added to filter paper disks placed in the Finn chamber. The two tapes containing the Finn chambers are then applied vertically to either side of the back. It is critical to remember that the right-left orientation of the tape is reversed upon application to the back. The marks in the upper left corners should help with orientation. Patches are then fastened down with additional Scanpore tape.

The patient is instructed to leave the patches in place and not wash the back for 2 days or until the patches are removed. These procedures are generally performed by a nurse or technician. Any patient who experiences severe pruritus under one of the patches is instructed to return to the office. The offending patch is removed and recorded, and the remaining patches are left in place for the full 2 days.

After 48 hours, the patient returns to the office, and the patches are removed. As the tape is slowly removed, the position of each patch is indicated with a mark. Reading of the patch sites must be delayed for 15 to 20 minutes, until the erythema secondary to pressure resolves.

Patch test reactions are graded on a standard scale from (+/−) to (3+). Criteria used to evaluate patch test reactions are erythema, edema, induration, vesicles, and bullae, as follows: (+/−) reactions are doubtful with mild erythema and no edema; (1+) reactions show erythema throughout the area of the patch test site with associated edema or induration; (2+) reactions exhibit erythema, edema, and isolated vesicles; (3+) reactions demonstrate a strong inflammatory response with erythema, edema, and confluent vesicles. Paraphenylenediamine is a dye that normally leaves a black residue at the patch test site, which must be distinguished from an inflammatory reaction. Both strong and weak reactions are potentially of clinical significance. Clinically significant reactions may appear at 72 hours, or (+/−) reactions may evolve to become more evident at 72 hours. For these reasons, it is routine to have the patient return for a 72-hour reading. This reading is dependent upon the reliability of the skin markings made at 48 hours, when the tapes were removed.

FALSE-POSITIVE REACTIONS

There are several types of false-positive reaction. The petrolatum vehicle may cause a mild folliculitis with perifollicular erythema and an occasional pustule. This can be distinguished from a positive patch test reaction because the erythema is localized to the hair follicles and is not distributed uniformly throughout the patch test site. This false-positive reaction can be seen with the petrolatum control.

Allergic or irritant reactions to the tape are distinguished by their distribution and lack of relationship to the patch test sites. Strong positive reactions may induce an "angry back syndrome," in which the inflammation induces false-positive reactions from most of the patches on the back.

Similarly, a strong (3+) positive reaction may induce a false (1+) reaction in surrounding patches. It may be necessary to repeat the patch test using several antigens separately or separated by greater distances.

TESTING WITH NONSTANDARDIZED ALLERGENS

The reliability of patch testing depends upon the ability of the method to distinguish irritation from allergic contact dermatitis. Standardized allergens have been tested on large numbers of people to arrive at a concentration that is neither irritating nor sensitizing. Patch testing with nonstandardized allergens is therefore problematic. Only substances designed for prolonged application to the skin can be safely tested in occluded patch tests (e.g., Finn chambers). Compounds that are generally safe for patch testing include cosmetics, moisturizers, and topical medications. Clippings of shoes and clothing can also be applied as occluded patch tests along with a small volume of water. Other nonstandardized compounds are generally not safe for patch testing because they may be irritating or sensitizing.

DETERMINING THE CLINICAL SIGNIFICANCE OF PATCH TEST RESULTS

All patch test results must be evaluated with respect to the morphology of the eruption and the patient's history. The evaluation is often a lengthy process in which additional history is obtained. Positive patch test results may not be relevant to the patient's condition and may reflect a previous sensitization. Sweat and moisture are important factors in allergic contact dermatitis, because it is often necessary to leach the allergen out of the responsible object. For this reason, allergic contact dermatitis may manifest only in hot weather. Evaluation of occupational dermatitis may require obtaining the ingredients and material safety data sheets (MSDSs) for many compounds (Table 36–6). There are several excellent reference books on allergic contact dermatitis that detail the distribution and uses of a large number of allergens, as well as the patch test concentrations for multiple additional antigens.[198, 233]

SIGNIFICANCE OF THE STANDARD PATCH TEST ALLERGENS

Nickel

Nickel is the most common cause of contact allergy in North America. It is present in most metal alloys, including 14-karat gold. The classic presentation is ear lobe dermatitis secondary to earrings,[240] but any site at which metal is in contact with the skin can be involved. Dermatitis of the wrists may be secondary to bracelets or watchbands, and neck dermatitis may result from a necklace. Eyeglass frames as well as the zippers, hooks-and-eyes, and snaps in clothing may represent additional metal contact with skin. In sensitive people, metal items that are handled (e.g., tools, keys) may cause hand dermatitis.[230]

The role of dietary nickel in skin eruptions in sensitive patients is controversial. Most nickel-sensitive patients can avoid problems by wearing 18-karat gold jewelry and testing suspect objects with the dimethylglyoxime test (Allertest NI, Allerderm Laboratories, P.O. box 931, Mill Valley CA 94941; or Delasco Dermatologic Lab & Supply, 608 13th Avenue, Council Bluffs, IA 51501).

TABLE 36–6
MAJOR ALLERGENS LISTED BY OCCUPATION

Occupation	Allergen(s)
Construction worker	Chromate (cement) Epoxy resins Formaldehyde resins *p*-Tertiary-butylphenol formaldehyde resin Sawdust (esp. cedar, redwood)
Hairdresser	Ammonium persulfate Formaldehyde Fragrances Glycerol thioglycolate Nickel (in instruments) Paraphenylenediamine
Machinist and mechanic	Lubricating and cutting oils Antioxidants (e.g., paraphenylenediamine) Biocides Oil additives (*p*-tertiary-butylphenol) Organic solvents
Medical and dental professions	Antimicrobials and disinfectants Formaldehyde (formalin) Glove dermatitis Rubber accelerators Latex allergy Topical exposure to antibiotics

Rubber Accelerators: Thiurams, Carbamates, Mercaptobenzothiazole

Allergic contact dermatitis to rubber is usually caused by sensitivity to rubber accelerators, such as mercaptobenzothiazole, thiurams, and carbamates. Rubber allergy may manifest as dermatitis at sites of elastic bands in undergarments, as shoe dermatitis, or as glove dermatitis. Other exposures to rubber are rubber garments, barrier contraceptives, and rubber cements.

Thiurams are the most common cause of rubber allergy. Thiuram mix includes tetramethylthiuram disulfide, tetramethylthiuram monosulfide, tetraethylthiuram disulfide, and dipentamethylenethiuram disulfide. Carbamate mix contains diphenylguanidine, diethyldithiocarbamate, and dibutyldithiocarbamate. Carbamates are used as both rubber accelerators and garden fungicides. Allergy to black rubber also may be mediated by the dye paraphenylenediamine.

Contact urticaria to latex rubber is caused by an IgE-mediated allergy to the latex rather than the rubber accelerators. Patients with a history of contact urticaria to rubber should not undergo patch testing because of the risk of anaphylaxis.

Paraphenylenediamine

Paraphenylenediamine is a black dye used in permanent oxidative hair dyes. It is also used as an antioxidant for oils and greases and as a dye for leather and rubber. This compound or related compounds are used along with cross-linkers to obtain all hair dye colors.[185, 232] Thus, no color permanent hair dye is safe in a paraphenylenediamine-sensitive patient. Semipermanent hair dyes generally do not contain paraphenylenediamine and are acceptable alternatives. However, some "semipermanent" dyes now contain low levels of paraphenylenediamine, so it is necessary to check ingredients by calling the help number supplied on the package by the company. Paraphenylenediamine is a major cause of allergic contact dermatitis in professional hairdressers.

There are many non–hair-related uses for paraphenylenediamine both as a dye and an antioxidant. Black rubber and leather products are dyed with paraphenylenediamine, which may cause dermatitis in a sensitive patient.[217] Many oils and greases used for lubrication, including automobile-lubricating oils, contain paraphenylenediamine as an antioxidant. A mechanic who is sensitive to paraphenylenediamine may be unable to work in this occupation. Paraphenylenediamine is also a component of color film developers.[183]

Fragrances: Balsam of Peru and Cinnamic Aldehyde

Balsam of Peru is a mixture used to screen for allergic contact allergy to fragrances. Cinnamic aldehyde, a component of balsam of Peru, is used extensively for fragrances and flavors. Fragrances containing balsam of Peru or cinnamic aldehyde are present in many topical preparations, cosmetics, soaps, perfumes, and toothpastes. Sensitive patients must use "fragrance free" products. Use of "unscented" products is not sufficient, because "unscented" products may contain a masking fragrance.

p-Tertiary-Butylphenol Formaldehyde Resin

p-Tertiary-butylphenol formaldehyde resin (PTBP) is a phenolic contact adhesive used in the manufacture of plastics, plywood, cardboard boxes, varnish, rubber cements, leather products, and lacquers. PTBP may be a factor in shoe dermatitis as well as in allergic contact dermatitis to plastic products. Sensitization is usually to the resin rather than the formaldehyde. PTBP is also an oil additive.

Epoxy Resins

Epoxy resins are widely used as adhesives in electronics, the construction industry, and boats.[190, 212, 263] Epoxys are also used in marine paints and varnishes.

Formaldehyde

Formaldehyde is one of the most widespread allergens in the environment.[182, 191, 198] Aside from its obvious use in fixatives, formaldehyde resins are among the most common adhesives. They are used in plywood, cardboard boxes, fiberboard, rubber cements, and shoes. Virtually any product requiring an adhesive may use a formaldehyde resin. Sensitivity to formaldehyde resin may not induce sensitivity to formaldehyde (see earlier discussion of PTBP).

A second use of formaldehyde is as a preservative and disinfectant. Almost all shampoos contain formaldehyde (exceptions: Neutrogena, Ionil). Many toiletry articles contain formaldehyde. Cosmetics, moisturizers, and creams generally do not contain formaldehyde as a listed ingredient but often do contain preservatives that release formaldehyde. Formaldehyde-releasing preservatives include quaternium-15 (Dowicil), imidazolidinyl urea (Germall), and methyl-chloro-isothiazolinone (Kathon). Many disinfectants contain either formaldehyde or formaldehyde releasers.

Formaldehyde is also used as a fabric treatment.[200] Textile treatments that use formaldehyde include Permanent Press, Durable Press, anti-cling, and other "care-free" type fabrics. This is usually only a problem for highly sensitive patients, because most formaldehyde-sensitive patients can tolerate garments that have been washed multiple times.

Preservatives (Imidazolidinyl Urea, Quaternium-15)

Both imidazolidinyl urea and quaternium-15 are preservatives commonly used in cosmetics, moisturizers, creams, and topical medications. They are formaldehyde releasers, and a reaction may reflect either allergy to the compound or an allergy to formaldehyde (Fig. 36–13). Sensitive patients must check ingredient lists.

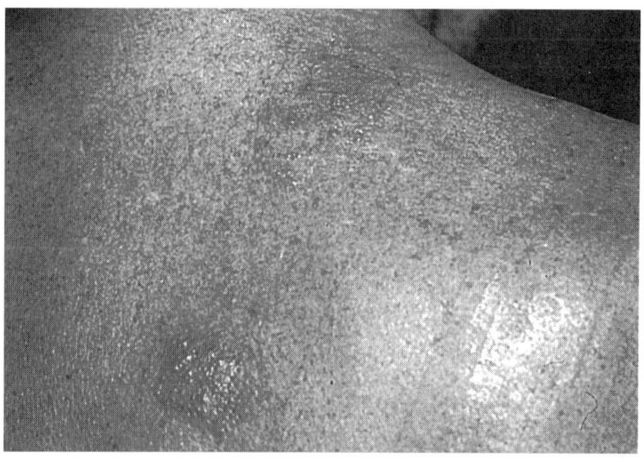

FIGURE 36–13. Positive patch test reactions to both formaldehyde and quaternium-15, which is a formaldehyde releaser.

Benzocaine

Benzocaine is a sensitizer, and topical benzocaine preparations should be avoided. Cross-reactions to procaine (Novocaine) are possible. Benzocaine is a common component of many over-the-counter products, including hemorrhoid preparations, burn products, and topical anesthetics.

Neomycin

The antibacterial agent neomycin is a common sensitizer. Bacitracin may also induce sensitization.

Chromates

The most common exposures to potassium dichromate result from its uses in the tanning of leather and in cement. Construction workers may exhibit chromate allergy as dermatitis on their arms after contact with cement. Chromate in leather can also have a role in shoe dermatitis. Contact dermatitis to chromate in leather shoes may be seasonal, because the allergen is leached out with sweat.

TABLE 36–7
CLASSIFICATION OF POTENCY OF CORTICOSTEROID PREPARATIONS*

Group 1	Clobetasol propionate 0.05% cream or ointment Diflurasone diacetate 0.05% ointment Betamethasone dipropionate 0.05% cream or ointment (optimized vehicle: Diprolene)
Group 2	Fluocinonide 0.05% cream or ointment
Group 3	Triamcinolone 0.1% ointment Amcinonide 0.1% ointment Betamethasone valerate 0.1% ointment
Group 4	Triamcinolone 0.1% cream Fluocinolone acetonide 0.025% ointment
Group 5	Hydrocortisone valerate 0.2% cream
Group 6	Hydrocortisone 1% & 2.5% cream and ointment

*Group 1, 2, and 3 steroids should not be used on the face. Group 4 steroids can be used on the face for acute dermatitis provided that the duration of treatment does not exceed 1 week. For longer applications to the face, hydrocortisone valerate 0.2% is usually tolerated. For young children, it is advised to use group 6 steroids. The penalty for the use of potent corticosteroids on the face is the development of acne vulgaris, rosacea, skin atrophy, and telangectasia.

Data from Stoughton RB: Vasoconstrictor assay—specific applications. In Maibach HI, Surber C (eds): Topical Corticosteroids. Karger, Basel, 1992.

TREATMENT OF CONTACT DERMATITIS

Treatment of contact dermatitis requires both avoidance of contact with the offending irritant or contact allergen and appropriate treatment of the dermatitis. Thus, identification of the responsible allergen through history, morphology, or patch testing is an essential element of treatment. The decision whether to treat with topical medications alone or to use systemic steroids is made on the basis of severity of the eruption as well as the medical condition of the patient. Because contact dermatitis resolves spontaneously with simple removal of the offending agent, it is important for the clinician to remember to "do no harm" in considering treatment options.

TOPICAL TREATMENT

Topical steroids are the basis of treatment of contact dermatitis. Acute dermatitis generally responds best to class I super–high-potency steroids (e.g., clobetasol propionate 0.05%) (Table 36–7). Chronic or subacute dermatitis can often be treated with class II steroids (e.g., fluocinonide 0.05%). These potent steroids should not be used on the face, axilla, breasts or genitalia. Except for the face, class III steroids (e.g., triamcinolone 0.1%) may be used in these locations, provided that the treatment is limited to 1 week. For longer treatments or for the face, class IV steroids (e.g., hydrocortisone valerate 0.2%) should be used. The vehicle is a significant consideration. Gels are drying and are preferred on acute vesicular dermatitis. Ointments are most effective on chronic lichenified dermatitis. Creams are often used when the patient does not tolerate ointments for aesthetic reasons. Topical steroids often reduce pruritus in several days and inflammation within 1 week. However, no treatment is likely to be effective if the patient does not avoid contact with the offending allergen.

Allergic contact dermatitis to topical medications is a significant problem, especially because topical medications contain many of the same preservatives as cosmetics (Fig. 36–14). If allergy to a topical cream is suspected, it is preferable to use a topical steroid preparation lacking preservatives until the offending chemical is identified by patch testing. Several steroid ointments (e.g., triamcinolone 0.1% ointment [Aristicort]) lack preservatives and are useful in such cases.

Tar has mild anti-inflammatory effects and can be a useful adjuvant to topical steroids for the treatment of chronic lichenified dermatitis. Tar may be used as 5% crude coal tar in petrolatum or as tar bath oil soaks (e.g., Balnetar). Tar is too irritating for treatment of acute dermatitis.

Palliative treatments for the pruritus associated with allergic contact dermatitis include calamine lotion, oatmeal baths, and milk soaks. These treatments may be very appropriate for children with self-limited allergic contact dermatitis to plants (e.g., poison ivy). Calamine preparations containing

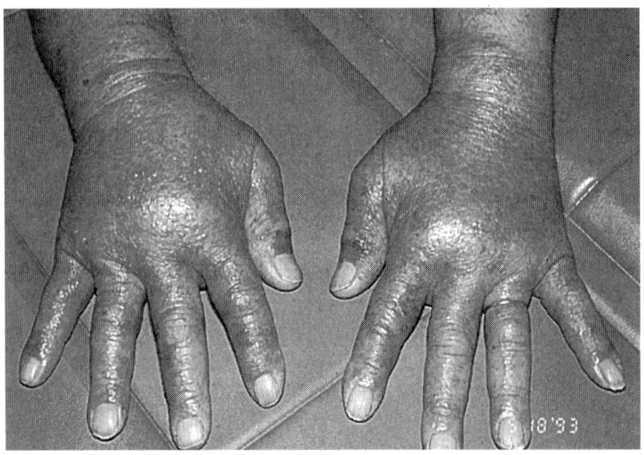

FIGURE 36–14. Allergic contact dermatitis to topical steroid preparation applied to hands. Note massive edema, erythema, and sparing of skin under watch band.

diphenhydramine should be avoided, because this agent is a contact sensitizer.

ANTIHISTAMINES IN ALLERGIC CONTACT DERMATITIS

There are multiple inflammatory mediators in allergic contact dermatitis (delayed hypersensitivity), and antihistamines have little or no effect on the inflammation or pruritus. However, diphenhydramine and hydroxyzine are both commonly prescribed for use at night to allow the patient to sleep.

SYSTEMIC STEROID TREATMENT

Severe cases of allergic contact dermatitis may justify treatment with systemic steroids. Indications include involvement of a large body surface area and interference with function. The decision to use systemic steroids must weigh the patient's medical condition and age. Untreated allergic contact dermatitis generally lasts approximately 2 weeks and is probably terminated by elimination of the allergen. This fact must be remembered in treatment planning. A common mistake is to use an insufficient dosage of steroids for an insufficient time. Termination of a severe generalized allergic contact dermatitis usually requires 1.0 mg/kg of prednisone as an initial daily dose. After 2 or 4 days, it is generally possible to decrease the daily dose to 0.66 mg/kg for the duration of treatment. It is not advised to further taper the prednisone. The total duration of treatment should be 14 days, at which time the prednisone is discontinued without tapering.

With prednisone therapy, it is necessary to monitor blood pressure and glucose levels. Patients should be informed of the side effects of prednisone and warned to watch for signs of infection. The decision to use systemic steroids requires a medical evaluation of the patient with respect to risks of steroid use—diabetes mellitus, hypertension, and history of infections, including tuberculosis.

SPECIAL CASES OF CONTACT DERMATITIS

AUTOECZEMATIZATION REACTIONS

Patients with a highly inflamed dermatitis may develop a generalized eczematous reaction. Possible inciting conditions include inflammatory tinea pedis, inflammatory stasis dermatitis, and acute eczematous allergic contact dermatitis. This generalized eruption is termed an *autoeczematization* or *id reaction*. It is postulated to result from either systemic spread of allergen or an autoimmune phenomenon triggered by the eczematous dermatitis.

Autoeczematization reactions often manifest as inflammatory edematous follicular papules with a generalized distribution, including the trunk. The condition is usually pruritic. Eruptions of the hands and feet often parallel each other, frequently with bullous eruptions. Autoeczematization reactions develop after the initial dermatitis and are common with severe allergic contact dermatitis, such as that seen with poison ivy.

Treatment of an autoeczematization reaction usually requires systemic steroids. If steroids are not medically contraindicated, it is preferable to initiate therapy with oral prednisone at 1 mg/kg daily. After 2 days, the dose is dropped to 0.66 mg/kg and maintained at this level for a total of 14 days of treatment. The initial dermatitis is simultaneously treated aggressively with topical steroids.

CONTACT DERMATITIS TO TOPICAL MEDICATIONS

Whenever a patient's rash becomes worse after the use of a topical medication, allergic contact dermatitis to that medication should be suspected (Fig. 36–15). The other common cause of medication-induced flares is the use of topical steroids to treat fungal disease. Inflamed skin is more likely to develop an allergic reaction than normal skin. Preservatives that have an excellent safety record on normal skin may induce sensitization on diseased skin. Patients with chronic stasis dermatitis or chronic ulcerations of the lower extremity are particularly prone to the development of allergic contact dermatitis to topical medications (Fig. 36–16).

Creams are emulsions of oil and water that contain multiple possible allergens, including preservatives, emulsifiers, antioxidants, propylene glycol, and stabilizers. Ointments do not contain water and may not require many of these ingredients. Contact dermatitis to topical medications generally results from sensitization to the preservative. There are reports that a small fraction (e.g., 10%) of patients reacting to a topical steroid preparation are allergic to the corticosteroid.[228, 251]

HAND AND GLOVE DERMATITIS

Hand and glove dermatitis must be distinguished from latex allergy. Chronic hand dermatitis is often difficult to treat. The relative roles of irritant contact dermatitis and allergic contact dermatitis in this disorder are often unclear. Dyshidrotic eczema, with vesicles along the lateral margins of the fingers, may result from irritant dermatitis but may be

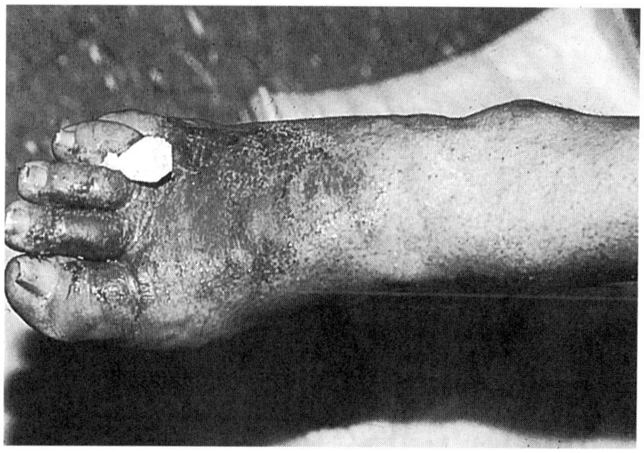

FIGURE 36–15. Application of antifungal cream to the feet induced this allergic reaction. Note the involvement between the toes. The patient also suffered an autoeczematization reaction from this acute eczematous reaction.

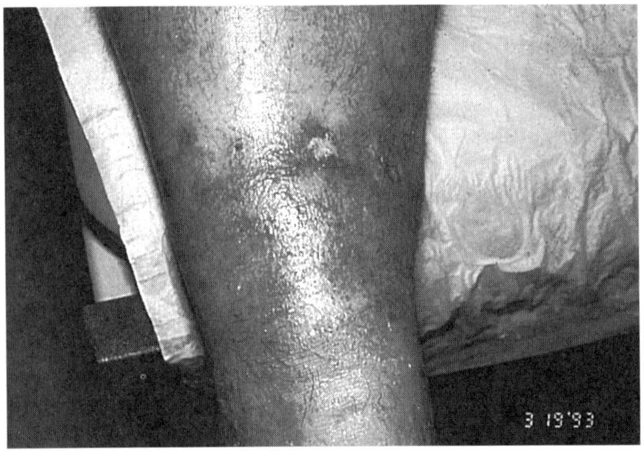

FIGURE 36–16. Chronic ulcerations on the lower extremity are particularly likely to develop allergic contact dermatitis. This eruption resulted from sensitization to bacitracin.

idiopathic. Psoriasis can often mimic hand dermatitis, as can tinea manum.

Examination of the feet is essential in the evaluation of hand dermatitis. Irritant or allergic contact dermatitis is unlikely to affect both hands and feet. Conditions that frequently involve both hands and feet are psoriasis, tinea, and dyshidrotic eczema. A sharp cutoff of the dermatitis at the wrist may indicate allergic contact dermatitis to gloves. Nickel allergy may induce hand dermatitis, because most metal items are made of alloys containing nickel. Allergic contact dermatitis often spares the palmar surface of the hand because of the thickness of the stratum corneum. When allergic contact dermatitis involves the palms, the dorsum of the hand is usually also involved. Nickel allergy may be an exception, because tools and other metal items are generally handled with the palmar surface of the hand.

With the adoption of universal precautions in the health care field, the use of gloves and incidence of glove dermatitis have increased greatly. Glove dermatitis may result from irritation by the powder, in which case powderless gloves are curative. Allergic contact dermatitis to latex gloves is most often mediated by rubber accelerators (e.g., thiurams, carbamates, mercaptobenzothiazole).[220] Gloves vary in the amount of extractable thiuram, and certain brands are less allergenic.

In contrast to allergic contact dermatitis to rubber accelerators, allergy to latex is IgE-mediated and may manifest as contact urticaria or anaphylaxis.[173, 187, 226, 272] Affected patients must avoid all latex exposure, including use of "hypoallergenic" latex gloves, and should not undergo patch testing. Skin prick tests and radioallergosorbent tests (RASTs) may be helpful in the evaluation of such patients. Latex-allergic patients must avoid latex completely and use vinyl gloves. Vinyl hypoallergenic nonsterile and surgical gloves are available from Allerderm Laboratories (P.O. Box 931, Mill Valley, CA 94942-0931, 1-800-365-6868).

SHOE AND LEATHER DERMATITIS

Shoe dermatitis usually manifests on the dorsum of the foot. Because of the thicker stratum corneum on plantar skin, isolated plantar involvement is less common. Sweat is an important factor, because moisture can leach the allergens from the shoe. For this reason, there can be a seasonal variation. Patients suspected of having shoe dermatitis should undergo patch testing. Responsible allergens include formaldehyde resins, chromate from leather, rubber accelerators (e.g., mercaptobenzothiazole, thiurams, and carbamates), rubber cement components (e.g., *p*-tertiary-butylphenol), epoxy resins, and dyes (e.g., paraphenylenediamine).[218] It is possible to patch-test with cuttings from shoes moistened with water and placed under occlusive bandaging. Patch test results can be used to plan hypoallergenic footwear. In some patients, shoe dermatitis can be managed by reducing moisture with frequent sock changes and avoidance of sneakers. Allergic contact dermatitis to leather may also be observed at sites under watchbands and belts (Fig. 36–17).

OCCUPATIONAL CONTACT DERMATITIS

Contact dermatitis is a major cause of occupational illness and loss of time from work.[193, 234, 235, 252] Approximately 40% of all occupational illness results from skin disease, and at least 90% of occupational skin disease is caused by contact dermatitis. Contactants commonly associated with several occupations are discussed here and listed in Table 36–6. (For more information, see also references 167, 232, and 233.)

Hairdressers are exposed to water, detergents, gloves, dyes, instruments, shampoos, and permanent wave solutions.[266, 267] They frequently develop hand dermatitis, which may be either irritant or allergic contact. Common allergens are glycerol thioglycolate in acid permanent wave solutions, paraphenylenediamine in hair dyes, formalin in shampoos, ammonium persulfate in oxidative boosters, fragrances in a multitude of products, and nickel in instruments.[202, 260]

Construction workers are exposed to epoxy and formaldehyde-based glues and resins.[190, 207, 236, 264] Additional contacts are rubber[189] and oils containing antioxidants, such as paraphenylenediamine. Cement exposure is associated with allergic contact dermatitis to chromate.[206, 211]

Machinists and mechanics are exposed to cutting oils containing biocides and antioxidants (e.g., paraphenylenediamine) which may induce both irritant and allergic contact

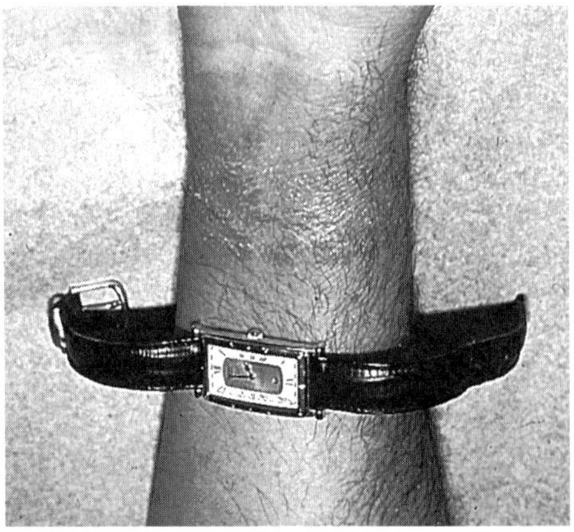

FIGURE 36–17. Allergic dermatitis from a black leather watch band. Possible allergens include chromates used to tan leather and the paraphenylenediamine dye.

dermatitis.[203, 242] An additional risk factor is exposure to organic solvents, which act as irritants.[223]

PLANT DERMATITIS (POISON IVY)

Many plants and plant products are contact sensitizers.[253] The most notorious in North America are the urushiol-containing plants poison ivy and poison oak of the Anacardiaceae family. Other contact sensitizers are tulip bulbs,[185] *Philodendron,*[219] and hydrangea.[209] Compositae plants (e.g., chrysanthemum) are reported to cause allergic contact dermatitis from both direct and airborne contact.[238, 245] The responsible allergens are sesquiterpene lactones.[244] With the growing use of "natural herbal" extracts in cosmetics and personal care items, allergic contact dermatitis to plants is likely to become a more important issue.

PHOTOALLERGIC REACTIONS

PHOTOTOXIC AND PHOTOALLERGIC REACTIONS

Both phototoxic and photoallergic reactions result from the interaction of ultraviolet light (UV) with skin components.[170, 197, 205, 249] UV is classified depending upon wavelength. UVB comprises wavelengths from 290 to 320 nm, and UVA wavelengths from 320 to 400 nm. Shorter wavelengths carry more energy but penetrate skin less deeply than longer wavelengths. Photosensitivity reactions depend on the photochemistry resulting from absorption of light by the sensitizing agent. Most photosensitizers absorb light in the UVA wavelengths. This has clinical significance, because unlike UVB, UVA is produced by fluorescent lights, can pass through window glass, and is not blocked by UVB sunscreens.

Phototoxic reactions are the direct result of photochemistry and do not depend on immune sensitization. There is significant individual variation, but all persons with a sufficient exposure to a phototoxic agent should have an increased photosensitivity. Psoralen is a photosensitizer. All persons exposed to sufficient psoralen develop erythema when exposed to UVA. Phototoxic reactions often resemble a bad sunburn. They differ from a UVB sunburn in that they may peak at 48 hours rather than 12 to 24 hours. The skin is usually tender and erythematous. Severe phototoxic reactions can produce bullae.

Photoallergic reactions result when the photochemical reaction of UV with a sensitizing agent generates an immunogenic hapten. Photoallergic reactions are thus dependent on both photochemistry and the immune response. Once the antigenic photoproduct is generated, the pathogenesis of photoallergic reactions is similar to that of allergic contact dermatitis. There is considerable variation between people in sensitization to photoallergens, and generally, only a small subset of exposed individuals become sensitized. Photoallergens tend to produce an eczematous, pruritic dermatitis with a photodistribution.

Photoallergic and phototoxic reactions may be either systemic or contact. Systemic reactions usually result from systemic drug exposure and are expressed symmetrically on most sun-exposed skin. Contact photosensitivities are a function of topical contact with the photosensitizer and are expressed only on skin that is exposed to both the photosensitizer and ultraviolet light.

DIAGNOSIS OF PHOTOALLERGIC REACTIONS

Recognition of an eczematous dermatitis in a photodistribution is the key to the diagnosis of photoallergic reactions. An archetypal photodistribution involves the extensor aspects of the forearms, much of the face, and the V region of the neck. The volar forearms are relatively spared, along with areas covered by clothing. Typically, there is relative sparing of the skin of the eyelids, beneath the chin, directly below the nose, and in the nasolabial folds. An eruption with this photodistribution can be seen with a large number of photosensitivity disorders.

The differential diagnosis of photosensitivity disorders includes autoimmune diseases such as lupus erythematosus, many of the porphyrias, polymorphic light eruption,[243] phototoxic reactions, and photoallergic reactions. Conditions that may be mistaken for a photosensitivity disorder are allergic contact dermatitis to aeroallergens,[172] rosacea, and allergic contact dermatitis to agents in contact with exposed skin. Chronic photosensitivity dermatitis can evolve into actinic reticuloid,[178] which does not resolve upon avoidance of the inciting agent. Actinic reticuloid, a variant of chronic actinic dermatitis, is associated with induration of the skin and a dense lymphocytic infiltrate often demonstrating atypical lymphocytes.

Evaluation of a photodistributed eruption should be directed by the results of history and physical examination. Photoallergic reactions are generally eczematous and pruritic. Phototoxic reactions resemble sunburns and usually lack an eczematous component (i.e., scaling, crust, lichenification). Solar urticaria manifests as urticaria (hives) within 15 minutes of sun exposure. The action spectrum can be UVA, UVB, visible light, or a combination of wavelengths (see Chapter 35). Pathogenesis may involve phototoxic reactions to drugs, erythropoietic protoporphyria, or sensitization to an endogenous photoallergen. *Porphyria cutanea tarda* is the only common acquired porphyria. It often manifests as blisters and milia on the dorsum of the hands associated with skin fragility. The porphyrias can be diagnosed by the findings of elevated urine and/or stool porphyrins. *Polymorphic light eruption* can be suspected from the history and examination, and diagnosed with skin biopsy. It manifests as a recurrent pruritic papular eruption of the sun-exposed skin of shoulders and upper extremities that flares with first sun exposure in the late spring. The condition abates with "harding" from continued sun exposure and often clears by late summer. *Autoimmune diseases* such as lupus erythematosus should be screened for by history, review of systems, and physical examination. If necessary, serology, biopsy, and direct immunofluorescence testing may be indicated.

As with contact dermatitis, photocontact dermatitis is suggested by linearity and lack of symmetry. The conclusive evidence for a photoallergic reaction is a positive photopatch test result (see later).

SYSTEMIC PHOTOSENSITIZERS

Most photosensitizers are drugs. Many photosensitizing drugs are capable of inducing both phototoxic and photoallergic reactions.[170, 249, 268] Categories of photosensitizing drugs are the tetracyclines (especially doxycycline),[227] sulfonamides, furosemide, thiazides, quinidine,[271] griseofulvin,[221] carbamazepine, chlorpromazine,[254] and nonsteroidal anti-inflammatory agents (NSAIDs).[242] Piroxicam is probably the most photosensitizing NSAID available in the United States, and it is capable of inducing both phototoxic and photoallergic reactions.[204, 208] Phototoxic reactions to ibuprofen have also been observed.[176] Patients with human immunodeficiency virus have an exceptionally high incidence of photosensitivity reactions to sulfonamides and NSAIDs.[175] The therapeutic function of the psoralens depends on their photosensitizing properties.

CONTACT PHOTOALLERGENS AND PHOTOSENSITIZERS

The principal contact photoallergens are fragrances, antimicrobials, and sunscreen agents.[194, 200, 233] The most significant fragrance photosensitizers are musk ambrette and 6-methylcoumarin. Musk ambrette is a common component of aftershave lotions and other fragrances marketed for men. 6-Methylcoumarin is used as a fragrance in cosmetics and can act as both a photoallergen and a phototoxic agent.

Plant-derived psoralens can induce phototoxic contact dermatitis. Lime, celery, and parsnip contain sufficient psoralens to result in dermatitis at sites exposed to both the juice of such a plant and light. Typically, the eruption leaves streaks of residual hyperpigmentation where the juice dripped onto the patient's face.

Photosensitizing antimicrobial agents have been a major problem but are now less commonly used. The principal culprits were the salicylanilide compounds (tetrachlorosalicylanilide, tribromosalicylanilide). Additional photosensitizing antimicrobial agents are triclosan, dichlorophen, hexachlorophene (pHisoHex), and chlorhexidine (Hibiclens).

Sunscreen agents obviously absorb ultraviolet light and are also capable of acting as photoallergens.[178, 261, 265] Photoallergic reactions have been reported to para-aminobenzoic acid (PABA), octyl dimethyl PABA (padimate O), and oxybenzone. PABA-sensitive patients may also react to sulfonamides, benzocaine, *p*-aminosalicylic acid (PAS), and paraphenylenediamine (hair dye). At present, sunscreens are probably the most significant photoallergens.

PHOTOPATCH TESTING

Photopatch testing is a variation of patch testing in which the skin is also exposed to UVA.[240] The allergen patches are applied in duplicate. One set is covered to prevent light exposure, and the second set is removed after 24 hours and exposed to UVA. The UVA-exposed patches are then recovered for 24 hours longer, and all patches are read at 48 and 72 hours.

Allergens suggested for photopatch testing and their standard diluents[197] include musk ambrette (1% petrolatum), PABA (5% alcohol), octyl dimethyl PABA (5% alcohol), oak moss (1% petrolatum), bithionol (1% petrolatum), 6-methylcoumarin (1% alcohol), and petrolatum control. Clinically relevant creams, sunscreens, and cosmetics intended for prolonged application can also be used for photopatch testing.

Photopatch testing requires appropriate UVA and UVB light sources along with UV monitoring equipment. UVA sources for photopatch testing must emit light throughout the UVA spectrum. Standard UVA fluorescent lights used for PUVA therapy are sufficient. The UVB light source can be a standard UVB fluorescent bulb (e.g., FS40 bulbs).

Prior to photopatch testing, the patient is tested for sensitivity to UVB and UVA. This is necessary to screen for other photosensitivity conditions (e.g., chronic actinic dermatitis) and as a preliminary for photopatch testing. Minimal erythema doses (MEDs) for UVB and UVA are determined. MED is the minimal dose of light that induces a uniform erythema in the test area of skin. Normal subjects should not develop erythema with 10 J/cm^2, of UVA. Following exposure to UV for the MED determinations, the photoallergen patches are applied to the back in duplicate. One set of patches is covered with aluminum foil as well as tape to prevent light exposure. To maintain its stability, 6-methylcoumarin should be applied separately on the second day, 30 minutes prior to UVA exposure.

The mechanics of patch application are similar to those for standard patch testing. On day 2 (24 hours), the MEDs for UVA and UVB are determined by reading the test site. One set of patches is then removed for UVA exposure and the sites are marked. Provided that the MED for UVA was greater than 10 J/cm^2, the exposed patches are irradiated with 5 J/cm^2. The patient returns on day 4, and all patch sites are examined.

Photopatch reactions are first scored from (+/−) to (3+), as described for standard patch testing. Interpretation requires comparison of the irradiated and nonirradiated sets of patches. Positive reactions to an allergen on both the irradiated and nonirradiated skin indicate allergic contact dermatitis. Photocontact dermatitis is diagnosed only if the reaction is observed on the irradiated skin, but not on the nonirradiated skin.

TREATMENT OF PHOTOALLERGIC REACTIONS

The key points in the treatment of a photoallergic reaction are identification of the responsible allergen, avoidance of the responsible allergen, photoprotection, and use of corticosteroids. Unfortunately, some patients develop a chronic photosensitivity despite removal of the initiating allergen, which may evolve into chronic actinic dermatitis or actinic reticuloid. Photoprotection should block both UVA and UVB wavelengths, because UVA is usually responsible for photoallergic and phototoxic reactions. Patients are exposed to UVA through window glass and from fluorescent lights. Both topical and systemic steroids have an important role in the treatment of photoallergic reactions. The guidelines for use of corticosteroids in photoallergic dermatitis are the same as those described in allergic contact dermatitis. However, corticosteroids are not likely to be effective unless the patient is protected from ultraviolet light and avoids the responsible allergen(s).

REFERENCES

1. Adinoff AD, Tellez P, Clark RAF: Atopic dermatitis and aeroallergen contact sensitivity. J Allergy Clin Immunol 81:736–742, 1988.
2. Amemiya T, Matsuda H, Uehara M: Ocular findings in atopic dermatitis with special reference to the clinical features of atopic cataract. Ophthalmologica 180:129–132, 1980.
3. Atherton DJ, Carabett F, Glover MT, et al: The role of psoralen chemotherapy (PUVA) in the treatment of severe atopic eczema in adolescence. Br J Dermatol 118:791–795, 1988.
4. Beck H-I, Korsgaard J: Atopic dermatitis and house dust mites. Br J Dermatol 120:245–251, 1989.
5. Besnier E: Piémière note et observations préliminares pour sévir d'introduction à l'étude des pruripos diatrhésiques. Ann Dermatol Syph 23:634–637, 1892.
6. Bieber T, de la Salle H, Wollenberg A, et al: Human epidermal Langerhans cells express the high affinity receptor for immunoglobulin E (Fc epsilon R1). J Exp Med 175:1285–1290, 1992.
7. Bock SA, Lee WY, Remigio LK, May CD: Studies of hypersensitivity reactions to food in infants and children. J Allergy Clin Immunol 62:327–334, 1978.
8. Bradding P, Feather IH, Howarth PH, et al: Interleukin 4 is localized and released by human mast cells. J Exp Med 176:1381–1386, 1992.
9. Brunsting LA, Reed WB, Bair HL: Occurrence of cataracts and keratoconus with atopic dermatitis. AMA Arch Dermatol Syphilol 72:237–241, 1955.
10. Burks AW, Mallory SB, Williams LW, Shirrell MA: Atopic dermatitis: clinical relevance of food hypersensitivity reactions. J Pediatr 113:447–451, 1988.
11. Burrows D, Penman RWB: Prognosis of the eczema-asthma syndrome. Br J Med 2:825–828, 1960.
12. Burton JL: Dietary fatty acids and inflammatory skin disease. Lancet 1:27–31, 1989.
13. Castrow FF: Atopic cataracts versus steroid cataracts. J Am Acad Dermatol 5:64, 1981.
14. Chan SC, Audrea C, Rocklin R, et al: Cyclic nucleotide regulation of T cell cytokine production and feedback control in atopic dermatitis [abstract]. Clin Res 41:5A, 1993.
15. Christensen JD: Frequency of cataract in atopic dermatitis. Acta Derm Venereol (Stockh) 61:76–77, 1981.
16. Clark RAF, Adinoff AD: Aeroallergen contact can exacerbate atopic dermatitis: patch tests as a diagnostic tool. J Am Acad Dermatol 21:863–869, 1989.
17. Clark RAF, Adinoff AD: The relationship between positive aeroallergen patch test reactions and aeroallergen exacerbations of atopic dermatitis. Clin Immunol Immunopathol 53(suppl):s132–s140, 1989.
18. Clemmensen OJ, Hjorth N: Treatment of dermatitis of the head and neck with ketoconazole in patients with type 1 sensitivity to *Pityrosporon orbiculare*. Semin Dermatol 2:26–29, 1983.
19. Cole WC, Roth HL, Sacks LB: Group psychotherapy as an aid in the medical treatment of eczema. J Am Acad Dermatol 18:286–291, 1988.
20. Coleman R, Trembath RC, Harper JI: Chromosome 11q13 and atopy underlying atopic eczema. Lancet 341:1121–1122, 1993.
21. Colloff MJ: Exposure to house dust mites in homes of people with atopic dermatitis. Br J Dermatol 127:322–327, 1992.
22. Colver GB, Symons JA: Soluble interleukin 2 receptor in atopic eczema. Br Med J 298:1426–1428, 1989.
23. Cooper K: Atopic dermatitis: recent trends in pathogenesis and therapy. Prog Dermatol 27:1–16, 1993.
24. Cooper KD, Kang K, Chan SC, Hanifin JM: Phosphodiesterase inhibition by Ro 20-1724 reduces hyper-IgE synthesis by atopic dermatitis cells in vitro. J Invest Dermatol 84:477–482, 1985.
25. Cronin E, Bandemann H-J, Calnan D, et al: Contact dermatitis in the atopic. Acta Derm Venereol (Stockh) 50:183–187, 1970.
26. Cronin E, McFadden JP: Patients with atopic eczema do become sensitized to contact allergens. Contact Dermatitis 28:225–258, 1993.
27. Czech W, Krutmann J, Schopf E, et al: Serum eosinophilic cationic protein (ECP) is a sensitive measure for disease activity in atopic dermatitis. Br J Dermatol 126:351–355, 1992.
28. DeGroot AC: The frequency of contact allergy in atopic patients with dermatitis. Contact Dermatitis 22:273–277, 1990.
29. Diepgen TL, Fartasch M, Hornstein OP: Evaluation and relevance of atopic basic and minor features in patients with atopic dermatitis and in the general population. Acta Derm Venereol Suppl (Stockh) 144:50–54, 1989.
30. Diepgen TL, Fartasch, M: Recent epidemiological and genetic studies in atopic dermatitis. Acta Derm Venereol Suppl (Stockh) 176:13–18, 1992.
31. Doherty V, Sylvester DGH, Kennedy CTC, et al: Treatment of itching in atopic eczema with antihistamines with a low sedative profile. Br Med J 298:96–97, 1989.
32. Drake LA, Fallon JD, Sober A: Relief of pruritus in patients with atopic dermatitis after treatment with topical doxepin cream: the Doxepin Study Group. J Am Acad Dermatol 31:613–616, 1994.
33. Epstein S, Moharjerin AH: Incidence of contact sensitivity in atopic dermatitis. Arch Dermatol 90:284–287, 1964.
34. Eriksson-Lihr Z: The incidence of allergic diseases in childhood. Acta Allergol 8:289–313, 1955.
35. Faulstich ME, Williamson DA, Duchmann EG, et al: Psychophysiologic analysis of atopic dermatitis. J Psychosom Res 29:415–417, 1985.
36. Feinberg SM: Seasonal atopic dermatitis: the role of inhaled atopens. Arch Derm Syph 40:200, 1939.
37. Fergusson DM, Horwood LJ, Shannon FT: Parental asthma, parental eczema, and asthma and eczema in early childhood. J Chronic Dis 36:517–524, 1983.
38. Fiocchi A, Sala M, Signoroni P, et al: The efficacy and safety of gamma-linoleic acid in the treatment of infantile atopic dermatitis. J Int Med Res 22:24–32, 1994.
39. Foster CS, Calogne M: Atopic keratoconjunctivitis. Ophthalmology 97:992–1000, 1990.
40. Frain-Bell W: The photoaggravated dermatoses. In Cutaneous Photobiology. Oxford University Press, New York, 1985, pp 60–61.
41. Frosch PJ, Schwanitz HJ, Macher E: A double-blind trial of H_1 and H_2 receptor antagonists in the treatment of atopic dermatitis. Arch Dermatol Res 276:36–40, 1984.
42. Garrie EV, Garrie SA, Mok T: Anxiety and atopic dermatitis. J Consult Clin Psychol 42:742, 1974.
43. Garrity JA, Liesegang TJ: Ocular complications of atopic dermatitis. Can J Ophthalmol 19:21–24, 1984.
44. Glover MT, Atherton DJ: A double-blind controlled trial of hyposensitization to *Dermatophagoides pteronyssinus* in children with atopic eczema. Clin Exp Allergy 22:440–446, 1992.
45. Grewe SR, Chan SC, Hanifin JM: Elevated leukocyte cAMP-phosphodiesterase in atopic disease: a possible mechanism for cyclic AMP agonist hyporesponsiveness. J Allergy Clin Immunol 70:452–457, 1982.
46. Guillet G, Guillet M: Natural history of sensitizations in atopic dermatitis—a 3 year follow-up in 250 children: food allergy and high risk of respiratory symptoms. Arch Dermatol 128:187–192, 1992.
47. Guenther L, Wexler D: Efamol and the treatment of atopic dermatitis. J Am Acad Dermatol 17:860, 1987.
48. Gurevitch AW, Heiner DC, Reisner R: IgE in atopic dermatitis and other common dermatoses. Arch Dermatol 107:712, 1973.
49. Gustafson D, Lowhagen T, Andersson K: Risk of developing atopic disease after early feeding with cow's milk based formula. Arch Dis Child 67:1008–1010, 1992.
50. Halpern SR, Sellars WA, Johnson RB, et al: Development of childhood allergy in infants fed breast, soy, or cow's milk. J Allergy Clin Immunol 51:139, 1973.
51. Hanifin JM: Phosphodiesterase and immune dysfunction in atopic dermatitis. J Dermatol Sci 1:1–6, 1990.
52. Hanifin JM, Rajka G: Diagnostic features of atopic dermatitis. Acta Derm Venereol Suppl (Stockh) 92:44–47, 1980.
53. Hanifin JM, Ray LF, Lobitz WC Jr: Immunologic reactivity in dermatophytosis. Br J Dermatol 90:1–8, 1974.
54. Heskel NS, Chan SC, Tiel ML, et al: Elevated umbilical cord blood leukocyte cyclic adenosine monophosphate-phosphodiesterase activity in children with atopic parents. J Am Acad Dermatol 11:422–426, 1987.
55. Holden CA, Chan SC, Hanifin JM: Monocyte localization of elevated cAMP phosphodiesterase activity in atopic dermatitis. J Invest Dermatol 87:372–376, 1986.
56. Jekler J, Larko O: Combined UVA-UVB versus UVB phototherapy for atopic dermatitis. J Am Acad Dermatol 22:49–53, 1990.
57. Jones HE: The atopic-dermatophytosis syndrome. Acta Derm Venereol (Stockh) 92:81–85, 1980.
58. Jones HE, Inouye JC, McGerity JL, Lewis CW: Atopic disease and serum immunoglobulin E. Br J Dermatol 92:17–25, 1975.
59. Jones HE, Lewis C, McMarlin SL: Allergic contact sensitivity in atopic dermatitis. Arch Dermatol 107:217–222, 1973.

60. Kang K, Cooper KD, Hanifin JM: Thymopentin pentapeptide (TP-5) improves clinical parameters and lymphocyte subpopulations in atopic dermatitis. J Am Acad Dermatol 8:372–377, 1983.
61. Kapp A, Czech W, Krutmann J, et al: Eosinophilic cationic protein in sera of patients with atopic dermatitis. J Am Acad Dermatol 24:555–558, 1991.
62. Kapsenberg ML, Wierenga EA, Bos JD, Jansen HM: Functional subsets of allergen-reactive human CD4+ T cells. Immunol Today 12:392–395, 1991.
63. Katavisto M: Prurigo diathesique Besnier and cataract. Acta Ophthalmol 27:581, 1949.
64. Kay AB: Allergen injection immunotherapy (hyposensitization) on trial. Clin Exp Allergy 119:591–596, 1989.
65. Kay J, Gawkrodger DJ, Mortimer MJ, Jaron AG: The prevalence of childhood eczema in a general population. J Am Acad Dermatol 30:35–39, 1994.
66. Kim J-W, Chan SC, Handerson WR, et al: Disordered prostaglandin E_2 control of cytokine production in atopic dermatitis [abstract]. J Invest Dermatol 98:610, 1992.
67. Kjellman NIM, Johansson SGO: Soy versus cow's milk in infants with a biparental history of atopic disease: development of atopic disease and immunoglobulins from birth to 4 years of age. Clin Allergy 9:347–358, 1979.
68. Koblenzer CS: Psychotherapy for intractable inflammatory dermatoses. J Am Acad Dermatol 32:609–612, 1995.
69. Koblenzer CS, Koblenzer PJ: Chronic intractable atopic eczema. Arch Dermatol 124:1673–1677, 1988.
70. Lammintausta K, Kalimo K: Does a patient's occupation influence the course of atopic dermatitis? Acta Derm Venereol (Stockh) 73:119–122, 1993.
71. Larsen FS: Atopic dermatitis: a genetic-epidemiologic study in a population-based twin sample. J Am Acad Dermatol 28:719–723, 1993.
72. Larsen FS, Hanifin JM: Secular change in the occurrence of atopic dermatitis. Acta Derm Venereol Suppl (Stockh) 176:7–12, 1992.
73. Larson FS, Holm NV, Hennigsen K: Atopic dermatitis: a genetic-epidemiological study in a population-based twin sample. J Am Acad Dermatol 15:487–494, 1986.
74. Latchman Y, Bungy GA, Atherton DJ, et al: Efficacy of traditional Chinese herbal therapy in vitro: a model system for atopic eczema: inhibition of CD23 expression on blood monocytes. Br J Dermatol 132:592–598, 1995.
75. Leiferman KM, Ackerman SJ, Sampson HA, et al: Dermal deposition of eosinophil-granule major basic protein in atopic dermatitis. N Engl J Med 313:282–285, 1985.
76. Leroy BP, Jacquemin MG, Lachapelle JM, et al: Allergen-sensitive atopic dermatitis is improved by injections of allergen combined with F(ab′)2 fragments of specific antibodies. Br J Dermatol 132:599–603, 1995.
77. Leung DYM, Geha RS, Schneeberger EE, et al: Characterization of the mononuclear cell infiltrate in atopic dermatitis using monoclonal antibodies. J Allergy Clin Immunol 71:47–56, 1983.
78. Leung DYM, Harbeck R, Bina P, et al: Presence of IgE antibodies to staphylococcal exotoxins on the skin of patients with atopic dermatitis: evidence for a new group of allergens. J Clin Invest 92:1374–1380, 1993.
79. Leung DYM, Hirsch RL, Schneider L, et al: Thymopentin therapy reduces the clinical severity of atopic dermatitis. J Allergy Clin Immunol 85:927–933, 1990.
80. Lever WF, Lever GS: Histopathology of the Skin. J.B. Lippincott, Philadelphia, 1990, pp 104–108.
81. Lever R, Turbitt M, Sanderson A, et al: Immunophenotyping of the cutaneous infiltrating and of mononuclear cells in the peripheral blood in patients with atopic dermatitis. J Invest Dermatol 89:4–7, 1987.
82. Leyden JJ, Marples RR, Kligman AM: *Staphylococcus aureus* in the lesions of atopic dermatitis. Br J Dermatol 90:525–530, 1974.
83. Linde YW: Dry skin in atopic dermatitis. Acta Derm Venereol Suppl (Stockh) 177:9–13, 1992.
84. Manku MS, Horrobin DF, Morse NL, et al: Essential fatty acids in the plasma phospholipids of patients with atopic eczema. Br J Dermatol 110:643–648, 1984.
85. Martin AJ, Landau LI, Phelan PD: Predicting the course of asthma in children. Aust Pediatr J 18:84–87, 1982.
86. May CD: Objective clinical and laboratory studies of immediate hypersensitivity reactions to foods in asthmatic children. J Allergy Clin Immunol 58:500–515, 1976.
87. McFadden JP, Noble WC, Camp RD: Superantigenic exotoxin-secreting potential of staphylococci isolated from atopic eczematous skin. Br J Dermatol 128:631–632, 1993.
88. Meenan FOC: The significance of Morgan's fold in children with atopic dermatitis. Acta Derm Venereol Suppl (Stockh) 92:42, 1980.
89. Mevorah B, Frenk E, Wietlisbach V, Carrel CF: Minor clinical features of atopic dermatitis; evaluation of their diagnostic significance. Dermatologica 177:360–364, 1988.
90. Mevorah B, Marazzi A, Frenk E: The prevalence of accentuated palmoplantar markings and keratosis pilaris in atopic dermatitis, autosomal dominant ichthyosis and control dermatological patients. Br J Dermatol 112:679–685, 1985.
91. Mihm MC, Soter NA, Dvorak HF, et al: The structure of normal skin and the morphology of atopic eczema. J Invest Dermatol 67:305–312, 1976.
92. Mitchell EB, Crow J, Williams G, et al: Basophils in allergen-induced patch test sites in atopic dermatitis. Lancet 1:127–130, 1982.
93. Morison WL, Parrish JA, Fitzpatrick TB: Oral psoralen photochemotherapy of atopic eczema. Br J Dermatol 98:25–30, 1978.
94. Mosmann TR, Cherwinski H, Bond MW, et al: Two types of helper T cell clone I: definition according to profiles of lymphokine activities and secreted proteins. J Immunol 136:2348–2357, 1986.
95. Mosmann TR, Moore KW: The role of IL-10 in crossregulation of Th1 and Th2 responses. Immunol Today 12:A49–53, 1991.
96. Mudde GC, Van Riejsen FC, Boland GJ, et al: Allergen presentation by epidermal Langerhans cells from patients with atopic dermatitis is mediated by IgE. Immunology 69:335–341, 1990.
97. Neuber K, Konig W: Effects of *Staphylococcus aureus* cell wall products (teichoic acid, peptidoglycan) and enterotoxin B on immunoglobulin (IgE, IgA, IgG) synthesis and CD23 expression in patients with atopic dermatitis. Immunology 75:23–28, 1992.
98. Nishioka K, Matsunaga T, Katayama I: Gamma-interferon therapy for severe cases of atopic dermatitis of the adult type. J Dermatol 22:181–185, 1995.
99. Norman PS: Immunotherapy. Progr Allergy 32:318–346, 1982.
100. Ohman S, Johansson SGO: Immunoglobulins in atopic dermatitis with special reference to IgE. Acta Derm Venereol (Stockh) 54:193–202, 1974.
101. Oka C, Ideta H, Nagasaki H, et al: Retinal detachment with atopic dermatitis similar to traumatic detachment. Ophthalmology 101:1050–1054, 1994.
102. Oshinskie L, Haine C: Atopic dermatitis and its ophthalmic complications. J Am Optom Assoc 53:889–894, 1982.
103. Peck SM, Salomon G: Eczema of infancy and childhood: contacts as etiologic agents, with particular reference to feathers. Am J Dis Child 46:1308, 1933.
104. Pene J, Rousset F, Briere F, et al: IgE production by normal human B cells induced by alloreactive T cell clones is mediated by IL-4 and suppressed by IFN-γ. J Immunol 141:1218–1224, 1988.
105. Prinz B, Nachbar F, Plewig G: Treatment of severe atopic dermatitis with extracorporeal photopheresis. Arch Dermatol Res 287:48–52, 1994.
106. Pryzbilla B, Ring J, Enders F, Winkelmann H: Stigmata of atopic constitution in patients with atopic eczema or atopic respiratory disease. Acta Derm Venereol (Stockh) 71:407–410, 1991.
107. Queille-Roussel C, Raynaud F, Saurat JH: A prospective computerized study of 500 cases of atopic dermatitis in childhood. Acta Derm Venereol Suppl (Stockh) 114:87–92, 1985.
108. Rajka G: Essential Aspects of Atopic Dermatitis. Springer-Verlag, Berlin, 1989.
109. Rasmussen JE: Advances in nondietary management of children with atopic dermatitis. Pediatr Dermatol 6:210–215, 1989.
110. Reitamo S, Visa K, Kahonen K, et al: Eczematous reactions in atopic patients caused by epicutaneous testing with inhalant allergens. Br J Dermatol 114:303–309, 1986.
111. Rich LF, Hanifin JM: Ocular complications of atopic dermatitis and other eczemas. Int Ophthalmol Clin 25:61–76, 1985.
112. Rocha C, Maubeuge J, Sarfati M, et al: Characterization of cellular infiltrates in skin lesions of atopic dermatitis by means of monoclonal antibodies. Dermatologica 169:330–338, 1984.
113. Roth HL, Kierland RR: The natural history of atopic dermatitis. Arch Dermatol 89:209–214, 1964.
114. Rotteveel FTM, Kokkelnik I, van Lien RAW, et al: Clonal analysis of functionally distinct human CD4+ T cell subsets. J Exp Med 168:1659–1673, 1988.

115. Rubin LA, Kurman CC, Fritz ME, et al: Soluble interleukin 2 receptors are released from activated human lymphoid cells in vitro. J Immunol 137:3172–3177, 1985.
116. Rystedt I: Factors influencing the occurrence of hand eczema in adults with a history of atopic dermatitis in childhood. Contact Dermatitis 12:185–191, 1985.
117. Rystedt I: Prognostic factors in atopic dermatitis. Acta Derm Venereol (Stockh) 65:206–213, 1985.
118. Salob SP, Atherton DJ: Prevalence of respiratory symptoms in children with atopic dermatitis attending pediatric dermatology clinics. Pediatrics 91:8–12, 1993.
119. Salob SP, Laverty A, Atherton DJ: Bronchial hyperresponsiveness in children with atopic dermatitis. Pediatrics 91:13–16, 1993.
120. Sampson HA: The immunopathogenic role of food hypersensitivity in atopic dermatitis. Acta Derm Venereol Suppl (Stockh) 176:34–37, 1992.
121. Sampson HA: The role of food allergy and mediator release in atopic dermatitis. J Allergy Clin Immunol 81:635–645, 1988.
122. Sampson HA, Broadbent KR, Bernhisel-Broadbent J: Spontaneous release of histamine from basophils and histamine-releasing factor in patients with atopic dermatitis and food hypersensitivity. N Engl J Med 312:228–232, 1989.
123. Sampson HA, Jolie PL: Increased plasma histamine concentrations after food challenges in children with atopic dermatitis. N Engl J Med 311:372–376, 1984.
124. Sampson HA, McCaskill CM: Food hypersensitivity and atopic dermatitis: evaluation of 113 patients. J Pediatr 107:669–675, 1985.
125. Sampson HA, Scanlon SM: Natural history of food hypersensitivity in children with atopic dermatitis. J Pediatr 115:23–27, 1989.
126. Sanford AJ, Shirakawa T, Moffat MF, et al: Localisation of atopy and β subunit of high-affinity IgE-receptor (FcεRI) on chromosome 11q. Lancet 341:332–334, 1993.
127. Sanda T, Yasue T, Oohashi M, Yasue A: Effectiveness of house dust-mite allergen avoidance through clean room therapy in patients with atopic dermatitis. J Allergy Clin Immunol 89:653–657, 1992.
128. Savin JA, Dow R, Harlow BJ, et al: The effect of a new nonsedative H1 receptor antagonist (LN 2974) on the itching and scratching of patients with atopic eczema. Clin Exp Dermatol 11:600–602, 1986.
129. Scholtz JR: Management of atopic dermatitis. Calif Med 102:210, 1965.
130. Schopf E, Baumgarten A: Patch testing in atopic dermatitis. J Am Acad Dermatol 21:860–862, 1989.
131. Service WC: The incidence of major allergic diseases in Colorado Springs. JAMA 112:2034–2037, 1939.
132. Sheehan MP, Atherton DJ: A controlled trial of traditional Chinese medicinal plants in widespread non-exudative atopic eczema. Br J Dermatol 126:179–184, 1992.
133. Sheehan MP, Atherton DJ: One-year follow up of children treated with Chinese medicinal herbs for atopic eczema. Br J Dermatol 130:488–493, 1994.
134. Sheehan MP, Rustin MH, Atherton DJ, et al: Efficacy of traditional Chinese herbal therapy in adult atopic dermatitis. Lancet 340:13–17, 1992.
135. Stephens RB, Lee ML, Cooper A: Cyclosporin treatment of atopic dermatitis: five case studies and literature review. Australas J Dermatol 35:55–59, 1994.
136. Stiller MJ, Shupack JL, Kenny C, et al: A double-blind, placebo-controlled trial to evaluate the safety and efficacy of thymopentin as an adjunctive treatment in atopic dermatitis. J Am Acad Dermatol 30:597–602, 1994.
137. Stone SP, Muller SA, Gleich GJ: IgE levels in atopic dermatitis. Arch Dermatol 108:806–811, 1973.
138. Svejgaard E, Faergeman J, Jemec G, et al: Recent investigations on the relationship between fungal skin diseases and atopic dermatitis. Acta Derm Venereol Suppl (Stockh) 144:140–142, 1989.
139. Svensson A, Edman B, Moller H: A diagnostic tool for atopic dermatitis based on clinical criteria. Acta Derm Venereol Suppl (Stockh) 114:33–40, 1985.
140. Tada J, Toi Y, Akiyama H, Arata J: Infra-auricular fissures in atopic dermatitis. Acta Derm Venereol (Stockh) 74:129–131, 1994.
141. Taylor RS, Baadsgaard O, Hammerberg C, et al: Hyperstimulatory CD1a+CD1b+CD36+ Langerhans cells are responsible for increased autologous T lymphocyte reactivity to lesional epidermal cells of patients with atopic dermatitis. J Immunol 147:3794–3802, 1991.
142. Taylor B, Wadsworth J, Wadsworth M, Peckham C: Changes in the reported prevalence of childhood eczema since the 1938–45 war. Lancet 2:1255–1257, 1984.
143. Tuft L: Importance of inhalant allergens in atopic dermatitis. J Invest Dermatol 12:211–219, 1949.
144. Tuft L, Heck VM: Studies in atopic dermatitis IV: importance of seasonal inhalant allergens, especially ragweed. J Allergy 23:528–540, 1952.
145. Uehara M: Infraorbital fold in atopic dermatitis. Arch Dermatol 117:627, 1981.
146. Uehara M, Amemiya T, Arai M: Atopic cataracts in a Japanese population with special reference to factors possibly relevant to cataract formation. Dermatologica 170:180–184, 1985.
147. Uehara M, Hayashi S: Hyperlinear palms. Arch Dermatol 117:490–491, 1981.
148. Uehara M, Izukura R, Sawai T: Blood eosinophilia in atopic dermatitis. Clin Exp Dermatol 15:264–266, 1990.
149. Uno H, Hanifin JM: Langerhans cells in acute and chronic epidermal lesions of atopic dermatitis observed by L-dopa histofluorescence, glycol methacrylate thin section, and electron microscopy. J Invest Dermatol 75:52–60, 1980.
150. van der Heijden FL, Wierenga EA, Bos JD, Kapsenberg ML: High frequency of IL-4 producing CD4+ allergen-specific T lymphocytes in atopic dermatitis lesional skin. J Invest Dermatol 97:389–394, 1991.
151. Van Joost T, Stolz E, Muele F: Efficacy of low dose cyclosporin in severe atopic disease. Arch Dermatol 123:166–167, 1987.
152. Vickers CFH: The natural history of atopic eczema. Acta Derm Venereol Suppl (Stockh) 92:113–115, 1980.
153. Walker RB, Warin RP: The incidence of eczema in early childhood. Br J Dermatol 68:182–183, 1956.
154. Wang B, Rieger A, Kilgus O, et al: Epidermal Langerhans cells from normal human skin bind monomeric IgE via FcεR1. J Exp Med 175:1353–1365, 1992.
155. Wierenga EA, Snoek M, deGroot C, et al: Evidence for compartmentalization of functional subsets of CD4+ T lymphocytes in atopic patients. J Immunol 144:4651–4656, 1990.
156. Williams H, Pottier A, Strachan D: Are viral warts seen more commonly in children with eczema? Arch Dermatol 129:717–720, 1993.
157. Williams HC: Is the prevalence of atopic dermatitis increasing? Clin Exp Dermatol 17:385–391, 1992.
158. Williams HC, Burney PGJ, Hay RJ, et al: The U.K. Working Party's Diagnostic Criteria for Atopic Dermatitis. I: derivation of a minimum set of discriminators for atopic dermatitis. Br J Dermatol 131:383–396, 1994.
159. Williams HC, Burney PGJ, Strachan D, et al: The U.K. Working Party's Diagnostic Criteria for Atopic Dermatitis II: observer variation of clinical diagnosis and signs in atopic dermatitis. Br J Dermatol 131:397–405, 1994.
160. Williams HC, Burney PGJ, Pembroke AC, et al: The U.K. Working Party's Diagnostic Criteria for Atopic Dermatitis. III: independent hospital validation. Br J Dermatol 131:406–416, 1994.
161. Wise F, Sulzberger MB: Editorial comment. In Year Book of Dermatology and Syphilology. Yearbook, Chicago, 1933, p 38.
162. Wolf R, Sandbank M, Krakowski A: Extensive pityriasis alba and atopic dermatitis. Br J Dermatol 112:247, 1985.
163. Wright S, Burton JL: Oral evening primrose seed oil improved atopic eczema. Lancet 2:1120–1122, 1982.
164. Yamamoto K, Korstanje M: Eczema in childhood. In Marks R (ed): Eczema. Martin Dunitz, London, 1992, pp 239–253.
165. Zachary CB, Allen MH, MacDonald DM: In situ quantification of T-lymphocyte subsets and Langerhans cells in the inflammatory infiltrate of atopic eczema. Br J Dermatol 112:149–156, 1985.
166. Zeiger RS, Heller S, Mellon MH, et al: Genetic and environmental factors affecting the development of atopy through age 4 in children of atopic parents: a prospective randomized study of food allergen avoidance. Pediatr Allergy Immunol 3:110–127, 1992.
167. Adams RM (eds): Occupational Skin Disease, 2nd edition. WB Saunders Co, Philadelphia, 1990.
168. Adams RM, Fisher AA: Contact allergen alternatives: 1986. J Am Acad Dermatol 14:951–969, 1986.
169. Aiba S, Katz SI: Phenotypic and functional characteristics of in vivo activated Langerhans cells. J Immunol 145:2791–2796, 1990.
170. Allen JE: Drug-induced photosensitivity. Clinical Pharmacy 12:580–587, 1993.
171. Alon R, Rossiter H, Wang X, et al: Distinct cell surface ligands mediate T lymphocyte attachment and rolling on P and E selectin under physiological flow. J Cell Biol 127:1485–1495, 1994.

172. Angelini G, Vena GA: Airborne contact dermatitis. Clin Dermatol 10:123–131, 1992.
173. Arellano R, Bradley J, Sussman G: Prevalence of latex sensitization among hospital physicians occupationally exposed to latex gloves. Anesthesiology 77:905–908, 1992.
174. Berg EL, Yoshino T, Rott LS, et al: The cutaneous lymphocyte antigen is a skin lymphocyte homing receptor for the vascular lectin endothelial cell-leukocyte adhesion molecule 1. J Exp Med 174:1461–1466, 1991.
175. Berger TG, Dhar A: Lichenoid photoeruptions in human immunodeficiency virus infection. Arch Dermatol 130:609–613, 1994.
176. Bergner T, Przybilla B: Photosensitization caused by ibuprofen. J Am Acad Dermatol 26:114–116, 1992.
177. Bigby M, Vargas R, Sy MS: Production of hapten-specific T cell hybridomas and their use to study the effect of ultraviolet B irradiation on the development of contact hypersensitivity. J Immunol 143:3867–3872, 1989.
178. Bilsland D, Ferguson J: Contact allergy to sunscreen chemicals in photosensitivity dermatitis/actinic reticuloid syndrome (PD/AR) and polymorphic light eruption (PLE). Contact Dermatitis 29:70–73, 1993.
179. Bjorkman PJ, Saper MA, Samraoui B, et al: Structure of the human class I histocompatibility antigen, HLA-A2. Nature 329:506–512, 1987.
180. Bjorkman PJ, Sapper MA, Samraoui B, et al: The foreign antigen binding site and T cell recognition regions of class I histocompatibility antigens. Nature 329:512–518, 1987.
181. Bos JD, de Boer OJ, Tibosch E, et al: Skin-homing T lymphocytes: detection of cutaneous lymphocyte-associated antigen (CLA) by HECA-452 in normal human skin. Arch Dermatol Res 285:179–183, 1993.
182. Bousquet J, Michel FB: Allergy to formaldehyde and ethylene-oxide. Clin Rev Allergy 9:357–370, 1991.
183. Brancaccio RR, Cockerell CJ, Belsito D, Ostreicher R: Allergic contact dermatitis from color film developers: clinical and histologic features. J Am Acad Dermatol 28:827–830, 1993.
184. Bruynzeel DP, de Boer EM, Brouwer EJ, et al: Dermatitis in bulb growers. Contact Dermatitis 29:11–15, 1993.
185. Burnett CM, Corbett JF: The chemistry and toxicology of hair dyes. pp 203–220. In Drill VA, Lazar P (eds): Cutaneous Toxicity. Academic Press, New York, 1977.
186. Caputo R, Peluchetti D, Monti M: Freeze-fracture of Langerhans granules: a comparative study. J Invest Dermatol 66:297–301, 1976.
187. Charous BL, Hamilton RG, Yunginger JW: Occupational latex exposure: characteristics of contact and systemic reactions in 47 workers. J Allergy Clin Immunol 94:12–18, 1994.
188. Chu A, Eisinger M, Lee JS, et al: Immunoelectron microscopic identification of Langerhans cells using a new antigenic marker. J Invest Dermatol 78:177–180, 1982.
189. Conde-Salazar L, del-Rio E, Guimaraens D, Gonzalez Domingo A: Type IV allergy to rubber additives: a 10-year study of 686 cases. J Am Acad Dermatol 29:176–180, 1993.
190. Conde-Salazar L, Gonzalez de Domingo MA, Guimaraens D: Sensitization to epoxy resin systems in special flooring workers. Contact Dermatitis 31:157–160, 1994.
191. Cronin E: Formaldehyde is a significant allergen in women with hand eczema. Contact Dermatitis 25:276–282, 1991.
192. Das PK, de Boer OJ, Visser A, et al: Differential expression of ICAM-1, E-selectin and VCAM-1 by endothelial cells in psoriasis and contact dermatitis. Acta Derm Venereol Suppl (Stockh) 186:21–22, 1994.
193. Davidson CL: Occupational contact dermatitis of the upper extremity. Occup Med 9:59–73, 1994.
194. DeLeo VA, Suarez SM, Maso MJ: Photoallergic contact dermatitis: results of photopatch testing in New York, 1985 to 1990. Arch Dermatol 128:1513–1518, 1992.
195. Dupuis G, Benezra C: Chemically reactive functions in haptens and in proteins. In Allergic Contact Dermatitis to Simple Chemicals: a Molecular Approach. New York, Marcel Dekker, 1982, pp 47–84.
196. Dustin LM, Singer KH, Tuck DT, Springer TA: Adhesion of T lymphoblasts to epidermal keratinocytes is regulated by interferon gamma and is mediated by intercellular adhesion molecule 1 (ICAM-1). J Exp Med 167:1323–1340, 1988.
197. Emmett EA: Phototoxicity and photosensitivity reactions. In Adams RM (ed): Occupational Skin Disease, 2nd edition. WB Saunders, Philadelphia, 1990, p 184.
198. Fisher AA: Contact Dermatitis. Lea & Febiger, Philadelphia, 1986.
199. Flyvholm MA, Menne T: Allergic contact dermatitis from formaldehyde: a case study focussing on sources of formaldehyde exposure. Contact Dermatitis 27:27–36, 1992.
200. Fotiades J, Soter NA, Lim HW: Results of evaluation of 203 patients for photosensitivity in a 7.3 year period. J Am Acad Dermatol 33:597–602, 1995.
201. Fowler JF Jr, Skinner SM, Belsito DV: Allergic contact dermatitis from formaldehyde resins in permanent press clothing: an underdiagnosed cause of generalized dermatitis. J Am Acad Dermatol 27:962–968, 1992.
202. Frosch PJ, Burrows D, Camarasa JG, et al: Allergic reactions to a hairdressers' series: results from 9 European centres: the European Environmental and Contact Dermatitis Research Group (EECDRG). Contact Dermatitis 28:180–183, 1993.
203. Goh CL, Gan SL: Efficacies of a barrier cream and an afterwork emollient cream against cutting fluid dermatitis in metalworkers: a prospective study. Contact Dermatitis 31:176–180, 1994.
204. Goncalo M, Figueiredo A, Tavares P, et al: Photosensitivity to piroxicam: absence of cross-reaction with tenoxicam. Contact Dermatitis 27:287–290, 1992.
205. Gould JW, Mercurio MG, Elmets CA: Cutaneous photosensitivity diseases induced by exogenous agents. J Am Acad Dermatol 33:551–573, 1995.
206. Halbert AR, Gebauer KA, Wall LM: Prognosis of occupational chromate dermatitis. Contact Dermatitis 27:214–219, 1992.
207. Handley J, Burrows D: Dermatitis from hexavalent chromate in the accelerator of an epoxy sealant (PR1422) used in the aircraft industry. Contact Dermatitis 30:193–196, 1994.
208. Hariya T, Osawa J, Kitamura K, Ikezawa Z: Piroxicam has at least two epitopes for contact photoallergy. Dermatol Sci 6:219–224, 1993.
209. Hausen BM: Hydrangenol, a strong contact sensitizer found in hydrangea (Hydrangea sp.; Hydrangeaceae). Contact Dermatitis 24:233–235, 1991.
210. Hauser C, Saurat JH, Schmitt A, et al: Interleukin 1 is present in normal human epidermis. J Immunol 136:3317–3321, 1986.
211. Irvine C, Pugh CE, Hansen EJ, Rycroft RJ: Cement dermatitis in underground workers during construction of the Channel Tunnel. Occup Med 44:17–23, 1994.
212. Jolanki R: Occupational skin diseases from epoxy compounds: epoxy resin compounds, epoxy acrylates and 2,3-epoxypropyl trimethyl ammonium chloride. Acta Derm Venereol Suppl (Stockh) 159:1–80, 1991.
213. Jones DA, McIntire LV, Smith CW, Picker LJ: A two-step adhesion cascade for T cell/endothelial cell interactions under flow conditions. J Clin Invest 94:2443–2450, 1994.
214. Kalish RS: Antigen processing: the gateway to the immune response [review]. J Am Acad Dermatol 32:640–652, 1995.
215. Kalish RS, Johnson KL: Enrichment and function of urushiol (poison ivy) specific T-lymphocytes in lesions of allergic contact dermatitis to urushiol. J Immunol 145:3706–3713, 1990.
216. Kalish RS, Wood JA, LaPorte A: Processing of urushiol (poison ivy) hapten by both endogenous and exogenous pathways for presentation to human T-cells. J Clin Invest 93:2039–2047, 1994.
217. Kaniwa MA, Isama K, Nakamura A, et al: Identification of causative chemicals of allergic contact dermatitis using a combination of patch testing in patients and chemical analysis: application to cases from industrial rubber products. Contact Dermatitis 30:20–25, 1994.
218. Kaniwa MA, Isama K, Nakamura A, et al: Identification of causative chemicals of allergic contact dermatitis using a combination of patch testing in patients and chemical analysis: application to cases from rubber footwear. Contact Dermatitis 30:26–34, 1994.
219. Knight TE: Philodendron-induced dermatitis: report of cases and review of the literature. Cutis 48:375–378, 1991.
220. Knudsen BB, Larsen E, Egsgaard H, Menne T: Release of thiurams and carbamates from rubber gloves. Contact Dermatitis 28:63–69, 1993.
221. Kojima T, Hasegawa T, Ishida H, et al: Griseofulvin-induced photodermatitis—report of six cases. J Dermatol 15:76–82, 1988.
222. Kripke ML, Munn CG, Jeevan A, et al: Evidence that cutaneous antigen-presenting cells migrate to regional lymph nodes during contact sensitization. J Immunol 145:2833–2838, 1990.
223. Kristensen O: A prospective study of the development of hand eczema in an automobile manufacturing industry. Contact Dermatitis 26:341–345, 1992.
224. Kupper TS: The activated keratinocyte: a model for inducible cytokine

production by non–bone marrow–derived cells in cutaneous inflammatory and immune responses. J Invest Dermatol 94:146S–150S, 1990.

225. Kupper TS, Ballard D, Chua AO, et al: Human keratinocytes contain mRNA indistinguishable from monocyte interleukin 1 alpha and beta mRNA. J Exp Med 164:2095–2100, 1986.
226. Kurup VP, Kelly KJ, Turjanmaa K, et al: Immunoglobulin E reactivity to latex antigens in the sera of patients from Finland and the United States. J Allergy Clin Immunol 91:1128–1134, 1993.
227. Layton AM, Cunliffe WJ: Phototoxic eruptions due to doxycycline—a dose-related phenomenon. Clin Exp Dermatol 18:425–427, 1993.
228. Lepoittevin JP, Drieghe J, Dooms-Goossens A: Studies in patients with corticosteroid contact allergy. Arch Dermatol 131:31–37, 1995.
229. Lever WF, Schaumburg-Lever G: Non-infectious vesicular and bullous diseases. In Histopathology of the Skin, 7th edition. JB Lippincott, Philadelphia, 1990, p 103.
230. Liden C: Occupational contact dermatitis due to nickel allergy. Science of the Total Environment 148:283–285, 1994.
231. Maibach HI, Gellin GA (eds): Occupational and Industrial Dermatology. Year Book Medical, Chicago, 1982.
232. Marcoux D, Riboulet-Delmas G: Efficacy and safety of hair-coloring agents. Am J Contact Dermatitis 5:123–129, 1994.
233. Marks JG, DeLeo VA: Contact and Occupational Dermatology. Mosby–Year Book, Boston, 1992.
234. Marrakchi S, Maibach HI: What is occupational contact dermatitis? An operational definition (review). Dermatol Clin 12:477–484, 1994.
235. Mathias CGT: Occupational dermatoses. J Am Acad Dermatol 19:1107–1114, 1988.
236. Mattison P: Dermatitis on construction sites. Occup Health 45:122–124, 1993.
237. Meuer SC, Schlossman SF, Reinherz EL: Clonal analysis of human cytotoxic T lymphocytes: T4+ and T8+ effector T cells recognize products of different major histocompatibility complex regions. Proc Natl Acad Sci USA 79:4395–4399, 1982.
238. Nandakishore T, Pasricha JS: Pattern of cross-sensitivity between 4 Compositae plants, *Parthenium hysterophorus, Xanthium strumarium, Helianthus annuus* and *Chrysanthemum coronarium,* in Indian patients. Contact Dermatitis 30:162–167, 1994.
239. Neumann NJ, Holzle E, Lehmann P, et al: Pattern analysis of photopatch test reactions. Photodermatol Photoimmunol Photomed 10:65–73, 1994.
240. Nielsen NH, Menne T: Nickel sensitization and ear piercing in an unselected Danish population: Glostrup Allergy Study. Contact Dermatitis 29:16–21, 1993.
241. Niklasson B, Bjorkner B, Sundberg K: Contact allergy to a fatty acid ester component of cutting fluids. Contact Dermatitis 28:265–267, 1993.
242. Ophaswongse S, Maibach H: Topical nonsteroidal antiinflammatory drugs: allergic and photoallergic contact dermatitis and phototoxicity. Contact Dermatitis 29:57–64, 1993.
243. Pao C, Norris PG, Corbett M, Hawk JL: Polymorphic light eruption: prevalence in Australia and England. Br J Dermatol 130:62–64, 1994.
244. Paulsen E: Compositae dermatitis: a survey. Contact Dermatitis 26:76–86, 1992.
245. Paulsen E, Andersen KE: Compositae dermatitis in a Danish dermatology department in 1 year (II): clinical features in patients with Compositae contact allergy. Contact Dermatitis 29:195–201, 1993.
246. Picker LJ: Regulation of tissue-selective T-lymphocyte homing receptors during the virgin to memory/effector cell transition in human secondary lymphoid tissues. Am Rev Respir Dis 148:S47–S54, 1993.
247. Picker LJ, Martin RJ, Trumble A, et al: Differential expression of lymphocyte homing receptors by human memory/effector T cells in pulmonary versus cutaneous immune effector sites. Eur J Immunol 24:1269–1277, 1994.
248. Piguet PF, Grau GE, Hauser C, Vassalli P: Tumor necrosis factor is a critical mediator in hapten induced irritant and contact hypersensitivity reactions. J Exp Med 173:673–679, 1991.
249. Potter TS, Hashimoto K: Cutaneous photosensitivity to medications. Compr Ther 20:414–417, 1994.
250. Rietschel RL: Patch testing for corticosteroid allergy in the United States. Arch Dermatol 131:91–92, 1995.
251. Romagnoli P, Sinigaglia F: Selective interaction of Ni with an MHC-bound peptide. EMBO J 10:1303–1306, 1991.
252. Rosen RH, Freeman S: Prognosis of occupational contact dermatitis in New South Wales, Australia. Contact Dermatitis 29:88–93, 1993.
253. Santucci B, Picardo M: Occupational contact dermatitis to plants. Clin Dermatol 10:157–165, 1992.
254. Srebrnik A, Hes JP, Brenner S: Adverse cutaneous reactions to psychotropic drugs. Acta Derm Venereol Suppl (Stockh) 158:1–12, 1991.
255. Stingl G, Gazze-Stingl LA, Aberer W, Wolff K: Antigen presentation by murine epidermal Langerhans cells and its alteration by ultraviolet B light. J Immunol 127:1707–1713, 1981.
256. Stingl G, Katz SI, Clement L, et al: Immunological functions of Ia-bearing epidermal Langerhans cells. J Immunol 121:2005–2013, 1978.
257. Stingl G, Katz SI, Shevach EM, et al: Detection of Ia antigens on Langerhans cells in guinea pig skin. J Immunol 120:570–578, 1978.
258. Stingl G, Tamaki K, Katz SI: Origin and function of epidermal Langerhans cells. Immunol Rev 53:149–174, 1980.
259. Stoughton RB: Vasoconstrictor assay—specific applications. In Maibach HI, Surber C (eds): Topical Corticosteroids. Karger, Basel, 1992, p 42.
260. Sutthipisal N, McFadden JP, Cronin E: Sensitization in atopic and non-atopic hairdressers with hand eczema. Contact Dermatitis 29:206–209, 1993.
261. Szczurko C, Dompmartin A, Michel M, et al: Photocontact allergy to oxybenzone: ten years of experience. Photodermatol Photoimmunol Photomed 10:144–147, 1994.
262. Toews GB, Bergstresser PR, Streilein JW: Epidermal Langerhans cell density determines whether contact hypersensitivity or unresponsiveness follows skin painting with DNCB. J Immunol 124:445–453, 1980.
263. Tosti A, Guerra L, Bardazzi F: Occupational contact dermatitis from exposure to epoxy resins and acrylates. Clin Dermatol 10:133–140, 1992.
264. Tosti A, Guerra L, Vincenzi C, Peluso AM: Occupational skin hazards from synthetic plastics. Toxicol Ind Health 9:493–502, 1993.
265. Trevisi P, Vincenzi C, Chieregato C, et al: Sunscreen sensitization: a three-year study. Dermatology 189:55–57, 1994.
266. van der Walle HB: Dermatitis in hairdressers (II): management and prevention. Contact Dermatitis 30:265–270, 1994.
267. van der Walle HB, Brunsveld VM: Dermatitis in hairdressers (I): the experience of the past 4 years. Contact Dermatitis 30:217–221, 1994.
268. Wainwright NJ, Collins P, Ferguson J: Photosensitivity associated with antibacterial agents. Drug Safety 9:437–440, 1993.
269. Walsh LJ, Murphy GF: Role of adhesion molecules in cutaneous inflammation and neoplasia. J Cutan Pathol 19:161–171, 1992.
270. Wildner O, Lipkow T, Knop J: Increased expression of ICAM-1, E-selectin, and VCAM-1 by cultured human endothelial cells upon exposure to haptens. Exp Dermatol 1:191–198, 1992.
271. Wolf R, Dorfman B, Krakowski A: Quinidine-induced lichenoid and eczematous photodermatitis. Dermatologica 174:285–289, 1987.
272. Wrangsjo K, Osterman K, van Hage-Hamsten M: Glove-related skin symptoms among operating theatre and dental care unit personnel (II): clinical examination, tests and laboratory findings indicating latex allergy. Contact Dermatitis 30:139–143, 1994.
273. Yago T, Tsukuda M, Yamazaki H, et al: Analysis of an initial step of T cell adhesion to endothelial monolayers under flow conditions. J Immunol 154:1216–1222, 1995.

37 Drug Allergy

PETER D. GOREVIC

The vaccinated individual reacts to the vaccine lymph, the syphilitic patient to the syphilis virus, the tuberculous patient to tuberculin, the individual injected with serum to such serum—each of them reacts in a different manner from that of an individual who has not yet been in contact with the agent in question. . . . For this general concept of an altered capacity to react I propose the term "allergy."

Von Pirquet, 1906

Drug allergy or hypersensitivity refers to a variety of clinical syndromes in which specific immunologic reactivity can be demonstrated. This reactivity may be directed to epitopes unique to the drug itself or cross-reactive with other chemically related drugs, to conjugates formed with host proteins, or to neoantigens of host proteins exposed during conjugation.[159] Alternatively, immune responses may be directed to a metabolite or metabolites of a drug or develop as a consequence of an immunomodulatory effect of the medication on the host's immune system. In some instances, such as penicillin allergy, specific immune mechanisms have been well defined in series of elegant experimental and clinical investigations; in many others, information is spotty, and much is conjecture.

Drug allergy has been termed hapten immunology in humans because immune responses are directed against the drug as a low molecular weight haptenic determinant covalently conjugated to a carrier, assumed to be normal serum or tissue proteins.[126] The type and intensity of the elicited immune response may be a function of the intrinsic reactivity of the drug with macromolecules and the density of haptenation. Distinct and occasionally multiple humoral and cell-mediated immune responses to these haptenic determinants may occur in the same individual, providing several potential handles for monitoring the allergic responses to a drug. The resulting pathology and clinical manifestations of the hypersensitivity reaction are determined in turn by the immunologic mechanisms that predominate, which may vary between drugs. The purpose of this chapter is to summarize current information regarding immunologic and nonimmunologic mechanisms of drug allergy. Several comprehensive reviews provide additional background information.[40, 41, 137, 144, 176]

The majority of drug-related adverse reactions (Table 37–1) are in fact not due to allergy. Non-allergic adverse reactions may be due to the expected pharmacology of the drug (overdosage, side effects, secondary effects, drug interactions) or reflect a susceptibility (intolerance or idiosyncrasy) that is qualitatively abnormal and unique to certain individuals (Table 37–2). Adverse drug reactions are particularly important in the geriatric population and in hospitalized patients because of the number of medications to which the person is exposed, the increased potential for drug interactions, and the presence of underlying diseases. Drug reactions are estimated to account for 19% of adverse reactions occurring in the hospital setting, with the incidence being particularly high for certain drugs, such as digitalis, anticoag-

TABLE 37–1
IMMUNOLOGIC MECHANISMS OF HYPERSENSITIVITY TO DRUGS

Anaphylaxis
IgE antibodies
Triggering by complement activation
Cytotoxic Antibodies
Hapten cell mechanism (e.g., penicillin)
Immune complex mechanism (e.g., phenacetin)
Induction of autoantibodies (e.g., methyldopa)
Immune Complex
Serum sickness
Cell Mediated
Contact dermatitis
Lymphokine mediated
?Granulomatous reactions

TABLE 37–2
ADVERSE DRUG REACTIONS

Overdosage (toxicity)
Side effects (at required dosage)
Secondary effects
Drug interactions
Intolerance (lowered threshold)
Idiosyncrasy (not immunologic)
Nonimmunologic histamine release
Allergy or hypersensitivity

ulants, cytotoxic agents, and corticosteroids.[95] In total, adverse reactions account for 2% to 6% of all hospital admissions in some series, a number that rivals common diseases, such as peptic ulcer or chronic obstructive lung disease, as causes for hospitalization.[28, 74, 105]

Allergic reactions occur in less than 2% to 3% of individuals receiving most drugs, but they include some of the most life-threatening of adverse drug reactions. In certain instances, such as asparaginase, the incidence of allergy has been found to be considerably higher in individuals who are receiving repeated courses of the medication and thus has prohibited usage of the drug. The exact incidence of anaphylactic reactions is unknown, with widely discrepant figures reported for commonly used drugs, such as the penicillins.[21, 76, 78, 147, 164] Patients most likely require multiple courses of a drug to develop sufficient sensitization for the severe hypersensitivity seen in many instances of anaphylaxis. Repeated exposure may be the most critical factor explaining the high incidence of IgE-mediated immune responses, including antibiotic allergy, among persons affected by cystic fibrosis.[136] With an ever-increasing pharmacopeia and the greater likelihood of interspersal of one class of medicines with other classes, such sensitization may in fact become increasingly common. The scope of the problem is outlined in Table 37–3.

Whereas genetic and environmental influences may alter the induction of an allergic response to a drug, the effect of these influences on the actual elicitation of drug allergy remains less clear (Table 37–4). The most important predisposing factor for drug allergy is a history of sensitization. Sensitization may be particularly difficult to assess if the initial exposure occurred without the patient's knowledge, such as via small amounts of antibiotics present in foodstuffs, vaccines, or combination medicines, or is elicited via cross-

TABLE 37–3
SCOPE OF THE PROBLEM

Three percent of all acute medical hospitalizations are for adverse drug reactions[28, 74, 105]
Allergic reactions account for less than 10% of all adverse drug reactions
About 10% of adults give a history of an allergic reaction to a drug, usually an antimicrobial
Six percent to 15% of in-hospital drug treatments result in an adverse reaction
Rashes are by far the most common allergic reactions seen (exanthemas > urticaria > other)[14, 145]
The true incidence of anaphylaxis is unknown and may be changing with patterns of drug usage
Allergic drug reactions are more common in females[14]

TABLE 37–4
GENETIC FACTORS IN DRUG ALLERGY

IgE immune response genes—no evidence
HLA associations—limited evidence for gold/penicillamine nephrotoxicity, toxic epidermal necrolysis due to sulfonamides, levamisole-induced agranulocytosis, and hydralazine-induced lupus[145]
Determinants of drug metabolism, such as acetylator polymorphism or the level of activity of microsomal enzymes, such as cytochrome P450[144]
Disease associations—cystic fibrosis, HIV infection, infectious mononucleosis
Other host factors[58, 75]

reaction with other drugs. In retrospective studies, severe immediate or anaphylactic reactions have been noted to occur with increased frequency in patients given medications intravenously compared with orally.[71, 76] Nevertheless, many well-documented case reports of anaphylaxis following oral administration of a drug exist in the literature. Retrospective studies also suggest a decreased incidence of anaphylaxis in children and older adults.[34, 76, 183] No such age variation has been shown for the vast majority of cutaneous reactions to drugs. The fact that cutaneous drug reactions seem more common in women may simply reflect drug usage or increased reporting.[21]

Some observations suggest that underlying disease or immunosuppression may significantly influence the expression of drug allergy by affecting normal suppressor mechanisms or simply by altering the host's ability to express an immune response. Examples include the development of drug allergy in patients on cytotoxic agents, the high incidence of ampicillin rash in infectious mononucleosis, and the frequency of rashes and other toxicities due to sulfa drugs in HIV infection.[31a, 138, 182] The role of genetic factors and atopy in the expression of drug allergy remains uncertain. Specific HLA associations have not been found among persons developing drug allergy to penicillin.[167] Similarly, anecdotal information that atopic individuals are more susceptible than nonatopics has not been substantiated by careful surveys of clinical penicillin allergy or drug skin test reactivity.[31, 72] Lastly, polymorphisms and variations in the levels of enzymes critical in drug metabolism may significantly influence the expression of hypersensitivity reactions.[144]

IMMEDIATE-TYPE HYPERSENSITIVITY

Immediate-type hypersensitivity reactions include urticaria, angioedema, anaphylaxis, laryngeal edema, flush reactions, and bronchospasm. These reactions generally occur within minutes to hours of drug administration, although occasionally delayed reactions of this sort may be seen if absorption and metabolism are important variables. The similarity of these symptoms to the hemodynamic and peripheral manifestations of histamine suggested a central role for the mast cell and basophil in the pathogenesis of these reactions. This has been confirmed by histamine infusion to volunteers, as well as by direct measurement of plasma histamine during drug and other allergic reactions (Fig. 37–1).[86, 117, 165]

Release of histamine, as well as other vasoactive mediators,

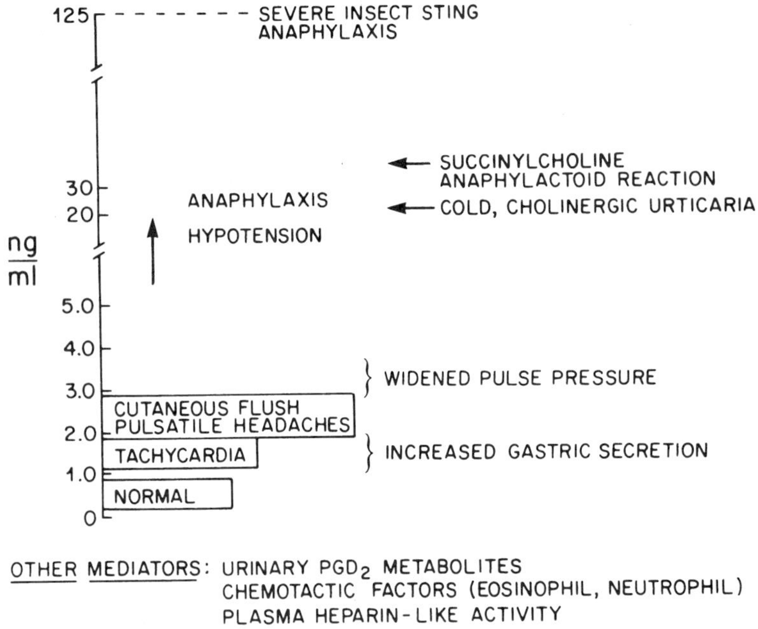

FIGURE 37–1. Correlation between clinical signs and symptoms of immediate hypersensitivity reactions and plasma histamine levels, determined by infusion of histamine into normal volunteers or measurements of blood samples collected during drug or other allergic reactions. The contribution of other vasoactive mediators released from mast cells or basophils to clinical drug allergy is not known; however, their measurement or assays of their metabolites may eventually provide other ways by which allergic reactions to drugs might be assessed.

from basophils and mast cells may be a consequence of immunologic, nonimmunologic, and cytotoxic triggers (Fig. 37–2, Tables 37–5 and 37–6). Immunologic triggering may occur via specific receptors for IgE antibody or complement cleavage products with anaphylatoxin activity (C5a, C4a, C3a) on the surface of these cells. In addition, various lymphokines and monokines have been shown to have histamine-releasing activity. Specific reaginic (IgE) hypersensitivity has been demonstrated in penicillin and insulin allergy, as well as certain instances of allergy to anesthetics and other drugs. Hapten-protein conjugates bridge adjacent IgE molecules with specificity to the eliciting allergen so as to cause lateral aggregation of Fc_ϵ receptors. This initiates a series of biochemical events leading to mediator release. In drug allergy, the size and degree of conjugation of the hapten-carrier conjugate are important determinants of clinical allergy.[100] Prior exposure or an induction period is necessary for the development of IgE antibodies of high affinity, and the reaction characteristically occurs with exposure to minute amounts of antigen.

Anaphylactoid reactions with characteristics of histamine reactions may follow challenge of susceptible individuals with radiographic contrast media, aspirin and related nonsteroidal agents, opiates, or local anesthetics. Although in some instances, such as intravenous anesthetics, direct measurement of plasma histamine has correlated with clinical symptomatology following challenge, the correlation is inexact in others, such as contrast dye reactions.[117] More specific indicators for mast cell involvement are measurements of release of tryptase or prostaglandin D_2 (PGD_2) during allergic reactions.[20, 153] Nonimmunologic triggers do not require prior exposure for elicitation, generally occur at higher concentra-

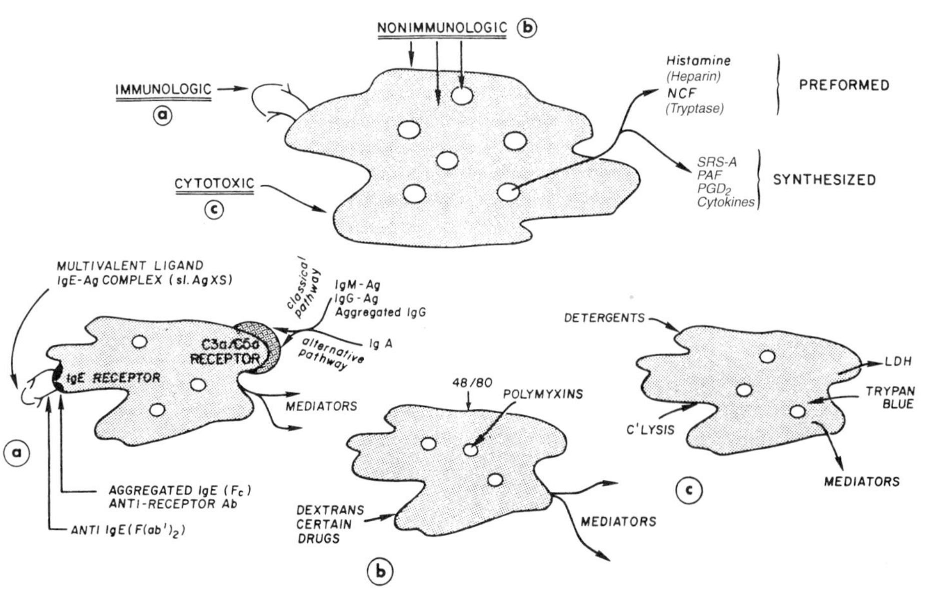

FIGURE 37–2. Immunologic, nonimmunologic, and cytotoxic triggers of mediator release from mast cells and basophils. Pharmacologic differences between basophils and mast cells, or between subsets of mast cells, may exist in regard to specific triggers.

TABLE 37–5
IMMUNOLOGIC VERSUS NONIMMUNOLOGIC MECHANISMS OF IMMEDIATE-TYPE HYPERSENSITIVITY DRUG ALLERGY

Characteristic	Immunologic	Nonimmunologic
Occurs in a minority of patients	Yes	Yes
Prior exposure or induction period required	Yes	No
Required concentration of eliciting antigen	Minute	Higher
Cross reactions with similar chemical structures	Haptenic (structural)	Functional assays
Dose responsiveness of cross-reacting structures in a given test system	Restricted	Variable

tions of drugs, and show dose responsiveness that varies considerably depending on the test system, such as inhibition of prostaglandin synthetase activity in different tissues by nonsteroidals, mast cell degranulation, and depression of FEV_1 following bronchial challenge (see Table 37–5). Pseudoallergic reactions may be triggered by histamine-releasing drugs, potentiated by beta-blockers, and mimicked by enzyme inhibitors, such as captopril and nonsteroidal anti-inflammatory drugs (NSAIDs).[123]

TABLE 37–6
HISTAMINE RELEASE FROM BASOPHILS AND MAST CELLS

Immunologic Triggers
- Antibody (IgE, IgG4)
- Antigen (multivalent)
- Aggregates (polymerized IgG, IgE, antigen-antibody complexes)
- C3a, C4a, C5a
- Delayed hypersensitivity reactions (cutaneous basophil hypersensitivity)
- Lymphokines

Noncytotoxic Triggers[127]
- Proteolytic enzymes
  - Chymotryptic enzymes, pronase
  - Phospholipase A
  - Lysosomal cationic (band 2) protein
- Surface-active agents (concanavalin A, Tween, bile salts)
- Basic polypeptides (low molecular weight)
  - Compound 48/80 (mast cell)
  - Polymyxin, colistin, gramicidin
  - Venom polypeptides (cobra venom activator, mellitin, mast cell degranulating protein of bee venom)
- Calcium ionophores (A23187)
- High molecular weight compounds (certain dextrans)
- Vancomycin*
- Opiates
- Vitamins (B_{12}, thiamine)
- Local anesthetics
- Quaternary ammonium compounds (*d*-tubocurarine, hexamethonium)*
- Short-acting intravenous anesthetics (Thiopental)
- Polycations (protamine at high concentrations)*
- Radiographic contrast media
- ATP (0.01–0.1 mM)
- Certain foods (strawberries)

Cytotoxic Triggers
- IgG antibody to cell surface components: lysis by complement (C5b–C9)
- Destruction by surface-active agents: aliphatic amines, detergents
- Tissue damage

*May also trigger allergic reactions via specific IgE antibodies.

TABLE 37–7
COMMON DRUG ALLERGENS

Drug Allergen	Reaction Rate*
Amoxicillin	51.4
Trimethoprim-sulfamethoxazole	33.8
Ampicillin	33.2
Whole blood	21.6
Cephalosporins	21.1
Semisynthetic penicillins	20.7
Penicillin G	18.5
Allopurinol	7.7
Isoniazid	5.6
Barbiturates	4.0
Diazepam	0.4

*Relative cutaneous rates of allergic reactions.
From Bigby M, Jicks H, Arndt K: Drug-induced cutaneous reactions. JAMA 256:3358–3363, 1986. Copyright 1986. American Medical Association.

DRUG-INDUCED SKIN DISEASE

Relative rates of common drug allergens causing skin rashes seen in an inpatient setting, taken from the Boston Collaborative Drug Surveillance Program, are indicated in Table 37–7.[14] Antibiotics (sulfas, penicillins, cephalosporins) make up the majority of drugs associated with more than a 2% incidence of allergic skin reactions. In turn, cutaneous reactions constitute most of the drug allergies seen in clinical practice (Table 37–8). Most such reactions are exanthematous eruptions that may develop as relatively late manifestations in the course of therapy. Urticaria and angioedema occur with perhaps half the frequency of morbilliform rashes. Whereas many of the former are clearly IgE mediated, most of the latter have not yet been shown to be due to specific immunologic mechanisms. Angioedema due to use of angiotensin-converting enzyme (ACE) inhibitors may be more

TABLE 37–8
CUTANEOUS MANIFESTATIONS OF DRUG ALLERGY

- Exanthematous eruptions (most common)
  - Morbilliform
  - Maculopapular
- Urticaria/angioedema (most likely IgE mediated)
- Contact dermatitis (cell-mediated immunity, delayed hypersensitivity)
  - Localized
  - Systemic
- Erythema multiforme
  - Stevens-Johnson syndrome
- Exfoliative dermatitis
- Fixed drug eruptions
- Purpura/vasculitis
- Toxic epidermal necrolysis (adults)
- Erythema nodosum
- Photosensitivity eruptions
  - Phototoxic (complement activation, other)
  - Photoallergic (contact dermatitis)

frequent and severe than that associated with penicillins, particularly in patients with a history of idiopathic angioedema or on hemodialysis with high-flux dialysis membranes, and has been attributed to inhibition of kinin metabolism.[123, 145]

Contact dermatitis may be elicited by drugs applied directly to the skin and is an important occupational allergy for health care professionals and in the drug industry and certain industrial settings.[4, 8, 158] Examples of contact allergens include antibiotics, such as penicillin, sulfonamides, or neomycin; local anesthetics; antihistamines; and additives, such as parabens, in certain topical medications, cosmetics, and creams. Contact allergies characteristically become evident 48 to 72 hours after exposure, manifesting as an intensely pruritic, papular eruption at the site of exposure, progressing with time and reexposure to eczema. Systemic exposure to a contact allergen may cause flare-ups of dermatitis at previous sites of reactivity or elicit a systemic drug eruption. An example of this phenomenon is a generalized reaction to ethylenediamine that may occur in a person given aminophylline intravenously who has been sensitized to this drug as a component of Mycolog cream.[131] In certain photoallergic reactions, such as to griseofulvin, sulfa drugs, or phenothiazines, contact allergens arise in skin de novo after exposure to radiant energy, and clinical allergy may be elicited later when the drug is taken systemically.[49] (See Chapter 36.)

The immunologic mechanisms for other drug-induced skin reactions remain less clear. These include erythema multiforme and the Stevens-Johnson syndrome (sulfonamides, penicillin, barbiturates), fixed drug eruptions (phenolphthalein, sulfa, barbiturates, tetracycline, heavy metals, quinine), toxic epidermal necrolysis, erythema nodosum (contraceptives, halogens, sulfones or sulfa drugs, penicillin, gold), exfoliative erythroderma (gold compounds, antibiotics, phenothiazines), lichenoid eruptions, thrombocytopenic and nonthrombocytopenic purpura, cutaneous vasculitis, and photosensitivity reactions.[88, 146] A particularly severe form of hypersensitivity syndrome, manifesting as exanthematous, purpuric, or other rashes, often associated with fever and visceral involvement, has been well described with allopurinol and anticonvulsants, such as carbamazepine.[5, 39]

OTHER ORGAN SYSTEMS

Hematologic reactions to drugs include hemolytic anemia, neutropenia, and thrombocytopenia (Table 37–9).[56, 113, 133, 159, 171] Different immune mechanisms have been demonstrated in such reactions, including direct haptenation of the cell membrane by highly reactive derivatives, such as penicilloyl and penicillenate structures of penicillin; modification of the membrane by nonimmunologic absorption, such as cephalothin; drug-dependent antibodies directed against specific membrane constituents, such as antibodies to glycoproteins Ib/IX and IIb/IIIa in quinidine and quinine-induced thrombocytopenia; attachment of antibodies to cells via F_c-domain binding to specific receptors, such as one type of heparin-induced thrombocytopenia; and induction of autoantibodies that are not drug dependent, such as aldomet-associated anti-RBC antibodies. Although such drug hypersensitivity reactions are generally cell type specific, overlap does occur. For example, quinidine is a common cause of thrombocytopenia but may occasionally also cause hemolytic anemia or pancytopenia. Immunologic abnormalities may considerably exceed in prevalence clinically apparent cytotoxicity in several of these syndromes. However, when the latter occurs, the net result is the destruction of blood cells in the vascular space or the premature removal of cells by the liver or spleen at a rate exceeding the capacity of the bone marrow to compensate.

TABLE 37–9
HEMATOLOGIC REACTIONS TO DRUGS

Hemolytic Anemia	**Thrombocytopenia**
Hapten-penicillin (covalent binding), cephalosporins (absorption)	Quinidine/quinine
Immune complex-phenacetin, quinine/quinidine, PAS	Digoxin
Autoimmune-methyl/levodopa, procainamide, chlorpromazine	Sulfonamides
Agranulocytosis	*p*-Aminosalicylic acid
Phenothiazines	Gold salts
Sulfonamides	Heparin
Penicillin	Aspirin
Barbiturates	Thiazides
Thiouracil	Meprobamate
Gold salts	Cimetidine
Chloramphenicol	**Eosinophilia**
p-Aminosalicylic acid	Allopurinol
Antihistamines	Aminoglycosides
Anticonvulsants	Phenothiazines
	Penicillamine
	Gold

Drug-induced hepatic or pulmonary hypersensitivity reactions are generally inferred on the basis of clinical presentation (latency; presence of manifestations, such as a rash, fever, or eosinophilia; recurrence on rechallenge with small doses of drug) or on histologic grounds (mononuclear cell infiltrates, vasculitis, eosinophilia) (Table 37–10).[80, 137] Specific antibodies to enzymes critical in drug metabolism have been implicated in the pathogenesis of halothane-induced hepatitis and drug-specific lymphocyte responsiveness described in some instances of hypersensitivity associated with the use of anticonvulsants.[137, 144, 145, 163]

To a great degree, current concepts regarding the patho-

TABLE 37–10
DRUG-INDUCED HEPATIC AND PULMONARY REACTIONS

Hepatic	**Pulmonary**
Hepatocellular	Hypersensitivity pneumonitis
Halothane	Bleomycin
Isoniazid	Methotrexate
Methyldopa	Pulmonary infiltrates/eosinophilia
Allopurinol	Penicillin
Hydantoins	Sulfonamides
Gold salts	Cromolyn
Cholestatic	Mediastinal and hilar changes
Phenothiazines	Dilantin
Erythromycin	Pleural effusion
Granulomatous	Nitrofurantoin
Allopurinol	Methysergide
Quinidine	Bronchoconstriction
	Aspirin
	Pituitary snuff
	Cromolyn
	Polymyxin

TABLE 37–11
DRUGS ASSOCIATED WITH HYPERSENSITIVITY ANGIITIS (ARMED FORCES INSTITUTE OF PATHOLOGY)

Allopurinol	Griseofulvin
Ampicillin	Penicillin
Bromides	Potassium iodide
Thiazides	Quinidine
Chlorpropamide	Spironolactone
Cromolyn	Sulfonamides
Colchicine	Tetracycline
Dextrans	Trimethadione
Dilantin	

From Mullick FG, McAllister HA Jr, Wagner BM, Fenoglio JJ Jr: Drug-related vasculitis. Hum Pathol 10:313, 1979.

genesis of serum sickness–like syndromes (fever, urticarial or maculopapular rashes, arthralgias or frank arthritis, neuropathy, glomerulonephritis, vasculitis) in drug allergy have been influenced by assumptions derived from animal studies as to the phlogistic potential of circulating immune complexes, as well as by early clinical observations in human serum sickness due to the administration of heterologous sera. In fact, the full serum sickness syndrome may be quite rare as a manifestation of drug allergy, possibly because the concentrations of both antigen and antibody formed are insufficient to cause clinical immune complex disease.[135] Systemic hypersensitivity angiitis involving multiple major organs, often with prominent cutaneous manifestations, has been associated with various drugs, unaccompanied by other features of the serum sickness syndrome (Table 37–11).[46, 120, 145] Similarly, drug fever may be a concomitant of pyrogen-releasing inflammatory reactions, necrosis, or cellular hypersensitivity without having to invoke immune-complex disease as a mechanism (Table 37–12).[30]

Drug hypersensitivity affecting the kidney is far less common than is toxic nephropathy.[3] In addition to presumed immune-complex glomerulonephritis in serum sickness–like syndromes, renal involvement may complicate vasculitic syndromes, such as with sulfonamides, or manifest primarily as interstitial nephritis (Table 37–13). The latter is a well-described manifestation of penicillin (primarily methicillin) hypersensitivity, although recent observations have broadened the spectrum of drugs implicated to include a variety of agents, notably some of the newer NSAIDs.[45, 97]

DRUG-INDUCED AUTOIMMUNE DISEASE

A variety of autoantibodies have been associated with drugs. In general, the incidence of clinical autoimmune disease is much lower than that of seroreactivity. Examples

TABLE 37–12
MECHANISMS OF DRUG FEVER

Release of pyrogens (exogenous, endogenous)
Cytotoxic tissue damage with necrosis
Central and hormonal effects
Cell-mediated immunity
Serum sickness

From Cluff LE, Johnson JE II: Drug fever. Prog Allergy 8:149, 1964. Karger, Basel.

TABLE 37–13
DRUG-INDUCED RENAL DISEASE

Acute Interstitial Nephritis	
Strong association	
Methicillin[45]	NSAIDS
Penicillin	Cimetidine
Cephalothin	
Probable association	
Carbenicillin	Sufonamides
Oxacillin	Rifampin
Ampicillin	Thiazides
Furosemide	
Weak association	
Phenytoin	Captopril
Tetracycline	Allopurinol
Probenecid	
Clinical features	
Morbilliform rash	
Fever	
Leukocytosis	
Eosinophilia	
Renal effects	
Azotemia	
Tubular abnormalities	
Pyuria, eosinophiluria	
Casts	
Hematuria	
Proteinuria (mild)	
Immunologic effects	
High total IgE	
IgM and IgG anti-BPO antibodies[9]	
Positive lymphocyte transformation to methicillin	
Antitubule basement membrane antibodies[17]	
Pathology	
Interstitial nephritis	
Tubular penicilloyl antigen[9]	
Tubular IgG ? IgM ?C′	
Immunologically Mediated Glomerular Injury	
Strong association	
Penicillamine	Mercury
Gold	NSAIDS
Captopril	
Weak association	
Dilantin	Probenecid
Penicillin	Allopurinol
Thiazides	Sulfonamides
Heroin	

include positive antinuclear antibodies in patients chronically on procainamide and IgG antibodies with Rh specificity in patients on methyldopa. Only a minority of these patients actually develop clinical lupus (10%–20%) or frank hemolytic anemia (<10%). Conversely, such serologies may persist for long periods after discontinuation of the drug. A variety of generally dissimilar medications have been associated with the development of lupus-like syndromes, the main three being hydralazine, procainamide, and isoniazid (Table 37–14). Widely divergent incidence rates may reflect a heterogeneity of mechanisms leading to clinical disease. Direct interaction with polynucleotides or components of the complement system, genetically determined differences in the rate of acetylation, the generation of cytotoxic metabolites in cells such as polymorphonuclear leukocytes, and immunomodulatory effects in uncovering autoreactivity have all been implicated in the pathogenesis of drug-induced lupus.[186]

TABLE 37–14
DRUG-INDUCED AUTOIMMUNE DISEASES[85]

Lupus Erythematosus–like
Hydralazine
Procainamide
Isoniazid
Anticonvulsants (various classes)
Chlorpromazine
D-Penicillamine
Sulfa drugs
Scleroderma-like
Eosinophilia-myalgia syndrome (L-tryptophan)
Vinyl chloride disease
Bleomycin
Pentazocine
Polymyositis, Myasthenia Gravis, Pemphigus
Penicillamine
Retroperitoneal Fibrosis
Methysergide
Polyarteritis
Amphetamines
Sjögren's Syndrome
Practolol
Rheumatoid-like
Thiouracils

TABLE 37–15
CLASSIFICATION OF ALLERGIC REACTIONS TO PENICILLIN

Reaction	Incidence (%)	
Immediate (2–30 minutes)		
Anaphylaxis	~0.004	
Hypotension, shock	~0.5–2	
Laryngeal edema		
Wheezing		
Accelerated (1–72 hours)		
Urticaria/angioedema	~1	
Pruritus		
Wheezing, laryngeal edema		
Late (>72 hours)	~3–5	Overall incidence 4–8
Morbilliform rash		
Maculopapular rash		
Unusual Late Allergic Reactions		
Serum sickness[50]		
Drug fever[30]		
Hemolytic anemia[56]		
Agranulocytosis[171]		
Renal effects (interstitial nephritis)[152]		
Recurrent urticaria/arthralgias		
Bleeding disorders[89]		
Erythema multiforme/Stevens-Johnson syndrome[146]		

Modified from Gorevic PD, Levine BB: Penicillin allergy: prediction, prevention, diagnosis, treatment, and desensitization. In Rosse W (ed): Clinical Immunology Update. Elsevier Science Publishing Co, Inc, New York, 1985, p 117.

D-Penicillamine is of particular interest in that it has been associated with the development of not only lupus-like disease but also myasthenia gravis, pemphigus foliaceus, polymyositis, immune-complex nephropathy, and Goodpasture's syndrome. A variety of symptoms suggestive of drug hypersensitivity, including febrile reactions and drug rashes, have also been noted.

PENICILLIN ALLERGY

Contact hypersensitivity to penicillin became apparent in early attempts to rub the mold filtrate into festering sores. The first case of anaphylaxis was reported in 1946. Subsequent series and case reports have documented a broad spectrum of hypersensitivity syndromes due to penicillin (Table 37–15).[63]

SKIN TEST REAGENTS

Initial hopes that allergic reactions to the β-lactam antibiotics would be reduced with purer preparations or the advent of the semisynthetic penicillins were not substantiated by longitudinal studies of the incidence of penicillin allergy reported from venereal disease clinics.[147] During the early 1960s, studies in the laboratories of Eisen[41, 170] and Levine[104] established that the principal antigenic determinant of penicillin allergy was the penicilloyl moiety covalently bound to ϵ-amino groups of lysine residues of protein. From this work, a skin test reagent, penicilloyl polylysine, was developed that was specific for the moiety.[24] This reagent was found to be nonimmunogenic in experimental animals if the penicilloyl group was maximally conjugated to a low molecular weight carrier. A high incidence of skin test reactivity to this antigenic determinant was substantiated in early studies in patients with a history of penicillin allergy and specificity established by hapten inhibition studies.[98] This antigenic determinant, benzylpenicilloyl polylysine (BPL), has been termed "major" because the majority of benzylpenicillin that reacts irreversibly with proteins forms this group. The term "major," however, does not refer to the relative immunologic importance of this hapten.

Many patients with a history of penicillin allergy do not react positively to BPL. Passive transfer studies established that this included individuals who had recently experienced severe anaphylactic reactions.[161] These persons have presumably developed antibody specificity for other antigenic determinants. Initially, it was considered that the immunogenicity of penicillin in some of these instances may be due to trace contaminants, such as polymers of penicillin in combination with its degradation products, foreign proteins, or additives (Table 37–16).[44] These mechanisms for penicillin allergy appear to be rare, if they occur at all. Many of these patients have shown positive skin reactivity when tested with penicil-

TABLE 37–16
POTENTIAL DRUG ALLERGENS

Hapten-protein conjugates (skin, serum, etc., proteins; covalent bonding)
Native drug
Reactive degradation product
Metabolite
Impurities (proteinaceous material from fermentation)
Additives (e.g., carboxymethylcellulose)
Polymers (ampicillin)

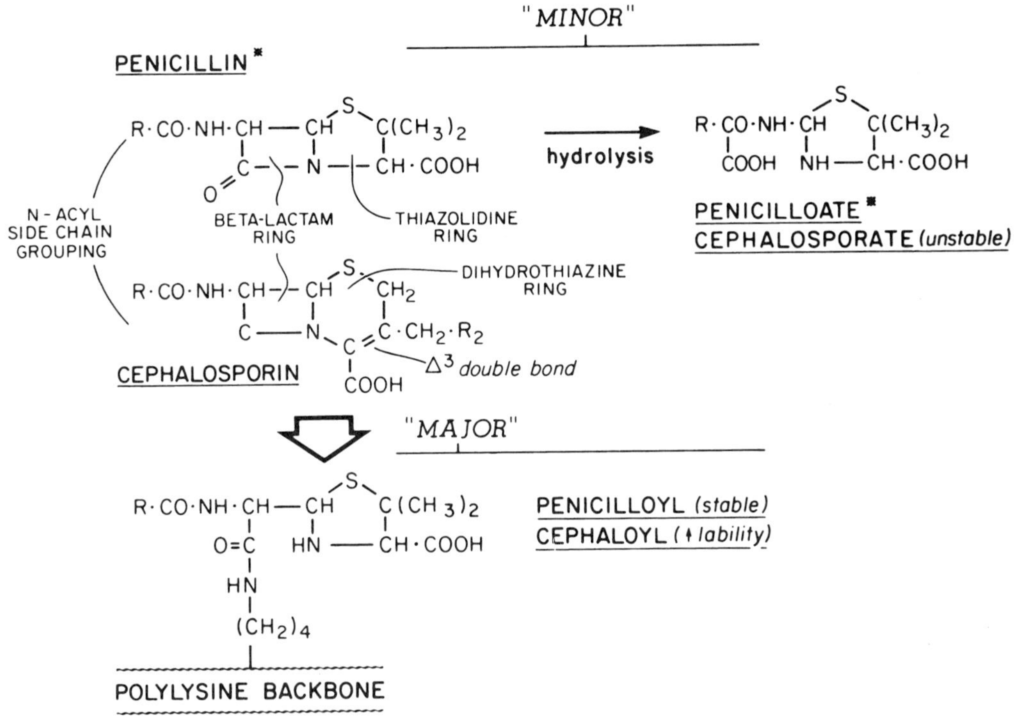

FIGURE 37–3. Haptenic determinants in penicillin and cephalosporin allergy. Major determinants are formed by reaction with protein to form BPO (penicilloyl)-protein conjugates. Skin test reagents used to test for minor determinant hypersensitivity include penicillin, penicilloate, and (in an NIAID cooperative study) benzylpenicilloyl-N-propylamine (not shown). The contribution of the cephaloyl determinant or cephalosporate to cephalosporin allergy is unknown, as these compounds are unstable in vitro and undergo proteolysis. (From Gorevic PD, Levine BB: Penicillin allergy: prediction, prevention, diagnosis, treatment, and desensitization. In Rosse W (ed): Clinical Immunology Update. Elsevier Science Publishing Co, Inc, New York, 1985, p 117.)

lin itself, penicilloic acid, or other degradation products. These haptenic determinants, collectively termed the "minor" determinants, are responsible for many immediate reactions to both penicillin and the semisynthetic penicillins (Fig. 37–3).[102]

The most reliable means for assessing IgE antibodies to penicillin determinants to predict anaphylactic reactions is the direct skin test using both major and minor determinants (Table 37–17).[104] At low concentrations irritant reactions are rarely seen, although some reactions may be indeterminate or equivocal. Intradermal testing is preceded by a prick test, which introduces about 1/1,000 the concentration of antigen, and this in turn may be diluted an additional 1:100 in the presence of a history of recent or severe hypersensitivity. Controls include diluent and histamine (0.01% or 0.275 mg/ml).[2]

The predictive value of penicillin skin testing was established in a large cooperative study involving 3,000 patients conducted under the auspices of the American Academy of Allergy.[65] This study showed that the majority of patients giving a history of penicillin allergy are not skin test positive (Table 37–18). A detailed history documenting the severity and allergic nature of the previous reaction, as well as how recently the previous episode occurred, is most important. Skin tests were positive in 45% of patients with a history of anaphylaxis, 17% of patients with a history of urticaria, and only 7% of those with a history of maculopapular rash.[65]

Although this study demonstrated the safety and predictive value of skin testing in a large group of patients, it was flawed because penicillin G was the only minor determinant tested. Earlier studies of small groups of penicillin-allergic individuals had shown that a significant proportion reacted to the penicilloate determinant (Table 37–19).[102] Most importantly, some of these individuals were negative

TABLE 37–17
REQUIREMENTS FOR A SKIN TEST REAGENT

Low molecular weight (usually <100,000)
Physiologic pH and ionic strength
Low concentrations
  Minor determinants 10^{-2} M
  BPL × 10^{-6} M
  Insulin 10^{-5} M or lower
Should not degranulate mast cells nonimmunologically
Carrier should not be immunogenic (e.g., polylysine)

TABLE 37–18
AMERICAN ACADEMY OF ALLERGY STUDY (1977)

3,000 patients
BPL, penicillin G only
  Eighty-five percent of history-positive patients have negative skin tests
  Forty-five percent of those with a history of anaphylaxis have positive skin tests
  Six percent of history-positive and 2% of history-negative and skin test–negative patients will develop allergic reactions on challenge (none immediate)
  Sixty-six percent of skin test–positive patients will develop allergic reactions on challenge (many immediate)

TABLE 37–19
SKIN REACTIVITY OF 26 MINOR DETERMINANT MIXTURE REACTORS*

Drug		No.	Percent of Total
Penicillin G alone		2	
Penicilloate alone		8	
BPL plus penicillin G		1	
BPL plus penicilloate		2	
Penicillin G plus penicilloate		4	
BPL plus penicillin G plus penicilloate		9	
BPL	Total reactors	12	46
Penicillin G	Total reactors	16	62
Penicilloate	Total reactors	23	88

*Patients were selected on the basis of MDM sensitivity; no patient had only reactivity to BPL. One patient reacted to penicilloate and penicilloylamine but not to the other determinants.

Modified from Levine BB, Redmond AP: Minor haptenic determinant-specific reagins of penicillin hypersensitivity in man. Int Arch Allergy Appl Immunol 35:445, 1969. Karger, Basel.

when tested with BPL and penicillin G. Whereas penicillin G and its principal hydrolysis product penicilloic acid cannot directly conjugate to protein as the penicilloyl moiety, they are presumed to undergo reactions in vivo, yielding distinct haptenic determinants capable of combining with protein and eliciting penicillin allergy. The chemical nature of these eliciting haptenic determinants has yet to be determined.

The general validity of the American Academy of Allergy study has been corroborated in other clinical surveys that have employed the full minor determinant mixture (MDM).[13, 53, 54, 65, 166, 173, 179] Up to 10% of the general population report a history of penicillin allergy, with the incidence being higher in those exposed to repeated courses of antibiotic treatment, such as patients with spina bifida or cystic fibrosis. However, overall, the incidence of positive skin tests among history-positive patients is only 7% to 18% (Table 37–20). The most extensive cooperative study to date, sponsored by the National Institutes of Health, used an MDM that also included penicilloyl-*N*-propylamine based on unpublished studies showing specific reactivity to this determinant in some MDM reactors.[166] By contrast, the incidence of positive skin tests among people giving no history of penicillin allergy has been 1.7% to 4% (Table 37–21).[1, 53, 65]

Although most people found to have positive skin tests react to BPL, MDM reactivity correlates more closely with immediate reactions (Table 37–22). The overwhelming majority of people with documented anaphylactic hypersensitivity react to one or more minor determinants (Fig. 37–4). In two large series, 84% to 85% of skin test–positive patients were reactive when tested with BPL, and 16% to 25% were reactive when tested with MDM; 10% to 15% of skin test–positive patients react with MDM alone. Among the MDM reactors, 80% reacted with only a single component of the mix, and 9% would have been missed if tested with BPL and penicillin G alone, observations that underscore the importance of full testing with all components in the complete diagnostic work-up for penicillin allergy.[166]

The clinical validity of skin testing for IgE antibodies to penicillin haptenic determinants has been shown by challenging skin test–negative and skin test–positive patients with penicillin G itself or other semisynthetic penicillins.[1, 54, 104, 147, 166, 173, 179] Zero to 4% of skin test–negative patients given full therapeutic doses of the drug experience adverse effects, most being mild late reactions not requiring treatment. Among these skin test–negative patients, the incidence of reactions thought to be allergic was slightly higher among

TABLE 37–20
POSITIVE SKIN TESTS IN PATIENTS GIVING A HISTORY OF PENICILLIN ALLERGY

Year	Reagents	No. Tested	No. Positive: Total	No. Positive: Major/Minor	Percent	Comment
1965	BPL PCN G	120	120	44/18	37/15	↓ On serial testing
1969	BPL "Old" PCN	120	17	16/10	10.6	Children
1976	BPL MDM	218	33	—	15.1	—
1977	BPL PCN G	1,718	325	253/154	18.9	Allergy clinics
1978	BPL MDM	253	29	—	11.5	2/3 children
1981	BPL MDM	740	469	250/193	63.4	—
1982	BPL MDM	778	108	79/55	13.9	Included testing to semisynthetic penicillins
1983	BPL	606	85	—	14.0	—
1992	BPL MDM	825	146	*	18.0	Hospitalized patients
1993	BPL MDM	776	55	*	7.1	STD clinic

*See text.

PCN G = penicillin G.

Updated from Gorevic PD, Levine BB: Penicillin allergy: prediction, prevention, diagnosis, treatment, and desensitization. In Rosse W (ed): Clinical Immunology Update. Elsevier Science Publishing Co, Inc, New York, 1995, p 117.

Data from references 13, 53, 54, 65, 166, 173, and 179.

TABLE 37–21
POSITIVE SKIN TESTS IN PATIENTS WITH NO HISTORY OF PENICILLIN ALLERGY

Year	Skin Test Reagents	Patient Population	No. Tested	No. Positive Total	No. Positive Major/Minor	Percent
1965	BPL PCN G	Allergy clinic	97	6	5/1	6.2
1971	BPL MDM	Inpatients	163	10	9/6	6.1
1972	BPL MDM	Inpatients Outpatients	555 160	47 6	— —	8.5 3.8
1977	BPL PCN G	Outpatients	1,229	87	65/39	7.1
1983	BPL MDM	Outpatients	567	38	—	6.7
1992	BPL MDM	Inpatients	610	25	—	4.0
1993	BPL MDM	STD clinic	4,287	73	—	1.7

Data from references 53, 54, 63, 65, and 166.

those with a history of adverse reactions to penicillin. On the other hand, 22% to 73% of history-positive and skin test–positive patients challenged with penicillins developed reactions, many while receiving minute doses for desensitization of clinical allergy (Table 37–23). Most of these reactions were immediate, and some were life threatening and required therapeutic intervention.

OTHER TESTS FOR HYPERSENSITIVITY TO PENICILLIN

IgE antibodies can also be demonstrated by passive transfer of patient serum to the skin of an unsensitized recipient, with subsequent challenge of the site with antigen (Prausnitz-Küstner reaction) (Table 37–24). This method measures circulating rather than basophil-bound or mast cell–bound IgE antibodies and is less sensitive than direct skin testing.[140]

In vitro assays for antibodies to specific penicillin haptenic determinants are of interest because they provide alternatives to the potential hazards of skin testing a highly sensitive individual, as well as the ability to do retrospective studies (Table 37–25). Two approaches that have been taken include challenge of sensitized basophils with multivalent ligands and measurements of subsequent histamine release and radio- or enzyme-linked immunoassays.[2, 33, 35, 70] Because the actual eliciting haptens responsible for MDM hypersensitivity remain unknown, such assays have been applicable only to major determinant hypersensitivity. Longitudinal studies have shown that 10% to 20% of patients who have completed a recent course of penicillin without adverse reactions will have positive skin tests or IgE antibodies demonstrable by radioallergosorbent test (RAST). There follows a rapid diminution in titer over the ensuing months, such that the majority of patients are negative when retested 6 to 12 months later.[53, 125] Thus skin testing is most useful predictively and is of little value immediately following a recent course of treatment.

Specificity for the penicilloyl antigen may also be detected in other immunoglobulin classes (IgG, IgM, IgA, IgD) utiliz-

TABLE 37–22
PENICILLIN SKIN TEST REAGENTS

Major determinant
BPL 10^{-6} M
Minor determinants
Penicillin, Penicilloate, Penicilloyl-*N*-propylamine — 10^{-2} M (8,000 U/ml)

Intradermal = 0.01 ml (80 U penicillin G)
Prick = 1/1,000 intradermal

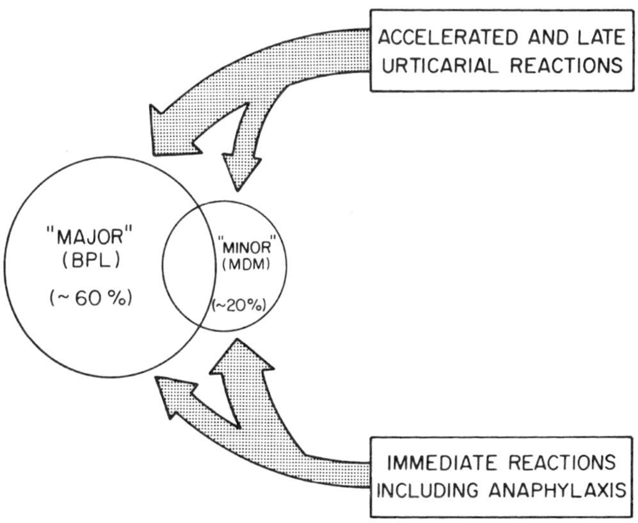

FIGURE 37–4. Relative incidence of major and minor skin test reactivity among both history-positive and history-negative patients. Sixty percent to 80% of all skin-test positive patients react to benzylpenicilloyl polylysine alone and 15% to 25% react to one or more minor determinants; the remainder in several series react to both or give indeterminate skin test results. Immediate reactions, including anaphylaxis, correlate more closely with MDM reactivity, whereas BPL reactivity is more prevalent among accelerated and late reactions (both urticarial and exanthematous eruptions).

TABLE 37–23
INCIDENCE OF ALLERGIC REACTIONS DEVELOPING IN PATIENTS TREATED WITH PENICILLIN

Year	History	No. Challenged	Patients With Allergic Reaction No.	Patients With Allergic Reaction Percent	Comments
History only*					
1973	–	24,906	155	0.6	½-hour observation
	+	78	10	12.8	
1968	+	75	3	4.0	⅓ required treatment
1971	–	54	1	1.9	1 accelerated reaction
1976	–	185	7	3.8	6 late exanthems
1977	–	346	12	3.5	3/12 had early reactions
Skin test negative†					
1978	–	169	2	1.2	2 urticarial, 1 systemic
1982	–	290	12	4.1	5/12 urticarial
	+	83	2	2.4	Both late reactions
1983	–	529	6	1.1	Not attributed to PCN
	+	443	35	7.9	1 early urticarial reaction 15 late reactions
1992	–	568	0	0	
	+	726	7	1.2	8 maculopapular rashes also noted
1993	–	4,201	40	1.0	18 felt to be IgE reactions
	+	649	17	2.7	9 immediate; 8 accelerated; 8 delayed
Skin test positive†					
1969	+	11	8	72.7	8 immediate reactions; 3 also had late reactions
1977	+	9	6	66.6	3/6 immediate reactions
1982	+	8	4	50.0	Urticaria or rash
1992	+	9	2	22.0	

*Data from references 1, 63, 65, 147, 173, and 179.
†Data from references 54, 65, 104, and 166.

ing sensitive hemagglutination assays.[56, 101] Although IgM or IgG antibodies to the benzylpenicilloyl (BPO) group can be demonstrated in a large percentage of individuals experiencing immediate and late reactions to penicillin, their diagnostic utility has been limited.[103] High-titer IgM hemagglutinating antibodies are found in one fourth to one third of penicillin-induced exanthematic eruptions.[103] IgG anti-BPO antibodies have been associated with serum sickness, as well as with Coombs-positive hemolytic anemia.[50, 101] The latter complication may occur in patients receiving high doses of penicillin intravenously, usually for endocarditis.[56, 101] Immune mechanisms have also been implicated in neutropenia or agranulocytosis and thrombocytopenia secondary to penicillin, as well as rare cases of factor VIII deficiency due to induction of an acquired inhibitor of this protein.[89, 121]

TABLE 37–24
DIAGNOSTIC TESTS IN PENICILLIN ALLERGY

- Direct immediate skin test[2]
  - BPL major
  - MDM (penicillin G, penicilloic acid, other determinants)
- Passive transfer (Prausnitz-Küstner)[140]
  - Has 50%–75% sensitivity of the direct immediate skin test
- Hemagglutination assays[101]
  - IgG, IgM, anti-BPO
  - ? Other haptens
- Total IgE[119]
- RAST[70] or ELISA[33]
  - Available only for penicilloyl major determinant
- Cell-mediated immunity
  - In vitro reactivity[22, 178]
  - Patch testing (penicillin G)[139]
- Basophil degranulation/histamine release[2, 35]
  - Challenge with BPL multivalent haptens (D_2O required)

Modified from Gorevic PD, Levine BB: Pencillin allergy: prediction, prevention, diagnosis, treatment, and desensitization. In Rosse W (ed): Clinical Immunology Update. Elsevier Science Publishing Co, Inc, New York, 1985, p. 117.

Delayed hypersensitivity to penicillin has been shown by patch testing, blastogenesis assays, and measurement of specific lymphokine activity.[139, 178] Cloned T cells manifesting proliferative responses to penicillin antigens have been isolated from peripheral blood mononuclear cells of allergic individuals and found to be heterogeneous as to antigen specificity, phenotype, major histocompatibility complex (MHC) restriction, and cytokine profile.[22]

Two types of serum sickness–like reactions have been described in patients receiving or who have recently received penicillin (Table 37–26). Levine and colleagues[103] described the clinical and immunologic features of 16 patients who developed recurrent urticaria and arthralgias as a late reaction 3 to 21 days after the drug was discontinued. All of these patients had MDM reactivity, most frequently to penicilloate, and only about 20% reacted to BPL. A second group of patients studied by Fellner and Baer[50] had clinical signs and symptoms suggestive of serum sickness developing during a course of penicillin therapy. Skin test reactivity was

TABLE 37–25
IMMUNE RESPONSE TO PENICILLIN HAPTENS IN THE VARIOUS LATE ALLERGIC REACTIONS

	Percent Incidence				
	IgE		Anti-BPO		
Response	**BPL**	**MDM**	**IgM**	**IgG**	**Delayed Hypersensitivity**
Immediate	40	100	Low titer	60	Yes
Accelerated/late urticaria	100	40	100	100	60
Morbilliform	25*	0	25–33 ↑	Low titer	15
Hemolytic anemia	Rare	Rare	Low titer	High titer	Unknown
Urticaria/arthralgias (16 cases)	30	100	Low titer	Low titer	0
Methicillin nephritis[9]	Yes	No	Yes	Yes	Yes

*Developed late in the course of the reaction.
From Levine BB, Redmond AP, Fellner MJ, et al: Penicillin allergy and the heterogeneous immune responses of man to benzylpenicillin. J Clin Invest 45:1895, 1966. Reproduced from The Journal of Clinical Investigation, by copyright permission of The American Society for Clinical Investigation.

primarily to penicillin G but did not develop until after the reaction in 7 of 11 cases studied; 45% of these patients also reacted to BPL.

Over 70 cases of acute allergic interstitial nephritis due to penicillin and its analogues, most notably methicillin, have been described.[45] In one well-studied patient who underwent a renal biopsy, the penicilloyl hapten was detected by direct fluorescence on the tubular basement membrane and could not be eluted with univalent penicilloyl hapten. This patient also was found to have IgE, IgM, and IgG anti-BPO antibodies after methicillin was discontinued, as well as a positive tuberculin-type skin test to methicillin.[9]

THERAPEUTIC MODALITIES

As indicated, the proper management of penicillin allergy begins with a careful history, particularly noting the severity and type of prior reaction, as well as the time since it occurred. If an alternative antibiotic will not pose a management problem, it may be reasonable to utilize it regardless of skin test reactivity in the face of a history of clear-cut life-threatening allergic reaction, such as anaphylaxis or exfoliative dermatitis. A history of maculopapular rash developing during a previous course of penicillin therapy may not be a contraindication to subsequent treatment with penicillin, as these late reactions do not appear to be mediated by IgE antibodies and, at least in children, are not associated with an increased risk on subsequent rechallenge with penicillin.[99, 183]

Treatment of severe immediate and accelerated reactions consists of discontinuing the drug, administering epinephrine if there is laryngeal edema or vascular compromise, and prescribing antihistamines for urticarial reactions or angioedema and to relieve pruritus (Table 37–27). Corticosteroids have little utility in the management of the acute IgE antibody reaction but may inhibit the late cellular phase of an allergic reaction if it is particularly severe and sustained. High-dose (60 mg prednisone/day) steroids have also been used for the management of serum sickness–like reactions (fever, arthralgias, nephropathy, neuropathy), as well as exfoliative dermatitis. Maculopapular rashes generally do not require therapy. Most resolve spontaneously within a week after discontinuation of the drug. In some cases, resolution has also been noted despite continued administration. However, continued therapy does pose a risk of generalized erythroderma or exfoliative dermatitis.

Skin testing with BPL and MDM may be used to establish reaginic hypersensitivity in patients for whom penicillin is the drug of choice or who have had questionable past reactions. As noted previously, skin testing may be positive in some asymptomatic persons who have completed a recent course of the drug.[125] Skin tests may be negative in severely

TABLE 37–26
SERUM SICKNESS–LIKE REACTIONS TO PENICILLIN

Recurrent urticaria and arthralgias[103]
- Begins 3–21 days after drug is discontinued
- Recurrent urticaria/erythema annulare/angioedema lasting 2–15 weeks
- Eighty percent have arthralgias with periarticular edema and erythema
- Terminates spontaneously in 75%; may respond to milk-free diet
- Minor determinant reactivity; primarily to the penicilloate-derived hapten-protein conjugate

Serum sickness–like[50]
- Occurs 1–3 weeks after onset of penicillin therapy
- Rash (usually urticaria/arthralgia plus fever, proteinuria, or edema)
- Perivascular eosinophilic infiltrates
- Skin reactivity to minor determinants develops later and may be persistent
- Positive lymphocyte stimulation with penicillin G

TABLE 37–27
TREATMENT

Immediate reactions
- Discontinue drug
- Epinephrine and antihistamines
- Desensitization

Accelerated and late reactions
- Antihistamines only
- Steroids for exfoliative dermatitis and erythema multiforme

Maculopapular eruptions
- Antihistamine as needed
- Wait (up to 3 weeks)

Contact allergy
- Topical steroids

TABLE 37–28
THERAPEUTIC APPROACHES TO THE ABROGATION OF ANAPHYLACTIC HYPERSENSITIVITY

Induction of IgG-blocking antibodies
- Accelerated urticarial reactions to penicillin[51, 177]
  - BPO-specific IgE ± MDM
  - IgM and low levels of IgG hemagglutinating (HA) antibodies to BPO
  - IgG HA antibody levels increase dramatically with resolution of desensitization
- Insect venom immunotherapy[73]
  - Venom and phospholipase-specific IgG
- Certain cases reported of desensitization for insulin allergy[184]

True desensitization
- Immediate penicillin reactors
- MDM-specific IgE; no HA antibodies yet demonstrated
- Certain cases reported of desensitization for insulin allergy[111]

Monovalent hapten inhibitors[42, 43]

Hapten-specific tolerance
- Copolymer of D-glutamic acid and D-lysine[29]
- Isologous IgG[18]

debilitated patients or in desensitized patients who are tested after a severe immediate reaction.

Drug desensitization is reserved for clinical situations in which no alternative antibiotic of equivalent efficacy is available or in which alternative antibiotics have failed or cannot be administered because of severe intolerance.[130] It must be preceded by complete skin testing to establish specific sensitivities that may be followed during the procedure. Two immunologic mechanisms for desensitization have been documented. The first has occurred in patients experiencing accelerated urticarial reactions and who have primarily BPL reactivity. Here, resolution of urticaria with continuance of the drug has been associated with a striking anamnestic response monitored as a dramatic increase of IgG hemagglutinating antibodies to the penicilloyl antigen from initially low levels. There is no loss of BPL skin reactivity during desensitization. It has been suggested that BPO-specific IgG antibody may function as a blocking antibody to prevent reaction of antigen with IgE antibodies that remain on the mast cell surface.[51, 177]

True desensitization (Table 37–28) for MDM-specific IgE responders is a potentially dangerous procedure that should be performed only with informed consent in an intensive care setting; it may be particularly hazardous in patients with cystic fibrosis.[48] Clinical details have been reported in case reports and small series (Table 37–29).[19, 26, 59, 62, 64, 122, 134, 141, 168] Several of these patients have isolated reactivity to the penicilloate antigen. Complete cross-reactivity with other semisynthetic penicillins has been demonstrated by success-

TABLE 37–29
REPORTS OF DESENSITIZATION IN PATIENTS WITH MDM-SPECIFIC REACTIVITY

Year	Age	Sex	History of Penicillin Allergy	Skin Tests	Premedication	Route of Administration	Clinical Course
1962	27	F	Urticaria 2 months prior	PCN G +	Yes	IM	No side effects; skin test negative after premedication
1967	1		—	Penicilloate	—	IV	Transient flare skin test reactivity prior to flush
1972	47	F	Rash 20 years prior	BPL + MDM − → +	Yes	IM IV	Two challenges; hypotension
1974	53	M	Urticaria 17 years prior (PCN); recent reactions to cephalothin	BPL − PCN G +	Yes	IV	Immediate reactions; late urticaria
1981	68	M	Morbilliform rash 9 months prior	BPL − PCN G − Penicilloate +	Yes	IV	Flush with carbenicillin
1982	16 14 (mean 52 years)	M F	—	BPL + 21 (5 only) PCN G + 17 (2 only) Penicilloate + 17 (3 only)	No	PO	10 mild early reactions 9 urticaria > 6 hours later 1 nephritis 65% skin tests → negative 35% ↓ intensity
1982	11	M	Immediate reactions 3 months prior	BPL + MDM +	—	IV PO	Ticarcillin, PCN G } mild reactions
1983	47	F	Reactions 27, 16, 5, and 3 years prior	BPL + Penicilloate + PCN G +	No	ID	Immediate reactions; late urticaria
1987	18 8 (2 children)	M F	Anaphylaxis (6); Angioedema (3); Urticaria (7); Rash (4); 1 serum sickness	BPL +16 PCN G +18 Penicilloate + 18	No	PO	13/26 reactions; urticaria (5); angioedema (1); rash (1); pruritus (4); serum sickness (2); bronchospasm (1); 6-all skin tests negative; 5-at least one skin test negative

PCN G = penicillin G.

Updated from Gorevic PD, Levine BB: Penicillin allergy: prediction, prevention, diagnosis, treatment and desensitization. In Rosse W (ed): Clinical Immunology Update. Elsevier Science Publishing Co, Inc, New York, 1985, p 117.

Data from references 19, 26, 59, 62, 64, 122, 141, and 168.

ful desensitization with the latter. In other instances, differential skin test reactivity between semisynthetic penicillins has been reported, suggesting in turn specific IgE antibodies to side chain groupings (see Figure 37–3).[162] Clinical, laboratory, and immunologic data regarding one case previously reported are summarized in Table 37–30 and Figure 37–5.[62] Generally, patients are not premedicated with antihistamines or epinephrine prior to the procedure so as not to interfere with skin test reactivity. Successful desensitization is usually associated with a marked decrease or loss of skin reactivity to the specific haptenic determinant, including BPL.[134] Patients have been desensitized by intravenous injection of gradually increasing doses of penicillin or by oral desensitization (Table 37–31).[168]

Alternative modalities of therapy have been suggested, grounded mostly in animal studies. These include the use of monovalent hapten inhibitors or the induction of specific tolerance.[18, 29, 42, 43, 57, 96] The former has not proved successful in limited trials, and the latter has been achieved only in animals and in human lymphocytes made tolerant in vitro for the penicilloyl major haptenic determinant.[10, 18, 29, 57] Applicability of these alternative approaches to the treatment of penicillin allergy awaits further delineation of the eliciting haptenic determinants responsible for minor determinant reactivity.

CEPHALOSPORINS

First-generation cephalosporins differ from penicillins in the presence of a dihydrothiazine instead of the thiazolidine ring (see Fig. 37–3). Allergic reactions include immediate hypersensitivity reactions such as urticaria (1%–2%) or anaphylaxis, rashes, cytopenias, drug fever, and interstitial nephritis.[56, 67, 151, 152] Cephalosporins resemble the penicillins in the spectrum of allergic reactions seen and the elicitation of specific immune responses demonstrable as IgG, IgM, and IgE antibodies, as well as in cell-mediated immunity.[132]

Cross-reactivity between first-generation cephalosporins and penicillins was initially shown by parallel rises in antibodies to penicilloyl and cephalosporin antigenic determinants in rabbits immunized with these drugs.[23] It was also shown in clinical studies in which the antibody response to both determinants was monitored and in hemagglutination cross-inhibition experiments using either antigen.[56] Anaphylactic cross-reactivity between penicillin and first-generation cephalosporins (cephalothin or cephaloridine) has been described in eight case reports.[67, 151] The exact incidence of this important entity, as well as its immunologic basis, is unknown. This is due in large part to lack of knowledge regarding the exact cephalosporin haptenic determinants that elicit IgE responses in humans. Most clinical studies in which skin testing to cephalosporins has been performed have utilized the native drug as a reagent. However, in vitro studies suggest that the cephalosporoyl moiety and cephalosporate may not be stable entities and thus are incapable of eliciting IgE antibodies (see Fig. 37–3). Whereas early clinical studies suggested that the incidence of cross-reactivity to cephalosporins (cephaloridine, cephalothin, cephalexin, cefazolin, cefamandole) among history-positive penicillin-allergic individuals may approach 50%, this has not been substantiated in later surveys (Tables 37–32 and 37–33).[16, 132, 149, 179] Some of the apparent increase in reactions to cephalosporins has been attributed to a general and nonspecific increase in drug reactions among penicillin-allergic patients, and some to a contamination of early cephalosporin preparations by penicillin.[164] Regardless of cause, it seems likely that cephalosporins may be well tolerated, even in a large number of patients with documented IgE antibodies to penicillin haptenic determinants.

TABLE 37–30
CASE STUDY OF DESENSITIZATION

Patients

- 68-year-old male; long history of chronic obstructive lung disease
- February 1976: Right upper lobe pneumonia; generalized rash 3 days after intravenous penicillin
- March 1976: Right upper lobectomy, thoracoplasty, bullectomy
- April–July 1976: Tolerates several courses of cephalosporin without incident
- October 1976: New left lower lobe infiltrate
- November 1976: Drainage of empyema
- December 1976: *Serratia marcescens* septicemia; no response to adequate gentamicin, clindamycin; sensitive to carbenicillin

Desensitization Protocol

- Informed consent; intensive care unit
- Epinephrine and lidocaine on standby
- Central line
- Serial monitoring: vital signs, central venous pressure, electrocardiogram, skin test
- First dose 0.1 ml of concentration giving a 2+ skin test
- Dose given intravenously and doubled every 15 minutes
- Follow the skin test serially

Subsequent Course

- Tolerates carbenicillin without incident for 7 days
- Dies of Brown-Séquard's syndrome due to metastatic carcinoma of the lung
- Mitral and tricuspid endocarditis found at postmortem

Conclusion

- Isolated penicilloate sensitivity explains cross-reactivity to carbenicillin, lack of cross-reactivity with cephalosporins, and true desensitization

TABLE 37–31
FEATURES OF TRUE DESENSITIZATION

- Specific loss of skin test reactivity (no change in response to other allergens)[172]
- No effect on skin mast cell receptor sensitivity (still degranulate with anti-IgE); not due to depletion of mediators (still degranulate on stimulation with compound 48/80 and polymyxin)[172]
- Basophil histamine release is unaffected (still activated by penicilloyl antigen and anti-IgE)[134]
- Not likely to be due to IgG blocking antibody* (no change in penicilloyl-specific IgE and IgG, although levels may increase after desensitization)[122]; serum does not block degranulation in vitro[134]
- No evidence of complement activation (C3, C4, CH50) or de novo formation of IgG immune complexes[62]
- Subsequent elevation in total IgE[122]
- No increase in blood histamine in the absence of adverse reactions[62]
- Skin reactivity may return within days if drug is discontinued
- No information as to
  - Actual eliciting of hapten-protein conjugates responsible for minor determinant hypersensitivity
  - Locus (loci) of desensitization in terms of sequence of biochemical events leading to mast cell degranulation

*Decreased insulin-specific and total IgE has been noted during desensitization for insulin allergy.[111]

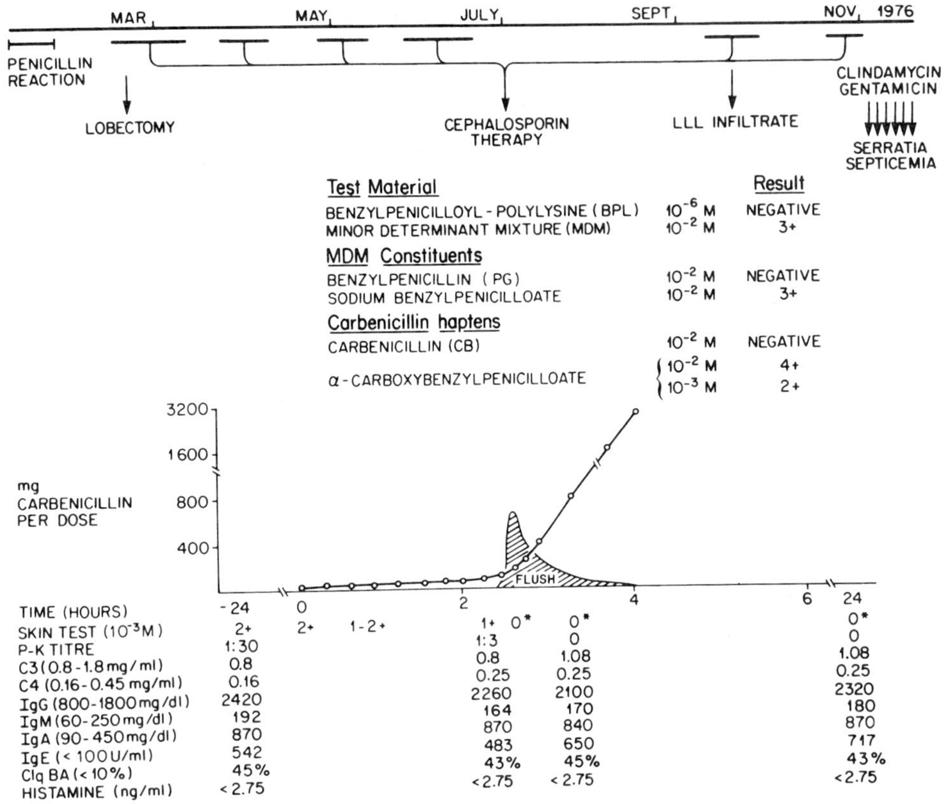

FIGURE 37–5. Clinical course and immunologic studies of a patient desensitized for anaphylactic hypersensitivity to the penicilloate minor determinant of penicillin and carbenicillin. (From Gorevic PD, Levine BB: Penicillin allergy: prediction, prevention, diagnosis, treatment, and desensitization. In Rosse W (ed): Clinical Immunology Update. Elsevier Science Publishing Co, Inc, New York, 1985, p 117.)

The situation regarding the newer classes of cephalosporins (monobactams, carbapenems, clavams, oxacephems) is more complex, reflecting significant variation in both ring structure and side chain groupings. Whereas the carbapenems, such as imipenem, cross-react with antipenicillin IgE on skin testing, the monobactams (aztreonam) generally do not and thus appear to be safe for administration to penicillin-allergic individuals.[81, 149] Occasional instances of cross-sensitization have been described, however, in the setting of cystic fibrosis.[118]

AMPICILLIN

The incidence of ampicillin rashes significantly exceeds that seen with penicillin, semisynthetic penicillins, or the cephalosporins (see Table 37–7).[12, 14, 27, 156] Prospective studies carried out during the Boston Collaborative Drug Surveillance Program showed that the difference in incidence from penicillin is due largely to an increased number of late cutaneous reactions, occurring more than 7 days after exposure to the drug (Fig. 37–6).[156] The majority of these late reactions are maculopapular exanthematous eruptions, often self-limited, occurring in patients who do not have skin test reactivity to standard penicillin skin test reagents.[12, 32] The incidence of these rashes is significantly increased in patients who have chronic lymphocytic leukemia or mononucleosis due to Epstein-Barr virus or cytomegalovirus and has also been reported to approach 90% in patients with glandular fever.[25, 27, 107, 138] Some studies have suggested that ampicillin rashes may be due to homopolymer formation by reaction of the free amino group in the molecule, to specific IgM and IgG antibody responses, to specific IgE responses not shared with other β-lactams, or to a cellular immune response to the antibiotic.[109a, 114, 124, 135, 162]

TABLE 37–32
CEPHALOSPORINS

Anaphylactic reactions to cephalosporins in patients with a history of penicillin allergy have been well described[67, 151]
Clear-cut cross-reactivities have been shown by hemagglutination assays[132]
Increased lability of the cephaloyl and cephaloate moieties compared with penicilloyl groups and penicilloate has been shown in vitro[149]
The incidence of allergic reactions to cephalosporins among penicillin-allergic patients has been reported to be up to four times that among persons with no history of penicillin allergy[132]
The actual incidence of cephalosporin allergy in penicillin-allergic patients may be quite low (see Table 37–33)
Some second- and third-generation cephalosporins may be less cross-reactive because bulky side chains are more immunogenic and block access to the β-lactam ring[16]

SULFONAMIDE ALLERGY

Studies during the 1940s associated sulfonamide therapy with vasculitic syndromes resembling polyarteritis nodosa.[142] The major hypersensitivity reactions to sulfa drugs seen more recently in clinical practice are a variety of cutaneous eruptions, including urticaria/angioedema, morbilliform rashes, contact sensitivity, photoallergic reactions, erythema multiforme/Stevens-Johnson syndrome, and toxic epidermal necrolysis (TEN).[145, 146] Other manifestations of hypersensitivity include hepatotoxicity, drug fever, serum sickness,

TABLE 37–33
ALLERGIC REACTIONS TO CEPHALOSPORINS IN PATIENTS WITH POSITIVE SKIN TESTS TO PENICILLIN DETERMINANTS OR A HISTORY OF PENICILLIN ALLERGY

Authors	Year	No. of Patients	No. of Reactions	Percent	Comments
Thoburn et al.[175]	1966	11	2	18.2	History
Girard[60]	1968	23	2	8.7	History
Assem and Vickers[6]	1974	3	3	100.0	History
Petz[132]	1978	24	11	45.8	+ Skin test
		701	57	8.11	
Warrington et al.[179]	1978	3	0	0	+ Skin test
Solley et al.[166a]	1982	178	2	1.1	History
		24	0	0	+ Skin test
Saxon et al.[149]	1989	62	1	1.6	+ Skin test
Blanca et al.[16]	1989	19	2	10.5	+ Skin test

blood dyscrasias, nephritis, and cardiotoxicity.[135] Significant cross-reactivities for some of these reactions may occur with sulfonylureas, thiazide diuretics, and sulfasalazine. Whereas the overall prevalence of drug rash from sulfonamide-containing medications is 3% to 6%, this figure rises considerably in the HIV-infected population, reaching up to 28% in children and 50% in adults.[155, 183]

Several mechanisms have been suggested to explain sulfonamide hypersensitivity (Table 37–34). Sulfamethoxazole has been shown to be particularly reactive with serum proteins. IgE antibodies have been demonstrated in some patients with immediate hypersensitivity-type reactions, both by solid-phase assay and skin testing with a poly-L-tyrosine conjugate.[115] Similar to observations in some forms of drug-induced lupus, an increased incidence of slow acetylator phenotype has been noted among patients manifesting systemic hypersensitivity reactions.[144, 157, 186] Sulfonamides are one of a group of drugs, including dapsone and rifampin, primarily metabolized by *N*-acetylation that may be associated with up to a 10-fold increase in adverse reactions in HIV-infected patients.[90] Abnormalities in *N*-acetylation may in turn shift metabolism to the cytochrome P450 system, leading in turn to the generation of hydroxylamines and nitrosometabolites that are cytotoxic to lymphocytes (Fig. 37–7).[143] A deficiency in glutathione, which inactivates hydroxylamine metabolites, has been suggested as one potential mechanism to explain the increased incidence of drug toxicity in AIDS patients.[90, 155] Lastly, a direct role for T-cell reactivity to sulfa antigens has been implicated by proliferative cell assays in patients manifesting systemic reactions such as TEN.[87, 112]

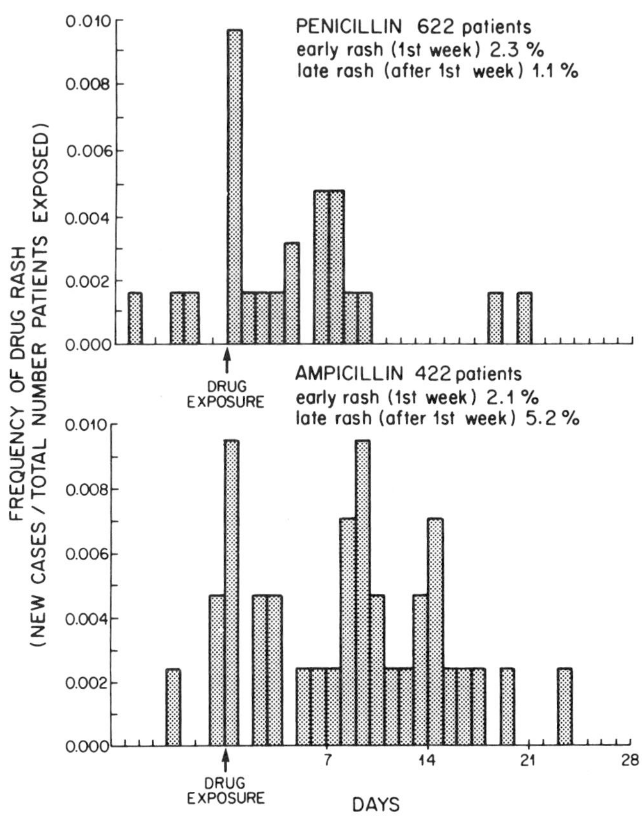

FIGURE 37–6. Relative incidence of cutaneous reactions to penicillin and ampicillin, assessed prospectively, reported as part of the Boston Collaborative Drug Surveillance Program. (From Shapiro S, Siskin DV, Sloane D, et al: Drug rash with ampicillin and other penicillins. Lancet 2:969, 1969. The Lancet Limited, 1969.)

Management of sulfonamide allergy involves considering this diagnosis in the setting of a cutaneous reaction, such as Stevens-Johnson syndrome, or of an HIV-infected patient and being alert to possible cross-reactivities or shared sensitivities with other drugs that are similarly metabolized. Desensitization regimens similar to those employed in the management of β-lactam allergy have been successfully used in patients manifesting immediate hypersensitivity reactions to bactrim or sulfasalazine, but the immunologic basis for this drug tolerance remains to be defined.[130, 182]

INSULIN ALLERGY

IgE-mediated immediate hypersensitivity reactions may occur after administration of a variety of low molecular

TABLE 37–34
MECHANISMS IN SULFONAMIDE HYPERSENSITIVITY

- IgE antibodies to N^4-sulfamethoxazole determinant[115]
- T-cell response to sulfonamide antigens (haptenated proteins, reactive metabolites)[87, 112]
- Slow acetylator status[157]
- Toxicity of hydroxylamine metabolites generated by hepatic microsomes for lymphocytes and possibly other cells[143]
- ? Deficient glutathione synthetase (inactivation of hydroxylamine metabolites)

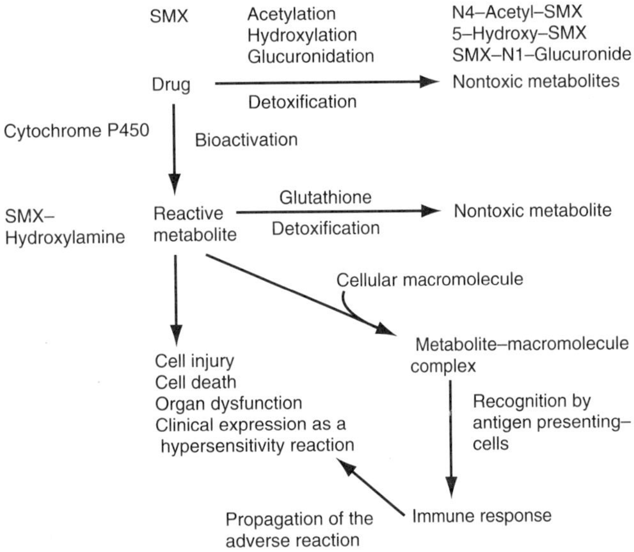

FIGURE 37–7. Metabolic pathways of sulfonamide (and related) drugs via N-acetylation and the cytochrome P450 mixed-function oxidase system in relation to potential mechanisms relevant to clinical hypersensitivity reactions. SMX = sulfamethoxazole. (From Shapiro LE, Knowles SR, Shear NH: Sulfonamide allergies—management in the '90s. Allergy Clin Immunol Int 8:5–12, 1996.)

weight polypeptide hormones, including adrenocorticotropic hormone (ACTH), insulin, and calcitonin. Although it has been considered in each case that reactivity may be directed to a contaminant, immunologic studies have shown that the major immune response is directed to the hormone itself. To a great extent in past years, this has been due to the need to obtain these hormones from animal sources. The intensity of the antibody response is to a great degree a function of interspecies differences in amino acid sequence. Thus the availability of human (recombinant DNA) hormone preparations (insulin, calcitonin) has led to a reduction of immunologic phenomena, although it remains likely that the extraction process itself may continue to cause the development of allergenic (conformational) determinants.

Local reactions to insulin are far more common than systemic reactions (Table 37–35).[93] These generally develop during the first 2 to 3 weeks after initiation of therapy and resolve spontaneously within 3 to 4 weeks, even in the face of ongoing insulin treatment. Many patients experience a hive at the site of injection, and others develop a biphasic

TABLE 37–35
ALLERGIC REACTIONS TO INSULIN

Local
- Clinical: immediate, delayed, dual, or biphasic
- Dermatopathology: late-phase, vasculitic, delayed hypersensitivity

Systemic (1%–2%)
- Urticaria/angioedema
- Serum sickness
- Purpura
- Other

The overall incidence was 5%–10%. Reductions in allergic phenomena, as well as immunologic improvement, have been noted when patients were transferred from conventional to purified or human (recombinant DNA) insulin.

TABLE 37–36
INSULIN ALLERGY AND RESISTANCE

- Positive skin test or insulin-binding IgE antibodies to insulin are common during therapy and may not correlate with insulin allergy[106]
- Systemic reactions usually occur in individuals who have interrupted or intermittent therapy and then resume insulin; many are preceded by local reactions[129]
- Anti-insulin antibodies of all five immunoglobulin classes (G, M, A, E, D) have been found in insulin-treated diabetic patients
- High levels of IgG anti-insulin antibodies are associated with the insulin resistance syndrome (> 200 U/day requirement)[84]
- Concomitance of insulin allergy and insulin resistance may be as high as 25%–35%[84]

or late reaction, with painful swelling developing at 4 to 6 hours and lasting days. It has been suggested that some of the latter reactions may be analogous to IgE-mediated late-phase reactions. However, detailed histopathologic studies have shown that some of these late dermal reactions are vasculitic or have histologic features of tuberculin-type delayed hypersensitivity reactions.[36] Local reactions rarely require treatment; if they cause discomfort, H_1 blockers may be used.

In early studies, some diabetics were found to develop anti-insulin antibodies, often in low titer, within months of starting therapy (Table 37–36).[84] Many of these patients also were found to mount lymphocyte proliferative responses, which were specific for beef or pork insulin, C peptide, or protamine, linked to different histocompatibility loci.[108] Correlation of these measures of immune responsiveness with clinical symptomatology and allergic reactions was inexact. In those rare patients in whom local reactions become worse or are followed by systemic reactions, it may be necessary to define the IgE response by testing with different insulin preparations. This is best accomplished by skin testing, beginning at 10^6 U/ml and increasing by 10-fold serial dilutions until full concentration of U-100 insulin is achieved.[130] RAST assays for species-specific IgE anti-insulin antibodies are also commercially available but are less sensitive and more expensive than skin testing.[68] Beef insulin is more immunogenic by virtue of three amino acid substitutions (two in the A chain, one in the B chain) compared with one (B chain) for pork (Table 37–37). The availability of human (recombinant DNA, Humulin) insulin has reduced the need for testing species differences, although skin reactivity and clinical reactions may still occur.[150]

Although it has been considered that other immunogens may be present in some insulin preparations, it appears that these must be rare causes of clinical allergy (Table 37–38).[150]

TABLE 37–37
AMINO ACID SEQUENCE DIFFERENCES OF INSULINS

Source	A Chain: Residue 8	A Chain: Residue 10	B Chain: Residue 30
Human	Thr	Ile	Thr
Pig	Thr	Ile	Ala
Rabbit	Thr	Ile	Ser
Cow	Ala	Val	Ala

TABLE 37–38
POTENTIAL IMMUNOGENS

Insulin
  Polymer > single component
  Beef > pork > human
  IgE response to Humulin demonstrable in some instances
Proinsulin
  May have cross-reactivity with insulin
Other hormones
Contaminating proteins
Protamine, zinc (antigen or adjuvant effects)

Lymphoproliferative responses to both proinsulin (C peptide) and protamine may be demonstrated in vitro.[108] RAST inhibition studies, however, have shown complete cross-reactivity of IgE antibodies between insulin and proinsulin.[91] IgE-mediated systemic reactions to protamine have been well documented in patients receiving this agent for reversal of anticoagulation with heparin or diabetics administered NPH protamine zinc insulin to prolong absorption.[181] It should also be recalled that this drug is able to degranulate basophils nonimmunologically because of its polycationic properties.[127] It has also been suggested that protamine may have adjuvant properties and that inorganic zinc (protamine zinc and crystalline zinc) may alter insulin antigenicity in some instances and provide a novel cause of allergy.[38, 150]

Systemic reactions to insulin are uncommon and generally occur in clinical settings in which insulin has been interrupted and restarted. Rare syndromes of lymphadenopathy, Coombs-positive hemolytic anemia, vasculitis, and the development of eosinophilia and hypergammaglobulinemia have been described.[93] However, the more usual clinical picture is that of generalized urticaria, angioedema, or frank anaphylaxis. If the reaction is very severe and has occurred within 24 to 48 hours, the patient may in effect be desensitized, as previously described for penicillin. This may be determined by skin testing; in this situation, it has been suggested that the dose be reduced to one third to one fourth and then gradually increased over several days while the patient is observed in the hospital.[111] If more than 48 hours has elapsed, it is likely that reaginic hypersensitivity is again present, and the patient should be retested and desensitized. A representative schedule for rapid desensitization is shown in Table 37–39.[83, 130] Generally, patients are not pretreated with H_1 blockers so that clinical reactions and skin test reactivity can be followed serially through the procedure.

Immunologic insulin resistance is a rare clinical entity characterized by a requirement for very high doses of insulin due to the development of high-titer IgG anti-insulin antibodies.[128] It has been estimated that the incidence of combined insulin allergy and resistance is 25% to 35%. Initial treatment consists of switching insulin preparations, as previously described. If this is unsuccessful, a large number (~75%) of patients will respond to high-dose steroid therapy (60 mg prednisone/day) or, in rare cases, cytotoxic agents either with or without plasmapheresis. Both treatment modalities must be monitored carefully for exacerbation of diabetes, side effects, or consequences of immunosuppression, such as infection by opportunistic organisms. As the majority of patients developing insulin resistance remit within 6 months, however, such treatment is required for only a minority of individuals on a short-term basis.[83] Rapid tapering is usually possible after 2 to 3 weeks, or the patient is switched to alternate-day steroids.

TABLE 37–39
DESENSITIZATION FOR INSULIN ALLERGY

Day	Time*	Insulin Dose (U)†	Route‡
1	7:30 AM	0.00001	Intradermal
	Noon	0.0001	Intradermal
	4:30 PM	0.001	Intradermal
2	7:30 AM	0.01	Intradermal
	Noon	0.1	Intradermal
	4:30 PM	1.0	Subcutaneous
3	7:30 AM	2.0	Subcutaneous
	Noon	4.0	Subcutaneous
	4:30 PM	8.0	Subcutaneous
4	7:30 AM	12.0	Subcutaneous
	Noon	16.0	Subcutaneous
5	7:30 AM	20.0	Subcutaneous
6	7:30 AM	35.0	Subcutaneous

*In ketoacidosis, injections can be given every 10–15 minutes.
†Regular insulin days 1–4; NPH or lente insulin days 5–6.
‡All doses may be given subcutaneously.
Adapted from Patterson R: General principles of prevention of allergic drug reactions. Allergy Proc 15:239–264, 1994.

ANESTHETIC ALLERGY

The great majority of adverse reactions occurring to local anesthetics are not immunologically mediated. These include a variety of toxic effects on the central nervous system (stimulation or depression, vertigo, nausea, convulsions), vasovagal episodes, syncope, and cardiovascular effects (hypotension, cardiac failure, shock). Contact dermatitis is an occupational hazard among health care professionals and is occasionally seen in individuals sensitized by any of a variety of topical medications that contain anesthetics, such as sunburn lotions and lozenges (Table 37–40).[8] Patch testing of such individuals has indicated that there is little cross-reactivity between the para-aminobenzoic acid esters and those lacking the para-aminophenyl group. This has predictive value in the evaluation of contact dermatitis developing after the administration of a topical medicine, such as procaine in

TABLE 37–40
LOCAL ANESTHETICS

Benzoic Acid Esters	Others
Procaine (Novocain)	Lidocaine (Xylocaine)
Tetracaine (Pontocaine)	Mepivacaine (Carbocaine)
Ethylaminobenzoate (benzocaine)	Prilocaine (Citanest)
Chloroprocaine (Nesacaine)	Dibucaine (Nupercainal)
Butethamine (Monocaine)	Pramoxine (Tronothane)
Meprylcaine (Oracaine)	Dyclonine (Dyclone)
Cocaine	(Phenacaine (Holocaine))
Butacaine (Butyn)	Antihistamines
Cyclomethycaine (Surfacaine)	(Bipinocacaine (Manzacaine))
(Myrilacaine (Oracaine))	
Piperocaine (Metycaine)	
(Amydricaine (Alypine))	

eye drops, although some of these individuals may be found on further testing to be sensitive to parabens or other additives commonly found in such medications.[4]

Extrapolation from patch testing to an immediate-type hypersensitivity reaction, such as generalized urticaria, angioedema, bronchospasm, or anaphylaxis, is fraught with hazards. In the face of a severe prior reaction, avoidance, use of an alternative class of medication, such as 1% benadryl infiltrated locally, or even general anesthesia may need to be considered. Some studies have advocated the use of provocative test dosing, in which the patient is challenged with increasing doses of the anesthetic beginning with prick and intradermal testing of 1% solutions of procaine and lidocaine as representative of the two classes of anesthetics. Negative tests are followed at 15- to 20-minute intervals by repeat testing at 10 times the concentration, continuing to full dose, and observing at 24 to 48 hours for the development of late reactions possibly indicative of delayed hypersensitivity.[37, 55, 77]

Allergic reactions may develop during anesthesia after injection of barbiturates, narcotics, ketamine, Althesin, propanidid, or muscle relaxants, such as succinylcholine, D-tubocurarine, or gallamine.[15] In the United States, thiopental and thioamylal are major agents responsible for allergic reactions, causing anaphylactic or anaphylactoid reactions, with an incidence of 1/14,000 to 1/30,000 injections. In Great Britain, Althesin and propanidid have been reported to cause milder allergic reactions in as many as 1/150 to 1/1,000 injections.[7, 116]

Mechanisms implicated in these reactions include IgE antibodies (quaternary or tertiary ammonium ions, protamine, latex) and nonimmunologic release of histamine (see Fig. 37–2). As noted previously, histamine levels have been found to be elevated in blood of individuals experiencing anaphylactoid reactions to succinylcholine (see Fig. 37–1).[117] In vitro studies have shown that some of these drugs can degranulate mast cells and basophils.[11] Cutaneous hypersensitivity, positive passive transfer, and in vitro release of histamine by basophils have been reported for several muscle relaxants, as has the presence of specific IgE antibodies.[15, 69] An increased incidence of reactions has been noted in individuals previously exposed to the drug or who have a history of atopic disease, particularly asthma. Based on these observations, skin testing has been advocated in some series, as well as pretreatment with H_1 or H_2 blockers and possibly steroids. Few controlled studies have been performed to assess the efficacy of such pretreatment.

ASPIRIN SENSITIVITY

Hypersensitivity symptoms following ingestion of aspirin and other NSAIDs are commonly seen, largely as a result of the huge amounts of these medications consumed by the general population. Four types of hypersensitivity reactions have been described: urticaria/angioedema, rhinoconjunctivitis/bronchospasm, anaphylactoid reactions, and hypersensitivity pneumonitis.[169] Interestingly, these syndromes rarely coexist in the same individual. Aspirin/NSAID idiosyncrasy generally has onset in the middle years and affects 1% to 5% of the general population, 10% to 15% of the asthmatic population, up to 23% of patients with urticaria, and 30% to 40% of asthmatics with polyposis/pansinusitis.

Clinical features typical of the upper respiratory syndrome are hyperplastic vasomotor rhinitis with chronic nasal blockade (>90%); rhinorrhea; anosmia; x-ray evidence of sinusitis (>90%); purulent sinus drainage; nasal and/or paranasal polyps (>90%), which often recur after polypectomy; <20% incidence of atopy; bronchial asthma (20% mild; 30% dependent on topical steroids; 50% oral steroid dependent); and eosinophilia (bronchial, nasal, blood >20%).[169] Urticaria may present de novo after taking aspirin or another NSAID or as a worsening of a chronic urticaria. Anaphylactoid reactions are usually specific for a particular NSAID and present as hypotension/shock and syncope/unconsciousness.[169]

In spite of the presence of demonstrable immunogenic contaminants in aspirin preparations, the bulk of evidence is that salicylate hypersensitivity is not mediated by immunologic mechanisms. This conclusion is based on failure to demonstrate clinically significant skin test reactivity or circulating IgE antibodies to aspirin in these patients, as well as cross-reactivity with NSAIDS, most of which are structurally dissimilar to aspirin and share only the property of inhibiting prostaglandin synthesis. The finding of a loose correlation between the degree of airway obstruction, number of patients responding to oral challenge, minimum inducing dose, and IC_{50} (in vitro concentration inhibiting prostaglandin synthetase by 50%) of various NSAIDs in aspirin-sensitive asthmatics challenged with various NSAIDs has provided a basis for this pathogenic mechanism.[174] Against this is the observation of cross-reactivity with high (>1,000 mg) doses of acetaminophen in occasional aspirin-sensitive individuals.[154] It remains unclear whether the net effect is selective depression of some classes of prostaglandins, loss of a normal feedback effect of prostaglandins on mast cells mediated by specific receptors, a concomitant increased elaboration of or shunting to lipoxygenase pathway metabolites with bronchoconstrictive activity, or enhanced airway sensitivity to leukotrienes (Table 37–41).[79]

The most definitive diagnostic modality for suspected aspirin sensitivity is oral challenge, beginning with doses of 15 mg or lower and monitoring the FEV_1 for up to 4 hours after ingestion; urticarial reactions occur at 2 to 6 hours after challenge. Following a negative response, the dose is increased progressively up to a 650-mg tablet dose. For accurate results, the patient should be in remission before

TABLE 37–41
POSSIBLE MECHANISMS IN ASPIRIN IDIOSYNCRASY

Immunologic mechanisms (IgE, IgG)
  Salicyloyl or aspiryl (anhydride) conjugates
  No evidence for complement activation
Direct degranulation of lung mast cells
  Blockade by cromolyn
  Little evidence for increased histamine, NCF, etc.
Abnormal receptors
  PGE inhibition of histamine/SRS-A release
Cyclooxygenase inhibition
  Inhibition of PGE > $PGF_{2\alpha}$ (?tissue specific)—little evidence
Increased levels of lipoxygenase bronchoconstrictors
Enhanced airway sensitivity to leukotrienes—blocked by lipoxygenase receptor inhibitor

challenge testing, and this may require aggressive drug therapy before the procedure is carried out.[110]

Avoidance of aspirin, aspirin-containing compounds, and NSAIDs is of prime importance. Ancillary treatment modalities include adequate treatment of sinus infections and sinusitis with antibiotics and drainage, regular use of decongestants and inhaled steroids as indicated, polypectomy if necessary, and aggressive treatment of asthma, often with systemic and topical corticosteroids. Desensitization regimens have been advocated based on the observation of a refractory period of 2 to 7 days after oral challenge. Cross-desensitization with other nonsteroidals has also been observed.[169] However, this has not been shown to be an immunologic desensitization, as described previously. Moreover, the procedure is tedious and potentially dangerous and is usually not warranted unless there is an absolute need for these drugs.

REACTIONS TO RADIOGRAPHIC CONTRAST MEDIA

A variety of adverse effects may occur following administration of radiographic contrast media (RCM), with an overall incidence of up to 8%. Severe reactions occur with a frequency of about 1/1,000, and fatal reactions occur with an incidence ranging from 1/3,000 for intravenous cholangiography to 1/40,000 to 1/110,000 for intravenous urography.[185] Nonidiosyncratic effects are often mild and include fluid shifts secondary to hyperosmolarity, chemotoxicity, vasodilation, flush and myocardial effects, neurotoxicity (headache, convulsions), or renal effects. Some of the most severe adverse reactions have features of anaphylaxis (1%–2%), including urticaria, bronchospasm, respiratory arrest, or vascular collapse, and were noted a number of years ago to resemble histamine reactions.[109] Predisposing factors include age (increased incidence over age 50), a history of prior RCM reactions (10-fold increase in risk), dehydration, and underlying disease, such as cardiac disease, multiple myeloma, homocystinuria, and pheochromocytoma. An increased incidence of respiratory symptoms has been reported among asthmatics.[185]

RCM are low molecular weight 2,4,6-triiodinated benzoic acid compounds (Fig. 37–8).[61] Older RCM are weak acids and must be administered as a salt with varying percentages of sodium or methylglucamine. Introduction of large amounts of sodium may precipitate pulmonary edema in

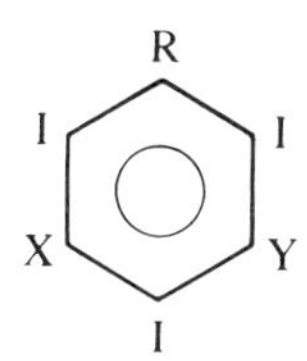

FIGURE 37–8. General structure for 2,4,6-triiodinated substituted benzoic acid compounds. They are weak acids by virtue of a carboxyl group at R and are given as a salt with varying percentages of sodium or methylglucamine. Full substitution (X and Y) is associated with poor albumin binding and primary glomerular filtration. Patients may receive 30 to 50 ml at concentrations greater than 1 molar, in boluses of 35 to 120 g. (From Gorevic PD, Kaplan AP: Contrast agents and anaphylactic-like reactions. J Allergy Clin Immunol 63:225, 1979.)

TABLE 37–42
CONTRAST DYE REACTIONS

Histamine
In vitro triggering
Histamine release in animal models
Similarity of hemodynamic/peripheral signs to histamine effects[109]
Elevated histamine and/or metabolites in blood and urine[47]
Complement
Decreased CH_{50}
Nonsequential activation of complement components
Depression of C1 INH, activation of kallikrein[94]
Hyperosmolar Triggering of Basophils[52]

patients with a history of cardiac disease. Newer RCM have the same iodine concentrations but are nonionic. These agents cause less hypertonicity, as they do not dissociate, and bind calcium to a lesser degree. The incidence of immediate reactions has dropped from 2% to 3% to 0.5% with these agents, but they are not yet sufficiently cost effective for general use.[185]

Because RCM do not form covalent conjugates with protein, they are unlikely to form immunogenic hapten-carrier conjugates. Thus adverse reactions may occur on initial exposure, do not generally change in severity, and are inconsistently seen on repeat exposure. The bulk of evidence is that RCM do not elicit a significant immune response in either humans or experimental animals.[61] Direct and indirect mechanisms have thus been invoked to explain histamine release in anaphylactoid reactions due to RCM. These include direct nonimmunologic triggering of basophils or mast cells (see Fig. 37–2), activation of complement by a variety of mechanisms, such as to generate anaphylatoxins, and hyperosmolar triggering, which has been demonstrated in vitro with human basophils (Table 37–42).[52, 61]

The incidence of second reactions on challenge in patients with a history of a reaction to RCM is 25% to 35%. This increase in incidence over 5% to 8% in the general population has suggested that RCM reactions may be idiosyncratic, perhaps related to congenitally determined host factors. In this sense, such reactors may be similar to the slow acetylator who develops drug lupus or the glucose-6-phosphate dehydrogenase-deficient person who develops a hemolytic anemia on challenge with primaquine. The exact basis for this effect in contrast dye reactors is unknown.

Several studies have established the efficacy of pretreatment in reducing the risk of reactions among high-risk patients who require contrast procedures. Various regimens have been shown to reduce the incidence of reactions in such patients from 25% to 35% to as low as 3%, with the majority of reactions that still occur being mild and not requiring treatment. In all instances, alternative diagnostic modalities should be sought, the absolute need for the contrast dye study determined, the risk explained, and informed consent obtained. Pretreatment regimens include prednisone, benadryl, and ephedrine (Table 37–43).[66]

SUMMARY

Allergic responses to drugs may develop owing to immunologic or nonimmunologic mechanisms. The immune re-

TABLE 37–43
TREATMENT APPROACH TO PATIENTS WITH A HISTORY OF RADIOGRAPHIC CONTRAST MEDIA REACTIONS

Determine need for study and advise patient of risk involved (~30% incidence of repeat reactions)
Premedicate with
Prednisone 50 mg every 6 hours, 13, 7, and 1 hour before
Benadryl 50 mg intramuscularly 1 hour before
Ephedrine 25 mg or albuterol 4 mg 1 hour before (omit with angina, arrhythmia, or cardiac risk)

From Greenberger PA, Patterson R: The prevention of immediate generalized reactions to radiocontract media in high-risk patients. J Allergy Clin Immunol 87:867–872, 1991.

sponse to a drug may be heterogeneous in terms of the haptenic determinants to which it is directed and the cell-mediated responses elicited. Genetic factors determine the intensity of the immune response and cell-cell interactions, as well as the polymorphism of individual enzymes and enzyme systems responsible for metabolizing the drug or indirectly affected by it. The form of consequent immunopathology may vary with the predominant type of immune response that results, as well as the organ or cell types against which it is directed. In those instances in which detailed information and good experimental models for drug allergy exist, reliable methods are available for assessing it, as well as for specific immunologic intervention. With the accumulation of additional information, the ability of the clinician to accurately predict, diagnose, and treat drug allergies will continue to improve.

ACKNOWLEDGMENTS

This chapter is dedicated to my wife, Judy. I thank Allen Kaplan for useful discussions and for sustaining my interest in this important subject.

REFERENCES

1. Adkinson NF Jr, Thompson WL, Maddrey WC: Routine use of penicillin skin testing on an inpatient service. N Engl J Med 285:22, 1971.
2. Adkinson NF Jr: Tests for immunological drug reactions. In Rose NR, de Macario EC, Fahey JL, et al (eds): Manual of Clinical Laboratory Immunology, 4th edition. American Society of Microbiology, Washington, DC, 1992, p 717–722.
3. Adler SG, Cohen AH, Border WA: Hypersensitivity phenomena and the kidney: role of drugs and environmental agents. Am J Kidney Dis 5:75–96, 1985.
4. Andersen KE, Maibach HI: Allergic reactions to drugs used topically. Clin Toxicol 16:415, 1980.
5. Arellano FA, Sacristan JA: Allopurinol hypersensitivity syndrome: a review. Ann Pharmacother 27:337–343, 1993.
6. Assem E-SK, Vickers MR: Tests for penicillin allergy in man. The immunological cross-reaction between penicillins and cephalosporins. Immunology 27:255, 1974.
7. Assem E-SK (ed): Allergic reactions to anesthetics. Monogr Allergy 30:24–53, 1992.
8. Baer RL, Ramsey DL, Biondi E: The most common contact allergens. J Am Acad Dermatol 108:74, 1973.
9. Baldwin DS, Levine BB, McCluskey RT, Gallo GR: Renal failure and interstitial nephritis due to penicillin and methicillin. N Engl J Med 279:1245, 1968.
10. Basomba A, Pelaez A, Villalmanzo IG, Campos A: Allergy to penicillin unsuccessfully treated with a haptenic inhibitor (benzyl-penicilloyl-N_2-formil lysine: BPO-FLYs)—a case report. Clin Allergy 8:341, 1978.
11. Beaven MA: Anaphylactoid reactions to anesthetic drugs. Anesthesiology 55:3, 1981.
12. Bierman CW, Pierson WE, Zeitz ST, et al: Reactions associated with ampicillin therapy. JAMA 220:1098, 1972.
13. Bierman CW, Van Ardsdel PP Jr: Penicillin allergy in children: the role of immunological tests in its diagnosis. J Allergy Clin Immunol 43:267, 1969.
14. Bigby M, Jick S, Jick H, Arndt K: Drug-induced cutaneous reactions. JAMA 256:3358–3363, 1986.
15. Birnbaum J, Porri F, Pradal M, et al: Allergy during anesthesia. Clin Exp Allergy 24:915–921, 1994.
16. Blanca M, Fernandez J, Miranda A, et al: Cross reactivity between penicillins and cephalosporins: clinical and immunological studies. J Allergy Clin Immunol 83:381–385, 1989.
17. Border WA, Lehman DH, Egan JD, et al: Antitubular basement membrane antibodies in methicillin-associated interstitial nephritis. N Engl J Med 291:381, 1974.
18. Borel Y, Kilham L, Loyslop N, Borel H: Isologous IgG-induced tolerance to benzyl penicilloyl. Nature 261:49, 1976.
19. Borish L, Tamir R, Rosenwasser LJ: Intravenous desensitization to beta-lactam antibiotics. J Allergy Clin Immunol 80:314–319, 1987.
20. Bosso JV, Schwartz LB, Stevenson DD: Tryptase and histamine release during aspirin-induced respiratory reactions. J Allergy Clin Immunol 88:830, 1991.
21. Boston Collaborative Drug Surveillance Program: Drug-induced anaphylaxis: a cooperative study. JAMA 224:613, 1973.
22. Brander C, Mauri-Hellweg D, Bettens F, et al: Heterogeneous T-cell responses to β lactam modified self-structures are observed in penicillin-allergic individuals. J Immunol 155:2670–2678, 1995.
23. Brandriss MW, Smith JW, Steinman HG: Common antigenic determinants of penicillin G, cephalothin, and 6-aminopenicillanic acid in rabbits. J Immunol 94:696, 1965.
24. Brown BC, Price EV, Moore MD: Penicilloyl-polylysine as an intradermal test of penicillin sensitivity. JAMA 189:599, 1964.
25. Brown GL, Kanwar BS: Drug rashes in glandular fever. Lancet 2:1418, 1967.
26. Brown LA, Goldberg ND, Shearer WT: Long-term ticarcillin desensitization by the continual administration of penicillin. J Allergy Clin Immunol 69:51, 1982.
27. Cameron SG, Richard J: Ampicillin hypersensitivity in lymphatic leukemia. Scott Med J 16:425, 1971.
28. Caranasos GJ, Stewart BB, Cluff LE: Drug-induced illness leading to hospitalization. JAMA 228:713, 1974.
29. Chiorazzi N, Eschar Z, Katz DH: Induction of immunological tolerance to the major antigenic determinant of penicillin: a therapeutic approach to penicillin allergy. Proc Natl Acad Sci USA 73:2091, 1976.
30. Cluff LE, Johnson JE II: Drug fever. Prog Allergy 8:149, 1964.
31. Cooke RA: Allergy in drug idiosyncrasy. JAMA 73:759, 1919.
31a. Coopman SA, Johnson RA, Platt R, Stern RS: Cutaneous disease and reactions in HIV infection. N Engl J Med 328:1670–1674, 1993.
32. Croyden CAP, Wheeler AW, Grinshaw JJ, et al: Prospective study of ampicillin rash: report from a collaborative study group. Br Med J 1:7, 1973.
33. Dehaan P, Boorsma DM, Kalsbek GI: Penicillin hypersensitivity determination and classification of anti-penicillin antibodies by enzyme-linked immunosorbent assay. Allergy 34:111, 1979.
34. Delage C, Irey NS: Anaphylactic deaths: a clinicopathologic study of 43 cases. J Forensic Sci 17:525, 1972.
35. Dembo M, Goldstein B, Sobotka AK, Lichtenstein LM: Degranulation of human basophils: quantitative analyses of histamine release and desensitization due to a bivalent penicilloyl hapten. J Immunol 123:1864, 1979.
36. De Shazo RD, Boehm TM, Kumar D, et al: Dermal hypersensitivity reactions to insulin: correlations of three patterns to their histopathology. J Allergy Clin Immunol 69:229, 1982.
37. De Shazo RD, Nelson HS: An approach to the patient with a history of local anesthetic hypersensitivity: experience with 90 patients. J Allergy Clin Immunol 63:387, 1979.
38. DeShazo R, Galloway JA: Insulin allergy. Ann Allergy 76:217–218, 1996.
39. De Vriese ASP, Philippe J, Van Renterghem DM, et al: Carbamazepine hypersensitivity syndrome: report of four cases and review of the literature. Medicine (Baltimore) 74:144–151, 1995.
40. Dewdney JM: Immunology of the antibiotics. In Sela M (ed): The Antigens. Vol 4. Academic Press, New York, 1977, pp 73–245.

41. De Weck A, Bundgaard H: Allergic Reactions to Drugs. Springer-Verlag, Berlin, 1983.
42. De Weck AL, Girard JP: Specific inhibition of allergic reactions to penicillin by a monovalent hapten. II. Clinical studies. Int Arch Allergy Immunol 42:798, 1972.
43. De Weck AL, Schneider CH: Specific inhibition of allergic reactions to penicillin in man by a monovalent hapten. 1. Experimental immunologic and toxicologic studies. Int Arch Allergy Immunol 42:782, 1972.
44. De Weck AL, Schneider CH, Gutershon J: The role of penicilloylated protein impurities, penicillin polymers and dimers in penicillin allergy. Int Arch Allergy Appl Immunol 33:535, 1968.
45. Ditlove J, Weidmann P, Bernstein M, Massry SG: Methicillin nephritis. Medicine (Baltimore) 56:483, 1977.
46. Dubost JJ, Souteyrand P, Sauvezie B: Drug-induced vasculitides. Baillieres Clin Rheumatol 5:119–138, 1991.
47. Dyer J, Merlin S, Greenhill A, et al: Urine histamine after intravenous contrast studies. J Allergy Clin Immunol 71:148, 1983.
48. Earl HS, Sullivan TJ: Acute desensitization of a patient with cystic fibrosis allergic to both beta-lactam and aminoglycoside antibiotics. J Allergy Clin Immunol 79:477–481, 1987.
49. Epstein JH: Photoallergy. Arch Dermatol 106:741, 1972.
50. Fellner MJ, Baer RL: Immunologic studies in patients with serum sickness–like reactions following penicillin therapy. J Invest Dermatol 48:384, 1967.
51. Fellner MJ, Hecke EV, Rozan M, Baer RL: Mechanisms of clinical desensitization in urticarial hypersensitivity to penicillin. J Allergy 45:55, 1970.
52. Findlay SR, Dvorak AM, Kagey-Sobotka A, Lichtenstein LM: Hyperosmolar triggering of histamine release from human basophils. J Clin Invest 67:1604, 1981.
53. Finke SR, Grieco MH, Connell JT, et al: Results of comparative skin tests with penicilloyl-polylysine and penicillin in patients with penicillin allergy. Am J Med 38:71, 1965.
54. Gadde J, Spence M, Wheeler B, Adkinson NF Jr: Clinical experience with penicillin skin testing in a large inner-city STD clinic. JAMA 270:2456–2463, 1993.
55. Gall H, Kaufmann R, Kalveram CM: Adverse reactions to local anesthetics: analysis of 197 cases. J Allergy Clin Immunol 97:933–937, 1996.
56. Garratty G: Immune cytopenia associated with antibiotics. Transfus Med Rev 7:255–267, 1993.
57. Geha RS, Fruchter L, Borel Y: Hapten-specific T-cell unresponsiveness induced by benzylpenicilloyl autologous gammaglobulin conjugates in human lymphocytes in vitro. J Clin Invest 65:1950, 1980.
58. Gennis MA, Vemuri R, Burns EA, et al: Familial occurrence of hypersensitivity to phenytoin. Am J Med 91:631–634, 1991.
59. Gillman SA, Korotzer JL, Haddad ZH: Penicillin desensitization: correlation of clinical and immunologic events using an in vitro model. Clin Allergy 2:63, 1972.
60. Girard JP: Common antigenic determinants of penicillin G, ampicillin and the cephalosporins demonstrated in man. Int Arch Allergy Appl Immunol 33:428, 1968.
61. Gorevic PD, Kaplan AP: Contrast agents and anaphylactic-like reactions. J Allergy Clin Immunol 63:225, 1979.
62. Gorevic PD, Levine BB: Desensitization of anaphylactic hypersensitivity specific for the penicilloate minor determinant of penicillin and carbenicillin. J Allergy Clin Immunol 68:267, 1981.
63. Gorevic PD, Levine BB: Penicillin allergy: prediction, prevention, diagnosis, treatment, and desensitization. In Rosse W (ed): Clinical Immunology Update. Elsevier, New York, 1985, pp 117–139.
64. Graybill JR, Sande MA, Reinarz JA, Shapiro JR: Controlled penicillin anaphylaxis leading to desensitization. South Med J 67:62, 1974.
65. Green GR, Rosenblum AH, Sweet LC: Evaluation of penicillin hypersensitivity: value of clinical history and skin testing with penicilloyl-polylysine and penicillin G. J Allergy Clin Immunol 60:339, 1977.
66. Greenberger PA, Patterson R: The prevention of immediate generalized reactions to radiocontrast media in high-risk patients. J Allergy Clin Immunol 87:867–872, 1991.
67. Grieco MH: Cross allergenicity of the penicillins and cephalosporins. Arch Intern Med 119:141, 1967.
68. Hamilton RG, Rendell M, Adkinson NF Jr: Serological analysis of human IgG and IgE anti-insulin antibodies by solid-phase radioimmunoassays. J Lab Clin Med 96:1022, 1980.
69. Harle DG, Baldo BA, Fisher MM: Detection of IgE antibodies to suxamethonium after anaphylactoid reactions during anesthesia. Lancet 1:930, 1984.
70. Harle DG, Baldo BA: Identification of penicillin allergenic determinants that bind IgE antibodies in the sera of subjects with penicillin allergy. Mol Immunol 27:1063–1071, 1990.
71. Herman R, Jick H: Cutaneous reaction rates to penicillin—oral vs. parenteral. Cutis 24:232, 1979.
72. Horowitz L: Atopy as a factor in penicillin reactions. N Engl J Med 292:1243, 1975.
73. Hunt KJ, Valentine MD, Sobotka AK, et al: Controlled trial of immunotherapy in insect hypersensitivity. N Engl J Med 299:157, 1978.
74. Hurwitz N: Predisposing factors in adverse reactions to drugs. Br Med J 1:536, 1969.
75. Hutchin T, Haworth I, Higashi K, et al: A molecular basis for human hypersensitivity to aminoglycoside antibiotics. Nucleic Acids Res 21:4174–4179, 1993.
76. Idsoe O, Guthe T, Willcox RA, DeWeck AL: Nature and extent of penicillin side-reactions with particular reference to fatalities from anaphylactic shock. Bull World Health Organ 38:159, 1968.
77. Incaudo G, Schatz M, Patterson R, et al: Administration of local anesthetics to patients with a history of prior adverse reaction. J Allergy Clin Immunol 61:339, 1978.
78. International Rheumatic Fever Study Group: Allergic reactions to long-term benzathine penicillin prophylaxis for rheumatic fever. Lancet 337:1308–1310, 1991.
79. Israel E, Fischer AR, Rosenberg MA, et al: The pivotal role of 5-lipoxygenase products in the reaction of aspirin-sensitive asthmatics to aspirin. Am Rev Respir Dis 148:1447–1451, 1993.
80. Israel-Biet D, Labrune S, Huchon GJ: Drug-induced lung disease: 1990 review. Eur Respir J 4:465–478, 1991.
81. Jensen T, Pedersen S, Hoiby N, Koch C: Safety of aztreonam in patients with cystic fibrosis and allergy to beta-lactam antibiotics. Rev Infect Dis 13(suppl)7:S594–597, 1991.
82. Jung A, Paauw D: Management of adverse reactions to trimethoprim-sulfamethoxazole in human immunodeficiency virus–infected patients. Arch Intern Med 154:2402–2406, 1994.
83. Kahn CR: Insulin allergy and resistance. In Fauci AS, Lichtenstein LM (eds): Current Therapy in Allergy, Immunology and Rheumatology. CB Decker, Philadelphia, 1983, pp 315–318.
84. Kahn CR, Rosenthal AS: Immunologic reactions to insulin: insulin allergy, insulin resistance, and the autoimmune insulin syndrome. Diabetes Care 2:283, 1979.
85. Kahn MF (ed): Drug-induced rheumatic diseases. Baillieres Clin Rheumatol 5:1–191, 1991.
86. Kaliner M, Shelhamer J, Otteson EA: Effects of infused histamine: correlation of plasma histamine levels and symptoms. J Allergy Clin Immunol 69:283, 1982.
87. Kalish RS, LaPorte A, Wood JA, et al: Sulfonamide-reactive lymphocytes detected at very low frequency in the peripheral blood of patients with drug-induced eruptions. J Allergy Clin Immunol 94:465–472, 1994.
88. Kaplan AP: Drug-induced skin diseases. J Allergy Clin Immunol 74:573, 1984.
89. Klein KE, Parkin JD, Madaras F: Studies on an acquired inhibitor of factor VIII induced by penicillin allergy. Clin Exp Immunol 26:155, 1976.
90. Koopmans PP, van der Ven AJAM, Vree TB, van derMeer JWM: Pathogenesis of hypersensitivity reactions to drugs in patients with HIV infection: allergic or toxic? AIDS 9:217–222, 1995.
91. Kumar D, Rosenquist RJ, Parameswaran V: Insulin allergy: reaginic antibodies to insulin and proinsulin. J Clin Endocrinol Metab 49:252, 1979.
92. Lafaye P, Lapresle C: Fixation of penicilloyl groups to albumin and appearance of anti-penicilloyl antibodies in penicillin-treated patients. J Clin Invest 82:7–12, 1988.
93. Lamkin N, Lieberman P, Hashimoto K, et al: Allergic reactions to insulin. J Allergy Clin Immunol 58:213, 1976.
94. Lasser EC, Lang JH, Lyon SG, Hamblin AE: Complement and contrast material reactors. J Allergy Clin Immunol 64:105, 1979.
95. Leape LL, Brennan TA, Laird N, et al: The nature of adverse events in hospitalized patients: results of the Harvard Medical Practice Study II. N Engl J Med 324:377–384, 1991.
96. Lee WY, Sehon AH: Suppression of reaginic antibody formation. IV. Suppression of reaginic antibodies to penicillin in the mouse. J Immunol 117:927, 1976.

97. Levin ML: Patterns of tubulo-interstitial damage associated with nonsteroidal anti-inflammatory drugs. Semin Nephrol 8:55–61, 1988.
98. Levine BB: N(α-D-penicilloyl) amines as univalent hapten inhibitors of antibody-dependent allergic reactions to penicillin. J Med Pharm Chem 5:1025, 1962.
99. Levine BB: Skin rashes with penicillin therapy: current management. N Engl J Med 286:42, 1972.
100. Levine BB, Fellner MJ: The nature of immune complexes initiating allergic wheal-and-flare reactions. J Allergy 36:342, 1965.
101. Levine BB, Redmond AP: Immune mechanisms of penicillin-induced immunohemolytic anemia. Int Arch Allergy Immunol 21:594, 1967.
102. Levine BB, Redmond AP: Minor haptenic determinant-specific reagins of penicillin hypersensitivity in man. Int Arch Allergy Appl Immunol 35:445, 1969.
103. Levine BB, Redmond AP, Fellner MJ, et al: Penicillin allergy and the heterogeneous immune responses of man to benzylpenicillin. J Clin Invest 45:1895, 1966.
104. Levine BB, Zolov DM: Prediction of penicillin allergy by immunological tests. J Allergy 43:231, 1969.
105. Levy M, Lipshitz M, Eliakim M: Hospital admissions due to adverse drug reactions. Am J Med Sci 277:49, 1979.
106. Lieberman P, Patterson R, Metz R, Lucena G: Allergic reactions to insulin. JAMA 215:1106, 1971.
107. Lund BMA, Bergan T: Temporary skin reactions to penicillins during acute stage of infectious mononucleosis. Scand J Infect Dis 7:21, 1975.
108. Mann DL, Mendell N, Kahn CB, et al: In vitro lymphocyte proliferation response to therapeutic insulin components: evidence for genetic control by the human major histocompatibility complex. J Clin Invest 72:1130, 1983.
109. Mann ME: The pharmacology of contrast media. Proc R Soc Med 54:473, 1961.
109a. Martin JA, Igea JM, Frai J, et al: Allergy to amoxicillin in patients who tolerated benzylpenicillin, aztreonam and ceftidime. Clin Infect Dis 14:592, 1992.
110. Mathison DA, Stevenson DD: Hypersensitivity to nonsteroidal anti-inflammatory drugs: indications and methods for oral challenge. J Allergy Clin Immunol 64:669, 1979.
111. Mattson R, Patterson R, Roberts M: Insulin therapy in patients with systemic insulin allergy. Arch Intern Med 135:818, 1975.
112. Mauri-Hellweg D, Bettens F, Mauri D, et al: Activation of drug-specific CD4+ and CD8+ T cells in individuals allergic to sulfonamides, phenytoin and carbamazepine. J Immunol 155:462–472, 1995.
113. McFarland JG: Laboratory investigation of drug-induced immune thrombocytopenias. Transfus Med Rev 7:275–287, 1993.
114. McKenzie H, Parrats D, White RG: IgM and IgG antibody levels to ampicillin in patients with infectious mononucleosis. Clin Exp Immunol 26:214, 1976.
115. Meekins CV, Sullivan TJ, Gruchalla RS: Immunochemical analysis of sulfonamide drug allergy: identification of sulfamethoxazole-substituted human serum proteins. J Allergy Clin Immunol 94:1017–1024, 1994.
116. Moscicki RA, Sockin SM, Corsello BF, et al: Anaphylaxis during induction of general anesthesia: subsequent evaluation and management. J Allergy Clin Immunol 86:325–332, 1990.
117. Moss J, Fahmy NR, Sunder N, Beaven MA: Hormonal and hemodynamic profile of an anaphylactic reaction in man. Circulation 63:210, 1981.
118. Moss RB: Sensitization to aztreonam and cross-reactivity with other beta-lactam antibiotics in high-risk patients with cystic fibrosis. J Allergy Clin Immunol 87:78–88, 1991.
119. Muller V, Morell A, Hoigne R: IgE in allergic drug reactions. Int Arch Allergy Appl Immunol 44:667, 1973.
120. Mullick FG, McAllister HA Jr, Wagner BM, Fenoglio JJ Jr: Drug-related vasculitis. Hum Pathol 10:313, 1979.
121. Murphy MF, Riordan T, Minchinton RM, et al: Demonstration of immune-mediated mechanisms of penicillin-induced neutropenia and thrombocytopenia. Br J Haematol 55:155, 1983.
122. Naclerio R, Mizrahi EA, Adkinson NF Jr: Immunologic observations during desensitization and maintenance of clinical tolerance to penicillin. J Allergy Clin Immunol 71:294, 1983.
123. Orfan N, Patterson R, Dykewicz MS: Severe angioedema related to ACE inhibitors in patients with a history of idiopathic angioedema. JAMA 264:1287–1289, 1990.
124. Parker AC, Richmond J: Reduction in the incidence of rash using polymer-free ampicillin. Br Med J 1:998, 1976.
125. Parker TJ, Parrinello JT, Condemi JJ, et al: Penicillin resensitization among hospitalized patients. J Allergy Clin Immunol 88:213–217, 1991.
126. Parker CW: Hapten immunology and allergic reactions in humans. Arthritis Rheum 24:1024, 1981.
127. Paton W: Histamine release by compounds of simple chemical structure. Pharmacol Rev 9:269, 1957.
128. Patterson R, Mellies CJ, Roberts M: Immunologic reactions against insulin. II. IgE anti-insulin, insulin allergy and combined IgE and IgG immunologic insulin resistance. J Immunol 110:1135, 1973.
129. Patterson R, Roberts M, Grammer LC: Insulin allergy: reevaluation after two decades. Ann Allergy 64:459–462, 1990.
130. Patterson R: General principles of prevention of allergic drug reactions. Allergy Proc 15:239–264, 1994.
131. Petrozzi JW, Shore RN: Generalized exfoliative dermatitis from ethylenediamine. Arch Dermatol 112:525, 1976.
132. Petz LD: Immunologic cross-reactivity between penicillins and cephalosporins: a review. J Infect Dis 137:574, 1978.
133. Petz LD: Drug-induced autoimmune hemolytic anemia. Transfus Med Rev 7:242–254, 1993.
134. Pienkowski MM, Kazmier WJ, Adkinson NF Jr: Basophil histamine release remains unaffected by clinical desensitization to penicillin. J Allergy Clin Immunol 82:171–178, 1988.
135. Platt R, Dreis M, Kennedy D, et al: Serum sickness–like reactions to amoxicillin, cefaclor, cefalexin and trimethoprim-sulfamethoxazole. J Infect Dis 158:474, 1988.
136. Pleasants RA, Walker TR, Samuelson WM: Allergic reactions to parenteral beta-lactam antibiotics in patients with cystic fibrosis. Chest 106:1124–1128, 1994.
137. Pohl LR, Satoh H, Christ DD, Kenna JG: The immunologic and metabolic basis of drug hypersensitivities. Annu Rev Pharmacol 28:367–387, 1988.
138. Pullen H, Wright N, Murdoch J: Hypersensitivity reactions to antibacterial drugs in infectious mononucleosis. Lancet 2:1176, 1967.
139. Redmond AP, Levine BB: Delayed skin reaction to benzylpenicillin in man. Int Arch Allergy Appl Immunol 33:193, 1968.
140. Redmond AP, Levine BB: The relationship between direct immediate skin tests and passive transfer tests in man. J Allergy 39:51, 1967.
141. Reisman RE, Rose NR, Witebsky E, Arbesman CE: Penicillin allergy and desensitization. J Allergy 33:178, 1962.
142. Rich AR: The role of hypersensitivity in periarteritis nodosa as indicated by seven cases developing during serum sickness and sulfonamide therapy. Bull Johns Hopkins Hosp 71:123, 1942.
143. Rieder MJ, Uetrech NH, Shear M, et al: Diagnosis of sulfonamide hypersensitivity reactions by in-vitro "rechallenge" with hydroxylamine metabolites. Ann Intern Med 110:286, 1989.
144. Riley RJ, Leeder JS: In vitro analysis of metabolic predisposition to drug hypersensitivity reactions. Clin Exp Immunol 99:1–6, 1995.
145. Roujeau J-C, Stern R: Severe cutaneous adverse reactions to drugs. N Engl J Med 331:1272–1285, 1994.
146. Roujeau J-C, Kelly JP, Naldi L, et al: Medication use and the risk of Stevens-Johnson syndrome or toxic epidermal necrolysis. N Engl J Med 333:1600–1607, 1995.
147. Rudolph AH, Price EV: Penicillin reactions among patients in venereal disease clinics: a national survey. JAMA 223:499, 1973.
148. Samter M: Intolerance to aspirin. Hosp Pract (Off Ed) Dec:85, 1973.
149. Saxon A, Beall GN, Rohr AS: Immediate hypersensitivity reactions to beta-lactam antibiotics. Ann Intern Med 107:204–215, 1987.
150. Scherthaner G: Immunogenicity and allergenic potential of animal and human insulins. Diabetes Care 16 (suppl 3):155–165, 1993.
151. Scholand JF, Tennenbaum IL, Cerilli GJ: Anaphylaxis to cephalothin in a patient allergic to penicillin. JAMA 206:130, 1968.
152. Schrier RW, Bulger RJ, Van Ardsdel PP: Nephropathy associated with penicillin and homologs. Ann Intern Med 64:116, 1966.
153. Schwartz LB, Yunginger JW, Miller J, et al: Time course of appearance and disappearance of human mast cell tryptase in the circulation after anaphylaxis. J Clin Invest 83:1551–1555, 1989.
154. Settipane RA, Schrank PJ, Simon RA, et al: Prevalence of cross-sensitivity with acetaminophen in aspirin-sensitive asthmatic patients. J Allergy Clin Immunol 96:480–485, 1995.
155. Shapiro LE, Knowles SR, Shear NH: Sulfonamide allergies—management in the '90s. Allergy Clin Immunol Int 8:5–12, 1996.
156. Shapiro S, Siskin DV, Sloane D, et al: Drug rash with ampicillin and other penicillins. Lancet 2:969, 1969.
157. Shear NH, Spielberg SP, Grant DM, et al: Differences in metabolism

of sulfonamides predisposing to idiosyncratic toxicity. Ann Intern Med 105:179–184, 1986.

158. Shimines E, Tayler JS, Petz LD, et al: Immunologic reactions in penicillin factory workers. Ann Allergy 36:313, 1976.
159. Shulman NR, Reid DM: Mechanisms of drug-induced immunologically mediated cytopenias. Transfus Med Rev 7:215–229, 1993.
160. Siegel BB: Hidden contacts with penicillin. Bull World Health Org 21:703, 1959.
161. Siegel BB, Levine BB: Antigenic specificities of SSA in sera from patients with immediate systemic reactions to penicillin. J Allergy 35:488, 1964.
162. Silviu-Dan F, McPhillips S, Warrington RJ: The frequency of skin test reactions to side-chain penicillin determinants. J Allergy Clin Immunol 91:694, 1993.
163. Smith GCM, Kenna JG, Harrison DJ, et al: Autoantibodies to hepatic microsomal carboxyesterase in halothane hepatitis. Lancet 342:963–964, 1993.
164. Smith JW, Johnson JE, Cluff LE: Studies on the epidemiology of adverse drug reactions. II. An evaluation of penicillin allergy. N Engl J Med 274:998, 1966.
165. Smith PL, Kagey-Sobotka A, Bleecker ER, et al: Physiologic manifestations of human anaphylaxis. J Clin Invest 66:1072, 1980.
166. Sogn DD, Evan R, Shepherd GM, et al: Results of the National Institutes of Allergy and Infectious Diseases Collaborative Clinical Trial to test the predictive value of skin testing with major and minor penicillin derivatives in hospitalized adults. Arch Int Med 152:1025–1032, 1992.
166a. Solley GO, Gleich GJ, van Dellen RG: Penicillin allergy: clinical experience with a battery of skin test reagents. J Allergy Clin Immunol 69:238, 1982.
167. Spengler H, De Weck AL: Evaluation of genetic control of the immune response. Monogr Allergy 11:116, 1977.
168. Stark BJ, Earl HS, Gross GN, et al: Acute and chronic desensitization of penicillin-allergic patients using oral penicillin. J Allergy Clin Immunol 79:523–532, 1987.
169. Stevenson DD, Simon RA: Sensitivity to aspirin and nonsteroidal antiinflammatory drugs. In Middleton E Jr, Reed CE, Ellis EF, et al (eds): Allergy: Principles and Practice, 4th edition. Vol II. C.V. Mosby, St. Louis, 1993, pp 1747–1765.
170. Stewart GT, McGovern JP: Penicillin Allergy: Clinical and Immunologic Aspects. Charles C Thomas, Springfield, Ill, 1970.
171. Stroncek DF: Drug-induced immune neutropenia. Transfus Med Rev 7:268–274, 1993.
172. Sullivan TJ: Antigen-specific desensitization of patients allergic to penicillin. J Allergy Clin Immunol 69:500, 1982.
173. Sullivan TJ, Wedner HJ, Shatz GS, et al: Skin testing to detect penicillin allergy. J Allergy Clin Immunol 68:171, 1981.
174. Szczeklik A: Analgesics, allergy and asthma. Drugs 32 (suppl 4):148–163, 1986.
175. Thoburn R, Johnson JE, Cluff LE: Studies of the epidemiology of adverse drug reactions. IV. The relationship of cephalothin and penicillin allergy. JAMA 198:111, 1966.
176. Van Ardsdel P (ed): Drug allergy. Immunol Allergy Clin North Am 11:461–700, 1991.
177. Voss HE, Redmond AP, Levine BB: Clinical detection of the potential reactor to penicillin by immunologic tests. JAMA 196:679, 1966.
178. Warrington RJ, Sander PJ, Rutherford WI: Studies of migration inhibition tests in penicillin hypersensitivity. Clin Exp Immunol 38:148, 1979.
179. Warrington RJ, Simons FER, Ho HW, et al: Diagnosis of penicillin allergy by skin testing: the Manitoba experience. Can Med Assoc J 118:787, 1978.
180. Webster AW, Thompson RA: The ampicillin rash: lymphocyte transformation by ampicillin polymer. Clin Exp Immunol 18:513, 1974.
181. Weiss ME, Nyhan D, Peng Z, et al: Association of protamine IgE and IgG antibodies with life-threatening reactions to intravenous protamine. N Engl J Med 320:886–892, 1989.
182. Weiss RB: Hypersensitivity reactions. Semin Oncol 19:458–477, 1992.
183. Wilson NW: Antibiotic allergy in children. Adv Pediatr Infect Dis 10:307–335, 1995.
184. Witters LA, Ohman JL, Weir GC, et al: Insulin antibodies in the pathogenesis of insulin allergy and resistance. Am J Med 63:703, 1977.
185. Wolf GL, Mishkin MM, Roux SG, et al: Comparison of rates of adverse drug reactions: ionic contrast agents, ionic agents combined with steroids, and nonionic agents. Invest Radiol 26:404–410, 1991.
186. Young RL, Johnson KJ, Richardson BC: New concepts in the pathogenesis of drug-induced lupus. Lab Invest 73:746–759, 1995.

38 *Erythema Multiforme and Stevens-Johnson Syndrome*

NICHOLAS A. SOTER

Erythema multiforme and Stevens-Johnson syndrome are episodic, self-limited inflammatory disorders of the skin and mucous membranes, which are characterized by a variety of morphologic cutaneous lesions. The clinical manifestations vary in degree from mild to severe, and various diagnostic appellations have been applied to the different degrees of severity. Traditionally, the mild form has been termed erythema multiforme minor and the severe form erythema multiforme major or Stevens-Johnson syndrome.[142, 152]

A recent classification of severe erythema multiforme recognizes five categories: erythema multiforme with involvement of less than 10% body surface area and localized target lesions; Stevens-Johnson syndrome with involvement of less than 10% body surface area and widespread target or atypical target lesions; overlap Stevens-Johnson syndrome–toxic epidermal necrolysis with involvement of 10% to 30% body surface area and widespread cutaneous lesions; toxic epidermal necrolysis with involvement of greater than 30% body surface area and discrete lesions; and toxic epidermal necrolysis with involvement of greater than 10% body surface area and large epidermal sheets without discrete lesions.[8] Stevens-Johnson syndrome, Stevens-Johnson syndrome–toxic epidermal necrolysis overlap syndrome, and toxic epidermal necrolysis are probably variants of a single disorder with evolution from one category to another. They are mainly caused by drugs.[5] Erythema multiforme minor primarily is caused by herpes simplex virus, sometimes by other infectious agents, and rarely by drugs.[5]

In this chapter, the terms erythema multiforme minor, erythema multiforme major (Stevens-Johnson syndrome), and toxic epidermal necrolysis will be used.

EPIDEMIOLOGY

The prevalence of erythema multiforme minor among patients attending dermatologic clinics is approximately 1%.[57, 67] Erythema multiforme minor occurs with equal frequency in both sexes, achieves peak prevalence in the second and third decades, and occurs less frequently in infancy and old age.[3] Erythema multiforme minor accounts for most of the cases of erythema multiforme.

There is no geographic or racial predilection. A majority of cases occur during the first half of the year.[89] Reported epidemics of erythema multiforme may be related to associated infectious diseases or the introduction of new chemicals into the environment.

Erythema multiforme major (Stevens-Johnson syndrome) is more common in men.[3, 31] After exposure to drugs, the reaction rates vary from 1 per 10,000 to 1 per 100,000 exposed individuals.[27] Erythema multiforme major has an incidence rate ranging from 2.6 to 7.1 cases per one million population per year.[144]

PATHOGENESIS

Erythema multiforme minor and major are reactions of the skin and mucous membranes to a variety of agents, usually infections and drugs. Although many factors have been implicated as causes, the evidence is convincing for relatively few.

A genetic predisposition to the development of erythema multiforme minor is suggested by an association with HLA class I antigens Aw33 and B15 and HLA class II antigens DRw53, DQw3, and the DQB1 allele DQB1*0301 that encodes for the DQ β chain of HLA-DQw7.[37, 70, 76, 81] Recurrent postherpetic erythema multiforme has been associated with HLA-DQw3.[70] Erythema multiforme major has been associated with HLA-Bw44, a subgroup of HLA-B12.[100] An increased expression of HLA-B12 was noted in toxic epidermal necrolysis.[119]

A relation to infection is supported by reports of epidemics occurring after infections with *Streptococcus*, adenovirus, and histoplasmosis,[83, 130, 145, 149] as well as by sporadic cases occurring in patients with tuberculosis.[154] Elevated titers of specific antibodies to herpes simplex virus,[45, 105] influenza type A,[156] psittacosis,[40] *Mycoplasma pneumoniae*,[22, 71, 88, 125, 135] and histoplasmosis[83] have been detected.

The association between erythema multiforme and primary atypical pneumonia was first noted in 1945 in a report of 17 cases of a new entity termed the mucosal respiratory syndrome.[139] Subsequently, *M. pneumoniae* has been associated with erythema multiforme minor and major.[82, 97, 137] Elevated titers of complement-fixing antibodies to *M. pneumoniae* were detected, and *M. pneumoniae* was isolated from blister fluids. However, *M. pneumoniae* infection cannot be detected in most patients whether or not pulmonary involvement is present.[50]

Recurrent erythema multiforme minor occurs after flares of herpes simplex virus, which has become the most common etiologic agent in children and adults.[18, 47, 65, 79, 158] The lag period between the onset of herpes virus infection and the appearance of erythema multiforme minor is a mean of 11 days.[79] Not all recurrences of herpes simplex virus infection are followed by an episode of erythema multiforme, and not all episodes of erythema multiforme minor are preceded by a clinically apparent herpes simplex virus infection.[62, 65]

Herpes simplex virus has been cultured from cutaneous lesions.[92] Herpes simplex virus antigens have been detected in keratinocytes and endothelial cells in lesional sites.[94, 104] The herpes glycoprotein antigen gB from the viral envelope has been demonstrated by direct immunofluorescence techniques in the epidermis of lesional but not uninvolved skin of herpes-associated erythema multiforme.[65, 104] Herpes simplex virus DNA has been detected in lesional epidermis of herpes-associated erythema multiforme and recurrent erythema multiforme minor of unknown cause by the polymerase chain reaction and by in situ hybridization.[17, 34, 99, 158] The demonstration of herpes simplex virus DNA in biopsy specimens from patients without preceding herpes simplex virus lesions supports a role for herpes simplex virus infection in the etiology of idiopathic erythema multiforme minor. Herpes simplex virus was also detected by immunoperoxidase techniques in the oral lesions of erythema multiforme.[93]

The intradermal injection of a formaldehyde-inactivated herpes simplex virus preparation in a patient with recurrent episodes of erythema multiforme occurring after herpes simplex virus infection produced a cutaneous reaction that was clinically and histologically interpreted as erythema multiforme.[132]

A role for immune complexes has been suggested by hypocomplementemia with decreased levels of C1q, C4, C2, and C3, as well as by C1q binding substances in sera and blister fluids.[66, 124] Circulating immune complexes containing herpes simplex virus antigen have been detected in sera and blister fluids of some patients.[68, 72, 147, 165] Cryoglobulins were present in the sera of some patients.[66] Circulating antibodies to epidermal or basement-membrane zone antigens have not been detected by indirect immunofluorescence techniques.[108] IgM and C3 were detected in the superficial dermal microvasculature and along the basement-membrane zone in early lesions.[61, 73, 152] Since similar tissue alterations have been noted after injury induced by trauma, the specificity and relevance of the deposition of these immunoreactants are unclear.[98]

Circulating antibodies that bind in vivo to lesional skin and mucosa along the cytoplasmic membranes of keratinocytes and are directed against the desmosomal plaque proteins desmoplakin I and II have been detected in patients with erythema multiforme major. No discriminating clinical features exist in patients with and without the antibodies.

Only patients with these antibodies show histologic suprabasal acantholysis in skin biopsy specimens. Since these antibodies bind to the portions of the desmosomal plaque where keratin filaments assemble, these antibodies may interfere with the assembly of keratin filaments and lead to alterations of cell-cell adhesion and acantholysis.[43, 44]

Histologic studies of the evolution of clinical lesions of erythema multiforme minor have shown a resemblance to the alterations in allergic contact dermatitis.[94, 152] The sequential appearance of immune reactants, lymphocytes, and basophils; the microvascular abnormalities; and the interstitial deposition of fibrin suggest roles for immune complex–mediated tissue injury and cell-mediated immunologic reactions in erythema multiforme. The cells of the dermal inflammatory infiltrate and keratinocytes display HLA-DR, which is an alteration observed in cell-mediated immune responses.[167]

The detection of herpes simplex virus DNA in the keratinocytes and the immunopathologic findings reminiscent of the changes in allergic contact dermatitis suggest that erythema multiforme minor may result from a cell-mediated immunologic response directed against herpes simplex virus antigens in keratinocytes, with the lymphocyte as the predominant effector cell.[94]

The administration of drugs has been implicated as a cause of erythema multiforme major, Stevens-Johnson syndrome–toxic epidermal necrolysis overlap syndrome, and toxic epidermal necrolysis.[120] In a retrospective review of 426 patients with Stevens-Johnson syndrome, the eruption was ascribed to drugs in 58%, to infections in 15%, and to unknown causes in the remainder. In approximately one half of 138 cases, drugs were used to treat initial symptoms that may have represented the prodrome of Stevens-Johnson syndrome. In a small percentage of cases, no apparent exogenous factors were present. In over 50% of patients, two or more drugs had been used.

Although the evidence associating drugs with erythema multiforme major is often circumstantial, recurrences after challenge with the suspected drug have been documented with phenolphthalein, nitrogen mustard, and certain sulfonamides.[6, 10, 16, 143] Sulfonamides, nonsteroidal anti-inflammatory agents, penicillins, cephalosporins, hydantoin derivatives, phenobarbital, and allopurinol are prominent causes.[10, 23, 27, 53, 118, 120, 146]

In toxic epidermal necrolysis, the most frequently implicated drugs were sulfonamides, anticonvulsants, and nonsteroidal anti-inflammatory agents, notably phenylbutazone and oxicam derivatives.[55] Toxic epidermal necrolysis develops frequently in patients with human immunodeficiency virus infection, owing perhaps to the large number of drugs being administered.[30]

Erythema multiforme has also been reported to occur after topical exposure to medicaments and other chemicals. It has developed after the topical application of sulfacetamide,[48, 51] in burn patients treated with mafenide acetate cream,[166] and in organic chemistry students who prepared 9-bromofluorene.[25, 35] It has appeared after x-ray therapy for internal malignant disorders and after immunizations.[26, 78, 101]

Although precipitating etiologic factors can at times be identified in erythema multiforme major, its pathogenesis remains speculative. An immune hypothesis suggests that a cell-mediated immune reaction that leads to the tissue damage is directed against foreign antigens, which are derived from drugs or infectious agents and located at mucocutaneous sites.

An alternative hypothesis proposed to explain drug-associated erythema multiforme major and toxic epidermal necrolysis is based on a toxic effect on the epidermis.[131, 138, 162] Keratinocytes may have a role in the detoxification of certain chemicals and drugs that may cause cell damage if not detoxified. Some individuals with a genetically determined inability to detoxify drug metabolites may be predisposed to develop drug-induced toxic epidermal necrolysis. Support for such a hypothesis for the pathogenesis of the epithelial damage has been demonstrated with anticonvulsants and sulfonamides.[131, 138]

Drug-induced and idiopathic forms of toxic epidermal necrolysis are assumed to be immunologically mediated disorders. Supporting evidence includes an association with graft-versus-host disease, the development of sicca syndromes, the deposition of immunoreactants in the skin, the demonstration of drug-dependent antiepidermal antibodies, and altered lymphocyte subsets in the peripheral blood and dermal inflammatory cell infiltrate.[59, 96, 107, 121, 122, 140]

The pathophysiology of the staphylococcal scalded skin syndrome, a form of toxic epidermal necrolysis, has been examined in 3-day-old mice after the administration of the toxin, which alters the intercellular substance between epidermal cells with the distention of the intercellular spaces followed by alterations of desmosomes.[95] The skin lesions in patients and the mouse model are similar histologically.[84] The toxin does not require an intact complement system or immunocompetent thymocytes in mice.[161]

CLINICAL DESCRIPTION

ERYTHEMA MULTIFORME MINOR

The clinical pattern is the sudden onset of a symmetric erythematous eruption with a predilection for the dorsal aspects of the hands and feet and the extensor surfaces of the forearms and legs. The diagnostic cutaneous sign is known as the target or iris lesion (Fig. 38–1). It appears as a central, dusky, erythematous area surrounded by a pale edematous ring with a peripheral erythematous margin. A bulla that may become hemorrhagic may develop. The lesions are not extended if the skin is subjected to a shearing force (negative Nikolsky's sign). Other skin lesions include erythematous macules and papules, wheals, and bullae (Fig. 38–2). Erosions of the oral mucous membranes involve the labial and buccal mucosae (Fig. 38–3).[42]

The eruption is often symptomless, but occasionally a burning sensation or pruritus is present. The eruption appears in crops, persists for 1 to 2 weeks, and recedes in 4 to 6 weeks. Erythema multiforme minor is a self-limited condition and never evolves to widespread cutaneous involvement. Most of the cutaneous damage occurs in the first 4 to 6 days; the healing phase is slow. The eruption may occur at sites of physical trauma or sunburn.[41, 63, 64] Hyperpigmentation may be a sequela. Recurrences may occur in one third of individuals.[74, 153] A persistent form of erythema multiforme that occurs continually over weeks to months has been described.[36, 79]

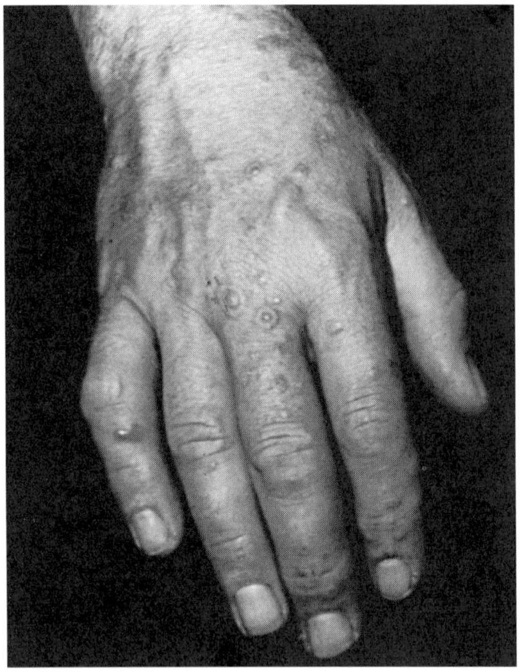

FIGURE 38–1. Erythema multiforme minor. Target (iris) lesions over the dorsum of the hand.

ERYTHEMA MULTIFORME MAJOR

Erythema multiforme major is a term that has been defined in the literature in different ways. It has been used as a synonym for Stevens-Johnson syndrome or as a term to embrace a spectrum of conditions that includes Stevens-Johnson syndrome, bullous erythema multiforme, and overlap with toxic epidermal necrolysis.[8]

Erythema multiforme major often begins with prodromal symptoms that include fever, malaise, cough, sore throat,

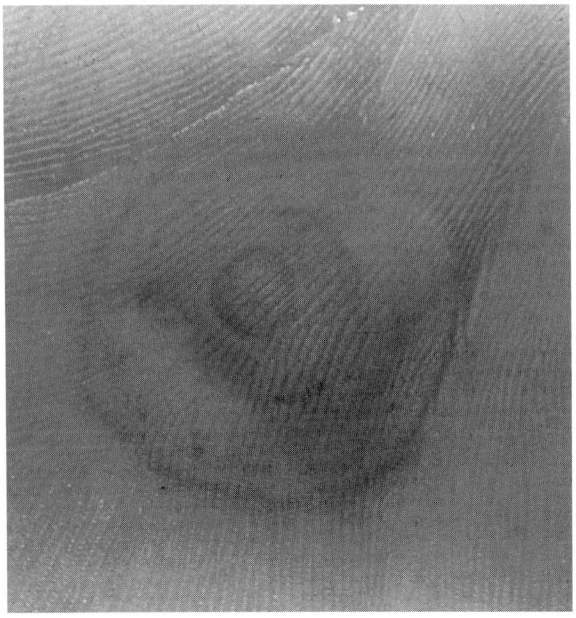

FIGURE 38–2. Erythema multiforme minor. Bullous target (iris) lesion over the palm.

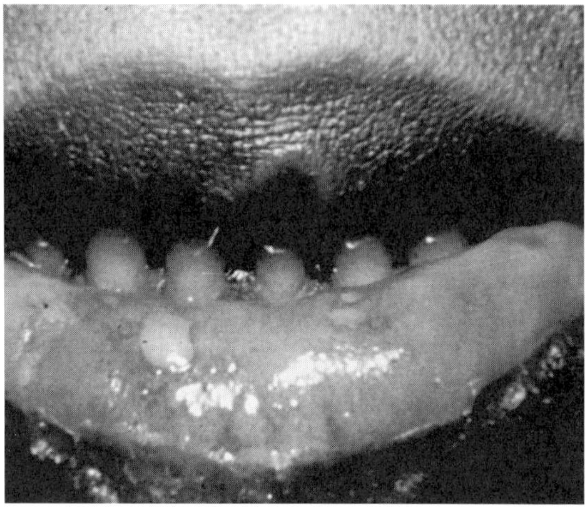

FIGURE 38–3. Erythema multiforme minor. Erosions of the labial mucosa. Note target (iris) lesion of the upper lip.

vomiting, myalgias, and arthralgias. Target lesions and atypical target lesions that are described as having two zones of color and a poorly defined border may be present.

Mucosal lesions involving at least two mucosal surfaces are present in 20% to 45% of patients with erythema multiforme major. The oropharyngeal mucosae, lips, and conjunctivae are frequently affected.[3, 10, 28, 69, 75, 85, 163] Erosions of the oral cavity are common (Fig. 38–4). The lips may develop hemorrhagic crusts.

The evolution of oral lesions has been studied over a 15-day period.[163] A small erythematous macule, 1 to 3 mm in size, lasts a few hours and develops into a clear or hemorrhagic bulla. Within 2 days, the epithelium overlying the bulla is sloughed, and a painful erosion covered by a gray or white membrane develops, which upon removal exposes a hemorrhagic base.

In severe cases of erythema multiforme major, the eyes, external nares, pharynx, larynx, trachea, bronchi, and esophagus may be affected.[15, 141] Although ocular involvement is usually mild, it may be extensive, with swollen lids, chemosis, photophobia, subconjunctival hemorrhages, adhesions between the tarsal and bulbar conjunctivae, vesicles on the cornea, and iritis with ciliary injection.[7, 161] Complications include keratitis sicca, corneal opacification, and blind-

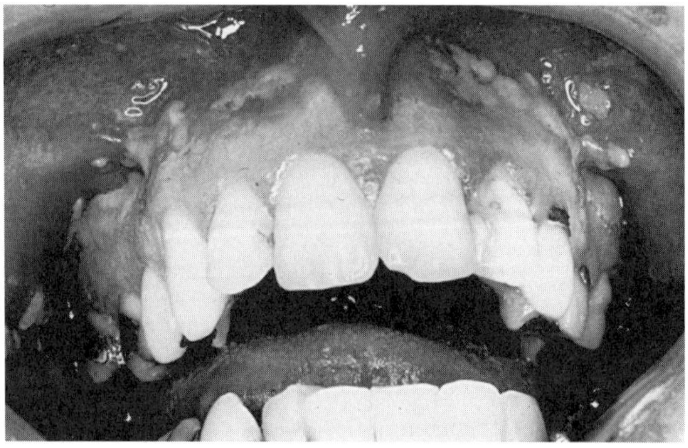

FIGURE 38–4. Erythema multiforme major (Stevens-Johnson syndrome). Buccal mucosal erosions with sparing of the gingiva.

ness.[60, 106] The tracheobronchial tree is involved in 50% of patients.[28, 31, 49] Inasmuch as primary atypical pneumonia due to *M. pneumoniae* has been known to induce erythema multiforme, it may be difficult to determine whether the pulmonary involvement is a complication or a cause of the disease. Balanitis and vulvovaginitis may result in scars and stenosis. The anus is infrequently affected. Generalized lymphadenopathy is often present.[74]

Involvement of the kidneys, heart, gastrointestinal tract, and central nervous system is rare. Renal alterations similar to those observed in acute glomerulonephritis, acute tubular necrosis, and proximal tubule damage have been reported.[13, 14, 29] Myocardial injury may lead to arrhythmias, pericarditis, and congestive heart failure.[12, 126] Abdominal pain, hematemesis, and melena may develop. Central nervous system involvement may lead to confusion, irritability, drowsiness, coma, or seizures. Permanent anonychia has been reported.[155]

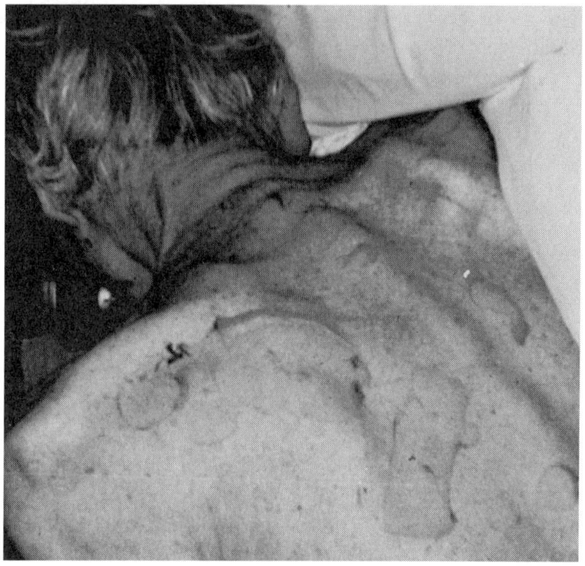

FIGURE 38–6. Toxic epidermal necrolysis. Sheets of denuded skin.

TOXIC EPIDERMAL NECROLYSIS

Severe cases of erythema multiforme have been reported to evolve into a clinical syndrome resembling toxic epidermal necrolysis.[102, 116, 124] Alternatively, it has been proposed that erythema multiforme major and the overlap syndromes with toxic epidermal necrolysis are a spectrum of evolution of a single disorder.[8] Toxic epidermal necrolysis can be divided into two distinct etiologic categories. In children and immunosuppressed adults, the eruption is caused by infection with *Staphylococcus aureus* and is known as the staphylococcal scalded skin syndrome (Fig. 38–5). This disorder will not be discussed further. In adults, toxic epidermal necrolysis is related to the administration of therapeutic agents or is idiopathic.

The skin lesions appear as erythematous macules with flaccid bullae that lead to sheets of necrotic epidermis after mechanical trauma, resulting in large, denuded areas (Fig. 38–6). The occurrence of mucosal disease of the mouth and genital area may be high.[87] In a study of 87 patients, erosive mucous membrane lesions identical to those of the severe form of erythema multiforme were present, supporting the suggestion that toxic epidermal necrolysis is an expression of the severe form of erythema multiforme.[114] In patients with toxic epidermal necrolysis, the principal cause of death was infection with *Staphylococcus aureus* or *Pseudomonas aeruginosa*. The age of the patient and percentage of denuded skin were associated with the prognosis.[114]

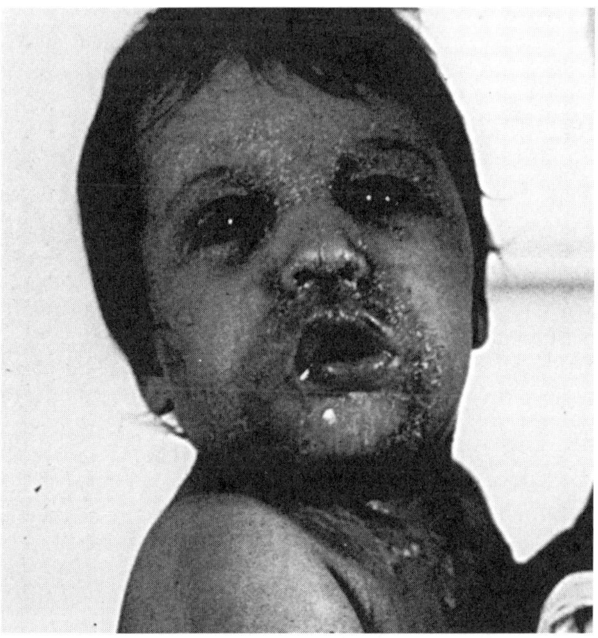

FIGURE 38–5. Staphylococcal scalded skin syndrome.

Data for mortality and recurrences in patients with erythema multiforme major and toxic epidermal necrolysis are difficult to interpret, owing to lack of precise clinical criteria for diagnosis. Reported mortality figures of hospitalized cases vary from 3% to 19%.[10, 28, 31] The mortality may be as high as 18% especially in patients with pneumonia.[117] These figures appear to be high and are not in line with current clinical experiences. Recent mortality rates of 1% or less have been reported for erythema multiforme major.[129, 144] The mortality in toxic epidermal necrolysis has been reported to be 20% to 25%.[87, 114]

LABORATORY FINDINGS

Evaluation of patients with erythema multiforme minor, erythema multiforme major, and toxic epidermal necrolysis should concentrate on a careful history seeking recent drug exposures and infections.

Laboratory findings usually are normal in erythema multiforme minor. In erythema multiforme major, leukocytosis, an elevated erythrocyte sedimentation rate, albuminuria, and hematuria may be present. Neutropenia and lymphopenia are harbingers of a poor outcome. Serologic studies for *M. pneumoniae* infection, cold agglutinins, a chest radiograph, and cultures of skin and blood may be obtained. Herpes simplex virus and *M. pneumoniae* have been cultured only rarely from blister fluids.[45, 88, 90, 127] Skin or mucous membrane biopsy specimens will aid in confirming the diagnosis.

The two types of toxic epidermal necrolysis can be differentiated from each other on the basis of history, age of the patient, and examination of skin biopsy specimens.[1] The drug-associated form shows a separation at the basal cell layer, whereas the infection-associated disease shows a separation at the granular layer of the epidermis.

Tzanck smears can be performed to search for multinucleate giant cells, and herpes simplex virus cultures can be obtained.

PATHOLOGIC FINDINGS

Pathologic alterations of erythema multiforme minor in skin biopsy specimens have been correlated with the appearance of the clinical lesion (Fig. 38–7).[94, 103, 151] The early changes in erythematous, papular, cutaneous lesions consist of epidermal and dermal alterations.[9, 109] The epidermis exhibits intercellular edema (spongiosis) and focal necrosis of individual cells or groups of keratinocytes. Epidermal necrosis predominates in bullous and iris lesions. Endothelial cells of venules exhibit enlargement, vacuolization, and necrosis, with edema of the papillary dermis (Fig. 38–8).[152] Increased expression of a vascular permeability factor (vascular endothelial cell growth factor mRNA) was detected in lesional skin, suggesting a role for increased microvascular permeability.[19]

The basement membrane may form the bulla roof or its floor and become thin or fragmented.[24, 91, 103] Fibrin deposits occur in the vesicle and dermal connective tissue.[152] A dermal perivascular cellular infiltrate contains lymphocytes with basophils and rarely eosinophils, neutrophils, and erythrocytes (see Fig. 38–8). At times, the infiltrate may be lichenoid.[32] The major infiltrating cells of the epidermis are $CD8^+$ T lymphocytes.[94] Large granular lymphocytes have also been noted in the epidermis.[46] $CD4^+$ T lymphocytes are the predominant cell in the dermis.[94]

Biopsy specimens of Stevens-Johnson syndrome show necrosis of the epidermis and a minimal inflammatory cell infiltrate.[32]

The oral lesions of erythema multiforme in the macular

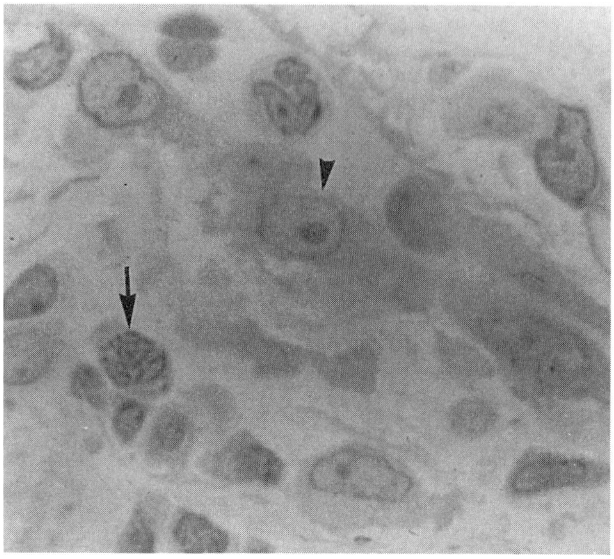

FIGURE 38–8. Erythema multiforme minor. Target (iris) lesion: dermal venule with activated endothelial cells (arrow). Note hypogranulated basophil (arrowhead) (1-μm section, Giemsa, original magnification ×1,000).

stage show vascular engorgement, a dermal infiltrate, and epidermal vacuolar changes of keratinocytes.[20, 133, 134, 163] Bullous lesions are characterized by separation of the epithelium from the lamina propria. A fibrinous exudate with leukocytes overlies areas of tissue repair and is associated with a dermal inflammatory cell infiltrate.

Immunofluorescence studies of skin biopsy specimens taken from lesions of erythema multiforme of less than 24 hours' duration show C3 protein, either alone or with IgM, in the superficial microvasculature.[21, 39, 61, 73] C3 may be deposited along the dermoepidermal junction. A common finding is the fluorescent keratinocyte that correlates with the necrotic keratinocyte detected on light microscopy.[38]

Electron microscopic studies of undefined skin lesions show enlargement and vacuolization of endothelial cells, as well as abnormalities of the vascular basal lamina.[24, 103]

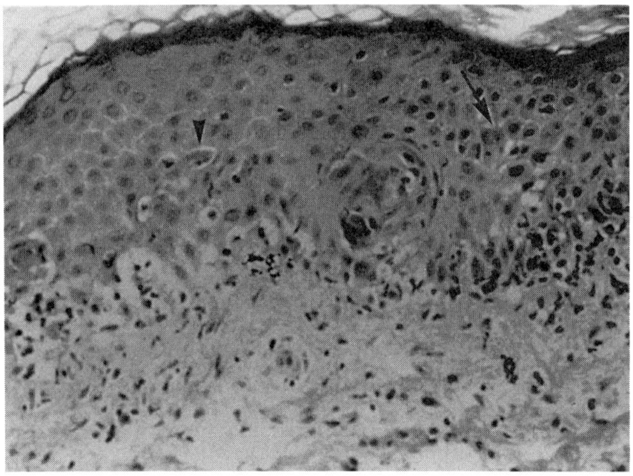

FIGURE 38–7. Skin biopsy specimen with a dermal infiltrate of lymphocytes. Note necrotic keratinocytes (arrowhead) and spongiosis (arrow) of the epidermis (hematoxylin-eosin, original magnification ×400).

DIFFERENTIAL DIAGNOSIS

Proposed diagnostic criteria for erythema multiforme minor include a self-limited, episodic disease of less than 4 weeks' duration; symmetrically distributed, discrete, cutaneous lesions, some of which evolve with concentric color changes to form target (iris) lesions; and mucosal involvement absent or limited to one mucosal surface.[65]

Criteria for erythema multiforme major are a self-limited disease of less than 6 weeks' duration; symmetrically distributed, discrete, cutaneous skin lesions; concentric color changes in some lesions causing target lesions or atypical target lesions; prodrome of fever, cough, sore throat, and malaise; and mucosal involvement of at least two mucosal surfaces.[8, 65]

Erythema multiforme must be differentiated from urticaria, toxic erythemas resulting from infection or drug hypersensitivity, meningococcal and gonococcal septicemia, hypersensitivity angiitis, systemic lupus erythematosus, bullous impetigo, bullous pemphigoid, herpes gestationis, the mucocutaneous lymph node syndrome (Kawasaki syndrome), Behçet's syndrome, Reiter's syndrome, and hand-foot-and-mouth disease.[11, 111, 123, 150, 159] When erythema multiforme is limited to the oral cavity, the differential diagnosis includes cicatricial pemphigoid, pemphigus vulgaris, lichen planus, Behçet's syndrome, aphthous ulcers, and herpetic stomatitis.

TREATMENT

In the treatment of erythema multiforme minor and major and toxic epidermal necrolysis, elimination of suspected etiologic factors is of importance. Suspected drugs should be discontinued unless the hazard from this maneuver is life threatening.[113] They are not readministered, owing to the risk of a more serious recurrence. Underlying infection should be treated. Other therapeutic maneuvers are symptomatic and include hydration to maintain fluid balance, antihistamines to decrease pruritus, analgesics to relieve pain, wet dressings to debride crusted erosions, and baths to minimize discomfort.

In erythema multiforme major, systemic corticosteroids have been conventionally used. However, the evidence that corticosteroid administration is efficacious is anecdotal, and no controlled prospective studies proving the efficacy or safety of systemic corticosteroids are available.[157] On the contrary, retrospective reviews of patients admitted to the hospital with Stevens-Johnson syndrome suggested a prolonged recovery, with an increased incidence of medical complications in the systemic steroid–treated group compared with the group receiving only supportive care.[38, 48, 112] Of interest is the fact that long-term corticosteroid therapy may delay the onset of toxic epidermal necrolysis but does not halt its progression.[54]

The use of oral acyclovir as either a 5-day course or prolonged therapy for 6 months for the treatment of herpes simplex virus has prevented the recurrence of herpes virus–associated erythema multiforme.[52, 80, 128] A placebo-controlled double-blind trial of the administration of continuous acyclovir therapy decreased episodes of recurrent erythema multiforme and in some cases may have induced remission.[148] If acyclovir is administered after the onset of herpes simplex virus infection, it fails to prevent the subsequent episodes of erythema multiforme.[52] Dapsone, azathioprine, cyclophosphamide, levamisol, and cyclosporine have been reported to be of value without controlled studies.[53, 58, 85, 128, 160]

The systemic administration of antibiotics is indicated for underlying infection. Without data obtained from controlled trials, erythromycin has been suggested as the initial antibiotic in all patients with Stevens-Johnson syndrome and pulmonary involvement.[137] In some cases of Stevens-Johnson syndrome and toxic epidermal necrolysis, care in a burn unit may be required.[38, 56, 77] Control of infection and fluid balance are important, inasmuch as sepsis and hypovolemia are major causes of death.[115]

For painful mouth erosions, topical anesthetics such as lidocaine, diphenhydramine elixir, and dyclonine may be used. A liquid or soft diet may be used as tolerated.

In those patients with eye involvement, close observation by an ophthalmologist is essential. Warm compresses, irrigation, and frequent topical application of antibiotic and corticosteroid preparations may be of benefit. The severity of the ophthalmologic complications correlates with the severity of the disease rather than with the local treatment regimen.[2] Ocular sequelae may require artificial tears, a moisture chamber, or surgical intervention.

REFERENCES

1. Amon RB, Dimond RL: Toxic epidermal necrolysis: rapid differentiation between staphylococcal and drug-induced disease. Arch Dermatol 111:1433, 1975.
2. Arstikaitis MJ: Ocular aftermath of Stevens-Johnson syndrome. Arch Ophthalmol 90:376, 1973.
3. Ashby DW, Lazar T: Erythema multiforme exudativum major (Stevens-Johnson syndrome). Lancet 1:1091, 1951.
4. Assaad D, From L, Ricciatti D, et al: Toxic epidermal necrolysis in Stevens-Johnson syndrome. Can Med Assoc J 118:154, 1978.
5. Assier H, Bastuji-Garin S, Revuz J, et al: Erythema multiforme with mucous membrane involvement and Stevens-Johnson syndrome are clinically different disorders with distinct causes. Arch Dermatol 131:539, 1995.
6. Azinge NO, Garrick GA: Stevens-Johnson syndrome (erythema multiforme) following ingestion of trimethoprim-sulfamethoxazole on two separate occasions in the same person: a case report. J Allergy Clin Immunol 62:125, 1978.
7. Bailey JH: Lesions of the cornea and conjunctiva in erythema exudativum multiforme (Hebra). Arch Ophthalmol 6:362, 1931.
8. Bastuji-Garin S, Rzany B, Stern RS, et al: Clinical description of cases of toxic epidermal necrolysis, Stevens-Johnson syndrome, and erythema multiforme. Arch Dermatol 129:92, 1993.
9. Bedi TR, Pinkus H: Histopathological spectrum of erythema multiforme. Br J Dermatol 95:243, 1976.
10. Bianchine JR, Macaraeg PVJ Jr, Lasagna L, et al: Drugs as etiologic factors in the Stevens-Johnson syndrome. Am J Med 44:390, 1968.
11. Bitter JJ, Friedman SA, Paltzik RL, et al: Kawasaki's disease appearing as erythema multiforme. Arch Dermatol 115:71, 1979.
12. Bloom A, Lovel TWI: Erythema multiforme with renal and myocardial injury. Proc R Soc Med 57:175, 1964.
13. Bluefarb SM, Szanto P: Erythema multiforme associated with acute renal tubular necrosis. Arch Dermatol 92:367, 1965.
14. Blum L, Chosidow O, Rostoker G, et al: Renal involvement in toxic epidermal necrolysis. J Am Acad Dermatol 34:1088, 1996.
15. Boe J, Dalgaard JB, Scott D: Mucocutaneous-ocular syndrome with intestinal involvement. Am J Med 25:857, 1958.
16. Brauer MJ, McEvoy BF, Mitus WJ: Hypersensitivity to nitrogen mustards in the form of erythema multiforme: a unique adverse reaction. Arch Intern Med 120:499, 1967.
17. Brice SL, Krzemien D, Weston WL, et al: Detection of herpes simplex virus DNA in cutaneous lesions of erythema multiforme. J Invest Dermatol 93:183, 1989.
18. Britz M, Sibulkin D: Recurrent erythema multiforme and herpes genitalis (type 2). JAMA 233:812, 1975.
19. Brown LF, Harrist TJ, Yeo K-T, et al: Increased expression of vascular permeability factor (vascular endothelial growth factor) in bullous pemphigoid dermatitis herpetiformis, and erythema multiforme. J Invest Dermatol 104:744, 1995.
20. Buchner A, Lozada F, Silverman S Jr: Histopathologic spectrum of oral erythema multiforme. Oral Surg Oral Med Oral Pathol 49:221, 1980.
21. Bushkell LL, Mackel SE, Jordon RE: Erythema multiforme: direct immunofluorescence studies and detection of circulating immune complexes. J Invest Dermatol 74:372, 1980.
22. Cannell H, Churcher GM, Milton-Thompson GJ: Stevens-Johnson syndrome associated with *Mycoplasma pneumoniae* infection. Br J Dermatol 81:196, 1969.
23. Carroll OM, Bryan PA, Robinson RJ: Stevens-Johnson syndrome associated with long-acting sulfonamides. JAMA 195:691, 1966.
24. Caulfield JB, Wilgram GF: An electron microscopic study of blister formation in erythema multiforme. J Invest Dermatol 39:307, 1962.
25. Cavendish A: A case of dermatitis from 9-bromofluorene and a peculiar reaction to a patch test. Br J Dermatol 52:155, 1940.
26. Chalmers D: A fatal case of erythema multiforme following deep x-ray therapy. Br J Dermatol 71:256, 1959.

27. Chan H-L, Stern RS, Arndt KA, et al: The incidence of erythema multiforme, Stevens-Johnson syndrome, and toxic epidermal necrolysis: a population-based study with particular reference to reactions caused by drugs among outpatients. Arch Dermatol 126:43, 1990.
28. Claxton RC: Review of 31 cases of Stevens-Johnson syndrome. Med J Aust 1:963, 1963.
29. Comaish JS, Kerr DNS: Erythema multiforme and nephritis. Br Med J 2:84, 1961.
30. Correia O, Chosidow O, Ph S, et al: Evolving pattern of drug-induced toxic epidermal necrolysis. Dermatology 186:32, 1993.
31. Costello MJ: Erythema multiforme exudativum (erythema bullosum malignans-pluriorificial type): personal observations of cases in Willard Parker Hospital for Contagious Diseases (1932–1946). J Invest Dermatol 8:127, 1947.
32. Côté B, Wechsler J, Bastuji-Garin S, et al: Clinicopathologic correlation in erythema multiforme and Stevens-Johnson syndrome. Arch Dermatol 131:1268, 1995.
33. Crosby SS, Murray KM, Marvin JA, et al: Management of Stevens-Johnson syndrome. Clin Pharmacy 5:682, 1986.
34. Darragh TM, Egbert BM, Berger TG, et al: Identification of herpes simplex virus DNA in lesions of erythema multiforme by polymerase chain reaction. J Am Acad Dermatol 24:23, 1991.
35. DeFeo CP Jr: Erythema multiforme bullosum caused by 9-bromofluorene. Arch Dermatol 94:545, 1966.
36. Drago F, Perodi A, Rebora A: Persistent erythema multiforme: report of two new cases and review of literature. J Am Acad Dermatol 33:1366, 1995.
37. Duvic M, Reisner EG, Dawson DV, et al: HLA-B15 association with erythema multiforme. J Am Acad Dermatol 8:493, 1983.
38. Esterly NB (ed): Special symposium: corticosteroids for erythema multiforme? Pediatr Dermatol 6:229, 1989.
39. Finan MC, Schroeter AL: Cutaneous immunofluorescence study of erythema multiforme: correlation with light microscope patterns and etiologic agents. J Am Acad Dermatol 10:497, 1984.
40. Finland M, Jolliffe LS, Parker F Jr: Pneumonia and erythema multiforme exudativum: report of four cases and three autopsies. Am J Med 4:473, 1948.
41. Fitzpatrick JE, Thompson PB, Aeling JL, et al: Photosensitive recurrent erythema multiforme. J Am Acad Dermatol 9:419, 1983.
42. Fletcher MWC, Harris RC: Erythema exudativum multiforme (Hebra)—bullous type. J Pediatr 27:465, 1945.
43. Foedinger D, Anhalt GJ, Boecskoer B, et al: Autoantibodies to desmoplakin I and II in patients with erythema multiforme. J Exp Med 181:169, 1995.
44. Foedinger D, Sterniczky B, Elbe A, et al: Autoantibodies against desmoplakin I and II define a subset of patients with erythema multiforme. J Invest Dermatol 106:1012, 1996.
45. Foerster CW, Scott LV: Isolation of herpes-simplex virus from a patient with erythema multiforme exudativum (Stevens-Johnson syndrome). N Engl J Med 259:473, 1958.
46. Ford MJ, Smith KL, Croker BP, et al: Large granular lymphocytes within the epidermis of erythema multiforme lesions. J Am Acad Dermatol 27:460, 1992.
47. Forman L, Whitwell GPB: The association of herpes catarrhalis with erythema multiforme (Hebra). Br J Dermatol 46:309, 1934.
48. Geavert GI, Cohen EJ, Donnenfeld ED, et al: Erythema multiforme after use of topical sulfacetamide. Am J Ophthalmol 99:465, 1985.
49. Genieser NB, Becker MH, Rothman J: Mediastinal emphysema complicating Stevens-Johnson syndrome. Arch Dermatol 105:421, 1972.
50. Gordon AM, Lyell A: Mycoplasmas and erythema multiforme, letter. Lancet 1:1314, 1969.
51. Gottschalk HR, Stone OJ: Stevens-Johnson syndrome from ophthalmic sulfonamide. Arch Dermatol 112:513, 1979.
52. Green JA, Spruance SL, Wenerstrom G, et al: Post-herpetic erythema multiforme prevented with prophylactic oral acyclovir. Ann Intern Med 102:632, 1985.
53. Gruppo Italiano Studi Epidemiologici in Dermatologia (GISED): Cutaneous reactions to analgesic-antipyretics and nonsteroidal anti-inflammatory drugs: analysis of reports to the spontaneous reporting system of the Gruppo Italiano Studi Epidemiologici in Dermatologia. Dermatology 186:164, 1993.
54. Guibal F, Bastuji-Garin S, Chosidow O, et al: Characteristics of toxic epidermal necrolysis in patients undergoing long-term glucocorticoid therapy. Arch Dermatol 131:669, 1995.
55. Guillaume J-C, Roujeau J-C, Revuz J, et al: The culprit drugs in 87 cases of toxic epidermal necrolysis (Lyell's syndrome). Arch Dermatol 123:1166, 1987.
56. Halebian PH, Madden MR, Finklestein JL, et al: Improved burn center survival of patients with toxic epidermal necrolysis managed without corticosteroids. Ann Surg 204:503, 1986.
57. Hellgren L, Hersle K: Erythema multiforme: statistical evaluation of clinical and laboratory data in 224 patients and matched healthy controls. Acta Allergol 21:45, 1966.
58. Heng MCY, Allen SG: Efficacy of cyclophosphamide in toxic epidermal necrolysis: clinical and pathophysiological aspects. J Am Acad Dermatol 25:778, 1991.
59. Hensen EJ, Claas FJH, Vermeer BJ: Drug-dependent binding of circulation antibodies in drug-induced toxic epidermal necrolysis. Lancet 2:151, 1981.
60. Howard GM: The Stevens-Johnson syndrome: ocular prognosis and treatment. Am J Ophthalmol 55:893, 1963.
61. Howland WW, Golitz LE, Weston WL, et al: Erythema multiforme: clinical, histopathologic, and immunologic study. J Am Acad Dermatol 10:438, 1984.
62. Huff JC: Erythema multiforme and latent herpes simplex infections. Semin Dermatol 11:207, 1992.
63. Huff JC, Weston WL: The photodistribution of erythema multiforme. Arch Dermatol 116:477, 1980.
64. Huff JC, Weston WL: Isomorphic phenomena in erythema multiforme: clinical, pathologic, and immunologic studies. Clin Exp Dermatol 8:409, 1983.
65. Huff JC, Weston WL: Recurrent erythema multiforme. Medicine 68:133, 1989.
66. Huff JC, Weston WL, Carr RI: Mixed cryoglobulinemia, ^{125}IC1q binding and skin immunofluorescence in erythema multiforme. J Invest Dermatol 74:375, 1980.
67. Huff JC, Weston WL, Tonnesen MG: Erythema multiforme: a critical review of characteristics, diagnostic criteria, and causes. J Am Acad Dermatol 8:763, 1983.
68. Imamura S, Yanase K, Taniguchi S, et al: Erythema multiforme: demonstration of immune complexes in the sera and skin lesions. Br J Dermatol 102:161, 1980.
69. Jensen JL, Rhyne RR, Correll RW, et al: Acute episodic inflammatory lesions of the mucous membrane and skin. J Am Dent Assoc 100:896, 1980.
70. Kampgen E, Burg G, Wank R: Association of herpes simplex virus–induced erythema multiforme with human leukocyte antigen DQw3. Arch Dermatol 124:1372, 1988.
71. Katz HI, Wooten JW, Davis RG, et al: Stevens-Johnson syndrome: report of a case associated with culturally proven *Mycoplasma pneumoniae* infection. JAMA 199:504, 1967.
72. Kazmierowski JA, Peizner DS, Wuepper KD: Herpes simplex antigen is present in immune complexes obtained from patients with erythema multiforme after recurrent herpes simplex infection. JAMA 247:2547, 1982.
73. Kazmierowski JA, Wuepper KD: Erythema multiforme: immune complex vasculitis of the superficial cutaneous microvasculature. J Invest Dermatol 71:366, 1978.
74. Keil H: Erythema multiforme exudativum (Hebra): a clinical entity associated with systemic features. Ann Intern Med 14:449, 1940.
75. Kennet S: Erythema multiforme affecting the oral cavity. Oral Surg Oral Med Oral Pathol 25:366, 1968.
76. Khalil I, Lepage V, Douay C, et al: HLA DQB1*0301 allele is involved in the susceptibility to erythema multiforme. J Invest Dermatol 97:697, 1991.
77. Kim PS, Goldfarb JW, Gaisford JW, et al: Stevens-Johnson syndrome and toxic epidermal necrolysis: a pathophysiological review and recommendations for a treatment protocol. J Burn Care Rehabil 4:91, 1983.
78. Lane JM, Ruben FL, Neff JM: Complications of smallpox vaccination, 1968: results of ten statewide surveys. J Infect Dis 122:303, 1970.
79. Leigh IM, Mowbray JF, Levene GM, et al: Recurrent and continuous erythema multiforme—a clinical and immunological study. Clin Exp Dermatol 10:58, 1985.
80. Lemak MA, Duvic M, Bean SF: Oral acyclovir for the prevention of herpes-associated erythema multiforme. J Am Acad Dermatol 15:50, 1986.
81. Lepage V, Douay C, Mallet C, et al: Erythema multiforme is associated to HLA-Aw33 and Drw53. Tissue Antigens 32:170, 1988.

82. Levy M, Shear NH: *Mycoplasma pneumoniae* infection and Stevens-Johnson syndrome: report of eight cases and review of the literature. Clin Pediatr 30:42, 1991.
83. Leznoff A, Frank H, Telner P, et al: Histoplasmosis in Montreal during the fall of 1963, with observations on erythema multiforme. Can Med Assoc J 91:1154, 1964.
84. Lillibridge CB, Melish ME, Glasgow L: Site of action of exfoliative toxin in the staphylococcal scalded-skin syndrome. Pediatrics 50:728, 1972.
85. Losada-Nur F, Gorsky M, Silverman S Jr: Erythema multiforme: clinical observations and treatment of 95 patients. Oral Surg Oral Med Oral Pathol 67:36, 1989.
86. Ludlam GB, Bridges JB, Benn EC: Association of Stevens-Johnson syndrome with antibody for *Mycoplasma pneumoniae*. Lancet 1:958, 1964.
87. Lyell A: A review of toxic epidermal necrolysis in Britain. Br J Dermatol 79:662, 1967.
88. Lyell A, Gordon AM, Dick HM, et al: *Mycoplasma* and erythema multiforme. Lancet 2:1116, 1967.
89. Lynch FW: Erythema multiforme: a review. South Med J 48:279, 1955.
90. MacDonald A, Feiwel M: Isolation of herpes simplex virus from erythema multiforme. Br Med J 2:570, 1972.
91. MacVicar DN, Graham JH, Burgoon CF Jr: Dermatitis herpetiformis, erythema multiforme, and bullous pemphigoid: a comparative histopathological and histochemical study. J Invest Dermatol 41:289, 1963.
92. Major PP, Morisset R, Kurstak C, et al: Isolation of herpes simplex virus type 1 from lesions of erythema multiforme. Can Med Assoc J 118:821, 1978.
93. Malmström M, Ruokonen H, Konttinen YT, et al: Herpes simplex virus antigens and inflammatory cells in oral lesions in recurrent erythema multiforme: immunoperoxidase and autoradiographic studies. Acta Derm Venereol (Stockh) 70:405, 1990.
94. Margolis RJ, Tonnesen MG, Harrist TJ, et al: Lymphocyte subsets and Langerhans cells/indeterminate cells in erythema multiforme. J Invest Dermatol 81:403, 1983.
95. McKay ALC, Arbuthnott JP, Lyell A: Action of staphylococcal epidermolytic toxin in mouse skin: an electron microscopic study. J Invest Dermatol 65:423, 1975.
96. Merot Y, Gravallese E, Guillén FJ, et al: Lymphocyte subsets and Langerhans' cells in toxic epidermal necrolysis: report of a case. Arch Dermatol 122:455, 1986.
97. Mesegver MA, DeRafael L, Vidal ML: Stevens-Johnson syndrome with isolation of *Mycoplasma pneumoniae* from skin lesions. Eur J Clin Microbiol 5:167, 1986.
98. Miller RAW, Griffiths WAD: Experimentally induced complement and immunoglobulin deposition along the basement membrane zone (BMZ) and in the dermal blood vessels. Br J Dermatol 106:275, 1982.
99. Miura S, Smith CC, Burnett JW, et al: Detection of viral DNA within skin of healed recurrent herpes simplex infection and erythema multiforme lesions. J Invest Dermatol 98:68, 1992.
100. Mondino BJ, Brown SI, Rabin BS: HLA antigens in Stevens-Johnson syndrome with ocular involvement. Arch Ophthalmol 100:1453, 1982.
101. Nawalkha PI, Mathus NK, Malhotra YK: Severe erythema multiforme (Stevens-Johnson syndrome) following telecobalt therapy. Br J Radiol 45:768, 1972.
102. Øhlenschlaeger K: Toxic epidermal necrolysis and Stevens-Johnson's disease. Acta Derm Venereol (Stockh) 46:204, 1966.
103. Orfanos CE, Schaumburg-Lever G, Lever WF: Dermal and epidermal types of erythema multiforme. Arch Dermatol 109:682, 1974.
104. Orton PW, Huff JC, Tonnesen MG, et al: Detection of herpes simplex virus antigen in skin lesions of erythema multiforme. Ann Intern Med 101:48, 1984.
105. Pandi DN: Herpetic erythema multiforme. Br Med J 1:746, 1964.
106. Patz A: Ocular involvement in erythema multiforme. Arch Ophthalmol 43:244, 1950.
107. Peck G, Herzig GP, Elias PM: Toxic epidermal necrolysis in a patient with graft-vs-host reaction. Arch Dermatol 105:561, 1972.
108. Peck SM, Osserman KE, Weiner LB, et al: Studies in bullous diseases: immunofluorescent serologic tests. N Engl J Med 279:951, 1968.
109. Pierard J, Whimster I: The histopathological diagnosis of dermatitis herpetiformis, bullous pemphigoid and erythema multiforme. Br J Dermatol 73:253, 1961.
110. Prendiville JS, Hebert AA, Greenwald MJ, et al: Management of Stevens-Johnson syndrome and toxic epidermal necrolysis in children. J Pediatr 115:881, 1989.
111. Rallison ML: Lupus erythematosus and Stevens-Johnson syndrome. Am J Dis Child 101:725, 1961.
112. Rasmussen JE: Erythema multiforme in children: response to treatment with systemic corticosteroids. Br J Dermatol 95:181, 1976.
113. Rasmussen JE: Erythema multiforme: should anyone care about the standards of care? Arch Dermatol 131:726, 1995.
114. Revuz J, Penso D, Roujeau J-C, et al: Toxic epidermal necrolysis: clinical findings and prognosis factors in 87 patients. Arch Dermatol 123:1160, 1987.
115. Revuz J, Roujeau J-C, Guillaume J-C, et al: Treatment of toxic epidermal necrolysis: Créteil's experience. Arch Dermatol 123:1156, 1987.
116. Robinson HJ Jr, Samorodin CS: Thiabendazole-induced toxic epidermal necrolysis. Arch Dermatol 112:1757, 1976.
117. Rostenberg A, Fagelson HJ: Life threatening drug eruptions. JAMA 194:660, 1965.
118. Roujeau J-C: Clinical aspects of skin reactions to NSAIDs. Scand J Rheumatol Suppl 65:131, 1987.
119. Roujeau J-C, Huynh TN, Bracq C, et al: Genetic susceptibility to toxic epidermal necrolysis. Arch Dermatol 123:1171, 1987.
120. Roujeau J-C, Kelly JP, Naldi L, et al: Medication use and the risk of Stevens-Johnson syndrome or toxic epidermal necrolysis. N Engl J Med 333:1600, 1995.
121. Roujeau J-C, Koso M, Andre C, et al: Sjögrens-like syndrome after drug-induced toxic epidermal necrolysis. Lancet 1:609, 1985.
122. Roujeau J-C, Moritz S, Guillaume JC, et al: Lymphopenia and abnormal balance of T-lymphocyte subpopulations in toxic epidermal necrolysis. Arch Dermatol Res 277:24, 1985.
123. Rowell NR, Beck JS, Anderson JR: Lupus erythematosus and erythema multiforme–like lesions. Arch Dermatol 88:176, 1963.
124. Safai B, Good RA, Day NK: Erythema multiforme: report of two cases and speculation on immune mechanisms involved in the pathogenesis. Clin Immunol Immunopathol 7:379, 1977.
125. Sanders DY, Johnson HW: Stevens-Johnson syndrome associated with *Mycoplasma pneumoniae* infection. Am J Dis Child 121:243, 1971.
126. Schartum S: Stevens-Johnson syndrome with cardiac involvement. Acta Med Scand 179:729, 1966.
127. Schmidt H: Isolation of herpes simplex virus from blisters of a patient with Stevens-Johnson's syndrome. Acta Derm Venereol (Stockh) 41:53, 1961.
128. Schofield JK, Tatnall FM, Leigh IM: Recurrent erythema multiforme: clinical features and treatment in a large series of patients. Br J Dermatol 128:542, 1993.
129. Schöpf E, Stühmer A, Rzany B, et al: Toxic epidermal necrolysis and Stevens-Johnson syndrome: an epidemiologic study from West Germany. Arch Dermatol 127:839, 1991.
130. Sellers TG Jr, Price WN Jr, Newberry WM Jr: An epidemic of erythema multiforme and erythema nodosum caused by histoplasmosis. Ann Intern Med 62:1244, 1965.
131. Shear NH, Spielberg SP, Grant DM, et al: Differences in metabolism of sulfonamides predisposing to idiosyncratic toxicity. Ann Intern Med 105:179, 1986.
132. Shelley WB: Herpes simplex virus as a cause of erythema multiforme. JAMA 201:153, 1967.
133. Shklar G: Oral lesions of erythema multiforme. Arch Dermatol 92:495, 1965.
134. Shklar G, McCarthy PL: Oral manifestations of erythema multiforme in children. Oral Surg Oral Med Oral Pathol 21:713, 1966.
135. Sieber OF, John J, Fulginiti YA, et al: Stevens-Johnson syndrome associated with *Mycoplasma pneumoniae* infection. JAMA 200:79, 1967.
136. Smith RG: Erythema multiforme exudativum: recurrent oral lesions. Review of the literature and a case history. J Dent 1:223, 1973.
137. Sontheimer RD, Garibaldi RA, Krueger GG: Stevens-Johnson syndrome associated with *Mycoplasma pneumoniae* infections. Arch Dermatol 114:241, 1978.
138. Spielberg SP, Gordon GB, Blake DA, et al: Anticonvulsant therapy *in vitro:* possible role of arene oxides. J Pharmacol Exp Ther 217:386, 1981.
139. Stanyon JH, Warner WP: Mucosal respiratory syndrome. Can Med Assoc J 53:247, 1945.
140. Stein KM, Schlappner OLA, Heaton CL, et al: Demonstration of basal cell immunofluorescence in drug-induced toxic epidermal necrolysis. Br J Dermatol 86:246, 1972.
141. Stein MR, Thompson CK Jr, Sawicki JE, et al: Esophageal stricture complicating Stevens-Johnson syndrome: a case report. Am J Gastroenterol 62:435, 1974.

142. Stevens AM, Johnson FC: A new eruptive fever associated with stomatitis and ophthalmia: report of two cases in children. Am J Dis Child 24:526, 1922.
143. Straus DA: Generalized bullous eruption following testing for sulfonamide hypersensitivity. N Engl J Med 239:956, 1948.
144. Strom BL, Carson JL, Halpern AC, et al: A population-based study of Stevens-Johnson syndrome: incidence and antecedent drug exposures. Arch Dermatol 127:831, 1991.
145. Ström J: Febrile mucocutaneous syndromes (ectodermosis erosiva pluriorificialis, Stevens-Johnson's syndrome, etc.) in adenovirus infections. Acta Derm Venereol (Stockh) 47:281, 1967.
146. Stügen G: Toxic epidermal necrolysis provoked by barbiturates. Br J Dermatol 88:291, 1973.
147. Swinehart JM, Weston WL, Huff C: Identification of circulating immune complexes in erythema multiforme. J Invest Dermatol 70:219, 1978.
148. Tatnall FM, Schofield JK, Leigh IM: A double-blind placebo-controlled trial of continuous acyclovir therapy in recurrent erythema multiforme. Br J Dermatol 132:267, 1995.
149. Telner P, Leznoff A, Frank H: A relationship between erythema multiforme and histoplasmosis. J Invest Dermatol 45:135, 1965.
150. Tokora Y: Skin lesions in Behçet's disease. Int J Dermatol 16:227, 1977.
151. Tonnesen MG, Harrist TJ, Wintroub BU, et al: Erythema multiforme: microvascular damage and infiltration of lymphocytes and basophils. J Invest Dermatol 80:282, 1983.
152. Tonnesen MG, Soter NA: Erythema multiforme. J Am Acad Dermatol 1:357, 1979.
153. Ustvedt HJ: Erythema exudativum multiforme. I. The clinical picture. Acta Med Scand 131:32, 1948.
154. Ustvedt HJ: Erythema exudativum multiforme. II. Relations to tuberculosis. Acta Med Scand 131:226, 1948.
155. Wanscher B, Thormann J: Permanent anonychia after Stevens-Johnson syndrome. Arch Dermatol 113:970, 1977.
156. Wasserman E, Glass WI: Stevens-Johnson syndrome. Arch Intern Med 104:787, 1959.
157. Weeks VT, Lehmann WX: Erythema multiforme exudativum (Stevens-Johnson syndrome) treated with cortisone or ACTH. J Pediatr 44:508, 1954.
158. Weston WL, Brice SL, Jester JD, et al: Herpes simplex virus in childhood erythema multiforme. Pediatrics 89:32, 1992.
159. Weston WL, Huff JC: The mucocutaneous lymph node syndrome: a critical re-examination. Clin Exp Dermatol 6:167, 1981.
160. Wilkel CS, McDonald CJ: Cyclosporine therapy for bullous erythema multiforme. Arch Dermatol 126:397, 1990.
161. Wilkins J, Morrison L, White CR Jr: Oculocutaneous manifestations of the erythema multiforme/Stevens-Johnson syndrome/toxic epidermal necrolysis spectrum. Dermatol Clin 10:571, 1992.
162. Wolkenstein P, Charue D, Laurent P, et al: Metabolic predisposition to cutaneous adverse drug reactions: role in toxic epidermal necrolysis caused by sulfonamides and anticonvulsants. Arch Dermatol 131:544, 1995.
163. Wooten JW, Katz HI, Hoffman S, Link JF: Development of oral lesions in erythema multiforme exudativum. Oral Surg Oral Med Oral Pathol 24:808, 1967.
164. Wuepper KD, Dimond RL, Knuston DD: Studies of the mechanism of epidermal injury by staphylococcal epidermolytic toxin. J Invest Dermatol 68:191, 1975.
165. Wuepper KD, Watson PA, Kazmierowski JA: Immune complexes in erythema multiforme and the Stevens-Johnson syndrome. J Invest Dermatol 74:368, 1980.
166. Yaffee HS, Dressler DP: Topical applications of mafenide acetate: its association with erythema multiforme and cutaneous reactions. Arch Dermatol 100:277, 1969.
167. Zaim MT, Giorno RC, Golitz LE, et al: An immunopathological study of herpes-associated erythema multiforme. J Cutan Pathol 14:257, 1987.

39 *Insect Sting Allergy*

DAVID F. GRAFT MARTIN D. VALENTINE

HISTORICAL PERSPECTIVE

Certain individuals are susceptible to a generalized allergic response when stung by insects of the order Hymenoptera. In some, the reaction is so severe that prevention of future reactions is a physician's principal concern. Although counseling avoidance of stings is the cornerstone of prevention, it is not always sufficient to prevent potentially fatal stings. Braun[10] was the first to employ a regimen of immunization with an extract prepared from the posterior 1/8 inch of the insect. Later, Benson[3] thought he had found an intrinsic bee protein throughout the entire insect bodies. Benson's studies led to the practice of immunization of sting-allergic patients with an extract of mixed stinging insects made from a filtrate of crushed whole insect bodies. Most allergists were content to use this crude preparation of whole insect bodies, ignoring the logic of Loveless,[67] who advocated the use of unadulterated venom either collected and administered from a syringe or from naturally delivered stings.

Venom collection from honeybees was facilitated by the development of an electric stimulation technique in 1964.[4] With this method, large quantities of honeybee venom could be collected without great injury to the bees, which reflexively expelled droplets of venom onto an electrically charged collecting plate. The dried venom droplets were eventually gleaned from the collecting plate. Attempts at modifying the honeybee venom collection technique to allow collection of vespid venoms resulted in increased numbers of people, and even pet cats and dogs, being stung in the vicinity of the collectors. Apparently, an attractant pheromone in honeybee venom that leads other honeybees to deposit their venom at a single, focused site has no counterpart in the vespid venoms: the insects attempted to sting everything indiscriminately.

Benton[98] perfected a separation process that allowed centrifugal extraction of high-purity venom from vespid venom sacs using a β-alanine buffer. Using venom collected by these methods, researchers found that peripheral blood basophils from venom-allergic patients exposed to nontoxic concentrations of venom would release histamine in a dose-dependent fashion.[101] The importance of this observation was the recognition that high concentrations of venom will cause nonspecific toxic histamine release from all mast cells and basophils, but lower concentrations are able to elicit histamine release only from the cells of sensitized individuals. It was then shown that this reaction was dependent on the presence and participation of venom-specific IgE antibodies. Other clinical observations have been made regarding toxic,[8] rather than immunologic, effects in humans.

Researchers subsequently demonstrated the safety and efficacy of skin testing with dilute venom solutions in human volunteers.[45, 109] Schwartz[89] noted the ambiguity of test results when he used the irritating extracts made from whole insect bodies. Treatment failures—failure of whole body extract (WBE) immunotherapy to prevent major or even fatal sting reactions—also were reported in the medical literature.[104, 80] That the majority of practicing and academic allergists accepted the idea that WBE extract was curative for insect sting allergy was reflected by the results of a poll of the membership of the American Academy of Allergy, which showed that practicing allergists were satisfied with the efficacy of WBE therapy. Yet less than a decade later, the need for a radical reassessment of WBE treatment efficacy was brought to the fore in the first contemporary report of venom treatment. A child who was treated had been a WBE failure, as had his deceased sister before him.[59] After 3 months of honeybee venom immunotherapy, the immunized child had developed a titer of venom-specific blocking antibody comparable to that of his immune father (a professional beekeeper who received as many as 200 stings in a normal workweek with impunity). This was the first instance in which the development of blocking IgG antibodies was correlated with the development of immunity to a sting. An in-hospital challenge sting was then administered to the child, resulting in a few shed tears but no allergic reaction.

The criterion for the quantity of blocking antibody that was expected to be protective was empirically derived from the values found in patients who were immunized with venoms and then successfully stung (without systemic reaction) and amounted to a doubling of the individual's baseline antibody. Later, the functional assay for the measurement of blocking antibody was replaced by an immunoassay for venom-specific IgG.[25, 40, 100] A study in 1978 showed that venom immunotherapy (VIT) was 97% effective in reducing the risk of future sting reactions and that WBE therapy was no more effective than placebo.[46]

Venoms were licensed for commercial use in 1979. Subsequent research has focused on selection of patients for VIT, tests for determining efficacy of VIT, and how long VIT should be continued. As discussed later, the means by which immunotherapy protects patients from sting reactions is by no means certain and is a subject of great interest.

There is now a consensus that immunotherapy with specific venoms reduces the risk and severity of future reactions to insect stings in patients who have previously experienced systemic allergic reactions to similar stings.[106] Insect venoms that have been evaluated include those from the honeybee, yellow jacket, white-faced hornet (black hornet), yellow hornet, and Polistes paper wasp.[103] Sensitivity to stings from the imported fire ant *(Solenopsis)*[14, 15] has been successfully treated with extracts prepared from whole ant bodies, presumably because the ratio of relevant venom protein to irrelevant body protein in these extracts is relatively large. In all of the Hymenoptera, only females can sting. The males are relegated to more mundane tasks, the term drone being applied to male honeybees.

PATHOPHYSIOLOGY

The insects most frequently responsible for allergic reactions in humans are yellow jackets, honeybees, wasps, hornets, and ants. An abbreviated classification showing the taxonomic relationship of the insects of most importance in venom allergy is shown in Figure 39–1. The relationships are reflected by immunochemical relationships of the constituents of the venoms of these insects, which are discussed later.

Hymenoptera venoms contain a number of biologically interesting constituents. The protein and peptide constituents of the more common insect venoms are shown in Table 39–1. The allergens in the venoms are mostly proteins

ORDER	Hymenoptera (Bees, wasps, hornets, ants)					
SUPERFAMILY	Apoidea			Vespoidea		Scoliodea
FAMILY	Apidae		Halictidae **Sweat bees**	Vespidae		Formicidae
SUBFAMILY	Apinae			Vespinae	Polistinae	Myrminicae
TRIBE	Apini **Honeybees**	Bombini **Bumblebees**		**Yellow jackets Hornets**	**Paper-nest wasps**	**Fire ants Harvester ants**

FIGURE 39–1. Abridged classification of stinging insects.

TABLE 39–1
PROTEIN AND PEPTIDE COMPONENTS IN HONEYBEE AND VESPID VENOMS

	Honeybee		Vespid	
	MW	*% of Venom*	*MW*	*% of Venom*
Proteins				
Phospholipase A_2	15,800	12		
Phospholipase A_1		0	37,000	6–14
Hyaluronidase	45,000	2	43,000	1–3
Antigen 5		0	23,000	3–10
Acid phosphatase	49,000	?	49,000	?
Peptides				
Mellitin	2,840	50		0
Apamin	2,038	2		0
Mast cell degranulating peptide	2,593	2	1,600	?
Kinin		0	1,200	?

with enzyme activity. Although honeybees originated in Europe and have both phospholipase and hyaluronidase activities in their venom, the proteins bearing the same enzymatic functions in vespid venoms are immunochemically different. This may be an example of convergent evolution, since these functional activities represent proteins with little structural homology (for example, between honeybee and yellow jacket hyaluronidase). Antibody inhibition studies on sera from mice immunized with purified venom allergens show that extensive cross-reactivity exists between white-faced hornet, yellow hornet, and yellow jacket for hyaluronidase and antigen 5, but not phospholipase.[52, 53, 68, 69] Thus although a degree of cross-sensitization to hyaluronidase and antigen 5 is observed between the vespids, and to a lesser extent with Polistes wasp (between wasp, yellow hornet, and white-faced hornet for hyaluronidase and between wasp and yellow jacket for antigen 5), there is limited cross-reactivity between honeybee, vespid, and fire ant venoms.

The dried weight of the venom deposited by a honeybee, induced to sting a plastic film, is approximately 50 μg.[47] A single sting from one of the Vespoidea is thought to deliver between 10 and 100 μg. Estimates of the protein content of venoms are probably overstated because the micro-Kjeldahl assay usually performed to estimate protein in such materials does not discriminate between proteins and small polypeptides that may be present. Thus if one adds up the individually assayed proteins, such as hyaluronidase and phospholipase, the sum obtained in this way falls far short of the overall protein found by the micro-Kjeldahl estimate. Thus the individual, larger protein allergens in a vial of commercially prepared venom may represent as little as 10% of the stated content on the vial label (T.P. King, personal communication).

The barbs along the shaft of the honeybee stinger cause it to remain embedded in the sting recipient's flesh. Thus as it flies away, the honeybee that has stung kills itself through evisceration. The eviscerated bee's venom sac, still attached to the stinger in the victim's skin, seems to contract spasmodically as it flies away. Contrary to common wisdom, there is no evidence that the agonally contracting sac is anything but empty. Leaving the stinger behind at the sting site is called autotomy.[71] This process distinguishes the honeybee from the other stinging Hymenoptera, whose stingers are rarely left at the sting site and that therefore sting repeatedly. Other interspecies differences are seen not only in behavior but also in the chemical constituents of their venoms.

SPECTRUM OF REACTIONS

A sting from one of the Hymenoptera usually will result in local redness, swelling, pruritus, and/or pain, all of which are transient and caused by proinflammatory chemicals or substances in the venoms. This reaction arrives in seconds or minutes and fades within a few hours. It is distinguished from the large local reaction, which begins hours after a sting, peaking 12 to 48 hours later.

Systemic allergic reactions come in many shapes and sizes. Those that occur within seconds or minutes after allergen exposure are regarded as one or another variety of anaphylaxis, even though the clinical manifestations may be mild and non–life threatening, such as in a reaction consisting solely of generalized urticaria. An unwarranted forecast often made by emergency physicians or other health care providers when evaluating a sting victim is that the severity of ensuing reactions will inevitably be worse than prior reactions. Thus the patient who appears in an emergency room covered with hives is usually told that the next reaction may be fatal. This assumption is contrary to observations made during both in-hospital sting challenges and natural stings. Only between 25% and 60% of patients with histories of prior systemic sting reactions will react again on deliberate sting challenge.[46, 63] When an unimmunized patient experiences a reaction from a subsequent sting, it most likely is similar qualitatively and in severity to previous reactions. Obviously, a small proportion of sting reactions are sufficiently worse to be fatal, but this is a tiny fraction of all patients who are sensitive.

Types of Systemic Reactions

Cutaneous. Generalized urticaria, angioedema, or flushing, usually with pruritus, are recognized as varieties of cutaneous sting reactions. The pattern of eruption and pruritus may conform to the pattern of increased skin mast cell distribution seen at skin folds in the wrist, elbow, axilla, neck, knee, and inguinal area.

Vascular. The commonest vascular reactions to stings appear as hypotension, usually with tachycardia. This may be difficult to distinguish from a vasovagal reaction. However, the latter is usually accompanied by bradycardia. Rarely, hypertension may occur, presumably because of release of endogenous sympathomimetic amines.[64]

Respiratory. Dyspnea and wheezing may result from bronchospasm; inspiratory stridor may signal laryngeal edema.

Delayed Systemic Reactions. Rarely, in a patient without an immediate reaction, a significant systemic allergic reaction may be seen hours after a sting. No explanation has been found for this sort of event.

Serum Sickness. Urticaria, fever, proteinuria, lymphadenopathy, and arthropathy have occurred as a result of a sting, usually after an acute systemic reaction. This has been termed serum sickness, despite the imperfect analogy with classic serum sickness. Although one might be concerned lest serum sickness recur when venom immunotherapy is initiated in such patients (to prevent anaphylaxis), this has not been reported. However, a patient treated with WBE experienced fever, arthralgia, malaise, and lymphadenopathy after each injection.[44] These symptoms did not occur when the patient was later immunized with venom.

Other Reactions After Stings. A variety of atypical reactions have been described after insect stings, including nausea, vomiting, diarrhea, myasthenia gravis, and peripheral neuropathies.[62, 70] The mechanism of these reactions is unclear. When considering whether to employ immunotherapy in such cases, one must always consider the possibility of immunotherapy causing harm rather than a good result.

Large Local Reactions. Delayed cutaneous reactions, areas of erythema, and firm induration, contiguous with the site of a sting and generally peaking 48 to 72 hours after a sting, are termed large local reactions. Although at one time they were considered examples of Arthus reactions, in which the participation of IgG antibodies and complement caused a local inflammatory response, they are now considered IgE mediated and examples of late-phase reactions.[35] As such, the inflammatory tissue component is responsive to the administration of corticosteroids, whereas purely immediate reactions are unaffected by corticosteroids. Approximately 10% of patients with this type of reaction history will have a systemic allergic reaction with a future sting. Most physicians do not employ immunotherapy unless such a patient has also experienced a systemic reaction. However, it is considered appropriate to equip such patients with emergency epinephrine self-treatment kits. Some have suggested that emergency medical technicians who work in remote areas be equipped with epinephrine kits for unexpected anaphylactic reactions.[17]

EPIDEMIOLOGY

There are no data regarding the number of people who have been stung in the past, those who are stung in any given season, or what proportion of those who are stung experience any reaction out of the ordinary. Attempts to derive such data from population samples were undertaken in Rhode Island, where allergists examined the frequency of Hymenoptera sensitivity in college students, patients in their office practices,[12, 96] and boys in summer Boy Scout encampments.[94] The Boy Scout figures probably should be regarded as incidence, since they reflect how many youngsters reacted in a given time period. The answers to these questions have been pursued worldwide.[7, 13, 97] Settipane found a figure of about 0.4%, which is a much smaller number than the one arrived at by Golden in his evaluation of a random sample of workers at a factory in a Baltimore suburb.[24, 32, 95] Golden found that nearly 5% of a randomly selected sample of workers had a history of more than a normal reaction to a sting. Moreover, he found that there was evidence with skin tests and/or radioallergosorbent tests (RAST) of the presence of venom-specific IgE antibodies in nearly 25% of his sample, even in workers without a history of unusual sting reactions.

MORTALITY FROM STING REACTIONS

In the United States, about 50 deaths each year are attributed to insect sting reactions.[2] Additional deaths have been reported abroad.[16, 85] More men than women die from insect sting reactions. The risk of death increases with age. Despite the observation that the typical individual who experiences a systemic reaction is a male child, most systemic reactions in childhood consist predominantly of urticaria, and only one or two children experience fatal reactions each year. In 50% of those who die from sting reactions, there may be no prior history of difficulty with insect stings.

Stinging insect allergy is a worldwide problem. About 20 sting-induced deaths occur in Europe each year, and fewer occur in Asia. In all countries, an unknown number of additional deaths may be incorrectly attributed to an acute cardiovascular or central nervous system event. In a survey of postmortem sera from individuals dying from no known cause, a significant number had clinically relevant levels of IgE antibodies to one or more Hymenoptera.[91, 108]

INSECT MORPHOLOGY AND BEHAVIOR

Honeybees are small, fuzzy-appearing insects with alternating tan and dark brown stripes. To the person just stung or the casual observer, they may be indistinguishable from the yellow- and black-striped yellow jackets or some striped wasps. They are often seen gathering nectar from attractive flowers, while the hairs on their back legs accumulate pollen grains. Although one can find pollen allergens in honey, there are none in venom; nor are there any venom allergens in honey. Although they may become aggressive or excessively defensive in very wet or very dry weather, they are relatively noncombative while they are grazing for nectar and generally sting only when caught underfoot.

All of the honeybees in the United States were at one time of European descent (imported deliberately by colonists from Europe). Africanized honeybees (so-called killer bees) are the result of escaped offspring from interbreeding between established colonies of European honeybees and African honeybees brought to Brazil to improve honey production. The killer bees do not have unusual venom potency but do have a tendency to attack en masse.[18, 87] They have steadily advanced northward and in 1994 reached the middle of Texas. Bumblebees are large, slow-moving, noisy bees with hairy bodies of alternating yellow and black stripes. They are nonaggressive and account for only a small fraction of stings but have been reported to cause problems in certain occupations.[55] Sweat bees belong to another family (Halictidae) but also are capable of causing anaphylaxis with stings.[76]

Ground-nesting yellow jackets are identified by alternating yellow and black body stripes. Although they too appreciate a sip of nectar, they are omnivorous scavengers. They are often seen darting around picnic tables and garbage cans. Some regard the yellow hornets as aerial-nesting yellow jackets. Their globular nests may be found hanging from low tree branches or in shrubs. The black (white or bald faced) hornets are found in similar locations. A single entrance to the nest usually can be seen in a dependent location. The nest is constructed of a paper-like material made from wood masticated by the insects; the color of the paper reflects the color of the wooden source, but all are shades of grey. The yellow jacket nest is typically subterranean and formed at the site of an old mouse or other animal burrow.

Although not visible until unearthed, the yellow jacket nest is also made of paper manufactured by the insects. Rows of cells, where eggs are laid and develop into pupae, are neatly arranged in layers in a roughly spherical form. This nest is similar to the hornet nest, with the exception that the hornet nests have an extra paper sheath around the entire structure. The locations of the nests pose particular problems to lawn cutters, landscapers, and tree and bush trimmers, who may unwittingly come upon a nest and be subjected to dozens of stings. The nests of the narrow-waisted paper wasps (Polistinae) are built in the eaves of buildings, under air conditioners, in outdoor light sockets, or in mail boxes and have a characteristic appearance in which the hexagonal cells where eggs are laid, hatch, and pupate are not enclosed in a paper envelope.

The imported fire ants appear to have been inadvertently launched from a visiting freighter at the port of Mobile, Alabama, earlier this century. They have gradually extended their distribution in the Gulf States and continue to enlarge their territory.[20] Although they cannot tolerate cold temperatures, they have been found tunneling north under the warm pavement of interstate highways. They build 2- to 3-foot-high mounds containing thousands of ants, which are very aggressive.[14] When they sting, they seize the skin of their victim with their jaws and pivot about, inflicting a circle of stings with their abdominal stinger. The pain of their stings probably results from the piperidine alkaloid content of their venom. Sterile pustules form at sting sites in 1 to 2 days.[15] Fire ants present a special hazard to children, who may fall upon a mound and receive dozens or even hundreds of stings. Their venoms also contain traces of the immunogenic proteins found in vespid venoms and thus may contribute to the allergic reactions seen. Atypical (neurologic) sequelae to stings have also been reported.[11]

DIAGNOSIS AND THERAPY

Anaphylaxis is a term generically applicable to a spectrum of systemic allergic reactions ranging from mild, cutaneous reactions, such as urticaria, to potentially fatal bronchospasm, obstructive edema of the upper airway, and hypotension refractory to treatment with simple measures. Schwartz[90] and others have found significant levels of mast cell tryptase in serum after anaphylaxis. Blood eosinophilia may also be present, and urinary metabolites of histamine may be increased.[102] Blood histamine has been elevated in patients with hypotensive sting reactions.[99]

TESTS FOR INSECT- OR VENOM-SPECIFIC IgE ANTIBODIES

Skin Test Techniques and Concentrations

Cautious titration of skin reactivity to a panel of venoms usually helps to narrow the field of suspects.[99] Although an epicutaneous test (prick/puncture) is usually recommended before intradermal tests are performed, most allergists have never seen a positive epicutaneous test with venom, possibly because most individuals would react on prick or puncture only to a concentration of venom of 1,000 μg/ml or greater. Since commercially prepared venoms can be successfully reconstituted only to about 200 μg/ml, this is not feasible.

In practice, intracutaneous skin tests are begun with a concentration in the range of .001 to 0.1 μg/ml, the weaker concentrations being preferable for those whose reactions have been fairly recent and/or extremely severe. Approximately 0.02 ml (enough to raise a tiny bleb) is placed very superficially on the flexor aspect of the forearm, with positive and negative controls on the same arm. If the lower concentrations are negative, 10-fold increases in concentration, up to a maximum of 1.0 μg/ml, are tested. Although the argument has been made that the 1.0 μg/ml concentration is too strong for highly specific results (positive tests that are correlated with the severity of a patient's reaction),[21] the 0.1 μg/ml concentration is not sufficiently sensitive to detect more than 80% of patients with prior systemic reactions.[45] Furthermore, some have pushed the maximum skin test concentration of venom to 3.0 μg/ml. Even at this concentration, not enough antigen is introduced in the skin testing procedure to result in an increase in serum or cell-bound IgE venom antibodies.

There is some question about choosing a suitable time for skin testing. The theory has been advanced that a systemic allergic reaction may result in a temporary refractory state, such that tests performed soon after a reaction may be falsely negative. This refractory state is believed to resemble the condition of a patient after a successful, rapid desensitization procedure (such as might be done with penicillin in a penicillin-allergic patient). In the case of rapid desensitization, it is thought that the subject becomes desensitized (or refractory to allergen challenge) by one or more of several mechanisms: (1) saturation of all cell-bound antigen-specific IgE antibodies with antigen tightly bound from the prior reaction; (2) depletion of intracellular mediators during the preceding reaction, so that the quantity of mediators that remain is not sufficient to support a clinically apparent reaction; and (3) down-regulation of the signal transduction mechanisms, resulting in failure of the mediator secretory process. It is thought that one or more of these conditions may exist in a patient who has recently experienced a systemic allergic reaction.

Crossed Sensitization and Shared Antigens Among Venoms

As noted previously, the venoms of different members of the vespid superfamily contain structurally homologous proteins that have extensive immunologic cross-reactivity. Whether crossed sensitization can result in clinically relevant cross-reactivity has not been established. Patients whose sting reactions were caused by yellow jackets may exhibit positive skin tests when tested with other vespid venoms, presumably because of the homology of the authentic with the cross-reacting antigens. Whether this degree of cross-reactivity is sufficient to result in clinically relevant cross-reactivity to accidental stings is not really known. However, it is known that patients with positive skin tests to yellow jacket and to Polistes, and whose Polistes RAST is inhibited by the addition of yellow jacket venom, fail to react to a Polistes challenge after immunization solely with yellow jacket venom.[34]

RAST Inhibition to Detect Cross-Sensitivity

RAST is a legitimate serologic test that may be applied to venom allergy if appropriate reagents, duplicates, and controls are used. Hamilton and Adkinson[40] have developed a variant of this test that provides the clinician with information that is not only qualitative but also quantitative and reproducible.

The technique of RAST inhibition, in which authentic antigen (e.g., yellow jacket venom) is allowed to react with a patient's antibody-containing serum prior to addition of the possibly cross-reacting venom (e.g., Polistes wasp), has been used to enable the practitioner to eliminate one or more venoms from a patient's immunotherapy prescription.[41] In the example given, Polistes antigen would be prevented from binding to the patient's serum because of prior binding of yellow jacket antigens to the antibodies in the test mixture. In other words, if the binding of patient serum to the Polistes venom-labeled substrate in the performance of the Polistes RAST could be reduced by 90% or more through the addition of yellow jacket venom, this result could be interpreted to mean that the vast majority of the binding of Polistes antigen to patient serum was due to cross-reactivity.

Positive History and Negative Skin Test

It has been reported that a small number of patients with negative venom skin tests but positive histories for insect sting reactions have subsequently reacted to accidental stings.[93] It is not known whether these patients would have had a positive RAST at the time of their negative skin tests. In other reports, up to 10% of history-positive, skin-test negative patients had a positive RAST or venom-induced basophil histamine release in vitro. In general, venom-induced basophil histamine release correlates well with skin testing.[101]

ACUTE TREATMENT OF STING REACTIONS

Minor local swelling and pruritus is expected and can be treated with ice and antihistamines. If present, the imbedded stinger should be flicked off with a scraping motion. Some authorities believe that one should not grasp the fleshy venom sac to extract the stinger since more venom might then be injected through the stinger. However, Schumacher and colleagues[88] showed that essentially the entire honeybee venom load is injected in less than 20 seconds.

If a generalized reaction occurs, epinephrine is the keystone of management. Epinephrine halts the further release of mediators and reverses many of the effects of released mediators. Other measures commonly employed in the treatment of anaphylaxis include oxygen, inhaled sympathomimetics, intravenous fluids, pressor agents, and antiarrhythmics.

Epinephrine

Most systemic allergic reactions will be reversed promptly after the administration of a single, subcutaneously injected dose of epinephrine. The adult dose is 0.3 mg (0.3 cc of a 1:1,000 dilution). Although a larger dose may be required if the patient is taking a β-receptor blocking agent, it is usually better to repeat the 0.3 mg dose in 10 to 15 minutes if the first dose does not appear effective or if there is no effect on the pulse rate. Larger initial doses usually add nothing except unpleasant side effects, which may lead patients to claim that they are allergic to epinephrine. Epinephrine, even administered intravenously in a 1:10,000 concentration, may be ineffective in profound anaphylactic shock, unless the functional hypovolemia of this state is corrected with intravenous fluid.[99] Some authorities have suggested that military anti-shock trousers, which help to reverse peripheral blood pooling, may be useful if epinephrine is ineffective.[37] The pediatric dose of epinephrine, based on weight, is .01 mg/kg, up to a maximum of 0.3 mg. Over-the-counter epinephrine inhalers are sold for self-treatment of self-diagnosed asthma. Although inhaled epinephrine may reach the systemic circulation, it is doubtful whether the 0.1 mg (per puff) inhaled dose, or two or three puffs, would be sufficient to reverse the signs of systemic anaphylaxis. Glucagon administration, which stimulates secretion of endogenous catecholamines, has been suggested for patients with pharmacologic blockade of their β receptors and patients unresponsive to subcutaneous epinephrine.[78]

Risk/Benefit Analysis

In older adults, who may have significant, sometimes undiagnosed, cardiovascular disease, the potential risk of adverse cardiovascular side effects from the administration of epinephrine must be weighed against the consequences of inadequately treated anaphylaxis. Well-meaning but misguided medical personnel may try to save a patient the cost of a commercially prepared kit by preparing a disposable plastic syringe with a premeasured dose of epinephrine. This is inadvisable, as the epinephrine in such kits will likely oxidize within minutes or hours; the epinephrine in commercial kits is packed under nitrogen to prevent premature spoilage. Pharmacologic β-receptor blockade presents a problem: the patient who needs a β-blocker often also needs immunotherapy, and epinephrine might be required in the event of a reaction to therapy.[54]

Kits Available

Center Laboratories distributes the Epi-Pen (0.3 mg epinephrine) and Epi-Pen Jr (0.15 mg dose); these are spring-actuated autoinjectors manufactured by Survival Technology, a firm experienced in the manufacture of autoinjectors of various types. The Ana-Kit and Ana-Guard (Miles/Hollister-Stier) provide a syringe loaded with two doses of 0.3 mg of epinephrine. Although these kits require self-injection, they also permit the administration of fractional doses. Physicians who prescribe a self-injectable epinephrine kit should ensure that patients understand the indications and technique for its use.

PREVENTION OF FUTURE STING REACTIONS

Although one would think it unnecessary, sensitized individuals should be advised to take positive steps to avoid stings. Common sense measures include avoidance of areas where insect nests are known to exist, use of fragrance-free cosmetics and toiletries, and avoidance of uniformly dark clothing or clothing with floral prints. Patients should avoid eating outdoors, in picnic areas, and in garbage disposal areas. Hands, feet, and other body parts should not be placed where patients have not first looked for insects or insect nests. Closed shoes are preferred to bare feet, open-toed shoes, or sandals. Nests near a patient's residence should be removed or exterminated professionally.

SELECTION OF PATIENTS FOR VIT

Evidence for the presence of IgE antibody, either in vivo by skin test or in vitro by RAST, is a prerequisite for recommending VIT.

Challenge Stings

Because not every patient with IgE antibody to venom and a prior history of a sting reaction will react when subjected to a challenge sting from a relevant insect, some authorities (notably Europeans) favor including a positive response to a challenge sting in the list of treatment prerequisites.[63] Although sharp differences of opinion still exist on this topic, most physicians believe that a challenge sting presents too great a risk, even if omitting this procedure leads to the treatment of an excess of patients.[60, 65, 74, 81]

Systemic Reaction History

Patients selected for prophylactic VIT should have had at least one prior systemic reaction to a sting. The use of VIT should be considered in patients with a history of a sting-induced systemic reaction and skin test or in vitro evidence of venom-specific IgE.

Age

Valentine and colleagues[105] demonstrated that children who have had mild reactions (cutaneous symptoms such as itching, hives, or angioedema of lips) have only a 5% to 10% risk of any reaction to a future sting and thus do not generally require VIT. Many physicians believe that it is unnecessary to offer immunotherapy to such individuals. However, most feel that if a child's prior reaction has been vascular or respiratory, immunotherapy should be employed. Some practitioners have applied the pediatric experience to young adults and recommend withholding VIT from young, otherwise healthy adults whose systemic reactions to stings have been limited to the skin. This practice, however, is not based on controlled observation but is simply an application of data obtained in a population of children to a biologically different group of subjects, in which the outcome may eventually be unanticipated.

Multiple Stings

Individuals reacting systemically only after multiple stings may react because of the large allergen burden and might not react to the amount of venom in a single sting. There are no hard data on this point, but this seems to have occurred in patients who have done well without the intervention of immunotherapy.

The controlled trial of VIT in 1976 demonstrated that 60% of adults with a history of sting-induced anaphylaxis and positive venom skin tests (VST) treated only with placebo injections experienced a recurrent reaction when subjected to a challenge sting. As noted previously, van der Linden and colleagues[63] reported the results of a 10-year study in which individuals were stung intentionally; a systemic reaction was used as the criterion for initiating VIT. Of 272 patients with a history of anaphylaxis after a yellow jacket sting, only 68 (25%) reacted to the in-hospital challenge sting. The recurrence rate was somewhat higher (27 of 52, 52%) for honeybee-sensitized patients. However, other Dutch investigators employing a similar protocol found that a significant proportion of patients who tolerated a first challenge sting without a systemic reaction subsequently reacted to a second challenge.[19] Furthermore, although it may be safe to intentionally sting individuals who have a history of mild or moderate reactions, the procedure appears to be too risky for patients who have had more severe reactions in the past. In van der Linden's study, patients with histories of the most severe type of anaphylaxis (involving hypotension) had the highest recurrence rate of systemic reactions following challenge stings (32%), and more than half of these were again rated as severe.

Sting-induced large local reactions probably involve an allergic mechanism (85% have positive VST). However, VIT is rarely recommended for these patients because the risk of subsequent systemic reactions is low (2%–10%) and the morbidity of large local reactions is usually not severe enough to warrant the attendant risks of VIT.

A positive VST or RAST without a history of a sting-induced generalized allergic reaction is not an indication for therapy. Golden has found that as many as one fourth of the population may have evidence for IgE antibodies to venom. This situation is probably transient, but the appropriate prospective studies that would predict risk have not been done.

SELECTION OF VENOMS FOR IMMUNOTHERAPY

Formerly, immunotherapy was carried out with WBE. The standard of practice changed when it was shown that WBE treatment was no more effective than placebo. Since the immune response to insect stings is relatively specific for the venom proteins of particular species of Hymenoptera, it is appropriate medically and financially to narrow the choice of venoms as much as possible.

Although H. Mueller (personal communication) was fond of relating anecdotes that illustrated how difficult it may be for patients to identify the type of insect that stung them, the detailed history of the sting may help incriminate a specific species. The geographic locale of the sting, as well as the appearance and location of the insect nest, may be useful in classifying the type of insect responsible for a sting reaction. For example, honeybees are common causes of stings among agricultural workers and where commercial or amateur gardens are located. House painters and air-conditioner service workers often disturb nests of Polistes wasps. Yellow jacket nests are usually found buried in soil, compost, or mulch or in niches in masonry walls; hornet nests are found in shrubs or suspended from the lower branches of trees. Polistes wasp stings are more common in the deep South, as are fire ant stings. Other stinging insects are found in more exotic locations, such as Polistes metricus on the island of Kwajalein in the Pacific and in southern Asia (M. Guralnick, personal communication). Of course, positive identification by an entomologist is most helpful whenever possible.

The exception to the statement made previously about the usefulness of venom therapy versus treatment with WBE is that extracts of imported fire ant bodies are effective in treating individuals with anaphylactic sensitivity to stings from these aggressive insects.

REGIMENS OF IMMUNOTHERAPY

The venom package insert suggests a series of 15 weekly injections commencing at 0.05 μg, progressing gradually to the usual maintenance dose of 100 μg of each venom prescribed. All venoms are administered separately except for mixed vespid venom, which is a combination of equal amounts of yellow jacket, yellow hornet, and white-faced hornet venoms; the usual maintenance dose for the mixture of three vespid venoms is 300 μg. Hunt and colleagues[44–46] employed a modified rush protocol in which several doses were given at each of the first two visits. This protocol was well tolerated and served to shorten the buildup phase; the maintenance dose was achieved in 6 weeks. Subsequently, the interval between maintenance injections is increased by 1-week increments to 4 weeks, after which the injections are given every 4 weeks for the first 6 to 12 months. A modification of this schedule is shown in Table 39–2. Generally, the interval between venom injections is lengthened to 6 or 8 weeks in the second year. In Israel, Goldberg and colleagues[22] studied 28 children and adults in whom the VIT injection interval was increased to 3 months after receiving monthly injections for a mean duration of 17 months. Nineteen honeybee-allergic subjects tolerated a challenge sting after 6 to 38 months (mean 18 months) of 3-month injection intervals. In another study, Golden[34] found greater immunity to sting challenge with yellow jackets and higher levels of serum IgG antibody against yellow jacket venom in patients immunized with mixed vespid venoms than in those immunized with yellow jacket venom alone.

Although Yunginger[5] reported unsatisfactory results with a rush VIT protocol in which 11 of 20 patients required

TABLE 39–2
MODIFIED PROTOCOL FOR VENOM IMMUNOTHERAPY

Day	Venom Concentration (μg/ml)	Volume (ml)	Dose (μg)
1	1.0	0.1	0.1
	20 minutes later if negligible local reaction:		
	10.0	0.1	1.0
8	10.0	0.5	5.0
	20 minutes later if local reaction negligible:		
	100.0	0.1	10.0
15	100	0.2	20.0
22	100	0.4	40.0
29	100	0.7	70.0
36	100	1.0	100
43	100	1.0	100*
	Skip 1 Week		
57	100	1.0	100
	Skip 2 Weeks		
71	100	1.0	100
	Skip 3 Weeks		
92	100	1.0	100

*Check venom-specific IgG. If ≥3.5 μg/ml, proceed with schedule. If not, consider gradually increasing venom dose to 150 or 200 μg. Continue giving maintenance doses every 4 weeks. Recheck IgG antibody levels at 6 months, when schedule can be renegotiated.

Courtesy of Johns Hopkins Asthma and Allergy Center.

treatment with epinephrine for injection-induced reactions,[107] variations on this theme have been popular in Europe, particularly when a patient presents for evaluation shortly before the next stinging season. Some protocols have combined the administration of venom antibody–rich sera with rush VIT.[9, 56, 57, 73] Bernstein and colleagues[6] extended their observations on rush VIT. Seventy-seven patients received a cumulative dose of 58.55 μg of venom on treatment day 1, followed by doses of 70, 80, 90, and 100 μg on days 3, 7, 14, and 21, respectively. Only four patients had reactions on day 1, and all were mild.

The maintenance dose of venom has been the subject of some debate.[82, 83] The notion that 100 μg of venom is an appropriate maintenance or target immunotherapy dose was originally based on observations made in preparation for immunization of the child described by Lichtenstein and colleagues.[59] When dried stings from honeybees were collected after bees were individually induced to deposit their venom on plastic wrap by the patient's father (a professional beekeeper), the dried droplets had a mean weight of 50 μg. It had been reasoned that if immunized patients could tolerate twice the venom in a single sting, then they could be considered relatively immune. Considering Reisman's opinion that satisfactory results are obtained with a 50 μg top dose, it seems apparent that there must be a range of IgG responses elicited in different patients by different venom doses. Indeed, Golden and colleagues[23] found that only 79% of subjects who were brought to a 50 μg target dose were protected from challenge sting–induced systemic reactions.

Antigen (venom)-specific IgG blocking antibodies appear in the serum of most venom-immunized patients. Binding of venom antigens to IgG antibodies in the circulation, and thus de facto inactivation of venom proteins as circulating antigens, remains the most likely mechanism by which venom immunotherapy leads to lessening of a patient's susceptibility to a reaction to a sting, at least early in the course of treatment.[23] Other theories have been advanced dealing with the possibility that the development of autoantibodies[50] and anti-idiotypic antibodies[51] during the course of venom immunotherapy might be beneficial. Studies of passive immunotherapy support the IgG hypothesis. Lessof and colleagues[56] identified five honeybee-allergic individuals who suffered systemic reactions, ranging from angioedema to respiratory distress, when subjected to subcutaneous injections of honeybee venom in doses of 10 to 100 μg. Soon after intramuscular or intravenous administration of the gamma globulin fraction of pooled beekeepers' serum containing a high antihoneybee venom blocking antibody titer, the same subjects tolerated 1.5 to 5 times the previous symptom-eliciting venom dose without reactions.

EFFICACY OF TREATMENT AND MECHANISM OF PROTECTION

Ninety-seven percent of patients treated with venoms are protected from significant systemic allergic reactions as judged by their response to a challenge sting. However, a placebo-controlled trial of immunotherapy found that more than half of previously reacting patients will fail to react to challenge stings without benefit of immunotherapy. Among immunized patients, those who continue to react to stings generally have exceptionally small increases in their venom-specific IgG antibodies.[26] Such a paucity of IgG antibodies can usually be remedied by an increase in venom dosage (1.5–2 times the usual dose) or frequency of administration. Since there are so few treatment failures with VIT, it may not be cost effective to perform venom IgG antibody assays on all immunized patients.[84] Even so, most patients prefer to know whether they are at greater risk of reactions to stings despite venom immunotherapy. Patients occasionally wish to have a challenge sting in the clinic setting to demonstrate immunity. If undertaken, this should be done with all the necessary precautions as if it were assumed the challenge would result in a life-threatening reaction. Several investigators have observed that neither skin-test reactivity to venom nor serum IgE or IgG antivenom antibodies bear any relation to immunity to stings in patients who have undergone prolonged (>4 years) VIT.[50] In immunized patients, there is a gradual shift toward the selective production of IgG4 antibodies.[1]

DURATION OF THERAPY

The optimal duration of venom treatment for prophylaxis of recurrent sting-induced systemic reactions has not been determined. When VIT was first introduced and found to be extremely effective, it was assumed that it would be administered indefinitely. However, it was eventually observed that there might be a relatively favorable outcome of stings in individuals who had stopped VIT for reasons of cost or inconvenience. Those reports suggest an intermediate risk of sting-induced systemic reactions of about 25% in patients who prematurely discontinue VIT. This contrasts with the 1% to 3% risk in patients treated for 4 or more years and the 40% to 60% risk in patients never treated.

Various indications for stopping VIT have been considered. Loss of allergic sensitization determined by either VST or measurement of venom-specific IgE levels occurs in some patients. Over time, VST may become negative in 5% to 29% of patients. Randolph and Reisman[79] discontinued VIT in patients whose venom-specific IgE levels had fallen to insignificant levels; they experienced a 5% reaction rate per sting. Most authorities consider the ablation of allergic sensitization the most obvious indication for stopping VIT. However, as noted, only a minority of patients develop a negative VST or unmeasurable levels of venom-specific IgE. Therefore, many researchers have selected a duration of treatment as a parameter for discontinuing VIT.

Golden and colleagues at Johns Hopkins prospectively studied 30 patients who agreed to stop VIT after 5 or more years of injections. Sting challenges performed after 12 months without VIT resulted in no systemic reactions to 29 yellow jacket and 3 honeybee stings.[23] A follow-up report of 74 patients who had been treated with venom injections for 5 to 8 years and then repeatedly subjected to challenge stings every 1 to 2 years noted sting reactions in 7 (10%) of the patients. An update provided further data on these patients.[30, 33] Of the 74 patients who were stung after stopping VIT of 5 or more years duration, systemic symptoms occurred in 8 of 270 stings (3% of stings) and 7 (9%) of the patients. All of the eight systemic reactions included pruritus and erythema, one had urticaria and angioedema, one had scattered urticaria, and two had solitary urticarial lesions. Seven patients had subjective symptoms only.[31] Schuberth and colleagues[86] reported similar results in children.

Mayo Clinic researchers studied 51 patients aged 9 to 67 years who stopped VIT after 2 to 10 years (mean 5 years) of treatment. All patients had tolerated challenge stings at the conclusion of therapy. One year later, challenge stings caused systemic reactions in 2 of the 51 patients. One patient had only itching of the face and neck, but the other suffered hypotension and difficulty breathing. VIT was resumed in both. Both patients who reacted had the most severe grade of reaction before VIT and received VIT for a shorter than average length of time (2 and 4 years). Subsequently, 16, 11, 2, and 2 patients underwent sting challenges 2, 3, 4, and 5 years, respectively, after VIT was discontinued. No further reactions occurred.[48]

European researchers have also investigated the outcome of deliberately discontinuing VIT.[75] Haugaard and colleagues[42] studied 25 primarily yellow jacket–sensitive adults treated with VIT for 36 to 83 months (mean 43 months). No systemic reactions resulted from 21 yellow jacket and 7 honeybee challenge stings administered 12 to 36 months (mean 25 months) after the conclusion of VIT. Müller and colleagues[72] reported on 86 honeybee-sensitive children and adults with severe reactions before VIT who received VIT for 3 to 10 years. A challenge sting 10 to 24 months (mean 13 months) later resulted in only normal local reactions in 71 patients (83%).

Currently, there are no accepted guidelines for practicing allergists concerning discontinuation of VIT. A report from a multispecialty group practice setting suggests that VIT should be continued indefinitely in only a small minority of patients.[36] Of 204 patients in whom VIT was initiated between 1978 and 1986 only 12 (6%) were still receiving venom injections in 1992 when the population was surveyed. Approximately equal proportions of patients had discontinued VIT because of patient preference or physician recommendation. Several researchers have found that patients with severe reactions before VIT are more likely to react to stings after VIT has been discontinued. Some observers have suggested that VIT should be continued indefinitely, especially for patients with a history of more severe reactions. If venom maintenance injections can be spaced every 2 to 3 months, this would greatly diminish the associated inconvenience. When VIT is stopped after 5 or more years, the risk of a subsequent sting reaction increases from 1% to 3% to about 5% to 10%. Whether that degree of an increased reaction rate warrants further administration of VIT is best decided jointly by the patient and physician, considering the severity of the reaction before VIT, age, occupation, and other factors.

REACTIONS TO IMMUNOTHERAPY

Although many expect venom to result in more frequent or more severe reactions when employed in immunotherapy, the range of reactions to VIT is no different from that to immunotherapy with other allergens, nor are reactions more frequent.[58] Although some allergists seem to fear reactions to VIT more than reactions to pollen immunotherapy, this may be because there is too little awareness of the potential severity of the latter.[66] The safety of VIT during pregnancy was studied by Schwartz and colleagues,[92] who found that neither mother nor fetus was compromised by the treatment. However, although it seems safe and probably even desirable for pregnant women to maintain their venom immunity by continuing an established regimen of venom injections, it is probably wise to avoid initiating any type of immunotherapy during a known pregnancy in order to avoid the occasional systemic allergic reactions that may occur with any immunotherapy regimen.

Occasionally, a patient may seem to react adversely and objectively to nearly every attempt at venom immunotherapy. If the reactions are systemic and severe, one must decide whether to continue attempts at immunotherapy. In general, if any immunotherapy reaction is potentially life threatening, very careful consideration must be given to discontinuing therapy and placing reliance instead on sting avoidance and prompt use of an emergency kit if an accidental sting occurs. Before therapy is stopped, the treatment regimen may be modified to provide smaller increases in venom dosage than those seen in the usual regimen. Both slow and fast dosage schedules are eventually associated with immunity to sting reactions. Although there is no ultimate advantage to any particular regimen, there are fewer total reactions to therapy if the faster regimen is used.

An intermediate position is to adopt the tactic of attempting to block the symptoms of a reaction by pretreatment of the patient with mediator antagonists and steroids, as is recommended in anticipation of a reaction to the intravenous administration of iodinated radiographic contrast materials. Essentially, H_1 and H_2 histamine receptor blockers, with or without prednisone, are given 13 hours before treatment, 60 minutes before treatment, and 11 hours later if needed.[38, 39, 61] Another tactic employed in special circumstances in patients sensitive only to honeybees was suggested by the studies of combined active and passive immunotherapy, utilizing IgG antibodies from beekeepers' serum. After the beekeepers' antivenom IgG was given to patients sensitive to bee stings, honeybee venom was administered to patients who previously had not tolerated venom alone. When such measures fail to prevent reactions, one must weigh the benefit against the risk of morbidity from VIT.

REFERENCES

1. Ameno S, Ameno K, Fuke C, et al: Hymenoptera sting anaphylaxis: detection and clinical significance of individual bee and wasp venoms specific IgE and IgG4 antibodies. Nippon Hoigaku Zasshi 47(3):207–212, 1993.
2. Barnard JH: Studies of 400 Hymenoptera sting deaths in the United States. J Allergy Clin Immunol 52:259, 1973.
3. Benson RL, Semenov H: Allergy in its relation to the bee sting. J Allergy 1:105, 1930.
4. Benton AW, Morse RA, Stewart JD: Venom collection from honeybees. Science 142:228, 1963.
5. Berchtold E, Maibach R, Müller U: Reduction of side effects with rush-immunotherapy with honeybee venom by pretreatment with terfenadine. Clin Exp Allergy 22:59–65, 1992.
6. Bernstein DI, Mittman RJ, Kagen SL, et al: Clinical and immunologic studies of rapid venom immunotherapy in Hymenoptera-sensitive patients. J Allergy Clin Immunol 84:951–959, 1989.
7. Birnbaum J, Vervloet D, Charpin D: Atopy and systemic reactions to Hymenoptera stings. Allergy Proc 15:49–52, 1994.
8. Bousquet J, Huchard G, Michel FB: Toxic reactions induced by Hymenoptera venom. Ann Allergy 52:371–374, 1984.
9. Bousquet J, Fontez A, Aznar R, et al: Combination of passive and active immunization in honeybee venom immunotherapy. J Allergy Clin Immunol 79:947–954, 1987.
10. Braun LIB: Notes on desensitization of a patient hypersensitive to bee stings. S Afr Med Rec 23:408, 1925.
11. Candiotti KA, Lamas AM: Adverse neurologic reactions to the sting of the imported fire ant. Int Arch Allergy Immunol 102(4):417–420, 1993.
12. Chafee FH: The prevalence of bee sting allergy in an allergic population. Acta Allergol (Copenh) 25:292, 1970.
13. Charpin D, Birnbaum J, Lanteaume A, Vervloet D: Prevalence of allergy to Hymenoptera stings in different samples of the general population. J Allergy Clin Immunol 90:331–334, 1992.
14. deShazo RD, Butcher BT, Banks WA: Reactions to the stings of the imported fire ant. N Engl J Med 323:462–466, 1990.
15. deShazo RD, Griffing C, Kwan TH, et al: Dermal hypersensitivity reactions to imported fire ants. J Allergy Clin Immunol 74:841–847, 1984.
16. Fernandez J, Rodes F, Marti J, Blanca M: Wasp sting anaphylaxis as a cause of death: A case report. Allergol Immunopathol (Madrid) 20:40–41, 1992.
17. Fortenberry JE, Laine J, Shalit M: Use of epinephrine for anaphylaxis by emergency medical technicians in a wilderness setting. Ann Emerg Med 25:785–787, 1995.
18. Franca FO, Benvenuti LA, Fan HW, et al: Severe and fatal mass attacks by 'killer' bees (Africanized honey bees—Apis mellifera scutellata) in Brazil: clinicopathological studies with measurement of serum venom concentrations. Q J Med 87(5):269–282, 1994.
19. Franken HH, Dubois AEJ, Minkena ITJ, et al: Lack of reproducibility of a single negative sting challenge response in the assessment of anaphylactic risk in patients with suspected yellow jacket sensitivity. J Allergy Clin Immunol 93:431–436, 1994.
20. Freeman TM: Imported fire ants: the ants from hell! Allergy Proc 15(1):11–15, 1994.
21. Georgitis JW, Reisman RE: Venom skin tests in insect-allergic and insect-nonallergic populations. J Allergy Clin Immunol 76:803–807, 1985.
22. Goldberg A, Confino-Cohen R, Mekori YA: Deliberate bee sting challenge of patients receiving maintenance venom immunotherapy at 3-month intervals. J Allergy Clin Immunol 93:997–1001, 1954.
23. Golden DBK, Johnson K, Addison BI, et al: Clinical and immunologic

observations in patients who stop venom immunotherapy. J Allergy Clin Immunol 77:435–442, 1986.
24. Golden DB: Epidemiology of allergy to insect venoms and stings. Allergy Proc 10:103–107, 1989.
25. Golden DBK, Valentine MD: Allergen-specific IgG antibody measurements in the management of immediate hypersensitivity to Hymenoptera venoms. J Clin Immunoassay 6:172–176, 1983.
26. Golden DB, Lawrence ID, Hamilton RG, et al: Clinical correlation of the venom-specific IgG antibody level during maintenance venom. J Allergy Clin Immunol 90:386–393, 1992.
27. Golden DB, Kagey-Sobotka A, Valentine MD, Lichtenstein LM: Dose dependence of Hymenoptera venom immunotherapy. J Allergy Clin Immunol 67(5):370–374, 1981.
28. Golden DBK, Valentine MD: Allergen-specific IgG antibody measurements in the management of immediate hypersensitivity to Hymenoptera venoms. J Clin Immunoassay 6:172–176, 1983.
29. Golden DB, Meyers DA, Kagey-Sobotka A, et al: Clinical relevance of the venom-specific immunoglobulin G antibody level during immunotherapy. J Allergy Clin Immunol 69:489–493, 1982.
30. Golden DBK, Kwiterovich KA, Kagey-Sobotka A, et al: Discontinuing venom immunotherapy (VIT): outcome after five years. J Allergy Clin Immunol 97:579–587, 1996.
31. Golden DBK, Kwiterovich KA, Valentine MD, et al: Risk and benefit of discontinuing venom immunotherapy (VIT) after 5 years. J Allergy Clin Immunol 87:237, 1991. Abstract.
32. Golden DB, Marsh DG, Kagey-Sobotka A, et al: Epidemiology of insect venom sensitivity. JAMA 262:240–244, 1989.
33. Golden DBK, Kwiterovich KA, Kagey-Sobotka A, et al: Discontinuing venom immunotherapy (VIT): determinants of clinical reactivity. J Allergy Clin Immunol 83:273, 1989. Abstract.
34. Golden DB: Guidelines for venom immunotherapy. Ann Allergy 61:159–161, 1988.
35. Graft DF, Schuberth KC, Kagey-Sobotka A, et al: A prospective study of the natural history of large local reactions after Hymenoptera stings in children. J Pediatr 104:664–668, 1984.
36. Graft DF, Schoenwetter WF: Insect sting allergy: analysis of a cohort of patients who initiated venom immunotherapy from 1978 to 1986. Ann Allergy 73:481–485, 1994.
37. Granata AV, Halickman JF, Borak J: Utility of military anti-shock trousers (MAST) in anaphylactic shock—a case report. J Emerg Med 2(5):349–351, 1985.
38. Greenberger PA: Contrast media reactions. J Allergy Clin Immunol 74:600–605, 1984.
39. Greenberger PA, Halwig JM, Patterson R, Wallemark CB: Emergency administration of radiocontrast media in high-risk patients. J Allergy Clin Immunol 77:630–634, 1986.
40. Hamilton RG, Adkinson NF Jr: Clinical laboratory methods for the assessment and management of human allergic diseases. Clin Lab Med 6:117–138, 1986.
41. Hamilton RG, Wisenauer JA, Golden DB, et al: Selection of Hymenoptera venoms for immunotherapy on the basis of patient's IgE antibody cross-reactivity. J Allergy Clin Immunol 92:651–659, 1993.
42. Haugaard L, Norregard OFH, Dahl R: In-hospital sting challenge in insect venom-allergic patients after stopping venom immunotherapy. J Allergy Clin Immunol 87:699, 1991.
43. Hoffman DR, Dove DE, Moffitt JE, Stafford CT: Allergens in Hymenoptera venom. XXI. Cross-reactivity and multiple reactivity between fire ant venom and bee and wasp venoms. J Allergy Clin Immunol 82:828–834, 1988.
44. Hunt KJ, Sobotka AK, Valentine MD, et al: Sensitization following Hymenoptera whole body extract therapy. J Allergy Clin Immunol 61:48–53, 1978.
45. Hunt KJ, Valentine MD, Sobotka AK, Lichtenstein LM: Diagnosis of allergy to stinging insects by skin testing with Hymenoptera venoms. Ann Intern Med 85:56–59, 1976.
46. Hunt KJ, Valentine MD, Sobotka AK, et al: A controlled trial of immunotherapy in insect hypersensitivity. N Engl J Med 299:157–161, 1978.
47. Kagey-Sobotka A: Personal communication.
48. Keating MU, Kagey-Sobotka A, Hamilton RG, Yunginger JW: Clinical and immunologic follow-up of patients who stop venom immunotherapy. J Allergy Clin Immunol 88:339–348, 1991.
49. Kemeny DM, Tomioka H, Tsutsumi A, et al: The relationship between anti-IgE auto-antibodies and the IgE response to wasp venom during immunotherapy. Clin Exp Allergy 20:67–69, 1990.
50. Kemeny DM, Lessof MH, Patel S, et al: IgG and IgE antibodies after immunotherapy with bee and wasp venom. Int Arch Allergy Appl Immunol 88:247–249, 1989.
51. Khan RH, Szewczuk MR, Day JH: Bee venom anti-idiotypic antibody is associated with protection in beekeepers and bee sting-sensitive patients receiving immunotherapy against allergic reactions. J Allergy Clin Immunol 88(2):199–208, 1991.
52. King TP: Insect venom allergens. Monogr Allergy 28:84–100, 1990.
53. King TP, Valentine MD: Allergens of hymenopteran venoms. Clin Rev Allergy 5:137–148, 1987.
54. Kivity S, Yarchovsky J: Relapsing anaphylaxis to bee sting in a patient treated with beta-blocker and Ca blocker. J Allergy Clin Immunol 85:669–670, 1990.
55. Kochuyt AM, Van Hoeyveld E, Stevens EA: Occupational allergy to bumble bee venom. Department of Internal Medicine, University Hospital of Leuven, Belgium. Clin Exp Allergy 23:190–195, 1993.
56. Lessof MH, Sobotka AK, Lichtenstein LM: Effects of passive antibody in bee venom anaphylaxis. Johns Hopkins Med J 142(1):1–7, 1978.
57. Lessof MH, Sobotka AK, Lichtenstein LM: Protection against anaphylaxis in Hymenoptera-sensitive patients by passive immunization. J Allergy Clin Immunol 57:246, 1976.
58. Levine MI: Systemic reactions to immunotherapy. J Allergy Clin Immunol 63:209, 1979.
59. Lichtenstein LM, Valentine MD, Sobotka AK: A case for venom treatment in anaphylactic sensitivity to Hymenoptera sting. N Engl J Med 290:1223–1227, 1974.
60. Lichtenstein LM: Comment on Reisman RE [letter] Insect sting challenges: Do no harm. J Allergy Clin Immunol 96:702–703, 1995.
61. Lieberman P: The use of antihistamines in the prevention and treatment of anaphylaxis and anaphylactoid reactions. J Allergy Clin Immunol 86:684–686, 1990.
62. Light WC, Reisman RE, Shimizu M, Arbesman CE: Unusual reactions following insect stings. Clinical features and immunologic analysis. J Allergy Clin Immunol 59:391–397, 1977.
63. van der Linden PW, Hack CE, Struyvenberg A, van der Zwan JK: Insect-sting challenge in 324 subjects with a previous anaphylactic reaction: current criteria for insect-venom hypersensitivity do not predict the occurrence and the severity of anaphylaxis. J Allergy Clin Immunol 94:151–159, 1994.
64. van der Linden PWG, Struyvenberg A, Kraaijenhagen RJ, et al: Anaphylactic shock after insect-sting challenge in 138 persons with a previous insect-sting reaction. Ann Intern Med 11:161–168, 1993.
65. van der Linden PWG, Hack CE, Struyvenberg A, van der Zwan JC: Comment on Novey HS [letter] Sting challenges as criteria for venom immunotherapy. J Allergy Clin Immunol 96:702–703, 1995.
66. Lockey RF, Benedict LM, Turkeltaub PC, Bukantz SC: Fatalities from immunotherapy and skin testing. J Allergy Clin Immunol 79:660–677, 1987.
67. Loveless MH: Wasp venom allergy and immunity. Ann Allergy 1956;14:347.
68. Lu G, Kochoumian L, King TP: Sequence identity and antigenic cross-reactivity of white face hornet venom allergen, also a hyaluronidase, with other proteins. J Biol Chem 270:4457–4465, 1995.
69. Lu G, Villalba M, Coscia MR, et al: Sequence analysis and antigenic cross-reactivity of a venom allergen, antigen 5, from hornets, wasps, and yellow jackets. J Immunol 150:2823–2830, 1993.
70. Mazza JA, Moote DW, Gamble JB, Young GB: Memory loss and pneumonitis after anaphylaxis due to an insect sting. Can Med Assoc J 144:175–176, 1991.
71. Mulfinger L, Yunginger J, Styer W, et al: Sting morphology and frequency of sting autotomy among medically important vespids (Hymenoptera: Vespidae) and the honey bee (Hymenoptera: Apidae). J Med Entomol 29:325–328, 1992.
72. Müller U, Berchtold E, Helbling A: Honeybee venom allergy: results of a sting challenge 1 year after stopping successful venom immunotherapy in 86 patients. J Allergy Clin Immunol 87:702–709, 1991.
73. Müller U, Morris T, Bischof M, et al: Combined active and passive immunotherapy in honeybee-sting allergy. J Allergy Clin Immunol 78:115–122, 1986.
74. Novey H: Sting challenges as criteria for venom immunotherapy. J Allergy Clin Immunol 96:703, 1995.
75. Oei HD, Stroes ES, Beukema WP, van der Zwan JC: When can desensitization with bee and wasp venom be stopped? Ned Tijdschr Geneeskd 135:719–720, 1991.
76. Pence HL, White AF, Cost K, et al: Evaluation of severe reactions to sweat bee stings. Ann Allergy 66:399–404, 1991.

77. Perkin RM, Anas NG: Mechanisms and management of anaphylactic shock not responding to traditional therapy. Ann Allergy 54:202–208, 1985.
78. Pollack CV Jr: Utility of glucagon in the emergency department. J Emerg Med 11:195–205, 1993.
79. Randolph CC, Reisman RE: Evaluation of decline in serum venom-specific IgE as a criterion for stopping venom immunotherapy. J Allergy Clin Immunol 77(6):823–827, 1986.
80. Reisman RE: Stinging insect allergy—treatment failures. J Allergy Clin Immunol 52:257–258, 1973.
81. Reisman RE: Insect sting challenges: do no harm. J Allergy Clin Immunol 96:702, 1995.
82. Reisman RE, Livingston A: Venom immunotherapy: 10 years of experience with administration of single venoms and 50 micrograms maintenance doses. J Allergy Clin Immunol 89:1189–1195, 1992.
83. Reisman RE: Venom hypersensitivity. J Allergy Clin Immunol 94:651–658, 1994.
84. Reisman RE: Should routine measurements of serum venom-specific IgG be a standard of practice in patients receiving venom immunotherapy? J Allergy Clin Immunol 90:282–284, 1992.
85. Sasvary T, Müller U: Fatalities from insect stings in Switzerland 1978 to 1987. Schweiz Med Wochenschr 124:1887–1894, 1994.
86. Schuberth KC, Kwiterovich KA, Kagey-Sobotka A, et al: Starting and stopping venom immunotherapy (VIT) in children with insect allergy. J Allergy Clin Immunol 81:200, 1988. Abstract.
87. Schumacher MJ, Schmidt JO, Egen NB, Lowry JE: Quantity, analysis, and lethality of European and Africanized honey bee venoms. Am J Trop Med Hyg 43(1):79–86, 1990.
88. Schumacher MJ, Tveten MS, Egen NB: Rate and quantity of delivery of venom from honeybee stings. J Allergy Clin Immunol 93:831–835, 1994.
89. Schwartz HJ: Skin sensitivity in insect allergy. JAMA 194:113, 1965.
90. Schwartz LB, Yunginger JW, Miller J, et al: Time course of appearance and disappearance of human mast cell tryptase in the circulation after anaphylaxis. J Clin Invest 83:1551–1555, 1989.
91. Schwartz HJ, Squillace DL, Sher TH, et al: Studies in stinging insect hypersensitivity: postmortem demonstration of antivenom IgE antibody in possible sting-related sudden death. Am J Clin Pathol 85:607–610, 1986.
92. Schwartz HJ, Golden DB, Lockey RF: Venom immunotherapy in the Hymenoptera-allergic pregnant patient. J Allergy Clin Immunol 85:709–712, 1990.
93. Selcow JE, Mendelson LM, Rosen JP: Anaphylactic reactions in skin test-negative patients. J Allergy Clin Immunol 65:400, 1980.
94. Settipane GA, Boyd GK: Prevalence of bee sting allergy in 4992 Boy Scouts. Acta Allergol 25:286, 1970.
95. Settipane GA, Chafee FH: Natural history of allergy to Hymenoptera. Clin Allergy 9:385–390, 1979.
96. Settipane GA, Newstead GJ, Boyd GK: Frequency of Hymenoptera allergy in an atopic and normal population. J Allergy Clin Immunol 50:146, 1972.
97. Shimizu T, Hori T: Evaluation of venom specific IgE and total serum IgE among forest administration workers. Arerugi 39:654–661, 1990.
98. Simon RP, Benton A: A method for mass collection of wasp venoms. Ann Entomol Soc Am 62:277–278, 1969.
99. Smith PL, Kagey-Sobotka A, Bleecker ER, et al: Physiologic manifestations of human anaphylaxis. J Clin Invest 66:1072, 1980.
100. Sobotka AK, Valentine MD, Ishizaka K, Lichtenstein LM: Measurement of IgG blocking antibodies: development and application of a radioimmunoassay. J Immunol 117:84–90, 1976.
101. Sobotka AK, Valentine MD, Benton AW, Lichtenstein LM: Allergy to insect stings. I. Diagnosis of IgE-mediated Hymenoptera sensitivity by venom-induced histamine release. J Allergy Clin Immunol 53:170–184, 1974.
102. Stephan V, Zimmermann A, Kuhr J, Urbanek R: Determination of N-methylhistamine in urine as an indicator of histamine release in immediate allergic reactions. J Allergy Clin Immunol 86:862–868, 1990.
103. Thueson DO, Rahr R, Findlay SR, et al: Diagnosis of Polistes sensitivity. J Allergy Clin Immunol 63:136, 1979.
104. Torsney PJ: Treatment failures: insect desensitization. J Allergy Clin Immunol 52:303–306, 1973.
105. Valentine MD, Schuberth KC, Kagey-Sobotka A, et al: The value of immunotherapy with venom in children with allergy to insect stings. N Engl J Med 323:1601–1603, 1990.
106. Valentine MD: Allergy to stinging insects. Ann Allergy 70(6):427–432, 1993.
107. Yunginger JW, Paull BR, Jones RT, Santrach PJ: Rush venom immunotherapy program for honeybee venom sensitivity. J Allergy Clin Immunol 63:340–347, 1979.
108. Yunginger JW, Nelson DR, Squillace DL, et al: Laboratory investigation of deaths due to anaphylaxis. J Forensic Sci 36(3):857–865, 1991.
109. Zeleznick LD, Hunt KJ, Sobotka AK, et al: Diagnosis of Hymenoptera hypersensitivity by skin testing with Hymenoptera venoms. J Allergy Clin Immunol 59:2–9, 1977.

IV Therapeutic Modalities

40 Sympathomimetic and Cholinergic Agents and Antagonists

ALBERT L. SHEFFER JONATHAN P. ARM LAWRENCE M. DU BUSKE

This chapter addresses the specific employment of adrenergic agents, including the nature of adrenergic receptors, use of β-agonists in asthma therapy, and routes of administration and adverse effects of such therapy, as well as the particular role of β_2-agonists. The parasympathetic innervation of the lung and use of anticholinergic agents in the treatment of asthma are then considered.

MOLECULAR STRUCTURE OF ADRENERGIC RECEPTORS

The classification of adrenergic receptors is based upon the physiologic effects of various agonists, studies of the activity and binding of agonists and antagonists, and the subsequent cloning of the cDNAs and elucidation of the deduced amino acid sequence of each receptor. Interest in asthma has focused mostly on the β_2-adrenergic receptor, which is widely distributed in the airways and principally mediates bronchodilatation of the airways.

STRUCTURE AND FUNCTION OF β_2-ADRENERGIC RECEPTORS

The adrenergic receptors are members of the large superfamily of G protein–coupled receptors, exemplified by rhodopsin, which are characterized by seven hydrophobic transmembrane domains (Fig. 40–1).[57] The function of the β_2-adrenergic receptor depends on its coupling to Gs, which in turn stimulates adenyl cyclase, leading to increased levels of cyclic AMP (cAMP) that acts as a second messenger mediating the physiologic functions of the receptor. At least part of the action of the β_2-adrenergic receptor on smooth muscle is to open large-conductance, calcium-activated potassium channels, via cAMP or directly through Gs.[157] Site-directed mutagenesis and deletional mutagenesis studies suggest that ligands bind within the hydrophobic core of the receptor (reviewed in ref. 135). Aspartic acid 113 (*D* in Fig. 40–1) in the third transmembrane domain is critical for ligand binding. Serines at positions 204 and 207 in the fifth transmembrane domain likely participate in ligand binding. Coupling to G proteins is mediated through the third cytoplasmic (Cyt) loop and the fifth and sixth transmembrane (TM) domains. The most carboxyl terminal portion of the third cytoplasmic loop confers G protein specificity.

DESENSITIZATION

Following receptor/ligand binding and signal transduction, the β_2-adrenergic receptor, in common with many other receptors, exhibits a period of reduced sensitivity to further stimulation.[91, 92] This process of desensitization has two principal phases. First, within seconds or minutes, there is un-

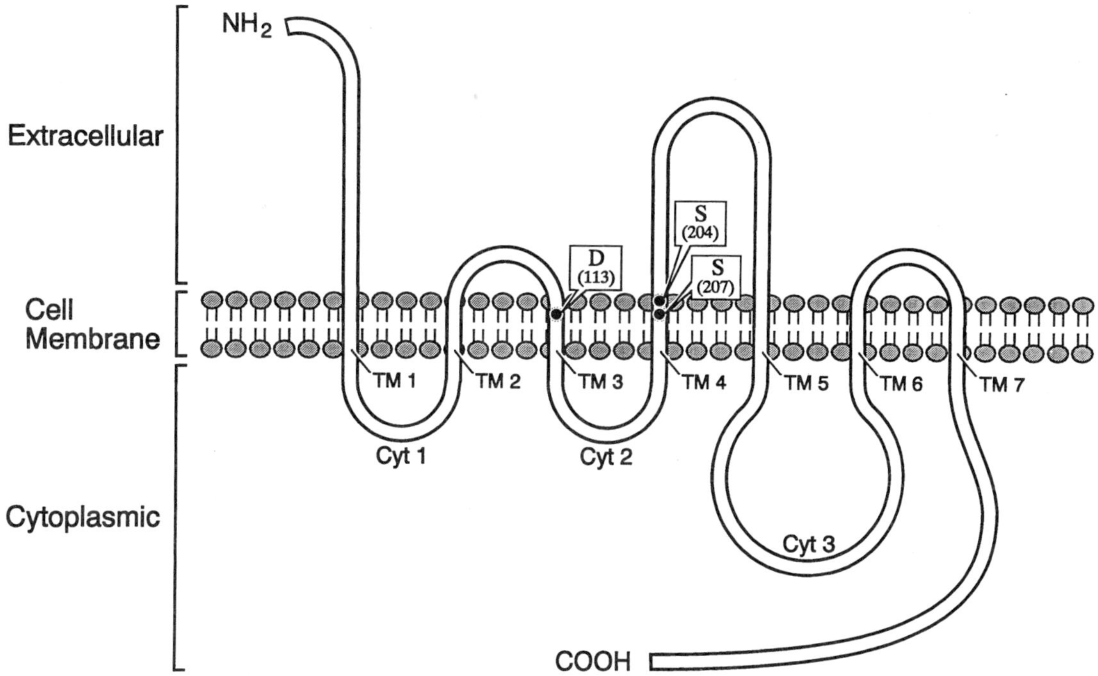

FIGURE 40–1. Molecular structure of β_2-adrenergic receptor.

coupling of the β_2-adrenergic receptor from Gs through phosphorylation of cytoplasmic residues.[91] This phosphorylation is mediated by cAMP-dependent protein kinase A and a receptor-specific kinase termed β_2-adrenergic receptor kinase (βARK) that is analogous to a specific rhodopsin kinase.[19] The activity of these specific kinases is dependent on binding of another protein termed arrestin—β_2 arrestin in the case of the β_2-adrenergic receptor.[18] Rapid uncoupling is rapidly reversible upon removal of the activating stimulus.

The second process of desensitization is termed down-regulation and requires continuous exposure to agonist for several hours. This process of down-regulation involves the internalization of the receptor and proteolytic digestion through a largely cAMP-independent mechanism.[46] cAMP may also contribute to down-regulation through decreasing the stability of the mRNA transcript for the β_2-adrenergic receptor, with a reduction in steady-state levels of the transcript.

Mechanisms also exist for inducing new synthesis of receptors.[46, 168] Short-term agonist stimulation increases β_2-adrenergic receptor transcription through the action of cAMP acting upon distinct cAMP response elements in the promotor/enhancer region of the gene. Thus cAMP may act to modulate expression of the β_2-adrenergic receptor, influencing both down-regulation and new synthesis of the receptor. A glucocorticoid response element has also been defined in the 5′ upstream sequence of the β_2-adrenergic receptor gene, mediating increased transcription of the gene in response to glucocorticoids, thus preventing homologous down-regulation of β_2 receptors.

DISTRIBUTION

β_2-Adrenergic receptors are widely distributed throughout the airways and are present on smooth muscle cells, epithelium, submucosal glands, alveoli, and prejunctional nerves, as well as numerous inflammatory cells that participate in the asthmatic process.[168] Although there is no direct innervation of human smooth muscle by adrenergic nerves, β_2-adrenergic receptors are plentiful. In contrast, pulmonary blood vessels have a rich sympathetic innervation. The principal effect of β_2-adrenergic receptor agonists is to stimulate β_2-adrenergic receptors on smooth muscle, leading to bronchodilatation. Although β_2-agonists may act to increase mucociliary clearance, increase airway mucus secretion, stimulate surfactant production, and modulate cholinergic neurotransmission, these effects are likely of minor importance compared with their action on smooth muscle.[11, 168]

PHARMACOLOGY OF β_2-ADRENERGIC RECEPTORS

Adrenergic receptors have been identified throughout the body. β-Adrenergic receptors execute a variety of functions. Originally classified by physiologic and pharmacologic assessments, recent cloning of the receptors has provided new insight into their pharmacology.

Ahlquist[1] proposed that adrenergic receptors could be classified into two types: α receptors, responding to epinephrine > norepinephrine > isoproterenol, and β receptors, responding to isoproterenol > epinephrine > norepinephrine. Stimulation of the α receptor induces smooth muscle contraction, whereas β-receptor stimulation induces relaxation.[108] Lands[124] further differentiated β-agonists into β_1 and β_2 subtypes. β_1 Receptors have an equal affinity for epinephrine and norepinephrine, whereas β_2 receptors have a greater affinity for epinephrine. These β_2 receptors occur throughout the body, whereas β_1 receptors are mainly in the myocardium.[27, 31] However, 50% of the atrial and ventricular β receptors are of the β_2 subtype.[27, 31]

In vitro selectivity is based on the measured effects on isolated guinea pig atrial (β_1) and tracheal (β_2) preparations. Potency is the concentration of the β-agonists producing 50% of the maximal response (EC50) assessed via dose response curves, whereas selectivity can be derived by comparing EC50 values of an agent on β_1- or β_2-mediated responses.[5]

Data emphasize in vitro assessment of β_2-agonists on cAMP modulation of mast cell mediator release. Anti-inflammatory effects have been ascribed to salmeterol and formoterol.[141] In vitro, these agents inhibit the release of inflammatory mediators from chopped, passively sensitized lung tissue and from stimulated alveolar macrophages.[156] Similar studies demonstrated a decrease in eosinophil activity.[51] Primary assessment by bronchial biopsy showed no effect of salmeterol on airway inflammation; however, other data suggest down-regulation of various cytokines following β_2-agonist therapy. These observations have been inconsistent, and confirmatory studies are lacking.

Bronchial β_2-receptor stimulation leads to bronchial smooth muscle relaxation. The naturally occurring catecholamines, norepinephrine and epinephrine, compete with exogenously administered adrenergic drugs for β_2-receptor site occupancy. Epinephrine is derived from the adrenal medulla, whereas norepinephrine arises from the postsynaptic sympathetic nerve endings. Thus smooth muscle relaxation is mediated by circulating ephinephrine, but not norepinephrine, since bronchial smooth muscle receives no direct sympathetic innervation.[5]

The β-adrenoreceptor agonists can be classified, in general, into the catecholamines and noncatecholamines, isoproterenol and albuterol, respectively.[136] The noncatecholamine agonists differ in their N-substitution on the phenylethanolamine nucleus, as well as the hydroxyl substitutions on the benzene ring (Fig. 40–2).[136] By modifying the major structure in the 3,4-hydroxyl groups on the benzene ring, resistance to catechol-O-methyltransferase (COMT) can be achieved. Alteration in this position prolongs bronchodilator activity. The second major alteration is achieved by enlarging the carbon side chain. This enhances β_2 specificity and protects against monoamine oxidase (MAO) degradation, thus enhancing duration of the bronchodilatation. The long-acting β_2-agonists that possess long lipophilic side chains are thought to be anchored at an exosite adjacent to the β_2-receptor site, prolonging the effectiveness of these drugs.[140] The objective of β_2-agonist therapy is to achieve maximal bronchodilatation with the least adverse effects.

EPHEDRINE

Ephedrine was the first β-agonist to be used therapeutically. An oral preparation derived from the Chinese herb ma huang, ephedrine is rapidly inactivated by COMT. Initially, ephedrine was used in combination with low doses of theophylline plus phenobarbital or hydroxyzine to overcome the central nervous system (CNS) side effects of ephedrine. It had been used for thousands of years and was synthesized in 1923. Its bronchodilator effects are mainly indirect via norepinephrine release from adrenergic nerve ending storage sites.[243] Ephedrine is a weak bronchodilator and requires dosages considerably higher (2.5–10 times higher) than more direct-acting, newer oral sympathomimetic agents. At such large doses, troublesome CNS side effects occur, such as tremulousness, hypertension, and urinary retention. Because of the adverse side effects, this drug is seldom used.

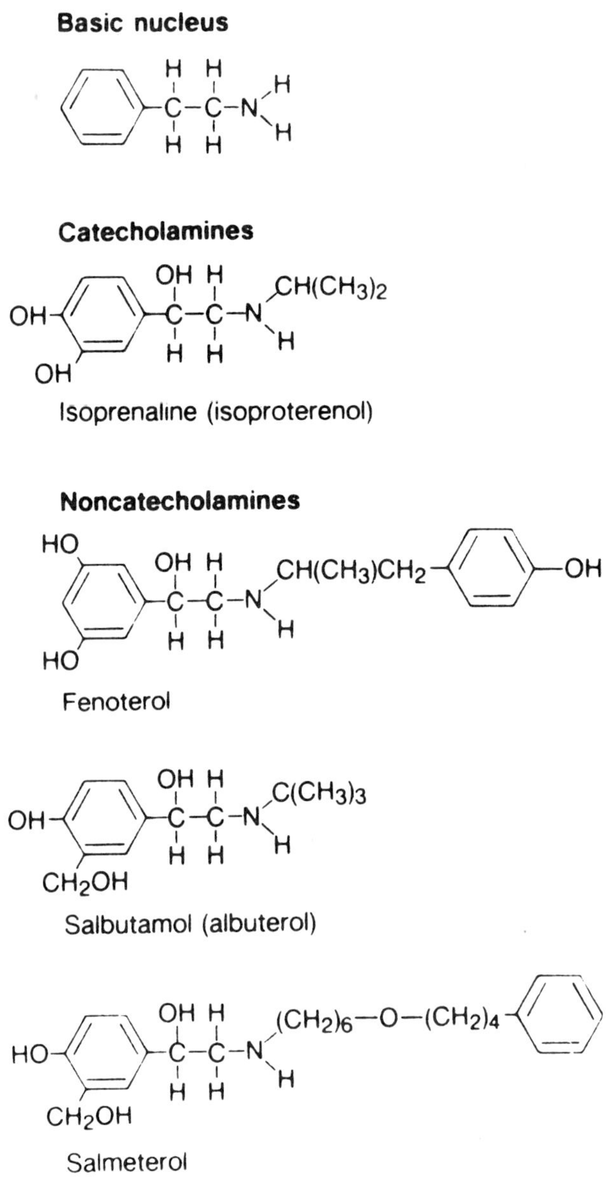

FIGURE 40–2. Molecular structure of β-adrenoreceptor agonists.

EPINEPHRINE

Epinephrine is most effective by systemic administration and exerts α, β_1, and β_2 effects. Epinephrine was the first synthetic β-agonist and was introduced early in the 20th century.[10] Used by both subcutaneous injection and aerosol, this drug is mainly reserved for the treatment of anaphylaxis. When administered subcutaneously, aqueous epinephrine has a rapid onset of action but short duration.[72, 201, 205] Adverse side effects include CNS stimulation, cardiovascular stimulation with headache, tachycardia, and hypertension. Parenteral administration of epinephrine is indicated only for cardiovascular emergencies. In older patients particularly, epinephrine must be administered cautiously because of its adverse cardiac effects. When administered by aerosol using metered-dose inhalers (160–300 μg/puff) or nebulization of a 1% solution, the effect is short, and CNS and cardiovascular side effects develop at dosages required for bronchodilatation.

ISOPROTERENOL

Isoproterenol was the first drug developed to resist metabolism by COMT. It is administered by aerosolization, by nebulization, and sublingually. Metered-dose inhalers of isoproterenol in solution or dry crystalline powder in suspension generally deliver 75 to 125 μg per actuation. Nebulization of a 5% solution was a standard therapy for acute asthma.[63, 152, 198] Isoproterenol has been administered intravenously, usually for impending respiratory failure due to asthma.[96, 177, 249] However, cardiac toxicity, even at lower dosages of intravenous infusions of isoproterenol, has made this modality of therapy unpopular.

Electrocardiographic changes indicating myocardial ischemia and/or focal myocardial necrosis, as well as elevations of serum creatine phosphokinase (CPK) MB isoenzymes, have occurred.[144] It became apparent, particularly in high concentrations, that the cardiotoxic effects of isoproterenol contribute significantly to asthma mortality.[214] In adult patients with impending respiratory failure, gradually increasing doses administered intravenously over 2 hours led to progressive bronchodilatation with little cardiovascular adverse side effects.[117] However, isoproterenol's potential serious cardiovascular toxicity required careful monitoring with continuous electrocardiograph and serial CPK-MB levels. With enhanced patient education, recognition of earlier symptoms, use of inhaled steroids, early introduction of systemic steroids, and availability of more selective β_2-adrenergic receptor agonists and because of adverse effects, isoproterenol is no longer recommended.

ISOETHARINE

Isoetharine was the initial β_2-agonist susceptible to COMT and resistant to MAO.[229] It is always administered by aerosol. Peak effect is attained within 15 minutes and sustained for less than 2 hours.[194] It is more β_2 selective and has less cardiac stimulatory effects than isoproterenol.[97, 132]

METAPROTERENOL

Metaproterenol is not susceptible to COMT inactivation and is therefore amenable to aerosol, oral, and parenteral administration. It is a resorcinol derivative of isoproterenol, whose major advantage is its prolonged duration of action. Its pharmacologic effects are similar to those of isoproterenol, and it exhibits similar cardiotoxicity.[229, 151] When orally administered, its bronchodilator effect is noted at 30 minutes and persists for 4 to 5 hours. CNS side effects and tachycardia are infrequent. Metered-dose inhaler aerosol preparations deliver 650 μg per puff, with bronchodilatation occurring within 5 minutes and persisting for 5 hours. The preparation is available in a 5% aerosol solution for nebulization.

TERBUTALINE

Terbutaline is a β_2-selective drug with oral, parenteral, and aerosolized forms. This compound is resistant to both COMT and MAO, permitting it to be administered orally, parenterally, and by inhalation. The dose-limiting effect is the tremor. A dose of 400 μg nebulized induces bronchodilatation in 15 minutes that is sustained for 2 hours, whereas oral administration has an onset at 2 hours and persists for 4 to 8 hours.[247a, 62, 197] Subcutaneous administration of 500 μg of terbutaline elicited bronchodilatation within 5 minutes, which persisted for 3 to 4 hours.[205, 211] Frequent administration of subcutaneous doses of terbutaline has not been associated with adverse cardiovascular complications.[232] It is well tolerated without significant tachyphylaxis of its bronchodilator effect or production of clinically significant cardiovascular effects.[246]

Administered subcutaneously, terbutaline has little therapeutic advantage over epinephrine.[72, 170, 202] Subcutaneous administration of 250 μg of terbutaline produces bronchodilatation that is similar in onset and duration to 250 μg of epinephrine, but without CNS or cardiovascular side effects.[72] When administered orally, terbutaline (5 mg) is more effective than ephedrine (25 mg), with an earlier onset (30 minutes), a duration of effect of nearly 7 hours,[70] and similar cardiovascular side effects. Metered-dose inhalers of terbutaline (500 μg) and metaproterenol (1,500 μg) produced equivalent peak bronchodilatation, although the effect of terbutaline persisted longer. Because terbutaline is used to interrupt labor, it is now recognized by the Food and Drug Administration as a class B drug for use in pregnancy.

ALBUTEROL

Albuterol (salbutamol), available since 1968, has oral, aerosol, metered-dose inhaler, and dry powder forms. When it is administered orally, bronchodilatation occurs within 15 minutes, peaks at 2 to 4 hours, and lasts for 5 hours.[131] Greater bronchodilatation is attained by inhalation than by ingestion. Inhalation of 200 μg of albuterol produces bronchodilatation at 1 minute that lasts for 6 hours. Adverse side effects are slight, and there is no tachycardia. Albuterol can be nebulized as a wet aerosol for the treatment of persistent, severe asthma, using dosages of 2,500 μg.[165] Intravenous administration of albuterol has been associated with cardiovascular and systemic side effects.[22]

PIRBUTEROL

Pirbuterol produces bronchodilatation and cardiac effects equivalent to those of albuterol when administered by metered-dose inhaler.[21] The duration of the effect is 6 hours. Pirbuterol has been administered via breath-activated inhaler. A 400-μg dose is the lowest dose producing maximum bronchodilatation without significant cardiovascular alterations.[139] Since pirbuterol is not a catecholamine, neither COMT nor MAO affects this drug.

FENOTEROL

Fenoterol, a resorcinol derivative of metaproterenol, is not available in the United States. It has been associated with increased asthma mortality in New Zealand, particularly when administered on a regular versus an as-needed basis.[206, 216, 227] Oral fenoterol of 5,000 μg is considered comparable to 4,000 μg of albuterol and 5,000 μg of terbutaline.[93] Fenoterol of 200 to 400 μg administered by metered-dose inhaler induces bronchodilatation within a few minutes that peaks at 60 to 120 minutes and persists for 5 hours. Fenoterol induces ionotropic and chronotropic cardiovascular effects comparable to those of isoproterenol[37, 48] and greater than those induced by albuterol and terbutaline[248] when administered in equivalent doses. The reduced β_2 specificity and particularly the greater potency of fenoterol, leading to use of a higher dose equivalent, have been proposed as factors contributing to asthma mortality in New Zealand.[49, 216]

BITOLTEROL

Bitolterol is an inactive pro-drug, 3,4-diester colterol, that undergoes hydrolysis to the active drug colterol following inhalation. It is an effective bronchodilator with a duration of 8 hours and minimal side effects.[242]

PROCATEROL

Procaterol is effective at a low dosage of 50 to 100 μg. Oral preparations of 100 μg have provided bronchodilatation persisting for 12 hours.[209, 253] However, transient CNS stimulation occurs.[209] Procaterol is thought to be more potent than isoproterenol.[223, 251] Tremor and headache were the most common adverse side effects with oral and metered-dose inhaler therapy.

FORMOTEROL

Formoterol is a highly selective β_2-agonist with rapid onset of bronchodilatation. Administered by aerosol, 12 μg provides maximum bronchodilatation at 5 minutes, persisting for 12 hours.[138] In studies up to 1 year after regular therapy, there was no change in bronchodilatation or inhibition of histamine-induced bronchospasm. Formoterol has been used as both a rescue and maintenance inhaled bronchodilator.[6] Formoterol provides significant protection against methacholine-induced bronchospasm for at least 12 hours[16] and also inhibits exercise- and hyperventilation-induced bronchospasm for at least 4 hours following inhalation.[146, 150]

SALMETEROL

Salmeterol is a long-acting selective β_2-agonist. There is a delayed onset to peak bronchodilatation with 50 μg requiring 2 hours for maximum bronchodilatation, which then persists for 12 hours. Structurally similar to albuterol, it has a long lipophilic side chain, which is believed to anchor the compound firmly to an exosite in the vicinity of the β receptor. This permits a more prolonged duration of action.[28] At 50 and 100 μg, salmeterol causes little cardiovascular effect, with a mild tremor comparable to that noted with albuterol 250 μg. Salmeterol 200 μg produces significant, although modest, increments in heart rate and tremor. On a twice-daily regimen, salmeterol reduces nocturnal asthma.

BAMBUTEROL

Bambuterol is a lipophilic pro-drug of terbutaline with sustained bronchodilator action.[171] Administered once daily in an oral dose of 20 mg, it has a duration of effect of 24 hours.

ROUTES OF ADMINISTRATION

Administration of a β_2-agonist may be oral, inhaled, or parenteral.[108] Inhalation via metered-dose inhaler or nebulizer delivers optimal pharmacologic dosages. Oral administration is appropriate when airway hyperresponsiveness or age preclude inhaled medication. Although oral preparations have been prescribed for nocturnal asthma, tachyphylaxis and long-acting inhaled β_2-agonists preclude their use in adults. Supervised administration of β_2-agonist metered-dose inhalers with spacers delivers dosages equivalent to nebulizers.[115, 44, 25, 47]

Because of the ozone-depleting effects of chlorofluorocarbons, the delivery system of metered-dose inhalers is being changed to include only agents that are not ozone depleting. These include either dry powder systems or the propellants using hydrofluoroalkanes (HFA) 134a or 227. The conversion mandated by the United Nations Environmental Program at the Montréal Agreement requires implementation when such delivery systems are safe and effective.

SYSTEMIC EFFECTS OF β_2-AGONISTS

Systemic effects of β_2-agonist therapy may accompany dose-related improvements in airway response following inhalation of β_2-agonists. Systemic absorption occurs via the lung-vascular bed; lipophilic compounds are more rapidly absorbed by the gastrointestinal tract.

HYPOKALEMIA

Administration of β-agonists is often associated with reduction in serum potassium concentration.[48, 60, 88, 120, 133, 166, 204, 208] Hypokalemia is greatest with systemic administration but also occurs by inhalation. Hypokalemia results from the intracellular shift of potassium (K) into skeletal muscle when β_2-agonists are inhaled, due to stimulation of membrane-bound sodium/potassium-ATPase.[33] There is some evidence that the intracellular shift of potassium (K^+) is through stimulation of pancreatic β_2 receptors, leading to increases in serum insulin concentration.[187, 204, 212, 228] Regardless of cause, the increased cellular uptake of potassium results in a reduction in the extracellular potassium concentration.[121]

The extracellular potassium ion concentration is the most important determinant of myocardial membrane stability.[195] Administration of high doses of β_2-agonist and arrhythmias appear to be associated.[98] A link with hypokalemia, arrhythmia, and fatal asthma has not been established.[206] Hypokalemic effects of the β_2-agonist can be further accentuated by concomitant administration of corticosteroids, diuretics, and theophylline.[137] Therapeutic administration of terbutaline led to a decline in serum potassium concentrations within 15 minutes, with a maximum 14% reduction at 30 minutes, which remained depressed for 2 hours. Similar hypokalemic responses were observed by other routes of administration. Furthermore, the magnitude of hypokalemia could be correlated with the degree of prolongation of the electrocardiographic QTc interval. Hypoxemia with associated electrolyte disturbance could potentiate the hypokalemia and myocardial irritability.[158, 216]

HYPOXIA

Bronchodilator administration accentuates hypoxia.[89, 104, 145, 176, 175, 185, 223] Such decreases in PaO_2 occur within 5 minutes after administration of the bronchodilator.[114] Although transient and modest, such hypoxia can aggravate hypoxia in severe asthma and potentiate myocardial irritability.[45] This reduction in PaO_2 following β-agonist administration in asthma patients has been attributed to a ventilation-perfusion defect.[176] α-Agonists induce arteriolar vasoconstriction, further accentuating this ventilation-perfusion mismatch.

METABOLIC EFFECTS

Decreases in serum magnesium, calcium, and phosphate possibly related to increased circulating insulin levels[184, 212] have been observed with β_2-agonist administration. Increments in blood sugar have been observed following administration of aerosolized β-agonist.[166] Such elevations are transient and of significance mainly in diabetic patients.[230] High-density lipoprotein cholesterol levels have also been observed to increase in patients receiving β-agonist therapy,[228, 100] a potentially beneficial side effect.

MYOCARDIAL TOXICITY

β-Agonists increase the force of cardiac contractility (ionotropic effect) and cardiac rate (chronotropic effect) through their action at the β_1 receptor.[29] Consequently, increments in cardiac output, cardiac work, and myocardial oxygen consumption occur.[220] The cardiac effects can be minimized by use of more selective β_2-agonists administered by metered-dose inhaler.[180] With abuse, hemodynamically significant effects may occur, such as increases in cardiac output, stroke volume, left ventricular mean velocity, and fiber shortening.[40]

Contraction band necrosis has been observed in animals administered isoproterenol and aminophylline, particularly fat female Sprague-Dawley rats.[15, 196] Similar lesions have been described in individuals dying of asthma.[59] Pretreatment with corticosteroids prevented such lesions,[86, 59] which have been observed in humans receiving intravenous isoproterenol.[59] CPK-MB elevations in cardiac muscle have also occurred in individuals with severe asthma who were administered intravenous isoproterenol. Arrhythmias have been noted after inhalation of fenoterol, but not with comparable doses of albuterol.[224] β-Agonists delivered by nebulizer may not be completely safe, as they induced arrhythmias in older patients who underwent Holter monitoring.[98] This is a controversial point, as other studies with 24-hour Holter monitoring failed to demonstrate any potentially dangerous arrhythmias.[85]

CENTRAL NERVOUS SYSTEM

At conventional dosage, β-agonists fail to significantly stimulate the CNS, since these polar compounds fail to cross the blood-brain barrier. The apparent CNS stimulation may result from peripheral cardiovascular-metabolic effects.[243]

SKELETAL MUSCLE

Tremor is a dose-dependent phenomenon following systemic administration of β_2-agonists, particularly terbutaline.[127]

MICTURITION

Stimulation of the detrusor bladder muscle induces relaxation of this muscle, thus decreasing pressure for micturition. Obstruction may occur, particularly in individuals with prostatism.

VASCULAR SMOOTH MUSCLE

β_2-Agonists may reduce diastolic arterial blood pressure, especially after systemic administration.

PARADOXICAL BRONCHOSPASM

Paradoxical bronchospasm occurring after β-agonist use is increasingly recognized in individuals abusing β-agonist metered-dose inhalers. It can also occur following spirometry-induced bronchospasm related to deep inhalation preceding a forced exhalation maneuver or even during forced exhalation.[24, 143, 217] Reflex bronchospasm may be consequent to the irritant effect of the aerosol vehicle or a result of β-adrenergic tachyphylaxis. Airway hypersensitivity to the β-agonist or vehicle itself may cause such reactions, induced possibly by sulfites.[118]

CLINICAL PHARMACOLOGY

As first-line therapy, the β_2-agonists provide prompt reversal of bronchospasm in mild, moderate, and even severe asthma. When β_2-agonist therapy is required more than three times weekly, concomitant anti-inflammatory therapy is required.[163] In the stepwise zonal therapy program, even mild asthma may require β_2-agonist bronchodilator therapy with early introduction of anti-inflammatory medication. With the advent of long-acting β_2-agonists, it is now recommended that concomitant anti-inflammatory therapy be administered. The efficacy of the β_2-agonists, particularly long-acting agents, often provides patients with a false sense of improvement, leading them to discontinue the anti-inflammatory therapy.

β_2-Agonists are the most predictable and effective bronchodilators available for asthma therapy. However, there is concern as to the wisdom of using β_2-agonists on a regular basis in treating asthma.[206] These concerns arise from the suggestion that there may be tachyphylaxis to the bronchodilator effects of β_2-agonists or to the reduction in the ability of β_2-agonists to protect against bronchospasm induced by other stimuli.[13] As noted previously, such tachyphylaxis may arise from receptor desensitization. Nevertheless, the effects of β_2-agonists on receptor expression and coupling are complex and may include increased synthesis of receptors mediated through cAMP-response elements on the β_2-adrenergic receptor gene.

Tolerance to β_2-agonists can be caused by rapid desensitization, uncoupling of the receptor from the signal transduction mechanism, or gradual down-regulation of the receptors.[17, 169] Thus it is important to consider the effect of long-term therapy with β_2-agonists and their ability to elicit acute bronchodilatation or protect against bronchoconstricting agents.[13] Fatal asthma has been reported in patients abusing regular β_2-agonist therapy.[206] In most instances, such patients were not being administered concomitant anti-inflammatory therapy. Thus the role of regular versus intermittent or on-demand β_2-agonist therapy is controversial.[206]

The protective effects of inhaled β_2-agonist against nonspecific pharmacologic challenge by histamine, methacholine, adenosine, and cold air have been used to evaluate other parameters of efficacy of the drugs.[13] β_2-Agonist–induced protection against induced bronchospasm is attenuated with long-term albuterol therapy.[71] In this study, following regular oral administration of β_2-agonist, a single inhaled dose of albuterol failed to protect against exercise challenge as well as inhaled β_2-agonist did prior to regular oral therapy. Regular terbutaline administered for 7 days lost the protective effect of a single dose of terbutaline against the bronchoconstriction induced by adenosine monophosphate and methacholine.[172] In these studies, the inhibition to the bronchoconstricting agent was reduced by 2.1 and 1.5 doubling doses, respectively; the route of the regularly administered drug differed from that used to treat the induced bronchospasm.

In mild asthma, salmeterol administered in a parallel double-blind study during an 8-week trial versus placebo demonstrated an increase in FEV_1 1 hour after inhalation of the salmeterol, which failed to change significantly during the study period.[43] However, on the first day, salmeterol afforded significant protection against methacholine-induced bronchoconstriction. Following 4 to 8 weeks of treatment, the salmeterol-induced change in peak expiratory flow rate was attenuated to only a two-fold increase compared with a ten-fold increase at baseline. Thus the effect diminished with time. Two to four days following treatment cessation, the PC20 was similar to pretreatment values.[43]

As previously noted, there is increasing concern regarding the repeated use of inhaled β_2-agonists, with deterioration in asthma control and lung function and an increase in airway hyperresponsiveness.[239, 119, 116] Regularly scheduled or frequent use of short-acting β_2-agonists for prolonged management of asthma fails to adequately control asthma symptoms, peak flow variability, and/or airway hyperresponsiveness.[206] Treatment of patients with mild asthma for 3 weeks with regular β-agonist was associated with an increase in peak expiratory flow variability and following cessation of treatment with a 10% baseline fall in FEV_1 and an increase in bronchial reactivity to histamine compared with pretreatment. A modest dose of albuterol can subsequently lead to a 10% reduction in FEV_1 after only 3 weeks of treatment. This increase in bronchial reactivity after cessation of β_2-agonist treatment persists at least 59 hours.[241] Such changes have been observed with terbutaline,[119, 116, 239] fenoterol,[206] and albuterol,[238] suggesting a class effect of β-agonists.

The mechanism contributing to the increase in bronchial reactivity and deterioration in asthma control after β_2-agonist treatment is unclear. Desensitization of β-receptors has been postulated,[239, 226] with reduction in smooth muscle relaxation and enhanced mediator release. β-Agonist receptors are reduced in numbers and functions,[148] but other studies argue against β-receptor desensitization.[238, 90] Furthermore, protection against histamine-induced bronchoconstriction has been reduced.[239, 71] Other proposed causes of accentuated airway hyperresponsiveness include an increase in airway inflammation resulting from enhanced airway exposure to allergen following bronchodilatation[160] and inhibition of mast cell heparin release.[173]

Although the precise mechanism underlying airway hyperresponsiveness in asthma remains to be established, it is generally considered that airway inflammation is a major factor in inducing and sustaining hyperresponsiveness. For this reason, it has been suggested that anti-inflammatory agents such as cromolyn and nedocromil be used for mild asthma and that steroids be used for mild to moderate or even severe asthma.[163] Successful asthma therapy should include anti-inflammatory agents to reduce the underlying pathologic process and bronchodilator drugs to abruptly relieve the bronchospastic response.

Thus asthma therapy invariably includes a β-agonist for rescue medication and prophylactic anti-inflammatory therapy to reduce the inflammatory component and prevent episodes of bronchoconstriction. Methylxanthines can also be used for long-term bronchodilator protection. Whatever medication schedule is used, it is critical for both the physician and the patient to realize that inadequate and short-lasting responses to treatment occur with short-acting β-agonists and that progressively worsening asthma dictates immediate intensive therapeutic intervention. Indications of diminished control of asthma by increased use of the β-adrenergic agents, failure to appreciate the severity of asthma, or an inadequate response of therapy with β-agonist are major risk factors of asthma morbidity and mortality.

EXERCISE-INDUCED ASTHMA

Exercise is a common stimulus for asthma, particularly when it is conducted in the cold. An asthma attack will occur in 90% of patients after 6 to 8 minutes of vigorous exercise. One of the goals of therapy is for patients to resume gainful activity, including exercise. β_2-Adrenergic agents are the most effective in modifying exercise-induced asthma when administered 5 to 60 minutes prior to exercise.[4] The selection of the drug to prevent exercise-induced asthma should include a pharmacologic assessment of the drugs. The rapidity of the onset of bronchodilatation and the site and duration of the drugs are of considerable importance. Aerosolized β_2-adrenoreceptors will prevent exercise-induced asthma attacks in 98% of patients. The duration of protection is usually 1 to 2 hours[3, 250] and can be increased when the dosage is increased[250, 128] or used during exercise.[236] The protection provided by salmeterol 50 μg 30 minutes prior to exercise is effective in most subjects and will last several hours.[2] Similar results were obtained with formoterol.

In summary, effective management of asthma requires both nonpharmacologic and pharmacologic interventions to attain the goals of therapy. Four components of therapy must be included:

1. Education of the patient and the patient's family
2. Environmental control: avoidance of triggers such as allergens, cold, and respiratory infections
3. Use of objective measures of assessment to determine severity or deterioration of asthma
4. Pharmacologic therapy of asthma aimed at achieving maximal reversal of air flow obstruction and reducing airway hyperresponsiveness by preventing and reversing airway inflammation

β_2-Agonists are the most predictable and powerful bronchodilator agents available for relieving the bronchospasm of asthma and preventing exercise-induced asthma. The rapid relief produced by such agents often promotes overuse or abuse. Considerable attention has been directed, therefore, to the appreciation of the molecular basis of the β_2-receptor physiology, the pharmacology of each agent, and the therapeutic indications for β_2-agonist use.

Whatever medication schedule is used, it is critical for both the physician and the patient to appreciate that inadequate or short-lasting response to therapy in the face of progressively worsening asthma dictates immediate, intensive therapy. Increased use of β-adrenergic agents, failure to appreciate the severity of asthma, or inadequate response to therapy are major risk factors for asthma morbidity and mortality. Anti-inflammatory therapy is a major component of the pharmacotherapy of asthma and should be introduced in patients having daily symptoms. β_2-Agonists are safe and effective bronchodilators and should be used to relieve acute asthma.

ASTHMA THERAPY

ANTICHOLINERGIC AGENTS

Parasympathetic Innervation of the Lung

The autonomic nervous innervation of the normal human airway is predominantly provided by the parasympathetic nervous system via fibers of the vagus nerve, which supplies branches throughout the lungs at peribronchial ganglia most commonly found near larger airways. Innervation of mucous glands, smooth muscle cells, and pulmonary arterial and ciliated epithelial cells occurs through postganglionic fibers, which supply acetylcholine-containing postganglionic nerves capable of activating muscarinic receptors within the lungs.[193] Activation of these receptors induces enhanced mucus production, smooth muscle contraction, and increased ciliary beating. Chronic cholinergic tone is a prominent controlling factor of normal lung physiology.[193]

A smaller number of efferent autonomic nerves arises from the nonadrenergic, noncholinergic, or purinergic branch of the autonomic nervous system. The mediators of this nervous system, including vasoactive intestinal peptide and peptide histidine methionine, are present concomitantly with acetylcholine within nerve terminals. Mediators released by purinergic nerve stimulation counteract smooth muscle contraction, having a bronchodilator effect opposing the activity of acetylcholine released from the parasympathetic nerve endings.[245]

Vagal Reflexes

The vagus nerve plays an important role in a variety of reflexes that induce bronchospasm. Irritant receptors and nonmyelinated C fibers located within respiratory airways, as well as receptors found within the esophagus and upper airways, may initiate a reflex consequent to irritation induced by inhaled stimuli, including cold air, histamine, and respiratory irritants. These reflex axons involve afferent vagal nerves, which travel centrally to the brain stem and then return as vagal efferents to the airways.[84] Potentially, vagal reflexes could be completely mitigated through the use of anticholinergic agents. Anticholinergics compete with or inhibit the activity of acetylcholine at muscarinic receptors and thereby limit the cholinergic activity responsible for bronchomotor tone.

Generally, anticholinergics will only partially reverse air flow obstruction in most airway diseases, suggesting that cholinergic pathways are not solely responsible for most bronchoconstriction.[245] In instances of bronchospasm induced by exercise, hyperventilation, and cold air, anticholinergic agents have been moderately effective but generally less effective than β_2-agonists.[74] In contrast to asthma, wherein inflammatory mechanisms are not affected by the use of anticholinergic therapy, patients with chronic obstructive lung disease may demonstrate some degree of reversibility that is likely related to inhibition of cholinergic nervous activity.[75] In these patients, anticholinergic activity may be one of the few forms of therapy yielding significant bronchodilatation.

Muscarinic Receptors

Five muscarinic receptors (M1 through M5) have been identified through cDNA cloning.[38] Like the adrenergic receptors, they are members of the G protein–linked superfamily, with an extracellular $-NH_2$ terminus, seven transmembrane domains, and a cytoplasmic -COOH terminus. The muscarinic receptors fall into two functional categories: (1) the M1, M3, and M5 receptors, which are associated with the pertussis toxin (PTX)-insensitive family of G proteins and stimulate phosphatidyl inositol hydrolysis; and (2) the M2 and M4 receptors, which couple to the PTX-sensitive family of G proteins to inhibit adenyl cyclase activity. These receptors are formed by the activity of at least nine muscarinic receptor genes, which produce polypeptide subtypes having the capability of inducing membrane-based ion channels, in addition to possessing G-protein activities and phosphoinositol activation.[79] Typically, these receptors are also found in larger airways, suggesting that the major clinical effects of anticholinergic agents will take place therein.[14]

M1 receptors are localized in parasympathetic ganglia, alveoli, and possibly submucosal glands of human airways.[12] Their presence at parasympathetic ganglia may facilitate neurotransmission. Thus pirenzipine, a specific M1 receptor antagonist, could be administered at a dose that inhibits reflex cholinergic bronchoconstriction due to inhalation of sulfur dioxide (SO_2) and have no effect on bronchoconstriction elicited by direct cholinergic stimulation with methacholine.[123] The role of M1 receptors in alveoli is unclear, as there is no direct parasympathetic innervation of the lung periphery.

M2 receptors are present on the prejunctional region of the postganglionic cholinergic nerves and inhibit cholinergic neurotransmission.[19] Thus the stimulatory effects of cholinergic neurotransmission may be autoregulated by the action of acetylcholine on M2 receptors, thereby providing negative feedback. Activation of M2 receptors inhibits cholinergic nerve-induced contraction of human airway muscle in vitro. Selective stimulation of prejunctional M2 receptors by pilocarpine inhibits reflex bronchoconstriction induced by SO_2; but pilocarpine was without effect in asthmatic subjects, indicating possible dysregulation of prejunctional M2 receptors in asthma.[155] Animal studies and in vitro studies indicate that viral infection through the action of viral neuraminidase, inflammation induced by ozone or allergen, and eosinophil granule proteins may all contribute to the loss of function of the M2 receptor.[67] Agents could be developed that specifically inhibit M1 and M3 receptors without affecting M2 receptors. These agents, if developed, would be more effective than the currently available anticholinergic agents that act against all three receptor subtypes.[79]

M3 receptors[12] are localized in airway smooth muscle. Their stimulation elicits sequential phosphatidylinositol (PI) hydrolysis, formation of inositol triphosphate, Ca^{2+} flux, and smooth muscle contraction. M3 receptors are also present on submucosal glands, and M3 receptor antagonists inhibit mucus secretion from human airways in vitro. Weak expression is observed on airway epithelial cells and endothelial cells. No functional M4 or M5 receptors have been described in human lung.

Physiologic Effects of Anticholinergic Therapy

The main functions of the cholinergic fibers within the airways are to enhance bronchomotor tone through smooth muscle contraction, increase release of submucosal gland secretions, and enhance ciliary activity of epithelial cells. Although anticholinergic agents enhance air flow in normal subjects, in disease states where increased cholinergic airway tone is noted, such as chronic obstructive lung disease and asthma, even further enhancement of air flow is noted using anticholinergic therapy.[80]

In contrast to the effects of anticholinergics on airway tone, under normal conditions, anticholinergic agents do not affect airway secretion except in situations when secretion is increased. The effects of anticholinergic agents on both secretions and ciliary activity, however, are less marked than effects noted on bronchomotor tone.[80] Clinically, the effects of anticholinergic agents thus appear largely related to modulation of smooth muscle tone. As the majority of muscarinic receptor activity and cholinergic innervation occurs in the larger central airways, the effects of anticholinergic agents tend to be largely related to diminution of central airway contraction. Deposition of inhaled anticholinergic agents also tends to favor activity in the central airway sites.[83]

Atropine

The oldest anticholinergic agents included a variety of plant-derived alkaloids, including atropine, which had been used in traditional herbal remedies for centuries throughout Asia and Europe. In the last century, atropine derivatives were the most widely used bronchodilators in the world. It was not until the discovery of epinephrine early in the century that adrenergic drugs replaced the use of anticholinergic therapies.[69]

The anticholinergic alkaloids that are derived from plants are all tertiary ammonium compounds occurring as tropine ring structures (Fig. 40–3). When converted to salts, these compounds, including atropine and hyoscine (scopolamine), are well absorbed, being both water and lipid soluble.[82] Tertiary ammonium salts are orally active and capable of inhibiting muscarinic receptors selectively throughout the body, although they affect these muscarinic receptors in a nonselective manner.[82] Consequent to the widespread normal physiologic activity of the cholinergic nervous system in the body and the easy passage of these agents across the brain

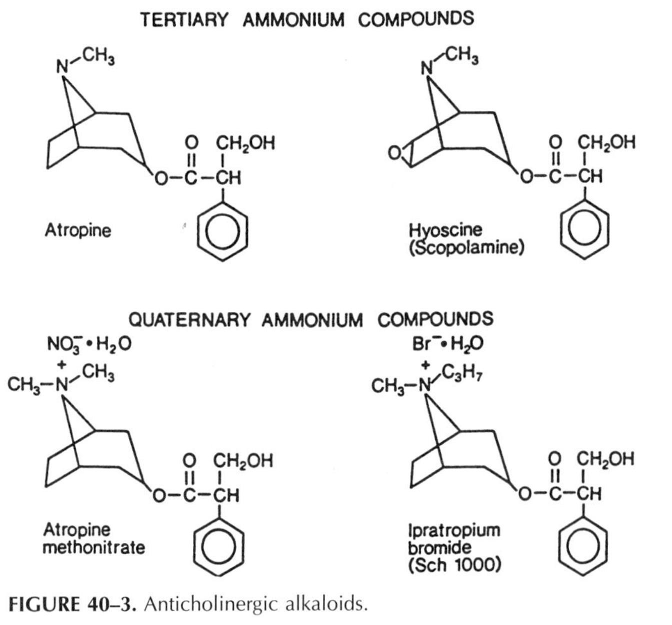

FIGURE 40–3. Anticholinergic alkaloids.

barrier, minute doses of tertiary ammonium salts (as little as 1 to 2 mg) may produce significant systemic toxicity.

Ipratropium Bromide

PHARMACOLOGY

Newer developments in anticholinergic therapy include the formulation of quaternary ammonium compounds, including atropine methonitrate and ipratropium bromide (Atrovent). Within the tropine ring, these quaternary ammonium compounds contain a positively charged nitrogen ionically bound to either methonitrate or bromide, resulting in lack of their absorption from mucosal surfaces.[74] Such compounds are only effective at the site of direct delivery, such as delivery to the central airways. As minimal absorption occurs even at these sites, the systemic effects induced are minimal.

Ipratropium bromide is a synthetic quaternary isopropyl derivative of atropine acting through interruption of vagally mediated bronchoconstriction through inhibition of the cyclic guanosine 3′5′-monophosphate system at parasympathetic nerve endings. The activity of ipratropium bromide is partially dependent on a decrease in cyclic guanosine monophosphate. Ipratropium bromide, when inhaled at a dose of two puffs containing 18 μg each puff, results in a very low blood level that peaks within 2 hours, the half-life in the circulation being 4 hours.[74] When delivered by nebulizer, a 500 μg dose of ipratropium bromide is considered optimal. When it is administered by a metered-dose inhaler, asthmatics have been reported to respond to between 40 and 80 μg per administration. In chronic obstructive lung disease, however, up to 160 μg per administration may be required.[82] Those patients having the most severe chronic air flow obstruction tend to require the higher dosing regimen.

Tolerance to ipratropium bromide is not believed to be a significant problem, as use of antagonist receptors typically does not down-regulate but rather up-regulates receptor activity, in contrast to the situation in which a β-agonist is administered.[207] Confirming this hypothesis, increased methacholine receptor responsiveness has been noted in some patients treated with ipratropium bromide.[167] The low serum concentration achieved after ipratropium bromide inhalation results in this agent being well tolerated and generally free of significant adverse side effects.[149]

PHYSIOLOGIC EFFECTS IN BRONCHOPROVOCATION

In experimental studies of the effects of anticholinergic agents, such as ipratropium bromide, a range of efficacy has been noted dependent on the stimulus employed to induce bronchospasm. Typically, ipratropium bromide and atropine are very protective against bronchospasm induced by cholinergic agents, including methacholine and carbachol.[74] Bronchospasm induced by mast cell–derived mediators, such as prostaglandins and histamine, is only partially inhibited through the use of anticholinergic agents. Furthermore, nonspecific irritant-induced bronchospasm, including that induced by dust and chemical gases, is only partially alleviated through the use of anticholinergic therapy, the effects being less than that provided by β_2-agonist therapy.[74]

Clinically, the effects have been variable, with the efficacy of anticholinergic agents in allergen-induced bronchospasm definitely being less than that of β_2-agonist therapy.[74] Studies of antigen-induced histamine release from sensitized human lung in vitro have demonstrated that acetylcholine has a modest effect in increasing the responsiveness of mast cells to antigen. Pretreatment with ipratropium bromide prior to acetylcholine challenge competitively abolishes the acetylcholine-induced augmentation of histamine release.[161]

CLINICAL UTILITY

Most studies employing ipratropium bromide fail to show a definitive difference in responsiveness between nonatopic and atopic asthmatic patients. Greater responsivity to the anticholinergic agents compared with β-agonists, however, appears to be clearly demonstrated with bronchitis and emphysema.[203]

Anticholinergic agents are very effective in inhibiting bronchospasm induced by β_1-blocking agents, which may be employed for treatment of cardiovascular disease.[55] In selected patients, such β-blocker therapy may allow for essentially unopposed activity of the cholinergic nervous system, making drugs such as ipratropium bromide the treatment of choice.[103, 102] In instances of bronchospasm induced by psychogenic factors, anticholinergic agents have also demonstrated clinical superiority compared with β_2-agonists.[191]

An early double-blind placebo-controlled crossover trial demonstrated that ipratropium bromide in both asthmatics and chronic bronchitic patients resulted in more than a 15% increase in FEV_1 within 5 minutes of treatment, with persistent efficacy noted for up to 5 hours and effects continuing throughout the 2-week duration of therapy. Treatment with ipratropium bromide did not affect sputum volume, nor were adverse events noted, suggesting the potentially favorable role for this agent in both asthma and chronic bronchitis.[42]

Although significant variations may occur with increasing dosage of ipratropium bromide, most patients will exhibit maximal response within 24 hours of therapy, tolerating high doses without significant adverse side effects.[153] Typically, anticholinergic agents require a longer time to be efficacious than do β_2-agonists, often not peaking until 2 hours after inhalation.[200] Peak bronchodilatation of anticholinergic therapy is also generally less than that induced by β_2-agonists, but the peak activity of certain agents, such as ipratropium bromide, is sustained longer than that of β_2-agonists, such as albuterol or metaproterenol.

However, even when very high doses of anticholinergic agents are given, subsequent administration of β_2-agonists results in further enhancement of bronchodilation, substantiating the greater potency of β_2-agonists as bronchodilators when compared with anticholinergic agents.[234] Curiously, clinical variability exists among asthmatics, with some responding better to anticholinergic therapy than to β_2-agonists, and others responding poorly to anticholinergic therapy and responding only to β_2-agonist therapy.[36] In general, it is believed that older asthmatics with long-standing disease have a better clinical response than do younger asthmatics or asthmatics with a more clearly defined allergic etiology of the disease.[234, 111] Atopic asthmatics are distinguished from other cohorts of asthmatics by their younger age of presentation, family history of asthma and other atopic disease, lower instance of mucus hypersecretion, and history of allergic provocation of wheezing.[111]

SAFETY

In the past, adverse side effects related to the administration of anticholinergic therapies, including atropine sulfate, were numerous. Atropine sulfate doses of more than 2 mg may induce skin flushing, dryness of the mouth, tachycardia, disturbance of mentality, and some visual effect. An absolute contraindication to the use of atropine includes the presence of benign prostatic hypertrophy or glaucoma.[76]

Ipratropium bromide typically lacks atropine-like side effects, as it is not significantly absorbed. As long as it is not administered directly into the eye, ipratropium bromide can be given to patients with glaucoma. Ipratropium bromide does not affect prostate function in men with prostatic hypertrophy.[76] No significant changes have been noted in mucus production or viscosity in patients treated with ipratropium bromide as contrasted to the effects induced by atropine.[182] Ipratropium bromide also does not increase hypoxemia and has no significant effect on the pulmonary circulation or hemodynamics in contrast to adrenergic agents.[78]

When compared with β_2-agonists, which can induce cardiac positive inotropic effects and reduce plasma potassium levels, ipratropium bromide is remarkable for being free of extrapulmonary adverse side effects.[247] Adverse side effects related to ipratropium bromide include cough, nausea, palpitations, dry mouth, nervousness, gastrointestinal distress, and dizziness, all of which are usually mild.[147] The major clinical adverse side effect noted with ipratropium bromide use is coughing, which occurs in up to 10% of patients.[218] The etiology of this cough remains unclear, although it may be related to more effective blockade of the M2 receptor in selected individuals, thereby augmenting cholinergic tone, or related to a reaction to the propellant in the inhalation aerosol. In some early studies, paradoxical bronchoconstriction induced by ipratropium bromide nebulization may have been related to the preservatives EDTA and benzalkonium chloride, which had been used as preservatives in such solutions.[99] Severe bronchoconstriction has been reported in less than 0.3% of patients treated with nebulized ipratropium bromide therapy and may be related to the preservative in the nebulization solution or to heightened selectivity of this agent for the M2 receptor in some patients.[81]

SUMMARY

To be maximally efficacious, ipratropium bromide should be administered at a dosing interval four times daily, as the clinical half-life of efficacy is between 4 and 5 hours, with peak bronchodilation typically occurring 60 minutes after administration. As ipratropium bromide is a slow-acting bronchodilator, it should not be used as the primary treatment for acute exacerbations of asthma. Ipratropium bromide should be used mainly as an adjunct in the treatment of chronic stable asthma, with efficacy noted in cases of β-adrenergic antagonist-induced, irritant-induced, and nocturnal-exacerbated asthma. It also may be employed in combination with β_2-adrenergic agents for treatment of acute severe asthma.[26]

ALPHA-ADRENERGIC AGENTS

Pulmonary Effects

Previous studies of α-adrenergic responsiveness in asthma focused on α-adrenergic stimulation inducing bronchoconstriction. In one such study, asthmatic subjects required considerably lower amounts of phenylephrine to constrict the cutaneous vascular bed and dilate pupillary sphincter muscle when compared with normal controls, suggesting significantly enhanced α-adrenergic responses in allergic asthmatics.[95]

Clinical Effects

Clinically, α-adrenergic agonists do not appear to significantly affect asthma. In studies employing pretreatment with either inhaled atropine or inhaled propranolol to exclude cholinergic and β_2 effects, inhalation of phenylephrine did not differ significantly from inhalation of saline with regard to change in FEV_1.[231] Addition of the α-adrenergic agonist phenylephrine neither potentiates nor prolongs the activity of β_2-agonists isoetharine or isoproterenol. Peak activity of isoetharine or isoproterenol effects occurring within 15 minutes after inhalation is not prolonged by concomitant administration of phenylephrine. In addition, phenylephrine has no effect on specific airway resistance and fails to increase air flow rates.[112]

In a study of patients with exercise-induced bronchospasm who received intravenous infusions of the nonselected α-agonist noradrenaline or the α-1–selective agonist phenylephrine, both agents induced elevation in systolic and diastolic blood pressure. However, neither agonist altered lung function as assessed by specific airway compliance, peak expiratory flow, and end expiratory flow rates. A similar finding was noted in healthy individuals, suggesting that α-agonist therapy failed to alter basal bronchial tone in patients with exercise-induced asthma or in healthy controls.[126]

Pseudoephedrine administered in doses of 60 or 180 mg demonstrated no significant bronchodilatory effect following administration or exertion. Ephedrine in 25 mg dosage demonstrated only weak bronchodilatory effect for up to 2 hours after administration, further demonstrating lack of clinical effect of α-adrenergic agonists on pulmonary function.[122]

The role of α-adrenergic receptors in the regulation of human lung airways is less well defined than in certain animal models, wherein α-receptor activation has been noted to mediate bronchoconstriction. α-Receptor antagonists do not have significant efficacy in humans as bronchodilators. Although α-receptors may be present in the airways, it is likely that α-receptor activation is more important in modulating airway blood flow than in regulating airway caliber.[215, 13]

REFERENCES

1. Ahlquist RP: A study of adrenotropic receptors. Am J Physiol 153:586, 1948.
2. Anderson SD, Rodwell LT, Du Toit J, et al: Duration of protection by inhaled salmeterol in exercise-induced asthma. Chest 100(5):1254–1260, 1991.

3. Anderson SD, Rozea PJ, Dolton R, et al: Inhaled and oral bronchodilator therapy in exercise-induced asthma. Aust N Z J Med 5:544–550, 1975.
4. Anderson SD, Seale JP, Ferris L, et al: An evaluation of pharmacotherapy for exercise-induced asthma. J Allergy Clin Immunol 64:612–624, 1979.
5. Ariens EJ, Simonis AM: Physiological and pharmacological aspects of adrenergic receptor classification. Biochem Pharmacol 32:1539–1545, 1983.
6. Arvidsson P, Larsson S, Lofdahl CG, Melander B, et al: Formaterol, a new long-acting bronchodilator for inhalation. Eur Respir J 2:325, 1989.
7. Ashutosh K, Dev G, Steele D: Nonbronchodilator effects of pirbuterol and ipratropium in chronic obstructive pulmonary disease. Chest 107:173–178, 1995.
8. Baba Y, Hayashida M, Yasunami J, et al: Bronchoconstrictive effect of ultrasonic nebulized distilled water on asthmatic children. J Asthma 26:299–307, 1989.
9. Baigelman W, Chodosh S: Bronchodilator action of the anticholinergic drug, ipratropium bromide (Sch 1000), as an aerosol in chronic bronchitis and asthma. Chest 71:324–328, 1977.
10. Barger G, Dale HH: Chemical structure and sympathomimetic action of amines. J Physiol (Lond) 41:19, 1910.
11. Barnes PJ: β-adrenoceptors in smooth muscle, nerves and inflammatory cells. Life Sci 52:2101, 1993.
12. Barnes PJ: Muscarinic receptor subtypes in airways. Life Sci 52:521, 1993.
13. Barnes PJ: Neural mechanisms in asthma. In Holgate ST, Austen KF, Lichenstein LM, et al (eds): Asthma Physiology, Immunopharmacology and Treatment—4th International Symposium. Academic Press, San Diego, 1993, pp 259–273.
14. Barnes PJ, Basbaum CB, Nadel JA: Autoradiographic localization of autonomic receptors in airway smooth muscle: marked differences between large and small airways. Am Rev Respir Dis 127:758, 1983.
15. Beamish RW, Singal PK, Dhalla NS: Stress and heart disease. In: Proceedings of the International Symposium on Stress and Heart Disease, June 26–29, 1984, Winnipeg, Canada. Martinus-Nijhoff, Boston, 1984.
16. Becker AB, Simons FER: Formaterol, a new long-acting selective beta$_2$-adrenergic receptor agonist: double blind comparison with salbutamol and placebo in children with asthma. J Allergy Clin Immunol 84:891, 1989.
17. Bel EH, Timmers MC, Zwinderman AH, et al: The effect of inhaled corticosteroids on the maximal degree of airway narrowing to methacholine in asthmatic subjects. Am Rev Respir Dis 143:109–113, 1991.
18. Benovic JL, Kuhn H, Weyland I, et al: Functional desensitization of the isolated β-adrenergic receptor by the β-adrenergic receptor kinase: potential role of an analog for the retinal protein arrestin (48-kDa protein). Proc Natl Acad Sci USA 84:8879, 1987.
19. Benovic JL, Mayor F Jr, Staniszewski C, et al: Purification and characterization of the β-adrenergic receptor kinase. J Biol Chem 262:9026, 1987.
20. Berdel D, Berg AV: Use of parasympatholytics. Acta Paediatr Sin 30:378–388, 1989.
21. Beumer HM: Pirbuterol aerosol vs. salbutamol in placebo aerosols in bronchial asthma. Drugs Exp Clin Res 2:77, 1980.
22. Bohn D, Kalloghlian A, Jenkins J, et al: Intravenous salbutamol in the treatment of status asthmaticus in children. Crit Care Med 12:892, 1984.
23. Boner AL, Spezia E, Piovesan P, et al: Inhaled formoterol in the prevention of exercise-induced bronchoconstriction in asthmatic children. Am J Respir Crit Care Med 149:935–939, 1994.
24. Bouhuys A, van de Woestijne KP: Mechanical consequences of airway smooth muscle relaxation. J Appl Physiol 30:670, 1971.
25. Bowton DL, Goldsmith WM, Haponik EF: Substitution of metered-dose inhalers for hand-held nebulizers. Success in cost-saving in a large acute care hospital. Chest 101:305–308, 1992.
26. Braun SR, McKensie WN, Copeland C, et al: A comparison of the effect of ipratropium and albuterol in the treatment of chronic obstructive airway disease. Arch Intern Med 149:544–547, 1989.
27. Bristow MR, Ginsburg R: Beta-2 receptors on myocardial cells in human ventricular myocardium. Am J Cardiol 57:3F-6F, 1986.
28. Brittain RT: Approaches to a long-acting, selective beta$_2$-adrenoceptor stimulant. Lung 168(suppl):111, 1990.
29. Brittain RT, Dean CM, Jack D: Sympathomimetic bronchodilator drugs. Pharmacol Ther Bull 2:423, 1976.
30. Brodde OE, Howe U, Egerszegi S, et al: Effect of prednisolone and ketotifen on β_2-adrenoreceptors in asthmatic patients receiving β_2-bronchodilators. Eur J Clin Pharmacol 34:145–150, 1988.
31. Brodde OE, Karad K, Zerkowski HR, et al: Coexistence of beta-1 and beta-2 adrenoreceptors in human right atrium: direct identification by (-)-[^{125}I]-iodocyanopindolol binding. Circ Res 53:752–758, 1983.
32. Brown IG, Chan CS, Kelly CA, et al: Assessment of the clinical usefulness of nebulized ipratropium bromide in patients with chronic airflow limitation. Thorax 39:272–276, 1984.
33. Brown MJ, Brown DJ, Murphy MB: Hypokalemia from beta-2 receptor stimulation by circulating epinephrine. N Engl J Med 309:1414–1419, 1983.
34. Bruderman I, Cohen-Aronovski R, Smorzik JA: A comparative study of various combinations of ipratropium bromide and metaproterenol in allergic asthmatic patients. Chest 83:208, 1983.
35. Bryant DH, Rogers P: Effects of ipratropium bromide nebulizer solution with and without preservatives in the treatment of acute and stable asthma. Chest 102:742, 1992.
36. Burge PS, Harries MG, l'Anson E: Comparison of atropine with ipratropium bromide in patients with reversible airways obstruction unresponsive to salbutamol. Br J Dis Chest 74:259, 1980.
37. Burgess CD, Windom HH, Pearce N, et al: Lack of evidence for β_2 receptor selectivity: a study of metaproterenol, fenoterol, isoproterenol, and epinephrine in patients with asthma. Am Rev Respir Dis 143:444, 1991.
38. Caulfield MP: Muscarinic receptors—characterization, coupling and function. Pharmacol Ther 58:319, 1993.
39. Chapman KR: The role of anticholinergic bronchodilators in adult asthma and chronic obstructive pulmonary disease. Lung 168:295–303, 1990.
40. Chapman KR, Smith DL, Rebuck AS, Leenen FH: Hemodynamic effects of an inhaled beta-2 agonist. Clin Pharmacol Ther 35:762, 1984.
41. Chervinsky P: Concomitant bronchodilator therapy and ipratropium bromide. Am J Med 81:67–73, 1986.
42. Chervinsky P: Double-blind study of ipratropium bromide, a new anticholinergic bronchodilator. J Allergy Clin Immunol 59:22–30, 1977.
43. Cheung D, Timmers MC, Zwinderman AH, et al: Long-term effects of a long-acting β_2-adrenoreceptor agonist, salmeterol, on airway hyperresponsiveness in patients with mild asthma. N Engl J Med 327(17):1198–1203, 1992.
44. Colacone A, Afilalo M, Wolkobe N: A comparison of albuterol administered by metered-dose inhaler (and holding chamber) or wet nebulizer in acute asthma. Chest 104:835–841, 1993.
45. Collins JM, McDevitt DG, Shanks RG, Swanton JG: The cardio-toxicity of isoprenaline during hypoxia. Br J Pharmacol 36:35, 1969.
46. Collins S: Recent perspectives on the molecular structure and regulation of the β_2-adrenergic receptor. Life Sci 52:2083, 1993.
47. Connor WT, Dolovich MB, Frame RA, et al: Reliable salbutamol administration in 6- to 36-month-old children by means of a metered-dose inhaler and aerochamber with mask. Pediatr Pulmon 6:263–267, 1989.
48. Crane J, Burgess C, Beasley R: Cardiovascular and hypokalemic effects of inhaled salbutamol, fenoterol and isoprenaline. Thorax 44:136, 1989.
49. Crane J, Pearce N, Flatt A, et al: Prescribed fenoterol and death from asthma in New Zealand, 1981–1983: case-control study. Lancet 1:917–922, 1989.
50. Crimi N, Palermo F, Oliveri R, et al: Influence of antihistamine (astemizole) and anticholinergic drugs (ipatropium bromide) on bronchoconstriction by substance P. Ann Allergy 65:115–120, 1990.
51. Dahl R, Pedersen B, Venge P: The influence of inhaled salmeterol on bronchial inflammation: a bronchoalveolar lavage study in patients with bronchial asthma. Am Rev Respir Dis 143(suppl):A649, 1991. Abstract.
52. Davis PB: Pupillary responses and airway reactivity in asthma. J Allergy Clin Immunol 77:667–673, 1986.
53. Davis PB, Lieberman P: Normal alpha 2-adrenergic responses in platelets from patients with asthma. J Allergy Clin Immunol 69:35–38, 1982.
54. Davis PB, Paget GL, Turi V: Alpha-adrenergic responses in asthma. J Lab Clin Med 105:164–169, 1985.
55. De Vries K: The protective effect of inhaled Sch 1000 MDI on bronchoconstriction induced by serotonin, histamine, acetylcholine and propranolol. Postgrad Med J 51(suppl. 7):106, 1975.

56. Deckers W: The chemistry of new derivatives of tropane alkaloids and the pharmacokinetics of a new quaternary compound. Postgrad Med J 51(suppl. 7):76, 1975.
57. Dixon RAF, Kobilka BK, Strader DJ, et al: Cloning of the gene and the cDNA for mammalian β-adrenergic receptor and homology with rhodopsin. Nature 32:75, 1986.
58. Djukanovic R, Roche WR, Wilson JW, et al: Mucosal inflammation in asthma. Am Rev Respir Dis 142:434–457, 1990.
59. Drislane FW, Samuels MA, Kozakewich H, et al: Myocardial contraction band lesions in patients with fatal asthma: possible neurocardiologic mechanisms. Am Rev Respir Dis 135:498, 1987.
60. D'Silva JL: The action of adrenaline on serum potassium. J Physiol (Lond) 82:393, 1934.
61. Eichler HG, Blochl-Daum B, Eichler I, et al: Normal responsiveness of superficial hand veins to alpha- and beta-adrenergic stimuli in allergic asthma: effects of terbutaline and prednisolone on beta-adrenergic responsiveness. J Allergy Clin Immunol 86:714–725, 1990.
62. Fairshter RD, Novey HS, Wilson AF: Site and duration of bronchodilatation in asthmatic patients after oral administration of terbutaline. Chest 95:50, 1981.
63. Fanta CH, Rossing TH, McFadden ER Jr: Treatment of acute asthma. Is combination therapy with sympathomimetics and methylxanthines indicated? Am J Med 80(1):5, 1986.
64. Fontana G, Mugnai M, Cresci F, et al: Histamine-induced bronchial response after administration of placebo, salbutamol and a combination of a beta-2-adrenergic drug (fenoterol) with an anticholinergic agent (ipratropium bromide) in asymptomatic asthma patients. Respiration 50:201–205, 1986.
65. Fraser CM, Nelson HS, Middleton E Jr: Adrenergic agents. In Middleton E Jr, Reed C, Ellis E, et al (eds): Allergy Principles and Practice, 4th edition. St. Louis, Mosby, 1993, pp 778–815.
66. Friberg S, Graff-Lonnevig V: Ipratropium bromide (Atrovent) in childhood asthma: a cumulative dose-response study. Ann Allergy 62:131–134, 1989.
67. Fryer AD, Jacoby DB: Effect of inflammatory cell mediators on M_2 muscarinic receptors in the lungs. Life Sci 52:529, 1993.
68. Fujimura M, Azuma H, Uotani K, et al: Additive effects of isoproterenol-phenylephrine aerosol following ipratropium bromide on airway obstruction in older patients with intrinsic asthma and chronic bronchitis. JPN Med J 25:122–126, 1986.
69. Gandevia B: Historical review of the use of parasympatholytic agents in the treatment of respiratory disorders. Postgrad Med J 51(suppl 7):13, 1975.
70. Geumei AM, Miller WF, Miller J, Gast LR: Bronchodilator effect of a new oral beta-adrenoceptor stimulant TH1165a. A comparison with metaproterenol sulfate. Chest 70:460, 1976.
71. Gibson GJ, Greenacre JK, Konig P, et al: Use of exercise challenge to investigate possible tolerance to beta-adrenoceptor stimulation in asthma. Br J Dis Chest 72:199–206, 1978.
72. Glass P, Dulfano NJ: Evaluation of a new β_2 adrenergic receptor stimulant, terbutaline, in bronchial asthma. I. Subcutaneous comparison with epinephrine. Curr Ther Res Clin Exp 15(4):141, 1973.
73. Grainger J, Woodman K, Pearce N, et al: Prescribed fenoterol and death from asthma in New Zealand, 1981–7: a further case-control study. Thorax 46:105–111, 1991.
74. Gross NJ: Anticholinergic agents. In Weiss EB, Stein M (eds): Bronchial Asthma. Little, Brown and Co, Boston, 1993, pp 876–883.
75. Gross NJ: COPD: a disease of reversible airflow obstruction. Am Rev Respir Dis 133:725, 1986.
76. Gross NJ: Ipratropium bromide. N Engl J Med 319:486, 1988.
77. Gross NJ: The influence of anticholinergic agents on treatment for bronchitis and emphysema. Am J Med 91:11S–12S, 1991.
78. Gross NJ, Bankwala Z: Effects of an anticholinergic bronchodilator on arterial blood gases of hypoxemic patients with COPD. Am Rev Respir Dis 136:1091, 1987.
79. Gross NJ, Barnes PJ: A short tour around the muscarinic receptor. Am Rev Respir Dis 138:765, 1988.
80. Gross NJ, Co E, Skorodin MS: Cholinergic bronchomotor tone in COPD: estimates of its amount in comparison to normal. Chest 96:984, 1989.
81. Gross NJ, Petty TL, Friedman M, et al: Dose-response to ipratropium nebulized solution in COPD: a 3-center study. Am Rev Respir Dis 139:1188–1191, 1989.
82. Gross NJ, Skorodin MS: Anticholinergic agents. In Jenne JW, Murphy S (eds): Drug Therapy for Asthma. Lung Biology in Health and Disease. Vol 31. Dekker, New York, 1987, pp 615–668.
83. Gross NJ, Skorodin MS: Anticholinergic, antimuscarinic bronchodilators. Am Rev Respir Dis 129:856, 1984.
84. Gross NJ, Skorodin MS: Role of the parasympathetic system in airway obstruction due to emphysema. N Engl J Med 311:421, 1984.
85. Grossman J: The occurrence of arrhythmias in hospitalized asthmatic patients. J Allergy Clin Immunol 57:310, 1976.
86. Guideri G, Barletta M, Lehr D: Extraordinary potentiation of isoproterenol cardiotoxicity by corticoid pretreatment. Cardiovasc Res 8:775, 1974.
87. Haahtela T, Ahokas I, Ahonen A, et al: Inhaled bronchodilators in asthma: low or high dose? Ann Allergy 66:175–180, 1991.
88. Haalboom JRE, Deenstra M, Struyvenberg A: Hypokalemia induced by inhalation of fenoterol. Lancet 1:1125, 1985.
89. Harris L: Comparison of the effect on blood gases, ventilation, and perfusion of ioproterenol-phenylephrine and salbutamol aerosols in chronic bronchitis with asthma. J Allergy Clin Immunol 49:63, 1972.
90. Harvey JE, Tattersfield AE: Airway response to salbutamol: effect of regular salbutamol inhalation in normal, atopic and asthmatic subjects. Thorax 37:280–287, 1982.
91. Hausdorff WP, Bouvier M, O'Dowd BF, et al: Phosphorylation sites on two domains of the β_2-adrenergic receptor are involved in distinct pathways of receptor desensitization. J Biol Chem 264(21):12657–12665, 1989.
92. Hausdorff WP, Caron MG, Lefkowitz RJ: Turning off the signal: desensitization of β-adrenergic receptor function. FASEB J 4:2881, 1990.
93. Heel RC, Brogden RN, Speight TM, Avery GS: Fenoterol: a review of its pharmacological properties and therapeutic efficacy in asthma. Drugs 15:3, 1978.
94. Heimer D, Brami JL, Liberman D, et al: Comparison of a B2 adrenergic agonist and an anticholinergic agent given by sequential inhalation in patients with severe chronic obstructive pulmonary disease. Isr J Med Sci 27:307–310, 1991.
95. Henderson WR, Shelhamer JH, Reingold DB, et al: Alpha-adrenergic hyper-responsiveness in asthma. N Engl J Med 300:642–647, 1979.
96. Herman JJ, Noah ZL, Moody RR: Use of intravenous isoproterenol for status asthmaticus in children. Crit Care Med 11(9):716, 1983.
97. Hershfus JA, Bresnick E, Levinson L, Segal MS: A new sympathomimetic amine (neusuprel) in the treatment of bronchial asthma. Ann Allergy 9:769–773, 1951.
98. Higgins RM, Cookson WO, Lane DJ, et al: Cardiac arrhythmias caused by nebulized beta-agonist therapy. Lancet 2:863, 1987.
99. Holgate ST: Anticholinergics in acute bronchial asthma. Postgrad Med J 63:35–39, 1987.
100. Hooper PL, Woo W, Visconti L, Pathak DR: Terbutaline raises high-density-lipoprotein cholesterol levels. N Engl J Med 305:1455, 1981.
101. Hughes DT: The use of anticholinergic drugs in nocturnal asthma. Postgrad Med J 63:47–51, 1987.
102. Ind PW, Barnes PJ, Brown MJ, et al: Plasma histamine concentration during propranolol induced bronchoconstriction. Thorax 40:903–909, 1985.
103. Ind PW, Dixon CM, Fuller RW, et al: Anticholinergic blockade of beta-blocker induced bronchoconstriction. Am Rev Respir Dis 139:1390–1394, 1989.
104. Ingram RH Jr, Krumpe PE, Duffell GM, Maniscalco B: Ventilation-perfusion changes after aerosolized isoproterenol in asthma. Am Rev Respir Dis 101:364, 1970.
105. Inman WHN, Adelstein AM: Rise and fall of asthma mortality in England and Wales in relation to use of pressurised aerosols. Lancet 2:279–283, 1969.
106. International Consensus Report on Diagnosis and Treatment of Asthma: National Heart, Lung, and Blood Institute, US Department of Health and Human Services publication 92-3091, 1992.
107. Jackson RT, Beaglehole R, Rea HH, et al: Mortality from asthma: a new epidemic in New Zealand. Br Med J 285:771–774, 1982.
108. Jenne JW, Taskin DP: Beta-adrenergic agonists. In Weiss EB, Stein M (eds): Bronchial Asthma, 3rd edition. Lippincott, Philadelphia, 1993, pp 700–748.
109. Jeppsson AB, Löfdahl CG, Waldeck B, et al: On the predictive value of experiments in vitro in the evaluation of the effect of duration of bronchodilator drugs for local administration. Pulm Pharmacol 2:81–85, 1989.
110. Johnson M: The pharmacology of salmeterol. Lung 168(suppl):115, 1990.
111. Jolobe OM: Reversible airflow obstruction: clinical spectrum and responsiveness to anticholinergic drugs. Respiration 45:232–236, 1984.

112. Kaimel J, Schwartz HJ, Chester EH: Aerosol bronchodilator therapy: a comparison of the effects of bronkometer with isoetharine, isoproterenol and phenylephrine. Ann Allergy 43:151–154, 1979.
113. Karpel JP, Pesin J, Greenberg D, et al: A comparison of the effects of ipratropium bromide and metaproterenol sulfate in acute exacerbations of COPD. Chest 98:835–839, 1990.
114. Keltz H, Stone DJ, Samortin T: Nebulization of saline and isoproterenol in chronic bronchitis. Arch Intern Med 130:44, 1972.
115. Kelly HW, Murphy S: Beta-adrenergic agonists for acute severe asthma. Ann Pharmacother 26:81–91, 1992.
116. Kerrebijn KF, van Essen-Zandvliet EEM, Neijens HJ: Effect of long-term treatment with inhaled corticosteroids and beta-agonists on the bronchial responsiveness in children with asthma. J Allergy Clin Immunol 79:653–659, 1987.
117. Klaustermeyer WB, Di Bernardo RL, Hale FC: Intravenous isoproterenol: rationale for bronchial asthma. J Allergy Clin Immunol 55(5):325, 1975.
118. Koepke JW, Selner JC, Dunhill AL: SO_2 derived from bronchodilator solutions. J Allergy Clin Immunol 71(suppl):147, 1983.
119. Kraan J, Koëter GH, Mark TW, et al: Changes in bronchial hyperreactivity induced by 4 weeks of treatment with antiasthmatic drugs in patients with allergic asthma: a comparison between budesonide and terbutaline. J Allergy Clin Immunol 76:628–636, 1985.
120. Kung M: Parenteral adrenergic bronchodilation and potassium. Chest 89:322, 1986.
121. Kung M, White JR, Burki NK: The effect of subcutaneously administered terbutaline on serum potassium in asymptomatic adult asthmatics. Am Rev Respir Dis 129:329, 1984.
122. Laitinen LA, Empey DW, Bye C, et al: A comparison of the bronchodilator action of pseudoephedrine and ephedrine in patients with reversible airway obstruction. Eur J Clin Pharmacol 23:107–109, 1982.
123. Lammers JW, Minette P, McCusker M, et al: The role of pirenzipine-sensitive (M_1) muscarinic receptors in vagally mediated bronchoconstriction in humans. Am Rev Respir Dis 139:446, 1989.
124. Lands AM, Arnold A, McAuliff JP, et al: Differentiation of receptor systems activated by sympathomimetic amines. Nature 214:597–598, 1967.
125. Larsson K, Bevegard S, Mossberg B: Posture-induced airflow limitation in asthma: relationship to plasma catecholamines and an inhaled anticholinergic agent. Eur Respir J 1:458–463, 1988.
126. Larsson K, Martinsson A, Hjemdahl P: Influence of circulating alpha adrenoceptor agonists on lung function in patients with exercise induced asthma and healthy subjects. Thorax 41:552–558, 1986.
127. Larsson S, Svedmyr N, Thiringer G: Lack of bronchial beta adrenoceptor resistance in asthmatics during long-term treatment with terbutaline. J Allergy Clin Immunol 59:93, 1977.
128. Latimer KM, O'Byrne PM, Morris MM, et al: Bronchoconstriction stimulated by airway cooling: better protection with combined inhalation of terbutaline sulphate and cromolyn sodium than with either alone. Am Rev Respir Dis 128:440–443, 1983.
129. Leak A, O'Connor T: High dose ipratropium—is it safe? Practitioner 232:9, 1988.
130. Lefcoe NM, Toogood JH, Blennerhassett G, et al: The addition of an aerosol anticholinergic to an oral beta agonist plus theophylline in asthma and bronchitis. Chest 82:300–305, 1982.
131. Legge JS, Gaddie J, Palmer K: Comparison of the two oral selected β_2-adrenergic stimulating drugs in bronchial asthma. Br Med J 1:637, 1971.
132. Leifer K, Wittig H: The β_2 sympathomimetic aerosols in the treatment of asthma. Ann Allergy 35:69, 1965.
133. Leitch AG, et al: Effect of intravenous infusion of salbutamol on ventilatory response to carbon dioxide and hypoxia on heart rate and plasma potassium in normal men. Br Med J 1:365, 1976.
134. Liggett SB: β-adrenergic receptor structure and function. J Respir Dis 15(4):S28–S38, 1994.
135. Liggett SB, Raymond JR: Pharmacology and molecular biology of adrenergic receptors. In Bouloux PM (ed): Catecholamines. Ballière's Clinical Endocrinology and Metabolism. Vol 7. WB Saunders Co, London, 1993, p 279.
136. Lipworth BJ: Risks vs benefits of inhaled β_2-agonists in the management of asthma. Drug Safety 7(1):54–70, 1992.
137. Lipworth BJ, McDevitt DJ, Struthers AD: Prior treatment with diuretic augments the hypokalemic and electrocardiographic effects of inhaled albuterol. Am J Med 86:653–657, 1989.
138. Littner MR, et al: Double-blind comparison of acute effects of inhaled albuterol, isoproterenol or placebo on cardiopulmonary function and gas exchange in asthmatic children. Ann Allergy 50:309, 1983.
139. Littner MR, Tashkin DP, Calvarese B, et al: Acute bronchial and cardiovascular effects of increasing doses of pirbuterol acetate aerosol in asthma. Ann Allergy 48(1):14–20, 1982.
140. Löfdahl CG: Basic pharmacology of new long-acting sympathomimetics. Lung 168(suppl 1):21, 1990.
141. Löfdahl CG, Chung KF: Long-acting β_2-adrenoceptor agonists: a new perspective in the treatment of asthma. Eur Respir J 4:218–226, 1991.
142. Löfdahl CG, Svedmyr N: Beta-agonists—friends or foes? Eur Respir J 4(10):1161–1165, 1991.
143. Lonky SA, Tisi GM: Determining changes in airflow caliber in asthma: the role of submaximal expiratory flow rates. Chest 77:741, 1980.
144. Maguire JF, Geha RS, Umetsu DT: Myocardial-specific creatine phosphokinase isoenzyme elevation in children with asthma treated with intravenous isoproterenol. J Allergy Clin Immunol 78:631, 1986.
145. Maguire WC, Nair S: Ventilation and perfusion effects of inhaled alpha and beta agonists in asthma patients. Chest 73(suppl):983, 1978.
146. Malo J-L, Cartier A, Trudeau C: Formaterol, a new inhaled beta-2 adrenergic agonist has a longer blocking effect than albuterol on hyperventilation-induced bronchoconstriction. Am Rev Respir Dis 142:1147, 1990.
147. Mann KV, Leon AL, Tietze KJ: Use of ipratropium bromide in obstructive lung disease. Clin Pharm 7:670–680, 1988.
148. Martinsson A, Larsson K, Hjemdahl P: Studies in vivo and in vitro of terbutaline-induced beta-adrenoceptor desensitization in health subjects. Clin Sci (Colch) 72:47–54, 1987.
149. Massey KL, Gotz VP: Ipratropium bromide. Drug Intell Clin Pharm 19:5–12, 1985.
150. McAlpine LG, Thomas NC: Prophylaxis of exercise-induced asthma with inhaled formaterol, a long-acting beta$_2$-adrenergic agonist. Respir Med 84:293, 1990.
151. McEvoy JDS, Vall-Spinosa A, Paterson JW: Assessment of orciprenaline and isoproterenol infusions in asthmatic patients. Am Rev Resp Dis 108:490, 1973.
152. McFadden ER Jr, Kiser R, DeGroot WJ: Acute bronchial asthma. Relations between clinical and physiologic manifestations. N Engl J Med 288(5):221, 1973.
153. Millar AB, Bush A, al-Hillawi H, et al: Ipratropium bromide: are patients treated with optimal therapy? Postgrad Med J 66:1040–1042, 1990.
154. Milner AD: Ipratropium bromide and airways obstruction in childhood. Postgrad Med J 63:53–56, 1987.
155. Minette PA, Lammers JW, Dixon CM, et al: A muscarinic agonist inhibits reflex bronchoconstriction in normal but not in asthmatic subjects. J Appl Physiol 67:2461, 1989.
156. Mita H, Shida T: Anti-allergic activity of formoterol, a new beta-adrenoceptor stimulant, and salbutamol in human leukocytes and human lung tissue. Allergy 38:547–552, 1983.
157. Miura M, Belvisi MG, Stretton CD, et al: Role of potassium channels in bronchodilator responses in human airways. Am Rev Respir Dis 146:132, 1992.
158. Moler FW, Hurwitz ME, Custer JR: Improvement in clinical asthma score and $PaCO_2$ in children with severe asthma treated with continuously nebulized terbutaline. J Allergy Clin Immunol 81:1101, 1988.
159. Moore PF, Constantine JW, Baith WE: Pirbuterol, a selective β_2-adrenergic bronchodilator. J Pharmacol Exp Ther 207:410, 1978.
160. Morley J, Sanjar S, Newth C: Viewpoint: untoward effects of beta-adrenoceptor agonists in asthma. Eur Respir J 3:228–233, 1990.
161. Morr H: Immunological release of histamine from human lung. II. Studies on acetylcholine and the anticholinergic agent ipratropium bromide. Respiration 38:273–279, 1979.
162. Morris HG: Review of ipratropium bromide in induced bronchospasm in patients with asthma. Am J Med 81:36–44, 1986.
163. National Asthma Education Program: Guidelines for the Diagnosis and Management of Asthma. National Heart, Lung, and Blood Institute. US Department of Health and Human Services publication 91-3042, 1991.
164. Nelson HS: Adrenergic therapy of bronchial asthma. J Allergy Clin Immunol 77:771–785, 1986.
165. Nelson HS, Spector SL, Whitsett TL, George RB: The bronchodilator response inhalation of increasing doses of aerosolized albuterol. J Allergy Clin Immunol 72:371, 1983.
166. Neville A, Palmer JB, Gaddie J, May CS: Metabolic effects of salbutamol: comparison of aerosol and intravenous administration. Br Med J 1:413, 1977.

167. Newcomb R, Tashkin DP, Hui KK, et al: Rebound hyperresponsiveness to muscarinic stimulation after chronic therapy with an inhaled muscarinic antagonist. Am Rev Respir Dis 132:12–15, 1985.
168. Nijkamp FP: β-adrenergic receptors in the lung: an introduction. Life Sci 52:2073, 1993.
169. Nijkamp FP, Engels F, Henricks PAJ, et al: Mechanisms of β-adrenergic receptor regulation in lungs and its implications for physiological responses. Physiol Rev 72:323–367, 1992.
170. Nou E: A clinical comparison of subcutaneous doses of terbutaline and adrenaline in bronchial asthma. Scand J Respir Dis 52:192, 1971.
171. Nyberg L: Pharmacokinetic properties of bambuterol in solution and tablet—basis for once daily dosage in asthma. Acta Pharmacol Toxicol 59(suppl 5):229, 1986.
172. O'Connor BJ, Aikman SL, Barnes PJ: Tolerance to the non-bronchodilator effects of inhaled B2-agonists in asthma. N Engl J Med 327:1204–1208, 1992.
173. Page CP: One explanation of the asthma paradox: inhibition of natural anti inflammatory mechanism by $beta_2$ agonists. Lancet 337:171–720, 1991.
174. Pakes GE, Brogden RN, Heel RC, et al: Ipratropium bromide: a review of its pharmacological properties and therapeutic efficacy in asthma and chronic bronchitis. Drugs 20:237–266, 1980.
175. Palmer KNV: Effect of bronchodilator drugs on arterial blood gas tensions in bronchial asthma. Postgrad Med J 47(suppl):75, 1971.
176. Palmer KNV, Hamilton WF, Lge JS, Diament ML: Effect of a selective beta-adrenergic blocker in preventing falls in arterial oxygen tension following isoprenaline in asthmatic subjects. Lancet 2:1092, 1969.
177. Parry WH, Martorano F, Cotton EK: Management of life-threatening asthma with intravenous isoproterenol infusions. Am J Dis Child 130(1):39, 1976.
178. Pasterkamp H, Tal A, Leahy F, et al: The effect of anticholinergic treatment on postexertional wheezing in asthma studied by phonopneumography and spirometry. Am Rev Respir Dis 132:16–21, 1985.
179. Paterson JW, Conolly ME, Davies DS, et al: Isoprenaline resistance and the use of pressurised aerosols in asthma. Lancet 2:426–429, 1968.
180. Paterson JW, Woolcock AJ, Shenfield GM: Bronchodilator drugs. Am Rev Respir Dis 120:1149, 1979.
181. Patrick DM, Dales RE, Stark RM, et al: Severe exacerbations of COPD and asthma. Incremental benefit of adding ipratropium to usual therapy. Chest 98:295–297, 1990.
182. Pavia D, Bateman JR, Sheahan NF, et al: Effect of ipratropium bromide on mucociliary clearance and pulmonary function in reversible airways obstruction. Thorax 34:501–507, 1979.
183. Pearce N, Grainger J, Atkinson M, et al: Case control study of prescribed fenoterol and death from asthma in New Zealand 1977–1981. Thorax 45:170–175, 1990.
184. Phillips PJ, Vedig AE, Jones PL, Chapman MG: Metabolic and cardiovascular side effects of the β_2-adrenoceptor agonists salbutamol and rimterol. Br J Clin Pharmacol 9:483, 1980.
185. Pierson RN Jr, Grieco MH: Isopreterenol aerosol in normal and asthmatic subjects. Am Rev Respir Dis 100:533, 1969.
186. Polosa R, Phillips GD, Rajakulasingam K, et al: The effect of inhaled ipratropium bromide alone and in combination with oral terfenadine on bronchoconstriction provoked by adenosine 5′-monophosphate and histamine in asthma. J Allergy Clin Immunol 87:939–947, 1991.
187. Porte D: Beta adrenergic stimulation of insulin release in man. Diabetes 16:150, 1964.
188. Ramsdale EH, Otis J, Kline PA, et al: Prolonged protection against methacholine-induced bronchoconstriction by the inhaled β_2-agonist formoterol. Am Rev Respir Dis 143:998–1001, 1991.
189. Rebuck AS, Chapman KR, Abboud R, et al: Nebulized anticholinergic and sympathomimetic treatment of asthma and chronic obstructive airways disease in the emergency room. Am J Med 82(1):59–64, 1987.
190. Rebuck AS, Gent M, Chapman KR: Anticholinergic and sympathomimetic combination therapy of asthma. J Allergy Clin Immunol 71:317–323, 1983.
191. Rebuck AS, Marcus HI: Sch 1000 in psychogenic asthma. Scand J Respir Dis 103(suppl):186, 1979.
192. Reisman RE: Asthma induced by adrenergic aerosols. J Allergy 46:162–170, 1970.
193. Richardson JB: Innervation of the lung. Eur J Respir Dis Suppl 117:13, 1982.
194. Riker JB, Cacace LG: Double-blind comparison of metaproterenol and isoetharine-phenylephrine solutions in intermittent positive pressure breathing in bronchospastic conditions. Chest 78:723–725, 1980.
195. Roden DM, Iansmith DHS: Effects of low potassium or magnesium concentration on isolated cardiac muscle. Am J Med 82(suppl 3A):18–23, 1987.
196. Rona G: Catecholamine cardiotoxicity. J Mol Cell Cardiol 17:291, 1985.
197. Rosen JP, Chervinsky P, Renald RL, et al: Duration of action of oral albuterol in an asthmatic population. Ann Allergy 56:28, 1986.
198. Rossing TH, Fanta CH, Goldstein DH, et al: Emergency therapy of asthma: comparison of the acute effects of parenteral and inhaled sympathomimetics and infused aminophylline. Am Rev Respir Dis 122(3):365, 1980.
199. Rudolf M: Combination therapy—a review of clinical studies. Postgrad Med J 60:9–12, 1984.
200. Ruffin RE, McIntyre E, Crockett AJ, et al: Combination bronchodilator therapy in asthma. J Allergy Clin Immunol 69:60–65, 1982.
201. Sackner MA, Dougherty R, Watson H, Wanner A: Hemodynamic effects of epinephrine and terbutaline in normal men. Chest 68:616–624, 1975.
202. Sackner MA, Greeneltch N, Silva G, et al: Bronchodilator effects of terbutaline and epinephrine in obstructive lung disease. Clin Pharmacol Ther 16:499, 1974.
203. Schleuter DP: Ipratropium bromide in asthma. A review of the literature. Am J Med 81:55–60, 1986.
204. Schnack C, Podolsky A, Watzke H: Effects of somatostatin and oral potassium administration on terbutaline-induced hypokalemia. Am Rev Respir Dis 139:176–180, 1989.
205. Schwartz HJ, Trautlein JJ, Goldstein AR: Acute effects of terbutaline and epinephrine on asthma. J Allergy Clin Immunol 58(4):516, 1976.
206. Sears MR, Taylor RD, Print CG, et al: Regular inhaled B-agonist treatment in bronchial asthma. Lancet 336:1391–1396, 1990.
207. Shifrin GS, Klein WL: Regulation of acetylcholine receptor concentration in cloned neuroblastoma cells. J Neurochem 34:993, 1980.
208. Shires R, et al: Metabolic studies in acute asthma before and after treatment. Br J Dis Chest 73:66, 1979.
209. Siegel SC, Katz RM, Rachelefsky GS, et al: A placebo-controlled trial of procaterol: a new long-acting oral beta 2-agonist in bronchial asthma. J Allergy Clin Immunol 75:698, 1985.
210. Silverman M: The role of anticholinergic antimuscarinic bronchodilator therapy in children. Lung 168:304–309, 1990.
211. Sly RM, Badiei B, Faciane J: Comparison of subcutaneous terbutaline with epinephrine in the treatments of asthma in children. J Allergy Clin Immunol 59:128, 1977.
212. Smith SR, Kendall MJ: Metabolic responses to $beta_2$ stimulants. J R Coll Physicians Lond 18:190, 1984.
213. Smolensky MH, McGovern JP, Scott PH, et al: Chronobiology and asthma. II. Body-time-dependent differences in the kinetics and effects of bronchodilator medications. J Asthma 24:91–134, 1987.
214. Speizer FE, Doll R, Heaf P, et al: Investigation into use of drugs preceding death from asthma. Br Med J 1:339–343, 1968.
215. Spina D, Rigby PJ, Paterson JW, et al: α-adrenoceptor function and autoradiographic distribution in human asthmatic lungs. Br J Pharmacol 97:701–708, 1989.
216. Spitzer WO, Buist AS: Case-control study of prescribed fenoterol and death from asthma in New Zealand 1977–81. Thorax 45:645, 1990.
217. Stamm AM, Clausen JL, Tisi GM: Effects of aerosolized isoproterenol on resting myogenic tone in normals. J Appl Physiol 40:525, 1976.
218. Storms WW, Bodman SF, Nathan RA, et al: Use of ipratropium bromide in asthma: results of a multi-clinic study. Am J Med 81(suppl 5A):61–66, 1986.
219. Storms WW, DoPico GA, Reed CE: Aerosol Sch 1000. An anticholinergic bronchodilator. Am Rev Respir Dis 111:419–422, 1975.
220. Strauss MH, Reeves RA, Smith DL, Leenen FH: The role of cardiac beta-1 receptors in the hemodynamic response to a beta-2 agonist. Clin Pharmacol Ther 40:108, 1986.
221. Summers QA, Tarala RA: Nebulized ipratropium in the treatment of acute asthma. Chest 97:425, 1990.
222. Suzuki S, Miyashita A, Matsumoto Y, et al: Bronchoconstriction induced by spirometric maneuvers in patients with bronchial asthma. Ann Allergy 65:315–320, 1990.
223. Tai E, Read J: Response of blood gas tensions to aminophylline and isoprenaline in patients with asthma. Thorax 22:543, 1967.
224. Tandom MK: Cardiopulmonary effects of fenoterol and salbutamol aerosols. Chest 77:129, 1980.
225. Tashkin DP, Ashutosh K, Bleecker ER, et al: Comparison of the anticholinergic bronchodilator ipratropium bromide with metaprotere-

nol in chronic obstructive pulmonary disease. A 90 day multiceneter study. Am J Med 81(suppl 5A):81–90, 1986.
226. Tattersfield AE: Tolerance to β-agonists. Bull Eur Physiopathol Respir 21:1s–5s, 1985.
227. Taylor DR, Sears MR: Regular beta-adrenergic agonists: evidence, not reassurance, is what is needed. Chest 106(2):552–559, 1994.
228. Taylor MW, Gaddie J, Murchison LE, Palmer KN: Metabolic effects of oral salbutamol. Br J Med 1:22, 1976.
229. Thiringer G, Bergh NP, Svedmyr N: A comparative study of the effects of isoetharine and some other adrenergic beta-stimulators in chronic obstructive lung disease. Scand J Respir Dis 52:183, 1971.
230. Thomas DJB, Gill B, Brown P, Stubbs WA: Salbutamol-induced diabetic ketoacidosis. Br Med J 2:438, 1977.
231. Thomson NC, Daniel EE, Hargreave FE: Role of smooth muscle alpha 1-receptors in nonspecific bronchial responsiveness in asthma. Am Rev Respir Dis 126:521–525, 1982.
232. Tipton WR, Nelson HS: Frequent parenteral terbutaline in the treatment of status asthmaticus in children. Ann Allergy 58:252, 1987.
233. Twentyman OP, Finnerty JP, Harris A, et al: Protection against allergen-induced asthma by salmeterol. Lancet 336:1338–1342, 1990.
234. Ullah MI, Newman GB, Saunders KB: Influence of age on response to ipratropium and salbutamol in asthma. Thorax 36:523, 1981.
235. Ullman A, Hedner J, Svedmyr N: Inhaled salmeterol and salbutamol in asthmatic patients: an evaluation of asthma symtoms and the possible development of tachyphylaxis. Am Rev Respir Dis 142:571–575, 1990.
236. Ullman A, Svedmyr N: Salmeterol: a new long acting inhaled beta2 adrenoceptor agonist: comparison with salbutamol in adult asthmatic patients. Thorax 43:674–678, 1988.
237. van Schayck CP, Dompeling E, van Herwaarden CL, et al: Bronchodilator treatment in moderate asthma or chronic bronchitis: continuous or on demand? BMJ 303:1426–1431, 1991.
238. van Schayck CP, Graafsma SJ, Visch MB, et al: Increased bronchial responsiveness after inhaling salbutamol during 1 year is not caused by subsensitization to salbutamol. J Allergy Clin Immunol 86:793–800, 1990.
239. Vathenen AS, Knox AJ, Higgins BG, et al: Rebound increase in bronchial responsiveness after treatment with inhaled terbutaline. Lancet 1:554–558, 1988.
240. Virtanen R, Kanto J, Iisalo E, et al: Pharmacokinetic studies on atropine with special reference to age. Acta Anaesthesiol Scand 26:297–300, 1982.
241. Wahedna I, Wong CS, Wisniewski AFZ, et al: Asthma control during and after cessation of regular beta$_2$-agonist treatment. Am Rev Respir Dis 148:707–712, 1993.
242. Walker SB, Kradjan WA, Bierman CW: Bitolterol mesylate: a beta-adrenergic agent. Chemistry, pharmacokinetics, pharmacodynamics, adverse effects and clinical efficacy in asthma. Pharmacotherapy 5:127, 1985.
243. Weiner N: Norepinephrine, epinephrine, and the sympathomimetic amines. In Gillman AG, Goodman LD, Gillman A (eds): The Pharmacologic Basis of Therapeutics, 6th edition. Macmillan, New York, 1980.
244. Wess J: Mutational analysis of muscarinic acetylcholine receptors: structural basis of ligand/receptor/G protein interactions. Life Sci 53:1447, 1993.
245. Widdicombe JG: The parasympathetic nervous system in airways disease. Scand J Respir Dis Suppl 103:38–43, 1979.
246. Wilson AF, Novey HS, Cloninger D, Davis J: Cardiopulmonary effects of long-term bronchodilator administration. J Allergy Clin Immunol 58:204, 1976.
247. Windom HH, Burgess CD, Siebers RW, et al: The pulmonary and extrapulmonary effects of inhaled beta-agonists in patients with asthma. Clin Pharmacol Ther 48:296–301, 1990.
247a. Wolfe JD, Yamate M, Biederman AS, et al: Comparison of the acute cardiopulmonary effects of oral albuterol, metaproterenol, and terbutaline in asthmatics. JAMA 253:2068, 1985.
248. Wong CS, Pavord ID, Williams J, Britton JR: Bronchodilator, cardiovascular, and hypokalemic effects of fenoterol, salbutamol, and terbutaline in asthma. Lancet 336:1396, 1990.
249. Wood DW, Downes JJ, Scheinkopf H, et al: Intravenous isoproterenol in the management of respiratory failure in childhood status asthmaticus. J Allergy Clin Immunol 50(2):75, 1972.
250. Woolley M, Anderson SD, Quigley BM: Duration of protective effect of terbutaline sulfate and cromolyn sodium alone and in combination on exercise-induced asthma. Chest 97:39–45, 1990.
251. Yagura T, Yamamura Y: A new selective beta-adrenoceptor stimulant (procaterol): its bronchodilator potency and characteristics in asthmatic patients. Curr Ther 10:45, 1979.
252. Yang SC, Yang SP, Lee TS: Nebulized ipratropium bromide in ventilator-assisted patients with chronic bronchitis. Chest 105:1511–1515, 1994.
253. Zanetti CL, Rotman HH, Dresner AJ: Efficacy and duration of action of procaterol, a new bronchodilator. J Clin Pharmacol 22:250, 1982.

41 Antihistamines

F. ESTELLE R. SIMONS

Antihistamines (H_1-receptor antagonists) have been used for five decades in the treatment of symptoms of allergic disorders. This chapter reviews new information about H_1-receptor antagonist basic science, including the molecular basis for action, mechanisms of action (H_1-receptor blockade, and antiallergic effects); and clinical science, including pharmacokinetics, pharmacodynamics, efficacy, and adverse effects.

BASIC SCIENCE

MOLECULAR BASIS FOR ACTION OF H_1-RECEPTOR ANTAGONISTS

H_1-receptors have been defined pharmacologically by the actions of their respective agonists and antagonists.[11] Although there is little evidence that peripheral and central H_1 receptors differ, isoforms of H_1 receptors or perhaps different subtypes of H_1 receptors may exist.

The gene encoding the histamine H_1 receptor has been cloned from bovine, guinea pig, rat, and human tissue and expressed in heterologous cell lines. The human histamine H_1 receptor is located on the short arm of chromosome 3. It shows 70 to 80% homology with the H_1 receptors from other species, approximately 45% homology with the muscarinic receptor, and no homology with the H_2 receptor (Fig. 41–1).[5] Histamine receptors belong to a family of G-protein coupled receptors; the G proteins function essentially as on/off switches for cellular signaling. The histamine H_1 receptor has been linked to multiple signaling events, including phosphoinositol hydrolysis, cyclic AMP accumulation, arachidonic acid release, and calcium flux.

Histamine mediates a variety of physiologic and pathologic responses in different tissues and cells and is an important chemical mediator of inflammation in allergic disease (Table 41–1).[19] Acting via H_1 receptors and inositol phospholipid hydrolysis, histamine plays an important role in causing smooth muscle contraction in the respiratory and gastrointestinal tracts and in causing pruritus and sneezing via sensory nerve stimulation. Histamine induces vascular endothelium to release nitric oxide that stimulates guanylate cyclase and increases cyclic guanosine monophosphate (GMP) levels in vascular smooth muscle, causing vasodilation. Acting via H_1 and H_2 receptors, it causes hypotension, tachycardia, flushing, and headache. Activation of H_2 receptors alone causes an increase in gastric acid secretion and numerous other pharmacologic responses. H_3-receptor stimulation may have negative modulatory effects. Representative agonists and antagonists of histamine receptors are listed in Table 41–2.

In the central nervous system, histamine is a neurotransmitter and can be readily demonstrated by immunohistochemical techniques. It is synthesized in situ from L-histidine by specific L-histidine decarboxylase and metabolized exclusively by specific histamine *N*-methyltransferase. Studies of human cerebrospinal fluid suggest that brain histaminergic activity increases with age.

MECHANISMS OF ACTION OF H_1-RECEPTOR ANTAGONISTS

The three important structural features of H_1-receptor antagonists are the basicity of the nitrogen group, the presence of multiple aromatic or heterocyclic rings and alkyl substituents, and the nature of the linkage between the rings and substituents, which historically was used to categorize H_1-receptor antagonists into six groups: ethanolamines, ethylene diamines, alkylamines, piperazines, piperidines, and phenothiazines (Fig. 41–2, Table 41–3). Medications within each class may vary in their efficacy and adverse effect profiles. Some of the newer second-generation H_1-receptor antagonists do not fit readily into the traditional classification system; for example, terfenadine, astemizole, and levocabastine each contain a piperidine ring but are not typical piperidines. Acrivastine is structurally similar to triprolidine, cetirizine is an active human metabolite of hydroxyzine, and loratadine is structurally similar to azatadine and cyproheptadine.

Histamine H_1-receptor antagonists are highly selective for H_1 receptors, having little effect on H_2 or H_3 receptors.[4] First-generation H_1-receptor antagonists may also block muscarinic cholinergic, 5-hydroxytryptamine (serotonin), or α-adrenergic receptors, whereas few of the second-generation

	Transmembrane 3	Transmembrane 5
H-H_1R	RPLCLFWLSMDYVASTASIFSVFILCIDRY	WFKVMTAIINFYLPTLLMLWFYA
B-H_1R	RPLCLFWLSMDYVASTASIFSVFILCIDRY	WFKVMTAIINFYLPTLLMLWFYA
R-H_1R	RPLCLFWLSMDYVASTASIFSVFILCIDRY	WFKVMTAIINFYLPTLLMLWFYV
GP-H_1R	RPLCLFWLSMDYVASTASIFSVFILCIDRY	WFKVMTAIINFYLPTLLMLWFYI
H-H_2R	KVFCNIYTSLDVMLCTASILNLFMISLDRY	VYGLVDGLVTFYLPLLIMCITYY
C-H_2R	KVFCNIYTSLDVMLCTASILNLFMISLDRY	VYGLVDGLVTFYLPLLVMCITYY

A

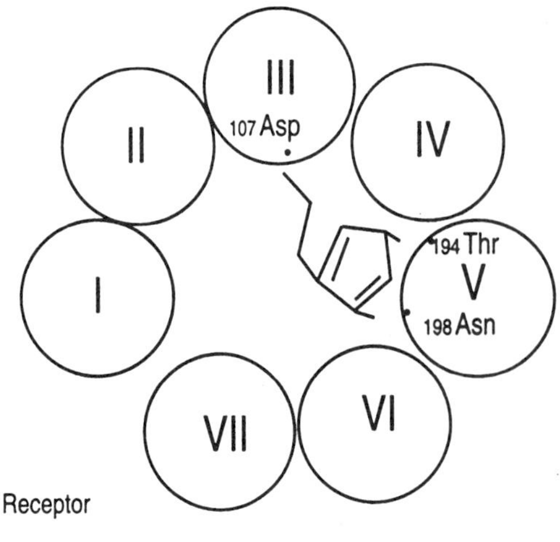

B H_1 Histamine Receptor

FIGURE 41–1. Amino acid alignment of the third and fifth transmembrane domains of the H_1 and H_2 receptors of different species. **(A)** Transmembrane domains in the receptors' sequences are identified by a line above the sequence. Residues shown in bold are presumed to bond with the ligand. H = human; B = bovine; R = rat; GP = guinea pig; C = canine. **(B)** A model illustrates the binding site of the H_1 receptor. The view of the receptor is from the extracellular face of the plasma membrane. Seven transmembrane helixes are numbered I through VII. Binding to Asp^{107}, Thr^{194}, and Asn^{198} by histamine is shown and corresponds to the bold D, T, and N shown above. (Chowdhury BA, Kaliner MA: Molecular cloning and characterization of the human histamine H_1-receptor gene. ACI News 7:24–8, 1995.)

TABLE 41–1
ACTIVITIES MEDIATED THROUGH HISTAMINE RECEPTORS IN HUMANS

	H_1 Receptor	H_2 Receptor	H_3 Receptor
Location	Bronchial and gastrointestinal smooth muscle, brain	Gastric mucosa, uterus, brain	Brain, bronchial smooth muscle
Function	Constrict smooth muscle (vascular and bronchial) ↑ Vascular permeability ↑ Pruritus ↑ Pain ↑ Cyclic GMP ↑ Prostaglandin generation ↓ Atrioventricular node conduction time Activation of airway vagal afferent nerves ↑ Glycoprotein secretion (bronchial mucosa goblet cells) Stimulation of cough receptors ↑ Histidine uptake ↑ Hypotension ↑ Flushing ↑ Headache ↑ Tachycardia ↑ Release of mediators of inflammation ↑ Recruitment of inflammatory cells	↑ Vascular permeability ↑ Gastric acid secretion Activates adenylate cyclase, ↑ cyclic AMP Chonotropic action in atrial muscle Inotropic action in ventricular muscle Bronchial smooth muscle relaxation ↑ Mucous secretion Lipolytic effect in fat cells Stimulation of T-suppressor cells ↓ Basophil histamine release ↓ Neutrophil and basophil chemotaxis and enzyme release Inhibit cytotoxicity and proliferation of lymphocytes Inhibit natural killer cells ↑ Hypotension ↑ Flushing ↑ Headache ↑ Tachycardia	Vasodilation of cerebral vessels Prevents excessive bronchoconstriction Negative feedback ↓ Neurogenic microvascular leakage ↓ Sympathetic transmission in perivascular nerves

H_1-receptor antagonists have any of these properties. First-generation H_1-receptor antagonists also cross the blood-brain barrier readily.[30] Whereas H_1-receptor selectivity may contribute to the low central nervous system (CNS) toxicity of the second-generation H_1-receptor antagonists, H_1-receptor antagonism alone may cause sedation. Lack of central nervous system toxicity likely is due primarily to their inability to cross the tightly fused outer membranes of the endothelial cells lining the brain capillaries.

The precise structural requirements for H_1-receptor selectivity and affinity are being elucidated. For example, the α,α-diphenyl-4-piperidino-methanol moiety is the pharmacophore for H_1-receptor activity of terfenadine, and the phenylbutanol moiety prevents terfenadine from crossing the blood-brain barrier.[32]

H_1-RECEPTOR BLOCKADE

At low concentrations, H_1-receptor antagonists are competitive antagonists of histamine. They bind to H_1 receptors but do not activate them, thus preventing histamine binding and action. At higher concentrations, some second-generation H_1-receptor antagonists, such as astemizole, loratadine, and terfenadine, also exhibit noncompetitive inhibition. The binding of most H_1-receptor antagonists is readily reversible, but some, such as astemizole and terfenadine, do not readily dissociate from H_1 receptors.

During the immediate hypersensitivity reaction, after histamine is released from mast cells, tissue histamine concentrations theoretically reach 10^{-5} to 10^{-3} M. The concentration of an H_1-receptor antagonist achieved in tissue varies with its physicochemical properties, pharmacokinetics, and dose; however, peak concentrations seldom exceed 10^{-6} M. For H_1-receptor antagonists, such as terfenadine, astemizole, and loratadine, tissue concentrations of active H_1-receptor antagonist metabolites may be more relevant than those of the parent compound.

ANTIALLERGIC EFFECTS

In vitro, many H_1-receptor antagonists prevent release of mediators of inflammation from human basophils and mast

TABLE 41–2
HISTAMINE AGONISTS AND ANTAGONISTS*

	H_1 Receptor	H_2 Receptor	H_3 Receptor
Agonists	2-Methylhistamine, betahistine, 2-pyridylethylamine	4-Methylhistamine, betahistine, dimaprit, impromidine	α-Methylhistamine
Antagonists	Chlorpheniramine, diphenhydramine, hydroxyzine, terfenadine, astemizole, loratadine, cetirizine	Burimamide, tiotidine, metiamide, cimetidine, ranitidine, famotidine, nizatidine, etintidine	Thioperamide, impromidine, betahistine, burimamide

*Partial list.

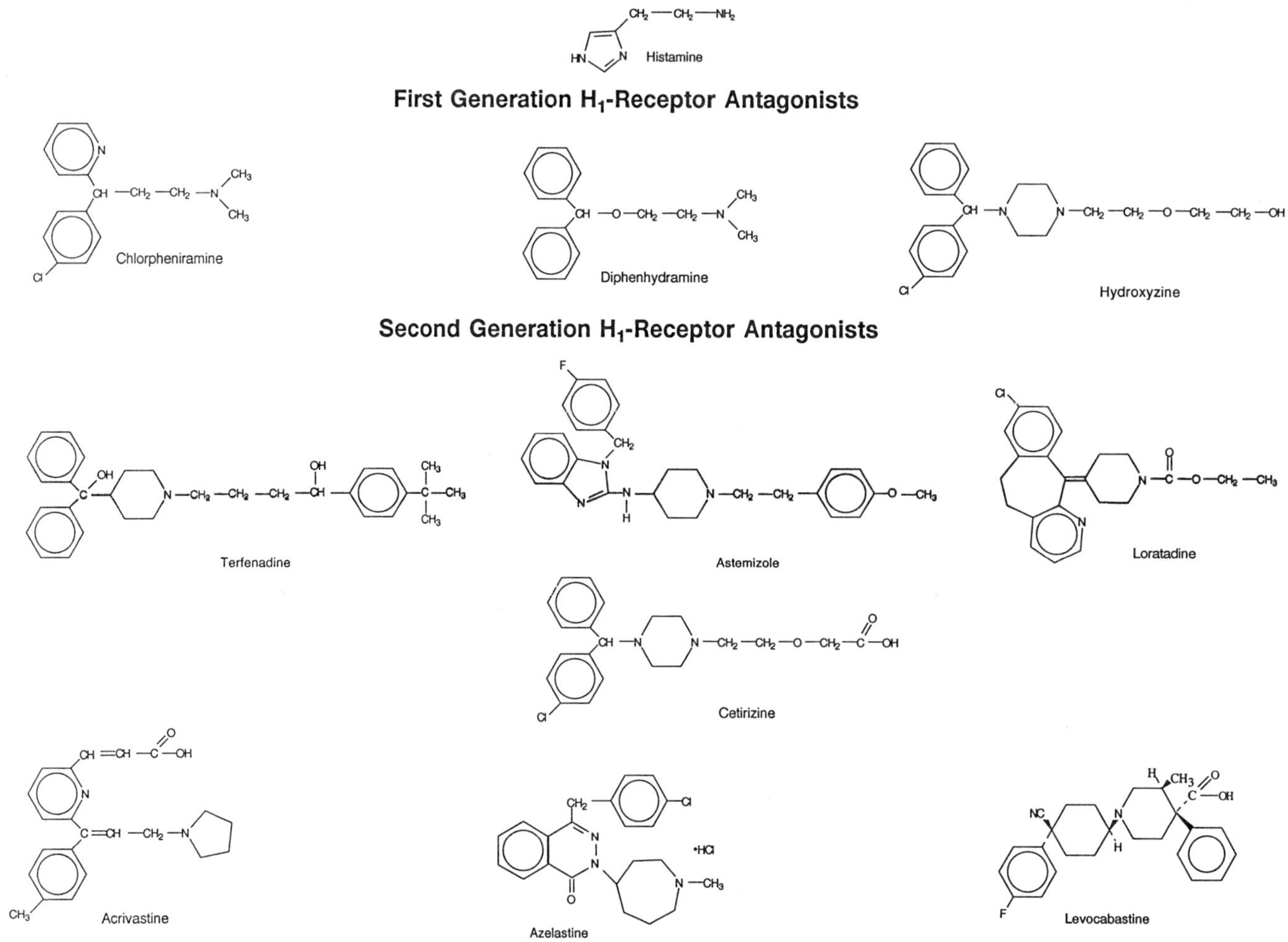

FIGURE 41–2. Chemical structure of histamine and chemical structures of selected first- and second-generation H_1-receptor antagonists.

cells.[2, 21] These effects vary with the stimulus for mediator release, the mediator being measured, and the H_1-receptor antagonist concentration. For some H_1-receptor antagonists, the concentrations required are up to 1,000 times higher than can be achieved in vivo after usual doses. The biochemical mechanisms by which H_1-receptor antagonists inhibit mediator release do not involve H_1-receptor antagonism. Rather, the H_1-receptor antagonists form ionic associations with cell membranes, prevent calcium binding, and inhibit membrane-related activities.

TABLE 41–3
STRUCTURE-BASED CLASSIFICATION OF H_1-RECEPTOR ANTAGONISTS, WITH EXAMPLES

Class	Old, First Generation	New, Second Generation
Alkylamine	Triprolidine	Acrivastine
Ethanolamine	Diphenhydramine	
Ethylenediamine	Tripelennamine	
Phenothiazine	Promethazine	
Piperazine	Hydroxyzine	Cetirizine
Piperidine	Cyprohepatadine	Loratadine
Other		Terfenadine, astemizole azelastine, levocabastine (topical)

In vivo, pretreatment with some second-generation H_1-receptor antagonists decreases mediator release after antigen challenge on the nasal mucosa or skin of subjects naturally sensitized to the antigen.[2, 21] For example, in allergic rhinitis, pretreatment with terfenadine or loratadine reduces histamine and prostaglandin D_2 (PGD_2) release into nasal secretions. An H_1-receptor antagonist may inhibit mediator release more effectively in one organ than in another. In the skin, pretreatment with cetirizine decreases histamine, platelet-activating factor (PAF), and PGD_2 release after antigen challenge and inhibits eosinophil, neutrophil, and basophil migration induced by antigen or by PAF. In allergic rhinitis, however, cetirizine is less effective in inhibiting mediator release and does not inhibit eosinophil migration. In allergic conjunctivitis, cetirizine reduces ICAM-1 levels after antigen challenge in vivo (Fig. 41–3).[6]

In addition to inhibition of mediator release, decreased migration and activation of inflammatory cells, and reduced adhesion protein expression, H_1-receptor antagonists inhibit proinflammatory cell activation and generation of products such as superoxide radicals, LTB_4, LTC_4, neutrophil elastase, and eosinophilic cationic protein. They also down-regulate mononuclear cells.

The contribution of the antiallergic and anti-inflammatory effects of H_1-receptor antagonists to their overall clinical

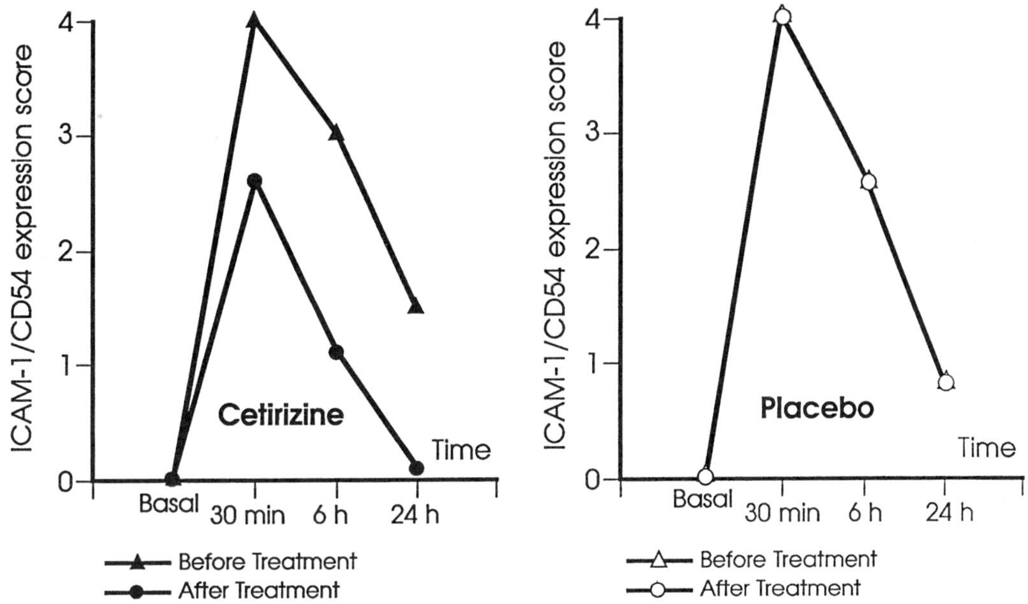

FIGURE 41–3. Ten mg of cetirizine twice daily for 3.5 days in contrast to matched placebo, decreased intercellular adhesion molecule-1 (ICAM-1/CD54 expression) on epithelial cells, 30 minutes (early-phase reaction), 6 hours, and 24 hours (late-phase reaction) after out-of-pollen season, allergen-specific conjunctival challenge. Median values of total scores of ICAM-1/CD54 expression on epithelial cells before and after treatment and before and after allergen-specific conjunctival challenge are shown. Deviation of individual values from the median was less than 1. ICAM-1/CD54 expression on conjunctival epithelium was significantly increased in all subjects 30 minutes, 6 hours, and 24 hours after challenge before treatment versus after treatment and after placebo. Cetirizine also suppressed itching, hyperemia, lacrimation, and swelling of the eyelids and reduced the number of inflammatory cells in conjunctival scrapings (not shown). (Ciprandi G, Buscaglia S, Pesce G, et al: Cetirizine reduces inflammatory cell recruitment and ICAM-1 (or CD54) expression on conjunctival epithelium in both early- and late-phase reactions after allergen-specific challenge. J Allergy Clin Immunol 95:612–621, 1995.)

efficacy is unknown. Most studies are narrowly focused on a few H_1-receptor antagonists and a few tests; no broad spectrum studies are available. Few investigators have attempted to correlate in vitro and in vivo antiallergic and anti-inflammatory effects.

CLINICAL SCIENCE

EFFICACY

There are interesting and clinically important differences among the pharmacokinetic and pharmacodynamic profiles of H_1-receptor antagonists (Table 41–4).[25, 26]

H_1-receptor antagonists are medications of first choice for allergic rhinoconjunctivitis sufferers and are widely used for self-medication in this disorder (Fig. 41–4, Table 41–5). They are less effective for relief of nasal blockage than of sneezing, itching, rhinorrhea, ocular itching, tearing, and erythema.[26] If they fail to relieve these symptoms, doubling the dose or substituting one H_1-receptor antagonist for another is a less helpful option than adding a topical intranasal glucocorticoid to the treatment regimen for long-term relief of mucosal inflammation.

There is considerable interest in the effect of H_1-receptor antagonists on the quality of life in people suffering from allergic rhinoconjunctivitis. In one study, although the H_1-

FIGURE 41–4. In a double-blind, parallel-group, placebo-controlled, 6-week study during the grass pollen season, 118 subjects received 10 mg of loratadine daily or placebo. Total symptom-free days occurred more frequently in those receiving loratadine. At the end of the study, 65% of those receiving loratadine and 49% of those receiving placebo had no symptoms or mild symptoms. The differences in symptom scores between loratadine and placebo were not significant. Adverse effects did not differ. (Dolovich J, Moote DW, Mazza JA, et al: Efficacy of loratadine versus placebo in the prophylactic treatment of seasonal allergic rhinitis. Ann Allergy 73:235–239, 1994.)

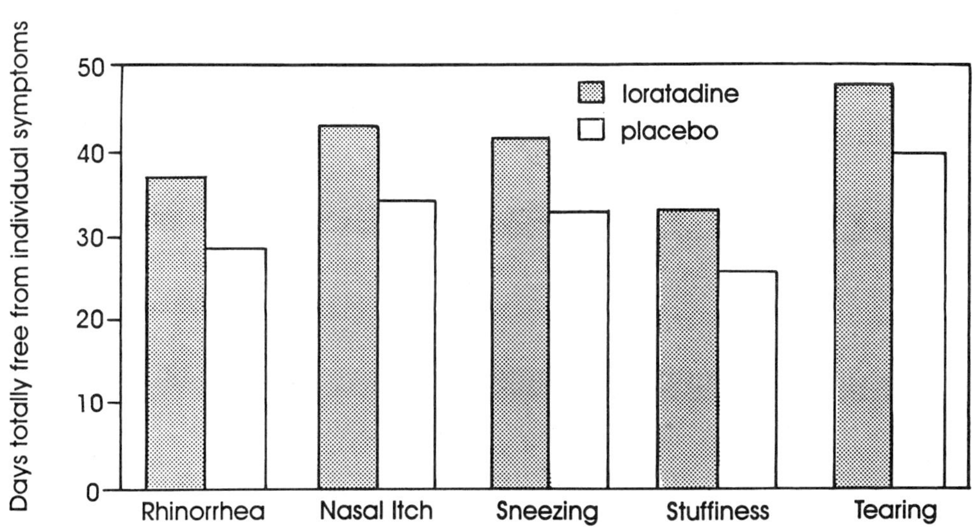

TABLE 41–4
H_1-RECEPTOR ANTAGONISTS: IMPORTANT PHARMACOKINETIC AND PHARMACODYNAMIC CONCEPTS

First-Generation H_1-Receptor Antagonists	Pharmacokinetics	Pharmacodynamics
Chlorpheniramine	Long t1/2	Single dose suppresses wheal and flare and signs and symptoms for 24 hours
Diphenhydramine	Relatively short t1/2	Does not suppress the wheal and flare for 24 hours
Hydroxyzine	Long t1/2, well studied in different populations	Single dose suppresses wheal and flare for 24 or more hours; high skin concentrations are achieved
Acrivastine	Renal elimination, very short half-life	Rapid onset of action; short duration of action
Astemizole	Long t1/2 of active metabolite; potential for medication interactions	Single dose ± effective; multiple doses very effective and effects last for weeks after a short course is discontinued
Azelastine	Long t1/2; oral or topical use	Few pharmacodynamic studies
Cetirizine	Renal elimination, small volume of distribution	Most effective H_1-receptor antagonist in suppressing the histamine- or allergen-induced wheal and flare
Levocabastine	Renal elimination, long t1/2; used topically, little systemic absorption	Few pharmacodynamic studies
Loratadine	Eliminated by more than one enzyme in the cytochrome P_{450} system, active metabolite	Single 10 mg dose suppresses wheal and flare for up to 24 hours
Terfenadine	No terfenadine measurable in plasma under usual circumstances; active metabolite; medication interactions are a potential problem	Single dose suppresses wheal and flare and signs and symptoms for 24 hours

t1/2 = terminal elimination half life.

receptor antagonist being tested did not improve nasal symptoms as much as did the topical intranasal glucocorticoid with which it was being compared, the two classes of medications were comparably effective for nonallergic rhinitis symptoms, eye symptoms, effect on emotions and activities, and overall quality of life.[14]

In mild, chronic asthma, H_1-receptor antagonists, such as astemizole, azelastine, cetirizine, loratadine, and terfenadine, give some relief of symptoms, but doses higher than those recommended for allergic rhinoconjunctivitis are generally needed.[26]

In chronic urticaria, H_1-receptor antagonists are first-line medications for relief of pruritus and reduction of number, size, and duration of urticarial lesions. There is some rationale for administering an antihistamine, such as doxepin, which has combined H_1- and H_2-receptor antagonist effects, or for concurrent administration of an H_1- and H_2-receptor antagonist in the treatment of refractory urticaria. H_2-receptor antagonists such as cimetidine decrease vascular leakage and may also inhibit the metabolism of a concomitantly administered H_1-receptor antagonist in the hepatic cytochrome P_{450} system, leading to elevated plasma and tissue

TABLE 41–5
HISTAMINE-MEDIATED SYMPTOMS POTENTIALLY RELIEVED BY ANTIHISTAMINES IN ALLERGIC DISORDERS

Disease	Symptoms	Pathophysiology	Comment
Allergic rhinitis	Pruritus (H_1-)	Sensory nervous stimulation	Histamine is quantitatively an important mediator in allergic rhinitis. It plays little role in hyperirritability and congestion
	Sneezing (H_1-)	Sensory nervous stimulation	
	Rhinorrhea (H_1-)	↑ Mucus secretion	
	Obstruction (H_1-)	Mucosal edema	
Asthma	Bronchospasm (H_1-)	Smooth muscle constriction	Histamine plays an indirect role in causing airway inflammation
	Mucosal edema (H_1-)		
	Mucus secretion (H_2-)		
Urticaria	Wheal (H_1-)	↑ Vascular permeability	Histamine is involved in producing all symptoms
	Erythema (H_1-)	Vasodilation	
	Pruritus (H_1-)	Sensory nerve stimulation	
Anaphylaxis	Urticaria, angioedema (H_1-)	↑ Vascular permeability	Histamine is involved in producing all symptoms; other vasoactive substances may contribute as well
	Laryngeal edema (H_1-)	↑ Vascular permeability	
	Intestinal edema (H_1-)	↑ Vascular permeability	
	Flushing (H_1-)(H_2-)	Vasodilation	
	Headache (H_1-)(H_2-)	Vasodilation	
	Hypotension (H_1-)(H_2-)	Vasodilation	
	Palpitations (H_1-)		
	Rhinorrhea (H_1-)(H_2-)	Mucus secretion	
	Bronchorrhea (H_1-)(H_2-)	Mucus secretion	
Atopic dermatitis	Pruritus (H_1-)	Sensory nerve stimulation	In addition to histamine, serotonin, proteases, peptides; and prostaglandins may cause pruritus
	Erythema (H_1-)	Vasodilation	

concentrations of the H_1-receptor antagonist. In this context, there is probably little rationale for combining an H_2-receptor antagonist with an H_1-receptor antagonist such as cetirizine, which is eliminated primarily by the renal route (Fig. 41–5).[27]

In anaphylaxis, H_1- and H_2-receptor antagonists are used concurrently to reduce the effect of histamine on the peripheral vasculature and the myocardium.[15] Older H_1-receptor antagonists, such as diphenhydramine, chlorpheniramine, and hydroxyzine, are still widely used in the treatment of anaphylaxis as, in contrast to the newer medications, they are available for parenteral use.

Second-generation H_1-receptor antagonists, like their predecessors, are effective in the treatment of atopic dermatitis but may be required in doses higher than those generally recommended for allergic rhinoconjunctivitis.[9]

SAFETY

The adverse effects of H_1-receptor antagonists are summarized in Tables 41–6 and 41–7.[18, 22–24] Most of the second-generation medications are relatively free from adverse CNS effects,[28] primarily because they do not cross the blood-brain

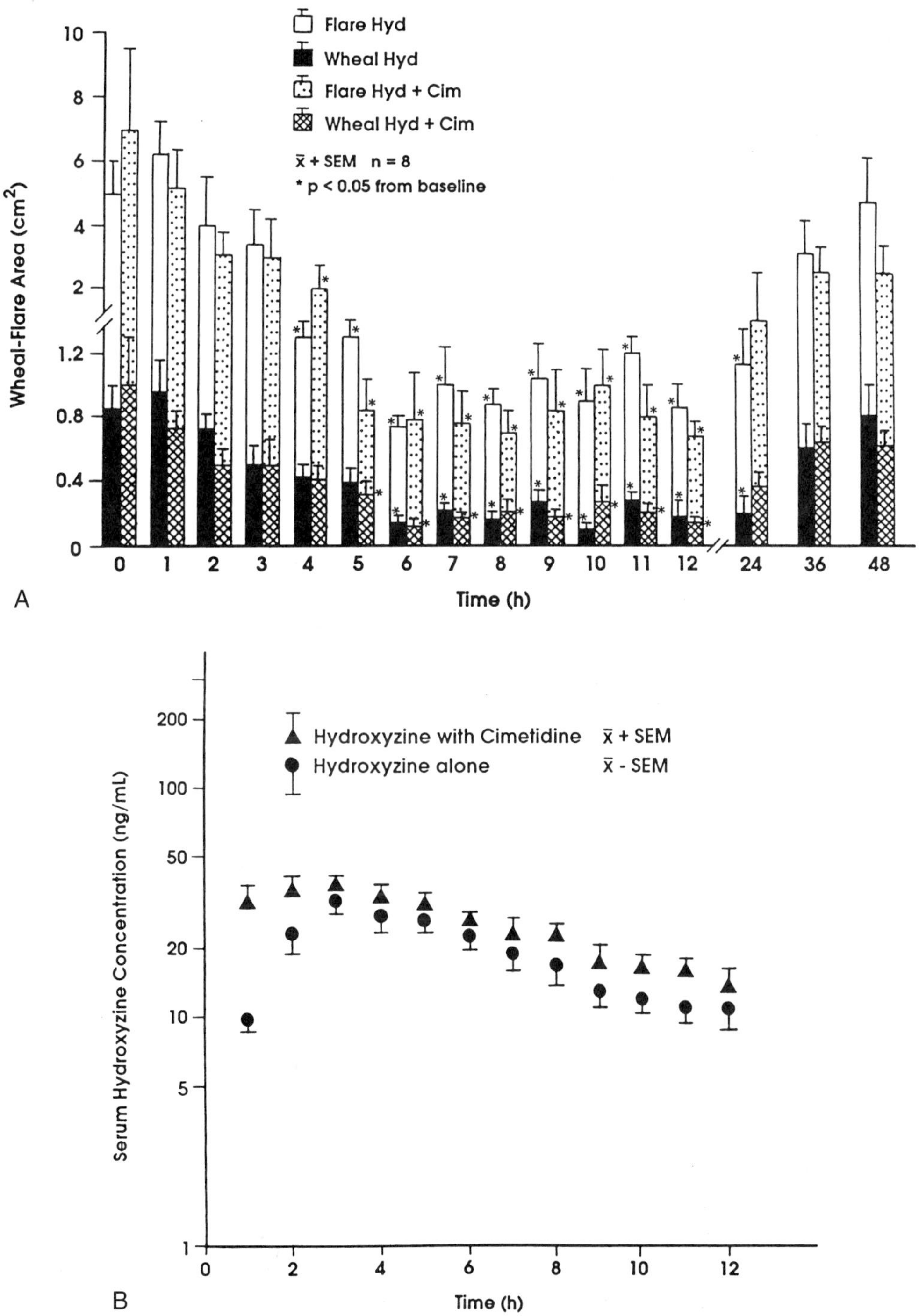

FIGURE 41–5. In a randomized, double-blind, parallel-group study in 16 subjects with chronic urticaria, the suppressive effect of 25 mg of hydroxyzine before and after treatment with 600 mg of cimetidine twice daily for 10 days was examined.

(A) When hydroxyzine was given with cimetidine, wheal-and-flare suppression increased compared with when hydroxyzine was given alone, although the difference was not statistically significant ($p>0.05$). **(B)** Coadministration of hydroxyzine with cimetidine also resulted in significantly increased serum hydroxyzine concentration and a significantly increased partial hydroxyzine area under the curve ($p<0.05$). There may be some rationale for a trial of concomitant administration of cimetidine in people suffering from chronic urticaria unresponsive to treatment with an H_1-receptor antagonist alone.

In the same study, there was no therapeutic rationale for coadministration of cetirizine with cimetidine (not shown). (Simons FER, Sussman GL, Simons KJ: Effect of the H_2-receptor antagonist cimetidine on the pharmacokinetics and pharmacodynamics of the H_1-receptor antagonists hydroxyzine and cetirizine in patients with chronic urticaria. J Allergy Clin Immunol 95:685–693, 1995.)

TABLE 41–6
CENTRAL NERVOUS SYSTEM EFFECTS OF H_1-RECEPTOR ANTAGONISTS: DOUBLE-BLIND, PLACEBO-CONTROLLED, OBJECTIVE STUDIES*

Second-Generation H_1-Receptor Antagonist (dose range, mg)	First-Generation H_1-Receptor Antagonist Comparators (dose range, mg)	Tests	Comments
Acrivastine (4–60)	Triprolidine (2 and 5)	Performance: RT, adaptive tracking Subjective: VAS	Acrivastine did not impair adaptive tracking or reaction time, but in doses >8 mg, does impair CNS function
Astemizole (10–40, 10 used in most studies)	Mequitazine (4), diphenhydramine (50)	Performance: RT, CFF, DSS, pursuit rotor Subjective: VAS	Astemizole did not impair performance, in contrast to comparators; peripheral H_1-blockade measured in one study; serum concentrations measured in one study
Azelastine†			
Cetirizine (5–20)	Hydroxyzine (25–50), diphenhydramine (50), triprolidine (5 bid)	Performance: DSS, driving simulator, simulated assembly line EEG: spectrum analysis, quantified EEG: P300, MSLT Subjective: VAS	Cetirizine 5–10 mg caused less CNS dysfunction than all first-generation comparators; peripheral blockade measured in most studies
Levocabastine (0.5 mg/mL, 2 drops in each eye/2 drops, each nostril)	Triprolidine (10)	Performance: RT, CFF, simulated car-tracking, memory, word recognition Subjective: VAS	Levocabastine administered topically in healthy adults did not cause CNS dysfunction
Loratadine (10–40)	Triprolidine (10), diphenhydramine (50)	Performance: RT, DSS, coordination, DVA, short-term memory, flight simulation, learning ability EEG: MSLT Subjective: SSS	Loratadine 10–20 mg did not cause CNS dysfunction or somnolence in contrast to its comparators
Terfenadine (20–240, 60 used in most studies)	Chlorpheniramine (4–8), clemastine (1–3), promethazine (10), triprolidine (10), diphenhydramine (25–150), hydroxyzine (25–50)	Performance: RT, CFF, DSS, etc., including flight simulation, simulated and actual driving tests EEG: P3, P300, MSLT Subjective: VAS, SSS	Terfenadine caused less CNS dysfunction than did all comparators

*Most of the studies have been conducted in healthy subjects.
†Little published information
Performance: CFF = critical flicker fusion; DSS = digit-symbol substitution; DVA = dynamic visual acuity; EEG: P3 or P300 = P3 or P300 event-related potential; MSLT = multiple sleep latency test; Subjective: VAS = visual analog scale; SSS = Stanford Sleepiness Scale; LARS = line analog rating scale (subjective sedation).
From Simons FER: The therapeutic index of newer H_1-receptor antagonists. Clin Exp Allergy 24:707–723, 1994.

TABLE 41–7
RISK FACTORS ASSOCIATED WITH ASTEMIZOLE- OR TERFENADINE-INDUCED QTc PROLONGATION, TORSADE DE POINTES, AND OTHER CARDIAC DYSRHYTHMIAS

Risk Factors	H_1-Receptor Antagonist Dose (mg/day)	Comments
Large dose or overdose	Astemizole 10–200 or 2.5–16.7 mg/kg (child), or terfenadine 120–360	Many people with dysrhythmias had no CNS effects; seizures occurred in one person, lethargy in four
Other disorders: cardiac abnormalities, such as congenital increased QTc, ischemic heart disease	Astemizole 10–20 or terfenadine 120–180	Some people also had other risk factors, such as concomitant ingestion of CYP3A4 inhibitors, or electrolyte imbalance
Hepatic dysfunction (cirrhosis)	Terfenadine 240*	
Concomitant adminstration of other CYP3A4 inhibitors, such as macrolide antibiotics or imidazole antifungals, or of medications that prolong the QTc interval	Terfenadine 120	Some people also had ischemic heart disease or prolonged QT interval by history
Severe hypokalemia, hypomagnesemia, or hypocalcemia	Terfenadine 120–900	Some people also had ischemic heart disease, congestive heart failure, history of ethanol abuse, or concomitant ketozonazole ingestion

From Simons FER: The therapeutic index of newer H_1-receptor antagonists. Clin Exp Allergy 24:707–723, 1994.
*Fexofenadine, a terfenadine metabolite, may lack cardiac side effects at 7240.

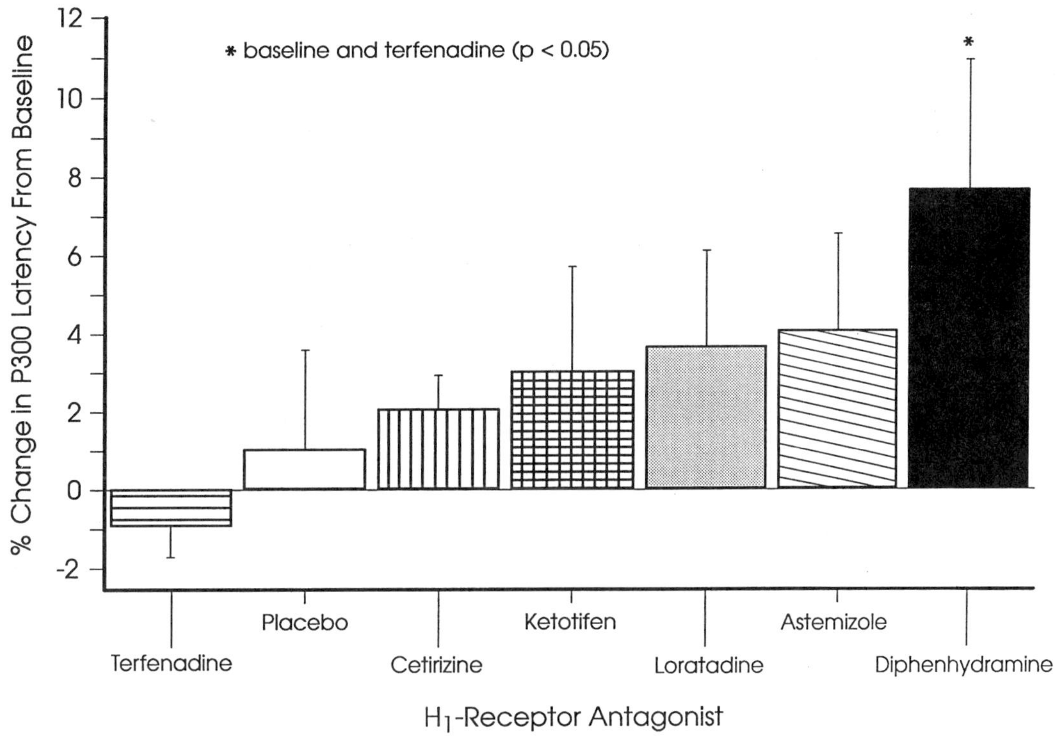

FIGURE 41–6. Fifteen healthy subjects received 10 mg of cetirizine, 60 mg of terfenadine, 10 mg of astemizole, 10 mg of loratadine, 2 mg of ketotifen, 50 mg of diphenhydramine, or placebo before and 2–2.5 hours after measurement of an evoked potential on the electroencephalogram (the P300 event-related potential). In rank order from least effects to greatest effects on this test, the medications were terfenadine, placebo, loratadine, cetirizine, astemizole, ketotifen, and diphenhydramine. Diphenhydramine had a significantly greater effect than placebo and baseline. The newer medications had a similar effect to placebo and to each other. (Simons KJ, Fraser TG, Reggin JD, Simons FER: Comparison of the central nervous system effects and peripheral H_1-blockade produced by six H_1-receptor antagonists. Clin Exp Allergy (in press).)

barrier to the extent that their predecessors do but also because they are more selective for H_1 receptors, rather than muscarinic, serotoninergic, or other receptors, than are their predecessors (Fig. 41–6). After astemizole and terfenadine had been widely used for many years, they were reported to cause prolongation of the QTc interval, torsade de pointes, and other cardiac arrhythmias (Fig. 41–7).[20] These adverse cardiovascular events occur rarely, following overdose or after administration to people with hepatic or cardiac dysfunction or those receiving concomitant treatment with macrolide antibiotics such as erythromycin or with oral antifungals such as ketoconazole.

During pregnancy, most second-generation H_1-receptor antagonists are classified by the Food and Drug Administration as having a category C risk and should be used only if the benefit to the mother justifies the unknown risk to the fetus. Loratadine and cetirizine have been assigned a category B risk, implying that they are safer for use during pregnancy. All H_1-receptor antagonists enter breast milk. These new medications are widely believed to be safe for use in infants and young children, but to date, they are not well studied in this age group.

Some selected H_1-receptor antagonists will be reviewed in detail, including a few first-generation medications still in widespread use. For each of these H_1-receptor antagonists, important attributes will be summarized with regard to pharmacokinetics, pharmacodynamics, clinical efficacy, and safety. Although newer medications such as astemizole, cetirizine, loratadine, and terfenadine are considerably more expensive than generic formulations of older medications such as chlorpheniramine or diphenhydramine, they may actually be similar in cost to some brand name chlorpheniramine or diphenhydramine formulations. These newer medications may be less expensive than other older medications such as clemastine and azatadine, which in addition to causing adverse CNS effects in some patients, have not been as widely studied.[1] Recommended doses of H_1-receptor antagonists are listed in Table 41–8.

FIRST-GENERATION H_1-RECEPTOR ANTAGONISTS

Chlorpheniramine

Chlorpheniramine terminal elimination half-life values are surprisingly long, with mean values of 21 to 28 hours in adults and up to 13 hours in children.[25] The duration of action of a single dose of chlorpheniramine as assessed by suppression of the histamine-induced wheal and flare and allergic rhinitis symptoms is at least 24 hours. There is a direct correlation between mean serum chlorpheniramine concentrations and effect on symptom relief ($r = 0.75$) and an inverse correlation between mean serum chlorpheniramine concentrations and mean histamine-induced wheal and flare diameters ($r = -0.68$ and $r = -0.92$, respectively). The rationale for using time-release or repeat-action formulations of chlorpheniramine is primarily to reduce peak serum and

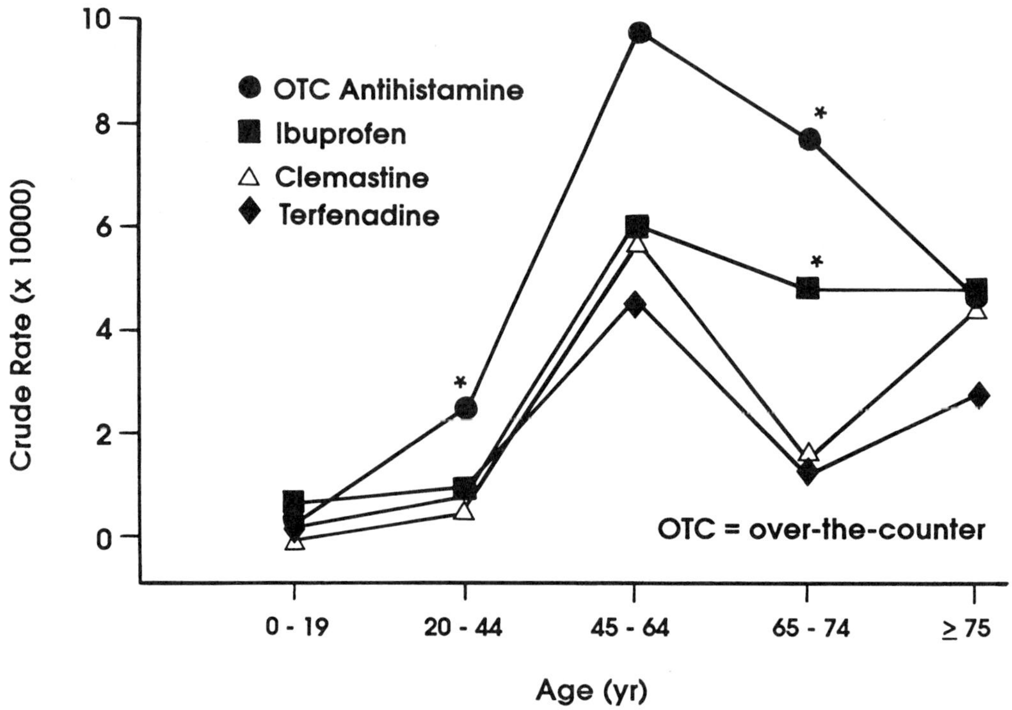

FIGURE 41–7. Investigators tested the hypothesis that terfenadine exposure increased the risk of arrhythmias, using an observational historical cohort study design and a medication exposure period of 30 days in people receiving terfenadine (n = 181,672), OTC (over the counter, nonprescription) antihistamines (n = 150,689), ibuprofen (n = 181,672), and clemastine (n = 83,156). Ibuprofen was studied as a control because it is free from cardiovascular effects. The incidence of ventricular arrhythmias and cardiac arrest was higher in the OTC antihistamine group than in the terfenadine, ibuprofen, and clemastine groups. Crude rates per 10,000 prescription exposures of developing a life-threatening ventricular arrhythmia are represented for the four medication cohorts over the age categories assessed in the study. Interaction (↑ relative risk) between terfenadine and ketoconazole was identified (n = 648, relative risk = 26.08, $p < 0.001$). There was a trend toward interaction between terfenadine and erythromycin (n = 41,308, relative risk = 1.36, p = NS) (not shown). (Reprinted by permission of the publisher. Pratt CM, Hertz RP, Ellis BE, et al: Risk of developing life-threatening ventricular arrhythmias associated with terfenadine in comparison with over-the-counter antihistamines, ibuprofen and clemastine. Am J Cardiol 73:346–352, 1994. Copyright 1994 by Excerpta Medica Inc.)

CNS concentrations and thus reduce CNS adverse effects. So-called tachyphylaxis to chlorpheniramine may be related to decreased compliance rather than to induction of hepatic metabolism of the medication.

Chlorpheniramine remains in widespread use for the treatment of allergic rhinitis and, less appropriately, upper respiratory tract infections. It is frequently combined with a decongestant or other medications.

The adverse CNS effects of chlorpheniramine are well documented. In manufacturers' recommended doses, it causes somnolence, decreased performance, and changes in the electroencephalogram. In overdose, it may produce coma or, paradoxically, seizures and other evidence of CNS stimulation.

Diphenhydramine

The terminal elimination half-life value of diphenhydramine in young adults is 9 hours.[25] The half-life is prolonged in people with chronic liver disease and in the elderly but is shorter in children. Significant suppression of the histamine-induced wheal and flare and symptoms induced by nasal allergen challenge lasts at least 10 to 12 hours.

Diphenhydramine is still widely used for treatment of allergic rhinitis, urticaria, and, with little rationale, upper respiratory tract infections. It is used orally and parenterally for the prevention or ancillary treatment of anaphylactic and anaphylactoid reactions.

The adverse CNS effects of diphenhydramine have been repeatedly confirmed, as it has been used frequently as the positive control in comparative studies with newer H_1-receptor antagonists (see Fig. 41–6).[28] In people suffering from allergic disorders, the CNS effects are generally considered undesirable. Under some circumstances, however, these effects are considered therapeutic. Worldwide, diphenhydramine is still the most commonly used nonprescription medication for insomnia.

Hydroxyzine

The pharmacokinetics and pharmacodynamics of hydroxyzine have been well studied. Its terminal elimination half-life ranges from 7 hours in young children and 14 to 20 hours in healthy adults to 37 hours in adults with hepatic dysfunction secondary to primary biliary cirrhosis.[25] The pharmacokinetics of hydroxyzine do not change over time. It enters the skin rapidly, and sustained high concentrations in the skin can be found after single and multiple doses. A single dose suppresses the histamine-induced wheal and flare significantly for at least 36 hours in healthy adults.

Hydroxyzine is still used in the treatment of chronic urticaria and atopic dermatitis, in which its sedative effects may

TABLE 41–8
FORMULATIONS AND DOSAGES OF REPRESENTATIVE H_1-RECEPTOR ANTAGONISTS

	Formulation	Recommended Dose
First Generation		
Chlorpheniramine maleate (Chlortrimeton)	Tablets 4 mg, 8 mg†, 12 mg† Syrup 2.5 mg/5 mL Parenteral solution 10 mg/mL	Adults: 8–12 mg bid† Pediatric*: 0.35 mg/kg/24 hr
Diphenhydramine hydrochloride (Benadryl)	Capsules 25 or 50 mg Elixir 12.5 mg/5 mL Syrup 6.25 mg/5 mL Parenteral solution 50 mg/mL	Adult: 25–50 mg tid Pediatric: 5 mg/kg/24 hr
Hydroxyzine hydrochloride (Atarax)	Capsules 10, 25, 50 mg Syrup 10 mg/5 mL	Adult: 25–50 mg qd (hs) bid Pediatric: 2 mg/kg/24 hr
Second Generation		
Acrivastine (Semprex)	Tablets 8 mg‡	Adult: 8 mg tid‡
Astemizole (Hismanal)	Tablets 10 mg Suspension 10 mg/5 mL**	Adult: 10 mg qd Pediatric: 0.2 mg/kg/24 hr
Azelastine (Astelin)	Nasal solution 0.1% (0.137 mg/spray) Tablets 2 mg**	Topical: 2 sprays in each nostril qd or bid Adult: 2–4 mg bid**
Cetirizine (Reactine)	Tablets 10 mg	Adult: 5–10 mg qd
Levocabastine (Livostin)	Microsuspension 50 μg/mL	Topical: two drops in each eye bid-qid
Loratadine (Claritin)	Tablets 10 mg Syrup 1 mg/mL	Adult: 10 mg qd Pediatric: 2–12 yrs, 5 mg/day; >12 yrs and >30 kg, 10 mg/day
Terfenadine (Seldane)	Tablets 60 mg, 120 mg** Suspension 30 mg/5 mL**	Adult: 60 mg bid *or* 120 mg qd** Pediatric: 3–6 yrs, 15 mg bid; 7–12 yrs, 30 mg bid

*For children weighing ≤40 kg.
**Not approved in the United States at time of publication.
†Timed release.
‡With pseudoephedrine 60 mg.
qd = once daily; bid = twice daily; tid = three times daily; qid = four times daily.

contribute to its efficacy in relief of pruritus. Its CNS effects have been well documented objectively and subjectively. Except in urticaria or atopic dermatitis sufferers unable to sleep because of severe pruritus, these effects are generally considered undesirable.

SECOND-GENERATION H_1-RECEPTOR ANTAGONISTS

Acrivastine

Acrivastine is a metabolite of triprolidine and is excreted largely unchanged in the urine.[3] It has a terminal elimination half-life of 1 to 3 hours, and its metabolite has a half-life of 2 hours. It suppresses the histamine-induced wheal and flare response promptly, within 15 minutes for the flare and 25 minutes for the wheal, with peak effects at 90 and 120 minutes, respectively. It also reduces the response to histamine challenge in the nose, conjunctivae, and lower airways.

Acrivastine 8 mg three times daily is effective in the treatment of allergic rhinoconjunctivitis or chronic urticaria. In the United States, it is marketed only for rhinoconjunctivitis, in a fixed-dose combination with pseudoephedrine.

It causes less drowsiness than first-generation H_1-receptor antagonists but in doses greater than 8 mg may cause some adverse CNS effects. It may also potentiate the effect of alcohol. It does not produce dysrhythmias or other adverse cardiovascular system effects.

Astemizole

Astemizole is metabolized in the cytochrome P_{450} system to desmethylastemizole (DMA), which has significant antihistaminic activity.[12] Steady-state plasma concentrations of unchanged astemizole are reached within 1 week, and those of astemizole plus metabolites within 4 weeks. After a single 30 mg astemizole dose, the terminal elimination half-life is 1.1 days and the terminal elimination half-life of DMA is 9.5 days. In human liver microsome preparations in vitro, the metabolism of astemizole to DMA is less sensitive to the effects of ketoconazole than is the metabolism of terfenadine to hydroxyterfenadine.

The recommended dose of astemizole is 10 mg daily. An initial dose or a single dose may not have a significant beneficial effect, so this medication is probably not ideal for sporadic use. After a short course of astemizole, the effects on suppression of the histamine-induced wheal-and-flare and of histamine-induced bronchoconstriction may last for 4 to 6 weeks.

When administered on a regular basis, astemizole is highly effective in the treatment of seasonal allergic rhinoconjunctivitis, perennial allergic rhinitis, and chronic urticaria. Adverse CNS effects have not been attributed to astemizole. Prolongation of the QTc interval, torsade de pointes, and other dysrhythmias may occur after astemizole overdose or when astemizole is administered concurrently with cytochrome P_{450} inhibitors. Some people complain of inappropriate weight gain during astemizole treatment.[22–24]

Azelastine

Azelastine has a half-life of 22 hours and is metabolized by hepatic oxidation.[17] Its major metabolite, desmethylazelastine, which is pharmacologically active, has a half-life of 54 hours. Further studies of azelastine pharmacokinetics in subjects of different ages or with different diseases and of azelastine interactions with other medications are needed. The antiallergic effects of azelastine have been studied extensively in vitro and in the guinea pig asthma model.

It is administered in a dose of 2 to 4 mg by mouth twice daily or as two sprays of a topical nasal solution daily or twice daily. After oral azelastine, wheal and flare suppression is dose related, peaking at about 4 hours and persisting for 1 week after the last dose of a short course of treatment. Few comparative studies of the effect of azelastine and other H_1-receptor antagonists have been performed. Azelastine significantly inhibits the response to intranasal histamine. In asthmatics, it protects against bronchial challenge with histamine and produces dose-related bronchodilation.

Orally administered azelastine in doses up to 4 mg per day consistently relieves seasonal allergic rhinoconjunctivitis or perennial allergic rhinitis symptoms and has a modest beneficial effect in mild, chronic asthma. Azelastine nasal spray is as effective as orally administered H_1-receptor antagonists, such as terfenadine 120 mg daily, in relieving rhinitis symptoms.

Azelastine may cause dysgeusia or altered taste perception, even if administered topically in the nose. It has been reported to cause drowsiness, but its potential adverse CNS and cardiovascular effects have not yet been optimally investigated.[22–24]

Cetirizine

Cetirizine is the carboxylic acid metabolite of hydroxyzine.[29] Its elimination has been well studied in subjects of different ages and with different disorders; 40 to 60% of a single dose is excreted unchanged in the urine. Cetirizine elimination is decreased in subjects with renal impairment. It is not eliminated to any extent by hemodialysis. It has a small volume of distribution compared with that of other H_1-receptor antagonists. Skin cetirizine concentrations are similar to or exceed serum concentrations 24 hours after a single dose and at steady-state.

Cetirizine is the most effective H_1-blocker currently available for wheal and flare suppression. In contrast to other H_1-receptor antagonists, it will significantly decrease the wheal and flare even if high concentrations of histamine phosphate, such as 500 mg/mL, are used in the test. It has a significant effect within 1 hour of administration and a peak effect 4 to 8 hours after administration. Significant suppression lasts for at least 24 hours after a single dose. Cetirizine should be discontinued for 3 to 4 days before skin tests with histamine or allergen. No tachyphylaxis or clinically important adverse interactions of cetirizine with other medications have been reported.

Cetirizine 10 mg once daily is an effective treatment for seasonal allergic rhinoconjunctivitis, perennial allergic rhinitis, chronic idiopathic urticaria, and reactions to mosquito bites. In higher doses, it is effective in atopic dermatitis treatment.[9] In asthmatics, cetirizine 5 to 20 mg provides a dose-dependent protective effect against histamine-induced bronchospasm. It has a modest bronchodilator effect in mild chronic asthma.

In most objective studies, cetirizine 10 mg does not impair CNS functions significantly. In this dose, however, it may produce more subjective feelings of sedation than does placebo or manufacturers' recommended doses of astemizole, loratadine, or terfenadine. Even in doses as high as 60 mg, it does not prolong the QTc interval and has not been reported to cause torsade de pointes or other cardiac dysrhythmias.[22–24]

Levocabastine

Levocabastine is a cyclohexyl piperidine derivative that has been developed for nasal and ocular topical administration.[7] It has a half-life of 35 to 40 hours and is eliminated primarily unchanged by the kidneys. When administered topically, it does not inhibit the wheal and flare reaction to histamine significantly, suggesting that little systemic absorption occurs. Topically applied levocabastine prevents histamine or allergen challenge-induced nasal or ocular symptoms.

In controlled trials, levocabastine is effective in the treatment of allergic rhinoconjunctivitis when compared with placebo. It has a rapid onset of action. Applied topically to the nasal mucosa or conjunctivae, it has comparable efficacy to that of sodium cromoglycate but is less effective than topical glucocorticoids for rhinitis treatment.

After topical levocabastine administration, local adverse effects are uncommon, and sensitization has not been reported. CNS effects are uncommon, and cardiovascular effects have not been noted.[22–24]

Loratadine

Loratadine, a piperidine, is rapidly metabolized in the cytochrome P_{450} CYP3A4 system into an active metabolite, descarboethoxyloratadine (DCL).[10] After a single dose, the terminal elimination half-life ranges from 8 to 11 hours, and the elimination half-life of DCL is 17 to 23 hours. Although the terminal elimination half-life values of loratadine and DCL tend to be prolonged in healthy elderly subjects and in those with alcoholic liver disease, values in both of these populations may still fall within the wide range seen in normal healthy subjects. In children, the half-life of DCL is 14 hours. Hemodialysis has a negligible effect on the clearance of loratadine and DCL.

Loratadine may also be metabolized by cytochrome P_{450} CYP2D6. No important interactions of loratadine and other medications have been noted.

The magnitude and duration of suppression of the histamine-induced wheal and flare by loratadine are dose related. Significant wheal suppression occurs within a few hours of administration and lasts for 12 to 24 hours after a dose of 10 mg. After 10 mg daily for 1 week, the residual effect on wheal-and-flare suppression or on bronchial challenge with histamine or allergen lasts for 7 days. Regular treatment with loratadine 10 mg daily for 3 months does not result in tachyphylaxis.

Loratadine is an effective H_1-receptor antagonist for the treatment of seasonal allergic rhinoconjunctivitis (see Fig. 41–4),[8] perennial allergic rhinitis, and chronic urticaria. In the recommended dose of 10 mg daily, it does not cause adverse CNS or cardiovascular effects.[22–24]

Terfenadine

Terfenadine has a terminal elimination half-life of 16 to 24 hours and is rapidly and extensively metabolized by the cytochrome P_{450} CYP3A4 isoenzyme on first pass through the liver.[16] Unmetabolized terfenadine is not generally found in the plasma after the usual 60 mg dose. The active human metabolite of terfenadine, terfenadine acid metabolite, has a half-life of approximately 17 hours and is being developed as an H_1-receptor antagonist in its own right.

Potentially serious medication interactions may occur when terfenadine is coadministered with a macrolide antibiotic, such as erythromycin or clarithromycin, imidazole antifungals, such as ketoconazole or itraconazole, or other medications that inhibit the cytochrome P_{450} CYP3A4 system. During concomitant administration, terfenadine parent compound may accumulate in serum and cardiac tissue and lead to prolongation of the QTc interval and ventricular arrhythmias, such as torsade de pointes. Terfenadine acid metabolite does not cause adverse CNS or cardiovascular system effects.[31]

Terfenadine 60 mg produces prompt suppression of the histamine-induced wheal and flare, which lasts for 24 hours. Terfenadine pretreatment also protects against histamine- or allergen-induced nasal symptoms or bronchoconstriction in a dose-related manner. The histamine blockade produced by a 7-day course of terfenadine persists for a further 7 days after the medication is stopped. Tachyphylaxis to terfenadine does not occur.

Terfenadine is an effective medication for seasonal allergic rhinoconjunctivitis, perennial allergic rhinitis, and chronic urticaria. In recommended doses, it does not impair CNS function or produce somnolence. It does not enhance the CNS effects of concomitantly administered alcohol or benzodiazepines. Rarely, it causes adverse cardiovascular effects (see Fig. 41–7).[22–24]

SUMMARY

This chapter reviewed new basic science information about H_1-receptor antagonists: the molecular basis for their action, their mechanisms of action, and their ability to produce H_1-blockade and antiallergic effects. An up-to-date overview of the clinical science of H_1-receptor antagonists was presented, with particular emphasis on 10 of the most commonly used H_1-receptor antagonists worldwide. These medications differ remarkably with regard to their pharmacokinetics, pharmacodynamics, and safety but are rather similar in terms of efficacy.

There is renewed interest in the topical use of H_1-receptor antagonists. Many promising new H_1-receptor antagonists are being studied in phase I, II, and III trials.[13] In the future, we can expect greatly improved H_1-receptor antagonists: enantiomers of currently used H_1-receptor antagonists that will lack CNS adverse effects, active metabolites of currently used H_1-receptor antagonists that will lack adverse cardiovascular system effects,[31] and new doxepin-like medications that have both H_1- and H_2-receptor antagonist properties. Now that the gene encoding the H_1 receptor has been cloned in humans and the molecular configuration required to bind to the H_1 receptor competitively and produce H_1-receptor blockade is being identified,[32] safer and more effective H_1-receptor antagonists may eventually become available.

REFERENCES

1. Anonymous: New advertisements for an old antihistamine. Med Lett 35:9–10, 1993.
2. Bousquet J, Campbell A, Michel F-B: Antiallergic activities of antihistamines. In Church MK, Rihoux J-P (eds): Therapeutic Index of Antihistamines. Hogrefe & Huber Publishers, Lewiston, NY, 1992, pp 57–96.
3. Brogden RN, McTavish D: Acrivastine. A review of its pharmacological properties and therapeutic efficacy in allergic rhinitis, urticaria and related disorders. Drugs 41:927–940, 1991.
4. Casy AF: Antagonists of H_1 receptors of histamine: recent developments. In Uvnäs B (ed): Histamine and Histamine Antagonists. Springer-Verlag, Berlin, 1991, pp 549–572.
5. Chowdhury BA, Kaliner MA: Molecular cloning and characterization of the human histamine H_1-receptor gene. ACI News 7:24–28, 1995.
6. Ciprandi G, Buscaglia S, Pesce G, et al: Cetirizine reduces inflammatory cell recruitment and ICAM-1 (or CD54) expression on conjunctival epithelium in both early- and late-phase reactions after allergen-specific challenge. J Allergy Clin Immunol 95:612–621, 1995.
7. Dechant KL, Goa KL: Levocabastine. A review of its pharmacological properties and therapeutic potential as a topical antihistamine in allergic rhinitis and conjunctivitis. Drugs 41:202–224, 1991.
8. Dolovich J, Moote DW, Mazza JA, et al: Efficacy of loratadine versus placebo in the prophylactic treatment of seasonal allergic rhinitis. Ann Allergy 73:235–239, 1994.
9. Hannuksela M, Kalimo K, Lammintausta K, et al: Dose ranging study: cetirizine in the treatment of atopic dermatitis in adults. Ann Allergy 70:127–133, 1993.
10. Haria M, Fitton A, Peters DH: Loratadine. A reappraisal of its pharmacological properties and therapeutic use in allergic disorders. Drugs 48:617–637, 1994.
11. Hill SJ: Distribution, properties, and functional characteristics of three classes of histamine receptor. Pharmacol Rev 42:45–83, 1990.
12. Janssens MM-L: Astemizole. A nonsedating antihistamine with fast and sustained activity. Clin Rev Allergy 11:35–63, 1993.
13. Janssens MM-L, Howarth PH: The antihistamines of the nineties. Clin Rev Allergy 11:111–153, 1993.
14. Juniper EF, Guyatt GH, Dolovich J: Assessment of quality of life in adolescents with allergic rhinoconjunctivitis: development and testing of a questionnaire for clinical trials. J Allergy Clin Immunol 93:413–423, 1994.
15. Lorenz W, Duda D, Dick W, et al: Incidence and clinical importance of perioperative histamine release: randomised study of volume loading and antihistamines after induction of anaesthesia. Lancet 343:933–940, 1994.
16. McTavish D, Goa KL, Ferrill M: Terfenadine: an updated review of its pharmacological properties and therapeutic efficacy. Drugs 39:552–574, 1990.
17. McTavish D, Sorkin EM: Azelastine: a review of its pharmacodynamic and pharmacokinetic properties, and therapeutic potential. Drugs 38:778–800, 1989.
18. Meltzer EO: Comparative safety of H_1 antihistamines. Ann Allergy 67:625–633, 1991.
19. Pearce FL: Biological effects of histamine: an overview. Agents Actions 33:4–7, 1991.
20. Pratt CM, Hertz RP, Ellis BE, et al: Risk of developing life-threatening ventricular arrhythmia associated with terfenadine in comparison with

over-the-counter antihistamines, ibuprofen and clemastine. Am J Cardiol 73:346–352, 1994.
21. Rimmer SJ, Church MK: The pharmacology and mechanisms of action of histamine H_1-antagonists. Clin Exp Allergy 20:3–17, 1990.
22. Rombaut NEI, Hindmarch I: Psychometric aspects of antihistamines: a review. Human Psychopharmacol Clin Exp 9:157–169, 1994.
23. Simons FER: H_1-receptor antagonists. Comparative tolerability and safety. Drug Saf 10:350–380, 1994.
24. Simons FER: The therapeutic index of newer H_1-receptor antagonists. Clin Exp Allergy 24:707–723, 1994.
25. Simons FER, Simons KJ: Pharmacokinetic optimisation of histamine H_1-receptor antagonist therapy. Clin Pharmacokinet 21:372–393, 1991.
26. Simons FER, Simons KJ: The pharmacology and use of H_1-receptor antagonist drugs. N Engl J Med 330:1663–1670, 1994.
27. Simons FER, Sussman GL, Simons KJ: Effect of the H_2-antagonist cimetidine on the pharmacokinetics and pharmacodynamics of the H_1-antagonists hydroxyzine and cetirizine in patients with chronic urticaria. J Allergy Clin Immunol 95:685–693, 1995.
28. Simons KJ, Fraser TG, Reggin JD, Simons FER: Comparison of the central nervous system effects and peripheral H_1-blockade produced by six H_1-receptor antagonists. Clin Exp Allergy (in press).
29. Spencer CM, Faulds D, Peters DH: Cetirizine. A reappraisal of its pharmacological properties and therapeutic use in selected allergic disorders. Drugs 46:1055–1080, 1993.
30. ter Laak AM, Tsai RS, Donné-Op den Kelder GM, et al: Lipophilicity and hydrogen-bonding capacity of H_1-antihistaminic agents in relation to their central sedative side-effects. Eur J Pharm Sci 2:373–384, 1994.
31. Woosley RL, Chen Y, Freiman JP, Gillis RA: Mechanism of the cardiotoxic actions of terfenadine. JAMA 269:1532–1536, 1993.
32. Zhang MQ, ter Laak AM, Timmerman H: Structure-activity relationships within a series of analogues of the histamine H_1-antagonist terfenadine. Eur J Med Chem 28:165–173, 1993.

42 Cromolyn Sodium and Nedocromil Sodium

RONI GRAD SHIRLEY MURPHY

Asthma is widely recognized as a lung disease characterized by reversible airway obstruction, airway inflammation, and increased airway responsiveness to a variety of stimuli. Because of the inflammatory nature of asthma, treatment should include efforts to reduce the underlying inflammation. Although inhaled glucocorticoids are effective in reducing airway inflammation and airway hyperreactivity in asthma, side effects such as growth retardation and adrenal suppression are being increasingly reported. Thus the need for safer anti-inflammatory agents, particularly for long-term use, exists. Cromolyn sodium and nedocromil sodium have gained increasing use as long-term anti-inflammatory agents in asthma, and their mechanisms of action and clinical use are the subjects of this chapter. Their structure is shown in Figure 42–1.

CROMOLYN SODIUM

Cromolyn sodium was discovered by Roger Altounyan, a physician and asthma patient, during the course of research in the United Kingdom in the mid 1960s. Altounyan was studying the naturally occurring antispasmodic agent khellin. While performing inhalation challenges on himself, he discovered that khellin derivatives in which the 2-methyl group had been replaced by a carboxylic acid moiety had no bronchodilator properties but when taken prophylactically, inhibited the bronchoconstriction induced by antigen inhalation.[3] On January 19, 1965, disodium cromoglycate, or cromolyn sodium, was synthesized and became available for use in the United Kingdom in 1968 and in the United States in 1973.

PHARMACOKINETICS

Cromolyn sodium consists of two monochromone nuclei linked by an alkyl residue. The molecule is lipophobic, highly polar, and acidic, with a molecular weight of approximately 500 and a pKa of approximately 2. At physiologic pH, cromolyn sodium exists almost exclusively in ionized form and is therefore not absorbed from the gastrointestinal tract. The ionized state, however, does confer several advantages. The slow absorption of the ionized drug from the surface of the lung results in prolonged duration of action. Clearance from the lungs is nevertheless fairly rapid, and approximately 75% is removed within 2 hours. Additionally, the ionized state of cromolyn sodium limits its entry into cells and any interference with intracellular function. Because of its ionized form, cromolyn sodium is not metabolized and is excreted unchanged in the urine and bile. The ionized state of cromolyn sodium at physiologic pH thus explains its very low incidence of side effects.[23]

After intravenous administration, cromolyn sodium is

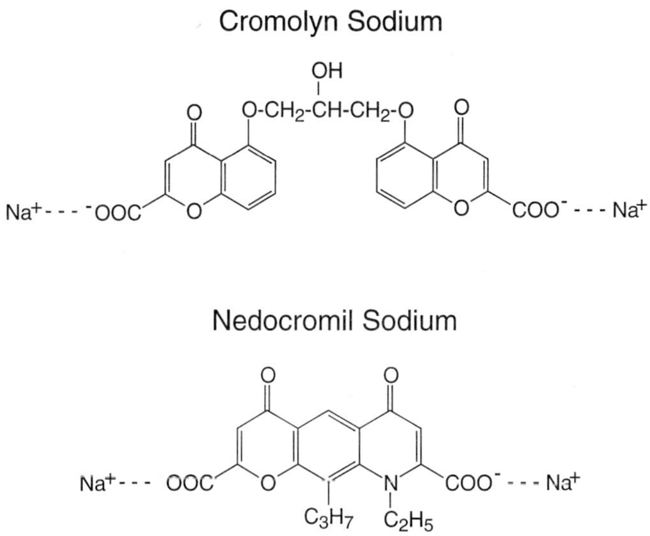

FIGURE 42–1. Molecular structure of cromolyn sodium and nedocromil sodium.

cleared rapidly from the plasma and excreted unchanged, with approximately equal amounts excreted in the urine and bile. Oral absorption of cromolyn sodium is less than 1%. When 1 mg of cromolyn sodium is injected directly into a second-order bronchus, the initial half-life in minutes is 1.9±0.4, the terminal half-life in minutes is 64±10, the time of maximal concentration in minutes is 15±4, and the maximal concentration in ng/ml is 9±0.7. The area under the curve in ng/ml/min is 804±112.[67] Approximately 10% of a 20 mg dose delivered by the Spinhaler delivery system reaches the airways, and the drug shows absorption rate-limited disposition kinetics after inhalation.

MECHANISMS OF ACTION

Numerous mechanisms have been proposed to explain the efficacy of cromolyn sodium (Table 42–1). The principal mode of action has long been thought to involve the stabilization of lung mast cells and prevention of the release of mediators after challenge. Cromolyn sodium has been shown to prevent the release of histamine up to 30% and prostaglandin D_2 up to 85% in human dispersed lung mast cells.[20] Pretreatment with cromolyn sodium prior to the inhalation of ragweed in ragweed-sensitive asthmatics blocks both the

TABLE 42–1
PROPOSED MECHANISMS OF ACTION OF CROMOLYN SODIUM

Stabilizes mast cells
Blocks NCF-A release
Decreases number of lung inflammatory cells
Inhibits protein kinase C
Inhibits activation of inflammatory cells
Decreases bronchial hyperreactivity
Blocks early and late asthmatic reactions
Decreases airway permeability
Inhibits pulmonary neuronal reflexes
Prevents down-regulation of β_2 receptors
Inhibits bronchoconstrictor effects of tachykinins

antigen-induced bronchospasm and the increase in neutrophil chemotactic activity.[4] Cromolyn sodium 20 mg four times daily (q.i.d.) administered for 4 weeks in asthmatics diminishes the number of eosinophils recovered in bronchoalveolar lavage, suggesting that cromolyn sodium may block the release from mast cells of eosinophil chemotactic substances, such as RANTES, platelet activating factor, and leukotriene B_4.[30] Interestingly, IgE-mediated histamine release is more effectively inhibited by cromolyn sodium from mast cells obtained from the mucosal surface by bronchoalveolar lavage than from mast cells dispersed from human lung tissue by enzymatic digestion, suggesting that there are subpopulations of mast cells with differing sensitivities to the effects of cromolyn sodium.[37] This mucosal mast cell is likely the first to make contact with inhaled allergen.

The exact cellular site of the action of cromolyn sodium is not well understood. Because it is ionized, cromolyn sodium remains in the extracellular fluid and thus likely interacts with a cell surface receptor. When linked to fluorescent polyacrylamide gel beads, cromolyn sodium has been shown to bind to mast cell membranes. In rat peritoneal mast cells, cromolyn sodium induces the phosphorylation of a 78 kD molecular weight protein, which coincides with the inhibition of the release of histamine following the stimulation of the cells with anti-IgE and compound 48/80.[76] Furthermore, evidence in lizards suggests that cromolyn sodium may inhibit protein kinase C activity, thus inhibiting cell activation.[52] It therefore appears likely that cromolyn sodium works on mast cells by binding to a cell surface receptor, with subsequent effects upon intracellular messenger molecules.

In addition to its effects on mast cells, cromolyn sodium also affects the function of other inflammatory cells. At low concentrations and in a time-dependent manner, cromolyn sodium directly inhibits the in vitro activation of human neutrophils, eosinophils, and monocytes, possibly explaining its effect in decreasing the airway permeability in experimental models of asthma and in blocking the late asthmatic response.[34, 45]

Cromolyn sodium may also inhibit neuronal reflexes within the lung. Experiments in dogs have demonstrated that prophylactic cromolyn sodium is effective in blocking the reflex-induced bronchospasm that follows the stimulation of C fiber sensory nerve endings with capsaicin. Additionally, cromolyn sodium is effective in blocking the response to sulfur dioxide challenge, a nonimmunologically driven system. In addition to the inhibition of neuronal influences, other effects of cromolyn sodium include the prevention of down-regulation of β_2 receptors on lymphocytes and the inhibition of the bronchoconstrictor effect of tachykinins.[43, 49]

CLINICAL EFFECTS

Inhalation of 2.0 to 40 mg of cromolyn sodium inhibits allergen-induced bronchoconstriction. This protection is noted at 30 minutes and 5 hours after the inhalation of the cromolyn sodium but not at 24 hours. Cromolyn sodium also blocks the antigen-induced reduction in mucociliary clearance. In addition to its effect on allergen-induced bronchoconstriction, cromolyn sodium has been shown to inhibit the effects of sulfur dioxide, toluene diisocyanate, western red cedar, laboratory animals, metabisulfite, and aspirin challenge.[58, 59] When administered prior to exercise, total inhibition of bronchospasm has been demonstrated in 66% of patients, and significant protection in 87%.[58] Additionally, pretreatment with 40 mg cromolyn sodium has been shown to prevent cold air induced bronchoconstriction.[12] The dose required to block challenges varies with the challenge, and the duration of the blockage varies with the dose. For example, with sulfur dioxide, 200 mg is more protective than 40 mg, which in turn is more protective than 20 mg.[59] During exercise, at 150 minutes, 20 and 40 mg are equally effective; at 270 minutes, 20 and 40 mg are partially effective, whereas 2 mg is ineffective.[64]

Cromolyn sodium blocks both early and late responses in contrast to albuterol, which blocks only early responses, and inhaled corticosteroids, which block only late responses.[21] Cromolyn sodium also blocks the increase in nonspecific airway hyperresponsiveness following antigen inhalation and in this respect may be more potent than inhaled corticosteroids. For example, Cockroft[21] found protection of 100% of patients with cromolyn sodium as opposed to 60% with steroids. Cromolyn sodium has also been shown to prevent the seasonal rise in airway reactivity in asthmatics during pollen season and to decrease nonspecific reactivity in long-term clinical trials.[58]

DELIVERY FORMS OF CROMOLYN SODIUM

Three forms of delivery of cromolyn sodium are available in the United States: a capsule containing 20 mg of the drug in powder form delivered by Spinhaler, a 1% nebulizer solution containing 20 mg of the drug in 2 ml solution, and a metered-dose inhaler delivering 1 mg per actuation, of which 800 mcg reaches the airways.[81]

Spinhaler

Spinhalers were initially developed to overcome the coordination problems in aerosol therapy and are coming into widespread use with the worldwide reduction in the usage of aerosols containing chlorofluorocarbon. The Spinhaler is composed of a small open plastic tube and a propeller-like device that rotates at high speed while air is inhaled through the device. A gelatin capsule containing a mixture of cromolyn sodium and lactose is inserted into a cup in the propeller. A plastic sleeve is slid down the Spinhaler, resulting in two perforations being made in the capsule. When air is inhaled through the mouthpiece, the action of the propeller causes the drug to be dispersed into the inhaled air through the perforations in the capsule wall. The powder breaks up into particles of varying sizes. The small fine particles are deposited in the lower respiratory tract, and the larger particles are retained in the mouth and upper airways.

The drug is released early in inhalation and continues while adequate air flow is maintained, distributing cromolyn sodium over the surface of the airways. The distribution of the powder is determined by the air flow through the device and by the length of breath holding. As it is a breath-activated system, it requires no coordination or the use of spacers and has been used successfully by children above the age of 4 years.

Studies using the Spinhaler delivery system have demonstrated its efficacy in improving symptoms, school performance, exercise tolerance, and sleep efficiency.[42, 54] In one worldwide study, the effects were especially obvious in patients with moderate or severe asthma, with increases in evening peak flow rates in patients receiving cromolyn sodium.[33]

Nebulizer Solution

The nebulizer solution contains 20 mg of cromolyn sodium in 2 ml of purified water with no preservatives and is packaged in 2 ml unit-dose ampules. The solution is delivered by a nebulizer driven by compressed air or oxygen. The solution is compatible for 60 minutes with metaproterenol sulfate solution, isoproterenol hydrochloride solution, isoetharine hydrochloride (0.25%) inhalation solution, epinephrine hydrochloride solution, terbutaline sulfate solution, albuterol solution, and 20% *N*-acetyl cysteine solution. Thus cromolyn sodium may be mixed with a number of medications simultaneously to facilitate delivery.

Cromolyn nebulizer solution is especially useful for children under 4 years of age, patients unable to tolerate the powder formulation because of extremely hyperreactive airways, and patients requiring the simultaneous administration of bronchodilator and cromolyn sodium. The nebulizer solution has similar clinical efficacy to the Spinhaler.[16, 22] Very young children treated with nebulizer solution have been demonstrated to have fewer symptoms, less bronchodilator usage, fewer emergency visits and hospitalizations, and fewer corticosteroid courses.[41, 55]

Metered-Dose Inhaler

The metered-dose inhaler form of cromolyn sodium became available in the United States in 1986. The canisters contain micronized cromolyn sodium and sorbitan trioleate, with dichlorotetrafluoroethane and dichlorodifluoromethane as propellants. Each metered spray contains 1 mg cromolyn, of which 800 mcg is delivered to the patient; most of the particles have a mass median diameter of less than 5 microns. The recommended dose of 2 mg q.i.d. has been shown to be equivalent to cromolyn sodium 20 mg q.i.d. delivered by Spinhaler.[33] Cromolyn sodium by metered-dose inhaler has been shown to improve asthma symptoms and peak flow rates.[7, 39, 70]

COMPARISON WITH OTHER AGENTS

Theophylline

In nonsteroid-dependent chronic asthma patients, 60 to 70% can be controlled with the use of either theophylline or cromolyn sodium as first-line therapy. Studies comparing the two agents have demonstrated similar efficacy but a higher frequency of gastrointestinal and central nervous system side effects in patients treated with theophylline.[32, 38, 60] Additionally, cromolyn sodium decreases bronchial hyperreactivity and thus is more likely to alter the course of asthma than is theophylline.

Corticosteroids

Early clinical studies demonstrated that corticosteroid usage could be reduced in some patients following the addition of cromolyn sodium to their therapeutic regimen.[18, 73] Subsequent studies have failed to show a significant steroid-sparing effect in severe steroid-dependent asthmatics. In general, inhaled steroids are considered a more potent agent. Nevertheless, one study in adults demonstrated that cromolyn sodium 10 mg q.i.d. is as effective as beclomethasone 100 mcg q.i.d. in controlling mild to moderate asthma.[35]

SAFETY

Due to its ionized form at physiologic pH, side effects from cromolyn sodium are extremely rare. In a prospective study of 375 patients, investigators reported a 2% rate of side effects, all of which were mild and easily reversible.[72] Cromolyn sodium has a pregnancy category B rating, and no reports of drug-related fetal malformations exist. Rarely, type 1–like adverse reactions to cromolyn sodium have been reported. In one case, specific anti–cromolyn sodium IgE antibodies have been demonstrated in serum.[80]

NEDOCROMIL SODIUM

Nedocromil sodium was approved for use in the United States in 1994. Its development was a natural outgrowth from the previous work with cromolyn sodium and the attempt to develop a nonsteroidal anti-inflammatory agent more potent than cromolyn sodium.

CHEMISTRY AND PHARMACOKINETICS

Nedocromil sodium is the disodium salt of a pyranoquinolone dicarboxylic acid. After inhalation of nedocromil sodium, peak plasma concentrations are achieved within a mean of 20 minutes and decline with a half-life of 85 minutes. After inhalation, nedocromil sodium remains in the circulation approximately 129 minutes, and following intravenous administration, 48 minutes. The difference in these times, 81 minutes, represents the absorption time; thus nedocromil sodium is absorbed very slowly from the lungs.[74]

Exercise and the rapid performance of FEV_1 maneuvers increase the plasma concentration of nedocromil sodium after inhalation, suggesting that stretching of the lungs during inhalation is responsible for the absorption of nedocromil sodium into the plasma.[75] Approximately two thirds of the drug is excreted unchanged in the urine, and one third in the feces.[5] Urinary excretion is a helpful measure of total lung absorption.

MECHANISM OF ACTION

As is the case with cromolyn sodium, a precise mechanism explaining the clinical activity of nedocromil sodium has not been delineated. In vitro studies have suggested that nedocromil sodium exerts anti-inflammatory effects by inhibiting the release of mediators from mast cells, eosinophils, and neutrophils, and modulating their migration.[13] Nedocromil sodium inhibits chemotaxis of neutrophils and eosinophils stimulated by various chemoattractants, including platelet activating factor, zymosan-activated serum, *N*-formyl-methionyl-leucyl-phenylalanine, and leukotriene B_4.[14, 15]

There is evidence that nedocromil sodium may inhibit the response of neutrophils and eosinophils to chemotactic agents, as well as the release of leukotriene C_4 from eosinophils.[15, 71, 79] Nedocromil sodium has been shown to inhibit interleukin-6 (IL-6) production by allergen-stimulated alveolar macrophages from asthmatics and IL-8 production by human bronchial epithelial cells stimulated by IL-1.[11, 78] It has been shown to inhibit the release of IL-3, IL-6, IL-10, and tumor necrosis factor-alpha from conjunctival epithelium in a guinea pig model of allergic conjunctivitis.[56]

Nedocromil sodium has also been shown to inhibit the release of histamine from mast cells and is more potent than cromolyn sodium in this respect.[51, 57, 62] Furthermore, nedocromil sodium has been shown to inhibit the release of granulocyte-macrophage colony-stimulating factor from bronchial epithelium.[53] Finally, nedocromil sodium has been shown to inhibit the cytotoxic activity of neutrophils, eosinophils, macrophages, and platelets.[57, 77] Its effect is more potent on the granulocytes than on the mast cells.[57]

Data indicate that nedocromil sodium, like sodium cromoglycate, modulates chloride transport in different cell types, suggesting that the effect of nedocromil sodium may be mediated by its inhibition of chloride channels in mast cells. Immune activation is thought to cause an influx of this chloride ion, which hyperpolarizes the cell membrane. This leads to calcium influx and degranulation. These compounds reverse this process.[60a] There is therefore abundant and increasing evidence that nedocromil sodium exerts its clinical effect through its anti-inflammatory properties. Tachyphylaxis to the effect of nedocromil sodium is seen in mast cells derived from lung parenchyma but not from the airway lumen, suggesting that the agent works primarily on cells in the airway lumen.[51]

DELIVERY FORMS OF NEDOCROMIL SODIUM

Nedocromil sodium is available in the United States as a pressurized metered-dose aerosol suspension containing micronized nedocromil sodium and sorbitan trioleate, with dichlorotetrafluoroethane and dichlorodifluoromethane as propellants. Each actuation delivers 1.75 mg nedocromil sodium. Each 16.2 g canister provides 112 metered inhalations.

CLINICAL PHARMACOLOGY

Inhalation of 6 mg nedocromil sodium prior to challenge with house dust mite antigen inhibits the early and late reactions and improves the postchallenge bronchial hyperresponsiveness.[1] When administered after recovery from the early response, the later response was delayed but still occurred.[25] The later response could be abolished if nedocromil sodium was inhaled 30 to 90 minutes before the onset of the late reaction. In addition to its inhibition of allergen-induced bronchoconstriction, nedocromil sodium has been shown to inhibit bronchoconstriction induced by various nonallergic stimuli. These include sulfur dioxide, substance P, capsaicin, neurokinin A, adenosine monophosphate, ultrasonically nebulized distilled water, and cold dry air.[27–29, 31, 44, 65, 68, 69]

Nedocromil sodium inhalation protects against exercise-induced bronchoconstriction.[2, 10] A dose of 4 mg by metered-dose inhaler or cromolyn sodium 20 mg by Spinhaler provides similar inhibition when inhaled 20 minutes before exercise, although cromolyn sodium has a longer duration of action.[47]

CLINICAL TRIALS

Numerous trials have shown that nedocromil sodium is superior to placebo in reducing asthma symptoms, decreasing the requirement for additional inhaled β-agonists, and improving lung function.[13] A double-blind study has shown that nedocromil sodium 4 mg q.i.d. is more effective than placebo at reducing asthma severity, asthma cough, sleep difficulty, and bronchodilator use and increases morning peak flow rates.[36] Nedocromil sodium 4 mg q.i.d. is modestly effective in improving symptoms in patients with severe asthma whose symptoms persist in spite of optimal doses of inhaled corticosteroids.[66] The addition of 8 mg q.i.d. nedocromil sodium in patients taking up to 1,000 mcg daily of inhaled corticosteroids significantly improved daytime symptoms, but not nighttime symptoms or morning tightness, in a study of 24 adult asthmatics.[61]

Nedocromil sodium 4 mg q.i.d. has been shown to be effective at controlling daytime asthma symptoms after withdrawal of oral methylxanthines.[19] This effect is noted within the first 3 days of therapy.[19] Treatment with nedocromil sodium for several weeks may allow the reduction in dosage of oral corticosteroids in those patients chronically treated with these agents.[46] Use of nedocromil sodium also may allow a reduction in dosage of inhaled corticosteroid treatment, but this effect is not seen in patients on high-dose (1,000–2,000 mcg/day) beclomethasone.[9]

Several uncontrolled trials have been performed involving the addition of nedocromil sodium 4 mg q.i.d. to the regimen of patients with uncontrolled asthma. At the end of 12 months, 75% of patients as rated by themselves and 48% of patients as rated by their clinicians considered nedocromil sodium to be at least moderately effective.[17] By the end of 30 months, clinical well-being is maintained in spite of withdrawal of inhaled corticosteroids or inhaled bronchodilators in some patients. Long-term use of nedocromil sodium has also been shown to improve quality of life.[24, 48]

COMPARISONS WITH OTHER PHARMACOLOGIC AGENTS

Theophylline

Nedocromil sodium 4 mg q.i.d. has been shown to be equivalent to theophylline at serum concentrations of 10 to 20 mg/l in improving symptoms and peak flows and diminishing inhaled bronchodilator use.[26]

Beta$_2$-Agonists

Nedocromil sodium was shown to be superior to salbutamol (albuterol) in improving asthma symptoms and peak flows in a multicenter trial of 212 asthma patients whose symptoms were not adequately controlled by oral theophylline and β_2-agonists taken as needed.[13]

Inhaled Corticosteroids

Several trials have compared nedocromil sodium 4 mg b.i.d. or q.i.d. with beclomethasone dipropionate 400 mcg daily when added to maintenance therapy consisting of β_2-agonists or methylxanthines.[13] Neither agent has been found to significantly affect lung volumes, whereas both agents significantly improved peak flows.[6, 40] Beclomethasone has been found to be somewhat more effective in alleviating symptoms.[40] Thus nedocromil sodium 4 mg q.i.d. is equivalent to beclomethasone 100 mcg q.i.d. and has promise as an alternative to the use of inhaled corticosteroids as anti-inflammatory agents.

Cromolyn Sodium

In patients requiring low to moderate dosages of inhaled corticosteroids, nedocromil sodium 4 mg q.i.d. was more effective than cromolyn sodium 2 mg q.i.d. as substitution therapy in reducing symptoms and the use of bronchodilators.[50] A nonblinded 12-week study of nedocromil sodium and cromolyn sodium suggested that nedocromil sodium 4 mg q.i.d. was more effective than cromolyn sodium 10 mg q.i.d. in decreasing asthma symptoms.[63] However, a study comparing nedocromil sodium 4 mg q.i.d. with cromolyn sodium 20 mg q.i.d. showed no difference.[8] One, 2, and 4 mg of nedocromil sodium were as effective as 10 mg cromolyn sodium in protecting against hyperventilation-stimulated airway constriction.[44] Four mg nedocromil sodium is more potent than 10 mg cromolyn sodium in inhibiting adenosine-induced bronchoconstriction.[27, 28]

The average diameter of cromolyn sodium crystals is 1.7 micrometers, and that of nedocromil sodium is 1.4 micrometers. Cromolyn sodium crystals are shaped like rods, and nedocromil sodium like rhombohedra. Both crystals are isometric, with blunt corners and edges, explaining the lack of tissue irritation from these drugs. Both substances are hydrophilic and dissolve rapidly in the lung lining fluid but are absorbed slowly and thus remain in the lung for prolonged periods.

SAFETY

Nedocromil sodium is well tolerated and the side effects are few. The most common side effects reported have been unpleasant taste in 12% of patients, nausea in 4%, vomiting in 1.7%, sore throat in 5.7%, cough in 7%, and headache in 6%. The side effects are similar in nature and frequency to those of cromolyn sodium, and the gastrointestinal and central nervous system side effects are fewer than with theophylline. The unpleasant taste with nedocromil sodium may necessitate the withdrawal of therapy and the use of other agents, particularly in children.

REFERENCES

1. Aalbers R, Kauffman HF, Groen H, et al: The effect of nedocromil sodium on the early and late reaction and allergen-induced bronchial hyperresponsiveness. J Allergy Clin Immunol 87:993–1001, 1991.
2. Albazzaz MK, Neale MG, Patel KR: Dose-response study of nebulized nedocromil sodium in exercise induced asthma. Thorax 44:816–819, 1989.
3. Altounayan REC: Inhibition of experimental asthma by a new compound—disodium cromoglycate (Intal). Acta Allergol 22:487, 1967.
4. Atkins PC, Norman ME, Zweiman B: Antigen-induced neutrophil chemotactic activity in man: correlation with bronchospasm and inhibition by disodium cromoglycate. J Allergy Clin Immunol 62:149–155, 1978.
5. Auty RM: The clinical development of a new agent for the treatment of airway inflammation, nedocromil sodium (Tilade). Eur J Respir Dis 147:120–131, 1986.
6. Bergmann K-C, Bauer CP, Overlack A: A placebo-controlled blind comparison of nedocromil sodium and beclomethasone dipropionate in bronchial asthma. Curr Med Res Opin 11:533–542, 1989.
7. Blumenthal MN, Selcow J, Spector S: A multicenter evaluation of the clinical benefits of cromolyn sodium aerosol by metered-dose inhaler in treatment of asthma. J Allergy Clin Immunol 81:681–687, 1988.
8. Boldy DA, Ayrew JG: Nedocromil sodium and sodium cromoglyate in patients over 50 years with asthma. Resp Med 87:517–523, 1993.
9. Bone MF, Kubik MM, Keaney NP, et al: Nedocromil sodium in adults with asthma dependent on inhaled corticosteroids: a double blind, placebo controlled study. Thorax 44:654–659, 1989.
10. Boner AL, Vallone G, Bennati D: Nedocromil sodium in exercise-induced bronchoconstriction in children. Ann Allergy 62:38–41, 1989.
11. Borish L, Williams J, Johnson S, et al: Anti-inflammatory effects of nedocromil sodium: inhibition of alveolar macrophage function. Clin Exp Allergy 22:984–990, 1992.
12. Breslin FJ, McFadden ER, Ingram RH: The effects of cromolyn sodium on the airway response to hyperpnea and cold air in asthma. Am Rev Respir Dis 122:11–16, 1980.
13. Brogden RN, Sorkin EM: Nedocromil sodium: an updated review of its pharmacological properties and therapeutic efficacy in asthma. Drugs 45:693–715, 1993.
14. Bruijnzeel PL, Warringa RA, Kok PT: Inhibition of platelet-activating factor and zymosan-activated serum-induced chemotaxis of human neutrophils by nedocromil sodium BN 52021 and sodium cromoglycate. Br J Pharmacol 97:1251–1257, 1989.
15. Bruijnzeel PL, Warringa RA, Kok PT, et al: Inhibition of neutrophils and eosinophil induced chemotaxis by nedocromil and sodium cromoglycate. Br J Pharmacol 99:798–802, 1990.
16. Bundgaard A, Pedersen JZ, Schmidt A, et al: Should stable asthma be treated with nebulizer or pressurized metered dose spray? Ugeskr Laeger 143:2878–2880, 1981.
17. Carrasco E, Sepulveda R: The acceptability, safety and efficacy of nedocromil sodium in long-term clinical use in patients with perennial asthma. J Int Med Res 16:394–401, 1988.
18. Chai H, Molk L, Falliers CJ, et al: Steroid-sparing effects of disodium cromoglycate (DSC) in children with severe clinical asthma. In Serafini U (ed): New Concepts in Allergy and Clinical Immunology. Excerpta Medica, Amsterdam, 1971.
19. Cherniack RM, Wasserman SI, Ramsdell JW, et al: A double-blind multicenter group comparative study of the efficacy and safety of nedocromil sodium in the management of asthma. Chest 97:1299–1306, 1990.
20. Church MK, Hiroi J: Inhibition of IgE-dependent histamine release from human dispersed lung mast cells by anti-allergic drugs and salbutamol. Br J Pharmacol 90:421–429, 1987.
21. Cockcroft DW, Murdock KY: Comparative effects of inhaled salbutamol sodium cromoglycate and beclomethasone dipropionate on allergen-induced early asthmatic responses, late asthmatic responses, and increased bronchial responsiveness to histamine. J Allergy Clin Immunol 79:734–740, 1987.
22. Corkey C, Mindorff C, Levinson H, et al: Comparison of three different preparations of disodium cromoglycate in the prevention of exercise-induced bronchospasm. Am Rev Respir Dis 125:623–626, 1982.
23. Cox JSG: Review of chemistry, pharmacology, toxicity, metabolism, specific side-effects, antiallergic properties in vitro and in vivo of disodium cromoglycate. In Frankland AW (ed): Disodium Cromoglycate in Allergic Airway Disease. Butterworth's, London, 1970.
24. Creticos P, Bark J, Smith L, et al: The use of twice daily nedocromil sodium in the treatment of asthma. J Allergy Clin Immunol 95:829–836, 1995.
25. Crimi E, Brusasco V, Crimi P: Effect of nedocromil sodium on the late reaction to bronchial antigen challenge. J Allergy Clin Immunol 83:985–990, 1989.
26. Crimi E, Voltolini S, Troise C, et al: Local immunotherapy with *Dermatophagoides* extract in asthma. J Allergy Clin Immunol 87:721–728, 1991.
27. Crimi N, Palermo F, Oliveri R, et al: Effect of nedocromil on bronchospasm induced by inhalation of substance P in asthmatic subjects. Clin Allergy 18:375–382, 1988.
28. Crimi N, Palermo F, Oliveri R, et al: Bronchospasm induced by inhalation of substance P: effect of sodium cromoglycate. Respiration 1:95–99, 1988.
29. del Bufalo C, Fasano L, Patalano F, et al: Inhibition of fog-induced bronchoconstriction by nedocromil sodium and sodium cromoglycate in intrinsic asthma: a double-blind, placebo-controlled study. Respiration 55:181–185, 1989.
30. Diaz P, Galleguillos FR, Gonzalez MC, et al: Bronchoalveolar lavage in asthma: the effect of disodium cromoglycate (cromolyn) on leukocyte counts, immunoglobulins, and complement. J Allergy Clin Immunol 74:41–48, 1984.
31. Dixon CMS, Fuller RN, Barnes PJ: Effects of nedocromil sodium on sulfur dioxide induced bronchoconstriction. Thorax 42:462–465, 1987.
32. Edmunds AT, Carswell F, Robinson P, et al: Controlled trial of cromoglycate and slow-release aminophylline in perennial childhood asthma. Br Med J 281:842, 1980.
33. Eigen H, Reid JJ, Dahl R, et al: Evaluation of the addition of cromolyn sodium to bronchodilator maintenance therapy in the long-term management of asthma. J Allergy Clin Immunol 80:612–621, 1987.
34. Erjefalt I, Persson CG: Anti-asthma attenuates inflammatory leakage of plasma into airway lumen. Acta Physiol Scand 128:653–654, 1986.
35. Faurschou P, Bing J, Edman G, et al: Comparison between sodium cromoglycate (MIP: metered-dose inhaler) and beclomethasone dipropionate (MDI) in treatment of adult patients with mild to moderate bronchial asthma. A double-blind, double-dummy randomized, parallel-group study. Allergy 49:659–663, 1994.
36. Fink JN, Forman S, Silvers WS, et al: A double-blind study of the efficacy of nedocromil sodium in the management of asthma in patients using high doses of bronchodilators. J Allergy Clin Immunol 94:473–481, 1994.
37. Flint KC, Leung KBP, Pearce FL, et al: Human mast cells recovered by bronchoalveolar lavage: their morphology, histamine release and the effects of sodium cromoglycate. Clin Sci (Colch) 68:427–432, 1985.
38. Furukawa CT, Shapiro GC, Bierman CW: A double-blind study comparing the effectiveness of cromolyn sodium and sustained-release theophylline in childhood asthma. Pediatrics 74:453–459, 1984.
39. Geller-Bernstein C, Levin S: Sodium cromoglycate pressurized aerosol in childhood asthma. Curr Ther Res 34:345–349, 1983.
40. Harper GD, Neill P, Vathenenen AS, et al: A comparison of inhaled beclomethasone dipropionate and nedocromil sodium as additional therapy in asthma. Respir Med 84:463–469, 1990.
41. Hiller EJ, Milner AD, Lenney W: Nebulized sodium cromoglycate in young asthmatic children. Arch Dis Child 52:875–876, 1977.
42. Hyde JS, Isenberg PD, Floro LD: Short- and long-term prophylaxis with cromolyn sodium in chronic asthma. Chest 63:875–880, 1973.
43. Joos G, Pauwels R, Van Der Straeten M: The effect of sodium cromoglycate and nedocromil sodium on neuropeptide-induced bronchoconstriction in the rat. Presented at the Annual Meeting of the European Academy of Allergology, 1987, .
44. Juniper EF, Kline PA, Morris MM, et al: Airway constriction by isocapnic hyperventilation of cold, dry air: comparison of magnitude and duration of protection by nedocromil sodium and sodium cromoglycate. Clin Allergy 17:523–528, 1987.
45. Kay AB, Walsh GM, Moqbel R, et al: Disodium cromoglycate inhibits activation of human inflammatory cells in vitro. J Allergy Clin Immunol 80:1–8, 1987.

46. Keenan JM, Bielory L, Famion PC, et al: Nedocromil in the outpatient management of asthma. Arch Fam Med 4:835–842, 1995.
47. Konig P: Inhaled corticosteroids—their present and future role in the management of asthma. J Allergy Clin Immunol 82:297–306, 1988.
48. Konig P: Clinical overview of nedocromil sodium. Allergy Proc 16:67–71, 1995.
49. Kusenbach G, Reinhardt D: Effect of sodium cromoglycate on alpha and beta 2 receptors of platelets and lymphocytes. Atem Lugnenkrkh 12:86–88, 1986.
50. Lal S, Dorow PD, Venho KK, et al: Nedocromil sodium is more effective than cromolyn sodium for the treatment of chronic reversible obstructive airway disease. Chest 101:438–447, 1993.
51. Leung KBP, Flint KC, Brostoff J, et al: Effects of sodium cromoglycate and nedocromil sodium on histamine secretion from human lung mast cells. Thorax 43:756, 1988.
52. Lucas AM, Shuster S: Cromolyn inhibition of protein kinase C activity. Biochem Pharmacol 36:562–565, 1987.
53. Marini M, Soloperto M, Zheng Y, et al. Protective effect of nedocromil sodium on the IL1-induced release of GM-CSF from cultured human bronchial epithelial cells. Pulm Pharmacol 5:61–65, 1992.
54. McLean WL, Lozano J, Hannaway P: Cromolyn treatment of asthmatic children. Am J Dis Child 125:332–337, 1973.
55. Mellon H, Harden K, Zeiger RS: The effectiveness and safety of nebulizer cromolyn solution in the young childhood asthmatic. Immunol Allergy Prac 4:168–172, 1982.
56. Merayo-Lloves J, Calonge M, Foster CS: Experimental model of allergic conjunctivitis to ragweed in guinea pig. Curr Eye Res 14:487–494, 1995.
57. Moqbel R, Cromwell O, Walsh GM, et al: Effects of nedocromil sodium (Tilade) on the activation of human eosinophils and neutrophils and the release of histamine from mast cells. Allergy 43:268–276, 1988.
58. Murphy S: Cromolyn sodium. In Jenne J, Murphy S (eds): Drug Therapy for Asthma: Research and Clinical Practice. Marcel Dekker, New York, 1987.
59. Myers DJ, Bigby BG, Boushey HA: The inhibition of sulfur dioxide-induced bronchoconstriction in asthmatic subjects by cromolyn is dose dependent. Am Rev Respir Dis 13:1150–1153, 1986.
60. Newth CJ, Newth CV, Turner JA: Comparison of nebulized sodium cromoglycate and oral theophylline in controlling symptoms of chronic asthma in preschool children; a double-blind study. Aust N Z J Med 12:232–348, 1982.
60a. Norris AA: Pharmacology of sodium cromoglycate. Clin Exp Allergy 26(Suppl 4):5–7, 1996.
61. O'Hickey SP, Rees PJ: High-dose nedocromil sodium as an addition to inhaled corticosteroids in the treatment of asthma. Respir Med 88:499–502, 1994.
62. Okayama Y, Benyon RC, Rees PH, et al: Inhibition profiles of sodium cromoglycate and nedocromil sodium on mediator release from mast cells of human skin, lung, tonsil, adenoid and intestine. Clin Exp Allergy 22:401–409, 1992.
63. Orefice U, Struzzo P, Dorigo R, et al: Long-term treatment with sodium cromoglycate, nedocromil sodium and beclomethasone dipropionate reduces bronchial hyperresponsiveness in asthmatic subjects. Respiration 59:97–101, 1992.
64. Patel KR, Kerr W: The dose-duration effect of sodium cromoglycate in exercise-induced asthma. Clin Allergy 14:87–91, 1984.
65. Phillips GD, Scott VL, Richards R, et al: Effect of nedocromil sodium and sodium cromoglycate against bronchoconstriction induced by inhaled adenosine 5′-monophosphate. Eur Respir J 2:210–217, 1989.
66. Rebuck AS, Kesten S, Boulet LP, et al: A 3-month evaluation of the efficacy of nedocromil sodium in asthma: a randomized, double-blind, placebo-controlled trial of nedocromil sodium conducted by a Canadian multicenter study group. J Allergy Clin Immunol 85:612–617, 1990.
67. Richards R, Dickson CR, Renwick AG, et al: Absorption and disposition kinetics of cromolyn sodium and the influence of inhalation technique. J Pharmacol Exp Ther 241:1028–1032, 1987.
68. Richards R, Phillips GD, Holgate ST: Nedocromil sodium is more potent than sodium cromoglycate against AMP-induced bronchoconstriction in atopic asthmatic subjects. Clin Exp Allergy 19:285–291, 1989.
69. Robuschi M, Vaghi A, Simone P, et al: Prevention of fog-induced bronchospasm by nedocromil sodium. Clin Allergy 17:69–74, 1987.
70. Rubin AE, Alroy G, Spitzer S: The treatment of asthma in adults using sodium cromoglycate pressurized aerosol: a double-blind controlled trial. Curr Med Res Opin 8:553–558, 1983.
71. Sedgwick JB, Bjornsdottir U, Geiger KM, et al: Inhibition of eosinophil density change and leukotriene C_4 generation by nedocromil sodium. J Allergy Clin Immunol 90:202–209, 1992.
72. Settipane GA, Klein DE, Boyd GK, et al: Adverse reactions to cromolyn. JAMA 241:811–813, 1979.
73. Smith JM, Devey GF: Clinical trial of disodium cromoglycate in the treatment of asthma in children. Br Med J 2:340–344, 1968.
74. Summers QA, Honeywell R, Renwick AG, et al: The protective efficacy of inhaled, oral and intravenous adenosine-5′-monophosphate-induced bronchoconstriction in asthmatic volunteers. Pulm Pharmacol 3:190–197, 1990.
75. Summers QA, Singh S, Honeywell RG, et al: The effects of respiratory maneuvers and pharmacological agents on the pharmacokinetics of nedocromil sodium after inhalation. Br J Clin Pharmacol 33:431–438, 1992.
76. Theoharides TC, Sieghart W, Greengard P, et al: Anti-allergic drug cromolyn may inhibit histamine secretion by regulating phosphorylation of a mast cell protein. Science 207:800–882, 1980.
77. Thorel T, Joseph M, Vorng H, et al: Regulation of IgE-dependent antiparasite functions of rat macrophages and platelets by nedocromil sodium. Int Arch Allergy Appl Immunol 85:227–231, 1988.
78. Vittori E, Sciacca F, Colotta F, et al: Protective effect of nedocromil sodium on the interleukin-1-induced production of interleukin-8 in human bronchial epithelial cells. J Allergy Clin Immunol 90:76–84, 1992.
79. Warringa RAJ, Mengelers HJJ, Maikoe T, et al: Inhibition of of cytokine-primed eosinophil chemotaxis by nedocromil sodium. J Allergy Clin Immunol 91:802–809, 1993.
80. Wass U, Plaschke P, Bjorklander J, et al: Assay of specific IgE antibodies to disodium cromoglycate in serum from a patient with an immediate hypersensitivity reaction. J Allergy Clin Immunol 81:750–757, 1988.
81. Watanabe H: The effect of disodium cromoglycate against bronchial hyperresponsiveness in asthmatic children. J Asthma 29:117–120, 1992.

43 Theophylline: Role of Importance in the Treatment of Asthma

RICHARD J. MARTIN

In spite of over 60 years of experience using theophylline preparations in clinical practice, we still do not fully understand how this medication works. The use of theophylline in clinical practice is extensive but appears to be decreasing. The recommendation for the use of theophylline in asthma has had a cyclical history. Currently many people are recommending that treatment with theophylline be relegated to a third-line drug status or not be used at all. This type of statement is most unfortunate and not supported by available data. In fact, information suggests that theophylline has anti-inflammatory properties that help in the control of asthma.

MECHANISMS OF ACTION

PHOSPHODIESTERASE INHIBITION

The suggested mechanisms of action attributed to theophylline are listed in Table 43–1. Most attention has been focused on theophylline as a phosphodiesterase (PDE) inhibitor. In the past, there was some question about whether in vivo levels are adequate to produce this type of effect. However, the levels used in clinical practice more than likely produce PDE inhibition, with resultant bronchodilatation at the smooth muscle site or alternatively nonsmooth muscle intracellular effects. This latter mechanism is similar to prostaglandin E_2 (PDE_2) action of increasing cyclic adenosine 3′,5′-monophosphate (AMP) and blocking cellular mediator release such as histamine and leukotrienes from mast cells.[21]

TABLE 43–1
POTENTIAL MECHANISMS OF ACTION FOR THEOPHYLLINE

- Phosphodiesterase inhibition
  —As more specific phosphodiesterase inhibition agents are developed, the undesirable side effects will be minimized
- Improved respiratory muscle function
  —Possibly more important in COPD
- Decrease in trapped gas volume
- Respiratory stimulation
  —Minimal effect
- Improved ciliary function
  —Secretions and plugs play a prominent role in asthma
- Anti-inflammatory
  —Occurs at relatively low serum levels

Theophylline does this by PDE inhibition, and PDE_2 by increasing the conversion of adenosine triphosphate (ATP) to cyclic AMP. This possibility begins to suggest that theophylline may provide beneficial anti-inflammatory activity. Similarly, in the smooth muscle cell, these same reactions can cause relaxation of the muscle.

The PDE enzyme is not a singlet, and molecular characterization has shown that it has multiple forms. This has lead to the development of selective inhibitors for some of these forms.[12] Using these agents has led to the identification of PDE isoenzymes in different tissues and cells.[3, 10, 31, 32] Specific inhibitors can then affect only certain tissues. Thus studies involving in vitro human airway smooth muscle have identified specific PDE isoenzymes and specific inhibitors that produce bronchorelaxation. Whether site-specific PDE inhibitors will work in vivo remains to be established.

EFFECT ON RESPIRATORY MUSCLES

Theophylline also improves contraction of respiratory muscles. This effect has been studied extensively in patients with chronic obstructive pulmonary disease (COPD) and probably plays a greater role in that disease. However, improvement of respiratory muscle function, both strength and endurance, could aid the asthmatic patient at night when muscle activity normally decreases. Theophylline theoretically could delay muscle fatigue during acute severe exacerbations, allowing time for other interventions to take effect.

DECREASING TRAPPED GAS VOLUME

Another effect that theophylline has on respiratory muscles is to decrease trapped gas volume, thereby allowing the diaphragm to work at a better mechanical advantage.[8] Trapped gas volume is the difference between the volume of air in the lungs measured by a body plethysmograph (patient totally inside a box so all volume is measured) and a mouth measurement of volume by helium dilution technique, in which only the volume of gas in open connecting airways is measured (Fig. 43–1). Again, the difference between these two volume measurements is referred to as the trapped gas volume. In normals, these measurements are virtually the

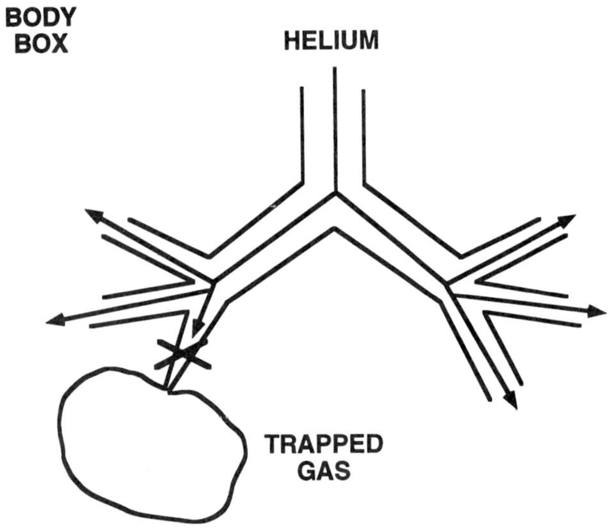

FIGURE 43–1. An example of trapped gas volume, which is the air within the lungs that is not communicating with larger airways.

same. In patients with a disease such as COPD, the difference can be very significant and place the diaphragm at a mechanical disadvantage by flattening the diaphragm and thus producing muscle weakness. Theophylline in this situation will decrease the trapped gas volume, improve mechanical functioning of the diaphragm, and result in better muscle contraction. For the asthmatic patient, the lungs become progressively hyperinflated as bronchoconstriction worsens, resulting in flattening of the diaphragm and producing this mechanical disadvantage. Theophylline has the potential to reverse this mechanical defect.

RESPIRATORY STIMULATION

Overall, theophylline is a minor stimulant of the respiratory system and has very little effect in this capacity in asthma. Perhaps in children this effect may be of benefit if there is a dual problem of asthma associated with the apneas of infancy or childhood. Apneas in children (not so for adults) respond well to theophylline.[27] It has been demonstrated for both children and adults that if a respiratory sleep disorder, sleep apnea, is improved by the use of nasal continuous positive airway pressure (CPAP), then the associated asthma improves not only during the night but also during the daytime.[7, 42] Therefore, if respiratory sleep disturbances are improved by theophylline, this would aid in the treatment of asthma.

SECRETIONS

Airway secretions play a prominent role in asthma. Our pathology colleagues continue to remind us that asthmatic airways are packed with secretions in autopsy studies.[15] Perhaps the use of an agent with ciliary stimulatory properties, such as theophylline, can improve the clearance of these secretions and help maintain intraluminal patency.[2] This is particularly important at night, when ciliary function normally decreases and asthma often worsens.[22]

ANTI-INFLAMMATORY AGENT

What is the evidence that theophylline is a potential anti-inflammatory agent? Neclerio and colleagues[28] used a nasal allergen challenge model to determine if theophylline protects against mediator release into the nose. Their findings demonstrated that theophylline produced a rightward shift in the dose-response curve to nasal allergen. That is, when these patients were on theophylline, it took a significantly higher dose of allergen to produce the same amount of TAME esterase activity as well as histamine and kinin release compared with a placebo. This was expressed clinically by the marked reduction in the symptom of sneezing while on theophylline.

Pauwels[30] has shown in asthmatic individuals that the late asthmatic response to an allergen challenge is inhibited by theophylline. If asthmatic individuals are sensitive to an aeroallergen, they will have an immediate asthmatic response following inhalation of the allergen. Depending on the time of day the allergen challenge is given, for example, 8:00 AM vs 8:00 PM, the incidence of a late asthmatic response is between 40% and 90%.[5, 26] The immediate asthmatic response is considered to reflect acute bronchoconstriction, whereas the late asthmatic response is believed to be caused by inflammation and edema. Inhaled corticosteroids will have very little effect on the immediate asthmatic response but will block the late asthmatic response. In Pauwels' study, theophylline had virtually the same effect on the immediate and late asthmatic response as did inhaled corticosteroids. Again, this suggests that there are anti-inflammatory properties related to theophylline.

Sullivan and colleagues[36] also demonstrated that theophylline attenuates the late asthmatic response. They additionally biopsied the airways 24 hours after allergen challenge and showed that the number of eosinophils beneath the epithelial basement membrane and the number of EG2-positive activated eosinophils were significantly lower on theophylline compared with placebo. This study strongly suggests that the eosiniphilic response to an inhaled allergen and the physiologic response were both inhibited by theophylline. The serum theophylline concentrations were on the lower side, being in the 5 to 6 μg/mL range.

Although we consider the inflammatory aspect of asthma to be related mainly to the eosinophil and perhaps the neutrophil, these are among the effector cells in a complex array of factors contributing to the inflammatory cascade. Evidence supports that the lymphocyte is indeed at least one of the primary controller cells of the late phase. Specifically, the T-lymphocyte population seems to be of great importance in asthma. Daytime studies in acute asthma have shown that the CD4 (helper) T lymphocyte is a marker of severity.[4, 18] Two studies looking at the effect of theophylline on T lymphocytes in asthma patients further our information base that theophylline may function, at least partially, as an anti-inflammatory agent.

Fink and colleagues[16] looked at normals and at asthmatic patients both on and off theophylline. The percent of T

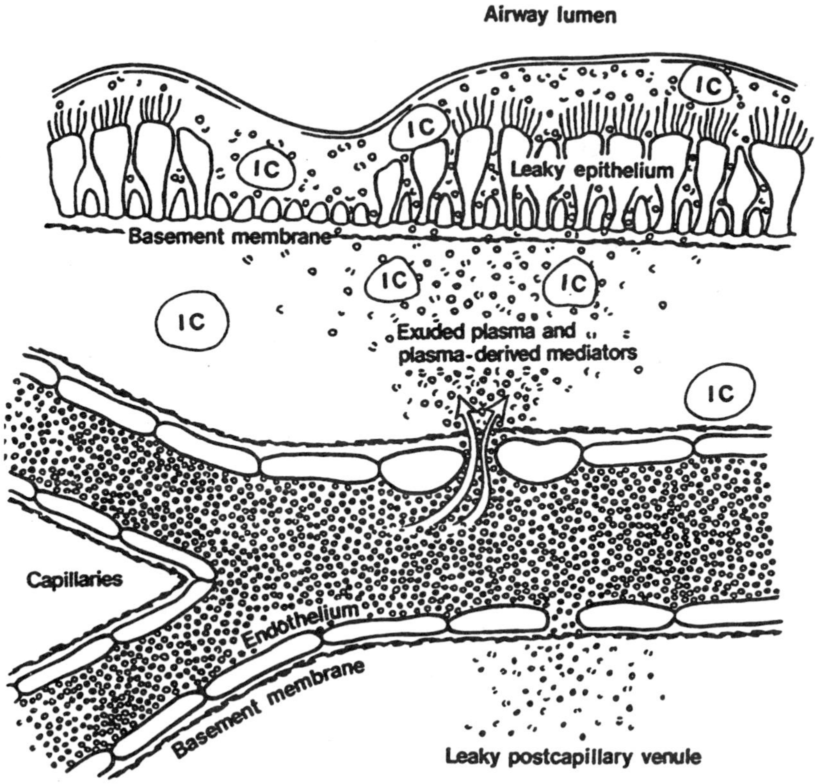

FIGURE 43–2. A schematic illustration showing leakage of inflammatory cells, mediators, and fluid from the postcapillary venules. Theophylline may act at this site to prevent the leakage. IC = inflammatory cells. (From Persson CGA: Xanthines as anti-inflammatory drugs. J Allergy Clin Immunol 81:615–617, 1988.)

lymphocytes overall was the same in the three groups, being about 60%. However, the CD4 cell population of T lymphocytes was significantly higher in those asthmatics not taking theophylline than in those asthmatics on theophylline. Conversely, the CD8 (suppressor cell) T-lymphocyte population was significantly lower in those asthmatics off theophylline. It has been shown in children that asthma improves as the CD8 T-lymphocyte population is increased.[35] This is consistent with the aforementioned study showing both the CD4 T-lymphocyte population being lower and the CD8 population higher in those asthmatics taking theophylline.

Shohat and colleagues[35] studied asthmatic children on and off theophylline for a month. The CD8 T lymphocytes again were increased on theophylline compared with when those children came off the medication. This was related to the significant improvement in the clinical asthma score on theophylline compared with being off this medication. Theophylline withdrawal studies showed that tissue lymphocytes are increased when patients are removed from theophylline.[20]

Of interest, Thorne and colleagues[37] demonstrated an inhibition of the cytotoxic activity of eosinophils by theophylline (in vitro), which also occurred with prednisolone and beclomethasone. This inhibition was caused by a decreased production of an eosinophil activating factor from blood monocytes and not by a direct effect on the eosinophil itself. Two other cells that theophylline appears to alter and are important in asthma are neutrophils and alveolar macrophages. McDonald[25] demonstrated that neutrophil oxidant production and neutrophil-dependent lung injury were reduced on pentoxifylline. Dent and colleagues[11] showed that human alveolar macrophages are altered by the PDE inhibition of the respiratory burst; that is, production of hydrogen peroxide falls in the presence of theophylline.

The airway edema that is seen with an inflammatory response is due to an increase in vascular permeability. Figure 43–2 shows conceptually where the leakage of inflammatory cells, mediators, and fluid occurs in the postcapillary venules. It is believed that one of the potential effects of theophylline is to block this permeability from occurring and thus to inhibit, at least to a certain extent, the influx of inflammatory cells and mediators into the lung. This is not a proven effect of theophylline but if correct may indeed be an important therapeutic benefit.

How these nonbronchodilating aspects of theophylline play a role in the treatment of asthma is not yet clearly delineated. However, two interesting clinical studies show that theophylline has properties that can improve symptoms of patients on inhaled or oral corticosteroids, as well as actually reduce the dose of oral steroids.[6, 29] In a study by Nassif and colleagues,[29] theophylline was compared with a placebo in 21 patients taking inhaled beclomethasone. While continuing the inhaled corticosteroids, the symptoms of asthma at night and during the day, cough, and wheeze were significantly improved on theophylline compared with the placebo. Similarly, 10 individuals being maintained on oral prednisone also had the same symptomatic improvement on theophylline compared with the placebo.

Brenner and colleagues[6] demonstrated in severe oral corticosteroid-dependent children the need to increase oral prednisone dose when these patients were on placebo compared with theophylline. The increase was not trivial and averaged 20.7 mg of prednisone. As shown in Figure 43–3, an example of two patients in that study have not only higher but much more consistent lung function over a month on theophylline and oral steroids compared with when they were on placebo and a higher oral steroid dose. In fact, the

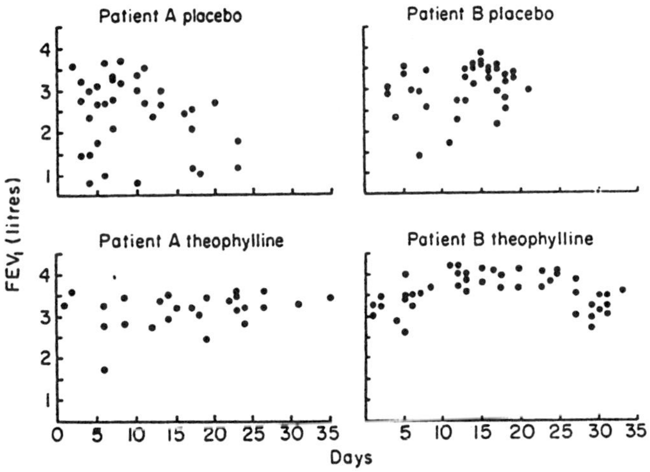

FIGURE 43–3. Two oral steroid-dependent asthmatic patients who have better stability of lung function at a lower steroid dose when on theophylline than placebo. (From Brenner M, Berkowitz R, Marshall N, Strunk R: Need for theophylline in severe steroid-requiring asthmatics. Clin Allergy 18:143–150, 1988.)

study was mandated to stop after only five patients were studied because three developed status asthmaticus when theophylline was eliminated in spite of increased steroid dosage.

USE OF THEOPHYLLINE: HOW AND WHEN

TOXICITY

Since the major critique with regard to theophylline use is adverse events, toxicity will be discussed initially in this section. The three main objectives regarding its use are high morbidity/mortality, adverse behavioral effects in children, and disruption of sleep. These issues are important, and the data to support or reject the perceived adverse theophylline effects are interesting.

Two commonly quoted studies demonstrate the severe consequences of exceptionally high theophylline blood levels. Woolcock and colleagues[40] found a mortality rate of 1.4% in hospitalized patients with theophylline levels greater than 35 mg/l. Of the four patients with toxic manifestations in this study, two had seizure-associated mortality, one survived a seizure episode, and one had a nonlethal cardiac arrest. In a study in which the mean theophylline level was 57 mg/l, there was a higher mortality rate of 7%.[1] Of the four patients who died, three had underlying renal disease and one had congestive heart failure. Thus when a patient's theophylline level is inappropriately allowed to climb to exceptionally high levels, mortality can occur. However, this is physician error and not a primary drug problem.

In one of the largest studies involving theophylline, Derby and colleagues[13] showed that the overall risk for hospitalization due to theophylline toxicity is a rare event. This HMO-based study analyzed 35,909 outpatients who filled more than 220,000 prescriptions for theophylline over 9 years. They found only 30 hospitalizations for toxicity due to theophylline. The age range was 3 to 82 years, and the serum theophylline concentration ranged from 21 to 61 μg/ml. There were no deaths in the hospitalized patients. Confusion and anxiety occurred in two patients and was associated with theophylline levels of approximately 45 to 50 μg/ml. Two patients had associated seizures with levels in the upper 50 to low 60 μg/ml range. Other associated symptoms were considered minor. These investigators concluded that the overall hospitalization incidence rate was 7.8 per 10,000 person years, which is exceedingly low.

Looking specifically for electrocardiographic alteration in an elderly patient population (mean age 66 years) with toxic theophylline levels of 23 to 67 μg/ml, Sessler and colleagues[34] found that tachyarrhythmias requiring therapy were uncommon. Arrhythmias that did not need intervention included supraventricular ectopy and ventricular premature beats and ventricular tachycardia. Only one elderly patient with heart disease developed sustained ventricular tachycardia associated with a theophylline level of 66 μg/ml, which responded to intervention.

Thus it appears that if used appropriately, theophylline is a very safe drug with minimal side effects. However, as with any medication, if the blood level is allowed to climb to very high levels (greater than 35 mg/l), then dire consequences can occur. In fact, Schiff and colleagues[33] found that recurring management errors contributed to inpatient theophylline toxicity. They believed that most toxicity and morbidity could have been prevented. Thus the problem with the risk-benefit ratio of theophylline is due to management error and not a narrow therapeutic window.

EMERGENCY TREATMENT

All studies comparing theophylline (aminophylline) with a β-agonist in the emergency room show the superiority or equality of the β-agonist in this situation, with the end point being the improvement in the FEV_1. However, one study sheds some new information in this area. Wrenn and colleagues[41] in a double-blind placebo-controlled study in the emergency room used either theophylline or a placebo in conjunction with the standard β-agonist and IV steroid therapy. As in other studies, the improvement in lung function was similar comparing the placebo group with the theophylline group. That is, the inhaled β-agonist was working promptly, and side effects were essentially the same in the two groups.

Of great interest, the percent of admissions from the emergency room to the hospital was threefold less on theophylline than for the placebo group. Since this was a double-blind controlled trial, the physicians did not know which patients were receiving theophylline. The exact reason for this marked improvement with aminophylline (less hospitalization) is not known. If this study holds up, there is a potential for a tremendous savings in medical costs with regard to the treatment of asthma in the emergency room. An example of this cost savings is as follows. The average emergency room cost in this study was $350, including doctors' fees. The hospital cost for those admitted was $1,750, excluding doctors' fees. Taking this savings across the United States, there would be a one-half billion dollar yearly savings in medical costs.

Huang and colleagues[19] questioned whether theophylline

would benefit asthmatic patients once they were admitted to the hospital from the emergency room. All patients received nebulized albuterol and intravenous steroids, plus aminophylline or placebo. The improvement in FEV_1 at 3 hours was significantly greater in the aminophylline group (29 ± 23%) compared with placebo (10 ± 10%). At 48 hours, the FEV_1 percent of predicted was 75 ± 19%, whereas the placebo group was only at 58 ± 15%.

Thus in the acute situations, β_2-adrenergic agents are the drug of choice for immediate bronchodilation. However, it appears that theophylline is exerting additional positive effects with regard to fewer hospitalizations from the emergency room and better improvement in lung function if admitted to the hospital.

CHRONIC ASTHMA AND THEOPHYLLINE USE

Asthma is affected by many normally occurring circadian (24 hours) biologic rhythms, which set up an environment for worsening of bronchoconstriction at night. Nocturnal symptoms arising from bronchial asthma were recognized as far back as 1698 by John Floyer[17] when describing his own asthma: "I have observed the fit always to happen after sleep in the night where nerves are filled with windy spirits and the heat of the bed has rarefied the spirits and humors." To determine the frequency of nocturnal asthma in an outpatient population, Turner-Warwick[39] conducted a survey of 7,729 asthmatic outpatients in the United Kingdom. Seventy-four percent awoke symptomatic at least one night a week, 64% awoke at least three nights a week, and 39% awoke every night. In a washout phase of a large pharmacologic study, 1,525 out of 1,631 dyspneic episodes in 3,129 patients occurred between 10:00 PM and 7:00 AM, with the peak at 4:00 AM.[14] Thus the incidence of this potentially serious problem is higher than previously realized. With these facts in mind, one must treat asthma more intensely at night, when it is worse. This concept is termed chronotherapeutics and has worked well for many disease states. Drug tolerance and toxicity appear to be markedly lower when not giving a patient the standard consistent 24-hour daily blood levels that we all have been taught.

Zwillich and colleagues[43] showed the superiority of a sustained-released theophylline preparation (Theo-Dur) in treating asthmatic patients with mild to moderate nocturnal asthma compared with a long-acting (8-hour duration) inhaled β_2-agonist (bitolterol, Tornalate). Sleep quality and architecture were unchanged between the different preparations, demonstrating that the presence of theophylline did not alter sleep compared with the β_2-agonists. Additionally, not only was the FEV_1 improved in the morning, but there was less nocturnal oxygen desaturation while on theophylline.

In patients with more significant nocturnal asthma, higher serum theophylline concentrations (STC) during the night and lower STC during the daytime, when it is easier to control the bronchoconstriction (chronotherapeutics), have been demonstrated to be successful. Comparing two theophylline preparations with different pharmacokinetics, Martin and colleagues[23] showed that higher STC (about 16 μg/ml) from 3:00 to 5:00 AM produced a marked improvement in the overnight worsening of lung function versus lower therapeutic levels (about 11.5 μg/ml). During the daytime, the agent that gave a higher nocturnal STC (Uniphyl, given once daily at 7:00 PM) had a progressive decline in the STC, reaching a nadir before the next dose. The other agent (Theo-Dur, given twice a day) had higher daytime STC levels compared with nighttime. The FEV_1 levels measured every 2 hours during the daytime were not significantly different between the agents even though the STCs were different. With a higher STC during sleep, there was approximately a 9% decrease in the FEV_1 compared with a 28% decrement on the lower STC. D'Alonzo and colleagues[9] also showed a significant relationship between increasing STC and improvement in FEV_1 from 2:00 to 6:00 AM, but not from 2:00 to 6:00 PM. These studies document chronotherapeutic principles that higher therapeutic levels are needed when the disease is worse, that is, during the night. It also helps to explain why previous studies on the efficacy of theophylline performed during the daytime have not shown that increasing the STC above approximately 10 μg/ml improves lung function any more than do lower levels. Furthermore, sleep quality and architecture are not altered between higher and lower therapeutic STC, but there is less oxygen desaturation with higher STCs.[23, 43]

One does not need to get an STC at 4 AM. If patients are started on theophylline, several things can be done. Start patients on a low dose and tell them that it is a low dose and will take a short period of time to build up to where it will be an adequate dose. In this manner, patients will be able to tolerate the theophylline better versus being given a jolt in the beginning. Additionally, patients can take a once-a-day theophylline preparation with their evening meal, some time between 6 and 7 PM, to give a peak effect about 3 to 5 AM, when it is most needed. To see how patients are progressing in regard to the desired level of theophylline in the middle of the night, they can come into the physician's office or the laboratory around 7 to 8 AM and have their blood drawn. If the STC is 13 to 14 μg/ml at this time, then at approximately 4 AM the STC will be about 16 μg/ml. The STC will fall during the daytime, so the patient can better tolerate the lower levels during the waking hours. A trough level of 8 to 9 μg/ml would be most appropriate.

FIRST-LINE THERAPY FOR ASTHMA

The overwhelming consensus for asthma treatment is to focus on the inflammatory aspect of asthma. This concept is exceedingly important and is supported by legions of editorials and articles on the potential beneficial effects of inhaled corticosteroids. Yet there are still questions to be answered in regard to first-line therapy for asthma. In fact, two articles demonstrate equal efficacy of theophylline to inhaled corticosteroids in the treatment of mild to moderate asthma from 6 weeks to 1 year of investigation.[24, 38]

Matthys and colleagues[24] compared theophylline with inhaled budesonide in mild to moderate asthma in 8 patients. This was a double-blind randomized crossover study of 6 weeks' duration. The theophylline preparation was given twice daily, with the mean level of 11.9 ± 4.6 μg/ml. Budesonide was given two puffs twice daily (0.8 mg/d). The outcome variables were as follows:

	Theophylline	Budesonide
PEFR (L/min)		
AM	460 ± 133	439 ± 127
PM	483 ± 118	483 ± 125
β-Agonist use (# puffs)		
Day	1.2 ± 2.9	1.97 ± 3.0
Night	0.1 ± 0.39	0.1 ± 0.5
Mucociliary clearance		
(scintillation %)	32 ± 15	33 ± 14
FEV_1 (L)	3.27 ± 1.32	3.32 ± 1.11
FEV_1 (following 0.01 mg carbachol)	2.92	2.87

After 6 weeks, there were no significant differences in bronchoalveolar fluid cell differential between inhaled corticosteroids and theophylline.

Tinkelman and colleagues[38] compared the benefits and adverse reactions of theophylline (n = 93) and beclomethasone (BDP) (n = 102) in the long-term (1 year) control of mild to moderate asthma in a pediatric population (6–16 years). BDP dosing was 84 mcg (two puffs) four times daily versus theophylline twice daily. The theophylline blood levels were overall very low. Twenty-eight to 45% of the subjects had levels of 0 to 4.0 μg/ml at various times over the study period, 24 to 44% had levels of 4.1 to 7.9 μg/ml, and 19 to 33% had levels of 8.0 to 15.0 μg/ml. Only 7% had levels at any time during the year greater than 15 μg/ml.

The results of this study were intriguing. Over the year, the findings were virtually identical for theophylline and inhaled corticosteroid groups with regard to symptoms; peak flow rates measured in the AM, PM, or mean daily value or as a percent change between the AM and PM; and FEV_1 before and after bronchodilator. One could argue that the inhaled corticosteroid group had fewer side effects (various reported side effects significantly greater on theophylline compared with BDP). However, a major adverse effect, linear bone growth velocity, was inhibited on inhaled corticosteroids. Perhaps the most interesting result was that 7.8% of the BDP children were terminated from the study by the parents due to lack of benefit, while this occurred in only 1.1% of the theophylline group (p = 0.02). The investigators conclude: "Both theophylline and beclomethasone are effective therapy for mild to moderate asthma. Caution must be used with the administration of beclamethasone in children because of possible growth velocity suppression."

TREATMENT REVIEW (Table 43–2)

For the symptomatic mild asthmatic, starting with an inhaled corticosteroid is preferred. In children, there are advantages of using cromolyn or nedocromil instead of steroids because there are fewer side effects, such as growth suppression. The majority of the studies of the benefits of inhaled corticosteroids in asthma have been carried out in mild asthmatics. Using an inhaled steroid in the mild asthma patient has some theoretic advantage. If inflammation is a major cause of the remodeling of the airway histology that can be seen on biopsy, perhaps this can be prevented by initially using inhaled corticosteroids. It appears that in more moderate or severe asthma, inhaled steroids are not as effective. The mild asthmatic patient can use an inhaled β-agonist as needed for events such as an upper respiratory infection or exercise. If nocturnal problems are not eliminated by the inhaled steroids, then theophylline should be added to the regimen.

TABLE 43–2
USE OF MEDICATIONS IN ASTHMA

Mild Asthma

- Inhaled steroids*
- $β_2$-agonists used intermittently (with triggers, such as upper respiratory infection or exercise)
- Theophylline (if nocturnal worsening not controlled by inhaled steroids)

Moderate Asthma

- Inhaled steroids*
- Theophylline doses appropriately to time and varying levels
- $β_2$-agonists used intermittently (with triggers, such as upper respiratory infection or exercise) or long-acting β-agonist

Severe Asthma

- Inhaled steroids
- Theophylline doses appropriately to time and varying levels
- β-agonists as needed (daily basis, long duration preparation)
- Oral steroids (if needed)

*In children, cromolyn/nedocromil appears to be effective, with minimal side effects.

If the patient has more moderate or severe asthma, theophylline can be added to the inhaled corticosteroids. As discussed, theophyllines actually may have synergism with the inhaled corticosteroids, improving both symptoms and lung function. The asthmatic patient with moderate asthma can use the inhaled β-agonist as needed, as was indicated for the mild patient, or a very long-acting inhaled β-agonist may be of benefit.

For the more severe patient, inhaled steroids and theophylline are used as described. However, the β-agonist will probably need to be used on a daily basis, such as salmeterol (12–16 hours). As the patient's asthma becomes more difficult to control, then oral steroids may be needed.

REFERENCES

1. Aitken M, Martin T: Life-threatening complications of theophylline toxicity are not predicted by serum theophylline levels. Am Rev Respir Dis 139:A68, 1989.
2. Bateman J, Pavia D, Clarke S: The retention of lung secretions during the night in normal subjects. Clin Sci Mol Med 55:523–527, 1978.
3. Belvisi M, Miura M, Peters M, et al: Effect of isoenzyme—selective cyclic nucleotide phosphodiesterase inhibitors on human smooth muscle tone. Br J Pharmacol 107:53p, 1992.
4. Bentley A, Menz G, Storz C, et al: Identification of T lymphocytes, macrophages, and activated eosinophils in the bronchial mucosa in intrinsic asthma. Am Rev Respir Dis 146:500–506, 1992.
5. Booij-Noord H, DeVries K, Sluiter H, Orie N: Late bronchial obstructive reaction to experimental inhalation of house dust extract. Clin Allergy 2:43–61, 1972.
6. Brenner M, Berkowitz R, Marshall N, Strunk R: Need for theophylline in severe steroid-reauiring asthmatics. Clin Allergy 18:143–150, 1988.
7. Chan C, Woolcock, Sullivan C: Nocturnal asthma: role of snoring and obstructive sleep apnea. Am Rev Respir Dis 137:1502–1504, 1988.
8. Chrystyn H, Mulley B, Peake M: Dose response relation to oral theophylline in severe chronic obstructive airways disease. Br Med J 297:1506–1510, 1988.
9. D'Alonzo G, Smolensky M, Feldman S, et al: Twenty-four hour lung function in adult patients with asthma. Am Rev Respir Dis 142:84–90, 1990.

10. deBoer J, Philpott A, VanAmsterdam G, et al: Human bronchial cyclic nucleotide phoshodiesterese isoenzyme. Br J Pharmacol 106:1028–1034, 1993.
11. Dent G, Gienbycz M, Rabe K, et al: Theophylline suppresses human macrophage respiratory burst through phosphodiesterase inhibition. Am J Respir Cell Mol Biol 10:565–572, 1994.
12. Dent G, Magnussen H, Rabe K: Cyclic nucleotide phosphodiesterases in the human lung. Lung 172:129–146, 1994.
13. Derby L, Jick S, Langlois J, et al: Hospital admission for xanthine toxicity. Pharmacotherapy 10:112–114, 1990.
14. Dethlefsen U, Repgas R: Ein neues therapieprinzip bei nachtlichen asthma. Klin Med (Mosk) 80:44–47, 1985.
15. Dunnill M: The pathology of asthma in allergy, principles and practice. In Middleton E Jr, Rees C, Elto E (eds): CV Mosby, St Louis, 1978, pp 678–686.
16. Fink G, Mittelman M, Shohat B, Spitzer S: Theophylline-induced alterations in cellular immunity in asthmatic patients. Clin Allergy 17:313–316, 1987.
17. Floyer J: A Treatise on Asthma. Richard Witkin, London, 1698, pp 7–8.
18. Gerblich A, Salik H, Schuyler M: Dynamic T-cell changes in peripheral blood and bronchoalveolar lavage after antigen bronchoprovocation in asthmatics. Am Rev Respir Dis 143:533–537, 1991.
19. Huang D, O'Brien R, Harman E, et al: Does aminophylline benefit adults admitted to the hospital for an acute exacerbation of asthma? Ann Intern Med 119:1155–1160, 1993.
20. Kidney J, Dominguez M, Taylor P, et al: Airway lymphocyte infiltration in asthma increases after withdrawing chronic theophylline treatment. Am J Respir Crit Care Med 149:A280, 1994.
21. Kuehl F Jr, Zanetti M, Soderman D, et al: Cyclic AMP-dependent regulation of lipid mediators in white cells; a unifying concept for explaining the efficacy of theophylline in asthma. Am Rev Respir Dis 136:210–213, 1987.
22. Martin R: Nocturnal asthma: an overview. In Martin R (ed): Nocturnal Asthma: Mechanisms and Treatment. Futura Publishing Co, Inc, Mount Kisco, NY, 1993, pp 71–115.
23. Martin R, Cicutto L, Ballard R, et al: Circadian variations in theophylline concentrations and the treatment of nocturnal asthma. Am Rev Respir Dis 139:475–478, 1989.
24. Matthys H, Muller S, Herrog R: Theophylline vs budesonide in the treatment of mild-to-moderate bronchial asthma. Respiration 61:241–248, 1994.
25. McDonald R: Pentoxifylline reduces injury to isolated lungs perfused with human neutrophils. Am Rev Respir Dis 144:1347–1350, 1991.
26. Mohiuddin A, Martin R: Circadian basis of the late asthmatic response. Am Rev Respir Dis 142:1153–1157, 1990.
27. Myers T, Milsap R, Krduss A: Low-dose theophylline therapy in idiopathic apnea of prematurity. J Pediatr 96:99–103, 1980.
28. Naclerio R, Bartenfelder D, Proud D, et al: Theophylline reduces histamine release during pollen-induced rhinitis. J Allergy Clin Immunol 78:874–876, 1986.
29. Nassif E, Weinberger M, Thompson R, Huntley W: The value of maintenance theophylline in steroid-dependent asthma. N Engl J Med 304:71–75, 1981.
30. Pauwels R, VanReuterghem D, VanDer Staeton V, et al: The effect of theophylline and enprofylline on allergen induced brochoconstriction. J Allergy Clin Immunol 76:583–589, 1985.
31. Rabe K, Tenor H, Dent G, et al: Effects of selective phosphodiesterase inhibitors on human pulmonary artery tone in vitro. Am Rev Respir Dis 147:A183, 1993.
32. Rabe K, Tenor H, Dent G, et al: Phosphodiesterase isoenzymes modulating inherent tone in human airways; identification and characterization. Am J Physiol 264:L458–464, 1993.
33. Schiff G, Hegde H, LaCloche L, Hryhorczuk D: Inpatient theophylline toxicity: preventable factors. Ann Intern Med 114:748–753, 1991.
34. Sessler C, Cohen M: Cardian arrhythemias during theophylline toxicity: a prospective continuous electrocardiographic study. Chest 98:672–678, 1990.
35. Shohat B, Volovitz B, Varsano I: Induction of suppressor T-cells in asthmatic children by theophylline treatment. Clin Allergy 13:487–493, 1983.
36. Sullivan P, Bekir S, Jaffar Z, et al: Antiinflammatory effects of low-dose oral theophylline in atopic asthma. Lancet 343:1006–1008, 1994.
37. Thorne K, Richardson B, Butterworth A, et al: Effect of drugs used in the treatment of asthma on the production of eosinophil-activating factor by monocytes. Int Arch Allergy Appl Immunol 85:257–259, 1988.
38. Tinkelman D, Reed C, Nelson H, Offord K: Aerosol beclomethasone dipropionate compared with theophylline as primary treatment of chronic, mild to moderate severe asthma in children. Pediatrics 92:64–77, 1993.
39. Turner-Warwick M: Epidemiology of nocturnal asthma. Am J Med 85(suppl 1B):6–8, 1988.
40. Woolcock A, Johnson M, Geddes D: Theophylline prescribing, serum concentratins and toxicity. Lancet 2:610–612, 1983.
41. Wrenn K, Slavis C, Murphy F, Greenberg R: Aminophylline therapy for acute bronchospastic disease in the emergency room. Ann Intern Med 115:241–247, 1991.
42. Zaragoza R, Szefler S, Bratton D: Therapeutic manipulations in severe nocturnal asthma. A nonconventional approach in a severe high-risk asthmatic. J Asthma 29:281–287, 1992.
43. Zwillich C, Neagley S, Cicutto L, et al: Nocturnal asthma therapy. Am Rev Respir Dis 139:470–474, 1989.

44 Corticosteroids and Anti-Metabolites

JOHN H. TOOGOOD NIGEL A.M. PATERSON FREDERICK A. WHITE

The properties that account for the physiologic and potentially therapeutic effects of the glucocorticoid hormones are almost all expressed through a specific intracellular receptor common to all of the steroid-responsive cells located in different target tissues.[10]

To act, the glucocorticoid must first be transported to its target cell. In the case of the naturally occurring hormone cortisol, or prednisolone, most of the glucocorticoid is bound in transit to a carrier macroglobulin, transcortin. Other synthetic steroids bind loosely to albumin instead of transcortin.[14] On reaching a target cell, this carrier-hormone complex dissociates, leaving the lipophilic steroid molecule free to penetrate the cell wall.

Inside the cell, the glucocorticoid receptors are present in the cytosol in a form that may be visualized as an acorn nestled in its protecting cap. When the glucocorticoid combines with the acorn (receptor), this activates the receptor to jettison its cap, which then splits into its constituent parts: two heat shock proteins (HS90) plus the immunophyllin P59. These remain in the cytoplasm to be recycled. The activated steroid receptor, on the other hand, promptly pairs with an adjacent one to form a homodimer, which is then transported to the nucleus. The specific DNA-binding configuration of the homodimer binds to its matching site in the nuclear chromatin. There it interacts with a pair of transactivating regions, one on the ligand-binding domain and the other on the modulatory domain, to activate a signal that allows RNA polymerase to begin transcribing the gene.[20] This may result in up- or down-regulation of the formation of transcription factors, depending on which gene is affected.[30]

The clinically useful anti-inflammatory and immunosuppressive effects of glucocorticoids are thought to largely reflect their inhibitory effects on the transcription of the cytokines, growth factors, and enzymes that are normally involved in the inflammatory process. Mechanistically, these inhibitory effects may be accomplished by at least five distinguishable processes:[30]

1. The activated glucocorticoid receptor binds in the genome to negative glucocorticoid response elements (nGRE) that act to repress the ability of the promoter region of the gene to produce cytokines, such as IL-6.[155]
2. In addition, the activated glucocorticoid receptor can bind directly to the transcription factor activating protein (AP_1) and in this way prevent AP_1 from binding to its recognition site on the target gene.
3. Furthermore, the activated glucocorticoid receptor can up-regulate the transcription of ribonucleases that break down the mRNA for cytokines, such as IL-1β, IL-6, granulocyte-macrophage colony-stimulating factor (GM-CSF), and interferon-α (IFN-α). GM-CSF appears particularly susceptible to this action of glucocorticoids.[149, 203]
4. Steroid treatment may also diminish the expression and availability of the transcription factor, nuclear factor kappa B (NFkB), in the lung tissue, thereby attenuating subsequent cytokine-mediated events.[3]
5. Finally, the activated glucocorticoid receptor may combine with a domain on the gene that overlaps other sites that normally have an up-regulating action and thus physically interfere with the up-regulating action of the latter sites. This has been shown for the IL-6[155] and osteocalcin genes.[191]

Aside from these inhibitory effects on the production of proinflammatory cytokines and enzymes and in accord with the behavior of other hormones, chronic exposure to excess amounts of endogenously produced or exogenously administered glucocorticoid may down-regulate the expression of its own specific receptor by as much as 50%.[137, 161] This does not appear to carry any important adverse clinical implications.[32]

CORTICOSTEROIDS FOR CHRONIC ASTHMA

RATIONALE FOR INHALED STEROID TREATMENT

Untreated or suboptimally treated patients with chronic asthma, including those with mild disease and few symptoms, show histologic evidence of chronic inflammatory edema and a diffuse leukocyte infiltration that thickens the walls of the pulmonary airways. This thickening alters the physics of the airways so as to exaggerate the rise in airway resistance that normally occurs in response to bronchial smooth muscle contraction.[103] Thus the thickening acts as a signal amplifier (Fig. 44–1). If this intramural thickening could be resolved, the same amount of smooth muscle con-

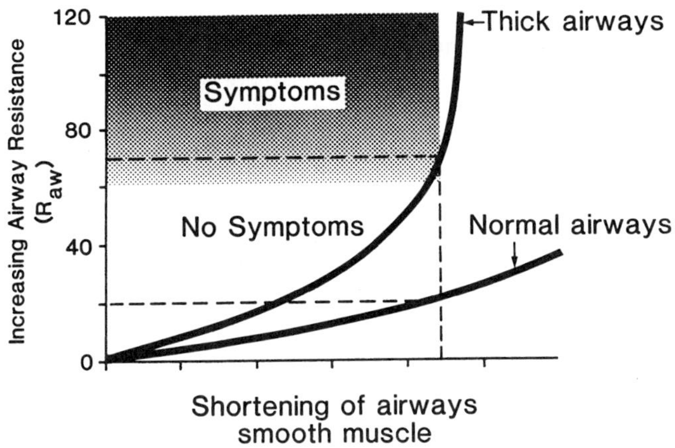

FIGURE 44–1. The schema compares the rise in airways resistance (R_{aw}) that results from contraction of the bronchial smooth muscle in normal airways (below) or airways thickened by chronic inflammation (above). If the thickening can be resolved, the same degree of smooth muscle contraction may occur without evoking a sufficient rise in R_{aw} to cause respiratory distress (see intercept of dashed vertical with the curves). (From Toogood JA: First-line management of asthma with anti-inflammatory agents. Pract Allergy Immunol 7:149–153, 1992.)

traction in response to a bronchospastic stimulus would exert a reduced effect on airway resistance. Consequently, asthma symptoms and the need for bronchodilators would be expected to diminish and possibly disappear entirely.

Anti-inflammatory agents have the potential to resolve this airway thickening, but bronchodilators do not. Therefore, anti-inflammatory therapy constitutes a more logical primary approach to the treatment of chronic asthma than do bronchodilators, which are relegated to a supporting role for the relief of symptoms that break through the preventive regimen. Furthermore, this primary role for anti-inflammatory treatment is equally logical at all levels of asthma severity—mild, moderate, or severe.

The glucocorticosteroids are the most effective anti-inflammatory agents available to treat asthma. Among these, the topically active agents formulated for inhalation delivery are the most efficient, since they have a much more favorable ratio of antiasthmatic to systemic glucocorticoid potencies than do oral or parenterally administered corticosteroid drugs. Because of these properties, inhaled steroids now occupy a pivotal position in the treatment of chronic asthma.

RECOMMENDED USAGE OF INHALED STEROIDS

Accepted practice in the United States endorses the use of an inhaled steroid as primary maintenance therapy for asthma, with the proviso that the nonsteroidal anti-inflammatory agents cromolyn and nedocromil remain the preventive agents of choice in children.[227, 228] However, if a preliminary 8- to 12-week trial of either of the latter drugs fails to reduce the need for inhaled β-agonist usage to less than four doses per week, conversion to an inhaled steroid formulation is recommended. Inhaled steroid is not recommended for the treatment of acute exacerbations of asthma or for asthmatic bronchitis.[228] Additionally, the use of dexamethasone aerosol, the first topically active corticosteroid formulation marketed for asthma treatment in the United States, is no longer

TABLE 44–1
GOALS OF TREATMENT FOR PATIENTS WITH CHRONIC ASTHMA

1. Unrestricted activities consistent with the patient's lifestyle
2. No asthma symptoms most of the time
3. Infrequent need for β-agonist aerosol
4. Air flow rates as close to normal as possible
5. No need for emergency room treatment
6. Minimal or no drug toxicity

From Hargreave FE, Dolovich J, Newhouse MT (eds): The assessment and treatment of asthma: a conference report. J Allergy Clin Immunol 85:1098–1111, 1990.

recommended in light of the availability of alternative topically active corticosteroid drugs that have a more favorable ratio of antiasthmatic to systemic potencies.[228]

The overall aims of asthma management are briefly stated in Table 44–1. These therapeutic objectives derive from a series of Canadian consensus conferences convened in 1989[84] and agree closely with those subsequently developed in Europe and the United States and published in various national and international guidelines.[115, 185, 226, 227]

In clinical practice, the patient's requirement for a short-acting inhaled β-agonist to relieve bronchospasm provides a useful indicator of the need to initiate preventive inhaled steroid therapy. However, different sets of treatment guidelines vary with respect to the particular level of β-agonist usage that they designate as indicating the need to step up to regular inhaled steroid usage (Table 44–2). This variability presumably reflects attitudinal differences among physicians and patients about the efficiency of inhaled steroid compared with β-agonist usage and/or the risk of adverse effects accruing insidiously from the long-term use of an inhaled steroid.

To the extent that the newly introduced long-acting β-agonists salmeterol or formoterol succeed in supplanting the clinical use of short-acting bronchodilators, such as albuterol, they can be expected to vitiate the usefulness of this simple and sensitive early warning sign that alerts the physician or patient to changes in the activity of the disease process. This, in turn, is likely to delay recognition of the need for changes in the patient's anti-inflammatory regimen, such as an increase in daily dosage or a switch to a more effective drug, or for a more aggressive search for respirable irritants or allergens in the patient's environment that may be avoidable. Such delays are undesirable in light of evidence indicating that irreversible damage to the airways may accrue if inhaled steroid treatment is not initiated early in the course of the disease (Fig. 44–2).[4, 58, 82, 83, 113]

It would appear reasonable to limit the use of salmeterol

TABLE 44–2
INHALED BRONCHODILATOR USAGE AS A CUE TO INITIATE INHALED STEROID THERAPY

Published Guidelines	β-Agonist Usage	
	Dose per Day	*Days per Week*
Canada[84]	> 0	
International[227]		> 3
United Kingdom[185]	> 1	
Canadian Pediatrics[115]	> 2–3	
United States[226]	> 3–4	

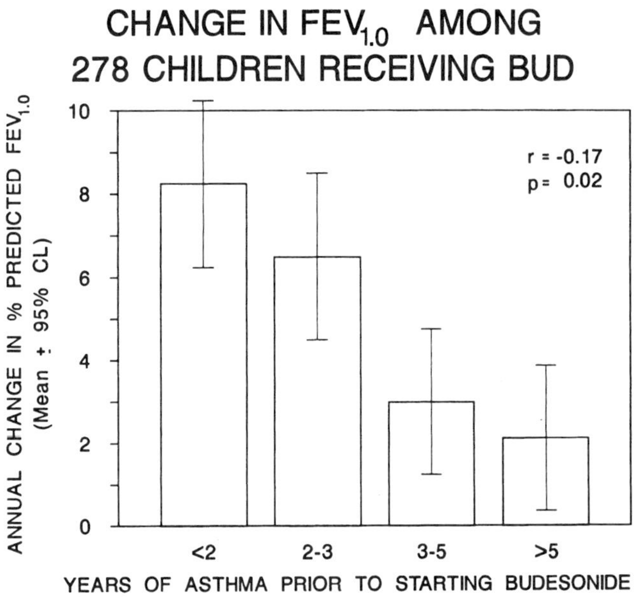

FIGURE 44–2. In children receiving budesonide treatment, the annual increment in FEV_1 after they began inhaled steroid therapy was found to be inversely related to the duration of their asthma prior to commencing the inhaled steroid. (From Agertoft L, Pedersen S: Effects of long-term treatment with an inhaled steroid on growth and pulmonary function in asthmatic children. Respir Med 88:373–381, 1994.)

or formoterol to a few well-defined clinical circumstances, such as in patients in whom there is a manifest need to improve symptom control because they have failed to respond satisfactorily to environmental control measures and low doses of inhaled steroid. In these circumstances, regular salmeterol therapy may be added as one alternative to increasing the dose of inhaled steroid. This approach has been shown to be effective for this purpose, at least in the short term.[78] However, the long-term outcome of this regimen remains to be determined, particularly in regard to the risk of allowing insidiously progressive chronic air flow limitation to proceed unchecked.

Salmeterol may also be indicated in some patients with well-controlled asthma to facilitate down-titrating the dosage of inhaled steroid or theophylline because their dose requirements appear sufficiently high to arouse concern about their future toxicity. The potential usefulness (if any) of salmeterol in these circumstances needs to be validated by systematic study.

BENEFITS OF INHALED STEROIDS

Inhaled steroid treatment has been shown to reduce all aspects of asthma morbidity[4, 82, 101, 164, 202, 205, 232] and the associated health care costs.[48, 164] It is more effective than nonsteroidal anti-inflammatory agents, such as cromolyn or nedocromil.[4, 91, 133, 163, 206] In addition, the regular use of an inhaled steroid, such as beclomethasone, has been associated with a significant reduction in asthma mortality,[63] an advantage that has not been demonstrated (or claimed) for nonsteroidal agents, such as cromolyn or nedocromil.

These favorable outcomes reflect the capacity of inhaled steroid therapy to improve pulmonary impairment and the accompanying airway hyperresponsiveness. Some aspects of the hyperresponsiveness begin to respond within 6 hours,[231] but months or years of regular treatment may be required to achieve a maximal response, and few patients attain fully normal values (Fig. 44–3).[101, 248] Symptom and air flow indexes normally respond much more quickly, within days or weeks, provided that the dose is high enough.

Both the benefits and adverse effects of inhaled steroid are dose dependent,[54, 89, 205, 206, 210, 215–217, 219] and one's concept of what constitutes an effective or toxic dose depends on the response index chosen to measure the drug's effect. For the purposes of an initial therapeutic trial of short duration, high doses have been found to give more accurately predictable results than have lower doses.[213] Tachyphylaxis has not been seen in patients started on high doses and subsequently down-titrated to minimum effective levels.[4, 83] If too low a daily dose of inhaled steroid is used in patients with moderate to severe disease, the therapeutic response may be slow[159] and plateau well short of normal.[230] The latter observation indicates that prolonged low-dose treatment cannot offset the therapeutic inadequacies of a suboptimal daily dosage of inhaled steroid.

In addition to the normalizing effect of inhaled steroid therapy on asthmatic pulmonary impairment, several long-term controlled studies indicate that these drugs, given at low[113] or high dosage,[44, 83] may decelerate or possibly prevent the progress of the obstructive impairment of asthmatic patients toward nonreversible chronic air flow limitation. Furthermore, the earlier in the clinical course the inhaled steroid is started, the more effective it appears to be in this regard (see Fig. 44–2).[4, 83]

All of these benefits are deemed to flow from the normalizing effect of inhaled steroids on the primary inflammatory process in the airways. This effect is manifested by significant reductions in inflammatory cell numbers,[57, 98, 113] the local production of proinflammatory cytokines,[83] plasma exudation,[27] and the goblet cell hyperplasia, excess mucus secretion, and epithelial shedding that characterize the asthmatic airway.[113, 173] On the other hand, once established, the submucosal fibrosis and smooth muscle hyperplasia appear to be nonreversible with inhaled steroid therapy,[113, 121] although some contrary observations have been reported.[223]

Inhaled steroid therapy does not cure asthma. Although some investigators have observed that many patients can sustain control of their asthma for longer than 1 month after abrupt cessation of their inhaled steroid therapy, indicating a strong carry over of the drug's anti-inflammatory effect,[25] others report a high relapse rate.[83, 230, 233] In patients treated with budesonide, prior use of higher daily doses was associated with a longer remission.[25]

In a group of 31 adult patients pretreated aggressively to optimize control of their mild to moderate asthma, abrupt replacement of their beclomethasone with a therapeutically inert agent under double-blind conditions resulted in an objectively documented asthma relapse in 50% of the group within 10 days and in 100% within 48 days.[204] Fourteen of these patients had received regular inhaled steroid therapy for more than 5 years. One had been virtually symptom free and vigorously active in competitive athletics for 10 years while using beclomethasone or budesonide regularly. In clinical practice, the longest remissions we have observed in patients who continued regular clinical surveillance after

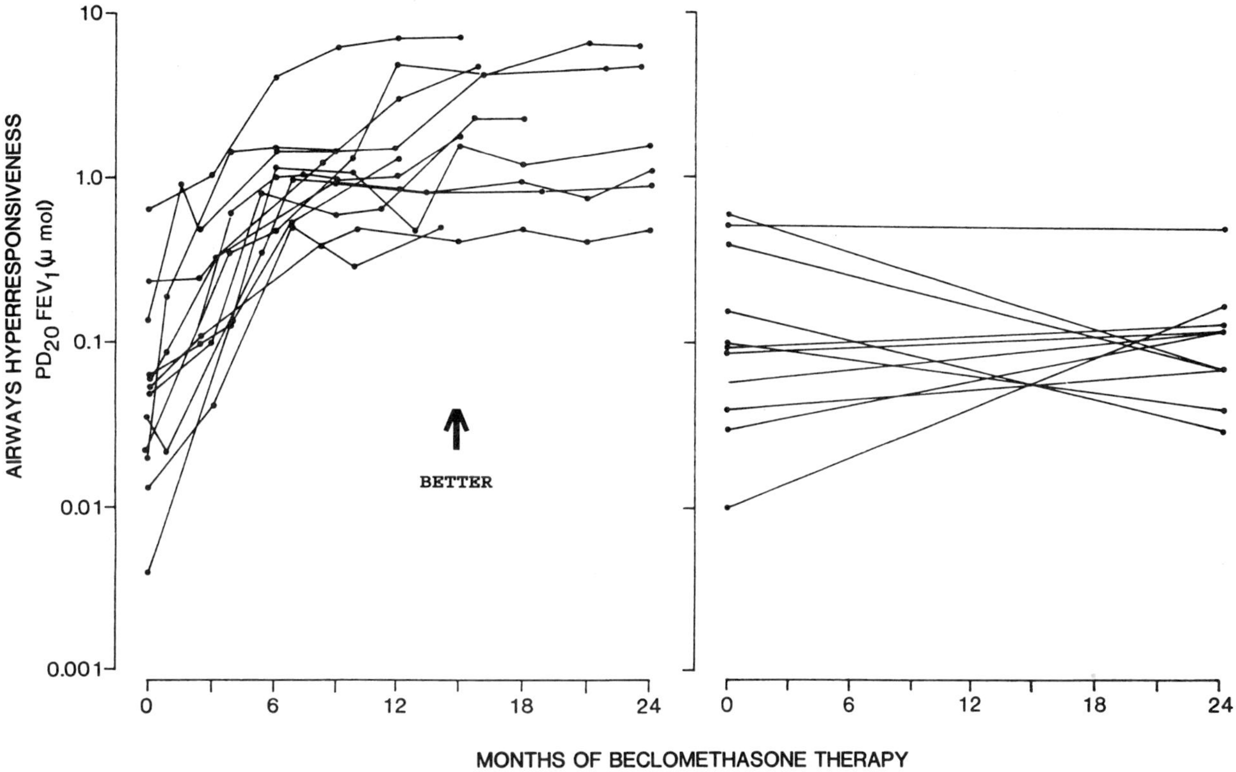

FIGURE 44–3. Graph on the left shows the gradual improvement of airways hyperresponsiveness in response to low-dose beclomethasone in a group of patients who participated in a structured treatment plan that included daily recording of peak expiratory flow rate. PD_{20} values above 4.0 are normal. In the patients on the right, who received the same drug without a structured plan for therapy, airways hyperresponsiveness failed to improve despite 2 years of treatment. The results of inhaled steroid therapy are critically dependent on the clinical management system used by the physician to ensure good patient compliance. (From Woolcock AJ, Yan K, Salome CM: Effect of therapy on bronchial hyperresponsiveness in the long-term management of asthma. Clin Allergy 18:165–176, 1988.)

withdrawal from previously effective inhaled steroid were 12 and 16 months, respectively.

It would appear that once started, the need for regular inhaled steroid therapy is likely to continue indefinitely, except in those patients in whom a dominant causative factor, typically an inhaled allergen or irritant, can be identified in the home or workplace and removed. In light of this prospect for prolonged usage and evidence that the cumulative dose of the drug might be an important determinant of its systemic toxicity,[31, 207] it is essential that the daily dose be kept as low as is consistent with maintaining optimal control of the asthma. Ancillary measures also should be used to minimize the daily dose requirements. In view of this prospect for extended and indefinite usage, the risks of inhaled steroid treatment, as well as the potential benefits, need to be considered.

SIDE EFFECTS OF INHALED STEROIDS

Inhaled steroid therapy for asthma carries less risk of complicating morbidity or mortality than that associated with other antiasthmatic drugs, such as prednisone, theophylline, or β-agonist bronchodilators. However, inhaled steroids are not entirely risk free. Some of the potential adverse effects that merit consideration are discussed here.

Infections

Increases in bacterial, viral, or fungal lung infections have not been a problem in patients treated with inhaled steroids, at least not in North America or Europe. However, prudence dictates that inhaled steroids be avoided or used with great caution in asthmatic patients who also have structural lung lesions that may harbor a mycetoma or in patients who have coexisting drug-resistant tuberculosis or atypical tuberculosis or are immunosuppressed.

Disseminated infection and death have been observed in a few patients who experienced a varicella or measles infection during treatment with an oral corticosteroid. Severe varicella has complicated the intranasal use of corticosteroids for chronic sinusitis.[1] To date, no such cases have been reported in patients treated for asthma with inhaled steroid. Nevertheless, because a fraction of each dose of the inhaled drug is systemically bioavailable, because patients vary widely in their susceptibility to the systemic activities of glucocorticoids, and because it is not known how the route of administration, daily dose, or duration of inhaled steroid treatment may affect the risk of developing these complications, physicians are cautioned to take appropriate preventive action in patients who may be exposed to these infections while receiving steroid therapy. Depending on the circumstances, this may include the use of varicella zoster immunoglobulin or pooled gamma globulin and temporary withdrawal from the oral or inhaled steroid.

Use During Pregnancy and Lactation

No adverse effects of low-dose beclomethasone treatment on the pregnant mother or fetus have been found in several large surveys.[71, 74, 225] Because of the well-documented risks of poorly controlled asthma to the fetus and mother,[12, 225] coupled with the absence of published evidence of damage to the fetus from conventional doses of oral or parenteral corticosteroids in general and of inhaled steroids in particular,[71, 74, 225] an inhaled steroid should be used in pregnant asthmatic women if they have a manifest clinical need.

Low levels of some systemically administered corticosteroids are known to be distributed in human milk. It is conceivable that they might suppress the growth of nursing infants, although this has not been documented in humans. There are no relevant data regarding breast milk disposition for any of the inhaled steroids currently used to manage asthma.

Local Effects in the Airways

Light and electron microscopy studies of bronchial biopsies taken before and after long-term inhaled steroid treatment have shown no deleterious effect on airway tissues.[120, 121, 200] On the contrary, they show ciliogenesis and repair of preexisting epithelial damage.[113, 120] However, the hypertrophy and hyperplasia of smooth muscle appear to be nonreversible once established.[113, 121] Contrary reports have appeared with respect to the potential reversibility of subepithelial fibrosis.[223]

The oropharyngeal complications of inhaled steroid use (thrush or dysphonia) are fairly common.[208, 209] However, they are easily avoidable and easily treated in most cases,[208, 210] being more of a nuisance than a threat. Physicians' concerns about these drugs center mainly on their possible adverse effects on the hypothalamic-pituitary-adrenal (HPA) axis, the eye, and growth and bone density.

HPA Axis Effects

A few case reports have been published of children and adults who developed cushingoid features of hypercortisonism or a significant drop in cortisol production while using low-dose beclomethasone, triamcinolone acetonide, or budesonide[92, 201, 249] or high-dose beclomethasone.[33, 40] Accompanying adrenal atrophy or acute adrenal insufficiency (addisonian crisis) has also been documented in a few cases,[35, 244] including one child who had been receiving 0.5 mg/day for intranasal and asthma treatment.[249] It is not clear whether such individuals metabolize glucocorticoids more slowly than normal or whether they used more than the prescribed dose, or perhaps both.

Besides the dose per day, the cumulative dose of inhaled steroid may be an important determinant of toxicity.[31, 207] Among a group of patients undergoing systematic surveillance of budesonide's long-term safety, a few individuals tolerated high daily dosage for several years without adverse systemic effect but eventually dropped their morning cortisol significantly after the cumulative dose of budesonide reached 1g. In one of these individuals, an episode of addisonian crisis was triggered by an acute enteric viral infection. Each of these patients had required high-dose budesonide to control their asthma, and most used intermittent or low-dose prednisone on alternate mornings as well.[207]

Judged by the paucity of cases reported, stress-induced addisonian crisis appears to be a very rare complication of inhaled steroid treatment. However, it is prudent to routinely administer a preventive oral or intravenous glucocorticoid supplement to all patients receiving an inhaled steroid if they experience major trauma, surgery, or a severe prostrating illness.

In such circumstances, it is our practice to administer 25 mg of oral prednisone (which is effective after approximately 1 hour) or 100 mg of intravenous hydrocortisone (which is effective immediately). It may be advisable to add 4 mg intravenous dexamethasone to prolong the effectiveness of the first agent. If the patient's blood pressure drops, the intravenous hydrocortisone is repeated as frequently as needed.

This preventive approach is advisable because patients vary markedly in their tolerance of glucocorticoid drugs, and a few may show suppression of HPA axis function even with low daily doses of inhaled steroid. It is less expensive and more expeditious to provide such prophylaxis routinely to all patients taking an inhaled steroid than to perform preliminary tests of HPA axis function in an attempt to determine which ones are at risk for the development of stress-induced addisonian crisis.

Adverse effects, such as clinically important HPA axis suppression, may be encountered occasionally in patients receiving inhaled steroid therapy. Regardless of the daily dosage of inhaled steroid and whether or not it suppresses HPA axis function, the systemic activity of the inhaled steroid is consistently less than that of the dose of oral prednisone that would be required to achieve the same level of asthma control in the same patient.[89, 205, 208]

Ocular Involvement

Posterior subcapsular cataracts have been observed in a few patients treated with beclomethasone or dexamethasone aerosol.[7, 72, 104, 108] However, these isolated case reports do not allow the issue of causality to be resolved, since they cannot adequately take into account the confounding influences of past or current oral steroid therapy or nonsteroidal risk factors for posterior subcapsular cataract that may also have been present in these patients. Posterior subcapsular cataracts have been observed to resolve in some asthmatic children after they converted from their previous oral prednisone regimen to low-dose beclomethasone.[160]

In a large multicenter trial that compared beclomethasone with theophylline in asthmatic children, no posterior subcapsular cataracts were found in the steroid treated group after 1 year of treatment at a dose of 0.4 mg/day (nominal dose).[202] The most rigorous evaluations of this particular risk that have been published to date derive from two cross-sectional surveys by slit lamp, one in adults[211] and the other in children.[179] Both patient groups had been exposed for an extended period to daily doses of inhaled steroid averaging 0.75[179] and more than 1.0 mg/day.[211] Neither survey found any evidence that inhaled steroid treatment causes posterior subcapsular cataracts.

The design of the adult study allowed the effects of inhaled and oral steroids to be compared with one another over a wide range of exposure to each drug since most patients had received both agents.[211] The amount of prednisone exposure was found to correlate significantly with the prevalence of posterior subcapsular cataract. Indeed, after 20 years of prednisone use, 50% of the group had posterior subcapsular cataracts. However, there was no indication that the inhaled steroid used by these patients contributed to this risk by acting either alone or in conjunction with prednisone or other nonsteroidal risk factors, such as age or the presence of coexisting disease, such as diabetes mellitus or arthritis.

On the contrary, the negative correlation between the cumulative lifetime dose of inhaled steroids and the prevalence of posterior subcapsular cataracts that was observed in these patients, despite their use of exceptionally high daily doses of inhaled steroids for an average of 9.1 years (extending up to 21 years), suggests that inhaled steroid treatment may actually reduce the risk of posterior subcapsular cataract formation, presumably by facilitating partial or complete withdrawal from prednisone. This would be consistent with the observation that posterior subcapsular cataracts may resolve after converting from prednisone to beclomethasone treatment.[160] This reduction in the risk of cataracts may reflect the fact that inhaled steroids, unlike their oral or systemic counterparts, exhibit little or no adverse effect on carbohydrate metabolism.[109, 134] Abnormalities of carbohydrate metabolism have been thought to play an important role in the pathogenesis of glucocorticoid-induced cataract.

These studies cannot rule out the possibility that posterior subcapsular cataracts might complicate inhaled steroid usage if a particular patient has exceptionally high susceptibility. However, taken together, the combined results of the two cross-sectional surveys (143 patients and 670 patient years of exposure to the drug) indicate that the risk is negligible in the asthmatic population at large; that inhaled steroid usage is more likely to reduce than increase the risk of posterior subcapsular cataracts, inasmuch as it can replace the need for prednisone; and that routine ophthalmologic surveillance for posterior subcapsular cataracts in all patients treated with inhaled steroid is not warranted. This probably applies to all inhaled steroids as a class, although the only data that provide an adequate basis for assessing the magnitude of this particular risk derive from patients treated with budesonide or beclomethasone.[179, 211]

Incipient glaucoma may be exacerbated by inhaled steroid therapy for asthma, even at low dosage.[60] The magnitude of this risk as a function of the choice of drug or daily dosage is not known but merits prospective study.

Effects on Growth

The possibility of growth inhibition as a complication of inhaled steroid therapy is a concern to the pediatrician and pediatric respirologist or allergist. All of the early studies of the effect of inhaled steroid treatment on growth relate to the use of doses less than 1 mg/day (nominal dose). Among those performed prior to 1991, only one study found evidence of inhibition of growth.[118] Nevertheless, a clinically important degree of stunting has been documented in a few children treated with beclomethasone or budesonide at various dose levels.[201, 234] The stunting would appear to have been related to the drug rather than to the severity of the asthma, because it promptly reversed after the drug was withdrawn.[201, 234]

In addition to these isolated case reports, controlled studies in Europe[22, 59, 241, 242] and the United States[202] have shown that either budesonide[4, 241] or beclomethasone[59, 202] can inhibit growth velocity. The effect of short-term treatment with 0.8 mg/day of budesonide[242] or long-term treatment with more than 0.8 mg/day,[4] although statistically significant, appears to be clinically unimportant. On the other hand, in a large group of children treated with 0.4 mg beclomethasone per day (nominal dose) for 1 year, growth velocity averaged 1.6 cm/yr less than in the theophylline-treated controls.[202] Unless offset by catch-up growth at maturity, such retardation of growth could prove clinically important. The only study published to date that actually followed the growth of beclomethasone-treated children through to adulthood found that they ultimately attained their predicted normal height.[13] Additional long-term studies of this issue are needed.

Few studies of the effect of high doses of inhaled steroid on growth have been reported. This is important since the growth-inhibitory effect of the drug is dose dependent, and the increasingly widespread use of concentrated formulations of inhaled steroid facilitates the use of higher daily doses. Because of dose-related differences in the mechanisms by which glucocorticoids may influence growth, high-dose treatment could result in permanent stunting, whereas the growth retardation associated with low-dose treatment is likely to be offset at maturation by catch-up growth.[190] Triamcinolone acetonide and flunisolide are the only concentrated formulations currently marketed in the United States. The data available for flunisolide show no growth inhibition with doses of up to 1.0 mg/day used for 1 year.[114]

Children vary in their susceptibility to glucocorticoid-induced growth inhibition.[156, 201] A proportion of asthmatic children seem to be unusually susceptible to this complication, and this susceptibility appears to apply selectively to growth, and not to other organ systems normally targeted by glucocorticoid activity.[156]

Skeletal Changes

In asthmatic patients treated long term with oral or parenteral glucocorticoids, such as prednisone or prednisolone, skeletal complications are a much more frequent cause of major morbidity than is the rare but dramatic occurrence of acute adrenocortical insufficiency. Furthermore, controlled studies have shown that the risks to bone cannot be avoided by giving prednisone on alternate days.[162] It is surprising therefore that few data existed to document the effects of inhaled steroid therapy on skeletal metabolism and the risk of fracture.

Both budesonide and beclomethasone are capable of interfering with bone turnover. These metabolic effects are dose and drug related and appear to be greater with beclomethasone than with budesonide.[6, 89, 99] Nevertheless, the magnitude of these effects is much less, at least with inhaled budesonide, than that of prednisone when the two drugs are compared at dose levels in which the inhaled steroid is equally or more effective than the oral steroid.[89] No similar data are available for flunisolide or triamcinolone acetonide.

To determine the clinical importance of these laboratory abnormalities, it is necessary to determine the effects of inhaled steroid therapy on bone mineral density and the incidence of fracture. To date, published reports of cross-sectional surveys of bone mineral density have given conflicting results in patients treated with inhaled steroid.[96, 110, 146, 158, 186, 240] In those that found a reduction in bone density, the causal relationship to the inhaled steroid per se remains unclear because of the effects of past or current oral steroid usage or by coexisting nonsteroidal factors that may also reduce bone density.[52, 96, 146, 150, 186]

To address this question, we measured bone density and the prevalence of vertebral fracture in 69 adult asthmatic patients.[212] The survey was specifically designed to differentiate between any effect of the inhaled steroid that might be observed and that due to past or current oral steroid therapy or nonsteroidal factors, such as age, physical activity, or the postmenopausal state. The key observations from this survey are as follows:

1. Inhaled steroid treatment was associated with a dose-dependent and statistically significant reduction in bone density. Density dropped by an average of 0.5 standard deviations for each increment of inhaled steroid dosage by 1 mg/day (nominal dose).
2. This bone-depleting effect was offset to a clinically valuable degree by an opposing effect that related to the cumulative lifetime dose of inhaled steroid. This resulted in increased bone density and reduced risk of fracture. We hypothesize that this reflects bone reconstitution consequent to withdrawal of the patients from previously used prednisone after they switched to inhaled steroid. This repair process was not prevented by the use of beclomethasone or budesonide in doses averaging 1.2 mg/day.
3. The postmenopausal women in this group who had received prolonged inhaled steroid therapy, as evidenced by a lifetime dose exceeding 3 g (plus an estrogen supplement), had normal bone density on average. Furthermore, this applied regardless of how much prednisone they had used in the past and despite their current use of inhaled budesonide or beclomethasone at an exceptionally high daily dose, averaging 1.6 mg/day.
4. The prevalence of vertebral fracture in these patients decreased significantly with increasing exposure to inhaled steroid, as quantified by their cumulative lifetime dose.

In summary, these data indicate that the daily dose but not the duration of inhaled steroid therapy may adversely affect bone density and that estrogen therapy may offset this bone-depleting effect in postmenopausal women. Further studies are needed to test the hypotheses generated from this study: (1) the existence of two opposing effects of inhaled steroid therapy on bone density, one a direct effect of the daily dose and the other an indirect effect of prolonged use of the drug, with an accompanying abstention from oral or parenteral steroid use; and (2) the apparent capacity of supplemental estrogen therapy to prevent or correct glucocorticoid-induced osteoporosis in women, in addition to its expected effect on involutional osteoporosis.

The only pediatric studies published to date found no reduction in bone density in cross-sectional surveys of asthmatic children treated with low[15] or intermediate[110] doses of beclomethasone for several years. However, in one of these studies,[15] the average increment in bone density observed prospectively over the 6 months subsequent to the survey was materially less than that observed in control children not receiving an inhaled steroid. This suggests an inhibitory effect of the treatment on bone formation, which was not large enough to attain statistical significance, given the small number of patients studied, but could be a harbinger of future problems.

It remains to be determined whether the maximal bone density achieved by young adults may be adversely affected if they receive substantial amounts of inhaled steroid prior to 30 years of age. This information is needed because failure to achieve maximal bone density during youth could materially increase the risk of osteoporotic fracture when those individuals reach 60 years of age and older.

MINIMIZING RISKS

Since concern about the potential risks of inhaled steroid drugs is perhaps the single most important impediment to their use and since their systemic toxicity is a function of the daily dose, the latter should regularly be titrated down to minimum effective levels after optimal control has been established by an initial period of more aggressive dosing. Several measures may facilitate such dose titration.

Equivalent levels of antiasthmatic effect may be achieved at lower and less toxic doses if the daily dose of inhaled steroid is given more rather than less frequently.[214] The differences in potency are large enough to be clinically important.[125, 214] Therefore, when feasible, especially in patients who require relatively high doses to control their asthma, the inhaled steroid should be administered in four rather than two doses. This probably applies to any of the inhaled steroids currently used to treat asthma, although the most definitive data are derived from studies of budesonide.

If the daily doses of inhaled steroid are scheduled for the forenoon rather than diurnally, significantly higher morning levels of serum cortisol and osteocalcin may be seen.[215] However, there is no parallel sparing of the steroid-induced eosinopenia, and the inhibitory effect on cortisol production integrated over 24 hours is the same with either regimen.[215] Thus it is unlikely that any clinically useful reduction in the overall risk of adverse systemic effects can be achieved by using a morning dose schedule. This would be consistent with earlier studies of patients treated with oral steroids. These found that the clinical signs of chronic glucocorticoid excess consequent to long-term prednisone treatment occur as frequently when the drug is administered as a single morning dose as when the doses are divided throughout the day, when the same daily dosages are compared.[94, 142]

Cotreatment with theophylline (if tolerated) can facilitate reductions in inhaled and oral steroid dosage to lower and less toxic levels. Cromolyn or nedocromil may also be considered as adjunct therapy for such patients. However, the evidence that either of these drugs is sufficiently effective to facilitate a clinically worthwhile reduction in corticosteroid use in patients with severe asthma remains equivocal at best.[91, 143, 206, 243]

It is advisable to minimize the use of inhaled β-agonists as much as possible because of the potential risks of increased morbidity and mortality.[171, 193] This is a practical option, as evidenced by our experience that one half of all patients who attend our adult asthma clinic for ambulatory care require an inhaled β-agonist less than once per month, and many others use it only a few times per week (73% currently receive an inhaled steroid).[126]

A number of comparative trials have shown that better asthma control can be achieved if patients are treated with an inhaled steroid regimen supplemented by a β-agonist as needed rather than regularly scheduled doses of β-agonist used as an alternative or adjunct to the inhaled steroid.[82, 101, 171, 232] In patients receiving both drugs, any increase in symptoms that may occur as a consequence of regular β-agonist usage might lead to the daily doses of both the β-agonist and inhaled steroid being gradually escalated in a vain attempt to correct a problem that appears not to be preventable by steroid therapy.[171] Severe examples of such an escalation of β-agonist usage were described years ago under the sobriquet locked-lung syndrome as a complication of treatment with the unselective β-agonist isoproterenol.[106] However, this course of events was observed in a few patients treated with more selective β-agonists, such as albuterol or fenoterol, plus gradually escalating doses of oral or inhaled steroid. The need for high doses of steroid fell promptly after the excessive use of inhaled β-agonist was abruptly terminated.

Environmental control measures ought to be ancillary to any drug regimen chosen for asthma, and inhaled steroid therapy cannot adequately substitute for these important avoidance measures. In appropriately selected patients, environmental control of allergenic house dust exposure or the elimination of household pets has been shown to reduce asthma morbidity and drug requirements and to significantly improve airway hyperresponsiveness, provided that the control measures are rigorously applied and sustained for many months.[138, 152, 233] Avoidance of nonallergic trigger factors, such as tobacco smoke in the home and workplace, is also very important.[183]

SAFETY SURVEILLANCE

At present, no system of safety surveillance is formally sanctioned for use in patients receiving inhaled steroid treatment. The system outlined below and currently used in our clinic is essentially empiric, having evolved from personal observations made during 20 years of clinical studies of beclomethasone and budesonide.

In every patient, whether a low or high dose of inhaled steroid is used, we record at each follow-up visit the presence or absence of easily discernible features of hypercortisonism, such as steroid purpura or cushingoid facial features, and body weight. In children, height is recorded as well.

In those patients who require a dose of beclomethasone or budesonide greater than 1.6 mg/day to control their asthma (about 10% of our inhaled steroid users), we check their morning serum cortisol level once or twice a year, especially if they require daily, alternate-day, or intermittent prednisone as well. If the cortisol level is suppressed on two successive tests, the inhaled steroid dosage is reduced to try to restore the cortisol level to normal and to resolve any accompanying manifestations of chronic hypercortisonism. Nonsteroidal medications are added, as required, to maintain control of the asthma.

The serum cortisol level provides not only a direct measure of endogenous cortisol production but also indirect evidence about the systemic effects of inhaled steroid treatment on bone. If the serum cortisol level is significantly reduced (less than 210 nmol/L by the immunoassay technique used in our hospital laboratory), one can reasonably assume that the serum osteocalcin level (a measure of osteoblast function and bone formation) is reduced significantly as well.[215]

Furthermore, if a postmenopausal woman has a morning serum cortisol of less than 210 nmol/L, our data indicate that her adrenocortical output of androgens approximates zero.[216] Because estrogen deficiency is a major risk determinant of osteoporosis and fracture in postmenopausal women and because their residual estrogen supply is entirely dependent on biotransformation of these androgens of adrenocortical origin, the reduction in androgen output may augment the risk of bone complications in some older women if they are treated for asthma with high-dose inhaled steroid or a combined inhaled, and oral steroid regimen in the absence of an estrogen supplement. An analogous situation was observed in a young man with primary testicular failure and inadequate testosterone replacement after treatment with high-dose beclomethasone for 2 years.[40]

It is our practice to restrict bone densitometry to selected patients, such as elderly men and women or postmenopausal women who complain of back or hip pain or demonstrate persistent laboratory or conspicuous clinical evidence of chronic hypercortisonism. Steroid purpura may be a useful sign, since some clinical studies have found that it correlates significantly with the presence of steroid-induced osteoporosis.[212]

Since our experience in adults and that of others who have studied children indicate that inhaled steroid therapy appears to be a negligible risk factor for the occurrence of posterior subcapsular cataract,[179, 211] we believe that routine surveillance for cataracts is not warranted in patients receiving inhaled steroid therapy. Ophthalmologic examination is therefore limited to patients who complain of impaired visual acuity. Similarly, our clinical experience and available metabolic data indicate that it is unnecessary to monitor patients receiving inhaled steroid therapy for possible adverse effects on serum glucose, electrolyte, or lipid levels.

COMPARISONS OF EFFICACY, TOXICITY, AND EFFICIENCY

The choice of one inhaled steroid formulation over another is fraught with many uncertainties. To compare gravimetrical doses of different inhaled steroids, it is useful to consider both nominal and labeled dosage. Nominal dosage implies the amount of drug released by each activation of the valve of the pressurized metered-dose inhaler. For some, but not all, inhaled steroid formulations marketed in the United States, the labeled dosage reflects the nominal dosage adjusted to allow for losses estimated to occur within the delivery device. Logically, similar adjustments ought to be made for every combination of a metered-dose inhaler with the many different add-on spacer devices now widely used in clinical practice, but this is impractical.

Because the regulatory requirements for labeling vary from one formulation to another and one jurisdiction to another, as shown in Table 44–3 column C, nominal dosage provides the only readily accessible common denominator for comparing different formulations of inhaled steroid. Therefore, the daily doses cited in the accompanying text refer to nominal dosage. The number of valve activations required to release a nominal dose of 1 mg/day of the inhaled steroid formulations marketed in the United States and Canada are shown in Table 44–3 column A.

To compare different inhaled steroids in terms of equivalent anti-inflammatory doses, the volumetric doses shown in column A may be adjusted to allow for differences in anti-inflammatory activity, as quantified by their respective affinities for the glucocorticoid receptor. Such anti-inflammatory equivalents provide a basis for rank ordering the different drugs but do not fully take into account such factors as their lipophilicity and retention time within the lung, which also influence the therapeutic potency of these drugs in clinical practice.

To determine therapeutically equivalent doses for different inhaled steroids, clinical trials are essential. It is feasible to do this, but the confidence limits for the estimated therapeutically equivalent doses are wide,[54] and their reproducibility may vary with the trial design and the response index chosen to measure the effect of the treatment (Fig. 44–4).[54, 65]

The therapeutic index (ratio of topical anti-inflammatory to systemic activities) provides a useful and clinically relevant basis for comparing inhaled steroid drugs. For example, data indicate that budesonide has about the same antiasthmatic potency as beclomethasone but less systemic toxicity and fluticasone may have about twice the antiasthmatic potency of beclomethasone and less systemic activity than either beclomethasone or budesonide. If further studies confirm these findings and quantify their relative toxicities, particularly with respect to their effects on bone, fluticasone (which is currently an investigational new drug for asthma) may emerge as the drug with the most favorable therapeutic index. Factors other than the therapeutic index also influence the performance of these agents in clinical practice. One of these is intrapulmonary drug delivery.

The intrapulmonary delivery of inhaled steroid drugs is a function of (1) various characteristics of the aerosol, such as the percent of the aerosolized particles of active drug that fall within the respirable range; (2) the delivery device used to inhale the drug, such as a metered-dose inhaler with or without a spacer (and the size and design of the spacer) or a breath-actuated inhaler or dry powder delivery device instead of the conventional pressurized metered-dose inhaler; and (3) the individual patient's inhalation technique.

Interactions among this multiplicity of factors will determine the clinical efficiency of any particular inhaled steroid formulation in any particular patient and the efficiency of one formulation relative to another if any pair of these drugs is compared by clinical trial. Efficiency may be defined as the increase in therapeutic efficacy achieved per unit increase in unwanted systemic activity.

Given these practical difficulties and the absence of a generally accepted standard methodology for making such comparisons, it is important that the clinical practitioner consider the questions of cost, convenience, and patient preference. These factors are likely to be major determinants of the patient's long-term compliance with the treatment. Compliance is the most important single determinant of treatment success or failure—more important, for example, than the age of the patient, disease severity, or pathogenesis of the asthma.[218]

Having selected an agent appropriate to the circumstances, the factors that have been shown by controlled trials to influence the therapeutic response to inhaled steroid may then be manipulated to the best advantage of each patient. These include the dose per day,[217, 219] dosing frequency,[125, 214] drug delivery system,[220] duration of treatment,[248] and (most important) management plan used by the physician to encourage long-term patient compliance (see Figs. 44–3 and 44–4).[248]

ANTIMETABOLITES FOR CHRONIC ASTHMA

A variety of alternative anti-inflammatory drugs have been proposed for use in those asthmatic patients whose disease

TABLE 44–3
COMPARISON OF INHALED STEROID FORMULATIONS FOR ASTHMA

	A	B	C	
			Labeled Dose per Puff (mg)	
Drug (Generic)	*Puffs per Day to Release a 1.0 mg Nominal Dose*	*Nominal Dose per Puff (mg)*	*United States*	*Canada*
Vanceril or Beclovent (beclomethasone)	20	.05	.042	.05
Azmacort (triamcinolone acetonide)	5	.20	.10	.10
Pulmicort (budesonide)	5	.20	—	.20
AeroBid (flunisolide)	4	.25	.25	.25
Beclovent (beclomethasone)	4	.25	—	.25

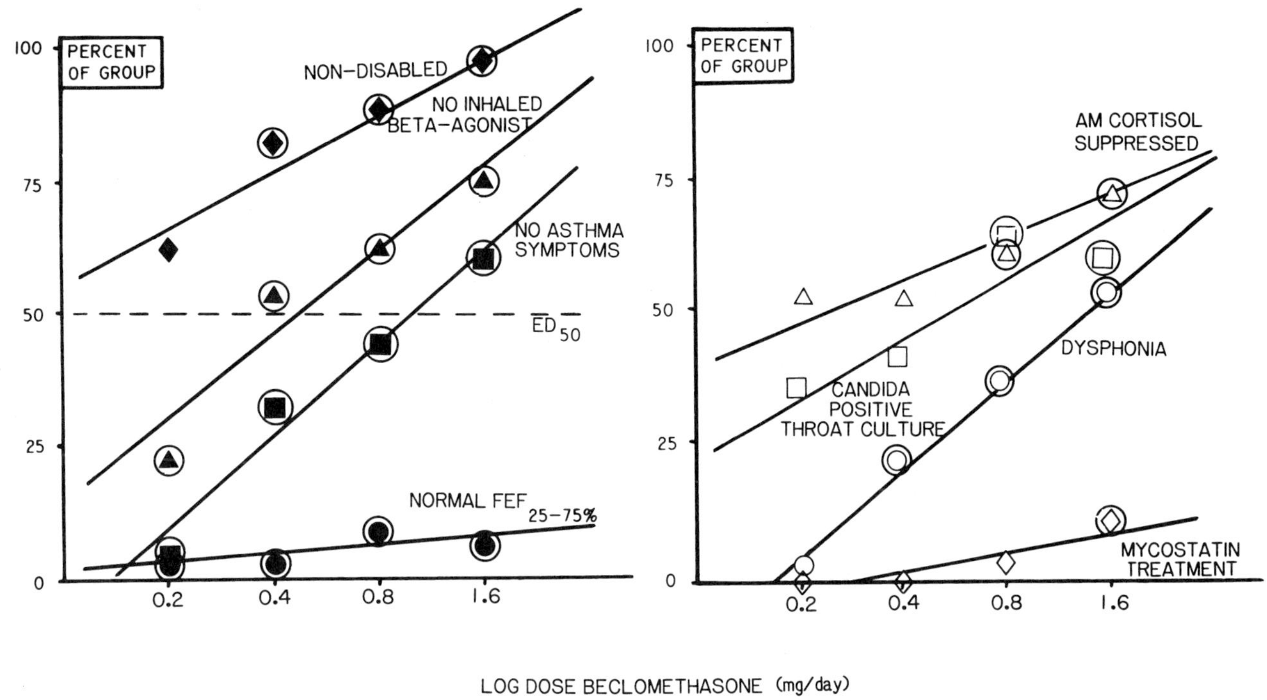

FIGURE 44–4. Response of 34 prednisone-dependent adult asthmatics to graded dosages of beclomethasone dipropionate (BDP). At each encircled point, the mean change from the pre-BDP baseline value was significant ($p < 0.05$ or better). The effective BDP dose for 50% of group (ED_{50}) may be determined by relating the intercepts of the dashed line with each regression line to the abscissa scale. The antiasthmatic effects, and the systemic and oropharyngeal complications of inhaled BDP, are all dose dependent. The prednisone dosage was held stable in this study, and the stepwise BDP increments were added as shown. Mean prednisone dosage was 11 mg/day. The high incidence of adrenal suppression in the group reflects their past systemic steroid therapy plus the effect of the combined oral and inhaled steroid treatment. (From Toogood JH: Corticosteroids. In Jenne JW, Murphy S (eds): Drug Therapy for Asthma: Research and Clinical Practice. Marcel Dekker Inc., New York, 1987, pp 719–759. Reprinted by courtesy of Marcel Dekker Inc.)

is inadequately controlled despite steroid therapy. The evidence for therapeutic benefit from these steroid-sparing agents is reviewed herewith.

When contemplating the use of one of these agents, the need for such intervention must be evaluated carefully since in many, perhaps most, asthmatic patients, careful reevaluation of the patient's prior and current clinical course will obviate the need. For example, Szefler and coworkers[196] found that only 6 of 125 asthmatic children referred to a national asthma center for consideration of treatment with an alternative or steroid-sparing agent actually received this additional therapy.

Table 44–4 summarizes some of the important reasons for apparent steroid failure in asthma. First, the diagnosis needs to be accurate. Upper airway disorders, such as vocal cord dysfunction, often masquerade as asthma. The distinction between asthma and less reversible lower airway disorders, such as chronic bronchitis and bronchiolitis, may also be difficult. Second, opportunities to reduce exposure to triggers or exacerbating factors, such as environmental irritants and allergens, drugs, and esophageal reflux, may not have been fully exploited and should be reviewed. Third, the patient may not have been receiving the intended regimen because of incomplete compliance, errors in timing of the steroid administration, such as the need for an afternoon steroid dose, or inefficient inhaler technique. Fourth, it may be possible to increase the intensity of the conventional antiasthmatic regimen by increasing the dose of inhaled steroid, adding a long-acting inhaled or oral bronchodilator, or adding a nonsteroidal antiallergic agent. Last, mechanisms of pharmacologic steroid resistance may be amenable to dose or regimen adjustment. These include abnormal steroid pharmacokinetics (increased clearance) and cellular resistance (e.g., monocytes, T lymphocytes).[53]

TABLE 44–4
REASONS FOR INEFFECTIVENESS OF STEROIDS IN ASTHMA TREATMENT

- Wrong diagnosis
- Avoidable or modifiable triggers
- Inadequate patient compliance or education
- Submaximal therapy
- Steroid resistance

Despite careful attention to these considerations, there remains a small subset of asthmatic patients in whom inadequate asthma control or the presence of serious steroid side effects indicates a need for an effective alternative drug. The proposed alternatives include methotrexate, gold, cyclosporin A, dapsone,[18] intravenous immunoglobulin,[128] hydroxychloroquine,[43] and colchicine[170] (Table 44–5). Of these, methotrexate, gold, and cyclosporin A have been most studied and are therefore reviewed here in detail.

METHOTREXATE

The successful use of low-dose methotrexate as an anti-inflammatory agent in rheumatoid arthritis and psoriasis prompted consideration of its use in asthma. Its anti-

TABLE 44–5
POSSIBLE STEROID-SPARING AGENTS FOR ASTHMA TREATMENT

- Methotrexate
- Gold
- Cyclosporin A
- Immunoglobulins
- Hydroxychloroquine
- Colchicine
- Dapsone

inflammatory effect at doses of about 15 mg weekly is probably unrelated to its inhibition of dihydrofolate reductase and may reflect other properties demonstrable in vitro, such as inhibition of neutrophil chemotaxis in response to LTB_4, inhibition of IL-1 release from macrophages or its subsequent action, and possibly inhibition of histamine release from basophils.[37] Methotrexate does not alter glucocorticoid pharmacokinetics.[73]

Most clinical trials of methotrexate in asthma have focused on steroid sparing as the major end point. The findings are discordant. Whereas Mullarkey and coworkers[136] found that methotrexate permitted an approximate one-third reduction in oral steroid requirement (corresponding to about 10 mg of prednisone daily), several subsequent studies report less steroid sparing[61, 188] or none at all.[45, 64, 199, 224]

Restriction of the methotrexate trial to 3 months or less in three of the negative studies may be pertinent,[45, 64, 224] since Shiner and colleagues[174] report that significant steroid sparing was not demonstrable in their double-blind parallel trial until 24 weeks of therapy had elapsed. In uncontrolled studies, further steroid sparing (including complete withdrawal in some cases) occurred after the methotrexate continued for up to 2 years.[175] Unfortunately, the steroid requirements rise rather promptly when the methotrexate is eventually discontinued,[174, 181] as might be expected since methotrexate has not been shown to reduce airway hyperresponsiveness.[64]

In the studies published to date, methotrexate has been generally well tolerated. Nevertheless, its potential side effects are a concern. These range from hematologic abnormalities, gastrointestinal intolerance, alopecia, and rash to the less common teratogenicity, marrow aplasia, and serious hepatic and pulmonary toxicity. The risk of hepatotoxicity can be minimized by patient selection and monitoring. A paradoxical increase in airway responsiveness induced by methotrexate has been reported.[100] The possibility of uncommon consequences of long-term methotrexate treatment, such as pneumocystic pneumonia (particularly if used in conjunction with corticosteroids) or cirrhosis, cannot be discounted.

In summary, the currently available evidence does not permit a firm conclusion about the role of methotrexate in asthma. The studies published to date suffer from one or more biases, both positive (submaximal inhaled steroid therapy, inadequate baseline observation, open-label studies) and negative (small numbers of test subjects, brief observation periods). Methotrexate appears unlikely to assume a major role in asthma therapy since its steroid-sparing efficacy has been modest on average, prospective identification of a responder subgroup has not been possible, long-term toxicity remains a concern, and there is no evidence of clinical benefit persisting after withdrawal of the drug.

GOLD

The documented benefit of gold treatment (chrysotherapy) in rheumatoid arthritis prompted detailed examination of its anti-inflammatory properties. Its actions with antiasthmatic potential include inhibition of neutrophil activation and monocyte chemotaxis, inhibition of mediator release from basophils and mast cells, and a reduction in the responsiveness of sensitized tracheal smooth muscle.[19, 51, 53] Adverse effects of chrysotherapy, commonly occurring in the first few months of treatment, include nephrotoxicity, mucocutaneous reactions, and hematologic abnormalities. Rarer side effects include neuropathies, hepatitis, and pneumonitis. Gold appears to be less toxic if given orally, but it is also less effective.

The first suggestion that gold therapy might be beneficial in asthma came from Japanese studies in asthmatic patients of varying severity, with or without controls. A response was seen in about one third of recipients and, as with methotrexate, was typically delayed by several months after initiation of therapy. In addition, however, these studies suggest that, in contrast to methotrexate, gold offers the potential of a remittent response, with a long-term reduction in airway hyperresponsiveness.

Further experience, albeit limited, has been with the oral formulation of gold, auranofin, given at a dose of 3 mg twice daily to steroid-dependent asthmatics. In an open trial in 18 patients, Bernstein and coworkers[19] observed an approximate 40% reduction in prednisone requirement (corresponding to about 6 mg daily). Nierop and coworkers[141] found in a double-blind parallel group trial of 32 steroid-dependent asthmatics that the auranofin-treated group achieved both a small reduction in the daily prednisone dose (by 4 mg) and improvement in several indexes of asthma control.

In summary, the effects of gold therapy appear similar to those of methotrexate in that a minority of patients with steroid-dependent asthma exhibit improved asthma control and reduced steroid requirement after a delay of several months. In contrast to methotrexate, gold may have a remittive effect, coupled with a sustained reduction in airway hyperresponsiveness. As with methotrexate, side effects are substantial and require close monitoring. Further studies are required to determine the role, if any, of gold in asthma treatment.

CYCLOSPORIN A

The rationale for examination of cyclosporin A as a potential antiasthmatic agent lies in its ability to inhibit T-lymphocyte activation and lymphokine release (IL-2, IL-4, IL-5). These are attractive properties in view of the known correlation between activated CD4 T lymphocytes and chronic asthma severity. Additional and potentially useful antiasthmatic effects include the inhibition of mediator release from basophils and lung mast cells, suppression of experimental eosinophilia, and inhibition of macrophage activation.[38] As with methotrexate and gold, adverse effects, notably nephrotoxicity, hypertension, and neuropathy, are an important consideration.

The experience with cyclosporin A treatment of asthma is extremely limited. In an open study, Szczeklik and coworkers[195] demonstrated a reduction in prednisone requirements (from 30 mg to 11 mg daily) in 6 of 12 asthmatics after 9 months of cyclosporine therapy. Alexander and coworkers[5] conducted a double-blind crossover trial in 33 steroid-dependent asthmatics. No attempt was made to reduce the maintenance steroid dose. During the 12-week cyclosporine arm, mean peak flows rose, and the number of asthma exacerbations requiring additional steroid use fell. Toxicity was generally mild.

In summary, although cyclosporin A is an attractive therapeutic alternative, studies to date are extremely limited, and its role as an adjunct or alternative to steroids in the treatment of asthma remains to be determined.

SUMMARY

In most patients with severe asthma that is apparently steroid unresponsive, careful consideration of the diagnosis, environmental triggers, and factors known to augment or facilitate the efficiency of conventional antiasthmatic agents will lead to improved asthma control. For the small minority of patients in whom steroid toxicity or resistance remains a problem, as evidenced by incomplete asthma control, the usefulness of agents such as methotrexate, gold, and cyclosporine is currently being explored. However, each of these agents carries a substantial risk of side effects, and their role as steroid-sparing or alternative agents for asthma treatment remains to be established.

CORTICOSTEROIDS FOR ACUTE ASTHMA

Placebo-controlled trials have clearly demonstrated the efficacy of steroid therapy for acute asthma.[66, 150] A ventilatory response may become discernible after an hour but is not prominent until 5 to 9 hours later. Therefore, it is not possible to demonstrate a significant response to steroid treatment in a clinical trial unless observation continues for more than 6 hours after the start of the steroid therapy and concomitant bronchodilator is either withheld[47] or maintained at a stable level while the steroid treatment is added.[66] Failure to attend to these exigencies of trial design has generated controversy about the usefulness of steroids for acute asthma,[119, 187] whereas the value of prompt and aggressive bronchodilator treatment is generally conceded.

The rationale for treating acute severe asthma with a systemic steroid rests on the following considerations:

1. It is not possible to accurately predict which patient presenting with severe asthma may suddenly die.[123, 239]
2. Failure to use steroids early and in adequate dosage has been cited as a frequent correlate of sudden death or near death during severe asthma.[102, 157]
3. The risks from using steroids in conventional dosage to treat asthma are negligible.
4. Steroids exert an early normalizing effect on the arterial oxygen tension in acute asthma that is not attainable with bronchodilators alone.[150, 62] Since hypoxemia is an important determinant of the risk of death during asthma, this effect may be clinically valuable.
5. In patients who have become refractory to β-agonist drugs due to down-regulation of adrenoreceptors, steroids may correct this refractory state within a few hours.[194]
6. In some patients with severe acute asthma, iatrogenic adrenocortical insufficiency may contribute to the risk of death.[182] Replacement steroid treatment could be critical in such patients.
7. The use of steroids to supplement bronchodilators in the emergency treatment of severe asthma has been shown to significantly reduce hospital admission[167, 198] and the incidence of asthma relapse soon after hospital discharge[41, 66] in comparison with what can be achieved with bronchodilators alone.

ORAL VERSUS PARENTERAL

The oral and intravenous routes of administration differ little with respect to the onset of their antiasthmatic effects. Prednisolone has approximately equivalent bioavailability by either route, and oral doses achieve peak blood levels in an hour or less. Either prednisone or prednisolone may be used since they are rapidly interconvertible and the peak levels achieved are influenced more by interpatient differences in the conversion ratio than by which drug was administered.[88, 130]

DOSAGE

A review of the results of 10 different dose-ranging studies indicates that an adult dose below 40 mg methylprednisolone per day may be suboptimal for some patients with acute asthma and that 80 to 160 mg methylprednisolone per day can achieve optimal results.[222] No additional benefit accrues if larger doses are used. A better result can be achieved in a shorter time by assuring prompt aggressive bronchodilator treatment than by pushing the steroid dose to heroic levels. Furthermore, sudden death may accompany high-dose intravenous prednisolone therapy, presumably as a consequence of arrhythmias triggered by electrolyte shifts.[24] High-dose systemic steroid treatment for more than 1 week can produce a protracted generalized myopathy.[79] Fatal varicella zoster is a rare complication of concern in children.[105, 178]

As a general rule, after the initial 24 to 48 hours of treatment, the intravenous steroid (if used) may be switched to oral prednisone in divided doses ranging from 50 to 150 mg/day, depending on the severity of the asthma and the patient's tolerance. We generally use 60 to 80 mg/day (0.85–1.5 mg/kg/day) because adverse neuropsychiatric effects are less of a problem if the prednisone dose does not exceed 80 mg/day.

At this dose, normalization of the air flow may occur as quickly as 3 days,[86] although patients vary widely in their rate of recovery. Using 0.85 mg/kg prednisone per day, we found that 10 to 14 days are generally required for improvement in the middle forced expiratory flow ($FEF_{25-75\%}$) to plateau in adult asthmatics with associated chronic obstructive pulmonary disease, who constitute the majority of our hospital admissions. This recovery period will appear shorter if a less sensitive index of the therapeutic response is chosen, such as symptoms alone or peak expiratory flow rate. Serial spirometry provides the most reliable guide as to how long the high-dose regimen should continue, because the signs and symptoms of asthma clear well before the pulmonary functional improvement reaches a plateau.[131, 237]

TAPERING

The rate at which the high-dose steroid is withdrawn after clinical recovery remains empiric. Abrupt withdrawal may be associated with a high rate of relapse and an increased risk of mortality during the 14 days following hospital discharge.[107] These risks can be diminished by tapering the steroid dose slowly. However, if high-dose inhaled steroid is introduced at this point, tapering may be unnecessary. The oral steroid may be stopped abruptly without incurring serious risk, assuming that patients comply with the inhaled steroid treatment and that an adequate system of patient surveillance is in place.[144, 166]

CORTICOSTEROIDS FOR VASCULITIS

(See Chapter 52)

HYPERSENSITIVITY VASCULITIS

Hypersensitivity vasculitis comprises a heterogeneous group of clinical syndromes in which the prominent lesion is located in small vessels and usually limited to the skin. Corticosteroid therapy is seldom required but is highly effective when the disease is severe or involves other organ systems.[39] In patients with severe serum sickness type of reactions, prednisone 40 to 60 mg/day for a few days is helpful.[68] In Schönlein-Henoch purpura, corticosteroids are reserved for patients with severe joint or gastrointestinal symptoms or renal involvement.

POLYMYALGIA RHEUMATICA

Corticosteroid therapy is highly effective for the symptoms, but many patients can be controlled satisfactorily with a nonsteroidal anti-inflammatory drug, thus avoiding the adverse effects of prolonged corticosteroid usage. When clinically necessary, prednisone 20 mg/day is an effective initial dose in most cases.[111]

TEMPORAL ARTERITIS

Among the vasculitis syndromes, the efficacy of systemic corticosteroid treatment is best documented for temporal arteritis.[140] If symptoms of ocular or cerebral involvement are present, corticosteroid should be started immediately. Confirmatory biopsy can be secured any time in the first week of steroid therapy with little loss in diagnostic potential.[8] Therapy should begin with 40 to 60 mg of prednisone, tapering gradually to 7.5 to 10 mg/day, with dose adjustments if symptoms recur.[68] This may take months to achieve. The corticosteroid should continue for 1 to 2 years.[17]

TAKAYASU'S ARTERITIS

Perhaps 50% of patients with Takayasu's arteritis are corticosteroid sensitive.[172] Although 40 to 60 mg of prednisone per day can alleviate symptoms, there is no evidence that it substantially improves life expectancy.[97]

POLYARTERITIS NODOSA

After the introduction of corticosteroid therapy for polyarteritis, 5-year survival rates improved to approximately 60%.[165] Studies suggest that better results may be achieved in polyarteritis nodosa patients who are hepatitis B surface antigen positive if they are also treated with plasmapheresis and antiviral therapy.[81] Polyarteritis nodosa without hepatitis B surface antigen positivity continues to have a poor prognosis, despite corticosteroid and cyclophosphamide therapy.[46, 69]

WEGENER'S GRANULOMATOSIS

Corticosteroid alone can rapidly resolve the nonrenal or pulmonary manifestations of Wegener's granulomatosis and increase survival, whereas previously it was uniformly fatal. However, corticosteroid should be considered an adjunct to cyclophosphamide,[70] since the combined use of cytotoxic and corticosteroid drugs leads to marked improvement in 90% and complete remission in 75% of patients.[90] Trimethoprim-sulfamethoxazole may be used as an adjunct in refractory cases or as monotherapy for mild disease or for maintenance of remission.[132, 229] The long-term complications of cytotoxic therapy are of increasing concern.[90]

OTHER VASCULITIDES

Biopsy-proven vasculitis not uncommonly falls outside the defined nosologic categories. However, the principles of corticosteroid use are essentially the same, regardless of categorization.

When corticosteroid treatment is clinically necessary for active vasculitis, prednisone 1 mg/kg/day is a reasonable starting regimen.[67] Initially, this is administered daily in three or four divided doses. This is continued until the acute manifestations subside, generally 7 to 10 days or longer if necessary.[87] The divided doses are then consolidated to a single morning dose, which continues until the symptoms and signs fully resolve. Dose tapering then begins with decrements of 5 to 10 mg every week or two, followed by smaller decrements as the dose declines. Conversion to alternate-day prednisone may reduce the drug's systemic toxicity but may be less efficacious than daily dosing.[67]

If fulminant pulmonary or renal involvement is present, cyclophosphamide is used in conjunction with high-dose corticosteroid. Corticosteroid acts promptly, whereas cyclophosphamide may require as long as 14 days for its effect to become apparent.[87]

The duration of corticosteroid therapy in the systemic vasculitides syndromes is controversial. Among systemic vasculitis patients treated with corticosteroid for more than a year, up to two thirds may be affected by complications, which may relate more to the treatment than to the primary disease.[46, 112]

A variety of vasculitides may occur in association with the human immunodeficiency virus.[36] Therefore, the HIV status of patients with vasculitis should be investigated prior to the use of potent immunosuppressive agents.

CORTICOSTEROIDS FOR ANAPHYLAXIS

Injectable epinephrine is the drug of choice for anaphylaxis, and maintenance of an effective airway and circulatory system is the primary therapeutic goal. There are no controlled data to support the use of corticosteroid in acute anaphylaxis. Systemic corticosteroids do not suppress the primary phase of anaphylaxis and would not be expected to play a role in its acute management since many of the anti-inflammatory effects of corticosteroid require hours, days, or weeks to achieve maximal expression.[34, 80] Nevertheless, corticosteroids continue to be used clinically in the hope of averting late sequelae.

Biphasic anaphylaxis is being recognized increasingly.[154, 184] Although the second phase may occur despite steroid treatment of the acute phase,[154, 184] the corticosteroid may moderate its severity by increasing β-adrenoreceptor responsiveness and inhibiting cell activation and mediator release.[55, 168] In the cutaneous model of the late-phase allergic response, a single dose of prednisolone immediately prior to antigen challenge may reduce the 6-hour lesion diameter by 50%.[153] Therefore, the administration of intravenous hydrocortisone (4–8 mg/kg) or methylprednisolone (2 mg/kg) seems prudent, with repetition every 6 hours as needed.

RECURRENT IDIOPATHIC ANAPHYLAXIS

In addition to its use for acute anaphylaxis, oral corticosteroid may be useful for the prevention of recurrent exacerbations of idiopathic anaphylaxis.[29, 245] Prednisone 60 to 100 mg is administered each morning for 7 to 14 days, along with oral albuterol or hydroxyzine. Following this, the patient is converted to alternate-day prednisone and then titrated down by 5 mg every 2 to 4 weeks as symptoms permit.[77] This regimen is reportedly effective in achieving remission rates of 30% to 50% in patients with recurrent idiopathic anaphylaxis.[246] A subset of such patients may require regular preventive corticosteroid,[77, 238] and a small number are corticosteroid resistant.[147]

REACTIONS TO RADIOCONTRAST MEDIA

In patients with a history of previous anaphylactoid reaction to iodinated radiocontrast media, corticosteroid premedication may reduce the incidence of reaction about sixfold.[75, 76, 127] If a noninvasive diagnostic procedure cannot be substituted, it is prudent to pretreat any patient with a history of previous anaphylactic reaction to radiocontrast media. Three 50 mg doses of prednisone are recommended at 6-hour intervals, with the third dose scheduled 1 hour before the procedure (along with diphenhydramine 50 mg intramuscularly and ephedrine 25 mg orally, when not contraindicated).[148] The use of a low osmolar contrast agent will further reduce the reaction rate if the previous reaction involved a high osmolar agent. The combination of prophylaxis and a low osmolar agent has been estimated to reduce the expected recurrence rate from 16% to 30% to 0.6%.[116] Although this pretreatment protocol is highly effective in reducing the frequency and severity of anaphylactoid reactions, it has not been shown to prevent life-threatening nonanaphylactoid reactions, such as those due to noncardiogenic pulmonary edema.[26, 124]

CORTICOSTEROIDS FOR OTOLARYNGOLOGIC DISEASE

Because of the potential for systemic complications, long-term oral steroid therapy is reserved for patients with severe disease, whereas the topically active intranasal steroids are increasingly used for rhinitis, often as first-line therapy. Controlled clinical trials have documented the efficacy of intranasal steroids for seasonal and perennial atopic rhinitis,[9, 28, 95, 129, 189, 236] nonallergic hyperplastic rhinitis with eosinophilia (NARES syndrome),[135] and nasal polyposis.[42, 85]

Beclomethasone, flunisolide, triamcinolone, and fluticasone are marketed in the United States and Canada as pressurized aerosol suspension or aqueous sprays for intranasal use. Comparative studies of the different drugs and formulations demonstrate equal efficacy, although a few suggest that budesonide (BUD) may be marginally more effective than beclomethasone (BDP).[177]

INTRANASAL STEROIDS RELATIVE TO OTHER THERAPIES

Most studies comparing intranasal steroids with intranasal cromolyn in seasonal or perennial allergic rhinitis have demonstrated that intranasal steroids are more effective.[23, 236] Few studies have directly compared intranasal steroids with antihistamines. Some suggest that intranasal steroids and long-acting antihistamines may provide equal benefit[176, 247]; others found that intranasal steroids are more effective.[21] In practice, these therapies are complementary and may provide the most effective relief if used in combination.[11] There are no studies comparing intranasal steroids with immunotherapy with respect to long-term cost benefits or efficacy.

SYSTEMIC CORTICOSTEROIDS

In seasonal allergic rhinitis, the therapeutic role of oral steroids is limited to patients who present with severe symptoms and nasal obstruction at the peak of seasonal pollination. Such patients are at risk for developing complicating infective sinusitis, eustachian tube dysfunction, and potentially, sleep apnea.[2, 250] Intranasal steroids are not effective at this stage because of poor access to the nasal passages. A 1- or 2-week course of prednisone will carry the patient through the peak of the season and allow the intranasal steroid to be introduced later if needed.

Patients with chronic allergic rhinitis are sometimes treated with intraturbinal depot injections of steroid. Although effective for symptom relief, this practice should be abandoned because it is occasionally complicated by permanent blindness due to retinal vessel spasm.[122]

Intranasal steroids may be effective in the management of small nasal polyps for both treatment and prevention of recurrence following surgical resection.[85] However, intranasal steroids are much less effective than oral steroids for large polyps, which obstruct the airway and prevent successful application of the topical agent. It has been our experience that large polyps and the acute exacerbations of polyps commonly triggered by viral respiratory infection respond promptly and consistently to 3 to 4 weeks of prednisone commencing at 40 mg/day (adult dose). The remission can usually be sustained with an intranasal steroid.[221]

INTRANASAL STEROIDS FOR OTHER CONDITIONS

There are no published trials of the effectiveness of oral or intranasal steroids in the treatment of rhinitis medicamentosa. In our clinical experience, a 2- to 4-week course of prednisone is predictably effective for relieving symptoms, facilitating abrupt withdrawal from the causative agent, and preventing the recurrence of previous dependence on vasoconstrictor nose sprays. Others report success with intranasal steroids.[177]

The response of primary vasomotor rhinitis to oral or intranasal steroids is variable, reflecting the pathogenetic diversity of patients with this nonspecific diagnosis.

Early suggestions of the value of preventive intranasal steroids for chronic serous otitis media complicating chronic allergy have not been substantiated by a subsequent double-blind controlled study.[117]

ADVERSE EFFECTS

The systemic toxicity of all the intranasal steroid formulations appears to be negligible when they are used in conventional doses. This is evidenced by the results of tests of HPA axis function, the absence of symptoms of hypercortisonism in intranasal steroid-treated patients, and the resolution of preexisting signs of hypercortisonism after previous prednisone therapy has been substituted with intranasal steroids. In children younger than 6 years, neither safety nor efficacy data are available.

Routine nasal swabs for candida during long-term treatment with intranasal steroids are very rarely positive, and there are no reported cases of nasal thrush in immunocompetent patients. As with systemic steroids, intranasal steroids should be avoided or used with caution in immunocompromised patients because of the risk of opportunistic infection.

The commonest complication of chronic intranasal steroid use is a small erosion of the nasal septum, whose presence is usually signaled by epistaxis. The problem is easily resolved by applying petrolatum to the ulcerated area immediately before using the intranasal steroid. Habitual nose picking may prevent healing and could lead to septal perforation. Perforation has been observed in a few patients treated with intranasal steroids.[169, 180] It is prudent therefore to document whether the nasal septum is intact before starting intranasal steroid therapy.

Nasal biopsies studied by light and electron microscopy have not shown atrophic changes or other evidence of cumulative damage similar to the connective tissue atrophy that the same topically active steroids produce when applied chronically to the skin.[93,139, 151] The rapid clearance of the drug from the respiratory tract presumably accounts for this difference.

Animal safety data suggest that the steroids prescribed for inhalation into the nose or lower airways probably do not have carcinogenic or mutagenic potential in humans. Very large doses of these drugs are teratogenic and fetotoxic in rabbits and rats, but conventional doses of beclomethasone inhaled by pregnant mothers with severe asthma did not increase the incidence of congenital malformations in the newborn.[74] Some steroids are known to be distributed in human milk and might conceivably suppress growth in nursing infants, but there are no relevant data for the steroids prescribed for inhalation. Because of the absence of data from controlled studies in humans, intranasal steroids should be used with caution in pregnant or nursing women.

CORTICOSTEROIDS FOR DERMATOSES

Systemic or topical corticosteroids are useful in the treatment of allergic dermatoses. Their mechanism of action is incompletely understood but relates to their anti-inflammatory effects. They are available in a great variety of formulations whose effects and adverse effects have been reviewed.[145, 197] In general, the more potent formulations are indicated for use over thick skin (palms and soles), and low-potency formulations should be used on the thin skin of the face or groin.

ADVERSE EFFECTS

Prolonged or intensive topical corticosteroid therapy may lead to cutaneous or systemic adverse effects, particularly if applied to large areas under occlusion and in infants and children. Iatrogenic Cushing's syndrome occurs rarely. Suppression of normal HPA axis function is more common.[49]

Localized cutaneous effects include dermal atrophy, striae, hypopigmentation, hypertrichosis, impaired wound healing, and local infection. Contact dermatitis is increasingly reported.[50] Inhaled steroid therapy for rhinitis or asthma rarely causes similar adverse effects on the perioral skin.[56]

FORMULATIONS

Corticosteroid stronger than 1% hydrocortisone or 0.5% desonide should be avoided on the face in order to prevent corticosteroid-induced rosacea or perioral dermatitis. Because of the potential for these complications, patients should be monitored closely, and the frequency of application or potency of the drug reduced when possible. The standard frequency of application is controversial; two to three times per day is usually recommended, but once daily may be sufficient for mild to moderate dermatitis.[192] The choice of a particular agent varies with the severity and location of the dermatitis and patient preference. It is important to consider the latter so as to ensure patient compliance. Creams spread more easily than an ointment and are more cosmetically acceptable. However, creams require a preservative in the formulation that may cause allergic sensitization. Ointments are preferred for dry areas and fissured or scaling lesions on the hand or feet. Gels and lotions are convenient for hairy areas, but the alcohol may be drying.

ATOPIC DERMATITIS

Skin hygiene and topical corticosteroid therapy are the mainstays of atopic dermatitis therapy. Chronic systemic corticosteroid use should be avoided, but an occasional short course may be needed to control a severe exacerbation and restore responsiveness to topical therapy. For milder exacerbations, 1 to 2 weeks of treatment with a moderate to high-potency topical agent (avoiding face and body folds) is indicated, switching thereafter to maintenance therapy with a low-potency agent to avoid a corticosteroid withdrawal rebound in severity.

URTICARIA

In chronic urticaria, systemic corticosteroid therapy should be restricted to intermittent short-term use to control disabling exacerbations resistant to other therapy, including combinations of H1 and H2 antihistamines. Prolonged oral daily steroid treatment should not be given for chronic urticaria unless it is associated with other disorders for which such treatment is indicated, such as systemic vasculitis. Alternate day steroid therapy with gradual tapering over months may become the standard for severe chronic urticaria alone or with concomitant angioedema (see Chapter 35).

OTHER DERMATOSES

High-dose systemic corticosteroid is the treatment of choice for acute pemphigus vulgaris or bullous pemphigoid.[16] It is often used in erythema multiforme, although in the absence of controlled trials, the indications for its use remain empiric and controversial.

Prednisone 20 to 40 mg/day for 1 week is rapidly and consistently effective for acute dermatitis caused by drug allergy or widespread allergic contact dermatitis, such as poison ivy; 40 to 60 mg/day for 10 days may be required for disseminated involvement or severe facial rash. Chronic contact dermatitis is appropriately treated with topical corticosteroid, provided that a diagnostic allergy assessment and appropriate avoidance procedures have been undertaken.

REFERENCES

1. Abzug MJ, Cotton MF: Severe chickenpox after intranasal use of corticosteroids. Pediatrics 123:577–579, 1993.
2. Ackerman MN, Friedman RA, Doyle WJ, et al: Antigen-induced eustachian tube obstruction: an intranasal provocative challenge test. J Allergy Clin Immunol 73:604–609, 1984.
3. Adcock IM, Gelder CM, Shirasaki H, et al: Effects of steroids on transcription factors in human lung. Am Rev Respir Dis 145:A834, 1992.
4. Agertoft L, Pedersen S: Effects of long-term treatment with an inhaled corticosteroid on growth and pulmonary function in asthmatic children. Respir Med 88:373–381, 1994.
5. Alexander AG, Barnes NC, Kay AB: Trial of cyclosporine in corticosteroid-dependent chronic severe asthma. Lancet 339:324–328, 1992.
6. Ali NJ, Capewell S, Ward MJ: Bone turnover during high dose inhaled corticosteroid treatment. Thorax 46:160–164, 1991.
7. Allen MB, Ray SG, Leitch AG, et al: Steroid aerosols and cataract formation. Br Med J 299:432–433, 1989.
8. Allison MC, Gallagher PJ: Temporal artery biopsy and corticosteroid treatment. Ann Rheum Dis 43:416–417, 1984.
9. Arbesman C, Bernstein IL, Bierman CW, et al: Multicenter, double-blind, placebo-controlled trial of fluocortin butyl in perennial rhinitis. J Allergy Clin Immunol 71:597, 1983.
10. Baxter JD, Funder JW: Hormone receptors. N Engl J Med 301:1149, 1979.
11. Backhouse CI, Finnamore VP, Gosden CW: Treatment of seasonal allergic rhinitis with flunisolide and terfenadine. J Int Med Res 14:35–40, 1986.
12. Bahna SL, Bjerkedal T: The course and outcome of pregnancy in women with bronchial asthma. Acta Allergol (Kbh) 27:397, 1972.
13. Balfour-Lynn L: Growth and childhood asthma. Arch Dis Child 61:1049–1055, 1986.
14. Ballard PL: Delivery and transport of glucocorticoids to target cells. Monogr Endocrinol 12:25, 1979.
15. Baraldi E, Bollini MC, De Marchi A, Zacchello F: Effect of beclomethasone dipropionate on bone mineral content assessed by X-ray densitometry in asthmatic children: a longitudinal evaluation. Eur Respir J 7:710–714, 1994.
16. Becker BA, Gaspari AA: Pemphigus vulgaris and vegetans. Dermatol Clin 11:429–451, 1993.
17. Beevers JDG, Harpur JE, Turk KAD: Giant cell arteritis—the need for prolonged treatment. J Chron Dis 26:571–584, 1973.
18. Berlow BA, Liebhaber MI, Dyer Z, Spiegel TM: The effect of dapsone in steroid-dependent asthma. J Allergy Clin Immunol 87:710–715, 1991.
19. Bernstein DI, Bernstein IL, Bodenheimer SS, Pietrusko RG: An open study of auranofin in the treatment of steroid-dependent asthma. J Allergy Clin Immunol 81:6–16, 1988.
20. Besedovsky J, Del Rey A, Sorkin E, Dinarello C: Immunoregulatory feedback between IL-1 and glucocorticoid hormones. Science 233:652–654, 1986.
21. Beswick KBJ, Kenyon GS, Cherry JR: A comparative study of beclomethasone dipropionate aqueous nasal spray with terfenadine tablets in seasonal allergic rhinitis. Curr Med Res Opin 9:560–567, 1985.
22. Bisgaard H: Systemic activity of inhaled topical steroid in toddlers studied by knemometry. Acta Paediatr 82:1066–1071, 1993.
23. Bjerrum P, Illum P: Treatment of seasonal allergic rhinitis with budesonide and disodium cromoglycate. Allergy 40:65–69, 1985.
24. Bocanegra TS, Castaneda MO, Espinoza LR, et al: Sudden death after methylprednisolone pulse therapy. Ann Intern Med 95:122, 1981.
25. Boe J, Rosenhall L, Alton M, et al: Comparison of dose-response effects of inhaled beclomethasone dipropionate and budesonide in the management of asthma. Allergy 44:349–355, 1989.
26. Borish L, Matloff SM, Findlay SR: Radiographic contrast media–induced noncardiogenic pulmonary edema: case report and review of the literature. J Allergy Clin Immunol 74:104–107, 1984.
27. Boschetto P, Rogers DF, Fabbri LM, Barnes PJ: Corticosteroid inhibition of airway microvascular leakage. Am Rev Respir Dis 143:605–609, 1991.
28. Bousquet J, Chanal I, Alquie MC, et al: Prevention of pollen rhinitis symptoms: comparison of fluticasone propionate aqueous nasal spray and disodium cromoglycate aqueous nasal spray: a multicenter, double-blind, double-dummy, parallel group study. Allergy 48:327–333, 1993.
29. Boxer MB, Greenberger PA, Patterson R: The impact of prednisone in life-threatening idiopathic anaphylaxis: reduction in acute episodes and medical costs. Ann Allergy 62:201–204, 1989.
30. Brattsand R, Selroos O: Current drugs for respiratory diseases. Glucocorticoids. In Page CP, Metzger WJ (eds): Drugs and the Lung. Raven Press, Ltd, New York, 1994, pp 101–220.

31. Brown PH, Blundell G, Greening AP, et al: Hypothalamo-pituitary-adrenal axis suppression in asthmatics inhaling high dose corticosteroids. Respir Med 85:501–510, 1991.
32. Brown PH, Teelucksigh S, Matusiewicz SP, et al: Cutaneous vasoconstrictor response to glucocorticoids in asthma. Lancet 337:576–580, 1991.
33. Brown PH, Greening AP, Crompton GK: Hypothalamo-pituitary-adrenal axis suppression in asthmatic adults taking high dose beclomethasone dipropionate. Br J Clin Pract 46:102–104, 1992.
34. Burge PS, Efthimiou J, Turner-Warwick M, Nelmes PTJ: Double-blind trials of inhaled beclomethasone dipropionate and fluocortin butyl ester in allergen-induced immediate and late asthmatic reactions. Clin Allergy 12:523–531, 1982.
35. Busuttil A: Adrenal atrophy at autopsy in two asthmatic children. Am J Forensic Med Pathol 12:36–39, 1991.
36. Calabrese LH, Estes M, Yen-Lieberman B, et al: Systemic vasculitis in association with human immunodeficiency virus infection. Arthritis Rheum 32 (5) :569–576, 1989.
37. Calderon E, Coffey RG, Lockey RF: Methotrexate in bronchial asthma. J Allergy Clin Immunol 88:274–276, 1991.
38. Calderon E, Lockey RF, Bukantz SC, et al: Is there a role for cyclosporine in asthma? J Allergy Clin Immunol 89:629–636, 1992.
39. Callen JP, Ekenstam EAF: Cutaneous leukocytoclastic vasculitis: clinical experience in 44 patients. South Med J 80:848–851, 1987.
40. Chalkley SM, Chisholm DJ: Cushing's syndrome from an inhaled glucocorticoid. Med J Aust 160:611–615, 1994.
41. Chapman K, Verbeek R, White JG, Rebuck A: Effect of a short course of prednisone in the prevention of early relapse after the emergency room treatment of acute asthma. N Engl J Med 324:788–794, 1991.
42. Charlton R, Mackay I, Wilson R, Cole P: Double blind, placebo controlled trial of betamethasone nasal drops for nasal polyposis. Br Med J 291:788, 1985.
43. Charous BL: Open study of hydroxychloroquine in the treatment of severe symptomatic or corticosteroid-dependent asthma. Ann Allergy 65:50–53, 1991.
44. Chung KF: Long-term inhaled corticosteroid therapy in chronic airways obstruction. Eur Respir J 5:913–914, 1992.
45. Coffey MJ, Sanders G, Eschenbacher WL, et al: The role of methotrexate in the management of steroid-dependent asthma. Chest 105:117–121, 1994.
46. Cohen RD, Conn DL, Ilstrup DM: Clinical features, prognosis, and response to treatment in polyarteritis. Mayo Clin Proc 55:146–155, 1980.
47. Collins FV, Clark TJH, Brown D, Townsend J: The use of corticosteroids in the treatment of acute asthma. Q J Med 174:259–273, 1975.
48. Connett GJ, Lenney W, McConchie SM: The cost effectiveness of budesonide in severe asthmatics aged one to three years. Br J Med Econ 6:127–134, 1993.
49. Cook LJ, Freinkel RK, Zugerman C, et al: Iatrogenic hyperadrenocorticism during topical steroid therapy: assessment of systemic effects by metabolic criteria. J Am Acad Dermatol 6 (6):1054–1060, 1982.
50. Coopman S, Degreef H, Dooms-Goossens A: Identification of cross-reaction patterns in allergic contact dermatitis from topical corticosteroids. Br J Dermatol 121:27–34, 1989.
51. Cott GR: Current studies of alternative anti-inflammatory therapy in asthma: critical re-appraisal. Semin Respir Crit Care Med 15:136–146, 1994.
52. Crompton GK: Corticosteroids and bone mass in asthma. Br Med J 294:123, 1987.
53. Cypcar D, Busse WW: Steroid-resistant asthma. J Allergy Clin Immunol 92:362–372, 1993.
54. Dahl R, Lundback B, Malo J-L, et al: A dose-ranging study of fluticasone propionate in adult patients with moderate asthma. Chest 104:1352–1358, 1993.
55. Davies AO, Lefkowitz RJ: Regulation of B-adrenergic receptors by steroid hormones. Annu Rev Physiol 46:119–130, 1984.
56. Degreef H, Dooms-Goossens A: The new corticosteroids: are they effective and safe? Dermatol Ther 11:155–160, 1993.
57. Djukanovic R, Wilson JW, Britten KM, et al: Effect of an inhaled corticosteroid on airway inflammation and symptoms in asthma. Am Rev Respir Dis 145:669–674, 1992.
58. Dompeling E, van Schayck CP, Van Grunsven PM, et al: Slowing the deterioration of asthma and chronic obstructive pulmonary disease observed during bronchodilator therapy by adding inhaled corticosteroids. Ann Intern Med 118:770–778, 1993.
59. Doull IJM, Freezer NJ, Holgate ST: Growth of asthmatic children on inhaled corticosteroids. Am Rev Respir Dis 147:A265, 1993.
60. Dreyer EB: Inhaled steroid use and glaucoma. N Engl J Med 329:1822, 1993.
61. Dyer PD, Vaughan TR, Weber RW: Methotrexate in the treatment of steroid-dependent asthma. J Allergy Clin Immunol 88:208–212, 1991.
62. Ellul-Micallef R, Borthwick RC, Hardy GJR: The effect of oral prednisolone on gas exchange in chronic bronchial asthma. Br J Clin Pharmacol 9:479–482, 1980.
63. Ernst P, Spitzer WO, Suissa S, et al: Risk of fatal and near-fatal asthma in relation to inhaled corticosteroid use. JAMA 268:3462–3464, 1992.
64. Erzurum SC, Leff JA, Cochran JE, et al: Lack of benefit of methotrexate in severe, steroid-dependent asthma. Ann Intern Med 114:353–360, 1991.
65. Fabbri L, Burge PS, Croonenborgh L, et al: Comparison of fluticasone propionate with beclomethasone dipropionate in moderate to severe asthma treated for one year. Thorax 48:817–823, 1993.
66. Fanta CH, Rossing TH, McFadden ER Jr: Glucocorticoids in acute asthma: a critical controlled trial. Am J Med 74:845–851, 1983.
67. Fauci AS, Dale DC, Balow JE: Glucocorticoid therapy: mechanisms of action and clinical considerations. Ann Intern Med 84:304–315, 1976.
68. Fauci AS, Haynes BF, Katz P: The spectrum of vasculitis. Ann Intern Med 89 (1) :660–676, 1978.
69. Fauci AS, Katz P, Haynes BF, Wolff SM: Cyclophosphamide therapy of severe systemic necrotizing vasculitis. N Engl J Med 301:235–238, 1979.
70. Fauci AS, Haynes BF, Katz P, Wolff SM: Wegener's granulomatosis: prospective clinical and therapeutic experience with 85 patients for 21 years. Ann Intern Med 98:76–85, 1983.
71. Fitzsimons R, Greenberger PA, Patterson R: Outcome of pregnancy in women requiring corticosteroids for severe asthma. J Allergy Clin Immunol 78:349–353, 1986.
72. Fraunfelder FT, Meyer SM: Posterior subcapsular cataracts associated with nasal or inhalation corticosteroids. Am J Ophthalmol 109:489–490, 1990.
73. Glynn-Barnhart AM, Erzurum SC, Leff JA, et al: Effect of low-dose methotrexate on the disposition of glucocorticoids and theophylline. J Allergy Clin Immunol 88:180–186, 1991.
74. Greenberger PA, Patterson R: Beclomethasone dipropionate for severe asthma during pregnancy. Ann Intern Med 98:478–480, 1983.
75. Greenberger PA, Patterson R, Radin RC: Two pretreatment regimens for high-risk patients receiving radiographic contrast media. J Allergy Clin Immunol 74:540–543, 1984.
76. Greenberger PA, Patterson R, Tapio CM: Prophylaxis against repeated radiocontrast media reactions in 857 cases. Arch Intern Med 145:2197–2200, 1985.
77. Greenberger PA: Idiopathic anaphylaxis. Immunol Allergy Clin North Am 23:571–583, 1992.
78. Greening AP, Ind PW, Northfield M, Shaw G: Added salmeterol versus higher-dose corticosteroid in asthma patients with symptoms on existing inhaled corticosteroid. Lancet 344:219–224, 1994.
79. Griffin D, Coursin D, Grossman JE: Acute myopathy during treatment of status asthmaticus with corticosteroids and steroidal muscle relaxants. Chest 102:510–514, 1992.
80. Gronneberg R, Strandberg K, Stalenheim G, Zetterstrom O: Effect in man of anti-allergic drugs on the immediate and late phase cutaneous allergic reactions induced by anti-IgE. Allergy 36:201–208, 1981.
81. Guillevin L, Lhote F, Leon A, et al: Treatment of polyarteritis nodosa related to hepatitis B virus with short term steroid therapy associated with antiviral agents and plasma exchanges. A prospective trial in 33 patients. J Rheumatol 20:289–298, 1993.
82. Haahtela T, Järvinen M, Kava T, et al: Comparison of a beta$_2$-agonist, terbutaline with an inhaled corticosteroid, budesonide, in newly detected asthma. N Engl J Med 325:388–392, 1991.
83. Haahtela T, Jarvinen M, Kava T, et al: Effects of reducing or discontinuing inhaled budesonide in patients with mild asthma. N Engl J Med 331:700–705, 1994.
84. Hargreave FE, Dolovich J, Newhouse MT (eds): The assessment and treatment of asthma: a conference report. J Allergy Clin Immunol 85 (6) :1098–1111, 1990.
85. Hartwig S, Linden M, Laurent C, et al: Budesonide nasal spray as prophylactic treatment after polypectomy. J Laryngol Otol 102:148–151, 1988.
86. Haskell RJ, Wong BM, Hansen JE: A double-blind, randomized clinical trial of methylprednisolone in status asthmaticus. Arch Intern Med 143:1324–1327, 1983.
87. Haynes BF, Allen NB, Fauci AS: Diagnostic and therapeutic approach to the patient with vasculitis. Med Clin North Am 70 (2):355–368, 1986.

88. Hill MR, Szefler SJ, Bartoszek M, Brenner Am: Monitoring glucocorticoid therapy: a pharmacokinetic approach. Clin Pharmacol Ther 48:390–398, 1990.
89. Hodsman AB, Toogood JH, Jennings B, et al: Differential effects of inhaled budesonide and oral prednisolone on serum osteocalcin. J Clin Endocrinol Metab 72 (3) :530–540, 1991.
90. Hoffman GS, Kerr GS, Leavitt RY, et al: Wegener granulomatosis: an analysis of 158 patients. Ann Intern Med 116:488–498, 1992.
91. Holgate ST: Clinical evaluation of nedocromil sodium in asthma. Br J Clin Pract 41 (1) :13–19, 1987.
92. Hollman GA, Allen DB: Overt glucocorticoid excess due to inhaled corticosteroid therapy. Pediatrics 81:452–455, 1988.
93. Holopainen E, Malmberg H, Binder E: Long-term follow-up of intranasal beclomethasone treatment. A clinical and histologic study. Acta Otolaryngol (Stockh) 386:270–273, 1982.
94. Hunder GG, Shops SG, Allen GL, Joyce JW: Daily and alternate-day corticosteroid regimens in treatment of giant cell arteritis. Ann Intern Med 82:613–618, 1975.
95. Incaudo G, Schatz M, Yamamoto F, et al: Intranasal flunisolide in the treatment of perennial rhinitis: correlation with immunologic parameters. J Allergy Clin Immunol 65:41–49, 1980.
96. Ip M, Lam K, Kung A, Ng M: Decreased bone mineral density in premenopausal asthma patients receiving long-term inhaled steroids. Chest 105:1722–1727, 1994.
97. Ishikawa K: Natural history and classification of occlusive thromboaortopathy (Takayasu's disease). Circulation 57 (1) :27–35, 1978.
98. Jeffery PK, Godfrey RW, Adelroth E, et al: Effects of treatment on airway inflammation and thickening of basement membrane reticular collagen in asthma. Am Rev Respir Dis 145:890–899, 1992.
99. Jennings BH: A comparison of budesonide and beclomethasone dipropionate in healthy volunteers. In: The Assessment of Systemic Effects of Inhaled Glucocorticoids. Department of Clinical Pharmacology, University of Lund, Sweden, 1990, Thesis. VII:1 –14.
100. Jones G, Mierins E, Karsh J: Methotrexate-induced asthma. Am Rev Resp Dis 143:179–181, 1991.
101. Juniper EF, Kline PA, Vanzieleghem MA, et al: Effect of long-term treatment with an inhaled corticosteroid (budesonide) on airway hyperresponsiveness and clinical asthma in nonsteroid-dependent asthmatics. Am Rev Respir Dis 142:832–836, 1990.
102. Kallenbach JM, Frankel AH, Lapinsky SE, et al: Determinants of near fatality in acute severe asthma. Am J Med 95:265–272, 1993.
103. Kamm RD, Drazen JM: Airway hyperresponsiveness and airway wall thickening in asthma. A quantitative approach. Am Rev Respir Dis 145:1246–1250, 1992.
104. Karim AKA, Thompson GM, Jacob TJC: Steroid aerosols and cataract formation. BMJ 299:918, 1989.
105. Kasper WJ, Howe PM: Fatal varicella after a single course of corticosteroids. Pediatr Infect Dis J 9:729–732, 1990.
106. Keighley JF: Iatrogenic asthma associated with adrenergic aerosols. Ann Intern Med 65:989–995, 1966.
107. Kelsen SG, Kelsen DP, Fleegler BF, et al: Emergency room assessment and treatment of patients with acute asthma. Am J Med 64:622–627, 1978.
108. Kewley GD: Possible association between beclomethasone dipropionate aerosol and cataracts. Aust Paed J 16:117–118, 1980.
109. Kiviranta K, Turpeinen M: Effect of eight months of inhaled beclomethasone dipropionate and budesonide on carbohydrate metabolism in adults with asthma. Thorax 48:974–978, 1993.
110. Konig P, Hillman L, Cervantes C, et al: Bone metabolism in children with asthma treated with inhaled beclomethasone dipropionate. J Pediatr 122:219–226, 1993.
111. Kyle V, Hazleman BL: Treatment of polymyalgia rheumatica and giant cell arteritis. I. Steroid regimens in the first two months. Ann Rheum Dis 48:658–661, 1989.
112. Kyle V, Hazleman BL: Treatment of polymyalgia rheumatica and giant cell arteritis. II. Relation between steroid dose and steroid associated side effects. Ann Rheum Dis 48:662–666, 1989.
113. Laitinen LA, Laitinen A, Haahtela T: A comparative study of the effects of an inhaled corticosteroid, budesonide, and a beta$_2$-agonist, terbutaline, on airway inflammation in newly diagnosed asthma: a randomized, double-blind, parallel-group controlled trial. J Allergy Clin Immunol 90:32–42, 1992.
114. Le Bourgeois M, Benoist MR, de Blic J, et al: One year treatment with two doses of inhaled flunisolide (250 and 500 mcg bid): effects on growth of asthmatic children. Am Rev Respir Dis 147:A265, 1993.
115. Levison H: Canadian consensus on the treatment of asthma in children. Can Med Assoc J 145 (11) :1449–1455, 1991.
116. Lieberman P, Siegle RL, Treadwell G: Radiocontrast reactions. Clin Rev Allergy 4:229–245, 1986.
117. Likeholdt T, Kortholm B: Beclomethasone nasal spray in the treatment of middle ear effusion—a double-blind study. Int J Pediatr Otorhinolaryngol 4:133, 1982.
118. Littlewood JM, Johnson AW, Edwards PA, Littlewood AE: Growth retardation in asthmatic children treated with inhaled beclomethasone dipropionate. Lancet 1:115–116, 1988.
119. Luksza AR: A new look at adult asthma. Br J Dis Chest 76:11–15, 1982.
120. Lundgren R: Scanning electron microscopic studies of bronchial mucosa before and during treatment with beclomethasone dipropionate inhalation. Scand J Respir Dis 101:179–187, 1977.
121. Lundgren R, Soderberg M, Horstedt P, Stenling R: Morphological studies of bronchia mucosal biopsies from asthmatics before and after ten years of treatment with inhaled steroids. Eur Respir J 1:883–889, 1988.
122. Mabry RI: Intraturbinal steroid injection: indications, results and complications. South Med J 71:78, 1978.
123. Macdonald JB, Seaton A, Williams DA: Asthma deaths in Cardiff 1963–74: 90 deaths outside hospital. Br Med J 1:1493–1495, 1976.
124. Madowitz JS, Schweiger MJ: Severe anaphylactoid reaction to radiographic contrast media. JAMA 241:2813–2815, 1979.
125. Malo J-L, Cartier A, Merland N, et al: Four-times-a-day dosing frequency is better than a twice-a-day regimen in subjects requiring a high-dose inhaled steroid, budesonide, to control moderate to severe asthma. Am Rev Respir Dis 140:624–628, 1989.
126. Markov AE, Toogood JH: Search for adverse effects of inhaled beta adrenergics (IBA) on therapeutic outcome of chronic asthma. J Allergy Clin Immunol 89:177, 1992.
127. Marshall C, Lieberman P: Analysis of 3 pretreatment procedures to prevent anaphylactoid reactions to radiocontrast in previous reactors. J Allergy Clin Immunol 83:254, 1989.
128. Mazer BD, Gelfand EW: An open-label study of high-dose intravenous immunoglobulin in severe childhood asthma. J Allergy Clin Immunol 87:976–983, 1991.
129. McAllen MK, Portillo PR, Parr EJ, et al: Intranasal flunisolide, placebo and beclomethasone dipropionate in perennial rhinitis. Br J Dis Chest 74:32–36, 1980.
130. McAllister WAC, Winfield CR, Collins JV: Pharmacokinetics of prednisolone in normal and asthmatic subjects in relation to dose. Eur J Clin Pharmacol 20:141–145, 1981.
131. McFadden ER Jr, Kiser R, deGroot WJ, et al: A controlled study of the effects of single doses of hydrocortisone on the resolution of acute attacks of asthma. Am J Med 60:52–59, 1976.
132. McRae D, Buchanan G: Long-term sulfamethoxazole-trimethoprim in Wegener's granulomatosis. Arch Otolaryngol Head Neck Surg 119:103–105, 1993.
133. Molema J, van Herwaarden CLA, Folgering H Th M: Effects of long-term treatment with inhaled cromoglycate and budesonide on bronchial hyperresponsiveness in patients with allergic asthma. Eur Respir J 2:308–316, 1989.
134. Monson JP: Systemic effects of inhaled corticosteroids. Thorax 48: 955–956, 1993.
135. Mullarkey MF: Eosinophilic nonallergic rhinitis. J Allergy Clin Immunol 82:941–949, 1988.
136. Mullarkey MF, Blumenstein BA, Anddrade WP, et al: Methotrexate in the treatment of corticosteroid-dependent asthma. N Engl J Med 603–607, 1988.
137. Muller M, Renkawitz R: The glucocortiocid receptor. Biochim Biophys Acta 1088:171–182, 1991.
138. Murray AB, Ferguson AC: Dust-free bedrooms in the treatment of asthmatic children with house dust or house dust mite allergy: a controlled trial. Pediatrics 71:418–422, 1983.
139. Mygind N, Sorensen H, Pedersen CB: The nasal mucosa during long-term treatment with beclomethasone dipropionate aerosol. Acta Otolaryngol (Stockh) 85:437–443, 1978.
140. Myles AB, Perera T, Ridley MG: Prevention of blindness in giant cell arteritis by corticosteroid treatment. Br J Rheumatol 31:103–105, 1992.
141. Nierop G, Gijzel WP, Bel EH, et al: Auranofin in the treatment of steroid-dependent asthma: a double blind study. Thorax 47:349–354, 1992.
142. Nugent CA, Ward J, MacDiarmid WD, et al: Glucocorticoid toxicity: single contrasted with divided daily doses of prednisolone. J Chron Dis 18:323–332, 1965.

143. O'Byrne PM, Cook D: Is nedocromil sodium effective treatment for asthma? Eur Respir J 6:5–6, 1993.
144. O'Driscoll BR, Kalra S, Wilson M, et al: Double-blind trial of steroid tapering in acute asthma. Lancet 341:324–327, 1993.
145. Ortonne JP: Clinical potential of topical corticosteroids. Drugs 36(suppl 5):38–42, 1988.
146. Packe GE, Douglas JG, McDonald AF, et al: Bone density in asthmatic patients taking high dose inhaled beclomethasone dipropionate and intermittent systemic corticosteroids. Thorax 47:415–417, 1992.
147. Patterson R, Wong S, Dykewicz MS, Harris KE: Malignant idiopathic anaphylaxis. J Allergy Clin Immunol 85:86–88, 1990.
148. Patterson R, DeSwarte RD, Greenberger PA, Grammer LC: Drug allergy and protocols for management of drug allergies NER. Allergy Proc 7:325–342, 1986.
149. Peppel K, Vinci JM, Baglioni C: The AU-rich sequences in the 3′-untranslated region mediate the increased turnover of interferon mRNA induced by glucocorticoids. J Exp Med 173:349–355, 1991.
150. Pierson WE, Bierman CW, Kelley VC. A double-blind trial of corticosteroid therapy in status asthmaticus. Pediatrics 54:283–287, 1974.
151. Pipkorn U, Pukander J, Suonpaa J, et al: Long term safety of budesonide nasal aerosol: a 5.5-year follow-up study. Clin Allergy 18:253–259, 1988.
152. Platts-Mills TAE, Tovey ER, Mitchell EB, et al: Reduction of bronchial hyperreactivity during prolonged allergen avoidance. Lancet 2:675–677, 1982.
153. Poothullil J, Umemoto L, Dolovich J, et al: Inhibition by prednisone of late cutaneous allergic responses induced by antiserum to human IgE. J Allergy Clin Immunol 57:164–167, 1976.
154. Popa VT, Lerner SA: Biphasic system anaphylactic reaction: three illustrative cases. Ann Allergy 53:151–155, 1984.
155. Ray A, Laforge KS, Sehgal PB: On the mechanisms of efficient repression of the interleukin-6 promotor by glucocorticoids: enhancer TATA box and RNA start site occlusion. Mol Cell Biol 10:5736–5746, 1990.
156. Redfearn A, O'Connor M, Holland FJ, et al: Correlates of reduced linear growth in asthmatics treated with inhaled corticosteroids. J Allergy Clin Immunol 91:168, 1993.
157. Renato S, Canny GJ, Bohn D, et al: Severe acute asthma in a pediatric intensive care unit: six years' experience. Pediatrics 83:1023–1028, 1989.
158. Reid DM, Nicoll JJ, Smith MA, et al: Corticosteroids and bone mass in asthma: comparisons with rheumatoid arthritis and polymyalgia rheumatica. Br Med J 293:1463–1466, 1986.
159. Ribeiro LB: Budesonide: safety and efficacy aspects of its long-term use in children. Pediatr Allergy Immunol 4:73–78, 1993.
160. Rooklin AR, Lampert SI, Jaeger EA, et al: Posterior subcapsular cataracts in steroid-requiring asthmatic children. J Allergy Clin Immunol 63(6):383–386, 1979.
161. Rosewicz S, McDonald AR, Maddux BA, et al: Mechanism of glucocorticoid receptor down-regulation by glucocorticoids. J Biol Chem 263:2581–2584, 1988.
162. Ruegsegger P, Medici T, Anliker M: Corticosteroid-induced bone loss: a longitudinal study of alternate-day therapy in patients with bronchial asthma using quantitative computed tomography. Eur J Clin Pharmacol 25:615–620, 1983.
163. Ruffin JRE, Rubinfeld AR, Alpers JH, et al: The efficacy of nedocromil sodium (Tilade) in asthma. Aust NZ J Med 17:557–561, 1987.
164. Rutten-van Molken MPMH, Van Doorslaer EKA, Jansen MCC, et al: Cost effectiveness of inhaled corticosteroid plus bronchodilator monotherapy in children with asthma. Pharmacoeconomics 4:257–270, 1993.
165. Sack M, Cassidy JT, Bole GG: Prognostic factors in polyarteritis. Rheumatol 2(4):411–420, 1975.
166. Salmeron S, Guerin J-C, Godard P, et al: High doses of inhaled corticosteroids in unstable chronic asthma: a multicenter, double-blind, placebo-controlled study. Am Rev Respir Dis 140:167–171, 1989.
167. Scarfone RJ, Fuchs SM, Nager AL, Shane SA: Controlled trial of oral prednisone in the emergency department treatment of children with acute asthma. Pediatrics 92:513–518, 1993.
168. Schleimer RP, Davidson DA, Lichtenstein LM, Adkinson NF: Selective inhibition of arachidonic acid metabolite release from human lung tissue by antiinflammatory steroids. J Immunol 136:3006–3011, 1986.
169. Schoelzel EP, Menzel ML: Nasal sprays and perforation of the nasal septum. JAMA 253:2046, 1985.
170. Schwartz YA, Kivity S, Ilfeld DN, et al: A clinical and immunological study of colchicine in asthma. J Allergy Clin Immunol 85:578–582, 1990.
171. Sears MR, Lake DC, Yates DM, et al: Regular inhaled beta-agonist treatment in bronchial asthma. Lancet 336:1391–1396, 1990.
172. Shelhamer JH, Volkman DJ, Parrillo JE, et al: Takayasu's arteritis and its therapy. Ann Intern Med 103:121–126, 1985.
173. Shimura S, Sasaki T, Ikeda K, et al: Direct inhibitory action of glucocorticoid on glycoconjugate secretion from airway submucosal glands. Am Rev Respir Dis 141:1044–1049, 1990.
174. Shiner RJ, Nunn AJ, Chung KF, Geddes DM: Randomised, double-blind, placebo-controlled trial of methotrexate in steroid-dependent asthma. Lancet 336:137–140, 1990.
175. Shiner RJ, Katz I, Shulimzon T, et al: Methotrexate in steroid-dependent asthma: long-term results. Allergy 49:565–568, 1994.
176. Sibbald B, Hilton S, D'Souza M: An open cross-over trial comparing two doses of astemizole and beclomethasone dipropionate in the treatment of perennial rhinitis. Clin Allergy 16:203–211, 1986.
177. Siegel SC: Topical intranasal corticosteroid therapy in rhinitis. J Allergy Clin Immunol 81:984–991, 1988.
178. Silk HJ, Perez-Atayde AR: Fatal varicella in steroid-dependent asthma. J Allergy Clin Immunol 81:47–51, 1988.
179. Simons FER, Persaud MP, Gillespie CA, et al: Absence of posterior subcapsular cataracts in young patients treatment with inhaled glucocorticoid. Lancet 342:776–778, 1993.
180. Soderberg-Warner ML: Nasal septal perforation associated with topical corticosteroid therapy. J Pediatr 105:840–841, 1984.
181. Sorkness CA, Bush RK: Alternatives to corticosteroids in the treatment of asthma. Immunol Allergy Clin NA 13:917–938, 1993.
182. Speizer FE, Doll R, Heaf P, Strang LB: Investigation into use of drugs preceding death from asthma. Br Med J 1:339–343, 1968.
183. Spitzer W, Lawrence V, Dales R, et al: Links between passive smoking and disease: a best-evidence synthesis. Clin Invest Med 13:17–42, 1990.
184. Stark BJ, Sullivan TJ: Biphasic and protracted anaphylaxis. J Allergy Clin Immunol 78:76–83, 1986.
185. Statement by the British Thoracic Society: Guidelines for management of asthma in adults: I— chronic persistent asthma. Research Unit of the Royal College of Physicians of London, King's Fund Centre, National Asthma Campaign. Br Med J 301:651–653, 1990.
186. Stead RJ, Horsman A, Cooke NJ, Belchetz P: Bone mineral density in women taking inhaled corticosteroids. Thorax 45:792, 1990.
187. Stein LM, Cole RP: Early administration of corticosteroids in emergency room treatment of acute asthma. Ann Intern Med 112:823–827, 1990.
188. Stewart GE, Diaz JD, Lockey RF, et al: Comparison of oral pulse methotrexate with placebo in the treatment of severe glucocorticosteroid-dependent asthma. J Allergy Clin Immunol 94:482–489, 1994.
189. Storms W, Bronsky E, Findlay S, et al: Once daily triamcinolone acetonide nasal spray is effective for the treatment of perennial allergic rhinitis. Ann Allergy 66:329–334, 1991.
190. Storr JNP: Growth of asthmatic children. Br Med J 303:719, 1991.
191. Strömstedt P-E, Poellinger L, Gustafsson J-Å, Carlstedt-Duke J: The glucocorticoid reeptor binds to a sequence overlapping the TATA box of the human osteocalcin promotor: a potential mechanism for negative regulation. Mol Cell Biol 11:3379–3383, 1991.
192. Sudilovsky A, Muir JG, Bocobo FC: Topical corticosteroids. The need (?) for frequent applications. Int J Dermatol 20:594–596, 1981.
193. Suissa S, Ernst P: Boivin J-F, Horwitz RI, Habbick B, et al: A cohort analysis of excess mortality in asthma and the use of inhaled β-agonists. Am J Respir Crit Care Med 149:604–610, 1994.
194. Svedmyr N: Action of corticosteroids on beta-adrenergic receptors: clinical aspects. Am Rev Respir Dis 141:S31–S38, 1990.
195. Szczeklik A, Nizankowska E, Dworski R, et al: Cyclosporine for steroid-dependent chronic severe asthma. Lancet 339:324–328, 1992.
196. Szefler SJ, Kamada AK, Hughes D, et al: Alternative treatments for asthma: assessing the need. J Asthma 29:91–97, 1992.
197. Takeda K, Arase S, Takahashi S: Side effects of topical corticosteroids and their prevention. Drugs 36 (suppl 5):15–23, 1988.
198. Tal A, Levy N, Bearman JE: Methylprednisolone therapy for acute asthma in infants and toddlers: a controlled clinical trial. Pediatrics 86:350–356, 1990.
199. Taylor DR, Flannery EM, Herbison GP: Methotrexate in the management of severe steroid-dependent asthma. NZ Med J 106:409–411, 1993.
200. Thiringer G, Eriksson N, Malmberg R, et al: Bronchoscopic biopsies

of bronchial mucosa before and after beclomethasone dipropionate therapy. Scand J Respir Dis Suppl 101:173–177, 1977.
201. Thomas BC, Stanhope R, Grant DB: Impaired growth in children with asthma during treatment with conventional doses of inhaled corticosteroids. Acta Paediatr 83:196–199, 1994.
202. Tinkelman DG, Reed CE, Nelson HS, et al: Aerosol beclomethasone dipropionate compared with theophylline as primary treatment of chronic, mild to moderate severe asthma in children. Pediatrics 92:64–77, 1993.
203. Tobler A, Meier R, Seitz M, et al: Glucocorticoids down-regulate gene expression of GM-CSF, NAP-1/IL-8 and IL-6, but not M-CSF in human fibroblasts. Blood 79:45–51, 1992.
204. Toogood JH, Frankish CW, Jennings BH, et al: A study of the mechanism of the antiasthmatic action of inhaled budesonide. J Allergy Clin Immunol 85:872–880, 1990.
205. Toogood JH, Baskerville J, Jennings B, et al: Bioequivalent doses of budesonide and prednisone in moderate and severe asthma. J Allergy Clin Immunol 84:688–700, 1989.
206. Toogood JH, Jennings B, Lefcoe NM: A clinical trial of combined cromolyn/beclomethasone treatment for chronic asthma. J Allergy Clin Immunol 67:317–324, 1981.
207. Toogood JH, Josephson D, Dervish G, Toogood PB: Safety of long term budesonide (BUD) therapy. Clin Invest Med 12(4):B5, 1989.
208. Toogood JH: Complications of topical steroid therapy for asthma. Am Rev Respir Dis 141(2):S89–S96, 1990.
209. Toogood JH, Jennings B, Greenway RW, Chuang L: Candidiasis and dysphonia complicating beclomethasone treatment of asthma. J Allergy Clin Immunol 65(2):145–153, 1980.
210. Toogood JH, Jennings B, Baskerville J, et al: Dosing regimen of budesonide and occurrence of oropharyngeal complications. Eur J Respir Dis 65:35–44, 1984.
211. Toogood JH, Markov AE, Baskerville J, Dyson C: Association of ocular cataracts with inhaled and oral steroid therapy during long-term treatment of asthma. J Allergy Clin Immunol 91:571–579, 1993.
212. Toogood JH, Baskerville JC, Markov AE, et al: Bone mineral density and the risk of fracture in patients receiving long-term inhaled steroid therapy for asthma. J Allergy Clin Immunol 96:157–166, 1995.
213. Toogood JH, Baskerville J, Errington N, et al: Determinants of the response to beclomethasone aerosol at various dosage levels: a multiple regression analysis to identify clinically useful predictors. J Allergy Clin Immunol 60:367–376, 1977
214. Toogood JH: Concentrated aerosol formulations in asthma. Lancet 2:790–791, 1983.
215. Toogood JH, Jennings B, Hodsman AB, et al: Effects of dose and dosing schedule of inhaled budesonide on bone turnover. J Allergy Clin Immunol 88:572–580, 1991.
216. Toogood JH, Crilly RG, Jones G, et al: Effect of high dose inhaled budesonide on calcium and phosphate metabolism and the risk of osteoporosis. Am Rev Respir Dis 138:57–61, 1988.
217. Toogood JH, Lefcoe NM, Haines DSM, et al: A graded dose assessment of the efficacy of beclomethasone dipropionate aerosol for severe chronic asthma. J Allergy Clin Immunol 59:298–308, 1977.
218. Toogood JH, Jennings B, Baskerville J, Lefcoe NM: Aerosol corticosteroids. In Weiss EB, Stein M (eds): Bronchial Asthma Mechanisms and Therapeutics, 3rd edition. Little, Brown and Company, Boston, MA, 1993, pp 818–841.
219. Toogood JH, Lefcoe NM, Haines DSM, et al: Minimum dose requirements of steroid-dependent asthmatic patients for aerosol beclomethasone and oral prednisone. J Allergy Clin Immunol 61:355–364, 1978.
220. Toogood JH, Baskerville J, Jennings B, et al: Use of spacers to facilitate inhaled corticosteroid treatment of asthma. Am Rev Respir Dis 129:723–729, 1984.
221. Toogood JH: Role of inhaled steroids in the management of chronic rhinitis. Contemporary Allergies 1:4–19, 1991.
222. Toogood JH: Bronchial asthma and glucocorticoids. In Schleimer RP, Claman HN, Oronsky A (eds): Antiinflammatory Steroid Action: Basic and Clinical Aspects. Academic Press Inc, San Diego, CA 1989, pp 423–468.
223. Trigg CJ, Manolitsas ND, Wang J, et al: Placebo-controlled immunopathologic study of four months of inhaled corticosteroids in asthma. Am J Respir Crit Care Med 150:17–22, 1994
224. Trigg CJ, Davies RJ: Comparison of methotrexate 30 mg per week with placebo in chronic steroid-dependent asthma: a 12-week double-blind, cross over study. Resp Med 87:211–216, 1993.
225. Turner ES, Greenberger PA, Patterson R: Management of the pregnant asthmatic patient. Ann Intern Med 93:905, 1980.
226. US Department of Health and Human Services: Guidelines for the Diagnosis and Management of Asthma. National Asthma Education Program. Expert Panel Report. Publication #91-3042 and 91-3042A, 1–135, 1991
227. US Department of Health and Human Services: International Consensus Report on Diagnosis and Management of Asthma. Publication #92-3091, 1992, pp 1–71.
228. Corticosteroids, Inhalation Local monograph. In Drug Information for the Health Care Professional, 15th edition. The US Pharmacopeial Convention, Inc, 1:840–846, 1995.
229. Valeriano-Marcet J, Spiera H: Treatment of Wegener's granulomatosis with sulphamethoxazole-trimethoprim. Arch Intern Med 151:1649–1652, 1991.
230. van Essen-Zandvliet EE, Hughes MD, Waalkens HJ, et al: Remission of childhood asthma after long-term treatment with an inhaled corticosteroid (budesonide): can it be achieved? Eur Respir J 7:63–68, 1994.
231. Vathenen AS, et al: Time course of change in bronchial reactivity with an inhaled corticosteroid in asthma. Am Rev Respir Dis 143:1317–1321, 1991.
232. Waalkens HJ, Gerritsen J, Koëter GH, et al: Budesonide and terbutaline or terbutaline alone in hyperresponsiveness and diurnal variation in peak flow. Thorax 46:499–503, 1991.
233. Waalkens HJ, Van Essen-Zandvliet EE, Hughes MD, et al: Cessation of long-term treatment with inhaled corticosteroid (budesonide) in children with asthma results in deterioration. Am Rev Respir Dis 148:1252–1257, 1993.
234. Wales JKH, Barnes ND, Swift PGF: Growth retardation in children on steroids for asthma. Lancet 338:1535, 1991.
235. Walshaw MJ, Evans CC: Allergen avoidance in house dust mite sensitive adult asthma. QJ Med 58:199, 1986.
236. Welsch PW, Stricker WE, Chu C-P, et al: Efficacy of beclomethasone nasal solution, flunisolide, and cromolyn in relieving symptoms of ragweed allergy. Mayo Clin Proc 62:125–134, 1987.
237. Whyte MKB, Choudry NB, Ind PW: Bronchial hyperresponsiveness in patients recovering from acute severe asthma. Respir Med 87:29–35, 1993.
238. Wiggins CA, Dykewicz MS, Patterson R: Corticosteroid-dependent idiopathic anaphylaxis: a report of five cases. J Allergy Clin Immunol 84:311–315, 1989.
239. Wilson JD, Sutherland DC, Thomas AC: Has the change to beta-agonists combined with oral theophylline increased cases of fatal asthma? Lancet 1:1235–1237, 1981.
240. Wolff AH, Adelsberg B, Aloia J, Zitt M: Effect of inhaled corticosteroid on bone density in asthmatic patients: a pilot study. Ann Allergy 67:117–121, 1991.
241. Wolthers OD, Pedersen S: Controlled study of linear growth in asthmatic children during treatment with inhaled glucocorticosteroids. Pediatrics 89:839–842, 1992.
242. Wolthers OD, Pederson S: Growth of asthmatic children during treatment with budesonide: a double blind trial. Br Med J 303:163–165, 1991.
243. Wong CS, Cooper S, Britton Jr, Tattersfield AE: Steroid sparing effect of nedocromil sodium in asthmatic patients on high doses of inhaled steroids. Clin Exp Allergy 23:370–376, 1993.
244. Wong J, Black P: Acute adrenal insufficiency associated with high dose inhaled steroids. Br Med J 304:1415, 1992.
245. Wong Sansan, Yarnold PR, Yango C, et al: Outcome of prophylactic therapy for idiopathic anaphylaxis. Ann Intern Med 114:133–136, 1991.
246. Wong S, Dykewicz MS, Patterson R: Idiopathic anaphylaxis: a clinical summary of 175 patients. Arch Intern Med 150:1323–1328, 1990.
247. Wood SF: Oral antihistamine or nasal steroid in hay fever: a double-blind double-dummy comparative study of once daily oral astemizole vs twice daily nasal beclomethasone dipropionate. Clin Allergy 16:195–201, 1985.
248. Woolcock AJ, Yan K, Salome CM: Effect of therapy on bronchial hyperresponsiveness in the long-term management of asthma. Clin Allergy 18:165–176, 1988.
249. Zwaan CM, Odlnk RJH, van De Waal HAD, et al: Acute adrenal insufficiency after discontinuation of inhaled corticosteroid therapy. Lancet 340:1289–1290, 1992.
250. Zwillich CW, Pickett C, Hanson FN, Weil JV: Disturbed sleep and prolonged apnea during nasal obstruction in normal men. Am Rev Respir Dis 124:158–160, 1981.

45 Immunotherapy

PETER S. CRETICOS

When exposed to a relevant aeroallergen, the patient with allergic rhinitis typically experiences itchy watery eyes, sneezing, rhinorrhea, nasal congestion, and postnasal drip and cough. The allergic asthmatic may present with cough, chest tightness, shortness of breath, and wheezing.

Immunotherapy involves administering to the patient increasing doses of an extract, consisting of the respective allergens to which that patient has been demonstrated to be allergic, in an attempt to significantly attenuate or eliminate this symptomatology through modulation of the patient's immune response.

PATHOPHYSIOLOGY OF THE ALLERGIC REACTION

The pathogenesis of an allergic reaction involves a combination of humoral and cellular events evoked by allergen exposure. The acute allergic response (e.g., exposure to a cat) results in IgE-dependent mast cell activation, inducing cellular activation, arachidonic acid metabolism, and mediator release.[29, 32, 69] Before development of this antigen-antibody interaction, allergen is processed by antigen-presenting cells (e.g., dendritic cells, macrophages, Langerhans cells), and specific peptide sequences (termed epitopes) are presented to a T lymphocyte.[50, 51] If this presentation meets appropriate receptors in the presence of costimulatory signals, then clones of $CD4^+$ ($Th2^+$ type) T cells are induced to express cytokines (interleukin (IL)-3, IL-4, IL-5) that can have direct effects on inflammatory cells (e.g., mast cells, basophils, eosinophils) and antibody-producing B cells to influence further cell-to-cell interactions, antibody (IgE) production, and inflammatory responses.[21, 56]

On the one hand, acute exposure to an intense allergic trigger (e.g., petting a cat) triggers immediate symptoms in the allergic patient. Perhaps of more relevance to the underlying allergic diathesis is the recognition that in many patients, because of persistent exposure (e.g., a cat in the home), this develops into a smoldering process that reflects not only an immediate phase of reactivity but also the development of a late phase of clinical symptomatology as a result of cellular recruitment, mediator release, and inflammation.[47] This inflammation often leads to the development of nonspecific airway reactivity whereby not only the relevant allergens but also nonspecific irritants (e.g., pollutants, smoke, cold air) are capable of triggering symptoms.[47, 49]

Laboratory procedures employing skin, nasal, or bronchial provocation provide the opportunity to characterize the clinical allergic response, as well as the underlying cellular and biochemical inflammatory mediator process. The accessibility of the skin provides the opportunity to readily obtain biopsy material to study the allergen-induced cellular response. Studies of grass-allergic rhinitics demonstrate classic immediate- and late-phase skin responses to provocative skin tests with grass extract. Biopsy specimens from the allergen-induced late-phase cutaneous response have demonstrated an infiltration of $CD4^+$ T lymphocytes; increased expression of IL-3, granulocyte-macrophage colony-stimulating factor (GM-CSF), and $Th2^+$-type cytokines (IL-4, IL-5); and recruitment and activation of eosinophils.[24, 67]

Utilizing a model of grass nasal provocation, Varney and colleagues[22] demonstrated an analogous cellular infiltration and cytokine mRNA expression during allergen-induced late-phase nasal responses. Likewise, various investigators have induced acute symptoms of allergic rhinitis with nasal challenge that correlates with the appearance of various preformed (histamine, kinins) as well as newly generated (prostaglandins, leukotrienes) inflammatory mediators in the nasal secretions.[15, 19, 48, 55] In a significant percentage of these allergic patients, a recrudescence of symptoms can be demonstrated approximately 6 to 11 hours following the allergen provocation. This late-phase response is characterized by a secondary wave of inflammatory mediators elicited from cells recruited into the inflammatory site—eosinophils, basophils, and neutrophils (Fig. 45–1).[49] The resultant allergen-induced mucosal inflammation appears to play a role in the development of a heightened responsiveness of the nasal mucosa to various nonspecific irritant stimuli (e.g., histamine).[46]

In a similar vein, employing a ragweed bronchial provocation model, it is again possible to demonstrate the same characteristic pattern of an immediate allergen-induced response, followed by a late-phase bronchial response with a similar profile of inflammatory mediators measurable in the bronchial lavage fluids.[10, 39] As in the nose, the allergic asthmatic's airways can be shown to develop a heightened

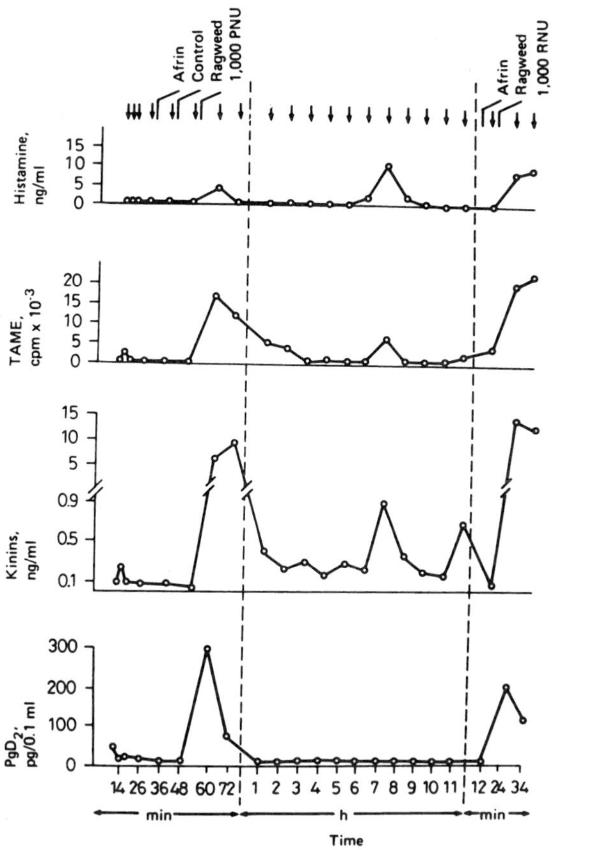

FIGURE 45–1. Mediators in nasal secretions during early, late, and rechallenge responses of allergic patients subjected to nasal challenge with ragweed extract. Vertical dashed lines represent changes in time units; minutes are expressed from beginning of interval, and hours represent time elapsed from first challenge. Large arrows indicate administration of specified material; small arrows indicate performance of nasal lavage. PGD_2 = prostaglandin D_2; TAMe = tosyl-L-arginine methyl esterase; AFRIN = oxymetazoline; PNU = protein nitrogen unit. (From Naclerio RM, Proud D, Togias A, et al: Inflammatory mediators in late antigen-induced rhinitis. N Engl J Med 313:65, 1985.)

responsiveness to an irritant stimulus (e.g., methacholine) during the relevant allergen season.[5]

Immunotherapy has been shown to favorably influence each of the relevant components of the allergic reaction—the cellular response, inflammatory mediator production, humoral response, and respective clinical end points.

MECHANISMS OF IMMUNOTHERAPY

CYTOKINES

As discussed, T cells play a major role in the unfolding of the allergic inflammatory response. Studies of peripheral blood from allergic individuals in which lymphocytes were incubated with allergen have shown enhanced lymphocyte proliferation with lymphokine production.[57] As these same patients underwent immunotherapy, these lymphocyte responses were noted to decrease, and an increase in the activity of antigen-specific suppressor cells was observed in their peripheral blood.[58]

Histamine-releasing factors (HRF) have been measured in early- and late-phase nasal lavages, late-phase bronchoalveolar lavage fluids, and late-phase skin blister fluids.[42, 59, 68] Several of these cytokines (RANTES, monocyte chemoattractant protein (MCP)-1, MCP-3, and IL-3) have been identified that are capable of inducing both mast cell and basophil histamine release through non-IgE mechanisms.[4, 43, 44] Alam and colleagues[2] studying asthmatics demonstrated a correlation between the spontaneous production of non–IgE-dependent HRF from peripheral blood mononuclear cells and the concentration of histamine required to produce a 20% fall in forced expiratory volume (FEV_1). Kuna and colleagues[31] demonstrated the clinical relevance of this in grass-allergic patients who showed a significant shift in spontaneous HRF production from their mononuclear cells that was paralleled by an improvement in their tolerance to histamine provocation following 2 years of grass immunotherapy.

MacDonald and colleagues[45] identified and purified an IgE-dependent HRF produced by lymphocytes of atopic individuals. This provides an important link for the IgE-mediated late-phase response in allergic individuals. A significant correlation between the severity of symptoms observed during the late-phase nasal reaction and IgE-dependent, HRF-induced basophil histamine release has been shown by Iliopoulos.[27]

Varney and colleagues studied the effects of grass immunotherapy in 40 patients with grass-induced rhinoconjunctivitis previously shown to be poorly controlled with pharmacotherapy. Their findings demonstrated significant clinical improvement as measured by a reduction in clinical symptoms and a reduced need for supplemental rescue medications during the grass pollen season (Fig. 45–2).[66] Their studies, employing provocative skin testing to assess the effects of immunotherapy on skin reactivity, showed a reduction in both the immediate- and late-phase intradermal skin test responses.[67]

Furthermore, using immunohistology staining techniques on skin biopsy material, the investigators showed a reduction in the number of T lymphocytes ($CD4^+$ cells) and activated eosinophils ($EG2^+$ cells) recruited into the dermis following allergen stimulation.[67] The placebo-injected group, however, showed significant increases in T lymphocytes, macrophages, total leukocytes, and eosinophils.[67] In situ hybridization techniques employed to study the effects of immunotherapy on the expression of various cytokines and lymphokines associated with allergic inflammation showed no effect of immunotherapy on down-regulating the expression of $Th2^+$ inflammatory cytokines (e.g., IL-4, IL-5) upon allergen exposure but did enhance the expression of mRNA for $Th1^+$-type cytokines (IL-2, interferon (IFN)-γ) in the majority of patients studied (Fig. 45–3).[67]

As a corollary to their skin biopsy findings, the investigators reported the results from their nasal biopsy studies in these same patients. A significant reduction in allergen-induced $CD4^+$ T cells and in total and activated eosinophils and a significant increase in message for IFN-γ and IL-12 were observed (Fig. 45–4).[22]

In contrast to these findings, Secrist and colleagues[60] studying cultured peripheral blood mononuclear cells from allergic patients receiving maintenance allergen immunotherapy demonstrated a significant decrease in allergen-induced IL-4 synthesis when their cells were exposed to allergen in vitro. However, no demonstrable effect on IL-2 or IFN-γ

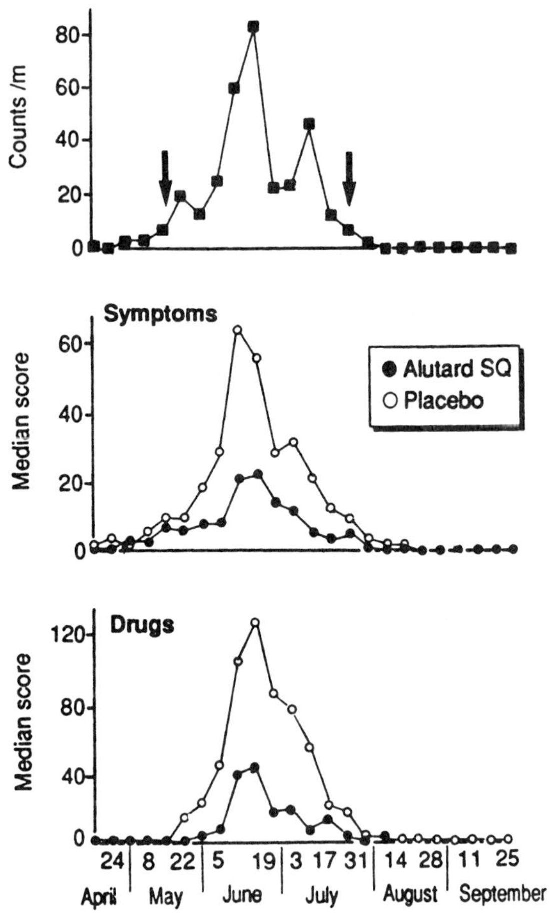

FIGURE 45–2. Average weekly grass pollen counts (1989) and symptom and drug scores for Alutard SQ and placebo groups. Arrows represent the beginning (15 May) and end (25 July) of pollen season. Data between these time points were used to calculate confidence intervals and p values for symptoms and drug scores. (From Varney VA, Gaga M, Freu AJ, et al: Usefulness of immunotherapy in patients with severe summer hay fever uncontrolled by antiallergen drugs. Br Med J 302:265–269, 1991. The BMJ Publishing Group.)

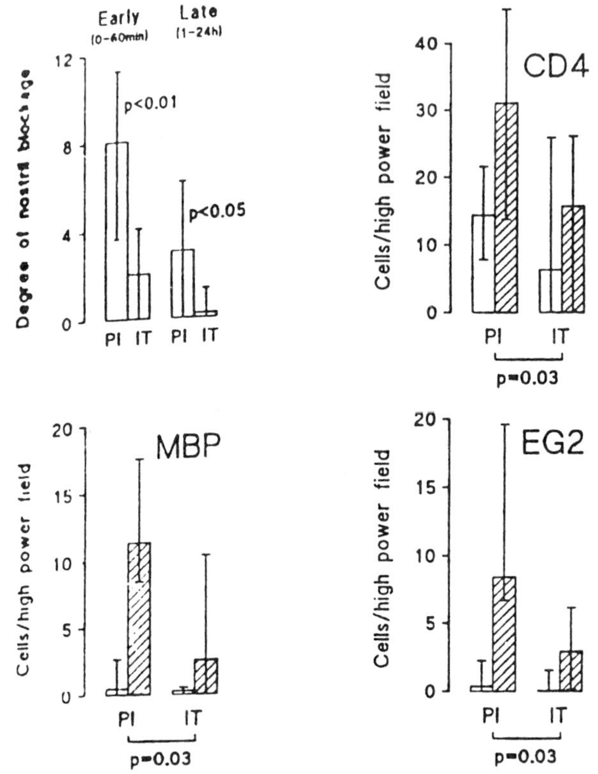

FIGURE 45–4. Effect of immunotherapy on allergen-induced early and late nasal responses (top left) and the associated recruitment of $CD4^+$ T lymphocytes and total major basic protein (MBP)–containing and activated cationic protein–secreting (EG2+) eosinophils (APAAP [alkaline phosphatase antialkaline phosphatase] techniques) 24 hours after control (□) and allergen (▨) challenge. Values represent median values and interquartile ranges. Between-group comparisons were performed using the Mann-Whitney U test. PI = placebo-treated patients (n = 13); IT = patients who have received 12 months of treatment with grass pollen immunotherapy (n = 15). (From Durham SR, et al: Changes in allergic inflammation associated with successful immunotherapy. Int Arch Allergy Immunol 107:282–284, 1995. Kargen, Basel.)

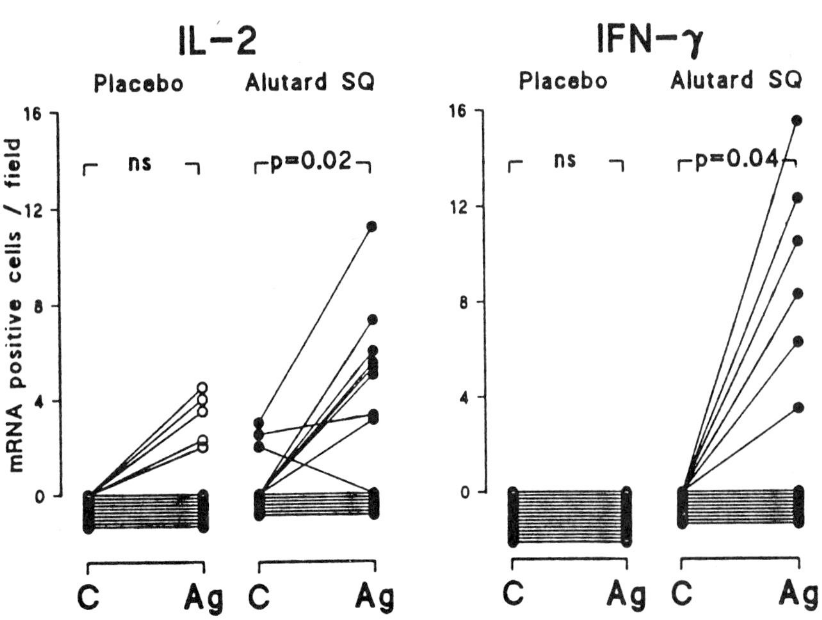

FIGURE 45–3. Expression of cytokine mRNA expression for IL-2 and IFN-γ in the dermis in placebo (open circles) and Alutard SQ (closed circles) groups after 9 months of treatment. Results are expressed as mRNA+ cells per field (× 100) 24 hours after intradermal 30 BU (biologic units) grass pollen extract (Ag) compared with counts after the control allergen diluent solution (C). NS = not significant. (From Varney VA, Hamid QA, Gaga M, et al: Influence of grass pollen immunotherapy on cellular infiltration and cytokine mRNA expression during allergen-induced late-phase cutaneous responses. J Clin Invest 92:644–651, 1993.)

synthesis was observed in these immunized patients. Jutel and colleagues[30] studying honey bee–allergic individuals demonstrated that venom immunotherapy resulted in decreased IL-4 and IL-5 secretion and increased IFN-γ secretion when their peripheral blood mononuclear cells were stimulated with phospholipase A, the primary allergen from honey bee venom.[30]

The clinical implications of these findings suggest that through immunotherapy it may be possible to induce an up-regulation of specific benign T-cell processes, effected through Th1-type helper cells, with the production of IFN-γ– and IL-2–specific cytokines that are capable of arresting the untoward inflammatory response. It may also be possible to directly down-regulate the specific Th2-induced inflammatory process that otherwise results in the production of various inflammatory cytokines.

CELLULAR EVENTS

The nasal provocation model can be used to study the effects of immunotherapy on the various components of the allergic reaction—the immediate-phase reaction, the late-phase reaction, cellular recruitment, and nonspecific reactivity. An initial study by Creticos and colleagues[15] provided an opportunity to assess the effects of immunotherapy on the mast cell– and basophil-induced immediate phase of an allergic reaction. In this study, 12 ragweed-allergic patients who had been on immunotherapy for 3 to 5 years (median dose: 6 μg ragweed Amb a 1/injection) were compared by the technique of nasal pollen challenge with 26 patients who had not been previously immunized. As had been previously demonstrated, the nonimmunized patients experienced clinical symptoms and demonstrated mediator release (histamine, tosyl-L-arginine methyl esterase (TAMe), prostaglandins, leukotrienes) in their nasal secretions. However, significantly fewer of the immunized patients demonstrated inflammatory mediator release in their nasal secretions or experienced sneezing to nasal pollen challenge (Fig. 45–5). Furthermore, the absolute concentrations of inflammatory mediators measurable in the nasal secretions upon allergen challenge were significantly lower in the immunized patients—a 5- to 10-fold difference in mediator release was observed at each point of the dose response curve (0.03–16.5 mg, 10,000–5,000,000 pollen grains)—compared with the nonimmunized patients (Fig. 45–6).[15]

Subsequent studies have demonstrated that ragweed immunotherapy not only influenced the immediate-phase reaction but also attenuated the late-phase inflammatory reaction. In a double-blind placebo-controlled study by Iliopoulos and colleagues,[27] of 41 ragweed-allergic patients undergoing ragweed immunotherapy (median dose: 2 μg Amb a 1/injection), a significant reduction in histamine, TAMe, kinins, and prostaglandin D_2 (PGD_2) was demonstrated in their late-phase nasal secretions after nasal provocation (see Fig. 45–6).

Our understanding of the late-phase reaction suggests that it is dependent on the recruitment of various cell types into

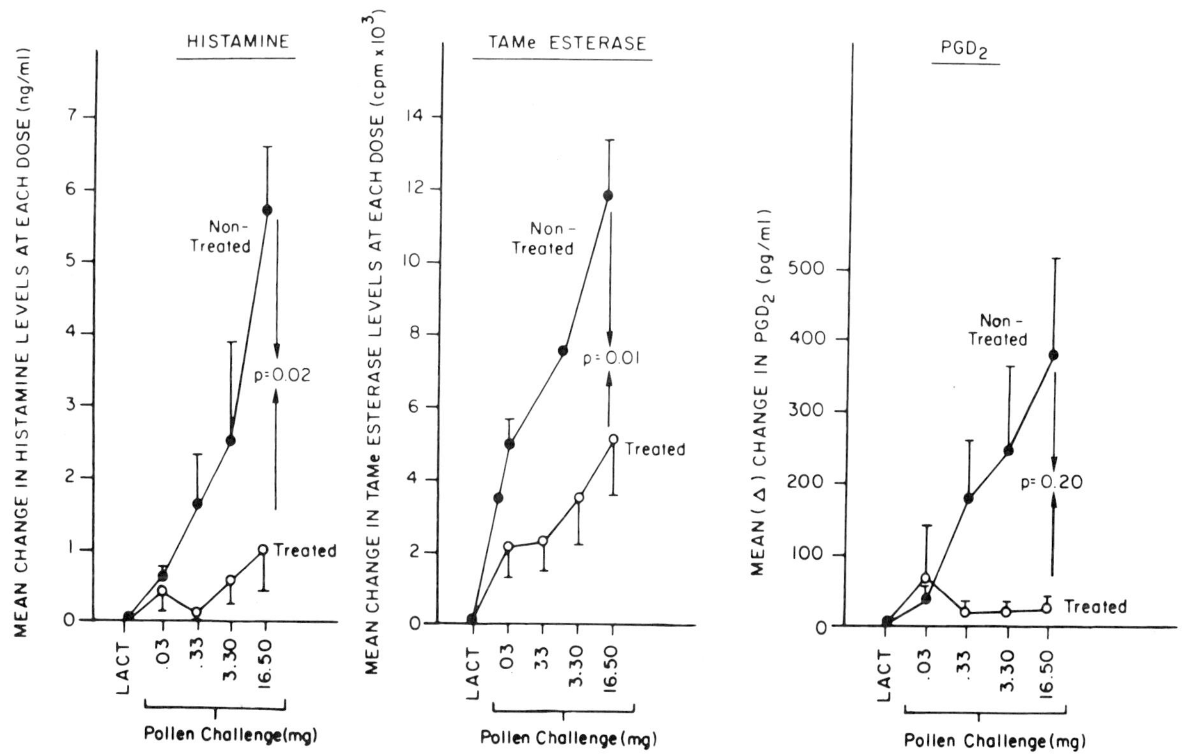

FIGURE 45–5. Differences in absolute amount of mediator released over baseline levels for nontreated (n = 26) (solid circles) and treated (n = 12) (open circles) groups of patients. Horizontal axis reflects 0.03/0.33/3.3/16.5 mg of pollen (10/100/1000/5000 × 10^3 of pollen grains, respectively). LACT = lactose; TAMe = tosyl-L-arginine methyl esterase; PGD_2 = prostaglandin D_2. (From Creticos PS, Adkinson NF, Kagey-Sobotka A, et al: Nasal challenge with ragweed pollen in hay fever patients: effect in immunotherapy. Clin Invest 76:2247–2253, 1985.)

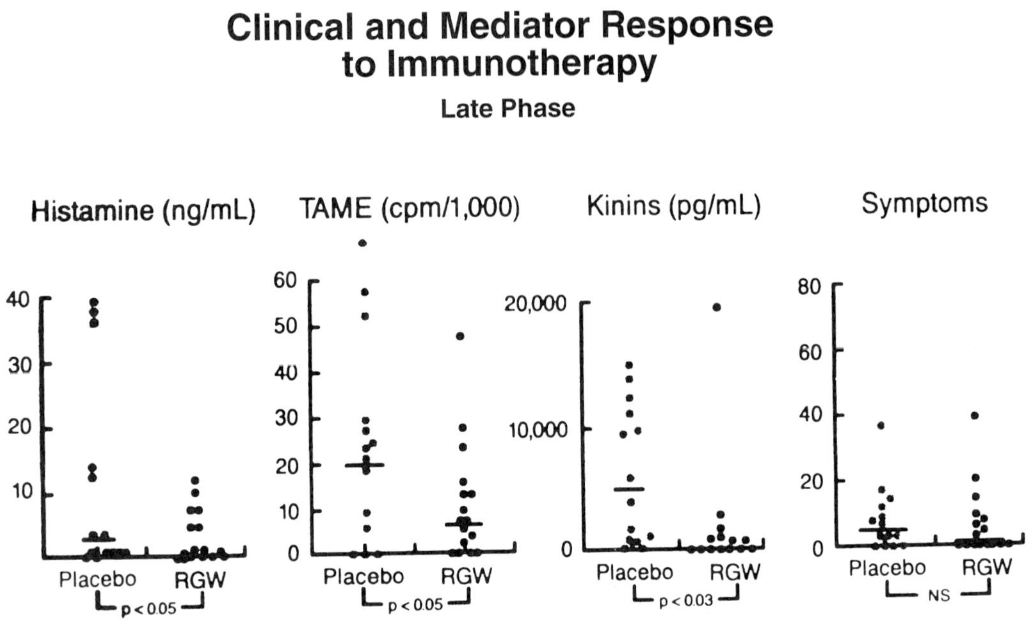

FIGURE 45–6. Comparison between histamine, tosyl-L-arginine methyl esterase (TAMe) activity, kinins, and symptoms generated using the late-phase reaction in the ragweed (RGW)-treated versus the placebo-treated group. Horizontal bars indicate median values; ordinates indicate net change. NS = nonsignificant difference. (From Iliopoulos O, Proud D, Adkinson NF Jr, et al: Effects of immunotherapy on the early, late, and rechallenge nasal reaction to provocation with allergen: changes in inflammatory mediators and cells. J Allergy Clin Immunol 87:855, 1991.)

the inflammatory site (eosinophils, basophils, neutrophils), which results in further inflammatory mediator release and a perpetuation of the clinical response.[49] Studies have demonstrated that eosinophil recruitment occurs over the course of 2 to 10 hours after antigen provocation. A similar influx of basophils has also been observed.[3, 11, 49] Furin and colleagues[25] showed that immunotherapy resulted in a decrease in the antigen-induced eosinophil migration into the nasal mucosa. Furthermore, immunotherapy blunted the typical seasonal influx of eosinophils into the nasal mucosa (Fig. 45–7).

The effects of immunotherapy on the nonspecific component of nasal reactivity have also been studied. Majchel and colleagues[46] employed histamine challenge to demonstrate that immunotherapy prevented the increased responsiveness of the nasal mucosa to histamine during the ragweed pollen season. Sundin and colleagues[61] demonstrated a similar effect in the lower respiratory tract, whereby immunotherapy not only ablated the specific allergen-induced bronchial hyperresponsiveness but also significantly attenuated hyperresponsiveness to a nonspecific irritant (histamine) in cat-allergic asthmatics.

These studies have provided conclusive data on the effects of immunotherapy at the cellular level, with a resultant down-regulation of the allergic inflammatory process as evidenced by a reduction in the immediate-phase allergic reaction, late-phase allergic reaction, specific allergen-induced sensitivity, and nonspecific airway reactivity.

ANTIBODY CHANGES

In 1921, Prausnitz and Kustner[54] recognized that a substance in the serum of an allergic patient could transfer the wheal and flare skin reaction seen in the allergic patient to the nonsensitized individual. Not until 1968 did the Ishizakas demonstrate that the factor responsible for this passive transfer phenomenon was a separate class of antibody, which they termed IgE.[28]

Subsequently, various studies of patients receiving allergen immunotherapy demonstrated that this form of treatment likewise induced an antibody response (Fig. 45–8).[12, 41] This was subsequently shown to be an IgG antibody response that was capable of blocking the passive transfer reaction.[33] Lichtenstein and colleagues[34] further showed that immunotherapy was capable of blunting the typical seasonal rise in IgE antibody observed in allergic rhinitic patients, and with sustained therapy often resulted in a fall in IgE titer to below the pretreatment IgE levels. This drop in IgE antibody was shown by Yunginger and colleagues[70] to be inversely correlated with the rise in blocking IgG antibody.

The clinical relevance of these observations was elucidated by Lichtenstein and colleagues,[36] who demonstrated in ragweed-immunized patients that those with high levels of IgG blocking antibodies often reported low symptom scores on symptom diary cards kept during the ragweed season compared with those patients who produced little or no blocking antibody. Although this general observation has held up through the years, specific antibody titers do not necessarily predict clinical success in individual patients. Nonetheless, an immunotherapeutic dose that fails to induce an increase in IgG antibody will be unlikely to result in any measurable clinical relief.[17]

Detailed studies of the IgG subclass response have demonstrated that IgG1 is the dominant antibody induced during the early therapeutic response to immunotherapy, whereas

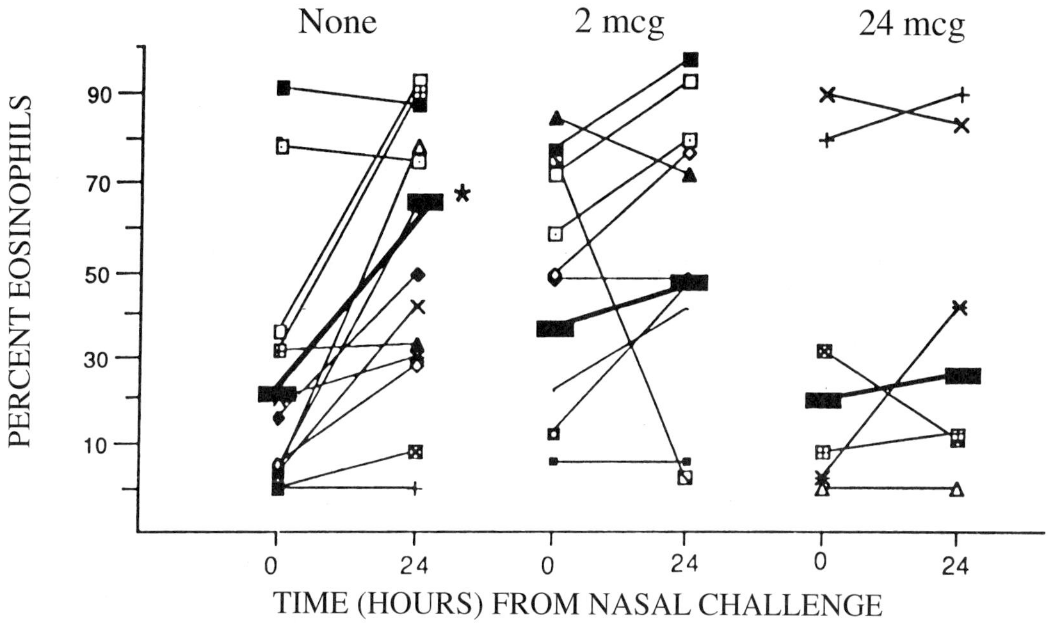

FIGURE 45–7. Immunotherapy decreases antigen-induced eosinophil migration into the nasal cavity. The figure shows the percentage of eosinophils recovered in nasal lavages performed immediately before and 24 hours after nasal provocation with ragweed antigen extract. Each symbol represents a single patient who was studied on two occasions, except in the case of the solid rectangle, which represents the mean of patient values. Three groups of subjects were studied: those not receiving immunotherapy (none), those receiving 1 year of immunotherapy with a maintenance dose of 2 μg, and those receiving immunotherapy for 2 years at a dose of 24 μg. The asterisk represents a significant ($p < 0.008$) increase in the percentage of eosinophils before and after provocation. Solid bars represent median value. (From Furin MJ, Norman PS, Creticos PS, et al: Immunotherapy decreases antigen-induced eosinophil cell migration into the nasal cavity. J Allergy Clin Immunol 88:27–32, 1991.)

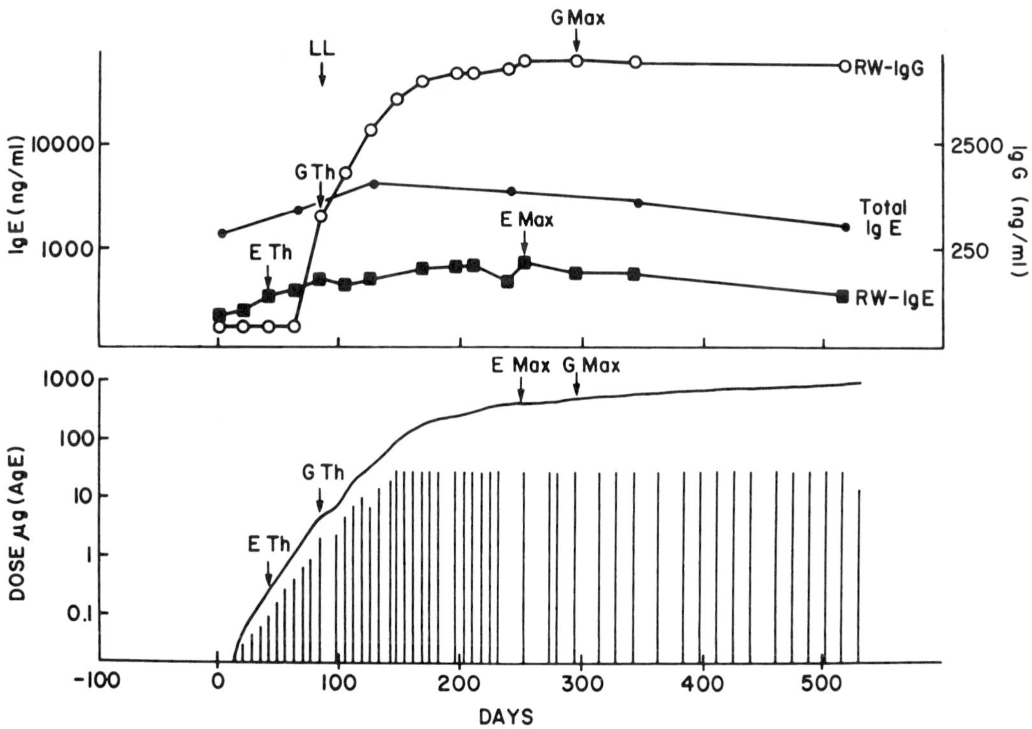

FIGURE 45–8. Profile of a typical patient illustrating the dose regimens for immunotherapy and the IgE and IgG antibody responses. Plotted are the relationships between time expressed in days, individual and cumulative doses of ragweed (RW) pollen extract expressed in nanograms of antigen E (AgE), and serum levels of RW-IgE, RW-IgG, and total IgE. Top panel shows RW-IgE, RW-IgG, total IgE data. Bottom panel shows progressive cumulative dose (line) over respective single doses (bars) over time in days. LL = large local reactions; G max = observations at maximum IgG response; E max = observations at maximum IgE response; G Th = threshold dose for IgG response; E Th = threshold dose for IgE response. (From Creticos PS, Van Metre TE, Mardiney MR, et al: Dose response of IgE and IgG antibodies during ragweed immunotherapy. J Allergy Clin Immunol 73:94–104, 1984.)

IgG4 begins to appear in significant quantities only after prolonged immunotherapy. Furthermore, with discontinuation of immunotherapy, IgG4 rapidly disappears.[52]

Although Platts-Mills and colleagues[53] have shown that immunotherapy is also associated with an increase in IgG and IgA antibody titers in the nasal secretions of immunized patients, this has not been shown to correlate with clinical symptom improvement.

In summary, studies of immunotherapy have demonstrated (1) a rise in serum IgG blocking antibodies, (2) a suppression of the usual seasonal rise in IgE antibodies followed by a slow decline in the level of specific IgE through the course of immunotherapy, and (3) an increase in IgG and IgA antibody levels in nasal secretions.

NONSPECIFIC CHANGES

Tissue mast cells and blood-borne basophils are capable of releasing histamine upon antigen exposure. A positive correlation has been shown between symptom diary scores and basophil sensitivity in allergic patients. Lichtenstein and colleagues[35, 37, 38] have demonstrated that immunotherapy is associated with a decrease in both cellular sensitivity (the amount of allergen required to induce 50% basophil histamine releasing ability) and cellular reactivity (the ability of basophils to release 100% of their cellular histamine). Related to this are the observations of Brunet and colleagues[8] that this cellular sensitivity and releasing ability of basophils are enhanced in patients as they go through an allergen season. These investigators subsequently showed that ragweed immunotherapy resulted in a blunting in basophil histamine releasing ability during the pollen season in immunized compared with placebo-injected patients.[7]

CLINICAL ISSUES

WHO SHOULD BE IMMUNIZED

Environmental control measures to reduce the patient's exposure to the allergen burden, in conjunction with the judicious use of appropriate pharmacotherapy, can often provide excellent control of the allergic patient's symptoms. At issue is when to consider immunotherapy, since it is a form of treatment that has the potential to modulate the underlying allergic inflammatory component of the disease process and thereby induce a prolonged clinical remission in selected patients. At task is a consideration of cost, compliance, and safety, as well as efficacy. With these considerations in mind, a practical set of guidelines can be constructed.

Immunotherapy should be considered in those allergic patients with substantial disease who have inadequate or only partial response to environmental control measures and pharmacotherapy; who have experienced side effects with medications; in whom compliance with the use of daily medications is a factor; or who have persistent symptoms as a result of exposure to relevant allergens on a persistent basis throughout the year.[17]

Identifying the patient who would most likely benefit from immunotherapy first requires the demonstration of a clinically relevant sensitivity to a prevalent allergen in the patient's environment. Skin tests or a radioallergosorbent test (RAST) may indeed detect evidence of IgE-mediated sensitivity, but a thorough clinical history, corroborated by physical examination, is essential in determining the clinical relevance of a particular allergen to the patient.

EXTRACT QUALITY

A major advancement in the field of allergy has been the development of techniques of immunologic standardization that have resulted in the characterization of the major protein moieties for a number of important aeroallergens. This has led the Allergen Standardization Subcommittee of the International Union of Immunologic Societies[1] to develop extract standards for some of these aeroallergens—certain pollens (short ragweed, timothy grass, birch), dust mites (*Dermatophagoides pteronyssinus*), and animals (cat, dog). These extracts have undergone extensive immunologic testing for specific allergenic protein content. Further work is being done to develop standards for other important aeroallergens (alternaria mold, cockroach, various other pollens) (Table 45–1).

In the United States, the Bureau of Biologics of the Food and Drug Administration has attempted to further characterize allergen extracts based on their total biologic activity. This is an attempt to provide the clinician with a measure of the overall activity of an allergenic extract based on an in vitro laboratory measurement of major protein content as correlated with the in vivo measure of skin test sensitivity to the particular standardized allergen extract.[18]

This work has led to the introduction of high-quality, well-characterized, and in many instances, standardized extracts into the marketplace. This has allowed the clinician to administer a precisely defined allergen dose to the allergic patient, hence taking the guesswork out of the treatment process.

Although usually well tolerated, allergy injections can

TABLE 45–1
SOURCE AND MAJOR PROTEIN FOR CERTAIN PRINCIPAL AEROALLERGENS

Source	Major Protein
Trees	
Birch*	Bet v 1
Grasses	
Rye*	Lol 1–4
Blue	Poa p 9
Timothy†	Phl p5, p6
Bermuda*	Cyn d 1
Weeds	
Ragweed*†	Amb a 1
Mites	
Dpt*†	Der p 1–2
Df†	Der f 1–3
Animals	
Cat†	Fel d 1
Dog*	Can f 1
Molds	
Alternaria	Alt 1

*World Health Organization standardized preparation.
†U.S. Food and Drug Administration standardized preparation.

sometimes cause an allergic reaction—hives, respiratory difficulties, and rarely a fatal allergic reaction. In the United States, safety concerns have been largely averted because the allergy subspecialist prepares the patient's extract and uses carefully developed guidelines for the administration of these newer high-quality or standardized extracts.

OPTIMAL DOSE RANGE

A successful therapeutic response with immunotherapy requires that an optimal dose of the respective allergens be administered for an appropriate length of time. Generally, empiric studies with immunotherapy have pushed to a maximally tolerated dose as the end point for gauging a therapeutic response. However, this underscores the potential risk of a more serious systemic reaction in patients undergoing immunotherapy. In this context, the art of immunotherapy has been advanced immeasurably by studies employing nasal pollen challenge, which have provided a model with which to evaluate the protection afforded from various dose levels of immunotherapy. Indeed, a more optimal target dose range, which is reflective of both the single dose given and the cumulative dosage received, can be predicted that will be likely to consistently result in clinical improvement.

As previously cited, Creticos and colleagues[15] clearly demonstrated that both the clinical and underlying inflammatory mediator responses to allergen provocation were significantly different in ragweed-allergic subjects who had been on maintenance immunotherapy (6 μg Amb a 1/injection) compared with patients who had never been immunized.

Furthermore, the 27 ragweed-allergic subjects, never previously immunized, were then randomized in a double-blind prospective study to two different immunotherapy regimens. In the patients randomized to a conventional extract of ragweed (an aqueous extract that contained all the relevant protein moieties and was characterized based on Amb a 1 content), the same principal findings were demonstrated as in the previously noted retrospective study. Specifically, as these patients progressed from low-dose immunotherapy (0.6 μg Amb a 1/injection) to moderate dose immunotherapy (12.4 μg Amb a 1/injection) to high-dose immunotherapy (24.8 μg Amb a 1/injection), a distinct stepwise attenuation (reduction) in nasal responsivity to pollen challenge was observed (Fig. 45–9).[16]

Specifically, low-dose immunotherapy (0.6 μg Amb a 1/injection) afforded no evidence of protection when this group of allergic subjects underwent nasal pollen challenge with ragweed. However, once these patients had achieved a therapeutic dose of 12.4 μg Amb a 1/injection, a significant reduction in the number of patients demonstrating mediator release, as well as the actual amount of mediator released, upon nasal challenge was clearly demonstrated (Fig. 45–10). A further, but nonsignificant, positive effect was observed as these patients were advanced to a dose of 24.8 μg Amb a 1/injection.

Symptom diaries recorded by these patients over the three respective ragweed seasons under observation demonstrated significant clinical improvement during the 2 years that the patients were on active immunotherapy compared with the pretreatment year (Fig. 45–11).[16] These studies suggest that therapeutic doses of 6 to 24 μg Amb a 1/injection provide demonstrable evidence of clinical relief in ragweed-allergic individuals.

Interestingly, studies have shown inconsistent results with lower immunizing doses. A study of 41 ragweed-allergic individuals receiving ragweed immunotherapy (2 μg Amb a 1/injection) or placebo injections demonstrated a difference between the immunized and placebo-injected groups upon nasal challenge after their first year of therapy. However, during the next phase of the study, those advancing to a dose of 2 μg Amb a 1/injection demonstrated no evidence of clinical relief on symptom diaries compared with a newly recruited placebo group. Furthermore, the same group of patients receiving 2 μg Amb a 1/injection as a maintenance dose over a 2-year treatment period also did not demonstrate statistically significant evidence of clinical relief on their symptom diaries that were completed during the respective

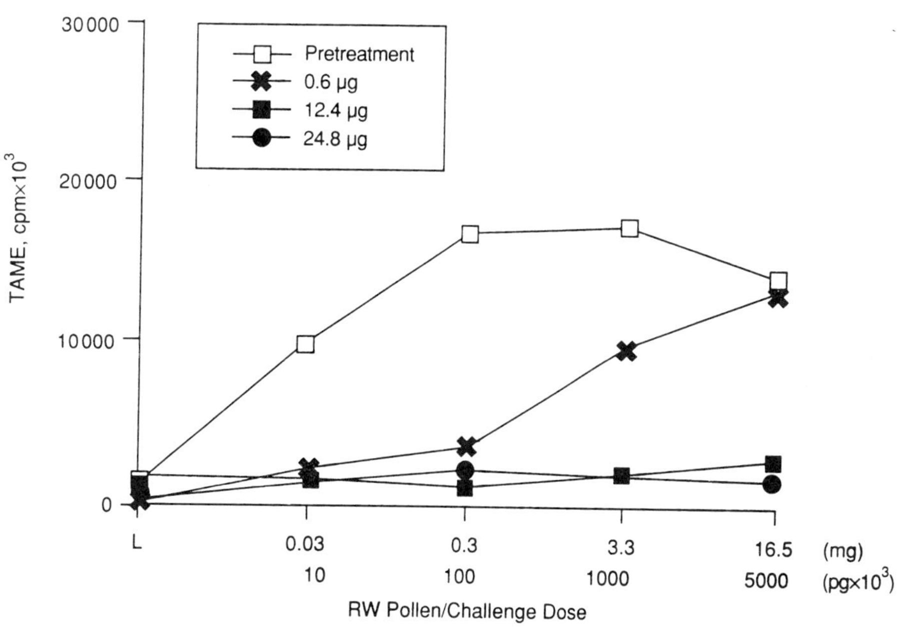

FIGURE 45–9. Effect of increasing therapeutic doses of ragweed (RW) immunotherapy (0.6, 12.4, 24.8 μg of AgE) on nasal challenge response. Vertical axis plots tosyl-L-arginine methyl esterase (TAMe) mediator amount; horizontal axis plots pollen challenge dose in milligrams and corresponding pollen grains in picograms (pg). (From Creticos PS: Immunologic changes associated with immunotherapy. Immunol Allergy Clin North Am 12:13–37, 1992.)

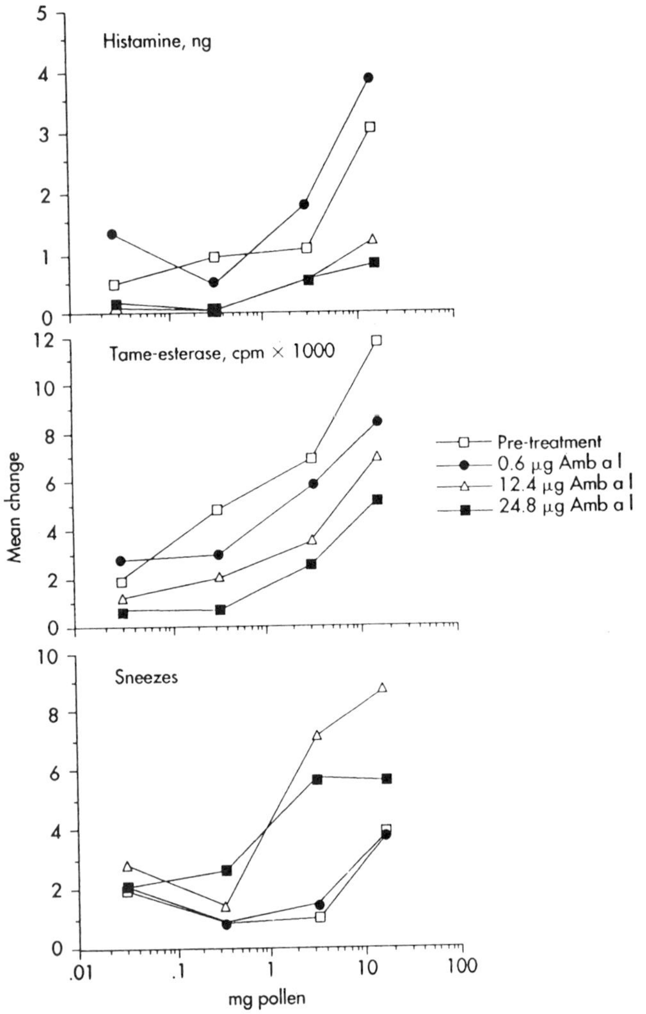

FIGURE 45–10. Effects of increasing therapeutic doses of ragweed immunotherapy (0.6, 12.4, 24.8 μg of AgE) on nasal challenge response in 11 patients. Dose-response curves demonstrate the mean of the increases from prechallenge levels for histamine, tosyl-L-arginine methyl esterase (TAMe), and sneezes. Vertical axis plots the mean change in mediator; horizontal axis plots dose of pollen (in μg) challenge. (From Creticos PS, Marsh DG, Proud D, et al: Responses to ragweed pollen nasal challenge before and after immunotherapy. J Allergy Clin Immunol 84:197–205, 1989.)

ragweed seasons.[27] The necessity of using an adequate immunizing dose is further elucidated in the previous work by Van Metre and colleagues,[63] which conclusively demonstrated that very low immunizing doses (0.006 μg Amb a 1/injection) provided no evidence of clinical efficacy in double-blind placebo-controlled studies (Fig. 45–12).

These studies of ragweed, a carefully defined (standardized) allergen, have allowed us to determine a more precisely defined optimal dose of immunotherapy for ragweed-allergic patients. Indeed, rather than basing the maintenance dose on a maximally tolerated end point, it is now possible to target an optimal therapeutic dose. These studies indicate that a maintenance dose between 6 and 12 μg of Amb a 1/injection should consistently result in clinical benefits in ragweed-allergic rhinitis.[14, 16]

Similar findings have been demonstrated in patients with ragweed-induced asthma. Bruce and colleagues[6] employing a dose of 2 μg of Amb a 1/injection failed to demonstrate clinical improvement in seasonal nasal or chest symptoms or in bronchial reactivity (specific airway conductance measurements). However, Creticos and colleagues[20] demonstrated that a maintenance dose of 10 μg of Amb a 1/injection resulted in a significant reduction in specific bronchial sensitivity to ragweed (PC_{20} FEV_1), which was paralleled by favorable effects on the clinical indexes that were measured (symptoms/peak flow measurements/medication needs) (Fig. 45–13).

Studies with other standardized allergens have also demonstrated similar findings with cat (major protein moiety: Fel d 1) and dust mites (major protein moiety: Der p 1). Van Metre and colleagues[65] studied cat-allergic asthmatics and contrasted a cat room exposure model to cat bronchoprovocation. This study demonstrated that a median single maintenance dose of 8 to 16 μg of Fel d 1 resulted in improvement in these clinical end points.

Haugaard and colleagues[26] utilized the bronchial provocation model to study mite-allergic asthmatics. The investigators demonstrated a significant dose-dependent improved tolerance to Der p 1 on bronchial allergen challenge in each of the immunized groups (group a: 21 μg Der p 1/injection, fourfold to fivefold change; group b: 7 μg Der p 1/injection, fivefold to ninefold change; group c: 0.7 μg Der p1/injection, twofold change), with no change in bronchial sensitivity in the control group. Interestingly, both the immunized groups and the control group demonstrated a significant reduction in nonspecific bronchial hyperresponsiveness (histamine PC_{20}). However, the authors noted a stepwise increase in the systemic reaction rate (0.56%, 3.30%, and 7.10%, respectively) as the immunizing dose was increased from 0.7 to 21 μg/injection. Although the higher dose regimens (7 and 21 μg Der p 1/injection) were demonstrated to be more effective compared with the 0.7 μg/injection regimen, the higher reaction rate with the 21 μg/injection regimen made the authors conclude that a maintenance dose of 7 μg Der p 1/injection was the appropriate target dose. These findings are consistent with those results observed with ragweed immunotherapy.

In summary, empiric studies with a variety of allergens have shown evidence of clinical relief within a wide dosing range (2–46 μg of the major protein/injection). These challenge studies have been able to narrow this maximally tolerated dosage to a more feasible target dose range for immunotherapy employing from 6 to 12 μg of the major protein/injection. In terms of standardized extracts that are available in each of these products, this corresponds to approximately 2,000 to 4,000 biologic allergy units (BAU)/injection for ragweed, cat, and dust mite. Although not every patient can achieve these doses, our studies suggest that the majority of patients will be able to achieve this maintenance dose without difficulty in clinical practice.

METHOD OF ADMINISTRATION

The typical immunotherapy protocol is based on immunizing a patient with a series of injections, given once or twice weekly, starting at a dose low enough to minimize any risk of an untoward allergic reaction (Table 45–2).[40, 62, 64] An initial starting dose should be selected based on the general sensitivity of the patient as judged by skin test reactivity. A

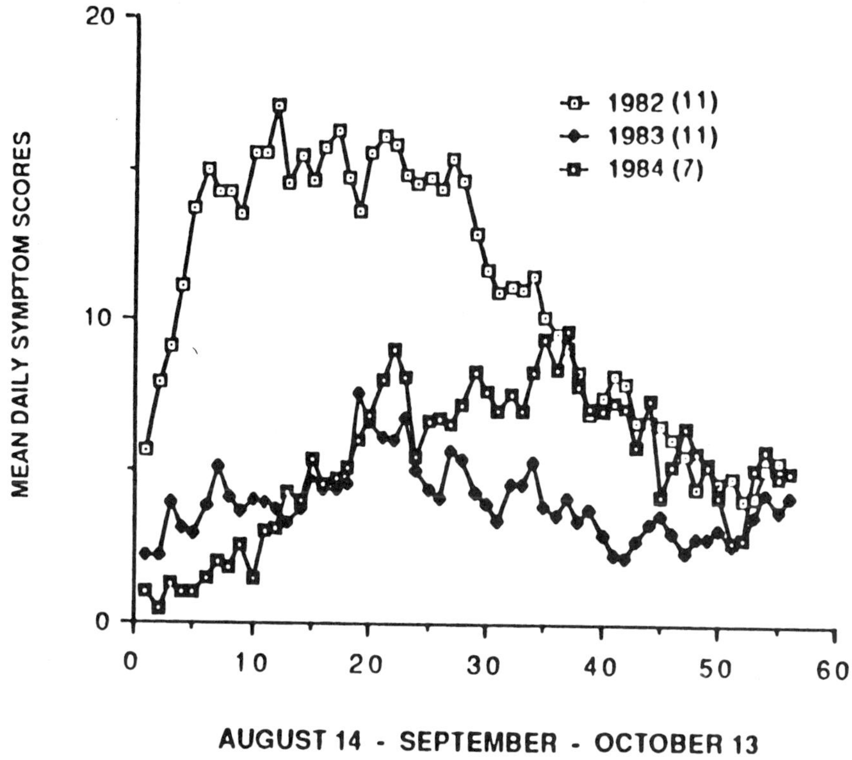

FIGURE 45–11. Daily symptom diary scores plotted for the three ragweed seasons of observation. (From Creticos PS, Marsh DG, Proud D, et al: Responses to ragweed-pollen nasal challenge before and after immunotherapy. J Allergy Clin Immunol 84:197–205, 1989.)

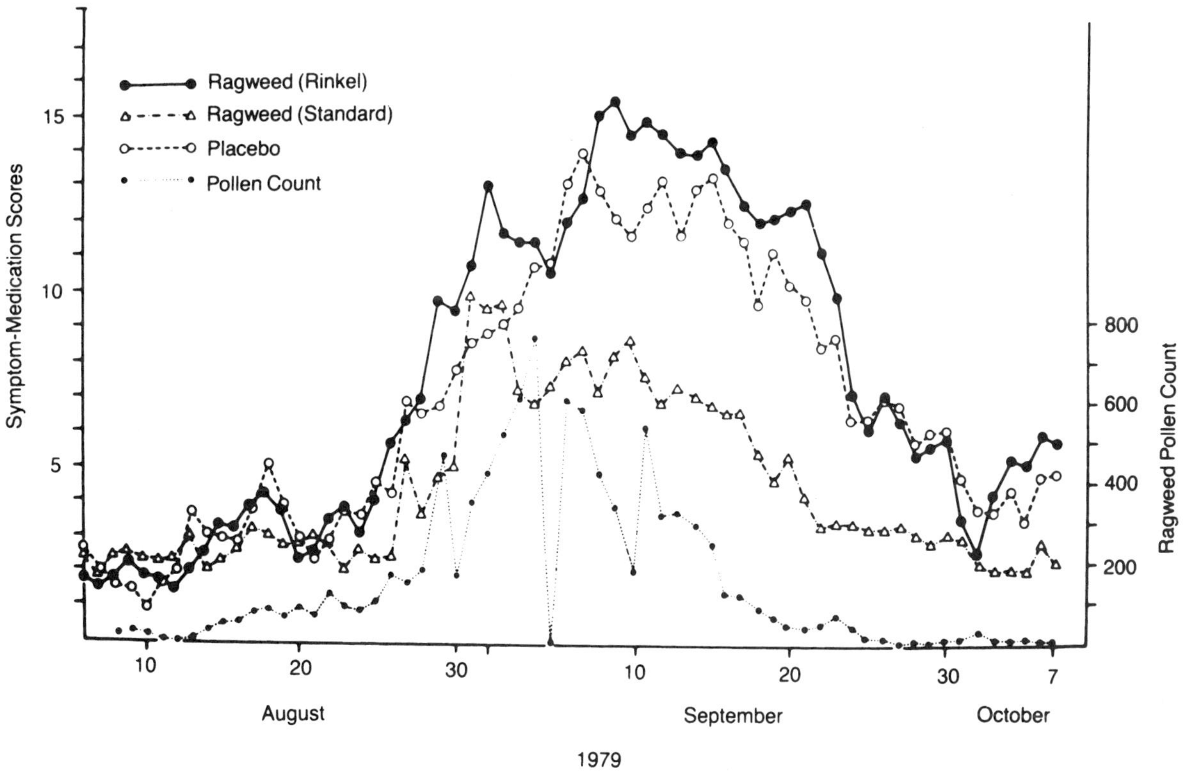

FIGURE 45–12. Arithmetic mean of daily symptom-medication scores for groups indicated, compared with pollen count reported as ragweed pollen grains per square centimeter of rotoslide (small closed circles). Symptom-medication scores of standard group (closed triangles) were significantly less ($p < .01$) than those of Rinkel immunotherapy group (large closed circles) and placebo group (open circles); those of Rinkel immunotherapy group (large closed circles) and placebo group (closed triangles) were not significantly different ($p < .30$). (From Van Metre TE, Atkinson NF Jr, Lichtenstein LM, et al: A controlled study for the effectiveness of the Rinkel method of immunotherapy for ragweed pollen hay fever. J Allergy Clin Immunol 65:288–297, 1980.)

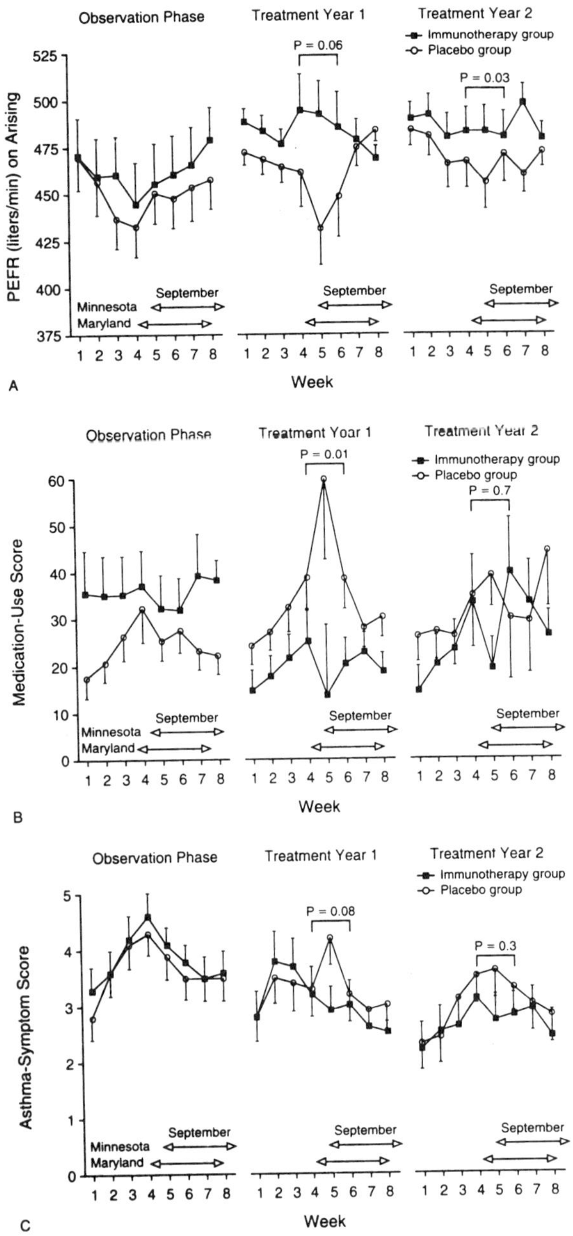

FIGURE 45–13. Evaluations of asthma. Data from Baltimore have been shifted by 1 week to make the times of ragweed exposure coincide for the Baltimore and Rochester, MN, areas. The brackets show the significance of the difference between the placebo and the immunotherapy groups in daily measurements or scores for the 3 weeks of greatest pollen exposure, with the use of an analysis of variance to correct for differences during the observation phase.

Panel A shows the weekly mean (±SE) peak expiratory flow rate (PEFR) measured in the morning before, during, and after the ragweed-pollination season. Measurements of peak expiratory flow were recorded (with a mini Wright peak flow meter) as the highest of three successive readings of peak flow when the patients arose.

Panel B shows the daily mean (±SE) medication scores for each week before, during, and after the ragweed-pollination season. Each of the following was scored as 1 unit: 200 mg of short-acting xanthine, 100 mg of long-acting xanthine, one puff from a sympathomimetic inhaler, a 2 mg albuterol tablet, a 2.5 mg terbutaline tablet, a 10 mg metaproterenol tablet, one puff of ipratropium, a half puff of inhaled corticosteroid, one puff of a nasal corticosteroid, a half puff of cromolyn, 0.5 mg of prednisone, and 0.4 mg of methylprednisolone. An injection of a bronchodilator was scored as 4 units, and respiratory therapy with a bronchodilator was scored as 4 units plus 1 unit for each 0.25 ml of medication. Antihistamines were not scored.

Panel C shows daily mean (±SE) asthma symptom scores. Symptoms were scored on a 6-point scale: 0 = none; 1 = trivial or doubtful; 2 = mild and causing little or no discomfort; 3 = annoying but causing no marked discomfort; 4 = moderately severe and causing marked discomfort; 5 = severe and interfering with sleep or activities but not incapacitating; 6 = incapacitation. (From Creticos PS, Reed CE, Norman PS, et al: Ragweed immunotherapy in adult asthma. N Engl J Med 334:501–506, 1996. Copyright (1996), Massachusetts Medical Society.)

useful guide is the assessment of the wheal and erythema response to an intradermal skin test with the mixture anticipated for injection therapy; in general, if this produces more than a 2+ skin test response, consideration should be given to formulating another 1:10 dilution of the immunotherapy mix and retesting to help determine a starting dose. Van Metre and colleagues[64] demonstrated that patients will usually tolerate a dose that is equal to 0.1 cc of the end point dilution that induces a skin reaction.

Doses are gradually increased at a set rate, such as doubling the dose at each visit, although the rate of increase commonly slows as the dosage nears the expected maximum. The increase may have to be slowed further if allergic symptoms develop with injection. Continuation of injections at a slower rate of increase in those patients who exhibit an adverse reaction usually results in an alteration of reactivity to the point where the projected final dose can be reached with no more than minor symptoms. A small number of patients persist in having allergic reactions even with repeated doses of a reduced concentration, and abandonment of immunotherapy or acceptance of a dose considered less than optimal may be necessary.[13]

After a maintenance dose of immunotherapy is achieved, the interval between booster injections may vary from 1 to 4 weeks depending on the dose and the apparent clinical response. Benefit is usually obvious during the first 6 months to 1 year of therapy and is usually maximal by 3 years with continued therapy. No guidelines exist as to how long therapy should continue. Many physicians will attempt to stop injections after 5 years of a successful treatment program. A few studies suggest that after discontinuation of maintenance immunotherapy, efficacy will fade, and it may be necessary

TABLE 45–2
ILLUSTRATIVE WEEKLY DOSE SCHEDULE FOR A SHORT RAGWEED ALLERGEN

Dose	Vial	Dilution* of 1:20 w/v Concentrate†	w/v	Dose			Amb a 1 (AgE) (μg)
				ml	*AU*	*PNU*	
1	D	1:10,000	1:200,000	0.1	0.5	0.4	0.002
2				0.2	1.0	0.8	0.004
3				0.4	2.0	1.6	0.008
4				0.8	4.0	3.2	0.016
5	C	1:1000	1:20,000	0.15	5.0	4.0	0.03
6				0.3	10.0	8.0	0.06
7				0.6	12.0	12.0	0.12
8	B	1:100	1:2000	0.1	50	40	0.2
9				0.15	75	60	0.3
10				0.25	125	100	0.5
11				0.35	175	140	0.7
12				0.5	250	200	1.0
13				0.7	350	280	1.4
14	A	1:10	1:200	0.1	500	400	2
15				0.15	750	600	3
16				0.25	1250	1000	5
17				0.35	1750	1400	7
18				0.5	2500	2000	10
19				0.7	3500	2800	14

*For this extract, 1:10 w/v contains 100,000 antitoxin units (AU)/ml, 80,000 protein nitrogen units (PNU)/ml, and 400 μg Amb a 1 (AgE)/ml.
†Many allergists use 1:20 w/v for their concentrated solution, because this is the strongest concentration made from a 1:10 w/v aqueous extract that contains 50% glycerin (see text).

to readminister immunotherapy. Thus any decision to discontinue immunotherapy should be carefully discussed with the patient, and the alternatives weighed.[13]

CLINICAL STUDIES

Properly controlled clinical studies have demonstrated the efficacy of immunotherapy in patients with allergic rhinitis and allergic asthma (see Table 45–2). In allergic rhinitis, controlled studies have demonstrated distinct symptom improvement in patients with seasonal pollinosis induced by the birch tree, mountain cedar, grass, and ragweed.[9, 17, 23] Favorable effects have also been shown in patients with dust mite, cat, and alternaria mold sensitivity.[9, 17, 23]

These studies in patients with symptoms of allergic rhinitis have provided objective evidence of the positive effects of immunotherapy on the immediate phase of the allergic reaction, late-phase allergic reaction, and underlying cellular and inflammatory components of the disease process. These studies provide solid evidence of the ability of immunotherapy to modulate the underlying allergic inflammatory component of allergic rhinitis.

Various studies have also suggested the benefit of immunotherapy in asthma induced by animals, dust mite, mold, and pollen. However, the majority of these studies have primarily focused on only subjective measures of symptom relief or laboratory challenge procedures to assess improvement.[9, 17, 23] In this context, a multicenter study was of particular importance, because it combined subjective clinical parameters and objective laboratory measurements to ascertain the effectiveness of immunotherapy in treating patients with seasonal ragweed-induced asthma.[20]

In this study, both placebo-injected and ragweed-immunized patients demonstrated significant improvement in their asthmatic symptoms, but for very different reasons. Careful follow-up and the judicious use of anti-inflammatory medications and bronchodilator drugs resulted in meaningful symptom improvement in both treatment groups over the 2-year treatment period compared with their pretreatment observation season. However, the protection afforded the ragweed-immunized group against both bronchial challenge and the seasonal reduction in peak expiratory flow measurements provided evidence for a specific benefit of immunotherapy.

The ragweed-immunized patients demonstrated an approximate 40% improvement in their asthmatic symptoms, required less medication to control their asthma, and had a measurable increase (30–35 liters/minute) in their peak flow readings, a measurement indicating a meaningful reduction in the underlying asthmatic inflammation in these patients. In contrast, the placebo-injected patients' asthma improved with a twofold to threefold increase in medication requirements. Their airway inflammation was still present, however, as indicated by their peak flow measurements, which continued to drop during the peak of each ragweed season.

The results of this study show that in carefully selected asthmatics, immunotherapy demonstrates positive clinical benefits in the treatment of seasonal ragweed-induced asthma. In fact, the improvement was comparable to that achieved in studies with moderate dose inhaled steroids and superior to that seen with other anti-inflammatory drugs (cromolyn, nedocromil) or maintenance bronchodilator medication (salmeterol, theophylline).

These findings are especially important considering the cost savings potentially afforded by reducing medication requirements. However, further outcome studies need to be done to determine the benefits of immunotherapy in reducing the morbidity of chronic asthma (emergency room visits, hospitalizations, overall economic costs). Completed studies of immunotherapy in patients with perennial dust mite sensitivity and multiple allergic sensitivities should further our understanding of the type of patients who should be considered for immunotherapy.

REFERENCES

1. Gershwin ME (editor-in-chief), Lockey RF (topic editor): Clinical Reviews in Allergy—Standardization of Allergenic Extracts and Immunotherapy, Part I. Elsevier Science Publishing Company, Inc, New York, vol. 4, no. 4:353–434, 1986.
2. Alam R, Kuna P, Rozniecki J, et al: The magnitude of the spontaneous production of histamine-releasing factor (HRF) by lymphocytes in vitro correlates with the state of bronchial hyperreactivity in patients with asthma. J Allergy Clin Immunol 79:103, 1987.
3. Bascom R, Wachs M, Naclerio R, et al: Basophil influx occurs after nasal antigen challenge: effects of topical corticosteroid pretreatment. J Allergy Clin Immunol 81:580–589, 1988.
4. Bochner BS, Charlesworth EN, Lichtenstein LM, et al: Interleukin-1 is released at sites of human cutaneous allergic reactions. J Allergy Clin Immunol 86:830–839, 1990.
5. Boulet L-P, Cartier A, Thomson NC, et al: Asthma and increases in nonallergic bronchial responsiveness from seasonal pollen exposure. J Allergy Clin Immunol 71:399–406, 1983.
6. Bruce AA, Norman PS, Rosenthal RR, et al: The role of ragweed pollen in autumnal asthma. J Allergy Clin Immunol 59:449–459, 1977.
7. Brunet C, Bédard PM, Lavoie A, et al: Allergic rhinitis to ragweed pollen. I. Reassessment of the effects of immunotherapy on cellular and hormonal responses. J Allergy Clin Immunol 89:76–86, 1992.
8. Brunet C, Bédard PM, Lavoie A, et al: Allergic rhinitis to ragweed pollen. II. Modulation of histamine releasing factor production by specific immunotherapy. J Allergy Clin Immunol 89:87–94, 1992.
9. Bush RK, Ritter MW: Allergen immunotherapy for the patient with allergic rhinitis. In Greenberger PA (ed): Immunology and Allergy Clinics of North America—Immunotherapy of IgE-Mediated Disorders. Vol 12. WB Saunders Company, Philadelphia, 1992.
10. Casale TB, Wood D, Richerson HB, et al: Direct evidence of a role for mast cells in the pathogenesis of antigen-induced bronchoconstriction. J Clin Invest 80:1507–1511, 1987.
11. Charlesworth EN, Iliopoulos O, MacDonald SM, et al: Cells and secretagogues involved in the human late-phase response. Int Arch Allergy Appl Immunol 88:50, 1989.
12. Cooke RA, Barnard JH, et al: Serologic evidence of immunity with coexisting sensitization in a type of human allergy (hay fever). J Exp Med 62:733–750, 1935.
13. Creticos PS: Immunotherapy with allergens. JAMA 268:2834–2839, 1992.
14. Creticos PS: Efficacy parameters. In Creticos MPS (ed): Immunotherapy: A Practical Guide to Current Procedures. Miles, Inc, West Haven, CT, 1994, pp 1–19.
15. Creticos PS, Adkinson NF, Kagey-Sobotka A, et al: Nasal challenge with ragweed pollen in hay fever patients. J Clin Invest 76:2247–2253, 1985.
16. Creticos PS, Marsh DG, Proud D, et al: Responses to ragweed pollen nasal challenge before and after immunotherapy. J Allergy Clin Immunol 84:197–205, 1989.
17. Creticos PS, Norman PS: Immunotherapy with allergens. JAMA: Primer on Allergic and Immunologic Diseases, 258:2874–2880, 1987.
18. Creticos PS, Norman PS, Anderson MC, et al: Standardization of allergenic extracts and immunotherapy, Part I. Clin Rev Allergy 4:353, 1986.
19. Creticos PS, Peters SP, Adkinson NF Jr, et al: Demonstration of peptide-leukotriene release following nasal antigen challenge in vivo. N Engl J Med 310:1626–1630, 1984.
20. Creticos PS, Reed CE, Norman PS, et al: Ragweed immunotherapy in adult asthma. N Engl J Med 334:501–506, 1996.
21. Durham SR, Ying VAS, Varney MR, et al: Cytokine messenger RNA expression for IL3, IL4, IL5, and granulocyte/macrophage colony-stimulating factor in the nasal mucosa after local allergen provocation: relationship to tissue eosinophilia. J Immunol 14:2390–2394, 1992.
22. Durham SR, Varney VA, Jacobson MR, et al: Effect of grass pollen immunotherapy on allergen-induced early and late nasal responses (abstract 598). J Allergy Clin Immunol 91:290, 1993.
23. Dykewicz MS: Allergen immunotherapy for the patient with asthma. In Greenberger PA (ed): Immunology and Allergy Clinics of North America—Immunotherapy of IgE-Mediated Disorders. Vol 12. WB Saunders Company, Philadelphia, 1992, pp 125–144.
24. Frew AJ, Kay AB: The relationship between infiltrating CD4+ lymphocytes, activated eosinophils, and the magnitude of the allergen-induced late phase cutaneous reaction in man. J Immunol 141:4158–4164, 1988.
25. Furin MJ, Norman PS, et al: Immunotherapy decreases antigen-induced eosinophil migration into the nasal cavity. J Allergy Clin Immunol 88:27–32, 1991.
26. Haugaard L, Dahl R, Jacobsen L, et al: A controlled dose-response study of immunotherapy with standardized, partially purified extract of house dust mite: clinical efficacy and side effects. J Allergy Clin Immunol 91:709–722, 1993.
27. Iliopoulos OD, Proud D, Adkinson NF Jr, et al: Effects of immunotherapy on the early, late, and rechallenge nasal reaction to provocation with allergen: changes in inflammatory mediators and cells. J Allergy Clin Immunol 87:855–866, 1991.
28. Ishizaka K, Ishizaka T: Human reaginic antibodies and immunoglobulin E. J Allergy 42:333–363, 1968.
29. Ishizaka T, Hirata F, Ishizaka K, et al: Stimulation of phospholipid methylation, Ca^{2+} influx, and histamine release by bridging of IgE receptors on rat mast cells. Proc Natl Acad Sci USA 77:1903–1906, 1980.
30. Jutel M, Pilcher WJ, Skrbic D, et al: Bee venom immunotherapy results in decrease of IL-4 and IL-5 and increase of IFN-g secretion in specific allergen-stimulated T cell cultures. J Immunol 95:4188–4194, 1995.
31. Kuna P, Alam R, Kuzminska B, et al: The effect of preseasonal immunotherapy on the production of histamine releasing factor (HRF) by mononuclear cells from patients with seasonal asthma: results of a double-blind, placebo-controlled randomized study. J Allergy Clin Immunol 83:816, 1989.
32. Lewis RA, Austen KF: Mediation of local homeostasis and inflammation by leukotrienes and other mast cell dependent compounds. Nature 293:103–108, 1981.
33. Lichtenstein LM, Holtzman NA, Burnett LS, et al: A quantitative in vitro study of the chromatographic distribution and immunoglobulin characteristics of human blocking antibody. J Immunol 101:317–324, 1968.
34. Lichtenstein LM, Ishizaka K, Norman PS, et al: IgE antibody measurements in ragweed hay fever: relationship to clinical severity and the results of immunotherapy. J Clin Invest 52:472–482, 1973.
35. Lichtenstein LM, Norman PS, Winkenwerder WL, et al: Clinical and in vitro studies on the role of immunotherapy in ragweed hay fever. Am J Med 44:514–524, 1968.
36. Lichtenstein LM, Norman PS, Winkenwerder WL, et al: A single year immunotherapy for ragweed hay fever: immunologic and clinical studies. Ann Intern Med 75:663–671, 1971.
37. Lichtenstein LM, Norman PS, Winkenwerder WL, et al: In vitro studies of human ragweed allergy: changes in cellular and humoral activity associated with specific desensitization. J Clin Invest 45:1126–1136, 1966.
38. Lichtenstein LM, Osler AG: Studies on the mechanism of hypersensitivity phenomena. IX. Histamine release from human leukocytes by ragweed pollen antigen. J Exp Med 120:507–530, 1964.
39. Liu MC, Hubbard WC, Proud D, et al: Immediate and late inflammatory responses to ragweed antigen challenge of the peripheral airways in allergic asthmatics. Am Rev Respir Dis 144:51–58, 1991.
40. Lockey RF, Portnoy JM, Creticos PS: Forms use for skin testing and immunotherapy. In Creticos MPS (ed): Immunotherapy: A Practical Guide to Current Procedures. Miles, Inc, West Haven, CT, 1994, pp 7–15, 49–50.
41. Loveless MH: Immunological studies of pollinosis: IV. The relationship between thermostable antibody in the circulation and clinical immunity. J Immunol 47:165–180, 1943.
42. MacDonald SM, Kagey-Sobotka A, Proud D, et al: Histamine-releasing factor release mechanism and responding population. J Allergy Clin Immunol 79:248, 1987.
43. MacDonald SM, Lichtenstein LM: Histamine-releasing factors and heterogeneity of IgE. Springer Semin Immunopathol 12:415–428, 1990.
44. MacDonald SM, Lichtenstein LM, Proud D, et al: Studies of IgE-dependent histamine releasing factors: heterogeneity of IgE. J Immunol 506:139, 1987.
45. MacDonald SM, Rafner T, Langdon J, et al: Molecular identification of an IgE-dependent histamine-releasing factor. Science 269:688, 1995.
46. Majchel AM, Proud D, Freidhoff L, et al: The nasal response to hista-

mine challenge: effect of the pollen season and immunotherapy. J Allergy Clin Immunol 90:85–91, 1992.
47. Naclerio RM: Allergic rhinitis. N Engl J Med 325:860–869, 1991.
48. Naclerio RM, Meier HL, Kagey-Sobotka A, et al: Mediator release after nasal challenge with allergen. Am Rev Respir Dis 128:597–602, 1983.
49. Naclerio RM, Proud D, Togias AG, et al: Inflammatory mediators in late antigen-induced rhinitis. N Engl J Med 313:65–70, 1985.
50. O'Hehir RE, Garman RD, Greenstein JL, et al: The specificity and regulation of T cell responsiveness to allergen. Annu Rev Immunol 9:676–695, 1991.
51. O'Hehir RE, Young DB, Kay AB, et al: Cloned human T lymphocytes reactive with *D. farinae* (house dust mite): a comparison of T and B cell antigen recognition. Immunology 62:635–640, 1987.
52. Peng Z, Naclerio RM, Norman PS, et al: Quantitative IgE and IgG subclass responses during and after long-term ragweed immunotherapy. J Allergy Clin Immunol 89:519–529, 1992.
53. Platts-Mills TAE, von Maur RK, Ishizaka K, et al: IgA and IgG anti-ragweed antibodies in nasal secretions. J Clin Invest 57:1041–1050, 1976.
54. Prausnitz C, Kustner H: Studies on supersensitivity. Zentralbl Bakteriol 86:160–169, 1921.
55. Proud D, Togias A, Naclerio RM, et al: Kinins are generated in vivo following nasal airway challenge of allergic individuals with allergen. J Clin Invest 72:1678–1685, 1983.
56. Robinson DS, Hamid Q, Ying S, et al: Predominant TH2-like bronchoalveolar T-lymphocyte population in atopic asthma. N Engl J Med 30:724–726, 1984.
57. Rocklin RE, Pence H, Kaplan H, et al: Cell-mediated immune response of ragweed-sensitive patients to ragweed antigen E: in vitro lymphocyte transformation and elaboration of lymphocyte mediators. J Clin Invest 53:735–744, 1974.
58. Rocklin RE, Sheffer AL, Greineder DK, et al: Generation of antigen-specific suppressor cells during allergy desensitization. N Engl J Med 302:1213–1219, 1980.
59. Schulman ES, Proud D, Liu MC, et al: Human lung macrophages induce histamine release from basophils and mast cells. Am Rev Respir Dis 131:230, 1985.
60. Secrist H, Chelen CJ, Yan W, et al: Allergen immunotherapy decreases interleukin 4 production in CD4+ T cells from allergic individuals. J Exp Med 178:2123–2130, 1993.
61. Sundin B, Lilja G, Graff-Lonnevig V, et al: Immunotherapy with partially purified and standardized animal dander extracts, 1. Clinical results from a double-blind study on patients with animal dander asthma. J Allergy Clin Immunol 77:478–487, 1986.
62. Van Metre TE Jr, Adkinson NF Jr: Immunotherapy for aeroallergen disease. In Middleton JE, Reed CE, Ellis EF, et al (eds): Allergy Principles and Practices, 4th edition. Mosby–Year Book, Inc, St Louis, 1993.
63. Van Metre TE Jr, Adkinson NF Jr, Amodio FJ, et al: A comparative study of the effectiveness of the Rinkel method and the current standard method of immunotherapy for ragweed pollen hay fever. J Allergy Clin Immunol 66:500–513, 1980.
64. Van Metre TE Jr, Adkinson NF Jr, Amodio FJ, et al: A comparison of immunotherapy schedules for injection treatment of ragweed pollen hay fever. J Allergy Clin Immunol 69:181–193, 1982.
65. Van Metre TE Jr, Marsh DG, Adkinson NF Jr, et al: Immunotherapy for cat asthma. J Allergy Clin Immunol 82:1055–1068, 1988.
66. Varney VA, Gaga M, Frew AJ, et al: Usefulness of immunotherapy in patients with severe summery hay fever uncontrolled by antiallergic drugs. Br Med J 302:265–269, 1991.
67. Varney VA, Hamid QA, Gaga M, et al: Influence of grass pollen immunotherapy on cellular infiltration and cytokine mRNA expression during allergen-induced late-phase cutaneous responses. J Clin Invest 92:644–651, 1993.
68. Warner JA, Pienkowski MM, Plaut M, et al: Identification of histamine-releasing factor(s) in the late phase of cutaneous IgE-mediated reactions. J Immunol 136:2583, 1986.
69. Wasserman SI: Mediators of immediate hypersensitivity. J Allergy Clin Immunol 372:101–115, 1983.
70. Yunginger JW, Gleich GJ: Seasonal changes in IgE antibodies and their relationship to IgG antibodies during immunotherapy for ragweed hay fever. J Clin Invest 52:1268–1275, 1973.

V Immunologic Diseases

46 Primary Immunodeficiency Diseases

REBECCA H. BUCKLEY

In the 44 years since Ogden Bruton[9] discovered agammaglobulinemia, more than 50 additional primary immunodeficiency syndromes have been described.[137] These defects involve one or more components of the immune system, including T, B, and natural killer (NK) lymphocytes; phagocytic cells; and complement proteins. Most are recessive traits, some of which are caused by mutations in genes on the X chromosome, others in genes on autosomal chromosomes. The descriptions of specific diseases in this chapter do not include all of the currently recognized immunodeficiency states. Those selected were chosen because of new information about them, their frequency, recent recognition, or relevance to allergic diseases.

Immunodeficiency diseases are characterized by an unusual susceptibility to infection. Knowledge of the predominant infectious agents and the body sites most often affected in a given patient can provide clues as to the most likely host deficit. Patients with antibody, phagocytic cell, or complement deficiencies have recurrent infections with high-grade encapsulated bacterial pathogens. By contrast, patients with deficiencies in T-cell function usually manifest opportunistic infections with viral and fungal agents and often have persistent or intractable diarrhea. These patients begin to fail to thrive shortly after these problems develop.

Some immunodeficiency diseases surprisingly are accompanied by excessive production of immunoglobulin E (IgE) antibodies or of autoantibodies. Because of the frequent use of antibiotics by primary care physicians, allergic or autoimmune problems may be the presenting manifestation in patients with these diseases. There is also an increased incidence of malignancy in patients with immunodeficiency diseases, particularly those that involve deficiencies of B- or T-cell function.[93] Whether this is due to defective tumor immunosurveillance or merely to increased susceptibility to infection with agents predisposing to malignancy is unknown.

When compared with acquired immunodeficiency disorders, genetically determined immunodeficiency is rare.[137] B-cell defects far outnumber those affecting T cells, phagocytic cells, or complement proteins. Selective IgA deficiency is the most common B-cell defect, with reported incidences ranging from 1 in 333 to 1 in 700.[24] Primary immunodeficiency is seen more often in childhood (60%) than in adult life (40%). Early in life, these disorders occur predominantly in males. Among adults, however, females are affected slightly more often than males.

Until recently, there was little insight into the fundamental problems underlying a majority of these conditions. Many of the primary immunodeficiency diseases have now been mapped to specific chromosomal locations, and their fundamental biologic errors have been identified.[11, 38, 53, 98, 105] These remarkable accomplishments were possible through a combination of new knowledge of molecular components involved in cell signaling, mechanisms of communication between cells of the immune system, and greatly improved approaches to mapping disease loci within the human genome.

The molecular bases of four X-linked immunodeficiency disorders have been reported: X-linked agammaglobulinemia, X-linked immunodeficiency with hyper-IgM, the Wiskott-Aldrich syndrome, and X-linked severe combined immunodeficiency.[11, 38, 98, 105] The abnormal gene in X-linked chronic granulomatous disease (CGD) had been identified earlier.[41] The faulty genes in X-linked lymphoproliferative disease and properdin deficiency have been localized to specific sites on the X chromosome.[124]

Autosomal recessive immunodeficiencies for which the molecular bases have been discovered include leukocyte adhesion deficiency type 1 (LAD1),[55] adenosine deaminase (ADA) deficiency,[64] purine nucleoside phosphorylase (PNP) deficiency,[77] ataxia-telangiectasia,[108] DiGeorge syndrome,[19] major histocompatibility complex (MHC) antigen deficiency,[35, 102, 120] Zap 70 deficiency,[48] and Janus kinase 3 (Jak3) deficiency.[107] The identification and cloning of the genes for these diseases have obvious implications for the potential of gene therapy. The rapidity of these discoveries suggests that there will soon be many more.

A committee of the World Health Organization (WHO) has published several versions of a classification of primary immunodeficiency diseases, the most recent in 1995.[137] Tables 46–1 and 46–2 list the conditions for which the molecular bases are currently known.

TABLE 46–2
AUTOSOMAL CHROMOSOME MAP LOCATIONS FOR FAULTY GENES IN PRIMARY IMMUNODEFICIENCY DISEASES

Chromosome	Disease
1q25	Chronic granulomatous disease ($gp67^{phox}$)*
2p11	Kappa chain deficiency*
2q12	CD8 lymphocytopenia (Zap 70)*
6p21.3	(?)Common variable immunodeficiency and selective IgA deficiency
7q11.23	Chronic granulomatous disease ($gp47^{phox}$)*
9p21–p13	Cartilage-hair hypoplasia
11	CD3 gamma chain deficiency*
11q22.3	Ataxia-telangiectasia (PIP-like kinase)*
14q13.1	Purine nucleoside phosphorylase deficiency*
14q32.3	Immunoglobulin heavy chain deletion*
16q24($gp22^{phox}$)*	Chronic granulomatous disease
19p13.3	Janus kinase 3 deficiency*
20q13-ter	Adenosine deaminase deficiency*
21q22.3	Leukocyte adhesion deficiency I (CD18)*
22q11.2	DiGeorge syndrome

*Gene cloned and sequenced and gene product known.

X-LINKED DEFECTS

X-LINKED AGAMMAGLOBULINEMIA

X-linked agammaglobulinemia (XLA) was the first recognized human immunodeficiency disorder.[9] Most patients with this or other B-cell defects are recognized because they have recurrent infections with high-grade bacterial pathogens.

Clinical Features

By virtue of maternally transmitted IgG antibodies, boys afflicted with XLA usually remain well during the first 6 to 9 months of life, except for occasional problems with bacterial conjunctivitis or otitis. Thereafter, they are highly susceptible to infections with extracellular pyogenic organisms, such as pneumococci, streptococci, and *Haemophilus influenzae*.[74] Infections with other organisms, such as meningococci, staphylococci, *Pseudomonas*, and various mycoplasmal species, may also occur. However, frequent use of antibiotics for respiratory infections may alter the typical pattern of presentation.

TABLE 46–1
X-CHROMOSOMAL MAP LOCATIONS FOR FAULTY GENES IN PRIMARY IMMUNODEFICIENCY DISEASES

Chromosome	Disease
Xp21.1	Chronic granulomatous disease ($gp91^{phox}$)*
Xp11.22–11.23	Wiskott-Aldrich syndrome protein*
Xp11.3–p21.1	Properdin deficiency*
Xq13	Severe combined immunodeficiency (common gamma chain deficiency)*
Xq22	X-linked agammaglobulinemia (Bruton tyrosine kinase)*
Xq34–26	X-linked lymphoproliferative syndrome
Xq26	Immunodeficiency with hyper-IgM (CD40 ligand, gp39)*

*Gene cloned and sequenced and gene product known.

The infections not only involve mucous membrane surfaces (sinusitis, pneumonia, otitis, and conjunctivitis) but also include skin infections (cellulitis, abscesses) and life-threatening systemic infections (septic arthritis, meningitis, and septicemia). Growth and development are usually normal despite chronic or recurrent bacterial infections, unless such patients develop bronchiectasis or persistent enteroviral infections.[79, 138] Chronic fungal infections are not usually present, and *Pneumocystis carinii* pneumonia rarely occurs unless there is an associated neutropenia. Viral infections are also usually handled normally, with the notable exceptions of the hepatitis viruses and enteroviruses.[138]

Meningoencephalitis or paralysis has occurred after live poliovirus (an enterovirus) vaccine administration due to failure of immune elimination of the vaccine virus by secretory IgA antibodies, postulated mutation of the vaccine virus to a more neurotropic form, and viremia followed by central nervous system infection because of a lack of circulating IgG antibody. Similarly, various echoviruses and coxsackieviruses have caused chronic, progressive, and eventually fatal central nervous system infections in more than 40 such patients.[79, 138] These observations suggest a primary role for secretory IgA antibody in host defense against this group of viruses, since T-cell function is normal in XLA.

Patients with this condition may have either septic arthritis or a rheumatoid-like arthritis.[74] Septic arthritis is rare after intravenous immune serum globulin (IVIG) replacement therapy is initiated. Infections with *Ureaplasma urealyticum*[81] and viral agents, such as echoviruses, coxsackieviruses, and adenovirus, however, have been identified from joint fluid cultures of patients even on IVIG replacement therapy.[74] Synovial biopsies have revealed a mononuclear round cell infiltrate but no deposition of immune complexes. Rheumatoid factor is absent in the serum due to the absence of antibody formation.

Immunologic Defects

A diagnosis of XLA is suspected if concentrations of all serum immunoglobulins are extremely low (usually <100 mg/dl). Tests for antibodies to blood group substances and to vaccine antigens, such as diphtheria, tetanus, *H. influenzae*, and pneumococcus, are useful in distinguishing this disorder from transient hypogammaglobulinemia of infancy or from protein-losing states, since antibody formation is profoundly impaired in this condition. Polymorphonuclear functions are usually normal if opsonizing IgG antibodies are provided by IVIG replacement therapy. However, some patients with this condition have had transient neutropenia in the early stages of serious infections or without any obvious cause.

Few if any B cells can be detected in the circulation of these patients, regardless of the method used. Variable numbers of pre–B cells can be found in the bone marrow, but this is strongly biased to a fetal-like repertoire of V-D-J gene usage.[80] Adenoids, tonsils, and peripheral lymph nodes are very small due to the absence of germinal centers. The numbers of circulating T cells and NK cells are usually normal or slightly increased in Bruton's patients. The percentages of T-cell subsets have been found to be normal in most. T- and NK-cell functions are normal, as is the morphology of the thymus and thymus-dependent areas of peripheral lymphoid tissues.

Molecular Basis

XLA had been precisely mapped to position Xq22 when two groups of investigators independently and almost simultaneously discovered the mutated gene. One group used the technique of positional cloning.[129] The other group sought and found a B-cell–specific tyrosine kinase important in B lymphocyte signaling.[128] The latter proved to be encoded by a gene in the region where XLA had been mapped. The tyrosine kinase has been named Bruton tyrosine kinase (Btk). Btk is a member of the Src-related nonreceptor tyrosine kinase family, which includes Lck, Fyn, and Lyn, thought to be involved in signal transduction in many hematopoietic cells (Fig. 46–1).[128, 129] Btk is expressed at high levels in all B-lineage cells, including pre–B cells.[37] It has not been detected in any cells of T lineage but has been found in cells of the myeloid series.[128]

Thus far, all males with known XLA (by family history)

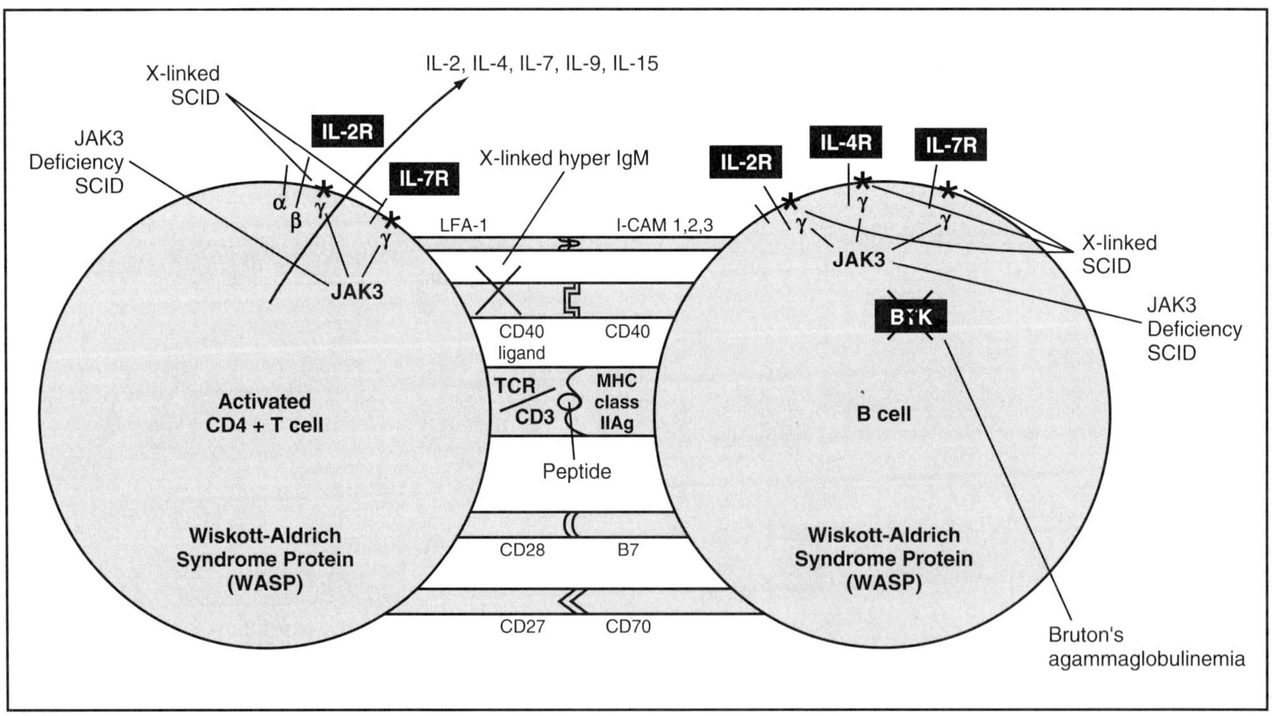

FIGURE 46–1. Schematic of molecules involved in T- and B-cell interaction and signal transduction, showing the location of newly defined molecular defects in three X-linked primary immunodeficiency diseases. Mutations in the gene encoding the cytoplasmic nonreceptor tyrosine kinase (Btk) lead to Bruton's or X-linked agammaglobulinemia (XLA) by preventing B-cell maturation beyond the pre–B-cell stage. Mutations in the gene for the CD40 ligand, or gp39, prevent expression of this crucial molecule necessary for T cells to activate B cells by interaction with CD40 on their surface. These mutations are responsible for the defect in X-linked immunodeficiency with hyper-IgM that prevents the B cells from isotype switching. Mutations in the common gamma chain (γ_c) for several cytokine receptors (IL-2, IL-4, IL-7, IL-9, and IL-15) in infants with X-linked severe combined immunodeficiency disease (XSCID) prevent the binding of those cytokines to their receptors, resulting in profound deficiencies in T-cell, B-cell, and natural killer (NK) cell development and function. Mutations in Janus kinase 3 (Jak 3), the primary signal transducer for γ_c, result in similar profound functional deficiencies in an autosomal recessive form of SCID. (From Buckley RH: Primary immunodeficiency diseases. In Bennett JC, Plum F (eds): Cecil Textbook of Medicine, 20th edition. WB Saunders Co, Philadelphia, 1996.)

have had low or undetectable Btk mRNA and kinase activity. Mutations in the gene-encoding Btk have also been shown to be the basis for the B-cell defect in CBA/N mice. Since such mice have a much milder antibody deficiency than do boys with XLA, speculation had been made that humans with mutations in the same part of the *Btk* gene might have a less severe immunodeficiency. However, many different mutations of the human *Btk* gene (122 in 157 kindreds) have already been described. These have encompassed most parts of the coding portions of the gene, and there has not been any clear correlation between the location of the mutation and the clinical phenotype.[116, 130]

Carriers of XLA can be detected by the finding of nonrandom X chromosome inactivation in their B cells.[98] Prenatal diagnosis of affected or nonaffected male fetuses has also been accomplished using closely linked probes and restriction fragment length polymorphism (RFLP) analysis. Such studies have also permitted identification of X-linked inheritance in some agammaglobulinemic boys with no family history.[98] The fact that Btk is also expressed in cells of myeloid lineage is of interest in light of the well-known occurrence of intermittent neutropenia in boys with XLA, particularly at the height of an acute infection.[13] It is conceivable that Btk is only one of the signaling molecules participating in myeloid maturation and that neutropenia would be observed in XLA only when rapid production of such cells is needed. XLA has been reported in association with growth hormone deficiency in nine patients.[27]

A condition that resembles XLA phenotypically and functionally has been reported in girls, that is, there is an absence of circulating B cells.[31] The molecular basis for this apparently autosomal recessive defect is under intense investigation.

Treatment and Prognosis

Except in those unfortunate patients who develop polio, persistent enteroviral infections, rheumatoid arthritis, or lymphoreticular malignancy (an incidence as high as 6% has been reported), the overall prognosis is reasonably good if IVIG replacement therapy is instituted early. Systemic infection can be prevented by administration of IVIG at a dose of 400 mg/kg every 3 to 4 weeks.[15] Many patients develop persistent enteroviral infections or crippling sinopulmonary disease despite IVIG therapy, since no effective means exists for replacing secretory IgA at the mucosal surface. Chronic antibiotic therapy is usually necessary in addition to monthly IVIG infusions for the management of patients with pansinusitis or bronchiectasis.

X-LINKED IMMUNODEFICIENCY WITH HYPER-IgM

Clinical Features

Similar to patients with XLA, those with the hyper-IgM syndrome may become symptomatic during the first or second year of life with recurrent pyogenic infections, including otitis media, sinusitis, pneumonia, and tonsillitis.[90] In contrast to patients with XLA, however, the frequent presence of lymphoid hyperplasia in hyper-IgM patients often leads to a delayed diagnosis. Coexistent neutropenia is considered a possible explanation for the occurrence of *Pneumocystis carinii* pneumonia and extensive verruca vulgaris lesions in some such patients.

Immunologic Defects

Hyper-IgM is characterized by very low serum IgG and IgA concentrations but either a normal or, more frequently, a markedly elevated concentration of polyclonal serum IgM. Some patients have low molecular weight IgM molecules that give falsely high IgM values in radial immunodiffusion assays. High titers of IgM antibodies to blood group substances and to *Salmonella* O antigen have been found in some patients, but very low titers or no IgM antibodies have been noted in others. However, there is an increased frequency of autoantibody formation in the hyper-IgM syndrome.[90] Hemolytic anemia and thrombocytopenia have been seen in several patients and transient, persistent, or cyclic neutropenia is a common feature.

Even though normal numbers of B lymphocytes are usually present in the blood of these patients, this condition was until recently classified as a B-cell defect, since only IgM is produced. Moreover, since crude tests of T-cell functions were usually normal in such patients, most immunologists did not consider that this could be a T-cell defect. However, B cells from some such patients demonstrated the capacity to synthesize IgM, IgA, and IgG normally when cocultured with a switch T-cell line, suggesting that in those patients the defect lay in T lineage cells.[78]

Molecular Basis

The abnormal gene in X-linked hyper-IgM was localized to Xq26 and has been identified (see Table 46–1).[91] The gene product is the gp39 ligand (CD40L) present on activated T helper cells, which interacts with CD40 molecules on B cells.[1, 86] CD40 is a type I integral membrane glycoprotein expressed on B cells, monocytes, some carcinomas, and a few other types of cells. It belongs to the tumor necrosis factor (TNF)/nerve growth factor receptor family. Cross-linking of CD40 on either normal or hyper-IgM B cells by reacting them with a monoclonal antibody to CD40 or allowing CD40 to interact with normal T-cell CD40L in the presence of certain cytokines (IL-2, IL-4, or IL-10) causes the B cells to undergo proliferation and isotype switching and to secrete various types of immunoglobulins.

CD40L is a type II integral membrane glycoprotein with significant sequence homology to TNF and is found only on activated T cells, primarily of the CD4 phenotype.[86] Thus mutations in the gene encoding the CD40L on activated T cells from hyper-IgM patients result in failure of signaling of B cells to undergo isotype switching; therefore, they produce only IgM (see Fig. 46–1). Many distinct point mutations or deletions in the gene encoding the CD40L have been identified, giving rise to frame shifts, premature stop codons, and single amino acid substitutions, most of which were clustered in the TNF homology domain located in the carboxy-terminal region.[1] A highly polymorphic microsatellite dinucleotide (CA) repeat region has been identified in the 3′ untranslated end of the gene for the CD40 ligand.[44] Approximately 80% of women are heterozygous for this polymorphism, consisting of eight alleles. Therefore, this marker can be used to detect carriers of X-linked hyper-IgM and has been used to make a prenatal diagnosis of this condition.[44]

The facts that not all males with hyper-IgM have had a mutation in the CD40L and that there are several examples in females indicate that this condition has more than one genetic cause. In such patients, the B cells are not able to switch from IgM-secreting to IgG-, IgA-, or IgE-secreting cells, even when cocultured with monoclonal antibodies to CD40 and a variety of cytokines.[29] Thus in those patients, the condition truly is a B-cell defect. CD40 has been present on the surfaces of the B cells in such patients, ruling out deficiency of that protein as the defect. However, there is currently an intense search for a B-cell–specific, CD40-associated signaling molecule defect in those patients.

Treatment and Prognosis

Because these patients have an inability to make IgG antibodies, the treatment for this condition is the same as for agammaglobulinemia, namely, monthly IVIG infusions,[15] The prognosis is reasonably good for many patients. However, there is an increased incidence of both autoimmunity and malignancy in this condition.

IMMUNODEFICIENCY WITH THROMBOCYTOPENIA AND ECZEMA (WISKOTT-ALDRICH SYNDROME)

The Wiskott-Aldrich syndrome is an X-linked recessive syndrome characterized clinically by the triad of eczema, thrombocytopenic purpura with normal-appearing megakaryocytes but small defective platelets, and undue susceptibility to infection.[104, 137] Often there is prolonged bleeding from the circumcision site or bloody diarrhea during infancy. The thrombocytopenia appears to be caused by an intrinsic platelet abnormality. Survival times of homologous but not autologous ^{51}Cr-labeled platelets have been normal in these patients.

Atopic dermatitis and recurrent infections usually also develop during the first year of life. In younger patients, infections are commonly those produced by pneumococci and other bacteria having polysaccharide capsules, resulting in episodes of otitis media, pneumonia, meningitis, and sepsis. Later, infections with agents such as *Pneumocystis carinii* and the herpes viruses become more frequent. Autoimmune cytopenias and vasculitis are common in those who live beyond infancy. Survival beyond the teens is rare. Infections and bleeding are major causes of death, but there is also a 12% incidence of fatal malignancy in this condition.

Immunologic Defects

Patients with this syndrome uniformly have an impaired humoral immune response to polysaccharide antigens, as evidenced by absent or markedly diminished isohemagglutinins and poor or absent antibody responses after immunization with polysaccharide antigens.[137] Antibody titers to protein antigens also fall with time, and anamnestic responses are often poor or absent. Studies of immunoglobulin metabolism have shown an accelerated rate of synthesis, as well as hypercatabolism of albumin, IgG, IgA, and IgM, resulting in highly variable concentrations of different immunoglobulins, even within the same patient. The predominant pattern is a low serum IgM, elevated IgA and IgE, and a normal or slightly low IgG concentration. Analyses of blood lymphocytes have shown moderately reduced percentages of T cells reacting with monoclonal antibodies to CD3, CD4, and CD8. Lymphocyte responses to mitogens are moderately depressed, and cutaneous anergy is a frequent finding.

Molecular Basis

The abnormal gene responsible for this defect was shown to be closely linked to the novel hypervariable locus DXS255 on the proximal arm of the X chromosome between DXS7 (p11.3) and DXS14 (Xp11) and was mapped to Xp11.22–11.23.[36] The mutated gene was recently isolated and found to be limited in expression to lymphocytic and megakaryocyte lineages.[38, 73] The gene product, a 501 amino acid proline-rich protein that lacks a hydrophobic transmembrane domain, has been designated Wiskott-Aldrich syndrome protein (WASP). It has been shown to be an effector for CDC42H2, a member of the Rho family of GTPases important in actin polymerization.[125a] Carriers can be detected by nonrandom X chromosome inactivation in several hematopoietic cell lineages.[134]

Treatment and Prognosis

Several patients who required splenectomy for uncontrollable bleeding had impressive rises in their platelet counts and have done well clinically while on long-term antibiotics and antibody replacement therapy with IVIG.[83] A number of patients with this disorder have had complete corrections of both the platelet and immunologic abnormalities by HLA-identical sibling bone marrow transplants after being conditioned with irradiation or busulfan and cyclophosphamide.[12] Success has been minimal with T-cell–depleted haploidentical stem cell transplants in this condition, primarily because of the requirement for pretransplant immunosuppression to permit engraftment, the long time course to immunoreconstitution when T cells are depleted, resistance to engraftment, and a high mortality from preexisting opportunistic infections in that setting.[12] Unless immunologic reconstitution can be achieved, patients with this condition rarely reach adulthood. The most common cause of death currently is EBV-induced lymphoreticular malignancy.

CHRONIC GRANULOMATOUS DISEASE

X-linked chronic granulomatous disease (CGD) is a condition characterized by defective intracellular killing of bacterial and fungal organisms.[40, 113]

Clinical Features

During infancy, patients with CGD begin to have infections with catalase-positive organisms, such as *Staphylococcus aureus, Serratia marcescens, Pseudomonas* species, and *Salmonella*, but not with catalase-negative organisms, such as *Streptococcus pneumoniae*. These infections manifest most often as suppurative adenopathy, pneumonia, or visceral abscesses. The abscesses respond poorly to antibiotics and usually require surgical drainage. Osteomyelitis caused by bacteria (particularly *Serratia marcescens*) or fungi (especially *Aspergillus* species) is also frequent.

Immunologic Defects

The number of neutrophils is normal or elevated, and chemotactic, adherence, and phagocytic functions of neutrophils are normal. In CGD, the immunologic defects lie solely in an ability of the phagocyte to kill ingested organisms.[40] During normal phagocytosis, the hexose monophosphate shunt is activated and $NADP^+$ is converted to NADPH, which is then moved from the cytosol to an electron transport chain driven by NADPH oxidase in the cell membrane. A 66 kD flavoprotein appears to be the receptor for NADPH in the membrane and is linked to cytochrome b245, the terminal component of the electron transport chain. Cytochrome b245 is capable of directly reducing molecular oxygen to superoxide. Superoxide then dismutates to hydrogen peroxide, which is directly toxic to microorganisms or interacts with chloride ion to produce hypochlorite. Defects exist in this electron transport chain in CGD.

The diagnosis of CGD is made by demonstrating an inability of neutrophils from the patient to undergo a respiratory burst following phagocytosis or PMA stimulation, that is, to generate superoxide ions. The generation of superoxide ions can be demonstrated by measuring chemiluminescence, nitroblue tetrazolium (NBT) dye reduction, or by another type of dye test that detects this by flow cytometry. Alternatively, the ability of CGD neutrophils to kill bacteria, such as *Staphylococcus aureus* or gram-negative bacteria, can be assessed. As a result of ineffective destruction of phagocytized organisms in these conditions and compensatory responses by lymphoid cells, granulomatous lesions are formed, especially in the lung, liver, and gastrointestinal and urinary tracts.[40]

Molecular Basis

Approximately 65% of patients with CGD have an X-linked (X-CGD) mode of inheritance, and the remainder have autosomal recessive (AR-CGD) inheritance (see Table 46–4).[34, 40] The defect in X-CGD is due to mutations in the gene that encodes the heavy chain of the cytochrome b245 heterodimer. The latter chain is a glycoprotein of 91 kD, referred to as $gp91^{phox}$ (for phagocyte oxidase), and does not contain the cytochrome activity.[40, 41] The gene encoding $gp91^{phox}$ is at position Xp21.1 on the short arm of the X chromosome.[41]

Treatment and Prognosis

When CGD was first discovered, it was usually fatal in early childhood. In one early study, 50% of the patients died before 10 years of age. The prognosis has been much improved for patients diagnosed after 1978, even though morbidity and mortality are still significant. Aggressive treatment with antibiotics, especially trimethoprim-sulfamethoxazole, antistaphylococcic penicillins, and aminoglycosides, has reduced the frequency and severity of bacterial infections.[82] Fungal infections, especially with *Aspergillus*, have been a more important cause of death. Amphotericin B, with alternate day (nonirradiated) normal granulocyte transfusions, is the initial treatment of choice. Once *Aspergillus* infections are brought under control with the latter therapy, chronic therapy with itraconazole appears to be very effective in preventing recurrences.

A double-blind placebo-controlled study of the efficacy and safety of subcutaneous injections of interferon-γ (IFN-γ) in preventing serious infections was conducted in 128 patients with CGD. The investigators reported a significant reduction in the number of serious infections (as defined by requiring hospitalization) in those CGD patients who received IFN-γ subcutaneously three times a week compared with the number in placebo-treated CGD patients.[67] However, there was no improvement in phagocytic cell oxidative or microbicidal functions. Bone marrow transplantation has not been as successful in reconstituting phagocytic cell function in CGD patients as it has in restoring T-cell function in severe T-cell deficiency, primarily because full cytoreduction is necessary to gain graft acceptance by CGD patients, and many have chronic indolent bacterial or fungal infections that could not be controlled if such chemotherapy were given.[12] As with other defects for which the molecular bases are known, once gene therapy is perfected, patients with CGD will be candidates for this type of therapy.[96]

X-LINKED LYMPHOPROLIFERATIVE DISEASE

X-linked lymphoproliferative disease (XLP), also referred to as Duncan's disease, is a recessive trait characterized by an inadequate immune response to infection with EBV, resulting in fatal, malignant, or nonmalignant immune cell proliferation.[124] Affected individuals are apparently healthy until they experience infectious mononucleosis.[124] However, when males in susceptible families were studied prior to their contracting EBV infection, immunoglobulin class and subclass deficiencies were detected.[62] The mean age of presentation is less than 5 years. The most common form of presentation (75%) is severe fatal (80%) mononucleosis, primarily owing to extensive liver necrosis caused by polyclonally activated cytotoxic T cells that recognize EBV-infected autologous B cells.[124] Most patients surviving the primary infection developed global cellular immune defects involving T, B, and NK cells; lymphomas; or hypogammaglobulinemia.

There is a marked impairment in production of antibodies to the EBV nuclear antigen (EBNA), whereas titers of antibodies to the viral capsid antigen have ranged from zero to markedly elevated. Antibody-dependent cell-mediated cytotoxicity (ADCC) against EBV-infected cells has been low in many, and NK function is also depressed. There is also a deficiency in long-lived T-cell immunity to EBV. Studies of XLP T lymphocyte subpopulations with monoclonal antibodies have frequently revealed elevated percentages of CD8+ cells. Immunoglobulin synthesis in response to pokeweed mitogen stimulation in vitro is markedly depressed. Thus both EBV-specific and nonspecific immunologic abnormalities occur in patients with XLP. The defective gene in XLP has been localized to the Xq26–q27 region near DXS42 and DXS37.[124] The molecular defect in this condition has not yet been identified.

X-LINKED RECESSIVE SEVERE COMBINED IMMUNODEFICIENCY DISEASE

Clinical Features

Severe combined immunodeficiency (SCID) is a rare and fatal syndrome characterized by profound deficiencies of T- and B-cell function.[8, 52, 137] Since the initial description of SCID in 1950,[59] it has become evident that the genetic origins of this condition are quite diverse.[52] X-linked SCID (XSCID) is probably the most common form of SCID in the United States.[98] Table 46–3 lists the frequency of the various genetic forms of SCID evaluated by the author over the past 3 decades. Affected infants present in the first few months of life with frequent episodes of diarrhea, pneumonia, otitis, sepsis, and cutaneous infections. Growth may appear normal initially, but extreme wasting usually develops after infections and diarrhea begin. Persistent infections with opportunistic organisms such as *Candida albicans, Pneumocystis carinii*, varicella, measles, parainfluenzae 3, cytomegalovirus, EBV, and bacillus Calmette-Guérin lead to death. These infants also lack the ability to reject foreign tissue and are therefore at risk for graft-versus-host disease (GVHD). GVHD reactions can result from maternal immunocompetent cells crossing the placenta or from the administration of nonirradiated blood products or allogeneic bone marrow containing T lymphocytes.

Immunologic Defects

Infants with SCID have lymphopenia (Fig. 46–2)[61]; an absence of lymphocyte proliferative responses to mitogens, antigens and allogeneic cells in vitro; and delayed cutaneous anergy.[16, 52, 121] Serum immunoglobulin concentrations are diminished to absent, and no antibody formation occurs following immunization. Despite the uniformly profound lack of T- or B-cell function, patients with XSCID surprisingly have elevated percentages of B cells.[16, 26, 52, 121] However, these B cells do not produce immunoglobulin normally, even after immune reconstitution by bone marrow transplantation. By contrast, all but those with transplacentally acquired maternal T cells have few or no T cells. NK cells and function are usually very low or totally lacking in patients with XSCID.[110]

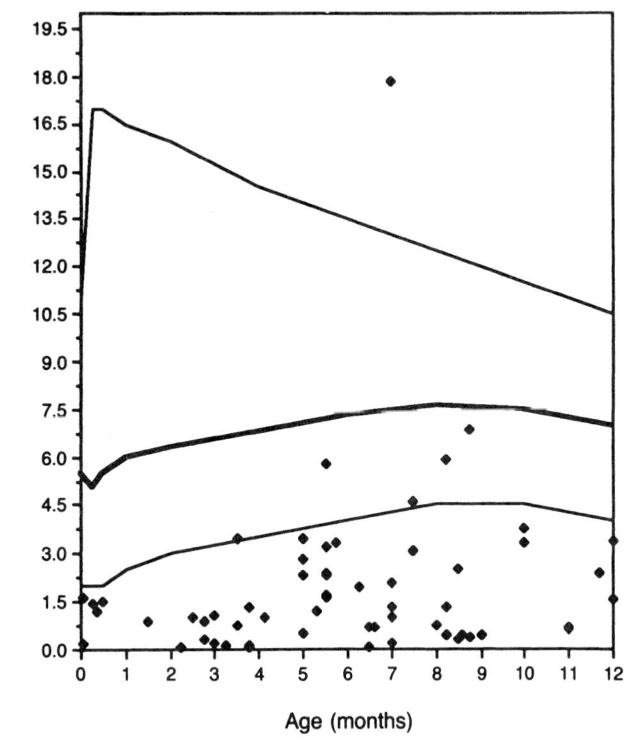

FIGURE 46–2. Absolute lymphocyte counts in 59 infants with severe combined immunodeficiency disease (SCID). The light lines indicate the normal 95% confidence limits, and the heavy line indicates the normal mean. (Normative data from Altman PL: Blood leukocyte values: man. In Dittmer DS (ed.): Blood and Other Body Fluids. Federation of American Societies for Experimental Biology, Washington, DC, 1961, pp 125–126. Adapted from Gossage DL, Buckley RH: Prevalence of lymphocytopenia in severe combined immunodeficiency. N Engl J Med 323:1422, 1990. Copyright (1990), Massachusetts Medical Society. All rights reserved.)

Typically, all SCID patients have very small thymuses (<1 g), which usually fail to descend from the neck, contain few thymocytes, and lack corticomedullary distinction and Hassall's corpuscles. Despite profound thymocyte depletion in SCID patients, thymic epithelium appears histologically normal. We know from the outcomes of bone marrow stem cell transplantation that these tiny thymuses can effect normal T-cell development. Both the follicular and paracortical areas of the peripheral lymph nodes are depleted of lymphocytes in SCID patients. Tonsils, adenoids, and Peyer's patches are absent or extremely underdeveloped.

TABLE 46–3
SCID: GENETIC DIVERSITY IN 98 PATIENTS

Adenosine deaminase deficiency	16 (16%)
Janus kinase 3 deficiency	6 (6%)
Cartilage-hair hypoplasia	1 (1%)
Reticular dysgenesis	1 (1%)
Other autosomal recessive defects	18 (18%)
X-linked due to γ_c mutations	40 (41%)
Unknown type (all males)	16 (16%)

Molecular Basis

The abnormal gene in XSCID was mapped by RFLP analysis to the Xq13 region[99] and identified as the gene encoding the common gamma chain (γ_c) shared by several cytokine receptors, including those for IL-2, IL-4, IL-7, IL-9, and IL-15.[88, 100] The author has examined the intrinsic capacity of

XSCID B cells to isotype switch and to produce IgE when cultured with anti-CD40 and IL-4 in vitro and found that they are capable of both, albeit with lesser amounts of IgE than with normal B cells.[85] Carriers can be detected by demonstration of the presence of nonrandom X-chromosome inactivation in T lymphocytes.[98] Results of X-chromosome inactivation studies had suggested that the genetic defect affects XSCID B-lineage cells, as well as those of NK and T lineage.[30, 135] The finding that the mutated gene results in faulty signaling through several cytokine receptors explains how multiple cell types can be affected by a single mutation (see Fig. 46–1).[42, 87, 106, 132]

Treatment and Prognosis

Unless immunologic reconstitution can be achieved through immunocompetent tissue transplants or germ-free isolation can be carried out, death usually occurs before the patient's first birthday and almost invariably before the second. Replacement therapy with IVIG fails to halt the progressively downhill course of SCID.[15] Conversely, transplantation of bone marrow cells from HLA-identical or haploidentical donors has resulted in correction of the immunologic defect in a large number of these patients, with more than 345 known long-term survivors.[12]

AUTOSOMAL DEFECTS FOR WHICH THE MOLECULAR BASES ARE KNOWN

AUTOSOMAL RECESSIVE SEVERE COMBINED IMMUNODEFICIENCY DISEASE

This was the first described of the SCID syndromes, reported initially by Swiss workers in 1958.[59] This pattern of inheritance is less common in the United States than in Europe (see Table 46–3).[121] The mutated genes on autosomal chromosomes have been identified in two forms of SCID, ADA deficiency and Jak3 deficiency.

Autosomal Recessive Severe Combined Immunodeficiency Disease Due to Adenosine Deaminase Deficiency

An absence of the enzyme ADA has been observed in approximately 15% of patients with SCID (see Table 46–3).[64] Patients with ADA deficiency have the same clinical problems of susceptibility to opportunistic bacterial, viral, and parasitic diseases described for XSCID and the same susceptibility to GVHD from allogeneic T cells in blood products or bone marrow. However, there are certain distinguishing clinical features of ADA deficiency, including the presence of rib cage abnormalities similar to a rachitic rosary and multiple skeletal abnormalities of chondro-osseous dysplasia on radiographic examination; these occur predominantly at the costochondral junctions, at the apophyses of the iliac bones, and in the vertebral bodies.

IMMUNOLOGIC DEFECTS

Such patients usually have a much more profound lymphopenia than do infants with other types of SCID, with mean absolute lymphocyte counts of approximately 500/mm^3, and they rarely have elevated percentages of B or NK cells. They have normal NK function and generally have excellent B-cell function after T-cell function is effected by bone marrow transplantation without pretransplant chemotherapy.[16] ADA deficiency affects primarily T-cell function, which is absent, as in all of the other forms of SCID. In further contrast to infants with other types of SCID, however, a few ADA-deficient patients have been found to have rare Hassall's corpuscles in their thymuses and changes suggestive of early thymic differentiation.

MOLECULAR BASIS

The gene encoding ADA was mapped to chromosome 20q13-ter, cloned, and sequenced. The ADA deficiency caused by mutations in this gene results in marked accumulations of adenosine, 2′-deoxyadenosine, and 2′-O-methyladenosine. The latter directly or indirectly lead to lymphocyte toxicity, which causes the immunodeficiency. Adenosine and deoxyadenosine are apparent suicide inactivators of the enzyme S-adenosylhomocysteine (SAH) hydrolase, resulting in the accumulation of SAH. SAH is a potent inhibitor of virtually all cellular methylation reactions.

TREATMENT AND PROGNOSIS

As with other types of SCID, ADA deficiency can be cured by HLA-identical or haploidentical T-cell–depleted bone marrow transplantation, which remains the treatment of choice.[12, 16, 17] Enzyme replacement therapy with polyethylene glycol–modified bovine ADA (PEG-ADA) administered subcutaneously once weekly has resulted in both clinical and immunologic improvement in more than 30 ADA-deficient patients.[63] However, the immunocompetence achieved is not nearly as effective as that with bone marrow transplantation. In view of this, PEG-ADA therapy should not be initiated if bone marrow transplantation is contemplated, because it will confer graft-rejection capability upon the infant. ADA deficiency is the first genetic defect in which gene therapy was attempted; the latter has not been very successful thus far.[7]

Autosomal Recessive Severe Combined Immunodeficiency Disease Due to Jak3 Deficiency

SCID patients with this defect resemble all other types in their susceptibility to infection and to GVHD from allogeneic T cells. However, they have lymphocyte characteristics most closely resembling those of patients with XSCID, including an elevated percentage of B cells and very low percentages of T and NK cells. Because Jak3 is the only signaling molecule known to be associated with γ_c, it was a candidate gene for mutations leading to autosomal recessive SCID not due to ADA deficiency. Thus far, ten patients have been identified who lack Jak3 (see Table 46–3).[76, 107] Like XSCID patients, they have very low or no NK activity. Even after successful T-cell reconstitution by transplantation of haploidentical stem cells, they fail to develop NK cells. Moreover, as with XSCID patients, they fail to develop normal B-cell function post-transplantation, despite their high number of B cells.

The reason for their failure to develop NK cells or B-cell function is unknown but is thought to be related to the defective function of the multiple types of cytokine receptors that share γ_c and its primary signal transducer, Jak3.

CD8 LYMPHOCYTOPENIA DUE TO ZAP 70 DEFICIENCY

Patients with this condition present during infancy with severe, recurrent, often fatal infections similar to those of SCID patients. Six cases have been reported, and a majority are Mennonites.[4, 48] They have normal or elevated numbers of blood T and B cells and low to elevated serum immunoglobulin concentrations. Their blood lymphocytes exhibit normal expression of the T-cell surface antigens CD3 and CD4, but CD8+ cells are almost totally absent. These CD4+ T cells fail to respond to mitogens or to allogeneic cells in vitro or to generate cytotoxic T lymphocytes. By contrast, NK activity is normal. The thymus of one patient exhibited normal architecture; there were normal numbers of CD4:CD8 double positive thymocytes but an absence of CD8 single positive thymocytes.

This condition has been shown to be due to mutations in the gene encoding Zap 70, a non-src family protein-tyrosine kinase important in T-cell signaling.[4, 48] The gene has been localized to chromosome 2q12. The hypothesis as to why there are normal numbers of CD4+ T cells is that thymocytes can use the other member of the same tyrosine kinase family, Syk, to facilitate positive selection of CD4+ cells. In addition, there is a stronger association of Lck with CD4+ than with CD8+ cells. Syk is present at fourfold higher levels in thymocytes than in peripheral T cells, possibly accounting for the lack of normal responses by the CD4+ blood T cells.

PURINE NUCLEOSIDE PHOSPHORYLASE DEFICIENCY

Clinical Features

Nearly 40 patients with cellular immunodeficiency with immunoglobulins (CID) have been found to have PNP deficiency.[77] The term CID is used to distinguish patients with low but not absent T-cell function from those with SCID. Although both ADA and PNP are purine salvage pathway enzymes, PNP deficiency does not lead to as severe an immunodeficiency as in ADA deficiency. In further contrast to ADA deficiency, no characteristic physical or skeletal abnormalities have been noted in PNP deficiency. Deaths have occurred from generalized vaccinia, varicella, lymphosarcoma, and GVHD mediated by T cells from nonirradiated allogeneic blood or bone marrow. Two thirds of patients have had neurologic abnormalities ranging from spasticity to mental retardation. One third of patients developed autoimmune diseases, the most common of which is autoimmune hemolytic anemia. Idiopathic thrombocytopenic purpura and systemic lupus erythematosus have also been reported.

Immunologic Defects

Most patients have normal or elevated serum concentrations of all classes of immunoglobulins, although there are exceptions. Like patients with ADA deficiency, PNP-deficient patients are profoundly lymphopenic, with absolute lymphocyte counts usually less than 1,000/mm^3. Analyses of lymphocyte subpopulations with monoclonal antibodies have demonstrated a marked deficiency of T cells and T-cell subsets but increased numbers of cells with NK phenotype and function. T-cell function is low but not absent and is variable with time.

Molecular Basis

The gene encoding PNP is on chromosome 14q13.1 and has been cloned and sequenced. A variety of mutations have been found in the PNP gene in patients with PNP deficiency. In contrast to patients with ADA deficiency, serum and urinary uric acid are markedly deficient, because PNP is needed to form the urate precursors, hypoxanthine and xanthine. Unlike most patients with CID, the thymuses of PNP-deficient patients have had occasional Hassall's corpuscles at postmortem examination, reminiscent of some patients with ADA deficiency. Prenatal diagnosis is possible.

Treatment and Prognosis

Attempts to correct the immunologic and enzymatic deficiencies of PNP-deficient patients by enzyme replacement or deoxycytidine therapy have not been successful. This condition is invariably fatal in childhood unless immunologic reconstitution can be achieved. Bone marrow transplantation is the treatment of choice but has thus far been successful in only three such patients. Gene therapy may be available in the future.

DEFECTIVE EXPRESSION OF THE T-CELL RECEPTOR–CD3 COMPLEX (Ti-CD3)

The first type of this disorder was found in two male siblings in a Spanish family.[3] The proband presented with severe infections and died at 31 months of age with autoimmune hemolytic anemia and viral pneumonia. His lymphocytes had responded poorly to mitogens and to anti-CD3 in vitro and could not be stimulated to develop cytotoxic T cells. However, his antibody responses to protein antigens had been normal, indicating normal T helper cell function. His 12-year-old brother is healthy but has almost no CD3-bearing T cells and has IgG2 deficiency similar to his sibling. The defect in this family was shown to be due to mutations in the CD3γ chain (see Fig. 3–4).[3]

The second type of this disorder was diagnosed in a 4-year-old French boy who had recurrent *Haemophilus influenzae* pneumonia and otitis media in early life but is now healthy. He has a partial defect in expression of CD3-Ti, and thus the percentage of CD3+ cells is about half normal but the level of expression is markedly decreased. His T cells do not proliferate in response to anti-CD3 or anti-CD2, nor do they express the IL-2 receptor or have normal calcium influx following these treatments. However, they do respond normally to stimulation with anti-CD28 or antigens, such as tetanus.[126] The defect has been shown to be due to two independent CD3ε gene mutations, leading to defective CD3ε chain synthesis and preventing normal association and membrane expression of the TCR/CD3 complex.[118]

DEFECTIVE EXPRESSION OF MHC ANTIGENS

There are two main forms: class I MHC antigen deficiency (bare lymphocyte syndrome) and class II MHC antigen deficiency.[72]

MHC Class I Antigen Deficiency

The isolated deficiency of MHC class I antigens is rare, and the resulting immunodeficiency is much milder than in SCID, contributing to a later age of presentation. Sera from affected patients contain normal quantities of class I MHC antigens and β_2-microglobulin, but class I MHC antigens are not detected on any cells in the body. There is a deficiency of CD8+ but not of CD4+ T cells. Two siblings from a Moroccan family presented with relatively late-onset recurrent, severe bacterial pulmonary infections and were found to have a nonsense mutation in one of two genes within the MHC locus on chromosome 6 that encode the antigenic peptide transporter protein known as TAP.[35, 45] The genes are designated *TAP1* and *TAP2*; the affected siblings had a nonsense mutation in *TAP2*. Both siblings had a deficiency of CD8+ cells and lacked MHC class I antigens on their lymphocytes. TAP functions to transport antigenic peptides from the cytoplasm across the Golgi apparatus membrane to join the α chain of MHC class 1 antigens and β_2-microglobulin, which are then assembled into an MHC class I complex that can then move to the cell surface. If the assembly of the complex cannot be completed because there is no antigenic peptide, the MHC class I complex is destroyed in the cytoplasm.

MHC Class II Antigen Deficiency

Many affected with this autosomal recessive syndrome are of North African descent.[72] Patients with the different genetic forms of this condition present with persistent diarrhea in early infancy. The latter is often associated with cryptosporidiosis, infections with enteroviruses (polio, Coxsackie), herpes or other viral agents, and oral candidiasis. They also experience bacterial pneumonia, pneumocystis, and septicemia. Nevertheless, their immunodeficiency is not as severe as in SCID, as evidenced by their failure to develop BCG-osis or GVHD from nonirradiated blood transfusions.[72]

IMMUNOLOGIC DEFECTS

MHC class II–deficient patients have a very low number of CD4+ T cells but normal or elevated numbers of CD8+ T cells. Lymphopenia is only moderate. The MHC class II antigens, HLA-DP, HLA-DQ, and HLA-DR, are undetectable on blood B cells and monocytes, even though B cells are present in normal number. The patients are nevertheless hypogammaglobulinemic due to impaired antigen-specific responses caused by the absence of these antigen-presenting molecules. In addition, MHC antigen–deficient B cells fail to stimulate allogeneic cells in mixed leukocyte culture and present antigen poorly.

Lymphocyte proliferation studies show normal responses to mitogens but no response to antigens. The thymus and other lymphoid organs are severely hypoplastic. The associated defects of both B- and T-cell immunity and HLA expression emphasize the important biologic role for HLA determinants in effective immune cell cooperation.

MOLECULAR BASES

MHC class II antigen deficiency is genetically heterogeneous, with three different complementation groups having been reported. The molecular defects thus far described affect the regulation of expression of class II genes rather than causing abnormalities of the coding regions for HLA-DP, HLA-DQ, or HLA-DR, and they do not segregate with any MHC genes on chromosome 6. Two different molecular defects have been defined, both of which cause impairment in the coordinate expression of MHC class II molecules on the surface of B cells and macrophages.[103] In one, there is a mutation in the gene on chromosome 2 that encodes a protein called RFX5, a promoter protein that binds to the MHC class II gene promoter region X-box.[102, 103] In the other, there is a mutation in the gene on chromosome 15 that encodes a novel MHC class II transactivator (CIITA), which coordinates the binding of proteins to the MHC class II gene promoter region.[103, 120] Twins with this syndrome were reported who did not have a regulatory defect in the coordinated control of MHC class II gene transcription.[139] Low levels of HLA-DRα- and HLA-DRβ-chain protein were detected. Cellular and humoral immune responses were induced in both infants after tetanus immunization. Both have had a benign clinical course.

LEUKOCYTE ADHESION DEFICIENCIES 1 AND 2 (LAD1 AND LAD2)

Leukocyte Adhesion Deficiency 1

This condition is due to mutations in the gene on chromosome 21q22.3 encoding the 95 kD β subunit (CD18) shared by three adhesive heterodimers: LFA-1 on B, T, and NK lymphocytes; complement receptor type 3 (CR3) on neutrophils, monocytes, macrophages, eosinophils, and NK cells; and p150,95, complement receptor type 4 (CR4) (see Table 46–2).[55, 71] The α chains of these three molecules (encoded by genes on chromosome 16) are not expressed because of the abnormal β chain. Those so affected have histories of delayed separation of the umbilical cord, omphalitis, gingivitis, recurrent skin infections, repeated otitis media, pneumonia, peritonitis, perianal abscesses, and impaired wound healing. Severe, widespread, and life-threatening bacterial and fungal infections account for the high mortality. Affected people do not have increased susceptibility to viral infections or malignancy.

Blood neutrophil counts are usually significantly elevated, even when no infection is present, owing to an inability of the cells to adhere firmly to vascular endothelium and migrate out of the intravascular compartment. All cytotoxic lymphocyte functions are markedly impaired because of a lack of the adhesion protein LFA-1. Deficiency of LFA-1 also interferes with immune cell interaction and immune recognition. CR3 binds fixed iC3b fragments of C3 and β-glucans; its absence causes abnormal phagocytic cell adherence and chemotaxis and a reduced respiratory burst with phagocytosis. Deficiencies of these glycoproteins can be screened for by cytofluorography of blood leukocytes with monoclonal antibodies to CD18 or any of the following commercially available monoclonal antibodies: anti-Mac-1, OKM1, Leu 15, or anti-Mo1, which react with the α chain of CR3, or with anti-Leu-M5, specific for the α chain of p150,95. Since the CD18 gene has been cloned and sequenced, this disorder is another candidate for gene therapy.[71]

Leukocyte Adhesion Deficiency 2

Another adhesion molecule deficiency state has been described, which is due to the absence of the neutrophil sialyl-Lewis X ligand of E-selectin on vascular endothelium.[49] This disorder was discovered in two unrelated Israeli boys, aged 3 and 5 years, each the offspring of consanguineous parents. Both have severe mental retardation, short stature, a distinctive facial appearance, and the Bombay (hh) blood phenotype and are secretor and Lewis negative. They both have had recurrent severe bacterial infections similar to those seen in patients with LAD1, including pneumonia, peridontitis, otitis media, and localized cellulitis. Similar to patients with LAD1, their infections have been accompanied by marked leukocytosis (30,000 to 150,000/mm^3) but an absence of pus formation at sites of recurrent cellulitis. In vitro studies revealed a marked defect in neutrophil motility. Because the genes for the red cell H antigen and secretor status encode for distinct α1,2-fucosyltransferases and the synthesis of sialyl-Lewis X requires an α1,3-fucosyltransferase, the authors have postulated a general defect in fucose metabolism as the basis for this disorder.[49]

ATAXIA-TELANGIECTASIA

Clinical Features

Ataxia-telangiectasia (AT) is a complex combined immunodeficiency syndrome with associated neurologic, endocrinologic, hepatic, and cutaneous abnormalities.[58, 137] The most prominent clinical features are progressive cerebellar ataxia, oculocutaneous telangiectasias, chronic sinopulmonary disease, a high incidence of malignancy, and variable humoral and cellular immunodeficiency. Ataxia typically becomes evident soon after the child begins to walk and progresses until he or she is confined to a wheelchair, usually by the age of 10 to 12 years. The telangiectasias develop between 3 and 6 years of age. Recurrent, usually bacterial, sinopulmonary infections occur in roughly 80% of these patients, but common viral exanthems have not usually resulted in untoward sequelae. Fatal varicella, however, occurred in one of the author's patients.

Immunologic Defects

The most frequent humoral immunologic abnormality is the selective absence of IgA, found in 50% to 80% of these patients. Hypercatabolism of IgA is also known to occur.[58] IgE concentrations are usually low, and the IgM may be of the low molecular weight variety. IgG2 or total IgG may be decreased. Specific antibody titers may be decreased or normal. In vivo, there is impaired (but not absent) cell-mediated immunity, as evidenced by delayed cutaneous anergy and prolonged allograft survival. In vitro tests of lymphocyte function have generally shown moderately depressed proliferative responses to T- and B-cell mitogens. There are moderately reduced percentages of CD3+ and CD4+ T cells, with normal or increased percentages of CD8+ T cells and elevated numbers of gamma/delta T-cell receptor-positive cells. Studies of immunoglobulin synthesis have shown both helper T-cell and intrinsic B-cell defects. The thymus is hypoplastic, exhibits poor organization, and is lacking in Hassall's corpuscles.

Cells from patients, as well as those from heterozygous carriers, have increased sensitivity to ionizing radiation, defective DNA repair, and frequent chromosomal abnormalities.[58, 125] The sites of chromosomal breakage involve chromosomes 7 and 14 in more than 50% of cases. The break points involve the genes that code for the T-cell receptor and immunoglobulin heavy chains, most likely accounting for the combined T- and B-cell abnormalities seen. Inversion of chromosome 7-inv (p14q35) is the most frequent rearrangement seen, although others involve chromosome 14 and the X chromosome. These rearrangements may be clonal and may either be stable or undergo malignant transformation. The malignancies reported in this condition have usually been of the lymphoreticular type, but adenocarcinoma and other forms have also been seen. There is also an increased incidence of malignancy in unaffected relatives.

Molecular Basis

Inheritance of AT follows an autosomal recessive pattern. The mutated gene (ATM) responsible for this defect was mapped by RFLP analysis to the long arm of chromosome 11 (11q22–23) and was cloned.[58, 108, 125] The gene product is similar to phosphatidylinositol-3′ (PI-3) kinases involved in mitogenic signal transduction, meiotic recombination, and cell cycle control.

Treatment and Prognosis

No satisfactory definitive treatment has been found.[58] The prognosis is exceedingly poor for patients with this condition, although a number have reached adulthood. The most common causes of death are lymphoreticular malignancy and neurologic incapacitation due to progressive cerebellar disease.

THYMIC HYPOPLASIA

Clinical Features

Thymic hypoplasia (DiGeorge syndrome) results from dysmorphogenesis of the third and fourth pharyngeal pouches during early embryogenesis, leading to hypoplasia or aplasia of the thymus and parathyroid glands.[65] Other structures forming at the same age are also frequently affected, resulting in anomalies of the great vessels (right-sided aortic arch), esophageal atresia, bifid uvula, congenital heart disease (atrial and ventricular septal defects), a short philtrum of the upper lip, hypertelorism, an antimongoloid slant to the eyes, mandibular hypoplasia, and low-set, often notched ears. The diagnosis is usually first suggested by the presence of hypocalcemic seizures during the neonatal period. Since the original description of the syndrome, it has become apparent that a variable degree of hypoplasia is more frequent than total aplasia of the thymus and parathyroid glands.

Some children have little trouble with life-threatening infections and grow normally; such patients are often referred to as having partial DiGeorge syndrome. Those with complete DiGeorge syndrome may resemble patients with SCID in their susceptibility to infections with opportunistic pathogens (fungi, viruses, and *P. carinii*) and to GVHD from nonirradiated blood transfusions. There are many clinical similarities between DiGeorge syndrome, velocardiofacial syndrome (VCFS), fetal alcohol syndrome, and retinoic acid toxicity.[65]

Immunologic Defects

Patients with DiGeorge syndrome are usually only mildly lymphopenic.[68] However, T-cell numbers are decreased; as a result, there is a relative increase in the percentage of B cells. B-cell function is impaired only to the extent of needing helper T cells. Immunoglobulin concentrations are usually normal, except for IgE, which is sometimes elevated; IgA may be low.[68] Monoclonal antibody analyses of blood lymphocytes have demonstrated that, despite a decreased number of CD3+ T cells, there are usually normal proportions of CD4 and CD8+ cells. Responses of blood lymphocytes following mitogen stimulation, like the intradermal delayed hypersensitivity response, have been absent, reduced, or normal, depending on the degree of thymic deficiency, suggesting that the T lymphocytes that are present are intrinsically normal. Thymic tissue, when found, contains Hassall's corpuscles and a normal density of thymocytes; corticomedullary distinction is present. Lymphoid follicles are usually present, but lymph node paracortical areas and thymus-dependent regions of the spleen show variable degrees of depletion.

Molecular Basis

DiGeorge syndrome has occurred in both males and females. It is rarely familial, but three cases of apparent autosomal dominant inheritance have been reported. Microdeletions of specific DNA sequences from chromosome 22q11.2, the DiGeorge chromosomal region (DGCR), have been shown in a majority of patients.[39, 46] A disrupted candidate gene has been identified in this region.[19]

Treatment and Prognosis

No immunologic treatment is needed for the partial form. If the patients do not have a severe cardiac lesion, they have few clinical problems, except that some experience seizures and developmental delay. Because of variability in the severity of the immunodeficiency, it is difficult to evaluate claimed benefits of fetal thymus transplantation.[25] Transplantation of HLA-DR matched cultured mature thymic epithelial explants has successfully reconstituted the immune function of some such infants. Three patients have experienced immunologic reconstitution following unfractionated HLA-identical bone marrow transplantation.[60]

AUTOSOMAL RECESSIVE CHRONIC GRANULOMATOUS DISEASE

Clinical Features

Patients with AR-CGD have infections similar to those in patients with X-CGD, namely, suppurative adenopathy, pneumonia, cutaneous and visceral abscesses, and osteomyelitis due to infections with catalase-positive bacterial organisms or fungi.

Immunologic Defects

As in X-CGD, the immunologic defects in the three forms of AR-CGD lie solely in inability of the phagocyte to kill ingested organisms. In the autosomal forms, defects exist in different components of the electron transport chain from that in X-CGD. However, as in the latter condition, a diagnosis of AR-CGD is made by demonstrating an inability of neutrophils from the patient to undergo a respiratory burst following phagocytosis or PMA stimulation, as measured by chemiluminescence, NBT dye reduction, or a flow cytometry dye test. Unlike X-CGD, however, carriers of AR-CGD cannot be detected by the latter methods.

Molecular Bases

Approximately 5% of patients with AR-CGD have a defect in the 22 kD subunit ($p22^{phox}$), or light chain, of the cytochrome b245 heterodimer, encoded by a gene on chromosome 16q24 (Table 46–4). However, in a majority of patients with AR-CGD, cytochrome b245 is intact.[34] Evaluation of cytochrome-positive AR-CGD patients led to the identifica-

TABLE 46–4
CHRONIC GRANULOMATOUS DISEASE: GENETIC DIVERSITY

X-linked due to mutations in cytochrome b245 heavy chain (gp91^{phox}) gene: 65%
Autosomal recessive due to mutations in cytosolic protein (gp67^{phox}) gene: 5%
Autosomal recessive due to mutations in cytosolic protein (gp47^{phox}) gene: 25%
Autosomal recessive due to mutations in cytochrome b245 light chain (gp22^{phox}) gene: 5%

tion of cytosolic proteins that participate in the respiratory burst. A majority (25% of all patients with CGD) lack a 47 kD phosphoprotein (gp47^{phox}) encoded by a gene on chromosome 7q11.23. In approximately 5% of patients, a 65 kD protein (gp67^{phox}) encoded by a gene on 1q25 is missing (see Table 46–4). Delineation of the specific molecular abnormality in any given patient with AR-CGD requires molecular techniques.

Treatment and Prognosis

The treatment and prognoses for AR-CGD are the same as for X-CGD.

AUTOSOMAL DEFECTS FOR WHICH THE MOLECULAR BASIS IS NOT KNOWN

COMMON VARIABLE IMMUNODEFICIENCY

Clinical Features

Common variable immunodeficiency (CVID), also known as acquired hypogammaglobulinemia or idiopathic late-onset immunoglobulin deficiency, may appear similar clinically in many respects to XLA.[32] The kinds of infections experienced and bacterial etiologic agents involved are generally the same for the two defects, except that echovirus meningoencephalitis is less common in patients with CVID.[79] However, patients with CVID generally have a later age of onset of infections, which may be somewhat less severe than in XLA. The sexes are almost equally affected with CVID.

CVID has been variably associated with a sprue-like syndrome, nodular follicular lymphoid hyperplasia of the intestine, thymoma, alopecia areata, hemolytic anemia, gastric atrophy, achlorhydria, and pernicious anemia. In addition, such patients have frequent thyroid abnormalities, vitiligo, keratoconjunctivitis sicca, and arthritis. The arthritis in such patients is usually mild to moderate in severity. Synovial biopsies have revealed capillary proliferation but an absence of lining cell hyperplasia and only variable infiltration by chronic inflammatory cells. Frequent complications include giardiasis (seen far more often here than in X-linked agammaglobulinemia), bronchiectasis, gastric carcinoma, lymphoreticular malignancy, and cholelithiasis. Lymphoid interstitial pneumonia, pseudolymphoma, amyloidosis, and noncaseating granulomata of the lungs, spleen, skin, and liver have also been seen. There is a 438-fold increase in lymphomas in affected women in the fifth and sixth decades.[33]

Immunologic Defects

The serum immunoglobulin and antibody deficiencies in CVID may be as profound as in the X-linked disorder. Despite normal numbers of circulating immunoglobulin-bearing B lymphocytes and the presence of lymphoid cortical follicles, blood lymphocytes from CVID patients do not differentiate into immunoglobulin-producing cells when stimulated with pokeweed mitogen in vitro, even when cocultured with normal T cells (Table 46–5).[32] From this it was concluded that the defect is intrinsic to the B cell.[32] However, studies have shown that CVID B cells can be stimulated both to isotype switch and to synthesize and secrete immunoglobulin when stimulated with anti-CD40 plus IL-4 or IL-10.[89]

T cells and T-cell subsets are usually present in normal percentages, but depressed T-cell function has been reported.[92, 119] Mitogen-activated T cells from some CVID patients were also found to be deficient in expression of genes for several lymphokines while retaining a normal capacity to proliferate.[47] In addition, a subset of patients with CVID was reported to have significantly depressed (but not absent) expression of CD40 ligand mRNA and surface protein in their activated T lymphocytes, suggesting that inefficient signaling by poorly expressed CD40 ligand on their T cells could account for failure of their B cells to differentiate.[50] Tonsils and lymph nodes are either normal sized or enlarged, and splenomegaly occurs in approximately 25% of patients with CVID. There is a tendency to autoantibody formation, and there are several cases of lupus erythematosus converting to CVID.[6] CVID rarely has been reported to resolve transiently or permanently when some such patients acquired HIV infection.[140]

Pathogenesis

Because this disorder occurs in first-degree relatives of patients with selective IgA deficiency (A Def) and in some

TABLE 46–5
CHARACTERISTICS OF SOME ANTIBODY DEFICIENCY DISORDERS

Disorder	Functional Deficiencies	Molecular Defect
X-linked agammaglobulinemia	B cells and their products	Mutations in Bruton tyrosine kinase
Common variable (acquired) hypogammaglobulinemia	Antibody	Unknown, ?in MHC class III region
Selective IgA deficiency	IgA antibody	Unknown, ?in MHC class III region
X-linked immunodeficiency with hyper-IgM	IgG and IgA antibodies	Mutations in CD40 ligand on activated T cells; non–X-linked types have intrinsic B-cell defects
Transient hypogammaglobulinemia of infancy	None: immunoglobulins low, but antibodies present	Unknown
Antibody deficiency with near-normal immunoglobulins	Antibody	Unknown; ?related to CVID
X-linked lymphoproliferative disease	Anti-EBV nuclear antigen antibody	Unknown, affects B cells; ?also T cells

patients with A Def later become panhypogammaglobulinemic, it had long been suspected that these diseases have a common genetic basis.[5] The high incidences of abnormal immunoglobulin concentrations, autoantibodies, autoimmune disease, and malignancy in families of both types of patients also suggested a shared hereditary influence.[57] This concept is supported by the finding of a high incidence of C4-A gene deletions and C2 rare gene alleles in the class III MHC region in individuals with either A Def[57, 109] or CVID,[66, 131] suggesting that there is a susceptibility gene in this region on chromosome 6 (see Tables 46–2 and 46–5). However, the abnormal gene has not yet been identified.

These studies also have shown that a small number of HLA haplotypes are shared by individuals affected with CVID and A Def, with at least one of two particular haplotypes being present in 77% of those affected.[131] In one large family with 13 members, two had A Def and three had CVID.[5] All of the immunodeficient patients in the family had at least one copy of an MHC haplotype shown to be abnormally frequent in A Def and CVID: HLA-DQB1 *0201, HLA-DR3, C4B-Sf, C4A-deleted, G11-15, Bf-0.4, C2a, HSP70-7.5, TNF-α5, HLA-B8, and HLA-A1. However, four immunologically normal members of the pedigree also possessed this haplotype, indicating that its presence alone is not sufficient for expression of the defects.[5] Environmental factors, particularly drugs such as phenytoin, have been suspected as providing the triggers for disease expression in individuals with the permissive genetic background.

Treatment and Prognosis

The treatment of patients with CVID is essentially the same as that for XLA.[15] The prognosis is reasonably good, unless severe autoimmune disease or malignancy develops.[33]

SELECTIVE IgA DEFICIENCY

An isolated absence or near absence (<10 mg/dl) of serum and secretory IgA is thought to be the most common well-defined immunodeficiency disorder, a frequency of 1 in 333 being reported among some blood donors.[10, 24]

Clinical Features

Although this disorder has been observed in apparently healthy individuals, it is commonly associated with ill health.[24] As would be expected when there is a deficiency of the major immunoglobulin of external secretions, infections occur predominantly in the respiratory, gastrointestinal, and urogenital tracts.[10] Bacterial agents responsible are essentially the same as in other types of antibody deficiency syndromes. There is no clear evidence that patients with this disorder have an undue susceptibility to viral agents.

Similar to CVID, there is a frequent association of A Def with collagen vascular and autoimmune diseases.[57] These include systemic lupus erythematosus, rheumatoid arthritis, ankylosing spondylitis, dermatomyositis, pernicious anemia, thyroiditis, diabetes mellitus, Addison's disease, Sjögren's syndrome, chronic active hepatitis, idiopathic thrombocytopenic purpura, Coombs'-positive hemolytic anemia, pulmonary hemosiderosis, regional enteritis, and ulcerative colitis. A sprue-like syndrome has occurred in adults with A Def, which may or may not respond to a gluten-free diet. In further similarity to patients with CVID, there is an increased incidence of malignancy.[93]

Immunologic Defects

Serum concentrations of other immunoglobulins are usually normal in patients with selective IgA deficiency, although IgG2 subclass deficiency may be present and IgM (often monomeric) may be elevated.[97] Children with IgA deficiency vaccinated with killed poliovirus intranasally produced local IgM and IgG antibodies. Several of them later contracted rubella, and IgM and IgG antirubella antibodies were found in their secretions during convalescence. Of possible etiologic and great clinical significance is the presence of antibodies to IgA in the sera of as high as 44% of patients with selective IgA deficiency.[24] IgG anti-IgA antibodies can fix complement and remove IgA from the circulation 4 to 20 times faster than the normal catabolic rate for IgA.

A number of IgA-deficient patients have had severe or fatal anaphylactic reactions after intravenous administration of blood products containing IgA, and anti-IgA antibodies (particularly IgE anti-IgA antibodies) have been implicated.[20] For this reason, only five times washed (in 200 ml volumes) normal donor erythrocytes or blood products from other IgA-absent individuals should be administered to these patients. Patients with A Def also frequently have IgG antibodies against cow milk and ruminant serum proteins. These antiruminant antibodies often falsely detect IgA in immunoassays that employ goat (but not rabbit) antisera.[10] A high incidence of autoantibodies has also been noted.[57]

Pathogenesis

The basic defect leading to selective IgA deficiency is unknown. In 10 of 11 IgA-deficient individuals studied, more than 80% of the IgA-bearing B cells also coexpressed surface IgM and IgD (similar to cord blood B cells) compared with less than 10% triple isotype-bearing IgA B cells in healthy persons, suggesting an IgA isotype-specific B-cell maturation arrest.[28] In others, treatment with phenytoin, D-penicillamine, sulfasalazine, or gold has been suspected as being the cause. The occurrence of IgA deficiency in both males and females and in families is consistent with autosomal inheritance; in some families, this appears to be dominant with variable expressivity. As already noted, this defect occurs in pedigrees with CVID patients, and genetic studies suggest that the susceptibility genes for these two defects may reside in the MHC class II region on chromosome 6 (see Table 46–5).[5, 131]

Treatment and Prognosis

Currently there is no treatment for A Def beyond the vigorous treatment of specific infections with appropriate antimicrobial agents. IVIG, which is greater than 99% IgG, is not indicated because most A Def patients make IgG antibodies normally.[15] Moreover, many IVIG preparations contain sufficient IgA to cause anaphylactic reactions.[15, 20] Even if serum IgA could be replaced (a dangerous thing to attempt), it could not be transported into the external secretions, because the latter is an active process involving only locally and endogenously produced IgA. In some A Def patients, the defect may spontaneously disappear with time, whereas in others it may evolve into CVID.[10]

IMMUNODEFICIENCY WITH THYMOMA

Patients with immunodeficiency with thymoma are adults who almost simultaneously develop recurrent infections, panhypogammaglobulinemia, deficits in cell-mediated immunity, and benign thymoma (see Table 46–5).[137] They may also have eosinophilia or eosinopenia, aregenerative or hemolytic anemia, agranulocytosis, thrombocytopenia, or pancytopenia. Antibody formation is poor, and progressive lymphopenia develops, although percentages of Ig-bearing B lymphocytes are usually normal. The thymomas are predominantly of the spindle cell variety, although other types of benign and malignant thymic tumors have also been seen.

IgG SUBCLASS DEFICIENCY

A number of patients have been reported to have deficiencies of one or more subclasses of IgG, despite normal total IgG serum concentrations.[97] Most of those with absent or very low concentrations of IgG2 have been patients with selective IgA deficiency. IgG2 deficiency would be suspected if patients had repeated problems with encapsulated bacterial pathogens, since a majority of the antipolysaccharide antibody molecules are of the IgG2 isotype.[112] However, it is difficult to know the biologic significance of the multiple moderate deficiencies of IgG subclasses that have been reported, particularly when completely asymptomatic individuals have been described who totally lacked IgG1, IgG2, IgG4, or IgA1 owing to gene deletion.[75]

A number of healthy children have been described who had low levels of IgG2 but normal responses to polysaccharide antigens when immunized.[114] Conversely, patients with the Wiskott-Aldrich syndrome, who have a profound antipolysaccharide antibody deficiency, have normal levels of IgG2.[84] Even in patients without this syndrome who have recurrent infections, marked deficiencies of antipolysaccharide antibodies have been noted in the presence of normal concentrations of IgG2.[2] When children with low IgG2 subclass levels who had histories of frequent infections were studied in depth, they were found to have broader and varied patterns of immunologic dysfunction, suggesting that they may have been in the process of evolving into frank CVID.[115]

From these observations, it can be concluded that IgG subclass measurement is not very helpful in the general assessment of immune function. Such assays provide no information about the patient's capacity to produce specific antibodies to protein, polysaccharide, or viral antigens. Moreover, there is considerable variability in values reported for the different subclasses when aliquots of the same serum sample are tested in different commercial laboratories. Thus when abnormalities are detected, one is still left with the more relevant question of what the patient's capacity is to make specific antibodies to protein and polysaccharide antigens. IVIG should not be given to patients with IgG subclass deficiency unless they are known to have a deficiency of antibodies to a broad array of antigens.[15]

ANTIBODY DEFICIENCY WITH NEAR-NORMAL IMMUNOGLOBULINS

Only scattered reports have appeared in the literature describing patients with apparently normal T-cell function and normal or near-normal immunoglobulin concentrations but deficient antibody responses (see Table 46–5).[2] Such individuals have recurrent pyogenic infections similar to those with agammaglobulinemia. Indeed, with time, serum immunoglobulin concentrations may decline to levels seen in CVID patients. This has led to speculation that this condition may be an early stage of CVID. Blood group antibody titers are frequently absent, and diphtheria, tetanus, *H. influenzae*, and pneumococcal antibody titers are significantly lower than normal. Primary immune responses to bacteriophage ϕX174 are far below the normal range. Because these patients do not have the ability to produce antibodies normally, they are candidates for monthly IVIG infusions.[15]

TRANSIENT HYPOGAMMAGLOBULINEMIA OF INFANCY

Unlike patients with XLA or CVID, patients with transient hypogammaglobulinemia of infancy (THI) can synthesize antibodies to human type A and B erythrocytes and diphtheria and tetanus toxoids.[127] Often these antibodies are found in normal titer by the time the infant is 6 to 11 months of age, long before their immunoglobulin concentrations become normal (see Table 46–5). Lymphocyte studies in vitro show no abnormalities in the percentages of cells in the different subpopulations or in their responses to mitogens. THI has been found in pedigrees of patients with other immune defects, including CVID and SCID. The finding of only 11 cases of THI among more than 10,000 patients whose sera were sent to the author for immunoglobulin studies over a 12-year period suggests that this is not a common entity.[127]

IVIG therapy is not indicated in this condition.[15] In addition to the known risk of inducing antiallotype antibodies, passively administered IgG antibodies could suppress endogenous antibody formation to infectious agents in the same manner that RhoGAM suppresses anti-D antibodies in Rh-negative mothers delivering Rh-positive infants. IVIG may also suppress immune responses by Fc-receptor interaction and the induction of anti-idiotypic antibodies.

CELLULAR IMMUNODEFICIENCY WITH IMMUNOGLOBULINS

Clinical Features

Like patients with PNP deficiency, other patients with CID also present during infancy with recurrent or chronic pulmonary infections, failure to thrive, oral or cutaneous candidiasis, chronic diarrhea, recurrent skin infections, gram-negative sepsis, urinary tract infections, or severe varicella, even though they have normal levels of PNP.[137]

Immunologic Defects

Serum immunoglobulins may be normal or elevated for all classes, but selective IgA deficiency, marked elevation of IgE, and elevated IgD levels have been found in some cases. Although antibody-forming capacity has been impaired in a majority, it has not been absent and has been apparently normal in roughly one third of the reported cases. Moreover, plasma cells are usually abundant in the lamina propria and lymph nodes. Other findings include neutropenia and eosinophilia. Studies of cellular immune function have shown delayed cutaneous anergy to ubiquitous antigens in all such patients, lymphopenia, and extremely low but not absent lymphocyte proliferative responses to mitogens, antigens, and allogeneic cells in vitro.

This syndrome is the primary immunodeficiency disorder most likely to be confused with AIDS in the pediatric age group. Patients with CID, however, have profound deficiencies of CD3+ T cells but usually normal proportions of CD4- and CD8-positive cells in contrast to patients with AIDS, who characteristically have a selective deficiency of CD4+ cells. Peripheral lymphoid tissues demonstrate paracortical lymphocyte depletion. The thymuses are very small and have a paucity of thymocytes and usually no Hassall's corpuscles. However, again in contrast to AIDS, thymic epithelium is intact.

Pathogenesis and Treatment

An autosomal recessive pattern of inheritance is usually seen. The molecular basis is unknown. Although patients with this disorder have been successfully reconstituted by matched sibling bone marrow transplants, most other forms of therapy have been unsuccessful. Despite the profound cellular immunodeficiency, however, patients with CID usually survive longer than do infants with SCID.

SEVERE COMBINED IMMUNODEFICIENCY

In addition to the patients with SCID for whom the molecular bases are known, there are many others (30%–40%) for whom the underlying cause has not yet been identified (see Table 46–3). These infants resemble all of the others in their extreme susceptibility to infections, profoundly deficient T and B lymphocyte functions, and death in infancy unless immunologic reconstitution can be achieved. However, there is heterogeneity in the phenotypes of circulating lymphocyte populations in infants with SCID of unknown type.[16, 26, 52, 64, 121] The lymphocyte phenotypes of some resemble those of patients with XSCID or Jak3-deficient SCID. In others, all or most of the circulating lymphocytes are large granular lymphocytes with NK-cell phenotype and function, similar to the lymphocyte phenotype of the SCID mouse.[111, 117]

SEVERE COMBINED IMMUNODEFICIENCY WITH LEUKOPENIA (RETICULAR DYSGENESIS)

In 1959, identical twin male infants were described who exhibited a total lack of both lymphocytes and granulocytes in their peripheral blood and bone marrow. Seven of eight infants reported with this defect died between 3 and 119 days of age from overwhelming infections; the eighth underwent complete immunologic reconstitution from a bone marrow transplant.[137] Mature normal-appearing granulocytes (although markedly reduced in number) were noted in three patients, and a normal percentage of E rosette T cells in the cord blood of a fourth patient, arguing against a total failure of stem cell differentiation in this defect. Despite the normal percentage of T cells in the latter patient's cord blood, however, the cells failed to give an in vitro proliferative response to mitogens. The thymus glands of all have weighed less than 1 g, no Hassall's corpuscles have been present, and few or no thymocytes have been seen. An autosomal recessive mode of inheritance seems most likely, but the molecular basis of this condition is not yet known.

CARTILAGE-HAIR HYPOPLASIA

Clinical Features

In 1965, an unusual form of short-limbed dwarfism with frequent and severe infections was reported among the Pennsylvania Amish; non-Amish cases have since been described.[95, 137] Features include short and pudgy hands with redundant skin, metaphyseal chondrodysplasia, hyperextensible joints of hands and feet but an inability to extend the elbows completely, and fine, sparse light hair and eyebrows. These features led to the name cartilage-hair hypoplasia (CHH). Radiographically, the bones show scalloping and sclerotic or cystic changes in the metaphyses. In contrast to ADA deficiency, in which the predominant changes are in the apophyses of the iliac bones, ribs, and vertebral bodies, the chondrodysplasia in CHH principally affects the limbs. Severe and often fatal varicella infections, progressive vaccinia, and vaccine-associated poliomyelitis have been observed. Associated conditions include deficient erythrogenesis, Hirschsprung's disease, and an increased risk of malignancies.

Immunologic Defects

Three patterns of immune dysfunction have emerged: defective antibody-mediated immunity, defective cellular immunity (most common form), and SCID. NK cells, however, are increased in number and function.

Pathogenesis, Treatment, and Prognosis

CHH is an autosomal recessive condition. The defective gene has been mapped to chromosome 9p21–p13 in Amish and Finnish families.[123] The gene has not been identified, however, so the fundamental molecular abnormality is unknown. In vitro studies have shown decreased numbers of T cells and defective T-cell proliferation, owing to an intrinsic defect related to the G1 phase, resulting in a longer cell cycle for individual cells.[94, 95] This abnormality also occurs in fibroblasts from these patients and in in vitro colony formation in erythroid, myeloid, and megakaryocytic lineages, suggesting a common cell proliferation defect in CHH.[69] Bone marrow transplantation has resulted in immunologic reconstitution in some CHH patients with the SCID phenotype. Those with milder types of immune deficiency have lived to adulthood, some even to old age.

HYPERIMMUNOGLOBULINEMIA E SYNDROME

Clinical Features

The hyperimmunoglobulinemia E (hyper-IgE) syndrome is a relatively rare primary immunodeficiency syndrome characterized by recurrent severe staphylococcal abscesses of the skin, lungs, and viscera and markedly elevated levels of serum IgE.[14, 18] The disorder was first reported by the author and her coworkers in two young boys in 1972.[18] She has since evaluated over 30 patients with the condition, and many other examples have been reported.[14] These patients all have histories of staphylococcal abscesses involving the skin, lungs, joints, and other sites from infancy (Fig. 46–3). Persistent pneumatoceles develop as a result of their recurrent pneumonias. The pruritic dermatitis that occurs is not typical atopic eczema and does not always persist. Respiratory allergic symptoms are usually absent.

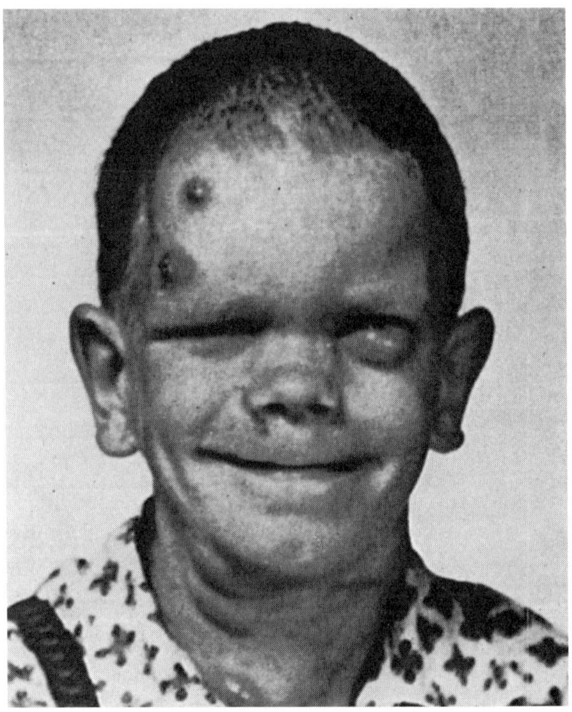

FIGURE 46–3. Patient with hyper-IgE syndrome, showing multiple abscesses of face and neck and coarse facial features. (From Buckley RH, Wray BB, Belmaker EZ: Extreme hyperimmunoglobulinemia E and undue susceptibility to infection. Pediatrics 49:59, 1972. Reproduced by permission of Pediatrics.)

Immunologic Defects

Laboratory features include exceptionally high serum IgE; elevated serum IgD; usually normal concentrations of IgG, IgA, and IgM; pronounced blood and sputum eosinophilia; abnormally low anamnestic antibody responses to booster immunizations; and poor antibody and cell-mediated responses to neoantigens. In vitro studies have shown normal percentages of CD2+, CD3+, CD4+, and CD8+ lymphocytes. There is no increase in the percentage of IgE-bearing B lymphocytes. Most have normal lymphocyte proliferative responses to mitogens but very low or absent responses to antigens or allogeneic cells from family members. Blood, sputum, and histologic sections of lymph nodes, spleen, and lung cysts show striking eosinophilia. Hassall's corpuscles and normal thymic architecture were observed at postmortem examination of one patient.

Phagocytic cell ingestion, metabolism, and killing and total hemolytic complement activity have been normal in all patients. Variable defects of mononuclear or polymorphonuclear chemotaxis have been present in some but not all patients and hence are not the basic problem in these patients.[14]

Pathogenesis and Genetics

The fundamental problem in this condition is unknown, despite intense study. Possibly related to these patients' impaired anamnestic antibody responses, impaired antigen-specific T-cell responses, and abnormal mixed leukocyte response is the observation by the author of a decreased percentage of T cells with the memory (CD45RO) phenotype in the blood of these patients. Paradoxically, B cells from these patients do not produce as much IgE as do normal or atopic B cells when they are cultured with IL-4 and anti-CD40 in vitro (Fig. 46–4).[23] The latter suggests that the B cells had already been exposed to IL-4 in vivo and were no longer sensitive to it, because they had already isotype switched in vivo. Due to the very short half-life of IL-4, serum levels cannot be detected. Therefore, it has been difficult to prove that the condition is caused by excessive IL-4 production. The presence of increased numbers of eosinophils in blood, sputum, and tissues suggests that some of the pathology seen may be eosinophil mediated. The fact that both men and women have been affected, as have members of succeeding generations, suggests an autosomal dominant form of inheritance with incomplete penetrance.

Treatment and Prognosis

The most effective management for this condition consists of long-term therapy with a penicillinase-resistant penicillin, with the addition of other antibiotics or antifungal agents as required for specific infections, and appropriate thoracic surgery for superinfected pneumatoceles or those persisting beyond 6 months. IFN-γ therapy has been tried but had no clinical benefit.[70] If the diagnosis is made early and antistaphylococcic antibiotic therapy is rendered in treatment doses continuously, the prognosis is good. The prognosis is poor in those who are not so treated, primarily because

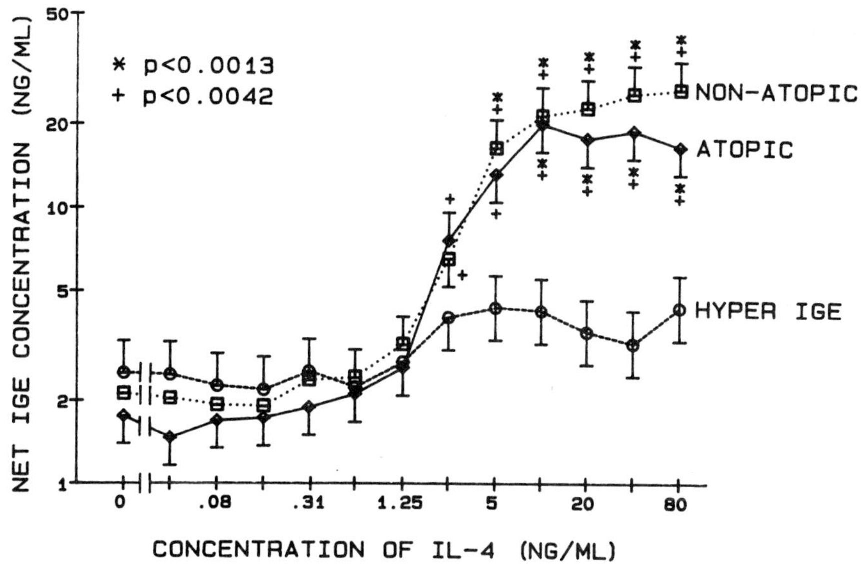

FIGURE 46–4. Geometric mean IL-4–induced IgE production by mononuclear cells from nine patients with the hyper-IgE syndrome compared with that by mononuclear cells from nine atopic patients and nine normal controls. Cultures were incubated for 18 days in Iscove's medium. Significantly less ($p<0.0013$) IgE was produced by B cells from hyper-IgE patients than by B cells from normal or atopic donors. (From Claassen JL, Levine AD, Schiff SE, et al: Mononuclear cells from patients with the hyper IgE syndrome produce little IgE when stimulated with recombinant interleukin 4 in vitro. J Allergy Clin Immunol 88:713, 1991.)

of recurrent staphylococcal pneumonia with pneumatocele formation. Three patients are known to have died of lymphoreticular malignancy, and three have experienced cryptococcal meningitis.

T-CELL ACTIVATION DEFECTS

These conditions are characterized by the presence of normal or elevated numbers of blood T cells that appear phenotypically normal but fail to proliferate or produce cytokines in response to stimulation with mitogens, antigens, or other signals delivered to the T-cell antigen receptor (TCR) due to defective signal transduction from the TCR to intracellular metabolic pathways.[22] These patients have problems similar to those of other T-cell–deficient individuals. Some with severe T-cell activation defects may resemble SCID patients clinically.

DEFECTIVE CYTOKINE PRODUCTION

Two main types of defects in cytokine production are known. The first is a selective inability to produce IL-2. In the two reported cases, patients had severe recurrent infections in infancy.[43, 133] The IL-2 gene was present in both, but no IL-2 message or protein was produced. Other T-cell cytokines were produced normally. The second type was seen in a single patient who also presented during infancy with severe recurrent infections and failure to thrive.[21] She had defective transcription of several lymphokine genes, including IL-2, IL-3, IL-4, and IL-5, possibly due to abnormal binding of nuclear factor of activated T cells (NF-AT) to response elements in the IL-2 and IL-4 enhancers.[21] She was treated with recombinant IL-2 with some clinical improvement. The molecular defects have not been identified in either type of cytokine deficiency.

CHÉDIAK-HIGASHI SYNDROME

This rare disease is characterized by oculocutaneous albinism and susceptibility to recurrent respiratory tract and other types of infections.[122] The hallmark of the disease is giant lysosomal granules, not only in neutrophils but also in most of the other cells of the body, including melanocytes, neural Schwann cells, renal tubular cells, gastric mucosa, pneumatocytes, hepatocytes, Langerhans cells of the skin, and adrenal cells. The granules in neutrophils are positive for peroxidase, acid phosphatase, and esterase. The abnormal lysosomes are unable to fuse with phagosomes, so that ingested bacteria cannot be lysed normally. In addition, there is nearly complete absence of NK-cell activity as a result of abnormal lysosomal granule function.

Abnormal chemotaxis has also been reported, and there is evidence of a profound alteration of the cytoskeleton of the neutrophils. There are reports of a decreased number of centriole-associated microtubules and abnormalities in tubulin tyrosinolation. The molecular defect in this autosomal recessive disorder was identified as being due to mutations in *LYST*—a gene on chromosome 1, at position q43. *LYST* encodes a protein with a carboxy-terminal prenylation motif and multiple potential phosphorylation sites. It is postulated to be a relay-integrating cellular signal response coupling protein.[5a] Approximately 85% of the patients develop an accelerated phase of the disease, with fever, jaundice, hepatosplenomegaly, lymphadenopathy, pancytopenia, bleeding diathesis, and neurologic changes. Once the accelerated phase occurs, the disease is usually fatal within 30 months, unless successful treatment with an unfractionated HLA-identical bone marrow transplant following cytoreductive conditioning can be accomplished.[12, 122]

COMPLEMENT COMPONENT DEFICIENCIES

Inherited deficiencies in almost all of the complement proteins have been discovered, and they have been summarized.[51] Complete deficiencies of complement proteins are rare, attesting to their importance in host defense. All but one of these proteins are encoded by genes on autosomal chromosomes; however, the gene encoding properdin is on the X chromosome. Complete deficiencies of the complement proteins (except properdin) require homozygous mutations, that is, they are autosomal recessive traits. Heterozygosity for complement protein deficiencies, relatively common, is not associated with a higher incidence of infections or autoimmune disease than that found in the general population. Complement protein deficiencies can be conveniently divided into those that involve the alternative pathway, the classic pathway, or late components of complement.[56]

CLINICAL FEATURES

Patients with either classic pathway or later component deficiencies tend to do relatively well, except when stressed by septicemia or any infection with a high-grade pathogen. By contrast, humans deficient in alternative pathway factors tend to have more frequent and severe infections, particularly early in life, because the alternative pathway is a very important host defense mechanism during the first exposure to an infectious agent. After such patients develop antibodies to the infectious agents, they become protected in part. A high incidence of autoimmune disease is also seen in patients with inherited complement deficiencies, possibly due to inadequate removal of immune complexes from the circulation because of a lack of opsonins derived from the complement pathway. These circulating immune complexes may then localize in the kidneys and other tissues and cause inflammatory reactions.[56]

C1q, C1r, C1s, C2, AND C4 DEFICIENCIES

Deficiencies of the classic pathway complement proteins C1q, C1r, C1s, C2, and C4 tend to result in less infection susceptibility than do those of the alternative pathway.[56] However, each of the classic pathway component deficiencies may be associated with an increased susceptibility to infections with encapsulated bacteria. The most common inherited complement deficiency is an absence of C2, affecting approximately 1 in 10,000 individuals. Clinically normal individuals with C2 deficiency have been described, but some have had recurrent septicemia, meningitis, or osteomyelitis.

Patients with each of the classic pathway component deficiencies may have symptoms resembling discoid lupus or systemic lupus erythematosus (SLE). In patients with the SLE-like syndrome, disease begins at an early age, with marked photosensitivity and a low but clinically significant incidence of renal disease; they may have negative ANA titers. Patients with C2 or C4 deficiency also have increased incidences of dermatomyositis, vasculitis, cold urticaria, inflammatory bowel disease, Hodgkin's disease, or Henoch-Schönlein purpura.[56] The association of CVID and IgA deficiency with rare alleles or deletions of C2 and C4 has been mentioned in those sections.

C3 DEFICIENCY

In general, alternative pathway defects lead to recurrent infections with high-grade encapsulated pathogens, including pneumonia, otitis media, and sinusitis. One example is C3 deficiency, which leads to abnormal classic pathway activation as well. It is a rare disorder due to either hypercatabolism or hyposynthesis of C3. Patients with hypercatabolism have absent C3b inactivator (factor I deficiency). The consequence is lack of control of the alternative complement pathway convertase so that C3b is not converted to C3bi. The enzyme PC3bBb acts to deplete native C3, so whatever C3 antigen remains is in the form of C3b. C3 deficiency is often associated with repeated infections of both low- and high-grade pathogens.[56] Deficiency of factor H, the cofactor for factor I and C4b inactivator, presents similarly but affects C4 as well as C3.

Properdin deficiency is an X-linked disorder that should be suspected in male patients with recurrent systemic meningococcal disease, systemic infection with a meningococcal strain of low virulence, or recurrent pyogenic infections. Properdin is a glycoprotein that up-regulates the alternative pathway of complement by stabilizing the C3b-Bb complex. More than 50 cases of properdin deficiency have been recorded in various ethnic origins. There are three subtypes, based on immunochemical and functional measurements of properdin: type I or total deficiency, type II or partial deficiency, and type III due to a dysfunctional molecule. Various point mutations were found in the properdin gene at Xp11.3–p21.1 in individuals with type I and type II properdin deficiency, showing for the first time that the properdin structural gene and properdin deficiency locus are one and the same.[136]

DEFICIENCIES OF TERMINAL COMPLEMENT COMPONENTS

Hereditary deficiency of one of the terminal complement components (C5, C6, C7, or C8) may be present in healthy individuals or is associated with an increased incidence of infection or autoimmune disease. Deficiencies of these late complement components lead to a high incidence of disseminated neisserial infections. Mere opsonization of neisserial organisms appears to be inadequate for their elimination, since C3, the principal opsonin generated by complement, is normal in these patients; lysis is required for the destruction of these organisms. Patients with C5 deficiency have been reported to have SLE and associated Raynaud's phenomenon, arthritis, diffuse membranoproliferative glomerulonephritis, recurrent pneumococcal pneumonia, and/or disseminated gonococcal infection. Deficiencies of C6, C7, or C8 have been associated with recurrent meningococcal meningitis or disseminated gonococcal infection. C7 and C8 deficiencies may also be associated with rheumatic diseases, such as SLE or rheumatoid arthritis.[56] C9-deficient persons may also have an increased incidence of neisserial infections; otherwise, most are normal.

DIAGNOSIS

A diagnosis of a congenital complement deficiency should be considered in anyone with recurrent infections with high-grade encapsulated organisms, with or without the concomitant presence of an autoimmune disease. The diagnosis of deficient terminal complement components should be suspected in any patient with recurrent neisserial infections. Total hemolytic complement determination (CH50) may be used as a screening procedure for all inherited complement protein deficiencies; in such patients, CH50 levels are extremely low or nondetectable. Individual complement components will need to be specifically quantified by specialized (usually research) laboratories.

TREATMENT

There is no specific treatment for complement component abnormalities. Acute infections are treated with antibiotics. Long-term management of these disorders often includes prophylactic antibiotics. Complement components cannot yet be replaced. In one patient with C3 deficiency, the infusion of 500 mL of normal plasma restored all complement-mediated functions for up to 17 days.[56] However, this approach is not likely to be useful as ongoing therapy, since in all likelihood an antibody would be induced to the missing protein. All of the complement protein and regulator genes have been sequenced, and many have been cloned. Gene therapy is therefore a potential future form of therapy for individuals with inborn errors of the complement system.

INTRAUTERINE DIAGNOSIS AND CARRIER DETECTION

Intrauterine diagnoses of ADA and PNP deficiencies can be made by enzyme analyses of amnion cells (fresh or cultured) obtained before 20 weeks of gestation.[64, 77] Diagnoses of several X-linked defects by RFLP studies of the X chromosome can be performed on amnion cells from male infants whose mothers have been identified as carriers and who are heterozygous for informative DNA polymorphisms.[101] Diagnosis of enzyme-normal SCID or other severe T-cell deficiencies, MHC class I or II antigen deficiencies, CGD, or Wiskott-Aldrich syndrome (by platelet size) can be made by appropriate tests of phenotype or function on small samples of blood obtained by fetoscopy at 18 to 22 weeks of gestation. In the case of those disorders for which the defective gene has been cloned and cDNA probes are available, the diagnosis can be made by analyses of chorionic villus samples obtained during the first trimester.

Carriers of ADA and PNP deficiency can be detected by quantitative enzyme analyses of blood samples. Carriers of XLA, XSCID, or the Wiskott-Aldrich syndrome can be identified by techniques designed to detect nonrandom X-chromosome inactivation in one or more blood cell lineages.[98, 134] These methods can be used successfully even when only one member of a family (or no previous members) has been affected, since neither of these methods depends on linkage analysis.

TREATMENT

The principal modes of therapy for the primary immunodeficiency disorders include protective isolation, use of antibiotics for the eradication or prevention of bacterial and fungal infections, and attempted replacement of missing humoral or cellular immunologic functions. The complexities of both the immunodeficiency diseases and their treatment emphasize the need for all such patients to be evaluated in centers where detailed studies of immune function can be conducted before therapy is selected or begun.

ANTIBODY DEFICIENCY DISORDERS

Judicious use of antibiotics and regular administration of antibodies are the only treatments that have proved effective for this group of disorders. Patients with agammaglobulinemia, X-linked immunodeficiency with hyper-IgM, antibody deficiency with near-normal immunoglobulins, Wiskott-Aldrich syndrome, and all forms of SCID are candidates for immunoglobulin replacement therapy.[15] The most common form of replacement therapy currently is with immune serum globulin (ISG) modified for safe intravenous use.

All seven IVIG preparations in the United States approved by the Food and Drug Administration consist primarily of IgG antibodies, with small amounts of antibodies of the other classes.[15] Experience suggests that 400 mg/kg/month of IVIG permits achievement of trough IgG levels close to the normal range. HIV is inactivated by the ethanol used in preparations of ISG and IVIG; current preparations are also free of hepatitis viruses. Systemic reactions to IVIG may occur but are rarely true anaphylactic reactions. Anaphylactic reactions caused by IgE antibodies (in the patient) to IgA (in the IVIG preparation), however, may occur in patients with common variable immunodeficiency who have absent serum IgA.[20] All newly diagnosed patients with the latter defect should be screened for anti-IgA antibodies through the American Red Cross before undergoing IVIG therapy. If such antibodies are detected, IVIG therapy may still be possible by use of IVIG containing almost no IgA, such as Gammagard (Baxter-Hyland) or a similar preparation from the American Red Cross.[15]

Immunoglobulin replacement therapy is contraindicated in patients with selective absence of serum and secretory IgA, owing to the high frequency of anti-IgA antibodies and because these patients usually have normal quantities of IgG antibodies.[15, 20, 24] IVIG should not be given to infants with transient hypogammaglobulinemia because it could suppress their innate capacity to form antibodies. There is no indication for the use of gammaglobulin therapy in patients with IgG subclass deficiencies unless they have been shown to have a broad defect in antibody-forming capacity. It is futile to give it to patients with low IgG, owing to protein-losing states, such as congenital lymphangiectasia or other protein-losing enteropathies.[15]

CELLULAR IMMUNODEFICIENCY

The only adequate therapy for patients with severe forms of cellular immunodeficiency is immunologic reconstitution by means of immunocompetent tissue transplantation.[12] Bone marrow cells that are MHC compatible or haploidentical with the recipient are the treatment of choice. There is no convincing evidence that whole fetal thymic gland transplants have caused immunologic reconstitution in patients with the complete DiGeorge syndrome. However, unfractionated HLA-identical bone marrow transplantation has been effective in all three complete DiGeorge syndrome patients in whom this was attempted.[60] For those unfortunate infants with complete DiGeorge syndrome who have no HLA-identical siblings, transplantation of HLA-DR matched, cultured mature thymic epithelial explants offers some promise. Such transplants have successfully reconstituted the immune function of three such infants.

The major risk to the recipient from transplants of bone marrow or fetal tissues is that of GVHD. The development of techniques to deplete all post-thymic T cells from donor marrow, however, has permitted the safe and successful use of haploidentical (half matched) bone marrow cells for the correction of SCID.[12] These techniques have employed initial incubation with soybean lectin followed by two rosette-depletion steps with sheep erythrocytes (the most successful approach) or incubation with monoclonal antibodies to T cells in the presence of fresh complement. Both methods enrich the final cell suspension for stem cells.

To date, more than 385 infants with SCID who lacked an HLA-identical donor have been treated with T-cell–depleted haploidentical parental bone marrow, with usually little or no GVHD; approximately 60% survive with successful immune reconstitution (see Table 46–3).[12] Patients with less severe forms of cellular immunodeficiency reject such grafts unless they are treated with immunosuppressive agents before transplantation. Even then, there has been a high incidence of resistance to engraftment of T-cell–depleted, half-matched marrow cells.[54]

Several patients with Wiskott-Aldrich syndrome and other forms of partial cellular immunodeficiency have been treated successfully with (usually HLA-identical) bone marrow transplants after immunosuppression.[12] Cytokine therapy has been considered a potential approach to the treatment of patients who for various reasons have not been candidates for bone marrow transplantation. Limited clinical trials with recombinant IL-2 (or T-cell growth factor) therapy have shown beneficial effects in some patients with T-cell activation defects. Finally, it is entirely possible that most of those genetic defects for which the molecular defects have been identified and the genes have been cloned and sequenced, such as ADA and PNP deficiencies, XLA, X-linked hyper-IgM, Wiskott-Aldrich syndrome, XSCID, Jak3 deficiency, ZAP 70 deficiency, LAD, and CGD, will be correctable by gene therapy in the future.

REFERENCES

1. Allen RC, Armitage RJ, Conley ME, et al: CD40 ligand gene defects responsible for X-linked hyper IgM syndrome. Sci 259:990, 1993.
2. Ambrosino DM, Umetsu DT, Siber GR, et al: Selective defect in the antibody response to *Haemophilus influenzae* type b in children with recurrent infections and normal IgG subclass levels. J Allergy Clin Immunol 81:1175, 1988.
3. Arnaiz-Villena A, Timon M, Corell A, et al: Brief report: primary immunodeficiency caused by mutations in the gene encoding the CD3− subunit of the T lymphocyte receptor. N Engl J Med 327:529, 1992.
4. Arpaia E, Shahar M, Dadi H, et al: Defective T cell receptor signaling and CD8+ thymic selection in humans lacking zap-70 kinase. Cell 76:947, 1994.
5. Ashman RF, Schaffer FM, Kemp JD, et al: Genetic and immunologic analysis of a family containing five patients with common variable immune deficiency or selective IgA deficiency. J Clin Immunol 12:406, 1992.
5a. Barbosa MDFS, Nguyen QA, Tchernev VT, et al: Identification of the homologous beige and Chédiak-Higashi syndrome genes. Nature 382:262, 1996.
6. Baum CG, Chiorazzi N, Frankel S, et al: Conversion of systemic lupus erythematosus to common variable hypogammaglobulinemia. Am J Med 87:449, 1989.
7. Blaese RM, Culver KW: Gene therapy for primary immunodeficiency disease. Immunodeficiency Rev 3:329, 1992.
8. Bortin MM, Rimm AA: Severe combined immunodeficiency disease. Characterization of the disease and results of transplantation. JAMA 238:591, 1977.
9. Bruton OC: Agammaglobulinemia. Pediatrics 9:722, 1952.
10. Buckley RH: Clinical and immunologic features of selective IgA deficiency. In Bergsma D, Good RA, Finstad J, et al (eds): Immunodeficiency in Man and Animals. Sinauer Associates, Inc, Stamford, CT, 1975, p 134.
11. Buckley RH: Breakthroughs in the understanding and therapy of primary immunodeficiency. Pediatr Clin North Am 41:665, 1994.
12. Buckley RH: Bone marrow transplantation in primary immunodeficiency. In Rich RR (ed): Clinical Immunology: Principles and Practice. Vol II. CV Mosby, St Louis, 1995, p 1813.
13. Buckley RH, Rowlands DR: Allergy rounds: agammaglobulinemia, neutropenia, fever and abdominal pain. J Allergy Clin Immunol 51:308, 1973.
14. Buckley RH, Sampson HA: The hyperimmunoglobulinemia E syndrome. In Franklin EC (ed): Clinical Immunology Update. Elsevier North-Holland, Inc, New York, 1981, p 147.
15. Buckley RH, Schiff RI: The use of intravenous immunoglobulin in immunodeficiency diseases. N Engl J Med 325:110, 1991.
16. Buckley RH, Schiff SE, Sampson HA, et al: Development of immunity in human severe primary T cell deficiency following haploidentical bone marrow stem cell transplantation. J Immunol 136:2398, 1986.
17. Buckley RH, Schiff SE, Schiff RI, et al: Haploidentical bone marrow stem cell transplantation in human severe combined immunodeficiency. Semin Hematol 30:92, 1993.
18. Buckley RH, Wray BB, Belmaker EZ: Extreme hyperimmunoglobulinemia E and undue susceptibility to infection. Pediatrics 49:59, 1972.
19. Budarf ML, Collins J, Gong W, et al: Cloning a balanced translocation associated with DiGeorge syndrome and identification of a disrupted candidate gene. Nature Genetics 10:269, 1995.
20. Burks AW, Sampson HA, Buckley RH: Anaphylactic reactions after gamma globulin administration in patients with hypogammaglobulinemia. N Engl J Med 314:560, 1986.
21. Castigli E, Pahwa R, Good RA, et al: Molecular basis of a multiple lymphokine deficiency in a patient with severe combined immunodeficiency. Proc Natl Acad Sci USA 90:4728, 1993.
22. Chatila T, Wong R, Young M, et al: An immunodeficiency characterized by defective signal transduction in T lymphocytes. N Engl J Med 320:696, 1989.
23. Claassen JL, Levine AD, Schiff SE, et al: Mononuclear cells from patients with the hyper IgE syndrome produce little IgE when stimulated with recombinant interleukin 4 in vitro. J Allergy Clin Immunol 88:713, 1991.
24. Clark JA, Callicoat PA, Brenner NA: Selective IgA deficiency in blood donors. Am J Clin Pathol 80:210, 1983.
25. Cleveland WW, Fogel BJ, Brown WR, et al: Fetal thymus transplant in a case of DiGeorge's syndrome. Lancet 2:1211, 1968.
26. Conley ME, Buckley RH, Hong R, et al: X-linked severe combined immunodeficiency. Diagnosis in males with sporadic severe combined immunodeficiency and clarification of clinical findings. J Clin Invest 85:1548, 1990.
27. Conley ME, Burks AW, Herrod HG, et al: Molecular analysis of X-linked agammaglobulinemia with growth hormone deficiency. J Pediatr 119:392, 1991.
28. Conley ME, Cooper MD: Immature IgA B cells in IgA deficient patients. N Engl J Med 305:495, 1981.
29. Conley ME, Larche M, Bonagura VR, et al: Hyper IgM syndrome associated with defective CD40-mediated B cell activation. J Clin Invest 94:1404, 1994.
30. Conley ME, Lavoie A, Briggs C, et al: Nonrandom X chromosome

inactivation in B cells from carriers of X chromosome-linked severe combined immunodeficiency. Proc Natl Acad Sci USA 85:3090, 1988.
31. Conley ME, Sweinberg SK: Females with a disorder phenotypically identical to X-linked agammaglobulinemia. J Clin Immunol 12:139, 1992.
32. Cunningham-Rundles C: Clinical and immunologic analyses of 103 patients with common variable immunodeficiency. J Clin Immunol 9:22, 1989.
33. Cunningham-Rundles C, Siegal FP, Cunningham-Rundles S, et al: Incidence of cancer in 98 patients with common varied immunodeficiency. J Clin Immunol 7:294, 1987.
34. Curnutte JT: Molecular basis of the autosomal recessive forms of chronic granulomatous disease. Immunodeficiency Rev 3:149, 1992.
35. de la Salle H, Hanau D, Fricker D: Homozygous human TAP peptide transporter mutation in HLA class I deficiency. Science 265:237, 1994.
36. de Saint Basile G, Fraser NJ, Craig IW, et al: Close linkage of hypervariable marker DXS255 to disease locus of Wiskott-Aldrich syndrome. Lancet 2:1319, 1989.
37. de Weers M, Verschuren MCM, Kraakman MEM, et al: The Bruton's tyrosine kinase gene is expressed throughout B cell differentiation, from early precursor B cell stages preceding immunoglobulin gene rearrangement up to mature B cell stages. Eur J Immunol 23:3109, 1993.
38. Derry JMJ, Ochs HD, Francke U: Isolation of a novel gene mutated in Wiskott-Aldrich syndrome. Cell 78:635, 1994.
39. Desmaze C, Scambler P, Prieur M, et al: Routine diagnosis of DiGeorge syndrome by fluorescent in situ hybridization. Hum Genet 90:663, 1993.
40. Dinauer MC: Leukocyte function and nonmalignant leukocyte disorders. Curr Opin Pediatr 5:80, 1993.
41. Dinauer MC, Orkin SH, Brown R: The glycoprotein encoded by the X-linked chronic granulomatous disease locus is a component of the neutrophil cytochrome b complex. Nature 327:717, 1987.
42. Disanto JP, Dautry-Varsat A, Certain S, et al: Interleukin-2 (IL-2) receptor chain mutations in X-linked severe combined immunodeficiency disease result in the loss of high-affinity IL-2 receptor binding. Eur J Immunol 24:475, 1994.
43. Disanto JP, Keever CA, Small TN, et al: Absence of interleukin 2 production in a severe combined immunodeficiency disease syndrome with T cells. J Exp Med 171:1697, 1990.
44. Disanto JP, Markiewicz S, Gauchat J, et al: Brief report: prenatal diagnosis of X-linked hyper IgM syndrome. N Engl J Med 330:969, 1994.
45. Donato L, de la Salle H, Hanau D, et al: Association of HLA class I antigen deficiency related to a TAP2 gene mutation with familial bronchiectasis. J Pediatr 127:895, 1995.
46. Driscoll DA, Budarf ML, Emanuel BS: A genetic etiology for DiGeorge syndrome: consistent deletions and microdeletions of 22q11. Am J Hum Genet 50:924, 1992.
47. Eisenstein EM, Jaffe JS, Strober W: Reduced interleukin-2 (IL-2) production in common variable immunodeficiency is due to a primary abnormality of CD4+ T cell differentiation. J Clin Immunol 13:247, 1993.
48. Elder ME, Lin D, Clever J, et al: Human severe combined immunodeficiency due to a defect in ZAP-70, a T cell tyrosine kinase. Science 264:1596, 1994.
49. Etzioni A, Frydman M, Pollack S, et al: Brief report: recurrent severe infections caused by a novel leukocyte adhesion deficiency. N Engl J Med 327:1789, 1992.
50. Farrington M, Grosmaire LS, Nonoyama S, et al: CD40 ligand expression is defective in a subset of patients with common variable immunodeficiency. Proc Natl Acad Sci USA 91:1099, 1994.
51. Figueroa JE, Densen P: Infectious diseases associates with complement deficiencies. Clin Microbiol Rev 4:359, 1991.
52. Fischer A: Severe combined immunodeficiencies. Immunodef Rev 3:83, 1992.
53. Fischer A, Arnaiz-Villena A: Immunodeficiencies of genetic origin. Immunol Today 16:510, 1995.
54. Fischer A, Landais P, Friedrich W: European experience of bone marrow transplantation for severe combined immunodeficiency. Lancet 336:850, 1990.
55. Fischer A, Lisowska-Grospierre B, Anderson DC, et al: Leukocyte adhesion deficiency: molecular basis and functional consequences. Immunodeficiency Rev 1:39, 1988.
56. Frank MM: Complement in disease: inherited and acquired complement deficiencies. In Frank MM, Austen KF, Claman HN, et al (eds): Samters Immunologic Diseases, Vol 1. Little, Brown and Company, Boston, MA, 1994, p 489.
57. French MA, Dawkins RL: Central MHC genes, IgA deficiency and autoimmune diseases. Immunol Today 11:271, 1990.
58. Gatti RA, Boder E, Vinters HV, et al: Ataxia-telangiectasia: an interdisciplinary approach to pathogenesis. Medicine (Baltimore) 70:99, 1991.
59. Glanzmann E, Riniker P: Essentielle lymphocytophtose. Ein neues krankeitsbild aus der Sauglingspathologie. Ann Paedit 174:1, 1950.
60. Goldsobel AB, Haas A, Stiehm ER: Bone marrow transplantation in DiGeorge syndrome. J Pediatr 111:40, 1987.
61. Gossage DL, Buckley RH: Prevalence of lymphocytopenia in severe combined immunodeficiency. N Engl J Med 323:1422, 1990.
62. Grierson HL, Skare J, Hawk J, et al: Immunoglobulin class and subclass deficiencies prior to Epstein-Barr virus infection in males with X-linked lymphoproliferative disease. Am J Med Genet 40:294, 1991.
63. Hershfield MS, Buckley RH, Greenberg ML, et al: Treatment of adenosine deaminase deficiency with polyethylene glycol-modified adenosine deaminase (PEG-ADA). N Engl J Med 316:589, 1987.
64. Hirschhorn R: Adenosine deaminase deficiency. Immunodeficiency Rev 2:175, 1990.
65. Hong R: The DiGeorge anomaly. Immunodeficiency Rev 3:1, 1991.
66. Howe HS, So AKL, Farrant J, et al: Common variable immunodeficiency is associated with polymorphic markers in the human major histocompatibility complex. Clin Exp Immunol 84:387, 1991.
67. International Chronic Granulomatous Disease Cooperative Study Group: A controlled trial of interferon gamma to prevent infection in chronic granulomatous disease. N Engl J Med 324:509, 1991.
68. Junker AK, Driscoll DA: Humoral immunity in DiGeorge syndrome. J Pediatr 127:231, 1995.
69. Juvonen E, Makitie O, Makipernaa A, et al: Defective in-vitro colony formation of haematopoietic progenitors in patients with cartilage-hair hypoplasia and history of anaemia. Eur J Pediatr 154:30, 1995.
70. King CL, Gallin JI, Malech HL, et al: Regulation of immunoglobulin production in hyperimmunoglobulin E recurrent infection syndrome by interferon. Proc Natl Acad Sci USA 86:10085, 1989.
71. Kishimoto TK, Springer TA: Human leukocyte adhesion deficiency: molecular basis for a defective immune response to infections of the skin. Curr Probl Dermatol 18:106, 1989.
72. Klein C, Lisowska-Grospierre B, LeDeist F, et al: Major histocompatibility complex class II deficiency: clinical manifestations, immunologic features, and outcome. J Pediatr 123:921, 1993.
73. Kwan SP, Hagemann TL, Radtke BE, et al: Identification of mutations in the Wiskott-Aldrich syndrome gene and characterization of a polymorphic dinucleotide repeat at the DXS6940, adjacent to the disease gene. Proc Natl Acad Sci USA 92:4706, 1995.
74. Lederman HM, Winkelstein JA: X-linked agammaglobulinemia: an analysis of 96 patients. Medicine (Baltimore) 64:145, 1985.
75. Lefranc MP, Hammarstrom L, Smith CIE, et al: Gene deletions in the human immunoglobulin heavy chain constant region locus: molecular and immunological analysis. Immunol Rev 2:265, 1991.
76. Macchi P, Villa A, Gillani S, et al: Mutations of Jak-3 gene in patients with autosomal severe combined immune deficiency (SCID). Nature 377:65, 1995.
77. Markert ML: Purine nucleoside phosphorylase deficiency. Immunodeficiency Rev 3:45, 1991.
78. Mayer L, Swan SP, Thompson C: Evidence for a defect in "switch" T cells in patients with immunodeficiency and hyperimmunoglobulinemia M. N Engl J Med 314:409, 1986.
79. McKinney RE, Katz SL, Wilfert CM: Chronic enteroviral meningoencephalitis in agammaglobulinemic patients. Rev Infect Dis 9:334, 1987.
80. Milili M, Le Deist F, de Saint-Basile G, et al: Bone marrow cells in X-linked agammaglobulinemia express pre-B-specific genes (λ-like and V pre-B) and present immunoglobulin V-D-J gene usage strongly biased to a fetal-like repertoire. J Clin Invest 91:1616, 1993.
81. Mohiuddin AA, Corren J, Harbeck RJ, et al: Ureaplasma urealyticum chronic osteomyelitis in a patient with hypogammaglobulinemia. J Allergy Clin Immunol 87:104, 1991.
82. Mouy R, Fischer A, Vilmer E, et al: Incidence, severity, and prevention of infections in chronic granulomatous disease. J Pediatr 114:555, 1989.
83. Mullen CA, Anderson KD, Blaese RM: Splenectomy and/or bone

marrow transplantation in the management of the Wiskott-Aldrich syndrome: long-term follow-up of 62 cases. Blood 82:2961, 1993.
84. Nahm MH, Blaese RM, Crain MJ, et al: Patients with Wiskott-Aldrich syndrome have normal IgG2 Levels. J Immunol 137:3484, 1986.
85. Nash DR, Levine AD, Buckley RH: B cells from most patients with either X-linked (XL) or autosomal recessive (AR) forms of severe combined immunodeficiency (SCID) produce IgE and other isotypes normally when stimulated with anti-CD40 mAb and IL-4. J Allergy Clin Immunol 93:273, 1994.
86. Noelle RJ, Roy M, Shepherd DM, et al: A 39-kDa protein on activated helper T cells binds CD40 and transduces the signal for cognate activation of B cells. Proc Natl Acad Sci USA 89:6550, 1992.
87. Noguchi M, Nakamura Y, Russell SM, et al: Interleukin-2 receptor gamma chain: a functional component of the interleukin-7 receptor. Science 262:1977, 1993.
88. Noguchi M, Yi H, Rosenblatt HM, et al: Interleukin-2 receptor gamma chain mutation results in X-linked severe combined immunodeficiency in humans. Cell 73:147, 1993.
89. Nonoyama S, Farrington M, Ochs HM: Activated B cells from patients with common variable immunodeficiency proliferate and synthesize immunoglobulin. J Clin Invest 92:1281, 1993.
90. Notarangelo LN, Duse M, Ugazio AG: Immunodeficiency with hyper IgM (HIM). Immunodeficiency Rev 3:101, 1992.
91. Padayachee M, Feighery C, Finn A, et al: Mapping of the X-linked form of hyper IgM syndrome (HIGM1) to Xq26 by close linkage to HPRT. Genomics 14:551, 1992.
92. Pandolfi F, Trentin L, San Martin JE, et al: T cell heterogeneity in patients with common variable immunodeficiency as assessed by abnormal T cell subpopulations and T cell receptor gene analysis. Clin Exp Immunol 89:198, 1992.
93. Penn I: Lymphoproliferative diseases in disorders of the immune system. Cancer Detect Prev 14:415, 1990.
94. Pierce GF, Polmar SH: Lymphocyte dysfunction in cartilage hair hypoplasia. II. Evidence for a cell cycle specific defect in T cell growth. Clin Exp Immunol 50:621, 1982.
95. Polmar SH, Pierce GF: Cartilage hair hypoplasia: immunological aspects and their clinical implications. Clin Immunol Immunopathol 40:87, 1986.
96. Porter CD, Parkar MH, Levinsky RJ, et al: X-linked chronic granulomatous disease: correction of NADPH oxidase defect by retrovirus-mediated expression of gp91-phox. Blood 82:2196, 1993.
97. Preud'Homme JL, Hanson LA: IgG subclass deficiency. Immunodeficiency Rev 2:129, 1990.
98. Puck JM: Molecular and genetic basis of X-linked immunodeficiency disorders. J Clin Immunol 14:81, 1994.
99. Puck JM, Conley ME, Bailey LC: Refinement of linkage of human severe combined immunodeficiency (SCIDXI) to polymorphic markers in Xq13. Am J Hum Genet 53:176, 1993.
100. Puck JM, Deschenes SM, Porter JC, et al: The interleukin-2 receptor gamma chain maps to Xq13.1 and is mutated in X-linked severe combined immunodeficiency, SCIDX1. Hum Mol Genet 2:1099, 1993.
101. Puck JM, Krauss C, Puck SM, et al: Prenatal exclusion of X chromosome linked severe combined immunodeficiency using maternal nonrandom T cell X inactivation and linkage analysis. N Engl J Med 321:1063, 1990.
102. Reith W, Barras E, Satola S: Cloning of the major histocompatibility complex class II promoter binding protein affected in a hereditary defect in class II gene regulation. Proc Natl Acad Sci USA 86:4200, 1989.
103. Reith W, Steimle V, Mach B: Molecular defects in the bare lymphocyte syndrome and regulation of MHC class II genes. Immunol Today 16:539, 1995.
104. Remold-O'Donnell E, Rosen FS: Sialophorin (CD43) and the Wiskott-Aldrich syndrome. Immunodeficiency Rev 2:151, 1990.
105. Rosen FS, Cooper MD, Wedgwood RJ: The primary immunodeficiencies. N Engl J Med 333:431, 1995.
106. Russell SM, Keegan AD, Harada N, et al: Interleukin-2 receptor gamma chain: a functional component of the interleukin-4 receptor. Science 262:1880, 1993.
107. Russell SM, Tayebi N, Nakajima H, et al: Mutation of Jak3 in a patient with SCID: essential role of Jak3 in lymphoid development. Science 270:797, 1995.
108. Savitsky K, Bar-Shira A, Gilad S, et al: A single ataxia telangiectasia gene with a product similar to PI-3 kinase. Science 268:1749, 1995.
109. Schaffer FM, Monteiro RC, Volanakis JE, et al: IgA deficiency. Immunodeficiency Rev 3:15, 1991.
110. Schiff SE, Buckley RH: Variation in natural killer (NK) lymphocyte function among the different molecular forms of severe combined immunodeficiency (SCID). J Allergy Clin Immunol 93:273, 1994.
111. Schwarz K, Hansen-Hagge TE, Knobloch C, et al: Severe combined immunodeficiency (SCID) in man: B cell negative (B−) SCID patients exhibit an irregular recombination pattern at the Jh locus. J Exp Med 174:1039, 1991.
112. Scott MG, Shackelford PG, Briles DE, et al: Human IgG subclasses and their relation to carbohydrate antigen immunocompetence. Diag Clin Immunol 5:241, 1988.
113. Seger RA, Berthet F, Hossle JP: Chronic granulomatous disease. Pediatr Allergy Immunol 3:1, 1992.
114. Shackelford PG, Granoff DM, Madassery JV, et al: Clinical and immunologic characteristics of healthy children with subnormal serum concentrations of IgG2. Pediatr Res 27:16, 1990.
115. Shackelford PG, Granoff DM, Polmar SH, et al: Subnormal serum concentrations of IgG2 in children with frequent infections associated with varied patters of immunologic dysfunction. J Pediatr 116:529, 1990.
116. Sideras P, Smith CIE: Molecular and cellular aspects of X-linked agammaglobulinemia. Adv Immunol 59:135, 1995.
117. Sindel LJ, Buckley RH, Schiff SE, et al: Severe combined immunodeficiency with natural killer cell predominance: abrogation of graft-versus-host disease and immunologic reconstitution with HLA-identical bone marrow cells. J Allergy Clin Immunol 73:829, 1984.
118. Soudais C, de Villartay J, Le Deist F, et al: Independent mutations of the human CD3− gene resulting in a T cell receptor/CD3 complex immunodeficiency. Nature Genet 3:77, 1993.
119. Spickett GP, Webster ADB, Farrant J: Cellular abnormalities in common variable immunodeficiency. Immunodeficiency Rev 2:199, 1990.
120. Steimle V, Siegrist CA, Mottet A, et al: Regulation of MHC class II expression by interferon—mediated by the transactivator gene CIITA. Science 265:106, 1994.
121. Stephan JL, Vlekova V, Le Deist F, et al: Severe combined immunodeficiency: a retrospective single-center study of clinical presentation and outcome in 117 cases. J Pediatr 123:564, 1993.
122. Stolz W, Graubner U, Gerstmeier J, et al: Chediak syndrome: approaches to diagnosis and treatment. Curr Probl Dermatol 18:93, 1989.
123. Sulisalo T, van der Burgt I, Rimoin DL, et al: Genetic homogeneity of cartilage-hair hypoplasia. Hum Genet 95:157, 1995.
124. Sullivan JL, Woda BA: X-linked lymphoproliferative syndrome. Immunodeficiency Rev 1:325, 1989.
125. Swift M: Genetic aspects of ataxia telangiectasia. Immunodeficiency Rev 2:67, 1990.
125a. Symons M, Derry JMJ, Karlak B, et al: Wiskott-Aldrich syndrome protein, a novel effector for the GTPase CDC42H2, is implicated in actin polymerization. Cell 84:723, 1996.
126. Thoenes G, Soudais C, Le Deist F, et al: Structural analysis of low TCR-CD3 complex expression in T cells of an immunodeficient patient. J Biol Chem 267:487, 1992.
127. Tiller TL, Buckley RH: Transient hypogammaglobulinemia of infancy: review of the literature, clinical and immunologic features of 11 new cases, and long-term follow-up. J Pediatr 92:347, 1978.
128. Tsukada S, Saffran DC, Rawlings DJ, et al: Deficient expression of a B cell cytoplasmic tyrosine kinase in human X-linked agammaglobulinemia. Cell 72:279, 1993.
129. Vetrie D, Vorechovsky I, Sideras P, et al: The gene involved in X-linked agammaglobulinaemia is a member of the src family of protein-tyrosine kinases. Nature 361:226, 1993.
130. Vihinen M, Cooper MD, de Saint Basile G, et al: BTKbase: a database of XLA-causing mutations. Immunol Today 16:460, 1995.
131. Volanakis JE, Zhu Z, Schaffer FM, et al: Major histocompatibility complex class III genes and susceptibility to immunoglobulin A deficiency and common variable immunodeficiency. J Clin Invest 89:1914, 1992.
132. Voss SD, Hong R, Sondel PM: Severe combined immunodeficiency, interleukin-2 (IL-2), and the IL-2 receptor: experiments of nature continue to point the way. Blood 83:626, 1994.
133. Weinberg K, Parkman R: Severe combined immunodeficiency due to a specific defect in the production of interleukin-2. N Engl J Med 322:1718, 1990.
134. Wengler G, Gorlin JB, Williamson JM, et al: Non-random inactivation of the X chromosome in early lineage hematopoietic cells in carriers of Wiskott-Aldrich syndrome. Blood 85:2471, 1995.

135. Wengler SG, Allen RC, Parolini O, et al: Nonrandom X chromosome inactivation in natural killer cells from obligate carriers of X-linked severe combined immunodeficiency. J Immunol 150:700, 1993.
136. Westberg J, Fredrikson GN, Truedsson L, et al: Sequence-based analysis of properdin deficiency: identification of point mutations in two phenotypic forms of an X-linked immunodeficiency. Genomics 29:1, 1995.
137. WHO Scientific Group: Primary immunodeficiency diseases: report of a WHO scientific group. Clin Exp Immunol 99:1, 1995.
138. Wilfert CM, Buckley RH, Mohanakumar T, et al: Persistent and fatal central nervous system echovirus infections in patients with agammaglobulinemia. N Engl J Med 296:1485, 1977.
139. Wolf HM, Hauber I, Gulle H, et al: Brief report: twin boys with major histocompatibility complex class II deficiency but inducible immune responses. N Engl J Med 332:86, 1995.
140. Wright JJ, Birx DL, Wagner DK, et al: Normalization of antibody responsiveness in a patient with common variable hypogammaglobulinemia and HIV infection. N Engl J Med 317:1516, 1987.

47 HIV-1 Infection, AIDS, and the Immune System

DAVID J. VOLKMAN JACK FUHRER RENEE E. FOX

Hints of the emergence of a new human pathogen began to surface in the late 1970s. During the next 15 years, the causative virus, human immunodeficiency virus (HIV), and its close relatives were isolated, characterized, and dissected.[8, 75, 135] The diseases it causes, acquired immunodeficiency syndrome (AIDS) and related illnesses, have been documented, carefully chronicled, and exhaustively approached therapeutically.

The rapid progress in characterizing HIV itself and the mechanisms it employs to ravage the human immune system has been unprecedented. Many chemotherapeutic agents and strategies have been developed to interfere with viral infection and to treat its clinical sequelae.[177] The genomes of numerous viral isolates have been meticulously sequenced. Moreover, several animal models have become available to study HIV infection and its treatment.[89] Despite these many advances, progress in treatment, prevention, vaccination, and public health measures has been frustratingly slow, and the worldwide pandemic has continued.

The rapid explosion in the breadth of our knowledge regarding HIV provides us with new strategies and therapeutic agents to attack this infection. Some of the concepts discussed here will evolve into important advances, and others will remain interesting potential clues. Our aim is not to anticipate correct directions but to provide a clear understanding of the mechanisms by which HIV establishes infection and decimates immunity. This chapter reviews the structure of the virus, the spectrum of clinical diseases it causes, its effects on the immune system, and therapeutic interventions aimed at its prevention and treatment.

STRUCTURE OF HIV

A brief description of the nature of HIV and its pathophysiology is essential to understand how it cripples the immune system and where the virus may be vulnerable to attack. HIV is a member of a viral group called lente viruses.[8, 75, 135, 173] These are retroviruses characterized by causing slowly progressive diseases in animals, such as leukemia, lymphoma, and aplastic anemia (feline leukemic virus). The members of this group that infect primates include HIV types 1 and 2, the closely related simian immunodeficiency virus (SIV), and human T-cell lymphotropic viruses (HTLV-I and HTLV-II). These are single-stranded RNA viruses that share a common structure and infectious strategy.

Figure 47–1 outlines the design of the HIV viral genome (reviewed in 84, 173). HIV carries at least nine genes capable of being expressed through differential splicing of the RNA genome. Understanding their function provides insights into the pathogenicity of HIV and clues into its treatment and prevention. The three major proteins common to RNA tumor

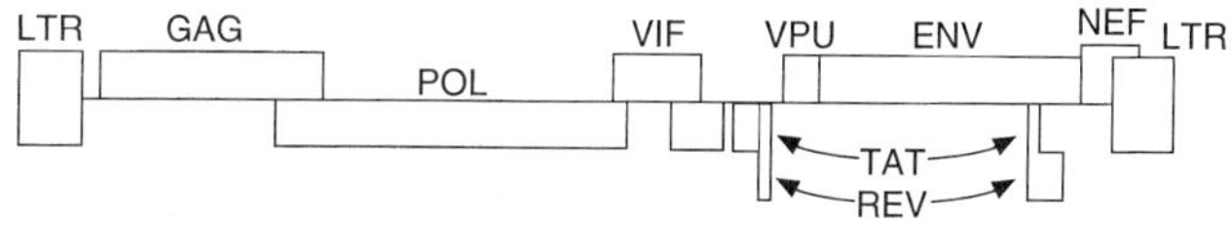

FIGURE 47-1. Schematic of HIV-1 genome. Abbreviations for the encoded genes are given in the text. LTR designates the long terminal repeats at either end. (From Greene W: Regulation of HIV-1 gene expression. Annu Rev Immunol 8:453–475, 1990. Reproduced with permission from the Annual Review of Immunology, volume 8, © 1990, by Annual Reviews Inc.)

virus are the (GAG), core structural proteins; the (POL), reverse transcriptase polymerase; and the (ENV), envelope proteins in the bipolar lipid layer encapsulating the virus.

ENV proteins are synthesized from a singly spliced mRNA translated into a 160-kD product. This is then cut into 41-kD and 120-kD proteins by a viral encoded protease. These proteins comprise the membrane-anchored stalk (via the 41-kD protein) and CD4 receptor (120-kD protein) on the outside of the virion. The 41-kD component spans the viral membrane and probably mediates both syncytia formation and part of the virus's cytopathic potential. The 120-kD component contains a peptide in its V3 loop homologous to nonpolymorphic regions of primate major histocompatibility complex (MHC) class II. This critical region binds to CD4 on cell surfaces and imparts the virus's tropism for CD4 cells. It is also the site against which the bulk of neutralizing antibodies are directed.[25, 27]

POL message generates reverse transcriptase, protease, and integrase. These viral proteins are all expressed, are critical to viral replication, and are thus potential targets of drugs aimed at reducing viral burdens. The transcriptase contains an RNase activity that destroys its RNA template after synthesizing a DNA strand. The protease is essential for packaging new virions to complete the infectious cycle. The viral-encoded integrase catalyzes the insertion of the newly synthesized viral DNA into the host cell's genome. The three required reactions are cleavage of the terminal dinucleotide, strand transfer, and disintegration, the reversal of the strand transfer reaction.[84]

GAG message produces a 53-kD precursor protein that is split into p24, p9, and p7 nucleocapsid proteins and a myristoylated p17. Concentrations of the major structural proteins p24 and p17 can be followed as surrogate markers of viral replicative activity.

Genes that regulate viral production by cellular machinery include TAT, REV, and NEF. TAT is an essential transactivating protein that strongly up-regulates the expression of genes linked to the virus. This probably works through the trans-activation response (TAR) site at the 5′ long terminal repeat (LTR) region of HIV (see Fig. 47–1). The REV gene is critical in triggering a switch to synthesizing structural genes, like GAG and ENV, for the assembly of new whole virus. This gene is also essential for infectivity of HIV. The NEF (negative factor) product appears to have a negative regulatory effect on several viral proteins and is not essential to viral replication, but it has a role in viremia and progression to AIDS. Studies have revealed a role for NEF in inducing apoptosis (programmed cell death) in infected cells. Other genes encoded in HIV, designated VIF, VPU, and VPR, also appear to have roles in regulation and assembly.

CELLULAR INFECTIOUS CYCLE

The steps by which HIV first infects single cells and then spreads to other susceptible cells and produces large numbers of progeny in rapidly succeeding generations are well characterized.[90, 91, 114, 125] The 120-gp protein on the outside of the viral envelope binds directly to CD4 molecules present on the surface of helper T cells and in smaller amounts on the surface of monocytes and similar antigen-presenting cells, such as dendritic cells. Once attached to a cell surface, the virus envelope fuses with the cell membrane and the viral RNA, and reverse transcriptase is carried into the cytoplasm using a cellular cofactor. Virus can infect cells by either free virions or contact with the membrane of an already infected cell. This second mechanism seems to be more efficient, so that HIV transmission from free virus is much less likely than from exposure to infected cells.

Once inside the cell, RNA is transcribed to a complementary DNA strand, destroying the viral RNA in the process. DNA is then translocated to the cell nucleus, where it is integrated into the cellular genomic DNA. At this stage, the state of activation of the infected cell seems to be important in determining whether the cell rapidly dies while synthesizing new viral particles, or whether the virus persists in cellular DNA, being triggered at a later time by appropriate conditions into virus assembly and release. Latter stages of viral production and assembly are mediated by the regulatory viral proteins mentioned previously.

Evidence points to early, widespread infection of susceptible cells.[52, 64, 90, 124, 126, 175] Active viral production is signaled by the presence of viral mRNA in infected cells. Viral-encoded protease is translated from this message and is critical for processing membrane and core structural components of new virions. Envelope proteins insert themselves directly into the cell membrane, whereas viral proteins constituting the core assemble around newly synthesized RNA on the inside of the cell membrane. Finally, the assembling virus completes its cycle by budding through the cell membrane, encasing itself in a bilipid membrane containing the viral envelope proteins. Agents that have been developed to interfere with several of these steps, especially polynucleotide synthesis and viral assembly, are discussed later.

IMMUNOLOGIC FEATURES OF HIV INFECTION

Profound changes occur in the immune systems of individuals infected with HIV.[125, 176] Long before the occurrence of overt clinical disease, marked abnormalities are apparent in lymphoid organs and at the cellular level. Tremendous amounts of viral replication are accompanied by enormous amounts of cell death, including the death of both infected and noninfected CD4 T cells. This cell turnover is reflected in the high rate of disintegrating CD4 T cells.[89, 90, 175] The high rates of viral replication coupled with parallel viral mutations continuously generate changes in viral progeny that blunt protective immune responses. Antibodies or cytotoxic T cells directed against critical sites on the gp120 of an infecting HIV often select for the emergence of new HIV species that have lost these specific epitope targets. Although the immune system can effectively limit, and in some cases eliminate, HIV infection, the majority of individuals progress to more severe disease and death.[88, 89, 168, 176]

Table 47–1 lists several of the immunologic abnormalities associated with HIV and subsequent AIDS. Soon after initial infection, virus is detectable in the germinal centers of hyperplastic lymphoid tissue. Although individuals often remain asymptomatic for more than 6 years, their lymph nodes reveal large numbers of CD4 T cells and macrophages pouring out copious amounts of new virus. New virus is produced by CD4 T cells, and to a lesser extent by macrophages,

TABLE 47–1
IMMUNOLOGIC SEQUELAE OF HIV INFECTION

Early
Increased CD8
Decreasing CD4/CD8 ratios
Anti-HIV antibodies (e.g., anti-gp120)
Increased cytotoxicity against HIV-infected cells
Circulating virally infected T cells (<1/1,000)
Circulating p24 antigen

Asymptomatic
Hyperplastic lymph nodes
Active viral replication and cellular destruction in lymphoid tissues
Hypergammaglobulinemia (primarily IgG anti-gp120/41)
Increased IgE
Declining CD4 numbers, marked decline in CD4/CD8 ratios
Decreased Th1/Th2 T CD4 cell ratio
Loss of cellular and humoral immunity
Loss of ability to respond to neoantigens
Changes in circulating levels of cytokines (increased IL-1, TNF, and IL-6; decreased IL-2, INF-α, and IL-12)

Late
CD4 cells <200/μm^3

expressing viral mRNA and located in germinal centers. Latently infected CD4 cells containing HIV DNA in their genomes are concentrated predominantly in the lymph node parenchyma, as are CD8 cytotoxic T cells.[64, 126, 172]

Viral particles are initially trapped on the tangle of follicular dendritic cells. As the dendritic cells are gradually destroyed, lymph node architecture and germinal centers fall apart. Other important host defenses begin to wane.[88, 176] Aggressive cytotoxic CD4 and CD8 responses that effectively contain viral infection and are detectable early in infection fall off. These failing immune defenses are accompanied by the appearance of increasing amounts of circulating viral antigen.

Evidence of immune dysregulation appears only gradually. T-cell functions, such as cell-mediated immunity evidenced by delayed-type hypersensitivity skin reactions and ability to mount cellular and humoral responses against recall antigens, are retained for many years.[16] Inability to mount immune responses against new antigens is manifested earlier.[16] In adults, vigorous humoral responses can be seen against both intercurrent bacterial infections and HIV itself.

Elevated levels of IgG occur. Much of the excess IgG is specific for HIV.[1, 174] Paradoxically, some of this IgG is neutralizing (directed against critical epitopes on the V3 loop of gp120) but fails to contain the progression of infection. This excess specific IgG production appears to be T-cell independent and may result from a combination of directly stimulating viral antigens, such as gp120; high levels of circulating cytokines, such as IL-6; and dysregulation of T-cell suppressive mechanisms.[43] IgE levels also increase in a subpopulation of HIV-infected individuals. The IgE is polyclonal, without a clear antigenic predilection. This increase does not seem to correlate to increased allergic symptoms and is probably also a result of abrogation of CD4 suppressor cells.

Increased skin eruptions have also been seen with advancing HIV infection. Inflammatory lesions worsen as clinical disease progresses and are generally characterized by CD8 involvement and folliculitis.[160] Pathologic findings typical of psoriasis vulgaris and seborrheic dermatitis have been described and occur more frequently in HIV patients than expected. These skin lesions have also been noted to share many characteristics of a graft-versus-host skin reaction, with aggressive CD8 invasion. Hypersensitivity reactions to drugs are another major skin morbidity in HIV infection. The most frequently observed reactions have been to sulfonamides, including trimethoprim-sulfamethoxazole, sulfadiazine, and trimethoprim-dapsone, and to some penicillins (discussed more fully in Chapter 37). These reactions occur significantly more frequently as immune functions, and CD4 counts deteriorate.

Even prior to the identification of HIV-1, one of the first observed immunologic features of HIV infection was the monotonous decrease in the number of CD4 T cells and its direct correlation with symptomatic disease.[16] We now understand that the decrease in CD4 T cells is a result of massive cell death and the eventual failure of the immune system to replace this cell loss, estimated at 10^9 cells per day.[90, 114] Two primary mechanisms behind this cell death have been implicated. The direct cytotoxic effect of HIV on infected cells clearly accounts for much cell death and CD4 turnover. After infection, debris from disintegrating CD4 gradually mounts. The number of circulating infected CD4 T cells and monocytes also gradually increases, although the actual percentage of infected cells remains small for some time (<1/1,000 for many years).

Since the amount of cell death far exceeds the number of cells directly infected, other mechanisms mediating this cell loss have received much attention.[69, 110] Evidence points to large-scale cellular apoptosis (programmed cell death) taking place. Once T cells are activated by triggering their T-cell receptor complex (including CD4 and CD8), they require a second signal from presenting cells, usually monocytes or dendritic cells, to begin proliferation and function. Lacking this second signal, cells commit suicide by apoptosis.

With advancing HIV infection, the percentage of activated CD4 and CD8 T cells expressing IL-2 receptors, as well as other surface activation markers such as CD28, mounts. Indeed, activation can be stimulated directly in CD4 cells by the viral gp120 (probably by engaging the CD4 receptor) and by increased levels of some proinflammatory cytokines, such as IL-1, tumor necrosis factor (TNF), and IL-6.[43] The necessary second signals, such as the surface protein B7 usually provided by monocytes and dendritic cells, are markedly attenuated or absent. Thus arrested in this state of activation, many T cells self-destruct. Although CD4 cells decrease more precipitously, both the number and protective cytotoxic potency of CD8 T cells also decline.

Finally, with infection, monokines and other cytokine functions are disturbed, and several have been implicated in HIV infection and the ensuing immunosuppression.[5, 164] IL-12 is a cytokine produced by stimulated monocytes and is a growth factor for CD4 T cells supporting important cytotoxic functions, T helper cells type 1 (Th1). Circulating levels of these cells dwindle with advancing infection. The lack of this factor probably accounts for the observation of the plummeting Th1/Th2 ratios and the disappearance of the very type of T cell that is essential for clearing viral infections and neoplasms.[56] Macrophage inflammatory proteins (MIP) have been identified as products of CD8 cells, which have a striking inhibitory effect on HIV replication.[46] Other cytokines that have generated considerable interest as potential therapeutic agents include RANTES, TNF-α, IL-2, and IL-1.[46, 164] The chemokine receptor, CCK-5, to which MIPIα, MIPIβ, and RANTES bind, has been shown to be required, with CD4, for HIV infection of cells. HIV-infected individuals exist who resist development of AIDS because of rare mutations of this receptor.

CLINICAL DISEASE

Clinical manifestations of HIV infection can be subdivided into three stages: acute retroviral syndrome, asymptomatic clinically latent infection, and symptomatic disease. Viral replication occurs in all three stages.[133]

The acute retroviral syndrome occurs within the first few months of infection and is seen in approximately 60% to 70% of patients. Because the symptoms are nonspecific, it is most often mistaken for infectious mononucleosis. Patients will often complain of marked fatigue and malaise, fevers, and generalized lymphadenopathy. Some patients develop a rash similar to a viral exanthem. Occasionally patients have a more severe initial course due to aseptic meningoencephalitis or interstitial pneumonitis. The diagnosis of an acute retroviral syndrome is often dependent on a high index of suspicion in an individual at risk. On presentation, a patient may not yet have seroconverted, and thus a negative HIV antibody test can be misleading. The use of HIV p24 antigen or polymerase chain reaction (PCR) HIV-RNA assays is more diagnostically sensitive in this setting.

In adults, an acute drop in $CD4^+$ lymphocyte counts is seen.[52] Within 1 to 12 weeks, antiviral immune responses develop and coincide with a dramatic decrease in circulating viral burden. Cytotoxic T lymphocytes appear before anti-HIV antibodies. With a decrease in circulating virus, a partial recovery of $CD4^+$ lymphocyte counts is seen.

The majority of patients then develop an asymptomatic infection. This phase can last from a few years to more than 15 years, with the typical range of 7 to 10 years. As previously mentioned, lymph node studies of asymptomatic individuals demonstrate that active viral replication is perpetually occurring. These patients often have generalized lymphadenopathy.

Although many patients may have near normal CD4 lymphocyte counts during the asymptomatic period, the majority have reduced CD4 numbers. However, the asymptomatic period may last in some patients until their CD4 counts are drastically reduced ($<50/mm^3$). A significant number of patients do not seek medical attention until they become symptomatic, sometimes in a markedly weakened immune state.

In the symptomatic stage, most patients develop signs and symptoms of immune dysfunction prior to the development of AIDS (Table 47–2). The Multicenter AIDS Cohort Study (MACS), which studied the natural course of HIV infection in a cohort of over 1,600 male homosexuals, identified oral thrush, oral hairy leukoplakia, and shingles as prognostic of imminent progression to AIDS within a few years.[72, 129] Shingles often precedes thrush and oral hairy leukoplakia by 12 to 18 months. Vaginal yeast infections can also precede oral thrush by several years.[139]

TABLE 47–2
AIDS-DEFINING CONDITIONS IN HIV-INFECTED INDIVIDUALS[37]

Candidiasis of bronchi, trachea, esophagus, or lungs
Cervical cancer, invasive
Coccidioidomycosis, disseminated or extrapulmonary
Cryptosporidiosis, chronic intestinal
Cytomegalovirus disease (other than liver, spleen, or nodes)
Cytomegalovirus retinitis
Encephalopathy
Herpes simplex: chronic ulcers, bronchitis, pneumonitis, or esophagitis
Histoplasmosis disseminated or extrapulmonary
Immunologic suppression (CD4 $<200/\mu m^3$)
Isosporiasis, chronic intestinal
Kaposi's sarcoma
Lymphoma: Burkitt's, immunoblastic, or primary brain
Mycobacterium avium complex or *M. kansasii*, disseminated or extrapulmonary
Mycobacterium tuberculosis
Mycobacterium: other species, disseminated or extrapulmonary
Pneumocystis carinii pneumonia
Pneumonia, recurrent
Progressive multifocal leukoencephalopathy
Salmonella septicemia, recurrent
Toxoplasmosis of brain
Wasting syndrome due to HIV

In addition, women with HIV infection seem to be at greater risk for cervical dysplasia and ultimate neoplastic disease.[108] Whether this is a function of simultaneous human papilloma virus (HPV) infection or a yet to be determined synergism between HIV and HPV is unknown.[151] Other less specific symptoms of HIV infection include fever, night sweats, weight loss, and diarrhea. In addition, some patients develop laboratory abnormalities secondary to immune dysregulation, such as idiopathic thrombocytopenic purpura (ITP).[12] Although ITP is not specific to HIV infection, diagnosing it in an individual who might engage in risky behavior warrants HIV antibody testing.

AIDS is classified in accordance with the criteria of the Centers for Disease Control (CDC) (see Table 47–2).[37] The syndrome can be divided into immunologic and clinical AIDS. Immunologic AIDS is defined by a CD4 lymphocyte count of $200/mm^3$ or less in an HIV-infected adult. Clinical AIDS is determined by the development of certain opportunistic infections, associated malignancies, a wasting syndrome, or dementia in an HIV-infected patient (see Table 47–2). As the scope of possible AIDS-defining illnesses is large, only the more common manifestations are discussed here.

Pneumocystis carinii pneumonia (PCP) is the most commonly encountered AIDS-defining illness. The organism, *P. carinii*, first thought to be a protozoa, was found to have the genetic makeup more closely resembling a fungus.[62, 132] Nonetheless, the organism responds to typical antiprotozoan medications and not to antifungal therapy. In addition to HIV-infected individuals, it occurs in other immunodeficient hosts, including persons with hematologic and lymphoreticular malignancies, transplant recipients, and patients taking immunosuppressive agents.

PCP presents as a subacute or chronic dry hacking cough associated with fevers, dyspnea (particularly on exertion), and occasionally atypical chest pain. Sputum production is typically scant and is described as white and foamy. The physical examination most commonly is unremarkable. In more severe cases, patients may have rapid labored breathing and may use accessory muscles. Typically, the chest radiograph reveals bilateral interstitial infiltrates, which can be present in all lung fields. Arterial blood gases are helpful in determining the extent of hypoxemia, which correlates with the severity of illness.[21] Similarly, serum lactic dehydrogenase levels are often elevated and correlate with the severity of illness.[11] With therapy, the serum LDH should decrease, which can be used as a marker of improvement.[179]

Diagnosis can be made with an open lung biopsy, but this is seldom required in an HIV-positive patient.[22, 163] Bronchoscopy with bronchoalveolar lavage (BAL) has a 90% to 95% yield in AIDS patients compared with a 70% yield in non–HIV-infected patients. The cysts of *P. carinii* can be readily identified in BAL fluid stained with Gomori's methenamine silver stain. Induced sputum examined with a modified Giemsa stain or with fluorescent or nucleotide tagged monoclonal antibodies is often more than 90% sensitive.[122] The differential diagnosis includes other causes of interstitial pneumonitis, including cytomegalovirus (CMV), varicella-zoster virus (VZV), herpes simplex virus (HSV), adenovirus, respiratory syncertial virus (RSV), mycobacteria (*Mycobacterium tuberculosis* and *M. avium-intracellulare*), fungi, toxoplasma, and noninfectious causes, such as lymphoma, Kaposi's sarcoma, vasculitis, and lymphoid interstitial pneumonitis. The drugs of choice for the treatment of PCP are trimethoprim-sulfamethoxazole (TMP-SMX) or pentamidine.

Three antibiotic regimens are effective in preventing either recurrent or primary PCP: low-dose TMP-SMX alone, dapsone alone or combined with either trimethoprim or pyrimethamine, and aerosolized pentamidine.[18, 34, 148] Patients with prior hypersensitivity to TMP-SMX may be desensitized (see Chapter 37).

Toxoplasma gondii is a protozoan, which in AIDS patients typically results in central nervous system (CNS) mass lesions and can cause global encephalopathy. The organism can be acquired by ingesting the oocyte that is excreted by the definitive host, the cat. It can also be acquired by ingesting undercooked or raw meats of animals infected with *Toxoplasma*. Vertical transmission from infected mother to fetus can occur at any trimester of pregnancy and can result in mental retardation, microcephaly, and chorioretinitis.

In otherwise immunocompetent patients, *Toxoplasma* infection usually results in subclinical infection, with about 10% developing a mononucleosis-like syndrome. Immunosuppressed hosts can develop more serious infection after newly acquired infection or reactivation of old infection, which can result in encephalitis, chorioretinitis, pneumonitis, and myocarditis. In AIDS patients, most active *Toxoplasma* infections are thought to occur after reactivation of prior infection.[106]

Patients with CNS toxoplasmosis usually present with neurologic deficits suggestive of localizing mass lesions, seizures, headaches, and mental status or personality changes.[121] The differential diagnosis for such lesions in HIV-positive patients includes primarily CNS lymphoma and less commonly bacterial brain abscess, tuberculous brain abscess, cryptococcal brain abscess, and occasionally multifocal leukoencephalopathy. Studies suggest a role for single-photon emission computed tomography (SPECT) scan imaging of the head, with increased uptake being seen in lymphoma but not in infectious etiologies like *Toxoplasma*.[147]

Definitive diagnosis is made with a brain biopsy, but this is often reserved for patients who have not responded to appropriate therapy for suspected *Toxoplasma* or who are seronegative for *Toxoplasma*.[136] Unfortunately, serology has limited utility in that it identifies only those who have been previously infected with *Toxoplasma* when immunocompetent and are thus at greatest risk for reactivation. Seronegative *Toxoplasma* has been reported to occur in less than 3% of AIDS patients with CNS toxoplasmosis. New infection may not elicit a reliable humoral response in these immunocompromised patients.

The therapy of choice remains a combination of pyrimethamine and sulfadiazine with leucovorin to protect host cells. A clinical or neuroradiologic response should be seen within 2 to 3 weeks of initiation of therapy. Clindamycin is a less effective alternative.[99] Adjunctive steroids should be considered only in patients with surrounding edema and mass effect.

Mycobacterial infections, particularly due to tuberculosis or the *Mycobacterium avium* complex (MAC), are very common in AIDS patients.[6, 93] MAC organisms are ubiquitous, and their mode of entry into humans is thought to occur by either the oral or respiratory route.[7] Although rarely a cause of serious pathology in immunocompetent hosts, MAC results in disseminated disease in AIDS patients, particularly those with CD4 lymphocyte counts less than 50/mm^3. These patients often suffer with high fevers, drenching night sweats, weight loss, intractable diarrhea, and marked fatigue. Signs may include hepatosplenomegaly, anemia, neutropenia, and thrombocytopenia, as well as an elevated alkaline phosphatase out of proportion to other liver function tests. Other less common manifestations include adrenalitis, pneumonitis, and sclerosing cholangitis. Although physical findings are often nonspecific, the organism can be recovered by culture.[6, 7]

The therapy of MAC infections ranges from two to five drug regimens, including newer macrolides (azalides) like clarithromycin or azithromycin, rifabutin, ethambutol, ciprofloxacin, clofazimine, and IV amikacin. Single drug therapy is likely to result in the development of drug resistance. Rifabutin or clarithromycin prophylaxis is recommended to reduce the incidence of MAC bacteremia in patients with CD4 lymphocyte counts below 100/mm^3. Although neither agent has been shown to extend life, both have clinical efficacy in preventing fever, night sweats, weight loss, and hospitalization due to MAC.[131]

Tuberculosis infection is a major complication of HIV infection.[7, 20, 138, 165] It is recommended that patients with HIV infection have annual tuberculin skin testing. As many immunosuppressed HIV-infected patients are anergic, assessing skin test reactivity to other common antigens, such as mumps, *Candida*, and *Trichophyton*, is recommended. A reaction of induration to tuberculin of 5 mm or greater is considered positive, although because of the prevalence of anergy, tuberculosis can be difficult to diagnose if not considered in the differential diagnosis.

Diagnosis of tuberculosis should be made by culture of appropriate tissue specimens or body fluids.[20] Confirmed cultures should be tested for drug sensitivity to eliminate the possibility of drug-resistant *M. tuberculosis*. As the HIV-infected patient with pulmonary tuberculosis can present atypically, it is recommended that HIV-infected patients with pulmonary infiltrates be placed in a respiratory isolation until tuberculosis is ruled out or an alternate diagnosis is made.[39]

A lack of appropriate infection control for tuberculosis has led to several outbreaks of multidrug-resistant tuberculosis in New York City and Miami hospitals and correctional facilities.[61, 127] Upon the diagnosis of tuberculosis, patients should be started on antituberculous therapy. In New York and other areas with high rates of multidrug-resistant tuberculosis, initial regimens of four to five drugs, including isoniazid, rifampin, ethambutol, pyrazinamide, and streptomycin, are recommended.[39]

Viral infections in HIV-infected patients are also common. The most frequently encountered viruses are HSV 1 and 2, VZV, and CMV. In addition, HIV itself can directly result in myopathies, neurologic disease, and enteropathies. The less commonly encountered JC virus can result in progressive multifocal leukoencephalopathy.

HSV 1 and 2 generally cause recurrent or chronic mucocutaneous infections in HIV-infected patients.[157] Less commonly encountered manifestations include esophagitis, resulting in odynophagia, as well as dysphagia, colitis, and rarely encephalitis. Successful treatment of HSV infections usually occurs with acyclovir, famciclovir, or valcyclovir. However, some patients develop strains that are resistant to these drugs.[3] In these patients with suspected or proven acyclovir-resistant strains, the drug of choice for serious HSV infections is foscarnet.[152]

VZV usually presents as shingles in a single or an adjacent dermatome. Many patients will describe shingles before the development of AIDS, and some authors suggest that it is an early manifestation of symptomatic HIV infection and a prognosticator of progression of disease.[72] Zoster ophthalmitis can result in keratitis.[4] Unless disseminated, zoster usually does not cause significant morbidity, with the exception of postherpetic neuralgia. Treatment with acyclovir, famciclovir, or valcyclovir reduces the incidence of postherpetic neuralgia, whereas adjunctive steroids do not have any beneficial effect. Unusual complications of zoster include transverse myelitis and encephalitis, a postzoster ophthalmitis, granulomatous vasculitis of the brain, progressive outer retinal necrosis, and acute retinal necrosis.[80, 94, 149] These latter eye infections are therapeutic dilemmas and inconsistently respond to therapeutic intervention.

CMV infection is prevalent among patients with HIV infection, with autopsy studies demonstrating active CMV disease in 40% to 90% of AIDS patients. Most disease is thought to occur as a result of reactivation of latently infected cells. Although CMV can result in infection in virtually any organ, the most common presentation in AIDS patients is retinitis.[74] Other less common CMV sites of infection include the esophagus, colon, gall bladder, lungs, and adrenals. In nonocular disease, the diagnosis is primarily made by pathologic examination of biopsied tissue

CMV retinitis usually presents as perivascular exudates with sheathing of the blood vessels and hemorrhages. Granular exudates without hemorrhage are also seen. Disease can be both central and peripheral. The goal of therapy is to prevent further progression and hopefully restore visual loss. Unfortunately, patients frequently develop relapsing retinitis while on maintenance therapies. At present, the therapies available include foscarnet and ganciclovir.

Fungal infection in AIDS patients is most commonly due to *Candida albicans*. Oral candidiasis (thrush) is an early manifestation of symptomatic HIV infection and is considered a prognosticator of progression of disease. Vaginal candidiasis is similarly encountered more frequently in HIV-infected women. With progression of disease, some patients develop esophageal involvement, resulting in symptoms of dysphagia and occasionally odynophagia.

Diagnosis can often be made on the basis of symptoms, on the finding of oral thrush, and by endoscopic biopsy. A response to appropriate antifungal therapy is highly suggestive of the diagnosis. In patients who fail to respond to antifungal therapy, one should consider alternate diagnoses, including drug-resistant candidiasis, HSV and CMV esophagitis, aphthous ulcerations, and malignancies. Successful therapy of candidiasis can usually be achieved with the imidazoles (ketoconazole, fluconazole, itraconazole). However, chronic use of these agents has led to resistant strains. Mild to moderate oral thrush is treated with topical therapy, such as clotrimazole and nystatin, and severe oral or esophageal candidiasis with imidazoles. In refractory disease, amphotericin B is used.

Other fungal infections described in AIDS patients include cryptococcosis, histoplasmosis, coccidioidomycosis, blastomycosis, aspergillosis, and sporotrichosis. Cryptococcosis and coccidioidomycosis usually present with a chronic meningitis. All of these infections can present with disseminated disease, although aspergillus and blastomyces have a greater predilection for lung involvement. The imidazoles have been shown to be effective against some of these fungi, but amphotericin B with or without 5-fluorocytosine remains the standard for serious infections.

Malignancies commonly associated with AIDS are Kaposi's sarcoma and non-Hodgkin's lymphoma (NHL). Kaposi's sarcoma is primarily seen in men who have sex with other men but has been described in HIV-infected patients with other risk behaviors. Investigators isolated a herpes-like virus from Kaposi's sarcoma tissue specimens, termed Kaposi's sarcoma–associated herpesvirus (KSHV), and have suggested that this virus is the etiologic agent.[42, 118] It has also been found in an unusual form of B-cell lymphoma involving serosal surfaces.[41] Curiously, the virus is also ubiquitous in the semen of normal, uninfected males.[117] Besides skin involvement, AIDS patients with Kaposi's sarcoma can typically have lymphatic, pulmonary, and gastrointestinal involvement. The diagnosis is usually made clinically when patients present with red violaceous lesions, which can be plaque-like or raised and indurated. A diagnosis is confirmed by biopsy.

Chemotherapeutic agents, including adriamycin, vincristine, VP-16, and bleomycin, used singly or in combination, are reserved for widely disseminated cutaneous disease or extracutaneous disease. Radiation therapy is suggested for patients who have significant local disease that causes marked edema or pain. Whether agents effective against other herpesviruses are effective against KSHV and useful in the management of Kaposi's sarcoma is yet to be determined.

The etiology of NHL in AIDS patients is not known, although herpesviruses, including Epstein-Barr virus (EBV) and KSHV, have been implicated.[41] The presentation of NHL can vary, as can the severity of immunosuppression among patients. Although primary CNS involvement is generally seen in more immunosuppressed patients (CD4 $< 50/mm^3$), peripheral lymphomas can be seen at earlier stages of HIV infection. Response to therapy similarly varies with location of disease and stage of immunosuppression. Pathologically, these lymphomas are high-grade (73%) or intermediate-grade (24%) B-cell types. Outcomes using multidrug chemotherapeutic regimens are not as favorable in AIDS patients as in non–HIV-infected patients. Although a complete response may be achieved in peripheral disease (53%), relapsing disease is frequent (54%).[73]

Patients with primary CNS lymphoma have an even worse response to chemotherapy, and are treated with palliative radiation therapy. The life expectancy for an AIDS patient with primary CNS lymphoma is 3 to 6 months.[9, 80]

Wasting has been noted in many patients with AIDS. This manifestation was initially described as slim disease in Africans with AIDS.[155] The etiologic factors contributing to AIDS-related wasting are probably multiple and include the release of excessive amounts of cytokines, hypermetabolism, enteropathies, and decreased oral intake. Cytokines, such as TNF-α (cachectin) and interferon-α, have been implicated in this weight loss.[71, 170] TNF is thought to inhibit lipoprotein lipase, thus interfering with normal lipid metabolism. Some studies have shown elevated levels of TNF in AIDS patients, whereas others have failed to demonstrate any relationship to alterations in lipid levels.[81] Interferon-α levels correlate with triglyceride levels and decreases in lean body mass.[82] In addition, there seems to be an increase in resting energy expenditure in patients with AIDS, particularly those with active infectious complications.[83] The wasting syndrome is likely a result of a combination of these factors.

PEDIATRIC CLINICAL DISEASE

The first reports of AIDS in children appeared in 1982.[36] Women and children now constitute the fastest-growing groups of newly infected individuals in the United States. Worldwide infant and child mortality rates will increase as much as 30% above previously projected rates as a direct consequence of perinatal HIV infection.[137] Thus the recognition and treatment of HIV-infected children are an extremely important aspect of this pandemic.

Vertical transmission (from infected mothers to their infants) will account for almost all new cases in young children in the future. Heterosexual acquisition of HIV-1 in developed countries has grown, so that women now represent 5 of every 11 newly infected adults worldwide, likely heralding increasing perinatal infection.[114a] Demographically, minority groups in the United States are disproportionally affected, with 54% of cases occurring in black, non-Hispanic children and 24% in Hispanics. Boys and girls are equally represented among children under 5 years. However, the finding that zidovudine (AZT) could significantly reduce the rate of mother-to-child transmission when administered to HIV-infected women during pregnancy and delivery and to their offspring for the first 6 weeks of life promises to reduce the numbers of HIV-infected children in countries where this therapy is available and broadly administered.[35, 50]

Adolescents are at risk from unprotected sexual intercourse or the use of contaminated needles. The magnitude of this risk is highlighted by the fact that 20% of people developing AIDS in the United States are aged 20 to 29 years and that AIDS is the leading cause of death in this age group. Given the prolonged incubation period, it is clear that a substantial proportion acquired their infection as teenagers.[76] Infection in this age group is similar to that in adults and will not be discussed separately.

HIV INFECTION

The viral life cycle, as outlined earlier in this chapter, is the same in children and adults, but the influence of growth and cellular differentiation on viral replication and pathogenesis remains to be delineated. These influences may help explain some of the differences in the course of disease between adults and children.

In children, acute infection by cell-associated or cell-free virus may occur parenterally (e.g., via a break in the integrity of the placental barrier) or across a mucosal surface (e.g., by ingestion of contaminated maternal blood during delivery). Although an acute mononucleosis-like illness is experienced by 50% to 70% of adults, clinical manifestations of primary infection are not as evident in infants.[168] This may be due to the timing of perinatal transmission, differences in transmitted viral burden or phenotype, or immaturities of the host immune response. Moreover, infants of infected mothers have preexisting (maternally derived) HIV-specific antibodies, which may attenuate the acute syndrome.

Unlike adults, it is difficult to document a pattern of decreasing $CD4^+$ lymphocyte counts in HIV-infected infants, as infants have much higher levels during the first 2 years of life.[68, 113] There appear to be a subset of children with more rapid disease progression and a second group that may follow a pattern of clinical latency, which is generally shorter than that in adult disease.

Throughout the course of infection, progressive destruction of $CD4^+$ T cells and of follicular dendritic cells (FDC) in lymph nodes occurs.[115, 124, 126, 172] The final breakdown of the germinal centers and FDC architecture and the profound impairment of HIV-specific host defenses are associated with decreased trapping of virus in lymphoid tissue and a high level of viremia. In both children and adults, late-stage disease is marked by a precipitous decline in $CD4^+$ lymphocyte counts and by the risk of opportunistic infections, neoplasms, and death.

$CD4^+$ LYMPHOCYTES

$CD4^+$ cells are depleted through several mechanisms. Apoptosis appears to be of considerable importance in both infants and adults. Thymic apoptosis of greater than 90% of T-cell clones occurs naturally, and the thymus is an important target organ of HIV-1.[60, 95] The thymus in HIV-infected children at autopsy shows extensive involvement, with thymusitis and precocious involution.[60, 95]

In addition to the numerical destruction of $CD4^+$ lymphocytes, functional abnormalities are also apparent. Both direct HIV-induced suppression of T helper function and the absence of T helper function resulting from the lack of maturation or immunologic priming may play roles in a child's immunodeficiency.[156] Critical subsets of CD4+ lymphocytes may be preferentially affected by HIV. CD4+/CD45RA+(naive) subset cells were significantly lower in the infected children.[134] This T-cell subset in cord blood suppresses immunoglobulin production. Disproportionate loss of these cells may be a factor in the polyclonal B-cell stimulation and hypergammaglobulinemia associated with both pediatric and adult HIV infection. The CD29+/CD45RO+(memory) subset, which provides helper functions and participates in responses to recall antigens, is also markedly reduced.[25]

CD8+ LYMPHOCYTES

Two separate CD8+ cell-mediated responses to HIV infection have been described.[105] The first is the classic cytotoxic T lymphocyte (CTL) response, which is MHC class I restricted and requires cell-to-cell contact. The second is mediated by a novel cytokine released by CD8+ cells, MIP-1α, which suppresses HIV replication in CD4+ lymphocytes.[5, 164] In children with vertically acquired infection, HIV-specific CTL responses are deficient.[107] Although specific CTL activity against HIV target proteins was detected in 24 of 25 perinatally infected children, responses were weaker than those in adults and diminished as children became symptomatic. Intrauterine infections could result in the presence of HIV antigens in the thymus and induce tolerance, which may contribute to the more rapid disease progression in these children compared with children infected intrapartum. HIV-specific CTL activities have also been reported in seroreverting infants of HIV-infected mothers.[45, 143] Whether these observations are the result of cross-reactivity with certain cellular proteins or represent triumphs of cellular immunity in controlling and possibly clearing virus remains controversial.

CYTOTOXIC NATURAL KILLER CELLS AND ANTIBODY-DEPENDENT CELLULAR CYTOTOXICITY

Natural killer (NK) cell activity is defective in advancing HIV disease.[33] Since NK cells and subpopulations of CD8 lymphocytes are mediators of antibody-dependent cellular cytotoxicity (ADCC), this non-MHC restricted killing of virus-infected cells could potentially be helpful in preventing perinatal transmission. However, studies have not shown any relationship between ADCC in mothers or their infants and subsequent infection status of the child.[23] A significantly higher frequency of ADCC was seen in asymptomatic HIV-infected children than in those with AIDS.[178]

NEUTRALIZING ANTIBODY

As noted, envelope protein epitopes are the primary targets for antibody neutralization.[105] Typically, HIV-1–infected individuals do not have strong neutralizing antibodies to their own virus strain. The clinical relevance of the humoral immune response remains uncertain.

NEUTROPHILS AND MONOCYTES

Bactericidal activity of neutrophils against *Staphylococcus aureus* in vitro was defective in 8 of 12 children with asymptomatic infection and 8 of 9 children with symptomatic HIV disease.[141]

Infection

Perinatal transmission encompasses the transmission of virus from an infected mother to her child either prenatally (intrauterine), during delivery (intrapartum), or following delivery through breast-feeding (postpartum). The term perinatal is used synonymously with vertical to describe mother-to-infant transmission.

Most infants born to infected mothers are themselves uninfected. Published transmission rates in infants born to untreated mothers vary from 13% in the European Collaborative Study to about 40% in Africa.[14, 66, 77, 86, 92, 150] Increased risk has been associated with higher levels of maternal viremia, lower CD4 counts, and more advanced maternal disease.[15, 17, 54, 150, 167] However, in the United States, most transmitting mothers are asymptomatic at delivery.[154] Intrapartum events that increase fetal exposure to maternal blood, such as amniocentesis, placenta previa, abruptio placentae, fetal scalp monitoring, episiotomy, and second-degree tears, are also associated with an increased risk of HIV transmission.[17]

The rate of disease progression in infants has been linked to the severity of disease in the mother at the time of delivery. Whether this is the result of a larger viral inoculum, earlier intrauterine transmission, or transmission of other pathogens that might influence disease progression is unclear.[13] The role of maternal immune factors is also controversial. Although some data suggested that higher maternal neutralizing antibody titers to autologous HIV isolates may correlate with decreased transmission, the role of maternal antibodies in preventing perinatal transmission is now discounted.[28, 153]

There is a well-documented discordance of transmission from one pregnancy to the next and between twins. A multinational study of 100 sets of twins born to seropositive mothers demonstrated that transmission is more common in the first-born twin; 50% of vaginally delivered and 38% of cesarean section–delivered first-born infants were infected as opposed to 19% of second-born twins delivered by either route. The first-born twin has more prolonged exposure to cervical and vaginal secretions. Intrapartum transmission is presumed to occur across the infant's mucous membranes, principally in the oropharynx and possibly in the esophagus and stomach. Field studies are being conducted to test whether cleansing of the birth canal during labor can reduce the risk of transmission.

Antiviral therapy appears to have a critical role in reducing perinatal HIV transmission. Zidovudine given to mothers during pregnancy and delivery and to their infants postnatally has demonstrated a highly significant reduction in transmission from 25.5 to 8.3%[50] This represents an important advance in the management of women who can be identified as infected during pregnancy. Treatment is started in the second trimester and extended throughout the perinatal period.

HIV infection can occur in utero, as well as intrapartum. In utero infection is defined as HIV being culturable or detectable by PCR from blood within 48 hours of birth.[26] In contrast, intrapartum infection is defined as having negative blood results within the first 48 hours, becoming positive from day 7 to 90. Breast-fed infants are excluded from this category. Large prospective studies using these definitions are in progress. Estimates indicate that in the absence of breast-feeding, 50% to 70% of transmission occurs around the time of delivery.[17]

Disease progression occurs more rapidly in children infected in utero.[27, 29, 102, 104] One explanation for this is that children infected in utero may have dissemination of virus to organs, such as the thymus, at a critical stage of development.[171] This may result in early and profound impairment of cellular and humoral immunity.

The additional risk of infection that occurs from HIV-positive mothers who breast-feed has been estimated to be 15% to 20%.[55, 59, 146, 165] The risk may be higher if the mother's primary infection occurs in the perinatal period, consistent with the viremia that occurs with initial infection and a lack of protective secretory IgA at the time of acute infection.[161] However, the benefits of breast-feeding may outweigh the risks of transmission in countries where safe water supplies and maintenance of sterility of bottle feeding equipment cannot be guaranteed.[103] The World Health Organization (WHO) encourages breast-feeding in countries where infectious diseases and malnutrition are the main causes of infant deaths and the infant mortality rate is high. The CDC and Public Health Service recommend that women who test positive for HIV antibody in the United States should avoid breast-feeding.[85]

DIAGNOSIS IN CHILDREN

For perinatally infected infants, the serologic tests for HIV-specific IgG antibodies are of no diagnostic value beyond confirming the serologic status of the mother. Almost 100% of infants of infected mothers acquire IgG antibodies to HIV transplacentally. These passively acquired antibodies gradually wane, with a median time to disappearance of 10 months. Positive ELISA and Western blots are therefore only diagnostic of infection in children over the age of 18 months.

The current approach to establishing the diagnosis in infants is to use tests that directly detect the virus or its components. The three most widely accepted methods are virus culture, detection of proviral genome by PCR, and detection of serum p24 antigen by ELISA. Despite the sensitivity of culture, PCR, and p24 antigen assays, between 50% and 70% of children who subsequently prove to be infected have negative results in the first few days of life.[102] This suggests peripartum transmission, with extremely low or absent circulating viral burden initially. Prenatal diagnosis has been attempted in a limited number of women, such as those undergoing cordocentesis for clinical indications.[51] HIV has also been cultured from amniotic fluid.[120] Any invasive procedure during the prenatal period runs a risk of carrying maternal blood to the infant and causing infections.

The differential diagnosis of HIV infection in symptomatic infants and children includes the primary combined immunodeficiency disorders, other congenital infections, such as syphilis, and the extensive list of causes of failure to thrive. A careful history that includes maternal risk factor may suggest HIV exposure. Initial laboratory tests should be performed, including an immunoglobulin profile and lymphocyte subsets using age-adjusted standards.

The classification system revised by the CDC in 1994 reflects the spectrum of clinical and immune abnormalities (see Table 47–2).[37] There are differences in HIV infection in children compared with adults. The most important difference is that disease progression may be more rapid in children. The period of latency is reduced compared with that of adults.[32, 169] Long-term survivors who do not develop PCP have a median survival of 8.4 years. The subtle initial symptoms in infants must be distinguished from problems associated with prematurity, intrauterine drug exposure, or congenital infections other than HIV. The incidence of encephalopathy is higher in children, ranging from 30% to 90% with advancing disease.[67] Failure to thrive, in particular the failure of normal linear growth, is considered a specific manifestation of pediatric HIV infection.[177]

Recurrent bacterial infections, particularly with polysaccharide encapsulated organisms, are more common, reflecting the immaturity of the humoral immune system, which normally develops the capacity to produce antipolysaccharide antibodies between 18 and 24 months. Toxoplasmosis and cryptococcoses are less common in children. Malignancies, in particular Kaposi's sarcoma, are also less common in children.

In contrast, lymphocytic interstitial pneumonitis (LIP) has been seen almost exclusively in the pediatric population. LIP is a chronic lung disorder of uncertain cause that affects up to 40% to 50% of vertically HIV-infected children.[49] It is less common in older children and hemophiliacs. The disorder is characterized by a diffuse, interstitial, reticulonodular infiltrate on chest x-ray. If it is associated with larger nodules and hilar or mediastinal lymphadenopathy, it is referred to as pulmonary lymphoid hyperplasia (PLH).

Clinically there is a wide spectrum of severity, from an asymptomatic individual in whom LIP is purely a radiologic diagnosis to severe exercise intolerance and oxygen dependency. A presumptive diagnosis may be made on the basis of suggestive radiographic changes that persist for months, are unresponsive to antimicrobial therapy, and are not the result of other specific infectious pathogens. PCP can coexist with LIP.

A definitive diagnosis of LIP may be made by lung biopsy, although this is rarely necessary. Characteristic findings are a diffuse lymphoid infiltration of the alveolar septa and peribronchiolar areas, with varying degrees of lymphoid aggregation that may show organization into early germinal centers. Both EBV DNA and HIV RNA have been identified by in situ hybridization in biopsy specimens from children with LIP.[2, 96, 100] The precise etiologic role of either is unclear, as is the reason why LIP is uncommonly seen in adults with HIV infection.

LIP may remit spontaneously. Treatment for LIP is only indicated in the presence of hypoxemia and shortness of breath. High-dose oral steroids are used for at least 6 weeks to suppress the lymphocytic proliferation. Symptoms frequently return on weaning steroids, and the lowest maintenance dose must be sought for each individual.

Neurologic problems occur frequently in symptomatic HIV-infected children. Estimates vary from 31% to 89% in different series.[10, 67] Lower CD4 percentages and positive p24 antigen levels are significantly associated with the presence of CNS abnormalities.

Only macrophage-tropic strains of HIV gain entry into the

CNS, which suggests that infected peripheral blood macrophages carry HIV across the blood-brain barrier.[105] HIV can be identified in the microglia and, to a lesser extent, astrocytes. Neurons are not directly infected. Activated macrophages may produce toxic factors, such as TNF-α, which has been implicated in demyelinization. Metabolic products, such as quinolinic acid, may mediate neuronal toxicity by binding to postsynaptic *N*-methyl-D-aspartate (NMDA) receptors, causing toxic calcium influx. Arachidonic acid metabolites, such as leukotrienes and prostaglandins, may cause toxicity by different mechanisms.

HIV encephalopathy is rarely evident at birth but may present in infancy with such signs as delayed acquisition of a social smile, poor head control, or truncal hypotonia. Subsequently, progressive motor abnormalities, such as spastic diplegia and oral motor dysfunction, become apparent.[10, 66] Expressive language is frequently more affected than receptive language. The course varies from static (developmental milestones acquired at a slower rate than normal) to progressive, with overt loss of previously acquired skills. Acquired microcephaly resulting from cerebral atrophy may be noted.

Computer tomography (CT) can demonstrate ventricular enlargement, cortical atrophy, or cerebral calcification, which is seen particularly in the basal ganglia in association with HIV infection.[57] Calcification is a hallmark of vertically acquired HIV infection and is rare in children with transfusion-acquired disease. Of the children with vertically acquired disease, 33% had calcifications, all of whom were encephalopathic. Postmortem findings include cerebral atrophy, calcification, focal necrosis, gliosis, reactive astrocytosis, vascular lesions, and inflammatory infiltrates, including multinucleated giant cells.

Therapeutically, the only currently licensed antiretroviral agent that penetrates the blood-brain barrier significantly is zidovudine. Striking improvements in motor abnormalities, neurophysiologic functioning, and radiographic finding have been associated with zidovudine therapy, particularly when given as a continuous infusion.[24, 133] Improvements in encephalopathic symptoms have been noted anecdotally with corticosteroid treatments.[162]

Growth failure is a common finding, and the cause is multifactorial. It may be a result of inadequate nutritional intake caused by suppressed appetite, oropharyngeal pathology, or neurologic disease; malabsorption due to HIV enteropathy or bacterial colonization of the small intestine; or increased metabolic requirements. Abnormalities of thyroid function, adrenal insufficiency, and growth hormone deficiency have been reported in HIV-infected children.

Infections of the gastrointestinal tract frequently contribute to the growth failure and wasting seen in HIV-infected children. *C. albicans* and HSV are the most common causes of oropharyngeal pathology.[159] Infectious pathogens associated with diarrhea in HIV-infected children include *Cryptosporidium, M. avium-intracellulare*, Microsporida, *Salmonella*, and *Shigella*.[130] HIV infection of enterochromaffin cells in the intestinal mucosa may dysregulate motility, and cytokines released by macrophages in the lamina propria may promote secretory diarrhea.[112]

Other abnormalities are similar to those seen in adults. Transaminase elevations are frequent and may be related to infections, including CMV, HSV, or *M. avium-intracellulare*, or drugs related to rifampin and antifungal azoles, as well as ceftriaxone and other antibiotics that may cause biliary sludging. Pancreatitis in HIV-infected children may be caused by CMV or a side effect of therapy with dideoxyinosine (ddI).[116]

The most common hematologic abnormality is anemia, seen in up to 94% of children.[31, 63, 133] Neutropenia (absolute neutrophil count < 500–$1,500$) is also common and is the major dose-limiting toxicity to zidovudine therapy in infants. Thrombocytopenia may be the presenting complaint of HIV infections.[140] It may be the result of direct effects of HIV, opportunistic infections of the bone marrow, autoimmune destruction, sequestration in the spleen, or antiretroviral medication.[178] A variety of coagulopathies have been described, including vitamin K deficiency.

Although the anticipated increased incidence of malignancies has not been observed in children under 13, there is a 360-fold increased risk of NHL in HIV-infected children. In addition, an increased incidence of leiomyomas and leiomyosarcomas, which have not been associated with immunodeficiency in adults, has been reported.[119]

INFECTIOUS SEQUELAE

Although the spectrum of infections in children with HIV is similar to that in adults reviewed earlier, their clinical features are sometimes distinctive. These include recurrent bacterial, mycobacterial, viral, protozoal, and fungal infections.

Recurrent bacterial infections are a hallmark of the B-cell defect in HIV-infected children, which may often manifest before evidence of a T-cell disorder. The most common bacterial pathogens are the polysaccharide encapsulated organism, particularly *Streptococcus pneumoniae*, when central venous catheter–associated infections are excluded.[101, 141] Excluding otitis media, soft tissue infections were most common (34%), followed by bacteremias, pneumonia, and sinusitis.[101] Neonatally acquired group B streptococcal disease can occur as late as 5 months of age.[58] *Pseudomonas* infections are not uncommon and are most commonly associated with central venous catheters, especially with a *Pseudomonas* species other than *P. aeruginosa*.

Viral infections carry a substantially greater risk for serious morbidity and mortality in HIV-infected children. Primary varicella may be associated with visceral dissemination and encephalitis.[97, 158] VZV may recur with increasing frequency as the immunodeficiency progresses. The lesion may be atypical, with hyperkeratosis and increased pigmentation or hypopigmentation without obvious vesiculation.[123]

HSV has been associated with severe herpetic gingivostomatitis, esophagitis, and chronic labial infection.[87] CMV may cause retinitis, pneumonitis, enterocolitis, hepatitis, and more rarely esophagitis, pancreatitis, or adrenal insufficiency.[87]

RSV, parainfluenza III, and adenoviruses may cause severe and even fatal pneumonitis. *P. carinii* pneumonia may be complicated by superinfection with any of these respiratory pathogens and carries a poor prognosis.

Measles is associated with a high incidence of pneumonitis and occasionally encephalitis.[98] Hepatitis viruses A, B, and C may be more fulminant. The B and C forms in particular may result in a chronic aggressive or frequently relapsing course.[19, 111]

Protozoal and fungal infections may present differently in children. *P. carinii* has been noted to be a cause of pulmonary disease in young children with HIV despite apparently high CD4 counts.[145] *P. carinii* pneumonia was the AIDS indicator disease in 38% of 3,471 reported pediatric AIDS cases through 1991. An early and frequently fatal peak is observed in infants around the age of 6 months. The presenting features of this disease are tachypnea, dyspnea, cough, and fever. As in adults, the presentation may be insidious rather than acute, with hypoxemia without frank infiltrate.

Treatment is identical to that discussed for adults. *P. carinii* pneumonia prophylaxis is currently recommended for all children with severe immunosuppression, as defined by low $CD4^+$ lymphocyte counts. All perinatally exposed infants and all proven HIV-infected infants younger than 1 year of age should receive prophylaxis through 12 months of age.[40] Any child with a history of *P. carinii* pneumonia, regardless of CD4 count, should receive secondary prophylaxis. The drug of choice is TMP-SMX.

The incidence of *T. gondii* infections in children is much lower than that in adults.[116] *C. albicans* may cause recurrent oropharyngeal candidiasis, including esophagitis. *Cryptococcus neoformans* is less prevalent in pediatric patients than in adults but may cause meningitis.

PREVENTIVE MEASURES

Prophylactic measures include the use of intravenous immunoglobulin and active and passive immunizations. Children with significant recurrent bacterial infections, hypogammaglobulinemia, or documented poor functional antibody development may be candidates for intravenous immunoglobulin 400 mg/kg every 28 days.[177] Higher doses may be useful in children with thrombocytopenia (500–1,000 mg/kg/day for 3-5 days).

Most childhood immunizations are currently recommended. Inactivated poliovirus vaccine should be substituted for oral polio vaccine, even after seroreversal, to prevent viral spread to immunodeficient family members.[177] The varicella vaccine recently licensed by the Food and Drug Administration is not yet recommended. Pneumococcal vaccine is recommended at age 2, and influenza vaccine is recommended annually in symptomatic children. Although bacille Calmette-Guérin (BCG) is not currently recommended in the United States, WHO recommends that it be given to asymptomatic children in areas of high prevalence.[100a]

Passive immunization is recommended for susceptible children with symptomatic HIV infection who are in contact with measles or VZV. Prophylaxis for *P. carinii* pneumonia has been previously discussed in this chapter.

Finally, prevention of perinatal transmission is of the highest priority. The results of the AIDS clinical trial protocol 076 study provide a major impetus to develop less complicated but equally effective interventions to eradicate HIV infection before it is well established. However, targeted prevention and treatment can be achieved only if HIV-infected mothers are identified prenatally.

ANTIVIRAL THERAPY

Antiviral therapy attempts to interfere with different steps in the HIV life cycle and hence interrupt viral replication. Although attempts at blocking many of the component steps have been made, only two classes of drugs are presently available: those inhibiting viral reverse transcriptase and those inhibiting protease enzymes.

REVERSE TRANSCRIPTASE INHIBITORS

This class of drugs can be subdivided into nucleoside and non-nucleoside agents. The prototype of the nucleoside analogues, zidovudine, was brought to market in 1987 for treatment of patients with AIDS, having demonstrated a significant advantage in morbidity and mortality when compared with a placebo.[70] Although initial studies also demonstrated an advantage in reducing the progression of disease in asymptomatic or minimally symptomatic HIV-infected individuals, this advantage was not apparent when patients were followed for more than 3 years.[48] Microbiologic, as well as clinical, resistance to zidovudine can be demonstrated.

Other nucleoside analogues, including didanosine (DDI), dideoxycytosine (DDC), stavudine (D4T), and lamivudine (3TC), were developed but showed the same limited benefit. Several studies have demonstrated that combination convergent (acting at same step) therapy had either additive or synergistic benefit. Most of these data have shown a beneficial effect on surrogate markers, such as viral loads and CD4 counts, suggesting a long-term clinical benefit. Perhaps the most interesting and potent convergent combination is zidovudine plus lamivudine. The latter induces a mutational change in the virus, which makes it more sensitive to zidovudine; hence, a synergistic effect is produced.[65] Whether lamivudine will confer a similar effect when used in combination with other nucleoside agents has yet be determined.

The nucleoside analogues can cause significant toxicity. Zidovudine's major toxicity is anemia and neutropenia, although gastrointestinal intolerance, headaches, and insomnia also are reported. Didanosine and stavudine can cause pancreatitis and peripheral neuropathy. Dideoxycytosine can result in peripheral neuropathy and, relatively uncommonly, large aphthous ulcers.

Several agents of the non-nucleoside transcriptase inhibitor group have been developed. Nevirapine and delaviridine are furthest along in development. Preliminary data are promising when these agents are used in combination with nucleoside analogues.

PROTEASE INHIBITORS

These agents are the newest and perhaps most potent drugs available. Saquinavir, the first inhibitor available, was released in the fall of 1995 and is most beneficial when used in combination with zidovudine and dideoxycytosine.[47] Saquinavir, although very potent in vitro, is poorly absorbed and thus not as active in vivo as the newer protease inhibitors. However, a new formulation of saquinavir that has improved absorption is presently being studied and should be available shortly.

Norvir and Crixivan were both released in the spring of 1996. Although both agents have been approved for either monotherapy or combination therapy with reverse transcriptase inhibitors, the most potent clinical effect, as determined by surrogate markers, occurs with combination therapy.[53, 109] Norvir is a strong inducer of hepatic enzymes and must be carefully used with other hepatically metabolized drugs. For the most part, only gastrointestinal intolerance is reported by patients, which often can be avoided by prescribing a rapid dose escalation. Crixivan is generally well tolerated, causing only a mild increase in bilirubin and renal stones in less than 5% of individuals.

SUMMARY

Following HIV-1 infection, the deterioration of the immune system takes place over many years and through several mechanisms. Its rate of destruction appears directly proportional to an increasing viral burden escaping immune control. On the other hand, the resilience of the immune system is demonstrated by the repeated observations that measures that decrease viral replication rapidly result in climbing CD4 numbers and some restoration of debilitated immune functions. This resilience, coupled with our rapidly expanding knowledge, offers hope for ameliorating the enlarging HIV pandemic.

REFERENCES

1. Amadori A, DeSilvestro G, Zamarchi R, et al: CD4 epitope masking by gp120/anti-gp120 antibody complexes; a potential mechanism for CD4+ cell function down-regulation in AIDS patients. J Immunol 148:2709–2716, 1992.
2. Andiman WA, Martin K, Rubinstein A, et al: Opportunistic lymphoproliferations associated with Epstein-Barr viral DNA in infants and children with AIDS. Lancet 2:1390–1393, 1985.
3. Balfour HH: Resistance to herpes simplex to acyclovir. Ann Intern Med 98:404–406, 1983.
4. Balfour HH Jr: VZV in immunocompromised hosts. Am J Med 85:68–73, 1988.
5. Balter M: Cytokines move from the margins into the spotlight. Science 268:205–206, 1995.
6. Barnes PF, Atrevado C: Blood culture positivity patterns in bacteremia due to *Mycobacterium avium intracellulare*. South Med J 81:1059, 1988.
7. Barnes PF, Bloch AB, Davidson PT, et al: TB in patients with HIV infection. N Engl J Med 324:1644, 1991.
8. Barre-Sinoussi F, Chermann JC, Rey F, et al: Isolation of a T-lymphotropic retrovirus from a patient at risk for acquired immune deficiency syndrome (AIDS). Science 220:868–871, 1983.
9. Baumgartner JE, Rachlin JR, Beckstead JH, et al: Primary CNS lymphomas: natural history and response to therapy in 55 patients with AIDS. J Neurosurg 73:206–211, 1990.
10. Belman AL: Acquired immunodeficiency syndrome and the child's central nervous system. Pediatr Clin North Am 39:691–714, 1992.
11. Benson CA, Spear J, Hines D, et al: Combined Apache II score and serum lactate dehydrogenase as predictors of in-hospital mortality caused by first episode *Pneumocystis carinii* pneumonia in patients with acquired immunodeficiency syndrome. Am Rev Respir Dis 144:319–323, 1991.
12. Bettaieb A, Oksenhandler E, Fromont P, et al: Immunochemical analysis of platelet autoantibodies in HIV-related thrombocytopenic purpura: a study of 68 patients. Por J Hematol 73:241–247, 1989.
13. Blanche S, Mayauz MJ, Rouzioux C, et al: French Pediatric HIV Infection Study Group. Relation of the course of HIV infection in children to the severity of the disease in their mothers at delivery. N Engl J Med 330:308–312, 1994.
14. Blanche S, Rouzioux C, Guihard Moscato M-L, et al: A prospective study of infants born to women seropositive for human immunodeficiency virus type 1. HIV Infection in Newborns French Collaborative Study Group. N Engl J Med 320:1643–1648, 1989.
15. Boue F, Pons JC, Keros L, et al: Risk for HIV-1 perinatal transmission varies with the mother's stage of HIV infection. Int Conf AIDS 6:1990.
16. Bowen DL, Lane HC, Fauci AS: Immunopathogenesis of the acquired immunodeficiency syndrome. Ann Intern Med 103:704–709, 1985.
17. Boyer P, Dillon M, Navaie M, et al: Factors predictive of maternal-fetal transmission of HIV-1. JAMA 271:1925–1930, 1994.
18. Bozzette SA, Sattler FR, Chiu J, et al: A controlled trial of early adjunctive treatment with corteosteroids for *Pneumocystis carinii* pneumonia in the acquired immunodeficiency syndrome. N Engl J Med 323:1451–1457, 1990.
19. Bodsworth NJ, Cooper DA, Donovan B: The influence of human immunodeficiency virus type 1 infection on the development of the hepatitis B virus carrier state. J Infect Dis 163:1138–1140, 1991.
20. Braun MM, Byers RH, Heyward WL, et al: AIDS and extrapulmonary TB in the US. Arch Intern Med 150:1913, 1990.
21. Brenner M, Ogribebe FP, Lack EE, et al: Prognostic factors and life expectancy of patients with acquired immunodeficiency syndrome and *Pneumocystis carinii* pneumonia. Am Rev Respir Dis 136:1199–1206, 1987.
22. Broaddus C, Dabe MD, Stulbarg MS, et al: Bronchoalveolar lavage and transbronchial biopsy for the diagnosis of pulmonary infections in the acquired immunodeficiency syndrome. Ann Intern Med 102:747–752, 1985.
23. Broliden K, Sievers E, Tovo PA, et al: Antibody-dependent cellular cytotoxicity and neutralizing activity in sera of HIV-1-infected mothers and their children. Clin Exp Immunol 93:56–64, 1993.
24. Brouwers P, Moss H, Wolters P, et al: Effect of continuous infusion zidovudine therapy on neuropsychologic functioning in children with symptomatic human immunodeficiency virus infection. J Pediatr 117:980–985, 1990.
25. Brunell P: Antibody in human immunodeficiency virus infection. Ann NY Acad Sci 693:9–13, 1990.
26. Bryson U, Luzuriaga K, Sullivan J, Wara D: Proposed definition for in utero versus intrapartum transmission of HIV-1. N Engl J Med 327:1246–1247, 1992.
27. Bryson Y, Lehman D, Garratty E, et al: The role of maternal autologous neutralizing antibody in prevention of maternal fetal HIV-1 transmission. J Cell Biochem Suppl 17E:95, 1993. Abstract.
28. Bryson Y, Dillon M, Garratty E, et al: The role of timing of HIV maternal-fetal transmission (in utero vs. intrapartum) and HIV phenotype on onset of symptoms in vertically infected infants. Int Conf AIDS 9:c10–c12, 1993.
29. Burgard M, Mayaux MJ, Blanche S, et al: HIV Infection in Newborns French Collaborative Study Group. The use of viral culture and p24 antigen testing to diagnose human immunodeficiency virus infection in neonates. N Engl J Med 327:1192–1197, 1992.
30. Buseyne F, Blanche S, Schmitt D, et al: Detection of HIV-specific cell-mediated cytotoxicity in the peripheral blood from infected children. J Immunol 150:3569–3581, 1993.
31. Butler KM, Husson RN, Balis FM, et al: Dideoxyinosine in children with symptomatic human immunodeficiency virus infection. N Engl J Med 324:137–144, 1991.
32. Byers B, Calwell B, Oxytoby M: Pediatric Spectrum of Disease Project. Survival of children with perinatal HIV infection: evidence for two distinct populations. Presented at the Ninth International Conference on AIDS, Berlin, June 6–11, 1993.
33. Cai Q, Huang XL, Rappocciolo G, Rinaldo CJ: Natural killer cell responses in homosexual men with early HIV infection. J Acquir Immune Defic Syndr 3:669–676, 1990.
34. Carr A, Tindall B, Penny R, et al: Trimethoprim-sulfamethoxazole appears more effective than aerosolized petamidine as secondary prophylaxis against *Pneumocystis carinii* pneumonia in patients with AIDS. AIDS 6:165– 171, 1992.
35. Centers for Disease Control: Zidovudine for the prevention of HIV transmission from mother to infant. MMWR Morb Mortal Wkly Rep 43:285–287, 1994.
36. Centers for Disease Control: Unexplained immunodeficiency and opportunistic infections in infants—New York, New Jersey, California. MMWR Morb Mortal Wkly Rep 31:665–667, 1982.
37. Centers for Disease Control: 1993 Revised classification system for HIV infection and expanded surveillance care definition for AIDS

among adolescents and adults. MMWR Morb Mortal Wkly Rep 41:RR-17, 1–19, 1992.
38. Centers for Disease Control: Guidelines for preventing transmission of TB in health care settings, with special focus on HIV-related issues. MMWR Morb Mortal Wkly Rep 39:RR-17, 1990.
39. Centers for Disease Control: Initial therapy for TB in the era of multidrug resistance: recommendations of the advisory council for the elimination of TB. MMWR Morb Mortal Wkly Rep 42:RR-7, 1993.
40. Centers for Disease Control: 1995 revised guidelines for prophylaxis against *Pneumocystis carinii* pneumonia for children infected with or perinatally exposed to human immunodeficiency virus. MMWR Morb Mortal Wkly Rep 44:1–11, 1995.
41. Cesarman E, Chang Y, Moore PS, et al: KS associated herpes virus–like DNA sequences in AIDS related body-cavity based lymphoma. N Engl J Med 332(18):1186–1191, 1994.
42. Chang Y, Cesarman E, Pessin MS, et al: Identification of herpes-like DNA sequences in AIDS-associated Kaposi's sarcoma. Science 266:1865–1869, 1994.
43. Chirmule N, Kalyanaraman VS, Lederman S, et al: HIV-gp 160–induced T cell–dependent B cell differentiation. Role of T cell–B cell activation molecule and IL-6. J Immunol 150:2478–2486, 1993.
44. Civitello L: Neurological complications of HIV infection in children. Pediatr Neurosurg 17:104–112, 1991.
45. Cheynier R, Langlade DP, Marescot MR, et al: Cytotoxic T lymphocyte responses in the peripheral blood of children born to human immunodeficiency virus-1–infected mothers. Eur J Immunol 22:2211–2217, 1992.
46. Cocchi F, DeVico AL, Garzino-Demo A, et al: Identification of RANTES, MIP-1 alpha, and MIP-1 beta as the major HIV-suppressive factors produced by CD8+ T cells. Science 270:1811–1815, 1995.
47. Collier AC, Coombs RW, Schoenfeld DA, et al: Treatment of HIV infection with saquinavir, zidovudine and zalcitabine. N Engl J Med 334(16):1011–1017, 1996.
48. Concorde Coordinating Committee: MRC/ANRS randomised double-blind controlled trial of immediate and deferred zidovudine in symptom-free HIV infection. Lancet 343:871–881, 1994.
49. Connor E, Marquis J, Oleske J: Lymphoid interstitial pneumonitis. In Pizzo PA, Wilfert CM (eds): The Challenge of HIV Infection in Infants, Children, and Adolescents. Williams & Wilkins, Baltimore, 1991, pp 343–354.
50. Connor EM, Sperling RS, Gelber R, et al: Pediatric AIDS Clinical Trial Group Protocol 076 Study Group. Reduction of maternal-infant transmission of human immunodeficiency virus type I with zidovudine treatment. N Engl J Med 331:1173–1180, 1994.
51. Cullen M, Viscarello R, Paryani S, Sanchez-Ramos L: Prenatal diagnosis of HIV infection: the use of cordocentesis, polymerase chain reaction and p24 antigen assay. Am J Obstet Gynecol 166:386, 1992.
52. Daar ES, Moudgil T, Meyer RD, Ho DD: Transient high levels of viremia in patients with primary human immunodeficiency virus type 1 infection. N Engl J Med 324:961–964, 1991.
53. Danner SA, Carr A, Leonard JM, et al: A short-term study of the safety, pharmacokinetics, and efficacy of ritonavir, an inhibitor of HIV-1 protease. European-Australian Collaborative Ritonavir Study Group. N Engl J Med 333:1528–1533, 1995.
54. D'Arminio Monforte A, Ravizza M, Muggiasca ML, et al: HIV-infected pregnant women: possible predictors of vertical transmission. Int Conf AIDS 7:1991.
55. Davis MK: Human milk and HIV infection: epidemiologic and laboratory data. In Symposium on Immunology of Milk and the Neonate. Plenum Press, New York, 1991, pp 271–280.
56. Del Prete G, Maggi E, Pizzolo G, Romagnani S: CD30, Th2 cytokines and HIV infection: a complex and fascinating link. Immunol Today 16:76–80, 1995.
57. DiCarli C, Civitello LA, Brouwers P, Pizzo PA: The prevalence of computed tomographic abnormalities of the cerebrum in 100 consecutive children symptomatic with the human immune deficiency virus. Ann Neurol 34:198–205, 1993.
58. DiJohn D, Krasinski D, Lawrence R, et al: Very late onset of group B streptococcal disease in infants infected with the human immunodeficiency virus. Pediatr Infect Dis J 9:925–928, 1990.
59. Dunn D, Newell M, Ades E, Peckham C: Risk of human immunodeficiency virus type 1 transmission through breastfeeding. Lancet 340:585–588, 1992.
60. Economides A, Anisman D, Schmid I, et al: Apoptosis in human HIV-1 infected thymocytes. J Cell Biochem Suppl 17E:62, 1993. Abstract.
61. Edlin BR, Tokars JI, Grieco MH, et al: An outbreak of MDRTB among hospitalized patients with AIDS. N Engl J Med 326:1514–1521, 1992.
62. Edman JC, Kovacs JA, Masur H, et al: Ribonsonial RNA sequence shows *Pneumocystis carinii* to be a member of the fungi. Nature 334:519–522, 1988.
63. Ellaurie M, Burns ER, Rubinstein A: Hematologic manifestations in pediatric HIV infection: severe anemia as a prognostic factor. Am J Pediatr Hematol Oncol 12:449–453, 1990.
64. Embretson J, Zupancic M, Ribas JL, et al: Massive covert infection of helper T lymphocytes and macrophages by HIV during the incubation period of AIDS. Nature 362:359–362, 1993.
65. Eron JJ, Benoit SL, Jemsek J, et al: Treatment with lamivudine, zidovudine, or both in HIV-positive patients with 200 to 500 CD4+ cells per cubic millimeter. North American HIV Working Party. N Engl J Med 333:1662–1669, 1995.
66. European Collaborative Study: Children born to women with HIV-1 infection: natural history and risk of transmission. Lancet 337:253–260, 1991.
67. European Collaborative Study: Neurologic signs in young children with human immunodeficiency virus infection. Pediatr Infect Dis J 9:402–406, 1990.
68. European Collaborative Study: Age-related standards for T lymphocyte subsets based on uninfected children born to human immunodeficiency virus 1-infected mothers. Pediatr Infect Dis J 11:1018–1026, 1992.
69. Fauci AS, Pantaleo G, Stanley S, Weissman D: Immunopathogenic mechanisms of HIV infection. Ann Intern Med 124:654–663, 1996.
70. Fischl MA: The efficacy of AZT in treatment of patients with AIDS and ARC. N Engl J Med 317:185–191, 1987.
71. Flores EA, Bistrian BR, Pomposelli JJ, et al: Infusion of TNF/cachectu promotes muscle catabolism in the rat: a synergistic effect with IL1. J Clin Invest 83:1614–1622, 1989.
72. Friedman-Kien AE, Lafleur FL, Gendler E, et al: Herpes zoster: a possible early clinical sign for development of acquired immunodeficiency syndrome in high risk individuals. J Am Acad Dermatol 14:1023, 1986.
73. Gall PS, et al: AIDS related malignant lymphoma: results of prospective treatment trial. J Clin Oncol 5:1322–1328, 1987.
74. Gallant JE, et al: Incidence and natural history of CMV disease in patients with advanced HIV disease treated with zidovudine. JID 166:1223–1227, 1992.
75. Gallo RC: The AIDS virus. Sci Am 256:46–56, 1987.
76. Gayle H, D'Angelo L: Epidemiology of acquired immunodeficiency syndrome and human immunodeficiency virus infections in adolescents. J Pediatr Infect Dis 10:322–328, 1991.
77. Goedert JJ, Drummond JE, Minkoff HL, et al: Mother-to-infant transmission of human immunodeficiency virus type 1: association with prematurity or low anti-gp120. Lancet 332:1351–1354, 1989.
78. Goedert JJ, Duliege A, Amos C, et al: The International Registry of HIV-exposed twins. High risk of HIV-1 infection for first-born twins. Lancet 338:1471–1475, 1991.
79. Golden DH, Gilden DH, Beinlich BP, Rubinstein EM, et al: Chronic progressive VZV encephalitis in an AIDS patient Neurology 38:1150–1153, 1988.
80. Goldstein JD, Dickson DW, Moser FG, et al: Primary central nervous system lymphoma in acquired immune deficiency syndrome. A clinical and pathologic study with results of treatment with radiation. Cancer 67:2756–2765, 1991.
81. Grunfeld C, Pang M, Doerrier W, et al: Lipids, lipoproteins, triglyceride clearance and cytolevels in HIV infection and AIDS. J Clin Endocrinol Metab 74:1045–1052, 1992.
82. Grunfeld C, Kotler DP, Shigenaga JK, et al: Circulating interferon and level and hypertriglycerdemia in AIDS. Am J Med 90:154–162, 1991.
83. Grunfeld C, Pang M, Shimizu L, et al: Resting energy expenditure, calorie intake, and short term weight change in HIV infection and AIDS. Am J Clin Nutr 55:455–460, 1992.
84. Greene W: Regulation of HIV-1 gene expression. Annu Rev Immunol 8:453–475, 1990.
85. Guidelines for Perinatal Care, 3rd edition. American Academy of Pediatrics, American College of Obstetricians and Gynecologists, Elk Grove Village, IL, 1992.
86. Gwinn M, Pappaioanou M, George J, et al: Prevalence of HIV infection in childbearing women in the United States: surveillance using newborn blood samples. JAMA 265:1704–1708, 1991.
87. Hanson I, Kaplan S: Opportunistic infections. Semin Pediatr Infect Dis 1:31–39, 1990.

88. Haynes BF, Pantaleo G, Fauci AS: Toward an understanding of the correlates of protective immunity to HIV infection. Science 271:324–328, 1996.
89. Heeney JL: AIDS: a disease of impaired Th-cell renewal? Immunol Today 16:515–520, 1995.
90. Ho DD: Viral counts in HIV infection. Science 272:1124–1125, 1996.
91. Ho DD, Neumann AU: Perelson AS, et al: Rapid turnover of plasma virions and CD4 lymphocytes in HIV-1 infection. Nature 373:123–126, 1995.
92. Hoff R, Berardi VP, Weiblen BJ, et al: Seroprevalence of human immunodeficiency virus among childbearing women. Estimation by testing samples of blood from newborns. N Engl J Med 318:525–530, 1988.
93. Horsburgh CR Jr: *Mycobacterium avium* complex infection in the AIDS. N Engl J Med 324:1332, 1991.
94. Jabs DA, Newman C, DeBustros S, et al: Presumed VZV retinitis in immunocompromised patients. Retina 7:9–13, 1987.
95. Jenkinson E, Kingston R, Smith C, et al: Antigen-induced apoptosis in developing T cells: a mechanism for negative selection of the T cell receptor repertoire. Eur J Immunol 19:2175–2177, 1989.
96. Joshi VV, Kauffman S, Oleske JM, et al: Polyclonal polymorphic B-cell lymphoproliferative disorder with prominent pulmonary involvement in children with acquired immune deficiency syndrome. Cancer 59:1455–1462, 1987.
97. Jura E, Chadwick EG, Josephs SH, et al: Varicella-zoster virus infections in children infected with human immunodeficiency virus. Pediatr Infect Dis J 8:586–690, 1989.
98. Kaplan LJ, Daum RS, Smaron M, McCarthy CA: Severe measles in immunocompromised patients. JAMA 267:1237–1241, 1992.
99. Katlama C, et al: Pyremethanine-Clindamycin vs. Pyromethamine-Sulfa CID. J Clin Invest 22(2):268–275, 1996.
100. Katz B, Berkman A, Shapiro E: Serologic evidence of active Epstein-Barr virus infection in Epstein-Barr virus associated lymphoproliferative disorders of children with acquired immunodeficiency syndrome. J Pediatr 120:228–232, 1992.
100a. Khouri YF, Mastrucci MR, Hutto C, et al: *Mycobacterium tuberculosis* in children with human immunodeficiency virus type 1 infection. Pediatr Infect Dis J 11:950–955, 1992.
101. Krasinski K, Borkowsky W, Bonk S, et al: Bacterial infections in human immunodeficiency virus-infected children. Pediatr Infect Dis J 7:323–328, 1988.
102. Krivine A, Firtion G, Cao L, et al: HIV replication during the first weeks of life. Lancet 339:1187–1189, 1992.
103. Lederman S: Estimating infant mortality from human immunodeficiency virus and other causes in breast-feeding and bottle-feeding populations. Pediatrics 89:290–296, 1992.
104. Levine M, Denamur E, Simon F, et al: Conversion of HIV viral markers during the first months of life in HIV infected children born to seropositive mothers. Presented at the Ninth International Conference on AIDS, Berlin, June 6–11, 1993.
105. Levy J: Pathogenesis of human immunodeficiency virus infection. Microbiol Rev 57:183–289, 1993.
106. Luft BJ: Toxoplasmic encephalitis in patients with acquired immunodeficiency syndrome. JAMA 252:913, 1984.
107. Luzuriaga K, McQuilken P, Alimenti A, et al: Early viremia and immune responses in vertical human immunodeficiency virus type 1 infection. J Infect Dis 167:1008–1013, 1993.
108. Maiman M, Frucher R, Serur E, et al: Human immunodeficiency virus and cervical neoplasia. Gynecol Obstet 38:377–382, 1990.
109. Markowitz M, Saag M, Powderly WG, et al: A prelim study of ritonavir. N Engl J Med 333(23):1534–1539, 1995.
110. Margolick JB, Volkman DJ, Lane HC, Fauci AS: Clonal analysis of T lymphocytes in the acquired immunodeficiency syndrome: evidence for an abnormality affecting individual helper and suppressor T cells. J Clin Invest 76:709–715, 1985.
111. Martin P, Di BA, Kassianides C, et al: Rapidly progressive non-A, non-B hepatitis in patients with human immunodeficiency virus infection. Gastroenterology 97:1559–1561, 1989.
112. Matsuyama T, Kobayashi N, Yamamoto N: Cytokines and HIV infection: is AIDS a tumor necrosis factor disease? AIDS 5:1405–1417, 1991.
113. McKinney R, Wilfert C: Lymphocyte subsets in children younger than 2 years old: normal values in a population at risk for human immunodeficiency virus infection and diagnostic and prognostic application to infected children. Pediatr Infect Dis J 11:639–644, 1992.
114. Mellors JW, Rinaldo CR, Gupta P, et al: Prognosis in HIV-1 infection predicted by the quantity of virus in plasma. Science 272:1167–1170, 1996.
114a. Merson M: The HIV pandemic: global spread and global response. Presented at the Ninth International Conference on AIDS, Berlin, June 6–11, 1993.
115. Michael N, Vahey M, Burke D, Redfield R: Viral DNA and mRNA expression correlate with the stage of human immunodeficiency virus (HIV) type 1 infection in humans: evidence for viral replication in all stages of HIV disease. J Virol 66:310–316, 1992.
116. Miller MJ, Remington JS: Toxoplasmosis in infants and children with HIV infection or AIDS. In Pizzo PA, Wilfert CM (eds): Pediatric AIDS. Williams & Wilkins, Baltimore, 1991, pp 299–307.
117. Monini P, DeLellia L, Fabris M, et al: Kaposi's sarcoma–associated herpesvirus DNA sequences in prostate tissue and human semen. N Engl J Med 334:1168–1172, 1996.
118. Moore PS, Chang Y: Detection of herpes virus–like DNA sequences in KS. N Engl J Med 332:1180–1185, 1995.
119. Mueller BU, Butler KM, Feuerstein IM, et al: Smooth muscle tumors in children with human immunodeficiency virus infection. Pediatrics 90:460–463, 1992.
120. Mundy D, Schinazi R, Gerber A, et al: Human immunodeficiency virus from amniotic fluid. Lancet 2:459–460, 1987.
121. Navia BA, Petito CK, Gold JW, et al: Cerebral toxoplasmosis complicating the AIDS: clinical and neuropathological findings in 27 patients. Ann Neurol 19:224, 1986.
122. Ng VL, Vrani NA, Chaisson RE, et al: Rapid detection of *Pneumocystis carinii* using direct fluorescent monoclonal antibody stain. J Clin Microbiol 28:2228–2233, 1990.
123. Pahwa S, Biron K, Lim W, et al: Continuous varicella-zoster infection associated with acyclovir resistance in a child with AIDS. JAMA 260:2879–2882, 1988.
124. Pantaleo G, Graziosi C, Demarest J, et al: HIV infection is active and progressive in lymphoid tissue during the clinically latent stage of disease. Nature 362:292–293, 1993.
125. Pantaleo G, Fauci AS: New concepts in the immunopathogenesis of HIV infection. Annu Rev Immunol 13:487–512, 1995.
126. Pantaleo G, Graziosi C, Demarest JF, et al: HIV infection is active and progressive in lymphoid tissue during the clinically latent stage of disease. Nature 362:355–358, 1993.
127. Pearson ML, et al: Nosocomial transmission of MDRTB: a risk to patients and to health care workers. Ann Intern Med 117:191–196, 1992.
128. Perelson AS, Neumann AU, Markowitz M, et al: HIV-1 dynamics in vivo: virion clearance rate, infected cell life-span, and viral generation time. Science 271:1582–1586, 1996.
129. Phau J, Munoz A, Detels R: Multicenter AIDS Cohort Study Group: the risk of *Pneumocystis carinii* pneumonia among men infected with human immunodeficiency virus type 1. N Engl J Med 322:161, 1990.
130. Pickering L, Cleary K: Problems of the digestive tract. In Pizzo PA, Wilfert CM (eds): Pediatric AIDS. Williams & Wilkins, Baltimore, 1991, pp 384–397.
131. Pierce M, Heifets L, Crampton S, et al: The effect of MAC and its prevention or survival in patients with advanced HIV infection. Presented at the 35th Interscience Conference in Antimicrobial Agents and Chemotherapy, San Francisco, September 17–20, 1995.
132. Pixley FJ, Wakefield AE, Banerji S, et al: Mitochondrial gene sequences show fungal homology for *Pneumocystis carinii*. Mol Microbiol 5:1347–1351, 1991.
133. Pizzo PA, Eddy J, Falloon J, et al: Effect of continuous intravenous infusion of zidovudine (AZT) in children with symptomatic HIV infection. N Engl J Med 319:889–896, 1988.
134. Plaeger-Marshall S, Hultin P, Bertolli J, et al: Activation and differentiation antigens of T cells of healthy, at-risk, and HIV-infected children. J Acquir Immune Defic Syndr 6:984–993, 1993.
135. Popovic M, Sarngadharan MG, Read E, Gallo RC: Detection, isolation, and continuous production of cytopathic retroviruses (HTLV-III) from patients with AIDS and pre-AIDS. Science 224:497–500, 1984.
136. Porter SB, Sande MA: Toxoplasmosis of the CNS in AIDS. N Engl J Med 327:1643–1648, 1992.
137. Quinn T: Population migration and the spread of types 1 and 2 human immunodeficiency viruses. Proc Natl Acad Sci USA 91:2407–2414, 1994.
138. Rieder HL, Cauthen GM, Kelly GD, et al: TB in the US. JAMA 262:385, 1989.
139. Rhoads JL, Wright DC, Redfield RR, Burke DS: Chronic vaginal candidiasis in women with HIV infection. JAMA 257:3105–3107, 1987.

140. Rigaud M, Leibovitz E, Sin Quee C, et al: Thrombocytopenia in children infected with human immunodeficiency virus: long-term follow-up and therapeutic considerations. J Acquir Immune Defic Syndr 4:450–455, 1992.
141. Roilides E, Marshall D, Venzon D, et al: Bacterial infections in human immunodeficiency virus type 1-infected children: the impact of central venous catheters and anti-retroviral agents. Pediatr Infect Dis J 10:813–819, 1991.
142. Roilides E, Mertins S, Eddy J, et al: Impairment of neutrophil chemotactic and bactericidal function in children infected with human immunodeficiency virus type 1 and partial reversal after in vitro exposure to granulocyte-macrophage colony-stimulating factor. J Pediatr 117: 531–540, 1990.
143. Rowland-Jones S, Nixon DF, Aldhous MC, et al: HIV-specific cytotoxic T-cell activity in and HIV-exposed but uninfected infant. Lancet 341:860–861, 1993.
144. Rose DN, Schechter CB, Sacks HS: Preventive medicine for HIV infected patients: an analysis of isoniazid prophylaxis for tubercular reactors and for patients. J Gen Intern Med 7:589–594, 1992.
145. Rubenstein A, Morecki R, Silverman B, et al: Pulmonary disease in children with acquired immune deficiency syndrome and AIDS-related complex. J Pediatr 108:498–503, 1986.
146. Ruff AJ, Halsey NA, Coberly J, Boulos R: Breast-feeding and maternal transmission of human immunodeficiency virus type 1. J Pediatr 121:325–329, 1992.
147. Ruiz A, Ganz WI, Post MJ, et al: Use of thallium-201 brain SPECT to differentiate cerebral lymphoma from toxoplasma encephalitis in AIDS patients. AJR Am J Roentgenol 15:1885–1894, 1994.
148. Ruskin J, LaRiviere M: Low dose co-trimoxazole for prevention of Pneumocystis carinii in human immunodeficiency virus disease. Lancet 337:468–471, 1991.
149. Ryder JW, Croen K, Kleinschmidt-DeMasters BK, et al: Progressive encephalitis 3 months after resolution of cutaneous zoster in a patient with AIDS. Ann Neurol 19:182–188, 1986.
150. Ryder RW, Nas W, Hassig SE, et al: Perinatal transmission of the human immunodeficiency virus type 1 to infants of seropositive women in Zaire. N Engl J Med 320:1637–1642, 1989.
151. Safrin S, Datsel BJ, Hauer L, Sweet RL: High frequency of latent and clinical human papillomavirus cervical infections in immunocompromised human immunodeficiency virus infected women. Obstet Gynecol 79(3):321–327, 1992.
152. Safrin S, Crumpacker C, Chatis P, et al: A controlled trial comparing foscarnet with vidarabine for acyclovir resistant mucocutaneous herpes simplex in AIDS. N Engl J Med 325:551–555, 1991.
153. Scarlatti G, Leitner T, Hodara V, et al: Neutralizing antibodies and viral characteristics in mother-to-baby transmission of HIV-1. AIDS 7:S45–S48, 1993.
154. Scott GB, Fischl MA, Klimas N, et al: Mothers of infants with the acquired immunodeficiency syndrome. Evidence for both symptomatic and asymptomatic carriers. JAMA 253:363–366, 1985.
155. Serwadda D, Mugerwa RD, Sewankambo NK, et al: Slim disease: a new disease in Uganda and its association with HTLV-III infection. Lancet 2:849–852, 1985.
156. Shearer G, Clerici M: Abnormalities of immune regulation in human immunodeficiency virus infection. Pediatr Res 33:S71–S74, 1993.
157. Siegal FP, Lopez C, Hammer GS, et al: Severe acquired immunodeficiency in male homosexuals, manifested by chronic perianal ulcerative herpes simplex lesions. N Engl J Med 305:1439–1444, 1981.
158. Silliman CC, Tedder D, Ogle JW, et al: Unsuspected varicella-zoster virus encephalitis in a child with acquired immunodeficiency syndrome. J Pediatr 123:418–422, 1993.
159. Smith PD, Eisner MS, Manischewitz JF, et al: Esophageal disease in AIDS is associated with pathologic processes rather than mucosal human immunodeficiency virus type I. J Infect Dis 167:547–552, 1993.
160. Solinger AM, Hess EV: Rheumatic diseases and AIDS—is the association real? J Rheumatol 20:678–683, 1993.
161. Stiehm ER, Vink P: Transmission of human immunodeficiency virus infection by breast-feeding. J Pediatr 118:410–412, 1991.
162. Stiehm ER, Bryson YJ, Frenkel LM, et al: Prednisone improves human immunodeficiency virus encephalopathy in children. Pediatr Infect Dis J 11:49–50, 1992.
163. Stover DE, Zama MB, Haydu I, et al: Bronchoalveolar lavage in the diagnosis of diffuse pulmonary infiltrate in the immunosuppressed host. Ann Intern Med 101:1–7, 1984.
164. Taub DD, Conlon K, Lloyd AR, et al: Preferential migration of activated CD4+ and CD8+ T cells in response to MIP-1 alpha and MIP-1 beta. Science 260:355–358, 1993.
165. Theuer CP, Hopewell PC, Elias D, et al: Human immunodeficiency virus infection in tuberculosis patients. J Infect Dis 162:8–12, 1990.
166. Thiry L, Sprecher G, Goldberger S, et al: Isolation of AIDS virus from cell-free breast milk of three healthy virus carriers. Lancet 2:891–892, 1985.
167. Tibaldi C, Tovo PA, Ziarati N, et al: Asymptomatic women at high risk of vertical HIV-1 transmission to their fetuses. Br J Obstet Gynaecol 100:334–337, 1993.
168. Tindall B, Cooper D: Primary HIV infection: host responses and intervention strategies. AIDS 5:1–14, 1991.
169. Tovo PA, De Martino M, Gabiano C, et al: Prognostic factors and survival in children with perinatal HIV-1 infection. Lancet 339:1249–1253, 1992.
170. Tredget EE, Yu YM, Zhong S, et al: Role of IL1 and TNF on energy metabolism in rabbits. Am J Physiol 255 (Endoc Metal 18):E760–E768, 1988.
171. Uittenbogaart C, Anisman D, Schmid I, et al: Role of HIV infection of thymocytes in the pathogenesis of pediatric AIDS. J Cell Biochem S17E:94, 1993. Abstract.
172. Vago L, Antonacci M, Cristina S, et al: Morphogenesis, evolution and prognostic significance of lymphatic tissue lesions in HIV infection. Appl Pathol 7:298–309, 1989.
173. Varmus H: Retroviruses. Science 240:1427–1435, 1988.
174. Volkman DJ, Craddock B, Gulla J, Steigbigel R: Immunization in HIV-infected patients: abrogation of spontaneous B cell anti-HIV production. Clin Research 42:156A, 1994.
175. Wei X, Ghosh SK, Taylor ME, et al: Viral dynamics in human immunodeficiency virus type 1 infection. Nature 373:117-122, 1995.
176. Westby M, Manca F, Dalgleish A: The role of host immune responses in determining the outcome of HIV infection. Immunol Today 17:120–126, 1996.
177. Working Group on Antiretroviral Therapy: National Pediatric HIV Resource Center. Antiretroviral therapy and medical management of the human immunodeficiency virus-infected child. Pediatr Infect Dis J 12:513–522, 1993.
178. Wong VK, Gillette SG, Roth MJ, et al: Plasma immunotherapy in a child with acquired immunodeficiency syndrome. Pediatr Infect Dis J 12:947–951, 1993.
179. Zaman MR, White DA: Serum lactic dehydrogenase levels and *Pneumocystis carinii* pneumonia: diagnostic and prognostic significance. Am Rev Respir Dis 137:796–800, 1988.

48 Autoimmunity

FREDERICK MILLER

The subject of autoimmunity has undergone major conceptual changes.[87, 115] As our understanding of the regulation of the immune system has improved, we have begun to realize that our initial ideas, dating to Erhlich, require substantial modification.[93, 140] Sensitive techniques have disclosed the presence of many autoantibodies in the general population, particularly in the older age group.[9, 96] Antibodies against cellular and intracellular constituents may facilitate the clearance of these substances from the circulation as cells become senescent and deteriorate.[44] Thus, it is not the occurrence of an autoantibody that leads to disease. Instead, its effector capabilities (such as fixing complement), the regulation of its synthesis, and the clearance of the products of its interaction with its antigen are more important.

It therefore follows that the previously held tenet that autoimmunity is necessarily harmful is no longer valid. Although the same scenario likely applies to cellular immune responses, there is not sufficient information to make this statement with the same assurance that one can with regard to humoral immunity. The distinction between responses to foreign determinants as opposed to self-molecules is also not so precise as formerly thought. Cross-reactivity between these two classes of epitopes and therefore degeneracy of the immune system are now accepted as a given. This concept is employed to explain how streptococcal pharyngitis might lead to rheumatic carditis.

Perhaps it would be advantageous to consider autoimmune disease as opposed to autoimmunity. As previously implied, antibodies to certain elements of self may not be abnormal. That is not to say that all antibodies directed against self are innocuous, even in minute concentrations.[98] Good examples are responses against critical cell surface molecules, such as the acetylcholine receptor (AChR). There may be some immune responses that are always deleterious and others that are so only if they exceed certain boundary conditions. The critical idea, in either case, is whether disease results. Autoimmune disease requires structural or functional abnormality, as well as a loss of self-tolerance.

TOLERANCE

It has become clear that the immune repertoire develops from seemingly random combinations of the V and J (and D in the case of heavy chain) germline gene segments, with additional diversity conferred by modifications at the combinatorial sites.[137] With some variation, the same processes apply to both B and T cells.[129] It is obvious that with such a mechanism of specificity generation many cells would arise bearing receptors reactive with self. It was formerly thought that all such clones must be extirpated and that autoimmune disease arose by a failure of the elimination to occur.[87] Several findings have greatly modified this thinking.

First, as noted previously, increased sensitivity in testing methodology has shown that normal individuals, particularly those of advanced age, have circulating antibodies that interact with autologous antigens.[96, 104] Indeed, a population of naive B cells can be stimulated in vitro with polyclonal activators, such as lipopolysaccharide, so that some clones produce immunoglobulins with specificity for nuclear antigens, such as DNA.[97] Second, as far as T cells are concerned, the concept of positive selection in the thymus implies that a T lymphocyte, in order to mature, must be able to recognize (interact with) the major histocompatibility complex (MHC) class I or class II molecules. This step is critical since the ability to separate self from other than self depends on a firm image of self. Balancing this is negative selection, the need to eliminate functional immunocytes whose interaction with one's own molecules would be damaging (tolerance of self). It is critical that we examine this paradox.

Central to these principles is that most immunologic learning occurs at a very early point in life. Imagine a point in time when the immune system of the fetus is developing and progenitor T cells are leaving the marrow to become wise in the thymus. The fetus is antigenically protected and ideally free from foreign cells or their products. The T cell is programmed to die via apoptosis unless its receptor interacts with an MHC molecule.[26] We believe that such an event may involve *bcl*-2, a gene that if activated rescues the T cell (or B cell) from suicide.[64, 99] Once this event occurs, cells that bind self-molecules in the context of the MHC must be inactivated or they would facilitate effector mechanisms that would injure the host. Since the fetus is isolated, the only determinants present in the thymus are those derived from self and not from pathogens.

Cells that react strongly to self-peptides expressed in the context of MHC in the thymus seem to trigger another gene, *fas*, which acts in a manner opposite to that of *bcl*-2.[50] *Fas* activates an apoptotic pathway and the cell dies. This apparent inconsistency is resolved when emphasis is placed on the strength and nature of the interaction, as well as the maturity of the interacting lymphocyte. Precursor cells, both B and T, handle signal transduction differently than do their adult counterparts. It also appears that the number of receptors they display is smaller. The signal expressed upon contact with an antigen is therefore slight relative to that in the mature cell. Thus tolerance, the state of immunologic unresponsiveness, is easier to induce in young animals than in adults.

Four outcomes are possible for a T cell as it enters the thymus (Fig. 48–1).[129] One, if it is unable to interact with the stromal cells expressing MHC, it undergoes apoptosis. Two, if it interacts with very modest force, differentiation occurs (*bcl*-2 is activated) and it moves deeper into the cortex. Three, if it interacts strongly (presumably with a self-peptide expressed in the groove of an MHC molecule), it dies (perhaps *fas* is expressed). Four, if the nature of the interaction is intermediate, not strong enough to kill but too

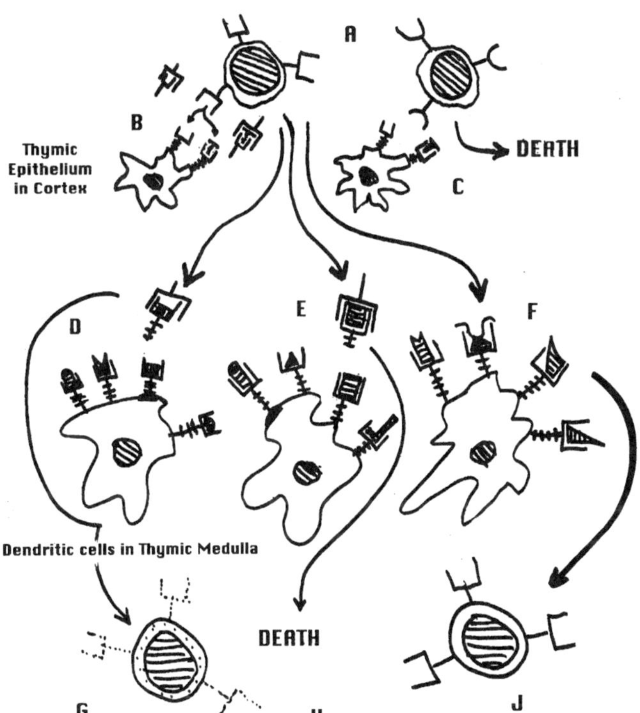

FIGURE 48–1. A hypothetical model for intrathymic positive and negative selection. Pre–T lymphocytes enter thymus (A) and with differentiation acquire their receptors (TCR). Thymic epithelial cells in the cortex display MHC molecules that either are empty or contain special peptides ('T') not expressed elsewhere (unsettled issue at this time). If the TCR binds (positive selection) to a suitable ligand, apoptosis is averted (B). If there is no 'match,' cell death occurs (C). A viable cell migrates inward, and three options are available as it encounters antigen-presenting cells having self-peptides in the context of MHC on their membranes. If there is a weak interaction (D), the cell is rendered nonreactive but enters the periphery (G). This is clonal anergy. There is uncertainty if this occurs in the thymus or peripherally, but it is convenient to hypothesize that it is an intrathymic alternative. If there is a strong interaction (E), that is, the TCR binds with high affinity to one or more self-peptides in the context of MHC molecules, apoptosis occurs. This is clonal deletion. Finally, if there is no interaction, the now immunocompetent T cell enters the blood and migrates to peripheral lymphoid tissue (negative selection).

much for differentiation, the T cell may survive but becomes anergic. This state implies that the cell is viable but incapable of responding to ordinary antigenic stimulation. This last may be critical to certain autoimmune disease because an anergic T cell has the capacity to foster a reaction against self if it encounters a strong enough costimulatory signal. Such a signal could arise if a nonspecific mitogen or superantigen were encountered by that cell.

The situation is similar in the case of B cells.[88] These lymphocytes, developing in the marrow, initially express IgM. If they contact an antigen during this period, they are either clonally deleted or rendered anergic. The terms clonal deletion and clonal anergy may be applied to both B and T cells and require clarification. By clonal deletion we mean that a cell with a given specificity (and its progeny, the clone) dies and that specificity is deleted from the repertoire. Clonal anergy implies that the clone of cells expressing a particular antigenic specificity is not eliminated but simply is rendered unresponsive to the usual stimuli (contact with antigen and presence of the costimulus or second signal). If appropriately prodded, they can express their product, such as an antibody, and therefore initiate an autoimmune reaction.

The developing B cells that continue their maturation (bearing IgM with activity against some nonself-peptide) next express IgD with the IgM and enter the periphery. On contact with an antigen, they then initiate usual humoral responses.

Studies with transgenic animals have provided additional insights.[77] Suppose we create mice with antibody genes that enable a reaction against a specific MHC class I molecule, Å, by producing anti–MHC-I-Å. In mice expressing Ä instead of Å, the presence of these cells has no effect since none of the cells express Å. However, if they develop in a mouse expressing Å, then B cells with anti-Å specificity do not develop. If they did, the mouse would destroy itself since all of its nucleated cells and platelets express all the MHC class I alleles that the mouse has inherited, would display Å, and be susceptible to anti-Å. There must be mechanisms that prevent the expression of antibody by these genetically programmed B cells.

If during development endogenous genes encoding heavy and light chains are rearranged or mutated so that their receptors do not react well (or at all) with Å, they are not deleted.[85] One can also construct mice that have cells that elaborate a particular antigen, X, and also have a large number of B cells committed to producing an antibody, anti-X. In such mice, no anti-X is detectable, yet B cells with the capability to produce anti-X reach peripheral lymphoid tissue.[1, 45] They bear reduced membrane levels of IgM anti-X and are anergic, even if immunized with X. Whether X is secreted or membrane bound is critical since if it is expressed on the membrane then reactive B lymphocytes are deleted.

In these two experimental models, we have created situations that allowed us to examine the mechanisms that bring about clonal deletion and clonal anergy. In coming years, we can expect that the molecular mechanisms will be clarified, which will permit the development of therapeutic strategies for dealing with autoimmune disease. If we were able to delete clonally or even render anergic cells reactive against self-constituents, many diseases would be cured or effectively treated.

Although there are many similarities in tolerance in B and T cells, there are well-established differences. As a general rule, it is considerably harder to tolerize B cells because larger amounts of antigen are required. Even after that is accomplished, B cells remain tolerant for substantially shorter periods of time. These points and the whole subject of tolerance are thoroughly reviewed by Schwartz.[109]

One important caveat underlies many of our assumptions about autoimmunity; namely, that they are based on relatively few studies with even fewer antigens. Inductive reasoning has been used to extend these ideas to the entire immune repertoire. We do not know if these conclusions will stand the test of more rigorous and extensive examination.

Before considering mechanisms, a final point must be made. Although emphasis has been placed on the learning of self in early life, it is clear that the immune repertoire does not shut down at birth. Marrow and thymic functions are largely but perhaps not entirely peripheralized. It is likely that many of the proteins and carbohydrates produced in the various organs do not enter the thymus. No inventory of self-derived peptides present in the thymus has been taken. The possibility exists that a substantial number of tissue-specific autoimmune diseases occur because the determinants involved in the responses that eventually occur were never expressed in the thymus and reactive cells were never deleted.

Many lymphocytes must leave the thymus selected for by low-order reactivity with MHC molecules but have the capacity to bind, presumably by virtue of cross-reactivity, to self-antigens. Such cells have been identified.[20] Since autoreactivity does not result, we could imagine that the epitopes are not exposed, that costimulation does not occur, or that peripheral tolerance can be achieved. Investigations have shown that the antigenic site on the self-molecule is available.[75] Studies with autoreactive T cells administered to transgenic mice (rendered capable of expressing the epitope) have resulted in disease. This would suggest that prior clonal deletion had occurred and the resulting immune deficiency had been repaired.[80, 84] Other work has disclosed that the problem could result from a failure of the antigen-presenting cells to deliver the costimulatory signal.

The implicit contradictions point to a current lack of understanding. There may be several mechanisms, or there may be problems inherent in the construction or interpretation of the experiments. There are a number of variables in transgenic studies[77]: whether the antigen is soluble or membrane bound; when it is expressed in terms of development; how much protein (antigen) is produced; the maturity of the reactive T cell when it encounters the antigen; how the state of the target cell, aside from the determinant it expresses, influences the outcome; whether the antigen-presenting cell is appropriate; whether the helper T cell has the correct repertoire; and how long the transgenic determinant persists (since transient exposures are not sufficient to initiate autoimmune disease).[75] Details remain unclear, and it is amazing that we understand as much of the phenomenon as we do. It is certain that this peripheral tolerization must occur and be significant. If such was not the case, it is hard to understand how adult immunization against newly evolving microorganisms could occur. It is also evident that recognition of self, at least in this context, must be ongoing. Possibly mechanisms that prevent fetal-maternal interaction can also operate on other systems in the adult.

Autoimmune disease does not likely result from spontaneous mutation in the recognition mechanism of lymphocytes in the majority of cases. One of the reasons cited will be the relative absence of such diseases in children. One could argue that mutation after peripheralization (a process that might enhance this likelihood) could explain such an event. In rebuttal, thymic atrophy and transfer of its functions to other lymphoid organs occur well before the peak incidence of autoimmune disease. Indeed, one of our considerations in accounting for the autoimmune process is that it is mainly confined to the period of reproductive activity. It is true that many diseases with suspected autoimmune causation, such as insulin-dependent diabetes mellitus (IDDM), juvenile rheumatoid arthritis (JRA), or rheumatic fever, frequently occur in young people. These rarely appear in infancy, and the mechanisms underlying them do not suggest random mutation for many reasons. For this discussion, specific mutation that might occur from viral infection is separated from alterations that occur through random processing of DNA or radiation effects.

MECHANISMS

Changes have occurred in much of the thinking about how autoimmune disease could develop as newer knowledge regarding immune regulation has accumulated.[79] We must consider two very different situations. In the first, disease results from an immune response directed against a well-defined moiety, commonly a cell surface or tissue-specific protein. Myasthenia gravis, in which the AChR is the target, and Goodpasture's syndrome, in which the globular domain of type IV collagen is the epitope, are good examples.[21, 74, 132] Attack may be cellular, as well as humoral, as in multiple sclerosis or certain forms of thyroiditis. In the second situation, disease results from an exuberant immune response that is more commonly humoral and broad in its targets. A number of autoantibodies are produced against antigens that come to circulate in the blood, and this leads to the formation of soluble immune complexes. The prototype of such a disorder is systemic lupus erythematosus.

The perennial issue we face is how these disorders arise. One question is whether the immune response is antigen driven or arises as a result of an aberrant cellular event. Consider a clone of cells that is released from feedback controls by a mutation and produces a protein product, say an antibody, that results in disease. The proliferation may approximate a neoplasm. There are excellent examples of such processes: certain cryoglobinopathies or even multiple myeloma may by chance have their specificities directed against a tissue component or circulating antigen. This would be very different from a normal immune response in which affinity maturation and class switching occur and the problem is not a mutagenic event but an impairment of normal control or loss of usual tolerance. Thus we shall see that autoimmune disease behaves more like an inflammatory response, such as to an infectious agent, that has gone astray in some manner rather than a neoplastic process. Although there may seem to be some overlap, the theme of a genetic substrate that fails in distinguishing clearly between a pathogen and self (and subsequently attacks self) will emerge as central in contemporary thought.[34]

What ideas have been advanced to account for a loss of

tolerance to self and how have they changed in recent years? Let us first list the possibilities, then consider evidence that supports or refutes them, and finally review specific examples that have come under careful study in the past few years. First, one can image a spontaneous mutation that might alter the specificity of a lymphocyte. Second, an antigen could fail to be represented in the thymus and therefore not be part of the self inventory (sequestered antigen) and subsequently be exposed and regarded as nonself. Third, the mechanisms that abort or render anergic certain clones might fail. For example, a defect might arise in the apoptotic pathway for a T-cell reactive with thyroglobulin.

Fourth, a suppressor circuit may be absent or defective. This supposes that one mechanism for controlling immune responses is the existence of specific cells that depress a specific response. Fifth, a helper T cell might be too stimulatory and enhance a response that would otherwise not occur. Sixth, there may be an intrinsic defect in the thymus such that resident cells do not properly educate immature T cells as to self. Note that B cells also mature and any that might have self-directed specificities must be lost or rendered unresponsive. Since most effector reactions involving B cells require IgG, for which T-cell help is needed, many investigators have avoided the issue of self-reacting B cells by assuming that they are controlled through their dependence on T-cell help.

Seventh, mechanisms exist to bypass the requirement for T-cell help. Perhaps a superantigen is introduced, or a polyclonal B cell stimulator, such as lipopolysaccharide, comes in contact with a self-reactive B cell. Eighth, the fault may lie not in the lymphocyte but in the antigen-presenting cell. Processing in macrophages or dendritic cells may be aberrant, or cells usually not expressing class II MHC molecules might be erroneously induced to do so. Under such a circumstance, a surface constituent might be presented in a context such that it is recognized as foreign. Ninth, the idiotypic network, a mechanism by which the immune system produces antibodies against idiotopes and in turn regulates itself, might be defective. Such a mechanism might explain how very high levels of antinuclear antibodies could occur and in turn lead to tissue injury.

ADJUVANT EFFECT (TWO-SIGNAL CONCEPT)

For many years, it has been known that optimal immune responses are achieved by the use of adjuvants. The best known of these was one composed by Jules Freund incorporating oil emulsion with tubercle bacilli. The effectiveness of such preparations was explained by the proposal of Bretscher and Cohn[19] that lymphocyte activation required two signals. The first required the binding of antigen by a specific receptor, whereas the second was a signal from the antigen-presenting cell to the lymphocyte by membrane contact or effete humoral message. The second signal would be nonspecific, but without it the lymphocyte, on contact with its antigen, would be inactivated, whereas with it stimulation would occur.

Subsequent work has substantiated this model. We term the second signal the costimulatory molecule. The state resulting from inactivation upon receiving only a single signal is referred to as clonal anergy.[53] We recognize that the costimulatory molecule may be endogenous (lymphokines) or exogenous (derived from microorganisms). The importance of this postulate to autoimmunity lies in the fact that many clones of self-reactive lymphocytes may be in a state of clonal anergy. An encounter with a sufficiently potent second signal may awaken them and result in tissue damage.

What evidence is there that such self-reactive cells may be normally present? It is evident that normal B lymphocytes can produce rheumatoid factor.[97] It is also known that sensitive assays detect antibodies against intracellular components, membrane proteins, and polypeptides. These do not depend on external stimuli since they may be demonstrated in embryos and neonates.[69, 126] Furthermore, such specificities commonly arise in lymphoid malignancies. Although usually of IgM isotype, low affinity, and little consequence, they may be IgG, have avidities of induced antibodies, and on occasion produce disease states.[17, 28] Sequence studies have shown that such autoantibodies are encoded in germline genes, and their common occurrence suggests a physiologic role.[15, 138] Although proof is lacking, it has been supposed that these serve to facilitate the clearance of cellular debris, to prevent autoimmune disease by interacting with cross-reactive (with self-) epitopes on foreign molecules, or both. This might prevent the development of IgG autoantibodies.

SPONTANEOUS MUTATION

Could autoimmune disease result from a spontaneous mutation (other than normal somatic hypermutation in B-cell responses), and if it did, in which component of the immune system might it reside? Consider the second part of the hypothesis first. The mutation could not simply involve professional antigen-presenting cells since regardless of the manner in which determinants were expressed, recognition lies with the B and T lymphocytes. For reasons considered under polyclonal B-cell activation, it is most probable that a T-cell mutation would be required. This type of alteration, involving a single clone, would only be applicable to tissue- or organ-specific autoimmune diseases.

Mutations are by their nature random. Therefore, if they were the cause of autoimmune disease, we would expect a great variety of epitopes and various effector mechanisms to be involved, with great variation among patients having the same target. This turns out not to be the case. In studied diseases, it appears that the same determinant is involved. Excellent examples are the myelin basic protein in experimental allergic encephalomyelitis, the Goodpasture antigen, or the antigen involved in pemphigus vulgaris.[3, 57, 128] Furthermore, studies of the T-cell antigen receptor (TCR) in a number of individuals with various autoimmune diseases disclose that the response is usually oligoclonal.[42] The exceptions appear to be the rare cases of lymphoproliferative disease in which the involved clone possesses autoimmune reactivity. In general, patients with these types of autoimmune injury are quite different from those that do not have an underlying lymphoid neoplasm.

There is one type of mutation that might be of real significance. Consider the consequences of a cell in a given tissue or organ acquiring the ability to express class II MHC molecules on its surface in the manner of a macrophage or dendritic cell. Peptides elaborated near that cell, some of which are undoubtedly tissue- or organ-specific, might be taken in, processed, and presented to T cells. Such a circumstance has been found to exist. There exists a model in which viral infection of glial cells in mice causes these cells to express MHC class II antigens, in turn to interact with T cells, and likely to contribute to the resulting demyelination.[123] This situation involves a virus, but such could occur, in all likelihood, as a result of spontaneous errors in DNA, radiation-induced changes, and so on.

According to current understanding, exogenous antigens are processed in the context of class II MHC molecules, whereas endogenous or cell-derived molecules (viral proteins, as well as self-components) are degraded and presented by class I MHC molecules (on the cell surface). Of particular interest are studies indicating that radiation of target organs does not induce autoimmune disease. Rather, radiation exerts its effect (in leading to reactions against self) by altering control mechanisms in T cells.[105]

Finally, although the data are scant in organ-specific autoimmune disease and only a bit better in diseases such as systemic lupus erythematosus (SLE), analysis of involved B-cell populations that have been clonally immortalized show minimal roles for somatic mutation. The heavy and light chain genes used are very similar to those in the germline, yet the response behaves as though it was driven by antigen. It is possible that mutational events are important in certain contexts. A normal B-cell response to a foreign antigen could be directed against self during affinity maturation. In this situation, somatic hypermutation occurs, and clones with reactivity against self might be produced (but without corresponding T helper cells).[39] It is not clear how these cells, being short lived and unstimulated, could survive to cause disease.

SEQUESTERED ANTIGENS—THE PRIVILEGED SITE HYPOTHESIS

There are anatomic regions of the body in which immune reactions do not usually occur or in which transplanted foreign grafts are not rejected. Tissues or their products from these sites are not represented in the fetal thymus. These areas have certain features in common: they are not normally exposed to blood, or a blood-tissue barrier exists; they lack cells expressing class II MHC molecules that could serve as antigen presenting cells; and they may have immune suppressing properties.[122] In some, there is no lymphatic drainage to regional lymphoid tissues, and thus antigenic components may not reach reactive cells. Examples of such tissues or organs are the eye, brain, gonads, and fetus developing in the uterus.

Two interesting features of some of these sites deserve notice. Their antigens can on occasion escape and elicit immune responses as though they were foreign. The antigens within them may escape the immune response, while at the same time identical antigens undergo immune elimination in traditional sites in the same animals.[8] This last phenomenon was recognized in the early days of transplantation when it was observed that allografts or even xenografts could be placed in certain sites, such as the anterior chamber of a rabbit's eye or a hamster's cheek pouch, and would not be rejected.[122]

The importance of the privileged site hypothesis to autoimmunity was that it led to the concept that if damage occurred to such a site and its antigens escaped, then an autoimmune disease could follow. An example often cited is that of sympathetic ophthalmia in which injury to an eye allows access by lymphocytes. The retinal or choroidal antigens are treated as foreign, antibodies then can be produced, and the other, intact eye may be damaged.[126] The concept extends readily to thyroid or even kidney. Tissue-specific determinants in the thyroid may face the follicle, a structure that lymphocytes would not normally be exposed to. In the case of the kidney, the antigen may lie proximate to the urinary space, a body component that is on the outside and therefore not under T lymphocyte surveillance. Unfortunately, although seemingly attractive, this hypothesis has been applicable in very few situations.

First and foremost, there is the clinical observation that breaching a privileged site and releasing a sequestered antigen does not invariably or even commonly lead to disease. When this occurs, the process is usually of short duration and therefore differs markedly from most autoimmune diseases that are chronic. The necessity for an adjuvant or prolonged exposure is an important element.[126] Second, in some instances, the theoretical assumptions have not been supported. Lymphocytes do, for example, enter tissues such as the brain.[89] Several other explanations for why they do not react have been offered.[18] It is still a strong possibility that many organs and tissues behave as sequestered sites because their critical determinants are not presented in the thymus and that migrating lymphocytes are not normally exposed to them in a suitable context.

FAILURE TO ELIMINATE SELF-REACTIVE CLONES

It is conceivable that autoimmune disease results from the failure to eliminate self-reactive T (or B) cells. Perhaps we should digress for a moment and focus on T cells. When one examines the naturally occurring autoantibodies, those that increase with advanced age and those that are represented in the germline genes, it is apparent that the antibodies produced are of relatively low avidity and invariably of IgM isotype. In contrast, when one looks at patients who suffer from autoimmune disease, either systemic or organ specific, it is clear that the antibodies are of higher affinity, show greater numbers of somatic mutations, and are commonly of IgG (and/or IgA) classes. Class switching and somatic mutation are signs of antigen-driven T-dependent reactions.[73] It therefore seems likely that T helper cells that can provide critical costimulatory signals to allow autoreactive B cells to mature are present. Such cells should have been eliminated but are obviously evident in patients with autoimmune diseases. Therein lies the reason for our attention.

Current concepts of T-cell differentiation hold the thymus to be central to educating T cells as to self. Three reasons for the failure to eliminate autoreactive thymic T cells come to mind: first, the antigen in question might not reach the thymus or may be in a form such that it cannot be degraded to an antigenic peptide; second, the antigen-presenting cells in the thymus may be incapable of expressing the particular antigen; and third, the machinery for eliminating the indiscriminate T cell may be defective. Let us consider each of these scenarios.

The antigen may not be expressed in the fetus at a time when thymic education is occurring. There may be a maturational delay in a particular organ. This seems unlikely for if such were the case, autoimmune diseases would be very common in early childhood. Disease would occur when the tissue in question caught up and expressed the antigen. The immune system would regard this as though it represented a foreign invader and would endeavor to destroy the tissue and thus cause disease.

In the second situation, an inborn error of metabolism might result in the absence of an enzyme activity, perhaps in the proteasome.[125] This is a large, multiple-subunit polyprotease structure, some of whose enzymes are encoded in the MHC. This suggests an important role for these enzymes in processing antigens to their immunodominant peptides. If the requisite enzyme or other component of the complex were absent, then the appropriate peptide would not be generated and could not be expressed in the context of the MHC class II molecule. Alternatively, we can imagine a defect in the MHC class II repertoire. This might derive from either somatic mutation or the inheritance of a complement of molecules that, although being able to express most foreign and self-peptides, could not bind a critical configuration.

Superficially, such postulates might be attractive because they link the known inheritance of certain MHC molecules associated with disease to a plausible mechanism (as with B27 and ankylosing spondylitis).[139] Closer examination leads to the rejection of both ideas. First, such defects have not been found. Second, if they existed, we would again wonder why disease waits for postadolescence to appear. Third, if the defect lay in thymic antigen-presenting cells, the same defect would be present peripherally and the self-antigen could never be presented to immunocompetent T helper cells needed to initiate the process.

Finally, there is the possibility of defective elimination of self-reactive lymphocytes. It has long been appreciated that enormous numbers of B and T cells enhance the repertoire on a daily basis. Most of these are eliminated. Work has shown that these cells have rearranged their antigen-specific receptors, and it is presumed that many (if not the great majority) are eliminated because they react with self. This is not surprising if one remembers that antigen-presenting cells process endogenous molecules as readily as exogenous ones and that many more of the former are available at any given time.

There is nothing to suggest any preference for a selection against self-molecules at the time of generation of specificity. It is known that clonal deletion results from apoptosis. We have noted the roles of *fas* and *bcl*-2. If a lymphocyte with a high-avidity receptor for the globular domain of type IV collagen activates *bcl*-2 inappropriately, then instead of dying, it persists. The circumstance necessary for Goodpasture's syndrome might then exist. We could postulate a spontaneous somatic mutation, a virus-induced transcriptional error, or a substance providing an aberrant signal to a cell surface receptor that can activate the gene. The effect is the same in each case. Similarly, *fas* has been shown to be altered in the MRL-lpr(homozygous) mouse.[131] This animal, which is subject to a lupus-like disease, has a vastly greater than normal peripheral complement of T cells.

ABNORMAL SUPPRESSOR CIRCUITRY

One of the major controversies in immunology has been whether there are suppressor cells. Were it not for the untimely death of Gershon, who with Kondo initially described the suppressor effect in a cell transfer setting, perhaps the issue might have been resolved by now.[38] There is no clear-cut marker for human suppressor cells nor has a suppressor cell been cloned. It is clear that in a number of situations, the only viable explanation is the existence of such cells or at least a property that resides in lymphocytes that can down-regulate a specific immune response. Indeed, a postulate underlying the use of cyclosporine as a treatment for autoimmune disease is that it can inhibit helper and effector T cells without impeding the suppressor cell pathway.[47] Advances in our knowledge have shown that these cells are induced by antigens administered intravenously and without adjuvants. These conditions are similar to those that lead to anergy.

It appears that cytokines such as TGFβ or IL-10 are mediators of the effect in certain cases, whereas in others that are more specific, a soluble secreted T-cell receptor has been suggested as the suppressor factor.[54, 106] Although most believe that the cells involved are CD8+, antigen-specific effects have been mainly documented in mice, and little concrete information from human material is available.[132] Attractive alternative hypotheses for T suppressor activity are an ability to bind critical maturation factors like IL-2 or to possess cytotoxic activity against specific T helper cells.[4, 109] The last idea has parallelism with the anti-idiotypic network proposed for B cells. It is probable that many combinations of suppressive activity exist. There is no evidence that nature has restrictive rules in this regard, and the very diversity of possibilities is the greatest impediment to our understanding.

Whatever the basis, antigen-specific and nonspecific suppressor activity seems likely. In turn, it is clear that if they restrict autoimmune responses, anything that might impair this activity could lead to autoimmune disease. Consider as one possibility a virus whose cellular binding site is the antigen-specific receptor on the suppressor T cell. Infection leads to selective destruction of that clone. Clearly this could result in the expression of antiself-effector responses and in turn organ-specific tissue damage.

INCREASED HELPER CELL ACTIVITY

Disturbed function of regulatory T cells has been postulated to be a cause of autoimmune disease, for example, an increase in Th1 cells or a deficiency in Th2 cells. One will recall that Th1 cells secrete IFN-γ and IL-2 in contrast to Th2 cells that elaborate IL-4, IL-5, and IL-10. Since large amounts of IL-2 will activate anergic cells, one can see how an inordinate response of Th1 cells might induce an antiself response. One difficulty exists, and that is how to account for specificity. Possibly one could have a somatic mutation in a single clone, but to imagine that the same exact events recurring in one and only one lymphocyte in every patient with a particular disease is very difficult. This means that a particular clone in every patient with Goodpasture's syndrome and different unique clones in patients with ankylosing spondylitis or Hashimoto's thyroiditis are specifically altered. At present, a mechanism by which this might occur is not known. The distinction between spontaneous alteration as induced by ionizing radiation and programmed change as occurs when viral infection introduces a uniform segment of DNA or RNA is important in this context. The latter are perfectly plausible but unproven.

In systemic autoimmune disease, one might simply say there is an imbalance that would generally favor activation of many tolerized clones. A genetic manipulation of the T-cell lineage in mice has produced an example of this.[105] The most telling argument against this mechanism is that no instance of its demonstration in spontaneous animal or human disease has been reported to our knowledge.

THYMIC DEFECTS

An interesting hypothesis is that autoimmune disease results when there is a failure to present a self-antigen in proper context (conjugated to an MHC molecule) on an antigen-presenting cell. This could represent a problem with the thymic epithelial or dendritic cells so that the antigen is not phagocytosed or endocytosed, not properly digested, not transported to the endoplasmic reticulum, or not in an environment that allows for proper interaction with MHC polypeptides. This concept embodies the same problems referred to in the failure to eliminate self-reactive clones and is closely allied to that idea.[104]

If, for example, a thyroid antigen was not able to be processed, because of an enzyme defect in the thymic antigen-presenting cell (APC), then developing thymocytes with receptors for epitopes on this tissue-specific peptide would not be eliminated. Later on, such cells could be central in causing autoimmune thyroiditis. There is little evidence to support this hypothesis other than the observation that autoimmune disease is more common in individuals with certain immunodeficiencies. In those cases, other defects in immunoregulation have been described.[79] Reports from animal studies suggest that rare exceptions may exist.[16, 114] Our review of studies to date indicates that they have not been described in humans.

BYPASSING THE REQUIREMENT FOR T-CELL HELP

One of the more attractive hypotheses for the development of autoimmune disease holds that circumstances exist in which a key element in tolerance, absence of helper T cells, might be circumvented. There are several ways this could come about. First, we know that there are polyclonal B-cell activators, such as lipopolysaccharide, that can activate B cells independent of T-cell help. In vitro, it has been shown that B cells can be induced to produce such autoreactive antibodies as rheumatoid factor and in vivo to initiate or accelerate disease in mice.[51, 113] Such a hypothesis would be untenable for organ-specific autoimmunity, because many different specificities, rather than a single one, would arise with polyclonal stimulation. For a disease such as lupus erythematosus, however, this situation is worthy of consideration.[61] Unfortunately, current evidence suggests that antibody production in lupus is T-cell dependent.

If B cells are not good targets for polyclonal stimulation, could specific help be circumvented by polyclonal activation of T cells? The idea here is that by providing a very strong stimulus, perhaps we could overcome clonal anergy. In patients with cancer who are treated with IL-2, autoantibodies appear.[108] Interestingly, anergic cells in culture can be sustained with this interleukin. When mice are infected with a retrovirus constructed to contain the IL-2 gene, pathologic changes akin to those in autoimmune disease have been observed.[83]

One observation could even provide some measure of specificity to polyclonal activation. Although in one model superantigens bind to the HLA molecule outside the peptide binding groove, their ability to bind is influenced by the state of occupancy of that receptor.[8, 29] One could imagine that only if the correct HLA-processed peptide pairing were present, a superantigen could interact. One major objection to the polyclonal activation hypothesis is the observation that in B cells the antibodies occurring in human and experimental autoimmune disease demonstrate the characteristics of an antigen-driven immune response.[73] Polyclonal activation produces mainly IgM antibodies, and the response does not show persistence, high avidity, or isotypic switching. All of these are present in both systemic and tissue-specific diseases whether naturally occurring or experimental.

A most attractive concept for bypassing T-cell requirements is that of molecular mimicry (Figs. 48–2 and 48–3). An infectious agent is thought to generate antibodies or T cells that cross-react with epitopes on self-constituents and result in tissue injury.[34, 91] The interest in this idea stems from the observation that infection frequently precedes an autoimmune disease, one of the best examples being rheumatic fever.[134] A clear experimental example is myelin basic protein (MBP) that causes encephalitis if combined with adjuvant and introduced into rabbits. The critical portion of MBP has been identified and found to contain six amino acids identical to a hexapeptide in the hepatitis B viral polymerase.[33]

Apparently, infectious agents may seek to evade the host response by approximating host structures to deceive the immune system. If a bacterium contains an antigenic group (S′) that is like a self-determinant (S) and one that is quite different from self (D) but on the same molecule (S′ is linked to D on the organism, either synthesized as a continuum or subsequently covalently linked), then the processed peptide may contain both S′ and D. T cells present that react against D can provide help to B cells capable of making anti-S′. This occurs although the host has had its anti-S′ T cells deleted or rendered anergic. Indeed, one could even imagine an S′ so that it would elicit a B- or T-cell response that would react with S.

It is necessary to keep in mind the degeneracy of the immune response and that with sensitive techniques cross reactions are detectable and specificity is rarely absolute. From an evolutionary perspective, it is inevitable that this would be the case. As parasites change to evade the human immune system, they must resemble human components more (at least as their surfaces are viewed from the perspec-

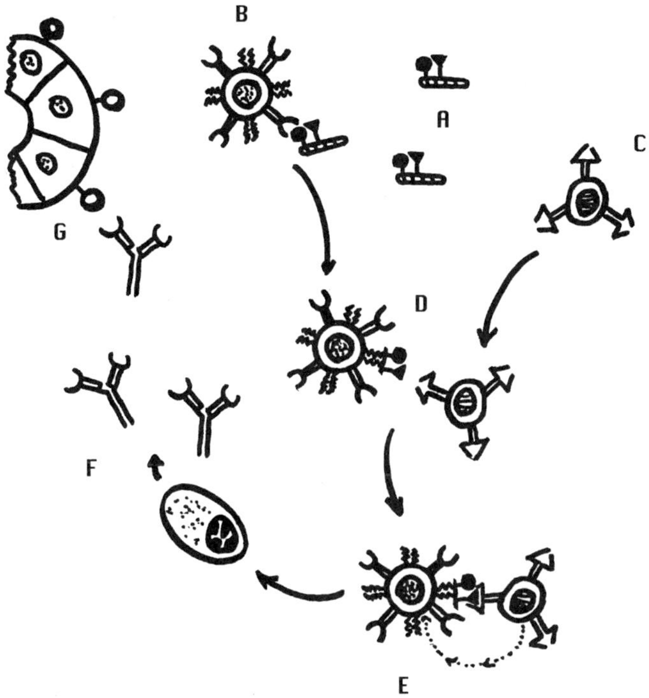

FIGURE 48–2. Bypassing the requirement for T-cell help. A B cell exists (B) that can react with a determinant on a thyroid follicle. It can never develop into a plasma cell and produce cytotoxic antibody because there is no T helper cell. An infection occurs caused by a bacteria (A) bearing an antigenic determinant that cross-reacts strongly with the B-cell receptor (IgM). On the same polypeptide, a determinant that corresponds to one in the T-cell repertoire is also expressed. The B cell processes and presents the bacterium (D) to the T lymphocyte (C). Now the T cell can respond to the epitope in the context of class II MHC and provide appropriate stimulation (costimulatory signals and interleukins) (E) so the B cell can proliferate and differentiate into a plasma cell (F). The resulting antibodies cause a thyroiditis (G).

tive of a human immunocyte). The immune system is therefore required to make finer and finer distinctions. The teleologic argument is that diversity of such cell surface molecules as MHC class I exists to protect the species at the expense of the individual. Consider the situation in which a particular MHC configuration is present on the cells of a specific individual. That molecular determinant may be the target for a particular parasite, enabling it to adhere to the surface of the cell and initiate infection. Alternatively, the bacteria or virus may have a surface that so closely resembles the MHC marker that the immune system cannot distinguish it from self. Cells of one person carrying a particular configuration, that is an organism's target or that it approximates to prevent the inflammatory reaction from recognizing it, are susceptible. Individuals who lack this MHC gene and its products are not susceptible to either infection or autoimmune disease. Therefore, the greater the diversity of the MHC, the greater the likelihood that some members of the species would survive the ravages of the organism or be less likely to lose tolerance to their constituents. If its subterfuge is sufficient, it can produce an infection that is not controlled. Alternatively, in destroying the invader, the host reacts and damages its own constituents by having tolerance breached. It is analogous to being between a rock (the pathogen) and a hard place (the need to maintain self-tolerance).

Another complication is the bystander phenomenon, which has become more common as our therapeutic armamentarium increases. In hemolytic anemia, caused by quinidine, chlorpromazine, and certain other drugs, an antibody formed against the drug has attached (presumably by nonspecific physicochemical interaction but also possibly by weak immune cross-reaction) to the erythrocyte surface.[63, 68] The antibody binds, complement is activated, and lysis follows. A variation would involve the immune complex forming first and then binding to the red cell surface.[107]

A perturbation of this idea involves a hapten-carrier (drug-erythrocyte) interaction. The circumstance is as follows: A drug, Rx, in its absorbed form or as modified by host metabolism (Rx′), binds as a hapten to the erythrocyte (or other cell, C, in the generalized form), which serves as a carrier. The product Rx′-C is antigenic. The immune response reacts to Rx′-C by forming antibodies or cytotoxic T cells. These now attack Rx′-C and destroy or damage the tissue. The individual remains tolerant to C in that transferring antibodies or lymphocytes to an isogeneic animal with C but not Rx′-C produces no ill effects. Such a mechanism occurs in autoimmune hemolytic anemia in patients given penicillin.[94, 107] Clearly, differences in certain blood groups might provide a binding site for Rx′, or the way in which Rx is metabolized might account for individual susceptibility. This would explain the genetic predisposition common in autoimmune disease.

Various drugs act in other ways. It is well known that

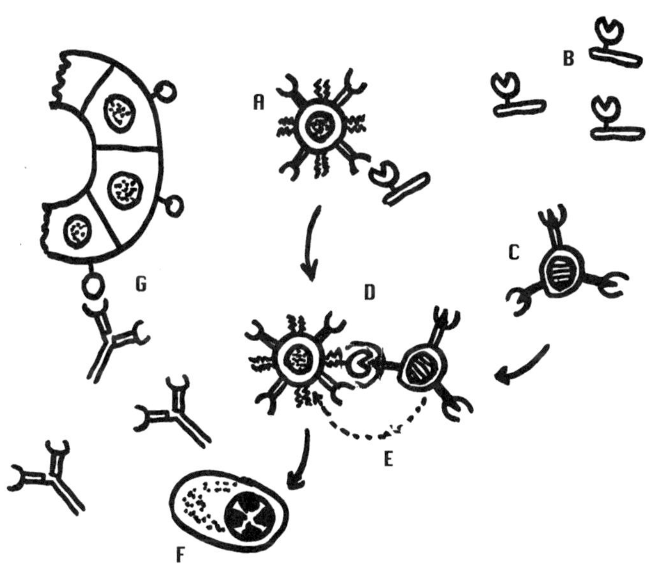

FIGURE 48–3. The situation is similar but simpler than that in Figure 48–2. In this case, the initial scenario is the same. A B cell exists that can react with a determinant on the surface of thyroid follicular cells. No T cell exists that can help this B cell since those that could were clonally deleted. The bacterium (B), however, has a determinant that mimics the thyroid follicle surface molecule (molecular mimicry). Although the T cell cannot respond to the determinant on the follicle (since that determinant cannot be accommodated in its receptor) (C), it can respond to that on the bacterium and in turn to the determinant presented by the B cell (D). Again, the B cell receives 'help' (E), plasma cells result (F), and antithyroid antibody results (G). Consider the situation if the bacterium were a virus that infected the follicle, or indeed, any cell. The same set of events could occur, but now the critical epitope would be presented in the context of class I MHC (since it is processed as an endogenous molecule by the infected cell). In this circumstance, the effector mechanism would be a cytotoxic T-cell response and the thyroiditis would be 'lymphocytic.'

agents such as procainamide, hydralazine, and methyldopa, among many others, produce lupus-like syndromes.[48] Certain metals, such as mercury or gold, can induce membranous nephropathy.[5] The list of agents that can function in one or more of the ways described is long ranging, from those noted to relatively simple compounds, such as hydrocarbons, that have been implicated in Goodpasture's syndrome.[14, 60] The mechanisms may be complex, and agents may act by altering lymphocytes directly, by changing the metabolism of cells so that their constituents are abnormal, or as discussed previously, by acting as haptens.

A fitting example, since we have touched on hemolytic anemia, occurs with α-methyldopa–associated reactions. In this case, it has been proposed that the drug acts by deregulating immunosuppression of the anergic but potentially reactive lymphocytes or by interfering with immune clearance.[58, 59] Of additional note, patients treated with α-methyldopa may also develop antinuclear antibodies. In lupus, the subject has been discussed by Hess,[47] and expanded discussions are found in standard texts.[32, 101] Figure 48–4 illustrates several of the mechanisms by which immune hemolysis might occur.

As protein or nucleic acid sequencing of microorganismal and human material becomes more commonplace, resemblances between sequences within processed peptides of self-origin and nonself-origin are detected more frequently.[33] When matched with autoimmune disease, they provide clues to basic mechanisms that can then be explored. Studies in type I diabetes mellitus suggest that such a situation might be operative.

For the heat shock proteins, there is a strong suggestion that molecular mimicry might be at work in adjuvant arthritis.[55, 127] A clone of T cells that reacts with a component of joint cartilage and the mycobacterial heat shock protein has been found. Many responsive cells are γ/δ T cells in the synovium, and the sets of V genes used in these receptors are expressed infrequently in other organs. This provides a basis for a localized response and limited (geographically speaking) disease. The concept is well discussed by Schwartz.[110]

ABNORMALITIES IN ANTIGEN PRESENTATION

It is obvious from the previous discussion that the immune response is a tightly regulated system. One could imagine that disturbances could arise at any point, and it is truly astounding that the human organism is as durable as it is. Since a critical step is the interaction between the APC and the helper T cell, there are two obvious ways that this interplay could be altered. Because the disturbance is not

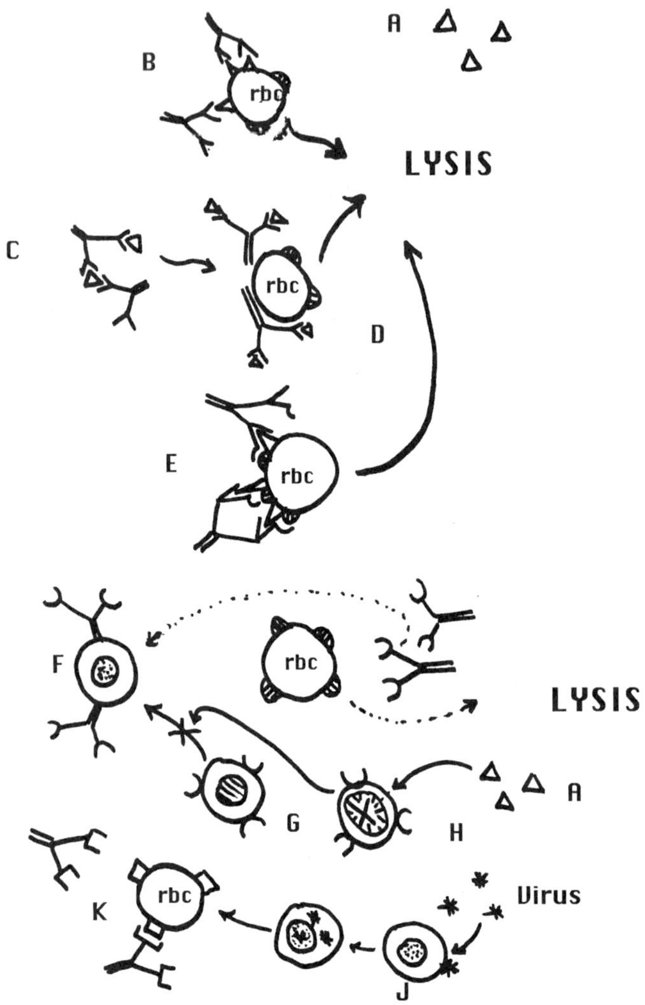

FIGURE 48–4. Mechanisms by which hemolytic anemia might result. A drug (A) may bind to the surface of erythrocytes (rbc). Antibody directed against the drug causes hemolysis (B), through complement activation or erythrophagocytosis (antibody-directed cell-mediated cytotoxicity), although the erythrocyte is just an innocent 'bystander'. In a like manner, immune complexes (C), involving the drug and antibody, interacting in the plasma, bind nonspecifically to the red cell surface and hemolysis follows (D). In the third example, the drug acts as a hapten. It reacts with the surface of the erythrocyte to form a covalent complex with a blood group (E). The red cell acts as a carrier and allows antibody formation. In the example shown, part of the erythrocyte is involved in the determinant but this need not be the case and antibody might be directed against only the haptenic configuration. One could also construct a situation in which the drug binds to MHC class I molecules. In such a case, we could have T-cell cytotoxic attack. The next example is more complex. Here, both a B cell (F) and a T helper cell (G) with receptors for a red cell determinant exist. A T suppressor cell (H) prevents the T helper cell from interacting. Now the drug (A) acts to block the suppressor effect. The drug is never part of the determinant against which the immune response is directed but acts indirectly; α-methyldopa may act in this manner. In the last example, a virus infects an erythroblast (J). A 'new' viral-derived antigen is expressed on the erythrocyte. A proper immune response destroys the infected red cell (K), causing hemolysis while eliminating a viral factory. Such a defensive mechanism could exist for any parasite infecting the red cells. In the last example, it should be noted that the agent does not cause autoimmune disease. Hemolysis results as a consequence of the infection, and the defense mechanism involves the immune system.

global, we cannot postulate general alterations because a given cell presents a very wide range of polypeptide (and perhaps other) determinants. Even diseases such as systemic lupus erythematosus are highly restricted as to which of the billions (or higher orders) of possible self-molecules they react with. It is more plausible to suggest that altered expression of costimulatory molecules may be a pathway to autoimmunity.

If many (or most) potentially self-reacting helper T cells exist in a state of clonal anergy, then if they were exposed to an inordinate stimulus because of overexpression by the APC, they might be activated. Their maturation could then result in tissue injury. The scenario is simple. APCs present self-peptides.[81] When an anergic T cell interacts with a self-peptide in the context of MHC class II, it usually does not receive a sufficient boost via costimulatory molecules to overcome the anergic state. If the APCs elaborated a molecule that would overcome this effect and stimulate the T cell, the consequences would be self-evident. Unfortunately, persuasive evidence for this has not been forthcoming.

Another possibility has been demonstrated in certain situations. One major safeguard against autoimmune reactions is the restricted expression of class II MHC molecules to professional APCs: macrophages, Langerhans cells, dendritic cells, thymic epithelial cells, and B cells.[120] Suppose another cell acquired the capacity to express these molecules on its surface. A helper T cell might see specific cell surface components of the potential target processed and expressed in the context of MHC class II, which is something that could never occur with the usual APC since it does not have activated genes encoding these tissue-specific markers. Macrophages, for example, do not make myelin and do not express it on their surfaces. If an oligodendroglial cell expressed class II molecules, the situation might be very different. Human endothelial cells possess the ability to express class II if appropriately stimulated, and this apparently plays an important role in graft rejection.[30] Some evidence that such might occur because of viral infection has been found in thyroid disease.[35] Again, there is a body of evidence that casts some doubt on the effectiveness of MHC class II expression in cells that are not professional APCs, at least to the extent that it has been studied.[71, 72]

DISTURBANCES IN THE IDIOTYPIC NETWORK

The idiotypic network refers to a postulated immunoregulatory system that has at its core the concept that since the combining sites of antibodies and TCRs are generated largely de novo and therefore represent unique configurations they themselves can serve as epitopes.[40] The actual determinant can be the product of one or both chains and need not lie specifically within the combining site. In turn, TCRs or antibodies that form in response to the idiotope (a designation given to the unique immunogenic configuration) can serve as targets for another set of anti-idiotypic responses, and so on. An idiotype is the aggregate of idiotopes on a given antigen receptor.[24]

Why don't these anti-idiotypes form all the time and in so doing block the immune response? First, there is the quantitative aspect. The concentration of any determinant must reach a level sufficient to cross-link its receptor before the determinant undergoes degradation. There also is the matter of timing. The initial immune response must be well underway before all of the components, the APC, helper cell, and effector cell, are coordinated. The resulting products may have competitive (canceling) effects. Antibodies may stimulate, inhibit, or destroy target cells depending on their isotype, affinity, and other factors.[62]

Several additional points require clarification. It is possible that T and B responses share an idiotype, but a few moments' reflection on the structures involved and their generation would suggest that this is not too likely. Next, since the idiotope may lie outside the binding site between the antibody and determinant, two antibodies with different specificities may have the same idiotope and be bound by identical anti-idiotypic antibodies. On the other hand, if the idiotopes in a network are all directed against the combining site proper, then the third set, the anti–anti-idiotype, will be an internal image of the initiating (foreign) antigen. This possibility leads to a remarkable possibility for immunization.[78] An antibody could so resemble a foreign determinant that if it could be produced by a hybridoma, it would be the perfect immunogen (entirely of human origin).[27]

Finally, the idiotypic network leads to a system of rising and falling levels of antibody. A particular bacterial antigen, B, induces an immune response anti-B with idiotope C. As anti-B rises, B undergoes immune elimination (and usual catabolism). In turn, the rise in anti-B is sufficient for C to trigger an anti-idiotypic response, anti-C. As anti-C rises, anti-B obviously falls. If anti-C had an idiotope D, there may be sufficient anti-C to initiate an anti-D response. A little thought will indicate that unless B persists, the limited life of antibodies and more importantly the cells that produce them will cause the network to decay and reset itself to the point in time before infection occurred. Of course all subsequent responses will be of secondary type. Since somatic mutation is typical of an antigen-driven immune response (and leads inexorably to affinity maturation), the idiotypic network generated on rechallenge might be different.

Suppose that a major function of the anti-idiotypic network is to suppress or contain anti-self reactions. It is common, particularly in the elderly, to encounter antibodies to nuclear antigens. These are potentially useful as garbage collectors. Their concentration might be regulated by an idiotypic network. Consider the consequences of an immune repertoire unable to mount an anti–anti-DNA response. Large amounts of high-affinity antibody might be formed and disease might result. Why isn't this a more popular model since besides everything else, it would nicely explain the occurrence of exacerbations and remissions so often hallmarks of autoimmune diseases?

Most of the work to date has dealt with unideterminant antigens, which are actually carrier-hapten conjugates. Little investigation of complex antigens, in which one idiotope may have a stimulatory effect and another one suppressive, has been done. If the level of each is not sufficient to be measurable, it is not easy to determine if they have a regulatory function. The administration of some anti-idiotypic antibodies specific for a particular monoclonal antibody (in the experimental situation, of course) may affect immune responses unrelated to the determinant in question.[92] This may be because they are directed against idiotopes outside the combining site and therefore may be present on other antigen receptors.[104]

There is some evidence to suggest that the network is more effective early in an immune response where they could affect the most important components, likely CD5+ B cells.[112] In mice, it has also been observed that stimulation is more common in young mice, whereas suppression is usually observed in older mice. Teleologically, if true in humans, this might explain why a defect in the system would be more likely to cause an antiself-response in mature as opposed to immature individuals. Unfortunately, it has not been easy to examine this interesting hypothesis because it is difficult to isolate a given anti-idiotypic response from all of the others the receptor elicits. Another difficulty stems from observations that an immune response may reach normal levels despite the presence of an anti-idiotypic antibody in a significant amount.[41]

One final observation warrants commentary. In an animal model, it has been noted that idiotypic responses can provoke rather than control an autoimmune response.[131] If rabbits are immunized with a compound, BisQ, which binds to the AChR, they develop myasthenia gravis. They also produce antibodies to the hapten and anti-idiotypic antibodies to anti-BisQ. It seems that the response to the anti-BisQ closely approximates the shape of AChR and therefore was an internal image of the receptor, the perfect immunogen discussed previously.[30] The idiotypic response to this second antibody (anti-anti-anti-BisQ) was specific for the receptor itself! It is this very multiphasic nature of the immune response that has prevented analysis to the point where prediction is possible.

GENES, VIRUSES, BACTERIA, AND HORMONES

Clearly genetics play a major role in autoimmune disease that may be heralded (perhaps initiated) by viral and bacterial infections. This group of diseases generally shows a strong predilection for women and therefore provokes an interest in hormonal influences.

Of all the genetic systems studied, only MHC has been successfully associated with autoimmunity.[111] The system is extremely polymorphic and shows ethnic, racial, and haplotypic (MHC alleles closely associated as a unit on each parental chromosome that resists recombination) predisposition. Until the development of molecular genetic technology, MHC has been difficult to analyze.[22, 76] MHC has certain important properties: the allelic pattern strongly affects the presentation of certain peptides to T cells[12, 136]; associations with other systems (close linkages) influence the immune response[52]; the nature of MHC plays a role in thymic selection[8]; and it shows strong linkage to diseases such as ankylosing spondylitis, rheumatoid arthritis, pemphigus, and many others.[43, 56, 86, 135] It seems that MHC plays a major role in controlling T-cell selection and stimulation. Work with mouse genetic lines has identified several genes that profoundly affect the development of lupus.[124] Twin concordance studies in humans have supported the importance of these observations.[13]

The importance of infectious agents has already been suggested. It is well known that many autoimmune disturbances are preceded by an infection. There is much interest in the heat shock proteins because of their conservation between bacteria and humans.[37] The anti-idiotypic network hypothesis suggests that products of the immune response might resemble the virus's cellular receptor and so induce damage.[46, 95] Interest in retroviruses and their possible relationship to non-MHC genes has also drawn attention.[83]

There is strong evidence that hormones are important in autoimmune disease. As noted, the bulk of those affected are female.[390] In systemic lupus erythematosus (SLE), excessive levels of certain metabolites of estrogen are produced.[65, 66] Administration of estrogen to certain strains of mice worsens their disease, whereas castration reduces its severity.[2] The effects of estrogen-androgen balance are not limited to SLE.[23] Prolactin hyperproduction has been implicated in adjuvant arthritis, iridocyclitis, SLE, and thyroid dysfunction of autoimmune origin.[11] The mechanisms involved have been elusive, and studies at the receptor level have been somewhat controversial.[90]

Let us look at two diverse and well-studied diseases to see how these varied mechanisms might apply. SLE and type I diabetes mellitus are common and have enjoyed much study. Although their basic mechanisms have not been established, much progress has been made.

SYSTEMIC LUPUS ERYTHEMATOSUS

This condition serves as the model for a circulating immune complex multisystem disease.[118] (See Chapter 50.) SLE involves skin, joints, brain, kidneys, blood, and other organs, but its hallmark is the presence of multiple antinuclear antibodies, most characteristically ones directed against dsDNA. It is marked by exacerbations and remissions, with very variable expression in the organs involved and also in severity. Many investigators have regarded this disease as a single entity with variable expression.

Steinberg[119] has contended that it is more plausible to consider SLE as a group of disorders. Much of his argument stems from studies on the mouse model. In that species, lupus erythematosus is mainly genetic, displays B- and T-cell abnormalities, and must have its origin in early precursor cells since transfer of stem cells can produce the disease in appropriate recipients.[103, 117] In one line, the NZB mouse, B cells are hyperactive from an early point in their development. The NZB mouse resists the induction of tolerance, and this can be hormonally modified.[67] There are strains in mice in which the sex incidence is equal (MRL-*lpr/lpr*), the males have more severe disease (BXSB), and hemolytic anemia (NZB) or lymphadenopathy (*lpr/lpr*) or nephritis (NZB/W/F_1) or arthritis predominate.[124]

In humans, no clear-cut defects in immunoregulation have been identified.[82, 116] If the SLE patient is poised on the edge of loss of self-tolerance, a B-cell stimulus could tip the balance. After tolerance is compromised, the pattern of disease expression seems dependent on the genetic makeup. There is one other interesting model that casts light upon possible interactions.

In graft-versus-host disease, in which immunocompetent cells are introduced into an immunoincompetent host of different genetic background, such as maternal cells introduced into a random-fathered offspring, pathology that bridges Sjögren's syndrome and SLE is observed. The response that damages the tissue is one in which the donor's T lymphocytes are stimulated (by the differences in the host's class II MHC molecules) and then stimulate host B cells (without exogenous autoantigen being required).[39, 70] Tissue injury follows. This supports ideas that the T cell is critical, although the disease is best recognized by the autoantibodies detected. The situation in a given patient with genes permitting autoimmune hemolytic anemia, nephritis, or arthritis might require multiple inductive events (viral infection, sunlight, certain drugs) to express the spectrum of potential symptoms.

As previously implied, considerable interest in the T-B–cell interaction has developed since it has also been shown that the immune response in SLE is antigen driven and therefore requires both B- and T-cell participation. It is evident that other factors influence the disease. For example, a deficiency in C4A, important in the clearance of immune complexes, is an order of magnitude more common in white females with SLE than in a comparable nonlupus population.[49] Thus not only are recognition and control critical, but also effector mechanisms play a role.

INSULIN-DEPENDENT DIABETES MELLITUS

Type I diabetes mellitus results from autoimmune destruction of the beta cells in the islets of Langerhans.[102] It is a common disease, usually has its inception in childhood, and shows racial and ethnic predilections that correlate with the presence of HLA-DR3 or HLA-DR4, with contributions by DR1, DR8, and DR16.[6] Protective alleles have also been described.[100]

Studies are well summarized by Atkinson and Maclaren[6] and are cited here. The reader is referred to their excellent review for details. Of interest is that other HLA-DR and HLA-DQ genes appear to protect. Susceptibility has been tied to TAP genes, which encode for a protein involved in antigen presentation.

In its early stages, the pathology is characterized by inflammation of the islets (insulitis) primarily by CD8 cells. The cells of the islets over express class I MHC, and endothelial cells, macrophages, and even beta cells themselves over express class II molecules. This form of diabetes is not only associated with a cellular immune response. Several antibodies to islet constituents have been found. The most important is one directed against a 64-kD protein that corresponds to the enzyme glutamate decarboxylase.[7, 10] Of note, for those supporting molecular mimicry, are homologies between coxsackie viral protein and this enzyme.[31] Other significant antigens may be carboxypeptidase H or beta cell sulfatides.[25] Another intriguing possibility arises from a homology between a 52-kD islet cell antigen and a rubella viral constituent associated with congenital diabetes.[6] A variety of studies have failed to resolve which immune mechanism is responsible for islet destruction: CD8 cells, lymphokines (beta cells can produce IL-6, and IFN-γ has been linked to aspects of the disease), and antibodies all have their champions.[6]

Possible initiation mechanisms include a viral infection with subsequent molecular mimicry, an environmental insult that causes the generation of cytokines and lymphocyte adhesion molecules on endothelium in the islets, or some other event that enables presentation of beta cell antigens in a way that initiates a sustained immune response is probable.[6] In all these situations, the presence of a genetic defect that impedes tolerance to beta cell determinants serves to establish and perpetuate the process. The release of inflammatory lymphokines or related molecules could augment the process by increasing HLA class I expression on beta cells. This would enhance their destruction by cytotoxic T cells. The importance of HLA-DR and HLA-DQ associations may relate to the way in which immunogenic peptides are bound, the likeness of viral and self-peptide configurational similarities, or even the ability of different HLA molecules to act as transducers.

SUMMARY

From the preceding discussion, autoimmune disease clearly depends on three fundamental conditions: a genetic predisposition; an inciting external event, likely infectious; and the responsiveness of the immune system that in part may be genetic but also may be determined by intercurrent events, such as unrelated disease, immunization, drug treatment unrelated to the immune system, and so on. Based on all available data, there is no single mechanism for initiation of autoimmune disease. As there is built-in redundancy in the immune system so that a single defect is not invariably lethal, so are there several ways the response can be turned against host tissue.

Considering the pressure resulting from the need to deal with varying antigenic challenge, especially in infectious agents, it is remarkable that even in its brief evolutionary span the human species has not already been eliminated by such pathogens as HIV. It must be a tribute to the design of the immune system that for the most part it maintains self-tolerance and that autoimmune disease does not exact an even greater price in morbidity and mortality than it does today. The most exciting aspect of this subject is that we seemed poised on the threshold of a fundamental grasp of the mechanisms involved.

REFERENCES

1. Adams E, Basten A, Goodnow CC: Intrinsic B cell hyporesponsiveness accounts for self-tolerance in lysozyme/anti-lysozyme doubletransgenic mice. Proc Natl Acad Sci USA 87:5687, 1990.
2. Ahmed SA, Dauphinee MJ, Talal N: Effects of short-term administration of sex hormones on normal and autoimmune mice. J Immunol 134:204, 1985.
3. Amagai M, Klaus-Koutun V, Stanley JR: Autoantibodies against a novel epithelial cadherin in pemphigus vulgaris, a disease of cell adhesion. Cell 67:869, 1991.
4. Ashwell JD, Fox BS, Schwartz RH: Use of receptor competition to explore the interaction of antigen-specific receptor with its ligands. Fed Proc 46:183, 1987.
5. Aten J, Veninga A, Bruijn JA, et al: Antigenic specificities of glomerular-bound autoantibodies in membranous glomerulopathy induced by mercuric chloride. Clin Immunol Immunopathol 63:89, 1992.
6. Atkinson MA, Maclaren NK: The pathogenesis of insulin-dependent diabetes mellitus. N Engl J Med 331:1428, 1994.
7. Atkinson MA, Maclaren NK, Scharp DW, et al: 64,000 M_r autoanti-

bodies are predictive of insulin-dependent diabetes. Lancet 335: 1357, 1990.

8. Avery AC, Markowitz JS, Gusby MJ, et al: Activation of T cells by superantigen in class II negative mice. J Immunol 153:4853, 1994.
9. Avrameas S: Natural autoantibodies—from horror autotoxicus to gnothi seauton. Immunol Today 12:154, 1991.
10. Baekkeskov S, Aanstoot HJ, Christgau S, et al: Identification of the 64K autoantigen in insulin-dependent diabetes as the GABA-synthesizing enzyme glutamic acid decarboxylase. Nature 34:151, 782 (erratum), 1990.
11. Berczi I: Prolactin, pregnancy and autoimmune disease. J Rheumatol 20:7, 1993.
12. Bjorkman PJ, Saper MA, Samraoui B, et al: Structure of the human class I histo-compatibility antigen, HLA-A2. Nature 329:506, 1987.
13. Block SR, Winfield JB, Lockshin M, et al: Studies of twins with systemic lupus erythematosus: a review of the literature and presentation of 12 additional sets. Am J Med 59:533, 1975.
14. Bombassei GJ, Kaplan AA: The association between hydrocarbon exposure and anti-glomerular basement membrane antibody-mediated disease (Goodpasture's syndrome). Am J Ind Med 21:141, 1992.
15. Bona CA: V genes encoding autoantibodies: molecular and phenotypic characteristics. Annu Rev Immunol 6:327, 1988.
16. Bonomo A, Kehn PJ, Shevack EM: Premature escape of double-positive thymocytes to the periphery of young mice. J Immunol 152:1509, 1994.
17. Borche L, Lim A, Binet JL, et al: Evidence that chronic lymphocytic leukemia B lymphocytes are frequently committed to production of natural autoantibodies. Blood 76:562, 1990.
18. Brent L: Immunologically privileged sites. In Johansson BB, Owman C (eds): Pathophysiology of the Blood-Brain Barrier. Elsevier, Amsterdam, 1990.
19. Bretscher PA, Cohn M: A theory of self-nonself discrimination. Science 163:1042, 1970.
20. Burns J, Rosenzweig A, Zweiman B, et al: Isolation of myelin basic protein-reactive T-cell lines from normal human blood. Cell Immunol 81:435, 1983.
21. Butkowski RJ, Shen G-Q, Weislander J, et al: Characterization of type IV collagen NC1 monomers and Goodpasture's antigen in human renal basement membranes. J Lab Clin Med 115:365, 1990.
22. Cambell RD, Milner CM: MHC genes in autoimmunity. Curr Opin Immunol 5:887, 1993.
23. Carlsten H, Tarkowski A, Holmdahl R, et al: Oestrogen is a potent disease accelerator in SLE-prone MRL lpr/lpr mice. Clin Exp Immunol 80:467, 1990.
24. Cerny J, Hiernaux J (eds): Idiotypic Networks and Diseases. American Society of Microbiology, Washington, DC, 1990.
25. Christie MR, Hollands JA, Brown TJ, et al: Detection of pancreatic islet 64,000 M_r autoantigens in insulin-dependent diabetes distinct from glutamate decarboxylase. J Clin Invest 92:240, 1992.
26. Cohen JJ, Duke RC, Fadok VA, et al: Apoptosis and programmed cell death in immunity. Annu Rev Immunol 10:267, 1992.
27. Cohen IR: Physiological basis of T-cell vaccination against autoimmune disease. Cold Spring Harb Symp Quant Biol LIV:879, 1989.
28. Dighiero G, Hart S, Lim A, et al: Autoantibody activity of immunoglobulins isolated from B cell follicular lymphomas. Blood 78:581, 1991.
29. Elliott T: How do peptides associate with MHC class-I molecules? Immunol Today 12:386, 1992.
30. Epperson DE, Pober JS: Antigen-presenting function of human endothelial cells. Direct activation of resting CD8 T cells. J Immunol 153:1502, 1994.
31. Fohiman J, Bohme J, Rask L: Matching of host genotype and serotypes of coxsackie B virus in the development of juvenile diabetes. Scand J Immunol 26:105, 1987.
32. Frank MM, Austen KF, Claman HN, Unanue ER (eds): Sampter's Immunologic Diseases, 5th edition. Little Brown & Co, Boston, 1994.
33. Fujinami RS, Oldstone MBA: Amino acid homology between the encephalitogenic site of myelin basic protein and virus: mechanism for autoimmunity. Science 230:1043, 1985.
34. Fujinami RS: Molecular mimicry. In Rose NR, Mackay IR (eds): The Autoimmune Diseases. II. Academic Press, London, 1992.
35. Gaulton GN, Stein ME, Safiko B, et al: Direct induction of Ia antigen on murine thyroid-derived epithelial cells by reovirus. J Immunol 142:3821, 1989.
36. Gelpi C, Rodriguez-Sanchez JL, Martinez MA, et al: Murine graft vs host disease: a model for study of mechanisms that generate autoantibodies to ribonucleoproteins. J Immunol 140:4160, 1988.
37. Georgopoulos C, McFarland H: Heat shock proteins in multiple sclerosis and other autoimmune diseases. Immunol Today 14:373, 1993.
38. Gershon RK, Kondo K: Infectious immunological tolerance. Immunology 21:903, 1971.
39. Giusti AM, Chien NC, Zack DJ, et al: Somatic diversification of S107 from an antiphosphocholine to an anti-DNA autoantibody is due to a single base change in its heavy chain variable region. Proc Natl Acad Sci USA 84:2926, 1987.
40. Greenspan NS, Bona CA: Idiotypes: structure and immunogenicity. FASEB J 7:437, 1992.
41. Hahn BH: Suppression of autoimmune diseases with antiidiotypic antibodies: murine lupus nephritis as a model. Springer Semin Immunopathol 7:25, 1984.
42. Hakoda M, Ishimoto T, Yamamoto K, et al: Clonal analysis of T-cell infiltrates in synovial tissue of patients with rheumatoid arthritis. Clin Immunol Immunopathol 57:387, 1990.
43. Hammer RE, Maika SD, Richardson JA, et al: Spontaneous inflammatory disease in transgenic rats expressing HLA-B27 and human β2m: an animal model of HLA-B27-associated human disorders. Cell 63:1099, 1990.
44. Hardin JA, Mimori T: Autoantibodies to ribonucleoproteins. Clin Rheum Dis 11:485, 1985.
45. Hartley SB, Crosbie J, Brink R, et al: Elimination from peripheral lymphoid tissues of self-reactive lymphocytes-B recognizing membrane-bound antigens. Nature 353:765, 1991.
46. Hemachudha T, Griffin DE, Giffels JJ, et al: Myelin basic protein as an encephalitogen in encephalomyelitis and polyneuritis following rabies vaccination. N Engl J Med 316:369, 1987.
47. Hess AD, Horwitz L, Beschorner WE, et al: Development of graft-vs-host disease-like syndrome in cyclosporine-treated rats after syngeneic bone marrow transplantation. I. Development of cytotoxic T lymphocytes with apparent polyclonal anti-la specificity, including autoreactivity. J Exp Med 161:718, 1985.
48. Hess E: Drug-related lupus. N Engl J Med 318:1460, 1988.
49. Howard PF, Hochberg MC, Bias WB, et al: Relationship between C4 null genes, HLA-D region antigens, and genetic susceptibility to lupus erythematosus in Causcasian and black Americans. Am J Med 81:187, 1986.
50. Itoh N, Yonehara S, Sihii A: The polypeptide encoded by the cDNA for human cell surface antigen Fas can mediate apoptosis. Cell 66:233, 1991.
51. Izui S, Lambert PH, Fournie GJ, et al: Features of systemic lupus erythematosus in mice injected with bacterial lipopolysaccharides. Identification of circulating DNA and renal localization of DNA-anti-DNA complexes. J Exp Med 145:1115, 1977.
52. Jacob CO, Lewis GD, McDevitt HO: MHC class II-associated variation in the production of tumor necrosis factor in mice and humans: relevance to the pathogenesis of autoimmune diseases. Immunol Res 10:156, 1991.
53. Jenkins MK, Pardoll DM, Mizuguchi J, et al: Molecular events in the induction of a non-responsive state in interleukin 2-producing helper T lymphocyte clones. Proc Natl Acad Sci USA 84:5409, 1987.
54. Karpus WJ, Swanborg RH: CD4+ suppressor cells inhibit the function of effector cells of experimental autoimmune encephalomyelitis through a mechanism involving transforming growth factor β. J Immunol 146:1163, 1991.
55. Kaufmann SHE, Schoel B, Vonembden JDA, et al: Heat-shock protein-60—implications for pathogenesis of and protection against bacterial infections. Immunol Rev 121:67, 1991.
56. Keat A: Reiter's syndrome and reactive arthritis in perspective. N Engl J Med 309:1606, 1983.
57. Kefalides NA, Ohno N, Wilson CB, et al: Identification of antigen epitopes in Type IV collagen by the use of synthetic peptides. Kidney Int 43:94, 1993.
58. Kelton JG: Impaired reticuloendothelial function in patients treated with methyldopa. N Engl J Med 313:596, 1985.
59. Kirtland HH III, Mohler DN, Horwitz DA: Methyldopa inhibition of suppressor-lymphocyte function: a proposed cause of autoimmune hemolytic anemia. N Engl J Med 302:825, 1980.
60. Kleinecht D, Morel-Maroger L, Callard P, et al: Antiglomerular basement membrane nephritis after solvent exposure. Arch Intern Med 140:230, 1982.
61. Klinman D, Steinberg AD: Systemic autoimmune disease arises from polyclonal B-cell activation. J Exp Med 165:1755, 1987.

62. Klinman DM, Steinberg AD: Idiotypy and autoimmunity. Arthritis Rheum 29:697, 1986.
63. Kopicky JA, Packman CH: The mechanisms of sulfonylurea-induced immune hemolysis: case report and review of the literature. Am J Hematol 23:283, 1986.
64. Korsmeyer S: Bcl-2 initiates a new category of oncogenes: regulators of cell death. Blood 80:879, 1992.
65. Lahita RG, Bradlow L, Fishman J, et al: Estrogen metabolism in systemic lupus erythematosus. Arthritis Rheum 25:843, 1982.
66. Lahita RG, Bradlow HL, Ginzler E: Low plasma androgens in women with systemic lupus erythematosus. Arthritis Rheum 30:241, 1987.
67. Lahita H: The importance of estrogen in systemic lupus erythematosus. Clin Immunol Immunopathol 63:17, 1992.
68. Lalezari P, Louie JE, Fadlallah N: Serologic profile of alpha methyldopa-induced hemolytic anemia: correlation between cell-bound IgM and hemolysis. Blood 59:61, 1982.
69. Levinson AI, Dalal NF, Haidar M, et al: Prominent IgM rheumatoid factor production by human cord blood lymphocytes stimulated in vitro with *Staphylococcus aureus* Cowan I. J Immunol 139:2237, 1987.
70. Lindholm L, Rydberg LA, Stannegard O: Development of host plasma cells during graft-versus-host reactions in mice. Eur J Immunol 3:511, 1973.
71. Lo D, Burkly LC, Widera G, et al: Diabetes and tolerance in transgenic mice expressing class II MHC molecules in pancreatic B cells. Cell 53:159, 1988.
72. Londei M, Lamb JR, Bottazzo GR: Epithelial cells expressing aberrant MHC class II determinants can present antigen to cloned human T cells. Nature 312:639, 1984.
73. Manser T, Gefter M: The molecular evolution of the immune response: idiotype specific suppression indicates that B-cells express germ-line-encoded V genes prior to antigenic stimulation. Eur J Immunol 16:1439, 1986.
74. McIntosh KR, Drachman DB: Induction of suppressor cells specific for AChR in experimental autoimmune myasthenia gravis. Science 232:401, 1986.
75. Miller JFAP, Morahan G: Peripheral T-cell tolerance. Annu Rev Immunol 10:51, 1992.
76. Moller E, Bohme J, Valugerdi MA, et al: Speculations on mechanisms of HLA associations with autoimmune diseases and the specificity of autoreactive T lymphocytes. Immunol Rev 118:5, 1993.
77. Möller G (ed): Transgenic mice and immunologic tolerance. Immunol Rev 122:1, 1992.
78. Möller G: Anti-idiotype antibodies as immunogens. Immunol Rev 90:5, 1987.
79. Möller G (ed): Models of autoimmunity. Immunol Rev 118:1, 1993.
80. Morahan G, Brennan FE, Bhathal PS, Allison J: Expression in transgenic mice of class I histocompatibility antigens controlled by the metallothionein promoter. Proc Natl Acad Sci USA 86:3782, 1989.
81. Moreno J, Vignali DAA, Nadimi F, et al: Processing of an endogenous protein can generate MHC class II–restricted T-cell determinants distinct from those derived from exogenous antigen. J Immunol 147:3306, 1992.
82. Morimoto C, Steinberg AD, Letvin NL, et al: A defect of immunoregulatory T cell subsets in systemic lupus erythematosus patients demonstrated with anti-2H4 antibody. J Clin Invest 79:762, 1987.
83. Mountz JD, Talal N: Retroviruses, apoptosis and autogenes. Immunol Today 14:532, 1993.
84. Murphy KM, Weaver CT, Elish M, et al: Peripheral tolerance to allogeneic class II histocompatibility antigens expressed in transgenic mice: evidence against a clonal-deletion mechanism. Proc Natl Acad Sci USA 86:10034, 1990.
85. Nemazee D, Buerki K: Clonal deletion of autoreactive B lymphocytes in bone marrow chimeras. Proc Natl Acad Sci USA 86:8039, 1989.
86. Nepom GT, Erhlich H: MHC class II molecules and autoimmunity. Annu Rev Immunol 9:493, 1991.
87. Nossal GJV: Cellular mechanisms of immunologic tolerance. Annu Rev Immunol 1:33, 1983.
88. Nunez G, Hockenbery D, McDonnell TJ, et al: Bcl-2 maintains B-cell memory. Nature 353:71, 1991.
89. Ohasi PS, Oehen S, Burki K, et al: Ablation of tolerance and induction of diabetes by virus infection in viral antigen transgenic mice. Cell 65:305, 1991.
90. Okuyama R, Abo T, Seki S, et al: Estrogen administration activates extrathymic T-cell differentiation in the liver. J Exp Med 175:66, 1992.
91. Oldstone MBA: Molecular mimicry and autoimmune disease. Cell 50:819, 1987.
92. Oudin J, Cazenave PA: Similar idiotypic specificities in immunoglobulin fractions with different antibody functions or even without detectable antibody function. Proc Natl Acad Sci USA 68:2616, 1971.
93. Peakman M, Vergani D: Autoimmune disease: etiology, therapy and regeneration. Immunol Today 15:345, 1994.
94. Petz LD: Drug-induced immune hemolysis. N Engl J Med 313:510, 1985.
95. Plotz PH: Autoantibodies are anti-idiotype antibodies to antiviral antibodies. Lancet 2:824, 1983.
96. Prabhakar BS, Saegusa J, Onodera J, et al: Lymphocytes capable of making monoclonal antibodies that react with multiple organs are a common feature of the normal B cell repertoire. J Immunol 133: 2815, 1984.
97. Primi D, Smith CI, Hammerström L, et al: Sera from lipopolysaccharide (LPS)-injected mice exhibit complement-dependent cytotoxicity against syngeneic and autologous spleen cells. Cell Immunol 32:252, 1977.
98. Protti MP, Manfredi AA, Straub C, et al: Immunodominant regions for T-helper-cell sensitization on the human nicotinic receptor α-subunit in myasthenia gravis. Proc Natl Acad Sci USA 87:7792, 1990.
99. Raff MC: Social controls on cell survival and cell death. Nature 356:397, 1992.
100. Reich ED-P, Sherwin RS, Kanagawa O, et al: An explanation for the protective effect of the MHC class II I-E molecule in murine diabetes. Nature 341:326, 1989.
101. Rose NR, MacKay IR (eds): The Autoimmune Diseases, 2nd edition. Academic Press, Orlando, 1992.
102. Rossini AA, Mordes JP: Like AA: immunology of insulin dependent diabetes mellitus. Annu Rev Immunol 3:289, 1985.
103. Russell AS: Genetic factors in systemic lupus erythematosus. Semin Arthritis Rheum 10:255, 1981.
104. Sakaguchi S, Sakaguchi N: Thymus and autoimmunity: capacity of the normal thymus to produce pathogenic self-reactive T cells and conditions required for their induction of autoimmune disease. J Exp Med 172:537, 1990.
105. Sakaguchi N, Miyai K, Sakaguchi S: Ionizing radiation and autoimmunity. J Immunol 152:2586, 1994.
106. Sakai K, Zamvil SS, Mitchell DJ, et al: Prevention of experimental encephalomyelitis with peptides that block interaction of T cells with major histocompatibility complex proteins. Proc Natl Acad Sci USA 86:9470, 1989.
107. Salama A, Mueller-Eckhardt C: On the mechanisms of sensitization and attachment of antibodies to RBC in drug-induced immune hemolytic anemia. Blood 69:1006, 1987.
108. Sauter NP, Atkins MB, Mier JW, et al: Transient thyrotoxicosis and persistent hypothyroidism due to acute autoimmune thyroiditis after interleukin-2 and interferon-α therapy for metastatic carcinoma—a case report. Am J Med 92:441, 1992.
109. Schwartz RS: Immunological tolerance. In Paul WE (ed): Fundamental Immunology, 3rd edition. Raven Press, Ltd, New York, 1993.
110. Schwartz RS: Autoimmunity and autoimmune disease. In Paul WE (ed): Fundamental Immunology, 3rd edition. Raven Press, Ltd, New York, 1993.
111. Shoenfeld Y, Schwartz RS: Immunologic and genetic factors in autoimmune diseases. N Engl J Med 311:1019, 1984.
112. Sidman CL, Shultz LD, Hardy RR, et al: Production of immunoglobulin isotypes by Ly-Ipl B cells in viable motheaten and normal mice. Science 232:1423, 1986.
113. Slack JH, Hang L, Barkley J, et al: Isotypes of spontaneous and mitogen-induced autoantibodies in SLE-prone mice. J Immunol 132:1271, 1984.
114. Smith H, Sakamoto Y, Kasai K, et al: Effector and regulatory cells in autoimmune oophoritis elicited by neonatal thymectomy. J Immunol 147:2928, 1991.
115. Smith HR, Steinberg AD: Autoimmunity: a perspective. Annu Rev Immunol 1:175, 1983.
116. Smolen JS, Chused TM, Leiserson WM, et al: Heterogeneity of immunoregulatory T-cell subsets in systemic lupus erythematosus. Am J Med 72:783, 1982.
117. Steinberg AD, Raveché ES, Laskin CA, et al: Systemic lupus erythematosus: insights from animal models. Ann Intern Med 100:714, 1984.
118. Steinberg AD, Gourley MF, Klinman DM, et al: Systemic lupus erythematosus. Ann Intern Med 115:548, 1991.
119. Steinberg AD: Concepts of pathogenesis of systemic lupus erythematosus. Clin Immunol Immunopath 63:19, 1992.

120. Steinman RM: The dendritic cell system and its role in immunogenicity. Annu Rev Immunol 9:271, 1991.
121. Streilein JW: Immune privilege as the result of local tissue barriers and immunosuppressive microenvironments. Curr Opin Immunol 5:428, 1993.
122. Streilein JW: Privileged sites. In Roitt IM, Delves PJ (eds): Encyclopedia of Immunology. Academic Press, London, 1992.
123. Suzumura A, Lavi E, Weiss SR, et al: Coronavirus infection induces H-2 antigen expression on oligodendrocytes and astrocytes. Science 232:991, 1986.
124. Theofilopoulos AN, Kofler R, Singer PA, et al: Molecular genetics of murine lupus models. Adv Immunol 46:61, 1989.
125. Trowsdale J, Cambell RD: Complexity in the major histocompatibility complex. Eur J Immunogen 19:45, 1992.
126. Underwood JR, Pedersen PJ, Chalmers PJ: Hybrids from normal, germ-free, nude and neonatal mice produce monoclonal autoantibodies to eight different intracellular structures. Clin Exp Immunol 60:417, 1990.
127. van Eden W: Heat shock proteins as immunogenic bacterial antigens with the potential to induce and regulate autoimmune arthritis. Immunol Rev 121:5, 1991.
128. van der Veen RC, Trotter JL, Hickey WF, et al: The development and characterization of encephalitogenic cloned T cells specific for myelin proteolipid protein. J Neuroimmunol 26:139, 1990.
129. Von Boehmer H: Developmental biology of T cells in cell receptor transgenic mice. Annu Rev Immunol 8:531, 1990.
130. Wasserman NH, Penn AS, Freimuth PI, et al: Anti-idiotypic route to anti-acetylcholine receptor antibodies and experimental myasthenia gravis. Proc Natl Acad Sci USA 79:4810, 1982.
131. Watanabe FR, Brannan CI, Copeland NG, et al: Lymphoproliferation disorder in mice explained by defects in Fas antigen that mediates apoptosis. Nature 356:314, 1992.
132. Wilcox N: Myasthenia gravis. Curr Opin Immunol 5:910, 1993.
133. Wilcox N, Baggi F, Batocchi A-P, et al: Approaches for studying the pathogenic T cells in autoimmune patients. Ann NY Acad Sci 681:219, 1993.
134. Williams RC Jr: Molecular mimicry and rheumatic fever. Clin Rheumatol Dis 11:573, 1985.
135. Winchester R, Dwyer E: MHC and autoimmune diseases: susceptibility to rheumatoid arthritis associated with a hydrophobic strip of α-helix encoded by several MHC alleles. In Bona C, Kaushik K (eds): Molecular Immunobiology of Selfreactivity. Marcel Dekker, New York, 1992.
136. Wraith DC, Smilek DE, Mitchell DJ, et al: Antigen recognition in autoimmune encephalomyelitis and the potential for peptide-mediated immunotherapy. Cell 59:247, 1989.
137. Yancopoulos GD, Alt FW: Regulation of the assembly and expression of variable-region genes. Annu Rev Immunol 4:339, 1986.
138. Young F, Tucker L, Rubinstein D, et al: Molecular analysis of a germ line encoded idiotypic marker of pathogenic human lupus autoantibodies. J Immunol 145:2545, 1990.
139. Yu DTY, Choo SY, Schaack T: Molecular mimicry in HLA-B27-related arthritis. Ann Intern Med 111:581, 1989.
140. Zouali M, Kalsi J, Isenberg D: Autoimmune diseases at the molecular level. Immunol Today 14:473, 1993.

49 Rheumatoid Arthritis

NATHAN J. ZVAIFLER

Rheumatoid arthritis (RA) is a common systemic inflammatory disorder of unknown etiology, characterized largely by the manner in which it involves joints. It is distributed worldwide, affecting approximately 1% of adult populations, and involves all racial and ethnic groups. Articular inflammation, the hallmark of the disease, may be remitting but if continuous results in characteristic deformities. Thus it is surprising that victims of RA cannot be clearly identified in ancient art or literature, unlike for instance, gouty arthritis, known since the time of Hippocrates in the fourth century B.C.[82] RA is not one of the rheumatic diseases definitely identified in ancient skeletons. Based on the evidence from paleopathology, RA of the severity seen today must have been uncommon in previous millennia, if present at all. Exceptions are reports from the United States and Mexico that pre-Columbian skeletons show joint erosions that might represent RA, suggesting that RA, like syphilis, was a New World disease that subsequently spread to Europe.[74]

In medieval times, joint afflictions were usually ascribed to gout, a term used as nonspecifically as arthritis is used today. It was not until the early 17th century that Sydenham attempted to distinguish specific diseases from the admixture of rheumatism. Gout was clearly recognized, and there were descriptions compatible with rheumatic fever. Sydenham also noted a chronic phase of arthritis in which the patient "became a cripple until the day of his death and wholly lose the use of his limbs while the knuckles of his fingers shall become knotty and protuberant." By the early 1800s, RA was well described in both the French and English literature, and in 1858, Garrod coined the term rheumatoid arthritis.[82]

Intensive investigation into the immunologic aspects of RA began after World War II, prompted by the discovery that the addition of RA serum to sheep red blood cells

Supported in part by a grant from NIH AR40770, Multipurpose Arthritis and Musculoskeletal Diseases Center.

coated or sensitized with rabbit antibodies produced marked agglutination. Waaler,[95] from Oslo, published his initial observations in 1940 and termed the serum material as agglutination activating factor.[95] In parallel studies, Rose and colleagues[73] identified a similar activity. Shortly thereafter, it was determined that the factor under study was a serum globulin and a member of the newly recognized antibody family. Because of the frequent disease association, it was termed the rheumatoid factor (RF).

The true significance of these observations and their relevance to the pathogenesis of RA awaited the incisive studies of Kunkel and his associates.[29, 51] In a series of landmark publications, they determined that RA serum contained a unique high molecular weight protein complex (sedimentation rate in an ultracentrifuge of 22 Svedberg units). This complex could be further dissociated into 19S and 7S components. The 19S component was identified as a high molecular weight antibody, now known as the IgM class of immunoglobulin. Subsequently, they showed that the high molecular weight material was present in both the blood and synovial fluid of patients with RA and defined the gamma globulin–antigammaglobulin nature of the immune complex.

Over the next three decades, investigations of RA paralleled the advances in our understanding of both humoral and cellular immunity. This information forms the basis of much of this chapter. These insights are beginning to modify the heretofore empirical nature of RA treatment and hopefully will be translated into effective, rational treatment for this chronic disabling disorder.

GENERAL DESCRIPTION—ANIMAL MODELS

Numerous manipulations can produce chronic inflammatory arthritis in laboratory animals. Most have in common a genetic component and an immune pathogenesis and thus may serve as surrogates for human rheumatic diseases. However, RA is a uniquely human disease, and no animal model accurately recapitulates both its clinical and pathologic features. Nevertheless, they provide valuable insights into the induction and perpetuation of inflammatory joint disease. Perhaps even more important, they allow the testing of new drugs and biologic intervention. A brief description of three forms of experimental arthritis that may have particular relevance to RA follows.

COLLAGEN-INDUCED ARTHRITIS

Immunization of certain strains of mice and rats with native type II collagen, the predominant form of collagen in cartilage, results in a symmetric synovitis reminiscent of RA.[11] Disease susceptibility is closely linked to specific class II major histocompatibility complex (MHC) genes.[103] Some experiments suggest that circulating antibodies to type II collagen play a role, since antibody titers increase dramatically after immunization and transient disease can be transferred with serum from affected animals.[39, 89] IgG2a and IgG2b antibodies, both of which activate complement, are present in high titer and might contribute to local complement activation. Other soluble factors produced by T cells have also been implicated.[37] The role of T cells is not as well defined, and transfer of disease with splenocytes is inconsistent. Anti-CD4 antibody treatment, prior to challenge with type II collagen, prevents arthritis but has no effect on established disease. Treatment with anti-TNF antibody causes a significant reduction in paw swelling. By combining the two reagents (anti-CD4 and anti-TNF), the collagen antibody responses are eliminated, and established joint disease is ameliorated.[100]

The relevance of type II collagen immunity to RA is not established. Although antibody- and cell-mediated immune responses are found at some time in many patients, the disease can begin prior to detection of antibodies to type II collagen, and similar antibodies are present in the circulation of patients with other forms of inflammatory arthritis. The failure to demonstrate antibody could be due to absorption by anti-idiotypic antibodies or rheumatoid factor in the circulation. This possibility is supported by a study demonstrating active synthesis of antibodies to type II collagen by RA synovial tissue cells in the absence of antibody in the circulation.[92] Although immunity to collagen is not a primary event in RA, it is still possible that synovial antibody production contributes to cartilage damage, either directly or via local complement activation.

ADJUVANT ARTHRITIS

Adjuvant arthritis is induced in Lewis rats after immunization with complete (containing *Mycobacterium butyricum*) Freund's adjuvant (CFA).[68] Over the ensuing weeks, the animals develop a self-limited polyarthritis that shares some histopathologic features with RA, including mononuclear cell infiltration of the synovium, pannus formation, destruction of cartilage, and erosion of bone. T cells are thought to play an important role in both the aggressive and regressive phases of the disease. Some T-cell clones have been isolated from rats immunized with CFA that can induce the disease, whereas others are protective.[10, 41] The critical antigens in CFA might be mycobacterial heat shock proteins (HSP).[94] Some evidence suggests that the link between the joint disease and HSP is an epitope shared between the 65-kD HSP and a fraction of cartilage proteoglycan.[94] It is also intriguing that synovial fluid mononuclear cells from patients with inflammatory arthritis proliferate in response to the 65-kD protein.[31]

STREPTOCOCCAL CELL WALL ARTHRITIS

Lewis rats develop streptococcal cell wall arthritis (SCWA) after intraperitoneal injection with cell wall fragments isolated from streptococci. The disease is biphasic: an initial nonspecific joint inflammation is replaced by a T-cell–specific, strain-specific progressive destructive arthritis. Control strains, such as Fischer rats, are resistant to this disease. Interestingly, the resistant strain develops a rapid increase in corticotropin-releasing factor (CRF), adrenocorticotropic hormone (ACTH), and cortisol after challenge with SCWA, whereas the Lewis rats have a blunted hypothalamic-pituitary-adrenal (HPA) response.[88] Steroid replacement in the Lewis rats decreases the initial nonspecific inflammatory arthritis, whereas pharmacologic inhibition of the HPA axis dramatically increases the incidence of arthritis in the usually resistant Fischer rats. Although the influence of the HPA on the immune phase of SCWA has not been defined, these intriguing data support the idea of a neuroendocrine role in immune-mediated diseases.

EPIDEMIOLOGY

INCIDENCE

Exact figures on incidence rates in RA vary somewhat because it is an uncommon disease, and there is difficulty ensuring that all cases are recognized at their inception. In addition, RA is sometimes difficult to distinguish from other forms of inflammatory arthritis, particularly early in the disease. The variable nature of its clinical course and presentation means that cross-sectional studies done at a particular point in time may fail to identify cases of RA that have remitted in the past. Despite these caveats, there is agreement that RA is a relatively uncommon disease, particularly in the young (15–30/100,000). It has a marked female excess in all populations studied and a homogeneous, worldwide geographic distribution. Table 49–1 confirms the rarity of the disease in males under the age of 45 and the increased incidence in women that becomes less apparent in older age groups.[91]

PREVALENCE

Because of its chronic nature, even an uncommon disorder like RA can accumulate large numbers of affected individuals. Thus prevalence figures between 0.5% and 1% of adult populations are reported in almost all studies. An interesting trend, which is still difficult to confirm, is an apparent decreasing incidence of RA, particularly in young women. Whether this reflects more stringent diagnostic criteria, the fact that the disease is becoming milder and less likely to reach medical attention, or a true reduction in incidence is

TABLE 49–1
INCIDENCE OF RHEUMATOID ARTHRITIS

	Incidence Rate per 100,000 Population	
Age	***Males***	***Females***
15–24	3.0	9.3
25–34	2.8	11.6
35–44	3.0	35.7
45–54	15.7	53.9
55–64	19.1	58.7
65–74	29.1	65.3
75–84	61.9	30.3
All ages	14.0	35.6
Adjusted all ages*	12.7	34.3

*Age and sex adjusted to 1991 population of England and Wales.
From Symmons DP, Barrett EM, Bankhead CR, et al: The incidence of rheumatoid arthritis in the United Kingdom: results from the Norfolk Arthritis Register. Br J Rheumatol 33:735–739, 1994.

not known.[86] Confirmation of these provocative findings might suggest a contribution from oral contraceptive pills or possibly a change in the inflammatory response to a putative pathogen.

GEOGRAPHY

Although RA is a worldwide disease, certain populations, such as some American Indians, have a very high rate of disease, whereas rural African and Chinese populations have very low rates. Of interest, when African natives move to the city, the prevalence of RA rises and approaches that seen in other populations.[83] Although there is no clear-cut explanation for population differences, the available epidemiologic evidence suggests genetic factors may explain the variation.

GENETICS

FAMILY SEGREGATION/TWIN STUDIES

As a rule, RA does not display any form of mendelian inheritance, although there are examples of families with multiple affected first-degree relatives (relative risk 0.8–4.3). Twin data provide better evidence of a genetic factor. One detailed study finds concordance rates for RA in dizygotic twins of 3.6% and in monozygotic twins of 15.2%.[84] The significance of such studies is always obscured by the problem that monozygotic twins are more likely than dizygotic twins to share a similar environment.

DISEASE MARKERS

The strongest evidence in support of genetic factors comes from an association between RA and certain HLA genes located on the short arm of chromosome 6 in humans. Initially, this was based on reports in Europeans of an association of RA with serologically defined HLA-DR4 specificities, especially Dw4 and Dw14. Subsequently, there was difficulty explaining the differences in HLA class II association in different populations with different subtypes of HLA-DR4.[104] For instance, certain American Indian tribes have a high frequency of RA in the absence of the DR4 haplotype; they have Dw16, a subtype of DR6.[101] Similar findings were observed in both the Japanese population and Israeli Jews (DR1 associated). Conversely, certain DR4 alleles have no association with RA (Dw10, Dw13).

These contradictions were reconciled by detailed molecular analysis of the MHC region, when it was found that the great majority of affected individuals shared an epitope present in the third allelic hypervariable region (3AHVR) of the HLA-DR β-1 chain regardless of the HLA haplotype. This distinct genetic element is found integrated into a number of alleles, including HLA-DR B1*0401 (former Dw4), B1*0404/8 (former Dw14), B1*0101 (former DR1), and B1*1402 (former DRw14/Dw16).

The shared amino acid sequence (known as the RA susceptibility epitope) resides in the α-helical segment of the DR β-1 chain between positions 67 and 74 (Fig. 49–1). This region is a critical binding site for foreign antigens and

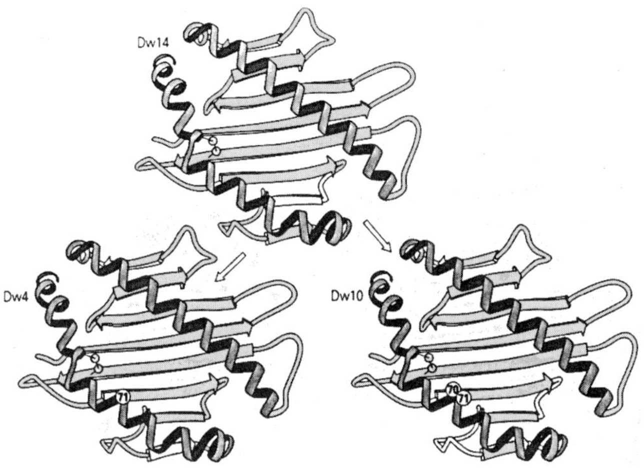

FIGURE 49–1. Hypothetical structure of HLA class II molecules associated with RA. (Based on the known crystallographic structure of the class I molecule, HLA-A2.) Dw4 and Dw14 are identical, except for the substitution of a lysine for an arginine at position 71. In contrast, the Dw10 molecule, which is not associated with RA, differs from Dw14 by the substitution of two acidic residues at positions 70 and 71. This has considerable implications for the types of antigens that can be bound. (From Wordsworth P, Pile K: Etiology: rheumatoid arthritis. In Klippel JH, Dieppe PA (eds): Rheumatology. Mosby–Year Book Europe Limited, London, 1994.)

supports the original notion that specific disease associations likely involve discrete disease-related epitopes immunologically relevant in terms of T-cell recognition. A search of computer-based data banks for peptides analogous to the RA amino acid sequence (QKRAA or QRRAA) has revealed homologies with sequences in bacterial HSP dnaJ and the 110-kD glycoprotein from the capsular antigen of the Epstein-Barr virus (EBV).[3, 75] It is probably not coincidental that both EBV and HSP have independently been implicated in the pathogenesis of RA.

Although it is true that the QKRAA sequence is associated with RA in almost all populations, there is a considerable variation in the strength of the association. In many European populations, the frequency of the shared epitope approaches 50%, but only 1% to 2% have the disease. So clearly, this sequence by itself is insufficient for the development of RA. Furthermore, 15% to 20% of patients who meet rigid criteria for the diagnosis of RA do not possess this sequence. Usually these are milder forms of RA. In a susceptibility model, the HLA-DR B1 allele product would be assumed to contribute to induction of disease. Of late, there has been an increased appreciation of a different role for these genes, namely, the progression of an established pathologic immune response. Hence evidence is accumulating that HLA-DR B1 genes represent severity markers and predict outcome in RA.[76]

The development of erosive and seropositive (rheumatoid factor) disease is almost invariably a consequence of the disease-associated gene sequences.[99] Patients with extra-articular disease generally carry two disease-linked HLA-DR B1 alleles, whereas those with only moderate disease show one copy of the disease-linked sequence. The proposed hierarchy of allelic HLA-DR B1 combinations in determining severity of rheumatoid arthritis is displayed in Figure 49–2. As can be seen, homozygous individuals, or those with two alleles, are at the greatest risk for both destructive joint disease and extra-articular manifestations. Patients with Felty's syndrome are almost always homozygous but also show a strong association with a DQ haplotype (DQw7).

Despite the strong evidence of the HLA-DR B1 associations, there is general agreement that RA is genetically heterogeneous and its etiology is likely to be multifactorial. HLA probably accounts for no more than 30% of the genetic contribution. Other genes of interest are those that code for various immunoglobulin segments, complement components and cytokines, and the β chain of the T-cell receptor. As yet, none of these approaches have yielded significant information about the pathogenesis of RA.

CLINICAL PRESENTATION—JOINT DISEASE

RA is a highly variable disease, ranging from a mild pauciarticular form of brief duration to a relentless, progressive, destructive polyarthritis associated with systemic features.[98] Frequently RA is heralded by prodromal symptoms, such as fatigue, anorexia, weakness, and generalized aching and stiffness that are not clearly localized to articular structures. Joint symptoms usually appear gradually and insidiously over a period of weeks to months. Occasionally there are brief remittent episodes prior to the development of more persistent arthritis. Approximately 20% of patients have an abrupt onset, with the rapid development of polyarthritis, often accompanied by fever, prostration, and severe constitutional symptoms.

Articular involvement is manifested clinically by joint pain, stiffness, limitation of motion, and signs of inflammation.[111] Morning stiffness lasting more than 30 minutes (and frequently several hours) is highly characteristic. Joint swelling results from a combination of synovial hypertrophy, angiogenesis, infiltration with inflammatory cells, and increase in the volume of synovial fluid (joint effusions). Although RA can affect any diarthrodial joint, symmetrical involvement of the small joints of the hands, wrists, knees,

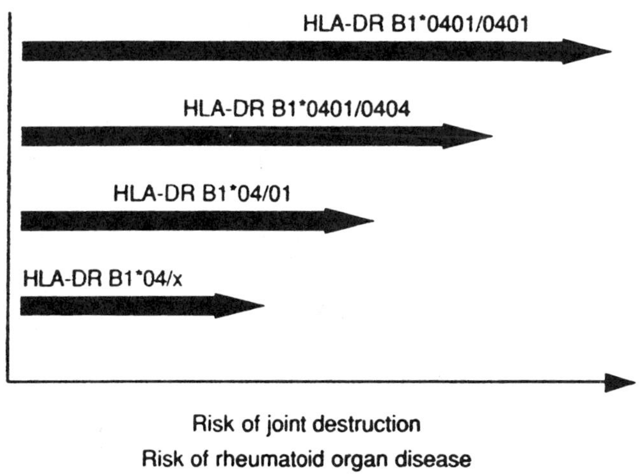

FIGURE 49–2. Hierarchy of allelic HLA-DR B1 combinations in determining disease severity of rheumatoid arthritis. (From Weyand CM, Goronzy JJ: HLA-DR B1 alleles as severity markers in RA. Bull Rheum Dis 43:5–8, 1994. Used by permission of the Arthritis Foundation.)

and feet is the most common distribution. As the disease becomes established, the arthritis spreads to the elbows, shoulders, hips, ankles, and subtalar and sternoclavicular joints.

Examination of the joints generally reveals characteristic abnormalities. Swelling of the proximal interphalangeal finger joints produces a fusiform- or spindle-shaped appearance. Bilateral and symmetrical soft tissue swelling of the metacarpal phalangeal joints, particularly the second and third, is a hallmark of rheumatoid arthritis. By contrast, the distal interphalangeal finger joints are usually spared. As the disease progresses, laxity of tissues increases. Under the pressure of regular use, characteristic hand changes develop, including ulnar deviation of the digits and hyperextension (swan neck) or flexion (boutonnière) deformities (Fig. 49–3). Wrist disease is an almost invariable accompaniment of RA, often complicated by carpal tunnel syndrome due to compression of the median nerve by hypertrophied synovium. Flexion contractures of the elbows are frequent, even at an early stage of the disease, and shoulder involvement is common.

In the lower extremities, RA can affect the hip joints, but usually only late in the illness. The knee, one of the most commonly involved joints, can develop contractures, deformities, and all degrees of ligamentous instability. Pain and limitation of flexion and extension of the foot result from disease of the ankle joint proper, whereas subtalar joint involvement causes pain and limitation of eversion and inversion. In the foot proper, synovitis of the metatarsal phalangeal joints is particularly common, resulting in ventral subluxation of the metatarsal heads and lateral deviation and clawing of the toes.

EXTRA-ARTICULAR MANIFESTATIONS

Low-grade fever, mild lymphadenopathy, anorexia, and weight loss are all evidence of the systemic nature of RA. Muscle atrophy is common and may be remarkable in its degree and rapidity of development. Subcutaneous nodules (rheumatoid granuloma) occur at some time in 20% to 25% of RA patients, almost always associated with rheumatoid factor in the blood.[111] Nodules usually appear in areas subjected to mechanical pressure, especially the olecranon and extensor surface of the forearms, Achilles tendon, and periarticular structures. Unusual locations include the pleura, meninges, occiput, pinna of the ears, and bridge of the nose. As a rule, the nodules are firm, nontender, oval or round masses in the subcutaneous or deeper tissues.

A spectrum of vascular lesions accompany RA. Inflamed capillaries and small venules participate in the development of rheumatoid nodules and synovitis. Other lesions include a bland intimal proliferation, commonly affecting digital and mesenteric vessels; subacute lesions of arterioles and venules; and occasionally a widespread necrotizing arteritis of small- and medium-sized arteries, which may be indistinguishable from polyarteritis nodosa. This form of rheumatoid vasculitis characteristically produces polyneuropathy, skin necrosis and ulceration, digital gangrene, perforation of the nasal septum, and visceral infarction. The prognosis in this fulminant vasculitis was exceedingly poor before the advent of immunosuppressive (cyclophosphamide) treatment. Much evidence supports a role for immune complexes in the pathogenesis of most vascular lesions.

Involvement of viscera, such as the eyes, heart, lungs, and peripheral nervous system, is well-recognized as a complication of RA.[111] The basic lesion in most is an admixture of a granulomatous response (analogous to the rheumatoid nodule) and some form of vascular injury. For instance, inflammatory microvascular lesions can be found throughout the myocardium in almost 40% of autopsied RA patients. Less common are granulomatous lesions involving the epicardium, myocardium, and valves. Interstitial pulmonary disease likely results from immune complex–mediated vascular abnormalities, whereas intrapulmonary nodules reflect granulomatous responses. Dryness of mucous membranes (the sicca complex), particularly dry eyes (xerophthalmia) and dry mouth (xerostomia), due to chronic inflammation of exocrine glands, occurs in about 15% of patients.

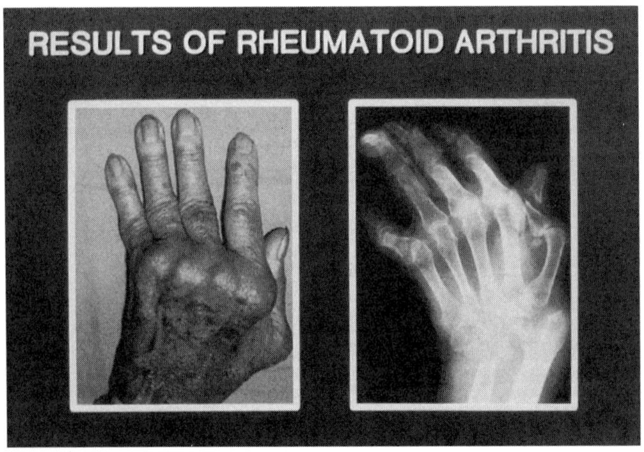

FIGURE 49–3. Chronic RA. Synovitis within the metacarpal phalangeal (MCP) joints produces swelling, inflammation, and tissue destruction, leading to volar subluxation and ulnar drift, the characteristic deformities in the RA hand. The accompanying radiograph shows the consequences of pannus formation, including cartilage loss, reduced bone density, erosions, and subluxations. These are most prominent in the MCP and pancarpal joints.

HISTOPATHOLOGY

The normal synovium is a delicate structure consisting of an intimal lining and a sublining layer. The former is usually one or two layers deep; the latter is comprised of occasional small blood vessels, loose stroma, fibroblasts, and fat cells. The lining cells (synoviocytes) can be divided into two separate populations based on conventional morphology, histochemical staining, and functional capacities. Type A cells (macrophage-like synoviocytes) possess phagocytic vacuoles, macrophage surface markers, surface HLA-DR, and Fc receptors. Type B cells (fibroblast-like synoviocytes) have features of secretory fibroblasts, including prominent rough endoplasmic reticulum and regular arrays of ribosomes.

Histopathologic changes in the RA joint vary considerably. Early on, sublining edema and proliferation of blood vessels are prominent. Fibrin deposits onto the surface of the lining facing the joint cavity, and there is a scant interstitial infiltrate with either neutrophils or lymphocytes. As the disease progresses, the lining becomes hyperplastic, and the sublining is infiltrated with mononuclear cells and lymphoid aggregates. The synoviocytes display high levels of HLA-DR molecules on their surface, particularly on macrophage-like cells, and large amounts of class II MHC mRNA are demonstrable in this region.[21] The lining layer is usually 5 to 10 cells deep as a result of an increase in both type A and B synoviocytes. This many hundred–fold increase in cellularity likely reflects both the local proliferation of fibroblast-like synoviocytes and increased migration of monocytes and macrophages into the joint.[112]

The sublining is often densely infiltrated with lymphocytes. These may be evenly dispersed throughout the tissue or collect into aggregates. T lymphocytes predominate in RA tissue, representing about 40% to 50% of the total number of synovial cells, along with immunoglobulin producing B cells and plasma cells. Most are CD4+ T helper cells, with a CD4:CD8 ratio ranging from 4:1 to 14:1. In synovial fluid (SF), CD8+ T cells equal or outnumber helper cells.[28, 46, 47, 57, 106] The CD8 infiltrate in the tissue is scanty and usually located at the periphery of the lymphoid aggregates, suggesting that within the aggregate, macrophages or dendritic cells are presenting antigen to the helper T cells and B cells. The relative absence of a CD8 population results in an unopposed immunoglobulin production.[42]

However, this model is somewhat simplistic and not without exceptions. For instance, synovial biopsies from some RA patients show equal numbers of CD4+ and CD8+ T cells in the subintimal region.[55, 106] In another study, lymphoid aggregates were identified in only a minority of patients. Occasionally the synovium displayed a stromal pattern made up almost exclusively of fibroblasts with only rare T cells. The peripheral blood cells of these RA patients tended to respond briskly to soluble recall antigens, such as purified protein derivative, whereas blood mononuclear cells from those with intense lymphocytic infiltrates failed to respond.[57] This reciprocal relationship between blood anergy and the degree of inflammatory infiltrate implies a different immunopathogenic mechanism in each subset. Finally, it should be appreciated that the classic histopathologic picture is not unique to RA, for it can be seen in a number of other forms of arthritis, including crystal-induced disease and even osteoarthritis, which are not likely antigen-driven processes.

IMMUNOLOGIC FEATURES AND MODELS FOR RA

The original notion that disordered immunity, particularly autoimmunity, is central to the pathogenesis of RA derives from the histopathologic findings in the joint and the discovery of an antibody, called RF, in the blood of most RA patients. This antibody, which binds to the Fc portion of human IgG, was taken as evidence for autoimmunity. Although most RF in the circulation is IgM, later studies demonstrated that an IgG RF is also produced.[72]

The importance of RF in the pathogenesis of RA was inferred from the fact that circulating B cells in RA spontaneously produce the antibody, and RF-producing plasma cells abound in the rheumatoid synovium.[63, 69] RF also is a major constituent of immune complexes in the blood and SF of RA patients, suggesting that local immune complex formation and complement fixation are involved in rheumatoid synovitis.[107] Chemotactic complement fragments (like C5a) recruit neutrophils, which ingest the complexes and release degradative enzymes and toxic O_2 products into the SF.[96] This model is supported by the observation that serum RF levels correlate positively with complement consumption in RA.[43] Another consequence of the immune complex–mediated intra-articular inflammation is cartilage damage and the release of additional antigens (such as type II collagen) that could contribute to local autoantibody production, complement fixation, and direct tissue injury.

Although RF undoubtedly contributes to synovitis and immune complex–mediated systemic vascular lesions, studies have focused on the importance of cellular immunity in RA. Three separate (but not mutually exclusive) paradigms have been invoked to explain the histologic findings of chronic rheumatoid synovitis (Fig. 49–4).

T-CELL–DRIVEN IMMUNE RESPONSE

RA is thought to begin when an arthrotropic pathogen enters the joint. The exact etiologic agent is not known but might be a virus or a nonbiodegradable product of bacteria, as in SCWA. Persistence in the synovial tissue would presumably result in a specific T-cell–mediated immune response involving the trimolecular complex of the T-cell receptor, antigen, and correct class II molecules. Much evidence has been advanced to support this sequence of events.[66] The class II–HLA–DR B1 associations discussed earlier are essential elements in this paradigm. An analogous situation might be the joint lesions of Lyme arthritis, in which spirochetal antigens are likely pathogenic; the histology is similar to RA, and persistence of the arthritis is determined by genetic factors.[54]

The T cells from RA synovial effusions and subintimal tissues appear activated and express cell surface markers, such as class II MHC antigens, transferrin receptors, and IL-2

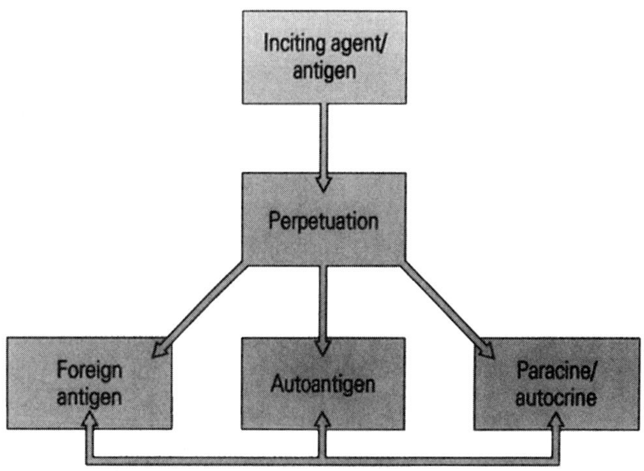

FIGURE 49–4. Pathways to rheumatoid arthritis. Theoretical steps involved in the conversion of an inciting event by an agent or antigen into a self-perpetuating chronic destructive disease. Both T-cell–dependent and T-cell–independent mechanisms are possible and not mutually exclusive. (Reprinted by permission of the publisher from Zvaifler NJ: New perspectives on the pathogenesis of rheumatoid arthritis. Am J Med 85:12–17, 1988. Copyright 1988 by Excerpta Medica Inc.)

receptors.[9, 46, 47] Synovial lining cells and interdigitating macrophages also display large amounts of class II antigens. Lymphocytes intimately associated with accessory cells should produce a variety of lymphokines that, along with macrophage-derived factors, can induce class II MHC expression and promote synoviocyte proliferation and the growth and differentiation of RF, producing B lymphocytes. Additional support for this scenario comes from studies showing that therapies directed at T cells, such as thoracic duct drainage, total nodal irradiation, and cyclosporin A, are modestly effective in RA.[66]

Thus a T-cell–driven specific immune response can explain many of the features of RA, but not all of the data are consistent with this hypothesis. For instance, most of the lymphocytes in the synovium appear small and quiescent. Little DNA synthesis is demonstrable, and the majority of dividing synovial T cells are CD8+ rather than CD4+.[22] Although present, IL-2 receptor expression is actually no different than on resting peripheral blood T cells.[24] Even infiltration of the synovium in RA with HLA-DR–positive T cells is nonspecific, since it also occurs in T-cell–independent forms of arthritis, like gout.[52] More troublesome, however, are two other important facts. The first is the surprising finding that the soluble mediators, cytokines produced in the joint, are primarily of non–T-cell origin. For instance, important T-cell cytokines, like IL-2, IL-3, IL-4, and IFN-γ, are barely detectable in RA tissue or SF.[23, 25, 59] However, in vivo production of these same lymphokines is easily demonstrated in a human T-cell–mediated response, such as tuberculous pleuritis.[5]

A second factor is the failure to consistently demonstrate restricted T-cell receptor (TCR) V gene usage, as would be anticipated in an antigen-driven T-cell response (reviewed in ref. 87). The possible explanations include the techniques used to assess TCR abundance, differences in study populations, and methods for selecting and expanding the cells under study. One can ask whether it is even realistic to anticipate finding TCR restrictions once the disease has become established and chronic, which is when most studies are performed. Early in RA, there might be some TCR homogeneity in the synovial lymphocyte population, reflecting a response to a specific antigen. Even then, it might only be one in several hundred T cells that would show the restriction.

As the disease progresses and other memory T cells enter the inflamed site under the influence of stimuli that are not antigen specific, the restricted population becomes greatly diluted, making identification of oligoclonality almost impossible. In addition, the majority of TCR gene analyses have focused on the β chain of the TCR. There are, however, a small percentage of peripheral blood T cells that express another TCR. These are γ/δ T cells, which have membrane CD3 but none of the other surface markers associated with functional subsets of α/β T cells, such as CD4 and CD8. In adjuvant arthritis, the γ/δ T cells are expanded in response to mycobacterial antigen, and a similar claim has been made in RA.[40, 41, 94]

Still another problem is the appreciation that antigens stimulate T cells in different ways. Conventional small peptides are presented by MHC molecules to a small number of T cells that have the appropriate receptor. Another class of antigens stimulate large numbers of T cells and hence are called superantigens.[30] An example is the staphylococcal enterotoxin responsible for the toxic shock syndrome. Superantigens do not require antigen processing, bind avidly to class II MHC molecules but show little MHC restriction, and are recognized by virtually all of the T cells that utilize a single or small group of the V-β gene family of the TCR. Superantigens bridge the antigen-presenting cell and lymphocyte by binding to the external aspect of the β chain of the class II molecule and the β chain of the TCR. Up to 10% to 20% of CD4+ and CD8+ T cells can be triggered by certain superantigens.

In the case of collagen-induced arthritis in the mouse, it has been shown that the mycoplasma superantigen (MAM) can clonally expand autoreactive T cells, resulting in an enhancement or triggering of arthritis. Furthermore, in these animals, resolved arthritis that had been inactive for months will recur upon systemic administration of superantigen, perhaps analogous to flares of RA thought to be induced by an infection. A superantigen recognized by the V-δ chain of γ/δ T cells is HSP. This is of interest because of the reported oligoclonal accumulation of γ/δ T cells in synovial tissue and the enhanced proliferation of T cells derived from synovial fluid when challenged with HSP. These findings, however, cannot explain the known HLA associations with RA.

AUTOREACTIVE T-CELL MODEL

Although it is usually assumed that the initiating agent in RA is responsible for both the early changes and the perpetuation of chronic synovitis, this need not be the case. The chronic rheumatoid lesion might be due to a response to antigens quite distinct from those responsible for starting the process. Such a scenario has been used to explain other chronic inflammatory lesions, like chronic thyroiditis, in which an appropriate response to a presumed viral insult results in the local elaboration of IFN-γ. This cytokine can induce HLA-DR expression on the surface of thyrocytes, rendering them targets for immune attack.[7]

The reaction between HLA-DR–bearing stimulator cells and autologous T lymphocytes is termed the autologous mixed leukocyte reaction (AMLR). Evidence that the synovial lesions in RA represent a localized AMLR is largely circumstantial but of interest.[24] First, the cytokine profile of RA synovitis is similar to an AMLR in that only small amounts of T-cell–derived factors, like IL-2 and IFN-γ, are present.[90] In contrast, allogeneic mixed leukocyte reactions produce high levels of these lymphokines. The cytotoxic T cells present in RA joint effusions are similar to the NK-like cells produced in the AMLR.[34] Finally, the articular cavity and synovium contain an abundance of HLA-DR–rich stimulator cells, including type A synoviocytes, macrophages, and dendritic cells.[113]

Autologous stimulation need not be limited to self-HLA-DR molecules. According to theories of molecular mimicry, a foreign antigen can closely resemble a self-antigen, and innocent bystanders become targets. This is one of the proposed mechanisms implicating EBV in the pathogenesis of RA. B lymphocytes are their primary target. Once infected, the B cells carry the EBV viral genome for life. Normal B cells that have been superinfected in vitro spontaneously proliferate and secrete immunoglobulins, including RF.[85]

In addition, rheumatoid patients are defective in controlling in vitro EBV infection, in part due to deficient IFN-γ secretion by RA T cells and a monocyte-derived IL-1 inhibitor.[36, 56] As noted earlier, there is a homology between the EBV glycoprotein gp110 and the amino acid sequence in the third allelic hypervariable region (3AHVR) of the HLA-DR B1 chain. It has been proposed that immune recognition of the antigens of a pathogen like EBV (or HSP of gram-negative bacteria) induces a high-affinity cross-reaction to the 3AHVR, which would normally be tolerated.[75] Hence immunity directed against the gp110 of EBV could inadvertently damage normal cells in hosts that express these surface MHC molecules. In the joint, high levels of class II molecules are sustained on a number of cell types, which could explain the perpetuation of synovitis. In a sense, EBV might initiate an AMLR-like reaction in genetically susceptible individuals, with HLA-DR B1 as the target.

Self-molecules, other than HLA-DR, have been proposed as targets for immune attack in arthritis. For instance, type II collagen can cause arthritis in susceptible animals and might contribute to chronic RA, probably as a perpetuating rather than an etiologic stimulus. Autoantibodies to proteoglycan, a macromolecule with a protein backbone and large glycosaminoglycan side chains, develop in the course of immune synovitis in rabbits, and the affected joint shows a loss of cartilage proteoglycan. The relevance of this model to human disease is not yet defined. As with type II collagen, if immunity to proteoglycan does contribute to cartilage damage, it is likely a secondary phenomenon.

Mycobacteria cause chronic inflammatory joint lesions and have long been implicated in the pathogenesis of RA. Evidence that mycobacteria could provide an important cross-reactive autoantigen comes from the recognition that an immunodominant antigen of the mycobacterium is a 65-kD protein with sequence homology to an intracellular stress protein present in all eukaryotic cells.[53] A massive increase in stress proteins was first demonstrated after cells were exposed to heat. Thus HSP and stress proteins are interchangeable terms. Because of the ubiquitous nature of these highly conserved proteins, the immune system is likely tolerant to them.

Repeated presentation of cross-reactive bacterial HSP or surface expression of similar proteins on T cells or macrophages might result in loss of tolerance and an autoimmune reaction. Several observations can be cited in support of this hypothesis. RA synovial fluid T cells, which do not proliferate when exposed to certain *Salmonella-Shigella* or *Ureaplasma* organisms, show an augmented reactivity to an acetone-precipitable fraction of mycobacterium tuberculosis. These same fractions of mycobacterium contain antigens that cross-react with antibodies to cartilage proteoglycan.[40, 94] Mycobacteria have been directly implicated in the pathogenesis of adjuvant arthritis, and T-cell clones from affected animals proliferate in the presence of a 65-kD HSP.[94] T-cell clones derived from RA synovial effusions recognize an epitope present in amino acids 1 to 15 of the HSP-65 molecule.[31] As previously noted, the QKRAA epitope on the HLA-DR4 B1 chain has complete homology with a sequence in a 70-kD stress proteins and could serve as an autoantigen in a manner similar to the EBV molecular mimicry.[77] In both of these models (EBV and HSP), the HLA associations would more likely be involved in the progression of RA rather than as a susceptibility or initiating factor. This is consistent with the concept of DR B1 alleles as markers for severity of RA.[99]

PARACRINE/AUTOCRINE MODEL

In the two previous models, T lymphocytes are assigned the major role for the perpetuation of rheumatoid synovitis. Products of these cells theoretically diffuse through the tissues, altering postcapillary venules, inducing the proliferation and differentiation of B cells, and directly influencing macrophages and synoviocytes in the joint lining. Unfortunately, as noted previously, this picture is not consistent with much of the data about T-cell activation in the joint.

In contrast, synovial macrophage-like and fibroblast-like cells appear highly activated based on their morphology, surface HLA-DR expression, and elaboration of cytokines. Table 49–2 shows a comparison of cytokine production by various synovial cells. Products of these cells, like IL-1,[27, 58, 64, 102] TNF-α,[78] IL-6,[35, 38] GM-CSF,[105] M-CSF (CSF-1),[23] prostaglandins, and collagenase, are abundant in synovial fluids and synovial tissues.

Studies using in situ hybridization to quantify cytokine production at the level of gene expression confirm experiments that detected high levels of secreted cytokines in culture supernatants of synovial tissue cells and in synovial effusions.[20] For instance, IL-1-β and TNF-α genes were expressed by large numbers of synovial macrophages. IL-6 probes also hybridized to a high percentage of RA synovial cells. Although T cells can produce IL-6 under some circumstances, in situ hybridization experiments show most of

TABLE 49–2
T-CELL AND MACROPHAGE/FIBROBLAST CYTOKINE PRODUCTION

Cellular Sources of Synovial Cytokines	
Cytokines	*Detected in RA Synovium/Synovial Fluid*
Products of T cells	
IL-2	±
IL-3	−
IL-4	−
IL-6	±
IFN-γ	−
TNF-α	−
TNF-β	−
GM-CSF	−
Products of macrophages/ type A synoviocytes	
IL-1	+ + +
IL-6	+
IL-8	+ + +
IL-10	+ +
TNF-α	+ +
M-CSF (CSF-1)	+
IFN-α	±
GM-CSF	+
TGF-β	+ +
MCP-1	+ +
Products of fibroblasts/ type B synoviocytes	
IL-6	+ + +
GM-CSF	+
MCP-1	+
TGF-β	+ +

− = negligible or no detection; ± = minimal amounts detected.

the IL-6 gene expression in the nonmacrophage, non–T-cell population, and that these cells are located mainly in the intimal lining of the joint. GM-CSF and TGF-β gene expression was observed in a lesser number of cells. As predicted from earlier studies on synovial IFN-γ production, the IFN-γ probe did not bind to synovial tissue cells.[25] Interestingly, the failure to detect cytokine mRNA, including IL-1, TNF-α, and IL-6 in mononuclear cells isolated from synovial fluid indicates that the synoviocytes are the source of most articular cytokines.

The cytokine profile of the rheumatoid synovium suggests that chronic articular inflammation is sustained by factors produced by neighboring macrophages and synovial fibroblasts in a paracrine or autocrine model.[26] This concept of a non–T-cell–driven pathogenesis of synovitis has support in some animal models. For instance, severe combined immunodeficiency (SCID) mice, which lack an immune system, when infected with *Borrelia,* develop a severe destructive arthritis that is much worse than that seen in normal mouse strains infected with the same organism. Likewise, when RA synovial tissues are transplanted into the joints of SCID mice, the resident T cells die, but the residual cells destroy the mouse articular cartilage.[32]

Many factors already identified in the joint could explain lining cell hyperplasia, class II display, and synovial angiogenesis. Figure 49–5 shows a simplified scheme of the complex cytokine circuits that could exist between synovial cells. For instance, IL-1 and TNF-α (synovial macrophage products) stimulate fibroblast-like synoviocyte proliferation and increase secretion of IL-6, GM-CSF, and collagenase.[13, 14, 44] GM-CSF, produced by synovial macrophages, can stimulate fibroblast-like synoviocytes, is a potent inducer of IL-1 secretion, and increases DR expression on macrophages.[4, 62] TNF-α can synergize with GM-CSF and probably also contributes to macrophage HLA-DR expression.[4] The local production of cytokines by macrophages and fibroblasts could also impact on T cells and contribute to the limited amount of T-cell activation observed. B-cell activation and rheumatoid factor production might result through T-cell–independent mechanisms or as yet undefined cell products.

A prediction of this alternative (paracrine) model is that T cells are not necessarily sequestered in the joint in response to a specific antigen but rather accumulate under the influence of factors made in the lining.[26] The RA synovium has an overrepresentation of mature memory helper cells (CD4-CD45RO), whereas naive CD45RA-bearing cells (the suppressor inducer subset) are conspicuously absent.[22] This could be explained by the fact that the movement of lymphocytes from the circulation into the joint is not a random process. Their sites of egress are the postcapillary venules, notably through those with high endothelium (HEV). Transendothelial migration is tightly regulated and involves specific molecules on the surface of the circulating cells and counterreceptors (ligands) for these molecules on the endothelium (reviewed in 45).

Three distinct steps account for T-cell adhesion to endothelium (Fig. 49–6). The process begins at sites where narrowing of the vascular bed leads to a diminished flow. Instead of rapidly moving down the center of the blood stream, lymphocytes marginate and begin to roll along the vessel wall. This allows for a loose tethering of lymphocytes to the vascular endothelial cells. The molecules that mediate tethering are members of the family of lectin-binding proteins, called selectins.

During its brief roll along the vascular endothelial surface (often less than a few seconds), a lymphocyte must decide whether to bind tightly at that site and migrate into tissue. This decision is strongly influenced by factors produced by the vascular endothelium at sites of inflammation or injury, such as cytokines (particularly IFN-γ, IL-1, and TNF-α), platelet activating factor (PAF), and chemokines. These factors deliver a triggering signal that up-regulates the amount or binding avidity of molecules normally present on the surface of the lymphocytes and their counterreceptors on the vascular endothelium.

The relevant lymphocyte molecules are members of two integrin families, the α_1/β_2 integrin (LFA-1 or $CD11_a$) and the α_4/β_1 integrin (VLA-4). Engagement by their opposite member on the vascular endothelium (ICAM-1 and VCAM-1, respectively) results in a dramatic change. The loose tethering becomes a strong adhesion to the endothelium. The lymphocyte spreads and then migrates through the en-

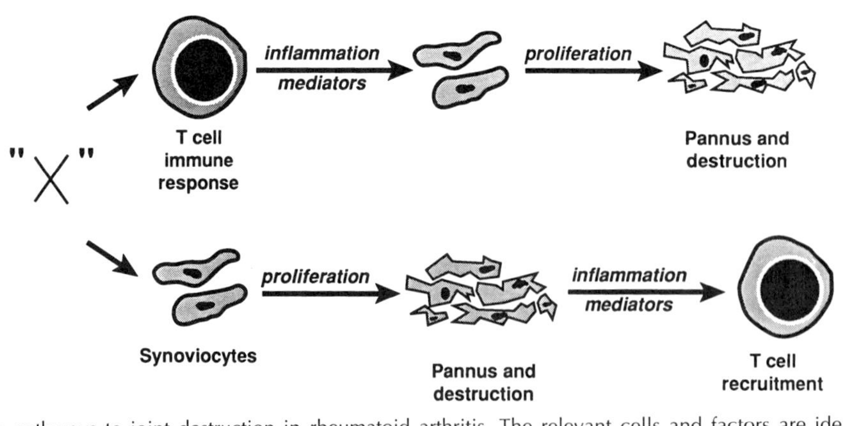

FIGURE 49–5. Alternative pathways to joint destruction in rheumatoid arthritis. The relevant cells and factors are identical in both schemes. In one, however, the unknown initiating factor (X) induces a T-cell immune response, and the consequences are mediator-driven proliferation of type A and B synoviocytes followed by pannus and joint destruction. Alternatively, X could modify either type A or type B synoviocytes, causing them to proliferate; pannus formation and joint destruction follows. Inflammatory mediators account for the accumulation of non–antigen-specific T cells in the synovium. (From Zvaifler NJ, Firestein GS: Pannus and pannocytes. Alternative models of joint destruction in rheumatoid arthritis. Arthritis Rheum 37:783–789, 1994.)

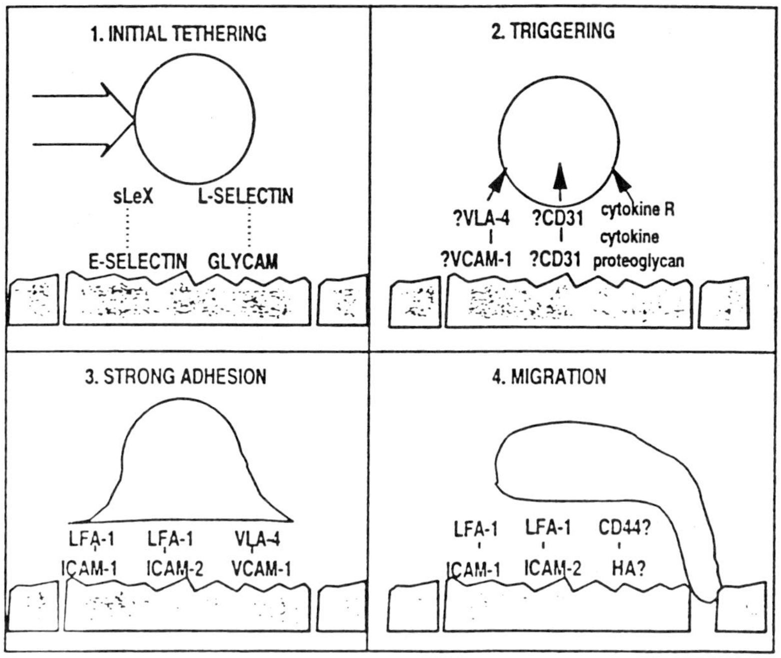

FIGURE 49–6. Steps involved in tethering, triggering, adhesion, and subsequent transmigration of T lymphocytes across the vascular endothelium. (From Tanaka Y, Adams DH, Shaw S: Regulation of leukocyte recruitment by proadhesive cytokines immobilized on endothelial proteoglycan. Curr Top Microbiol Immunol 184:99–106, 1993.)

dothelium into the surrounding tissues, where additional integrin-matrix interactions occur. It is noteworthy that neither antigen nor the TCR plays any role in this tissue localization (see Chapter 15).

Circulating memory-type lymphocytes express significantly greater amounts of LFA-1 and CD2 (the counterreceptors for ICAM-1 and LFA-3, found on postcapillary venules) than do naive lymphocytes. Thus the preferential accumulation of cells with a mature phenotype in the inflamed synovium is not surprising. The CD45RO cells also express greater amounts of VLA-4, whose ligands are VCAM-1 and the alternatively spliced form of fibronectin (CS-1), both of which are abundant in the synovial lining and subintimal regions.[16, 61] There is no information on the fate of memory lymphocytes once they enter into the tissues. Whether they are simply in transit or retained for long periods of time needs to be defined.

LABORATORY DIAGNOSIS

RA is a clinical diagnosis, but laboratory tests are useful to support the clinical assessment and monitor disease activity.[8] Acute phase reactants such as the erythrocyte sedimentation rate, serum orosomucoid, C-reactive protein (CRP), α_2 macroglobulins, and fibrinogen are all increased, likely reflecting the release from inflamed articular tissues of cytokines, particularly IL-1 and IL-6.[79] Anemia, usually associated with low serum iron, may be explained by similar factors.

RF (antigammaglobulins) are detected in the serum of approximately 70% of RA patients. Very high titers of IgM RF are usually associated with more aggressive, destructive arthritis and more extra-articular features, including vasculitis. Titers of RF fluctuate very little in the course of the disease and only occasionally fall in response to treatment. However, IgM RF are not specific for rheumatic diseases but are found in a variety of chronic and inflammatory conditions. RF of the IgG class, although probably important pathogenetically, particularly in the synovial space, are not measured in the conventional clinical laboratory tests because they are poor agglutinators.

Much information about the immunopathogenesis of RA comes from studies of cellular immunity in synovial tissues and fluids, but they are of limited clinical utility. Determinations of circulating lymphocyte numbers, subclasses, and surface markers have also been disappointing.[12, 22] Newer methods have been developed for assessing disease activity. The concentration of various cytokines; soluble cytokine receptors (like IL-2); molecules shed from activated lymphocytes or vascular endothelium (like soluble CD8 molecules, ICAM-1 or VCAM-1 molecules) have been measured in blood and synovial fluid samples. Although some definitely correlate with increased disease activity in RA, it is not clear that they perform significantly better than do conventional tests, such as the CRP and erythrocyte sedimentation rate.[17]

Inflammatory joint disease is associated with an accelerated metabolism of bone and cartilage matrix constituents. Connective tissue turnover can be quantified by measurements of proteoglycans, type II pro-collagen peptides, and hyaluronic acid in blood, and hydroxyproline, pyridinoline, and deoxypyridinoline cross-links in urine.[71] These studies are in their infancy, and their value as predictors of cartilage and bone destruction remains to be proven in longitudinal studies of RA. Preliminary data suggest that they may be helpful in predicting long-term disability.

SF analysis confirms that RA is an inflammatory joint disease.[110] The increased protein content is characteristic of an exudate. White blood cells range from 5 to 20,000 per mm^3, with counts in excess of 50,000 mm^3 occasionally encountered. Approximately two thirds of the cells are polymorphonuclear leukocytes, except in very early disease. Total hemolytic complement activity is reduced to less than one third of the serum values, especially in patients with seropositive RA, and early classic pathway components (C2 and C4) are most profoundly depressed. This is distinctly different in other inflammatory forms of joint disease in which the fluid C levels are proportional to their concentration in blood and supports a role for intra-articular immune complexes in the pathogenesis of RA.[107] Mononuclear cell surface antigens, cytokines, and constituents of the inflammatory reaction have all been measured in SF but are of limited utility. A possible exception is neopterin, a product of activated macrophages, whose concentration in SF appears to correlate directly with disease activity measurements.[49]

Roentgenograms, particularly of the hands and feet, remain the standard for assessing joint damage and progression in RA.[81] Erosions of articular cartilage and bone predict a poorer outcome and are used as an indication for aggressive drug treatment.

COURSE—NATURAL HISTORY

The course that RA will follow in any individual seen at the inception of the disease cannot be reliably predicted, but there are several recognized patterns of outcome. Approximately 10% of patients have a short-lived joint disease that remits without significant residua. In another 15% to 25%, arthritis persists for some time and then leaves, with only mild to moderate damage to the joints. Fifty percent of patients have persistent activity of the arthritis punctuated by exacerbations and remissions, but invariably leading to progressive deformity and disability. The remaining 10% to 15% have a relentless disease that is unresponsive to treatment and prior to the availability of joint replacement resulted in complete disability, with the patient restricted to a bed or wheelchair.

Clinical features that portend either a favorable or dismal outcome of RA have been identified. In general, remissions most likely occur during the first year of disease, especially after an acute onset with systemic manifestations. Factors that presage a less favorable disease course are an insidious onset, older age (>45 years old), female gender, a greater number of affected joints, development of nodules, persistence beyond 1 year without remission, and early appearance of bone erosions on radiologic examination of the joints.[19, 93] The presence of RF, particularly in high titers, is associated with a poor outcome. In retrospective studies, patients with certain DR-B1 alleles have increased frequency and severity of joint destruction and extra-articular manifestations of RA (see Fig. 49–2). Whether HLA typing of patients at the inception of disease will predict a particular outcome has not been formally proven. Rheumatoid patients may succumb to overwhelming sepsis or complications of drug or surgical therapy, but the majority generally die of the same diseases as age-matched cohorts, except 5 to 10 years sooner. In fact, the life expectancy for RA patients with advanced (stage IV) joint disease is similar to that for patients with Hodgkin's disease.[60] The dim outlook in these patients has been used to justify trials with toxic compounds, drug combinations, and experimental modalities.

TREATMENT

The natural course of RA is characterized by spontaneous remissions and exacerbations; therefore, the evaluation of therapy can be difficult. In this chapter, the discussion is limited to drug therapies, with an emphasis on classes of drugs. Any total management program for a patient with RA, however, requires the participation of a variety of medical and paramedical personnel: physiatrists, orthopedic surgeons, rheumatologists, visiting nurses, and other medical specialists when indicated. Successful treatment also depends on an empathetic doctor-patient relationship. Because it is impossible to present in detail the complexities and nuances of the treatment of RA in this chapter, interested readers are referred to several excellent rheumatologic texts for additional information.[1, 2]

A new classification of antirheumatic therapy also is being promulgated by the International League of Associations for Rheumatology and the World Health Organization.[15] Two major categories of drugs are proposed: (1) symptom-modifying antirheumatic drugs (SMARD), those that influence the symptoms and clinical features of inflammatory synovitis, and (2) a new category called disease-controlling antirheumatic therapy (DC-ART). To be included in the second category, a drug must change the course of RA by both improving and sustaining function in association with decreased inflammatory synovitis and preventing or significantly decreasing the rate of progression of structural joint damage. Although this latter category provides the basis for setting management objectives for RA, it is not clear whether any of the currently available treatments would meet these stringent DC-ART. Thus current nomenclatures are used in this discussion of treatment.

Nonsteroidal anti-inflammatory drugs (NSAID) are mainstays of RA therapy. The prototype is aspirin. Aspirin and the other NSAIDs have the capacity to inhibit prostaglandin and thromboxane synthesis by interfering with the cyclooxygenase enzyme. However, the fact that nonacetylated salicylates are poor inhibitors of prostaglandin synthesis and that the anti-inflammatory effect of NSAIDs requires doses in excess of those needed to inhibit prostaglandin synthesis suggest that these agents must have anti-inflammatory effects independent of arachidonic acid metabolism.[39] Indeed, they can influence neutrophil function and activation, interfere with the guanosine triphosphate–binding regulatory proteins (G protein), inhibit the activation of the nuclear transcriptions factor NFk-B, and probably have other effects through their ability to associate with the plasma membrane of certain cells.[48]

Many of these same pharmacologic properties likely account for important toxicities that develop in the course of NSAID use. Upper gastrointestinal injury occurs in many patients who take these compounds. Although infrequent (1%–2% per annum), upper gastrointestinal bleeding or perforation is recognized as a significant public health problem. Likewise, prostaglandins play an important role in renal blood flow. NSAID treatment introduces a significant risk for the development of renal impairment and congestive heart failure, particularly in elderly patients or those with decreased blood volume.

Glucocorticosteroids are used in RA to modify both inflammation and immune function. Their effects are multiple and complex.[33] Glucocorticoids alter leukocyte trafficking and recruitment of cells to sites of inflammation and modify neutrophil and monocyte functions. By interfering with the conversion of phospholipase A2 to arachidonic acid, they inhibit both the 5-lipoxygenase and cyclooxygenase pathways. Cellular responses to cytokines and cytokine production are reduced by steroids. Particularly important in this regard is the down-regulation of vascular endothelial cell expression of adhesion molecules.

Glucocorticoids are potent suppressors of collagenase production by cultured synoviocytes, in part by their ability to block the expression of c-*jun*, an important transcriptional regulator of the procollagenase gene. Higher concentrations diminish or block lymphocyte proliferation in vitro. Clinically, however, glucocorticoids are usually employed at small daily doses (prednisone 5.0–7.5 mg) in an attempt to minimize the side effects associated with their chronic use. They are seldom the exclusive therapeutic agent in RA. Rather, they are used in combination with NSAIDs or other slower acting drugs.

A second class of drugs used to treat RA have in common a slow onset of action, hence the acronym SAARD. Members of this group lack similar structural or pharmacologic properties but have serendipitously been observed to act as disease-modifying antirheumatic drugs (DMARD). They include intramuscular gold, oral gold (auranofin), penicillamine, sulfasalazine, and a number of aminoquinoline compounds, such as chloroquine and hydroxychloroquine. In contrast to NSAIDs, which act rapidly (often within hours or days) and lose their effects just as quickly, the second-line antirheumatic drugs often need to be taken for months before improvement is recognized, and their benefits may persist long after the drug is discontinued. Their exact mode of action is unknown.[6] Gold compounds appear to influence cells of the monocyte/macrophage lineage by interfering with lysosomal enzyme activity, antigen processing, or cytokine production. Penicillamine, on the other hand, seems to exert its effect on T-cell proliferation. Antimalarials have actions in both the nucleus and cytoplasm of cells. Their ability to interrupt the transport of intact HLA class II molecules from intracytoplasmic endosomes to the surface of monocytes theoretically could interfere with antigen presentation or T-cell activation.

Second-line drugs are considered in patients with persistent synovitis or progressive disability despite NSAID therapy. The appearance of periarticular erosions on radiographic evaluation and the development of extra-articular disease are additional indications.

There has been increasing skepticism about the long-term benefits of treatment with second-line drugs.[98] Most studies enforce the notion that even with treatment, RA is a relentlessly progressive disease. Conventional interventions appear to benefit a limited number of patients (one third to one half) in the short term (18–30 months). At the end of 5 to 7 years, however, there is less evidence for alteration in the natural history of the disease. This has evoked a number of responses, including appeals for the use of combination therapies.

Several second-line agents are given together based on the notion that there are multiple pathways in the pathogenesis of chronic synovitis and intervention at different points might improve effectiveness. An alternative approach is to introduce second-line agents earlier in the disease when a theoretic window of opportunity exists between the inception of RA and its subsequent perpetuation by autoimmune or chronic inflammatory processes. The problems inherent in these strategies have been detailed elsewhere.[109] A report showing that patients with RA (who failed on at least one DMARD) respond significantly better to the combination of methotrexate plus Plaquenil plus sulfasalazine than to either drug alone is promising. Whether these advantages will be maintained throughout long-term follow-up needs to be demonstrated.[65] It should also be appreciated that some DMARD combinations only increase toxicity without additional therapeutic benefit.[67]

Immunosuppressive treatment has been used in RA for more than 25 years. Initial enthusiasm for alkylating agents, such as nitrogen mustard, chlorambucil, and cyclophosphamide, was tempered by a high rate of toxicity and the development of skin and hematologic malignancies. Alkylating agents are usually reserved for patients with systemic, life-threatening complications of RA, such as necrotizing vasculitis. In contrast, azathioprine (Imuran) has a low incidence of side effects that are easily managed with appropriate attention to hematologic and hepatic testing. An increased incidence of malignancy can only be demonstrated by meta-analysis or very long follow-up of large numbers of patients. Thus the risks are very small and probably are offset by benefits in terms of the control of synovitis and the possibility of decreasing concomitant use of corticosteroids.

In the past decade, low-dose weekly methotrexate treatment of RA has become widespread despite substantial uncertainty regarding its mechanism of action. Patient acceptance is high and side effects are manageable. Fully 60% to 70% of patients remain on the drug for periods as long as 7 to 10 years compared with 20% for injectable gold, with a good clinical response.[97] Controversy exists whether methotrexate's action is immunosuppressive or anti-inflammatory. In the small doses used in RA (7.5–15 mg orally once a week), there is little effect on a variety of in vivo immunologic parameters.

Those who favor inhibition of inflammation as a mechanism of action cite a relatively rapid onset of beneficial effects (usually in 3–6 weeks), failure to halt the development of articular erosions on radiographic study, and rapid recurrence of the joint disease when the drug is stopped. Side effects usually consist of stomatitis and gastrointestinal disturbance; cytopenias are uncommon. The development of hepatotoxicity with chronic administration (as seen in patients treated for psoriasis) is only rarely observed in RA.[50] Occasional fatty infiltration and mild fibrosis are rare findings on a liver biopsy, but significant hepatic fibrosis or cirrhosis is only rarely encountered. Pulmonary hypersensitivity is rare, although it can be fatal. Despite these concerns, methotrexate alone or in combination with other second-line agents is currently the most effective and widely used treatment for severe active RA.

TREATMENT STRATEGIES FOR RHEUMATOID ARTHRITIS

With a greater appreciation of the importance of early recognition and intervention in RA and the availability of markers for severity and persistence of disease, it should be possible to improve on the poor results of treatment observed in the past. Basing his conclusion on the follow-up of a large group of patients (800) with early synovitis, Emery[18] has proposed that if patients at the inception of RA show only oligoarthritis or mild disease, they should begin treatment with sulfasalazine and switch to methotrexate or intramuscular gold if a response is not achieved within 3 months. He defined a response as a significant reduction in the indexes of joint inflammation plus normalization of the C-reactive protein (less than 20 mg/l).

The options for those with moderate or more severe disease would include intramuscular gold, low-dose oral corticosteroid, methotrexate and early administration of cyclosporin A. In the minority of patients who have a very poor prognosis, based on a rapid course, a high titer of blood RF, and the appropriate RA haplotype, a more radical approach may be required. This might include the early use of immunosuppressants or biologic agents. This approach, which is in its infancy, may be efficacious in the short term but needs to be substantiated by evaluation after 5 years.

The overall poor response to treatment and the shortened life expectancy in patients with advanced (stage IV) RA have encouraged trials of novel and experimental therapies and modalities. Cyclosporin A has benefits when compared with placebo, but only low doses can be used (2.5 mg/kg or less daily) because of nephrotoxicity.[80] Total nodal irradiation probably provides some relief, but the high rate of life-threatening infections has limited its utility.[108] Products of recombinant technology are currently under study.

In several large multiclinic trials, IFN-γ gives only modest benefit in RA. Small numbers of patients have been treated with monoclonal antibodies that eliminate T cells (anti-CD4, anti-CD5, anti-CD52). The results have been disappointing. In contrast, there are sometimes dramatic responses to maneuvers that neutralize TNF-α.[16a] Dietary manipulation, particularly of eicosapentaenoics, through the ingestion of fish oils also provides some benefit in some RA patients.[70] Of interest, the effects on cell function and leukotriene B4 release are more impressive than the modest clinical response. As understanding of the specific factors involved in the perpetuation of rheumatoid synovitis increases, it is hoped that the therapies available will become more specific and effective. It is no longer wishful thinking to believe that control of this devastating disease will be possible.

REFERENCES

1. Klippel JH, Dieppe PA (eds): Rheumatology. Mosby-Year Book Europe Limited, London, 1994.
2. Weisman MH, Weinblatt ME (eds): Treatment of the Rheumatic Diseases. WB Saunders Company, Philadelphia, 1995.
3. Albani S, Tuckwell JE, Esparza L, et al: The susceptibility sequence to rheumatoid arthritis is a cross-reactive B cell epitope shared by the *Escherichia coli* heat shock protein dnaJ and the histocompatibility leukocyte antigen DRB10401 molecule. J Clin Invest 89:327–331, 1992.
4. Alvaro-Gracia JM, Zvaifler NJ, Firestein GS: Cytokines in chronic inflammatory arthritis. IV. Granulocyte/macrophage colony-stimulating factor–mediated induction of class II MHC antigen on human monocytes: a possible role in rheumatoid arthritis. J Exp Med 170:865–876, 1989.
5. Barnes PF, Fong SJ, Brennan PJ, et al: Local production of tumor necrosis factor and IFN-gamma in tuberculous pleuritis. J Immunol 145:149–154, 1990.
6. Borigini MJ, Paulus HE: Rheumatoid arthritis. In Weisman MH, Weinblatt ME (eds): Treatment of the Rheumatic Diseases. WB Saunders Company, Philadelphia, 1994, pp 31–51.
7. Bottazzo GF, Pujol-Borrell R, Hanafusa T, et al: Role of aberrant HLA-DR expression and antigen presentation in induction of endocrine autoimmunity. Lancet 2:1115–1119, 1983.
8. Bull BS, Westengard JC, Farr M, et al: Efficacy of tests used to monitor rheumatoid arthritis. Lancet 2:965–967, 1989.
9. Burmester GR, Jahn B, Gramatzki M, et al: Activated T cells in vivo and in vitro: divergence in expression of Tac and Ia antigens in the nonblastoid small T cells of inflammation and normal T cells activated in vitro. J Immunol 133:1230–1234, 1984.
10. Cohen IR, Holoshitz J, van Eden W, et al: T lymphocyte clones illuminate pathogenesis and affect therapy of experimental arthritis. Arthritis Rheum 28:841–845, 1985.
11. Courtenay JS, Dallman MJ, Dayan AD, et al: Immunization against heterologous type II collagen induces arthritis in mice. Nature 283:666–668, 1980.
12. Cush JJ, Lipsky PE, Postlethwaite AE, et al: Correlation of serologic indicators of inflammation with effectiveness of nonsteroidal antiinflammatory drug therapy in rheumatoid arthritis. Arthritis Rheum 33:19–28, 1990.
13. Dayer J-M, Beutler B, Cerami A: Cachectin/tumor necrosis factor stimulates collagenase and prostaglandin E2 production by human synovial cells and dermal fibroblasts. J Exp Med 162:2163–2168, 1985.
14. Dayer JM, de Rochemonteix B, Burrus B, et al: Human recombinant interleukin 1 stimulates collagenase and prostaglandin E2 production by synovial cells. J Clin Invest 77:645–648, 1986.
15. Edmonds J: Proposed new classification of antirheumatic therapies: analysis of the DC-ART category. J Rheumatol 21(S1):1–63, 1994.
16. Elices MJ, Tsai V, Strahl D, et al: Expression and functional significance of alternatively spliced CS1 fibronectin in rheumatoid arthritis microvasculature. J Clin Invest 93:405–416, 1994.

16a. Elliott MJ, Maini RN, Feldmann M, et al: Randomized double-blind comparison of chimeric monoclonal antibody to tumour necrosis factor α (cA2) versus placebo in rheumatoid arthritis. Lancet 344:1105–1110, 1994.

17. Emery P, Chu CQ, Maini RN: The validity of surrogate markers in rheumatic diseases. Br J Rheumatol 32(S3):3–8, 1993.
18. Emery P, Luqmani R: Monotherapy in rheumatoid arthritis. Br J Rheumatol 32(S1):21–23, 1993.
19. Feigenbaum SL, Masi AT, Kaplan SB: Prognosis in rheumatoid arthritis. A longitudinal study of newly diagnosed younger adult patients. Am J Med 66:377–384, 1979.
20. Firestein GS, Alvaro-Gracia JM, Maki R: Quantitative analysis of cytokine gene expression in rheumatoid arthritis. J Immunol 144:3347–3353, 1990.
21. Firestein GS, Paine MM, Littman BH: Gene expression (collagenase, tissue inhibitor of metalloproteinases, complement, and HLA-DR) in rheumatoid arthritis and osteoarthritis synovium. Quantitative analysis and effect of intraarticular corticosteroids. Arthritis Rheum 34:1094–1105, 1991.
22. Firestein GS, Tsai V, Zvaifler NJ: Cellular immunity in the joints of patients with rheumatoid arthritis and other forms of chronic synovitis. Rheum Dis Clin North Am 13:191–213, 1987.
23. Firestein GS, Xu WD, Townsend K, et al: Cytokines in chronic inflammatory arthritis. I. Failure to detect T cell lymphokines (interleukin 2 and interleukin 3) and presence of macrophage colony-stimulating factor (CSF-1) and a novel mast cell growth factor in rheumatoid synovitis. J Exp Med 168(S):1573–1586, 1988.
24. Firestein GS, Zvaifler NJ: The pathogenesis of rheumatoid arthritis: a critical assessment of the role of autologous stimulation in the perpetuation of rheumatoid synovitis. Rheum Dis Clin North Am 13:447–461, 1987.
25. Firestein GS, Zvaifler NJ: Peripheral blood and synovial fluid monocyte activation in inflammatory arthritis. II. Low levels of synovial fluid and synovial tissue interferon suggest that gamma-interferon is not the primary macrophage activating factor. Arthritis Rheum 30:864–871, 1987.
26. Firestein GS, Zvaifler NJ: How important are T cells in chronic rheumatoid synovitis? Arthritis Rheum 33:768–773, 1990.
27. Fontana A, Hengartner H, Weber E, et al: Interleukin 1 activity in the synovial fluid of patients with rheumatoid arthritis. Rheumatol Int 2:49–53, 1982.
28. Forre O, Thoen J, Lea T, et al: In situ characterization of mononuclear cells in rheumatoid tissues, using monoclonal antibodies. No reduction of T8-positive cells or augmentation in T4-positive cells. Scand J Immunol 16:315–319, 1982.

29. Franklin EC, Holman HR, Muller-Eberhard HR, et al: An unusual protein component of high molecular weight in the serum of patients with rheumatoid arthritis. J Exp Med 105:425–438, 1957.
30. Friedman SM, Posnett DN, Tumang JR, et al: A potential role for microbial superantigens in the pathogenesis of systemic autoimmune disease. Arthritis Rheum 34:468–480, 1991.
31. Gaston JS, Life PF, Bailey LC, et al: In vitro responses to a 65-kilodalton mycobacterial protein by synovial T cells from inflammatory arthritis patients. J Immunol 143:2494–2500, 1989.
32. Geiler T, Kriegsmann J, Keyszer GM, et al: A new model for rheumatoid arthritis generated by engraftment of rheumatoid synovial tissue and normal human cartilage into SCID mice. Arthritis Rheum 37:1664–1671, 1994.
33. Goldstein RA, Bowen DL, Faucy AS: Adrenal corticosteroids. In Gallin JI, Goldstein IM, Snyderman R (eds): Inflammation: Basic Principles and Clinical Correlates, 2nd edition. Raven Press, New York, 1992, pp 1061–1081.
34. Goto M, Zvaifler NJ: Characterization of the killer cell generated in the autologous mixed leukocyte reaction. J Exp Med 157:1309–1323, 1983.
35. Guerne PA, Zuraw BL, Vaughn JH, et al: Synovium as a source of interleukin 6 in vitro. Contribution to local and systemic manifestations of arthritis. J Clin Invest 83:585–592, 1989.
36. Hasler F, Bluestein HG, Zvaifler NJ, et al: Analysis of the defects responsible for the impaired regulation of Epstein-Barr virus-induced B cell proliferation by rheumatoid arthritis lymphocytes. I. Diminished gamma interferon production in response to autologous stimulation. J Exp Med 157:173–188, 1983.
37. Helfgott SM, Dynesius-Trentham R, Brahn E, et al: An arthritogenic lymphokine in the rat. J Exp Med 162:1531–1545, 1985.
38. Hirano T, Matsuda T, Turner M, et al: Excessive production of interleukin 6/B cell stimulatory factor-2 in rheumatoid arthritis. Eur J Immunol 18:1797–1801, 1988.
39. Holmdahl R, Klareskog L, Andersson M, et al: High antibody response to autologous type II collagen is restricted to H-2q. Immunogenetics 24:84–89, 1986.
40. Holoshitz J, Klajman A, Drucker I, et al: T lymphocytes of rheumatoid arthritis patients show augmented reactivity to a fraction of mycobacteria cross-reactive with cartilage. Lancet 2:305–309, 1986.
41. Holoshitz J, Matitiau A, Cohen IR: Arthritis induced in rats by cloned T lymphocytes responsive to mycobacteria but not to collagen type II. J Clin Invest 73:211–215, 1984.
42. Janossy G, Panayi G, Duke O, et al: Rheumatoid arthritis: a disease of T-lymphocyte/macrophage immunoregulation. Lancet 2:839–842, 1981.
43. Kaplan RA, Curd JG, Deheer DH, et al: Metabolism of C4 and factor B in rheumatoid arthritis. Relation to rheumatoid factor. Arthritis Rheum 23:911–920, 1980.
44. Kaushansky K, Lin N, Adamson JW: Interleukin 1 stimulates fibroblasts to synthesize granulocyte-macrophage and granulocyte colony-stimulating factors. Mechanism for the hematopoietic response to inflammation. J Clin Invest 81:92–97, 1988.
45. Kishimoto TK, Anderson DC: The role of integrins in inflammation. In Gallin JI, Goldstein IM, Snyderman R (eds): Inflammation: Basic Principles and Clinical Correlates, 2nd edition. Raven Press, New York, 1992.
46. Klareskog L, Forsum U, Wigren A, et al: Relationship between HLA-DR-expressing cells and T lymphocytes of different subsets in rheumatoid synovial tissue. Scand J Immunol 15:501–507, 1981.
47. Konttinen YT, Reitamo S, Ranki A, et al: Characterization of the immunocompetent cells of rheumatoid synovium from tissue sections and eluates. Arthritis Rheum 24:71–79, 1981.
48. Kopp E, Ghosh S: Inhibition of NF-kappa B by sodium salicylate and aspirin. Science 265:956–959, 1994.
49. Krause A, Protz H, Goebel KM: Correlation between synovial neopterin and inflammatory activity in rheumatoid arthritis. Ann Rheum Dis 48:636–640, 1989.
50. Kremer JM, Phelps CT: Long-term prospective study of the use of methotrexate in the treatment of rheumatoid arthritis. Update after a mean of 90 months. Arthritis Rheum 35:138–145, 1992.
51. Kunkel HG, Franklin EC, Muller-Eberhard HJ: Studies on the isolation and characterization of the "rheumatoid factor." J Clin Invest 38:424–434, 1959.
52. Laffon A, Sanchez-Madrid F, Ortiz de Landazuri M, et al: Very late activation antigen on synovial fluid T cells from patients with rheumatoid arthritis and other rheumatic diseases. Arthritis Rheum 32:386–392, 1989.
53. Lamb JR, Bal V, Mendez-Samperio P, et al: Stress proteins may provide a link between the immune response to infection and autoimmunity. Int Immunol 1:191–196, 1989.
54. Lenjassen B, Strauss AF, Steere AC, et al: The T helper cell response in lyme arthritis—differential recognition: *Borrelia burgdorferi* outer surface protein A in patients with treatment-resistant or treatment-responsive lyme arthritis. J Exp Med 180:2069–2078, 1994.
55. Lindblad S, Klareskog L, Hedfors E, et al: Phenotypic characterization of synovial tissue cells in situ in different types of synovitis. Arthritis Rheum 26:1321–1332, 1983.
56. Lotz M, Tsoukas CD, Robinson CA, et al: Basis for defective responses of rheumatoid arthritis synovial fluid lymphocytes to anti-CD3 (T3) antibodies. J Clin Invest 78:713–721, 1986.
57. Malone DG, Wahl SM, Tsokos M, et al: Immune function in severe, active rheumatoid arthritis. A relationship between peripheral blood mononuclear cell proliferation to soluble antigens and synovial tissue immunohistologic characteristics. J Clin Invest 74:1173–1185, 1984.
58. Miossec P, Dinarello CA, Ziff M: Interleukin-1-lymphocyte chemotactic activity in rheumatoid arthritis synovial fluids. Arthritis Rheum 29:461–470, 1986.
59. Miossec P, Naviliat M, Dupuy AA, et al: Low levels of interleukin-4 and high levels of transforming growth factor beta in rheumatoid synovitis. Arthritis Rheum 33:1180–1187, 1990.
60. Mitchell DM, Spitz PW, Young DY, et al: Survival, prognosis, and causes of death in rheumatoid arthritis. Arthritis Rheum 29:706–714, 1986.
61. Morales-Ducret J, Wayner E, Elices MJ, et al: Alpha 4/beta 1 integrin (VLA-4) ligands in arthritis. Vascular cell adhesion molecule-1 expression in synovium and on fibroblast-like synoviocytes. J Immunol 149:1424–1431, 1992.
62. Morrissey PJ, Bressler L, Park LS, et al: Granulocyte-macrophage colony-stimulating factor augments the primary antibody response by enhancing the function of antigen-presenting cells. J Immunol 139:1113–1119, 1987.
63. Munthe E, Natvig JB: Immunoglobulin classes, subclasses and complexes of IgG rheumatoid factor in rheumatoid plasma cells. Clin Exp Immunol 12:55–70, 1972.
64. Nouri AME, Panayi GS, Goodman SM: Cytokines in the chronic inflammation of rheumatic disease. I. The presence of interleukin-1 in synovial fluids. Clin Exp Immunol 55:295–302, 1984.
65. O'Dell J, Haire C, Erikson N, et al: Triple DMARD therapy for rheumatoid arthritis: efficacy. Arthritis Rheum 37(9):S295. Abstract.
66. Panayi GS, Lanchbury JS, Kingsley GH: The importance of the T cell in initiating and maintaining the chronic synovitis of rheumatoid arthritis. Arthritis Rheum 35:729–735, 1992.
67. Paulus HE: The use of combinations of disease-modifying antirheumatic agents in rheumatoid arthritis. Arthritis Rheum 33:113–120, 1990.
68. Pearson CM: Experimental models in rheumatoid arthritis. Arthritis Rheum 7:80–86, 1964.
69. Petersen J, Heilmann C, Bjerrum OJ, et al: IgG rheumatoid factor-secreting lymphocytes in rheumatoid arthritis: evaluation of a haemolytic plaque-forming cell technique. Scand J Immunol 17:471–478, 1983.
70. Pike MC: Antiinflammatory effects of dietary lipid modification. J Rheumatol 16:718–720, 1989.
71. Poole R: Immunochemical markers of joint inflammation, skeletal damage and repair. Where are we now? Ann Rheum Dis 53:3–5, 1994.
72. Pope RM, Teller DC, Mannik M: The molecular basis of self-association of antibodies to IgG (rheumatoid factors) in rheumatoid arthritis. Proc Natl Acad Sci U S A 71:517–521, 1974.
73. Rose HM, Ragan C, Pearce E, Lipman MO: Differential agglutination of normal and sensitized sheep erythrocytes by sera of patients with rheumatoid arthritis. Proc Soc Exp Biol Med 68:1–6, 1948.
74. Rothschild BM, Turner KR, DeLuca MA: Symmetrical erosive peripheral polyarthritis in the Late Archaic Period of Alabama. Science 241:1498–1501, 1988.
75. Roudier J, Petersen J, Rhodes GH, et al: Susceptibility to rheumatoid arthritis maps to a T-cell epitope shared by the HLA-Dw4 DR beta-1 chain and the Epstein-Barr virus glycoprotein gp110. Proc Natl Acad Sci U S A 86:5104–5108, 1989.
76. Salmon M: The immunogenetic component of susceptibility to rheumatoid arthritis. Curr Opin Rheumatol 4:342–347, 1992.

77. Sargent CA, Dunham I, Trowsdale J, et al: Human major histocompatibility complex contains genes for the major heat shock protein HSP70. Proc Natl Acad Sci U S A 86:1968–1972, 1989.
78. Saxne T, Palladino J, Heidegard D, et al: Detection of tumor necrosis factor in rheumatoid arthritis synovial fluid and serum. Arthritis Rheum 31:1041–1045, 1988.
79. Scott DL, Spector TD: Value of ESR in assessment of RA. Lancet 2:1531–1532, 1989.
80. Shand N, Richardson B: Sandimmun (cyclosporin A): mode of action and clinical results in rheumatoid arthritis. Scand J Rheumatol Suppl 76:265–278, 1988.
81. Sharp JT: Radiologic assessment as an outcome measure in rheumatoid arthritis. Arthritis Rheum 32:221–229, 1989.
82. Short CL: The antiquity of rheumatoid arthritis. Arthritis Rheum 17:193–205, 1974.
83. Silman AJ: Epidemiology of rheumatoid arthritis. APMIS 102:721–728, 1994.
84. Silman AJ, MacGregor AJ, Thomson W, et al: Twin concordance rates for rheumatoid arthritis: results from a nationwide study. Br J Rheumatol 32:903–907, 1993.
85. Slaughter L, Carson DA, Jensen FC, et al: In vitro effects of Epstein-Barr virus on peripheral blood mononuclear cells from patients with rheumatoid arthritis and normal subjects. J Exp Med 148:1429–1434, 1978.
86. Spector TD, Hochberg MC: The protective effect of the oral contraceptive pill on rheumatoid arthritis: an overview of the analytic epidemiological studies using meta-analysis. J Clin Epidemiol 43:1221–1230, 1990.
87. Stamenkovic I, Stegagno M, Krane SM, et al: T lymphocytes in synovia of patients with rheumatoid arthritis. Springer Semin Immunopathol 10:169–180, 1988.
88. Sternberg EM, Hill JM, Chrousos GP, et al: Inflammatory mediator-induced hypothalamic-pituitary-adrenal axis activation is defective in streptococcal cell wall arthritis-susceptible Lewis rats. Proc Natl Acad Sci U S A 86:2374–2378, 1989.
89. Stuart JM, Dixon FJ: Serum transfer of collagen-induced arthritis in mice. J Exp Med 158:378–392, 1983.
90. Suzuki R, Suzuki S, Takahashi T, et al: Production of a cytokine with interleukin 3–like properties and cytokine-dependent proliferation in human autologous mixed lymphocyte reaction. J Exp Med 164:1682–1699, 1986.
91. Symmons DP, Barrett EM, Bankhead CR, et al: The incidence of rheumatoid arthritis in the United Kingdom: results from the Norfolk Arthritis Register. Br J Rheumatol 33:735–739, 1994.
92. Tarkowski A, Klareskog L, Carlsten H, et al: Secretion of antibodies to types I and II collagen by synovial tissue cells in patients with rheumatoid arthritis. Arthritis Rheum 32:1087–1092, 1989.
93. van der Heijde DM, van Leeuwen MA, van Riel PL, et al: Biannual radiographic assessments of hands and feet in a three-year prospective followup of patients with early rheumatoid arthritis. Arthritis Rheum 35:26–34, 1992.
94. van Eden W, Holoshitz J, Nevo Z, et al: Arthritis induced by a T-lymphocyte clone that responds to *Mycobacterium tuberculosis* and to cartilage proteoglycans. Proc Natl Acad Sci U S A 82:5117–5120, 1985.
95. Waaler E: On occurrence of factor in human serum activating specific agglutination of sheep blood corpuscles. Acta Pathol Microbiol Immunol Scand 17:172–188, 1940.
96. Ward PA, Zvaifler NJ: Complement-derived leukotactic factors in inflammatory synovial fluids of humans. J Clin Invest 50:606–616, 1971.
97. Weinblatt ME, Weissman BN, Holdsworth DE, et al: Long-term prospective study of methotrexate in the treatment of rheumatoid arthritis. 84-month update. Arthritis Rheum 35:129–137, 1992.
98. Weisman MH: Prognosis in rheumatoid arthritis. Curr Opin Rheumatol 2:458–462, 1990.
99. Weyand CM, Goronzy JJ: HLA-DRB1 alleles as severity markers in RA. Bull Rheum Dis 43:5–8, 1994.
100. Williams RO, Mason LJ, Feldmann M, et al: Synergy between anti-CD4 and anti-tumor necrosis factor in the amelioration of established collagen-induced arthritis. Proc Natl Acad Sci U S A 91:2762–2766, 1994.
101. Willkens RF, Nepom GT, Marks CR, et al: Association of HLA-Dw16 with rheumatoid arthritis in Yakima Indians. Further evidence for the "shared epitope" hypothesis. Arthritis Rheum 34:43–47, 1991.
102. Wood NC, Symons JA, Duff GW: Serum interleukin-2-receptor in rheumatoid arthritis: a prognostic indicator of disease activity? J Autoimmun 1:353–361, 1988.
103. Wooley PH, Luthra HS, Stuart JM, et al: Type II collagen-induced arthritis in mice. I. Major histocompatibility complex (I region) linkage and antibody correlates. J Exp Med 154:688–700, 1981.
104. Wordsworth BP, Bell JI: The immunogenetics of rheumatoid arthritis. Springer Semin Immunopathol 14:59–78, 1992.
105. Xu WD, Firestein GS, Taetle R, et al: Cytokines in chronic inflammatory arthritis. II. Granulocyte-macrophage colony-stimulating factor in rheumatoid synovial effusions. J Clin Invest 83:876–882, 1989.
106. Young CL, Adamson TC, Vaughan JH, et al: Immunohistologic characterization of synovial membrane lymphocytes in rheumatoid arthritis. Arthritis Rheum 27:32–39, 1984.
107. Zvaifler NJ: The immunopathology of joint inflammation in rheumatoid arthritis. Adv Immunol 16:265–336, 1973.
108. Zvaifler NJ: Fractionated total lymphoid irradiation: a promising new treatment for rheumatoid arthritis? Yes, no, maybe. Arthritis Rheum 30:109–114, 1987.
109. Zvaifler NJ: Rheumatoid arthritis: editorial overview. Curr Opin Rheumatol 2:421–422, 1990.
110. Zvaifler NJ: Synovial fluid analysis. In Stein JH (ed): Internal Medicine, 4th edition. Mosby–Year Book, St. Louis, 1994, pp 2357–2360.
111. Zvaifler NJ: Rheumatoid arthritis. In Stein JH (ed): Internal Medicine, 4th edition. Mosby–Year Book, St. Louis, 1994, pp 2407–2418.
112. Zvaifler NJ: Macrophages and the synovial lining. Scand J Rheumatol 24(S101):67–75, 1995.
113. Zvaifler NJ, Steinman RM, Kaplan G, et al: Identification of immunostimulatory dendritic cells in the synovial effusions of patients with rheumatoid arthritis. J Clin Invest 76:789–800, 1985.

50 Systemic Lupus Erythematosus

ALFRED D. STEINBERG

Idiopathic systemic lupus erythematosus (SLE) is an immune-mediated disorder characterized by the production of a variety of autoantibodies and disease manifestations in multiple organ systems.[136] Patients produce antibodies that react with nuclear, cytoplasmic, and cell-membrane antigens. Some of those antibodies contribute to disease. Individual patients with lupus may have any or all of the following: fatigue, fever, rash, joint pains, kidney disease, central nervous system disease, pneumonitis, cardiac disease, and hematologic problems. Although the etiology of SLE remains to be fully elucidated, this disorder appears to represent a syndrome in which immune dysregulation leads to the production of pathogenic autoantibodies. The pathway to disease may vary among patients. Environmental agents, especially certain drugs, can induce a lupus-like disorder. However, drug-induced lupus is generally distinguished from idiopathic SLE.[129]

Lupus is one of several classic diseases that exhibit a plethora of signs and symptoms able to mimic aspects of many other disorders. This syndrome is becoming better understood through advances in both immunology and molecular genetics. Studies of animals that develop lupus also have shed light on the pathogenesis. Advances in therapeutics have rendered SLE more treatable than it was in the past.

DIAGNOSIS

Patients with SLE often differ from one another in the clinical manifestations of their disease. The organ systems affected may vary among patients. There is also a marked variability in the severity of a clinical manifestation, ranging from very mild signs and symptoms to life-threatening disease. No single clinical finding or laboratory test alone can definitively determine the diagnosis of SLE, nor can a single observation rule it out. Typically, the diagnosis depends on a constellation of characteristic clinical and laboratory findings. A young woman who presents with pleurisy, butterfly rash, arthritis, glomerulonephritis, and high titers of antibodies that react with native DNA may be readily recognized to have SLE. However, the diagnosis is more difficult to make in an older individual who presents with a left hemiparesis without other features of SLE.

SLE researchers tend to include in clinical or epidemiologic studies patients who clearly have the disorder. This tendency has been codified in a set of criteria for the diagnosis of SLE for use in scholarly work (Table 50–1).[147] These criteria may also be used by practicing physicians to facilitate establishing a diagnosis but were not designed to provide definitive dictates for clinical practice. Although many patients diagnosed with SLE in clinical practice fulfill these criteria, some do not. For example, a young woman with SLE may have glomerulonephritis and high titers of anti-DNA antibodies without fulfilling the criteria. Another patient may have a rash, arthritis, pleurisy, and anti-nuclear antibodies and meet the criteria for SLE yet be suffering from leprosy rather than SLE. Therefore, the criteria should be seen as a statistical tool for use in scholarly work rather than as a definitive diagnostic test.

It is also interesting that one SLE patient may have a malar rash, discoid rash, photosensitivity, nasopharyngeal ulcers, arthritis, schizophrenia, and antiphospholipid antibodies and have no disease features overlapping with a second SLE patient manifesting pleuropericarditis, glomerulonephritis, leukopenia, thrombocytopenia, anemia, and anti-DNA antibodies. Despite having no signs, symptoms, or laboratory findings in common, both patients can be readily diagnosed as having SLE.

ETIOLOGY

It appears that both genetic and environmental factors may contribute to the development of SLE (Fig. 50–1). Their relative importance may vary greatly among individuals, however, and very few of the factors are defined.[136] It is believed that a consequence of genetic predisposition is impaired immune regulation, with increased humoral immune reactivity and impaired cell-mediated immunity.[66, 136, 137] Additional genes may mediate other steps of disease, for instance, by leading to increased production of specific autoantibodies, impaired clearance of immune complexes, or increased inflammatory responses to immune deposition.

Ultraviolet (UV) light can cause lupus flares and may trigger the initial disease expression. UV light impairs antigen handling by macrophages; interferes with the activation of suppressor T cells; allows immune complexes to persist, thereby increasing the burden of such complexes on target

TABLE 50–1
AMERICAN COLLEGE OF RHEUMATOLOGY CRITERIA FOR SLE[147]

Patients who satisfy 4 of the following 11 criteria either serially or simultaneously (during any period of observation) are deemed to have SLE for the purpose of inclusion in clinical reports.*

Criterion	Definition
1. Malar rash (60%)	Fixed erythema over the malar eminences (flat or raised), which tends to spare the nasolabial folds
2. Discoid rash (20%)	Erythematous raised patches with adherent keratotic scaling and follicular plugging; atrophic scarring (with hyperpigmentation or hypopigmentation) may be observed in older lesions
3. Photosensitivity (50%)	Skin rash resulting from an unusual reaction to sunlight (by patient history or observation by a health professional)
4. Mucosal ulcers (30%)	Oral or nasopharyngeal ulcers, usually painless, observed by a physician
5. Arthritis (90%)	Nonerosive arthritis involving two or more peripheral joints (tenderness, swelling, or effusion)
6. Serositis (40%)	Pleuritis (a convincing history of pleuritic pain, a rub heard by a health professional, or evidence of a pleural effusion) or pericarditis (documented by electrocardiogram, rub, or evidence of pericardial effusion)
7. Renal disorder (50%)	Persistent proteinuria (>0.5 G/d or 3+) or cellular casts (RBC, hemoglobin, granular, tubular, or mixed)
8. Neurologic disorder (45%)	Seizures or psychosis (must be in the absence of offending drugs or known metabolic abnormalities)
9. Hematologic disorder (50%)	Hemolytic anemia with reticulocytosis, leukopenia (<4,000/mm^3 on two or more occasions), lymphopenia (<1,500/mm^3 on two or more occasions), or thrombocytopenia (<100,000/mm^3 in the absence of offending drugs)
10. Immunologic disorder (95%)	Positive LE cell test, antibodies to native DNA (excessive amounts) or to the Sm antigen, or antibodies to phospholipids (e.g., cardiolipin) able to cause a false-positive serologic test for syphilis and confirmed by specific serologic testing
11. Antinuclear antibody (90%)	Excessive ANA titer in the absence of drugs known to induce ANA

*There are many additional clinical and laboratory signs in patients with SLE, including fatigue, alopecia, weight loss, anorexia, and findings that result from the involvement in specific organ systems. Although these may not be included in the criteria for diagnosis listed here, they are likely to be of concern to the patients affected.

organs; and triggers keratinocytes to secrete a variety of interleukins (IL), including IL-1, IL-3, and IL-6, granulocyte-macrophage colony-stimulating factor (GM-CSF), and tumor necrosis factor-α (TNF-α).[123] IL-1 in turn triggers lymphocytes to produce a variety of other cytokines, some of which stimulate unwanted immune responses. Sulfa drugs and tetracyclines may concentrate the effects of UV light in the skin to increase photosensitivity and predispose to lupus flares. The same is true of foods containing psoralens, such as celery, figs, parsley, and parsnips. Alfalfa (sprouts and

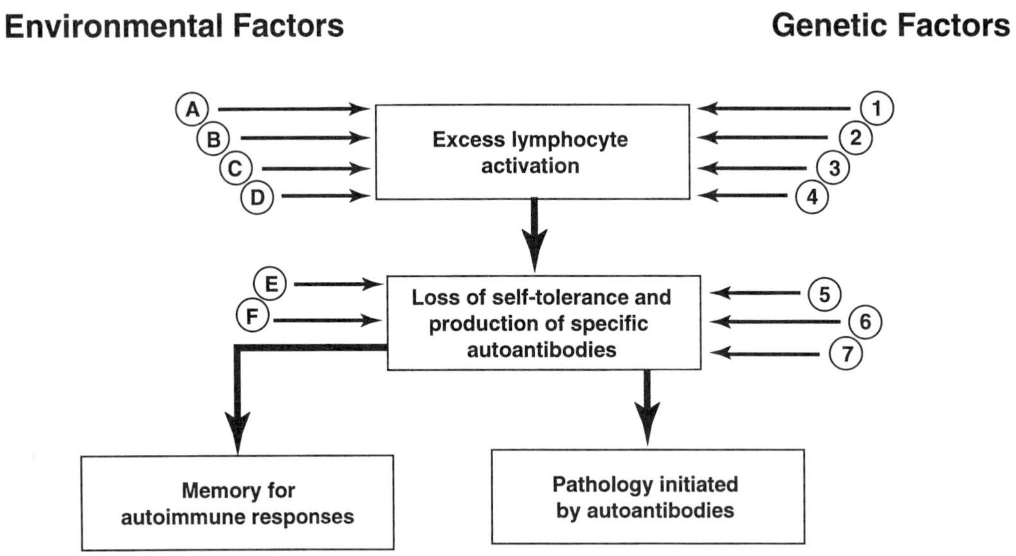

FIGURE 50–1. Diagram indicating the contribution of both genetic and environmental factors to the pathogenesis of the immune dysfunction that underlies SLE. Different genes (e.g., 1, 2, 3, 4) appear to stimulate lymphocyte activation, either directly or indirectly. Environmental factors (e.g., A, B, C, D) also may trigger such activation. It is likely that only some of these genetic and/or environmental factors are operative in a given individual. Lymphocyte activation, along with additional environmental factors (E, F) or genetic factors (5, 6, 7), induces a loss of self-tolerance and the development of autoantibodies. Ultimately, pathogenic autoantibodies and disease ensue. It must be stressed that we have only sketchy information regarding the possible genes and environmental factors indicated in this diagram. Exactly how the different genes work or the interactions of environmental factors with those genes remain largely unknown. There also may be genes that inhibit the expression of disease. The multigenic nature of lupus has been suggested by studies of murine lupus.[89, 111] A gene dosage effect of predisposing genes seen in murine lupus may also apply to humans.[113]

seeds) and other legumes that contain L-canavanine may trigger disease, as may mushrooms, containing hydrazines, and coloring agents containing tartrazine. Some of the genetic and environmental factors that are considered likely candidates for induction of SLE are listed in Table 50–2.

An infectious etiology for SLE has long been sought. Certain viral, bacterial, and parasitic diseases have been followed by features of lupus. For example, trypanosomiasis or mycobacterial infections may induce anti-DNA or even lupus-like signs and symptoms. Epstein-Barr virus infection may be followed by an autoimmune disease. In addition, lupus flares may be observed after infection. However, there has been no well-documented infectious cause of most instances of SLE, and an infectious etiology for SLE has remained elusive. If many different organisms can induce SLE in different subsets of people, however, current epidemiologic techniques would not have the power to uncover such infectious causes. Further, if multiple common organisms were able to induce SLE, it might be difficult in principle to make the connection, especially if genetic factors were also critical to disease expression. Thus the long sought lupus virus has been elusive and is likely to remain so.

PATHOGENESIS

Lupus is mediated by autoantibodies. Patients with SLE produce a great variety of autoantibodies (Table 50–3). Some of these bind to formed elements in the blood and participate in their elimination. Other autoantibodies contribute to vas-

TABLE 50–2
A FEW OF THE MANY FACTORS THAT MAY CONTRIBUTE TO SLE*

Genetic

HLA, including C4 null

Y chromosome

Various cytokines and their receptors—relative excess of Th2-type and relatively reduced Th1-type cytokine responses to immune stimuli, excess IL-6, excess IL-10, and impaired IFN-γ responsiveness

Sex hormone production, metabolism, and receptors—increased estrogenicity and reduced androgenicity

Endogenous retroviral sequences

Abnormal or impaired DNA repair mechanisms

Factors leading to impaired immune tolerance mechanisms—impaired apoptosis (as found in *lpr/lpr* and *gld/gld* mice) and others

Environmental

UV light

Foods—UV light enhancers (figs, celery, parsley, parsnips), L-canavanine containing (alfalfa sprouts and seeds, other legumes), and hydrazine containing (mushrooms and food dyes, e.g. tartrazine)

Hormones

Infections—parasitic (trypanosomes, other), bacterial (mycobacteria, any infection releasing bacterial DNA), bacterial products (superantigens), viral (EBV, other), and viral products (tat)

Toxins—aromatic amines, vinyl chloride, and silica, asbestos

Stress—Emotional and physical

Additional factors that impair immune tolerance

*This list is in flux to keep up with new discoveries and is neither complete nor definitive.

TABLE 50–3
PARTIAL LIST OF AUTOANTIBODIES FOUND IN THE SERA OF PATIENTS WITH SLE (ANTIGENS TO WHICH THE AUTOANTIBODIES REACT)

Specificity	Comment
Nuclear	Present in the great majority of patients with SLE
Native DNA	Historically, the hallmark of SLE
Denatured (single-stranded DNA)	Less specific for lupus than antinative DNA
DNA-histone complex	High specificity for SLE
Nucleosome	High specificity for SLE
Chromatin	High specificity for SLE
Histones H1, H3-4	Common in SLE
Histones H2A-H2B	More common in drug-induced lupus
Nuclear ribonucleoproteins (SnRPs)	Found in SLE, but highest amounts in mixed connective tissue disease (an overlap syndrome)
SS-B (La, Ha)	Sjögren's syndrome, SLE
SS-A (Ro)	Sjögren's syndrome, SLE
Ku	SLE
Proliferating cell nuclear antigen	SLE
DNA-RNA hybrids, double-stranded RNA	SLE
DNA : DNA binding proteins	SLE
Nucleolar antigens	Scleroderma, Sjögren's syndrome, SLE
RANA	Epstein-Barr virus, rheumatoid arthritis
Ribosomal RNA	SLE
t-RNA	SLE
Mitochondria	Biliary cirrhosis, SLE
Microsomal antigens	Chronic active hepatitis, malignancies
Lysosomes	SLE
Erythrocytes	May occur without major hemolysis in SLE
White cells	T cells, B cells, granulocytes in SLE
Platelets	Common in SLE without thrombocytopenia
Lipomodulin	SLE, rheumatoid arthritis
MHC class II	Interferes with immune function
Receptors	Antibodies to many different kinds of receptors are found in some SLE patients; some of these antibodies block the receptor, and others may stimulate (e.g., receptor for IL-2, insulin, leuteinizing hormone, Na/K pump)
Immunoglobulins	Rheumatoid arthritis, Sjögren's syndrome, SLE
Mitotic spindle	SLE, other rheumatic diseases
Intracellular supporting proteins	SLE, other rheumatic diseases
Clotting factors	SLE, others
Phospholipids bound to associated proteins	Antiphospholipid syndrome +/− SLE
Thyroid antigens	Thyroid diseases, Sjögren's syndrome, SLE

culitis or kidney pathology. Still others do not appear to cause disease signs or symptoms. Ordinarily, the body does not produce large amounts of pathogenic autoantibodies and is therefore said to be tolerant of its own antigens. Such immunologic tolerance must be breeched in lupus to permit autoantibody production. However, there may be many different ways by which the immune system can become so dysfunctional as to produce impaired immune tolerance, any of which may be responsible for the development of SLE. Different defects may underlie disease in different individuals, as has been observed in different strains of mice that develop lupus.

A further complication arises because SLE may be a multifactorial disorder. Even in one patient, several factors together may be responsible for the induction and perpetuation of disease. Such factors may be genetic or environmental, with more than one of each operative in a given patient. Some of the factors that appear to play a role in disease induction are discussed here.

B-CELL ACTIVATION IN SLE

The entire B-cell maturation pathway in SLE is expanded and activated, from the development of B cells in the bone marrow through the generation of mature B cells and their expansion and differentiation into mature antibody-forming cells.[136] In both murine and human SLE, there are increased numbers of B cells that produce antibodies reactive with self-antigens and foreign antigens, suggesting that many patients manifest multiclonal B-cell stimulation.[8, 15, 64–66] It is possible that an initial abnormality, which favors B-cell activation, is the first step in a multistep process that ultimately leads to the production of large amounts of IgG autoantibodies. Later steps in the process would include antigen-driven T-cell–dependent events.

The early multiclonal B-cell stimulation provides a positive feedback for the ultimate development of pathogenic autoantibodies. B cells that have their receptor for antigen engaged are resistant to programmed cell death.[118] Activated B cells are able to present antigen to T cells so as to activate them.[40] Thus stimulated B cells would be able to pick up antigen, avoid apoptosis, stimulate T cells, and divide. Their offspring would be further stimulated by the activated T cells and would also be protected from apoptosis as their antigen receptors became occupied. This fertile milieu of activated B cells may serve as a breeding ground for B cells in which a few mutate into those able to produce autoantibodies, many of which may initially be of low affinity and high cross-reactivity. Eventually, the mutated B cells would be selected to give rise to higher affinity, pathogenic IgG autoantibodies. Even the lupus IgG anti-DNA autoantibodies tend to cross-react with other determinants,[63, 66] which is a property that may be important in disease perpetuation.

AUTOANTIBODY PRODUCTION

Most pathogenic autoantibodies are IgG antibodies of high affinity, induced by an interaction between an antigen, a helper T cell, and a B cell.[26, 47, 48, 57, 66, 76, 109, 126, 136–138] Some of these antibodies react with nuclear antigens, including DNA. Indeed, antibodies reactive with native DNA have been the hallmark of lupus, although it is now recognized that these antibodies may be a subset of antibodies reactive with DNA-histone complexes, as found in chromatin, or nucleosomes.

Polymeric antigens that are mitogenic (able to induce replication of lymphocytes) are often unusually immunogenic because they can stimulate lymphocytes through the receptor for antigen and also provide a strong stimulus to cell division. The mitogenicity of an antigen may convert the antigenic signaling from tolerance to immunity. This is important for consideration of nucleic acids as antigens, because for many years it was believed that nucleic acids were not immunogenic. Subsequently, it was found that both mitogenic RNA and mitogenic DNA are able to stimulate the immune system.[41, 85, 104, 134, 135]

Low molecular weight DNA in DNA–anti-DNA complexes of lupus patients is enriched in cytosine-guanine (CG) content.[120] The CG content also determines the mitogenic properties of bacterial DNA.[86] The cytosine in CpG doublets of bacterial DNA is less often methylated than in CpG doublets in mammalian DNA, thereby increasing the mitogenicity of bacterial DNA. When oligomers of DNA contain unmethylated C in CpG, they are also more antigenic than when the C is methylated.[41, 69, 86] Therefore, bacterial DNA, characterized by unmethylated CpG motifs, might be immunogenic in lupus patients. This is also consistent with the observation that lupus flares may follow bacterial infections. Immunogenic human DNA might also be generated in patients if there is reduced methylation of the cytosines in an individual's CpGs.

Endogenous nucleosomes may provide another source of mitogenic DNA. The potential nucleosome specificity of many lupus antinuclear antibodies has long been suspected and was demonstrated.[4, 17, 56, 91, 110] Moreover, complexes of DNA with histones and DNA with DNA-binding proteins have been shown to uniquely engage the immune system.[17, 28] If nucleosomes are both mitogenic and immunogenic, they might trigger an immune response in a lupus-prone individual.

TOLERANCE AND LUPUS

Immunologic tolerance eliminates or temporarily inactivates lymphocytes capable of pathologic autoimmune responses. Such tolerance appears to be maintained through more than one mechanism. A defect in any of these might contribute to a loss of self-tolerance.[66, 137] For the T-cell compartment, intrathymic deletion, peripheral deletion, and peripheral tolerization without deletion all play a role in self-tolerance. B cells similarly may be tolerized or deleted early in development or inactivated/deleted later.[34, 44, 49, 96, 102] A defect in any one of these tolerance mechanisms may predispose to lupus. Indeed, despite markedly disparate genetics and disease expression, the various mouse strains that spontaneously develop lupus also manifest defects in experimental tolerance.[73–75, 90] Such abnormalities could be genetically determined, acquired, or due to some combination of genetic and environmental factors (see Fig. 50–1).

Resting B cells that bind antigen tolerize T cells that they contact. In contrast, activated B cells stimulate the T cells to which they present antigen.[40] Since B-cell activation is markedly increased in lupus, especially during flares, the immune system of such patients is shifted from tolerance to immunization. Moreover, activated B cells stimulate memory T cells, which causes a positive feedback loop, initially slow and gradually becoming a crescendo.[8, 10, 15, 64–66] Thus excess B-cell activation plus self-antigen presentation by the activated B cells may break tolerance and lead to, or perpetuate, autoimmunity (Fig. 50–2).

In lupus-prone New Zealand mice, T cells, perhaps through their excess Th2 cytokine production, actively interfere with tolerance.[74, 76, 90] These T cells are further stimulated by antigen-presenting activated B cells, causing a positive feedback loop in which the T cells produce more Th2 cytokines. From both animal and human studies, it appears that the loss of tolerance in lupus could result directly from the generalized immune activation that involves both T and B cells.[8, 15, 57, 62, 64–66, 136] In such a formulation, the B cells activate the T cells, which in turn help the B cells to produce autoantibodies.

APOPTOSIS AND LUPUS

Apoptosis (programmed cell death) is an energy-dependent process characterized by cell shrinkage; condensation

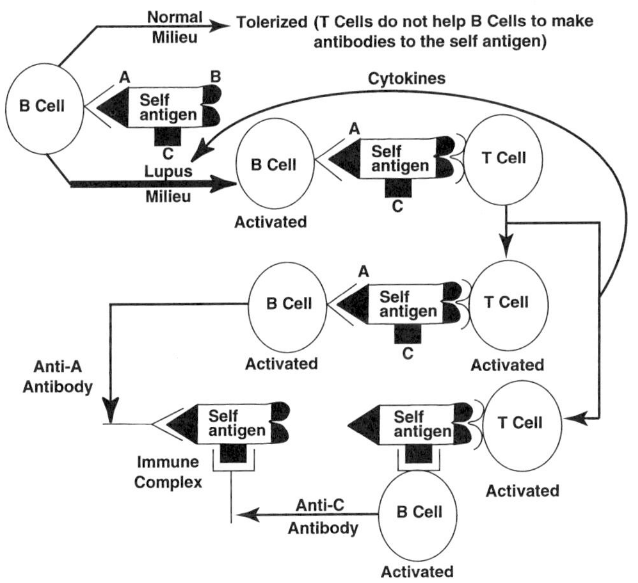

FIGURE 50–2. How the lupus milieu favors impaired immune tolerance and autoantibody production. The B cells in a person encounter a self-antigen with three epitopes (A, B, C). In a normal microenvironment, the B-cell receptor for antigen might bind the antigen at epitope A (a B-cell epitope) but would be unable to stimulate a T cell, and the individual would remain tolerant to the antigen and fail to mount an antibody response. In contrast, some of the B cells in a lupus milieu would be activated. An activated B cell would bind the self-antigen at epitope A and present that antigen to a T cell. The T cell would recognize epitope B (a T-cell epitope) and become activated. T cells so activated then would help a B cell recognizing epitope A to make anti-A antibodies and would help a B cell recognizing epitope C to make anti-C antibodies. These antibodies may bind to the self-antigen so as to form an immune complex, as shown in the lower left of the diagram. Moreover, the activated T cells produce Th2-type cytokines to perpetuate the lupus milieu so that additional autoimmune reactions may ensue.

of chromatin, which is compacted against the nuclear membrane; formation of nuclear and cytoplasmic clumps; and ingestion of the cell or cellular debris by macrophages.[98, 142, 150] It differs from necrosis, which is characterized by cellular swelling and induction of inflammation. Apoptosis occurs rapidly, so that the dying cells are usually not seen in tissue sections. Oxygen free radicals are not generated and inflammation does not occur.

Environmental factors that promote the accumulation of DNA strand breaks induce apoptosis, including ionizing radiation, oxygen free radicals, and alkylating agents, especially agents that interfere with DNA repair. In theory, defects in apoptosis could be a cause of impaired immunologic tolerance by preventing deletion of self-reactive lymphocytes. Defective apoptosis also would contribute to SLE induction by encouraging inflammation in association with nonapoptotic cell death, thereby promoting the presentation of intracellular macromolecules to the immune system, especially in particulate form.

In the peripheral immune system, the Fas:Fas ligand system appears to play an important role in apoptosis.[98, 150] Mice with mutations in Fas or the Fas ligand have defective apoptosis and develop both massive lymphadenopathy and autoantibodies characteristic of lupus.[2, 153, 155, 156, 159] In concert with these defects in Fas signaling, additional background genes may be necessary for certain specific lupus phenotypes. Although such gross defects in apoptosis have not been identified in humans, these mice illustrate how abnormalities in apoptosis can give rise to a lupus diathesis.

It is notable that the genetic defects in Fas and the Fas ligand (*lpr* and *gld* mutations) cause lupus-like disease, but the mutations are in genes that appear to have no direct connection to a self-antigen such as DNA and no connection to a subset of antigen-specific helper T cells. Rather, the mutations are in the Fas receptor for signals that trigger apoptosis and its own ligand.[2, 153, 155, 156, 159] Such a generalized defect is consistent with the generalized nature of the immune abnormalities observed in lupus. Thus the underlying mechanisms of the lupus diathesis appear to be antigen nonspecific. In a sense, autoantibody formation is a side effect of the *lpr* and *gld* mutations: the primary *lpr* and *gld* defects are in Fas:Fas ligand interactions. A secondary consequence is impaired apoptosis. This may provide an explanation for defects in tolerance and retention of self-reactive cells. A tertiary effect is autoantibody formation. If some of the autoantibodies induce disease, that would be a quaternary effect. This formulation suggests that for some instances of lupus, an antigen-nonspecific, multistep process may lead to disease (Fig. 50–3). For many individuals with lupus, the multistep process may start with antigen-nonspecific immune stimulation, followed by events that select for the production of specific autoantibodies in an antigen-specific manner.[62, 64–66, 134, 136–138]

ROLE OF CYTOKINES IN LUPUS

Cytokines are soluble factors that serve as intercellular signals for the immune system. Several cytokines induce lymphocytes to mature or proliferate.[25, 52, 95] $CD4^+$ helper T cells have been divided into those that produce Th1-type cytokines, including IL-2 and interferon-γ and Th2-type

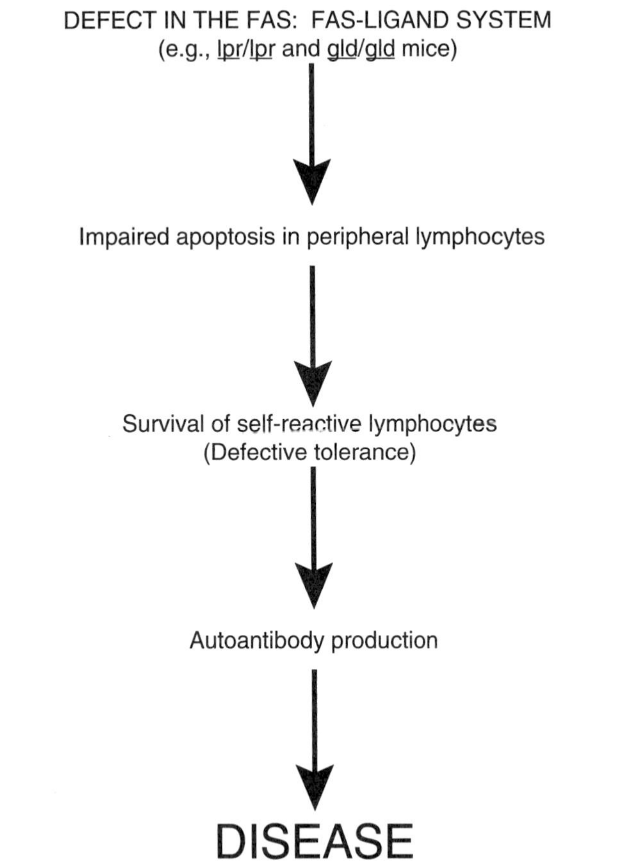

FIGURE 50–3. Genetic defects in Fas-dependent apoptosis induce murine lupus. A defect in the expression of Fas (e.g., mice homozygous for the *lpr* mutation) and a defect in the production of the ligand for Fas (e.g., mice homozygous for the *gld* mutation) have impaired Fas-dependent apoptosis in peripheral lymphocytes. This leads to survival of self-reactive lymphocytes (a manifestation of impaired self-tolerance) and autoantibody production. Pathogenic autoantibodies lead to disease; this occurs especially in the presence of additional "background genes" that predispose to autoimmunity (e.g., genes 1 to 7 in Figure 50–1).

cytokines, including IL-4, IL-6, and IL-10.[95] The Th1 cytokines tend to suppress the production of Th2-type cytokines and vice versa.[105] The balance between the mutually inhibitory cytokines affects the nature, strength, and duration of systemic immune responses.[52, 106]

One of the first and most interesting cytokine abnormalities discovered in lupus patients was the spontaneous production of what appeared to be an unusual (acid labile) interferon-α (IFN-α). This IFN-α was found to induce so-called viral-like particles (also called tubular reticular structures and lupus inclusions) in the cytoplasm of reticuloendothelial cells. The inclusions, which appear to be induced by chronic high levels of the unusual IFN-α in patients with active lupus, have been found in kidney biopsies and peripheral blood lymphocytes. These lupus inclusions are distinct from LE cells and hematoxylin bodies. They are composed of membranes and ribonucleoprotein, but not DNA. A unique 36-kD protein has been associated with the formation of the structures, which make contact with the outer nuclear membrane and the Golgi apparatus. It is possible that these structures could act as self-antigens.

It has been found that the IFN-α produced in SLE is normal but that another serum factor renders the IFN-α acid labile.[157] The quantity of this second serum factor varies with disease activity, but its nature and implications for disease pathogenesis remain uncertain. Nevertheless, patients who have received high doses of IFN-α as therapy for another disorder have occasionally been observed to develop an autoimmune disorder.

Lupus patients have additional, potentially pathogenic cytokine abnormalities. Indeed, many nonspecific constitutional symptoms of lupus patients may result from excess IL-1, IL-4, and IFN production. Moreover, the pathogenesis of the lupus immune diathesis may be favored by specific cytokine imbalances. Enumeration of cytokine-producing cells has shown that SLE patients have significantly fewer cells producing Th1-type cytokines, IFN-γ and IL-2, but significantly more cells secreting Th2-type cytokines, IL-6 and IL-10, than do normal controls.[66] Disease activity was inversely correlated with numbers of Th1-secreting cells.

These lupus cytokine data suggest that the increased ratio of Th2-type to Th1-type cytokine secreting cells may contribute to the increased B-cell activation characteristic of lupus patients and to disease perpetuation (Fig. 50–4). Such a cytokine imbalance might underlie the impaired self-tolerance discussed previously, because the Th2 cytokines stimulate B cells (see Fig. 50–2). Indeed, normal B cells will become hyperactivated and secrete autoantibodies if transferred into an autoimmune lupus environment.[65] Cytokines have been shown to interfere with tolerance.[14]

An imbalance in Th2:Th1 cytokine production could arise in one family from reduced Th1-type responses and in another family from excess Th2-type responses. An individual in a lupus-prone family not inheriting such a predisposition

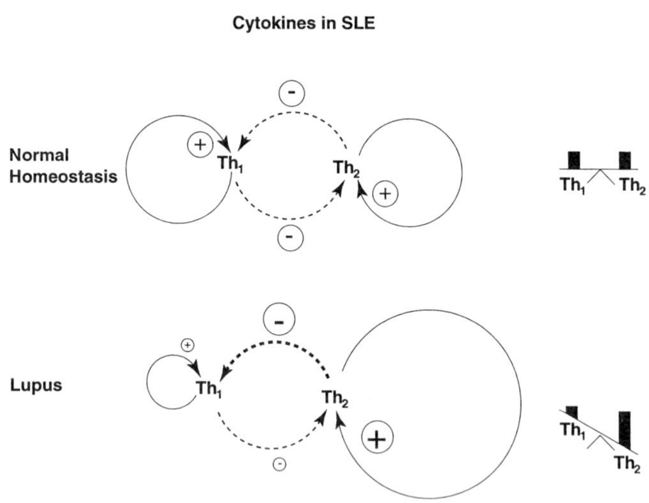

FIGURE 50–4. The Th2:Th1 cytokine imbalance in SLE. Normally, excess quantities of Th2 cytokines feed back to suppress Th1 cytokine production and vice versa. In normal physiology, corrective measures appear to operate to allow a balance in cytokine production—a steady state of adequate amounts of both Th1-type and Th2-type cytokines. Patients with SLE have an imbalance in their cytokine production such that there is a relative or absolute deficiency in Th1-type cytokines and a relative or absolute excess in Th2-type cytokines. Because of the feedback effects, and lack of a corrective force in SLE, once this imbalance becomes established, immune responses of the type shown in Figure 50–3 tend to perpetuate the cytokine imbalance as depicted here. Because of the positive feedback effects, this may become a self-perpetuating process in which the immune activation may exist until an immunosuppressive intervention occurs.

to excess Th2-type cytokine production might be spared disease induction despite other predisposing genetic defects or common environmental stimuli or might develop another autoimmune disorder, several of which are also increased in families of patients with SLE.

Lupus patients have excess IL-4 production, as well as increased numbers of IL-4 secreting cells.[31, 46, 66, 101] IL-4 appears to be the critical cytokine for positive feedback on $CD4^+$ T cells for the production of more Th2-type cytokines and for converting certain $CD8^+$ T cells into Th2-type cytokine producers (see Fig. 50–4).

IL-6 secretion may be more important for actually bringing about the SLE diathesis. Lupus patients have increased production of IL-6 and abnormalities of IL-6/IL-6 receptor interactions.[3, 77, 97, 130] These observations are especially important in light of the ability of IL-6 alone to induce a lupus-like illness. For example, IL-6 transgenic mice have increased humoral immunity and an autoimmune syndrome, and human cardiac myxomas both secrete IL-6 and induce a lupus-like autoimmune syndrome.[54, 144]

Despite relative and absolute increases in the production of Th2-type cytokines, lupus patients generally do not have marked expression of allergic phenomena. Approximately one third of patients with active lupus develop rashes with ampicillin therapy or sulfa drugs, such as Gantrisin. Otherwise, allergies have not been observed more commonly than in the general population, and most lupus patients do not have eosinophilia or excessive IgE production. It appears that excess production of IL-6 in SLE, rather than IL-4 and IL-5, may contribute to the skewing of their disorder toward lupus. Of course, those who are atopic also possess the genetic predisposition that links allergic rhinitis, asthma, and atopic dermatitis.

CLUES FROM COMPLEMENT DEFICIENCIES

An individual with a genetic deficiency in a complement (C) component may manifest a lupus-like disorder.[78, 107] This is especially true of deficiencies in C1q, C1r, C1s, and C4. The majority of individuals with these deficiencies appear to have lupus-like illnesses. More than a third of patients with C2 deficiency also manifest such a disease. This correlation between C deficiency and lupus could stem from either associated genetic factors or the C deficiencies themselves. That so many different C-deficiency states predispose to lupus-like signs and symptoms suggests that it is the C deficiency itself that is the cause. This view is supported by the successful therapy of a C2-deficient patient with C2.[141]

The strongest correlation between C deficiency and autoimmunity is found among deficiencies of the earliest components of the classical C pathway. This finding suggests that a defect in classical C function is causative. Among the many possible explanations, the especially appealing one is that failure of an early component of the C pathway to bind to immune complexes may alter the handling of those complexes to favor immunity. Indeed, under certain circumstances, immune complexes may be more immunogenic than antigen alone. The absence of early classical C components may also allow an antigen-antibody complex to become more immunogenic than would be the case if the C components bound to the complex. This may be mediated in part by abnormal clearance of complexes due to diminished deposition of C3b or C3bi. C deficiencies also may predispose to SLE simply by predisposing to certain infections that might trigger the disease.

A relative deficiency in C reactive protein has been observed in patients with active SLE. It is possible that failure to mount a good acute phase response to a variety of inflammatory stimuli might allow particles containing DNA to become immunogenic.[114]

T CELLS IN PATIENTS WITH SLE

Patients with SLE have activated T cells, some of which apparently are driven by autoantigens to divide and ultimately to stimulate self-reactive B cells to expand and produce autoantibodies.[57, 136, 137] As T cells divide, random somatic mutations occur in these cells. T cells in patients with SLE accumulate these mutations through multiple rounds of cell division.[43] The number of such T cells correlates with cumulative or past lupus disease activity, including the numbers of past disease flares, suggesting that each new disease flare is associated with T lymphocyte activation and proliferation; the longer the flare, the greater the magnitude of the flare.[27] It is thought that some of these mutant SLE T cells might represent self-reactive lymphocytes that have failed to undergo apoptosis. Indeed, a substantial fraction of these cells can help B cells to secrete autoantibodies.

A clinical finding that is strongly associated with mutant T cells is UV light–sensitive lupus skin disease.[27] Lupus disease activity is also associated with lymphocyte release of low molecular weight mitogenic DNA; such CG-enriched DNA is a potential immunogen in SLE. This release is increased by UV light.[24, 33, 120] Lupus patients also have impaired, unscheduled DNA repair after UV light exposure.[45, 115] These associations raise the possibility that patients with UV light–sensitive dermatitis may have exhibited impaired DNA repair during T-cell activation, thereby leading to higher mutation frequencies in surviving cells and to release of immunogenic, low molecular weight CG-enriched DNA.

SYNTHESIS OF PATHOGENETIC FACTORS

Many factors may induce the expression of systemic lupus, suggesting that lupus is not simply a disease but is a syndrome with multiple etiologies (see Fig. 50–1). Determining which pathogenetic factors are operative in a given patient will be an exciting challenge for the 21st century. At the moment, it appears that preclinical lupus may be characterized by excess lymphocyte activation and that the full-blown disorder exhibits the overproduction of specific pathogenic autoantibodies. The multiclonal immune activation seen in early lupus appears to compromise the host's ability to tolerize/suppress autoreactive lymphocytes, a process that is influenced by abnormal cytokine release. Once the lupus milieu is established, lymphocyte activation (rather than suppression) becomes favored and autoimmune responses ensue. The resultant immune-mediated destruction of target cells may then establish a positive feedback loop in which the release of self-antigens by injured cells induces further autoantibody production. During this process, the release of cytokines by activated lymphocytes creates an immunostimulatory milieu that facilitates further stimulation of cross-reactive B cells.

Figure 50–5 summarizes the various mechanisms of disease induction discussed in this section. Impaired immune regulation appears to be capable of giving rise to pathogenic autoantibodies. Sufficient stimulation by antigens or immunogenic immune complexes can also induce autoantibodies. C deficiencies may be associated with lupus in this manner, as may exposure to immunogenic microbial nucleic acids. The two abnormalities (impaired regulation and antigenic stimulation) most likely feed back on each other through secondary mechanisms to augment the process.

After lupus disease is well established, a variety of secondary and tertiary effects occur. Clinical findings may result from a small subset of all autoantibodies in a patient with lupus. At the time of clinical illness, the particular factors leading to specific autoantibodies may appear to be so critical that earlier, more generalized events may not seem to be relevant to the genesis of the phenotype.

The concepts expressed in this section are critical to therapeutic approaches to SLE, because attempts to modify the lupus diathesis itself may require suppression of the stimulatory cytokine milieu and the multiclonal activation that characterize the early stage of the disease. Thus therapy directed solely at a specific autoantibody-induced abnormality may not alter the underlying disorder.

DEMOGRAPHICS

Although the onset of SLE may be observed at birth, in childhood, and in older individuals, even those in their nineties, the majority of patients first present with the disease as teenagers or young adults.[6] Prior to puberty and after 40 years of age, the annual incidence of SLE in females is three times greater than in males. Between the ages of 13 and 40, the incidence in females is approximately 10 times that in males. These observations suggest a role of sex hormones in SLE expression.[59, 71, 136, 138] It appears that androgens suppress lupus expression, although that suppression may be overcome by strong enough stimuli to disease.[136, 138] An accelerated conversion of testosterone to estrogens may be a predisposing factor to SLE in some females.[71] Gonadotropin-releasing hormone accelerates lupus directly (not through sex hormones), suggesting a mechanism for lupus induction about the time of menopause in some women and the postmenopausal female predominance of lupus.[59]

Lupus, along with other immune-mediated diseases, tends to run in some families.[55] If one identical twin has lupus, the chance that the other twin will develop lupus is approximately 20%. If a first-degree relative, such as a parent or sibling, has lupus, the chance of developing SLE is approximately 5%. However, there are high-risk families in which several members have the disorder, and others with only a single affected individual. Despite the female predominance, father-to-son inheritance has occasionally been observed, suggesting that a Y chromosome factor may also predispose to disease, as has been found in a certain mouse strain (BXSB) that is predisposed to lupus.[138]

Caucasians originating in northern Europe have a lower annual incidence of lupus than do other racial groups and their disease tends to be milder.[37, 125] Africans, Polynesians, and Orientals appear to have a higher rate of lupus development than do Caucasians. The annual incidence of SLE among African Americans is approximately four times that of American Caucasians, and the disease in these African Americans tends toward the more serious end of the spectrum. An African American female in the United States has approximately a 0.4 to 0.5% chance of developing SLE in her lifetime. The greater Sioux family of Native Americans (Sioux, Crow, Arapaho) has a substantial predisposition toward SLE. The overall annual incidence of lupus is 2 new cases per 100,000 population for low-risk populations and approximately 35 new cases per 100,000 population for high-risk populations.[94]

The specific genes responsible for predisposition to lupus have not been elucidated in most instances, although some

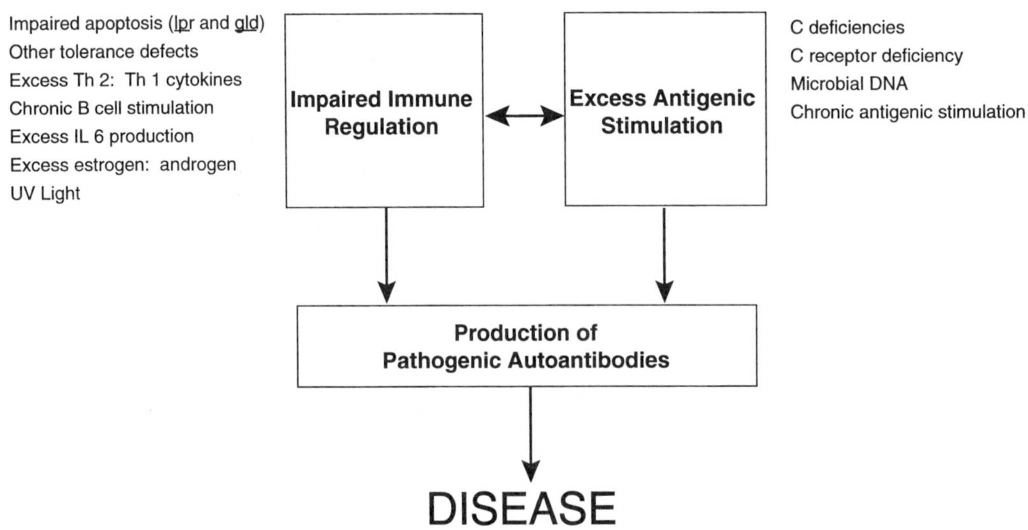

FIGURE 50–5. Factors in the pathogenesis of SLE. A number of genetic and environmental factors may be capable of causing sufficiently impaired immune regulation to predispose to autoantibody formation. Some of the factors are listed to the left of the figure. Excess antigenic stimulation also may predispose to production of pathogenic autoantibodies; some of the factors predisposing to excess antigenic stimulation are shown to the right of the figure. In addition, impaired immune regulation may predispose to excess antigenic stimulation and vice versa.

genetic information is available. Most impressive perhaps is the marked prevalence of lupus in individuals with several of the inherited C-deficiency states.[78, 107] Other genetic factors, such as specific haplotypes (e.g., HLA-A1, HLA-B8, and HLA-DR3) and the C4A null allele, also have been associated with a predisposition to SLE in Caucasians, Africans, and Asians.[32, 39, 50, 112, 113, 122] Both HLA-DR2 and HLA-DR3 have been reported to be associated with SLE. Lupus nephritis has been associated with HLA-DR2, DQw1 (mostly with DQβ1.AZH). Additional subsets of lupus patients, such as those without renal involvement, have been associated statistically with various clinical and genetic markers.[127, 128]

RELATIONSHIP BETWEEN CLINICAL FINDINGS AND IMMUNE ABNORMALITIES

Lupus is primarily an antibody-mediated disease. Antibodies can cause cellular destruction or elimination by acting on cellular targets, such as action of antiplatelet antibodies, anti-RBC antibodies, and antileukocyte antibodies. A deficiency of the cells may ensue as a result of such antibody activity. Antibodies cause a reduction in circulating erythrocytes and platelets. The reduction in formed elements with C receptors causes a relative deficiency of C receptors and thereby an increase in immune complexes able to induce inflammation throughout the body. Antibodies reactive with specific neurons may cause cerebellar disease. Other antibodies may cause cerebral disorders or lead to extrapyramidal syndromes. In all of these cases, the antibodies induce the problem by reacting with unique structures in the brain. Other antibodies reactive with clotting factors cause specific coagulation abnormalities. Antibodies to a sodium-potassium pump may cause electrolyte abnormalities. Antibodies to the receptor for the luteinizing hormone may cause breast swelling and even lactation. The lymphopenia observed in SLE, including reduction in specific T-cell subsets, results from the action of specific anti–T-cell antibodies.[92, 93] A loss of regulatory T cells results from such antibody effects and serves to allow the production of more autoantibodies so as to perpetuate the disease process.

Lupus antibodies also react against a variety of nuclear macromolecular targets (see Table 50–3). Some of these antibodies may not cause immunopathology. Others bind to antigen and deposit in the blood vessels of various organs, where they can induce an inflammatory process. Some immune complexes form in situ when antigen binds to a basement membrane or another structure, and then antibody binds secondarily. The binding of antibody to a macromolecular structure on a basement membrane (e.g., DNA or DNA-containing nucleosome or chromatin fragment) or the lodging of an immune complex on the vascular endothelium leads to C attachment and the production of C3a and C5a. These activated C components attract polymorphonuclear leukocytes and monocytes to the area and help to induce the release of inflammatory mediators from those cells and from basophils and mast cells. Oxygen free radicals, hydrolytic enzymes, and cytokines are produced locally, resulting in tissue destruction and additional stimulation of the process. In addition, platelets become activated, inducing formation of microthrombi and release of vasoactive substances, which induce vascular permeability.

Additional deposition of immune complexes or their persistence leads to a more chronic inflammatory process. This inflammatory process may occur in the blood vessels of any organ in which the antibodies or the immune complexes lodge, hence the variable and systemic nature of SLE. Almost any vascularized organ may be so affected. Some organs that are especially good at trapping antigen may manifest disease especially readily. For example, the basement membranes of the kidneys, skin, and choroid plexus may be especially efficient at trapping DNA or DNA bound to proteins. Antibodies reactive with the antigen then may preferentially induce the inflammatory processes at those sites.

Early lupus inflammatory lesions may be dominated by granulocytes, giving a leukocytoclastic angiitis picture. Late lesions tend to have chronic round cell infiltration. A mixed picture with acute and chronic lesions may be seen; however, granulomas are not a major feature of lupus immunopathology, and their prominence should suggest another disorder.

As might be expected in patients with excess immune complex–initiated immunopathology, patients with active SLE may manifest deficiencies in various C components and in Fc receptor function, leading to a vicious cycle of progressively more immune complex deposition and more immune-mediated pathology. Obviously, a variety of local factors, as well as the details of the composition and size of the immune complexes, may determine the extent of immune complex disease in various organs or parts thereof. Erythrocyte C receptors appear to play an important role in clearance of immune complexes.[53, 121] As a result, saturation of erythrocyte C receptors, a deficiency of such receptors, and anemia all predispose to more severe disease.

In addition to systemic signs and symptoms associated with specific autoantibodies, certain constitutional symptoms may be induced by cytokine abnormalities. For example, excess IL-1 or IL-6 causes suppressed libido, increase in sleep, appetite suppression, and stimulation of acute phase responses. These cytokines may also stimulate the sympathetic nervous system and the hypothalamic-pituitary-adrenal axis but suppression of the hypothalamic-pituitary-gonadal axis and the hypothalamic-pituitary-thyroid axis. Fatigue, such a prominent problem in some patients, may be largely due to cytokine actions.

THE ANTIPHOSPHOLIPID SYNDROME

The antiphospholipid syndrome is an example of the relationship between clinical findings and immune phenomena. This syndrome consists of venous and arterial thromboses (central nervous system thromboses and massive pulmonary emboli being among the most dread outcomes), excess fetal loss, and thrombocytopenia. Years ago, it was recognized that patients with SLE frequently had positive VDRL tests and other positive tests for syphilis. Patients with syphilis make antibodies reactive with a phospholipid dubbed cardiolipin, because it has been isolated from bovine hearts. Sera from lupus patients that have a false-positive test for syphilis also block an in vitro cardiolipin-dependent coagulation test (by inhibiting the conversion of prothrombin to thrombin). As a result of this in vitro finding, the lupus sera were said to contain a circulating anticoagulant. This was an especially unfortunate term because the patients did not have clinical bleeding but rather had clinical thromboses, sometimes pulmonary emboli or even massive strokes.[5, 42] Moreover, other SLE patients who had antibodies to a coagulation factor (e.g., factor VIII, IX, XI, or XII) did indeed have a predisposition to bleeding: they had true circulating anticoagulants.

Because patients with syphilis and some individuals with SLE made antibodies that caused a positive test for syphilis and interfered with an in vitro cardiolipin-dependent assay, it was assumed that the subset of lupus patients with these positive tests were making autoantibodies reactive with phospholipids, including cardiolipin. This turned out to be an oversimplification. Whereas patients with syphilis do make such antibodies, the SLE situation is slightly more complex.

Purified phospholipids in the absence of other serum factors do not readily bind to lupus antibodies. Rather, lupus antibodies bind to one or more other factors that also bind to the cardiolipin or other phospholipids.[9, 81, 84, 119] It is these other antibody specificities, or antibodies that recognize a combined epitope, that appear to be responsible for the antiphospholipid syndrome and the various in vitro test abnormalities. One of these other families of antibody specificities is directed against β_2 glycoprotein I, also called apolipoprotein H, either by itself or when bound to an anionic surface (e.g., activated platelet or endothelial cell) or phospholipid. Thus an antibody binds to β_2 glycoprotein I, which itself is bound to cardiolipin, causing a positive in vitro test for cardiolipin binding and in vivo consequences, the major one being thrombosis.

In addition to antibodies reactive with β_2 glycoprotein I, some individuals with lupus make antibodies to prothrombin. Studies suggest that phospholipid-bound prothrombin may be the target for antibodies of some patients with negative tests for cardiolipin-bound antibodies. Other patients may have antibodies reactive with other phospholipid-binding proteins, including antibodies reactive with protein C, protein S, and thrombomodulin, as well as antibodies reactive with vascular heparan sulfate proteoglycan.[103] Many patients with the antiphospholipid syndrome have more than one of these various specificities.

The effects of the antibodies involved in the antiphospholipid syndrome may be varied, but the final common pathway often is promotion of thromboses. These may occur in deep or superficial veins, and pulmonary embolization may ensue, especially following deep vein thrombosis. Chronic embolization or in situ clotting may lead to pulmonary hypertension. Arterial occlusion is most often manifested by strokes, which may be large. A patient may have several strokes if not treated. Smaller recurrent intracerebral infarcts may lead to dementia and loss of brain substance. There also may be fetal loss (with placental thrombosis/infarction), intrarenal blood vessel occlusion, and thrombosis of dermal vessels with ulceration. A diagnosis of the antiphospholipid syndrome should be considered in patients with a prolonged partial thromboplastin time (PTT), antibodies reactive with phospholipid complexes, or any evidence of thrombosis. The risk of thrombosis is approximately 10 times greater among patients with the causative antibodies than among patients without such antibodies.

Antibodies reactive with β_2 glycoprotein I (the factor that binds cardiolipin) bind to activated but not nonactivated platelets, leading to both thrombosis and thrombocytopenia. There is an increase in platelet interactions, promotion of microthrombus formation, and interference with fibrinolysis. The antibodies may also contribute to verrucous valvular disease (Libman-Sacks disease). Arterial embolization may occur from verrucous endocardial and valvular lesions. The antibodies reactive with vascular heparan sulfate proteoglycan may inhibit antithrombin III activity. Factors interfering with the protein C pathway might predispose especially to venous thromboses. Those that affect prostacyclin/thromboxane homeostasis may preferentially induce arterial thromboses.

CLINICAL PRESENTATION

The initial presentation of patients with lupus varies from nonspecific signs and symptoms, such as anorexia, fever, pharyngitis, and malaise, to more specific syndromes, such as butterfly rash, pleurisy, and nephritis. Arthralgia occurs in about three fourths of patients early in their illnesses and in approximately 90% eventually. It is common for patients to be sufficiently ill to seek medical attention when they have only one or two typical manifestations of lupus. Thus a patient may present with so few clinical signs and symptoms of disease that systemic lupus or even a rheumatic disorder may not be readily diagnosed, without a high index of suspicion.

Typically, the nature of the illness becomes clearer over several additional weeks of observation and as laboratory results become available. Even after the diagnosis is obvious, additional signs and symptoms of the disorder often occur as the time from onset increases. For example, patients may not have renal or central nervous system involvement in the first year of disease, but many develop one of those complications later. There is an old clinical saw: lupus patients tend to flare with the same spectrum of clinical findings with which they presented previously. However, there are sufficient examples to the contrary so that one should not hold too fast to that generalization.

Common laboratory findings are anemia, a high sedimentation rate, hypergammaglobulinemia, thrombocytopenia, lymphopenia, leukopenia, and one or more of a variety of autoantibodies, especially antinuclear antibodies (see Tables 50–1 and 50–3). Specific laboratory abnormalities result from involvement of specific organs.

Many manifestations of SLE, such as fever, arthralgia, central nervous system signs and symptoms, adenopathy, petichiae, vasculitis, malaise, rashes, and heart murmurs, are also found in one or more infectious diseases. As a result, even if a patient has a diagnosis of lupus and the clinical finding is consistent with a lupus manifestation, it is critical always to consider a possible infectious cause. This is especially true of patients with monoarthritis, pericarditis, pleural effusions, pneumonitis, central nervous system disease, and fever, even in the absence of a leukocytosis.

A variety of disorders may be confused with lupus, including rheumatic fever, juvenile rheumatoid arthritis, adult rheumatoid arthritis, autoimmune hemolytic anemia, autoimmune neutropenia, idiopathic autoimmune thrombocytopenia, thrombotic thrombocytopenic purpura, vasculitis, psychosis, lymphoma, secondary syphilis, drug reaction, porphyria, multiple sclerosis, myasthenia gravis, Schönlein-Henoch purpura, personality disorder, stroke, seizure disorder, polymyositis, Sjögren's syndrome, progressive systemic sclerosis (there may be overlaps between lupus and these last three diseases, as well as other autoimmune diseases), subacute bacterial endocarditis, bacterial peritonitis, gonococcal septicemia, meningococcal septicemia, tuberculosis, leprosy, sarcoidosis, serum sickness, angioimmunoblastic lymphadenopathy (AILD), Wegener's granulomatosis, leptospirosis, Lyme disease, Rocky Mountain spotted fever, and acquired immune deficiency syndrome (AIDS).

EARLY VERSUS LATE DISEASE

Lupus patients differ so much one from another that it is difficult to make generalizations. Some have the same kinds of recurring clinical problems over many decades. In general, however, the more acute systemic and immunologically fulminant problems tend to occur relatively early in a patient's course, and more degenerative problems are found later, especially in patients under treatment. The late problems include atherosclerosis (including coronary disease) various nervous system problems (including impaired mentation and loss of brain substance), osteoporosis, osteonecrosis, joint deformities, thrombophlebitis with or without pulmonary emboli, and pulmonary or cardiac dysfunction. It is this author's impression that patients treated with prolonged courses of corticosteroids in high dose suffer many of these late complications to a greater degree than do patients treated primarily with other medications, even cytotoxic agents. The premature aging observed late in SLE, especially in patients treated with high doses of corticosteroids, may represent a synergistic interaction between aspects of the disease and the treatment.

MAJOR VERSUS NONMAJOR ORGAN INVOLVEMENT

It often helps to separate signs and symptoms into prognostic and therapeutic categories. One useful approach is to determine whether a major organ is involved with disease, because there are important therapeutic implications of such a division. For example, pleurisy and arthralgia typically require less vigorous therapy than do nephritis and cerebritis. Table 50–4 provides a rough sorting of signs and symptoms into major and nonmajor organ involvement.

TABLE 50–4
DIVISION OF LUPUS FEATURES INTO ROUGH PROGNOSTIC AND THERAPEUTIC CATEGORIES*

Major Organ Lupus†	Nonmajor Organ Involvement
Kidney	Arthralgia/arthritis
Central nervous system*	Rash/skin vasculitis
Heart Lungs	Serositis—Pleurisy, pericarditis, peritonitis
Marrow-blood—thrombocytopenic purpura, hemolytic anemia (marked), severe granulocytopenia	Splenomegaly/lymphadenopathy Mucosal ulcers Hepatitis
Other—mesenteric vasculitis	Mucosal ulcers Episcleritis Peripheral neuropathy Myalgia Fever Fatigue Anorexia Alopecia Raynaud's phenomenon

*In general, the major organ involvement requires vigorous immunosuppressive therapy, whereas the nonmajor organ involvement usually does not. An occasional individual may have serositis or other nonmajor organ involvement sufficient to require vigorous therapy.
†The antiphospholipid syndrome might be considered a major organ manifestation if it involved the central nervous system or another major organ; however, the therapeutic implications would be different in that attention to anticoagulation rather than immunosuppression would be paramount.

CONSTITUTIONAL PROBLEMS

Fever, fatigue, malaise, anorexia, and weight loss are common presenting problems. However, these are nonspecific and do not point to a diagnosis of lupus. Indeed, even in a patient known to have SLE, such findings should stimulate a consideration of other causes of the problems, especially infection. Lupus patients are unusually predisposed to infection by both their illness and therapy; therefore fever should always trigger a search for infection.

MUSCULOSKELETAL PROBLEMS

The single most frequent manifestation of lupus is joint pain, occurring in more than 90% of patients. Arthralgia may be transitory in nature, lasting minutes, days, or weeks in a given joint. In other individuals, the joint pain may be constant and accompanied by frank arthritis. Although any joint may be affected, the most typical involvement occurs in the wrists, knees, and proximal interphalangeal joints of the hands. Morning stiffness, so often associated with rheumatoid arthritis, also is observed in lupus patients with serious joint disease. Lupus patients tend to have synovial fluid with better mucin clot formation than is found in rheumatoid arthritis, much lower synovial fluid leukocyte counts, and higher glucose levels.

The bony abnormalities found in rheumatoid arthritis are not a feature of systemic lupus. Nevertheless, 10% to 15% of patients may develop deformities, which resemble Jaccoud arthritis described in patients after rheumatic fever.[19] Such deformities initially tend to be reducible but can become less so with long-standing disease. The deformities may result from tendon slippage or chronic joint capsule swelling. Nodules do occur in some lupus patients. These have hematoxylin bodies in the center and differ histologically from rheumatoid nodules. Mild asymptomatic flexion contractures at the elbow often are a sign of active SLE early in disease. These may become less prominent as the disease remits, but may become fixed later.

Rupture of one or more tendons may occur in patients with lupus, even in the absence of corticosteroid therapy. Rupture of the Achilles' or quadriceps femoris tendons may occur suddenly, with substantial incapacity. Frequently, there is pain and swelling of the tendon, which heralds rupture and may be treated with immobilization.

Muscle pains occur in almost one third of lupus patients. Frank myositis, akin to muscle inflammation of polymyositis, is seen in only 5% of patients. Many patients with milder muscle disease may have elevated serum aldolase values with normal creatine kinases; they exhibit ultrastructural abnormalities.[38] Drugs, such as corticosteroids and antimalarials, given to lupus patients also may affect the muscles.

INTEGUMENT

SLE is a disease of blood vessels. Manifestations of vascular inflammation are most readily seen in the skin. Many of the acute lesions demonstrate vascular and perivascular inflammation (of arterioles or venules) with granulocytes; there may be necrosis. The acute inflammation is typically followed by mononuclear cell involvement. There are deposits of immunoglobulin and C at the dermal epidermal junction with or without inflammation there.

Some of the skin problems of lupus patients are thought to be more specific to the disorder, such as discoid lupus, a butterfly rash, lupus profundus, subacute cutaneous lupus, generalized erythema, and bullous disease.[20] Lesions less specific to lupus include livedo reticularis, vasculitis, alopecia, urticaria, mucosal lesions, and panniculitis. This division is not particularly helpful in caring for patients, because vasculitic lesions, which are not specific for lupus, occur in 20% of patients, whereas bullous lupus, which is specific for the disorder, occurs in 2% of patients.

Discoid lupus may occur alone or as part of systemic lupus. There is follicular plugging, erythema, hyperkeratosis, and later central atrophy with hyperpigmentation, hypopigmentation, and telangiectasia. The hypopigmentation may be especially disturbing to Africans. Scalp lesions, when severe and long standing, may lead to permanent local alopecia.

A butterfly rash is often observed in patients with SLE, aids in diagnosis, and may be an early sign of the disorder. Red cheeks vary from a slight blush to indurated, nonpapular erythema over both malar eminences and the bridge of the nose. This finding may precede other features of lupus or follow them. The rash may be pruritic or even painful. In some individuals, the butterfly rash varies with disease activity. The lesion may be found in patients who avoid ultraviolet light but is often induced or exacerbated by sun exposure.

Patients with SLE also may develop a maculopapular erythematous eruption, sometimes affecting even the palms and soles, which is indistinguishable from a drug eruption and may indeed be brought on by a drug, such as sulfisoxazole or another sulfa drug or ampicillin, or by UV light. Urticaria, angioedema, and subepidermal bullous disease are seen. Livedo reticularis occurs commonly in patients with SLE but is only rarely severe. Palmar erythema may be prominent in some patients and a sign of active lupus. The same is true of periungual erythema. Tender fingertip pulp lesions may occur, as well as splinter hemorrhages, findings that often cause concern about subacute bacterial endocarditis in nonlupus patients.

Purpura may be due to vasculitis, capillary fragility (often due to corticosteroid therapy), or thrombocytopenia. Approximately 20% of patients have vasculitic lesions of the skin. These are signs of active disease activity but do not necessarily imply an impending disaster. They are found on the fingertips, forearms, and lower legs, where they often ulcerate. Vasculitic lesions of mucosae lead to mucosal ulcers, such as on the hard and soft palates, nasal septum (rarely with perforation), other parts of the upper respiratory tract, and the vagina. Although mucosal ulcers are ordinarily without serious consequences, patients with upper airway lesions occasionally may require emergency tracheotomy.

Approximately 10% of patients may develop urticarial lesions, which often are vasculitic. In a rare patient, urticaria may be the dominant lesion (in some, it may be worsened by UV light exposure) and may be refractory to all but the most vigorous therapy. The pathology of these lesions consists of necrosis of vessel walls, especially in venules, infiltration with neutrophils, and deposition of immunoglobulin and C. Apparently, immune complexes deposit in small venules of the skin and cause sufficient inflammation for the production of C3a and C5a; histamine is then released from perivenular mast cells to cause the urticaria.

Raynaud's phenomenon occurs in patients with SLE, often without fingertip scarring, but may be severe in an occasional patient, leading to distal gangrene and loss of tissue. Superficial thrombophlebitis also is observed in lupus patients, which was discussed under the antiphospholipid syndrome.

Alopecia, except when in chronic discoid lesions, tends to be diffuse and temporary, often coming on with active disease and resolving with remissions. Patients often report increased hair on the comb or brush or pillow. Medication given for lupus also may induce alopecia.

Lupus profundus is an indurated inflammatory process characterized by skin lesions showing perivascular infiltration without fat necrosis. This lesion is often found in association with relapsing nonsuppurative panniculitis with fat necrosis and is reminiscent of Weber-Christian disease. There may be only superficial inflammation, often in a nodular form, or it can descend into the depths of the thighs and buttocks. The deeper lesions often calcify, and the overlying skin may ulcerate.

Subacute cutaneous lupus begins as erythematous papules or small plaques and is a nonscarring, remitting lesion intermediate between the common evanescent erythematous rash and the chronic scarring lesions. It may resemble lichen planus or psoriasis, or in an annular form, annular skin disorders. The most common serologic association is anti-Ro (anti-SS-A) antibodies in the serum and the lesions.[22]

UV light adversely affects many patients with lupus by either exacerbating skin disease or stimulating systemic flares. UV light is divided into UVA (320–400 nm) UVB (290–320 nm) and UVC (200–290 nm), which is screened out by the atmosphere of earth. It is thought that UVB and perhaps the more energetic parts of the UVA spectrum are especially deleterious, whereas the less energetic UVA rays may actually be beneficial.[83, 100] It is thought that UV light accelerates lupus by several mechanisms, including induction of cytokine production by keratinocytes and other cells in the skin, cell damage and release of DNA, and interference with antigen handling by mononuclear cells.

LIVER

A form of chronic hepatitis, once called lupoid hepatitis, appears to be unrelated to SLE. Lupus patients often have inconsequential hepatomegaly. They also may manifest liver enzyme elevations, sometimes in association with nonsteroidal anti-inflammatory drug (NSAID) therapy, especially aspirin. The enzyme abnormalities often resolve with corticosteroid therapy, disease remission, or withdrawal of the NSAID. A rare patient may have years of liver enzyme elevations. Patients who have received high doses of steroids for long periods may develop a fatty liver.

PANCREAS

Approximately 5% of lupus patients experience pancreatitis, due to either the underlying disease or corticosteroid therapy. The presentation is similar to that seen in patients without SLE. There is divided opinion regarding the approach to corticosteroid dosing in patients who develop the disorder while receiving substantial doses of corticosteroids. Corticosteroid-induced diabetes is common. When possible, nondiabetogenic drugs should be considered.

HEART

Any or all of the following may be found in a single individual: endocarditis, myocarditis, pericarditis, and coronary artery disease.[23] The most common electrocardiographic finding is nonspecific ST/T wave changes. There may be a prolonged PR interval or evidence of ischemia, infarction, or acute pericarditis.

Nonbacterial verrucous endocarditis (Libman-Sacks endocarditis) was quite a common clinical finding in the precorticosteroid era. Now, the diagnosis appears to be less commonly made in life, although it is frequent at autopsy.[16] Nonetheless, such vegetations may cause various degrees of valvular thickening from mild (seen on two-dimensional echocardiography) to marked (requiring surgical intervention). Bacterial endocarditis may occur on such roughened valves, suggesting the utility of prophylactic antibiotics for interventional procedures. The vegetations are especially found in the mitral valve at the forward flow edges but may be found on other valves, on the chordae tendineae and the endocardium. They consist of fibrin, mononuclear cells, cellular debris (including hematoxylin bodies), and platelet thrombi.

Myocarditis in patients with active lupus may be manifested by unexplained tachycardia and may resolve as other features of disease are treated. In some patients, the myocarditis stands out as a more discreet clinical problem. It may be associated with arrhythmias, conduction defects, or uncommonly, congestive heart failure. The latter is exacerbated by coexistent hypertension. Peripheral muscle disease need not be present.

Pericarditis is a clinical finding in about 30% of patients at some time in the course of their SLE but is more often found at autopsy.[16] It is recognized by precordial pain on lying down, which is partially or completely relieved by standing. Rubs are frequently heard when the patient is symptomatic. However, pericarditis may occur without symptoms, and evidence may be observed first on echocardiography. It is usually without consequence. In some individuals, chronic inflammation may lead to marked pericardial thickening. A patient with severe pericardial disease may experience tamponade.

It is not uncommon for a young, menstruating woman with SLE to develop a myocardial infarction. Indeed, as the time from onset of lupus increases, patients of both genders are at substantially increased risk of coronary occlusion. Coronary artery disease due to vasculitis occurs in SLE, typically in association with active multisystem disease. However, especially since the widespread use of corticosteroids in therapy, atherosclerotic disease is a more common cause of coronary narrowing.[12, 67] Patients who develop atherosclerosis often have had hypertension, hyperlipidemia, hyperglycemia, and prior inflammatory disease of the heart/pericardium. Coronary occlusion may also be associated with the antiphospholipid syndrome.

LUNG

Pleurisy occurs in up to 60% of lupus patients.[124] The pain on inspiration is more common than x-ray changes, and pleural rubs are even less frequently observed. As is the case with endocarditis and pericarditis, pleurisy is most frequently diagnosed at autopsy. Chronic pleural thickening can occur but is rare. Pleural biopsies may show varying degrees of fibrosis and inflammation. The pleural fluid is usually an exudate, and antinuclear antibodies may be found. The sugar is usually normal, in contrast to rheumatoid arthritis pleural fluid, in which it is characteristically low.

Because pneumonitis in lupus is infectious as often as it is due to the underlying disease, a careful search for infection is important. However, some of the more common vigorous search techniques carry their own hazards. There have been life-threatening responses to bronchoalveolar lavage in seriously ill lupus patients.

Pulmonary hemorrhage, when mild, may manifest as fleeting infiltrates. Moderately severe cases present with cough and hemoptysis, presumably due to vasculitis.[21] More fulminant pulmonary hemorrhage is extremely serious.

Acute lupus pneumonitis may resemble pneumonia. There is often fever, cough, dyspnea, and even hemoptysis and usually evidence of active lupus elsewhere. Chronic lupus pneumonitis resembles more diffuse interstitial lung disease. Patients exhibit dyspnea on exertion, nonproductive cough, and rales up the back. A rare syndrome of lymphocytic interstitial pneumonia typically occurs in active disease and may resemble one form of pseudolymphoma of Sjögren's syndrome or lymphangitic spread of malignancy. It is also seen in patients with AIDS.

Pulmonary hypertension may be characterized by dyspnea with a normal chest x-ray, mild hypoxia, reduced diffusing capacity, and restrictive pulmonary function tests. Some such patients have multiple pulmonary emboli or intrapulmonary thromboses in association with the antiphospholipid syndrome.

The shrinking lung syndrome is characterized by progressive dyspnea despite clear lung fields on chest x-ray, although high diaphragms are noted.[58] Pulmonary function tests demonstrate reduced lung volumes and a restrictive pattern. The syndrome is caused by impaired intercostal and diaphragmatic muscle function. In severe cases, the diaphragm may become atrophic and fibrotic.

GASTROINTESTINAL DISEASE

Acute active lupus commonly is characterized by anorexia, mild nausea, dyspepsia, or in severe cases, abdominal pain. It is often unclear whether these symptoms result from vascular disease of the bowel or moderate peritonitis. Typically, the complaints resolve with therapy for other manifestations of the disease.

The diagnosis of lupus peritonitis is made much more frequently at autopsy than in life, as is the case with pericarditis and pleuritis. It is likely that many of the acute constitutional signs and symptoms seen in untreated lupus patients, such as mild diffuse abdominal pain, anorexia, and nausea, result from peritonitis. Typically, the peritonitis follows the same course as other aspects of the lupus. Approximately 10% of cases have an associated ascites. In some of these patients, the ascites takes on a life of its own and may be a chronic problem when other manifestations of disease are quiescent. Of course, peritonitis could also be infectious. Spontaneous pneumococcal peritonitis and septicemia may occur in lupus patients, especially those who have undergone splenectomy. Prophylactic administration of pneumococcal vaccine is highly desirable to reduce the likelihood of that problem.

Mesenteric vasculitis is a serious manifestation of vasculitis in SLE.[160] It may occur in the absence of obvious vasculitis elsewhere, or there may be evidence of vasculitis. However, there commonly is other evidence of active disease. Patients experience lower abdominal pain that may not be of such a character as to call attention to a life-threatening problem. This is especially a problem in a patient under treatment who may have signs and symptoms masked by anti-inflammatory corticosteroids. Pain may be intermittent over several weeks or even longer and may develop or progress insidiously. The diffuse abdominal pain of peritonitis and mesenteric vasculitis may be difficult to distinguish by history or physical exam, and both may show rebound tenderness. Corticosteroid therapy may improve both. However, if bowel infarction has already occurred from mesenteric vasculitis, perforation may follow and be obscured by the therapy, and life-saving surgery delayed. If there is a suspicion of mesenteric vasculitis, the diagnosis may be confirmed by angiography. There may be rectal bleeding, and fiberoptic examination might show ulcerations of the small and large bowels. Avascular tissue may be recognized if infarction has occurred, necessitating prompt surgery.

SPLEEN AND LYMPH NODES

Lymphadenopathy is a common feature of early and untreated lupus and is especially common in younger patients.[127, 128] The nodes are typically soft and nontender, may be matted, and may change in size in relation to disease activity and corticosteroid therapy. The pathology shows reactive hyperplasia. Occasionally, lupus lymphadenopathy is so marked as to suggest a lymphoid malignancy.

Splenomegaly also is more common in younger patients and those with active disease. Indeed, a teenager may present with an autoimmune hematologic disorder without other features of SLE, have a splenectomy, and then be diagnosed with probable lupus on the basis of the splenic pathology. The typical splenic pathology is an onionskin lesion that represents periarteriolar and periarterial fibrosis. It is thought that circulating immune complexes in patients with SLE might overwhelm the reticuloendothelial system, thereby increasing the chance of deposition in vessel walls of a variety of tissues.

In addition to splenic hypertrophy, splenic atrophy and splenic lymphoma have been observed in lupus patients.[18, 29]

BONE MARROW–HEMATOLOGIC PROBLEMS

Anemia, leukopenia or lymphopenia, and thrombocytopenia are common features of SLE and are criteria for the diagnosis (see Table 50–1). Patients with lupus may have defective release of formed elements from the marrow, peripheral destruction, or both. In the absence of cytotoxic drug therapy, the bone marrow of a patient with active disease typically shows erythroid hyperplasia. A rare patient may have marrow hypoplasia and pancytopenia due to immune responses to precursor marrow elements.

Anemia is common in patients with active disease, is a negative prognostic indicator, and may contribute to disease perpetuation (there are fewer receptors for immune complexes). Anemia may be secondary to chronic inflammatory disease. A shortened erythrocyte survival is common and is often associated with erythrocyte-bound immunoglobulin and C. However, frank acute hemolytic anemia is uncommon.

Thrombocytopenia may occur in the patient with very active lupus disease and tends to follow the course of the lupus. It may also occur as a more isolated finding and present similarly to idiopathic thrombocytopenic purpura, with IgG antibody directed to platelet antigens, such as IIb/IIIa or Ib. There may be petichiae or purpura, but serious bleeding is uncommon unless other factors also are present, such as hypertension and vasculitis.

Leukopenia often varies with the clinical course. There is a rare syndrome of extreme granulocytopenia, which may respond to plasmapheresis/immunosuppressive therapy. Antibodies to coagulation factors are true lupus anticoagulants in that they cause bleeding. There may be antibodies to factors VIII, IX or XI with hemophilia-like presentation as well as uncommon anticoagulants directed to factors V, VII, or X. All patients so affected are at serious risk of bleeding during invasive procedures, such as biopsies, or surgery.

KIDNEY DISEASE

Lupus was once a prototype immune complex disease in which it was thought that preformed immune complexes deposited in the kidney and induced inflammation. Although such immune complex disease may well be a part of lupus kidney disease, that older view is believed to be simplistic in that considerable quantities of antibody may bind to antigen that itself has already bound to the renal basement membranes.

Renal deposition of immune complexes or binding of circulating antibody to antigen that had bound to renal basement membranes occurs in almost all patients. In many, there are no important consequences; in others, some degree of renal inflammation may ensue. Clinically evident kidney disease occurs in somewhat more than half of all patients, only some of which have sufficiently severe disease to require vigorous therapy.[30, 35, 116] When the renal disease worsens by changing from mesangial to capillary loop deposition, with inflammation, it carries a much greater threat of progression to renal failure. The prognosis of patients with substantial scarring is guarded. Nevertheless, early treatment of disease is efficacious, and progression to renal failure usually can be avoided.

Unlike the situation with most other manifestations of lupus, patients typically are not aware of kidney inflammation unless there is nephrotic syndrome or renal failure. The urinalysis may show proteinuria, hematuria, pyuria (in the absence of infection), or casts (RBC, WBC, mixed, granular). It is generally believed that crenated red cells, red cell casts, mixed cellular casts, and coarsely granular casts are evidence of renal inflammation. High-grade proteinuria also is seen as an adverse finding. However, the urinalysis may not be sufficiently specific to distinguish certain lesions. For example, an occasional patient with mesangial disease may have as many erythrocytes as one with diffuse proliferative disease. The distinction is important because the prognosis of the former is much better than that of the latter.

Although some students of lupus argue that the renal biopsy is of little utility in predicting outcome, most believe that the biopsy is of benefit in assessing prognosis and deciding upon therapy. Those with a special interest in lupus pathology have been developing progressively more complex histologic categorizations, an example of which is given in Table 50–5.[61] Although patients may change from one diagnostic category to another, this author believes that multiple biopsies generally are not needed to dictate therapy.[132] In contrast, multiple biopsies are the rule at some institutions and are frequently favored by renal pathologists and nephrologists with a strong histopathologic interest.[61] It is generally believed that the biopsy category shown in Table 50–5 helps to define prognosis and therefore should play a role in therapy. For example, a patient with rising serum creatinine and sclerosis on biopsy with little active disease might be treated less vigorously than another patient with a rising serum creatinine but substantial active inflammation on biopsy.

TABLE 50–5
MODIFIED WORLD HEALTH ORGANIZATION CLASSIFICATION OF LUPUS NEPHRITIS

I. Normal glomeruli on light microscopy
  a. Normal immunofluorescence and electron microscopy
  b. Deposits on immunofluorescence or electron microscopy

II. Pure mesangial disease
  a. Mesangial expansion and/or mild hypercellularity
  b. Moderate hypercellularity

IIIA. Focal segmental glomerulonephritis
  a. Active necrotizing lesions
  b. Active lesions and sclerosing lesions
  c. Sclerosing lesions

IIIB. Focal proliferative glomerulonephritis
  a. Active necrotizing lesions
  b. Active lesions and sclerosing lesions
  c. Sclerosing lesions

IV. Diffuse glomerulonephritis
  a. Without segmental lesions
  b. With active necrotizing lesions
  c. With active lesions and sclerosing lesions
  d. With sclerosing lesions

V. Diffuse membranous glomerulonephritis
  a. Pure membranous glomerulonephritis
  b. Associated with lesions of II
  c. Associated with lesions of III
  d. Associated with lesions of IV

VI. Advanced sclerosing glomerulonephritis

From Kashgarian M: Lupus nephritis: lessons from the path lab. Kidney Int 45: 928–938, 1994.

Clinical and laboratory findings also play an important role in the evaluation of patients with lupus nephritis. A falling C and rising anti-DNA commonly precede or are associated with a flare in lupus nephritis. At such times, a patient may need more careful observation and increased therapy. Hypertension is often a feature of lupus renal disease, even relatively early in the disorder. This is a special problem because the inflammatory disease and the hypertension can synergize in the destruction of renal tissue.

NERVOUS SYSTEM

Patients with SLE may develop a peripheral neuropathy (in up to 15%) or a mononeuritis multiplex picture, such as foot drop. The latter appears to be due to vasculitis of the vasa nervora but does not necessarily signal major vasculitis elsewhere.

It had been fashionable for many years to make a diagnosis of central nervous system lupus in lupus patients with central nervous system signs or symptoms. However, in view of the different causes of different central nervous system syndromes and the different approaches to therapy, that is now deemed an incomplete diagnosis. Central nervous system involvement in lupus is common. It may affect almost all patients subclinically and is clinically apparent in approximately half of patients.[1, 30, 36, 51, 72] For example, the antiphospholipid syndrome may predispose to stroke. The combination of mild thrombocytopenia, mild hypertension, and mild vasculitis may lead to intracerebral hemorrhage; NSAID therapy may be a further exacerbating factor.

Various antibodies reactive with neurones may cause any of a variety of psychiatric or organic mental problems. Antibodies to specific cerebellar cells may cause cerebellar disease. Other antineuronal antibodies may cause cerebral disorders, and still others may lead to extrapyramidal syndromes. In all of these cases, the antibodies induce the problem by reacting with unique antigenic determinants. Cerebellar disorders may occur as isolated phenomena or may be seen with other nervous system abnormalities. In occasional patients, an organic mental syndrome with impaired cognition may progress to coma and death. In addition to antineuronal antibody-mediated disease, deposits in the choroid plexus may alter the normal intracerebral milieu. Secondary central nervous system problems may arise from renal disease, other causes of metabolic abnormalities, or viral infections.

Multiple small infarcts due to the antiphospholipid syndrome, hypertension, corticosteroid therapy, or vasculitis may lead to formation of lacunae and loss of brain substance with irreversibly impaired cognition. Reversibly impaired cognition may be due to cerebritis, vasculitis, antineuronal antibodies, metabolic disturbances, viral or other infections, and various therapies. Cranial nerve abnormalities most frequently are manifested by defects in extraocular muscle movement.[36]

Lupus-related psychological problems can vary from mild alteration in personality to frank psychosis. Depression, mania, paranoid psychosis, and various forms of schizophrenia have been observed. It may be necessary to distinguish corticosteroid-induced psychologic problems, although the patient's recent therapeutic history usually provides a clue.

Seizures, including grand mal seizures, occur especially in younger patients with very active disease. Migraine headaches are common and may herald the onset of increased disease activity or be an isolated manifestation. They sometimes are preceded or accompanied by fortification spectra, a visual image of parallel lines resembling the plan for an ancient fort. Movement disorders, such as chorea, athetosis, and hemiballismus, are noted most commonly in younger patients.

NSAIDs may induce or exacerbate certain neurologic signs and symptoms, especially in patients with SLE. Some patients may appear to have features of multiple sclerosis, as well as SLE. Transverse myelitis in SLE may lead rapidly to permanent dysfunction unless vigorously treated.

CT scans, magnetic resonance imaging (MRI), and nuclear magnetic resonance (NMR) spectroscopy may be helpful in demonstrating lesions. The electroencephalogram typically shows nonspecific slow waves, although an occasional patient may have a spike and wave pattern. The cerebrospinal fluid may show mildly increased protein, increased gamma globulin, increased IgG, a moderate number of round cells, and normal sugar. Antineuronal antibodies are found in the cerebrospinal fluid of many patients with immunologically mediated disease. An association of CNS cerebritis with antibodies to ribosomal P component has been reported. It is appropriate to search for infection with bacteria, mycobacteria, fungi, spirochetes, and parasites in patients with diffuse or focal CNS disease (Table 50–6).

EYE

Patients with lupus may develop episcleritis or uveitis during active systemic disease. Occlusion of retinal arteries or veins may lead to visual impairment. Lupus retinopathy is a sign of active CNS involvement. There may be inflammation of the optic disc, hemorrhages, or cotton wool spots. Extraocular muscle abnormalities usually are due to cranial nerve defects. A variety of pupillary abnormalities may occur. Changes in the fluid content of the lens, perhaps due to changes in corticosteroid therapy, may lead to blurry vision. Chronic therapy leads to the formation of posterior subcapsular cataracts.

MANAGEMENT OF THE PATIENT WITH SYSTEMIC LUPUS

Although lupus was once a feared disorder, patients should be reassured that it is now eminently treatable and that the great majority of patients can live fulfilling and productive lives. Patients also should be educated about the manifestations of the disorder and the effects, including adverse effects, of the various therapies used so that the patient can be aware of the potential relevance of changes that occur and bring those to the attention of the physician. Psychologic problems occur from the diagnosis, the uncertainty of the course of SLE, the medication, and the disease itself. As a result, supportive psychotherapy often is an important part of management.

Patients should be told that many of the serious lupus problems do not affect most people and that there are therapies for them if they were to occur. Nevertheless, they also must understand that they have a chronic illness that has no cure and will require regular visits to physicians and, for most people, medication and some change in lifestyle. Early involvement with dieticians, physical therapists, educational programs, and support groups may be helpful.

Lupus patients often need more rest than average. When the disease is active, an afternoon nap may be useful. Exposure to UV light, especially UVB, should be avoided by religiously using sunscreen, remaining indoors during the middle of the day (10 AM–3 PM), wearing a broad-brimmed hat and long sleeves, and avoiding nonsolar sources of UV light, such as certain unshielded fluorescent bulbs. Patients should avoid drugs that augment the effects of UV light, such as tetracyclines, sulfa drugs, and psoralens. Foods that contain psoralens, such as parsley, figs, celery, and parsnips, should be avoided. It might also be prudent to avoid foods containing L-canavanine, such as alfalfa seeds and sprouts, and hydrazines, such as mushrooms and certain food dyes. It is not clear whether drugs that are able to induce a lupus-like syndrome, such as procainamide, hydralazine, and isoniazid, should be avoided by patients with idiopathic lupus.

Hypertension synergizes with the immune-mediated vascular disease. Therefore, the blood pressure should be kept in the middle of the normal range. It is necessary to repeatedly search for a possible infection causing the symptoms or inducing a lupus flare. This is especially a problem because lupus patients are unusually predisposed to infections because of their underlying immune dysfunction and the therapies they receive.

Patients should be told that they differ from one another, as the therapy of one individual with SLE might differ markedly from that of another. Moreover, the lay literature is capable of advancing new breakthroughs for lupus on a regular basis. Some of these are research advances not yet converted to clinical utility, and others are at best exaggerated and often groundless. Some may be detrimental for certain patients with lupus, and others may have evidence neither supporting nor denying their potential utility. It should be realized that natural substances contain chemicals just as do pills given by the pharmacist. The natural chemicals are neither better nor worse by virtue of their being natural and often have been less well studied and less well characterized. A natural therapy may contain a mixture of chemicals, including those that are beneficial, neutral, and harmful.

Patients with mild lupus often are adequately controlled with hydroxychloroquine and NSAIDs. Those with slightly more resistant disease may profit from the addition of low doses of corticosteroids for adequate symptomatic therapy. Patients with major organ involvement typically require vigorous therapy. The objective is preservation of function of the organ and prevention of organ failure.

Corticosteroids are extremely effective at rapidly reducing many of the signs and symptoms of patients with SLE. Unfortunately, many of the long-term complications that patients experience result from excess corticosteroid usage, including certain forms of heart and central nervous system disease, osteopenia, asceptic necrosis, metabolic abnormalities, posterior subcapsular cataracts, and infections. As a result, there must be careful consideration to risks, as well as potential disease-ameliorating benefits. Although the decision to start corticosteroids often is given great weight, the dosage and duration of therapy are far more important. Indeed, for patients who appear to require prolonged therapy, addition of an immunosuppressive drug and marked reduction in corticosteroid dosage may result in less long-term toxicity.

Immunosuppressive drugs found to be effective for different manifestations of lupus include azathioprine, cyclophosphamide, and methotrexate. Patients with life-threatening vasculitic complications of lupus, including mesenteric arteritis, cerebral vasculitis, and pulmonary vasculitis, or those with impending loss of critical functions, such as those with transverse myelitis, respond much more reliably to boluses of cyclophosphamide than to high doses of corticosteroids or other immunosuppressive drugs. Similarly, those with diffuse proliferative glomerulonephritis respond most reliably to cyclophosphamide-containing medications.[139]

Patients with thromboses should be evaluated for the antiphospholipid syndrome and given at least low-dose aspirin therapy to prevent serious thrombotic complications. Many physicians believe that anticoagulation is desirable to prevent pulmonary emboli, pulmonary thromboses, and thrombotic strokes in patients who have had evidence of past thromboses. Balancing the risks and benefits is sometimes difficult, but those with high titers of IgG antibodies may be especially predisposed to such thrombotic complications.

The treatment of proliferative and membranoproliferative lupus nephritis is a difficult and sometimes controversial area.[132] There is also much muddled thinking: a common practice is to treat patients with corticosteroids, add azathioprine if the patient flares, and then consider cyclophosphamide when renal failure becomes obvious. The withholding of cyclophosphamide until renal failure markedly decreases the likelihood that the drug will be effective and also may increase its toxicity. The drug works best when given early to a patient with proliferative glomerulonephritis. A common regimen is 500 to 1,000 mg/m^2 body surface area per month for 3 to 6 months, followed by drug every 2 to 3 months. It is given with ondansetron and decadron to minimize nausea.[133]

Patients with mesangial disease appear not to need vigorous therapy. Those with substantial focal proliferative disease appear to carry almost the same prognosis as those with diffuse proliferative disease.

Nonthrombotic central nervous system disorders may respond to corticosteroids but more reliably respond to cyclophosphamide. Serious seizures must be treated acutely with anticonvulsants, as well as corticosteroids, but long-term anticonvulsant therapy often is not be necessary.

Skin disease often responds to hydroxychloroquine 200 to 400 mg/d. Resistant skin disease often responds to azathioprine 150 to 250 mg/d. Hydroxychloroquine treatment requires periodic eye exams to detect potential retinal deposits, which could lead to seriously impaired vision. Azathioprine can cause idiosyncratic agranulocytosis in the first week of therapy. Thereafter, the white count tends to follow a dose-response pattern. Some patients experience nausea. A hepatitis picture is a known side effect.

In maintenance therapy, short-acting corticosteroids are preferred because they allow a switch to every other day therapy. The more often they are given, the greater the effectiveness and the greater the toxicity. For maintenance, every effort should be made to keep the patient's dose below 15 mg/m^2 body surface area every other day.

A variety of measures have been advanced to quantitate the degree of lupus activity. Although such measures may be useful in research efforts, this author has not found such indexes useful in the management of individual patients.

TABLE 50–6
CENTRAL NERVOUS SYSTEM ABNORMALITIES IN PATIENTS WITH SLE

Neurologic*	Psychiatric*
Thrombotic strokes	Personality disorder
Hemorrhagic strokes	Mania
Seizures	Depression
Movement disorders	Paranoid psychosis
Cranial neuropathies	Schizophrenia
Migraine headaches	
Cerebellar syndrome	
Cognitive dysfunction	
Organic mental syndrome	
Aseptic meningitis	
Optic neuritis and retinal hemorrhage	
Transverse myelitis	

*More than one may occur at the same time, and both neurologic and psychiatric abnormalities may be found together.

STRESS, EXERCISE, MARRIAGE, AND PREGNANCY

Stress may precede an exacerbation of disease activity. Therefore, avoidance of both physical and psychologic stress is recommended. Exercise should be consistent with the disease activity; exercise to the point of exhaustion is inadvisable. Marriage is perfectly consistent with lupus. The majority of patients marry, and it is useful to include the prospective spouse in the medical assessment so as to maximize understanding and cooperation. Withholding information about one's lupus from a prospective spouse may lead to feelings of duplicity and entrapment.

Patients with lupus experience decreased fertility and increased fetal loss. There is a strong association between the antiphospholipid syndrome and increased fetal loss. Pregnancy may not be advisable during active disease, especially active nephritis. Certain forms of active central nervous system disease, myocarditis, and pulmonary disease may be relative contraindications for pregnancy. Patients who once had severe lupus nephritis and then had been in remission for several years have become pregnant and delivered normal babies. Patients can be maintained on corticosteroids during pregnancy if they are necessary; immunosuppressive agents are best avoided.

HORMONAL ISSUES

Lupus flares may occur at any time in a woman's menstrual cycle. Mild symptomatology often is more common between ovulation and menstruation, and usually no change in therapy is needed for these minor fluctuations.[140] Although lupus is more common in women and sex hormones may play a role in pathogenesis, there is inconclusive evidence that sex hormone manipulation might be useful therapeutically. Indeed, in murine lupus, the major suppressive effects of androgens are observed when the androgens are started in the first 3 weeks of life. Comparable intervention is not possible in humans.

Excess prolactin effects may be important in some patients with lupus and may be an appropriate target for therapy in the future. Abnormal thyroid laboratory tests are common in patients with active lupus but do not necessarily require intervention.[88] Some patients with lupus develop autoimmune thyroiditis, which should be addressed as in patients without lupus.

The high doses of estrogen found in the older oral contraceptives were thought to precipitate lupus disease. This seems to be less of a problem with newer oral contraceptives, which contain much less estrogen. The question of estrogen replacement in lupus patients who have reached menopause is a controversial issue, primarily due to a lack of sufficient information. There is always the balance between the desire to prevent atherosclerosis and other estrogen deficiency problems with replacement and the desire not to induce lupus disease activity with the therapy.

FEVER, INFECTION, AND CUTANEOUS ANERGY

Patients with acute toxic lupus manifest fever, a variety of constitutional signs and symptoms, as well as specific lupus manifestations. This is a potentially fatal disorder if not treated with corticosteroids, but prolonged high-dose therapy usually is not necessary. In addition, many patients with active disease have fever as part of their lupus flares. Nonetheless, infections also are important causes of fever in lupus patients because of both the underlying immune disorder and the anti-inflammatory–immunosuppressive therapy given to patients. Indeed, only a little over half of the time will the fever be due to the lupus disease alone.[131] A fever should always induce a serious consideration of infection. Patients receiving corticosteroids may have some of the signs of infection masked. Moreover, lupus patients commonly have impaired skin tests due to the disease itself. Therefore, a skin test for tuberculosis may be negative in a lupus patient with that disease. In addition, leukocytosis may not be present, but there often is a shift to the left in the CBC with increased percentages of granulocytes, including immature forms.[131]

Many infections occur as a result of prolonged high-dose corticosteroid therapy. Such therapy should be avoided whenever possible. However, when an infection occurs in a patient receiving corticosteroids, a balance must be achieved between reduction in the offending corticosteroids and the need for corticosteroids during the stress of the infection.

FATIGUE

Fatigue is a common concomitant of early lupus and a frequent major complaint later in the course.[70] It tends to be undertreated early and overtreated late in disease. Because fatigue may be an isolated finding, as a result of excess cytokine production, the benefit of vigorous therapy late in disease may be outweighed by the potential adverse effects of such therapy. This is a major challenge to the physician following patients with lupus.

REFERENCES

1. Abel T, Gladmann D, Urowitz MB: Neuropsychiatric lupus. J Rheumatol 7:3, 1980.
2. Adachi M, Watanabe-Fukunaga R, Nagata S: Aberrant transcription caused by the insertion of an early transposable element in an intron of the Fas antigen gene of lpr/lpr mice. Proc Natl Acad Sci USA 90:1159–1163, 1993.
3. Al-Janadi M, Al-Balla S, Al-Dalaan A, Raziuddin S: Cytokine profile in SLE, RA and other rheumatic diseases. J Clin Invest 13:58, 1993.
4. Amoura Z, Chabre H, Koutouzov A, et al: Nucleosome-restricted antibodies are detected before anti-dsDNA and/or antihistone antibodies. Arthritis Rheum 37:1684–1688, 1994.
5. Asherson RA: The catastrophic antiphospholipid syndrome. J Rheumatol 19:508–512, 1992.
6. Ballou SP, Khan MA, Kushner I: Clinical features of SLE: differences related to race and age of onset. Arthritis Rheum 25:55, 1982.
7. Bastian D, Borel H, Sasaki T, et al: Immune response to nucleic acid antigens and native DNA by human peripheral blood lymphocytes in vitro. J Immunol 135:1772–1777, 1985.
8. Becker TM, Lizzio EF, Merchant B, et al: Increased multiclonal antibody-forming cell activity in the peripheral blood of patients with SLE. Int Arch Allergy Appl Immunol 66:293–303, 1981.
9. Bevers EM, Galli M, Barbui T, et al: Lupus anticoagulant IgG's (LA) are not directed to phospholipids only, but to a complex of lipid-bound human prothrombin. Thromb Haemost 66:629–632, 1991.
10. Blaese RM, Grayson J, Steinberg AD: Elevated immunoglobulin secreting cells in the blood of patients with active systemic lupus erythematosus: correlation of laboratory and clinical assessment of disease activity. Am J Med 69:345–350, 1980.
11. Bluestein HG, Williams GW, Steinberg AD: Cerebrospinal fluid antibodies to neuronal cells: association with neuropsychiatric manifestations of systemic lupus erythematosus. Am J Med 70:240–246, 1981.
12. Bonfiglio TA, Botti RE, Hagstrom JWC: Coronary arteritis, occlusion, and myocardial infarction due to lupus erythematosus. Am Heart J 83:153, 1972.
13. Boumpas DT, Austin HA III, Vaughan EM, et al: Severe lupus nephritis: controlled trial of pulse methylprednisolone versus two different regimens of pulse cyclophosphamide. Lancet 340:741–745, 1992.
14. Boussiotis VA, Barber DL, Nakarai T, et al: Prevention of T cell anergy by signaling through the gamma-c chain of the IL-2 receptor. Science 266:1039–1042, 1994.
15. Budman DR, Merchant EB, Steinberg AD, et al: Increased spontaneous activity of antibody-forming cells in the peripheral blood of patients with active systemic lupus erythematosus. Arthritis Rheum 20:829–833, 1977.
16. Bulkley BH, Roberts WC: The heart in systemic lupus erythematosus and the changes induced by corticosteroid therapy. Am J Med 58:243–264, 1975.
17. Burlingame RW, Boey ML, Starkebaum G, Rubin RL: The central role

of chromatin in autoimmune responses in histones and DNA in SLE. J Clin Invest 94:184, 1994.

18. Buskila D, Gladman DD, Hanna W, Kahn HJ: Primary malignant lymphoma of the spleen in systemic lupus erythematosus. J Rheumatol 16:993–996, 1989.
19. Bywaters EGL: Jaccoud's syndrome: a sequel to the joint involvement of systemic lupus erythematosus. Clin Rheum Dis 1:125–148, 1975.
20. Callen JP: Mucocutaneous changes in patients with lupus erythematosus. The relationship of these lesions to systemic disease. Rheum Dis Clin North Am 14:79–97, 1988.
21. Carette S: Cardiopulmonary manifestations of lupus erythematosus. Rheum Dis Clin North Am 14:135–147, 1988.
22. Casciola-Rosen LA, Abhalt G, Rosen A: Autoantigens targeted in systemic lupus erythematosus are clustered in two populations of surface structures on apoptotic keratinocytes. J Exp Med 179:1317, 1994.
23. Chang RW: Cardiac manifestations of SLE. Clin Rheum Dis 8:197, 1982.
24. Compton LJ, Steinberg AD, Sano H: Nuclear DNA degradation in lymphocytes of patients with systemic lupus erythematosus. J Immunol 133:213–216, 1984.
25. Croft M, Swain SL: B cell response to fresh and effector T helper cells: role of cognate T-B interaction and the cytokines IL-2, IL-4 and IL-6. J Immunol 146:4055, 1991.
26. Datta SK, Patel H, Berry D: Induction of a cationic shift in IgG anti-DNA autoantibodies: role of helper T cells with classical and novel phenotypes in three murine models of lupus nephritis. J Exp Med 165:1252, 1987.
27. Dawisha SM, Gmelig-Meyling F, Steinberg AD: Assessment of clinical parameters associated with increased frequency of mutant T cells in patients with systemic lupus erythematosus. Arthritis Rheum 37:270–277, 1994.
28. Desai OD, Krishnan MR, Swindle JT, Marion TN: Antigen-specific induction of antibodies against mammalian DNA in non-autoimmune mice. J Immunol 151:1614–1626, 1993.
29. Dillon AM, Stein HB, English RA: Splenic atrophy in SLE. Ann Intern Med 96:40–43, 1982.
30. Dubois EL, Tuffanelli DL: Clinical manifestations of systemic lupus erythematosus. Computer analysis of 520 cases. JAMA 190:104, 1964.
31. Dueymes M, Barrier J, Bescancenot JF, et al: Relationship of IL-4 to isotypic distribution of anti-DS DNA antibodies in SLE. Int Arch Allergy Appl Immunol 101:408, 1993.
32. Dunckley J, Gatenby PA, Hawkins B, et al: Deficiency of C4A is a genetic determinant of systemic lupus erythematosus in three ethnic groups. J Immunogenet 14:209–218, 1987.
33. Emerit I, Michelson AM: Mechanism of photosensitivity in systemic lupus erythematosus patients. Proc Natl Acad Sci USA 78:2537–2541, 1981.
34. Erikson J, Radic MZ, Camper SA, et al: Expression of anti-DNA immunoglobulin transgenes in non-autoimmune mice. Nature 349:331, 1991.
35. Estes D, Christian CL: The natural history of systemic lupus erythematosus by prospective analysis. Medicine 50:85, 1971.
36. Feinglass EJ, Arnett FC, Dorsch CA, et al: Neuropsychiatric manifestations of systemic lupus erythematosus: diagnosis, clinical spectrum, and relationship to other features of the disease. Medicine 55:323, 1976.
37. Fessel WJ: Systemic lupus erythematosus in the community. Arch Intern Med 134:1027, 1974.
38. Finol HR, Montagnani S, Marquez A, et al: Ultrastructural pathology of skeletal muscle in systemic lupus erythematosus. J Rheumatol 8:917–924, 1990.
39. Fronek A, Timmerman LA, Alper CA, et al: Major histocompatibility complex genes and susceptibility to systemic lupus erythematosus. Arthritis Rheum 33:1542–1553, 1990.
40. Fuchs EJ, Matzinger P: B cells turn off virgin but not memory T cells. Science 258:1156–1159, 1992.
41. Gilkeson GS, Grudier JP, Karounos DG, Pisetsky DS: Induction of anti-double stranded DNA antibodies in normal mice by immunization with bacterial DNA. J Immunol 142:1482, 1989.
42. Ginsburg KS, Liang MH, Newcomer L, et al: Anticardiolipin antibodies and the risk for ischemic stroke and venous thrombosis. Ann Intern Med 117:997–1002, 1992.
43. Gmelig-Meyling F, Dawisha S, Steinberg AD: Assessment of in vivo frequency of mutated T-cells in patients with systemic lupus erythematosus. J Exp Med 175:297–300, 1992.
44. Goodnow CC: Transgenic mice and analysis of B-cell tolerance. Annu Rev Immunol 10:489, 1992.
45. Golan TD, Foltyn V, Roueff A: Increased susceptibility to in vitro ultraviolet B radiation in fibroblasts and lymphocytes cultured from systemic lupus erythematous patients. Clin Immunol Immunopathol 58:289–304, 1991.
46. Hagiwara E, Gourley M, Klinman DM: Cytokine abnormalities in SLE. Arthritis Rheum In press.
47. Harada T, Suziki N, Mizushima Y, Sakane T: Usage of a novel class of germ-line Ig variable region gene for cationic anti-DNA autoantibodies in human lupus nephritis. J Immunol 153:4806–4815, 1994.
48. Hardin JA: The lupus autoantigens and the pathogenesis of SLE. Arthritis Rheum 29:457, 1986.
49. Hartley SB, Cooke MP, Fulcher DA, et al: Elimination of self-reactive B lymphocytes proceeds in two stages: arrested development and cell death. Cell 72:325, 1993.
50. Hartung K, Fontana A, Klar M, et al: Association of class I, II, and III MHC gene products with systemic lupus erythematosus. Rheumatol Int 9:13–18, 1989.
51. Harvey AM, Shulman LE, Tumulty A, et al: Systemic lupus erythematosus: review of the literature and clinical analysis of 138 cases. Medicine 33:291, 1954.
52. Heinzel FP, Sadick MD, Mutha SS, Locksley RM: Production of IFN gamma, IL-2, IL-4 and IL-10 by CD4+ lymphocytes in vivo during healing and progressive murine leishmaniasis. Proc Natl Acad Sci USA 88:7011, 1991.
53. Herbert L: The clearance of immune complexes from the circulation of man and other primates. Am J Kidney Dis 17:352–361, 1991.
54. Hirano T, Taga T, Yasukawa K, et al: Human B-cell differentiation factor defined by anti-peptide antibody and its possible role in autoantibody production. Proc Natl Acad Sci USA 84:228, 1987.
55. Hochberg MC: The application of genetic epidemiology to systemic lupus erythematosus. J Rheumatol 14:867–869, 1987.
56. Holman H, Deicher HR: The reaction of the lupus erythematosus (LE) cell factor with deoxyribonucleoprotein of the nucleus. J Clin Invest 38:2069, 1959.
57. Inghirami G, Simon J, Balow JE, Tsokos GC: Activated T lymphocytes in the peripheral blood of patients with systemic lupus erythematosus induce B cells to produce immunoglobulin. Clin Exp Rheumatol 6:269–276, 1988.
58. Jacobelli S, Moreno R, Massardo L, et al: Inspiratory muscle dysfunction and unexplained dyspnea in systemic lupus erythematosus. Arthritis Rheum 28:781–788, 1985.
59. Jacobson JD, Nisula BC, Steinberg AD: Modulation of the expression of murine lupus by gonadotropin-releasing hormone agonism and antagonism. Endocrinology 134:2516–2523, 1994.
60. Jungers P, Dougados M, Pelissier C, et al: Influence of oral contraceptive therapy on the activity of systemic lupus erythematosus. Arthritis Rheum 25:618, 1982.
61. Kashgarian M: Lupus nephritis: lessons from the path lab. Kidney Int 45:928–938, 1994.
62. Klinman DM: Polyclonal B cell activation in lupus-prone mice precedes and predicts the development of autoimmune disease. J Clin Invest 86:1249, 1990.
63. Klinman DM, Shirai A, Conover J, Steinberg AD: Cross-reactivity of IgG anti-DNA secreting B cells in patients with systemic lupus erythematosus. Eur J Immunol 24:53–58, 1994.
64. Klinman DM, Steinberg AD: Systemic autoimmune disease arises from polyclonal B cell activation. J Exp Med 165:1755, 1987.
65. Klinman DM, Steinberg AD: Similar in vivo expansion of B cells from normal DBA/2 and autoimmune NZB mice in xid recipients. J Immunol 139:2284, 1987.
66. Klinman DM, Steinberg AD: Inquiry into murine and human lupus. Immunol Rev 144:157–193, 1995.
67. Korbet SM, Schwartz MM, Lewis EJ: Immune complex deposition and coronary vasculitis in systemic lupus erythematosus. Am J Med 77:141–145, 1984.
68. Krieg AM, Steinberg AD: Analysis of thymic endogenous retroviral expression in murine lupus: genetic and immune studies. J Clin Invest 86:809–816, 1990.
69. Krieg AM, Yi A-K, Matson S, et al: B cell activation induced by oligodeoxynucleotides or DNA containing un-methylated CpG motifs. Arthritis Rheum 37, 5379. Abstract.
70. Krupp LB, LaRocca NG, Muir J, Steinberg AD: A study of fatigue in systemic lupus erythematosus. J Rheumatol 17:1450–1452, 1990.

71. Lahita RG, Kunkel HG, Bradlow HL: Increased 17 oxidation of testosterone in SLE. Arthritis Rheum 26:1517–1521, 1983.
72. Larson DL: Systemic Lupus Erythematosus. Little Brown, Boston, 1961.
73. Laskin CA, Taurog JD, Smathers PA, Steinberg AD: Studies of defective tolerance in murine lupus. J Immunol 127:1743–1747, 1981.
74. Laskin CA, Smathers PA, Reeves JP, Steinberg AD: Studies of defective tolerance induction in NZB mice: evidence for a marrow pre-T cell defect. J Exp Med 155:1025–1036, 1982.
75. Laskin CA, Smathers PA, Lieberman R, Steinberg AD: NZB T cells actively interfere with the establishment of tolerance to BGG in radiation chimeras. J Immunol 131:1121–1125, 1983.
76. Laskin CA, Haddad G, Soloninka CA: The regulatory role of NZB T lymphocytes in the production of anti-DNA antibodies in vitro. J Immunol 137:1867, 1986.
77. Linker-Israeli M, Deans R, Wallace D, et al: Elevated levels of endogenous IL-6 in systemic lupus erythematosus. J Immunol 147:117, 1991.
78. Liszewski MK, Kahl LE, Atkinson JP. The functional role of complement genes in systemic lupus erythematosus and Sjogren's syndrome. Curr Opin Rheumatol 1:347–52, 1989.
79. Llorente L, Richaud-Patin Y, Wijdenes J, et al: Spontaneous production of interleukin-10 by B lymphocytes and monocytes in systemic lupus erythematosus. Eur Cytokine Netw 4:421, 1993.
80. Mamula MJ, Lin R-H, Janeway CA Jr, Hardin JA: Breaking of T cell tolerance with foreign and self co-immunogens: a study of autoimmune B and T cell epitopes of cytochrome c. J Immunol 149:789, 1992.
81. Matsuura E, Igarashi Y, Yasuda T, et al: Anticardiolipin antibodies recognize beta 2-glycoprotein I structure altered by interacting with an oxygen modified solid phase. J Exp Med 179:457–462, 1994.
82. McCarty GA, Rice JR, Bembe ML, Pisetsky DS: Independent expression of autoantibodies in SLE. J Rheumatol 9:691, 1982.
83. McGrath H: UV-A1 light decreases disease activity and eliminates antibodies in patients with systemic lupus erythematosus. In Urbach F (ed): Biological Responses to Ultraviolet A Irradiation. Valdenmar Publishing Co, Overland Park, KS, 1992, pp 257–260.
84. McNeil HP, Simpson RJ, Chesterman CN, et al: Anti-phospholipid antibodies are directed against a complex antigen that includes a lipid-binding inhibitor of coagulation: beta 2-glycoprotein I (apolipoprotein H). Proc Natl Acad Sci USA 87:4120–4124, 1990.
85. Messina JP, Gilkeson GS, Pisetsky DS: Determinants of anti-DNA antibody responses. J Immunol 147:1759, 1991.
86. Messina JP, Gilkeson GS, Pisetsky DS, et al: The influence of DNA structure on the in vitro stimulation of murine lymphocytes by natural and synthetic polynucleotide antigens. Cellular Immunol 147:148–157, 1993.
87. Metsarinne K, Nordstrom D, Konttinen Y, et al: Plasma interleukin-6 and renin substrate in reactive arthritis, rheumatoid arthritis and systemic lupus erythematosus. Rheumatol Int 12:93, 1992.
88. Miller FW, Moore GF, Weintraub BD, Steinberg AD: Prevalence of thyroid disease and thyroid function test abnormalities in patients with systemic lupus erythematosus. Arthritis Rheum 30:1124–1131, 1987.
89. Miller ML, Raveche ES, Laskin CA, et al: Genetic studies in NZB mice. VI. Association of autoimmune traits in recombinant inbred lines. J Immunol 133:1325–1331, 1984.
90. Miller ML, Cowdery JS, Laskin CA, Steinberg AD: Studies of tolerance in autoimmune mouse strains. In Strober W, Lamm ME, McGhee JR, James SP (eds): Mucosal Immunity and Infections at Mucosal Surfaces. Oxford University Press, New York, 1988, pp 119–131.
91. Mohan C, Adams S, Stanik V, Datta SK: Nucleosome: a major immunogen for pathogenic autoantibody-inducing T cells of lupus. J Exp Med 177:1367, 1993.
92. Morimoto C, Reinherz EL, Schlossman SF, et al: Alterations of immunoregulatory T cell subsets in active systemic lupus erythematosus. J Clin Invest 66:1171–1174, 1980.
93. Morimoto C, Reinherz EL, Distaso JA, et al: Relationship between SLE T cell subsets, anti-T cell antibodies and T cell functions. J Clin Invest 73:689–700, 1984.
94. Morton RO, Gershwin ME, Brady C, Steinberg AD: Incidence of systemic lupus erythematosus (SLE) in North American Indians. J Rheumatol 3:186–190, 1976.
95. Mosmann TR, Coffman RL: Th1 and Th2 cells: different patterns of lymphokine secretion lead to different functional properties. Annu Rev Immunol 7:147–171, 1989.
96. Murakami M, Tsubata T, Okamoto M, et al: Antigen-induced apoptotic death of Ly-1 B cells responsible for autoimmune disease in transgenic mice. Nature 357:77, 1992.
97. Nagafuchi H, Suzuki N, Mizushima Y, Sakane T: Constitutive expression of IL-6 receptors and their role in the excessive B cell function in patients with systemic lupus erythematosus. J Immunol 151:6525, 1993.
98. Nagata S, Golstein P: The Fas death factor. Science 267:1449–1456, 1995.
99. Nemazee D: Immune complexes can trigger specific T cell-dependent autoanti-Ig antibody production in mice. J Exp Med 161:242, 1985.
100. Norris DA: Pathomechanisms of photosensitive lupus erythematosus. J Invest Dermatol 100 (suppl):58, 1993.
101. Ogawa N, Itoh M, Goto Y: Abnormal production of B cell growth factor in patients with systemic lupus erythematosus. Clin Exp Immunol 89:26, 1992.
102. Okamoto M, Murakami M, Shimizu A, et al: A transgenic model of autoimmune hemolytic anemia. J Exp Med 175:71, 1992.
103. Oosting JD, Derksen RHWM, Bobbink IWG, et al: Antiphospholipid antibodies directed against a combination of phospholipids with prothrombin, protein C, or protein S: an explanation for their pathogenic mechanism? Blood 81:2618–2625, 1993.
104. Parker LM, Steinberg AD: The antibody response to polyinosinic. polycytidylic acid. J Immunol 110:742–751, 1973.
105. Parronchi P, DeCarli M, Manetti R, et al: IL-4 and IFN (alpha and gamma) exert opposite regulatory effects on the development of cytolytic potential by TH1 or TH2 human T cell clones. J Immunol 149:2977, 1992.
106. Pearce EJ, Caspar P, Grzych JM, et al: Downregulation of Th1 cytokine production accompanies induction of Th2 responses by a parasitic helminth, Schistosoma mansoni. J Exp Med 173:159, 1991.
107. Perlmutter DH, Colten HR: Complement molecular genetics. In Gallin JI, Goldstein IM, Snyderman R (eds): Inflammation. Raven Press, New York, 1992, pp 81–102.
108. Pisetsky DS, Caster SA: The B-cell repertoire for autoantibodies: frequency of precursor cells for anti-DNA antibodies. Cell Immunol 15:294, 1982.
109. Rajagopalan S, Mao C, Datta SK: Pathogenic autoantibody-inducing gamma/delta T helper cells from patients with lupus nephritis express unusual T cell receptors. Clin Immunol Immunopathol 62:344–350, 1992.
110. Rekvig OP, Hannestad K: Lupus erythematosus (LE) factors recognize both nucleosomes and viable human leukocytes. Scand J Immunol 13:597, 1981.
111. Raveche ES, Novotny EA, Hansen CT, et al: Genetic studies in NZB mice. V. Recombinant inbred lines demonstrate that separate genes control autoimmune phenotype. J Exp Med 153:1187–1197, 1981.
112. Reinertsen JL, Klippel JH, Johnson AH, et al: B-lymphocyte alloantigens associated with systemic lupus erythematosus. N Engl J Med 299:515–518, 1978.
113. Reinertsen JL, Klippel JH, Johnson AH, et al: Family studies of B lymphocyte alloantigens in systemic lupus erythematosus. J Rheumatol 9:253–262, 1982.
114. Robey FA, Jones KD, Steinberg AD: C-Reactive protein mediates the solubilization of nuclear DNA by complement in vitro. J Exp Med 161:1344–1356, 1985.
115. Rosenstein BS, Rosenstein RB, Zamansky GB: Repair of DNA damage induced in systemic lupus erythematosus skin fibroblasts by simulated sunlight. J Invest Dermatol 98:469–474, 1992.
116. Rothfield NF: The kidney in systemic lupus erythematosus. Contrib Nephrol 7:128, 1977.
117. Rothfield NF, Stollar BD: The relation of Ig class, pattern of antinuclear antibody and complement fixing antibodies to DNA in sera from patients with SLE. J Clin Invest 46:1785, 1967.
118. Rothstein TL, Wang JKM, Panka DJ, et al: Protection against Fas-dependent Th1 mediated apoptosis by antigen receptor engagement in B cells. Nature 374:163–165, 1995.
119. Roubey RAS, Pratt CW, Buyon JP, Winfield JB: Lupus anticoagulant activity of autoimmune phospholipid antibodies is dependent upon beta 2-glycoprotein I. J Clin Invest 90:1100–1104, 1992.
120. Sano H, Imokawa M, Steinberg AD, Morimoto C: Accumulation of guanine-cytosine-enriched low M.W. DNA fragments in lymphocytes of patients with systemic lupus erythematosus. J Immunol 130:187–190, 1983.
121. Schifferli JA, Ng YC, Estreicher J, Walport MJ: The clearance of tetanus-antitetanus toxoid complexes from the circulation of humans.

Complement and erythrocyte complement receptor I-dependent mechanisms. J Immunol 140:899–904, 1988.
122. Schur PH, Marcus-Bagley D, Awdeh Z, et al: The effect of ethnicity on major histocompatibility complex complement allotypes in patients with systemic lupus erythematosus. Arthritis Rheum 33:985–992, 1990.
123. Schwarz T, Lugar TA: Effect of UV irradiation on epidermal cell cytokine production. J Photochem Photobiol B 4:1–13, 1989.
124. Segal AM, Calabrese LH, Ahmad M, et al: The pulmonary manifestations of systemic lupus erythematosus. Semin Arthritis Rheum 14:2020–224, 1985.
125. Serdula MK, Rhoads GG: Frequency of systemic lupus erythmatosus in different ethnic groups in Hawaii. Arthritis Rheum 22:328, 1979.
126. Shan H, Shlomchik MJ, Marshak-Rothstein A, et al: The mechanism of autoantibody production in an autoimmune MRL/lpr mouse. J Immunol 153:5104–5120, 1994.
127. Smolen JS, Morimoto C, Steinberg AD, et al: Systemic lupus erythematosus: delineation of subpopulations by clinical, serologic and T-cell marker analysis. Am J Med Sci 289:139–147, 1985.
128. Smolen JS, Klippel JH, Penner E, et al: HLA-DR antigens in systemic lupus erythematosus: association with specificity of autoantibody responses to nuclear antigens. Ann Rheum Dis 46:457–462, 1987.
129. Solinger AM: Drug-related lupus. Clinical and etiological considerations. Rheum Dis Clin North Am 14:187–202, 1988.
130. Spronk P, Ter Borg E, Limburg P, Kallenberg C: Plasma concentration of IL-6 in systemic lupus erythematosus: an indicator of disease activity? Clin Exp Immunol 90:106, 1992.
131. Stahl NI, Klippel JH, Decker JL: Fever in systemic lupus erythematosus. Am J Med 67:935, 1979.
132. Steinberg AD: The treatment of lupus nephritis. Kidney Int 30:769–787, 1986.
133. Steinberg AD: Cyclophosphamide. In Austin KF, Burakoff S, Rosen F, Strom T (eds): Therapeutic Immunology. Blackwell Scientific Pub Inc, Cambridge, MA, 1996, pp 23–43.
134. Steinberg AD, Baron S, Talal N: The pathogenesis of autoimmunity in New Zealand mice. I. Induction of anti-nucleic acid antibodies by polyinosinic.polycytidylic acid. Proc Natl Acad Sci USA 63:1102, 1969.
135. Steinberg AD, Chused TM, Jacobs ME, Talal N: Cyclophosphamide tolerance as a test for antigenicity of nucleic acids. Nature 228:1090, 1970.
136. Steinberg AD, Gourley MF, Klinman DM, et al: Systemic lupus erythematosus. Ann Intern Med 115:548–559, 1991.
137. Steinberg AD, Krieg AM, Gourley MF, Klinman DM: Theoretical and experimental approaches to generalized autoimmunity. Immunol Rev 118:129–163, 1990.
138. Steinberg AD, Raveche ES, Laskin CA, et al: Systemic lupus erythematosus: insights from animal models. Ann Intern Med 100:714–727, 1984.
139. Steinberg AD, Steinberg SC: Long-term preservation of renal function in patients with lupus nephritis randomized to receive cyclophosphamide-containing regimens as compared with prednisone only. Arthritis Rheum 34:945–950, 1991.
140. Steinberg BJ, Steinberg AD: Lupus disease activity associated with menstrual cycle. J Rheumatol 12:816–817, 1985.
141. Steinsson K, Erlendsson K, Valdimarsson H: Successful plasma infusion treatment of a patient with C2 deficiency and systemic lupus erythematosus. Clinical experience over forty-five months. Arthritis Rheum 32:906–913, 1989.
142. Steller H: Mechanisms and genes of cellular suicide. Science 267:1445–1449, 1995.
143. Stollar BD, Schwartz RS: Monoclonal anti-DNA antibodies: the targets and origins of SLE autoantibodies. Ann NY Acad Sci 465:192, 1986.
144. Suematsu S, Matsuda T, Aozasa K, et al: IgG 1 plasmacytosis in interleukin 6 transgenic mice. Proc Natl Acad Sci USA 86:7547, 1989.
145. Suzuki N, Sakane T, Engleman EG: Anti-DNA antibody production by CD5+ and CD5− B cells of patients with systemic lupus erythematosus. J Clin Invest 85:238, 1990.
146. Swaak AJG, van Rooyen A, Aarden LA: Interleukin-6 and acute phase proteins in the disease course of patients with systemic lupus erythematosus. Rheumatol Int 8:263, 1990.
147. Tan EM, Cohen AS, Fries JF, et al: The 1982 revised criteria for the classification of systemic lupus erythematosus. Arthritis Rheum 25:1271–1277, 1982.
148. Tanaka T, Hu-Li J, Seder RA, et al: IL-4 suppresses IL-2 and IFN-gamma production by naive T cells stimulated by accessory cell-dependent receptor engagement. Proc Natl Acad Sci USA 90:5914, 1993.
149. Tanaka Y, Kazuyoshi S, Shirakawa F, et al: Production of B-cell stimulatory factors by B cells in patients with SLE. J Immunol 141:3043, 1988.
150. Thompson CB: Apoptosis in the pathogenesis and treatment of disease. Science 267:1456–1462, 1995.
151. Umland S, Lee R, Howard M, Martens C: Expression of lymphokine genes in splenic lymphocytes of autoimmune mice. Mol Immunol 26:649, 1989.
152. Underwood JR, Pederson JS, Chalmers PJ, Toh BH: Hybrids from normal, germ free, nude and neonatal mice produce monoclonal autoantibodies to eight different intracellular structures. Clin Exp Immunol 60:417, 1985.
153. Watanabe-Fukunaga R, Brannan CI, Copeland NG, et al: Lymphoproliferation disorder in mice explained by defects in Fas antigen that mediates apoptosis. Nature 356:314–317, 1992.
154. Webb S, Morris C, Sprent C: Extrathymic tolerance of mature T cells: clonal elimination as a consequence of immunity. Cell 63:1249–1256, 1990.
155. Wu J, Zhou T, He J, Mountz JD: Autoimmune disease in mice due to integration of an endogenous retrovirus in an apoptosis gene. J Exp Med 178:461, 1993.
156. Wu J, Zhou T, Zhang J, et al: Correction of accelerated autoimmune disease by early replacement of the mutated *lpr* gene with the normal *fas* apoptosis gene in the T-cells of transgenic MRL-*lpr/lpr* mice. Proc Natl Acad Sci (USA) 91:2344–2348, 1994.
157. Yee AM, Yip YK, Fischer HD, Buyon JP: Serum activity that confers acid lability to alpha-interferon in systemic lupus erythematosus: its association with disease activity and its independence from circulating alpha-interferon. Arthritis Rheum 33:563–568, 1990.
158. Yokoyama H, Takabatake T, Takeeda M, Wada T: Up-regulated MHC-class II expression and gamma-IFN and soluble IL-2R in lupus nephritis. Kidney Int 42:755, 1992.
159. Zhou T, Bluthmann H, Zhang J, et al: Tolerance defect in SEB-induced T cells of MRL-lpr/lpr mice after neonatal SEB. J Exp Med 176:1063–1072, 1992.
160. Zizic TM, Classen JN, Stevens MB: Acute abdominal complications of systemic lupus erythematosus and polyarteritis nodosa. Am J Med 73:525–531, 1982.

51 Systemic Sclerosis (Scleroderma)

BARRY L. GRUBER

Systemic sclerosis represents a generalized connective tissue disorder with distinct autoimmune features. The pathology of systemic sclerosis is characterized by microvascular alterations and excessive fibrosis involving multiple organs. Most commonly the dermis is involved, hence the term scleroderma (hard skin), although cases of systemic sclerosis without skin involvement have been described (sine scleroderma). Scleroderma also may occur in the absence of systemic involvement. A classification system proposed by investigators in the field involves categorizing patients with disease restricted to the skin as localized scleroderma or systemic sclerosis (Table 51–1). The latter is further subdivided into limited or diffuse forms, defined by the extent of involved skin. This classification system has proven useful for purposes of clinical management, as well as prognosis.

Scleroderma refers to a process whereby cutaneous tissue thickens and represents the clinical hallmark of this disorder. Systemic involvement is absent in localized scleroderma, a clinically heterogenous group of dermatoses that may manifest as a patch of skin thickening (morphea), extensive bands of thickening (linear scleroderma), or in some cases, widespread generalized cutaneous thickening (generalized morphea). Systemic sclerosis, in contrast, affects particular internal organs, such as the heart, lungs, kidneys, or gastrointestinal tract. The skin involvement in systemic sclerosis invariably begins in the digits and progresses proximally over time. In the majority of patients, the development of scleroderma curiously halts as it ascends along the distal extremities without ever involving the trunk (limited). In others, the skin pattern becomes generalized (diffuse), distinguished by truncal involvement.

Recognizing these distinct patterns of skin involvement has proven of utmost significance, as the natural course of disease and prognosis tend to be divergent, especially over the first several years. The differences encompass distinct clinical manifestations, serologic findings, and associated morbidity and mortality, as described in detail later. These observations authenticate the concept of subdividing systemic sclerosis into limited and diffuse forms, which some even contend may represent different diseases.[46] Criteria for the diagnosis and classification of systemic sclerosis have been developed to ensure uniformity when comparing patients from one center to the next, especially important in the design of clinical trials, collecting epidemiologic data, and understanding the natural history of this disease (Table 51–2).[96]

EPIDEMIOLOGY AND NATURAL HISTORY

Many individuals view scleroderma as a rare disease; certainly many lay people are not familiar with the term. As mentioned previously, systemic sclerosis represents a broad spectrum of disease, especially if one includes the localized forms of scleroderma. Using the criteria set forth by the American Rheumatism Association (see Table 51–2), one can identify patients with 97% sensitivity and 98% specificity.[96]

The reported incidence of systemic sclerosis has varied considerably in the literature, in part due to differences in case definition and time periods of observation. Earlier studies suggested an incidence of 0.6 to 2.3 per million per year, based on hospital diagnoses.[55] Later surveys, including ambulatory and inpatient cases, indicate annual incidence rates of 6.3 to 12.0 per million per year.[93] A study at an academic center with a major interest in this disorder reported an incidence of 18.7 per million per year, based on data between 1973 and 1982.[89] These numbers suggest that the incidence of systemic sclerosis is likely to be on the rise, although enhanced physician awareness may partially account for the increase in reported cases.

The prevalence of systemic sclerosis can only be calculated based on incidence data available and life span of patients, since no study has been published to directly address this. A community-based prevalence estimated 253 per million at a particular point in time (1980), whereas other studies approximate 126 per million over a time interval.[56] An ongoing field study of individuals with Raynaud's phenomenon in South Carolina suggests that many cases are not being diagnosed.[51] There are probably at least 200,000 cases of systemic sclerosis in the United States.

Systemic sclerosis affects two to three times more females than males, with an increasing incidence peaking between ages 45 and 64. Rarely does the disease occur in children or males under age 30. The disease affects blacks and whites at similar rates but appears to be more severe in black women. The mortality from the disease may be rising, with age-adjusted mortality rates estimated at 3.08 per million.

Families have been reported with disease occurring in

first-degree relatives, although this remains a rare event. Perhaps more common is the finding of first-degree relatives with other autoimmune diseases, such as systemic lupus erythematosus or rheumatoid arthritis. This is often cited to support the concept of genetic factors but may also be evidence for environmental influences. Genetic influences are discussed in more detail later.

Environmental influences continue to intrigue investigators in the field.[28] Implicated agents include vinyl chloride, epoxy resins, organic solvents, silica and silicone implants, bleomycin, contaminants in denatured rapeseed oil associated with toxic oil syndrome, and certain lots of tryptophan associated with eosinophilia-myalgia syndrome. Each of these compounds can trigger a distinct clinical syndrome with varying degrees of fibrosis, which must be differentiated from idiopathic systemic sclerosis (Table 51–3).[28]

CLINICAL MANIFESTATIONS

Initial presentations of systemic sclerosis vary somewhat depending on the subset of disease, but Raynaud's phenomenon is characteristic. These individuals report that either cold or emotional stress leads to episodic, migratory vasospasm of distal digits, appearing initially with pallor, then cyanosis, and finally deep red discoloration. This triphasic response is secondary to ischemia, desaturation of hemoglobin, and then reactive hyperemia. Associated pain is common. Almost all patients who ultimately develop limited scleroderma have Raynaud's phenomenon, often for many years preceding any skin manifestations. Approximately three fourths of patients destined to develop diffuse scleroderma present with Raynaud's phenomenon, although typically the skin disease manifests shortly thereafter (within 2 years) or simultaneously. Very few individuals develop systemic sclerosis in the absence of Raynaud's phenomenon; this presentation should prompt the clinician to consider scleroderma-like conditions (see Table 51–3). If systemic sclerosis evolves in the rare patient without Raynaud's phenomenon, the prognosis is quite poor for unclear reasons.[106]

TABLE 51–1
CLASSIFICATION—CLINICAL SUBSETS

Systemic Sclerosis:

Often associated with constitutional symptoms, visceral and musculoskeletal involvement, and abnormal immune responses.

Diffuse disease: Cutaneous thickening involves the trunk, in addition to the face and extremities.

Limited disease: Cutaneous thickening limited to distal extremities and face, previously known as CREST-associated with calcinosis, Raynaud's, esophageal dysmotility, sclerodactyly, and telangiectasias.

Sine scleroderma: Systemic disease in the absence of cutaneous thickening, with characteristic fibrosis and vascular disease of viscera associated with typical serologic responses.

Localized Sclerosis:

Notably absent visceral involvement or constitutional symptoms.

Morphea: Sclerotic circumscribed patches with surrounding violaceous halo, occasionally becomes generalized with widespread involvement.

Linear scleroderma: Bands of cutaneous fibrosis, usually involving extremities; includes en coup de sabre (involvement of frontal or frontoparietal facial area).

TABLE 51–2
PRELIMINARY CRITERIA FOR CLASSIFICATION OF SYSTEMIC SCLEROSIS*

Major Criteria

Proximal scleroderma: Symmetric thickening, tightening, and induration of the skin of the fingers and proximal to the metacarpophalangeal or metatarsophalangeal joints. The changes may affect the entire extremity, face, neck, and trunk (thorax and abdomen).

Minor Criteria

Sclerodactyly: Skin changes limited to fingers.

Digital pitting scars or loss of substance from the finger pad: Depressed areas at tips of fingers or loss of digital pad tissue as a result of ischemia.

Bibasilar pulmonary fibrosis: Bilateral reticular pattern of linear or lineonodular densities most pronounced in basilar portions of the lungs on standard chest x-ray; may assume appearance of diffuse mottling or honeycomb. These changes should not be attributable to primary lung disease.

*These criteria were established for classifying patients in clinical trials, population surveys, and other studies. A person receives a diagnosis of systemic sclerosis if one major criterion or two or more minor criteria listed are present. Localized disease is excluded from this classification.
Subcommittee for Scleroderma Criteria of the American Rheumatism Association Diagnostic and Therapeutic Criteria Committee: Preliminary criteria for the classification of systemic sclerosis (scleroderma). Arthritis Rheum 23:581–590, 1980.
Alfonse T. Masi, MD, DRPH: Cochairman, Subcommittee for Scleroderma Criteria, ARA; Gerald P. Rodman, MD: Cochairman, Subcommittee for Scleroderma Criteria, ARA; Thomas A. Medsger, Jr., MD: Central Coordinator of the Scleroderma Criteria Cooperative Study; Roy D. Altman, MD; William A. D'Angelo, MD; James F. Fries, MD; E. Carwile LeRoy, MD; Allan B. Kirsner, MD; Allen H. MacKenzie, MD; Dennis J. McShane, MD; Allen R. Myers, MD; Gordon C. Sharp, MD.

It is now possible to assess an individual with Raynaud's phenomenon on initial encounter and predict those destined to evolve to systemic sclerosis or related connective tissue disease. Only those patients without any detectable clinical or serologic abnormalities should be classified as having a benign form of Raynaud's syndrome. From a practical standpoint, the most useful parameters to critically examine include the nailfold capillary beds and the presence of antinuclear and anticentromere antibodies. The nailfold capillary beds may reveal distorted architecture with characteristic patterns for systemic sclerosis.[50] The normal pattern of delicate, symmetric hairpin loops of capillaries is distinguished from either dilated, bushy, tortuous, thickened capillary loops (Fig. 51–1) or regions of capillary dropout (this latter finding being more specific for systemic sclerosis). These structural alterations are readily appreciated at the bedside with an inexpensive, small, hand-held illuminated microscope yielding 20- to 30-fold magnification (or even with an ophthalmoscope). If these abnormalities are detected, then prognostic insight has been gained, with recognition of this disease at its earliest stage. Nonetheless, many years may elapse before additional manifestations appear.

The early finding of Raynaud's phenomenon is frequently succeeded by puffy, edematous swelling of the fingers and hands. This presentation is not specific for systemic sclerosis and at this stage has been referred to as undifferentiated connective tissue disease.[47] This condition may evolve to systemic sclerosis or, alternatively, rheumatoid arthritis, systemic lupus erythematosus, overlap syndrome, or dermato-

TABLE 51–3
SCLERODERMA-LIKE CONDITIONS

Eosinophilic Fasciitis:

Inflammation and thickening involving the deep fascia; onset usually after vigorous exercise or trauma, especially in males. Rapid onset of pain and swelling of the extremities followed by progressive induration of skin and subcutaneous tissues of forearms, legs, and occasionally hands, feet, and face, leaving a thick orange-peel appearance with furrowing of the subcutis. Hematologic disorders, including aplastic anemia and myeloproliferative disorders, have been noted in association.

Scleredema (Buschke's scleredema):

Self-limited disease characterized by indurated edema of neck, shoulder girdle, and upper extremities (sparing hands); usually regresses within 12 to 18 months without sequelae. A second variety is recognized, manifesting as widespread cutaneous sclerosis with an extremely chronic course, in association with severe insulin-resistant diabetes. Absence of Raynaud's phenomenon and sparing of hands allow for differentiating from systemic sclerosis. The dermal histopathology reveals excessive collagen and proteoglycans.

Scleromyxedema:

Also known as papular mucinosis or lichen myxedematosus, this scleroderma-like condition presents as aggregated lichenoid papules, which may form generalized plaques with thickening and hardening of the skin. Excessive mucin deposition leads to immobile and mask-like facies and contracture of the fingers. The major difference with idiopathic scleroderma is that, in contrast to tight, thickened skin bound down to underlying structures, the skin becomes pendulous and folded. Systemic involvement is occasionally seen with Raynaud's phenomenon, esophageal dysmotility, and inflammatory myopathy. Paraproteinemia is frequently associated, usually of IgG γ type. Histopathology reveals excessive fibroblast proliferation, collagen, proteoglycan, and hyaluronic acid accumulation in the upper dermis.

Porphyria Cutanea Tarda (PCT):

Scleroderma-like changes seen in PCT are most like morphea or generalized morphea, with no visceral involvement. The usual areas affected include the chest, *V*-shaped area of the neck, face, and hands. Immunoglobulin deposition helps distinguish the histopathology from morphea.

Chronic Graft-Versus-Host Disease:

Rarely seen since the advent of cyclosporin usage in transplant settings, GVHD may cause scleroderma-like cutaneous changes.

Acrodermatitis Chronica Atrophicans:

Poorly demarcated, violaceous infiltrates on the distal parts of the extremities, which may spread proximally to the groin region or elbows. The skin becomes atrophied and wrinkled, with a mottled appearance and sclerodermatous changes. Most cases are caused by *Borrelia burgdorferi* and will respond to antibiotics.

Environmental Scleroderma-Like Conditions:

Toxic oil syndrome: An epidemic of acute pneumonitis associated with neuromyopathy, followed by scleroderma-like skin thickening, affected thousands of individuals in Spain in 1981; linked to a tainted rapeseed oil.

Eosinophilic myalgia syndrome: A similar syndrome, with a slightly different spectrum of clinical features, was linked to contaminated L-tryptophan in 1989 in the United States.

Other compounds: Vinyl chloride, epoxy resins, chlorinated hydrocarbons, pesticides, drugs such as bleomycin, pentazocine, or ethosuximide, silicon, and others may all stimulate sclerotic responses in skin or lung.

myositis. Symptoms at this stage often include morning stiffness, arthralgia, and parasthesias from carpal tunnel syndrome.

After several months, skin thickening begins on the digits, and the sensation of puffy edema (sausaging) becomes progressively less apparent. The skin appears taut, shiny, and indurated. Gradually the edematous phase is replaced by induration, and the dermis becomes firmly bound to underlying structures. Normal skin lines and creases, as well as hair appendages, disappear. The face and neck are frequently involved next. The face becomes mask-like, with loss of normal facial lines, thinning of the lips, and radial furrowing about the mouth (Fig. 51–2). As the skin thickening progresses, flexion of the digits becomes impaired and contractures develop. The ability to open the mouth may become progressively limited with the development of microstomia (see Fig. 51–2). Widespread areas of hyperpigmentation and hypopigmentation may develop. Mat-like telangiectasias, particularly on the face and upper trunk, may also develop. Over time, the skin changes spread at a variable rate in an ascending fashion over the distal extremities. The thickening may then spontaneously halt (limited scleroderma) or continue to involve the entire trunk, abdomen, and legs (diffuse scleroderma). At late stages, years after the onset of skin changes, atrophy predominates, with thin, fragile, and lax dermis.

The diagnosis of scleroderma is predicated on clinical grounds, with biopsy of the involved tissue rarely necessary. Monitoring skin changes is important, since the rate of progression and extent of involvement are related to overall prognosis and organ involvement. A variety of methods have been proposed, but perhaps the most widely used is the total Rodnan scoring system.[95] In this scheme, regions of the body are scored based on the degree of palpable thickening from 0 to 4 and recorded similar to a burn diagram. The total score is a useful parameter for assessing the response to therapy or progression of disease between visits. This scoring by experienced clinicians has been shown to correlate well with skin biopsy weights and hydroxyproline content.[73]

Internal organ involvement remains a dreaded complication of systemic sclerosis. Two processes affect organ functions: one is related to the vascular alterations, and the other results from progressive accumulation of extracellular matrix. Raynaud's phenomenon and capillary bed abnormalities are representative of a more widespread underlying vascular process. Structural changes in microvessels is perhaps the single most important early pathologic event in this disease.[66] The physiologic consequences of these abnormalities are illustrated with newer techniques that allow blood flow assessment in various internal organs during episodes of Raynaud's phenomenon. Cold-induced vasospasm leads to

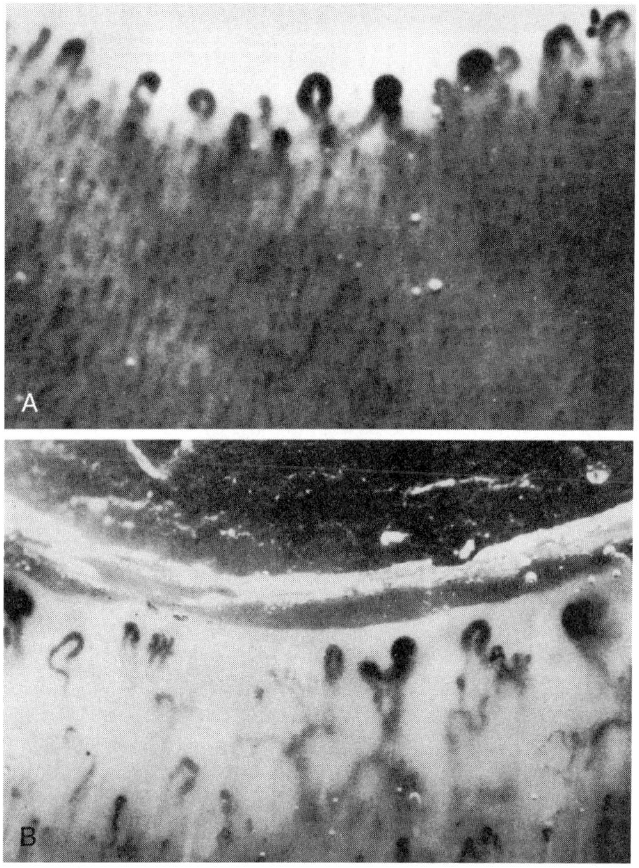

FIGURE 51–1. Nailfold capillary beds in two individuals with systemic sclerosis. **(A)** The normal delicate hairpin loops are mostly preserved or slightly thickened, with minimal disruption of the normal architecture. **(B)** An individual with more advanced disease, including a paucity of capillary loops (capillary dropout), vascular tortuosity, and gross dilatation of other loops. The latter findings are more disease specific for systemic sclerosis.

myocardial perfusion defects and transient wall abnormalities, as seen by scintigraphy or echocardiography. Alterations in pulmonary diffusing capacity and redistribution in pulmonary and renal blood flow have all been described with cold exposure in patients with systemic sclerosis.[80] These observations have their correlate with the clinical manifestation of renal crisis presenting more frequently during the winter.

Patients with systemic sclerosis often manifest generalized symptoms, such as fatigue, malaise, weight loss, hair loss, and rarely low-grade fevers. In addition, specific organ systems may be afflicted.

MUSCULOSKELETAL

Arthralgias are a common complaint, often in the absence of detectable synovitis. Careful studies, however, have documented erosive arthropathy in almost one third of patients.[3] The pattern of distribution is frequently symmetric, involving the fingers, wrists, knees, and ankles. Occasionally the synovitis may mimic rheumatoid arthritis. More common is the combined influence of skin changes, tenosynovial (periarticular) involvement, and moderate degrees of joint inflammation, all leading to impaired joint mobility, stiffness, pain, and swelling. Patients with diffuse scleroderma will commonly report a squeaking sensation when using afflicted joints. On examination, a palpable leathery crepitus can be appreciated with repetitive joint motion. This results from fibrinous deposits within tendon structures.[79] These tendon friction rubs are relatively specific for diffuse disease. Hence a patient with early and limited skin involvement, who demonstrates tendon friction rubs, will more often than not develop diffuse disease. It is not uncommon for these patients to rapidly progress to diffuse skin involvement. Carpal tunnel syndrome may also be seen, resulting from a similar process of fibrinous deposits and edema compromising the median nerve.

X-rays of affected areas may reveal calcific deposits within subcutaneous tissues (calcinosis) and resorption of the terminal tufts of distal phalanges. In advanced cases, the entire terminal phalanx undergoes dissolution (Fig. 51–3).

GASTROINTESTINAL

The entire intestinal tract can be affected by scleroderma, beginning with significant limitation in achieving adequate

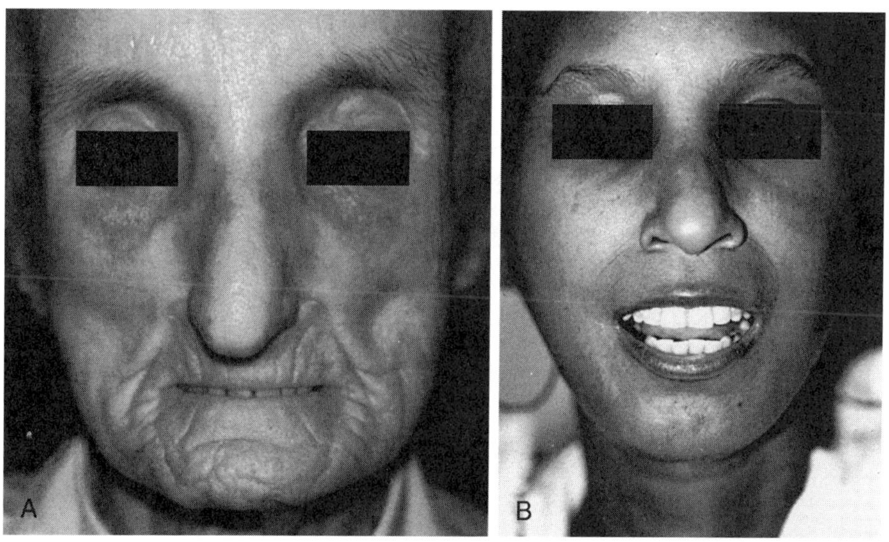

FIGURE 51–2. (A) A patient with long-standing scleroderma. Note the prominent telangiectasias on the nose and periorbital region. The perioral radial furrowing of skin about the lips is characteristic of scleroderma. **(B)** A younger individual with scleroderma demonstrating the marked restriction when maximally opening the mouth. The resultant microstomia, as demonstrated in this patient holding her mouth as wide open as possible, may interfere with normal eating. This patient was forced to nourish herself with a liquid diet using only straws.

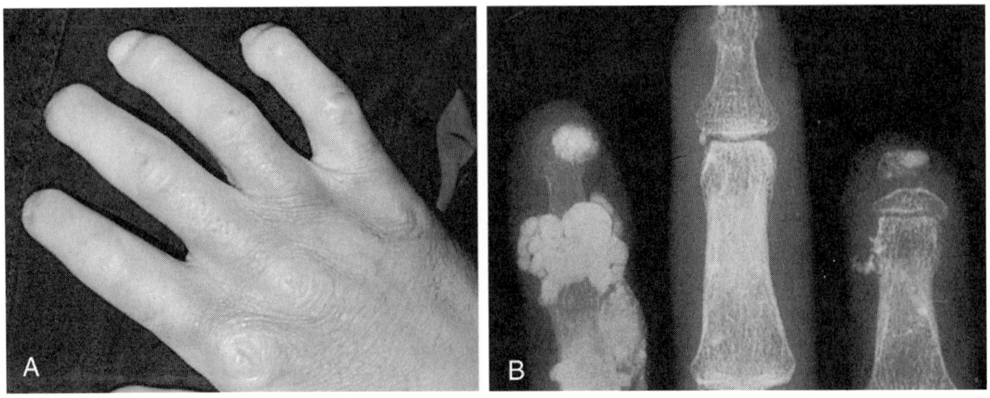

FIGURE 51–3. **(A)** Digits of a patient with long-standing systemic sclerosis and Raynaud's phenomenon. Over time, the patient experienced numerous pitting ulcerations at the tip of the digits and gradual loss of distal digital pulp tissue, especially in the index and middle fingers. **(B)** Radiographs of another individual with calcific deposits along the distal interphalangeal joints and other areas of punctate calcinosis. There is osseous resorption at the distal aspect in the digit on the far right.

nutrition because of difficulty opening the mouth.[84] This problem of nutrition and maintaining good oral hygiene is further complicated by the hand deformities and finger contractures. The oral cavity may also be affected by alterations in periodontal structures, leading to gingivitis and loosening of teeth, as well as associated Sjögren's syndrome in some patients.

Esophageal dysfunction is the most common visceral manifestation of systemic sclerosis, occurring in over 80% of patients. No difference in occurrence of esophageal involvement is noted between patients with limited or diffuse scleroderma. In some cases, esophageal dysfunction can be observed in the absence of skin findings (systemic sclerosis sine scleroderma). The fibrinous thickening that occurs in the submucosa and the muscularis leads to dysfunctional propulsive forces along the esophagus, with solid food lodging in the distal portion. The lower esophageal sphincter also becomes impaired, with acid reflux resulting in chronic esophagitis and subsequent strictures. Abnormalities are readily detected by cinefluoroscopic examination in the majority of patients or, alternatively, by radionuclide scintigraphy, pH monitoring, or esophageal manometry.

Some patients develop intestinal involvement, with complaints of bloating, cramps, and episodic diarrhea. Severe hypomotility may lead to malabsorption, weight loss, and profound wasting, often with bacterial overgrowth compounding the problem. The bowel atony may, at times, produce a pseudo-obstruction with a functional ileus. Another complication is pneumatosis cystoides intestinalis, in which air enters and tracks within the bowel wall.

Colonic involvement is common in systemic sclerosis, manifesting as constipation, often alternating with diarrhea. The fibrinous accumulation leads to functional hypomotility, similar to proximal portions of the alimentary tract. In addition, a peculiar finding is wide-mouthed diverticula as a result of patchy atrophy of mucosa along the antimesenteric border of the transverse and descending colon.

In addition to the abnormalities in the gastrointestinal tract, primary biliary cirrhosis may occur in patients with long-standing systemic sclerosis. Conversely, clinical evidence for systemic sclerosis exists in a portion of patients with primary biliary cirrhosis in association with anticentromere antibodies.[14]

PULMONARY

Whereas several years ago patients with systemic sclerosis succumbed to renal crisis, pulmonary manifestations have emerged as the leading cause of mortality. Lung disease occurs in nearly three quarters of individuals with systemic sclerosis,[61] with over half of the patients experiencing exertional dyspnea. Most patients have an insidious onset, frequently asymptomatic for some time, despite progressive involvement noted by pulmonary function testing or radiographs. The lack of symptoms is gradually replaced by diminished physical activity, nonproductive cough, and increasing exertional dyspnea. The examination may reveal dry bibasilar crackles or signs of pulmonary hypertension or be entirely normal.

Patients with diffuse disease are at highest risk for the development of interstitial fibrosis, especially in the earliest stages of progressive skin involvement. Patients with limited scleroderma may develop interstitial disease, but a unique feature observed after 10 to 30 years in these individuals is isolated pulmonary hypertension in the absence of interstitial changes.[77] The fibrotic process within the pulmonary interstitium is frequently accompanied by an inflammatory process, with accumulations of lymphocytes, macrophages, neutrophils, and variable numbers of eosinophils.

Chest radiographs are relatively insensitive for the detection of pulmonary involvement, although the addition of high-resolution computed tomography (CT) has proven quite useful.[99] In fact, the pattern of a ground-glass appearance on CT scan correlates well with inflammatory interstitial lung disease.[100] However, pulmonary function testing remains the mainstay of diagnostic tools. Restrictive defects are found in over two thirds of patients, regardless of disease subset. In addition, patients with late limited disease may develop isolated impaired diffusion capacity of carbon monoxide as a result of primary hypertension (in the absence of restrictive abnormalities). This dreaded complication occurs in a small percentage (less than 10%) of patients with limited scleroderma.

Based on several clinical series, it appears that not all patients with abnormal pulmonary function testing and established lung disease manifest progressive deterioration.[90] Patients with a poor outcome appear to include those who are young, black, or male.[90] Another concern is an apparent increased prevalence of lung cancer, especially in the setting of long-standing pulmonary fibrosis.[25, 54] The reported lung cancers are of varying histologic types, not merely alveolar cell carcinoma, which is frequently associated with advanced scar tissue.

CARDIAC

Myocardial dysfunction, with clinical evidence of congestive heart failure, occurs in less than 5% of patients with systemic sclerosis and almost always in the setting of diffuse disease.[61] More subtle involvement can be demonstrated by noninvasive radiologic techniques or continuous electrocardiography in nearly half of the patients. Pericardial effusions or thickening, usually asymptomatic, are commonly noted using echocardiography. Autopsy series reveal myocardial fibrosis in most patients, with contraction band necrosis suggesting episodic vascular spasm (intramyocardial Raynaud's disease). For the most part, coronary arteries are spared, but the small vasculature is affected, leading to patchy fibrosis. The fibrosis may involve the conduction system, causing complete heart block or arrhythmias.[69, 72]

Other causes of cardiac problems in systemic sclerosis relate to the secondary effects of advanced lung or renal disease. Cor pulmonale develops in the late stages of patients with pulmonary hypertension, with or without associated interstitial fibrosis. Renal crisis may produce myocardial dysfunction secondary to systemic hypertension.

RENAL

Before the advent of angiotensin-converting enzyme inhibitors to control hypertensive episodes, renal crisis in systemic sclerosis was almost always a fatal event. The syndrome was marked by abrupt onset of malignant hypertension, renal insufficiency, microangiopathic hemolysis, myocardial dysfunction, and rapid demise. Most commonly this would occur during the early stages of rapidly progressive skin involvement, often during the winter, and exclusively in patients destined to have diffuse cutaneous involvement. The mortality in early stages of diffuse disease is related largely to the occurrence of this complication. Fortunately, less than 20% of patients with the diffuse variety of systemic sclerosis manifest renal crisis. The accelerated hypertension is associated with hyperreninemia, but risk stratification is not predicted readily by quantifying plasma renin.[94] In addition, many patients have structural renal vascular disease who never manifest clinical renal disease.[16]

The underlying pathology reflects predominantly renal vascular alterations, which may lead to cortical necrosis. Most of these changes are nonspecific and may be observed in patients with idiopathic malignant hypertension, although adventitial fibrosis is more advanced in scleroderma renal disease.[9]

Some patients who develop renal disease may survive the initial crisis and be maintained on dialysis. With adequate control of blood pressure, renal function may return after several months of dialysis, with a favorable outcome.[92]

OTHER

Fibrosis may affect the thyroid gland, leading to hypofunction in about one fourth of patients with systemic sclerosis. Some patients have autoantibodies, suggesting coexistent Hashimoto's thyroiditis. In a similar fashion, fibrosis may spread to the salivary and lacrimal glands, leading to sicca symptoms. Sjögren's syndrome may also overlap with scleroderma, including the presence of autoantibodies typical of this syndrome (anti-Ro/La or SS-A/SS-B). The presence of the antibodies usually correlates with finding lymphocytic infiltrates in the salivary glands, rather than merely fibrosis. Impotence is a relatively frequent complaint of patients with scleroderma. Although the etiology must be individualized, penile vascular dysfunction is most common.[60]

NATURAL COURSE

The course of scleroderma is quite variable from one individual to the next. It has proven useful to divide patients not only into categories based on extent of cutaneous involvement (limited and diffuse) but also into stages of early and late disease. This staging process allows the patients, family, and physician to better anticipate certain clinical manifestations and complications (Table 51–4). Early disease is considered by some to be less than 3 years, and by others less than 5 years. Obviously the precise point to draw the line is arbitrary. For purposes of discussion, late disease will be considered as longer than 5 years.

In the diffuse variety, early disease is characterized by progressive skin involvement, tendon friction rubs and fibrous tenosynovitis, joint contractures, and visceral involvement, including cardiac, lung, gastrointestinal, and renal disease. Digital ulcerations are common. Skin thickening appears to reach a peak of severity within 3 years. Late disease is marked by a regression or plateau of skin thickening, with thinning of epidermis stretched over residual joint contractures. New visceral involvement is unusual. Alveolitis is replaced by bland fibrosis within the pulmonary interstitium. Constitutional symptoms are less prominent. Hence the term progressive systemic sclerosis generally applies only to the early stages of disease and has fallen out of favor.

In the limited variety, early disease is marked by prominent Raynaud's phenomenon and related local vascular complications. Puffy fingers become manifest, but constitutional symptoms are less problematic. Upper esophageal symptoms may dominate the clinical picture. Late disease is generally benign, but several complications may arise. Extensive calcinosis may lead to cutaneous ulcers and local infections, and digital ulcerations may become prominent. Repetitive ischemia leads to osteolysis and autoamputations. Esophageal strictures may develop. Small bowel complications arise (more commonly than in diffuse disease) and may result in malabsorption, weight loss, or episodic pseudo-obstructions. Sudden dyspnea heralds the onset of pulmonary hypertension and a uniformly fatal course.

SURVIVAL

Once thought to be a benign variant, limited cutaneous disease carries a mortality after 10 years, which exceeds the

TABLE 51–4
CLINICAL AND LABORATORY FEATURES OF SYSTEMIC SCLEROSIS

	Diffuse Scleroderma	Limited Scleroderma
Duration of Raynaud's phenomenon prior to skin changes	Short (months)	Long (years)
Organ involvement		
Telangiectasias	Scattered and small	Prominent and large
Skin thickening	Rapidly widespread	Limited
Joints, synovitis	Occurs	Rare
Tendon friction rubs	Common	Absent
Esophageal	Prominent	Prominent
Pulmonary fibrosis	Common	Rare
Pulmonary hypertension	Secondary	Late manifestation
Cardiac disease	Common	Rare
Renal disease	Occasional	Absent
Laboratory data		
ANA +	Common	Common
Anticentromere Ab	Rare	Frequent
Type I antitopoisomerase Ab	Occurs	Rare
Survival, limited	Early demise	Late demise
Early	Constitutional symptoms, fatigue, weight loss, etc. Rapid skin thickening Organ involvement, lung, cardiac, renal, GI Vascular complications, digital ulcers High mortality	Raynaud's phenomenon Minimal skin thickening No organ involvement, except esophageal Vascular complications, digital ulcers Low mortality
Late	Stable disease Constitutional symptoms rare Deformities of hands and joints predominate Low mortality	Esophageal strictures and malabsorption Calcinosis and digital ulcerations Pulmonary hypertension High mortality

Early disease = less than 5 years; late disease = more than 5 years.

diffuse variant. In diffuse disease, the prognosis is extremely variable but approaches 40% overall within the first 5 years.[81] Most investigators agree that male sex, older age, black race, and renal, cardiac, or lung involvement adversely affects outcome.[52] Nonetheless, long-term followup has revealed that patients with either limited or diffuse disease continue to exhibit excess mortality. Functional status may well prove to be another important predictor for survival. Other factors that have been examined to stratify risks for an individual with systemic sclerosis include serologic responses and HLA markers. In this regard, the finding of type I antitopoisomerase autoantibodies and HLA DR3/DR52a haplotype is associated with the development of pulmonary fibrosis and reduced survival.[2]

PATHOLOGY OF SYSTEMIC SCLEROSIS

The earliest pathologic changes can be demonstrated in otherwise clinically normal skin. These changes involve the endothelial cells and perivascular region. Endothelial cell alterations in nonlesional skin is reflected by decreased adenosine uptake, loss of detectable von Willebrand's factor (factor VIII–related antigen), and ultrastructural abnormalities.[66] The loss of stainable factor VIII-R antigen is consistent with the finding of elevated levels in the circulation. At the earliest stages, the endothelial cell alterations may reflect a highly activated state. With more advanced disease, however, ultrastructural changes suggest a regressive or degenerative process. Increased aggregation of cytoplasmic intermediate filaments, decreased pinocytotic vesicles, and at later stages, endothelial cell dehiscence with separation from the basement membrane and frank necrobiosis are seen.[66] These changes occur before the hallmark feature of this disease is present, that is, before excessive extracellular matrix accumulation and fibroblast activation.

As the disease progresses, the frank endothelial cell necrosis is associated with an overall decreased number of vessels. Perivascular edema is prominent. Within existing vessels, intravascular aggregation of platelets is evident. Another feature of advanced lesions is reduplication of basal lamina. In the vicinity of vessels, increased numbers of mast cells, CD4 and CD8 T cells, macrophages, and Langerhans cells are seen.[29, 66] At this stage, investigators have noted up-regulated fibroblast synthesis of mRNA for procollagen using in situ hybridization.[32, 42, 78] Most of the evidence suggests that increased expression of collagen mRNA, at least initially, involves perivascular fibroblasts.

The thickening of skin noted clinically is due to the accumulation of collagen and other extracellular matrix constituents, such as glycosaminoglycan and fibronectin. Edema also contributes to the skin thickening, especially appreciated in early disease. The etiology of edema is not known but is likely related to the microvascular disruption and hydrophobic effects exerted by the glycosaminoglycan accumulation. As the disease progresses, the vascular structural alterations and collagen accumulation dominate the pathologic picture (Fig. 51–4).

Digital arteries exhibit marked intimal hyperplasia with severe narrowing of the lumen and variable degrees of adventitial fibrosis. The luminal narrowing accentuates the physiologic effects of cold-induced vasospasm. Similar pathology emerges in the visceral organs, such as the myocardium. The resultant episodic ischemia leads to a peculiar pattern of myocardial contraction band necrosis. In the kidneys, the vascular hyalinization of intralobular arteries may result in numerous small cortical infarcts (Fig. 51–5). These changes may affect afferent arterioles and glomerular tufts. Notably, no evidence exists to suggest that these vascular changes emerge from vasculitis. Furthermore, immune deposits are scarce.

The finding of cellular infiltrates early in the course of disease has been noted not only in the dermis but also in organs, such as the lung. Variable degrees of alveolitis with mixed cellular infiltrates may accompany interstitial fibrosis, as demonstrated by bronchial lavage studies.[100] In the lung, the pathology and its functional consequences are most often related to the progressive accumulation of collagen, which gradually obliterates the vascular bed, impairing gas exchange (Fig. 51–6). However, as alluded to earlier, patients with long-standing limited scleroderma may develop cor pulmonale as a result of uniform narrowing of pulmonary arteries (pulmonary hypertension) in the absence of interstitial fibrosis. The vessels reveal medial smooth muscle hypertrophy without evidence of vasculitis.

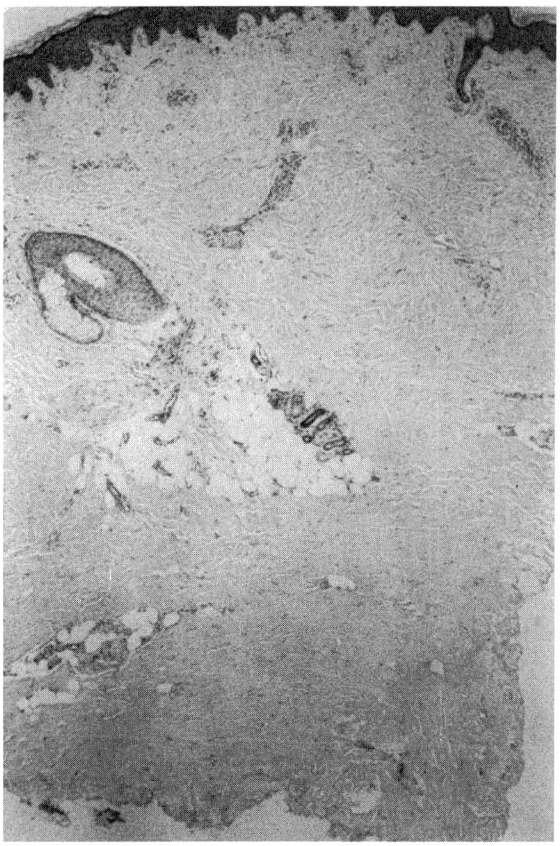

FIGURE 51–4. Photomicrograph of a skin biopsy from a patient with scleroderma (stained with hemotoxylin and eosin). Note the atrophy of the epidermis, loss of appendages, and extensive fibrosis involving the entire dermis into the underlying subcutaneous fat (magnification × 10). (Courtesy of Frederick Miller, State University of New York, Stony Brook, NY.)

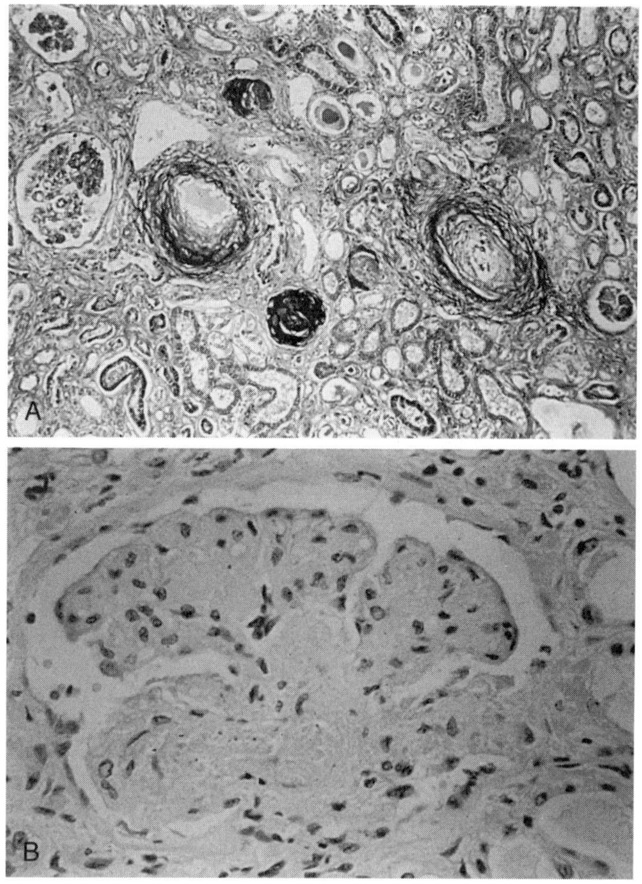

FIGURE 51–5. **(A)** Photomicrograph of a kidney biopsy from a patient with systemic sclerosis. Note the fibromuscular concentric sclerosis of arteries (onionskin) with secondary vascular atrophy of parenchyma (trichrome stain, magnification × 25). **(B)** Photomicrograph of a glomerulus showing acute microangiopathic alterations (hemotoxylin and eosin stain, magnification × 100). (Courtesy of Frederick Miller, State University of New York, Stony Brook, NY.)

Throughout the intestinal tract, the functional consequences of excessive collagen accumulation are evident. In the distal esophagus, the muscularis layer may become entirely replaced by collagen. Similar changes are found in the small and large intestine, often in association with mononuclear cell infiltrates. The intestinal walls become thickened with reduced motility.

IMMUNE EVENTS AND GENETIC FACTORS

That autoimmunity plays any role in systemic sclerosis stems primarily from two lines of evidence. First is the finding of distinct autoantibodies, which are relatively specific for limited and diffuse forms of this disease. Second is the histopathologic finding of lymphocytes in the vicinity of fibroblast activity. Additional support emerges with the frequent observation of familial clustering of other autoimmune diseases with systemic sclerosis. The immune abnormalities noted in systemic sclerosis will be reviewed under the catego-

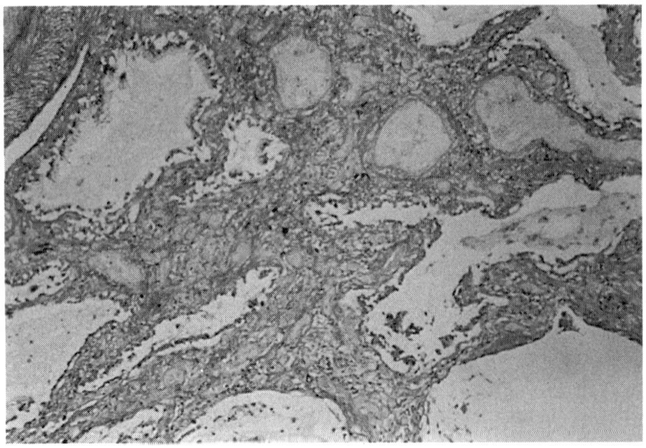

FIGURE 51–6. Photomicrograph of lung parenchyma obtained at autopsy from a middle-aged man with end-stage lung disease from systemic sclerosis. Note the diffuse interstitial fibrosis within what appeared grossly as a honeycombed lung (trichrome stain, magnification × 10). (Courtesy of Frederick Miller, State University of New York, Stony Brook, NY.)

ries of cellular immunity, humoral immunity, cytokine mediators, and immunogenetics.

CELLULAR IMMUNITY

Most studies in the literature report on lymphocyte abnormalities present in the peripheral circulation of patients with systemic sclerosis. The relevance of these findings to the organ-based pathology in this disease is questionable. Furthermore, the literature has been inconsistent, with findings of increased, decreased, and normal numbers and function of circulating T cells. T cells bearing γ/δ T-cell antigen receptors are normal, whereas the Vδ1+ subpopulation is increased.[58] Circulating T cells are activated with increased surface expression of HLA-DR and IL-2 receptor and increased soluble levels of IL-2 receptor.[40] In total, most of the studies suggest that in vivo T-cell function in systemic sclerosis is normal.[101]

As noted earlier, infiltration of skin with lymphocytes, activated eosinophils, mast cells, and scattered macrophages is characteristic.[21, 24, 27] The lymphocytes are predominately $CD4^+$, with B cells rarely found.[75] The mast cells are mostly of the MC_{TC} (tryptase, chymase) variety, as expected in the dermis. However, occasional patients have clusters of MC_T mast cells, a finding highly atypical in skin.[35] The T cells express class II major histocompatibility complex (MHC), suggesting activation.[75] These T cells are in juxtaposition to activated fibroblasts expressing mRNA for procollagen.[42] The linkage between T cells and fibroblasts, leading to fibrosis, is further illustrated in patients who develop graft-versus-host scleroderma-like disease. In this setting, $CD8^+$ cells predominate in the skin infiltrates.

In animal models of this disease, mast cells appear to degranulate immediately prior to the development of fibrosis.[12, 13] These highly degranulated mast cells have been noted in patients with rapidly progressive scleroderma.[10, 49] Animal models of scleroderma, however, negate the absolute requirement of mast cells for a sclerotic tissue response.[19] It is likely that mast cells serve to potentiate ongoing activation pathways, leading to sustained fibroblast activity. Both mast cells and lymphocytes adhere to stimulated fibroblasts in tissues actively forming scar tissue.[30]

The fibrosing alveolitis in systemic sclerosis lends itself to study, since lavaging lower airways allows analysis of cellular infiltrates. The investigations of bronchoalveolar lavage lymphocytes reveal reduced $CD4^+$, increased $CD8^+$ T cells, and a selective expansion of Vδ1+ γ/δ T cells compared with controls.[101]

The presence of inflammatory and immune cells in scleroderma tissue implies that homing responses, which require leukocyte adherence, transmigration, and retention, are activated. Indeed, the experimental data support this notion. Endothelium in both involved and uninvolved skin expresses E-selectin, fibroblasts express high levels of intercellular adhesion molecule 1 (ICAM-1), and the infiltrating leukocytes express the counterligand leukocyte function–associated antigen 1 (LFA-1).[11, 87] These molecules serve to recruit and retain inflammatory and immune cells to a perivascular vicinity. The presence of these cells may be key in stimulating fibroblast activity.

HUMORAL IMMUNITY

Modest hypergammaglobulinemia is noted in over one third of patients. Monoclonal gammopathy has been rarely described in scleroderma. Its presence should prompt consideration of either scleromyxedema or scleredema in the differential diagnosis.[37] Serum complement levels are typically normal, although circulating immune complexes are found in many patients. Rheumatoid factor is positive at low titer in approximately one third of patients. The lack of immune deposits within pathologic lesions raises a question as to the relevance of these findings.

Antinuclear antibodies can be demonstrated in over 98% of patients with the newer sensitive substrates.[15] Mostly, these occur in low titer with a speckled or nucleolar fluorescent pattern. Several specific autoantigens are recognized by sera from patients with systemic sclerosis, accounting for the majority of patients. Anticentromere antibodies are found in over 50% of patients with the limited form of scleroderma and are rarely seen with diffuse disease.[22] Although these antibodies are also observed in patients with only Raynaud's phenomenon, most longitudinal studies indicate that these individuals eventually develop a scleroderma-like illness.[97] The anticentromere antibodies recognize three specific centromeric proteins, CENP-A (19 kD), CENP-B (80 kD), and CENP-C (140 kD).[18] These proteins comprise centromeric antigens of the tritaminar kinetochore and do not consist of centromeric DNA.

Anti-Scl 70, now termed antitopoisomerase, is found in 20 to 50% of patients with diffuse disease. This antibody is found in association with patients at high risk for developing pulmonary fibrosis. The antibody was originally defined by immunoblotting revealing reactivity with a protein of 70 kD. It has now been shown that the 70 kD (Scl 70) is a degradation product of the 100 kD native type I topoisomerase, an enzyme involved in catalyzing relaxation of supercoiled DNA prior to transcription. Autoantibodies directed to type I topoisomerase are capable of neutralizing the enzyme's function, although multiple epitopes have been characterized.[101] Of interest is that a region of binding within the carboxyterminus of type I topoisomerase has homology to a retroviral p30gag protein, suggesting an etiology for the autoimmune features of this disease.[53]

Nucleolar fluorescence is noted in up to half of the patients with systemic sclerosis, with a high degree of specificity. Several of the responsible nucleolar antigens have now been characterized. PM-Scl is found in a small percentage of patients, usually with clinical features of limited scleroderma and polymyositis. Antibody to RNA polymerase I has been described in approximately 20% of patients, typically in women with diffuse scleroderma. Antibodies to U_3RNP are found in patients prone to develop pulmonary hypertension. Other nucleolar and nuclear antigens have been recognized and may relate to specific clinical subsets (see Table 51–3).

IMMUNOGENETICS

Most of the antibody systems described in systemic sclerosis are directed to some component of the chromosome or its processing enzymes. Considerable evidence exists, dating back many years, that patients with systemic sclerosis manifest chromosomal abnormalities.[34] Many such studies have demonstrated increased chromosomal breakage rate, deletions, and acentric fragments. There is evidence for a circulating clastogenic factor, capable of inducing chromosomal damage, in patients with systemic sclerosis.[105] Presumably these anomalies are acquired. Superoxide dismutase appears to neutralize the clastogenic activity, suggesting a role for oxygen radical damage to DNA.[2] These observations should also be considered in light of the increased prevalence of cancer found in patients with systemic sclerosis.[54]

Studies of MHC alleles in patients with systemic sclerosis have been conflicting and controversial. This may be explained in part by the heterogeneity of the disease, geographic differences, and ethnic variability.[2] The data have been the subject of reviews and suggest that weak and varied associations exist with class I MHC antigen HLA Bw35 and class II HLA-DR1, HLA-DR3, and HLA-DR5.[2] Newer molecular techniques probing the class II alleles suggest that DQA2 and the C4A null alleles may provide a strong correlation with systemic sclerosis in the United Kingdom, whereas B8-DR3-DRw52-DQB2 is an extended haplotype linked to the development of pulmonary fibrosis.[2, 7]

Perhaps the most exciting data forthcoming link the autoantibody responses in systemic sclerosis to HLA class II molecules. Anticentromere antibody responses in all Caucasians studied was found to be associated with a polar glycine or tyrosine in position 26 within the cleft region of the HLA-DQB1 molecule.[67] In patients displaying antitopoisomerase antibody responses, one finds a tyrosine residue at position 30 of the DQB1 chain or an acidic residue at position 69 of DPB1.[2, 68] The significance of these findings awaits further investigation.

CYTOKINES

With the explosion of knowledge concerning cytokines, it is not too surprising that many of these molecules retain the capacity to activate fibroblasts and have been purported to have significance in systemic sclerosis. Candidate molecules, such as interleukin (IL)-1 and tumor necrosis factor (TNF)-α, have been supplanted with reports of IL-2, IL-4, IL-6, transforming growth factor (TGF)-β, and platelet-derived growth factor (PDGF) in the tissue or sera of patients with systemic sclerosis.[20]

Perhaps no molecule has received more focus than TGF-β.[48] TGF-β is produced by a wide variety of cells, but platelets contain abundant quantities and presumably release this cytokine at sites of endothelial injury. TGF-β has the capacity to induce fibrosis when injected into subcutaneous tissue.[71] In vitro, TGF-β stimulates fibroblast chemotaxis, promotes the synthesis of extracellular matrix components, decreases levels of interstitial collagenase, and induces the release of tissue inhibitors of metalloproteinases, all of which would promote scar tissue formation.[70] Several studies have documented the presence of TGF-β mRNA and protein at sites of active procollagen (mRNA) production in systemic sclerosis.[26, 33, 44] Inhibitors of TGF-β have been administered to interfere with the fibrogenic effects of this peptide.[5]

IL-4 has effects on fibroblasts similar to those of TGF-β but has received considerably less attention as a potential fibrogenic molecule.[64, 65] Nonetheless, elevated levels of IL-4 have been detected in the sera of patients with systemic sclerosis.[59] Interferon (IFN)-γ, on the other hand, has the capacity to down-regulate fibroblast functions[39, 63] and, interestingly, has been undetectable in the circulation of patients with systemic sclerosis.[59] Stimulated peripheral blood mononuclear cells from patients also secrete less IFN-γ than do those from controls.[43] This suggests that an imbalance of cytokines that regulate fibroblast activity exists in systemic sclerosis. These findings also implicate Th2 lymphocytes as pathogenic in systemic sclerosis, rather than Th1 lymphocytes (elevated IL-4, low IFN-γ). However, the source of elevated IL-4 has not been elucidated and conceivably could involve mast cells.[24]

FIBROBLAST:MATRIX ALTERATIONS

Ultimately, the fibroblast becomes the major culprit in propagating the dramatic pathology of systemic sclerosis. Our understanding of fibroblast biology is still in its infancy. Many questions concerning the presence of fibroblast subpopulations and characterizing their phenotype remain unanswered. Considering that fibroblasts are critical for maintaining the normal architecture of tissue and can regulate the synthesis and removal of extracellular constituents, these cells have deservedly come under scrutiny in systemic sclerosis.[86]

Studies in systemic sclerosis have indicated that fibroblasts have an enhanced expression of matrix gene expression, at a transcriptional level, and little if any abnormalities of proteolytic activity to degrade matrix.[98] The observation that fibroblast subpopulations that differ in collagen synthetic activity can be depicted in culture has led to the concept that fibroblast selection and amplification occur in systemic sclerosis.[6] Unfortunately, investigation is hampered by the lack of specific markers that allow delineation of fibroblast subpopulations in vivo.

Whereas peripheral blood mononuclear cells serve a surveillance role, fibroblasts serve a role to maintain tissue integrity. In a resting healthy organ, fibroblasts have a low metabolic and proliferative rate. In contrast, when a wound is inflicted, fibroblasts respond to platelet products, serum factors, and other signals to escalate their rate of migration, proliferation, and synthetic activity. When the wound reaches a healed stage, either scar tissue is removed by fibroblasts, or a residual scar persists, and the resting state is resumed. In systemic sclerosis, this process goes awry, and the fibroblasts remain synthetically active in a milieu of excessive collagen.

The interaction of immune cells, including lymphocytes, monocytes, and mast cells, with fibroblasts to trigger an activated state is well established in culture systems.[24, 63] Evidence exists that mononuclear cells derived from patients with systemic sclerosis can stimulate scleroderma fibroblasts greater than do normal cocultures.[23] Cytokines released from these cells may be fibrogenic, as discussed earlier. Adhesive molecules expressed in vivo by scleroderma fibroblasts further facilitate interactions between the immune system and tissue fibroblasts.[63] However, the relationship between immune cells and fibroblasts is a relatively transient one and imperfect at best.

Fibroblasts continue to secrete increased amounts of extracellular matrix at later stages of disease, in the absence of inflammatory infiltrates. This has been interpreted and studied in different manners. Fibroblasts regulate themselves via the expression of integrin receptors. These molecules signal to the cell to coordinate function with surrounding environment.[76] The β_1 integrin family, involved in cell:matrix interactions, is particularly relevant for fibroblast behavior. Depending on which α subunit is expressed with β_1 to form a heterodimeric transmembrane receptor, the extracellular matrix can modulate fibroblast functions, such as adhesion, migration, proliferation, and collagen synthesis.[76]

Autonomous fibroblast matrix synthesis occurring in spite of surrounding excessive matrix accumulation, as observed in scleroderma, may result from alterations in integrin expression or function. For example, $\alpha_1\beta_1$ integrin on the surface of fibroblasts appears to normally regulate procollagen mRNA levels. Evidence suggests that there is abnormal expression of this integrin in systemic sclerosis.[36] As a result, fibroblasts continue to secrete excessive amounts of collagen because of faulty feedback and failure to down-regulate synthesis. This abnormality may reflect a general activation of otherwise normal fibroblasts.

An alternative, or possibly complementary, possibility is that clonal selection of high collagen–producing fibroblasts occurs.[57, 103] This would suggest that clones of fibroblasts evolve by a selection process that phenotypically could be identified by high collagen production. However, in situ hybridization studies of skin biopsies from patients with scleroderma have not confirmed nests of high collagen–producing fibroblasts (heterogeneity), but rather a uniform increase.[42] This suggests more of a general activation than an overrepresentation of a subpopulation. Further investigation using the newer molecular techniques will be necessary to provide adequate answers.

A PATHOGENIC SCHEME

The pathogenesis of systemic sclerosis must explain three key processes: vascular injury, immune abnormalities, and abundant deposition of extracellular matrix. It is probable that these individual events relate to each other in a complex manner. From careful pathologic studies, it appears that the vascular injury characteristic of this disease may be the initial detectable abnormality.[66] The cause of the vascular injury remains unknown. Early studies suggesting a serum proteolytic factor have not been confirmed.[8, 41] It is conceivable that immune cells directly mediate the endothelial damage, although the evidence for this is scanty. Exogenous toxins are receiving increased attention as potentiating fibrotic diseases.[28] Some have advanced the idea of retroviruses in systemic sclerosis.[38] Finding the cause of the vascular injury may not help in treating disease if irreversible alterations are established.

How the vascular injury is related to a fibrotic response also remains unanswered. Evidence has suggested that injured endothelial cells may initiate a cascade of events that lead to sclerosis.[45] Complex cytokine networks are involved, but convincing experimental evidence continues to emphasize the paramount role of TGF-β in orchestrating a sclerotic response.[5]

It has been proposed that endothelial cell injury leads to the release of factors such as angiotensinogen, which (converted to its active form, angiotensin II) stimulates the production of fibroblast TGF-β mRNA.[45] TGF-β is then capable of acting as an autocrine factor, up-regulating its own production and other fibroblast-activating factors,[88] to increase procollagen mRNA and collagen fibril formation. This novel hypothesis presumes that endothelial cells serve a critical role in normal physiology by maintaining fibroblasts in a quiescent state. Upon injury to the endothelial cells, this homeostatic function is lost.

The immune system, particularly Th2-type lymphocytes and mast cells, may further amplify this process by releasing fibrogenic cytokines. Ultimately, the fibroblasts behave autonomously, possibly because of altered integrin functioning, selective activation of a subpopulation, or sustained dysfunction of intracellular regulatory genes for matrix synthesis. In terms of the latter possibility, investigation using a mouse model (tsk, or tight-skin mice) of systemic sclerosis suggests that negative regulatory sequences along the promoter region of the procollagen α_1 (I) gene may be reduced in their activity, thus unleashing gene expression in fibroblasts.[62] The molecular basis of this involves an AP-1 transcription factor, which interacts and effectively dampens a negative promoter sequence upstream from transcription sites.[62]

Ongoing investigation with the tsk mouse model, which shares many of the autoimmune and sclerotic features of human disease,[4] will likely contribute to our understanding of the molecular biology of collagen dysregulation.[83] However, precise mapping of the human promoter region in procollagen α_1(I) and α_2(I) genes using transgenic models is revealing an extraordinarily complex array of enhancer elements, negative-regulatory sequences, and transactivating factors.[85] Nonetheless, relentless research in this area may eventually allow us to consider gene modulation in the treatment of fibrotic disorders.[98]

The finding of chromosomal anomalies and specific immune responses to chromosomal constituents is difficult to fit into a pathogenic scheme that unifies the pathologic features. More research is clearly needed to elucidate how every feature of this complex disease is related.

TREATMENT

No single disease-modifying agent or combination of drugs has been proven effective in prospective controlled trials. Most such trials have yielded disappointing results. However, many agents can be utilized to treat the complications of systemic sclerosis. It is of no value to approach the patient with undue pessimism. Although potentially life threatening, this disease usually can be adequately controlled. It is also impossible to predict the extent to which the disease will progress in any individual patient.

Glucocorticoids have essentially no role in the treatment of this disease, except for the rare patient with associated myositis. Corticosteroids do not slow the progress of the disease or benefit the skin disease. Some controversy remains concerning its judicious use for alveolitis at its earliest stages. High dosages have been associated with the development of renal failure.[31]

Considerable attention has been given to D-penicillamine for the treatment of this disease. Its use has been adopted by many rheumatologists, despite the lack of any controlled prospective data. Retrospective analyses at a large clinical center have supported its use for diffuse disease.[95] These data demonstrated a reduction in overall mortality, marked improvement in skin thickening, reduced renal involvement, and modest improvement in lung function when compared with controls receiving other therapies.[17, 95] Unfortunately, almost one third of patients experience adverse side effects, with up to one fourth of patients discontinuing the drug. A 2-year multicenter prospective controlled trial is now under way to evaluate this agent in diffuse scleroderma.

Immunosuppressive agents continue to be utilized in treating this disease. Azathioprine, 5-fluorouracil, and chlorambucil have been shown to be ineffective in prospective trials. Cyclosporin is being evaluated at some sites, with the initial enthusiasm mixed. Cyclophosphamide may have a specific role in treating interstitial lung disease in systemic sclerosis, although debate exists on this issue.[82, 91] Low-dose methotrexate may benefit certain aspects of the disease, such as the musculoskeletal manifestations, but its effect overall has been variable. IFN is under study in the United Kingdom, with inconsistent improvement noted. Extracorporeal photopheresis, used to treat cutaneous T-cell lymphomas, has been demonstrated to improve skin parameters in patients with diffuse scleroderma who have no evidence of visceral disease.[74] Clinical trials to further investigate this modality have been initiated.

Agents directed at the vascular features of this disease have been utilized. Dipyridamole and aspirin reduce levels of platelet aggregates and β-thromboglobulin but fail after 2 years to improve clinical parameters.[1] Vasodilators, including angiotensin-converting enzyme (ACE) inhibitors and serotonin antagonists, such as ketanserin, control episodes of Raynaud's phenomenon but appear to have little additional benefit. Raynaud's phenomenon can be controlled in about two thirds of individuals with the use of calcium channel blockers and conservative measures of avoiding cold exposure. Subjectively, some patients note improvement with the newer generation of calcium channel blockers, despite prior inefficacy. Occasionally, patients present with severe digital ischemia. Iloprost, an intravenous preparation of a stable prostaglandin analogue, appears efficacious in this setting.[104] The role of digital sympathectomy remains controversial.

Other organ complications often require aggressive therapy. Reflux esophagitis leads to intractable strictures and should be vigorously treated by reducing acid production. Proton pump inhibitors, such as omeprazole, appear useful in this regard and probably can be used chronically without problems. Elevating the head of the bed and avoiding recumbency immediately postprandial are other useful measures. Hypomotility will often respond to somatostatin inhibitors, such as cisapride.[84] Broad spectrum antibiotics are frequently necessary to reduce the bacterial overgrowth in the small bowels and prevent malabsorption.

Renal involvement may lead to hyperreninemic hypertensive crisis. Prompt recognition in patients at high risk is key to managing this complication. Blood pressure responds readily to ACE inhibitors or other newer vasodilators. Pulmonary hypertension, in contrast, responds poorly to antihypertensives and remains a major clinical problem in these patients. As mentioned earlier, these patients develop a rapidly detiorating course. Newer approaches, such as the use of intravenous prostanoids delivered continuously by implantable subcutaneous pumps, may be efficacious in stabilizing patients. Lung transplantations have now offered an alternative approach to advanced pulmonary disease.

Clinical treatment of systemic sclerosis remains a formidable challenge. The number of patients under care at any one site is small, and funding for properly designed trials has not been forthcoming. Clinicians committed to investigating this disease have formed a consortium to pool resources, establish guidelines for clinical trials, and organize therapeutic approaches.[102] The efforts of such groups, combined with an impressive number of scientists performing basic research on areas relevant to systemic sclerosis, should lead to more effective therapies.

REFERENCES

1. Beckett VL, Conn DL, Fuster V, et al: Trial of platelet inhibiting drugs in scleroderma. Arthritis Rheum 27:1137, 1984.
2. Black CM, Welsh KI: Genetics of scleroderma. Clin Dermatol 12:337–347, 1994.
3. Blocka KL, Bassett LW, Furst DE: The arthropathy of advanced progressive systemic sclerosis: a radiographic survey. Arthritis Rheum 24: 874, 1981.
4. Bocchieri MH, Christner PJ, Henriksen PD, Jimenez SA: Immunological characterization of (tight skin/NZB)F1 hybrid mice with connective tissue and autoimmune features resembling human systemic sclerosis. J Autoimmun 6:337–351, 1993.
5. Border WA, Ruoslahti E: Transforming growth factor-β in disease: the dark side of tissue repair. J Clin Invest 90:1–7, 1992.
6. Botstein GR, Sherer FK, LeRoy EC: Fibroblast selection in scleroderma: an alternative model of fibrosis. Arthritis Rheum 25:189–195, 1982.
7. Briggs DC, Vaughan RW, Welsh KL, et al: Immunogenetic prediction of pulmonary fibrosis in systemic sclerosis. Lancet 338:661–662, 1991.
8. Campbell PM, LeRoy EC: Pathogenesis of systemic sclerosis: a vascular hypothesis. Semin Arthritis Rheum 4:351–368, 1975.
9. Cannon PJ, Hassar M, Cararella WJ, et al: The relationship of hypertension and renal failure in scleroderma (progressive systemic sclerosis) to structural and functional abnormalities of the renal cortical circulation. Medicine (Baltimore) 53:1–46, 1974.
10. Claman HN: Mast cell changes in a case of rapidly progressive scleroderma: ultrastructural analysis. J Invest Dermatol 92:290–295, 1989.
11. Claman HN, Giorno RC, Seibold JR: Endothelial and fibroblastic activation in scleroderma—the myth of the uninvolved skin. Arthritis Rheum 34:1495–1501, 1991.

12. Claman HN, Jaffee BD, Huff JC, Clark RAF: Chronic graft-versus-host disease (GVHD) as a model for scleroderma. II: Mast cell depletion with deposition of immunoglobulins in the skin and fibrosis. Cell Immunol 94:73–84, 1985.
13. Claman HN, Lee Choi K, Sujansky W, Vatter AE: Mast cell "disappearance" in chronic murine graft-vs-host disease (GVHD)—ultrastructural demonstration of "phantom mast cells." J Immunol 137:2009–2013, 1986.
14. Clarke AK, Galbraith RM, Hamilton EBD, et al: Rheumatic disorders in primary biliary cirrhosis. Ann Rheum Dis 37:42–47, 1978.
15. Clegg DO, Williams HJ, Singer JZ, et al: Early undifferentiated connective tissue disease. II. The frequency of circulating antinuclear antibodies in patients with early rheumatic disease. J Rheumatol 18:1340–1343, 1991.
16. D'Angelo WA, Fries JF, Masi AT, et al: Pathologic observations in systemic sclerosis (scleroderma). A study of fifty-eight autopsy cases and fifty-eight controls. Am J Med 46:428, 1969.
17. De Clerck LS, Dequeker J, Francx L, et al: D-penicillamine therapy and interstitial lung disease in scleroderma. A long term follow-up study. Arthritis Rheum 30:643, 1987.
18. Earnshaw WC, Bordwell B, Marino C, Rothfield N: Three human chromosomal autoantigens are recognized by sera from patients with anti-centromere antibodies. J Clin Invest 77:426–430, 1986.
19. Everett ET, Pablos JL, Harley RA, et al: The role of mast cells in the development of skin fibrosis in tight-skin mutant mice. Comp Biochem Physiol A 110:159–165, 1995.
20. Fagundus DM, LeRoy EC: Cytokines and systemic sclerosis. Clin Dermatol 12:407–417, 1994.
21. Fleischmajer R, Perlish JS, Reeves JRT: Cellular infiltrates in scleroderma skin. Arthritis Rheum 20:975–984, 1977.
22. Fritzler MJ, Kinsella TD, Garbutt E: The CREST syndrome: a distinct serologic entity with anticentromere antibodies. Am J Med 69:520–526, 1980.
23. Gonzalez-Amaro R, Alarcon-Segovia D, Alcocer-Valers J, et al: Mononuclear cell-fibroblast interactions in scleroderma. Clin Immunol Immunopathol 46:412–420, 1988.
24. Gruber BL: The mast cell in the pathogenesis of scleroderma. Clin Dermatol 12:397–406, 1994.
25. Gruber BL, Miller F, Kaufman LD: Simultaneous onset of systemic sclerosis (scleroderma) and lung cancer: a case report and a provisional unifying hypothesis. Am J Med 92:705–707, 1992.
26. Gruschwitz M, Muller PU, Sepp N, et al: Transcription and expression of transforming growth factor beta in the skin of progressive systemic sclerosis: a mediator of fibrosis? J Invest Dermatol 94:197–203, 1990.
27. Gustafsson R, Fredens K, Nettelbladt O, Hallgren R: Eosinophil activation in systemic sclerosis. Arthritis Rheum 34:414–422, 1991.
28. Haustein U, Herrmann K: Environmental scleroderma. Clin Dermatol 12:467–473, 1994.
29. Hawkins RA, Claman HN, Clark RAF, Steigerwald JC: Increased dermal mast cell populations in progressive systemic sclerosis: a link in chronic fibrosis? Ann Intern Med 102:182–186, 1985.
30. Heard BE, Dewar A, Corrin B: Apposition of fibroblasts to mast cells and lymphocytes in normal human lung and in cryptogenic fibrosing alveolitis—ultrastructure and cell perimeter measurements. J Pathol 166:303–310, 1992.
31. Helfrich DJ, Banner B, Steen VD, et al: Normotensive renal failure in systemic sclerosis. Arthritis Rheum 25:241, 1989.
32. Herrmann K, Heckmann M, Kulozik M, et al: Steady-state messenger-RNA levels of collagen-I, collagen-III, fibronectin, and collagenase in skin biopsies of systemic sclerosis patients. J Invest Dermatol 97:219–222, 1991.
33. Higley H, Persichitte K, Waegell W, et al: Immunocytochemical localization and serologic detection of transforming growth factor β1. Arthritis Rheum 37:278–288, 1993.
34. Housset E, Emerit I, Baulon A, et al: Anomalies chromosomiques dans la sclerodemie generalisee. Etudes de 6 malades. Cr Hebd Seanc Acad Sci Paris 269:413–416, 1969.
35. Irani AA, Gruber BL, Kaufman LD, et al: Mast cell changes in scleroderma. Presence of MCt cells in the skin and evidence of mast cell activation. Arthritis Rheum 35:933–939, 1992.
36. Ivarsson M, McWhirter A, Black C, Rubin K: Impaired regulation of collagen pro-α1(I) mRNA and change in pattern of collagen-binding integrins on scleroderma fibroblasts. J Invest Dermatol 101:216–221, 1993.
37. Jablonska S, Blaszczyk M: Sclerodermalike diseases. Clin Dermatol 12:437–488, 1994.
38. Jimenez SA, Batuman O: Immunopathogenesis of systemic sclerosis: possible role of retroviruses. Autoimmunity 16:225–233, 1993.
39. Jimenez SA, Freundlich B, Rosenbloom J: Selective inhibition of human diploid fibroblast collagen synthesis by interferons. J Clin Invest 74:1112–1116, 1984.
40. Kahaleh MB: Soluble immunologic products in scleroderma. Clin Immunol Immunopathol 58:139–144, 1991.
41. Kahaleh MB, Sherer GK, LeRoy EC: Endothelial injury in scleroderma. J Exp Med 149:1326–1335, 1979.
42. Kahari VM, Sandberg M, Kalimo H, et al: Identification of fibroblasts responsible for increased collagen production in localized scleroderma by in situ hybridization. J Invest Dermatol 90:664–670, 1988.
43. Kantor TV, Friberg D, Medsger TA, et al: Cytokine production and serum levels in systemic sclerosis. Clin Immunol Immunopathol 65:278–285, 1992.
44. Kulozik M, Hogg A, Lankat-Buttgereit B, Krieg T: Co-localization of transforming growth factor β2 with alpha 1(I) procollagen mRNA in tissue sections of patients with systemic sclerosis. J Clin Invest 86:917–922, 1990.
45. Lee LK, Meyer TW, Pollack AS, Lovett DH: Endothelial cells injury initiates glomerular sclerosis in the rat remnant kidney. J Clin Invest 96:953–964, 1995.
46. LeRoy EC, Black C, Fleischmajer R: Scleroderma (systemic sclerosis): classification, subsets, and pathogenesis. J Rheumatol 15:202, 1988.
47. LeRoy EC, Maricq HR, Kahaleh MB: Undifferentiated connective tissue syndromes. Arthritis Rheum 23:341, 1980.
48. LeRoy EC, Smith EA, Kahaleh MB, et al: Current comment: a strategy for determining the pathogenesis of systemic sclerosis: is transforming growth factor beta the answer? Arthritis Rheum 32:817–825, 1989.
49. Lichtbroun AS, Sandhaus LM, Giorno RC, et al: Myocardial mast cells in systemic sclerosis: a report of three fatal cases. Am J Med 89:372–376, 1990.
50. Maricq HR, Spencer-Green G, Leroy EC: Skin capillary abnormalities as indicators of organ involvement in scleroderma (systemic sclerosis), Raynaud's syndrome and dermatomyositis. Am J Med 61:862, 1976.
51. Maricq HR, Weinrich MC, Keil JE: Prevalence of scleroderma spectrum disorders in the general population of South Carolina. Arthritis Rheum 32:998, 1989.
52. Masi AT: Clinical-epidemiological perspective of systemic sclerosis (scleroderma). In Jayson MIV, Black CM (eds): Systemic Sclerosis: Scleroderma Vol 1. John Wiley & Sons Ltd, New York, 1988, pp 7–31.
53. Maul GG, Jimenez SA, Riggs E, Ziemnicka-Kotula D: Determination of an epitope of the diffuse systemic sclerosis marker antigen DNA topoisomerase 1: sequence similarity with retroviral p30gag protein suggests a possible cause for autoimmunity in systemic sclerosis. Proc Natl Acad Sci USA 86:8492–8496, 1989.
54. Medsger TJ: Systemic sclerosis and malignancy—are they related? J Rheumatol 12:1041–1043, 1985.
55. Medsger TA, Masi AT: Epidemiology of systemic sclerosis (scleroderma) among male United States veterans. J Chronic Dis 31:73, 1978.
56. Michet CJ, McKenna CH, Elveback LR, et al: Epidemiology of systemic lupus erythematous and other connective diseases in Rochester, Minnesota, 1950 through 1979. Mayo Clin Proc 60:105–111, 1985.
57. Needleman B, Ordonez J, Taramelli D, et al: In vitro identification of a subpopulation of fibroblasts that produces high levels of collagen in scleroderma patients. Arthritis Rheum 33:842–852, 1990.
58. Needleman BW, Wigley FM, Stair RW: Vδ1 γ/δ T cells in scleroderma. Arthritis Rheum 34:S141, 1991.
59. Needleman BW, Wigley FM, Stair RW: Interleukin-1, interleukin-2, interleukin-4, interleukin-6, tumor necrosis factor-alpha, and interferon-gamma levels in sera from patients with scleroderma. Arthritis Rheum 35:67–72, 1992.
60. Nowlin NS, Brick JE, Weaver DJ, et al: Impotence in scleroderma. Ann Intern Med 104:794–798, 1986.
61. Owens GR, Follansbee WP: Cardiopulmonary manifestations of systemic sclerosis. Chest 91:118–127, 1987.
62. Philips N, Bashey RI, Jimenez SA: Increased alpha 1(I) procollagen gene expression in tight skin (TSK) mice myocardial fibroblasts is due to a reduced interaction of a negative regulatory sequence with AP-1 transcription factor. J Biol Chem 270:9313–9321, 1995.
63. Piela-Smith TH, Korn JH: Lymphocyte modulation of fibroblast function in systemic sclerosis. Clin Dermatol 12:369–377, 1994.
64. Postlethwaite AE, Holness MA, Katai H, Raghow R: Human fibroblasts synthesize elevated levels of extracellular matrix proteins in response to interleukin-4. J Clin Invest 90:1479–1485, 1992.

65. Postlethwaite AE, Seyer JM: Fibroblast chemotaxis induction by human recombinant interleukin-4. Identification by synthetic peptide analysis of two chemotactic domains residing in amino acid sequences 70–88 and 89–122. J Clin Invest 87:2147–2152, 1991.
66. Prescott RJ, Freemont AJ, Jones CJP, et al: Sequential dermal microvascular and perivascular changes in the development of scleroderma. J Pathol 166:255–263, 1992.
67. Reveille JR, Owerbach D, Goldstein R, et al: Association of polar amino acids at position 26 of the HLA-DQB1 first domain with the anticentromere autoantibody response in systemic sclerosis (scleroderma). J Clin Invest 89:1209–1213, 1992.
68. Reveille JR, Durban E, MacLeod-St Clair MJ, et al: Association of amino acid sequences in the HLA-DQB1 first domain with the antitopoisomerase I autoantibody response in scleroderma (progressive systemic sclerosis). J Clin Invest 90:973–980, 1992.
69. Ridolfi RL, Bulkley BH, Hutchins GM: The cardiac conduction system in progressive systemic sclerosis. Clinical and pathologic features in 35 patients. Am J Med 61:361–366, 1976.
70. Roberts AB, Mccune BK, Sporn MB: TGF-beta—regulation of extracellular matrix. Kidney Int 41:557–559, 1992.
71. Roberts AB, Sporn MB, Assoian RK, et al: Transforming growth factor β: rapid induction of fibrosis and angiogenesis in vivo and stimulation of collagen formation in vitro. Proc Natl Acad Sci USA 83:4167–4171, 1986.
72. Roberts NK, Cabeen WR: Atrioventricular nodal function in progressive systemic sclerosis. Electrophysiologic and morphologic findings. Br Heart J 44:529–533, 1980.
73. Rodnan GP, Lipinski E, Luksick J: Skin thickness and collagen content in progressive systemic sclerosis and localized scleroderma. Arthritis Rheum 22:130–136, 1979.
74. Rook AH, Freundlich B, Jegasothy BV, et al: Treatment of systemic sclerosis with extracorporeal photochemotherapy. Results of a multicenter trial. Arch Dermatol 128:337–346, 1992.
75. Roumm AD, Whiteside TL, Medsger TAJ, Rodnan GP: Lymphocytes in the skin of patients with progressive systemic sclerosis. Quantification, subtyping, and clinical correlations. Arthritis Rheum 27:645–651, 1984.
76. Ruoslahti E: Integrins. J Clin Invest 87:1–5, 1991.
77. Salerni R, Rodnan GP, Leon DF, et al: Pulmonary hypertension in the CREST syndrome variant of progressive systemic sclerosis. Ann Intern Med 86:394–399, 1977.
78. Scharffetter K, Lankat-Buttgereit B, Kreig T: Localisation of collagen mRNA in normal and scleroderma skin by in situ hybridization. Eur J Clin Invest 18:9–17, 1988.
79. Schumacher HR: Joint involvement in progressive systemic sclerosis (scleroderma). Am J Clin Pathol 60:593–600, 1973.
80. Seibold JR: Scleroderma. In Kelly WN, Harris ED, Ruddy S, Sledge CB (eds): Textbook of Rheumatology, 4th edition. WB Saunders, Philadelphia, 1993, pp 1113–1143.
81. Silman AJ: Scleroderma and survival. Ann Rheum Dis 50:267–269, 1991.
82. Silver RM, Warrick JH, Kinsella MB, et al: Cyclophosphamide and low dose prednisolone therapy in patients with systemic sclerosis (scleroderma) with interstitial lung disease. J Rheumatol 20:838–844, 1993.
83. Siracusa LD, Christner P, McGrath R, et al: The tight skin (tsk) mutation in the mouse, a model for human fibrotic diseases, is tightly linked to the beta 2-microglobulin (B2m) gene on chromosome 2. Genomics 17:748–751, 1993.
84. Sjogren RW: Review: gastrointestinal motility disorders in scleroderma. Arthritis Rheum 37:1265–1282, 1994.
85. Slack JL, Liska D, Bornstein P: Regulation of expression of type I collagen genes. Am J Med Genet 45:140–151, 1993.
86. Sollberg S, Mauch C, Eckes B, Krieg B: The fibroblast in systemic sclerosis. Clin Dermatol 12:379–384, 1994.
87. Sollberg S, Peltonen J, Uitto J, Jimenez SA: Elevated expression of beta 1 and beta 2 integrins, intercellular adhesion molecule 1, and endothelial leukocyte adhesion molecule 1 in the skin of patients with systemic sclerosis of recent onset. Arthritis Rheum 35:290–298, 1992.
88. Sporn MB, Roberts AB: Transforming growth factor-β: recent progress and new challenges. J Cell Biol 119:1017–1021, 1992.
89. Steen VD, Conte C, Medsger TA, et al: Twenty-year incidence of systemic sclerosis (scleroderma). Arthritis Rheum 31:S21, 1988.
90. Steen VD, Conte C, Owens GR, Medsger TAJ: Severe restrictive lung disease in systemic sclerosis. Arthritis Rheum 37:1283–1289, 1994.
91. Steen VD, Lanz JKJ, Conte C, et al: Therapy for severe interstitial lung disease in systemic sclerosis: a retrospective study. Arthritis Rheum 37:1290–1296, 1994.
92. Steen VS, Medsger TA: Outcome of scleroderma renal crisis in the pre- and postcaptopril eras. Arthritis Rheum 31:S21, 1988.
93. Steen VD, Medsger TA: Epidemiology and natural history of systemic sclerosis. In LeRoy EC (ed): Rheumatic Disease Clinics of North America: Scleroderma. Vol 16. WB Saunders, Philadelphia, 1990, pp 1–10.
94. Steen VD, Medsger TA, Osial TA, et al: Factors predicting development of renal involvement in progressive systemic sclerosis. Am J Med 76:779–786, 1984.
95. Steen VD, Medsger TA, Rodnan GP: D-penicillamine therapy in progressive systemic sclerosis (scleroderma). A retrospective analysis. Ann Intern Med 97:652, 1982.
96. Subcommittee for Scleroderma Criteria of the American Rheumatism Association Diagnostic and Therapeutic Criteria Committee: Preliminary criteria for the classification of systemic sclerosis (scleroderma). Arthritis Rheum 23:581–590, 1980.
97. Tramposch HD, Smith CD, Senecal JL, et al: A long-term longitudinal study of anticentromere antibodies. Arthritis Rheum 27:121–124, 1984.
98. Varga J, Jimenez SA: Modulation of collagen gene expression: its relation to fibrosis in systemic sclerosis and other disorders. Ann Intern Med 122:60–62, 1995.
99. Warrick JH, Bhalla M, Schabel SI, Silver RM: High resolution computed tomography in early scleroderma lung disease. J Rheumatol 18:1520–1528, 1991.
100. Wells AU, Hansell DM, Corrin B, et al: High resolution computed tomography as a predictor of lung histology in systemic sclerosis. Thorax 47:738–742, 1992.
101. White B: Immune abnormalities in systemic sclerosis. Clin Dermatol 12:349–359, 1994.
102. White B, Bauer EA, Goldsmith LA, et al: Guidelines for clinical trials in systemic sclerosis (scleroderma). I. Disease modifying interventions. Arthritis Rheum 38:351–360, 1995.
103. Whiteside TL, Ferrarini M, Hebda P, Buckingham RB: Heterogeneous synthetic phenotype of cloned scleroderma fibroblasts may be due to aberrant regulation in the synthesis of connective tissues. Arthritis Rheum 31:1221–1229, 1988.
104. Wigley FM, Wise RA, Seibold JR, et al: Intravenous iloprost infusion in patients with Raynaud phenomenon secondary to systemic sclerosis. A multicenter, placebo-controlled, double-blind study. Ann Intern Med 120:199–206, 1994.
105. Wolff DJ, White-Needleman B, Wasserman SS, Schwartz S: Spontaneous and clastogen induced chromosomal breakage in scleroderma. J Rheumatol 18:837–840, 1991.
106. Young EA, Steen VD, Medsger TA: Systemic sclerosis without Raynaud's phenomenon. Arthritis Rheum 29(suppl. 4):S51, 1986.

52 Vasculitis

ALLEN P. KAPLAN FREDERICK MILLER

Vasculitis implies inflammation of blood vessels with destruction of the vessel wall and altered function of organ systems supplied by those vessels. It may be the primary mechanism of tissue injury, such as polyarteritis nodosa; one of many inflammatory mechanisms present in a particular disorder, such as systemic lupus erythematosus; or secondary to some surrounding process, such as necrotizing pseudomonas pneumonia. The first category of disease in which vascular inflammation is primary will be the focus of this chapter. Other disorders will be addressed briefly, including some that are not truly vasculitis but resemble it because a diffuse angiopathy is an essential part of the process.

Although there are large gaps in our understanding of the mechanisms of vasculitis in individual diseases, in large part because the cause is often unknown, the prototypic presentation is that of an immune complex–mediated disorder, in which there is activation of complement, recruitment of inflammatory cells, and localized coagulation and fibrinolysis. Fibrinoid necrosis is the resultant pathologic finding, and scarring and organ destruction are often the end result unless the course is modified by therapy.

This mechanism evolved from early studies of the Arthus reaction in rabbits and its relationship to inflammation induced by immune complex deposition within blood vessels.[27] Experimental models of serum sickness produced by one or a small number of closely spaced injections of heterologous protein also served as a model of this process and led to the conclusion that protracted interaction of antigen and antibody in the circulation in an optimal environment of slight antigenic excess can cause the aforementioned cascade of events.[148] Many sites of such inflammation are possibly dependent on the deposition of immune complexes in particular tissues, such as the kidney, which receives a large percentage of cardiac output and functions as a natural filter, or within blood vessels that supply a wide variety of tissues. The first example in humans was serum sickness caused by the administration of horse serum, as was utilized in the 1940s to treat diphtheria with antitoxin. The resultant syndrome included fever, lymphadenopathy, skin rash (urticaria or urticarial vasculitis), joint pain or overt arthritis, proteinuria, and, in some subjects, additional manifestations of glomerulonephritis.[90]

PATHOGENIC MECHANISMS: GENERAL CONSIDERATIONS

IMMUNE COMPLEXES

Immune complexes are produced by two general mechanisms. They may be formed within the circulation to be subsequently deposited in tissues, or one component of the complex may first fix to a tissue site or receptor and then combine with the other component. In addition, antibody may be directed to a naturally occurring tissue component, combine with it, and create the complex in situ. For example, in the prodrome of hepatitis B infection in which a serum sickness–like syndrome is seen, circulating immune complexes consisting of hepatitis B surface antigen and IgG antibody may deposit in the kidney and cause glomerulonephritis.[28] Alternatively, the DNA and anti-DNA complexes that preferentially localize to the kidney in systemic lupus erythematosus may do so because glomerular basement membrane can serve as a binding site for circulating DNA to concentrate it within the kidney (planted antigen). IgG then can attach to the bound DNA to form a complex and cause glomerulonephritis.[3, 79] In Goodpasture's syndrome, the IgG antibody is directed to the naturally present basement membrane antigen consisting of the noncollagenous domain of type IV collagen.[147]

The presence of detectable immune complexes does not predict whether disease will result, or if it does, which manifestations will be seen. Some of the variables that determine whether disease will result are given in Table 52–1. The ratio of antigen to antibody is a critical parameter that determines the fate of immune complexes. With antibody excess, large complexes are formed, which are rapidly cleared by the reticuloendothelial system, and disease is less likely to result. If there is significant antigen excess, small complexes result, whose half-life in the circulation is substantial, but they may not deposit in tissues. At an extreme, with a molar ratio of antigen to IgG antibody of 2:1 (or more), both Fab sites can be bound by a single multivalent antigen so that no lattice results. Further, complement fixation will not occur, since cross-linking of at least two IgG molecules in close proximity is needed. Complement fixation by IgM is still possible. Slight antigen excess appears optimal both for

TABLE 52–1
VARIABLES DETERMINING DEPOSITION OF IMMUNE COMPLEXES

Size and charge of antigen
Dose (concentration, persistence) of antigen
Vigor of antibody response
Antibody affinity for antigen
Class and subclass of antibody response
Charge distribution of antibody molecules
Ability to fix complement—classic and alternative pathways
Blood flow to tissues
Tissue binding sites for antigen, antibody, complement components
Clearance of complexes by reticuloendothelial system
Ratio of antigen/antibody and lattice formation
Complex solubilization by complement components

tissue deposition and complement fixation, a condition that may be transiently met during an immune response or persistent if an autoantigen is involved.[32, 100]

The size of the complex, assuming it will deposit, can also affect where it deposits. For example, complexes of greater than 22S are rapidly cleared by hepatic Kupffer's cells, whereas intermediate-sized ones (11S–22S) persist longer, and the smallest complexes, longer still. Large complexes entering the glomerulus may pass through the endothelium but get no further and lodge in a subendothelial location. Smaller ones may lie within the basement membrane (intramembranous) or penetrate further and localize along the podocytes (renal epithelial cells) as a subepithelial complex. Localization can vary with the size and number of immunogenic epitopes of the antigen, the class or subclass of the antibody response, and the molar ratio of antigen and antibody. The valence of an antigen is also an important determinant of size. For example, larger proteins are typically multivalent, have multiple epitopes to which antibodies can bind, elicit vigorous antibody responses, and allow antibodies to cross-link multiple antigen molecules to form a lattice network.[139]

The net charge of the complex is also very important and is a function of the charge of the particular antigen and the nature of the antibody response. Since most tissue surfaces are negatively charged, binding is more likely by cationic (positive) complexes.[51, 52] Thus in the kidney, for example, the mobility through endothelium, basement membrane, and epithelial layers is really a complex function of the net charge, as well as the size.

The nature of the antibody response determines, among other things, whether complement is activated and if so, whether it will be via the classic pathway, the alternative pathway, or both. IgM and IgG subclasses 1 and 3 readily activate the classic pathway. IgG_2 is a weak activator, and IgG_4 is negative, as is IgA_1 and IgA_2. On the other hand, IgA complexes activate the alternative complement pathway, as do IgG complexes of all four subclasses.[109] However, IgG_4 is particularly effective on a molar basis, although its plasma concentration is low.

The status of the ability of the reticuloendothelial system to clear surrogate immune complexes, such as red cells coated with IgG anti-Rh, suggests that abnormal splenic clearance of such coated red cells in a disease such as systemic lupus erythematosus correlates with levels of circulating immune complexes.[49] FcγRIIIA appears to be the major IgG receptor involved.[25] The most prolonged clearance times are found in the subpopulation of patients with glomerulonephritis.[114] Clearance of aggregated albumin is normal, indicating that splenic macrophages are functional in general but that the abnormality relates specifically to their IgG receptors. With treatment and clinical improvement, the abnormality in clearance diminishes.[63] The reason for this abnormality is not clear. Saturation of receptors by circulating immune complexes is a tempting explanation, but receptor numbers of circulating monocytes exposed to such complexes are not reduced.[50] There may be functional differences between the fixed macrophages of the reticuloendothelial system when compared with circulating monocytes, or other factors that affect clearance may be operational, including a role for complement in immune complex clearance.

Lattice formation (complex size and stability) is dependent on the class of antibody, the valence of the antigen, and the ratio of the two. It is also a function of the affinity of antibody for antigen. One function of the alternative complement pathway is solubilization of immune complexes, in which activation of this cascade with deposition of C3b Bb somehow disrupts the lattice and lessens the inflammatory potential of the complex.[105] During the interaction of soluble antigens and their antibodies at or near equivalence, a factor B–dependent C3 convertase assembles on the immune precipitate and disrupts some of the primary bonds. Covalent binding of C3 to the Fd portion of IgG may be the relevant interaction that disrupts the lattice and sterically interferes with reassociation.[138] It has been shown that complement components from C5 to C9 are not needed for this phenomenon but that activation of the early components of the classic complement pathway augments this effect of the alternative pathway.[137] However, the classic complement cascade alone is far less efficient in disrupting the lattice. The affinity of antigen and antibody is an important determinant of the effectiveness of this potentially anti-inflammatory effect of complement activation.[135]

Receptors for antigen, antibody, or C3b can localize complexes to particular sites. For example, renal podocytes possess C3b receptors and can localize immune complexes that have fixed complement.[11, 120] Large complexes containing IgM antibody are cleared via receptors in the liver rather than the spleen.[126]

COMPLEMENT ACTIVATION

Activation of the classic cascade leads to the release of two major anaphylatoxins, C3a and C5a, and a minor anaphylatoxin, C4a.[26, 46, 57] Anaphylatoxins act via specific receptors on basophils and mast cells to release granular constituents, such as histamine.[19] The resultant increase in vascular permeability causes tissues to swell, localizes immune complexes, and facilitates their deposition within the vessel wall. Complement components and clotting factors also diffuse to the site.

C5a, or its cleavage product C5a des Arg, bound to vitamin D binding protein (plasma cochemotaxin), is the major complement-derived chemotactic factor and is active upon neutrophils, eosinophils, and monocytes.[47, 116, 142] However, as in the blood differential count, neutrophils predominate since there is little cell selectivity. The interaction of many of these vasoactive factors, such as histamine and platelet activating factor (PAF), or cytokines up-regulate adhesion molecules on migrating cells, as well as vascular endothelial cells, which are required for chemotaxis and transendothelial migration regardless of whether a cell lodges within the vessel wall, localizes around it, or migrates to a more distant site.

Neutrophils possess receptors for C5a, C3b (CRI), C3bi (CR3), and IgG ($F_c\gamma$RII, $F_c\gamma$RIIIB) and can attach to immune complexes (immune adhesion) and phagocytose them.[5, 47, 95, 97, 151] If the complex is too large or is attached to a nonphagocytosable surface, the cells will nevertheless secrete as a result of the interaction (frustrated phagocytosis). In some instances, activated monocytes (macrophages) may predominate and can also directly cause tissue damage by secretion of a similarly large array of proinflammatory substances, as well as procoagulant activity, including tissue factor and factor VII.[127]

RELEASE OF CELL CONSTITUENTS

Secretory products of neutrophils or monocytes can damage cells, including endothelial cells and other constituents of a vessel wall. Some of these products are toxic oxygen metabolites, such as H_2O_2, O_2^- and OH•, and neutral proteases, such as cathepsin G and elastase.[87] The latter enzyme can digest elastin and the link protein of proteoglycan (aggrecan) to yield hyaluronic acid and proteoglycan monomer.[84] Various metalloenzymes that are also secreted digest collagen (types I and III), further digest the core protein of proteoglycans, and degrade basement membrane.

Interstitial or neutrophil procollagenases (metalloproteinase I and VIII) are converted to collagenase by enzymes, such as plasmin or plasma kallikrein, or stromelysin (metalloproteinase III) and digest types I and III collagen. Gelatinases A and B degrade collagen further once it has been cleaved by collagenase and are among the proteases that degrade elastin, proteoglycans, and basement membrane collagen (type IV).[81] LTB_4 and PAF are additional chemotactic factors for neutrophils that are released from both neutrophils and monocytes. Prostaglandin E_2 (PGE_2), a potent vasodilator, is also released. Cytokines are produced; for example, neutrophils secrete IL-8 and tumor necrosis factor (TNF)-α, and monocytes secrete IL-1, TNF-α, IL-6, IL-8, and β chemokines, such as monocyte chemotactic protein (MCP)-1 and macrophage inflammatory peptide (MIPI)-α and MIPI-β.[18, 33]

PERTURBATION/INJURY TO ENDOTHELIAL CELLS

Endothelial cells can be activated to express class II major histocompatibility complex (MHC), up-regulate adhesion molecules so as to interact with blood cells, and become a thrombogenic surface. Histamine and thrombin are among the inflammatory products that up-regulate P-selectin.[6, 103] Integrins such as intercellular adhesion molecule (ICAM)-1 and (VCAM)-1 and the selectin (ELAM-1 are up-regulated by IL-1 and TNF-α.[15, 110, 118] Each of these latter cytokines also increases expression of tissue factor, decreases thrombomodulin-dependent activation of protein C, and increases secretion of plasminogen activator inhibitor, but decreases tissue plasminogen activator levels.[9, 65, 66] Further, TNF-α down-regulates the activated protein C cofactor, protein S.[73] The net result is to augment or initiate local blood coagulation and diminish fibrinolysis.

In the native state, endothelial cells do not express tissue factor but instead constitutively express thrombomodulin. This will complex with any local thrombin that may form and divert it from clotting fibrinogen. The thrombin-thrombomodulin complex also activates protein C. Protein Ca in complex with protein S inactivates any active factor Va or VIIIa that might facilitate clotting. In this manner, thrombomodulin acts as an anticoagulant. The stimulated endothelial cell, which now expresses tissue factor and down-regulates thrombomodulin, reverses this process, and the endothelial surface becomes thrombogenic. These reactions are fast, the process occurring within a few hours. The effects modulating fibrinolysis occur over 1 to 2 days, but the literature is less consistent on this point. For example, TNF-α has been reported to increase endothelial cell urokinase-type plasminogen activator, as well as plasminogen activator inhibitor (PAI)-1.[112]

INITIATION OF BLOOD COAGULATION AND FIBRINOLYSIS

The expression of tissue factor with endothelial cell damage and exposure of plasma to the subendothelium are sufficient to aggregate platelets and to initiate the extrinsic coagulation cascade (Fig. 52–1). Exposure to negatively charged proteoglycans can also activate the intrinsic coagulation cascade and liberate bradykinin (see Chapter 11). Figure 52–2 expands the final step in the conversion of fibrinogen to fibrin and adds the fibrinolytic pathway. At a later point in time, sufficient tissue plasminogen activator or urokinase-type plasminogen activator is produced to begin to lyse the clot. A circulating form of fibronectin known as cold-insoluble globulin binds to fibrin, is actually cross-linked to it by factor XIIIa, and is then degraded by plasmin to form intermediate-sized fibrin degradation products. The resultant material has the tinctorial properties and appearance of fibrinoid. A vessel or tissue with evident necrosis is said to have been subjected to fibrinoid necrosis (Fig. 52–3).

SPECIFIC DISORDERS

The various vasculitic disorders differ considerably in their histopathology in the following ways: demonstration of immune complexes within injured vessels or tissue, complement activation or tissue deposition, neutrophilic versus mononuclear cell infiltration, size and location of vessels, or eccentric versus concentric involvement. Table 52–2 compares the major systemic vasculitides in terms of these parameters on a 0 to +4 basis, in which +4 means that most, if not all, patients will demonstrate the finding and 0 or +1 means that none or only a relatively small percentage demonstrate the finding.

These observations must be tempered by the knowledge that the presence of immune complexes may be transient, that mononuclear cell infiltration can be seen as inflamma-

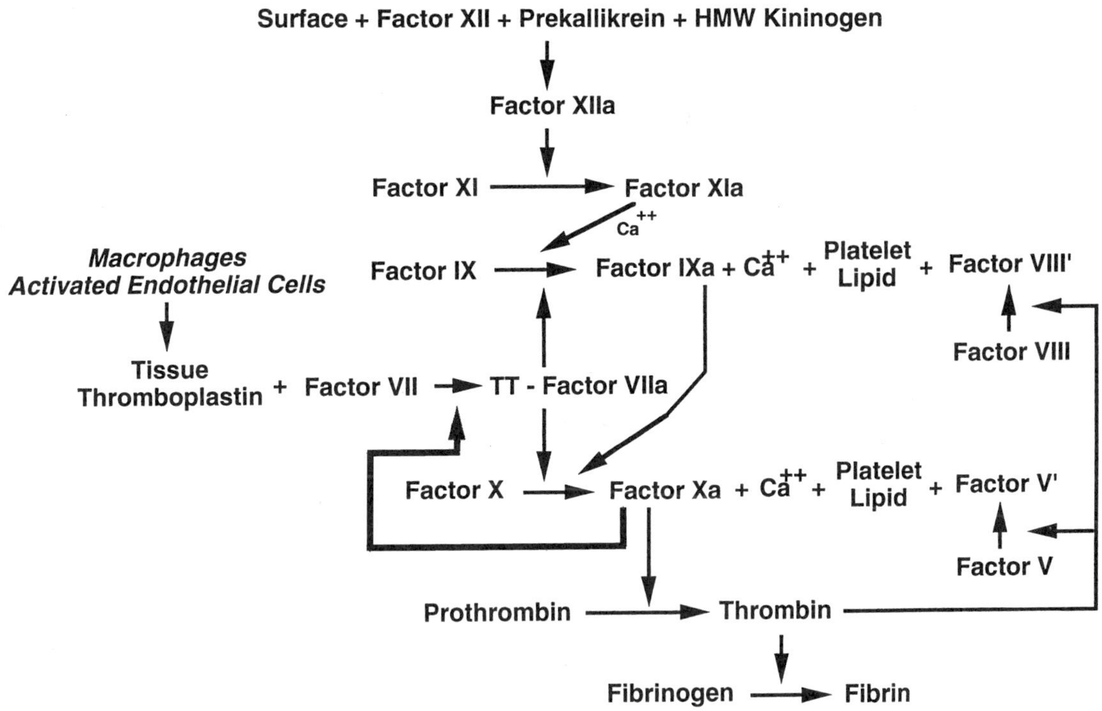

FIGURE 52–1. The intrinsic and extrinsic coagulation pathways for formation of fibrin.

tion mediated by neutrophils becomes quiescent, and that in many instances, the inciting antigen (if any) is not known. When complement is activated, the classic pathway predominates in all the listed disorders except Schönlein-Henoch purpura, which is dependent on IgA and the alternative complement pathway.

CLINICAL PRESENTATION AND THERAPY

The reader is referred to major reviews in other texts for details.[29, 82] Only brief consideration of each is given here.

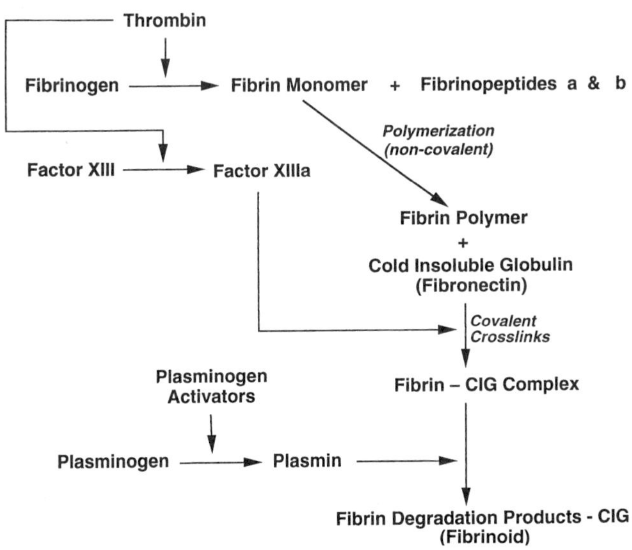

FIGURE 52–2. Formation and degradation of fibrinogen to form fibrinoid.

Polyarteritis Nodosa

This is a systemic vasculitis in which involvement of small and medium-sized arterial vessels predominates. However, damage to major abdominal vessels that derive from the celiac axis may be secondary to immune complex deposition within the much smaller nutrient vaso vasorum. This leads to fibrinoid necrosis of the wall of a much larger vessel and to the eccentric aneurysmal dilatation that is so characteristic (but not pathognomonic) of this disorder.[92, 152]

It is more commonly seen in men, with a mean age of onset of 45 years. There is often fever, malaise, myalgias, anthralgies, and occasionally frank arthritis. An antecedent association with hepatitis B infection is seen in approximately 20 to 30% of patients. Presentation of a hepatic disorder can vary from asymptomatic enzyme elevation to chronic active

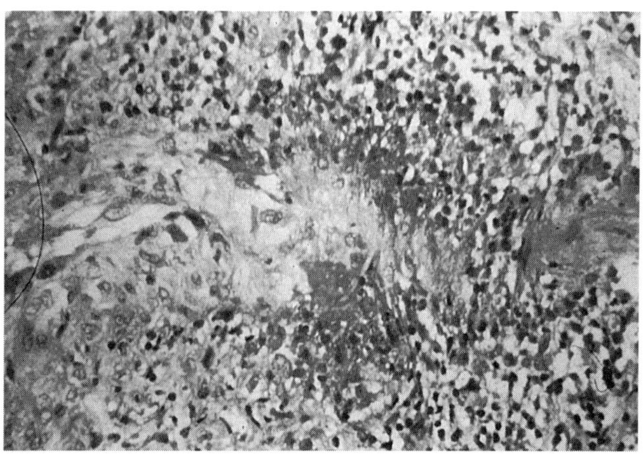

FIGURE 52–3. Positive stain for fibrin within an inflamed vessel wall indicative of fibrinoid necrosis.

TABLE 52–2
COMPARISON OF MAJOR SYSTEMIC VASCULITIDES

	Immune Complexes	Complement Activity	Neutrophils	Mononuclear Cells
Polyarteritis nodosa	+2	+2	+4	+1
Churg-Strauss syndrome	+2	+2	+3	+3
Wegener's granulomatosis	+1	±	+1	+4
Temporal arteritis	±	±	–	+4
Takayasu's arteritis	±	±	–	+4
Serum sickness	+4	+4	+4	–
Cryoglobulinemia	+4	+4	+4	–
Systemic lupus	+3	+3	+3	+1
Schönlein-Henoch purpura	+2	+2	+3	±
Behçet's disease	±	–	+3	±

hepatitis or cirrhosis.[130] In these cases, immune complexes of hepatitis B surface antigen and IgG antibody are thought to be the pathogenic immune complex.

The use of more sensitive assays that employ monoclonal antibodies against hepatitis B surface antigen or molecular probes for viral DNA in the peripheral blood lymphocytes of affected patients has been reported to increase the identification of hepatitis B infection in vasculitis patients who previously were negative using standard assays.[101] The prevalence of hepatitis B seropositively in polyarteritis may approach 75%.[21, 129] Additional evidence for infectious agents as the cause of systemic necrotizing vasculitis has included patients in whom the suspected agent was cytomegalovirus, parvovirus, and human immunodeficiency virus (HIV)-1.

Virtually any organ system of the body can be affected. However, a classic triad of renovascular hypertension, central nervous system (CNS) manifestations such as cerebral infarction, and abdominal pain (mesenteric angina or mesenteric thrombosis) is a common presentation. Weight loss, muscle pain, and myalgias or myositis can reflect vasculitis of muscles (Fig. 52–4). Cardiac involvement can include coronary arteritis with myocardial infarction, as well as hypertensive cardiovascular disease.[72] Pericarditis is less commonly seen. Gastrointestinal involvement is common and can be multifaceted. Mesenteric vasculitis (Fig. 52–5) can cause massive infarction or bowel perforation, whereas hepatic infarcts may reveal a friction rub upon deep inspiration during physical examination. Cholecystitis is very frequently seen at autopsy even if it is not diagnosed antemortem. Pancreatitis may also be evident. Isolated single organ involvement, particularly of the gastrointestinal tract, occurs.

The peripheral nervous system can be involved in two general ways. Vasculitis of vaso nervosum can cause infarction of nerves to cause a mononeuritis multiplex, or alternatively, a symmetric polyneuropathy may be seen.[107] CNS involvement can manifest as seizures, infarction, or cerebral hemorrhage. Cutaneous involvement can include a maculopapular rash, peripheral infarcts, livido reticularis, ulceration secondary to vasculitis, or subcutaneous nodules. Hypertension with elevated renin and aldosterone levels may be an independent early finding before renal disease (glomerulonephritis) is apparent and may dominate the clinical picture to cause nephrosclerosis, cardiac, and cerebrovascular manifestations.[146]

Laboratory data include an elevated sedimentation rate, leucocytosis, anemia, and thrombocytosis. The C1q binding assay or Raji cell assay is positive for immune complexes in at least two thirds of patients, and depressed C3 or C4 is often found. The rheumatoid factor may be positive in low titer, such as 1:160 or 1:320. Biopsy evidence of vasculitis is required to be certain of the diagnosis. Tissues often sampled include skin, muscle, sural nerve, or kidney. Angiographic evidence of characteristic aneurysmal dilatation of abdominal vessels (hepatic, renal, splenic, mesenteric) may be seen after

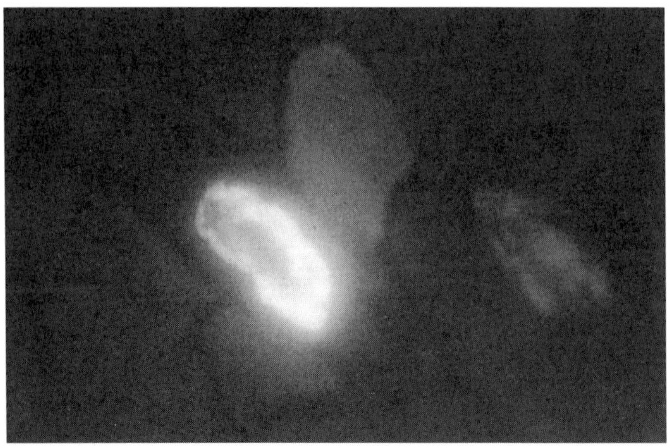

FIGURE 52–4. Positive immunofluorescence for IgG within the vessel wall of a small muscular artery.

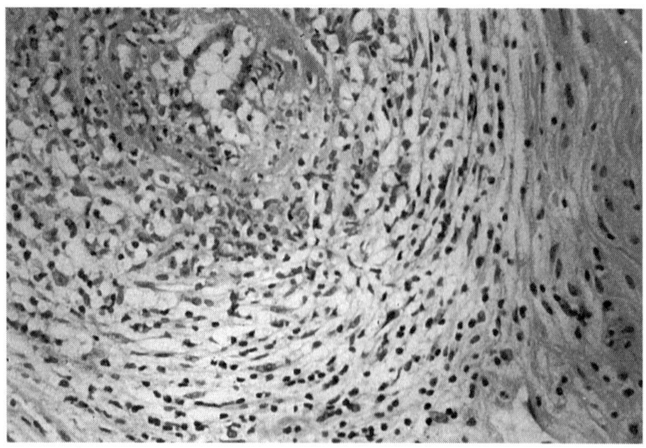

FIGURE 52–5. Classic vasculitis of a medium-size blood vessel in a patient with polyarteritis nodosa. There is disruption of the endothelium and media with evident inflammation throughout the entire vessel wall and surrounding connective tissue.

a celiac axis angiogram and is highly suggestive of polyarteritis nodosa if consistent with the clinical presentation. Lesions are commonly seen at branch points of vessels.

Therapy consists of daily corticosteroids in divided doses at 1 mg/kg for a period of months, depending on the clinical response. The dose is then consolidated to a single morning dose, with gradual conversion to alternate-day therapy. The dose is gradually decreased. If remission is achieved, therapy can be discontinued. Alternatively, a maintenance dose may be required. It is not unusual to require corticosteroids for 1 to 2 years.

Cytotoxic therapy with cyclophosphamide (cytoxan) is also utilized to treat polyarteritis nodosa because the incidence of induction of remission is higher with combined therapy.[40, 42] However, since steroids alone can be effective, use of cytoxan should be reserved for patients with more severe presentation, who worsen in spite of corticosteroids, or who show no objective improvement after 1 month of intensive corticosteroid therapy. These authors utilize combined therapy in most instances, as described by Fauci and Leavitt.[44] Cyclophosphamide is given orally at 2 mg/kg so as to maintain a white blood count of 3,000 to 3,500. The drug is continued for 1 year after remission is achieved and then tapered by 25 mg every 2 months. Steroids are given at 1 mg/kg for 1 month of therapy and then converted to alternate-day therapy and the dose tapered over 3 to 6 months. Exacerbations are treated with high-dose corticosteroids and again tapered. Potential complications of cytoxan used in this manner include an increased incidence of lymphoma, interstitial cystitis, bladder carcinoma, gonadal dysfunction, pulmonary fibrosis, bone marrow suppression, and myelodysplasia.

Churg-Strauss Syndrome

Churg-Strauss syndrome, or allergic angiitis and granulomatosis, is often described as a variant of polyarteritis nodosa but also has features of Wegener's granulomatosis.[89] Pulmonary manifestations are far more common than is seen in polyarteritis nodosa, although the histopathology of lesions seen may be identical. Pulmonary vessels are often involved, asthma is a common presenting complaint, and eosinophilia is associated. It is often described as a necrotizing vasculitis in an allergic asthmatic. However, some features are reminiscent of Wegener's granulomatosis since granuloma formation is typically seen.[102] There also is more prominent involvement of veins, venules, and arterioles. Eosinophil cationic protein deposition has been demonstrated within granulomas.[136] In contrast to polyarteritis nodosa, there is no association with hepatitis B antigenemia. The approach to therapy is essentially the same as that of classic polyarteritis nodosa.

Wegener's Granulomatosis

This disorder is primarily a pulmonary–renal syndrome in which there is a necrotizing vasculitis of arteries and veins of the upper or lower respiratory tracts and glomerulonephritis.[45, 69] The stimulus is unknown but appears to incite activated monocytes as a prominent feature in contrast to the predominance of activated neutrophils as seen in polyarteritis nodosa or neutrophils plus eosinophils as seen in Churg-Strauss syndrome. Release of neutral proteases, oxidants, metalloproteinases, prostaglandins, leukotrienes, and cytokines ensues with localized initiation of coagulation and fibrinolysis as described earlier. Involvement of the upper respiratory tract often involves severe rhinitis or rhinorrhea (20%), sinusitis (50%), nasal mucosal ulceration, and less frequently, otitis media. The symptoms can be confused initially with allergic or nonallergic rhinosinusitis. There may also be secondary infection with staphylococcal aureus requiring antibiotic treatment. Biopsy in this region is often not specific and rarely reveals either granulomas or clear-cut vasculitis. Granulomas with giant cell formation are best seen on lung biopsy.

Pulmonary symptoms may include cough, dyspnea, and hemoptysis. Pulmonary infiltrates are often nodular and cavitate. Distinction from other granulomatous disorders that may cavitate is important, such as pulmonary tuberculosis, sarcoidosis, or systemic fungal infection. Pleuritis with effusion may be seen, whereas hilar adenopathy and calcification are rarely, if ever, present. Renal involvement can include frank hematuria, proteinuria, and renal failure. Typical pathology includes a focal and segmental glomerulonephritis, but a diffuse fulminant (rapidly progressive) glomerulonephritis with crescent formation and renal failure may also be seen.[74] However, granulomas are not usually evident upon renal biopsy.

Other organs can also be involved. Retroorbital disease can cause proptosis. There may be skin rash, peripheral neuropathy, episcleritis, arthralgias or arthritis, or cranial neuropathy. Constitutional symptoms of fever and weight loss may be seen. Necrosis of the nasal septum with collapse of nasal cartilage can yield the saddle-nose deformity.

Laboratory data include a prominently elevated sedimentation rate, leucocytosis, anemia, and a positive test for antineutrophil cytoplasmic antibodies (ANCA). In 80% of patients, these are directed to proteinase 3 and are designated cytoplasmic ANCA (c-ANCA) (Fig. 52–6).[39, 61] A less specific ANCA with a perinuclear distribution (p-ANCA) is directed

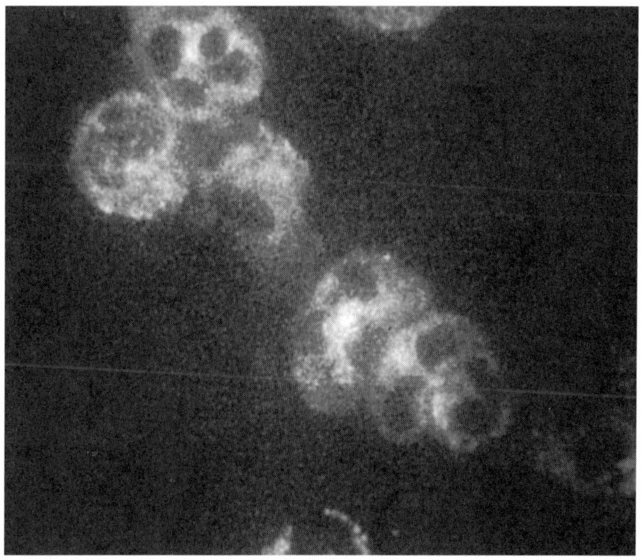

FIGURE 52–6. Positive c-ANCA in a patient with Wegener's granulomatosis.

to myeloperoxidase or elastase or cathepsin G and may be seen in a variety of other connective tissue disorders, including polyarteritis nodosa, Churg-Strauss syndrome, inflammatory bowel disease, systemic lupus erythematosus, and rheumatoid arthritis. Another systemic vasculitis variant called microscopic polyarteritis is defined by crescentic necrotizing glomerulonephritis in association with small vessel vasculitis but without granulomas and is associated with both c-ANCA and p-ANCA. ANCA may also be directly involved in causing the inflammation encountered in Wegener's granulomatosis.

Cytokines such as TNF-α can translocate ANCA-reactive proteases from the primary granules of neutrophils to the cell surface, thereby exposing the antigen to the cell surface and providing antigen for the immune system.[39] The antibodies may activate neutrophils or cause endothelial cell damage or lysis by primed neutrophils.[38, 85, 119] Active disease seems to be particularly associated with antibody of the IgG_3 subclass.[108] On the other hand, IL-I, TNF-α, and interferon (IFN)-γ may induce endothelial cells to express proteinase 3 on their surface.[132] Binding of antibody may induce antibody-dependent cell-mediated cytotoxicity mediated by mononuclear cells or neutrophils. Evidence from in vivo models to support one mechanism or another is lacking, however. These newer pathophysiologic studies have been reviewed and suggest an important and different kind of role for the neutrophil.[80]

Cytotoxic therapy is critical for the treatment of Wegener's granulomatosis. As with all necrotizing vasculitides very prompt intervention is essential to prevent irreversible scarring. The regimen outlined earlier in conjunction with corticosteroids is the standard approach.[43, 69] The mortality of the disease has been dramatically improved as a result. A combination of low-dose methotrexate and prednisone may provide a less toxic, acceptable alternative in patients whose disease is not life threatening.[71, 132] Therapy with trimethoprim/sulfamethoxazole has been reported to be effective in some patients, but these observations are unconfirmed.[143]

Lymphomatoid granulomatosis and lethal centrofacial midline granuloma resemble Wegener's granulomatosis but are invasive lymphomas with vascular inflammation or granulomatosus reaction.[41, 58, 115] Their prognosis is poor, and they should be treated utilizing chemotherapy protocols for highly invasive lymphomas.

Giant Cell Arteritides

These disorders include temporal or cranial arteritis, polymyalgia rheumatica, and Takayasu's arteriopathy. Temporal arteritis affects an older age group, usually over 55 years of age. In contradistinction to the aforementioned necrotizing arteritides, women are more commonly affected. Medium- to large-sized vessels are involved, most prominently the internal and external carotid system.[55, 57] Headache is common and can be unilateral or bilateral, often localized to the temporal areas. The temporal artery may be thickened, reddened, and tortuous. Occasionally, jaw or tongue claudication is reported. A particularly dangerous and not uncommon complication, which also can be the initial presentation, is sudden blindness due to occlusion of the ophthalmic artery to include the central retinal artery.

Severe proximal shoulder girdle pain and pain in the lower back, hips, and thighs may be seen, usually without true muscle weakness or evidence of elevated muscle enzymes. When these symptoms are present as an isolated muscular syndrome without overt vasculitis, it is called polymyalgia rheumatica.[23] There may be fever (usually low grade but occasionally prominent), malaise, arthralgias, and rarely frank arthritis.[20] The disorder generally runs a self-limited course whose duration is variously reported to be a mean of 1 to 3 years.[7] Temporal arteritis in some patients may be an even more widespread panarteritis and involve the cerebral vessels (stroke), renal vasculature (glomerulonephritis, renal infarction), and coronary arteries (myocardial infarction). Theoretically, virtually any artery can be involved; however, these are uncommon compared with isolated temporal artery involvement. Aortitis can lead to aortic insufficiency, thoracic aneurysms, or dissection.[37, 64, 88]

Fever, malaise, arthralgias, arthritis, a prominently elevated sedimentation rate, and anemia are commonly associated features of either temporal arteritis or polymyalgia rheumatica. Biopsy of the temporal artery, which should be serially sectioned, reveals infiltration with lymphocytes and macrophages. There may be a prominence of activated macrophages and epithelioid cells with giant cell formation located along the internal elastic lamina, with evident digestion by elastase, although giant cells are not always evident (Fig. 52–7). There may be skipped areas along the vessel, and the inflammation may be eccentric, that is, present along one side of the vessel but not circumferential. Thus serially sectioning a segment of the vessel is important. Temporal artery biopsy of patients presenting with polymyalgia rheumatica may reveal pathologic changes consistent with temporal arteritis in about 20% of patients, even though temporal arteritis is not clinically evident.

There are data pertaining to the role of the immune system in the pathogenesis of the lesions seen. Circulating immune complexes may be present, but it is uncommon to find immunoglobulin or complement deposition in biopsy material. Nevertheless, they are present in some patients.[35, 113] Both polymyalgia rheumatica and temporal arteritis are associated with an increased incidence of HLA-DR4 and perhaps HLA-DR3 and HLA-DR4 combined.[8, 14, 98] Association with the second hypervariable region of HLA-DRB1α, to include virtually all alleles, is seen in both polymyalgia rheumatica and giant cell arteritis.[145] This is in contrast to rheumatoid arteritis, in which the HLA-DR4 association is with the third hypervariable region, particularly alleles 0401 and 0404/8.

The predominant type of lymphocyte seen in biopsy material is the $CD4^+$ helper subset.[24] Production of IL-2 and IFN-γ by such lymphocytes is prominent in giant cell arteritis, whereas only IL-2 was found in positive biopsies of polymyalgia rheumatica patients.[144] Macrophages isolated from involved tissue produce large quantities of mRNA and protein for IL-Iβ, IL-6, and 72 kD type IV collagenase (metalloproteinase II).[141] Circulating blood cells also can be shown to be activated. Plasma IL-6 levels are high.[122] Both $CD4^+$ and $CD8^+$ T lymphocytes of patients with giant cell arteritis have selected usage of T-cell antigen receptor (TCR) V and J gene segments, indicative of oligoclonal expansion. Certain V_β-J_β combinations are favored, perhaps indicative of recognition of a putative disease-related antigen.[60]

Therapy of temporal arteritis requires high-dose (40–80

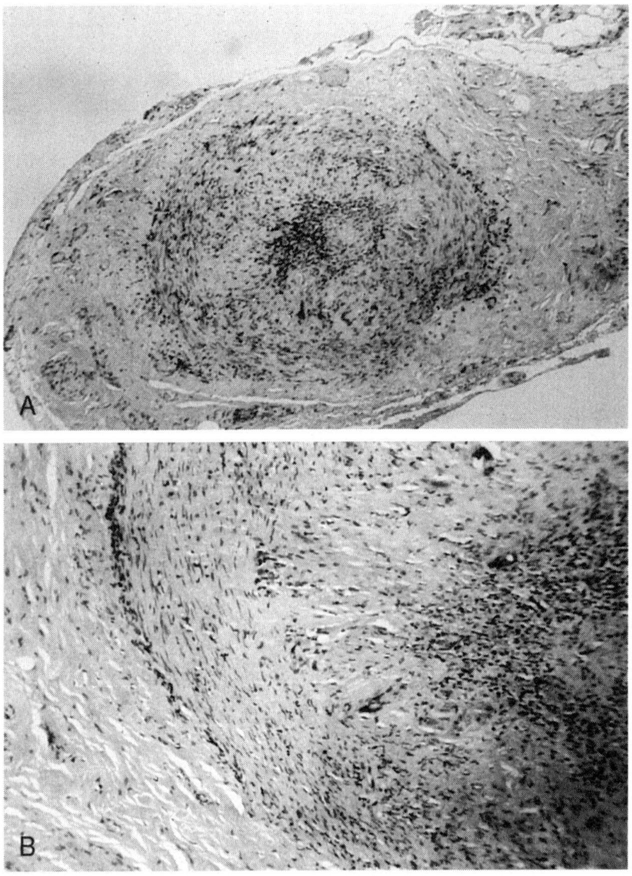

FIGURE 52–7. (A) Temporal artery biopsy in a patient with cranial arteritis, which reveals an inflammatory reaction within the media of the vessel that is eccentric. (B) High-power magnification reveals a mononuclear cell infiltrate with giant cells.

mg) prednisone therapy for many months (3–6 months) and then tapering to about 10 mg for 1 to 2 years. Polymyalgia rheumatica may be treated with 5 to 15 mg of prednisone daily, with dramatic amelioration of symptoms. Thus the clinical distinction from overt temporal arteritis is important.[75, 76] Biopsy of treated patients to confirm the diagnosis when in question can be done within 14 days and still be revealing, even after steroids have been started.[2]

By contrast, Takayasu's arteriopathy is an uncommon disorder but has very similar, if not identical, pathologic changes in affected blood vessels. It affects young women, often of Oriental descent, and also involves major blood vessels emanating from the aortic arch.[62] In a Japanese population studied, an increased incidence of HLA antigen Bw52 has been reported.[78] An association with B-cell alloantigens MB3 and DR4 was observed in a North American sample.[140]

Involvement of the external carotid arteries is uncommon, but involvement of the internal carotids, subclavian vessels, pulmonary branches, and coronary arteries may be seen, as well as involvement of abdominal vessels. Subclavian vessel involvement with ischemia or occlusion can lead to an absent peripheral pulse, hence the term pulseless disease. Cerebral vasculitis with stroke syndromes, myocardial infarction, pulmonary infarction, bowel infarction, renovascular hypertension, and congestive heart failure may all occur secondary to vasculitis. Arteriography usually reveals tapered vessels, an area of abrupt narrowing, and beading of vessels within the CNS. On physical examination, bruits are the most common physical finding.[86] Laboratory evaluation may reveal an elevated sedimentation rate, but there are no specific tests that can assist in this diagnosis. High-dose corticosteroids may be used to treat Takayasu's arteriopathy, but the response has been quite varied and less successful than for temporal arteritis. Cytoxan therapy or low-dose methotrexate has been tried either alone or with corticosteroids, particularly when the response to steroids alone has not been satisfactory.[70] Vascular reconstructive surgery to prevent ischemic injury to vital organs can improve the prognosis.[86]

Isolated CNS Vasculitis

This is a granulomatous vasculitis confined to the brain, with symptoms of infarction, seizures, delirium, dementia, personality change, and headache that require cerebral angiography for diagnosis and in some instances, brain biopsy (Fig. 52–8).[93] There is no evident involvement of other organs. Treatment is usually attempted with cytoxan plus corticosteroids.[13, 30]

Hypersensitivity Angiitis

This term is commonly used to describe a series of unrelated disorders in which small blood vessels are prominently involved (arteries, capillaries, venules) and larger muscular arteries or veins less so, with cutaneous manifestations particularly evident. The postcapillary venule is most commonly involved (Fig. 52–9). The disorders include serum sickness, Schönlein-Henoch purpura, cryoglobulinemia, small vessel vasculitis that can be associated with connective tissue diseases such as systemic lupus erythematosus, cutaneous vasculitis associated with malignancy, or isolated cutaneous vasculitis.[42, 149]

For the cutaneous manifestation, the term leucocytoclastic angiitis is often used because the histopathology consists of a neutrophilic vasculitis of small vessels, often with immune complex and complement deposition, and nuclear debris

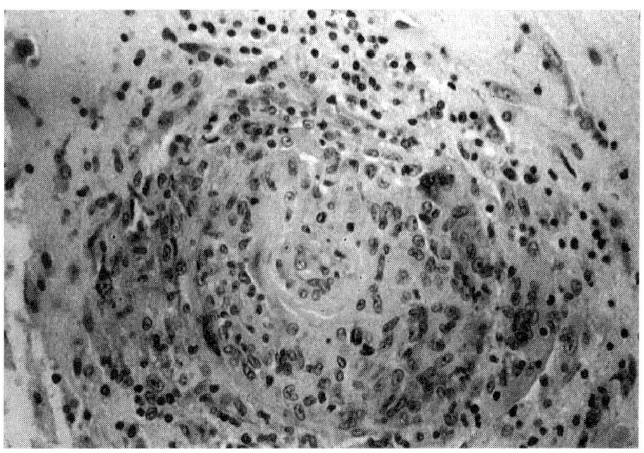

FIGURE 52–8. Brain biopsy of a patient with isolated vasculitis of the central nervous system demonstrates vasculitis with early granuloma formation.

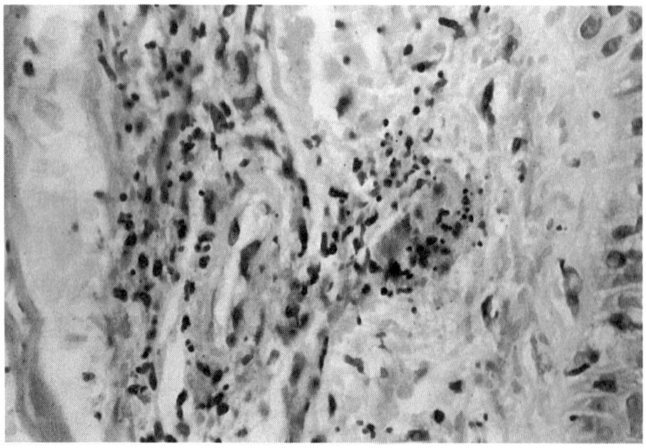

FIGURE 52–9. Leukocytoclastic vasculitis of cutaneous blood vessels seen in a patient with Henoch-Schönlein purpura.

derived from disintegrating neutrophils. The most common clinical manifestation is palpable purpura; this represents a small cutaneous infarct with surrounding hemorrhage, so that the lesions are elevated and an individual lesion will not blanch.[99] Although the inciting antigen is typically unknown, the pathology is suggestive of an immune complex–mediated disorder. However, cutaneous manifestations can include urticaria, ulceration, nodules, or papular rash.

Serum sickness is typically due to a drug reaction and consists of fever, lymphadenopathy, urticarial or maculopapular skin rash, arthralgias or overt arthritis, and, in as many as 50% of subjects, proteinuria indicative of a glomerulonephritis.[10] Uncommonly, a diffuse proliferative nephritis can be seen, which is associated with hematuria and red cell casts. Although self-limited, a brief course of corticosteroids can rapidly resolve symptoms and should be utilized in more severely affected persons.

Schönlein-Henoch purpura is typically a disease of childhood but can occur at any age.[68, 123] An association with prior streptococcal infection or a manifestation of a drug reaction has been reported but is not proven in terms of etiology.[104] The cutaneous reaction involves small and large purpuric areas, with a predilection for the lower extremities, particularly the buttocks and upper thigh. Although biopsy reveals a leucocytoclastic angiitis, IgA deposition and alternative complement pathway components are seen.[36, 54, 111] Plasma IgA levels may be elevated, and increased IgA-producing cells in the blood of such patients is demonstrable.[16]

Other organ systems may be affected, particularly the gastrointestinal tract, joints, and kidney. There may be abdominal pain or bloody stools due to a small vessel vasculitis of the gastrointestinal tract. Arthralgias and arthritis may be present, as well as a glomerulonephritis. A single, dramatic episode can occur and spontaneously resolve in 1 to 2 weeks, with no recurrence. In some patients, intermittent exacerbations may recur over a period of a few months. On rare occasion, there may be recurrences over a year or more. Treatment is usually supportive, but corticosteroid at 1 mg/kg is recommended for severe presentation or recurrent disease. It is difficult to assess the efficacy of therapy because of the remitting nature of the disease. Fever and an elevated sedimentation rate are commonly present.

Essential mixed cryoglobulinemia is an immune complex-mediated disease in which a monoclonal IgM rheumatoid factor is made that complexes with polyclonal IgG (type II cryoglobulin).[56, 117] The IgM is often of the V_k III b light chain variable region subgroup and the V_HI heavy chain variable region subgroup produced by a clonal expansion of B lymphocytes.[117] Although typical palpable purpura is seen, there may be many other systemic manifestations of the disease. It is strongly associated with hepatitis C infection, often with chronic active or progressive hepatitis.[1, 4, 91] A glomerulonephritis is commonly seen with marked depression of plasma C4 and C3 levels. Peripheral neuropathy is common, as is digital infarction, severe skin ulceration, and arthritis. Cold urticaria may occasionally be associated.[121] In theory, virtually any organ can be affected. Individual patients may have differing and sometimes unusual manifestations. It is poorly responsive to therapy. Often a combination of plasmapheresis, corticosteroids, and cytotoxic agents are utilized.[53] IFN-α may now be the treatment of choice, particularly in those who are hepatitis C positive.[17, 48, 106]

Vasculitis associated with systemic lupus erythematosus can include small vessels of the skin and present with a typical picture of leucocytoclastic angiitis.[22] There may be palpable purpura, urticaria (urticarial vasculitis), nodular lesions, skin ulceration, or digital infarction. Other connective tissue diseases, such as Sjögren's syndrome, occasionally can present similarly.[133, 134] Polyarteritis nodosa need not be exclusively related to larger blood vessels. Small vessels of the skin sometimes are also involved and may not be distinguishable from leucocytoclastic angiitis when present.

Rheumatoid arthritis can be associated with cutaneous vasculitis and palpable purpura. It can also be associated with a fulminant systemic vasculitis that resembles polyarteritis nodosa with circulating immune complexes and depressed C4 and C3 levels.[125] Systemic lupus patients may also have circulating cryoproteins, although they are typically a polyclonal IgM anti-IgG–type rheumatoid factor (type III cryoprotein).[56]

Cutaneous vasculitis has been associated with neoplasms and may represent an immune response to circulating tumor antigens.[59] It is most commonly seen with B-cell lymphoma or Hodgkin's disease. Isolated leukocytoclastic angiitis, with no association with any connective tissue disease or other manifestation, is an uncommon but well-described entity. In spite of the clear histopathology, the incidence of demonstrating immune complexes and complement deposition within involved cutaneous vessels is low.

Miscellaneous

Other forms of vasculitis may be considered a miscellaneous category. They are uncommon and less well characterized or understood. These include Behçet's disease, the hypocomplementemic urticarial vasculitis syndrome with C1q precipitins due to IgG anti-C1q, cutaneous nodular vasculitis, Degos' disease (malignant papulosis with gastrointestinal infarction), Buerger's disease (thromboangiitis obliterans), erythema elevatum diutinum, and Cogan's syndrome.[31, 67, 83, 94, 128, 133, 150] A group of embolic disorders with diffuse vasculopathy or in situ occlusion can mimic vasculitis and should be included in the differential diagnosis of vasculitis. These include subacute bacterial endocarditis, atrial myxoma, cholesterol emboli, and thrombotic thrombocytopenic purpura.[31]

REFERENCES

1. Abel G, Zhang Q-X, Agnello V: Hepatitis C virus infection in type II cryoglobulinemia. Arthritis Rheum 36:1341, 1993.
2. Achker AA, Lie JJ, Hunder GG, et al: How does previous corticosteroid treatment affect the biopsy findings in giant cell (temporal) arteritis. Ann Intern Med 120:987, 1994.
3. Adu J, Williams D: DNA-anti DNA circulating complexes in the nephritis of systemic lupus erythematosus. Clin Exp Immunol 43:605, 1981.
4. Agnello V, Chung RT, Kaplan LM: A role for hepatitis C virus infection in type II cryoglobulinemia. N Engl J Med 327:1490, 1992.
5. Ahearn JM, Fearon DT: Structure and function of the complement receptors CRI (CD35) and CR2 (CD21). Adv Immunol 46:183, 1989.
6. Asako H, Kurose I, Wolf R, et al: Role of H1 receptors and P selectin in histamine-induced leukocyte rolling and adhesion in post capillary venules. J Clin Invest 93:1508, 1994.
7. Ayoub WT, Franklin CM, Torretti D: Polymyalgia rheumatica. Duration of therapy and long term outcome. Am J Med 79:309, 1985.
8. Barrier J, Bignon JD, Soulillou JP, et al: Increased prevalence of HLA-DR4 in giant cell arteritis. N Engl J Med 305:104, 1981.
9. Bevilacque MP, Schleef RR, Gimbrone MA, et al: Regulation of the fibrinolytic system of cultured human vascular endothelium by interleukin 1. J Clin Invest 78:587, 1986.
10. Bielory L, Gasan P, Lawley TJ, et al: Human serum sickness: a prospective analysis of 35 patients treated with equine anti-thymocyte globulin for bone marrow failure. Medicine (Baltimore) 67:40, 1988.
11. Burkholder PM, Oberly TD, Barber TA, et al: Immune adherence in renal glomeruli: complement receptor sites in glomerular capillary epithelial cells. Am J Pathol 86:635, 1977.
12. Calabrese LH, Estes M, Yen-Lieberman B, et al: Systemic vasculitis in association with human immunodeficiency virus infection. Arthritis Rheum 32:569, 1989.
13. Calabrese LH, Mallek JA: Primary angiitis of the central nervous system. Medicine (Baltimore) 67:20, 1987.
14. Calamia KT, Moore SB, Elveback LR, et al: HLA-DR locus antigens in polymyalgia rheumatica and giant cell arteritis. J Rheumatol 8:993, 1981.
15. Carlos TM, Harlan JM: Leukocyte-endothelial adhesion molecules. Blood 84:2068, 1994.
16. Casanueva B, Rodriguez-Valverde V, Merino J, et al: Increased IgA-producing cells in the blood of patients with active Henoch-Schönlein purpura. Arthritis Rheum 26:854, 1983.
17. Casato M, Lagana B, Antonelli G, et al: Long-term result of therapy with interferon α for type II essential mixed cryoglobulinemia. Blood 78:3142, 1991.
18. Cassatella MA, Bazzoni F, Ceska M, et al: IL8 production by human polymorphonuclear leukocytes. The chemoattractant formyl-methionyl-leucyl-phenylalanine induces the gene expression and release of IL8 through a pertussis toxin-sensitive pathway. J Immunol 148:3216, 1992.
19. Chenoweth DE, Hugli TE: Demonstration of a specific C5a receptor on intact human polymorphonuclear leukocytes. Proc Natl Acad Sci USA 75:3943, 1978.
20. Chou C-T, Schumacher HR Jr: Arthritis Rheum 27:1107, 1984.
21. Christian CL: Hepatitis B virus (HBV) and systemic vasculitis. Clin Exp Immunol 9:1, 1991.
22. Christian CL, Sergent SS: Vasculitis syndromes: clinical and experimental models. Am J Med 61:385, 1976.
23. Chuang T-Y, Hunder GG, Ilstrup DM, et al: Ann Intern Med 97:672, 1982.
24. Cid MC, Campo E, Ercilla G, et al: Immunohistochemical analysis of lymphoid and macrophage cell subsets and their immunologic activation markers in temporal arteritis. Arthritis Rheum 32:884, 1989.
25. Clarkson SB, Kimberly RP, Valinsky JE, et al: Blockade of clearance of immune complexes by an anti Fc gamma receptor monoclonal antibody. J Exp Med 164:479, 1986.
26. Cochrane CG, Muller-Eberhard HJ: The derivation of two distinct anaphylatoxin activities from the third and fifth component of human complement. J Exp Med 127:371, 1968.
27. Cochrane CG, Weigle WO, Dixon FJ: The role of polymorphonuclear leukocytes in the initiation and cessation of the Arthus vasculitis. J Exp Med 110:481, 1959.
28. Combes B, Stastny P, Shorey J, et al: Glomerulonephritis with deposition of Australia antigen-antibody complexes in glomerulas basement membrane. Lancet 2:234, 1971.
29. Conn DL, Hunder GG, O'Duffy JD: Vasculitis and related disorders. In Kelley WN, Harris ED, Ruddy S, Sledge CB (eds): Textbook of Rheumatology, 4th edition. WB Saunders Co, Philadelphia, 1993, p 1077.
30. Cupps TR, Moore PM, Fauci AS: Isolated angiitis of the central nervous system. Prospective diagnostic and therapeutic considerations. Am J Med 74:97, 1993.
31. Degos R: Malignant atrophic papulosis. Br J Dermatol 100:21, 1979.
32. Dixon FJ: The role of antigen-antibody complexes in disease. Harvey Lect 58:21, 1963.
33. Djeu JY, Serbonsek D, Blanchard DK: Release of tumor necrosis factor alpha by human polymorphonuclear leukocytes. Blood 76:1405, 1990.
34. Doherty M, Bradfield JWB: Polyarteritis nodosa associated with acute cytomegalovirus infection. Ann Rheum Dis 40:419, 1981.
35. Espinoza LR, Bridgeford PH, Lowenstein MB, et al: Polymyalgia rheumatica and giant cell arteritis: circulating immune complexes. J Rheumatol 9:556, 1982.
36. Evans DL, William DG, Peters DK, et al: Glomerular deposition of properdin in Henoch-Schönlein syndrome and idiopathic focal nephritis. Br Med J 3:326, 1973.
37. Evans JM, Bowles CA, Bjornsson J, et al: Thoracic aortic aneurysm and rupture in giant cell arteritis. Arthritis Rheum 37:1539, 1994.
38. Ewert OH, Jennette JC, Falk RJ: The pathogenic role of anti-neutrophil cytoplasmic antibodies. Am J Kidney Dis 18:188, 1991.
39. Falk RJ, Terell RS, Charles LA, et al: Anti-neutrophil cytoplasmic autoantibodies induce neutrophils to degranulate and produce oxygen radicals in vitro. Proc Natl Acad Sci USA 87:4115, 1990.
40. Fauci AS, Doppman JL, Wolff SM: Cyclophosphamide-induced remissions in advanced polyarteritis nodosa. Am J Med 64:890, 1978.
41. Fauci AS, Haynes BF, Costa J: Lymphomatoid granulomatosis. Prospective clinical and therapeutic experience over 10 years. N Engl J Med 306:68, 1982.
42. Fauci AS, Haynes BF, Katz P: The spectrum of vasculitis: clinical, pathologic, immunologic, and therapeutic considerations. Ann Intern Med 89:660, 1978.
43. Fauci AS, Haynes BF, Katz P, et al: Wegener's granulomatosis: prospective clinical and therapeutic perspective over 85 patients for 21 years. Ann Intern Med 98:76, 1983.
44. Fauci AS, Leavitt RY: Systemic vasculitis. In: Current Therapy in Allergy, Immunology, and Rheumatology-3, BC Decker Inc, Philadelphia, 1988.
45. Fauci AS, Wolff SM: Wegener's granulomatosis. Studies of eighteen patients and a review of the literature. Medicine (Baltimore) 52:535, 1973.
46. Fernandez HM, Hugli TE: Primary structural analysis of the polypeptide portion of human C5a anaphylatoxin. J Biol Chem 253:6955, 1978.
47. Fernandez HN, Henson PM, Otani A, et al: Chemotactic response to human C3a and C5a anaphylatoxins I. Evaluation of C3a and C5a leukotaxis in vitro and understimulated in vivo conditions. J Immunol 120:109, 1978.
48. Ferri C, Marzo E, Longombardo G, et al: Interferon-α in mixed cryoglobulinemia patients: a randomized, crossover-controlled trial. Blood 81:1132, 1993.
49. Frank MM, Hamburger MI, Lawley TJ, et al: Defective reticuloendothelial system F_c-receptor function in systemic lupus erythematosus. N Engl J Med 300:518, 1979.
50. Fries LF, Mullins WW, Cho KR, et al: Monocyte receptors for the F_c portion of IgG are increased in systemic lupus erythematosus. J Immunol 132:685, 1984.
51. Gallo GR, Coulin-Glaser T, Lamm ME: Charge of circulating immune complexes as a factor in glomerular basement membrane localization. J Clin Invest 67:1305, 1981.
52. Gauthier VJ, Mannik M, Striker CE: Effect of cationized antibodies in preformed immune complexes on deposition and persistance in renal glomeruli. J Exp Med 156:766, 1982.
53. Geltner D, Kohn RW, Gorevic P, et al: The effect of combination therapy (steroids, immunosuppressives, and plasmapheresis) on 5

mixed cryoglobulinemia patients with renal, neurologic, and vascular involvement. Arthritis Rheum 24:1121, 1981.
54. Giangiacome J, Tsai CC: Dermal and glomerular deposition of IgA in anaphylactoid purpura. Am J Dis Child 131:981, 1977.
55. Goodman BW: Temporal arteritis. Am J Med 67:839, 1979.
56. Gorevic PD, Kassab HJ, Levo Y, et al: Mixed cryoglobulinemia; clinical aspects and long term follow up of 40 patients. Am J Med 69:287, 1980.
57. Gorski JP, Hugli TE, Muller-Eberhard HJ: C4a: the third anaphylatoxin of the human complement system. Proc Natl Acad Sci USA 76:5299, 1979.
58. Grange C, Cabane J, Dubois A, et al: Centrofacial malignant granulomas. Clinicopathologic study of 40 cases and review of the literature. Medicine (Baltimore) 71:179, 1992.
59. Green JM, Longley S, Edwards NL, et al: Vasculitis associated with malignancy. Experience with 13 patients and literature review. Medicine (Baltimore) 67:220, 1988.
60. Grunewald J, Andersson R, Rydberg L, et al: CD4(+) and CD8(+) J cell expansions using selected TCR V and J gene segments at onset of giant cell arteritis. Arthritis Rheum 37:1221, 1994.
61. Hagen CE, Bart EPB, Ballieux LA, et al: Antineutrophil cytoplasmic autoantibodies: a review of the antigen involved, the assays, and the clinical and possible pathogenetic consequences. Blood 81:1996, 1993.
62. Hall S, Barr W, Lie JT, et al: Takayasu's arteritis. A study of 32 North American patients. Medicine (Baltimore) 64:89, 1985.
63. Hamburger MI, Lawley TJ, Kimberly RP, et al: A serial study of splenic reticuloendothelial system F_c receptor functional activity in systemic lupus erythematosus. Arthritis Rheum 25:48, 1982.
64. Harris M: Dissecting aneurysm of the aorta due to giant cell arteritis. Br Heart J 30:840, 1968.
65. Hawroth PP, Handley DA, Esmon CT, et al: Interleukin 1 induces endothelial cell procoagulant while suppressing cell-surface anticoagulant activity. Proc Natl Acad Sci USA 83:3460, 1986.
66. Hawroth PP, Stern PM: Modulation of endothelial cell hemostatic properties by tumor necrosis factor. J Exp Med 163:740, 1986.
67. Haynes BF, Kaiser-Kupfer MI, Mason P: Cogan syndrome: studies in thirteen patients, long term follow up, and the review of the literature. Medicine (Baltimore) 59:426, 1980.
68. Heng MD. Henoch-Schönlein purpura. Br J Dermatol 112:235, 1985.
69. Hoffman GS, Kerr GS, Leavitt RY, et al: Wegener's granulomatosis: an analysis of 158 patients. Ann Intern Med 116:488, 1992.
70. Hoffman GS, Leavitt RY, Kerr GS, et al: Treatment of glucocorticoid-resistant or relapsing Takayasu arteritis with methotrexate. Arthritis Rheum 37:578, 1994.
71. Hoffman GS, Leavitt RY, Kerr GS, et al: The treatment of Wegener's granulomatosis with corticosteroids and methotrexate. Arthritis Rheum 35:1322, 1992.
72. Holsinger DR, Osmundson PJ, Edwards JE: The heart in periarteritis nosoda. Circulation 25:610, 1962.
73. Hooper WC, Phillips DJ, Ribeiro MJA, et al: Tumor necrosis factor α downregulates protein S secretion in human microvascular and umbilical vein endothelial cells but not in the Hep G-2 Hepatomia cell line. Blood 84:483, 1994.
74. Horn RF, Fauci AS, Rosenthal A: Renal biopsy pathology in Wegener's granulomatosis. Am J Pathol 74:423, 1974.
75. Hunder GG: Giant cell arteritis and polymyalgia rheumatica. In Kelley WN, Harris ED, Rudy S, Sledge CB (eds): Textbook of Rheumatology. WB Saunders, Philadelphia, 1993, pp 1103–1112.
76. Hunder GG, Sheps SG, Allen GI, et al: Daily and alternate-day corticosteroid regimens in treatment of giant cell arteritis: comparison in a prospective study. Ann Intern Med 82:613, 1975.
77. Huston KA, Hunder GG, Lie JT, et al: Temporal arteritis. A 25 year epidemiologic, clinical, and pathologic study. Ann Intern Med 88:167, 1978.
78. Isohisa I, Numano F, Maezawa J, et al: HLA-Bw52 in Takayasu's disease. Tissue Antigens 12:246, 1978.
79. Izui S, Lambert P-H, Miescher PA: In vitro demonstration of a particular affinity of glomerular basement membrane and collagen for DNA: a possible basis for a local formation of DNA-anti DNA complexes in systemic lupus erythematosus. J Exp Med 144:428, 1976.
80. Kallenberg CGM, Brouder E, Mulder HL: ANCA-pathophysiology revisited. Clin Exp Immunol 100:1, 1995.
81. Katsuda S, Okada Y, Okada Y, et al: Matrix metalloprotenase-9 (92 Kd gelatinase/type IV collagenase equals gelatenase B) can degrade arterial elastin, Am J Pathol 145:1208, 1994.
82. Katz P, Fauci AS: Systemic vasculitis. In Frank MM, Austen KF, Clamen HM, Unanue ER (eds): Samter's Immunological Diseases, 5th edition. Little Brown and Co, Boston, 1995, p 849.
83. Katz SI, Gallin JI, Hertz KC, et al: Erythema elevation diutinum: skin and systemic manifestations, immunologic studies and successful treatment with dapsone. Medicine (Baltimore) 56:443, 1977.
84. Keiser H, Greenwald RA, Feinstein G, et al: Degradation of cartilage proteoglycan by human neutral proteases—a model of joint injury II. Degradation of isolated bovine nasal cartilage proteoglycan. J Clin Invest 57:625, 1976.
85. Keogan MT, Esnault VLM, Green AJ, et al: Activation of human neutrophils by anti-neutrophil cytoplasm antibodies. Clin Exp Immunol 90:228, 1992.
86. Kerr GS, Hallahan CW, Giordino J, et al: Takayasu arteriopathy. Ann Intern Med 120:919, 1994.
87. Klebanolt SJ: Oxygen metabolites from phagocytes. In Gallin JI, Goldstein I, Synderman R (eds): Inflammation: Basic Principles and Clinical Correlates, 2nd edition. Raven Press, New York, 1992, pp 541–588.
88. Klinkhoff AV, Reid GD, Moscovich M: Aortic regurgitation in giant cell arteritis. Arthritis Rheum 28:582, 1985.
89. Lanham JC, Elkon KB, Pusey CD: Systemic vasculitis with asthma and eosinophilia. A clinical approach to the Churg-Strauss syndrome. Medicine (Baltimore) 63:65, 1984.
90. Lawley TJ, Bielory L, Gascon P, et al: A prospective clinical and immunologic analysis of serum sickness in man. N Engl J Med 311:1407, 1984.
91. Levey JM, Bjornsson B, Banner B: Mixed cryoglobulinemia in chronic hepatitis C infection. Medicine (Baltimore) 73:53, 1994.
92. Lie JT: Diagnostic histopathology of major systemic and pulmonary vasculitic syndromes. Rheum Dis Clin North Am 16:269, 1990.
93. Lie JT: Primary (granulomatous) angiitis of the central nervous system: a clinicopathologic analysis of 15 new cases and review of the literature. Hum Pathol 23:164, 1992.
94. Lie JT: Thromboangiitis obliterans (Buerger's Disease) in women. Medicine (Baltimore) 65:65, 1986.
95. Lieda E, Kinoshita T, Nojima J, et al: Different membrane anchors of Fc gamma RIII (CD16) on K/NK lymphocytes and neutrophils in protein vs. lipid anchor. J Immunol 143:1274, 1989.
96. LiLoong TC, Coyle PV, Anderson MJ, et al: Human serum parvovirus associated vasculitis. Postgrad Med J 62:493, 1986.
97. Looney RJ, Ryan DH, Takahashi K, et al: Identification of a second class of IgG F_c receptors on human neutrophils. A 40 kilodulton molecule also found on eosinophils. J Exp Med 163:826, 1986.
98. Lowenstein MB, Bridgeford PH, Vasey FB, et al: Increased frequency of HLA-DR3 and DR4 in polymyalgia rheumatica—giant cell arteritis, Arthritis Rheum 26:925, 1983.
99. Mackel SE, Jordan RE: Leukocytoclastic vasculitis. A cutaneous expression of immune complex disease. Arch Dermatol 118:296, 1982.
100. Mannick M, Haakenstad AD, Arend WP: The fate and detection of circulating immune complexes. Prog Immunol 5:91, 1974.
101. Marcellin P, Calmus Y, Takahashi H, et al: Latent hepatitis B virus (HBV) infection in systemic necrotizing vasculitis. Clin Exp Rheumatol 9:23, 1991.
102. Masi AT, Hunder GG, Lie JT, et al: The American College of Rheumatology 1990 criteria for the classification of the Churg-Strauss syndrome (allergic granulomatosis and angiitis). Arthritis Rheum 33:1094, 1990.
103. McEver RP, Beckstead JH, Moore KL, et al: GMP-140, a platelet alpha granule membrane protein is also synthesized by vascular endothelial cells and is localized in Weibel-Palade bodies. J Clin Invest 84:92, 1989.
104. Meadow R: Schönlein-Henoch syndrome. Arch Dis Child 54:822, 1979.
105. Miller GW, Nussenzweig V: A new complement function: solubilization of antigen-antibody aggregates. Proc Natl Acad Sci USA 72:418, 1975.
106. Misiani R, Bellavita P, Fenili D: Interferon alpha-2a therapy in cryoglobulinemia associated with hepatitis C virus. N Engl J Med 330:751, 1994.
107. Moore PM, Fauci AS: Neurologic manifestations of systemic vasculitis. A retrospective and prospective study of the clinicopathologic features and responses to therapy in 25 patients. Am J Med 71:517, 1981.
108. Mulder AHL, Stegeman CA, Kallenberg CGM: Activation of neutrophils by ANCA in active Wegener's granulomatosis: a predominant

note for the IgG 3 subclass of ANCA. Arthritis Rheum 37:5267, 1994. Abstract.

109. Müller-Eberhard HJ, Schreiber RD: Molecular biology and chemistry of the alternative pathway of complement. Adv Immunol 29:2, 1980.
110. Mulligan MS, Vaporciyan AA, Miyasaka M, et al: Tumor necrosis factor α regulates in vivo intrapulmonary expression of ICAM I. Am J Pathol 142:1739, 1993.
111. Nakamoto Y, Asano Y, Dohi K, et al: Primary IgA glomerulonephritis and Schönein-Henoch purpura nephritis: clinicopathological and immunohistological characteristics. Q J Med 188:495, 1978.
112. Niedbak MJ, Picarella MS: Tumor necrosis factor induction of endothelial cell urokinase-type plasminogen-activator mediated proteolysis of extracellular matrix and its antagonism by γ-interferon. Blood 79:678, 1992.
113. Papaioannou CC, Gupte RC, Hunder GC, et al: Circulating immune complexes in giant cell arteritis and polymyalgia rheumatica. Arthritis Rheum 23:1021, 1980.
114. Pareis TM, Kimberly RP, Inman RD, et al: Defective F_c receptor-mediated function of the mononuclear phagocyte system in lupus nephritis. Ann Intern Med 98:526, 1982.
115. Patton WF, Lynch JP: Lymphomatoid granulomatosis. Medicine (Baltimore) 61:1, 1982.
116. Perez HD, Kelly E, Chenworth DE, et al: Identification of the C5a des Arg cochemotaxin. Homology with vitamin D–binding protein L group specific component globulin. J Clin Invest 82:360, 1988.
117. Perl A, Gorevic PD, Ryan DH, et al: Clonal B cell expansions in patients with essential mixed cryoglobulinemia. Clin Exp Immunol 76:54, 1989.
118. Pober JS, LaPierre LA, Syolpan AY, et al: Activation of cultured human endothelial cells by recombinant lymphotoxin: comparison with tumor necrosis factor and interleukin 1 species. J Immunol 138:3319, 1987.
119. Purges AJ, Redecha PB, Kimberly WT, et al: Anti neutrophil cytoplasmic antibodies engage and activate human neutrophils via $F_{c\gamma}$ RIIa. J Immunol 153:1271, 1994.
120. Quigg RJ, Nicholson-Weller A, Cybulsky AV, et al: Decay accelerating factor regulates complement activation on glomerular epithelial cells. J Immunol 142:877, 1989.
121. Rawnsley HM, Shelley WB: Cold urticaria with cryoglobulinemia. Arch Dermatol 98:12, 1968.
122. Roche NE, Fulbright JW, Wagner AD, et al: Correlation of interleukin 6 production and disease activity in polymyalgia rheumatica and giant cell arteritis. Arthritis Rheum 36:1286, 1993.
123. Roth DA, Wilz DR, Theil GB: Schönlein-Henoch syndrome in adults. Q J Med 55:145, 1985.
124. Savage COS, Winearles CG, Evans DL, et al: Microscopic polyarteritis: presentation, pathology, and prognosis. Q J Med 56:467, 1985.
125. Schneider HA, Yonker RA, Katz P, et al: Rheumatoid vasculitis: experience with thirteen patients and review of the literature. Semin Arthritis Rheum 14:280, 1985.
126. Schreiber AD, Frank MM: The role of antibody and complement in the clearance and function of erythrocytes I. In vivo effects of IgG and IgM complement-fixing sites. J Clin Invest 51:575, 1972.
127. Schwartz BS, Levy GA, Curtiss LD, et al: Plasma lipoprotein induction and suppression of the generation of cellular procoagulant activity in vitro: two procoagulant activities are produced by peripheral blood mononuclear cells. J Clin Invest 67:1650, 1981.
128. Scully RE, Galdabini JJ, McNeeley BV: Case records of the Massachusetts General Hospital (Kohlmeier-Degos disease). N Engl J Med 303:1103, 1980.
129. Sergent JS: Vasculitis with hepatitis B antigenemia: long term observations in nine patients. Medicine (Baltimore) 67:354, 1976.
130. Sergent JS, Luckshin MD, Christian CL, et al: Vasculitis with hepatitis B antigenemia. Medicine (Baltimore) 55:1, 1976.
131. Sigal LH: Pseudovasculitis syndromes. In McCarty DJ, Koopman WJ (eds): Arthritis and Allied Conditions. Lea and Febiger, Philadelphia 1993, pp 1323–1330.
132. Sneller MC, Hoffman GS, Talar WC, et al: An analysis of forty-two Wegener's granulomatosis patients treated with methotrexate and prednisone. Arthritis Rheum 38:608, 1995.
133. Soter MA: Clinical presentation and mechanism of necrotizing angiitis of the skin. J Invest Dermatol 67:354, 1976.
134. Soter NA, Mihm MC Jr, Gigli I, et al: Two distinct cellular patterns in cutaneous necrotizing angiitis. J Invest Dermatol 66:334, 1976.
135. Stassen FL, Beck CJ: Complement-mediated solubilization of immune precipitates prepared with antibodies of different avidity. J Immunol 123:535, 1979.
136. Tai P, Holt ME, Denny P, et al: Deposition of eosinophil cationic protein in granulomas of allergic granulomatosis and vasculitis: the Churg-Strauss syndrome. Br Med J 289:400, 1984.
137. Takahashi M, Takahashi S, Hiroshi S: Solubilization of antigen-antibody complexes: a new function of complement as a regulator of immune reactions. Prog Allergy 27:134, 1980.
138. Takata Y, Tamura N, Fujita T: Interaction of C3 with antigen-antibody complexes in the process of solubilization of immune precipitates. J Immunol 132:2531, 1984.
139. Theofilopoulos AN, Dixon FJ: The biology and detection of immune complexes. Adv Immunol 28:89, 1980.
140. Volkman DJ, Mann DL, Fauci AS: Association between Takayasu's arteritis and a B cell alloantigen in North Americans. N Engl J Med 306:464, 1982.
141. Wagner AD, Guronzy JJ, Wayand CM: Functional profile of tissue-infiltrating and circulating CD68+ cells in giant cell arteritis. J Clin Invest 94:1134, 1994.
142. Ward PA, Newman LJ: A neutrophil chemotactic factor from human C5. J Immunol 102:93, 1969.
143. West BC, Todd JR, King JW: Wegener's granulomatosis and trimethoprim-sulfamethoxazole—complete remission after a twenty-year course. Ann Intern Med 106:840, 1987.
144. Weyand CM, Hicok KC, Hunder GG, et al: Tissue cytokine patterns in patients with polymyalgia rheumatica and giant cell arteritis. Ann Intern Med 121:484, 1994.
145. Weyand CM, Hunder NNH, Hicok KC, et al: HLA-DRB1 alleles in polymyalgia rheumatica, giant cell arteritis, and rheumatoid arthritis. Arthritis Rheum 37:514, 1994.
146. While RH, Schambelan M: Hypertension, hyperreninemia, and secondary aldosteronism in systemic necrotizing vasculitis. Ann Intern Med 52:199, 1980.
147. Wieslander J, Barr JF, Butkowski RJ, et al: Goodpasture antigen of the glomerular basement membrane: localization to noncollagenous regions of type IV collagen. Proc Natl Acad Sci USA 81:3838, 1984.
148. Wilson CB, Dixon FJ: Quantitation of acute and chronic serum sickness in the rabbit. J Exp Med 134:75, 1971.
149. Winkelmann RK, Ditto WB: Cutaneous and visceral syndromes of necrotizing or "allergic" angiitis. A study of 38 cases. Medicine (Baltimore) 43:59, 1964.
150. Wisnieski JJ, Naff GB: Serum IgG antibodies to C1q in hypocomplementemic urticarial vasculitis syndrome. Arthritis Rheum 32:1119, 1989.
151. Wright SD, Reddy PA, Jong MTC, et al: C3bi receptor (complement receptor type 3) recognizes a region of complement protein C3 containing the sequence Arg-Gly-Asp. Proc Natl Acad Sci USA 84:1965, 1987.
152. Zeek PM: Periarteritis nodosa and other forms of necrotizing angiitis. N Engl J Med 18:764, 1953.

53 Systemic Mastocytosis

PETER J. BIANCHINE DEAN D. METCALFE

Systemic mastocytosis is a rare disorder characterized by mast cell hyperplasia with infiltrates in tissues, including the skin, gastrointestinal tract, liver, spleen, lymph nodes, bone, and bone marrow.[2, 17, 49] Although it may occur at any age, mastocytosis most frequently presents in infancy and may disappear by late adolescence.[20] There is a second peak of onset in young adults, who then tend to have a persistent form of this disease.[26, 47] Mastocytosis is slightly more common in males than in females and appears to be more frequent in Caucasians.[4, 47] Following the accumulation of mast cells in various organs, the release of mast cell mediators results in a variety of symptom complexes, depending on the level and pattern of mediator release and the susceptibility of the individual to these mediators. Both preformed and newly synthesized mast cell mediators cause symptoms ranging from mild itching and flushing to severe systemic attacks with wheezing, vascular collapse, and even death.

Usually mastocytosis has a more indolent course, and the life expectancy of most patients is average. Unfortunately, mastocytosis may present with an associated hematologic disorder, which alters the overall prognosis to that of the specific hematologic disorder involved. Survival in these patients may be decreased to only a few years from the time of diagnosis. Assessment and prognosis are primarily based on the clinical presentation, organ system involvement, and pathology present on bone marrow biopsy and aspirate. These results are used to categorize patients into four specific categories of mastocytosis, each with a common pattern of mast cell involvement in the tissues. Of all the known forms of mastocytosis, the presence of leukemic mast cells circulating in the peripheral blood indicates the most grave prognosis. Although systemic mastocytosis is generally an isolated occurrence, rare familial cases have been reported with more than one family member affected.[48]

The etiology of mastocytosis remains unknown. However, advances in developmental biology and in understanding programmed cell death have revealed new insights into the biology of the mast cell. In contrast to the murine system, in which recombinant IL-3 alone promotes significant proliferation of mouse mast cells, neither IL-3 nor IL-4, alone or in combination, was sufficient to facilitate the development of mature human mast cells in vitro.[11, 24, 40, 53] Kirshenbaum and colleagues[21] studied the ontogeny of human mast cells in vitro and showed evidence that human mast cells arise from the $CD34^+$ pluripotent bone marrow stem cells when cocultured with 3T3 fibroblasts. It became clear that the supernatants of these 3T3 fibroblasts contained growth factors essential for human mast cells. This led to the discovery of a second mast cell growth factor, stem cell factor (SCF).[1, 8, 56, 57]

The proto-oncogene c-kit and its native ligand SCF have been found to play a crucial role in mast cell development and proliferation, as well as in vivo regulation of mast cell number.[1, 8, 14, 21, 53, 56–58] SCF is now identified as the principal growth factor for human mast cells.[21] The c-kit receptor is known to mediate signals for the development and maturation of mast cell progenitors. Single point mutations of c-kit in both murine and human mast cell lines lead to ligand-independent phophorylation of c-kit and constitutive activation of the tyrosine kinase function thought to lead to cellular transformation and tumorigenicity.[13, 51] Thus point mutations of the c-kit gene may play a pivotal role in mast cell transformation in some forms of mastocytosis. Advances also indicate that an altered metabolism of SCF may occur in the skin of patients with cutaneous forms of mastocytosis. This alteration may also play an etiologic role in some forms of the disease.[25]

In the murine system, SCF has been shown to rescue IL-3–dependent mast cells from undergoing apoptosis upon the removal of IL-3, demonstrating how these growth factors may act in concert to regulate mast cell number in vivo.[28] Thus it appears that several microenvironmental factors, such as the interaction between c-kit and SCF, control both mast cell proliferation and apoptosis. Taken together, these observations provide information regarding the physiology of mast cell proliferation and may provide insight into the pathophysiology of mastocytosis as well. Future discoveries may lead to the development of growth factor–specific therapy for certain forms of this disorder.

CLASSIFICATION OF MASTOCYTOSIS

Systemic mastocytosis is classified on the basis of pathologic findings, clinical presentation, and prognosis into four distinct clinicopathologic categories (Table 53–1).[29] The first category is called indolent mastocytosis. The clinical prognosis for patients in this category is good, whereas patients in the other three categories tend to do poorly. There are eight

TABLE 53–1
CONSENSUS REVISED CLASSIFICATION OF MASTOCYTOSIS

- I. Indolent mastocytosis
  - A. Syncope
  - B. Cutaneous disease
  - C. Ulcer disease
  - D. Malabsorption
  - E. Bone marrow mast cell aggregates
  - F. Skeletal disease
  - G. Hepatosplenomegaly
  - H. Lymphadenopathy
- II. Mastocytosis with an associated hematologic disorder
  - A. Myeloproliferative
  - B. Myelodysplastic
- III. Aggressive mastocytosis
  - Lymphadenopathic mastocytosis with eosinophilia
- IV. Mastocytic leukemia

possible associated findings in patients in category I, including those with an isolated skin involvement and those with evidence of systemic disease (Fig. 53–1). In most cases, category I patients gradually accumulate mast cells in the tissues, including the bone marrow, which may parallel an increase in symptoms (Fig. 53–2).[49] These patients are successfully managed for decades using combinations of medications designed to relieve symptoms caused by mast cell activation and degranulation.

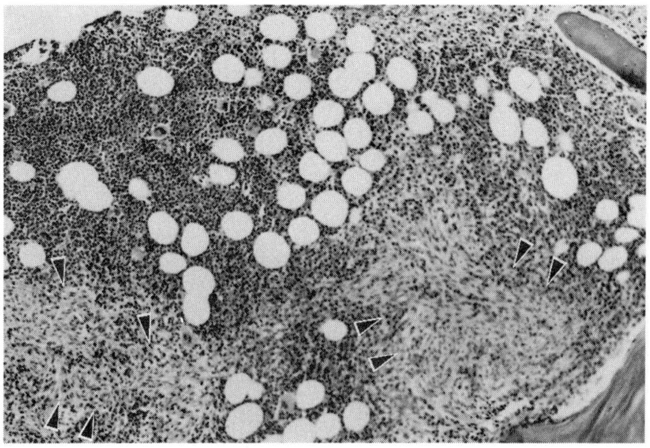

FIGURE 53–2. Indolent systemic mastocytosis. Focal aggregates of spindle-shaped mast cells (arrows) in peritrabecular and perivascular areas are surrounded by areas of normal hematopoiesis. Eosinophils help demarcate the infiltrates from the surrounding tissue, and a dense network of reticulin fibers and foci of lymphocytes accompanies the mast cell infiltrates. The noninfiltrated marrow shows a more normal hematopoiesis and fat distribution. These patients usually show involvement of the skin (urticaria pigmentosa). (Courtesy of Susan Tannenbaum, MD, Senior Staff, NIH Clinical Center.)

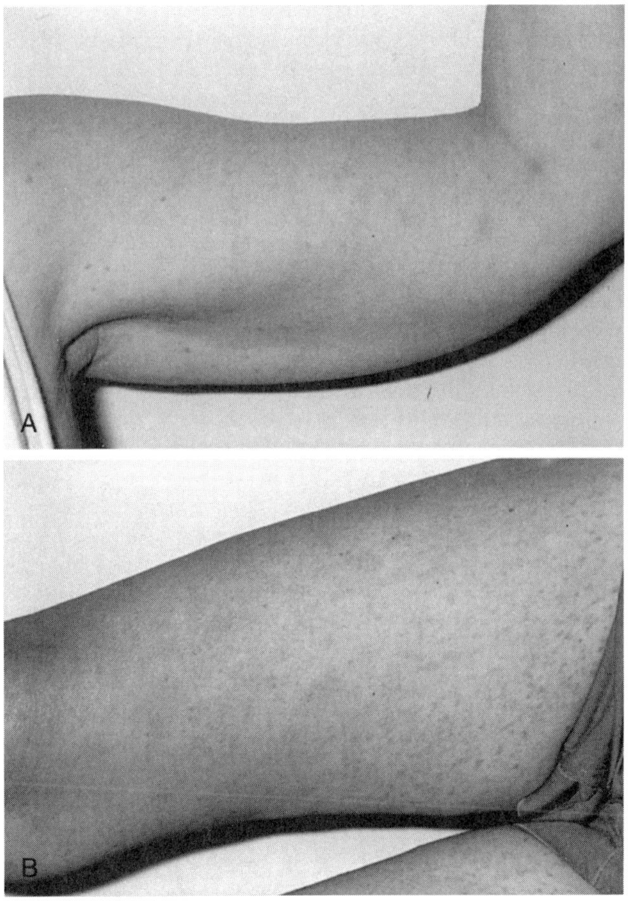

FIGURE 53–1. Urticaria pigmentosa lesions in indolent mastocytosis. **(A)** Small, reddish brown macules and papules in the left axilla of a patient with indolent mastocytosis. **(B)** Similar urticaria pigmentosa lesions on the medial aspect of the thigh of the same patient. Urticaria pigmentosa lesions are often clinically first identified in these areas. (Courtesy of Alexandra Worobec, MD, Clinical Associate, Allergic Diseases Section, LCI, NIH.)

The next category of patients includes the second most common form of mastocytosis, that associated with a hematologic disorder. In this group, examination of the bone marrow and peripheral blood reveals the hematologic abnormality, which may be classified as either myeloproliferative or myelodysplastic (Fig. 53–3).[49] Prognosis in category II is determined by the associated hematologic disorder.

Category III patients have what is termed aggressive mastocytosis (Fig. 53–4). These individuals have a poor prognosis but no distinctive hematologic disorder or mast cell leukemia present. A subset of patients with aggressive mastocytosis have a distinct syndrome that is called lymphadenopathic mastocytosis with eosinophilia because of the pronounced eosinophilia, hepatosplenomegaly, and lymphadenopathy. Patients with aggressive disease rapidly increase their mast cell burden and are difficult to manage. The prognosis in these patients is less optimistic than in those with indolent mastocytosis.

Mast cell leukemia defines the fourth category of mastocytosis. These individuals have the rarest and most fulminant form of mastocytosis.[49] Mast cell leukemia is distinguished from the other categories by its unique pathologic and clinical picture, with immature mast cells (greater than 10% of nucleated cells) present in the peripheral blood.

ETIOLOGY AND PATHOGENESIS

Although the pathophysiology of mastocytosis remains unknown, the regulation of mast cell number and mast cell differentiation is controlled by factors produced in the hematopoietic marrow, as well as by cells in the peripheral tissues in which mast cells finally reside. Several T-cell–derived cytokines exert effects on mast cell precursors, including IL-3, IL-4, IL-9, IL-10, and granulocyte-macrophage colony-stimulating factor (GM-CSF).[18] SCF is now accepted as a cytokine that stimulates both mast cell growth and differentiation in vitro.[1, 8, 56–58] SCF is the ligand for c-kit, a tyrosine kinase receptor, and is normally produced as both a membrane-bound form and a biologically active soluble form that is released by proteolytic cleavage.[1, 57]

SCF is present in normal human serum, but elevated levels have not been consistently detected in patients with mastocytosis.[14, 23] Both keratinocytes and interstitial cells produce SCF locally in normal skin, where it occurs predominantly in the membrane-bound form. Increased levels of the soluble form of SCF are found in the dermis of both normal and affected skin of some patients with cutaneous mastocytosis.[50] Since alterations in SCF gene transcription were not observed in these patients, it is possible that altered metabolism (increased proteolyic cleavage) of the membrane-bound form of SCF occurs and leads to increased levels of soluble SCF in the skin of patients with this disorder. Increased levels of soluble SCF would then lead to the accumulation of mast cells and the hyperpigmentation found in the epidermis of patients with cutaneous mastocytosis, indicating that some forms of mastocytosis represent a reactive hyperplasia rather than a mast cell neoplasia.

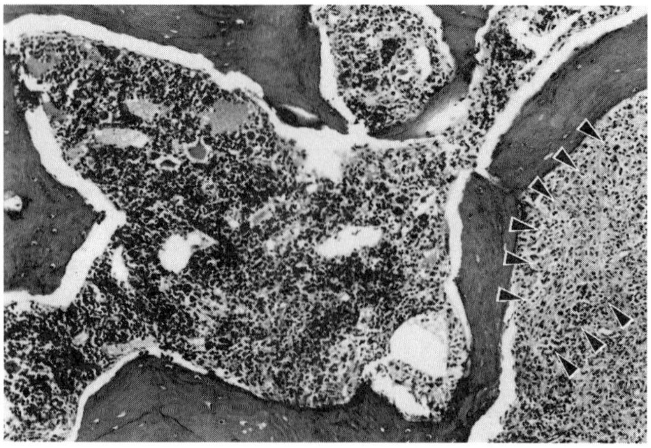

FIGURE 53–4. Aggressive systemic mastocytosis. Peritrabecular and perivascular sheets of spindle-shaped mast cells (arrows) with concomitant fibrosis and ostosclerosis. The noninfiltrated marrow areas show marked reduction in fat cell content and increased granulocytopoiesis. No primary skin involvement may be found in these cases. (Courtesy of Susan Tannenbaum, MD, Senior Staff, NIH Clinical Center.)

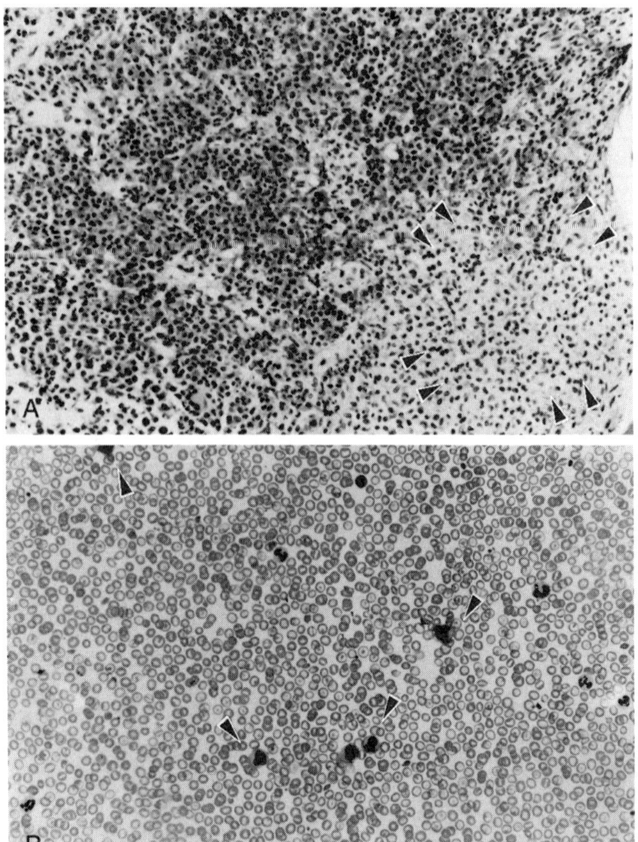

FIGURE 53–3. Mastocytosis with an associated hematologic disorder. **(A)** Atypical mast cells and myelomonocytic precursors (arrows) are observed, associated with hypoplasia of fat cells and normal blood precursors. **(B)** A peripheral blood smear of the same patient shows numerous circulating promonocytes, monocytes, and monoblasts (arrows) consistent with chronic myelomonocytic leukemia. (Courtesy of Susan Tannenbaum, MD, Senior Staff, NIH Clinical Center.)

SCF is known to have multiple effects on the biology of mast cells, both in vitro and in vivo. Injection of the recombinant form of SCF can induce mastocytosis in vivo.[27] Moreover, SCF is chemotactic for mast cells, activates them to release soluble mediators, and increases their responsiveness to FcεR1 activation.[5, 55, 27–33] Evidence also indicates that SCF is critical in the generation of mucosal mastocytosis in that in vivo administration of a monoclonal antibody against c-kit will completely prevent the normal intestinal mastocytosis that usually follows intestinal helminthic infections in rodents.[15]

Since both stem cells and mast cells express c-kit and proliferate following engagement of c-kit receptor with its ligand, it is logical to hypothesize that mutations in c-kit may enhance or interfere with mast cell proliferation. Studies have identified a point mutation in the catalytic domain of c-kit in the peripheral blood mononuclear cells of certain patients with mastocytosis.[30] Research to identify and characterize such mutations in c-kit is being actively pursued in patients with mastocytosis and may provide new information regarding the pathogenesis of mastocytosis, as well as a potential strategy for intervention. Taken together, these observations suggest that SCF–c-kit interactions regulate mast cell number in vivo and will provide the key to understanding the pathogenesis of systemic mastocytosis.

CLINICAL FEATURES

Mastocytosis is clinically identified by the effects of the distribution and activation of mast cells in the specific tissues where they reside, including bone marrow, spleen, liver, skin, and lymph nodes. These manifestations are best described by organ systems.

CUTANEOUS MANIFESTATIONS

The skin is most frequently involved in mastocytosis.[46] The most common cutaneous manifestation of mastocytosis is urticaria pigmentosa, a feature first recognized by Nettleship and Tay[31] in a 2-year-old girl in 1869. The term urticaria pigmentosa was later coined in 1878 by Sangster[41] for both the urtication and hyperpigmentation seen with these lesions. In 1887, Unna noted the presence of mast cells in urticaria pigmentosa lesions.[46] Urticaria pigmentosa is seen in over 90% of adult patients with indolent mastocytosis and in less than 50% of patients with mastocytosis with an associated hematologic disorder or those with lymphadenopathic mastocytosis with eosinophilia.

The lesions of urticaria pigmentosa appear usually as small, reddish-brown macules or slightly raised papules scattered over the body (see Fig. 53–1). However, the individual lesions may appear as macules, papules, or even nodules, with hyperpigmentation, vascular flare, and pruritis. Mild trauma, including scratching, rubbing, or stroking, may cause urtication and erythema around the macules, known as Darier's sign. Urticaria pigmentosa is associated with exacerbations induced by changes in temperature, skin friction, ingestion of hot beverages or spicy foods, alcohol, or certain drugs.

Urticaria pigmentosa, diffuse cutaneous mastocytosis, telangiectasia macularis eruptiva perstans, and solitary mastocytoma are the skin manifestations of mastocytosis.[10] Clinically, the cutaneous manifestations of mastocytosis usually present early in the disease course, with the development in time of pruritis, scattered macules, plaques, or nodules that contain a brownish pigment. In children, the most common cutaneous manifestation of mastocytosis is the solitary mastocytoma. Urticaria pigmentosa is the next most frequent manifestation. Young children with urticaria pigmentosa or diffuse cutaneous mastocytosis may also present with bullous lesions instead of the more classic macules, papules, or nodules. Diffuse cutaneous mastocytosis is the rarest form of this disorder. It presents with discoloration, dimpling, and peau d'orange in affected skin due to a diffuse dermal mast cell infiltration without discrete lesions.[45] A rare manifestation of mastocytosis known as telangiectasia macularis eruptiva perstans has been reported to occur exclusively in adults, with diffuse telangiectatic erythematous macules on a brown pigmented background that coalesce over time.

VASCULAR COLLAPSE

Patients in every category of systemic mastocytosis may experience flushing, wheezing, dyspnea, and cough, as well as systemic hypotension and vascular collapse. The latter may be provoked by alcohol, narcotic analgesics, exercise, or infections in susceptible individuals. Release of mast cell mediators into the systemic circulation may result in these findings.

GASTROINTESTINAL MANIFESTATIONS

Gastrointestinal disturbances often develop in patients with mastocytosis. These include gastric hypersecretion secondary to elevated plasma histamine levels, diarrhea, abdominal pain, peptic ulcer disease with the risk of gastrointestinal hemorrhage, and chronic diarrhea with malabsorption.

BONE MANIFESTATIONS

Bone pain, osteoporosis, fractures, and vertebral compression fractures may occur in systemic mastocytosis. Bone pain is the most common symptom in mastocytosis and is present in 19 to 28% of these patients. Bone disease occurs in the presence of marrow lesions containing mast cells associated with eosinophils, lymphocytes, plasma cells, histiocytes, and fibroblasts. Anemia, leukopenia, thrombocytopenia, and eosinophilia may all be observed in association with systemic mast cell disease. Radiographically detectable lesions are seen in up to 70% of patients with systemic mastocytosis. The proximal long bones are most often involved.

NEUROPSYCHIATRIC MANIFESTATIONS

Anxiety, depression, dementia, dementia with cerebral atrophy, and peripheral neuropathy have all been reported. Commonly reported problems include a decreased attention span, memory impairment, and irritability.

CARDIOVASCULAR MANIFESTATIONS

Congestive heart failure and acute myocardial infarction may result from mast cell degranulation. Perhaps cardiac mast cells participate in the disorder in some cases.[34a]

HEMATOLOGIC MANIFESTATIONS

Anemia, leukocytosis, leukopenia, thrombocytosis, thrombocytopenia, eosinophilia, basophilia, monocytosis, and circulating mast cells are all reported to occur in mastocytosis. These peripheral blood abnormalities are associated with bone marrow involvement. In a prospective study of 46 adult patients with clinical or pathologic evidence of mast cell proliferation, 74% had a bone marrow biopsy diagnostic of systemic mast cell disease.[24] The remaining 26% were considered to have cutaneous mast cell disease.

Univariate analysis showed that hepatosplenomegaly, alkaline phosphatase level, absolute lymphocyte count, and age at onset of symptoms positively correlated with systemic mast cell disease, whereas hemoglobin level was negatively correlated with systemic mast cell disease.[24] The following variables were identified by univariate analysis as significantly increasing the risk of death in patients with mastocytosis: later onset of symptoms, absence of cutaneous mastocytosis, thrombocytopenia, elevated lactate dehydrogenase (LDH), anemia, bone marrow hypercellularity, qualitative peripheral blood smear abnormalities, elevated alkaline phosphatase levels, and hepatosplenomegaly. Multivariate analysis revealed that the age at onset of symptoms and the LDH levels were significant independent predictors of survival. Eight of the 10 systemic mastocytosis patients in this study who died had myeloproliferative or myelodysplastic syndromes or acute nonlymphocytic leukemia.[24]

DIAGNOSIS

Systemic mastocytosis is extremely heterogeneous in its predilection for specific organs, including the skin, gut, bone marrow, skeleton, liver, spleen, and brain.

SKIN BIOPSY

Special mast cell stains, such as toluidine blue or Giemsa, are used to identify mast cells on skin biopsy and differentiate mastocytosis from other cutaneous lesions, such as pigmented nevi, xanthomas, or xanthogranulomas. Following the clinical appearance of cutaneous lesions, skin biopsies of affected areas will reveal extensive mast cell infiltrates around blood vessels and within the skin appendages, at times disrupting normal skin architecture.[20] In bullous lesions, skin biopsy of affected areas may differentiate bullous mastocytosis from bullous erythema multiforme or scalded skin syndrome, as well as other bullous diseases.

PLASMA HISTAMINE LEVELS

Plasma histamine levels are known to be elevated in the majority of patients with pediatric-onset mastocytosis.[19] Children with urticaria pigmentosa typically have plasma levels of histamine that range from normal to several times normal.

SERUM TRYPTASE

The release of tryptase, a tetrameric serine protease that is selectively concentrated in the secretory granules of human mast cells, is currently used as a clinical marker of mast cell activation in patients with anaphylaxis, sudden infant death syndrome, and systemic mastocytosis.[35, 42, 43, 54] The standard technique uses two monoclonal antibodies for enzyme-linked immunosorbent assay (ELISA), one called G5 for capture, and the other called G4 for detection, with an apparent sensitivity of 1 ng/ml for tryptase in serum or plasma. G5 recognizes a linear epitope on denatured tryptase, but not the tetrameric form of the active enzyme. In contrast, G4 recognizes the active tetrameric form of tryptase. With this test, normal controls show serum tryptase levels less than 5 ng/ml, with anaphylaxis patients ranging from 9 to 75 ng/ml and mastocytosis patients ranging from 4 to 88 ng/ml. Levels of tryptase in normal sera and plasma are undetectable at this level of sensitivity using these antibodies.

A new ELISA test has been developed using a mouse antihuman monoclonal antibody capable of detecting human tryptase in normal plasma and serum.[43, 44] The new immunoassay for tryptase is substantially more sensitive than previous assays since a greater portion of the total tryptase present in solution is detected. The lower limit of sensitivity for tryptase in serum with this assay is approximately 0.2 ng/ml. Since this immunoassay may be performed in less than 1 hour, this test may be used to influence therapy and disposition of patients in urgent clinical situations.

BONE SCAN

Lytic bone lesions are sometimes noted in systemic mastocytosis. Back pain secondary to vertebral compression factors due to osteoporosis is a presenting symptom in many cases.[2, 7, 12] Bone scanning provides an efficient, noninvasive method of assessing and following active bone and bone marrow involvement. The degree of bone scan abnormality in mastocytosis has been shown to correlate with urinary and plasma histamine levels and therefore, presumably, with disease activity.[38] In some instances, the bone scan will be abnormal despite a negative bone marrow. As the disease progresses, abnormalities on bone scan tend to become increasingly diffuse, reflecting the secondary marrow expansion associated with increasing marrow involvement.[3, 6]

SKELETAL SURVEY

Skeletal scintigraphy (bone scan) is more sensitive than radiographic surveys in detecting and locating active lesions of systemic mastocytosis.

BONE MARROW BIOPSY WITH ASPIRATE

In one review of 45 patients with systemic mastocytosis, the bone marrow findings were grouped into three distinct histologic patterns that differentiate the benign from the malignant variants of this disorder.[17] Patients with mast cell leukemia showed less than a 1% 5-year survival, whereas those with no evidence of associated hematologic disorders and normal hematopoiesis had approximately a 75% 5-year survival.[17]

TREATMENT

We currently lack the means to alter the disease process of systemic mastocytosis. No therapeutic approach offers a cure for this disorder. Thus current therapy for mastocytosis is almost exclusively directed toward relieving symptoms. H_1 and H_2 receptor antagonists are used to block the effects of histamine to try to alleviate pruritis, flushing, urticaria, diarrhea, bone pain, abdominal pain, and ulcer formation. Disodium cromoglycate is used to stabilize the mast cell membrane and to prevent mediator-induced signs and symptoms primarily in the gastrointestinal tract. Epinephrine is used to treat systemic hypotension. Despite these approaches, subjects often continue to have symptoms due to the inability to block high levels of histamine and other mast cell mediators. Oral and topical steroids have also been used to reduce bone pain, decrease malabsorption, and lighten skin lesions, but these effects are transient at best.

Clinical studies demonstrating the efficacy of IFN-α in the treatment of patients with chronic myelogenous leukemia (CML) prompted research into IFN-α's potential application to the treatment of patients with mastocytosis.[16, 32] IFN-α was hypothesized to have both antisecretory and antiproliferative effects on the mast cells found in mastocytosis. Preliminary studies of IFN-α reported mixed results for patients with mastocytosis. IFN-α was determined to be of benefit in a 63-year-old woman with systemic mastocytosis and chronic myelomonocytic leukemia (CMML), as well as in a 42-year-old man with aggressive (malignant) mastocytosis.[22, 36] In the former case, the patient demonstrated an initial response within 2 months of IFN-α therapy, with elimination of flushing, diarrhea, pleural effusions, and refractory anemia. Despite 10 months of treatment, the CMML continued, and the patient developed 20% circulating immature mast cells. The

TABLE 53–2
CONSENSUS DIAGNOSTIC WORK-UP

If mastocytosis is suspected on clinical grounds:
- Routine
  - Examine the skin—both gross and microscopic
  - Bone marrow biopsy and aspiration
  - 24-hour urine for mediators
  - Plasma for mast cell tryptase
- Additional studies
  - Bone scan/skeletal survey
  - GI work-up—upper GI series, small bowel x-ray, CT scan, endoscopy*
  - EEG, neuropsychiatric work-up

*May be adequate criteria for primary diagnosis.

patient was then treated with IFN-α at 6 million units three times a week, resulting in a complete remission in terms of circulating immature mast cells 6 weeks later. The course of the CMML is unclear, however. In our experience, mastocytosis often resolves as CMML progresses.

The male patient was treated for 12 months with IFN-α-2b at a dose of 5 million units subcutaneously three times a week. A remarkable bone marrow response was described, with decreased atypical mast cells and improved hematopoietic cellularity in the marrow, reduced transfusion requirements for refractory anemia, decreased number of urticaria pigmentosa lesions, decreased urinary excretion of histamine metabolites, and decreased hepatomegaly and ascites. However, conventional management with H_1 and H_2 antihistamines and oral cromolyn sodium had to be continued despite IFN-α therapy, along with 25 mg of daily prednisone to control the recurrent flushing, pruritus, diarrhea, and abdominal pain, which indicated that a substantial mast cell burden still remained during and following IFN-α treatment of this patient.

Other reports include the treatment of two patients with mastocytosis with IFN-α-2b (Intron A).[9] Although some symptom reduction occurred, including a decrease in the use of adrenaline sprays and the frequency of syncope, no significant improvement was noted overall. Objective data indicated that pigmented skin lesions in these patients did not fade. Histologic studies showed worsened mast cell infiltrates in one patient during the 8 weeks of therapy. At best, the modest improvements reported during this trial were transient. Careful evaluation of the overall results from these studies remain negative. In fact, reports in the literature indicate that IFN-α may induce anaphylactoid reactions with tachycardia, hypotension, bronchospasm, fever, and explosive diarrhea.[34]

In vitro studies show that IFN-γ inhibits the proliferation of murine mast cell progenitors whereas IFN-α does not.[39] However, in vivo clinical trials showing efficacy of IFN-γ in systemic mastocytosis are lacking for this form of therapy.

PROGNOSTIC INDICATORS

One prospective study followed 46 adult patients with mast cell disease to define clinically useful markers of prognostic value.[37] These patients were followed for up to 13 years. The Kaplan-Meier method was used to construct survival curves to examine the effects of several variables on the survival time. Thirty-two of the 46 patients had bone marrow biopsies diagnostic for systemic mastocytosis. The remaining 14 patients were considered to have cutaneous mastocytosis. Univariate analyses revealed that age at onset of symptoms, absence of cutaneous mastocytosis, thrombocytopenia, elevated LDH, anemia, bone marrow hypercellularity, qualitative peripheral blood smear abnormalities, elevated alkaline phosphatase, and hepatosplenomegaly significantly increased the risk of death in patients with systemic mastocytosis. Multivariate analysis showed that only the age at onset of symptoms and LDH levels were significant independent predictors of survival. The recommended studies to evaluate and diagnose patients for systemic mastocytosis are summarized in Table 53–2.[29]

REFERENCES

1. Anderson DM, Lyman SD, Baird A, et al: Molecular cloning of mast cell growth factor, a hematopoietin that is active in both membrane bound and soluble forms. Cell 63:235–243, 1990.
2. Andrew SM, Freemont AJ: Skeletal mastocytosis. J Clin Pathol 46:1033–1035, 1993.
3. Arrington ER, Eisenberg B, Hartshorne MF, et al: Nuclear medicine imaging of systemic mastocytosis. J Nucl Med 30:2046–2048, 1989.
4. Austen KF: Systemic mastocytosis. N Engl J Med 326:639–640, 1992.
5. Bischoff SC, Dahinden CA: c-Kit ligand. A unique potentiator of mediator release by human lung mast cells. J Exp Med 175:237–242, 1992.
6. Chen CC, Andrich MP, Mican JM, Metcalfe DD: A retrospective analysis of bone scan abnormalities in mastocytosis: correlation with disease category and prognosis. J Nucl Med 35:1471–1475, 1994.
7. Chines A, Pacifici R, Avioli LV, et al: Systemic mastocytosis presenting as osteoporosis: a clinical and histomorphometric study. J Clin Endocrinol Metab 72:140–144, 1991.
8. Copeland NG, Gilbert DJ, Cho BC, et al: Mast cell growth factor maps near the steel locus on mouse chromosome 10 and is deleted in a number of steel alleles. Cell 63:175–183, 1990.
9. Czarnetzki BM, Algermissen B, Jeep S, et al: Interferon treatment of patients with chronic urticaria and mastocytosis. J Am Acad Dermatol 63:500–501, 1994.
10. Demis DJ: The mastocytosis syndrome: clinical and biological studies. Ann Intern Med 59:194–206, 1963.
11. Dvorak AM, Saito H, Estrella P, et al: Ultrastructure of eosinophils and basophils stimulated to develop in human cord blood mononuclear cell cultures containing recombinant human interleukin-5 or interleukin-3. Lab Invest 61:116–132, 1989.
12. Fallon MD, Whyte MP, Teitelbaum SL: Systemic mastocytosis associated with generalised osteopenia. Hum Pathol 12:813–820, 1981.
13. Furitsu T, Tsujimura T, Tono T, et al: Identification of mutations in the coding sequence of the proto-oncogene c-kit in a human mast cell leukemia cell line causing ligand-independent activation of c-kit product. J Clin Invest 92:1736–1744, 1993.
14. Galli SJ, Iemura A, Garlick DS, et al: Reversible expansion of primate mast cell populations in vivo by stem cell factor. J Clin Invest 91:148–152, 1993.
15. Grencis RK, Else KJ, Huntley JF, Nishikawa SI: The in vivo role of stem cell factor (c-kit ligand) on mastocytosis and host protective immunity to the intestinal nematode *Trichinella spiralis* in mice. Parasite Immunol 15:55–59, 1993.
16. Griesshamer M, Hehlmann R, Hochhaus A, et al: Interferon in chronic myeloid leukemia. A workshop report. Ann Hematol 67:101–106, 1993.
17. Horny HP, Parwaresch MR, Lennert K: Bone marrow findings in systemic mastocytosis. Hum Pathol 16:808–881, 1985.
18. Ishizaka T, Mitsui H, Yanagida M, et al: Development of human mast cells from their progenitors. Curr Opin Immunol 5:937–943, 1993.
19. Kettelhut BV, Metcalfe DD: Plasma histamine concentration in evaluation of pediatric mastocytosis. J Pediatr 111:419–421, 1987.
20. Kettelhut BV, Metcalfe DD: Pediatric mastocytosis. Ann Allergy 73:197–206, 1994.

21. Kirshenbaum AS, Goff JP, Kessler SW, et al: Effect of IL-3 and stem cell factor on the appearance of human basophils and mast cells from CD34+ pluripotent progenitor cells. J Immunol 148:772–777, 1992.
22. Kluin-Nelemens HC, Jansen JH, Breukelman H, et al: Response to interferon alpha-2b in a patient with systemic mastocytosis. N Engl J Med 326:619–623, 1992.
23. Langley KE, Bennett LG, Wypych J, et al: Soluble stem cell factor in human serum. Blood 81:656–660, 1993.
24. Lawrence JB, Friedman BS, Travis WD, et al: Hematologic manifestations of systemic mast cell disease: a prospective study of laboratory and morphologic features and their relation to prognosis. Am J Med 91:612–624, 1991.
25. Longley BJ, Morganroth GS, Tyrrel L, et al: Altered metabolism of mast-cell growth factor (c-kit ligand) in cutaneous mastocytosis. N Engl J Med 328:1302–1307, 1993.
26. Longley J: Is mastocytosis a mast cell neoplasia or a reactive hyperplasia? Clues from the study of mast cell growth factor. Ann Med 26:115–116, 1994.
27. Meininger CJ, Yano H, Rottapel R, et al: The c-kit receptor ligand functions as a mast cell chemoattractant. Blood 79:958–960, 1992.
28. Mekori YA, Oh CK, Metcalfe DD: IL-3-dependent murine mast cells undergo apoptosis on removal of IL-3: prevention of apoptosis by c-kit ligand. J Immunol 151:3775–3784, 1993.
29. Metcalfe DD: Conclusions. J Invest Dermatol 96:64s–65s, 1991.
30. Nagata H, Worobec A, Oh C, et al: Identification of a point mutation in the catalytic domain of the proto-oncogene c-kit in peripheral blood mononuclear cells of patients who have mastocytosis with an associated hematologic disorder. Proc Natl Acad Sci USA 92:10560–10564, 1995.
31. Nettleship E, Tay W: Rare forms of urticaria: chronic urticaria, leaving brown stains; nearly two years duration. Br Med J 2:323–324, 1869.
32. Niederle N, Kloke O, Wnadl UB, et al: Long-term treatment of chronic myelogenous leukemia with different interferons: results from three studies. Leuk Lymphoma 9:111–119, 1993.
33. Nilsson G, Butterfield JH, Nilsson K, Siegbahn A: Stem cell factor is a chemotactic factor for human mast cells. J Immunol 153:3717–3723, 1994.
34. Pardini S, Bosincu L, Bonfigli S, et al: Anaphylactic-like syndrome in systemic mastocytosis treated with alpha-2-interferon. Acta Haematol 85:220, 1991.
34a. Patella V, Marino I, Lamparter B, et al: Human heart mast cells: isolation, purification, ultrastructure, and immunologic characterization. J Immunol 154:2855–2861, 1995.
35. Platt MS, Yunginger JW, Sekula-Perlman A, et al: Involvement of mast cells in sudden infant death syndrome. JACI 94:250–256, 1994.
36. Pulik M, Lionnet F, Petit A, et al: Long-term response to interferon-α in a patient with systemic mastocytosis and chronic myelomonocytic leukemia. Am J Hematol 47:66–66, 1994.
37. Rennick DM, Lee FD, Yokota T, et al: A cloned MCGF cDNA encodes a multilineage hematopoietic growth factor: multiple activities of interleukin 3. J Immunol 134:910–914, 1985.
38. Rosenbaum RC, Frieri M, Metcalfe DD: Patterns of skeletal scintigraphy and their relationship to plasma and urinary histamine levels in systemic mastocytosis. J Nucl Med 25:859–864, 1984.
39. Rottem M, Hull G, Metcalfe DD: Demonstration of differential effects of cytokines on mast cells derived from murine bone marrow and peripheral blood mononuclear cells. Exp Hematol 22:1147–1155, 1994.
40. Saito H, Hatake K, Dvorak AM, et al: Selective differentiation and proliferation of hematopoietic cells induced by recombinant interleukins. Proc Natl Acad Sci USA 85:2288–2292, 1988.
41. Sangster A: An anomalous mottled rash, accompanied by pruritis, factitious urticaria, and pigmentation, "Urticaria Pigmentosa(?)." Trans Clin Soc Lond 11:161–163, 1878.
42. Schwartz LB, Metcalfe DD, Miller JS: Tryptase levels as an indicator of mast cell activation in systemic anaphylaxis and mastocytosis. N Engl J Med 316:1622–1626, 1987.
43. Schwartz LB, Bradford TR, Lee DC, Chlebowski JF: Immunological and physico-chemical evidence for conformational changes occurring on conversion of human mast cell tryptase from active tetramer to inactive monomer: production of monoclonal antibodies recognizing active tryptase. J Immunol 144:2304–2311, 1990.
44. Schwartz LB, Bradford TR, Rouse C, et al: Development of a new, more sensitive immunoassay for human tryptase: use in systemic anaphylaxis. J Clin Immunol 190–204, 1994.
45. Shaw JM: Genetic aspects of urticaria pigmentosa. Arch Dermatol 97:137–138, 1968.
46. Soter NA: The skin in mastocytosis. J Invest Dermatol 96:32S–39S, 1991.
47. Stein DH: Mastocytosis: a review. Pediatr Dermatol 3:365–375, 1986.
48. Tay YK, Giam YC: Cutaneous mastocytosis in Singapore. Singapore Med J 34:425–429, 1993.
49. Travis WD, Li C-Y, Bergstralh EJ, et al: Systemic mast cell disease. Analysis of 58 cases and literature review. Medicine (Baltimore) 67:345–368, 1988.
50. Tsai M, Shih LS, Newlands GF, et al: The rat c-kit ligand, stem cell factor, induces the development of connective tissue-type and mucosal mast cells in vivo: analysis by anatomical distribution, histochemistry, and protease phenotype. J Exp Med 174:125–131, 1991.
51. Tsujimura T, Furitsu T, Morimoto M, et al: Ligand-independent activation of c-kit receptor tyrosine kinase in a murine mastocytoma cell line P-815 generated by a point mutation. Blood 83:2619–2626, 1994.
52. Valent P, Ashman LK, Hinterberger W, et al: Mast cell typing: demonstration of a distinct hematopoietic cell type and evidence for immunophenotypic relationship to mononuclear phagocytes. Blood 73:1778–1785, 1989.
53. Valent P, Spanblochl E, Sperr WR, et al: Induction of differentiation of human mast cells from bone marrow and peripheral blood mononuclear cells by recombinant human stem cell factor/kit ligand in long-term culture. Blood 80:2237–2245, 1992.
54. Wenzel S, Irani AM, Sanders JM, et al: Immunoassay of tryptase from human mast cells. J Immunol Methods 86:139–142, 1986.
55. Wershil BK, Tsai M, Geissler EN, et al: The rat c-kit ligand, stem cell factor induces c-kit receptor-dependent mouse mast cell activation in vivo. Evidence that signalling through the c-kit receptor can induce expression of cellular function. J Exp Med 175:245–249, 1992.
56. Williams DE, Eisenman J, Baird A, et al: Identification of a ligand for the c-kit proto-oncogene. Cell 63:167–174, 1990.
57. Zsebo KM, Wypych J, McNeice IK, et al: Identification, purification, and biologic characterization of hematopoietic stem cell factor from Buffalo rat liver-conditioned medium. Cell 63:195–201, 1990.
58. Zsebo KM, Williams DA, Geissler EN, et al: Stem cell factor is encoded at the Sl locus of the mouse and is the ligand for c-kit tyrosine kinase receptor. Cell 63:213–224, 1990.

54 Idiopathic Hypereosinophilic Syndrome

JOSHUA A. BOYCE WILLIAM F. OWEN, JR.

The idiopathic hypereosinophilic syndrome (IHES) is characterized by sustained (>6 months) peripheral blood eosinophilia (>1,500 cells/mm^3) in the absence of a definable cause and signs and symptoms of organ dysfunction referable to the hypereosinophilic state.[46] It is a nonmalignant disorder with selective eosinophil proliferation, separating IHES from leukemias with eosinophilic predominance.[25, 153] The etiology of IHES is unknown but likely involves diverse mechanisms. Therefore, IHES may not be a single disease, but a final common end point for a variety of disease processes.[268] This chapter reviews the clinical, pathologic, and laboratory features of IHES. The current treatment of IHES is reviewed, along with the features of eosinophil biology that are pertinent to this disorder.

EOSINOPHILS

MYELOPOIESIS

Eosinophils are bone marrow–derived granulocytes notable for their acidophilic granules.[185] They share many features in common with basophils, compatible with a relatively late myelopoietic divergence between them. For example, patients with basophilia often have eosinophilia, and a rare syndrome is characterized by the absence of both cell types solely.[10, 111] Basophilia is encountered occasionally in IHES, implying that there may be simultaneous selective hematopoiesis of these two granulocytes in some cases.[46, 80] These data suggest that both cell types may arise from a common progenitor. Indeed, experimental evidence based upon studies of hematopoiesis in vitro suggests that eosinophils arise from a progenitor cell that transiently possesses both eosinophil and basophil granules.[19, 60] Eosinophils and basophils continue to share biochemical and functional characteristics after their terminal differentiation, such as granules that contain major basic protein (MBP) and lysophospholipase, an intact 5-lipoxygenase pathway, and receptors for interleukin (IL)-3, IL-5, and granulocyte-macrophage colony-stimulating factor (GM-CSF).[2, 3, 138, 143, 266] Both cell types possess both low- and high-affinity receptors for IgE.[94, 144] Therefore, although differences between mature basophils and eosinophils include the presence of histamine in basophil granules, granule ultrastructure, staining properties of the granules, and nuclear morphology, there is ample evidence supporting a common lineage.[10, 60, 69]

Eosinophils arise from uncommitted and committed progenitors in the bone marrow under the control of T-cell–derived cytokines.[169, 212, 259] At least three hematopoietic cytokines have eosinophilopoietic bioactivity in vitro and in vivo: IL-3, IL-5, and GM-CSF.[72, 212, 215] These same three cytokines also are potent functional agonists for mature peripheral blood eosinophils.[180, 210, 211] Studies both in vitro and in vivo indicate that IL-3 and GM-CSF are nonselective hematopoietins that stimulate the production of all granulocyte species.[86, 212, 215] Only IL-5 is selective for eosinophils in its hematopoietic activity in humans.[47, 215] In IHES, there is a marked increase in the production of eosinophils and their progenitors.[56] IL-5 is detectable in the serum of some patients with IHES.[182] The bioactivity of IL-5 is therefore strongly implicated in the disordered selective production of eosinophils in these cases.

GRANULE PROTEINS AND FUNCTIONS OF EOSINOPHILS

MAJOR BASIC PROTEIN

The acidophilic granules of the eosinophil contain highly cationic proteins. MBP accounts for over 50% of the eosinophil granule contents by weight.[88] MBP is highly basic, with a calculated isoelectric point of 10.9, but is stored in secondary granules in an electroneutral pre-pro form.[261] The protein is localized to the secondary granule crystalline core.[191] MBP is cytotoxic to parasitic pathogens, such as *Schistosoma mansoni, Trichinella spiralis, Brugia malayi,* and *B. pahangi.*[35, 98, 99] MBP is also bactericidal to *Staphylococcus aureus* and *Escherichia coli,* causing permeabilization of both inner and outer membranes.[133] MBP may therefore be helminthocidal and bactericidal in vivo.

MBP may also exhibit dose-dependent toxicity to a variety of mammalian cell types in vitro and therefore be pathogenically important in human eosinophil-associated disorders.[88] In particular, MBP causes the ciliostasis and exfoliation of bronchial epithelial cells.[84] Similar changes are noted in the airway epithelium of asthmatic subjects. MBP is also demonstrated in the inflammatory lesions of acute necrotizing eosinophilic myocarditis by immunelectron microscopy, suggesting that it might be cardiotoxic as well.[59] This property of MBP may have pathogenic significance in IHES, in which endomyocarditis is prevalent. Other effects of MBP with potential pathobiologic relevance include the noncytotoxic degranulation with histamine release from mast cells and basophils, nonspecific activation of the classic complement pathway and dose-dependent stimulation of platelet functions, such as secretion of 5-hydroxytryptamine, other α-granule constituents, lysosomal constituents, and inhibition of Hageman factor activation.[135, 172, 203, 208] Therefore, MBP might promote thrombus formation and thromboembolic disease, another feature of IHES.

EOSINOPHIL CATIONIC PROTEIN

Like MBP, eosinophil cationic protein (ECP) is highly cationic, with an isoelectric point of 10.8. ECP exists as two isoforms, ECP1 and ECP2, as determined by acrylamide gel electrophoresis and liquid chromatography.[90, 178] ECP shares considerable homology with another cationic eosinophil granule protein, the eosinophil-derived neurotoxin (EDN), and pancreatic RNase.[90] ECP also possesses RNase activity in vitro.[90] Antigenically distinct storage and secreted forms of ECP can be differentiated by monoclonal antibodies. The former is recognized by the monoclonal antibody EG1 and found in peripheral blood eosinophils; the latter is recognized by EG2 antibody and found in eosinophils that have been activated by exposure to zymosan coupled to complement fragment C3b. It is also positive in eosinophils from patients with IHES.[241] The molecular basis for these antigenic differences is unknown. Unlike MBP, which localizes to the eosinophil granule core, ECP localizes to the matrix of the eosinophil's secondary granules by immunoelectron microscopy.[191]

Like MBP, ECP is a cytotoxin. It is potently toxic to the *schistosomula* of *S. mansoni;* newborn larvae of *B. pahangi, B. malayi,* and *T. spiralis;* and trypomastigotes of *Trypanosoma cruzi* in vitro.[156] ECP is also bactericidal, exhibiting toxicity to *E. coli* and *S. aureus* in vitro.[133] Like MBP, ECP is also cytotoxic to mammalian cells in vitro, causing exfoliation of respiratory epithelial cells.[84] ECP is tumoricidal and mediates neurotoxicity to rodents in vivo.[68, 109] The cytotoxic effects of ECP are mediated through its ability to form pores in target cell membranes and to cause osmotic lysis.[274] ECP also binds to and inactivates heparin. As with MBP, the latter effect may have relevance to the thromboembolic phenomena of IHES. ECP also prolongs clotting time and inhibits ellagic acid–induced activation of Hageman factor in vitro.[203]

EOSINOPHIL-DERIVED NEUROTOXIN

EDN is a third cationic granule protein of the eosinophil. It was named for its ability to provoke the Gordon phenomenon, a neuropathic syndrome occurring in rabbits or guinea pigs receiving intrathecal injections of ECP and EDN or extracts from eosinophil-rich lymph nodes from patients with Hodgkin's disease.[68, 92, 249] EDN has marked homology to ECP.[90] Both proteins have homology to pancreatic RNase, with the RNase activity of EDN being roughly 100-fold greater than that of ECP.[226] EDN colocalizes to the eosinophil secondary granule matrix with ECP.[191] Like ECP and MBP, EDN is helminthocidal but is less potent than the other two in this regard.[98, 99] The toxicity of EDN for the trypomastigotes of *T. cruzi* is inhibited by human placental RNasin, suggesting that the cytotoxic properties of EDN are dependent on its RNase activity.[156] Although EDN is clearly neurotoxic in experimental models, its role in the pathogenesis of human disease is unknown. Some have proposed that EDN and ECP may contribute to the nonthromboembolic neuropathic manifestations of IHES.[68]

EOSINOPHIL PEROXIDASE

Eosinophil granules contain an eosinophil peroxidase (EPO) that is antigenically and functionally distinct from neutrophil and monocyte myeloperoxidase (MPO).[176] EPO localizes to the eosinophil granule matrix and exists as a heterodimer.[37, 70] Unlike MPO, EPO preferentially utilizes bromide over chloride as a substrate in the production of hypohalous acids in vitro at physiologically relevant concentrations of the halides.[150] The products of halide + EPO + H_2O_2 reactions are toxic to bacteria, parasites, and certain mammalian cells.[109, 228, 229] These products also convert leukotriene C_4 (LTC_4) to biologically inactive subclass-specific sulfoxides and the diastereoisomers of LTB_4.[91, 128] However, EPO preferentially utilizes thiocyanate over either bromide or chloride. It is likely that hypothiocyanous acid is the major product of oxidation reactions catalyzed by EPO in vivo.[230] Thus the relevance in vivo of in vitro studies of products of halide + EPO + H_2O_2 reactions is uncertain.

EPO itself has cytotoxic properties, as it provokes ciliostasis, exfoliation, and blebbing of cultured guinea pig tracheal epithelial cells in vitro.[163] Like MBP, EPO induces granule protein and 5-hydroxytrypamine secretion from platelets.[208] Thus EPO may contribute directly to eosinophil pathogenicity.

EICOSANOID BIOSYNTHESIS

Eosinophils possess the enzymes of the 5-lipoxygenase and 15-lipoxygenase pathways.[125, 184] Eosinophils are the only human peripheral blood granulocytes exhibiting immunofluorescent staining for 15-lipoxygenase and produce 15-lipoxygenase products in response to stimulation with calcium ionophore A23187 in the presence of exogenous arachadonic acid.[142, 165] Eosinophils preferentially generate LTC_4 instead of LTB_4 in response to stimulation with calcium ionophore A23187 and other soluble stimuli.[107, 181] LTC_4, a product of the 5-lipoxygenase pathway product, is a potent modulator of vascular permeability, airway mucous secretion, and bronchomotor tone. Eosinophils primed in vitro with IL-3, IL-5, or GM-CSF exhibit augmented generation of LTC_4 compared with freshly isolated peripheral blood eosinophils, suggesting that cytokine priming in vivo may account for the observed differences in the biosynthetic capability of eosinophils in disease states, such as asthma.[181, 245]

Eosinophils produce the platelet activating factor (PAF) in vitro following stimulation by C5a, serum-treated zymosan, *N*-formyl-L-methionyl-L-leacyl-L-phenylalanine (fMLP), and calcium ionophore, particularly following priming with IL-3, IL-5, or GM-CSF.[29, 247, 248] PAF promotes superoxide production by neutrophils and has macrophage-activating properties.[103, 173, 223] It provokes increased vascular permeability of the skin and contraction of guinea pig ileum and lung parenchymal strips, and it causes anaphylactic-like reactions in rabbits.[152, 238–240] PAF also is potently chemotactic for eosinophils and causes superoxide generation and exocytosis in vitro.[120, 256] The treatment of eosinophils in vitro with a PAF antagonist, WEB2086, results in near complete inhibition of the serum-treated zymosan-induced respiratory burst, suggesting that PAF production by eosinophils may be important in regulating their generation of oxygen metabolites in an autocrine fashion.[247]

CYTOKINE PRODUCTION

Eosinophils produce several proinflammatory cytokines. The committed progenitors of eosinophils constitutively produce GM-CSF, which prolongs their viability and promotes their differentiation in vitro in an autocrine fashion.[19, 61] Eosinophils in the peripheral blood of patients with IHES, in intestinal tissues of patients with celiac sprue, and in nasal polyps synthesize transforming growth factor (TGF)-α and TGF-β as determined by immunohistochemistry and mRNA in situ hybridization.[175, 271, 272] This feature may enable eosinophils to participate in the remodeling and fibrosis of inflammatory tissue, such as in endomyocardial fibrosis or pulmonary fibrosis associated with IHES. When stimulated by calcium ionophore, peripheral blood eosinophils are capable of elaborating cytokines important in the autocrine regulation of function, including IL-3 and GM-CSF.[122, 160] Eosinophils at inflammatory foci express transcripts encoding IL-5, IL-3, and GM-CSF by mRNA in situ hybridization.[22, 62, 63, 66, 174] Peripheral blood eosinophils from IHES patients show granule localization of tumor necrosis factor (TNF)-α.[11] This cytokine activates endothelial cells and fibroblasts in vitro. In contrast, eosinophils from healthy donors do not have TNF-α in their granules.[11] Eosinophils also produce IL-1, a feature of potential importance in the eosinophil's capacity to present antigen to T cells.[267] Finally, eosinophils secrete both IL-6 and IL-8 in vitro.[100, 155] Eosinophils therefore have the capacity to influence their own function and that of neighboring cells through the elaboration of cytokines, both in vitro and in vivo.

MISCELLANEOUS FUNCTIONS

Although eosinophils are not generally thought of as phagocytic cells, peripheral blood eosinophils stimulated in vitro by GM-CSF phagocytize opsonized yeast.[137] Eosinophils also express the major histocompatibility class II antigen HLA-DR in vitro following priming with GM-CSF and the T-cell receptor CD4.[139, 140, 267] Eosinophils, like T lymphocytes, bear the receptor for IL-2.[201] These findings suggest that eosinophils in vivo could serve as antigen-presenting cells, respond chemotactically to IL-2 and lymphocyte chemoattractant factor, and bind other ligands for CD4, such as the human immunodeficiency virus protein, 1 gp 120.[140, 202, 267] Other chemotactic mediators with activity on eosinophils include complement fragments C5a and C3a, the chemokines RANTES, macrophage inflammatory protein (MIP)-1, monocyte chemotactic peptide (MCP)-3, and eotaxin.[54, 110, 115, 209, 274] The latter is selective for eosinophils for its bioactivity.

OTHER EOSINOPHIL-RELATED ENZYMES

Other eosinophil-associated enzymes include the Charcot-Leyden crystal protein, which is a distinctive lysophospholipase, arylsulfatase B, lysozyme, and an elastase similar to neutrophil elastase.[141, 161, 264, 265] The eosinophils associated with basal cell carcinoma reportedly express the mRNA for a type IV collagenase.[236]

EOSINOPHIL HETEROGENEITY

Peripheral blood eosinophils exhibit both physical and functional heterogeneity. When centrifuged through discontinuous gradients of percoll or metrizamide, peripheral blood eosinophils from donors with eosinophilia segregate into two groups. The first is a group of relatively dense eosinophils comprising the majority (>90%) of the circulating eosinophil population in healthy individuals (normodense eosinophils).[185] The second is a group of lighter density (hypodense) eosinophils.[196, 197] Although scarce in the peripheral blood of healthy individuals, hypodense eosinophils represent an increased proportion of peripheral blood eosinophils in patients with eosinophil-associated disorders. In IHES, most of the peripheral blood eosinophils are hypodense.[182]

There are significant functional differences between these two groups of eosinophils. Compared with normodense eosinophils, hypodense eosinophils have augmented generation of superoxide in response to the bacterial oligopeptide fMLP or antibody-coated sepharose beads, have an enhanced capacity for antibody-mediated and nonantibody-mediated cytotoxicity to schistosomes, and generate increased quantities of LTC_4 in response to fMLP or calcium ionophore A23187.[181, 182, 184, 221] Hypodense eosinophils from patients with IHES are morphologically altered, showing hypogranularity, cytoplasmic vacuolization, and reductions in granule core and matrix MBP.[41, 192] Hypodense eosinophils are therefore phenotypically distinct from normodense eosinophils, functionally primed, and capable of mediating damage to host tissue, as well as to invading parasites. Thus IHES is notable for not only increased eosinophil production but also phenotypically altered eosinophils.

Studies of eosinophil function in vitro provide insights into the cytokine regulation of eosinophil phenotypic characteristics. Normodense peripheral blood eosinophils may be converted in vitro to the hypodense phenotype with functional features similar to the hypodense eosinophils found in vivo. The culture of peripheral blood normodense eosinophils in the presence of the picomolar concentrations of IL-3, IL-5, or GM-CSF on a monolayer of murine 3T3 fibroblasts converts them to the hypodense phenotype over the course of 7 days.[180, 210, 211] Like their counterparts in vivo, these in vitro–derived hypodense eosinophils exhibit both augmented functional responses and morphologic changes.[41, 180, 184, 210, 211] Furthermore, the culture of peripheral blood eosinophils in the presence of IL-3, IL-5, or GM-CSF prolongs their viability for the duration of their cytokine exposure and protects them from corticosteroid-induced apoptosis in vitro.[105] The detection of serum IL-5 and hypodense peripheral blood eosinophils concurrently in some patients with IHES suggests that hypodense eosinophils may arise in vivo through cytokine-induced phenotypic conversion of normodense eosinophils.[182] Both serum IL-5 and hypodense eosinophils are also found in patients with the L-tryptophan–induced eosinophilia-myalgia syndrome (EMS) and episodic angioedema with eosinophilia.[33, 183] Thus although the stimuli responsible for inciting IHES are unknown, at least some cases may result from aberrantly increased production (or decreased clearance) of IL-5, the most selective eosinophilopoietic cytokine.

CLINICAL MANIFESTATIONS OF IHES: PATTERNS OF ORGAN SYSTEM INVOLVEMENT

IHES is predominantly a disease of adults. Most cases are reported between the ages of 20 and 50.[268] Infrequent pediatric cases are also reported.[177] There is a striking male predilection, with a male to female predominance of 9:1.[46, 268] Generally, the onset of symptoms in IHES tends to be insidious and gradually evolves over several months before diagnosis. In a series of 50 patients, their presenting symptoms included fatigue (26%), cough (24%), breathlessness (16%), myalgia or angioedema (14%), rash or fever (12%), and visual blurring (10%).[77] An additional 12% were detected incidentally with peripheral blood eosinophilia and no evident systemic disease at the time of presentation. Other series report presenting complaints that included weight loss in up to 40%, anorexia, fatigue, recurrent abdominal pain, night sweats, fever, cough, chest pain, pruritus, and signs of congestive heart failure.[46, 233] Alchohol intolerance is a presenting feature in some patients, with abdominal pain, nausea, flushing, or diarrhea.[126] Some patients experience aquagenic pruritus.[168] Rheumatologic complaints due to Raynaud's phenomenon, arthralgias, or large joint effusions with synovial fluid eosinophilia may occasionally be the presenting features.[46, 194, 233] Thus the presenting features of IHES are varied and nonspecific and may be referable to many organ systems (Table 54–1). The characteristic features of each organ system involved in IHES are discussed.

CARDIAC MANIFESTATIONS

Eosinophilic cardiac disease is the major cause of morbidity and mortality in IHES.[46] More than half of all patients with IHES develop manifestations of cardiovascular disease.[77, 233–235] Although the development of cardiac disease in IHES is generally insidious, some patients may present with the explosive onset of chest pain, dyspnea, and signs of left or right ventricular failure.[187]

The cardiac disease of hypereosinophilia evolves in three stages, based on chronicity.[21] In the first stage (0–10 weeks of eosinophilia, mean 5.5 weeks), there is an acute insult to the endocardium and myocardium. This stage may be clinically inapparent and escape detection. Pathologically, this stage is characterized by myocardial infiltration of eosinophils and mononuclear cells, with formation of eosinophilic microabscesses and focal myocardial necrosis.[216] Although patients are generally without symptoms during the acute necrotic stage, a few may die suddenly due to fulminant endomyocardial necrosis.[57, 58] Diagnosis is based upon biopsy of the right ventricle, as echocardiography and tests of cardiac function may be normal.[57] If recognized at the acute stage, the myocardial disease of IHES may respond favorably to corticosteroid treatment.[250]

The second stage of eosinophilic heart disease (mean duration of eosinophilia is 10 months) involves the formation of intraventricular thrombi.[21] Thrombosis is the likely result of endocardial damage occurring during the initial necrotic stage, with the possible contribution of the procoagulant activities of MBP and ECP. Thrombosis formation may involve any or all cardiac chambers.[21] Typically, pulmonic and aortic valves are spared.[268] Thrombi may be detectable by echocardiography at this stage.[71] Thromboembolic phenomena may result, with emboli from the left ventricle resulting in either transient cerebral ischemia or frank stroke or emboli from the right ventricle entering the pulmonary circulation and causing hypoxemia, pulmonary infarction, and other complications attendant to pulmonary emboli.[73, 96] Thromboembolic events during the second stage of eosinophilic carditis may be the presenting feature of IHES.[268] Peripheral veins may be involved as well, as indicated by the occurrence of deep venous thrombosis.[253] Unfortunately, anticoagulant therapy does not always prevent further embolic events in these patients.[234, 235, 268]

The third stage of eosinophilic heart disease is a late, fibrotic stage seen in patients with a protracted course of eosinophilia (mean duration of eosinophilia is 24.5 months).

TABLE 54–1
SIGNS AND SYMPTOMS OF IHES

Systemic	Cardiovascular	Neurologic	Pulmonary	Gastrointestinal
Fever	Chest pain	Memory loss	Cough	Abdominal pain
Weight loss	Dyspnea	Dementia	Dyspnea	Nausea
Night sweats	Orthopnea	Paraesthesia	Wheeze	Diarrhea
Anorexia	Hepatomegaly	Neuralgia		
Joint pains	S3 gallop	Weakness		
		Peripheral neuropathy		
Dermatologic	**Ocular**	**Rheumatologic**	**Miscellaneous**	
Rash (papular, nodular)	Blurred vision	Joint pain, effusions	Splenomegaly	

Histologically and pathophysiologically, this stage is similar to tropical endomyocardial fibrosis.[43] It is characterized by fibrotic, restrictive cardiomyopathy, with entrapment of the cordea tendinea and resultant regurgitation from both atrioventricular valves. Congestive heart failure ensues, with dyspnea, orthopnea, chest pain, and the development of regurgitant murmurs, hepatomegaly, and peripheral and pulmonary edema.[21] The most commonly associated EKG finding is T-wave inversion.[187] Other findings include ventricular premature beats, atrial fibrillation, nonspecific ST–T-wave changes, and left ventricular hypertrophy.[46, 187] Typical echocardiographic findings include thickening of the mitral valve and left ventricular posterior wall. There is increased intracardiac echogenicity from the fibrotic tissue.[57, 93] Cardiac catheterization may provide corroborative evidence of disease by demonstrating elevated right- and left-sided end-diastolic pressures.[58] Endomyocardial biopsy may show eosinophilic infiltrates or fibrotic changes only, depending upon tissue sampling and disease progression.

The cardiac disease of IHES is histopathologically similar to that caused by other diseases associated with hypereosinophilia.[6, 21, 235] Eosinophil granule MBP is detectable in the myocardium of patients dying of acute eosinophilic endomyocarditis, supporting the direct involvement of eosinophils and their granule proteins in the development of some eosinophilic heart diseases.[59] In instances where eosinophilia is linked with cardiac dysfunction, hypereosinophilia is essential, but not sufficient, for the development of cardiac disease. In a review of the clinical histories of patients with IHES, many did not develop heart disease.[102] There was no relationship between the risk of cardiac disease and the duration or severity of hypereosinophilia, but there was an association with the presence of peripheral blood hypogranular eosinophils.[102] In this series, male IHES patients with HLA-Bw 44, splenomegaly, and elevated serum vitamin B_{12} levels were more likely to have cardiac disease than were those who did not have these features.[102] Thus factors other than absolute eosinophil count influence the likelihood of cardiac damage.

Eosinophilic heart disease may respond to treatment with systemic corticosteroids, particularly if recognized at the early, inflammatory stage.[250] Alternatively, patients manifesting signs and symptoms of endomyocardial fibroelastosis may require treatment with diuretics or inotropes.[258] Valve replacement surgery is necessary for those with severe valvular dysfunction.

NEUROLOGIC MANIFESTATIONS

Next to cardiac disease, neurologic dysfunction is the predominant cause of morbidity in IHES, affecting greater than 50% of IHES patients.[77, 234] Neurologic manifestations are heralded by impaired cognition, memory loss, behavioral changes, confusion, or ataxia.[159] Peripheral neuropathy is common, and radiculopathy, painful paraesthesia, polyneuropathy, mononeuritis multiplex, and neuropathic muscle atrophy are reported.[12, 65, 157, 159, 269]

There are three distinct clinical patterns of IHES-related neurologic disease.[159] The first is manifested as either transient or permanent neurologic dysfunction secondary to embolic stroke. Damaged endocardial tissue due to eosinophilic heart disease is the origin of the embolus. This form of neurologic insult is most likely to manifest during the second stage of eosinophilic carditis, when the patient is at greatest risk for intracardiac thrombi.[58, 93] The second type is a primary central nervous system dysfunction of unclear origin. Encephalopathic features predominate, such as memory loss, behavioral changes, confusion, ataxia, dementia, seizures, and psychosis.[113, 159, 195] Encephalopathy may be accompanied by signs of upper motor neuron disease, including upgoing Babinski's reflexes, and may last for several weeks.[159] Dementia may persist for months. Cerebral hemorrhages and eosinophilic meningitis are rare but reported associations.[206, 263] The third type of neurologic dysfunction is peripheral neuropathy, which may be a presenting feature of IHES.[12] Peripheral neuropathy may be manifested as a symmetric or asymmetric polyneuropathy, with pain, paraesthesia, and motor or sensory deficits, or it may occur in a radicular distribution.[12, 65, 157, 269] Results of electromyography and nerve conduction studies are consistent with neuropathic disease, revealing reduction of motor unit action potentials during muscle contraction.[12, 65, 195]

The specific role of eosinophils and their products in the pathogenesis of the neuropathy of IHES is controversial. The eosinophil's granule proteins may participate directly in the neuropathy of IHES. Both EDN and ECP provoke neuropathic manifestations in rabbits when injected intrathecally.[68, 90, 92, 249] The clinical relevance of EDN and ECP in IHES neurotoxicity is unclear, however. Peripheral nerve biopsies from patients with IHES-related neuropathy do not exhibit the spongiform lesions characteristic of the Gordon phenomenon.[68] Capillary leakage, endothelial cell swelling, and secondary ischemia of nerve fibers are an alternative proposed mechanism for neuropathy in IHES.[159]

Other disorders associated with peripheral eosinophilia may cause neurologic disease. In particular, peripheral neuropathy is also a feature of Churg-Strauss syndrome, suggesting that a fundamental pathogenic eosinophil-mediated mechanism may be shared between these syndromes.[44, 148] However, the neuropathy of Churg-Strauss syndrome may be due to vasculitis, whereas peripheral nerve biopsies in IHES typically show axonal neuropathy without vasculitis.[12, 65, 148] Thus the pathogenesis of peripheral and nerve disease in IHES remains elusive.

PULMONARY DISEASE

Although the findings of cardiac or neurologic disease generally are predominant in IHES, pulmonary disease is also common, occurring in up to 40% of patients.[77, 233, 234] It is likely that the use of more sensitive diagnostic tests, such as diffusing capacity or high-resolution chest computed tomography (CT) scans, would detect more prevalent and widespread pulmonary disease than is evident on history, physical exam, and chest x-rays.

Persistent cough is the most common symptom of pulmonary disease in IHES.[233] Although wheezing is uncommon, airway involvement may occur in some individuals, causing an asthma-like syndrome.[132] IHES reportedly evolved in a patient with asthma.[124] IHES patients with isolated chronic cough generally have normal chest radiographs, although pulmonary infiltrates occur in up to one third of IHES patients.[46, 77, 268]

In contrast to the typical peripherally distributed infiltrates of chronic eosinophilic pneumonia, the radiographic abnormalities of IHES may be diffuse and interstitial in their distribution.[38, 46] Although little is written on the lung biopsy findings in IHES, the typical findings of eosinophilic pneumonia include a cellular interstitial and alveolar infiltrate consisting mainly of eosinophils, with involvement of the pulmonary vasculature and perivascular connective tissue reported as well.[106] Bronchoalveolar lavage fluid typically contains eosinophils.[224] Thus eosinophils can infiltrate the lung parenchyma in IHES and likely account for both the pulmonary symptoms and radiographic abnormalities. Pulmonary fibrosis may ensue, particularly in patients who have concomitant cardiac involvement.[77]

Pleural effusion is seen in IHES. Although most of these are transudative, eosinophilic pleural effusions have been described in association with an overlap syndrome between IHES and erythema elevatum diutinum.[51] IHES has been implicated as a cause of adult respiratory distress syndrome (ARDS) in one patient.[270] These features do not distinguish the lung disease of IHES from other diffuse eosinophilic lung diseases.

IHES patients may also have pulmonary symptoms secondary to underlying heart disease. Eosinophilic heart disease, particularly at the fibrotic stage, may produce dyspnea or wheeze due to congestive heart failure.[187] Pulmonary emboli emanating from the right ventricle may produce symptoms. Patients with congestive heart failure or pulmonary emboli have x-ray findings consistent with these entities.[73] Congestive heart failure may also be the origin of the pleural effusions of IHES.[46]

DERMATOLOGIC MANIFESTATIONS

Skin involvement occurs commonly in IHES, accounting for over 50% of patients, and may be the presenting sign of the disease.[77, 233] Two patterns predominate: angioedema with urticaria and erythematous pruritic papules and nodules. The description of a separate syndrome of episodic angioedema and urticaria with eosinophilia, with a different natural history and steroid response, might result in the reclassification of the former group of IHES patients into a separate category.[89] The distinction is important, since the latter disorder is typically characterized by a more benign prognosis and the absence of other organ system involvement.[89, 219] Punch skin biopsies from patients with papular or nodular skin lesions typically show a nonvasculitic lesion consisting of a mixed eosinophilic and mononuclear cellular infiltrate.[134]

Patients with IHES may also develop ulcers on virtually any mucosal surface.[5, 116, 134] These ulcers may be refractory to drug therapy.[5, 268] Mucosal ulcers may also be a prodrome to the fully blown systemic disease of IHES.[5] Experience with interferon (IFN)-α suggests that this agent may be especially beneficial for patients with refractory mucocutaneous ulcers.[34]

Other reported patterns of mucocutaneous involvement in IHES include generalized erythroderma, vesiculobullous lesions, cutaneous vesicles associated with bowel necrosis, and erythema annulare centrifugum.[27, 130, 189, 224] One unusual form of physical urticaria has been described, known as immediate pressure urticaria.[188] Cutaneous microthrombi are described in association with IHES.[79] As noted previously, aquagenic pruritus is reported in IHES.[170, 233]

With the notable exception of cutaneous ulcers, which may be refractory to conventional drug therapy, the cutaneous manifestations of IHES are responsive to various treatments. Systemic corticosteroid therapy is effective in patients with urticarial or papulonodular lesions.[116, 219] Corticosteroid-resistant skin disease may respond to dapsone or psoralen plus ultraviolet A (PUVA) therapy.[170, 254]

GASTROINTESTINAL MANIFESTATIONS

The reported frequency of gastrointestinal tract disease in IHES varies considerably, from over 50% in a British series to only 14% in an American series.[46, 234] The patterns of gastrointestinal tract involvement are varied. Chronic active hepatitis, sclerosing eosinophilic cholangitis, and pancreatitis are reported.[52, 74, 81, 95, 218] IHES may present with intrahepatic cholestatic jaundice.[64] Approximately 14% of IHES patients have elevated serum glutamic-oxaloacetic transaminase (SGOT) and serum glutamate pyruvate transaminase (SGPT).[46] Some patients with hepatic involvement have extensive eosinophilic hepatic infiltrates and may have centrilobular necrosis.[121] Nodular and variably echogenic lesions may be visualized by hepatic ultrasonography or CT scan in patients with eosinophilic hepatic infiltrates and may clear with prednisone therapy.[121] Diarrhea occurs in as many as 20% of IHES patients and may signify an underlying eosinophilic enteritis or colitis.[46, 218, 222, 233] Abdominal pain and nausea are frequent physical complaints in IHES.[46, 77] Abdominal pain may also occur with splenomegaly and resultant splenic capsular distention or infarction.[219]

OCULAR MANIFESTATIONS

Retinal emboli, thrombosis, and vasculitis may produce blurred vision in patients with IHES.[13, 42, 77] In one series, over half of IHES patients without visual symptoms had retinal vessel abnormalities detected with fluorescene angiograms.[42] Steroid-responsive keratoconjunctivitis sicca with episcleritis is also described.[20]

RHEUMATOLOGIC DISEASE

IHES is an uncommon cause of joint disease. However, large-joint arthritis with eosinophilic synovitis and arthralgia is reported.[23, 194] Raynaud's phenomenon is also reported, as is digital necrosis due to vascular compromise.[244] A syndrome resembling polymyositis may occur in association with IHES.[190, 199] In such cases, IHES must be differentiated from the L-tryptophan–induced EMS.[112]

LABORATORY FEATURES

The most striking and consistent laboratory feature of IHES is sustained (>6 months) peripheral blood eosinophilia. Peripheral leukocytosis is generally present, and total white cell counts of 25,000 or higher are common.[46] Eosinophils may be the predominant circulating leukocyte, although in some instances, absolute neutrophil counts are elevated as well.[80] Extremely high (>90,000/mm^3) white blood cell counts may indicate a poor prognosis.[46, 132] A mild basophilia may be present.[80] Platelet counts may be increased, decreased, or normal.[80] Anemia may occur, with nucleated red blood cells and teardrop cells present in the peripheral smears in some patients.[80] Leukocyte alkaline phosphatase may be elevated or decreased.[46] Elevated total IgE is found in almost 40% and may signify a subgroup of patients with a better prognosis and response to corticosteroid treatment.[186, 188] Elevated IgA, IgG, or IgM is found less frequently.[188] Erythrocyte sedimentation rates are elevated in a minority of patients.[188] Antinuclear antibodies (ANA), rheumatoid factor (RF), and mixed cryoglobulins are typically absent, which may be helpful in discriminating between IHES and collagen vascular disease with secondary eosinophilia.[188] Complement levels are normal.[188] Antineutrophil cytoplasmic antibodies (ANCA) are not detected. The latter may aid in the distinction between IHES and Churg-Strauss syndrome, in which ANCA may be detected.[148] Biochemical evidence of chronic active hepatitis or pancreatitis rarely is present, with 14% having transaminase abnormalities, as noted previously.[46, 52, 74, 81]

CLUES TO PATHOGENESIS

As noted previously, IHES probably is a shared end point for a variety of disorders that produce sustained, severe peripheral blood eosinophilia. Some clues to the pathogenesis of IHES come from studies of the associated features of the disease. For example, some patients with IHES have clinical features of myelodysplasia, including diminished (or elevated) leukocyte alkaline phosphatase, elevated levels of serum vitamin B_{12} and B_{12}-binding proteins, anemia, thrombocytopenia or thrombocytosis, splenomegaly, and myelofibrosis.[46, 77] IHES is also described concomitantly with polycythemia vera.[256] Chromosomal abnormalities are found in a minority of patients and are diverse, with some patients having aneuploidy and occasional patients having the Philadelphia chromosome; again, these abnormalities suggest an overlap with myeloproliferative diseases for some cases.[77]

It is not surprising that in a subset of patients, IHES may be confused with a leukemic or preleukemic state. Indeed, progression to blast crisis or myeloid leukemia is described occasionally.[24, 40, 77, 179] Thus a subgroup of IHES may be caused by pathogenic mechanisms common to myeloproliferative disease or stem cell disorders. Patients with myelodysplastic features account for 40 to 50% of all IHES patients. On retrospective analyses, these patients respond less favorably to prednisone alone and are more likely to require cytotoxic drugs.[77, 132, 219]

Another subset of patients with IHES have markedly elevated levels of serum IgE in the absence of demonstrable skin test reactivity to common environmental antigens; such patients account for 38% of the total population of one series.[188] These patients, in contrast to the patients having myelodysplastic features, are more likely to respond favorably to prednisone, less likely to present with cardiac or neurologic disease, and thus less likely to require therapy.[188] The concomitant elevation of IgE levels and eosinophil counts strongly suggests the elaboration of IL-4 and IL-5 by Th2-type helper T cells, such as has been demonstrated in atopic diseases accompanied by elevations of both IgE and total eosinophil count or in visceral leischmaniasis.[119, 205, 213] Elevated serum IL-5 was detected in three patients with IHES, although IL-4 was not concomitantly measured.[183] Proliferation of a CD4$^+$ CD3$^-$ T-cell clone was described in an IHES patient who had elevated serum IgE accompanied by markedly elevated serum IL-4 and IL-5.[48] Cloned CD4$^+$ T cells from other IHES patients also produce eosinophil viability-sustaining activities consistent with IL-5 or both IL-4 and IL-5.[200, 220, 243] Thus some cases of IHES may involve the clonal expansion of abnormal Th2-like CD4$^+$ T cells.

IHES may precede the development of T-cell lymphoma or acute lymphoblastic leukemia in some patients, suggesting a possible link to disordered lymphoproliferation.[117, 120, 166, 217, 242] Hypereosinophilia associated with T-cell lymphoma may produce endomyocardial disease similar to IHES.[158] In one patient with long-standing IHES, bone marrow biopsy revealed nonmalignant paratrabecular aggregates of T lymphocytes, with an eosinophil colony-stimulating activity, probably IL-5, detected in the serum.[154] Detection of the soluble IL-2 receptor, an index of T-cell activation, is described in IHES.[198] Hypereosinophilic syndromes are increasingly recognized as a complication of HIV infection, usually in association with cutaneous manifestations.[146, 149, 159, 162, 258, 262] In one such patient, the hypereosinophilia was associated with an elevated level of IL-5.[67] Thus in these instances, IHES may be the end result of an underlying abnormality of T-cell function, with abnormal T-cell proliferation of either neoplastic or non-neoplastic origin and dysregulated production of cytokines favoring eosinophilopoiesis, such as IL-5.

IHES rarely is recognized in association with autoimmune phenomena. An IHES-like syndrome has been reported as a prodrome of a facial Merkel cell carcinoma, a rare tumor associated with various endocrine paraneoplastic syndromes.[75] This patient also had an autoimmune hemolytic anemia. IHES is also described in association with insulin-resistant diabetes mellitus in a patient with high levels of anti-insulin antibodies. Both the hypereosinophilia and diabetes improved markedly on prednisone.[251] An acute peripheral neuropathy with demonstrable autoantibodies against the GM-1 ganglioside was reported in one patient with IHES.[129] Whether the autoimmune phenomena in these cases were also due to dysregulated T-cell function, and whether other cases of IHES-related neuropathy are also autoimmune in origin, is unknown.

DIFFERENTIAL DIAGNOSIS

By definition, IHES is a disease with no apparent clinical explanation for eosinophilia. It is therefore a diagnosis of exclusion. The diagnostic work-up of IHES should therefore have two objectives: excluding potential known causes for eosinophilia and establishing evidence for the end-organ involvement that is characteristic of IHES.

The initial evaluation of a suspected IHES patient must focus on any symptoms or signs consistent with systemic disease, such as fever, rash, night sweats, recent weight loss, chest pain, joint pain, memory loss, paraesthesias, difficulty ambulating, cough, shortness of breath, diarrhea, abdominal pain, and blurred vision. A careful history of recent drug use, travel outside the United States, or risk factors for HIV disease should be elicited. The physical examination should include a careful search for skin lesions, lymphadenopathy, and splenomegaly. Signs of cardiac disease or congestive heart failure, such as hepatomegaly, tachypnea, tachycardia, jugular venous distension, heart murmur, or gallop, should be sought. The evaluation should also include a careful neurologic examination, including tests of sensation and strength.

A laboratory work-up of a patient with persistent eosinophilia (>1,500 eosinophils/mm^3) must include a careful search for parasites, such as toxocariasis, trichinosis, and strongyloidiasis, using both serologic tests and stool examination.[39, 78, 82, 167, 171] If there is a recent travel history to Southeast Asia, India, or Africa, the serologic work-up should include complement fixation for microfilariae. Liver function abnormalities may signal hepatic involvement. An erythrocyte sedimentation rate, a serum protein immunoelectrophoresis, and an ANCA should be obtained. For patients presenting with rheumatologic complaints, the work-up should include a rheumatoid factor and antinuclear antibody. HIV serology should be performed on any hypereosinophilic patient with a history consistent with exposure. Chest radiography and lung function studies are useful to exclude eosinophilic lung diseases as primary diagnostic considerations. Any pulmonary infiltrate or pleural effusion should be investigated using appropriate diagnostic techniques, such as bronchoalveolar lavage, transbronchial biopsy, or pleural fluid analysis. A bone marrow biopsy should be included to exclude hematologic malignancy, such as leukemia or lymphoma.[117, 120, 158, 166, 217, 242] Echocardiography and electrocardiography are essential, although patients may have normal findings early in their course.[58] A CT scan of the abdomen and pelvis may be useful to detect malignancy or hepatic involvement.[121] Skin biopsy should be performed on patients with suspicious papular, nodular, or purpuric cutaneous lesions. Skin biopsy may also be useful in excluding skin diseases associated with peripheral blood eosinophilia, such as pustular folliculitis, Well's syndrome (a distinctive dermatosis resembling acute cellulitis with solid edema), and eosinophilic fasciitis.[1, 28, 76] Each of these have diagnostic biopsy findings that are distinct from those of IHES.

The diagnosis of IHES rests with the lack of other definable clinical causes for hypereosinophilia, the persistence of peripheral blood eosinophilia for 6 months or longer, and the demonstration of disease of the heart, lung, skin, peripheral or central nervous system, gastrointestinal tract, or hepatobiliary system (Fig. 54–1).

TREATMENT

The management of IHES patients with corticosteroids or other immunomodulatory therapies depends on the extent of organ involvement. In patients who are apparently well despite hypereosinophilia (benign hypereosinophilia), deferring treatment is acceptable, since they are likely to remain well and not develop organ damage over prolonged (one decade) periods of follow-up.[46, 77] In such patients, careful follow-up is warranted, since cardiac disease may develop insidiously, and echocardiography may be advisable at 3- to 6-month intervals.[21]

PREDNISONE

In patients with evidence of organ system involvement, such as neurologic abnormalities, pulmonary infiltrates, restrictive pattern of lung function, congestive heart failure, hepatosplenomegaly, abdominal pain, diarrhea, or weight loss, a trial of corticosteroids is warranted. Parrillo and colleagues[186] demonstrated that patients having a rapid suppression of peripheral blood eosinophilia in response to a single 60 mg dose of prednisone had a better overall prognosis than nonresponders, were likely to remain steroid responsive, and could be maintained on alternate-day prednisone or intermittent bursts of prednisone, as indicated for disease exacerbation. These steroid-responsive patients remained alive after an average follow-up of 3.5 years. For the treatment of steroid-responsive IHES, these investigators recommended prednisone therapy at 60 mg/daily for 1 week, followed by 60 mg every other day for 3 months. At that point, patients underwent an extensive reevaluation, including pulmonary function, urine analysis, EKG, bone marrow aspirate, and x-rays of any involved organ system. In patients with no sign of disease progression, prednisone was continued on an alternate-day basis for 1 year and then gradually tapered to the lowest possible dose that would control disease progression, with comprehensive reassessment every 3 to 6 months. Patients having urticaria and angioedema, elevated serum IgE, and eosinophilopenia in response to a single dose of prednisone were more likely to benefit from this regimen, whereas patients having splenomegaly, myelodysplastic features, congestive heart failure, or neurologic dysfunction at the time of presentation were less likely to benefit and more likely to require alternative drug therapy.[186, 187, 219] In all, at least two thirds of IHES patients can be expected to benefit from prednisone, with approximately one third having a complete remission for the duration of steroid therapy.[186]

The mechanisms responsible for corticosteroid-induced effects on eosinophils in vivo and for the efficacy of corticosteroids in the treatment of IHES are not clearly defined. Studies of eosinophilopoiesis in vitro suggest that corticosteroids may inhibit eosinophilopoiesis indirectly through effects on accessory cell function, possibly by inhibiting cytokine production by lymphocytes.[14, 32, 227] For example, corticosteroids inhibit the production of the eosinophilopoietic cytokines IL-3, IL-5, and GM-CSF by fibroblasts, human lung tissue, T cells, peripheral blood mononuclear cells, and cultured human tracheal epithelial cells in vitro.[45, 93, 97, 114, 118, 136, 207, 246] Additionally, corticosteroids rapidly (within 12 hours) induce the programmed cell death (apoptosis) of human peripheral blood eosinophils in vitro, whereas the eosinophilopoietic cytokines IL-3, IL-5, and GM-CSF protect eosinophils from the cytopathic effects of corticosteroids in a dose-dependent fashion.[105] The overproduction of eosinophilopoietic cytokines may result in corticosteroid resistance by eosinophils, as suggested in IHES associated with elevated serum IL-5.[182] Thus corticosteroid effects in eosinophil-asso-

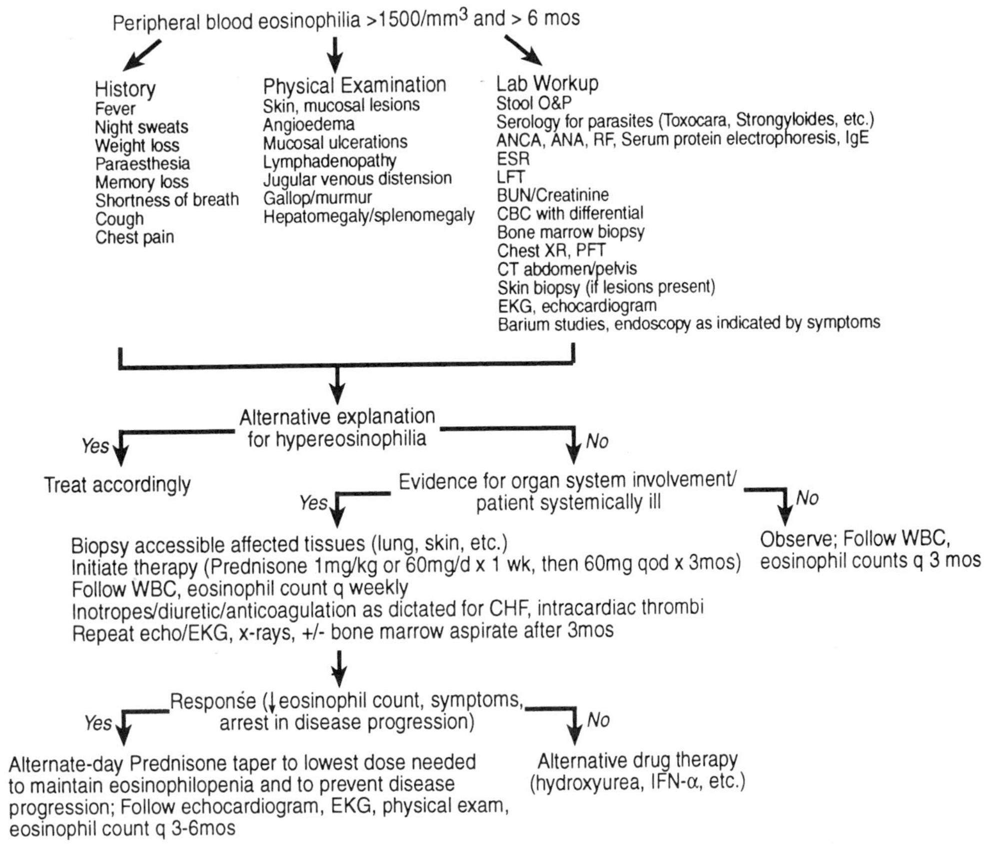

FIGURE 54–1. Algorithmic approach to the diagnostic work-up and therapy of a patient with persistent eosinophilia >1500/mm^3.

ciated diseases in vivo are likely to be diverse and may include inhibition of eosinophilopoietic cytokine production by accessory cells or by eosinophils themselves, with resultant inhibition of eosinophilopoiesis and induction of eosinophil apoptosis and subsequent clearance of eosinophils by macrophages.[237] Alternatively, corticosteroid-resistant cases of IHES may result from T-cell clones unresponsive to the suppressive effect of corticosteroids on cytokine production.

HYDROXYUREA

For patients without satisfactory responses to corticosteroids (persistent peripheral blood eosinophilopenia, symptoms of systemic disease, progression of organ system damage), hydroxyurea has been used successfully to control IHES.[186, 187, 256] Doses of 1 to 2 g daily are started, with a goal of reducing total leukocyte counts to normal range (5,000–10,000 cells/mm^3). Hydroxyurea acts by interfering with DNA synthesis; thus the fall in total eosinophil counts is delayed by 1 to 2 weeks. This differs from the time course of eosinophilopenia associated with prednisone, which occurs by a different mechanism and is more rapid in onset.

OTHER CHEMOTHERAPEUTIC AGENTS

Vincristine has been used successfully to treat IHES patients with corticosteroid-resistant disease.[49, 147] Doses of 1.5 to 2.0 mg every 2 weeks have proved beneficial. The expected onset of action (within 3 days) is more rapid than with hydroxyurea but more gradual than with corticosteroids. The vinca alkaloids have less marrow toxicity than does hydroxyurea. Neurotoxicity may limit therapy and may be confused with complications of the disease itself.[159]

Successful pulse therapy with chlorambucil for the long-term management of steroid-resistant IHES has been reported by Weller and colleagues.[268] The reported dose range is 4 to 10 mg/m^2 daily for 4 days each month on consecutive days. Etoposide, a podophyllotoxin derivative that mediates DNA damage, was used successfully in 1 patient to maintain disease control over an 18-month period.[231] Treatment was terminated because of myelosuppression. Cyclosporine was reported as adjunctive therapy for steroid-dependent IHES and as a single agent at 200 to 400 mg/daily for successful short-term induction of eosinophilopenia.[200, 275]

INTERFERON-α

There is increasing published experience using IFN-α for the treatment of steroid-resistant IHES. Its use was adopted based on experience with cell-mediated lympholysis. Initial case reports suggested the agent was effective in reducing peripheral eosinophil counts.[17, 30, 85, 164, 276] In the first published series of patients treated with recombinant IFN-α, all of whom had unsatisfactory therapeutic responses to prednisone, treatment was initiated at a dose of 1 to 6.25 million units daily.[31] All but one patient had a reduction in bone marrow eosinophils. All experienced dramatic reductions in peripheral blood eosinophil counts. Improvements were noted in echocardiographic parameters, including ejection fraction, in two patients who had measurements performed both before and during treatment. Both patients with mucosal ulcers had healing, and no new ulcers developed during IFN therapy. Systemic symptoms, such as fever and night sweats, improved. All patients were able to discontinue steroids and hydroxyurea over a minimum of 9 months of treatment. One patient, who discontinued therapy, had a rebound in eosinophil count to levels that exceeded his pre-IFN levels. One patient, with leukemoid features, died after developing multiple spinal cord chloromas.[34] Untoward effects reported included thrombocytopenia, watery stools, nausea, and vomiting.[31] Psychosis has also been reported in one patient.[104] Thus IFN-α may prove to be a feasible alternative to cytotoxic therapy in patients with steroid-resistant IHES, but longer term follow-up is necessary to determine the ultimate outcome for patients treated in this fashion.

Studies in vitro suggest that IFN-α acts by inhibiting the formation of early eosinophil progenitors.[26] One patient with IHES associated with high IgE, elevations of both IL-4 and IL-5, and an abnormal T-cell clone became steroid resistant after an initial satisfactory response to prednisone. IFN-α, started at a dose of 5 million units daily, markedly reduced his eosinophil count while leaving serum IL-5 levels unaffected.[48] Thus a direct effect on eosinophil progenitors appears likely in vivo as well.

ANCILLARY THERAPIES

In patients having exceedingly high eosinophil counts at risk for leukostasis (>100,000 cells/mm³), emergency leukapheresis may achieve a temporary reduction in eosinophilia.[15] Bone marrow transplant is employed only rarely and cannot be justified as a treatment for IHES.[7] Splenectomy may be beneficial for patients with overt hypersplenism, splenic infarctions, or splenic pain.[233] Emergency splenectomy is indicated only for splenic rupture, a rare complication of the disease.[234] Anticoagulant therapy with aspirin, coumadin, or heparin is often employed prophylactically in IHES, but the effectiveness of this therapy has not been rigorously established. Furthermore, many patients with IHES continue to suffer thromboembolic disease despite anticoagulant drug therapy.[159, 234] Higher doses of heparin may be required in IHES to achieve an equivalent degree of anticoagulation.[101]

Some patients suffering extensive endomyocardial disease, resulting in fibrosis, thrombosis, or valvar dysfunction, may require surgical intervention. Both mitral and tricuspid valve replacement has been successfully undertaken in IHES.[16, 18, 36] Concomitant replacement of the aortic and mitral valves is reported in one patient.[232] The treatment of mural thrombi may also be accomplished surgically.[83] Although thromboemboli may emanate from artificial valves in IHES, the satisfactory long-term outcome for many patients treated with valve replacement justifies the continued use of surgical modalities for cardiac disease not treated satisfactorily using medical approaches.

PROGNOSIS

The prognosis of IHES varies depending on several clinical criteria. Patients having features of myelodysplasia, such as splenomegaly or abnormal leukocyte alkaline phosphatase or vitamin B_{12} levels, have a worse prognosis and a poorer response to corticosteroids.[219] Congestive heart failure at the time of presentation and peripheral blood eosinophil counts greater than 90,000/mm³ also are indicative of a poorer prognostic group.[46, 186] Patients with elevated serum IgE and no splenomegaly, biochemical features, or myelodysplasia are more likely to respond favorably to prednisone and have a better prognosis.

Historically, most patients dying of IHES succumb to the cardiac complications of the disease.[46] However, many of the reported deaths occurred in patients with very advanced cardiac disease. The 1975 review by Chusid and colleagues[46] cited a 3-year survival of only 12%. Another series indicated a 5-year survival of 80% and 42% survival at 10 years.[132] Improved recognition and treatment of early cardiac disease, combined with advances in supportive measures for cardiac disease and alternative drug treatment for steroid-resistant cases, are likely to further modify the prognosis. Already, IHES patients have survived for decades with their disease.[204, 258] Recurrences of the disease are likely to occur off of therapy, necessitating reinitiation of therapy. Patients with an initially favorable response to prednisone are likely to respond to subsequent steroid courses.[186] Well-controlled long-term follow-up studies are necessary to better define the natural history of the disease, as well as the long-term benefits and risks of IFN-α therapy.

REFERENCES

1. Aberer W, Konrad K, Wolff K: Well's syndrome is a distinctive disease and not a histologic diagnosis. J Am Acad Dermatol 18:105, 1988.
2. Ackerman SJ, Weil GJ, Gleich GJ: Formation of Charcot-Leyden crystals by human basophils. J Exp Med 155:1597, 1982.
3. Ackerman SJ, Kephart GM, Habermann TM, et al: Localization of eosinophil granule major basic protein in human basophils. J Exp Med 158:946–961, 1983.
4. Ackerman SJ, Loegering DA, Venge P, et al: Distinctive cationic proteins of the eosinophil granule: major basic protein, eosinophil cationic protein, and eosinophil-derived neurotoxin. J Immunol 131:2977, 1983.
5. Akahoshi M, Hoshino S, Teramura M, et al: Recurrent oral and genital ulcers as the prodrome of the hypereosinophilic syndrome: report of a probable case. Nippon Naika Gakkai Zasshi 76:421, 1987.
6. Andy JJ, O'Connell JP, Daddario RC, Roberts WC: Trichinosis causing extensive ventricular mural endocarditis with superimposed thrombosis. Evidence that severe eosinophilia damages endocardium. Am J Med 63:824, 1977.
7. Archimbaud E, Guyotat D, Guillaume C, et al: Hypereosinophilic syndrome with multiple organ dysfunction treated by allogeneic bone marrow transplantation. Am J Hematol 27:302, 1988.
8. Ayars GH, Altman LC, Gleich GJ, et al: Eosinophil- and eosinophil granule-mediated pneumocyte injury. J Allergy Clin Immunol 76:595, 1985.
9. Ayars GH, Altman LC, McManus MM, et al: Injurious effects of the eosinophil peroxide-halide system and major basic protein on human nasal epithelium in vitro. Am Rev Respir Dis 140:125, 1989.
10. Bain BJ: Blood Cells—A Practical Guide. Lippincott, Philadelphia, 1988, pp 50–51.
11. Beil WJ, Weller PF, Tzizik DM, et al: Ultrastructural immunogold localization of tumor necrosis factor alpha to the matrix compartment of eosinophil secondary granules in patients with the hypereosinophilic syndrome. J Histochem Cytochem 41:1611, 1993.
12. Bell D, Mackay IG, Pentland B: Hypereosinophilic syndrome presenting as peripheral neuropathy. Postgrad Med J 61:429, 1985.
13. Binaghi M, Perrenoud F, Dhermy P, Coscas G: Syndrome hypereosinophilique avec atteinte oculaire. J Fr Ophthalmol 8:309, 1985.

14. Bjornsen BH, Harvey JM, Rose L: Differential effect of hydrocortisone on eosinophil and neutrophil proliferation. J Clin Invest 76:924, 1985.
15. Blacklock HA, Cleland JF, Tan P, Pillai VM: The hypereosinophilic syndrome and leukapheresis. Ann Intern Med 91:650, 1979.
16. Blake DP, Palmer TE, Olinger GN: Mitral valve replacement in idiopathic hypereosinophilic syndrome. J Thorac Cardiovasc Surg 89:630, 1985.
17. Bockenstedt PL, Santinga JT, Bolling SF: Alpha-interferon treatment for the idiopathic hypereosinophilic syndrome. Am J Hematol 45:248, 1994.
18. Boustany CWJ, Murphy GW, Hicks GLJ: Mitral valve replacement in idiopathic hypereosinophilic syndrome. Ann Thorac Surg 51:1007, 1991.
19. Boyce JA, Friend D, Matsumoto R, et al: Development in vitro of a hybrid eosinophil/basophil granulocyte: autocrine function of an eosinophil developmental intermediate. J Exp Med 182:49, 1995.
20. Bozkir N, Stern GA: Ocular manifestations of the idiopathic hypereosinophilic syndrome. Am J Ophthalmol 113:456, 1992.
21. Brockington IF, Olsen EGJ: Loeffler's endocarditis and Davie's endomyocardial fibroelastosis. Am Heart J 85:308, 1973.
22. Broide DH, Paine M, Firestein GS: Eosinophils express interleukin 5 and granulocyte-macrophage colony-stimulating factor mRNA at sites of allergic inflammation. J Clin Invest 90:1414–1424, 1992.
23. Brogadir SP, Goldwein MI, Schumacher HR: A hypereosinophilic syndrome mimicking rheumatoid arthritis. Am J Med 69:799, 1980.
24. Brown NJ, Stein RS: Idiopathic hypereosinophilic syndrome progressing to acute myelomonocytic leukemia with chloromas. South Med J 82:1303, 1989.
25. Bousser J: Eosinophilie et leucemie. Sang 28:533, 1957.
26. Broxmeyer HE, Lu L, Platzer E, et al: Comparative analysis of the influences of human alfa and beta interferons on human multipotential (CFU-GEMM), erythroid (BFU-E) and granulocyte-macrophage (CFU-GM) progenitor cells. J Immunol 131:1300, 1983.
27. Brugger F, Treuner J, Undeutsch W: Hypereosinophiliesyndrom (eosinophiles leukamoid) mit dermaler exanthematischer vesikulo-bulloser manifestation. Z Hautkr 55:855, 1980.
28. Buchness MR, Lim HW, Hatcher VA, et al: Eosinophilic pustular folliculitis in the acquired immunodeficiency syndrome. Treatment with ultraviolet B phototherapy. N Engl J Med 318:1183, 1988.
29. Burke LA, Crea AE, Wilkinson JR, et al: Comparison of the generation of platelet-activating factor and leukotriene C_4 in human eosinophils stimulated by unopsonized zymosan and by the calcium ionophore A23187: the effects of nedocromil sodium. J Allergy Clin Immunol 85:26–35, 1990.
30. Busch FW, Schmidt H, Steinke B: Alfa interferon for the hypereosinophilic syndrome. Ann Intern Med 114:338, 1991.
31. Butterfield JH, Gleich GJ: Interferon-α treatment of six patients with the hypereosinophilic syndrome. Ann Intern Med 121:648, 1994.
32. Butterfield JH, Ackerman SJ, Weiler D, et al: Effects of glucocorticoids on eosinophil colony growth. J Allergy Clin Immunol 78:450, 1986.
33. Butterfield JH, Leiferman KM, Abrams J, et al: Elevated serum levels of interleukin-5 in patients with the syndrome of episodic angioedema and eosinophilia. Blood 79:688, 1992.
34. Butterfield JH, Gleich GJ: Response of six patients with idiopathic hypereosinophilic syndrome to interferon alfa. J Allergy Clin Immunol 94:1318, 1994.
35. Butterworth AE, Wassom DL, Gleich GJ, et al: Damage to schistosomula of *Schistosoma mansoni* induced directly by eosinophil major basic protein. J Immunol 122:221–229, 1979.
36. Cameron J, Radford DJ, Howell J, O'Brien MF: Hypereosinophilic heart disease. Med J Aust 143:308, 1985.
37. Carlson MGCh, Peterson CGB, Venge P: Human eosinophil peroxidase: purification and characterization. J Immunol 134:1875, 1985.
38. Carrington CB, Addington WW, Goff AM, et al: Chronic eosinophilic pneumonia. N Engl J Med 280:787, 1969.
39. Carroll SM, Karthisgasu KT, Grove DI: Serodiagnosis of human strongyloidiasis by an enzyme-linked immunosorbent assay. Trans R Soc Trop Med Hyg 75:706, 1981.
40. Cassi E, De Paoli A, Fava S, et al: Idiopathic hypereosinophilic syndrome and "eosinophilic leukemia." Haematologica 77:430, 1992.
41. Caulfield JP, Hein A, Rothenberg ME, et al: A morphometric study of normodense and hypodense human eosinophils that are derived in vitro and in vivo. Am J Pathol 137:27, 1990.
42. Chaine G, Davies J, Kohner EM, et al: Ophthalmologic abnormalities in the hypereosinophilic syndrome. Ophthalmology 89:1348, 1982.
43. Chew CY, Ziady GM, Raphael MJ, et al: Primary restrictive cardiomyopathy. Non-tropical endomyocardial fibrosis and hypereosinophilic heart disease. Br Heart J 39:399, 1977.
44. Chumbley LC, Harrison EGJ, DeRemee RA: Allergic granulomatosis and angiitis (Churg-Strauss syndrome): report and analysis of 30 cases. Mayo Clin Proc 52:477, 1977.
45. Churchill L, Friedman B, Schleimer RP, Proud D: Production of granulocyte-macrophage colony-stimulating factor by cultured human tracheal epithelial cells. Immunology 75:189, 1992.
46. Chusid MJ, Dale DC, West BC, Wolff SM: The hypereosinophilic syndrome: analysis of fourteen cases with review of the literature. Medicine (Baltimore) 54:1, 1975.
47. Clutterbuck EJ, Sanderson CJ: Human eosinophil hematopoiesis studied in vitro by means of murine eosinophil differentiation factor (IL-5): production of functionally active eosinophils from normal human bone marrow. Blood 71:6346, 1988.
48. Cogan E, Schandene L, Crusiaux A, et al: Brief report: clonal proliferation of helper T-cells in a man with the idiopathic hypereosinophilic syndrome. N Engl J Med 330:535, 1994.
49. Cofrancesco E, Cortellaro M, Pogliani E, et al: Response to vincristine treatment in a case of idiopathic hypereosinophilic syndrome with multiple clinical manifestations. Acta Haematol 72:21, 1984.
50. Cook GC: Strongyloides stercoralis hyperinfection syndrome: how often is it missed? Q J Med 64:625, 1987.
51. Cordier JF, Faure M, Hermier C, Brune J: Pleural effusions in an overlap syndrome of idiopathic hypereosinophilic syndrome and erythema elevatum diutinum. Eur Respir J 3:115, 1990.
52. Croffy B, Kopelman R, Kaplan M: Hypereosinophilic syndrome. Association with chronic active hepatitis. Dig Dis Sci 33:233, 1988.
53. Culpepper JA, Lee F: Regulation of IL-3 gene expression by glucocorticoids in cloned murine T-lymphocytes. J Immunol 135:3191, 1985.
54. Daffern PJ, Pfeifer PH, Ember JA, Hugli TE: C3a is a chemotaxin for human eosinophils but not for neutrophils. I. C3a stimulation of neutrophils is secondary to eosinophil activation. J Exp Med 181:2119, 1995.
55. Dahl R, Venge P: Enhancement of urokinase-induced plasminogen activation by the cationic protein of eosinophil granules. Thromb Res 14:599, 1979.
56. Dale DC, Hubert RT, Fauci A: Eosinophil kinetics in the hypereosinophilic syndrome. J Lab Clin Med 87:487, 1976.
57. Davies J, Gibson DG, Foale R, et al: Echocardiographic features of eosinophilic endomyocardial disease. Br Heart J 48:434, 1982.
58. Davies J, Spry C, Sapsford R, et al: Cardiovascular features of 11 patients with eosinophilic endomyocardial disease. Q J Med 52:23, 1983.
59. de Mello DE, Liapis H, Jureidini S, et al: Cardiac localization of eosinophil-granule major basic protein in acute necrotizing myocarditis. N Engl J Med 323:1542, 1990.
60. Denburg JA, Telizyn S, Messner H, et al: Heterogeneity of human peripheral blood eosinophil-type colonies: evidence for a common basophil-eosinophil progenitor. Blood 66:312, 1985.
61. Denburg JA, Woolley M, Leber B, et al: Basophil and eosinophil differentiation in allergic reactions. J Allergy Clin Immunol 94:1135, 1994.
62. Desreumaux P, Janin A, Dubucquoi S, et al: Synthesis of interleukin-5 by activated eosinophils in patients with eosinophilic heart diseases. Blood 82:1553, 1993.
63. Desreumaux P, Janin A, Colombel JF, et al: Interleukin 5 messenger RNA expression by eosinophils in the intestinal mucosa of patients with coeliac disease. J Exp Med 175:293, 1992.
64. Dillon JF, Finlayson ND: Idiopathic hypereosinophilic syndrome presenting as intrahepatic cholestatic jaundice. Am J Gastroenterol 89:1254, 1994.
65. Dorfman LJ, Ransom BR, Forno LS, Kelts A: Neuropathy in the hypereosinophilic syndrome. Muscle Nerve 6:291, 1983.
66. Dubucquoi S, Desmereaux P, Janin A, et al: Interleukin 5 synthesis by eosinophils: association with granules and immunoglobulin dependent secretion. J Exp Med 179:703, 1994.
67. Drabick JJ, Magill AJ, Smith KJ, et al: Hypereosinophilic syndrome associated with HIV infection. Military Medical Consortium for Applied Retroviral Research. South Med J 87:525, 1994.
68. Durack DT, Sumi SM, Klebanoff SJ: Neurotoxicity of human eosinophils. Proc Natl Acad Sci USA 76:14373, 1979.
69. Dvorak AM, Saito H, Estrella P, et al: Ultrastructure of eosinophils and basophils stimulated to develop in human cord blood mononuclear

cell cultures containing recombinant interleukin-5 or interleukin-3. Lab Invest 61:116, 1989.

70. Egesten A, Alumets J, von Mecklenburg C, et al: Localization of eosinophil cationic protein, major basic protein, and eosinophil peroxidase in human eosinophils by immunoelectron microscopic technique. J Histochem Cytochem 34:1399, 1986.
71. Ejima J, Ohmura I, Kaji Y, et al: Diffuse endocardial thrombus associated with a case of hypereosinophilic syndrome. Jpn Heart J 32:267, 1991.
72. Ema H, Suda T, Nagayoshi K, et al: Target cells for granulocyte colony-stimulating factor, interleukin-3 and interleukin-5 in differentiation pathways of neutrophils and eosinophils. Blood 76:1956, 1990.
73. Epstein DM, Taormina V, Gefter WB, Miller WT: The hypereosinophilic syndrome. Radiology 140:59, 1981.
74. Eugene C, Gury B, Bergue A, Quevauvilliers J: Ictere relevant une atteinte pancreatique au cours d'un syndrome hypereosinophilique idiopathique. Gastroenterol Clin Biol 8:966, 1984.
75. Fain J, Frenkel EP: Autoimmune hemolytic anemia (AIHA) and hypereosinophilic syndrome (HES) preceding Merkel cell carcinoma (MCC) (Meeting abstract). Proc Annu Meet Am Soc Clin Oncol 13:A1379, 1994.
76. Falanga V, Medsger TAJ: Frequency, levels, and significance of blood eosinophilia in systemic sclerosis, localized scleroderma, and eosinophilic faciitis. J Am Acad Dermatol 17:648, 1987.
77. Fauci AS, Harley JB, Roberts WC, et al: NIH conference. The idiopathic hypereosinophilic syndrome. Clinical, pathophysiologic and therapeutic considerations. Ann Intern Med 97:78, 1982.
78. Feldman GJ, Parker HW: Visceral larva migrans associated with the hypereosinophilic syndrome and the onset of severe asthma. Ann Intern Med 116:838, 1992.
79. Fitzpatrick JE, Johnson C, Simon P, Owenby J: Cutaneous microthrombi: a histologic clue to the diagnosis of hypereosinophilic syndrome. Am J Dermatopathol 9:419, 1987.
80. Flaum MA, Schooley RT, Fauci AS, Gralnick HR: A clinico-pathologic correlation of the idiopathic hypereosinophilic syndrome. I. Hematologic manifestations. Blood 58:1012, 1981.
81. Foong A, Scholes JV, Gleich GJ, et al: Eosinophil-induced chronic active hepatitis in the idiopathic hypereosinophilic syndrome. Hepatology 13:1090, 1991.
82. Fourestie V, Douceron H, Brugieres P, et al: Neurotrichinosis. A cerebrovascular disease associated with myocardial injury and hypereosinophilia. Brain 116:603, 1993.
83. Fournial G, Schlanger R, Berthoumieu F, et al: Surgery for cardiac complications caused by endocardial mural thrombin deposits in a hypereosinophilic syndrome. Circulation 65:1010, 1982.
84. Frigas E, Loegering DA, Gleich GJ: Cytotoxic effects of the guinea pig eosinophil major basic protein on tracheal epithelium. Lab Invest 42:35, 1980.
85. Fruehauf S, Fiehn C, Haas R, et al: Sustained remission of idiopathic hypereosinophilic syndrome following alpha-interferon therapy. Acta Haematol 89:91, 1993.
86. Ganser A, Lindemann A, Ottmann OG, et al: Sequential in vivo treatment with two recombinant human hematopoietic growth factors (interleukin-3 and granulocyte-macrophage colony-stimulating factor) as a new therapeutic modality to stimulate hematopoiesis: results of a phase I study. Blood 79:2583, 1992.
87. Gleich GJ, Loegering DA, Kueppers F, et al: Physiochemical and biological properties of the major basic protein from guinea pig eosinophil granules. J Exp Med 140:313, 1974.
88. Gleich GJ, Frigas E, Loegering DA, et al: Cytotoxic properties of the eosinophil major basic protein. J Immunol 123:2925, 1979.
89. Gleich GJ, Schroeter AL, Marcoux JP, et al: Episodic angioedema associated with eosinophilia. N Engl J Med 310:1621, 1984.
90. Gleich GJ, Loegering DA, Bell MP, et al: Biochemical and functional similarities between human eosinophil-derived neurotoxin and eosinophil cationic protein: homology with ribonuclease. Proc Natl Acad Sci USA 83:3146, 1986.
91. Goetzl EJ: The conversion of leukotriene C_4 to isomers of leukotriene B_4 by human eosinophil peroxidase. Biochem Biophys Res Commun 106:270–205, 1982.
92. Gordon MH: Remarks on Hodgkin's disease: a pathogenic agent in the glands, and its application in diagnosis. Br Med J 1:641, 1933.
93. Gottdiener JS, Marn BJ, Schooley RT, et al: Two-dimensional echocardiographic assessment of the idiopathic hypereosinophilic syndrome. Anatomic basis of mitral regurgitation and peripheral embolization. Circulation 67:572, 1983.
94. Gounni AS, Lamkhioued B, Ochiai K, et al: High-affinity IgE receptor on eosinophils is involved in host defence against parasites. Nature 367:183–186, 1994.
95. Grauer L, Padilla VM 3rd, Bouza L, Barkin JS: Eosinophilic sclerosing cholangitis associated with hypereosinophilic syndrome. Am J Gastroenterol 88:1764, 1993.
96. Grisvold W, Jellinger K: Multifocal neuropathy with vasculitis in hypereosinophilic syndrome. An entity or drug-induced effect? J Neurol 231:301, 1985.
97. Guyre PM, Girard MT, Morganelli PM, Manganiello PD: Glucocorticoid effects on the production and actions of immune cytokines. J Steroid Biochem 30:89, 1988.
98. Hamann KJ, Barker RL, Loegering DA, Gleich GJ: Comparative toxicity of purified eosinophil granule proteins for newborn larvae of Trichinella spiralis. J Parasitol 73:523, 1987.
99. Hamann KJ, Gleich GJ, Checkel JL, et al: In vitro killing of microfilariae of *Brugia pahangi* and *Brugia malayi* by eosinophil granule proteins. J Immunol 144:3166, 1990.
100. Hamid Q, Barkans J, Menq Q, et al: Human eosinophils synthesize and secrete interleukin-6 in vitro. Blood 80:1496–1501, 1992.
101. Hanowell ST, Kim YD, Rattan V, MacNamara TE: Increased heparin requirement with the hypereosinophilic syndrome. 55:450, 1981.
102. Harley JB, Fauci AS, Gralnick HR: Noncardiovascular findings associated with heart disease in the idiopathic hypereosinophilic syndrome. Am J Cardiol 52:321, 1983.
103. Hartung H-P: Acetyl glyceryl ether phosphorylcholine (platelet-activating factor) mediates heightened metabolic activity in macrophages. FEBS Lett 160:209–212, 1983.
104. Hendrick A: Psychosis during interferon in eosinophilic leukaemia. Clin Lab Haematol 16:295, 1994.
105. Her E, Frazer J, Austen KF, Owen WF: Eosinophil hematopoietins antagonize the programmed cell death of eosinophils: cytokine and glucocorticoid effects on eosinophils maintained by endothelial cell conditioned medium. J Clin Invest 88:1982, 1992.
106. Hill R, Wang NS, Berry G: Hypereosinophilic syndrome with pulmonary vascular involvement. Angiology 35:238, 1984.
107. Holroyde MC, Altounyan RE, Cole M, et al: Bronchoconstriction produced in man by leukotrienes C and D. Lancet 2:17, 1981.
108. Horn BR, Robin ED, Theodore J, Van Kessel A: Total eosinophil counts in the management of bronchial asthma. N Engl J Med 292:1152, 1975.
109. Jong EC, Klebanoff SJ: Eosinophil-mediated mammalian tumor cell cytotoxicity: role of the peroxidase system. J Immunol 124:1949, 1980.
110. Jose PJ, Griffiths-Johnson DA, Collins PD, et al: Eotaxin: a potent eosinophil chemoattractant cytokine detected in a guinea pig model of allergic airways inflammation. J Exp Med 179:881, 1994.
111. Juhlin L, Michaelsson G: A new syndrome characterized by absence of eosinophils and basophils. Lancet 1:1233, 1977.
112. Kamb ML, Murphy JJ, Jones JL, et al: Eosinophilia-myalgia syndrome in L-tryptophan–exposed patients. JAMA 267:77, 1992.
113. Kaplan PW, Waterbury L, Kawas C, et al: Reversible dementia with idiopathic hypereosinophilic syndrome. Neurology 39:1388, 1989.
114. Kato M, Schleimer RP: Anti-inflammatory steroids inhibit granulocyte/macrophage colony-stimulating factor production by human lung tissue. Lung 172:113, 1994.
115. Kay AB, Shin HS, Austen KF: Selective attraction of eosinophils and synergism between eosinophil chemotactic factor of anaphylaxis (ECF-A) and a fragment cleaved from the fifth component of complement (C5a). Immunology 24:969, 1973.
116. Kazmierowski JA, Chusid MJ, Parillo JE, et al: Dermatologic manifestations of hypereosinophilic syndrome. Arch Dermatol 114:531, 1978.
117. Keidan AJ, Catovski D, Tavares de Castro J, Spry CJ: Hypereosinophilic syndrome preceding T cell lymphoblastic lymphoma. Clin Lab Haematol 7:83, 1985.
118. Kelso A, Munck A: Glucocorticoid inhibition of lymphokine secretion by alloreactive T cell clones. J Immunol 133:784, 1984.
119. Kemp M, Kurtzhals JAL, Bendtzen K, et al: Th-1 and Th-2–like T-cell clones from individuals who have recovered from visceral leischmaniasis. Infect Immun 61:1069, 1993.
120. Kim CJ, Park SH, Chi JG, et al: Idiopathic hypereosinophilic syndrome terminating as disseminated T-cell lymphoma. Cancer 67:1064, 1991.
121. Kim GB, Kwon JH, Kang DS: Hypereosinophilic syndrome: imaging findings in patients with hepatic involvement. AJR Am J Roentgenol 161:577, 1993.

122. Kita HT, Okubo Y, Weiler D, et al: Granulocyte/macrophage colony-stimulating factor and interleukin 3 release from human peripheral blood eosinophils and neutrophils. J Exp Med 174:745, 1991.
123. Kroegel C, Yukawa T, Dent G, et al: Stimulation of degranulation from human eosinophils by platelet-activating factor. J Immunol 142:3518, 1989.
124. Lauve RM: Hypereosinophilic syndrome in a bronchial asthmatic. J La State Med Soc 145:526, 1993.
125. Laviolette M, Picard S, Braquet P, Brogeat P: Comparison of 5- and 15-lipoxygenase activities in blood and alveolar leukocyte preparations from normal subjects and patients with eosinophilia. Prostaglandins Leukot Med 23:191, 1986.
126. Lederman J, Hasselbach H, Hippe E: Alcohol intolerance in the hypereosinophilic syndrome. Alcohol Clin Exp Res 12:147, 1988.
127. Lee CM, Changchien CS, Chen PC, et al: Eosinophilic gastroenteritis: 10 years' experience. Am J Gastroenterol 88:70, 1993.
128. Lee CW, Lewis RA, Tauber AI, et al: The myeloperoxidase-dependent metabolism of leukotrienes C_4, D_4, and E_4 to 6-trans-leukotriene B_4 diastereoisomers and the subclass-specific S-diastereoisomeric sulfoxides. J Biol Chem 258:15004, 1983.
129. Lee GH, Lee KW, Chi JG: Peripheral neuropathy as a hypereosinophilic syndrome and anti-GM1 antibodies. J Korean Med Sci 8:225, 1993.
130. Lee M-L, Fischer G, Gow E: Hypereosinophilic syndrome presenting with erythroderma. Australas J Dermatol 29:95, 1988.
131. Lee T, Lenihan DJ, Malone B, et al: Increased biosynthesis of platelet-activating factor in activated human eosinophils. J Biol Chem 259:5526, 1984.
132. Lefebvre C, Bletry O, Degoulet P, et al: Facteurs prognostiques du syndrome hypereosinophilique. Etude de 40 observations. Ann Med Interne (Paris) 140:253, 1989.
133. Lehrer RI, Szklarek D, Barton A, et al: Anti-bacterial properties of eosinophil major basic protein (MBP) and eosinophil cationic protein (ECP). J Immunol 142:4428, 1989.
134. Leiferman KM, O'Duffy JD, Perry HO, et al: Recurrent incapacitating mucosal ulcerations: a prodrome of the hypereosinophilic syndrome. JAMA 247:1018, 1982.
135. Lewis DM, Loegering DA, Gleich GJ: Antiserum to the major basic protein of guinea pig eosinophil granules. Immunochemistry 13:743, 1976.
136. Linden M, Brattsand R: Effects of a corticosteroid, budesonide, on alveolar macrophage and blood monocyte secretion of cytokines: differential sensitivity of GM-CSF, IL-1 beta, and IL-6. Pulm Pharmacol 7:43, 1994.
137. Lopez AF, Williamson DJ, Gamble JR, et al: Recombinant human granulocyte-macrophage colony-stimulating factor stimulates in vitro mature human neutrophil and eosinophil function, surface receptor expression, and survival. J Clin Invest 78:1220, 1986.
138. Lopez AF, Eglinton JM, Lyons AB, et al: Human interleukin-3 inhibits the binding of granulocyte-macrophage colony-stimulating factor and interleukin-5 to basophils and strongly enhances their functional activity. J Cell Physiol 145:69, 1990.
139. Lucey DR, Nicholson-Weller A, Weller PF: Mature human eosinophils have the capacity to express HLA-DR. Proc Natl Acad Sci USA 86:1348, 1989.
140. Lucey DR, Dorski DI, Nicholson-Weller A, Weller PF: Human eosinophils express CD4 protein and bind human immunodeficiency virus 1 gp 120. J Exp Med 169:327, 1989.
141. Lungarella G, Menegazzi R, Gardi C, et al: Identification of elastase in human eosinophils: immunolocalization, isolation, and partial characterization. Arch Biochem Biophys 292:128, 1992.
142. Maas RL, Turk J, Oates JA, Brash AR: Formation of a novel dihydroxy acid from arachadonic acid by lipoxygenase-catalyzed double oxygenation in rat mononuclear cells and human leukocytes. J Biol Chem 257:7056, 1982.
143. MacGrashan DW Jr, Peters SP, Warner J, Lichtenstein LM: Characteristics of human basophil sulfidopeptide leukotriene release: releasability defined as the ability of the basophil to respond to dimeric cross-links. J Immunol 136:2231, 1986.
144. Malveaux FJ, Conroy MC, Adkinson NF Jr, Lichtenstein LM: IgE receptors on human basophils. Relationship to serum IgE concentration. J Clin Invest 62:176, 1978.
145. Marolda M, Orefice G, Barbieri F, et al: The idiopathic hypereosinophilic syndrome. Clinical, electrophysiological and histological study of a case. Ital J Neurol Sci 10:70, 1989.
146. Marom Z, Shelhamer JH, Bach MK, et al: Slow-reacting substances, leukotrienes C_4 and D_4, increase the release of mucus from human airways in vitro. Am Rev Respir Dis 126:449, 1982.
147. Marshall GM, White L: Effective therapy for a severe case of the idiopathic hypereosinophilic syndrome. Am J Pediatr Hematol Oncol 11:178, 1989.
148. Masi AT, Hunder GG, Lie JT, et al: The American College of Rheumatology 1990 criteria for the classification of Churg-Strauss syndrome (allergic granulomatosis and angiitis). Arthritis Rheum 33:1094, 1990.
149. May LP, Kelley J, Sanchez M: Hypereosinophilic syndrome with unusual cutaneous manifestations in two men with HIV infection. J Am Acad Dermatol 23:202, 1990.
150. Mayeno AN, Curran AJ, Roberts RL, Foote CS: Eosinophils preferentially use bromide to generate halogenating agents. J Biol Chem 264:5660, 1989.
151. McLaren DJ, McKean JR, Olsson I, et al: Morphological studies on the killing of schistosomula of Schistosoma mansoni by human eosinophil and neutrophil cationic proteins in vitro. Parasite Immunol 3:359, 1981.
152. McManus LM, Hanahan DJ, Demopoulos CA, Pinckard RN: Pathobiology of intravenous infusion of acetyl glyceryl ether phosphorylcholine (AGEPC), a synthetic platelet-activating factor (PAF), in the rabbit. J Immunol 124:2919, 1980.
153. Meeker TC, Hardy D, Willman C, et al: Activation of the interleukin-3 gene by chromosome translocation in acute lymphocytic leukemia with eosinophilia. Blood 76:285, 1990.
154. Metz J, McGrath KM, Savoia HF, et al: T cell lymphoid aggregates in bone marrow in idiopathic hypereosinophilic syndrome. J Clin Pathol 46:955, 1993.
155. Miyamasu M, Harai K, Takahashi Y, et al: Chemotactic agonists induce cytokine generation in eosinophils. J Immunol 154:1339, 1995.
156. Molina HA, Kierszenbaum F, Hamann KJ, Gleich GJ: Toxic effects produced or mediated by human eosinophil granule components on *Trypanosoma cruzi*. Am J Trop Med Hyg 38:327, 1988.
157. Monaco S, Lucci B, Laperchia N, et al: Polyneuropathy in hypereosinophilic syndrome. Neurology 38:494, 1988.
158. Monsuez JJ, de Kerviler E, Barboteu M, et al: Non-Hodgkin's lymphoma related to eosinophilic endomyocardial disease. Eur Heart J 15:1423, 1994.
159. Moore PM, Harley JB, Fauci AS: Neurologic dysfunction in the idiopathic hypereosinophilic syndrome. Ann Intern Med 102:109, 1985.
160. Moqbel R, Hamid Q, Ying S, et al: Expression of mRNA for the granulocyte/macrophage colony-stimulating factor in activated human eosinophils. J Exp Med 174:749, 1991.
161. Moscinski LC, Kasnic G Jr, Saker A Jr: The significance of an elevated serum lysozyme value in acute myelogenous leukemia with eosinophilia. Am J Clin Pathol 97:195, 1992.
162. Morgan MB, Viloria J, Morgan JD, Suarez-Hoyos J: Human immunodeficiency virus infection and hypereosinophilic syndrome. An increasingly recognized association. J Fla Med Assoc 81:401, 1994.
163. Motojima S, Frigas E, Loegering DA, Gleich GJ: Toxicity of eosinophil cationic proteins for guinea pig tracheal epithelium in vitro. Am Rev Respir Dis 139:801, 1989.
164. Murphy PT, Fennelly DF, Stuart M, O'Donnell JR: Alfa-interferon in a case of hypereosinophilic syndrome. Br J Haematol 75:619, 1990.
165. Nadel JA, Conrad DJ, Ueki IF, et al: Immunocytochemical localization of arachadonate 15-lipoxygenase in erythrocytes, leukocytes, and airway cells. J Clin Invest 87:1139, 1991.
166. Nelken RP, Stockman J: The hypereosinophilic syndrome in association with acute lymphoblastic leukemia. J Pediatr 89:771, 1976.
167. Neva FA, Gam AA, Burke J: Comparison of larval antigens in an enzyme-linked immunosorbent assay for strongyloidiasis in humans. J Infect Dis 144:427, 1981.
168. Newton JA, Singh AK, Greaves MW, Spry CJ: Aquagenic pruritus associated with the idiopathic hypereosinophilic syndrome. Br J Dermatol 122:103, 1990.
169. Nielsen K, Fogh L, Andersen S: Eosinophil response to migrating *Ascaris suum* larvae in normal and congenitally thymus-less mice. Acta Pathol Microbial Immunol Scand 82:919, 1974.
170. Nir MA, Westfried M: Hypereosinophilic dermatitis. A distinct manifestation of the hypereosinophilic syndrome with response to dapsone. Dermatologica 162:444, 1981.
171. Nutman TB, Ottsen EA, Ieng S, et al: Eosinophilia in Southeast Asian refugees: evaluation at a referral center. J Infect Dis 155:309, 1987.
172. O'Donnell MC, Ackerman SJ, Gleich GJ, Thomas LL: Activation of basophil and mast cell histamine release by eosinophil granule major basic protein. J Exp Med 157:1981, 1983.

173. O'Flaherty JT, Miller CH, Lewis JC, et al: Neutrophil responses to platelet-activating factor. Inflammation 5:193, 1981.
174. Ohno I, Lea R, Finotto S, et al: Granulocyte/macrophage colony-stimulating factor (GM-CSF) gene expression by eosinophils in nasal polyposis. Am J Respir Cell Mol Biol 5:505, 1991.
175. Ohno I, Lea RG, Flanders KC, et al: Eosinophils in chronically inflamed upper airway tissues express transforming growth factor β 1 gene (TGF β 1). J Clin Invest 89:1662, 1992.
176. Olsen RL, Little C: Purification and some properties of myeloperoxidase and eosinophil peroxidase from human blood. Biochem J 209:781, 1983.
177. Olson TA, Virmani R, Ansinelli RA, et al: Cardiomyopathy in a child with the idiopathic hypereosinophilic syndrome. Pediatr Cardiol 3:161, 1982.
178. Olsson I, Persson A-M, Winqvist I: Biochemical properties of the eosinophil cationic protein and demonstration of its biosynthesis in vitro in marrow cells from patients with eosinophilia. Blood 67:498, 1986.
179. Owen J, Scott JG: Transition of the hypereosinophilic syndrome to myelomonocytic leukemia. Can Med Assoc J 121:1489, 1979.
180. Owen WF, Rothenberg ME, Silberstein DS, et al: Regulation of human eosinophil viability, density and function by granulocyte/macrophage colony-stimulating factor in the presence of 3T3 fibroblasts. J Exp Med 166:129, 1987.
181. Owen WF Jr, Soberman RJ, Yoshimoto T, et al: Synthesis and release of leukotriene C_4 by human eosinophils. J Immunol 138:3290, 1987.
182. Owen WF, Rothenberg ME, Petersen J, et al: Interleukin 5 and phenotypically altered eosinophils in the blood of patients with the idiopathic hypereosinophilic syndrome. J Exp Med 170:343, 1989.
183. Owen WF, Petersen J, Sheff DM, et al: Hypodense eosinophils and interleukin 5 activity in the blood of patients with the eosinophilia-myalgia syndrome. Proc Natl Acad Sci USA 87:8647, 1990.
184. Owen WF, Petersen J, Austen KF: Eosinophils altered phenotypically and primed by culture with granulocyte/macrophage colony-stimulating factor and 3T3 fibroblasts generate leukotriene C_4 in response to fMLP. J Clin Invest 87:1958, 1991.
185. Owen WF: Eosinophil heterogeneity. In C Chapman (ed): Immunopharmacology of Eosinophils. Academic Press, London, 1993.
186. Parrillo JE, Fauci AS, Wolff SM: Therapy of the hypereosinophilic syndrome. Ann Intern Med 89:167, 1978.
187. Parillo JE, Borer JS, Henry WL, et al: The cardiovascular manifestations of the hypereosinophilic syndrome: prospective study of 26 patients, with review of the literature. Am J Med 67:572, 1979.
188. Parrillo JE, Lawley TJ, Frank MM, et al: Immunologic reactivity in the hypereosinophilic syndrome. J Allergy Clin Immunol 64:113, 1979.
189. Parker CJ: Hypereosinophilic syndrome with cutaneous blisters and bowel necrosis. Australas J Dermatol 29:103, 1988.
190. Peison B, Benisch B, Lim M, Chin JC: Idiopathic hypereosinophilic syndrome with polymyositis. South Med J 81:403, 1988.
191. Peters MS, Rodriguez M, Gleich GJ: Localization of human eosinophil granule major basic protein, eosinophil cationic protein, and eosinophil-derived neurotoxin by immunoelectron microscopy. Lab Invest 54:656, 1986.
192. Peters MS, Gleich GJ, Dunnette SL, Fukuda T: Ultrastructural study of eosinophils from patients with the hypereosinophilic syndrome: a morphologic basis of hypodense eosinophils. Blood 71:780, 1988.
193. Pierce JR, Dyer EL: Extreme hypereosinophilia and strongyloidiasis: uncommon manifestation of a common disease. South Med J 74:995, 1981.
194. Prattichizzo FA, Bernini L: An idiopathic hypereosinophilic syndrome mimicking seronegative rheumatoid arthritis: 20-year follow-up with clinical and laboratory findings. Clin Exp Rheumatol 10:79, 1992.
195. Prick JJW, Gabreels-Festen AAWM, Korten JJ, van der Wiel TWM: Neurological manifestations of the hypereosinophilic syndrome (HES). Clin Neurol Neurosurg 90:269, 1988.
196. Prin L, Capron M, Tonnel AB, et al: Heterogeneity of human peripheral blood eosinophils: variability in cell density and cytotoxic ability in relation to the level and the origin of hypereosinophilia. Int Arch Allergy Appl Immunol 72:336, 1983.
197. Prin L, Charon P, Capron M, et al: Heterogeneity of human eosinophils. II. Variability of respiratory burst activity related to cell density. Clin Exp Immunol 57:735, 1984.
198. Prin L, Plumas J, Gruart V, et al: Elevated serum levels of soluble interleukin-2 receptor: a marker of disease activity in the hypereosinophilic syndrome. Blood 78:2626, 1991.
199. Pye M, Pope R, Jones JH, Williams G: Eosinophilic polymyositis presenting as a pseudotumor in the hypereosinophilic syndrome. Br J Rheumatol 26:384, 1987.
200. Raghavachar A, Fleischer S, Frickhofen N, et al: T lymphocyte control of human granulopoiesis: clonal analysis in an idiopathic hypereosinophilic syndrome. J Immunol 139:3753, 1987.
201. Rand TH, Silberstein DS, Kornfeld H, Weller PF: Human eosinophils express functional interleukin 2 receptors. J Clin Invest 88:825, 1991.
202. Rand TH, Cruikshank WW, Center DM, Weller PF: CD4-mediated stimulation of human eosinophils: lymphocyte chemoattractant factor and other CD4-binding ligands elicit eosinophil migration. J Exp Med 173:1521, 1991.
203. Ratnoff OD, Gleich GJ, Shurin SB, et al: Inhibition of the activation of Hageman factor (factor XII) by eosinophils and eosinophilic constituents. Am J Hematol 42:138, 1993.
204. Resnick M, Myerson RM: Hypereosinophilic syndrome. Report of two cases, with prolonged courses. Ann Intern Med 51:560, 1971.
205. Robinson DS, Hamid Q, Ying S, et al: Predominant Th-2-like bronchoalveolar T-lymphocyte population in atopic asthma. N Engl J Med 326:298, 1992.
206. Roche S, Cross S, Kauffman B: Intracranial hemorrhages occurring in the idiopathic hypereosinophilic syndrome. J Neurol Neurosurg Psychiatry 53:440, 1990.
207. Rolfe FG, Hughes JM, Armour CL, Sewell WA: Inhibition of interleukin-5 gene expression by dexamethasone. Immunology 77:494, 1992.
208. Rohrbach MS, Wheatley CL, Slifman NR, Gleich GJ: Activation of platelets by eosinophil granule proteins. J Exp Med 172:1271, 1990.
209. Rot A, Krieger M, Brunner T, et al: RANTES and macrophage inflammatory protein 1 alpha induce the migration and activation of normal human eosinophil granulocytes. J Exp Med 176:1489, 1992.
210. Rothenberg ME, Owen WF, Silberstein DS, et al: Human eosinophils have prolonged survival, enhanced function and become hypodense when exposed to human interleukin 3. J Clin Invest 81:1986, 1988.
211. Rothenberg ME, Petersen J, Stevens RL, et al: IL-5-dependent conversion of normodense eosinophils to the hypodense phenotype uses 3T3 fibroblasts for enhanced viability, accelerated hypodensity, and sustained antibody-dependent cytotoxicity. J Immunol 143:2311, 1989.
212. Saito H, Hatake K, Dvorak AM, et al: Selective differentiation and proliferation of hematopoietic cells induced by recombinant human interleukins. Proc Natl Acad Sci USA 85:2288, 1988.
213. Salgame P, Abrams JS, Clayberger C, et al: Differing lymphokine profiles of functional subsets of human CD4 and CD8 T cell clones. Science 254:279, 1991.
214. Sanchez JL, Padilla MA: Hypereosinophilic syndrome. Cutis 29:490, 1982.
215. Sanderson CJ: Control of eosinophilia. Int Arch Allergy Appl Immunol 94:122, 1991.
216. Sasano H, Virmani R, Patterson RH, et al: Eosinophilic products lead to myocardial damage. Hum Pathol 20:850, 1989.
217. Sato A, Kobayashi K, Okabe H, Fukuda S: A case of the hypereosinophilic syndrome complicated by malignant lymphoma. J Dermatol 10:75, 1983.
218. Scheurlen M, Mork H, Weber P: Hypereosinophilic syndrome resembling chronic inflammatory bowel disease with primary sclerosing cholangitis. J Clin Gastroenterol 14:59, 1992.
219. Schooley RT, Flaum MA, Gralnick HR, Fauci AS: A clinicopathologic correlation of the idiopathic hypereosinophilic syndrome. II. Clinical manifestations. Blood 58:1021, 1981.
220. Schrezenmeier H, Thome SD, Tewald F, et al: Interleukin-5 is the predominant eosinophilopoietin produced by cloned T lymphocytes in the hypereosinophilic syndrome. Exp Hematol 21:358, 1993.
221. Sedgwick JB, Geiger KM, Busse WW: Superoxide generation by hypodense eosinophils from patients with asthma. Am Rev Respir Dis 142:120, 1990.
222. Shah AM, Joglekar M: Eosinophilic colitis as a complication of the hypereosinophilic syndrome. Postgrad Med 63:485, 1987.
223. Shaw JO, Pinckard N, Ferrigni S, et al: Activation of human neutrophils with 1-*O*-hexa-dodecyl/octadodecyl-2-acetyl-sn-glyceryl-3-phosphoryl-choline (platelet-activating factor). J Immunol 127:1250, 1981.
224. Shelley WB, Shelley ED: Erythema annulare centrifugatum as the presenting sign of the hypereosinophilic syndrome: observations on the therapy. Cutis 35:53, 1985.
225. Slabbynick H, Impens N, Naegels S, et al: Idiopathic hypereosinophilic syndrome-related pulmonary involvement diagnosed by bronchoalveolar lavage. Chest 101:1178, 1992.

226. Slifman NR, Loegering DA, McKean DJ, Gleich GJ: Ribonuclease activity associated with human eosinophil-derived neurotoxin and eosinophil cationic protein. J Immunol 137:2913, 1986.
227. Slovick FT, Abboud CN, Brennan JK, Lichtman MA: Modulation of in vitro eosinophil progenitors by hydrocortisone: role of accessory cells and interleukins. Blood 66:1072, 1985.
228. Slungaard A, Vercellotti GM, Walker G, et al: Tumor necrosis factor alpha/cachectin stimulates eosinophil oxidant production and toxicity towards human endothelium. J Exp Med 171:2025, 1990.
229. Slungaard A, Mahoney JRJ: Bromide-dependent toxicity of eosinophil peroxidase for endothelium and isolated working rat hearts: a model for eosinophilic endocarditis. J Exp Med 173:117, 1991.
230. Slungaard A, Mahoney JR Jr: Thiocyanate is the major substrate for eosinophil peroxidase in physiologic fluids: implications for cytotoxicity. J Biol Chem 266:4903, 1991.
231. Smit AJ, van Essen LH, de Vries EG: Successful long-term control of idiopathic hypereosinophilic syndrome with etoposide. Cancer 67:2826, 1991.
232. Smith MD, Metcalfe M, DeMaria AN, et al: Hypereosinophilic syndrome resulting in aortic and mitral stenosis: a case requiring double valve replacement. Am Heart J 117:475, 1989.
233. Spry CJ: The hypereosinophilic syndrome: clinical features, laboratory findings and treatment. Allergy 37:539, 1982.
234. Spry CJ, Davies J, Tai PC, et al: Clinical features of fifteen patients with the hypereosinophilic syndrome. Q J Med 52:1, 1983.
235. Spry CJ, Take M, Tai PC: Eosinophilic disorders affecting the myocardium and endocardium: a review. Heart Vessels Suppl 1:240, 1985.
236. Stahle-Baeckdahl M, Sudbeck BD, Eisen AZ, et al: Expression of a 92-kDa type IV collagenase mRNA by eosinophils associated with basal cell carcinoma. J Invest Dermatol 99:497, 1992.
237. Stern M, Meagher L, Savill J, Haslett C: Apoptosis in human eosinophils. Programmed cell death in the eosinophil lead to phagocytosis by macrophages and is modulated by IL-5. J Immunol 148:3543, 1992.
238. Stimler NP, Bloor CM, Hugli TE, et al: Anaphylactic actions of platelet-activating factor. Am J Pathol 105:64, 1981.
239. Stimler NP, O'Flaherty JT: Spasmogenic properties of platelet-activating factor: evidence for a direct mechanism in the contractile response of pulmonary tissues. Am J Pathol 113:75, 1983.
240. Stimler-Gerard NP: Parasympathetic stimulation as a mechanism for platelet-activating factor-induced contractile responses in the lung. J Pharmacol Exp Ther 237:209, 1986.
241. Tai P-C, Spry CJ, Peterson C, et al: Monoclonal antibodies distinguish between storage and secreted forms of eosinophil cationic protein. Nature 309:182, 1984.
242. Takai K, Sanada M: Hypereosinophilic syndrome evolving to acute lymphoblastoid leukemia. Int J Hematol 54:321, 1991.
243. Takamizawa M, Iwata T, Wantanabe K, et al: Elevated production of interleukin-4 and interleukin-5 by T cells in a child with idiopathic hypereosinophilic syndrome. J Allergy Clin Immunol 93:1076, 1994.
244. Takekawa M, Imai K, Adachi M, et al: Hypereosinophilic syndrome accompanied with necrosis of the fingertips. Intern Med 31:1262, 1992.
245. Taniguchi N, Mita H, Saito H, et al: Increased generation of leukotriene C_4 from eosinophils in asthmatic patients. Allergy 40:571, 1985.
246. Tobler A, Meier R, Seitz M, et al: Glucocorticoids downregulate gene expression of GM-CSF, NAP-1/IL-8, and IL-6, but not of M-CSF in human fibroblasts. Blood 79:45, 1992.
247. Tool ATJ, Koenderman L, Kok PT, et al: Release of platelet-activating factor is important for the respiratory burst induced in human eosinophils by opsonized particles. Blood 79:2729, 1992.
248. Triggiani M, Schleimer RP, Tomioka K, et al: Characterization of platelet activating factor synthesized by normal and granulocyte-macrophage colony-stimulating factor-primed human eosinophils. Immunology 77:500, 1992.
249. Turner JC, Jackson HJ, Parker FJ: The etiologic relation of the eosinophil to the Gordon phenomenon in Hodgkin's disease. Am J Med Sci 195:27, 1938.
250. Uetsuka Y, Kasahara S, Tanaka N, et al: Hemodynamic and scintographic improvement after steroid therapy in a case with acute eosinophilic heart disease. Heart Vessels Suppl 5:8, 1990.
251. Urihara A, Morita S, Kuroda S, et al: Severe insulin-resistant diabetes mellitus associated with hyperesoinophilic syndrome. Intern Med 33:632, 1994.
252. Vadas MA, David JR, Butterworth AP, et al: A new method for the purification of human eosinophils and neutrophils, and a comparison of the ability of these cells to damage schistosomula of *Schistosoma mansoni*. J Immunol 122:1228, 1979.
253. Valente O, Scarpinella-Bueno MA: Deep venous thrombosis in hypereosinophilic syndrome. Am Fam Physician 50:921, 1994.
254. van den Hoogenband HM, van den Berg WH, van Diggelson MW: PUVA therapy in the treatment of skin lesions of the hypereosinophilic syndrome. Arch Dermatol 121:450, 1985.
255. Vargas CA, Maldonado O, Botero RC, et al: Budd-Chiari syndrome associated with the hypereosinophilic syndrome. Am J Gastroenterol 88:1802, 1993.
256. Varon D, Wetzler M, Berrebi A: Hypereosinophilic syndrome associated with polycythemia vera. Arch Intern Med 146:1440, 1986.
257. Venge P, Dahl R, Hallgren R: Enhancement of factor XII dependent reactions by eosinophil cationic protein. Thromb Res 14:641, 1979.
258. Volpi A, Rovelli GE, Maggoni AP: Benign course of endomyocardial fibrosis as a late complication of hypereosinophilic syndrome. G Ital Cardiol 15:238, 1985.
259. Walker C, Virchow J-C, Bruijnzeel PLB, Blaser K: T cell subsets and their products regulate eosinophilia in allergic and nonallergic asthma. J Immunol 146:1829, 1991.
260. Wardlaw AJ, Moqbel R, Cromwell O, Kay AB: Platelet-activating factor. A potent chemotactic and chemokinetic factor for human eosinophils. J Clin Invest 78:1701, 1986.
261. Wasmoen TL, Bell MP, Loegering DA, et al: Biochemical and amino acid sequence of human eosinophil granule major basic protein. J Biol Chem 263:12559, 1988.
262. Wattiaux MJ, Khalife J, Prin L, et al: Syndrome hypereosinophilique chez un sujet HIV 1+. Rev Med Interne 10:249, 1989.
263. Weingarten JS, O'Sheal SF, Margolis WS: Eosinophilic menigitis and the hypereosinophilic syndrome. Case report and review of the literature. Am J Med 78:674, 1985.
264. Weller PF, Goetzl EJ, Austen KF: Identification of human eosinophil lysophospholipase as the constituent of Charcot-Leyden crystals. Proc Natl Acad Sci USA 77:7440, 1980.
265. Weller PF, Austen KF: Human eosinophil arylsulfatase B. Structure and activity of the purified tetrameric lysosomal hydrolase. J Clin Invest 71:114, 1983.
266. Weller PF, Lee CW, Foster DW, et al: Generation and metabolism of 5-lipoxygenase pathway leukotrienes by human eosinophils: predominant production of leukotriene C_4. Proc Natl Acad Sci USA 80:7626, 1983.
267. Weller PF, Rand TH, Barrett T, et al: Accessory cell function of human eosinophils. HLA-DR-dependent, MHC-restricted antigen-presentation and IL-1 alpha expression. J Immunol 150:2554, 1993.
268. Weller PF, Bubley GJ: The idiopathic hypereosinophilic syndrome. Blood 83:2759, 1994.
269. Wichman A, Buchtal F, Pezeshkpour GH, Fauci AS: Peripheral neuropathy in hypereosinophilic syndrome. Neurology 35:1140, 1985.
270. Winn RE, Kollef MH, Meyer JI: Pulmonary involvement in the hypereosinophilic syndrome. Chest 105:656, 1994.
271. Wong DT, Weller PF, Galli SJ, et al: Human eosinophils express transforming factor α. J Exp Med 172:673, 1990.
272. Wong DT, Elovic A, Matossian K, et al: Eosinophils from patients with blood eosinophilia express transforming growth factor β 1. Blood 78:2702, 1991.
273. Ying S, Taborda-Barata L, Meng Q, et al: The kinetics of allergen-induced transcription of messenger RNA for monocyte chemotactic protein-3 and RANTES in the skin of human atopic subjects: relationship to eosinophil, T cell, and macrophage recruitment. J Exp Med 181:2153, 1995.
274. Young JD-E, Peterson CG, Venge P, Cohn ZA, et al: Mechanism of membrane damage mediated by human eosinophil cationic protein. Nature 321:613, 1986.
275. Zabel P, Schlaak M: Cyclosporin for hypereosinophilic syndrome. Ann Hematol 62:230, 1991.
276. Zielinski RM, Lawrence WD: Interferon-α for the hypereosinophilic syndrome. Ann Intern Med 113:716, 1990.

Index

Note: Page numbers in *italics* indicate figures; page numbers followed by t refer to tables.

ISBN 0-7216-4974-2

90038

9 780721 649740